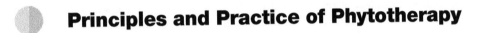

Principles and Practice of Phytotherapy

Dedication

This book is dedicated to the late Hein Zeylstra, a beloved colleague, and former Principal of the College of Phytotherapy in England, who through his enormous energy over 25 years inspired us both in our work.

About the Authors

Kerry Bone

Associate Professor Kerry Bone as the co-founder and Director of Research and Development is the innovation driver at MediHerb. He was an experienced research and industrial chemist before studying herbal medicine full-time in the UK where he graduated from the College of Phytotherapy in 1983 and joined the National Institute of Medical Herbalists. As a practising herbalist (28 years' experience) he still maintains a busy practice in Toowoomba in Queensland. As Associate Professor at the University of New England in Armidale, Australia, a position held for more than 7 years (currently adjunct), he developed their innovative programme, the Masters of Health Science (Herbal Medicine). Kerry is a prolific author, with six published herbal medicine books that are renowned as defining herbal texts in natural medicine schools throughout the world. A recent book, written in conjunction with Rob Santich, is *Healthy Children: Optimising Children's Health with Herbs*. He has also co-authored more than 30 scientific papers in the field of herbal research.

Simon Mills

Simon Mills is a Cambridge graduate in medical sciences who has been a herbal practitioner in the UK since 1977. In the intervening years he has had a leadership role in the field of herbal medicine, including as Chairman and President of the British Herbal Medicine Association, President of the National Institute of Medical Herbalists and President of the College of Practitioners of Phytotherapy. He has been a professional member of the Herbal Medicines Advisory Committee, the first UK government committee in this area, and since January 1997 Secretary of the European Scientific Cooperative on Phytotherapy (ESCOP), the lead European body working to ensure quality, safety and efficacy for herbal medicinal products in collaboration with the European Medicines Agency (EMA). He co-produced the 1996 edition of the authoritative *British Herbal Pharmacopoeia* and has written many books and articles in the scientific literature including controlled clinical trials and other primary research. In 2000 he founded the first MSc programme in herbal medicine in the USA at Tai Sophia Institute for the Healing Arts. More widely he has led large projects for the UK government and the European Union and has held academic posts at the University of Exeter and Peninsula Medical School in the UK. He pioneered many developments in complementary and alternative medicine in the UK and in 1999–2000 was Special Advisor to the seminal report from the British House of Lords Select Committee on Complementary and Alternative Medicine.

Content Strategist: Claire Wilson
Content Development Manager: Barbara Simmons
Project Manager: Sukanthi Sukumar
Designer: Russell Purdy
Illustration Manager: Jennifer Rose
Photographer: Martin Wall

Principles and Practice of Phytotherapy

Modern Herbal Medicine

SECOND EDITION

Kerry Bone MCPP FNHAA FNIMH FANTA DipPhyto BSc(Hons)
Director of Research and Development, MediHerb, Warwick, Queensland;
Associate Professor, University of New England, Armidale, Australia

Simon Mills MCPP FNIMH MA
Director, Centre for Complementary Health Studies, University of Exeter, UK;
Chairman, British Herbal Medicine Association; Secretary, European Scientific Cooperative on
Phytotherapy (ESCOP)

Forewords by

Michael Dixon OBE MA FRCGP
General Practitioner;
Chairman, College of Medicine, London, UK

Mark Blumenthal MA
Founder & Executive Director
American Botanical Council;
Editor, *HerbalGram*,
Austin, Texas, USA

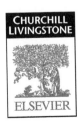

Edinburgh London New York Oxford Philadelphia St Louis Sydney Toronto 2013

CHURCHILL
LIVINGSTONE
ELSEVIER

First edition 2000
Second edition 2013
    Reprinted 2013, 2015 (twice), 2016, 2017 (twice), 2018 (twice)

ISBN 978-0-443-06992-5

British Library Cataloguing in Publication Data
A catalogue record for this book is available from the British Library

Library of Congress Cataloging in Publication Data
A catalog record for this book is available from the Library of Congress

Notices

Knowledge and best practice in this field are constantly changing. As new research and experience broaden our understanding, changes in research methods, professional practices, or medical treatment may become necessary.

Practitioners and researchers must always rely on their own experience and knowledge in evaluating and using any information, methods, compounds, or experiments described herein. In using such information or methods they should be mindful of their own safety and the safety of others, including parties for whom they have a professional responsibility.

With respect to any drug or pharmaceutical products identified, readers are advised to check the most current information provided (i) on procedures featured or (ii) by the manufacturer of each product to be administered, to verify the recommended dose or formula, the method and duration of administration, and contraindications. It is the responsibility of practitioners, relying on their own experience and knowledge of their patients, to make diagnoses, to determine dosages and the best treatment for each individual patient, and to take all appropriate safety precautions.

To the fullest extent of the law, neither the Publisher nor the authors, contributors, or editors, assume any liability for any injury and/or damage to persons or property as a matter of products liability, negligence or otherwise, or from any use or operation of any methods, products, instructions, or ideas contained in the material herein.

 ELSEVIER your source for books, journals and multimedia in the health sciences

www.elsevierhealth.com

Working together to grow libraries in developing countries

www.elsevier.com | www.bookaid.org | www.sabre.org

ELSEVIER   BOOK AID International   Sabre Foundation

The Publisher's policy is to use paper manufactured from sustainable forests

Printed in Great Britain
Last digit is the print number: 17

Contents

Family doctors working in the UK National Health Service know very well that their tools are not suitable for all their work. So many of their patients present conditions for which there are few effective prescription options. Most everyday viral infections are left for nature to take its course, with at best a little symptom relief; we check persistent headaches for pathologies and if absent send patients away to find their own analgesics; we are reluctant to prescribe much for children or add to the medication list of the elderly. Even where chronic long-term conditions are being medically well managed, many still come in with persistent tiredness, low mood, stress, distress and sleep problems, disabling joint and muscle pain, or a diversity of digestive problems that we tend to lump together as 'irritable bowel syndrome'. If we add the many menstrual and menopausal difficulties that women can face, we can quickly account for the bulk of family doctors' case loads and conclude that most of them are not appropriate for prescriptions.

What we can so often wish for is a range of remedies that are gently helpful, that will speed recovery without setting up new problems down the road, and can help patients feel part of their own treatment.

For over 15 years I have become aware that herbal medicines might address some of our daily 'effectiveness gaps'. Although they are not on my prescription pad, I will sometimes suggest that a patient go to the pharmacist for one of the reliable registered herbal medicines that we have available

in the UK. I have also worked with Simon Mills in the consulting room and have found the different herbal approaches he brings a very useful complement to mine.

In our new College of Medicine we bring together professionals from all areas of health care to work with patients towards a new vision of health care, in which all useful approaches may be integrated around the patient's experience. It has been notable how quickly herbal medicine has taken off as the area that has attracted particular interest in College events.

Prominently displayed above the desk in my consultation room are the two Mills and Bone classics, *Principles and Practice of Phytotherapy*, and the *The Essential Guide to Herbal Safety*. They have a unique rigour and scope in this field, processing thousands of published papers for clinical relevance. They make an ideal resource for someone tackling the diversity of conditions presenting to general practice, wanting sound evidence-based guidance and help in advising patients in their herbal self care. I am not surprised that they are the seminal texts around the world in herbal education.

As in all areas of health care, the science has moved enormously in the decade since the first *Principles and Practice* appeared and this new edition is a substantial reworking of the original. I very much look forward to having it on the shelf!

Dr Michael Dixon OBE, MA, FRCGP
General Practitioner;
Chairman, College of Medicine, London, UK

The use of herbs and herbal medicines has grown worldwide in the past several decades, creating an ever-increasing need for rational, authoritative, reliable information on the responsible use of these materials – like the information contained in this book. Since the publication of the first edition of this book in 2000, self-medication with herbs and phytomedicines, as well as the inclusion of herbs and phytomedicinal preparations in the clinical practice of herbal medicine (the practice frequently referred to as phytotherapy), has continued to expand and mature.

The growing interest in and demand for herbal medicine is a consumer-led phenomenon. In addition, there is also an increase in the numbers of clinically trained natural health practitioners who routinely employ herbs and phytomedicines in their clinical practices. These include naturopathic physicians who graduate from fully accredited 4-year post-graduate schools, and acupuncturists who have been extensively

trained in the subtleties of Traditional Chinese Medicine. And, there is an increase in the number of conventionally trained physicians, nurses, pharmacists and dietitians who are more receptive to the idea of including and/or recommending herbal products in their clinical practices. This maturation of the herbal marketplace is occurring worldwide – in North America, Europe, Australia, as well as in Asia, Africa, Central and South America – in both developed and developing nations.

Consumer use of and demand for herbs and herbal medicinal products continues what may be inexorable growth. This is evident in the market statistics for retail sales of herbal dietary supplements (as they are known and regulated in the United States) where sales increased by an estimated 4.8% in 2009 (the first full year of an economic recession) – a significant statistic given that the U.S. economy and many places around the world were experiencing the largest economic recession in about 70 years[1]. The rate of growth for herbal dietary supplements fell to just 0.2% in all sectors of the market in 2010 – still positive growth – according to the annual Herb Market Report published by the American Botanical Council in its journal *HerbalGram*.[2] The significance of this statistic is palpable: even in a down-cycle economy, with dwindling economic resources, millions of American consumers have 'voted for' the use of herbal products, and what they represent, as a form of natural nutrition and natural medicine with their even-more-precious funds! These market statistics include sales in health and natural food stores, mainstream retail stores (including drugstores and grocery stores), as well as via mail order, internet sales, sales by health practitioners (including naturopaths, chiropractors, herbalists, acupuncturists) and via direct sales and multi-level marketing companies. Similar trends are estimated for herb sales in other parts of the world.

The global increase in consumer demand for herbal products is also reflected by the growth in the publication of pharmacological and clinical research papers. In the 30-year period from 1977 to 2007 the number of articles dealing with pharmacological and human clinical research on herbs and phytomedicines rose from a yearly total of 739 in 1977 to 6,364 in 2007, with a significant number of these papers being review articles and randomized controlled clinical trials. And, fortunately, the authors of this book have kept up with much of this published research as reflected in the 50 monographs on leading herbs, citing thousands of articles from peer-reviewed scientific and clinical journals.[3]

So much for the old canard that 'there's no scientific research on herbal medicines', as often repeated by numerous critics, who are apparently inadequately familiar with the impressive body of herbal research. What's more, some of these same critics, after admitting that there are published scientific and clinical data supporting the overall safety and benefits of many popular herbs, still dismiss this research as having any compelling significance by claiming that the clinical trials are of inadequate design lacking appropriate controls, thus being inferior to clinical trials conducted on conventional pharmaceutical drugs. But, an independent research group at a Swiss university published a report in 2007 that compared randomly selected clinical trials on herbs/phytomedicines with trials on conventional medications.[4] They concluded that the controls and trial design in the herbal trials were equal to or even better on average than the conventional drug trials! And, to add another log on the fire, a pilot study conducted at Wake Forrest Medical School in the United States in 2008 determined, based on a review of advertising in the top 11 English-language medical journals that accept ads from pharmaceutical drug manufacturers, an inverse correlation between the level of coverage and the tone of that coverage compared to the number of drug ads in the journal.[5] In other words, the more ads for pharmaceutical drugs in a respected, leading English-language medical journal, the less coverage about herbs and other dietary supplements and whatever coverage was published was usually negative in its tone.

The relative safety of properly manufactured and responsibly used herbal medicinal products is well recognized. Data from numerous adverse event reporting databases shows a relatively low rate of reporting for herbal products, most reports being associated with relatively minor adverse effects. While it is a common truism that adverse events associated with the use of herbal medicinal products is probably under-reported, the existing data support their overall safety. An example is the database at the American Association of Poison Control Centers which reveals no deaths associated with herbal dietary supplements in the United States in 2007, 2008 or 2009.[6]

One of the key areas that differentiate many modern clinical herbalists is their willingness to include *both* the rich knowledge base of traditional use and ethnobotany, combined with modern scientific, chemical, toxicological, pharmacological, and clinical research – a position which some might consider under the term 'rational phytotherapy', distinguished from some herbal colleagues who, while embracing traditional use, frequently eschew modern scientific findings.

Bone and Mills are able to live in both worlds: they respect the robust body of traditional use of herbs in systems of traditional medicine, but they also believe that recommendations for use in modern clinical practice require whatever degree of scientific and clinical validation currently available from the growing body of such literature. These authors are eminently qualified to convey this information, and they do so in a lucid, non-dogmatic, rational manner.

The first edition of *Principles and Practice of Phytotherapy* (2000) is considered by many knowledgeable herbalists and others in the various fields of herbal medicine to be a landmark publication and it has achieved a status of a modern classic – a must-have volume for any competent phytotherapist's library. It is used as a primary textbook by many herb and naturopathic schools in the English-speaking world.

While some of my favourite herb books (and even my own previous books) have been primarily materia medica, this book combines some of the best elements of *both* a materia medica and a guide to the basic principles underlying the authors' approach to clinical herbal medicine, or as they call it by its more European term, phytotherapy. They provide up-to-date information in 50 monographs on popular herbs (there were 43 in the first edition) – many used globally. New monographs in this edition include Boswellia, gotu kola (*Centella asiatica*), myrrh gum (*Commiphora molmol*), and willow bark (*Salix* spp.), among others. But this is no mere materia medica; the authors also present their philosophy of herbal medicine/phytotherapy for practitioners. To Bone and Mills, phytotherapy is not simply the act of substituting an herbal remedy for a conventional pharmaceutical drug – as many so-called CAM physicians might tend to do. Phytotherapy transcends the standard, conventional mindset employed by most conventionally trained MDs et al. How? Well, perhaps it's almost time for the reader to explore the initial chapters to find out.

A few comments on the monographs in this book. They are quite extensive, representing some of the most up-to-date (and balanced) reviews of various medicinal herbs currently available in the literature. The monographs are obviously therapeutically oriented (as opposed to those which are published in pharmacopeias for identity and quality-control purposes), although the monographs in this book do mention which herbal materials are sometimes used as adulterants of the primary herb – an area of increased importance to the entire herb industry, as well as to those practitioners who are incorporating herbal products in their clinical practices.

The herb monographs probably contain more information than many busy clinicians will have time to read. This is understandable. And yet, it is important to provide to health practitioners the underlying substrate of the pharmacological, toxicological, and clinical literature that tend to support and validate the various clinical applications suggested here. If anyone ever doubted the growing body of scientific and clinical literature advancing the cause of phytotherapy, they need look no further than the pages of this remarkably well-researched tome.

The practice section of the book covers many areas of therapeutics, and in some cases may be an eye-opener to conventionally-trained practitioners, and even to some classically trained herbalists, regarding what the world of phytotherapy might be able to accomplish. As with the previous edition, the authors include chapters on the use of phytotherapy in cancer treatment, dermatological conditions, debilities, febrile conditions, infectious diseases, inflammatory conditions, and much more.

Given the inexorable increase in use in herbal products for health purposes and the eventual acceptance of appropriate herbal medicinal products in conventional and integrative medicine, this book and/or future iterations of it will no doubt become one of the key textbooks in conventional medical schools, whenever the time is prioritized for phytotherapy in the already-crowded medical education curriculum.

Mark Blumenthal MA
Founder & Executive Director
American Botanical Council;
Editor, *HerbalGram*,
Austin, Texas, USA

References

1. Cavaliere C, Rea P, Blumenthal M. Herb supplement sales rise in all channels in 2009. *HerbalGram*. 2009;86:62–65.
2. Blumenthal M, Lindstrom A, Lynch ME, Rea P. Herb sales continue to growth – up 3.3% in 2010. *HerbalGram*. 2010;90:64–67.
3. Hung S-K, Ernst E. Herbal medicine: an overview of the literature from three decades. *J Diet Suppl*. 2010;7(3):217–226.
4. Nartey L, Huwilder-muentener K, Shang A, Liewald K, Jueni P, Egger M. Matched-pair study showed higher quality of placebo-controlled trials in Western phytotherapy than conventional medicine. *J Clin Epidemiol*. 2007;60(8):787–794.
5. Kemper KJ, Hood KL. Does pharmaceutical advertising affect journal publication about dietary supplements? *BMC Complement Altern Med*. 2008;8:11.
6. Lindstrom A. Update: national poison control center database annual report reflects safety of dietary supplements. *HerbalGram*. 2011;91:18.

Having just completed the mammoth task of fully revising and updating the first edition, it is plainly evident we are witnessing an explosion of new information in the field of phytotherapy. By way of illustration, a quick search on the Medline database PubMed illustrates the onerous task faced these days by any author of herbal monographs. In the case of St John's wort (*Hypericum perforatum*), around 20% of the available research papers on PubMed were published in the past 3 years. The same applies for other well-researched herbs, such as *Ginkgo biloba*. For key phytochemicals, the situation is even more marked. More than 40% of the research papers on curcumin were published in the last 3 years and for berberine the amount is 24%. Keeping up with this new information is now a daunting challenge, certainly one that is beyond the time available to the herbal clinician. Hopefully, this speaks to the timeliness and utility of this second edition.

Given this exponential rise in new data, the need to be able to critically assess and discriminate the relevance and value of scientific information is more important than ever. This will definitely benefit patients, but will also help to allay concerns in the community in general, particularly with regard to the often-misplaced fears regarding herbal safety. However, it is equally important to acknowledge that just because a herb has been used traditionally for hundreds of years, this does not mean there is not a need for research into new applications and safety issues, for the latter particularly the phenomenon of potential interactions with conventional drugs.

This text, like the original, is divided into three key parts: the first defines the underlying principles and knowledge base of modern phytotherapy; the second explores the role of plants as therapeutic agents in a clinical setting; and the third contains the 50 detailed herbal monographs. What differentiates this book from many others (when it was first published it was relatively alone as a modern, comprehensive phytotherapy textbook in English) is the clinical focus of its authors (with a comprehensive and modern approach included for most disease states) and their skills in discerning the true value and relevance of the published research in the monographs, especially from the standpoint of applying this knowledge in clinical practice. Too many texts about herbs and herbal medicine contain misleading information because of excessive extrapolation from scientific publications, be they in vitro, animal or clinical studies, or because of vague allusions to traditional use. While it is appropriate to speculate on new uses for herbs, such speculation should be transparent. Hypotheses should not be presented as fact and all sources of information, be they traditional or scientific, should be clearly cited. Anecdotal information that has no traditional basis should be heavily discounted.

As noted above, one feature generally lacking from books about herbs or herbal medicine is adequate treatment of herbal therapeutics. To be fully effective in herbal therapy, it is not enough simply to know about the herbs themselves. Information must also be sought about how and when to use these herbs in response to the various therapeutic challenges. It is the therapeutic focus of this text, complete with actual case histories, which differentiates it from many other works and genuinely defines its audience as the student or professional reader.

The WHO has acknowledged that a form of herbal medicine is practised in every culture and in every country of the world, be it industrialised or not. Something deep within us recognises that there is healing power in the plant kingdom which, after all, is the nourishment of all animal life. Herbal medicine is not an anachronism practised by ignorant people. It is even more imperative to embrace the concept of phytotherapy and further develop its art and science for the benefit of all humanity.

Kerry Bone
Queensland, Australia, 2012

In the 12 years since writing for the first edition of *Principles and Practice in Phytotherapy*, there have been many events affecting herbal medicine. In the first preface there was an opportunity to look back to the pioneering steps in herbal medicine, the work of Hein Zeylstra (to whom this book is dedicated) and Fred Fletcher Hyde in developing herbal education and practice in the UK. Both of these leaders have sadly passed away since the first edition. We could also at that time reflect on other herbal cultures in Europe, North America and Asia and call for a more robust direction for phytotherapy based on the best of these legacies. We had the wind in our sails and were aspiring to great things for our work.

We may still look forward with promise. However there have been bumps in the road. There has certainly been much more academic study of herbal medicines, and the available literature we have had to process seems to be doubled in these intervening years! However, the large and more rigorous studies that we hoped for have not delivered strong messages of efficacy. In many cases it is possible to point to methodological shortcomings in the studies, particularly in relation to subject and treatment selection and outcome measures, but there is also a growing feeling that the more rigorous the study the less likely it is to come up with a positive conclusion. We have certainly had to trim the recommended uses for some of the monographs in this text in the face of these results.

There have also been less than promising developments from the UK and Europe to report. Immediately following the first edition I took on the role of Special Advisor to the House of Lords Science and Technology Committee report on Complementary and Alternative Medicine. Its seminal report in 2000 set out a substantial programme by which complementary approaches might become integrated with the wider community and with conventional health care provision in the UK. Surprisingly, the government accepted almost every recommendation. These included calls for better standards in the supply of herbal medicines and for the statutory regulation of herbal practitioners, both in the interests of public safety. In the former case the British medicines regulator, the Medicines and Healthcare Products Regulatory Agency (MHRA) led the way in Europe in framing a new European Directive, The Traditional Herbal Medicinal Products Directive. This started taking effect in 2004 and was fully implemented in 2011. Under its provisions it was possible to register a herbal product as a medicine on the basis of 30 years of traditional use rather than modern clinical studies to establish efficacy. On the other hand from 2011 it has been then illegal to supply a herbal product deemed medicinal without such a registration. It has proved too costly and difficult to register the vast majority of products that herbal practitioners use. For tinctures, extracts and other simple products it has been possible for the practitioner, under 1968 Medicines Act exemptions that still apply, to classify these as 'starting materials' in the production of individual formulations that are by definition not placed on the market. However finished products such as tablets are now considered as registrable medicines and these have been effectively withdrawn from supply to practitioners.

The way forward has been to pursue the statutory regulation of herbal practitioners, another recommendation from their Lordships. This would give herbal practitioners from many traditions, including China and Ayurveda, 'authorised health professional' status and the right to commission the supply of otherwise registrable medicines for the use of individual patients. However this path has been extremely slow and frustrating with the British government apparently awed by a few powerful voices against the proposal. Although in 2011 the Secretary of State for Health undertook in public statutorily to regulate herbal practice, the bureaucratic grind means this could be up to several years away still.

A key point of both regulatory measures is that there is no acknowledgement that herbs are effective, only that the public needs to be protected from poor quality provision. So although there is movement towards a stronger foundation in the modern community it is perhaps not for the reason we would wish. Our claim that phytotherapy can be recognised as an important contribution to health care in the UK is not much closer in this last decade.

So perhaps there is a lesson we can be learning here? Maybe the strength of what we do can be measured in other ways. As Mark Blumenthal points out in his foreword, the popular demand for herbal medicines has held up well in the USA, and the same is true elsewhere in the world. Other evidence points the same way, that when people are left to make their own devices they stubbornly reserve the right to try herbs in their health care, in spite of much negative media coverage. As conventional health care provision inflates itself beyond the capacity of public and even private budgets to support it, there is increasing interest in deferring the health care control to the patient (and even recognising that at that point they stop becoming patients).

Also in the last decade I helped set up and was first Director of a new Masters Program in Herbal Medicine at the Tai Sophia Institute in Maryland, USA. Here there is no State License available to practice as a herbalist, you cannot as a herbalist 'diagnose', 'prescribe', or even 'dispense' and one has 'clients' rather than 'patients'. Our graduates are taught to be advisors, guides, even coaches, helping their clients make the best herb choices for their particular health needs. For legal reasons our herbal practitioners become as much facilitators for self care as prescribers.

There is a promising pointer for our futures here. Our practitioners can be the experts that people turn to when they want to try herbs in their own self care. We may thus look for different ways to engage with our local communities, offering our specialist skills against a background of community-based self-care support, whether through local community gardening groups, yoga or relaxation classes, church groups, young parents or retired gatherings, or anywhere else where people might find herbal guidance helpful, especially if up till then they had not thought of that option. Then we may find ourselves translating the comprehensive information in this new book into something that makes sense to our communities.

Simon Y. Mills
Exeter, UK, 2012

Acknowledgments

The authors gratefully acknowledge the contributions of Margaret Bennett and Patricia Bone to the preparation of the manuscript. But above all the skills and tireless efforts of Vicki Matthews who contributed to and managed all the manuscript tasks involved in this huge project are particularly noted with gratitude.

Michelle Morgan

Michelle Morgan has a Bachelor of Science degree majoring in Chemistry, and worked as a laboratory technician and Quality Assurance Chemist before joining MediHerb in 1995. As Technical Writer she is responsible for literature searching, technical and marketing writing, editing and the organisation of technical publications including those on MediHerb's websites. She assisted in the research and writing of several herbal medicine text books including The Essential Guide to Herbal Safety, published by Elsevier in 2005. Michelle is a qualified herbalist and has practised part-time in Warwick, Queensland.

Michelle Morgan made a substantial contribution to most monographs in the first edition. In terms of the second edition, Michelle contributed to the update of around a dozen monographs in conjunction with Kerry Bone, wrote Appendices C and E and variously made small contributions to some of the chapters.

Berris Burgoyne

Berris Burgoyne is an experienced naturopath and phytotherapist with 20 years of clinical experience. She lectured for many years to undergraduate herbal students and in the past 10 years has become a well-known and popular presenter at seminars throughout Australia, New Zealand, South Africa and the United Kingdom. Berris has contributed to the writing of a number of herbal medicine courses and texts and updated the evening primrose monograph.

Jane Frawley

Jane is a practising herbalist, lecturer and author, is currently a PhD candidate (Gender and Health) at the University of Newcastle, and holds a Bachelor of Complementary Medicine from Charles Sturt University and a Master of Clinical Science from Southern Cross University. She has published numerous peer-reviewed articles and chapters on complementary medicine and serves on the editorial review board of Australian Journal of Medical Herbalism. Jane contributed to the updating of the barberry and golden seal, nettle and turmeric monographs in conjunction with Kerry Bone.

Camille Freeman

Camille received her Master's in herbal medicine from the Tai Sophia Institute in 2004, and is a professional member of the American Herbalist Guild. She is certified as a nutrition specialist through the American College of Nutrition, and is a licensed nutritionist in the State of Maryland. In 2007, Camille graduated with a Master of Science in physiology and biophysics from Georgetown University. Camille helped Simon Mills with contributions to the Valerian monograph and to the literature search in rewriting Chapters 8 and 9.

Roberta Hutchins

Roberta is a herbal practitioner in England who since graduating has taken a lead role in the herbal world. She is Secretary of the British Herbal Medicine Association and for many years has worked on the preparation of the European Scientific Cooperative on Phytotherapy (ESCOP) monographs that are published consensus reviews of medicinal products submitted formally to the European Medicines Agency. She is recently taken on the role of first editor of these monographs. She has worked in preparing draft monographs with Simon Mills.

Stefanie Oliver

Stefanie Oliver graduated with a Bachelor of Pharmacy in 1998 from Curtin University, WA and has been a practicing pharmacist since. In 2008 Stefanie completed the Graduate Diploma in Health Science (Herbal Medicine) from the University of New England (UNE), NSW and went on to complete a Master of Health Science (Herbal Medicine) from UNE in 2011, focussing her studies on research skills, indigenous health and traditional medicine in primary health care. Stefanie is based in south-west WA where she runs her own consultant business 'Botanical Perspectives'. Stefanie contributed to the updating of the kava and pau d'arco monographs in conjunction with Kerry Bone.

Jerome Sarris

Dr Jerome Sarris is an NHMRC Clinical Research Fellow at The University of Melbourne with a doctorate in the field of psychiatry from the University of Queensland. Jerome undertook post-doctoral training at The University of Melbourne, Department of Psychiatry; The Centre for Human Psychopharmacology, Swinburne University of Technology; and The Depression Clinic and Research Program at Harvard Medical School (MGH). He is co-editor of Clinical Naturopathy: an Evidence-based Guide to Practice, has over 50 publications and has been awarded $2.1 m in personal and study grants. Jerome is a founding member and Vice Chair of The International Network of Integrative Mental Health (INIMH). Jerome contributed to the updating of the Ginkgo and globe artichoke monographs in conjunction with Kerry Bone.

Diana van Die

Dr Diana van Die is a Melbourne-based medical herbalist, lecturer and researcher, who completed a PhD by research into phytotherapy. Her research involvements include women's health, breast cancer and prostate cancer. She has presented at international conferences, and received a scientific award in 2009 for her research on a herbal combination in menopause. Diana wrote the extensive and detailed updates of the St John's wort and St Mary's thistle monographs.

Hans Wohlmuth and Catherine Johnson

Dr Hans Wohlmuth is a Senior Research Fellow with Southern Cross Plant Science at Southern Cross University, Australia. He holds a PhD in pharmacognosy and has more than 25 years' experience with herbal medicines. He is the Curator of the University's Medicinal Plant Garden and Herbarium (PHARM) and a co-founder of its Herbal Authentication Service. Hans has taught extensively and has published in several areas including herbal quality, phytochemistry, phytopharmacology, herb–drug interactions and clinical trials. He currently leads a research group focused on plant compounds for wound healing and serves on the Therapeutics Goods Administration's Advisory Committee on Complementary Medicines.

Catherine Johnson first trained as a nurse, specialising in coronary and intensive care. She set up the Cardiac Rehabilitation Department at John Flynn Private Hospital in Queensland and has also worked extensively in cardiac stress testing. Over time she developed a keen interest in disease prevention and modification and completed a Bachelor of Naturopathy at Southern Cross University in 2001. She practices in the naturopathic clinic she co-owns in Ballina, New South Wales, and maintains an active interest in research. She also works as a technical writer and as a research assistant on clinical trials investigating herbal and nutritional supplements.

Hans and Catherine updated the black cohosh, licorice and thyme monographs in conjunction with Kerry Bone.

Eric Yarnell

Dr Eric Yarnell, ND is associate professor in botanical medicine at Bastyr University (Seattle, WA, USA). He is a clinician at the Bastyr Integrative Oncology Research Center focusing on urogenital cancers. He is vice president of Heron Botanicals and chief operations officer at Healing Mountain Publishing. He is author or co-author of Natural Approach to Gastroenterology 2nd ed, Naturopathic Approach to Urology and Men's Health, Clinical Botanical Medicine 2nd ed, and many other articles and textbooks. Dr Yarnell co-wrote the new gotu kola monograph with Kerry Bone, updated the Melilotus monograph and contributed to a few others including saw palmetto.

There are three conventions for naming herbal remedies. All are used freely in this book to reflect common parlance among herbal practitioners. Familiarity with all three will be useful for any reader.

The common name (here in English and occasionally pinyin Chinese) is the language used with patients and is rendered in this text in ordinary lower case as in 'dandelion'.

The botanical name, the most precise and globally applicable, used to define the plant scientifically and professionally, rendered here in the usual convention of the generic name starting with a capital letter and the specific name in lower case, all in italics, as in *Echinacea angustifolia* or *Taraxacum officinale*.

The abbreviated pharmaceutical name, the common shorthand terminology among practitioners and in the pharmaceutical sector, used especially where the generic name is sufficient (either because only one species is generally used or because the species used is not critical or one understands it to refer to the best species available); in this text the convention is to use an initial capital and no italics, as in 'Echinacea' or 'Taraxacum'.

Herbal medicine is a triumph of popular therapeutic diversity. Plants above all other agents have been used for medicines because they have fitted the immediate personal need: they are accessible and inexpensive, they speak to those who have used them in their own language and they are not provided from a remote professional or government apparatus. For these and other reasons, the use of plants for medicines around the world still vastly exceeds the use of modern synthetic drugs. Such activity is not completely dismissed in scientific society either: plants are increasingly appreciated in pharmaceutical research as a major resource for new medicines and an ever-growing body of medical literature supports the clinical efficacy of herbal treatments. Even where traditional use has largely died out in developed countries, there is an increasing yearning for a new deal in healthcare in which the old remedies feature strongly. To meet this demand, there is a growing number of well-educated herbalists and phytotherapists.

Most herbal use has been very parochial and empirical: local reputations have often been disparate; herbal lore has rarely travelled well. However, herbs have also provided the basis for the great medical systems in human history, of Hippocrates and Galen and the great Islamic medical eras, of the Ayurveda of the Indian subcontinent, of waves of Chinese systematisations over two millennia and the many smaller cultural traditions that were often hybrids of the foregoing. All these systems were formed in large part by the peculiar characteristics of their materia medica; plants have clearly demanded and been granted their own therapeutic approach.

The era of grand systems has probably passed but it is time to develop a new coherent approach to herb use for a scientific age. Apart from a general view that herbs are safer, there has been only a fragmentary rationale for using them as medicines in modern times. Now that there are increasing media attacks on herbal safety, mostly alarmist, there is the risk that even the perceived safety advantage is being whittled away. There is a pressing need to galvanise from the wealth of tradition, empirical practices and modern research a new positive, muscular and consistent pharmacological strategy that can meet the valid challenges of medical science, the safety and the placebo issues above all.

Four main sources of information were used in preparing the following text. Traditional use of herbs is both the largest and most difficult resource. The bewildering variety of folk practices around the world, the powerful confounding effect of social context and other non-specific or placebo effects make reliable conclusions from any one tradition difficult. However, evidence will be presented that in general, folk use and pharmacological activity are indeed closely correlated. More usefully, it will be shown that there are recurring themes in indigenous use: persistent therapeutic approaches and consistent use of 'archetypal' chemical groups within plants. These resonances will be identified and will provide the backdrop to discussions of modern use.

There is also the clinical experience of modern practitioners to consider. This has the advantages of being up to date and set in a modern medical context. It still suffers, however, from the confounding effect of non-specific effects of treatment: in many of the conditions for which modern phytotherapy is applied the placebo effect is likely to be high, sometimes very high, and without controlling for this effect the independent activity of the herbs themselves is hard to isolate. Nevertheless, there are ways in which the fog can be cleared and practitioners can often obtain quite reliable insights into the action of their prescriptions; where these accord more widely, they may also add usefully to a growing caseload.

The third data resource is less clinically relevant but is both substantial and scientifically sound. The available published literature on phytochemistry (the chemistry of plants) and preclinical pharmacology of plant extracts grows at an astounding pace, as noted earlier. There are several peer-reviewed scientific journals devoted to the subject and there is of course a powerful incentive for such work in the pharmaceutical industry's search for new drugs. Researchers have no doubt that nature is still the preeminent synthetic chemist and that in plants particularly, there are almost infinite reserves of fascinating chemical constituents with actual and potential effects on the human body. As such information accumulates, it is sometimes possible to understand better traditional uses of plants. Where such associations can be made, they will be posited in the text as leads for further exploration. They will not be used, however, as confirmation of a clinical effect; experience in practice is that the effect of the whole plant is rarely predicted by the effects of its parts. The pharmaceutical industry's own experience is that preclinical activity only occasionally translates into clinically useful benefits.

Finally, there is the evidence that counts most in the court of clinical judgement. There are still too few well-conducted, placebo-controlled, double blind clinical trials into the effect of herbal medicines. These are expensive to conduct and present methodological and logistical challenges (especially in satisfactorily measuring outcomes in the less pathologically defined conditions for which herbs are most often applied). Without patent protection, industry is less inclined to invest in such studies. However, the evidence is accumulating. A number of meta-analyses of clinical trial data have shown that for the few individual herbs most studied, the clinical evidence is indeed persuasive. In most such cases, the plants concerned are pharmacologically unremarkable; their survival through the most intense scrutiny reassures that other remedies could do the same. More importantly for this book, there are specific lessons that can be applied in judging likely efficacy of a wider range of plants.

No single source above can absolutely confirm that herbs are a rational treatment strategy. It is for this reason that herbs have sometimes been dismissed as the refuge of the romantic and the uncritical. However, when all sources of information are integrated something genuinely exciting emerges: traditionally based coherent treatment policies for a range of conditions are given new relevance in modern practice and resonate with new pharmacological insights into the activity of plant constituents. As most of the strategies developed are unique to herbal medicine and address clinical problems that are notoriously difficult to treat in modern times, they will repay further investigation.

The different data sources above are elaborated in the contents of this book. In Part One, traditional systematic approaches to herbal therapeutics from around the world are outlined first; this finishes with a brief review of modern insights into the behaviour of dynamic systems, which have lead to the development of chaos and complexity models and which incidentally provide new explanations for healing phenomena. There then follows an introduction to the pharmacological principles emerging from current knowledge of the activity of plant constituents. Many constituents are classified into 'archetypal' chemical groups with well-established pharmacological activities; understanding these activities allows for preliminary assessments of a plant's potential with only minimal information of its taxonomic group and constitution. The presence of prominent archetypal groups can often lead to fertile cross-referencing with traditional reputations to raise fascinating clinical prospects. This section extends to consideration of a radically new explanation for the effects of herbs on the body. It will be pointed out that most herbal constituents start with topical effects (i.e. locally at the site of application) and that they are particularly likely to stimulate the wide range of functions linked to trigger sites on the lining of the digestive tract. Traditional reputations will be linked to modern physiological insights to provide promising new strategies for a wide range of diseases.

There follow a number of sections which elaborate the practical implications of applying herbal remedies compared with other treatments. There is a section on the most persistent herbal therapeutic principles found in the traditional records, updated into modern terminology, and providing a basis for the more detailed discussions later. The most appropriate diagnostic information required for herbal prescription is discussed next, emphasising the importance of assessing functional performance in the body as much as morbid states; the ancient techniques of pulse and tongue diagnosis used around the world are reviewed in this context. Important discussions of the issues of validation and safety follow; in both areas herbal medicine is subject to challenge but in both reassuring progress is being made.

Part Two looks more closely at the herbal approach to particular clinical conditions. These are divided into two groups: general disease conditions that lead to the most common pathological states afflicting humanity and the more particular functional disturbances of the body's organ systems to which herbal medicine has so often been applied. Functional disturbances can have many causes; pathological processes are the most serious but probably not the most common. Herbal remedies have persistently been viewed as addressing what might be called 'misbehaviours' of body functions, a term that includes the notion of psychosomatic disorders but also all the other ways in which the living body finds it difficult to coexist smoothly with its environment.

No practical guide to using herbal remedies could be complete without a good review of the dosage issue and indeed this opens Part Two. There is much confusion abroad on this with widely varying dose regimes being recommended. The authors explore the relative cases for each approach, taking account of a wide range of sources, and make clear recommendations in all the following sections.

Part Three is devoted to individual remedies. Fifty plants most widely used in the Western herbal tradition, but including examples from around the world, are reviewed in considerable depth. Clinical imperatives still rule and the information most important to the practitioner opens each monograph – practical guides as to when to use and not to use each plant, cautions and doubts honestly raised as appropriate. However, there also follow comprehensive details of the current scientific information on each herb, fully referenced, so that the best available technical assessments can be made by each reader.

There are a number of reference guides for easy access. As well as a detailed general index, there is an index of symptoms and conditions and one for herb activities. All sections of the book are comprehensively supported with citations so that the reader can pursue further reading in depth.

Any new therapeutic framework needs broad agreement from current practitioners. There are now thousands of highly educated clinicians in the developed countries, many of them physicians, who prescribe herbal medicines regularly in their clinical work. Most of these have been bypassed by the vigorous scientific activity currently found at phytomedicine conferences or in the technical literature. They have obviously acquired valuable experience but rarely have the tools with which to separate the effects of the remedy from other clinical phenomena and still lack the institutional support that might underpin their aspirations. Nevertheless, they remain a vital community. Both authors of this book are experienced herbal practitioners and are guided in this work mainly by clinical priorities. They will aim to provide new information for debate among their colleagues, possible new rationales for their practices, even new approaches for difficult clinical problems.

The book should also reassure other healthcare workers, for example doctors, pharmacists, osteopaths and chiropractors, who are tempted to try herbal medicines themselves but want a sound basis first. Although many doctors in Europe prescribe phytomedicines, this is rare in English-speaking countries in which there is more scepticism about using crude historical folk remedies as a serious substitute for scientific medication. Although there is a growing interest in other complementary techniques, herbal medicine has not managed to persuade that it has a coherent strategy for treating difficult conditions. That patients increasingly resort to herbs is seen as something separate from medicine, unless a safety issue is perceived. This text will present a substantial and well-documented case for herbs as unique strategies in the treatment of some of the most intractable problems in modern healthcare.

In many developed countries, natural healthcare alternatives are provided by a range of naturopathic professional groups. As well as dietary treatment and various complementary disciplines, these practitioners frequently use herbal remedies. Sometimes, the herbal component has only a minor and adjunctive role in the overall treatment strategy. This text will surely persuade that there are many areas where informed application of herbs might transform the prospects of difficult conditions and that, in particular, dietary measures can be powerfully reinforced or amended by the established modulatory effects of herbs on the digestive processes. There is also a trend among complementary practitioners to favour herbal remedies from China and India, accompanied as these are by their own elaborate therapeutic system. This account should allow such practitioners better to understand the underlying principles and may reinstate indigenous remedies in their materia medica.

In the countries of Asia, Africa and South America, a much larger proportion of the population still choose or rely on herbal medicines for their day-to-day healthcare. The World Health Organisation and other international agencies have long recognised that traditional health practitioners and their remedies represent a vital resource to be encouraged, to more effectively maintain health in remote regions and better to maintain plant biodiversity and local communities and industries. As these practitioners work to develop their therapeutic approaches and integrate them better with Western delivery systems, they may welcome the insights of those with long experience of coexistence with Western medicine. The remedies will be different but the principles are likely to be the same.

The patient can also learn from this book. Anyone who wishes to be informed about the treatment of their personal condition, who wants to take responsibility for their own health, who is fascinated that there may be effective remedies provided freely in nature and who is able to grasp basic medical concepts will find this a treasure trove. All such readers must be reminded, however, that illness can often be complex and sometimes dangerous. They should never proceed far without expert advice and never stray from adequate supervision of any illness.

What follows is a contribution to a debate among those interested in herbal medicine. It will lay out as effectively as possible a realistic strategy in line with scientific evidence but based also on experience in practice and on the legacy of much longer traditions. It will inevitably be contentious in parts: some cherished beliefs will be challenged, but if this stimulates productive debate then nothing should be lost.

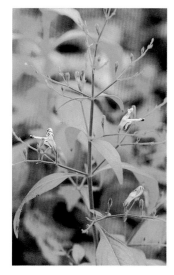

PLATE 1:
Andrographis
(*Andrographis paniculata*)

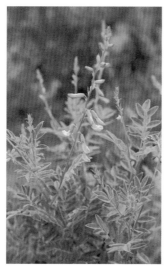

PLATE 2:
Astragalus
(*Astragalus membranaceus*)

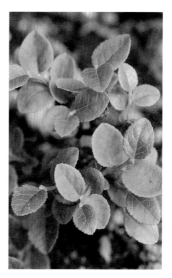

PLATE 3:
Bilberry
(*Vaccinium myrtillus*)

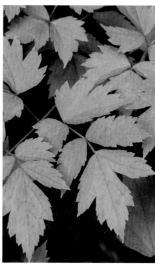

PLATE 4:
Black cohosh
(*Actaea racemosa*)

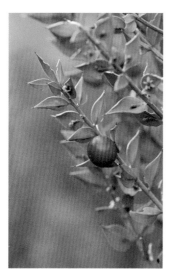

PLATE 5:
Butcher's broom
(*Ruscus aculeatus*)

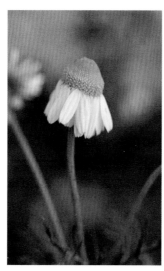

PLATE 6:
Chamomile, German
(*Matricaria recutita*)

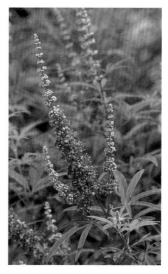

PLATE 7:
Chaste tree
(*Vitex agnus-castus*)

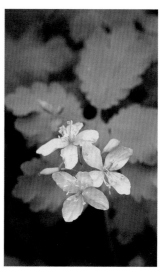

PLATE 8:
Chelidonium
(*Chelidonium majus*)

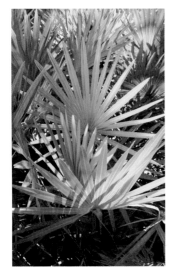

PLATE 25:
Saw palmetto
(*Serenoa repens*)

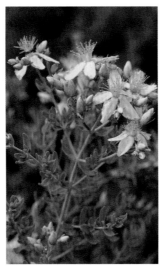

PLATE 26:
St John's wort
(*Hypericum perforatum*)

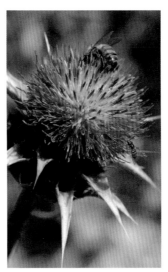

PLATE 27:
St Mary's thistle
(*Silybum marianum*)

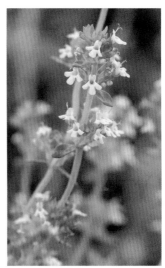

PLATE 28:
Thyme
(*Thymus vulgaris*)

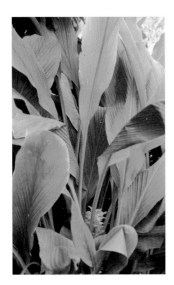

PLATE 29:
Turmeric
(*Curcuma longa*)

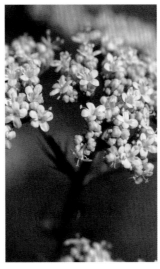

PLATE 30:
Valerian
(*Valeriana officinalis*)

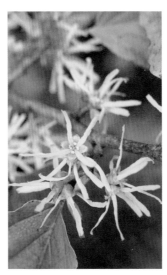

PLATE 31:
Witchhazel
(*Hamamelis virginiana*)

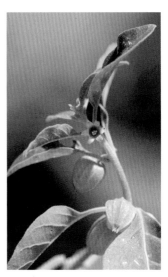

PLATE 32:
Withania
(*Withania somnifera*)

PART 1

Background and strategies

Herbal therapeutic systems

CHAPTER CONTENTS

From the beginning: popular practices

Plants and humans share many experiences. Humans are of course one species spread around the world with all individuals sharing essentially the same physiology and anatomy. However, even the myriad species of plants share more than they differ, with common mechanisms of primary metabolism and cell structure and many common strategies of regulation, reproduction and even defence. Although there are vast numbers of pharmacologically active 'secondary' metabolites in plants, they mostly classify into a small list of phytochemical groups (see Chapter 2). A review of human medical cultures shows that there are common themes that may arise from consistent experiences of consuming plants. When these themes are recast in the light of modern scientific enquiry one may glimpse therapeutic approaches that are radically different from those which underpin conventional medicine.

What also emerges again and again is that, contrary to modern prejudice, writers on medicine from the very earliest eras demonstrate a respect for rigorous observation and humane pragmatism that still may provide a valuable lesson for healthcare today. These sources are not to be dismissed lightly.

As it is now known that animals use plants for medicinal purposes,[1,2] it is unlikely that there was a time when humans did not use herbal remedies. There is prehistoric evidence of the use of medicinals from the USA[3] and medicinal plant traces found at neolithic sites.[4] There are also innumerable accounts of medicinal plants being used by small communities around the world, living wholly within the natural world and crafting their survival from the facilities around them.[5–7]

Most of what is known about herbal use from recorded history is provided by early texts, often among the earliest of all known books. However, one overwhelming gap in this record is that, although in its original mode herbal medicine was centred in local communities and practised largely by women, this is barely reflected in contemporary accounts.[8] After the demise of organised medicine with the collapse of the Roman empire, healthcare in Europe for most people was again provided at a very local level, probably including a mix of herbs and diet, together with faith and holy relics, as well as astrology, pagan incantation and ritual[9] (the Inquisition permitting – millions of women were killed for practising 'witchcraft' across Europe from the 13th to the 18th centuries).[10] Hildegarde von Bingen, one of the first prominent woman authorities in Europe, achieved particular renown through her medicinal text *Physica*. In it, she became the first woman publicly to discuss plants in relation to their medicinal properties.[11] She was, however, a solitary exception to the prevailing view that women were not in the forefront of academic, professional or literary efforts. Like her, however, most European writers of the time were from the monastic tradition, only moving into the popular arena around Chaucer's time. By then well-organised medicinal gardens and practices were recorded in England by authors such as Henry Daniel, John Arderne, John Bray and Chaucer himself, all reflecting on current medicinal practice across Europe in the 14th century.[12] Where systems were apparent in these texts, they appear to have been derived from the Graeco-Roman tradition with

DOI: http://dx.doi.org/10.1016/B978-0-443-06992-5.00001-3

varying amounts of astrology, especially in works by Culpeper and Gerard. It was only with the works of Paracelsus that scholarship began substantially to question the previous deference to Galen and medicine moved into the modern technological age, leaving folk practice way behind.

Such was the enormous variety of folk practices around the world that one must conclude that, while most rationales were based on empiricism, local shibboleths and traditions often acted as a brake on innovation. Nevertheless, there are likely to have been common features. A fascinating account of one remote group in Central America[13] shows significant similarities between their and other humoral approaches around the world. It is also certain that where therapeutic systems did develop, they were based on popular practices.

Graeco-Roman and Islamic medicine

The systematic development of medical ideas that started with the Hippocratic writings from the Greek island of Kos in the fifth and fourth centuries BC and climaxed in the work of Galen in the second century AD, laid the foundations for European medicine until the scientific era, and the framework for Islamic medicine until the present time. They were marked by almost modern standards of empiricism, logic and rigour.[14]

The Hippocratic writings,[15] a complex series of treatises from a school rather than from one individual, were an astonishing event. In passages of renaissant illumination, they evidenced an enlightened tradition that invoked dietary, lifestyle, environmental and psychotherapeutic means to encouraging health. The Hippocratic tradition is generally associated with the concept of the natural healing power of life, the *vis medicatrix naturae*. In fact, most of the texts are pragmatic guides to maintaining health and to the practice of medicine, with some passages (e.g. *The Art of Medicine*) being undisguised paeans to the importance of physicians in healthcare!

There were herbs included in the Hippocratic canon, but it was a wider doctrine of whole healthcare that was being formulated. It was left to others to formulate the materia medicae of the day. The Greek Dioscorides in the first century AD rigorously collected information about 500 plants and remedies in tours with the Roman armies and collated them in his seminal *Materia Medica*.[16]

Galen is widely regarded as the pivotal Graeco-Roman authority in medicinal matters. He wrote extensively about his subject, setting out comprehensive principles of sometimes surprising topicality. For example, he proposed a research agenda for establishing the 'powers' of a remedy, based on the observance of eight conditions:

1. The drug must be of good unadulterated quality.

2. The illness must be simple, not complex.

3. The illness must be appropriate to the action of the drug.

4. The drug must be more powerful than the illness.

5. One should make careful note of the course of illness and treatment.

6. One must ensure that the effect of the drug is the same for everybody at every time.

7. One must see that the effect of the drug is specific for human beings (in an animal it can have another effect).

8. One must distinguish the effect of drugs (working by their qualities) from foods (working by their substance).

In further passages (most have never been translated into English) he shows clear evidence of modern logical thought in setting out a series of experiments to prove that the kidneys were the source of urine into the bladder.[14]

The fundamental principle in Galen's work was that nature was an active dynamic force, and phenomena its expressed purpose. Treatments engaged these forces, either in the case of drugs through their own dynamic 'qualities', or in the case of foods by the qualities of their substance. In classifying the dynamic qualities of medicines, he refined the widely established view that they had 'temperaments' reflecting well-understood climatic influences.

In the Greek and Roman world the temperaments hot, cold, dampness and dryness were formed into paired combinations of the four elements that made up nature: earth, water, fire and air (heat is generated by fire and air, cold by earth and water and so on). The elements were associated with four fluids, 'juices' or humours in the body, respectively black bile, phlegm, yellow bile and blood (their more everyday manifestations were faeces, mucus, vomit and bleeding), with these being linked with personality types: the melancholic, phlegmatic, choleric and sanguine. As we will see elsewhere, the Old World had no problems in associating the most banal phenomenon with fundamental truths about human nature! Therapeutically the humours were the cornerstone and physicians moved to counteract excess (*plethora*) or deficiency (*kenos*) in any of them. For excess or toxic conditions 'diasthetic' remedies, sometimes alterants and eliminatives, were literally 'antidotes', primarily heating, cooling, drying and moistening accordingly, in degrees, with remedies in the 'first degree' milder than those in the third or fourth (which became increasingly dangerous). In deficiency conditions 'physic' remedies were replenishing, supportive or 'plerotic'.

A widely noted quality of remedies was the effect they appeared to have on the mobilisation of body heat, especially in relation to fevers. His authoritative definitions of these pharmaceutical qualities were widely used throughout medieval Europe:

> All medicines considered in themselves are either hot, cold, moist, dry or temperate.

> The qualities of medicines are considered in respect of man, not of themselves; for those simples are called hot which heat our bodies; for those cold which cool them; and those temperate which work no change at all …

> Such as are hot in the first degree, are of equal heat with our bodies, and they only add a natural heat to them, if it be cooled by nature or by accident thereby cherishing the natural heat when weak, and restoring it when wanting. Their use is: 1. To make the offending humours thin, that they may be expelled by sweat or perspiration; and 2. By outward application to abate inflammations and fevers by opening the pores of the skin.

> Such as are hot in the second degree, as much exceed the first, as our natural heat exceeds a temperature. Their use is to open the pores, and take away obstructions, by relaxing tough humours and by their essential force and strength, when nature cannot do it.

Such as are hot in the third degree, are more powerful in heating, because they tend to inflame and cause fevers. Their use is to promote perspiration extremely, and soften tough humours, and therefore all of them resist poison.

Such as are hot in the fourth degree, burn the body, if outwardly applied. Their use is to cause inflammation, raise blisters, and corrode the skin.

Such as are cold in the first degree, fall as much on the one side of temperate as doth hot on the other. Their use is: 1. To qualify the heat of the stomach and cause digestion; 2. To abate the heat in fevers; and 3. To refresh the spirits being almost suffocated.

Such as are cold in the third degree, are such as have a repercussive force. Their use is: 1. To drive back the matter, and stop defluctions; 2. To make the humours thick; and 3. To limit the violence of choler, repress perspiration, and keep the spirits from fainting.

Such as are cold in the fourth degree, are such as to stupefy the senses. They are used: 1. In violent pains; and 2. In extreme watchings, and the like cases, where life is despaired of.

This is a clinically elaborate classification. Heating remedies start as at 'equal heat with our bodies' (i.e. normalising a healthy body temperature), increasing in stages to those that are so hot that they must only be 'outwardly applied' in counter-irritation and blistering strategies (see p. 39). Their primary function is to thin 'offending humours', or toxic accumulations, a process that may have been likened to the effect of warming congealed meat stock, so that they may be expelled by perspiration (in fever). This strategy was clear: fevers were a healthy response and such remedies supported this response 'when nature cannot do it'. As they become stronger they are more forceful, till they actually 'cause fevers' and 'cause inflammations', taking over entirely from a failing constitution.

Cooling remedies are inherently more risky. The ultimate cold is the corpse. Nevertheless, they can be used to contain excessive vital responses such as pain, 'choler' and excessive eliminations ('defluctions'). Intriguingly, at the gentlest such level, the effect is to 'cause digestion'; the bitters (see p. 84) were included in this category, the attraction being that these cooled but did not depress, reducing heat by switching the physiology towards increased digestive activity (universally seen as cooling) and thus increased nourishment, a highly attractive tactic in many fevers. Also intriguing is the insight at the other end of the spectrum. Using powerful sedatives when all else fails and death is imminent ('in extreme watchings') is one of the less formally advisable clinical knacks from a more desperate age; it appears that the effect can be to wipe out the clamour of adversity at that stage of crisis so that new life might just flicker back. The works of the Graeco-Roman writers were most extensively remodelled by the medical writers of the Islamic era. Up to 100 authors on pharmaceutics and materia medica are identifiable in the Arabic bibliographies, most copying and adapting directly from Dioscorides and Galen. There were, however, notable developments, including the work of the Persians al-Majusi (Ali Abbas), ar-Rhazi (Rhazes) and Ibn-Sina (Avicenna), the Jew Maimonides and the Christian Hunayn ibn-Ishaq. However, not for the first time in reviews of classic texts (the Chinese canon is another example) there is a sense that much that was written was truly theoretical, with evidence of systematisation by rote, showing little regard for likely actual practices.[17]

Nevertheless, it is apparent that in Islamic pharmaceutics considerable respect was paid to the qualities of individual herbs (unlike the Chinese emphasis on formulations, these were seen as reflecting a secondary skill). Physicians were expected to understand intimately the nature of each remedy, its natural habitat, its specific energy pattern, actions, indications, specific relationships to the organs, duration of action, toxicity and contraindications, types of preparation, dosage, administration and antidotes.[18]

The Islamic medical tradition as Unani/Tibb has been maintained in its heartland until the present day and it also generated important benefits for the medicine of Europe. Montpellier and Salerno were among the first of the new medical centres of Europe. Rather than relying just on ancient texts, a new experimental culture led to reports of the tested effects of substances from identified plants. This advance was fostered by the foundation of universities and greatly aided by the later invention of the printing press, which also allowed wider dissemination of the classical texts.[19]

Chinese herbal medicine

The traditions of medicine that developed in China from prehistoric times have survived as a major part of healthcare provision to the present day and through this extraordinary continuity constitute the most comprehensive clinical strategy for the use of herbal medicines anywhere.

This text is not the place for an exhaustive overview of Chinese medicine. There are effective texts available in English, notably the essential work by Unschuld,[20] other classic texts,[21,22] one very accessible introduction,[23] a rigorous yet practical review,[24] and a summary designed to help the Western practitioner.[25] What will be attempted here is the distillation of uniquely herbal strategies and concepts from the vast corpus of Chinese medicine. There is much to choose from. Over the last 2000 years a number of seminal texts and systems have been developed, each incorporating the developments of their predecessors. These were often very intricate systems, reflecting perhaps the priorities of scholarship and portent lore (much theorising at the early stages was for the Imperial court[26]). At more than one stage, there appears to have been some difficulty in organising the empirical folk traditions into neat systems[20] and there is always a suspicion that realities may have been squeezed to justify the cosmology.

However, Chinese medicine was certainly not idle theorising. In one review of the medicine of early China,[27] it has been pointed out that among other 'modern' advances were the use of androgens and oestrogens (in placentas) to treat hypogonadism, the development of forensic medicine, the advocacy of hand washing to avoid infection and the association of hardening of the arteries with high salt intake. Qualifying examinations for physicians were conducted by the Chinese state as early as the first century AD and there was an elaborate system of medical ethics.

It is first important to emphasise that the Chinese world view has been fundamentally different from that in the West since the time of Aristotle. In Chinese thinking everything moves (the seminal classic, the *I Ching*, is translated as the 'Book of Changes'). Events are automatically described by their transient qualities in relation to other events and are manifestations of energies in ways that the West understood only after Einstein.[28] The generic term for these energies is *qi*, but in the case of the living body there are many forms of varying density, from *wei qi* as the most rarefied on the body surface, manifest in acute defensive reactions like fever and colds, through *ying qi*, the nourishing *qi* flowing through the meridians, to *xue* or blood, the most substantial aspect of *qi*, manifest in many somatic events. *Qi* is also manifest in *jing* (essence) and the body fluids. The comparison with modern physics is even more apposite as *qi* is simultaneously energy, movement and fluid (reminiscent of attempts to define light as waves and/or particles).

Transience continues: thus, in what has become known as Traditional Chinese Medicine (TCM – in fact the mainstream tradition in China after the Communist Revolution of 1948 and the one most widely used by Western practitioners), the framework by which diseases are addressed is made up of four sets of polar opposites, the 'eight conditions'.

Each pair denotes a spectrum of qualities onto which any illness can be placed; each implies that the aim of any therapeutic measure is to move extremes back towards a healthy mean. Although used as a diagnostic framework for acupuncture, it is widely agreed that TCM is primarily based on herbal therapeutics. Thus herbs are ascribed temperaments or tendencies accordingly: they may be *Yin* or *Yang*, tonic or dispersive, cooling or heating, eliminative or constructive. These manifestations are in turn aspects of fundamental properties of the remedies (see Table 1.1).

In Chinese medicine there is little regard for anatomy and the main entities upon which pathogenic or therapeutic forces act are essentially functional and physiological. There are six pairs of functions, often confusingly translated in the West as 'organs'. These, like all phenomena in the Chinese world, are ascribed to points on the five-phase cycle that further illuminate their qualities. The five phases (the frequently used term 'five elements' is clearly not appropriate here) are seasonal and cyclical transitions through which all the universe moves. They have a multitude of dynamic relationships with each

other and an array of more or less consistent qualities. The five phases, their attributes and their relationship with the six pairs of functions are illustrated in Table 1.2.

Following the strictures of Porkert,[21] words in this text which may be confused with their Western meanings are distinguished typographically (with capitals and italics though not, as he insisted, using completely new words altogether).

The five Tastes (Chinese pharmacology)

In days before laboratory investigations, taste was obviously a major arbiter of a plant's quality and it is easily seen how an association with pharmacological activity could be made. In the case of Chinese medicine the taste became a pharmacological force in its own right.

Two of the *Tastes* are primarily *yang* and tend to disperse upwards in the body. They are the pungent and sweet *Tastes* (the latter is usually yoked with a sixth non-taste quality, referred to here as the bland *Taste*).

Three *Tastes* are primarily *yin* and tend to flow downwards in the body. They are the sour, bitter and salty *Tastes*.

The *Tastes* were assigned to the five phases and their functional manifestations in the body, as below. In turn, this came to mean that the normal role of each *Function* included being a vehicle for the activity of its own *Taste* and depended on acquiring a quantum, primarily from food or medicine.

While a moderate amount of each *Taste* is necessary for its corresponding *Function*, there are also wider effects arising from their consumption. The relationships are expressed in Figure 1.1. (For a review of the implications of the four-phase nature of the relationships and the peculiar position of the *Spleen*, see Mills.[25])

Tonification

As well as being associated with one *Function*, each *Taste* is also seen to tonify, i.e. at moderate levels support, another *Function*.

Dispersing

Extra amounts of each *Taste* disperse excessive activity in the *Function* with which it is linked. This is straightforward except in the case of the *Spleen*, which is already tonified by sweet: it appears, therefore, to do a swap with the *Heart*.

Damaging

The effects of taking excessive amounts of any particular *Taste* follow a conventional destructive *ko* cycle pattern in the five-phase relationship.

A brief review of the properties of each *Taste* is instructive.

Salty

The taste of common salt and seafood, but is not well represented in the herbal materia medica. However, seaweeds are occasionally used in maritime cultures and in Japan. It is possible to classify the occasional remedy like celery seed in this

Table 1.1	
Condition	**Attributes**
Yang	Active, expanding, transforming, dispersive, centrifugal, aggressive, light
Yin	Constructive, sustaining, completing, condensing, centripetal, responsive, dark
Full	Repleted
Empty	Depleted
Hot	Active
Cold	Passive
External	Acute
Internal	Chronic

Table 1.2

Phase	*Fire*	*Earth*	*Metal*	*Water*	*Wood*
Attributes	Heating, attracting, burning, destructive, ascending, illuminative	Nourishing, stable, restful, central, fertile	Hard, strong but mouldable, cold but responsive to heat, lustrous, protective	Soaking, sinking, cold, still, deep, dark, potent, latent	Growing, spreading outward
Function (*yin*)	*Heart/Pericardium*	*Spleen*	*Lungs*	*Kidney*	*Liver*
Attributes	1) Sovereign, rules *xue*, stores *shen*, maintains individual integrity, seen in face, tongue, pleasure, sweating and laughter 2) Ambassador, origin of pleasure and social skills	Transformation, primary digestive function, in charge of upward movement, stores nourishing *qi*, rules flesh and limbs, seen also in lips, mouth, sympathy, saliva and singing	Prime minister, source of rhythm, directs movement outward (defence) and fluid downward, site of *qi* production, rules *qi*, seen also in nose, skin, sorrow, nasal secretions and crying	Root of life and will, stores *jing* (essence), rules birth, development and reproduction, source of *yin* and *yang*, heat and power, rules bones and marrow, seen also in hair, ears, fear, sputum and moaning	Allocation of resources, spreading, stores *xue*, rules sinews, also seen in nails, eyes, anger, tears, shouting
Function (*yang*)	*Small Intestine/Triple Heater*	*Stomach*	*Large Intestine*	*Bladder*	*Gallbladder*
Attributes	1) Rules separation of pure from impure 2) Smelting, distillation and condensation, regulates movement of fluids	Receives and digests food, in charge of downward movement, starts separation of pure from the impure	Rules elimination, continues separation of pure from impure	Rules fluid eliminations, confluence of fluids	Directs other functions, stores bile
Pharmacological attribute (*Taste*)	Bitter	Sweet	Pungent	Salty	Sour

category. In China, however, the main group of drugs classified as salty are animal tissues and the minerals.

The salty *Taste* is directed by the *Spleen* to the *Kidneys*. It is *yin* and tends to flow downwards in the body and particularly to the bones.

It is said to 'moisten' and 'soften' and salty remedies are used for 'dry, hard' pathologies, such as tumours, fibroses (e.g. liver cirrhosis), constipation and other abdominal swellings.

In moderation it tonifies the *Heart*, but damages it in excess. It is interesting to see how closely ancient observations tie in with current views on the influence of salt and electrolytes on the circulation.

Sour

This arises as the result of the stimulation of the sour taste buds by hydrogen ions. It is the taste of fruit acids, vinegar and tannins.

The sour *Taste* is directed by the *Spleen* to the *Liver*; it is *yin* and tends to move downwards in the body. It moves particularly to the muscle fibres (or 'sinews').

It is said to 'absorb' and 'bind' and is applied to discharges, excessive diuresis, incontinence, perspiration and premature ejaculation. Some of these indications recur in the discussion of the effect of tannins (see p. 35).

It disperses excess activity in the *Liver* and tonifies the *Lungs*. Among other roles, the latter is concerned with the maintenance of the body's defences against external pathogens. The role of fruit as protection, particularly against respiratory infections, was thus apparently not a new discovery.

In excess it damages the *Spleen*. Excessive consumption of tannins interferes with assimilation of foods.

Bitter

This taste is mediated by bitter taste buds in the mouth which are stimulated by a number of chemical structures. It is thus a quality recognised by the Chinese, and others, as being intrinsic to herbal remedies.

It is directed by the *Spleen* to the *Heart*; it is *yin* and tends to flow downwards in the body. It moves particularly to *xue* ('blood'). As the densest of the circulating energies in the body, *xue* is in effect the speculative force behind the more somatic events in the body. Compared to acupuncture, which is seen to primarily affect *qi*, the more rarefied circulating energy, the archetypal bitterness of herbal remedies is strongly associated with treating more substantial deep-seated clinical problems.

It is said to 'sedate', 'dry' and 'harden'. The first reflects bitter's cool temperament while 'drying' refers to bitter's use in 'damp-heat' conditions (e.g. hepatitis); 'harden' may be better translated by the term 'consolidate' to express the effect of improving assimilation and nourishment.

It disperses excess in the *Spleen*. A modern manifestation of such a condition is the excessive consumption of sweet

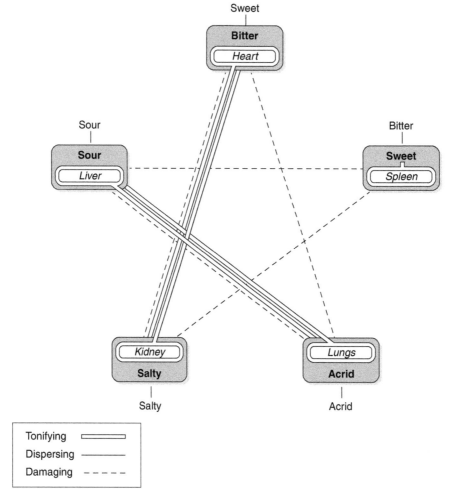

Figure 1.1 • The five Tastes and their relationships.

foods with the consequent possible disruptions in blood sugar levels. There is clinical experience of the benefits of bitter herbs in stabilising such disruptions.

It tonifies the *Kidneys*. As the repository of constitutional reserves, the *Kidneys* provide the greatest tonifying challenge, another example of the universal traditional reverence for bitters.

In excess it damages the *Lungs*. Excessive cooling suppresses vital defences.

Sweet

In a time when sugar was almost unknown, this was a far more subtle taste and was used to refer to the intrinsic sweetness of the rural diet: cereals, pulses, cooked root vegetables and those fruits suitable for drying and storing as winter food such as apricots, figs and prunes. In days when even honey was rare, the taste of extracted sugar would have been considered intrinsically excessive. In herbal remedies the sweet taste is exhibited particularly by the saponins, a chemical group often found in Chinese tonics and adaptogens.

The *Spleen* keeps the sweet *Taste* to itself; it is *yang* and tends to move upwards in the body, particularly to the soft tissues. Sweetness is nourishment: it is the quality of a simple

agrarian diet and has its most potent metaphor in mother's milk. It thus manifests in the soft tissues and in overall body shape.

It is said to 'tonify' and to 'balance'. As well as being the obvious tonic influence, a good stable agrarian diet is the most effective way to promote homeostasis; many saponin-rich adaptogenic remedies have a similar clinical reputation.

It disperses excess in the *Heart*, including symptoms of anxiety and nervous tension.

In excess it damages the *Kidneys*, a terminal effect in Chinese medicine, resulting in premature ageing. The Chinese in effect predicted an enfeeblement of general vitality through excessive sweet consumption.

Pungent

Sometimes also called 'acrid', this is the taste of the hot spices: cayenne, ginger, mustard, the peppers, horseradish, raw onions and garlic (both the latter become sweet when cooked) and generally all the 'heating' herbal remedies. Unlike the other four tastes, the effect is not linked to any special taste bud but simply follows direct irritation of any exposed tissues and sensory nerve fibres. The association with the *Metal* phase may have followed inhaling the fumes given off from smelting.

It is directed by the *Spleen* to the *Lungs*; it is *yang* and tends to move upward, particularly to *qi*. The heating properties of the pungent *Taste* are always its dominant feature.

It is said to 'move *qi*', 'disperse', 'activate the body fluids', 'cause expulsion from the *Lungs*' and 'open the pores'. It tends to be used therefore for superficial, external disease conditions, to counteract external pathogenic influences, especially *Wind* and *Cold*, and to mobilise stagnant body energies.

It disperses excess in the *Lungs*, notably that manifested by congested bronchial inflammations. It tonifies the *Liver*, the *Function* responsible for ensuring a balanced dispersal of all the body's energies and activities, but in excess also damages the *Liver*.

Bland

Is a substance seen as having no character and without dynamic action in the body. It is not, therefore, a typical *Taste* and is not recognised in all classical texts. Where it is, it is said to slip through the body without hindrance or interaction. It moves straight through from the *Spleen* to the *Bladder*, i.e. the urinary system, and thus out of the body.

Its only effect, therefore, is that it is a diuretic. Many of the diuretics used in herbal medicine have a characteristic blandness of taste.

Ayurvedic herbal medicine

The written record of the traditional medicine of India is less accessible than that for China, with few English texts from India itself[29–31] and few notable, though exceptional, texts written in the West.[32,33] Nevertheless, it is clear that this tradition includes significant systematising of medical practices in one of the major cultures in history. Medicines were classified, for example, by their *Tastes* and therapeutic categories, as in Chinese medicine, and their effects on illnesses linked to constitutional types (*doshas*) and humours.

The *doshas* provide the primary orientation. The word derives from the same root as the English 'dys-' as in 'dysfunction': the *dosha* is essentially a fault in the healthy state of the body. Three *doshas* are fundamental, each being a condensation of pairs of the five elements, waste products produced when the body replenishes its elements. The *doshas* support the body only as long as they continually flow out of it, as proper eliminations of urine, faeces and sweat.

Kapha is a condensation of water and earth (the damp and dry elements of matter) and it projects itself into the production of lubricant fluids in the body. It is the stabilising influence in the body and generally concentrates in the thorax to contain rising *vata*; it is associated with mucus. Illnesses of excessive *kapha* are marked by symptoms of cold, damp and heaviness (e.g. catarrh, oedema, abdominal congestion) and are relieved by warming, drying, stimulating remedies such as the pungent spices, warming diaphoretics and expectorants, emetics, aromatic and bitter digestives, and carminatives and, to a lesser extent, perhaps combined with the above, diuretics, laxatives and astringents.

Pitta collects fire and water elements into the production of bile and is associated with digestive juices more generally; it is in charge of transformation and processing, and concentrates in the mid-abdomen. Illnesses of excessive or obstructed *pitta* are marked by biliary disturbances and may include symptoms of heat, damp and excessive activity (e.g. fever, inflammation, infection, blood toxicities, bleeding); they are relieved as appropriate, and perhaps in combination, by cooling, drying, nutritive or calming remedies such as the bitters, purgatives, sweet tonic remedies, astringents, cooling diaphoretics, alteratives and diuretics.

Vata arises from condensation of air and space and is the (often unstable) windy form of *prana*, linked to the functions of the respiratory system. It is in charge of all movement in the body and it concentrates in the lower abdomen to help lift *kapha*. Illnesses of the *vata* type, marked by cold, dryness and excessive (especially nervous) activity, are of two types. Deficient *vata* (e.g. emaciation and constitutional dehydration) is treated with sweet and nutritive tonics, bulking laxatives, demulcents and salty remedies. Accumulated or obstructed *vata* is a congestive version that may include abdominal distension and gas, constipation and rheumatic and arthritic conditions. This is treated with modest pungent herbs in the short term only, moderate warming diaphoretics, carminatives and antispasmodics and temporary laxatives. All *vata* conditions are indications for traditional Ayurvedic enema therapy.

In a bias that often recurs in herbal medicine texts, the Ayurvedic tradition also sees many conditions as combinations of the *doshas* with toxicity, 'damp' or *ama*. This is a *kapha*-like influence, being generally cold, slimy, heavy and dense, with phlegm and mucus, loss of taste and appetite, indigestion, depression and irritability as common symptoms, and may arise from emotional difficulties as well as physical reasons. It lies at the root of much chronic disease and immune disturbance. Where there is evidence of *ama*, improving eliminations is the first priority of treatment, a universal theme in herbal therapeutics. The prime herbal influences in the elimination of *ama* are the bitter and pungent herbs, often in that sequential order, perhaps after a fast. (This is exactly the strategy for the Galenic elimination of 'damp'.) Sweet, salty and sour herbs can increase *ama*.

The treatment of *ama* is, however, complicated by its combinations with the *doshas* (in which case it has the suffix *sama*). Combined with *kapha* (*kapha sama*), it is marked by severe mucus conditions and is a clear indication for pungent with bitter herbs. *Pitta sama* is the classic Galenic damp-heat condition, with yellow tongue coating, urine and faeces, congestive anorexia, loss of thirst and biliousness. Bitter herbs lead the treatment, with modest amounts of pungent, as appropriate. *Vata sama* is associated with constipation, painful abdominal congestion and flatulence, anorexia and bad breath, and is treated with pungent herbs, warming aromatic digestives and carminatives combined with laxatives as required.

The six tastes (*rasas*)

As with the Chinese view, the effects of foods and the pharmacology of medicines were classified in terms of their immediate impact on the body. *Rasas* are not only subjective impressions but attributes of the body itself in its relationship with its environment: everyone craves the taste most lacking within. The choice of both medicines and foods is thus often determined by such assessments, the distinction between them again being a function of their effects on the body: foods nourish, medicines balance and poisons disturb.

The effects of *rasas* on the body are complex and rarely isolated. For example, the sweet, sour and salty tastes decrease *vata* and increase *kapha* but sour, salty and pungent tastes increase *pitta*. Bitter, pungent and astringent tastes increase *vata* and decrease *kapha*.

The primacy of cleansing

The Indian traditions of therapeutics concurred with most other older cultures in seeing disease as initially a toxic accumulation. The disease process is seen generally to start with an obstruction to the pathways and an accumulation of one or more of the *doshas* (one recalls that the healthy manifestations of *doshas* are as eliminations from the body) in their respective locales: the stomach for *kapha*, the intestine for *pitta* and the bowel for *vata*. It is easiest to combat diseases at this earliest stage and there are several cleansing routines that people are encouraged to observe to remove accumulations of *doshas* before they lead to the next stages of disease development.

If hygienic and other observances are insufficient to deal with the accumulations, a range of therapeutic measures are indicated. These may include an elaborate structure of procedures called *panchakarma*, designed to purify the body from the accumulations and pacify associated disturbances. Always the physician had to respect the relative strength of the patient and of the disease and adopt only those treatments that did not disturb or debilitate (there was little attraction in the 'healing crisis' of some more recent alternative traditions). Often a treatment would start with fasting, especially to promote removal of any *ama* or in acute outbreaks. Thereafter, there might be variously intense body massages with oils or heating and sweating to soften and loosen the *dosha* accumulations (as in the Galenic tradition referred to earlier).

Herbal or other remedies would be applied at any stage (or as a substitute for a stage of *panchakarma* where this was not indicated), with the most active tactics being those that led to the most vigorous eliminations (emetics for accumulated *vata* and *kapha*, purgatives for *pitta*) but because of the risks of depletion there were many approaches to consider, some being particularly gentle. For every purification treatment successfully completed, there would be a mandatory convalescence to allow recovery, perhaps augmented by appropriate rejuvenating remedies.

Ayurvedic prescribing

Ayurvedic texts provide considerable detail in their therapeutic recommendations. According to a recent English text,[34] Ayurvedic treatment is based on:

- correct diagnosis
- defined treatment principles
- understanding the disease process and the cause
- defined treatment strategies with an emphasis on the above
- developing a unique prescription.

Preparation of herbal remedies, for example, is most elaborate, with a wide range of methods designed to transform the original plant material in a variety of ways to match the typology of the disturbance being treated. The remedies were also applied to the body in many forms and at various times in the treatment according to its development.

As well as using the pulse, tongue and other traditional diagnostic methods, Ayurveda also invokes the 10 assessments: constitution, habits (lifestyle), state of balance in the body, mental state, quality of the tissues, digestive power, quality of the body, energy levels, body type and age.

From the above text again, the fundamental Ayurvedic treatment principles are:

- reducing excess: excess pathologies are either treated by purification or palliation
- tonifying deficiency with tonics (*rasayana*)
- drying therapy for excess dampness; diuretic and anticatarrhal herbs are Western examples
- lubricating dryness with oily or demulcent herbs
- fomentation or sweating therapy reduces coldness, heaviness, stiffness or trapped heat – using steam and diaphoretic herbs (very analogous to Thomsonian medicine)
- astringent herbs are used for excess flow of bodily fluids.

This approach translates into the following treatment strategy:

- Balance the humours
- Support digestion and correct imbalances
- Restore equilibrium to the tissues, focusing on where the disease is manifesting
- Treat the disease and disease manifestations
- Detoxify the whole body
- Select one or two herbs for each aspect of treatment.

Whatever the sophistication in Ayurvedic texts, it was clear, however, that they were meant to be enabling rather than a formulaic prescription; they encouraged a respect for diversity and complexity, for the individuality of the patient. Empiricism and pragmatism are essential features of any survival strategy but the repeated emphasis in the texts on judging a remedy or tactic by its effects on the body in clinical adversity rather than in theory, and the transparency of the therapeutic tactics, all provide an encouraging antidote to idle acquiescence to the elders.

Nineteenth-century North American herbal medicine

The majority of the early immigrants to North America were Europeans looking for a fresh chance in the vast spaces of the 'New World'. Although there were new towns and cities, significant numbers lived remotely from any organised services, for example often hundreds of miles from a doctor (who was often poorly qualified). These were hardy self-reliant people who had to find all resources on their doorstep. They had to rediscover their self-sufficiency in health terms as well, combining their (imported) old European home remedies with native North American flora and a considerable amount of Indian lore as well. Their experience provides the modern reader with a unique precedent: the rediscovery of traditional herbal medicine by a modern population.

A new group of practitioners emerged, sometimes referred to now as 'travelling medicine shows', more often contemporarily as 'white Indian doctors', often peripatetic, exploiting their claimed skills and usually their own patent nostrums. Many were opportunists with little to contribute in a lasting way to the development of healthcare (although one 19th-century herbal tonic was to become, as Coca-Cola, the most massively consumed product of all time). Nevertheless, there were also true pioneers among this group; some passionately keen to develop a self-reliant healthcare system based on what they knew of plant remedies.

One 'white Indian doctor' went into print. Samuel Thomson (1769-1843) was brought up as a shepherd boy in New Hampshire and introduced to herbs by a 'wise woman', Mrs Benton, who was versed in Indian lore. He very quickly became adept, being called upon by neighbours in competition with what may have been particularly poor service from the local doctor.

Thomson was horrified by the remedies used in 'regular physic', these being dominated by toxic minerals based on mercury, arsenic, antimony and sulphur. He also saw that there was a fundamental difference in therapeutic approach. He saw the objective of the doctors as being to stop the disease at all costs. The main conditions of the day were febrile infections and the regular approach was to use mineral products and bloodletting to stifle the symptoms and bring the temperature down (this was before germ theory redefined the objective as eliminating pathogens). Thomson had ministered to patients almost killed by the combination of calomel (mercurous chloride), antimony, bloodletting and fever. In native Indian tradition (as seen in the sweat lodge), Thomson treated fevers in the opposite way, by maintaining and supporting them. He saw the fever as a sign of healthy resistance: it was possible for damage to follow if the fever got out of hand but the main risk was failure of the febrile defence. Thus Thomson used Capsicum (cayenne) as a powerful support to the febrile mechanism, along with a range of other remedies including *Lobelia inflata* (lobelia), *Myrica cerifera* (bayberry), *Viburnum opulus* (cramp bark) and Zanthoxylum (prickly ash) to modulate and support various aspects of the febrile response.

Thomson was sufficiently enthused by the distinction between his and the regular approaches that he learned to read and write so that he could pass on his message. He set out a principle that at once encapsulated this tradition and fired the public imagination. The book in which he propagated his views[35] was a runaway publishing success across the East and Mid-West and at the time it was calculated that over half the population of Ohio were adherents of Thomsonian medicine.

Thomson's language was simple, even simplistic, and aimed at a God-fearing readership. However, he seemed to have touched a gut instinct that life and health are positive virtues, to be protected or recovered through personal self-sufficiency using the medicinal aids provided by the Maker. In one key passage he appears to have adopted some of the language of Graeco-Roman humoral medicine:

> I found that all animal bodies were formed of four elements. The Earth and Water constitute the solid; and the Air and Fire (or heat) are the cause of life and motion; that the cold, or the lessening of the power of heat, is the cause of all disease; that to restore heat to its natural state was the only way health could be produced, and that, after restoring the natural heat, by clearing the system of all obstruction and causing a natural perspiration, the stomach would digest the food taken into it, and the heat (or nature) be enabled to hold her supremacy.

To a readership versed in the Book of Genesis, the fact that Earth and Water (or clay) were the stuff of life, the dry and wet principles respectively, would have been readily appreciated. For those spending all their lives in the open, Air would have been easily equated with its original meaning, wind, a persistent metaphor for movement. The important vital principle, of course, was Fire or heat, the obvious difference between a living body and a corpse, the universal metaphor for life.

Thomson's message was simple. Heat is life. Disease and death are degrees of cold. Heating thus provides the fundamental principle of healing. Other measures, principally in improving eliminations and digestive performance, are often essential supports to this central measure. Cayenne is literally a life promoter.

In the case of fever this message was particularly appropriate in its radical emphasis. The battle lines between heat and cold are more clearly drawn. Thomson was of course essentially correct in his judgement: fevers are defence mechanisms and the symptoms of pyrexia, anorexia, nausea, vomiting, diarrhoea or convulsions are all side effects of this mobilisation, not to be confused with the underlying pathogen. Clinical experience is that a fever well fought, with a clear crisis and lysis, no hyperpyrexia and side effects prevented from causing collateral damage, can leave the body in a stronger position. Effective fever management can be a more helpful strategy than suppression.

The central point, of course, was that Thomson had articulated, with popular success, an essential feature of the herbal tradition: that the primary task was to support the body's own recuperative efforts. Everything else was secondary. He also sounded the essential difference between that tradition and what had already become conventional medicine. The fact that his relationship with the medical establishment was almost entirely acrimonious only served to reinforce his position as a fundamentalist.

Thomson highlighted common naturopathic and traditional principles in his principles of medicine (note, for example, similarities with the principles of Ayurvedic diagnosis and treatment listed above[34]). These included:[36]

1. Health follows from obeying natural laws
2. Disease is an obstruction or diminution of vital energy
3. Disease is caused by violation of natural laws such as:
   a. hereditary (violation by forefathers)
   b. lack or excess of exercise

c. sudden temperature changes

d. wrong diet and over-eating

e. poisons and pollutants

f. injury

4. Symptoms, such as fever, are due to the effect of the disease and are not the disease itself

5. Disease has only one basic type of cure – to remove obstructions or restore vital energy using substances that act in harmony with natural laws and the vital energy

6. In doing so one or more of the following effects should be accomplished:

a. relaxation

b. contraction

c. stimulation

d. soothing

e. nourishing

f. neutralisation.

There are some obvious and striking parallels between the Thomsonian strategies and Ayurveda. From the *Charaka Samhita Sutrasthana*[30] 1.53 and 22.4 we find 'The goal of Ayurveda is the equilibrium of the tissues' and 'One who knows how to reduce excess, nourish deficiency, dry, oleate (lubricate), sweat and astringe is a real Ayurvedic physician.'

Some of Thomson's followers were less keen on his simplicities. Much to the old man's disgust, several started developing variations on his teachings, recognising, for example, that there were conditions that could be diagnosed as excessive heat. There were different emphases on the need to control heat (in fact, circulation) and variations in the mechanisms for keeping the blood 'clean'. In the second half of the 19th century, at the same time as osteopathy and chiropractic emerged, Thomsonian approaches inspired both eclecticism and physiomedicalism. Unlike these former, however, the medicinal therapies did not fare well. The main colleges of physiomedicalism and eclecticism, along with those of homeopathy, were 'invited' to come within the umbrella of established medical training in talks held with the American Medical Association (AMA) at the turn of the century. This was an inspired example of the establishment eliminating radicalism by accommodation, the most notable of which was for osteopathy (the modern American osteopathic physician is to all intents a conventional medical practitioner).

Three figures stand out in physiomedicalism: the intellectual offshoot of Thomsonian medicine. TJ Lyle produced a superb herbal materia medica,[37] concentrating on the observed influence of each remedy on the human being rather than listing its symptomatic indications. JM Thurston produced the last authoritative physiomedical text, posing operational definitions of the vital force, health and disease and the distinctions between functional symptoms and those arising from organic ('trophic') origins, and elaborating on the need to use only such remedies as supported vitality. He also, rather prematurely, sought to classify remedies in terms of the newly discovered autonomic nervous system, reasoning that in its vasomotor activity control could be exerted on local circulation and thus on all tissue functions, including digestion, elimination and hormonal and nervous activity.[38]

Of the physiomedical theorists, WH Cook was particularly inspired. Like the others, Cook attempted to link the rapid new discoveries of medical science to traditional approaches. Through his arguments appears to run the theme that the living body is essentially a functional entity and that disease starts as a disturbance of normal functional rhythms, for example:

Regularity in periods of alternate labor and rest is characteristic of all vital action …

… the earliest departure of the tissues from under the full control of the vital force will be in the lack of ability either to relax or to contract some of the tissues as readily as in the healthy state …[39]

Like other physiomedicalists, Cook started with the principle that the ideal medicine should support recuperative functions, but added considerably to the view that thereafter they should have a gentle dynamism, helping to correct distorted functions, either 'relaxing' overstimulated tissues or functions, or 'contracting' those that are sluggish.

Thomsonian medicine and physiomedicalism both travelled to Britain to a welcome from the newly urbanised medical herbalists of the Industrial Revolution. Their approaches led to the birth of Anglo-American herbalism (which is largely reflected in this textbook) and formed the foundation of the oldest body of medical herbalism in the Western world, the National Institute of Medical Herbalists, established in 1864. Although the vigour of the American pioneers faded in the following century, their ideas at least survived on foreign shores while they singularly failed to do so after the AMA takeover at home.

Although the eclectics were a more intellectual and professional group than the Thomsonians, their system lacked an overall cohesive philosophy. Although they used their medicines in physical doses, their prescribing approach could be like homeopathy and many of their new remedies were adapted by homeopaths. However, their wealth of clinical experience was outstanding and they made substantial contributions to Anglo-American herbalism through the development of the materia medica. They introduced Echinacea and golden seal and discovered the immunostimulant action of the former (although they did not realise it at the time). Their innovations in pharmacy and chemical research on plants set the scene for modern phytochemistry. Some of their developments pre-empted modern drug medicine: in their development of 'Specific Medications' they rejected 'inert' plant material. The name of a leading eclectic figure John Uri Lloyd was preserved in the title of a major journal of plant research (*Lloydia*, now the *Journal of Natural Products*). The key eclectic texts are Ellingwood,[40] *King's Dispensatory*[41] and Felter.[42] *King's Dispensatory* (especially later versions written by Felter and Lloyd) provides the best traditional use data in existence for Western herbal medicine. Ellingwood also contains a wealth of clinical experience. Felter has extensive information on materia medica, including dosage charts. Subsequent developments with specific medications (and the costs involved) disenchanted the English herbalists who realigned themselves strongly with the physiomedicalists.

Middle European herbal medicine

Much of Western herbal therapeutics is imbued with the values of a healthcare tradition that arose in central Europe from the 18th century. Built on the philosophical foundations of Goethe and Schiller, a cultural view arose of health as a refinement, a separation of the pure from the greater impure.

The Goethian view achieved practical therapeutic form in Germany in the homeopathy of Samuel Hahnemann, the biochemic tissue salts of Schussler and, in the 20th century, the anthroposophical medicine that arose as one aspect of the holistic world view of Rudolph Steiner (and indirectly in the Flower remedies of Edward Bach in England). It also provided the founding principles of a variety of practices that have been grouped under the heading of naturopathy. The use of dietary changes (and in later years dietary supplements), hydrotherapy and a range of physical therapies in order to allow 'nature cure' has one of its strongest cultural roots in this tradition.

The European naturopathic tradition also developed Galenic concepts of heat and cold and notably (as a northern European phenomenon) that of damp. The concept of 'catarrh' and 'mucus' became a cornerstone of naturopathic treatment. Following the Graeco-Roman lead, many infectious and inflammatory diseases were seen as congestive toxicities to be warmed and dried. When germ theory established the role of bacteria in infections, these were seen as 'saprophytes' rather than pathogens; in other words, essentially beneficial cleansing organisms, like forest fungi breaking down dead wood, taking advantage of the catarrhal nutrients to effect extraordinary healing responses like inflammation and fever. As in all other foregoing traditions, herbal remedies were seen as important contributions to detoxifying damp conditions, although these were closely interwoven with dietary techniques in ways that have permeated much herbal practice in the West to this day.

The main impact of the Middle European tradition of herbal medicine was on dosage. Whereas the historical emphasis has always been on large 'heroic' doses of herbs, often single preparations for short-term use in acute diseases, the homeopathic initiative led to a general move towards smaller doses, often linked to the use of their 'mother tinctures' from fresh rather than dried plants. Some of today's leading German phytomedicine companies were formed by homeopaths and have provided plant products over a mixed range of doses and potencies, with the herbal remedies having sometimes tiny material doses. In some European countries, notably The Netherlands, the public perception of herbal or phytomedicine is that it uses homeopathic remedies. The significance of this is that the German industry makes up the largest single part of the European herbal market and the overwhelming part of the herbal clinical research literature. Much of this literature relates to products supplied in much lower doses than those commonly used elsewhere in the world, with chaste tree and black cohosh representing good examples.

The clinical implications, and possible limitations, of low-dose phytotherapy are reviewed in Chapter 6 on dosage. Whatever the pharmacological doubts, however, one beneficial effect is that it marked the move from primitive drastic short-term medication for acute conditions to a therapy that could, and did, take its place in the modern mainstream in the treatment of chronic disorders. Remedies changed their role when so transformed (for example, hawthorn moved from a fever management treatment in high doses to a gentle cardiovascular modulator, valerian from an alterative to a mild sedative, garlic from an antiseptic to a treatment for high plasma cholesterol). It can be argued that the Western fascination with Chinese and Ayurvedic herbal medicine is for traditions that have yet to be adequately exposed to the clinical realities of illnesses of a modern developed society.

Common elements: reading the body/mind as a natural phenomenon

Several themes emerge from the previous reviews of traditional herbal therapeutic systems, as already touched on in the comparison of Ayurvedic and Thomsonian treatment strategies:

1. Medicines, most of which were herbal, were seen as correcting internal disharmonies ('diseases') rather than targeting symptoms.
2. In the absence of modern instrumentation, internal disharmonies were understood as *subjective* matters, firstly manifested as body fluids or even excretions (the humours, *doshas*, *xue*, *jing* and *qi*) and then often described in climatic or emotional metaphors or by metaphysical constructs) that might be widely understood among the general population.
3. As most internal disharmonies involved disruptions of body fluids or humours most traditional medicine has been *humoral* medicine.
4. By definition the humours suffused equally the body and the mind (and often the spirit), so that one internal disharmony could affect all levels of experience. There was no Cartesian body/mind split in traditional medicine.
5. Herbal remedies were often classified by the internal disharmony they affected; thereafter many were used as allopathic remedies, in the strict sense of that term. Others were replenishing or tonic in effect, a role almost entirely lost in modern medicine, although as far as the Greeks were concerned supportive medicine was true 'physic'.

If modern herbal therapeutics is to be true to its traditions then it should be able to postulate modern versions of the above themes. Unfortunately, this language is lost among the modern population. Any postulates at this stage have to remain speculative and theoretical. They may form principles for the practitioner rather than an effective language for the patient.

It will also be difficult to arrive at acceptable modern versions of the humours. We no longer relish the language of body fluids and so lose the opportunity to create a modern metaphor that links both the bedpan and the spirit and our own personal experiences. At another level, however, modern systems analysis of body fluid dynamics may support the prospect for oceanic currents through the tissues rather than the mechanistic pipes and channels of Harvey,[43] so providing a possible rationale for meridianal movement. This is again not a substantial point.

There may still, however, be a future for a subjective physiology and pathology. Indeed, one of the concerns about the way modern medicine has developed is that its language has long left the patient behind. Doctors have become better and better at differentiating pityriasis alba from seborrhoeic eczema but are not as good at telling the patient what is wrong, especially if there is only superficial treatment available.

Again, there is a long way to go. However, there are few conceptual barriers to a new physiology that might become understood by anyone. Much of the theoretical ground has been broken in such disciplines as endocrinology and neuropeptide science, neurophysiology, immunology (and the radical North American hybrid of almost every human science: 'psychoneuroimmunology'). In embryology and developmental biology, researchers regularly think in four dimensions and of models of transience that are rare in the other medical sciences. For some time biology has been taking mathematics, physics and computer sciences into its domain. As will be seen in the next section, the fascinating insights that have followed a better understanding of the behaviour of complex living systems have also begun to affect the biomedical model, at least slightly. All these disciplines are still highly arcane, barely comprehensible even to other biologists, let alone the general public. However, they do offer opportunities for a functional physiology based on the insights of many cultures over many centuries.

The traditional herbal therapeutic systems reviewed in preceding sections were all constructed using empirical insights, honed by generations of observers of the human condition. Even without instrumentation, they were able to draw clinical connections between observed body functions in health and disease. As outlined earlier, there was an assumption that a principle applying at one level applied equally across others; there was also much more interest in function than anatomical structure, malfunctions rather than pathologies. Principles were often established with the acquiescence and knowledge of the wider population, using the common language. They were often workaday and pragmatic, with only occasional efforts to construct elaborate theoretical systems. The vast number of local cultures means that there are considerable diversity and even contradictions in the detail. Nevertheless, fundamental principles about vital functions were widely agreed. We can see the basis of a traditional physiology.[44]

All living organisms clearly:

- *perceive* and respond to their environment
- either *accommodate* to or *react* against each environmental stimulus
- on *ingestion* of environmental influences, either *assimilate* or *reject* them
- engage in a confusing and largely impenetrable triad of linked functions to *process* and *circulate* assimilated material and *remove* its metabolites

- *integrate* all these functions with an endogenous vital force that was manifest primarily as vital rhythms but was often also literal and material
- reproduce themselves, generally using functions analogous to the integrative functions.

Moreover, living organisms manifested these vital functions at every level of body, mind and spirit and in their social groups. In modern parlance, we would say equally at the cell, tissue, organ, body, psyche, society and wider ecosystem levels (the Gaia model develops similar principles). Importantly each of the vital processes above is a recognisable system that could be used to characterise a wide range of different functions. They lead to the thought that a systems analysis might be a fruitful language for the new physiology; that it is in the study of complex dynamic systems that the future may lie.

A new synthesis: the body/mind as complex dynamic systems

This theory of life's origins is rooted in an unrepentant holism, born not of mysticism, but of mathematical necessity.

Stuart Kauffman, *At Home in the Universe*[45]

One of the serious drawbacks of the science inspired by Galileo and Newton and developed mainly in the 19th century is that it was never designed to understand wholes. Its strength is in reduction of complexities to their parts. While modern science is, therefore, unprecedented in understanding the constituents of life and nature and building new edifices and realities with the results, it has been poor in understanding or predicting the behaviour of life and nature itself.

It is difficult to put this right. Scientific tools have not been readily available to understand patterns. Nevertheless, the study of complex systems has been tackled by leading scientific minds since computers provided the tools. Traditionally, the study has been one of high mathematics as the permutations and calculus of relationships between entities are worked through. However, application of often relatively simple mathematical formulae or simple modelling has shown that surprising things can happen in apparently random arrays. Programmed with only two simple instructions, dots on the screen behave spontaneously like flocks of birds, and a simple mathematical formula creates myriad self-similar fractal patterns of astonishing natural beauty that closely resemble natural patterns and structures. New properties that are genuinely more than the sum of the parts emerge from simple constituents.

All this has enormous implications for those who wish that there was another way to observe life and health rigorously, and the reader is strongly recommended to read the excellent early introductory texts.[46–48]

One of the most stunning proposals of complexity in the biological realm is the radical riposte to conventional views of the origin and, by inference, the mechanics of life. So far, the current view is that life formed once upon a time after the fortuitous combination of numbers of organic molecules in a primeval soup, perhaps aided by the odd burst of lightning.

The first key stage in reproducible life was the formation of strands of ribonucleic acid (RNA) that could provide the mechanism for protein synthesis and eventually replication. A mathematical review of this scenario shows how astonishingly improbable it is that such events could have happened by chance, even in the billion years or so that were available for this leap. Visions of monkeys producing not one but many Shakespearean texts by random play with a typewriter come to mind.

However, it is a principle of organic chemistry that molecules interact, tending to catalyse each other's transformations. If there are enough organic molecules together, catalytic loops may be closed (i.e. some catalysts are formed by transformations they themselves initiate), then the molecules in that loop become self-sustaining: they become an 'autocatalytic set'. Their levels will be built up within their locale, they will 'consume' building block molecules and 'excrete' metabolites and they will colonise any other locales into which they spill. This is not only possible; it is inevitable if there is sufficient diversity of organic molecules in the medium. Self-organisation is shown to happen spontaneously, simply out of the mathematical permutations of the events. This is 'order for free', as the leading proponent of this scenario, Stuart Kauffman, puts it.[45] It implies that organised structures arise spontaneously all the time. It resonates with a much wider finding that complex systems tend to self-organisation as an essential property of their complexity.

But this order is not fixed. If it were, it could not grow, move or adapt. It would be dead. It is important that there be some adaptability in self-organisation. Science and mathematics are now very familiar with the phenomena of chaotic behaviour in natural systems. The patterns of clouds or sand dunes or flames, the flow of water down pipes, the weather, all are manifestations of the behaviour of particles acted upon by natural forces. Chaos in this sense is not random; its patterns are deterministic, not actually predictable overall but made up of elements which at any one point follow a predictable trajectory. Chaotic behaviour also creates moving zones of minimum energy or 'attractors' (a 'point attractor' is reached by a ball dropped into a bowl) which behave in characteristic ways: these are the 'strange attractors'. The trajectories of activity to and from strange attractors mean that a small initial stimulus, if on the appropriate trajectory, could amplify to massive effects: the fabulous 'butterfly wing effect' where in theory a hurricane in the Gulf of Mexico could start with a butterfly flapping in the Amazon … or not.

Chaos, although sometimes manifest in familiar patterns (such as clouds), is not consistent with sustainable life and health. What appears to happen, however, in self-organised complex systems is that they spontaneously tend to a state just on the 'edge of chaos', a position where, in information theory terms, there is enough stability to store information, and enough fluidity to send it. It has been described as a 'phase transition' such as exists between the solid and fluid state of substances. Complexity therefore is seen as a state between fixed order and chaos, one to which complex systems seem gravitationally to revert. The cell sustains high potassium levels in a dissipative sea of sodium; the heart beats most effectively when it is neither too regular nor too sensitive but somewhere in between (and this behaviour may well be the inevitable dynamic effect of circulatory structures – the heart doesn't beat, it resonates); an ant colony appears automatically to adjust its boundaries so that its density is always at optimum levels for effective ant-to-ant interactions; human civilisations consume chaotic phenomena and construct stable systems from them before eventually decaying through too much order or too much chaos.

Without going through the many fascinating arguments, it really does appear possible that the hovering of complex systems on the edge of order and chaos is itself an attractor, a state of lowest energy for such systems. And this is the punch line: *health itself could be seen as a biological attractor, the state to which living systems revert, effortlessly!*

The interest of the herbalist in a science of wholes, of qualities rather than quantities, is obvious. Unlike conventional pharmaceutical medicine, even the remedy is a complex and unquantifiable thing. On the other hand isolated drugs produce unpredictable side effects because real people are also unfathomably complex. There may after all be a principle to be elucidated that one way to treat complexity is with an appropriate complexity – perhaps on some principle of pattern recognition (e.g. diagnosis or anamnesis).

This cannot be a thorough review of the impact of complexity theory on therapeutics; indeed, such a text has not yet been written. However, the subject is beginning to generate vigorous debate in some quarters and taking all the discussions in this chapter together, as well as reviewing the section on the placebo effect (see p. 89) it is possible to make the following tentative therapeutic propositions:

- Health in biological systems emerges out of an essential drive to self-organisation. Moves to self-correction are therefore the principal responses to pathogenic forces and the main origin of disease symptoms.
- System failure in adapting to disturbances is more likely to lead to ill health than pathogens as such.
- While a system is capable of adaptive self-organisation, including competent resistance to disturbance, selection of inputs from its environment and elimination of metabolites, therapeutic interventions are unnecessary except to steady the recovery (such healthy adaptations include fevers, inflammations and increased eliminations like coughing, vomiting and diarrhoea).
- Therapeutic measures are justified mainly in supporting self-organisation if it is failing; the value of any medication can be judged in relation to its effect on these adaptive processes.
- All recovery is self-repair. The placebo effect and spontaneous remission are merely examples of a principle that underpins all therapeutic efficacy – medicines in themselves do not heal.

Somewhere in this there is the basis of a truly rational therapeutic approach ideally suited to the use of herbal remedies.

References

1. Page JE, Balza F, Nishida T, Towers GH. Biologically active diterpenes from aspilia mossambicensis, a chimpanzee medicinal plant. *Phytochemistry*. 1992;10:3437–3439.

2. Jisaka M, Ohigashi H, Takegawa K, et al. Antitumoral and antimicrobial activities of bitter sesquiterpene lactones of Vernonia amygdalina, a possible medicinal plant used by wild chimpanzees. *Biosci Biotechnol Biochem*. 1993;57(5):833–834.

3. Leach JD, Holloway RG, Almarez FA. Prehistoric evidence for the use of chenopodium (goosefoot) from the hueco bolson of West Texas. *Texas J Sci*. 1996;48(2):163–165.

4. Litynska-Zajac M. Polish archaeobotanical studies in north Africa: Armant (Egypt). *Wiad Botaniczne*. 1993;37(3–4):171–172.

5. Crandon L. Grass roots, herbs, promotors and preventions: a re-evaluation of contemporary international health care planning. The Bolivian case. *Soc Sci Med*. 1983;17(17):1281–1289.

6. Ngilisho LA, Mosha HJ, Poulsen S. The role of traditional healers in the treatment of toothache in Tanga Region, Tanzania. *Community Dent Health*. 1994;11(4):240–242.

7. Le Grand A, Sri-Ngernyuang L, Streefland PH. Enhancing appropriate drug use: the contribution of herbal medicine promotion. A case study in rural Thailand. *Soc Sci Med*. 1993;36(8):1023–1035.

8. Petrucelli II RJ. Monastic incorporation of classical botanic medicines into the renaissance pharmacopeia. *Am J Nephrol*. 1994;14(4–6):259–263.

9. Sabatini S. Women, medicine and life in the middle ages (500–1500 AD). *Am J Nephrol*. 1994;14(4–6):391–398.

10. Trevor-Roper H. Medicine in the court of Charles I. In: Dickinson CJ, Marks J, eds. *Developments in Cardiovascular Medicine*. Lancaster, Engl: MTP Press; 1978. pp. 305–317.

11. Strehlow W, Hertzka G. *Handbuch der Hildegard-Medizin*. Freiburg: Verlag Hermann Bauer; 1987.

12. Harvey JH. *Mediaeval Gardens*. London: Batsford; 1981.

13. Messer E. Systematic and medicinal reasoning in Mitla folk botany. *J Ethnopharmacol*. 1991;33(1-2):107–128.

14. Singer PN (trans.).*Galen: Selected Works* UK: Oxford University Press; 1997.

15. Lloyd GER, ed. *Hippocratic Writings*. London: Pelican; 1978.

16. Scarborough J. Drugs and medicines in the roman world. *Expedition*. 1996;38(2):38–51.

17. Ullmann M. *Islamic Medicine*. Edinburgh: Edinburgh University Press; 1978. pp. 103–106.

18. Pormann PE, Savage-Smith E. *Medieval Islamic Medicine*. Edinburgh: Edinburgh University Press; 2007.

19. Nutton V. *Ancient Medicine*. Routledge; 2005.

20. Unschuld PU. *Medicine in China: A History of Pharmaceutics*. Berkeley: University of California Press; 1986.

21. Porkert M. *The Theoretical Foundations of Chinese Medicine*. Massachusetts: MIT Press; 1978.

22. Larre CSJ, Schatz J, Rochat de la Vallee E. *Survey of Traditional Chinese Medicine*. Paris: Institut Ricci; 1986.

23. Kaptchuk TJ. *The Web That Has no Weaver: Understanding Chinese Medicine*. New York: Congdon and Weed; 1983.

24. Wiseman N (trans.). *Fundamentals of Chinese Medicine*. Massachusetts: Paradigm Publications; 1994.

25. Mills SY. *Out of the Earth: The Essential Book of Herbal Medicine*. London: Viking; 1991. pp. 596–632.

26. Needham J. *Science and Civilisation in China*, Vol 2: *History of Scientific Thought*. Cambridge: University of Cambridge; 1956.

27. Chan ELP, Ahmed TM, Wang M, Chan JCM. History of medicine and nephrology in Asia. *Am J Nephrol*. 1994;14(4–6):295–301.

28. Capra F. *The Turning Point: Science, Society, and the Rising Culture*. London: Wildwood House; 1982.

29. Srikantha Murthy KR (trans.). *Vagbhata's Astanga Hridayam*. Varanasi: Krishnadas Academy; 1991.

30. Ray P, Gupta HN. *Charaka Samhita: A Scientific Synopsis*. New Delhi: National Institute of Sciences of India; 1965.

31. Savnur H. *Ayurvedic Materia Medica*. New Delhi: Sri Satguru Publications; 1984.

32. Wujastyk D, Meulenbeld GJ, eds. *Studies in Indian Medical history*. Groningen: Forsten; 1987.

33. Leslie C, ed. *Asian Medical Systems: A Comparative Study*. Berkeley: University of California Press; 1976.

34. Pole S. *Ayurvedic Medicine: The Principles of Traditional Practice*. Philadelphia: Elsevier Health Sciences; 2006.

35. Thomson S. *New Guide to Health; or the Botanic Family Physician*. Boston: 1835.

36. Colby B. *A guide to health: the principles and philosophy of Thomsonian Herbalism*. First published 1844. Queensland: Reprinted and revised by Mark Walker: Naturopathic Practice Newsletter Service; 2002.

37. Lyle TJ. *Physio-medical therapeutics, materia medica and pharmacy*. Ohio: 1897.

38. Thurston JM. *The philosophy of physiomedicalism*. Indiana: Nicholson; 1900.

39. Cook WH. *The science and practice of medicine*. Cincinnati: 1893.

40. Ellingwood F, Lloyd JU. *American materia medica, therapeutics and pharmacognosy*. 11th ed., Naturopathic medical series: botanical volume 2. Portland: First published 1898. Reprinted: Eclectic Medical Publications; 1983.

41. Felter HW, Lloyd JU. *King's American Dispensatory*. 18th ed., rev 3. Portland: First published 1905. Reprinted: Eclectic Medical Publications; 1983.

42. Felter HW. *The Eclectic Materia Medica, Pharmacology and Therapeutics*. Naturopathic Medical Series: Botanical volume 1. Portland: First published 1922. Reprinted: Eclectic Medical Publications; 1983.

43. Guyton AC. *Textbook of Medical Physiology*, 7th ed. Philadelphia: WB Saunders; 1986. pp. 230–236.

44. Mills SY. *Out of the Earth: The Essential Book of Herbal Medicine*. London: Viking; 1991. pp. 23–131.

45. Kauffman S. *At Home in the Universe: The Search for Laws of Self-Organisation and Complexity*. London: Viking Penguin; 1995.

46. Waldrop MM. *Complexity: The Emerging Science at the Edge of Order and Chaos*. London: Viking; 1992.

47. Lewin R. *Complexity: Life on the Edge of Chaos*. London: JM Dent; 1992.

48. Goodwin B. *How the Leopard Changed its Spots: The Evolution of Complexity*. London: Weidenfeld & Nicolson; 1994.

Principles of herbal pharmacology

CHAPTER CONTENTS

Defining our ground

Pharmacology can be defined as the study of the interaction of biologically active agents with living systems.[1] The study of pharmacology is further divided into two main areas. Pharmacodynamics looks at the effects of an agent at active sites in the body. In contrast, pharmacokinetics is concerned with the effects the body has on the medicine, and specifically the concentrations that can be achieved at active sites. The approach used in this chapter, and to some extent in the therapeutic chapters, is to examine the pharmacology of key chemical groups in plants, the 'archetypal plant constituents', as much as individual herbs. (For detailed information on the pharmacology of selected herbs see Part Three.)

The chemical nature and classification of these archetypal plant constituents are studied within the discipline known as phytochemistry. Hence, any discourse on herbal pharmacology must be founded on a sound knowledge of phytochemistry. A misconception about 'why medicinal plants work' sometimes occurs in lay and even in professional circles. This is that the various nutrients such as vitamins, minerals and so on are largely responsible for the pharmacological activity of plants. (It is perhaps supported by the fact that most herbal products in the United States are regulated as 'dietary supplements'.) Almost without exception, this is not the case. One notable exception is that certain plants, such as nettle leaf (*Urtica species*) and horsetail (*Equisetum species*), are rich sources of the trace element silicon. There is evidence that part of this silicon in horsetail is found intimately associated with cell wall polymers and can be released under mild extraction.[2] Another interesting exception comes from the clinical use of a leaf concentrate from alfalfa (*Medicago sativa*) as an efficacious iron and folate supplement.[3]

The archetypal plant constituents making up the vast majority of the pharmacological properties of plants generally come from the class of plant metabolites (phytochemicals) that are known as secondary metabolites. Primary metabolites are fundamental to the life of the plant and include enzymes and other proteins, lipids, carbohydrates and chlorophyll. In contrast, secondary metabolites do not appear to be necessary to sustain life at a fundamental biochemical level. However, they probably do have more subtle functions that increase the survival prospects of the plant in its natural environment. A brief general discussion of the functions of secondary metabolites (there are still many gaps in this knowledge) is provided below.

The phytochemistry of secondary metabolites is comprehensively covered in the relevant texts. Textbooks on pharmacognosy are especially relevant for the student of phytotherapy and two such texts have been drawn on for the phytochemistry content of this chapter:

- Bruneton J. *Pharmacognosy, Phytochemistry, Medicinal Plants*, 2nd ed. Paris: Lavoisier Publishing; 2008.
- Evans WC. *Trease and Evans' Pharmacognosy*, 16th ed. London: Saunders Elsevier; 2009.

The field of pharmacognosy (from the Greek *pharmacon* for medicine and *gnosis* for knowledge) is the study of the definition, description and phytochemistry of natural drugs (typically medicinal plants or preparations derived from them).[4] In fact, the term drug is derived from the old French word *drogue*, meaning to dry, referring originally to dried herbs. These days the application of pharmacognosy often extends to knowledge about the pharmacology of medicinal plants, and in some circles the term is used to specifically denote the study of herbal pharmacology, although this is technically incorrect.

DOI: http://dx.doi.org/10.1016/B978-0-443-06992-5.00002-5

There are also some primers in phytochemistry aimed at the herbal reader who does not have a strong background in natural products chemistry. In addition to this chapter, they represent a useful starting point for students of phytotherapy.[5,6]

Why should secondary metabolites have biological activity in animals? One suggestion put forward by Michael Baker is that enzymes in animals can share a common ancestry with enzymes or proteins in plants.[7] This evolutionary kinship, when combined with structural similarities between plant and animal substrates for these enzymes, could explain the hormone-like or hormone-modulating effects of several archetypal plant constituents in humans. (See the licorice monograph for one such example.)

The role of secondary metabolites

Before discussing the pharmacodynamics of the archetypal plant constituents, it is worthwhile to consider some examples of their value to the plant.

The immobility of plants in diverse and changing physical environments, along with the possibility of attack by animals and pathogens, has necessitated the development of numerous chemical mechanisms for protection and offence. Over the past few decades, considerable attention has been paid to the specific ecological roles of secondary metabolites, which were often formerly regarded as waste products.

However, there is still considerable debate on this complex issue. Even the line between primary and secondary metabolites can be arbitrary. They cannot be readily distinguished on the basis of precursor molecules, chemical structures or biosynthetic origins. For example, both primary and secondary metabolites are found among the diterpenes and triterpenes. In the diterpene series, both kaurenoic acid and abietic acid are formed by a similar sequence of related enzymatic reactions; the former is an essential intermediate in the synthesis of gibberellins. These are growth hormones found in all plants.[8] The latter is a resin component. Similarly, the essential amino acid proline is classified as a primary metabolite, whereas the six-carbon ring analogue pipecolic acid is considered an alkaloid and hence a natural product. Even lignin, the essential structural polymer of wood and second only to cellulose as the most abundant organic substance in plants, is considered a natural product (secondary metabolite) rather than a primary metabolite.[8]

It has been suggested that, in the absence of a valid distinction based on chemical structure and biochemistry, a functional definition becomes the logical choice.[8] Primary metabolites participate in nutrition and essential metabolic processes inside the plant, whereas secondary metabolites influence ecological interactions between the plant and its environment.

But even here, there is disagreement. Firn and Jones have recently argued that the terms primary and secondary metabolism as applied to plants are misleading and unsatisfactory.[9] They suggested that important metabolites such as lipids, polysaccharides and carotenoids do not fit into either class, and proposed that they be classified as supportive metabolites (with the remainder of secondary metabolites classified as speculative metabolites).

By way of elaboration, lipids are essential for the short-term functioning of the cell and all cells contain a mix of lipids. But there are some individual lipids made by only a few species and, when their synthesis is inhibited, the cell suffers no short-term disadvantage.[9]

Since there is no consensus yet on this issue, the term 'secondary metabolites' will still be employed in this chapter. Be they speculative, supportive or secondary metabolites, their specialised functions include:[10]

- defence against herbivores (insects, vertebrates)
- defence against plant pathogens
- defence against other plants
- signal compounds to attract pollinating and seed dispersing animals
- signals for communication between plants and symbiotic microorganisms
- protection against ultraviolet light, oxidation and other physical stressors.

Based on their biosynthetic origins, plant secondary metabolites (the archetypal plant constituents) can be divided into three major groups: the terpenoids, the alkaloids, and the phenylpropanoid and allied phenolic compounds.[8] All terpenoids, including the primary metabolites, are derived from the five-carbon precursor isopentenyl diphosphate. Alkaloids are biosynthesised principally from amino acids, and the phenolic compounds by either the shikimic acid pathway or the malonate/acetate pathway.[8]

According to Efferth and Koch, two large groups of secondary plant metabolites can be distinguished in terms of their biological/therapeutic activities:[11]

- A smaller group of highly active compounds possessing a high selectivity for cellular targets
- A larger group of moderately or weakly acting compounds that interact with a broad range of cellular targets (hence possessing molecular promiscuity).

These authors reflect that medicinal plants with highly active phytochemicals represent only a minority of those commonly used (probably because of potential toxicity). However, plants with highly active phytochemicals are sought after in natural products research because they represent prime candidates for new drug discovery. In contrast, 90% of all thoroughly described medicinal plants contain broad-spectrum phytochemicals with weak or moderate bioactivity. Efferth and Koch suggest that plants have learned to cope with the problem of resistance development by producing combinations of pleiotropic multi-targeted phytochemical complexes (see also the concept of intelligent mixtures discussed later).[11] They also note that those medicinal plants synthesising certain classes of highly active compounds might protect themselves by producing 'prodrug' phytochemicals that are activated only in predators or on damage to the plant.[11] Many such molecules are glycosides (for example, see the later discussion of cyanogenic glycosides and glucosinolates).[12,13]

Alkaloids can play a defensive role in plants against herbivores and pathogens.[8,14] Glucosinolates appear to have a role in protecting against insect attack.[15] Tannins act to preserve the wood in living trees from microbial decomposition and insects.[12] Several classes of secondary metabolites are induced by infection, wounding or grazing, which probably speaks to their defensive roles.[16] Variation in the speed and extent of such induction may account, at least in part, for the differences between resistant and susceptible plant varieties.[17] Both salicylic and jasmonic acids have been implicated as signals in such responses. Toxic chemicals formed in response to damage, especially from fungal attack, are called phytoalexins.[12] In legumes, secondary metabolites are involved in interactions with beneficial micro-organisms (flavonoids as inducers of the Rhizobium symbiosis) and in defence against pathogens (isoflavonoid phytoalexins).[8,18]

As noted above, plants have also developed chemical defences against other plants, a phenomenon known as negative allelopathy. Many compounds are implicated, including phenolics[19] and terpenoids.[20,21] Positive biochemical interaction, or facilitation, among plants is also becoming increasingly recognised (positive allelopathy).[22]

Confusing the use of the term is the fact that 'allelopathy' can be applied in a broader context to denote the interactions between plants and animals. In other words, the word is sometimes used to describe the field of study of the broader ecological functions of secondary metabolites, as discussed above. A recent allelopathy textbook reflects this wider application of the term.[21]

How do herbs differ from conventional drugs?

While many conventional drugs or their precursors are derived from plants, there is a fundamental difference between administering a pure chemical and the same chemical in a plant matrix. This issue of chemical complexity (and its possible advantage) is both rejected by orthodoxy as having no basis in fact and avoided by most researchers as introducing too many variables for comfortable research. Herein lies the fundamental difference between the phytotherapist, who prefers not just to prescribe chemically complex remedies, but often to administer them in complex formulations, and the conventional physician, who would rather prescribe a single agent.

Is there in fact any advantage in chemically complex medicines? Life is indeed chemically complex, so much so that science is only beginning to grasp the subtle and varied mechanisms involved in processes such as inflammation and immunity. It does seem logical that, just as our foods are chemically complex, so should be our medicines. But hard proof of this advantage has been difficult to establish. There are, however, several examples from the literature of how an advantage might arise from chemical complexity and some of these are discussed below.

Synergy and additive effects

'The body is not a one-note melody, but a symphony of many interactive components functioning synergistically ... the active ingredient model does not stem from a strength of the scientific method, as often supposed; rather, it stems from a

weakness – from the inability of the reductionist method to deal with complex systems.'[23]

Synergy is an important hypothesis in herbal pharmacology in the context of the advantage of chemical complexity. It applies if the action of a chemical mixture is greater than the arithmetical sum of the actions of the mixture's components: the whole is greater than the sum of the individual parts. In other words, there is a cooperative or facilitating effect between the components for a specific outcome. Another helpful definition of synergy is an effect seen by a combination of substances that is greater than would have been expected from a consideration of individual contributions.[24] A well-known example of synergy is exploited in the use of insecticidal pyrethrins. A synergist known as piperonyl butoxide, which has little insecticidal activity of its own, interferes with the insect's ability to break down the pyrethrins, thereby substantially increasing their toxicity. This example emphasises one important possible mechanism behind synergy as applied to medicinal plant components: increased or prolonged levels of key components at the active site. In other words, components of plants that are not active themselves can act to improve the stability, solubility, bioavailability or half-life of the active components. Hence a particular chemical might in pure form have only a fraction of the pharmacological activity that it has in its plant matrix. This key mechanism for synergy, therefore, has a pharmacokinetic basis.

Methods for assessing pharmacological synergy were proposed in an extensive paper by Berenbaum in 1989.[25] Later Williamson[26] and Houghton[27] elaborated on these in the context of medicinal plants. Essentially, there are four mathematical techniques for demonstrating synergy proposed and discussed in these works, but only the isobole method is truly rigorous, although it is not always undertaken because of its complexity. Hence, several of the examples of herbal synergy discussed below need to be viewed in the context that they are only possible examples of synergy, since the isobole method was not performed.

The isobole method has the advantage that it is independent of the mechanism of action involved. Although some explanations of the isobole method can be complex, a simple way to describe it follows. For a series of two-component mixtures, the concentration or dose of component A in each mixture required to give a defined effect (such as an ED_{50} or minimum inhibitory concentration, MIC) is plotted on the X axis against the concentration or dose of component B in the same mixture on the Y axis. The line joining all the points is then constructed. If there is no interaction between the effects of A and B, and their combination is merely additive, the line will be straight (Fig. 2.1). If there is a synergy between A and B, the line (the isobologram) will be concave. Alternatively, if antagonism exists the isobologram will be convex.

There are some published examples in the literature of the isobole method demonstrating synergy for mixtures of phytochemicals from the same herb. Williamson provides the example of ginkgolides A and B from ginkgo in terms of an anti-PAF (platelet activating factor) effect on platelets in vitro.[26] In much earlier work in mice, a potentiating effect of different concentrations sennoside C on the purgative activity

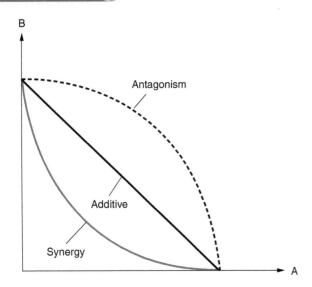

Figure 2.1 • The isobologram method for demonstrating synergy.

of sennoside A was observed.[28] In this study an isobologram of ED_{50} values for laxative activity was not plotted, but one can be readily constructed from the data provided showing a concave line. Interestingly, a mixture of these compounds in the ratio 3:7 (which somewhat reflects the relative levels in senna leaf) gave the lowest ED_{50} value.

In several published examples, only one mixture of two given phytochemicals from the same plant is tested, and hence an isobologram construct from just three points (A, B and A plus B) could be plotted. There is little point in doing this, however, since synergy is readily apparent from such a simple experimental design (if the activity of A plus B is greater than the expected activity calculated from the individual activities of A and B). Although this is a less robust means of demonstrating synergy than an isobologram constructed from four or more points, if there is a dramatic increase in activity from the mixture of A and B it is reasonable to assume that synergy has been demonstrated.

One example of where the combination of two components from the same plant has yielded a significantly greater effect than expected is a study on the upregulation of phase II detoxification enzymes in mice by the glucosinolate breakdown products from broccoli.[29] An orally administered mixture of crambene and indole-3-carbinol caused a significantly greater induction of glutathione S-transferase and quinone reductase that could be expected from the activity of oral doses of the individual treatments. Another example is the study where the three major curcuminoids from turmeric (*Curcuma longa*) were investigated for their in vitro nematocidal activity against second stage larvae of *Toxocara canis*.[30] Each of the three curcuminoids was ineffective on its own, whereas any combination of two, or all three together, was active. The combination of all three demonstrated the highest activity.

Another example identified in early research is the antibacterial activity of major components of lemongrass essential oil. While geranial and neral individually elicited antibacterial action, the third main component, myrcene, did not show any activity in vitro. However, when mixed with either of the other two main components, myrcene enhanced their activity.[31] As pointed out in one review[11] this example is technically not one of synergy, but rather exemplifies potentiation, where an inactive compound enhances the potency of a bioactive one.

In an interesting study, the impact on serum lipids of four active components of Chinese hawthorn (*Crataegus pinnatifida*), and their combination, was investigated in mice fed a high fat and cholesterol diet.[32] The four compounds (quercetin, hyperoside, rutin and chlorogenic acid), and their combination at percentages reflected in the berry, were each fed orally to the mice at a dose of 2.85 mg/kg. The greatest reduction in total cholesterol and LDL-cholesterol was found for the combination. For LDL-cholesterol, only the combination yielded a significant reduction versus the control group (p<0.01).

The above examples therefore demonstrate two types of synergistic interactions for phytochemicals within a plant. The first example is where the phytochemicals are all active in the test method used. The second example is where one or more of the phytochemicals are inactive, yet their inclusion in a mixture increases the observed effect.

Pharmacodynamic synergy has also been demonstrated for combinations of extracts or phytochemicals from different herbs. The in vitro antitumour activity for combinations of extracts of Corydalis and turmeric rhizomes (a traditional formulation) demonstrated a synergistic interplay, as determined using an isobologram.[33] Berberine from *Coptis chinensis* and evodiamine from *Evodia rutaecarpa* demonstrated synergistic antitumour activity in vitro against a human hepatocellular carcinoma cell line.[34] A pronounced convex curve was produced on an isobologram.

A recent review highlighted that two key developments are behind growing interest in synergy research in phytotherapy.[35] The first is the new methods of analytical chemistry and molecular biology that have become available in the 21st century. The second is an unexpected change of paradigm in chemotherapy that has appeared without drawing much attention as to its radical nature. This is the transition in chemotherapy towards a multi-drug approach. Multi-drug therapy is already widely practised in the treatment of AIDS and other infectious diseases, hypertension, cancer and many other diseases.

In particular, the review notes this multi-drug concept in cancer chemotherapy is often aimed at being biomodulatory, not just at direct destruction of the tumour.[35] Instead, suppression of different processes essential for the tumour's survival are also targeted (such as angiogenesis, oncogene expression, anti-apoptotic mechanisms, immunological tolerance and inflammation). This concept of multi-targeted or polyvalent therapy is not new to phytotherapy and is discussed further below.

There are several examples in the herbal research literature where synergistic interactions are strongly implied, although they have not been absolutely demonstrated using the isobologram method. One example is the research cited by Williamson[26] and several others where cannabis extract demonstrated higher antispastic activity in mice than the equivalent dose of pure tetrahydrocannabinol (THC). As pointed out by Houghton,[27] this might not represent an example of true synergy. Rather other components in the cannabis extract might also have antispastic activity. In other words, there could be an additive effect between THC and other phytochemical components in the extract. However, the increased activity is so striking that synergy is a very plausible explanation. Testing a THC-free cannabis extract in the same model would have provided clear proof, one way or another.

Another example of a striking result that strongly implies a synergistic interaction is provided by Williamson.[26] This is the research where the antiulcer activity of a fraction of ginger extract was found to be 66 times that calculated from the individual components of that fraction. More recent similar examples include:

• analysis of the in vitro butyrylcholinesterase inhibitory activities of essential oils of various *Salvia* species, which revealed that the activities of isolated major components could not account for the observed activity[36]
• tea tree oil (*Melaleuca alternifolia*), which exhibited pronounced in vitro antitumour activity against murine B16 melanoma cells.[37] However, a 'mock' tea tree oil (containing its five major phytochemical components at the same concentrations found in the oil, and representing 80% of its total content) was only half as active. Of these five major oil components, only terpinen-4-ol (about 40% of the oil) was active in this model.

There are several examples of a pharmacokinetic basis for synergy, where chemical complexity results in enhanced solubility or bioavailability of key phytochemical components in plant extracts. The basic issues were discussed by Eder and Mehnert.[38] The isoflavone glycoside daidzin given in the crude extract of *Pueraria lobata* achieves a much greater concentration in plasma than an equivalent dose of pure daidzin.[39] Ascorbic acid in a citrus extract was more bioavailable than ascorbic acid alone.[40] More recently, consumption of a preparation of fresh kiwi fruit resulted in up to five times more effective ascorbate delivery to tissues than when ascorbate was administered via the drinking water to vitamin C-deficient mice.[41] The kava lactones appear to increase each other's bioavailability, especially when given as the herbal extract. (For more details, see the kava monograph under Pharmacokinetics.)

Improved pharmacokinetic parameters can also apply to combinations of herbs, although this is not necessarily always the case. The traditional Chinese formulation Huangqin-Tang decoction, together with decoctions of its individual herbal components, were studied in rats after oral dosing.[42] The constituents/metabolites baicalin, wogonoside, oroxylin-A-glucuronide, risidulin I and liquiritin demonstrated higher overall bioavailability from the compound formulation than from the relevant single herb decoctions, due largely to a longer residence time.

Often synergy is invoked to explain experimental results that can be readily explained by additive effects. Synergy is not always necessary to justify the use of complex mixtures, be they single herbal extracts or herb combinations. Additive effects can be just as favourable to enhanced therapeutic activity and are probably more common in phytotherapy.

A team of German scientists headed by the late Dr Hilke Winterhoff discovered that the procyanidins in St John's wort extract (*Hypericum perforatum*) significantly increased the in vivo antidepressant activity of hypericin and pseudohypericin, probably by a solubilising effect (these compounds otherwise have poor solubility).[43] The same research team found that the flavonoids in St John's wort have activity in an animal model of depression, with hyperoside and isoquercitrin showing significant activity.[44] The flavonoid perspective was backed up by another in vivo study from Italy that found a flavonoid-enriched St John's wort extract exhibited a more significant influence on central neurotransmitters.[45] Later work from the German researchers demonstrated that a St John's wort extract free of both hypericin and hyperforin (another phytochemical in the herb thought to play a role in the antidepressant activity) still exerted an antidepressant activity in rodent models.[46] Hence, it seems that hypericin, procyanidins (indirectly), hyperforin and the flavonoids can all contribute to the clinically verified antidepressant activity of St John's wort.

Additive effects also apply to herb combinations. The reduction of amphetamine-induced hypermotility was studied in mice after a single oral dose of passionflower extract (*Passiflora incarnata*, 250 mg/kg), kava extract (100 mg/kg) or the two combined (250 mg/kg+100 mg/kg, respectively).[47] The combination yielded a much greater reduction in hypermotility over 2 hours than each individual herbal extract, which the authors attributed to a synergistic interaction. However, a careful analysis of the numbers suggests that the observed result is more likely to have been due to an additive effect (in terms of the differences observed from the control group). Additive benefits have also been observed at a clinical level. A combination of ginseng (*Panax ginseng*) and Ginkgo has been extensively investigated in volunteers for its acute and long-term impact on cognitive function. The effect of the combination appears to be significantly greater than either herb alone. This might be an example of synergy (which would be difficult to prove conclusively) but is at least an additive effect. (See the ginseng monograph for more details.)

Polyvalent or multifaceted activity

As touched on above, the concept of multi-agent medicines is a developing theme in modern drug therapy. However, it represents nothing new for phytotherapy. Due to their chemical complexity, even a single herbal extract is a nature-designed multi-agent medicine that can simultaneously target a range of desirable pharmacological effects. There are many examples of this provided in the herbal monographs in Part Three. This helps to explain why identifying the 'active constituent' in many herbal extracts has proved to be so difficult. For most if not all herbal extracts the 'active constituent' is the whole extract itself, as illustrated by the above discussion of the antidepressant activity of St John's wort. The potential for chemical complexity to confer polyvalent activity or polypharmacology can also explain the apparent therapeutic versatility of herbal extracts. As an example there is the rather large and novel range of clinical uses for Ginkgo, all somewhat supported by evidence from randomised, controlled trials.

It has also been argued that polyvalence may be behind some effects that have been attributed to synergy (although ultimately such a distinction is probably academic, as both explanations argue in favour of chemical complexity).[27] In whole organism or tissue studies, other compounds present in the mixture may be active against a range of targets, all acting to contribute to the observed outcome. Houghton goes on further to assert that:

> Polyvalence can be defined as the range of biological activities that an extract may exhibit which contribute to the overall effect observed clinically or in vivo. It is often confused with synergism but the distinction lies in the fact that synergism is strictly concerned with only one pharmacological function, rather than a range of activities resulting in an overall effect.[27]

As outlined by Houghton, polyvalence can occur at three key levels:

1. Several types of phytochemicals are present that each exert a different biological effect.
2. Phytochemicals of one particular chemical type are present that have more than one biological effect relevant to treating the disease and/or improving the health of the patient.
3. Phytochemicals are present that do not affect the cause or symptoms of the disease itself, but instead modify the side effects, absorption, distribution, metabolism or excretion of active constituents.

The third possibility overlaps with the concept of pharmacokinetic synergy underlining, as noted above, that the distinction between polyvalence and synergy might be quite arbitrary at times. There are many examples of these phenomena in the pharmacodynamic and pharmacokinetic sections of the monographs in Part Three of this book.

In a recent review, Gertsch observed that herbal extracts might be 'intelligent mixtures' of secondary plant metabolites that have been shaped by evolutionary pressures.[48] As such they could represent complex therapeutic mixtures possessing inherent synergy and polyvalence. Gertsch also notes that another important concept related to polyvalence is that of network pharmacology, as originally proposed by Hopkins.[49] In the context of plant extracts (which for commonly used herbs typically contain hundreds of potentially bioactive natural products with only mild activity) it is possible that different proteins within the same signalling network are only weakly targeted. However, this is sufficient to shut down or activate a given process by network pharmacology.[48] In other words, network pharmacology can explain how a number of weakly active plant secondary metabolites in an extract may be sufficient to exert a potent pharmacological effect without the presence of a highly bioactive compound.[48] In the context of herbal pharmacology, Paul Ehrlich's concept of the magic bullet is supplanted by one of a 'green shotgun', to paraphrase Gertsch and James Duke. However, the herbal research that can verify such theoretical constructs is only in its infancy.

The '-omic' technologies (genomics, transcriptomics, proteomics and metabolomics) are recent developments in molecular biology that have the potential to open new perspectives for our understanding of the multi-faceted activities of complex plant mixtures. However, their meaningful application to medicinal plant research poses several challenges.[50] The reviews of Wagner and colleagues and Efferth and Koch[11] provide a more complete discussion of the application of these techniques to natural product research.

Intelligent mixtures

Whether it is a manifestation of synergy or by other means, the hypothesis that herbal extracts might act at a pharmacological level as intelligent mixtures is intriguing. One such example could be the root of *Pelargonium sidoides*. Its phytochemical content is unremarkable, including oligomeric procyanidins (OPCs) and highly oxygenated simple coumarins.[51] Yet a liquid preparation of the herb has been shown to be effective in several clinical trials. A meta-analysis published in 2008 reviewed its efficacy for acute bronchitis.[52] Six randomised trials were included, providing results for a total of 1647 patients (treatment and control groups): one trial compared Pelargonium against a non-antibiotic treatment (N-acetylcysteine); the other five trials tested Pelargonium against placebo. In two trials the ages of the participants were 6 to 12 years, and 6 to 18 years. Adults were enrolled in the other trials. Key findings were:[52,53]

- all trials reported clinical results suggesting Pelargonium was beneficial in the treatment of acute bronchitis
- meta-analysis of the four placebo-controlled trials involving adults indicated that Pelargonium root significantly reduced bronchitis symptom scores by day 7
- the duration of illness was significantly shorter for patients treated with Pelargonium compared to placebo (Pelargonium-treated patients were able to return to work nearly 2 days earlier than placebo-treated patients)
- patients noticed a treatment effect earlier under Pelargonium than under placebo.

Moreover, the herb had previously developed a traditional reputation as a treatment for tuberculosis.

Another example of an intelligent mixture could be willow bark. Its phytochemical content cannot be reconciled against its impressive clinical results (see the willow bark monograph for more details).

Pharmacodynamics of the archetypal plant constituents

Simple phenols and glycosides

Phenols comprise the largest group of plant secondary metabolites. They range from simple structures with only one benzene ring to larger molecules such as tannins, anthraquinones, flavonoids and coumarins. Tannins and flavonoids are often referred to as polyphenolics. Phenols are defined as compounds that have at least one hydroxyl group attached to a benzene ring. They differ in their chemical properties from other tertiary alcohols because the presence of the benzene ring stabilises the phenolate ion; they are therefore more acidic and more reactive.

Glycosides are secondary metabolites that yield one or more sugars on hydrolysis. The most frequently occurring sugar is glucose (a glycoside yielding glucose is called a glucoside). The non-sugar component of the molecule, which may be a simple phenol, flavonoid, anthraquinone, triterpenoid or one of many other structures, is called the aglycone. If the glycosidic bond is via oxygen, the molecule is termed an O-glycoside; if it is via a carbon, it is a C-glycoside. The glycosidic linkage is somewhat resistant to human digestive enzymes (being a beta linkage) and glycosides are often poorly absorbed from the digestive tract. Hence, their usual fate is to travel to the distal ileum or large bowel. Here microbial activity forms the aglycone, which is less polar and can be absorbed into the bloodstream to a variable extent, depending on its structure (see Pharmacokinetics later in this chapter).

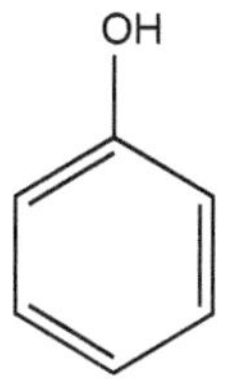

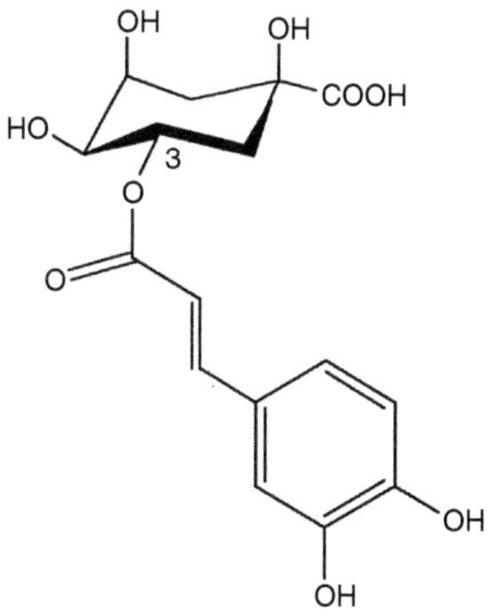

Chlorogenic acid
(3-caffeoylquinic acid)

Phenol

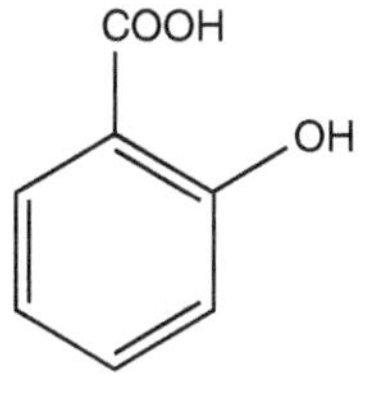

Salicylic acid

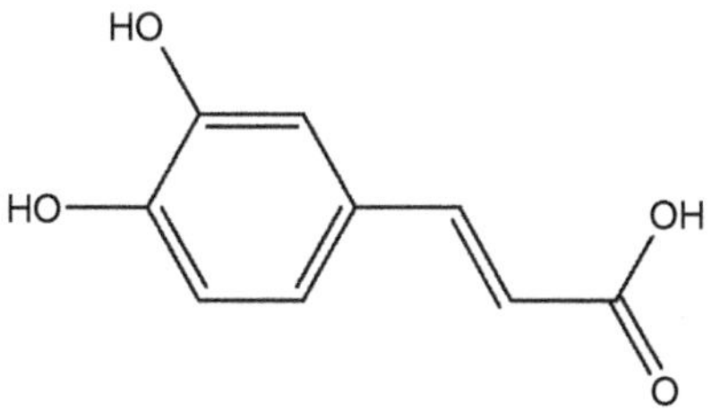

Caffeic acid also known as
3,4-dihydroxycinnamic acid

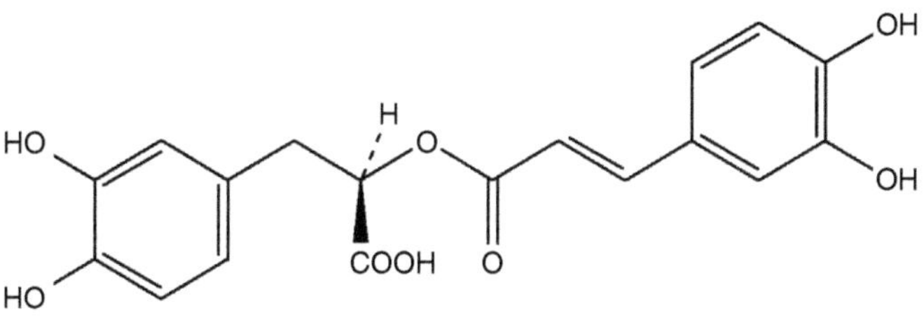

Rosmarinic acid

Phenolic acids are a special class of simple phenols that have in addition at least one carboxylic acid group. Phytochemists usually restrict this term to the benzoic and cinnamic acid derivatives only, such as gallic acid, salicylic acid, caffeic acid, vanillic acid and ferulic acid. Phenolic acids derived from cinnamic acid are usually found in plants as esters (phenolic acid esters). These include chlorogenic acid and rosmarinic acid. Caffeic acid esters of quinic acid, such as chlorogenic acid, are also known as caffeoylquinic acids (see the monograph on globe artichoke). Some of these compounds are sometimes called pseudotannins, since they have astringent characteristics, but lack all the properties of true tannins (see below).

From a pharmacological perspective, the best known simple phenol is salicylic acid. Its precursors are found in willow (*Salix* species) and poplar (*Populus* species) barks and salicylic acid is subsequently formed on ingestion (see Pharmacokinetics later). Salicylic acid has recognised antipyretic and anti-inflammatory properties that underlie the use of willow bark for fever and arthritis. Acetylsalicylic acid (aspirin) is a synthetic derivative of salicylic acid that in addition has pronounced antiplatelet properties due to the presence of the acetyl group.[54] Salicylic acid lacks this property and consequently willow bark is not suitable as a natural substitute for aspirin in cardiovascular patients. Simple phenols are also powerful antiseptics. Arbutin is a phenolic glycoside that confers bacteriostatic properties to urine (see the monograph on bearberry).

Several studies have shown that extracts of many members of the mint family (Lamiaceae or Labiatae) have considerable in vitro antioxidant activity due to the presence of phenolic acids such as rosmarinic acid. Highest antioxidant activity was found in *Prunella vulgaris*, which had a rosmarinic acid content of about 5%.[55]

Caffeic acid, as well as its derivatives such as rosmarinic acid and chlorogenic acid, were found to exert antithyroid activity after oxidation. This activity may form the basis of the clinical use of *Lycopus* species for hyperthyroidism (see the bugleweed monograph).[56] Similar oxidation products of caffeic acid inhibit protein biosynthesis in vitro and these compounds probably account for the clinically established antiviral activity of a topical preparation of *Melissa officinalis* (see also Chapter 8, p. 142).[57]

The simple phenol resveratrol is probably the most actively researched phytochemical worldwide, with many properties demonstrated in pharmacological models. There are more than 4000 studies on resveratrol. Resveratrol is a phytoalexin produced by several plants in response to fungal attack. However, well-known sources are grapes (*Vitis vinifera*) and the Chinese herb *Polygonum cuspidatum*. It has demonstrated an amazing array of (mainly in vitro) pharmacological activities including antioxidant, cardioprotective, antidiabetic, anticancer, antiviral, neuroprotective, antiplatelet, anti-inflammatory and modulation of fat metabolism.[58–60] Resveratrol inhibits cancer development at all the three known phases of chemical carcinogenesis, namely initiation, promotion and progression.[61] The development of other chronic diseases might also be reduced by resveratrol, based on the many laboratory studies. These diseases include cardiovascular disease, dementia, type 2 diabetes and osteoarthritis.[62,63] In addition to its indirect effects on the ageing process via SIRT1 (hence possibly acting as a calorie restriction mimetic), this one simple molecule has the potential to prevent most of the chronic diseases associated with ageing.[64] Resveratrol could well be the best example of the molecular promiscuity of common secondary metabolites: 'Considering the structural simplicity of this stilbene, the intensity of interest is phenomenal'.[61]

One important pharmacological study was published in *Nature* in 2006. Rather than administering resveratrol to normal mice to see if it simulated calorie restriction, the effect of resveratrol on a high calorie diet was studied. Middle-aged (1-year-old) male mice on a high calorie diet (HCD) were given resveratrol and compared to untreated mice on the same diet or a standard diet.[65] The administered doses of resveratrol were either 5.2 or 22.4 mg/kg/day for 6 months, but only results for the higher dose were reported.

The mice receiving the HCD become overweight, whether they were receiving resveratrol or not. However, a clear survival benefit from resveratrol was evident: survival rates for mice on the HCD plus resveratrol were the same as those for the mice on the standard diet (SD). Quality of life was determined by the rotarod test, which measures balance and coordination. Surprisingly, the resveratrol-fed mice on the HCD steadily improved their motor skills as they aged, to the point where they were indistinguishable from the SD group. Resveratrol also corrected the following parameters in the overfed mice to levels similar to those observed in the SD mice: plasma insulin, fasting glucose, plasma albumin, plasma amylase, liver weight, aortic elastic lamina morphology and mitochondria levels in liver tissue. Furthermore, resveratrol opposed the effects of the HCD on 144 out of 153 significantly altered metabolic pathways.

One of the issues with resveratrol is that it is rapidly metabolised and has limited bioavailability as such. However, resveratrol metabolites (mainly phase II conjugates) might also be bioactive, or act as a reservoir of resveratrol at target tissues. One study found that to maximise plasma resveratrol levels it should be taken with a standard breakfast and not with a high fat meal.[66] The high fat breakfast was observed to reduce its bioavailability by about 45%.

Cyanogenic glycosides

Cyanogenic glycosides are capable of generating hydrocyanic acid (prussic acid, cyanide). Structurally they are glycosides of 2-hydroxynitriles that can be hydrolysed by the enzyme beta-glucosidase into cyanohydrin. This is unstable and dissociates to hydrocyanic acid. Common cyanogenic glycosides include amygdalin found in bitter almonds and peach kernels (both used in Chinese medicine), and prunasin in wild cherry bark (*Prunus serotina*). The small quantities of cyanide generated from this bark are said to be responsible for its antitussive properties, although this has not been confirmed in modern pharmacological experiments. Both amygdalin and prunasin yield benzaldehyde on hydrolysis, which accounts for the characteristic almond-like aroma of wild cherry bark. The cyanogenic glycosides linustatin, neolinustatin and linamarin (trace) are found in linseeds (flax, *Linum usitatissimum*).[67]

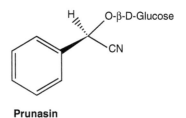

Prunasin

Amygdalin

Although hydrocyanic acid is a violent poison, oral intake of cyanogenic glycosides (for example via food, especially in primitive diets) is not necessarily toxic, particularly in the short-term. Hydrolysis of the glycosides in the digestive tract or by the liver leads to a slow release of hydrocyanic acid that is readily detoxified by the body. Addition of 10% apricot kernels to the diet of rats for 18 weeks showed only moderate toxic effects.[68] Amygdalin given orally to humans at 500 mg three times a day produced no toxic effects and only moderately raised blood cyanide levels.[69] However, co-administration of beta-glucosidase with amygdalin to rats substantially increased its toxicity.[70] Acute poisoning has occurred in grazing animals.[71]

Considerable interest arose in the 1970s regarding the use of a synthetic cyanogenic glycoside, patented as Laetrile (mandelonitrile beta-glucuronide), as an alternative anticancer compound.[72] However, most of what was subsequently sold as Laetrile was in fact amygdalin (which probably had similar properties on injection or ingestion).[73] The theory proposed was that cancer tissues contain beta-glucosidase and circulating cyanogenic glycosides can therefore act as selective cytotoxic agents. However, amygdalin did not prove to be an effective anticancer agent either in animals[74] or in humans,[75] presumably because the beta-glucosidase activity of cancer cells is quite low.[76] In an interesting development of the Laetrile theory, beta-glucosidase was conjugated to a tumour-associated antibody. When combined with amygdalin in vitro, the cytotoxicity of amygdalin to tumour cells was increased 36-fold.[77]

Longer periods of intake of subacute amounts of cyanogenic glycosides in daily food have led to chronic intoxication. Products of human detoxification processes, such as the formation of rhodanide and cyanocobalamine, lead to severe diseases, especially neurotoxic syndromes.[67] This is thought to be involved in tropical ataxic neuropathy in Nigeria. In other African countries, consumption of cassava root (*Manihot esculenta*, also known as tapioca) together with a diet deficient in sulphur amino acids is apparently responsible for an endemic upper motor neuron disease known as konzo.[67] The peeled root contains much lower levels of cyanogenic glycosides. Konzo typically occurs in epidemics in Mozambique, which may reflect inadequate processing of the root in times of drought or war.[78]

Mucilages

Although from a phytochemical standpoint mucilages are often considered a minor category of the group of large plant polysaccharides (a category that includes gums, the various mannans, hemicelluloses and pectins), they are highly prized by phytotherapists. Strictly speaking, the class of compounds that the phytotherapist considers as 'mucilages' are acidic heterogeneous polysaccharides or the 'acidic mucilages'.

Mucilages are generally not chemically well defined. They are large, highly branched polymeric structures built from many different sugar and uronic acid units (uronic acids are carboxylic acids derived from sugars). They are very hydrophilic (water loving) and are capable of trapping water (and other molecules) in their cage-like structures to form a gel. Consequently, when a mucilage is mixed with water it swells to many times its original volume as it absorbs water. The saccharide linkages are in a beta configuration, which means that human digestive enzymes cannot break down mucilages. However, they can at least be partially decomposed by bowel flora into beneficial metabolites such as short-chain fatty acids (SCFA). This may explain the traditional use of slippery elm bark (*Ulmus rubra*) as a food for convalescents. Not only would the mucilage soothe a disturbed digestive tract, the SCFA formed in the colon would provide a source of readily absorbed and assimilated nourishment. There are some clinical and experimental studies that support the concept that mucilages can act as prebiotics, especially after their partial processing by the upper gastrointestinal tract.[79–81]

Mucilaginous remedies have been primarily used for their topical emollient and internal demulcent properties and their direct, if temporary, benefits in the management of inflammatory conditions of the digestive tract. This anti-inflammatory effect is probably more than just mechanical, although the protective benefits of a layer of mucilage on the digestive mucosa are obvious, especially as an extra barrier to gastric acid. The protective effect of mucilage isolated from *Plantago major* leaves against aspirin-induced gastric ulcer has been demonstrated in rats.[82] Similar gastroprotective activity has been demonstrated for guar gum.[83] It has also been shown that guar gum forms a layer closely associated with the intestinal mucosal surface when given to rats, providing a protective barrier.[84]

In order to assess the activity of mucilages on epithelia, a test system based on porcine buccal membranes was devised.[85] While mucilages from marshmallow (*Althea officinalis*) and ribwort (*Plantago lanceolata*) showed moderate bioadhesion to epithelial tissue, polysaccharides from bladderwrack (*Fucus vesiculosus*) and Calendula exhibited strong adhesion. Histological studies of membranes indicated the presence of distinct polysaccharide layers on the apical membrane surface. In vitro investigations of an aqueous marshmallow root extract and its isolated mucilage on human epithelial KB cells (originating from the nasopharyngeal epithelia) and skin fibroblasts found a stimulating effect on the cell viability and proliferation of the former only.[86] The marshmallow mucilage was internalised into epithelial cells, but not into fibroblasts, although it did form a bioadhesive layer on the latter. Microarray analysis indicated an upregulation of genes related to cell adhesion proteins, growth regulators, extracellular matrix, cytokine release and apoptosis. The authors concluded that their findings were consistent with the traditional use of marshmallow root for irritated mucous membranes.

Mucilages are topically applied for an anti-inflammatory (demulcent) effect and for a drawing and healing effect on wounds and infected skin lesions. This latter application is analogous to the use of hydrocolloid dressings in modern medicine.

Mucilages can also function as bulk laxatives and the most widespread use in this regard is ispaghula or psyllium husks, widely sold as a number of proprietary products. These are derived from the seeds of *Plantago psyllium* or *P. ovata*. However, the traditional use of mucilages such as linseed (flaxseed) and fenugreek (*Trigonella foenum-graecum*) as bulk laxatives often provides a valuable alternative,[87] particularly where psyllium causes the characteristic side effects of bloating, abdominal pain and flatulence.[88] Slippery elm powder (*Ulmus rubra*) can also be useful here. Mucilages can also be employed as weight loss agents and presumably act by creating a sensation of fullness.[88] Since they are known to cause oesophageal obstruction, mucilages should be taken with plenty of water and not prescribed in tablet form.[89] Even then, Health Canada issued a 2010 warning that glucomannan (a fibre very similar to mucilage) as a powder or capsule needs to be taken with copious amounts of water as otherwise it may cause serious choking.[90]

Mucilages are also used by phytotherapists to create reflex demulcency, especially to ease irritable and ticklish dry coughs. It is clear that there is no readily recognised pharmacological model for the transfer of demulcent properties directly to the bronchial mucosa: mucilages are too large to be absorbed and transported to this remote site. The emetic effect in reverse, that is the reflex effects on the tracheobronchial musculature of a soothing effect on the upper digestive tract, is instead postulated, mediated by the vagus nerve. Similar associations are used to justify the use of mucilages in painful conditions of the urinary tract.

Reflex demulcency does have experimental support. An extract of marshmallow root and its isolated mucilage demonstrated significant antitussive activity in an animal test. Doses were administered orally (50 and 100 mg/kg of mucilage) and cough from both laryngopharyngeal and tracheobronchial stimulation was depressed.[91] The mucilage was as potent as some non-narcotic antitussive drugs. More recently, marshmallow mucilage was shown to be the most effective of a range of plant polysaccharides in terms of in vivo cough-suppressant activity.[92] There was no negative impact on expectoration, unlike for codeine. A mechanistic study in guinea pigs demonstrated that marshmallow root mucilage (25 and 50 mg/kg, oral) produced an antitussive effect that was comparable to codeine (10 mg/kg, oral) in the model used.[93] The effect was partially suppressed by a 5-HT$_2$ receptor antagonist, suggesting an involvement of these serotonergic receptors thought to participate in the cough reflex.

There is a complex association now recognised between gastro-oesophageal reflux (GORD) and chronic cough and asthma.[94-96] The link between reflux and asthma has long been suspected. In fact, there is quite long-standing evidence that reflux is an important cause of asthma in some asthmatics. Monitoring of oesophageal acidity revealed reflux in 7 out of 9 patients with persistent asthma.[97] In another early study 61% of patients with asthma had reflux.[98] Treatment of reflux by surgery or drugs can result in improvement or cure of asthma.[98,99]

While aspiration of gastric acid has been proposed as a possible cause, an effect from the reflux itself also has currency.[100] One paper reported an investigation into the link between acid reflux into the oesophagus and coughing or wheezing fits in asthmatic patients.[101] The scientists asked a question debated for some time among respiratory and gastrointestinal physicians: 'Does cough cause reflux or does reflux cause cough?' They studied more than 100 chronic adult asthmatics and found that half of all their coughs and wheezes occurred at the same time as when acid refluxed from the stomach into the oesophagus. But more importantly, they concluded that in the majority of cases it was the reflux that caused the coughing and not the other way around. The chronic cough that often follows a respiratory infection and seems to persist long after the infection is gone is probably due to acid reflux, which in turn is induced by the weakening of the oesophageal sphincter as a result of the violent coughing during the infection. Here the role of reflex demulcency is particularly valuable. Even further, if there is acid in the oesophagus, then the direct demulcent activity of the mucilage on the oesophageal wall will also soothe the irritation and thereby allay the very stimulus driving the cough or wheeze.

Animal models have confirmed that the association with GORD and cough is most likely a reflex mediated by the oesophageal afferent nerve fibres carried by the vagus nerve.[102] The nociceptive C-fibres are stimulated by the acid; however, multiple neural pathways are likely to be involved. In clinical studies, inhalation of a low concentration of a C-fibre stimulant leads to an irritating, itchy, urge-to-cough sensation that mimics the sensations associated with

cough linked to respiratory tract infection, post-infection, GORD and asthma.[103]

Mucilages are also a class of viscous soluble fibre and in this context the properties of psyllium husks have been well studied. In particular, the mucilage from psyllium is effective at lowering blood cholesterol, as evidenced by reviews of the clinical data.[104,105] Trial results suggest that it must be taken with food to be effective.[106] The effective dose is around 10 g/day, with recent trials suggesting more modest effects of around a 7% reduction in LDL-cholesterol.

Viscous soluble fibre helps to retain glucose in the gut and reduce blood insulin levels after eating. Probably the main effect here is delayed gastric emptying. Psyllium seed was shown to have particular benefits in this regard, with a clear dose-related response on the effects of a glucose challenge.[107] Results were not highly robust and obviously it needs to be taken with meals.[105]

Mucilages may compromise the absorption of nutrients and drugs (see Appendix C). However, the potential for psyllium to decrease the absorption of minerals is not proven.[105]

Since mucilages are water soluble and relatively insoluble in ethanol, liquid galenical preparations of mucilages are not appropriate (except for their use as reflex demulcents); for demulcent effects in the digestive tract, mucilages are best given as powders, capsules, or glycerol-based tinctures. In any case, an effectively made liquid extract of slippery elm, for example, would be so viscous that it could not be poured. Yet there are still some companies that sell this very thing (obviously not made well).

Essential oils

Phytochemistry

Essential oils (from the word 'essence') are mixtures of fragrant compounds that can be isolated from plants by the process of steam distillation. In this procedure, steam is driven through the plant material and then condensed, with the subsequent oil and water phases separating out. Since they are volatile in steam, and usually have pronounced aromas, essential oils are often referred to as volatile oils. However, this term is not accurate since they have boiling points well above 100°C. Often the oil is slightly modified by the steam distillation process, so that it does not exactly reflect what is found in the plant. In some cases, such as chamazulene produced from matricine in German chamomile, steam distillation actually produces substantial quantities of a new chemical.

Other processes are also used to produce essential oils and these include solvent extract using hexane or liquid or supercritical carbon dioxide, enfleurage (oil extraction of delicate essential oils in flowers) and expression (used to produce orange and lemon oils from the peel). Essential oils are important items of commerce, being used for perfumes, food flavourings and personal care and pharmaceutical products. They also comprise the medicines of the therapeutic system known as aromatherapy.

Essential oils are water-insoluble oily liquids that are usually colourless. Despite their being called oils, they are not related chemically to lipid oils (fixed oils) such as olive oil, corn oil and so on. Although often hydrocarbon in nature, they are unrelated to the hydrocarbon oils from the petrochemical industry. They will slowly evaporate if left in an open container, and placing a drop of oil on blotting paper can be used as a simple technique to test for adulteration with a fixed oil. If a fixed oil is present, an oily smear will remain on the paper a few days later.

Adulteration is an important issue in the trading of essential oils and many sophisticated techniques have been developed to imitate and extend essential oils. In some cases, such as oil of wintergreen, trade in the synthetic oil has completely supplanted the natural product. One survey found a large variability between the biological activities of different samples of oils and groups of oils under the same general name, for example lavender, eucalyptus or chamomile.[108] This reflected on the blending, rectification and adulteration that occurs with commercial oils. Of course, this issue does not apply for oils prescribed as part of the whole plant extract, as used by phytotherapists.

The synthesis and accumulation of essential oils are generally associated with the presence of specialised structures in the plant often located on or near the surface; for example, the delicate glandular trichomes (hairs) of the mint family (Lamiaceae or Labiatae). Essential oil composition can vary quite dramatically within a species and often distinct chemotypes are recognised. This means that the same plant species can produce quite different oils in terms of their chemistry, pharmacology and toxicology. From a biosynthetic perspective, components of essential oils can be classified into two major groups: the terpenoids and the phenylpropanoids. Any given essential oil might contain more than 100 of these components.

When the chemical structures of terpenoids are examined, they can be theoretically constructed from five-carbon isoprene units. Plants produce terpenoids using the mevalonic acid biosynthetic pathway. As mentioned earlier, the building block is actually isopentenylpyrophosphate, not isoprene, but the outcome is molecules based on the characteristic five-carbon units. Naming of terpenoids is based on multiples of 10 carbons (two isoprene units). Hence, molecules with 10 carbons are called monoterpenes; those with 15 are called sesquiterpenes (sesqui means one and a half) and so on. Only mono- and sesquiterpenes are found in essential oils. Higher terpenoids are too large and hence not volatile in steam. Diterpenes occur in resins as resin acids and triterpenes are found as saponins. Not even all mono- and sesquiterpenes are volatile in steam – the iridoids featured in the eyebright monograph are one example. Examples of monoterpenes in essential oils include limonene, geraniol, borneol and thujone. Bisabolol is a sesquiterpene.

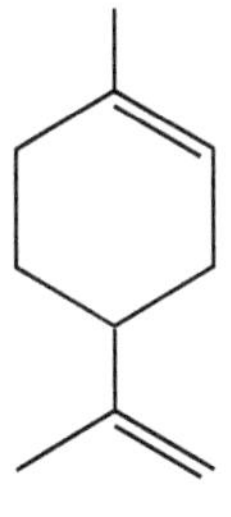

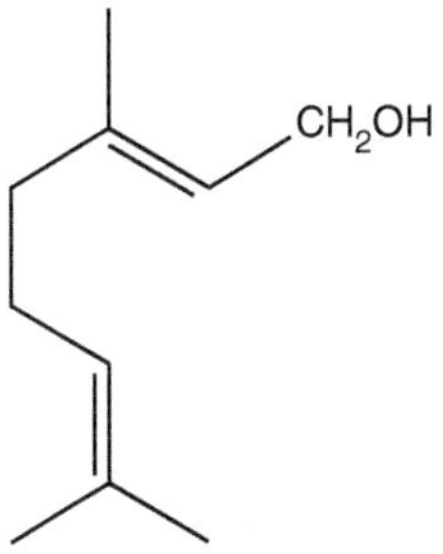

Geraniol

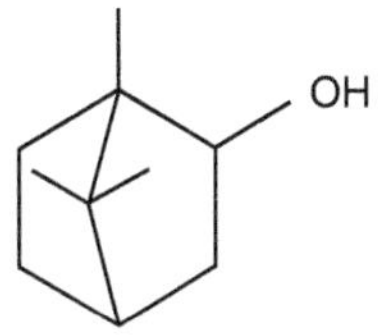

Borneol

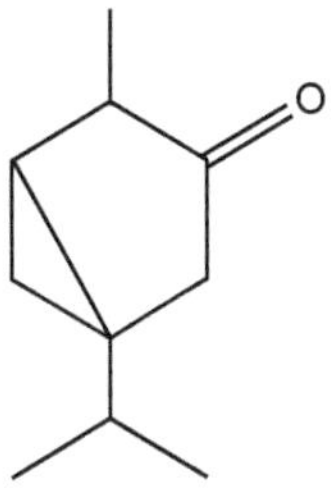

Thujone

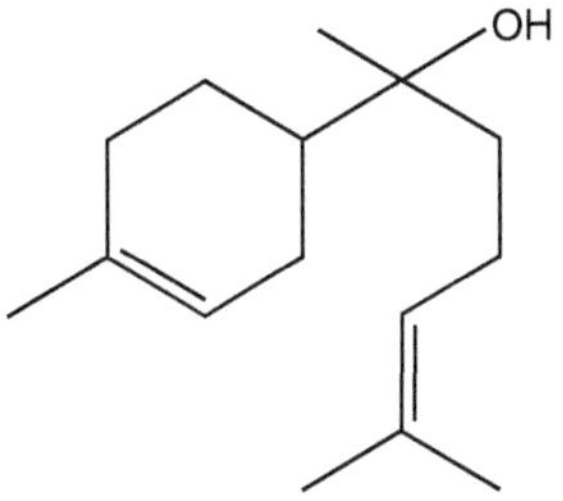

(–)-α-Bisabolol

Phenylpropanoids are far less common as components of essential oils. Their basic chemical skeleton is a three-carbon chain attached to a benzene ring. They are formed by the shikimic acid biosynthetic pathway and examples include anethole and eugenol.

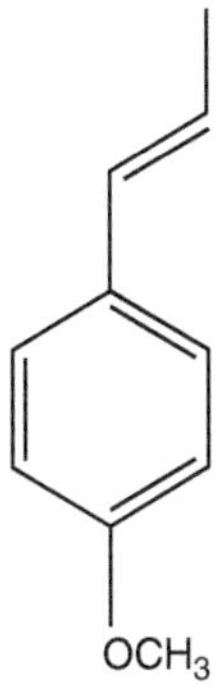

Limonene

trans-**Anethole**

OH

OCH₃

Eugenol

Essential oil components can also be classified according to their functional groups. The most common compounds found in essential oils are hydrocarbons, alcohols, aldehydes, ketones, phenols, oxides and esters. These functional groups play a large part in determining the pharmacology and toxicology of the essential oil component; for example, ketones are more active and toxic than alcohols, and alcohols and phenols are more potent as antimicrobial agents, with phenols being more irritant. Essential oil components often exhibit optical isomerism (where the two isomers are mirror images of each other). For example, (+)-carvone isolated from caraway oil has a caraway-like odour and (−)-carvone isolated from spearmint oil has a spearmint-like odour.

Pharmacodynamics

Aromatherapy is a treatment system based on the use of essential oils. The oils may be inhaled, applied to the skin or orifices, added to baths or ingested. There is no doubt that ingested oils or those applied to the skin or added to baths are absorbed into the bloodstream in significant quantities.[109] However, the use of essential oils by inhalation, mainly to influence mental function, is more controversial. In fact, in the German-speaking world, aromatherapy is typically defined as the therapeutic use of fragrances only by means of inhalation. Evidence is accumulating that this form of aromatherapy also has a pharmacological basis and is not placebo, nor is it a manipulation of emotions via the sense of smell. A recent review of the therapeutic properties of lavender essential oil exemplifies this, with 14 clinical studies demonstrating possible beneficial effects from its inhalation, including enhanced sleep, decreased anxiety and improved cognition.[110]

Given the great chemical diversity of essential oils, it is not surprising that they exhibit a wide variety of pharmacological activities. However, some common themes do emerge, notably antimicrobial (including antiviral) and spasmolytic actions.

Most of the evidence for the antibacterial and antifungal activities of essential oils comes from in vitro tests, although case reports and clinical trials are scattered throughout the literature (see below). A review of the published in vitro work between 1976 and 1986 found that results were difficult to compare.[111] Test methods used differed widely and important factors influencing results were frequently neglected. One of these factors was the composition of the essential oil being tested (given the existence of chemotypes and adulteration). This was highlighted in another study of commercial essential oils that found a wide variation in the antimicrobial activities of commercial samples of thyme oil, eucalyptus oil and geranium oil, among others.[108]

A review of more recent investigations summarised the antibacterial and antifungal activity data from around 50 studies.[112] Most tests assessed either MICs or the concentration required to kill 50% of the test micro-organism culture (EC_{50}). Many of the reviewed publications tested a range of oils and essential oil components. Wide variations in activity, depending on the test method, the essential oil tested and the test organism were tabulated.

Of 53 essential oils tested against four organisms, only a few oils exhibited remarkable activity, particularly thyme and origanum.[113] *Pseudomonas aeruginosa* was the least susceptible organism and *Candida albicans* the most susceptible. These oils stand out because they contain the highly active phenols thymol and carvacrol.[114]

Attempts have been made to identify the mechanisms behind the antifungal and antibacterial activities of essential oils and the key components responsible for this activity. Antimicrobial activity was said to parallel cytotoxic activity, suggesting a common mode of action, most probably exerted by membrane-associated reactions.[115] In simple terms, it appears that the mobile and lipophilic nature of essential oil components, especially the monoterpenes, enables them to penetrate and disrupt cell membranes. Concentrations of tea tree oil that inhibit or decrease growth of *Escherichia coli* also inhibit glucose-dependent respiration and stimulate the leakage of intracellular potassium.[116] According to a recent review, essential oils seem to have no specific cellular targets because of their great number of constituents.[112] This suggests a very low risk of the development of microbial resistance against essential oils. Being lipophilic (fat-soluble) they pass through the cell wall and membranes, disrupting their structures. In bacteria, permeabilisation of the membranes is associated with the loss of ions and a reduction of membrane potential, collapse of the proton pump and depletion of the ATP pool. Essential oils can also coagulate the cytoplasm and damage lipids and proteins. Damage to the cell wall and membrane can lead to the leakage of macromolecules and eventually to lysis.

In eukaryotic cells, essential oils can provoke depolarisation of mitochondrial membranes by decreasing the membrane potential, impact ionic calcium cycling and other ionic channels and reducing the pH gradient, affecting the proton pump and the ATP pool. Chain reactions from the cell wall or membrane invade the whole cell, leading to widespread oxidative damage.[112]

Of five components tested for antibacterial activity, cinnamic aldehyde was the most active, followed by citral, geraniol, eugenol and menthol.[117] Essential oils with high concentrations of thymol and carvacrol usually inhibit Gram-positive bacteria better than Gram-negative bacteria,[118] although they still possess a good broad-spectrum activity. In another study, linalool was the most active antibacterial agent and citral and geraniol were the most effective antifungal agents.[119] Essential oils with a high monoterpene hydrocarbon level were very active against bacteria but not against fungi, with the exception of dill.[108] There was a negative correlation observed between cineole content and antifungal activity. In the case of tea tree oil, terpinen-4-ol was identified as the most important antimicrobial compound[120,121] and cineole detracted from its antifungal activity.[121]

Recent research has highlighted the significant in vitro antiviral activity of essential oils.[122] Most of the studies have been conducted against herpes simplex virus (HSV)-1 and HSV-2, with quite potent activities (at the parts-per-million level) being observed. A viral envelope is necessary, as growth of non-enveloped (naked) viruses is not affected by essential oils. They appear to act on enveloped viruses by affecting the viability of the free virus (virion), probably by interfering with the viral envelope (which like the cell membrane is lipid in nature).[122]

Clinical studies of the antimicrobial activity of essential oils have been published, with a focus on Australian tea tree oil used only topically. In an early double blind trial, 10% tea tree oil cream reduced symptoms of tinea pedis but was not effective in eradicating the fungus.[123] However, a 5% tea tree oil gel was as effective as a 5% benzoyl peroxide lotion in the treatment of acne and patients experienced few side effects.[124]

A 2006 review of tea tree oil included published clinical trials.[125] In addition to the trials summarised above, tea tree oil demonstrated efficacy as an antibacterial mouthwash or gel in three trials (with a residual effect on oral bacteria), reduced methicillin-resistant *Staphylococcus aureus* (MRSA) carriage, and successfully treated fungal infections of the nails, mouth and skin. Since then, topical tea tree oil has demonstrated clinical efficacy in another randomised, double blind trial assessing its value in acne patients[126] and improved healing in recurrent herpes labialis after application of a 6% gel (although the results did not achieve statistical significance in this small trial).[127] Tea tree oil as a topical application is also quite effective for head lice infestation.[128,129]

One review noted that other essential oils show bactericidal activity against oral and dental pathogenic micro-organisms and have been incorporated into mouth rinses.[118]

Information about topical use is important, but phytotherapists also rely on essential oils to achieve antimicrobial effects within the body. In particular, the excretion of essential oils via the lungs or urine might be expected to exert at least a mild antimicrobial activity at these sites. This is the basis of the use of juniper and buchu for urinary tract infections and one of the reasons for the use of thyme in respiratory infections. However, essential oil components are excreted into the urine in metabolised forms, mainly as glucuronide and sulphate conjugates. Hence, any antibacterial activity may not be reflected in the urine. Studies are necessary to understand further this traditional use.

Essential oils certainly have a promising role in the management of intestinal pathogens, bacterial or otherwise. In an open label trial, oil of oregano was orally administered to 14 adult patients whose stools tested positive for the enteric parasites *Blastocystis hominis*, *Entamoeba hartmanni* and *Endolimax nana*.[130] After 6 weeks of 600mg/day of emulsified oil, there was a substantial reduction in detectable pathogens that correlated somewhat with an improvement in gastrointestinal symptoms. The clinical anthelmintic action of the (toxic) essential oil of wormseed (*Chenopodium ambrosioides*) is well documented, although this has been questioned.[131]

The spasmolytic activity of essential oils has been observed many times on isolated smooth muscle preparations and forms much of the basis of their use in functional gastrointestinal disorders.[132] The effects of essential oils from 22 plants and some of their constituents on tracheal and ileal smooth muscle were investigated in one study.[133] All of the oils had relaxant effects on tracheal smooth muscle, the most potent being angelica root, clove and elecampane root. Sixteen oils inhibited the phasic contractions of the ileal muscle preparation, the most potent being elecampane root, clove, thyme and lemon balm. Two oils (anise and fennel) increased the phasic contractions. Spasmolytic activity has also been confirmed clinically. For example, peppermint oil added to barium sulphate suspension significantly relieved colonic muscle spasm (p<0.001) during barium enema examination in a double blind, placebo-controlled study involving 141 patients.[134] For more examples of the clinical spasmolytic activity of peppermint oil and its value in irritable bowel syndrome, see the peppermint monograph.

Carminatives relax sphincters and assist in the expulsion of intestinal gas. Their activity is somewhat related to spasmolytic activity. Certain essential oils or essential oil-containing herbs have been traditionally used as carminatives over many years. Oils of peppermint, sage and rosemary all relaxed Oddi's sphincter, but peppermint was the most active.[135] The carminative activity of cardamom and dill was confirmed in human studies.[136] However, they were also shown to cause oesophageal reflux and should be used cautiously in susceptible patients.

Some essential oils are traditionally regarded as diuretics because they act as 'kidney irritants'. The infusion and essential oil of juniper berries as well as terpinen-4-ol were tested for diuresis response in rats.[137] On initial dosing, all three test substances exhibited an antidiuretic effect, but a significant diuretic effect was established on repeated doses, with the infusion having the strongest effect. The 'irritant' effect of juniper oil on the kidneys was also investigated, since there are concerns in the literature about its long-term use. No nephrotoxic effects were observed in an animal model and the authors suggested that provided high-quality oil is used (distilled from the ripe berries), concerns about the kidney irritant effects of juniper are unfounded.[138] Essential oil terpenes used orally had shown some promise in dissolving small kidney stones in small, uncontrolled trials in adult patients, but these findings were not supported by controlled trials.[139] However, a positive pilot trial in children suggests further investigations are desirable.

Certain essential oils (or the herbs that contain them) are used as expectorants. A proprietary product containing myrtle oil was popularly prescribed by doctors in Germany as an expectorant and mucolytic agent for acute and chronic bronchitis and sinusitis. The oil contains limonene, cineole and alpha-pinene. An expectorant activity for this oil was confirmed in a clinical trial in patients with chronic obstructive airways disease.[140] Earlier animal experiments by Boyd suggested an expectorant activity for essential oils probably via influencing goblet cells to secrete more respiratory tract fluid (RTF) and mucus.[141] In the 1940s, Boyd studied the effects of several essential oils in various experimental models.[142,143] The most pronounced increase of RTF was seen after ingestion of oil of anise. Interestingly ingestion of oil of eucalyptus had a moderate effect that was not eliminated by cutting efferent gastric nerves. This finding supports the premise that essential oils do not act as reflex expectorants (see later).

One intriguing aspect of Boyd's research is that he was able to demonstrate that inhaled essential oils also acted as expectorants. These results are summarised in Table 2.1.

Boyd found a biphasic effect in that high concentrations of essential oils suppressed RTF and mucin release, whereas lower doses (on the threshold of detection by the nose) had a pronounced stimulatory effect. A seasonal effect was also observed, with an increased activity in autumn (fall). These findings provide a rational basis for the hot lemon drink in respiratory infections, since active amounts of lemon oil would be inhaled while ingesting the hot drink.

The inhalation of essential oils into the lungs might exert a direct antimicrobial activity. A case report from Australia describes the successful use of inhaled eucalyptus oil to effect clinical improvement in a patient with tuberculosis.[144] A 28-year-old woman presented with cough, shortness of breath, fever, night sweats, weight loss and malaise. She had been unwell for 12 months. A sputum sample was positive for *Mycobacterium tuberculosis*. X-ray of the chest confirmed the diagnosis of pulmonary tuberculosis.

The patient initially refused conventional treatment and instead inhalation of a *Eucalyptus globulus* essential oil preparation (in an ethanol-water base) was initiated. A vapour inhaler was used to administer 3 mL of the preparation in 500 mL of boiling water 3 times a day for 3 weeks. After 10 days the patient reported reduced malaise, normal temperatures, improved appetite, absent cough and a gain of 4.5 kg in weight. Her sputum cultures were negative. The patient subsequently underwent conventional treatment.

A sedative activity following the ingestion of essential oils such as lavender is commonly recognised and was supported by early animal studies.[145] More recently, a proprietary essential oil of lavender at 80 mg/day was found to be clinically effective in sub-threshold anxiety disorder. Three randomised, controlled, double blind clinical trials were identified in a review, demonstrating significant improvements in anxiety scores after 10 weeks of treatment with the lavender oil.[146]

Stimulant activity has also been attributed to some essential oils. Inhalation and oral doses of rosemary oil increased locomotor activity in mice.[147] Infusions of essential oil-containing herbs are often taken as diaphoretics, especially during acute respiratory infections. In this context, it is interesting to note that a case report describes a patient who exhibited pronounced diaphoresis attributed to up to 10 cups a day of sassafras tea (not recommended because of potential carcinogenicity).[148]

Essential oils and essential oil components have been extensively studied in animal models for analgesic-like activity.[149] Overall, 43 bioactive essential oil components were identified in one review, mainly monoterpenes. However, these findings are yet to translate into clinical applications, apart from topical use of peppermint oil or menthol (for example) in headache and joint pain (see the peppermint monograph). In contrast, the local anaesthetic activity of oil of cloves is well described and the local anaesthetic activity of lavender oil has been demonstrated in an in vivo model.[150]

Given their cytotoxic properties on bacterial and fungal cells, it is not surprising that essential oils have exhibited a wide range of antitumour activities against cancer cell lines.[112,122] Essential oils exert cytotoxicity at levels considerably lower than their antibacterial activity (in the parts-per-million range). As in bacterial cells, the cell membrane is one of the sites of cytotoxic activity.[122] This antitumour research is particularly well developed (at least at the in vitro level) for thymoquinone, a component of the essential oil from the seeds of the black cumin (*Nigella sativa*).[151]

For more information about the pharmacology of essential oils and associated anti-inflammatory, antiulcer, spasmolytic,

Table 2.1 Expectorant effect of inhaled essential oils or their components

Year of study	Expectorants studied	Results
1968[580]	Thuja oil	RTF markedly increased, as was the soluble mucin content of RTF. Effect was most marked in fall
	Anise oil	No effect at normal doses
	Eucalyptus oil	No effect at normal doses
1969[581]	Menthol	No change in amount of RTF, but its soluble mucin content was increased
	Thymol	No effect at normal doses
1970[582]	Lemon oil	RTF and its soluble mucin content increased
1970[583]	Nutmeg oil	RTF and its soluble mucin content moderately increased. Effect most pronounced in fall
1970[584]	Citral, geraniol	RTF and its soluble mucin content moderately increased

RTF = respiratory tract fluid

oestrogenic, expectorant, antimicrobial and analgesic activities, see the monographs on chamomile, fennel, peppermint and thyme in Part Three.

Toxicology

Essential oils are highly concentrated from their original plant matrix and as a result can present specific safety issues when used as such. Their toxicology has already been comprehensively reviewed.[152] Nevertheless, a few issues are worth noting here. Certain toxic essential oils, notably pennyroyal, tansy and parsley, have been used as abortifacients. However, as early as 1913 it was found that these oils have absolutely no specific or direct stimulating action on the uterine muscle.[153] In fact, consistent with the known pharmacodynamics of essential oils, they were found to inhibit uterine contractions. Their abortifacient action was concluded to be due to general poisoning or gastrointestinal irritation, which makes their use not only uncertain, but also extremely dangerous.

Thujone is a constituent of commonly used herbs such as wormwood, yarrow, thuja and sage. This compound is neurotoxic and its presence in liqueurs such as absinthe apparently caused widespread toxicity and abuse syndromes in the early 20th century.[154] The first sign of toxicity is a headache. High and prolonged doses of the above herbs are hence best avoided, unless they are low-thujone varieties. It has been suggested that thujone intoxication may have played a part in Van Gogh's style of painting.[155] However, this has been recently challenged and it now appears that the syndrome known as *absinthism* is largely attributed to the toxic effects of ethanol.[156] Safrole, a major component of sassafras oil, is carcinogenic and its use should be avoided.

Topical use of essential oils can cause contact dermatitis, as one review of tea tree oil cases noted.[157] Oxidation, and hence the age of the oil, appears to increase the likelihood of a reaction.

Glucosinolates and isothiocyanates

Phytochemistry

Glucosinolates are sulphur- and nitrogen-containing glycosides responsible for the pungent properties of horseradish, nasturtium and mustard. The glucosinolate itself is not pungent. When it encounters the enzyme myrosinase, normally stored in another compartment of the cell, the aglycone is formed which then usually rearranges into a pungent and corrosive isothiocyanate. Isothiocyanates can also be formed from glucosinolates by steam distillation and so are called mustard oils. For this reason, they are sometimes classified as essential oils, but from a phytochemical perspective this is inappropriate. The structure of a typical glucosinolate is provided in the figure below. They are ionic in nature and occur in the plant as potassium salts.

Glucosinolate   **Isothiocyanate**

Glucosinolates are also found in brassicas such as cabbage, broccoli and Brussels sprouts. As such, they are frequently consumed as a normal part of human diet.

Pharmacodynamics

In traditional herbal and folk medicine, strong skin irritants and inflammatory substances were empirically used to combat inflammatory processes in tissues and organs remote from the site where the irritant was applied. This is the principle of counterirritation. This poorly understood effect is recognised in pharmacology and can often provide misleading anti-inflammatory effects in test models for substances with no pharmacological activity other than being irritants. The mode of action of such skin irritants is characterised by an ability to influence deeper regions of the body, probably by reflex responses mediated by the nervous system. The stinging of arthritic joints with nettles and the subsequent reduction in pain and inflammation is one such example. Hyperaemic medicines can be used in the form of ointments, compresses, liniments or plasters. The mustard compress or plaster is still used in Europe today, particularly for bronchial infections and detoxification in chronic diseases. Mustard oil is highly corrosive and if applied for too long will cause blistering and may even permanently scar the skin.

The main component of nasturtium oil (*Tropaeolum majus*) is benzyl isothiocyanate. This has potent antibacterial and antifungal activity. In Europe, enteric-coated capsules of the oil are used to treat bronchial and urinary tract infections.[158] Horseradish preparations are used in the treatment of bronchial and sinus conditions. Presumably, the sulphur compounds confer a mucolytic effect. Recent research interest in benzyl isothiocyanate relates to its potential role in cancer.[159]

Isothiocyanates and some of their products (such as goitrin) are goitrogenic and interfere with the function of the thyroid gland.[160] Goitrin inhibits iodine incorporation and the formation of thyroxin and its effects cannot be countered by iodine administration. Although this is a potentially toxic effect, it could possibly be exploited in cases of patients with hyperthyroidism.

The bulk of recent research attention on glucosinolates and their various transformation products (including sulforaphane, indole-3-carbinol and di-indoylmethane) has focused on their potential to prevent and modify cancer. This phenomenon has been known for more than 30 years. The anticarcinogenicity of these compounds, specifically in relation to brassica vegetables, has been recently reviewed for in vitro assays, animal experiments and various human studies.[161–163] Alterations in phase I, and particularly phase II, detoxification enzymes are suggested as mechanisms by which these plant constituents might inhibit chemical carcinogenesis or alter the level of cancer promoting hormones such as oestrogen. On the other hand, possible mutagenicity, tumour promotion and carcinogenicity are also discussed, indicating that caution should be exercised if recommending long-term intake of these compounds at doses well in excess of optimum dietary levels.

The following brief review of the data, especially for broccoli sprouts, is provided as a good example of the progress in this field of research. Epidemiological evidence suggests that diets containing vegetables from the Brassica genus (including broccoli, cabbage, Brussels sprouts and cauliflower) are associated with a reduced cancer risk. After reviewing the results of 7 cohort studies and 87 case-control studies, it was concluded that the association appears to be most consistent for lung, stomach, colon and rectal cancer.[164] A series of studies to find the active constituents and mechanisms of action began in the mid-1990s. As a result of this research, Brassica vegetables were found to be rich sources of inducers of phase II detoxification enzymes in vitro, with the isothiocyanate sulforaphane the main phase II inducer in broccoli.[165]

As noted above, glucosinolates in Brassica vegetables are broken down to form isothiocyanates (the aglycones) by the action of the enzyme myrosinase. This occurs when the plant is crushed, but also during cooking or in the human intestine by intestinal flora.[166] Glucoraphanin is the glucosinolate precursor of sulforaphane. Broccoli sprouts contain about 15 times more glucoraphanin than the mature broccoli plant.[167]

Sulforaphane was found to be a potent in vitro inducer of the phase II enzymes quinone reductase (QR) and glutathione S-transferase (GST).[168] Sulforaphane also induces phase II enzymes in vivo. In mice treated orally with sulforaphane, QR and GST were increased in many organs, including the liver.[168] It is a potent inducer of the multiorgan protector pathway and hence initiates the cytoplasmic transcription factor Nrf2 to migrate into the cell nucleus, where it activates the antioxidant response element, upregulating the production of antioxidant and phase II enzymes.

The induction of phase II enzymes is one of the main mechanisms by which sulforaphane exerts its chemopreventative activity. Orally administered sulforaphane has been shown to be protective against carcinogen-induced cancer at a variety of sites.[169] Taken together these findings suggest that sulforaphane can inhibit the development of cancer during the initiation and post-initiation stages.[169]

The chemopreventative activity of sulforaphane probably involves many mechanisms. These include:[169]

- inhibition of phase I enzymes
- induction of phase II enzymes
- antioxidant functions through increased tissue glutathione levels
- apoptosis-inducing properties
- induction of cell cycle arrest
- anti-inflammatory properties
- inhibition of angiogenesis.

A randomised, placebo-controlled trial found that sulforaphane exerted a phase II inducing effect in participants who achieved a good bioavailability (that is, who were able to convert glucoraphanin to sulforaphane in their intestine). Two hundred healthy volunteers from a region in China with a high risk for development of hepatocellular carcinoma were enrolled. Urinary levels of the markers of two environmental carcinogens were assessed. A strong, highly significant inverse association was observed when the marker levels were compared with levels of dithiocarbamate excretion (a measure of the metabolism of glucoraphanin).[170] Oral administration of a broccoli sprout homogenate over 3 days induced mucosal phase II enzyme expression in the upper airway of human volunteers.[171]

Flavonoids

Phytochemistry

Flavonoids are extremely common and widespread in the plant kingdom. They function as plant pigments and are responsible for the colours of many flowers and fruits. Being abundant in plants, flavonoids are commonly consumed in the human diet, especially if it is rich in fruits and vegetables.

The word 'flavonoid' is derived from the Latin word *flavus* meaning yellow and many flavonoids are indeed yellow in colour. However, many others are white and the special flavonoid-related anthocyanins are red, blue or purple. (For a discussion of the pharmacological properties of anthocyanins, see the bilberry monograph.) Flavonoids are also present in leaves, where they are said to protect the plant tissue against the damaging effects of ultraviolet radiation.

Flavonoids consist of a single benzene ring joined to a benzo-gamma-pyrone structure. They are formed from three acetate units and a phenylpropane unit (via the shikimic acid pathway). More than 2000 are known with nearly 500 occurring in the free (aglycone) state and the rest as O- or C-glycosides. Flavonoid glycosides are generally water-soluble. There are three main types, classified according to the state of oxygenation at carbon 3. These are flavones, flavonols and flavonones. The properties of isoflavonoids are discussed in the phyto-oestrogen section.

R = H: Apigenin
R = OH: Luteolin

Flavones

R = H: Naringenin
R = OH: Eriodictyol

Flavonones

R = H: Kaempferol
R = OH: Quercetin

Flavonols

Unfortunately, the term flavonoid is used rather loosely in the pharmacological literature. It is often applied as a collective term to describe any plant polyphenolic compounds, including anthocyanins, green tea polyphenolics, the flavonolignans in St Mary's (milk) thistle and oligomeric procyanidins and catechins, by way of example. None of these phytochemicals is actually flavonoids, and their bundling with flavonoids only serves to confuse any meaningful conclusions that can be drawn about the pharmacological properties of true flavonoids.

Pharmacodynamics

Most of the studies conducted on flavonoids have used in vitro models, often employing isolated enzyme systems. The findings of these studies need to be interpreted with caution, since it is uncertain that oral doses of flavonoid glycosides or even their aglycones can reach sufficient concentrations in living organisms to reproduce these effects. This reservation applies even more for oral doses of herbs containing flavonoids, since the flavonoid dose will be commensurately lower in the plant matrix. The issue was well illustrated by one early clinical pharmacology study that found, while quercetin and apigenin inhibited platelet aggregation in vitro, no significant effect was found in human volunteers.[172] Fortunately, clinical studies involving flavonoids (albeit at doses typically much higher than can be achieved by phytotherapy) and flavonoid-containing herbs are on the increase. (For a further discussion on the bioavailability of flavonoids, see the Pharmacokinetics section.) There are now tens of thousands of published studies on flavonoids. Hence, the brief section in this chapter serves only as a primer to this vast body of literature.

The original pharmacological interest in flavonoids arose during vitamin C research in the 1930s. Studies by Hungarian workers indicated that a number of vegetables and fruits (notably citrus) contained substances capable of correcting certain abnormalities associated with scurvy. In particular, this new factor, designated as vitamin P, corrected the capillary fragility associated with ascorbic acid deficiency. Vitamin P was subsequently found to be a mixture of flavonoids. Additional research disputed that vitamin P was essential to maintain human life and the term was dropped in the 1950s. However, research did confirm the therapeutic value of flavonoids for fragile capillaries (actually fragile connective tissue surrounding capillaries) and as extenders of vitamin C activity, possibly through improved absorption and protection from oxidation, and by partially substituting for some of its biological functions.[173]

Decreased capillary fragility denotes improved connective tissue tone and a reduced tendency for capillary contents to leak into surrounding tissue. This implies that flavonoids will prevent oedema associated with inflammation and stasis. Such effects from flavonoids are reasonably well established from clinical trials.

A proprietary mixture of micronised flavonoids consisting of 90% diosmin and 10% hesperidin, usually administered at a dose of 1000 mg/day, has been investigated in several clinical trials. Such double blind, placebo-controlled trials have shown that this flavonoid combination improves venous tone in normal volunteers,[174] enhances microcirculation in patients with venous insufficiency,[175] assists healing of venous ulcers[176] and relieves symptoms of acute haemorrhoids.[177] A recent critical review confirmed the benefits of this combination in patients with advanced venous disease.[178] A meta-analysis of clinical trials also supported its benefit in the treatment of haemorrhoids.[179] Of course, this is more a 'nutraceutical' therapy and it is arguable whether these doses have any relevance to phytotherapy, as they could not be realistically achieved by the administration of plant extracts.

Flavonoids are polyphenolic compounds (they contain several phenolic hydroxyl groups), some more so than others. The chemical properties that flow from this feature underlie many of the impressive in vitro pharmacological effects of these compounds. In particular, they are able to complex metal ions, act as antioxidants and bind to proteins such as enzymes and structural proteins (this last feature could also explain the ability of flavonoids to enhance the integrity of connective tissue).

The in vitro antioxidant properties of flavonoids were the focus of much early research.[180,181] The ability of flavonoids to complex pro-oxidant metallic ions such as iron probably augments their antioxidant effects in specific circumstances.[182] Of particular interest is the capacity of flavonoids to inhibit macrophage-mediated oxidation of LDL and thereby attenuate atherogenesis.[183] The antioxidant properties of flavonoids could also contribute to their observed anti-inflammatory and antiplatelet effects,[184] and are related not only to their structural characteristics, but also to their ability to interact with and penetrate the lipid bilayers of the cell membrane.[185] Flavonoids scavenge the nitric oxide radical,[186] the superoxide anion[187] and singlet oxygen.[188] Like most other antioxidants, flavonoids can also act as pro-oxidants in particular circumstances.[189]

The molecular promiscuity conferred by the phenolic groups of flavonoids is well demonstrated by the range of enzymes inhibited by them in vitro. Enzyme activities inhibited to varying degrees by flavonoids in vitro include cyclooxygenase,[190] lipoxygenase,[190] lens aldose reductase,[191] xanthine oxidase,[192] cGMP phosphodiesterase,[193] cAMP phosphodiesterase,[194] angiotensin-converting enzyme,[195] aromatase,[196] thyroid peroxidase,[197] hyaluronidase,[180] phospholipases[180] and protein phosphokinases.[180] However, more research is needed to determine which of these activities might realistically translate into clinical effects. Since enzyme-inhibiting activity depends on the structure of the flavonoid, some compounds are more likely than others to be clinically active.

Using isolated cells or organs in vitro, the activities demonstrated for flavonoids include antiviral activity, especially for the 3-methoxylated flavones,[181,195] anti-inflammatory activity,[198] antimicrobial activity,[195,199] inhibition of histamine release from mast cells,[200,201] antiplatelet activity,[195,202] tumour cell cytotoxicity, especially for highly methoxylated flavones,[195] and spasmolytic activity.[203,204] The flavonoid 8-isopentenylnaringenin (now 8-prenylnaringenin) isolated from the Thai herb *Anaxagorea luzonensis* was found to be an oestrogen agonist with an activity about 10 times greater than genistein.[205] This flavonoid, which also occurs in hops (*Humulus lupulus*), has now been extensively studied as a phyto-oestrogen.[206] It strongly activates oestrogen receptor alpha and at least partially accounts for the observed clinical value of hops in menopausal women experiencing mild vasomotor symptoms.[207]

Animal experiments (usually using high doses) have demonstrated a number of interesting pharmacological effects for flavonoids. One study found antioxidant effects in vivo for dietary flavonoids (quercetin and catechin), with reduced lipid peroxidation in rats.[208] Flavonoids have also demonstrated hepatoprotective, antiulcer (gastroprotective)[209] and analgesic activity in vivo.[180] Several flavonoids tested showed anti-inflammatory effects in acute and chronic animal models.[210,211] A favourable effect of quercitrin on experimentally induced diarrhoea was probably related to anti-inflammatory effects.[212]

Flavonoids have exhibited preventative activity against chemical carcinogens and tumour promotion in animal models,[213,214] although most of the speculation over their cancer preventative role is based on in vitro studies.[215] Anxiolytic properties have been demonstrated for some flavonoids (including chrysin and apigenin), which selectively bind with a high affinity to the central benzodiazepine receptor.[216,217]

The relationship between dietary flavonoid intake and cardiovascular disease was tested in several early epidemiological studies. The Zutphen Study in Holland found that flavonoid intake in elderly men (largely via tea, onions and apples) was significantly inversely associated with mortality and incidence of stroke.[218] A Finnish study also found that people with very low intakes of flavonoids had a higher risk of coronary disease,[219] but US studies found no significant association.[220] These investigations are confounded by the difficulties in isolating effects due to just the flavonoids and the loose use of the term, as discussed above.[221] This was well illustrated by another US study that found the observed non-significant inverse associations for broccoli, apples and tea on cardiovascular disease incidence in women were not mediated by flavonoids.[222] The same researchers later detected no protection from dietary flavonoids on incidences of insulin resistance, type 2 diabetes[223] and cancer,[224] all from epidemiological investigations in women.

In another interesting Finnish study, the total dietary intakes of 10 054 men and women during the year preceding the baseline examination were determined with a dietary history method.[225] Flavonoid intakes were estimated mainly on the basis of the flavonoid concentrations in Finnish foods. Participants with higher quercetin intakes exhibited lower mortality from ischaemic heart disease. The relative risk (RR) between the highest and lowest quartiles was 0.79 (95% CI: 0.63 to 0.99: p=0.02). The incidence of cerebrovascular disease was lower at higher kaempferol (0.70; p=0.003), naringenin (0.79; p=0.06) and hesperetin (0.80; p=0.008) intakes. Men with higher quercetin intakes had a lower lung cancer incidence (0.42; p=0.001), and men with higher myricetin intakes had a lower prostate cancer risk (0.43; p=0.002). Asthma incidence was lower at higher quercetin (0.76; p=0.005), naringenin (0.69; p=0.06) and hesperetin (0.64; p=0.03) intakes. A trend toward a reduction in risk of type 2 diabetes was associated with higher quercetin (0.81; p=0.07) and myricetin (0.79; p=0.07) ingestion.

Clinical studies of flavonoids (more as nutraceuticals than as herbal extracts) are yielding some interesting results. Citrus flavonoids have demonstrated promising results in patients with hypercholesterolaemia[226] and in combination appear to exert significant anti-inflammatory activity in patients with osteoarthritis.[227] Hesperidin, also from citrus, lowered diastolic blood pressure in a randomised, controlled trial.[228] Flavopiridol, a flavonoid-derived drug, is being developed as a treatment for cancer and inflammation.[229]

The flavonoid most widely studied as a clinical nutraceutical is quercetin, and doses of around 500 to 1000 mg/day are typical. Generally, the clinical findings are modest, possibly reflecting on its low and variable bioavailability.[230] Favourable effects were observed on endurance in a randomised, controlled trial,[231] although other trials have not been positive.[232–234] It did reduce blood pressure and oxidised LDL concentrations in overweight patients with a high cardiovascular disease risk phenotype at only 150 mg/day.[235]

For more information about the pharmacology of flavonoids, see the monographs on Astragalus, chamomile, Ginkgo, hawthorn, horsechestnut and licorice. In particular, the monographs on Ginkgo and hawthorn extensively review the cardiovascular effects of flavonoids, an area not emphasised in this chapter.

Toxicology

Flavonoid aglycones, but not their glycosides, are mutagenic in various assay systems. Quercetin is probably the most mutagenic (and most widespread) flavonoid. When glycosides are incubated with beta-glucosidase or bacteria possessing this enzyme, they acquire mutagenic properties.[236] However, the presence of methoxy groups markedly decreases the mutagenicity of the flavonoid.[237] Concerns about the mutagenicity and carcinogenicity of quercetin first arose among Japanese researchers who were searching for the carcinogenic compounds in bracken fern. However, those compounds were later identified to be ptaquilosides.[238] Dietary quercetin also enhanced pretumorous lesions in a model of rat pancreatic carcinogenesis, indicating possible promoting and progressing effects,[239] but lacked tumour-promoting effects in a different model.[240] On the other hand flavonoids, including quercetin, have shown antimutagenic effects and are widely considered to be antimutagens.[241,242]

With the initial discovery of the mutagenicity of quercetin and concerns about the carcinogenicity of bracken fern, tests were conducted to determine if quercetin was carcinogenic. While two studies were positive in rats, many other studies in rats, mice and golden hamsters failed to demonstrate carcinogenic activity.[243] This is reassuring since quercetin is the most common flavonoid in the human diet. Proposed reasons for the lack of carcinogenicity included poor absorption and rapid microbial degradation, as already discussed.

However, the lack of carcinogenicity of a massive exposure to quercetin at 10% of diet suggests that more active mechanisms might be at work. This was confirmed in a study that demonstrated the rapid metabolic inactivation of quercetin by catechol-O-methyltransferase to form non-mutagenic methoxy groups on the flavonoid.[243] This could be a major reason for the lack of carcinogenicity of other flavonoids in vivo. A more recent critical review of the data related to the safety of quercetin noted a lack of in vivo toxicity (including a lack of carcinogenic properties) and concluded that the weight of the available evidence supports the safety of this flavonoid.[244]

Tannins and oligomeric procyanidins

Tannins are defined as vegetable substances capable of tanning animal hides to produce leather. This is used as a method to preserve the hide, and at a molecular level is effected via the cross-linking of hide proteins by the tannins. This definition is prescriptive and powdered hide is still used as a phytochemical test for tannins. Like flavonoids, tannins are polyphenolic compounds that have an affinity for proteins. However, the higher number of phenolic groups and the larger molecular size of tannins mean that they are capable of binding strongly to proteins at several sites and can thereby precipitate them from solution.

The phytochemical classification of tannins can be complex, but two main groups are usually recognised: hydrolysable tannins and condensed tannins (the procyanidins or proanthocyanidins). Hydrolysable tannins usually consist of a central glucose molecule linked to molecules of gallic acid (gallotannins) or hexahydroxydiphenic acid (ellagitannins). They are readily hydrolysed, hence their name. Ellagitannins are found in herbs such as pomegranate, cranesbill, oak bark and meadowsweet. Oak bark (*Quercus robur*) also contains condensed tannins.

Geraniin – a hydrolysable tannin

Hexahydroxydiphenic acid

Gallic acid

Unlike hydrolysable tannins, condensed tannins are polymeric flavans and are not readily hydrolysable. They often consist of molecules of catechin and epicatechin joined by carbon-carbon bonds. Hence catechin and epicatechin are referred to as monomers and molecules containing 2 to 4 monomers are referred to as oligomeric (a few) procyanidins (OPCs). Protein-binding capacity increases markedly with the degree of polymerisation, so dimers are much less astringent than hexamers, for example. It is, however, difficult to define the point at which OPCs end and true tannins start. From a pharmacological perspective, OPCs and their monomers behave much like flavonoids (they also resemble them chemically) and they are sometimes incorrectly classified with them. Condensed tannins are known as proanthocyanidins (procyanidins) because they release coloured cyanidin compounds on boiling with acid, hence the prefix 'pro-' meaning 'forming'.

(+)-Catechin

Procyanidin B-2

(–)- Epicatechin

The polyphenolics in green tea (*Camellia sinensis*) are a class of pseudotannins known as catechins. These are smaller molecules than tannins. While they do possess some

astringency, they cannot tan hides, although they have been classified as condensed tannins in some publications. Green tea also contains condensed and hydrolysable tannins.[245]

Hydrolysable tannins generally decompose slowly when kept in aqueous solution. They may also be hydrolysed by acids or enzymes such as tannase into their component molecules. As noted above, condensed tannins are more resistant to decomposition into their monomeric components. However, they are readily oxidised over time, as shown by their colour change to purplish pink. These oxidised tannins are responsible for the reddish colour of many barks and roots. Prolonged storage of solutions of condensed tannins (such as tinctures and fluid extracts) induces extensive precipitation of condensate products known as phlobaphenes or phlobatannins. Glycerol was traditionally added to liquid galenicals to decrease this effect. Tannins complex with and precipitate alkaloids, and herbal extracts containing tannins should not be mixed with alkaloid-containing extracts.

Pharmacodynamics

When tannins encounter mucous membranes, they react with and crosslink proteins in both the mucus and epithelial cells of the mucosa. The mucosa is consequently bound more tightly and rendered less permeable, a process referred to as *astringency*. If this phenomenon occurs in the mouth, such as when eating an unripe banana, a puckering and drying sensation is experienced. Astringency affords increased protection to the subadjacent layers of the mucosa from micro-organisms and irritant chemicals. It also leads to an antisecretory effect on the mucous membrane.

Since tannins are large polar molecules, they are generally poorly absorbed through the skin or gastrointestinal tract. Hence, the pharmacological effects of tannins can be largely explained in terms of their local effects on these organs (such as astringency) or effects within the gastrointestinal lumen. However, decomposition products of tannins (and the monomers of condensed tannins) can be absorbed and thereby do exert systemic effects (see the Pharmacokinetics section). The poor bioavailability of tannins is fortunate, since they can be quite toxic if absorbed in large amounts. Being smaller molecules, the green tea catechins do show some intact bioavailability in humans. However, their polyphenolic nature ensures that this is still relatively low.

One of the most notable effects of tannins in the gut is their dramatic effect on diarrhoea. It can be proposed that the effect of tannins is to produce a protective (if temporary) layer of coagulated protein on the mucosa along the upper levels of the gut wall, so numbing the sensory nerve endings and reducing provocative stimuli to additional peristaltic activity. Supporting this central astringent activity, tannins will also inhibit the viability of infecting micro-organisms, check fluid hypersecretion and neutralise inflammatory proteins. Because of their affinity for free protein, they will concentrate in damaged areas.

Condensed tannins were able to bind to and inactivate the hypersecretory activity of cholera toxin.[246] At present, there are attempts to develop new therapies for cholera, and one approach showing promise is the inhibition of transport proteins involved in cAMP-activated chloride channels. One of these is the cystic fibrosis transmembrane conductance regulator protein (CFTR). (Mutations in CFTR cause cystic fibrosis, hence its name.) A hydrolysable tannin from the Chinese gallnut inhibited CFTR in vitro. Intraluminal placement of this tannin (0.6 mg/kg) in mice reduced cholera-toxin-induced intestinal fluid secretion by 75%, with no effect on intestinal fluid absorption.[247]

Roots from the genus Potentilla typically contain hydrolysable and condensed tannins.[248] In a randomised, double blind, placebo-controlled trial, an extract of tormentil root (*Potentilla erecta*) effectively treated rotavirus infection in children.[249] The duration of diarrhoea in the herbal group was 3 days, compared with 5 days in the control group (p<0.0001).

Tannins in herbs such as meadowsweet were traditionally regarded as beneficial in mild peptic ulceration and inflammation. This application is analogous to the use of the synthetic antiulcer drug known as sulcrafate. Sulcrafate is an astringent aluminium-based compound (aluminium is highly astringent). It is said to bind selectively to the exposed proteins at the ulcer base. The barrier thus created protects the ulcer crater from gastric contents. Antiulcer activity has been demonstrated for black tea extract[250] and for condensed tannins.[251] Ellagic acid suppresses acid secretion[252] and pomegranate prevented experimentally induced gastric ulcers.[253]

Tannins and pseudotannins can also affect bowel flora composition. For example, tea fed to chicks significantly changed the levels of particular microflora.[254] This may explain why rhubarb and other tannin-containing herbs reduced levels of uraemic toxins in rats with renal failure (perhaps at least in part by inhibition of the bowel flora production of some of these compounds).[255] Whatever the mechanism, tannin-containing herbs such as rhubarb have been used in China to treat renal failure.

Local use of tannins on bleeding surfaces renders a styptic or haemostatic effect due to localised vasoconstriction and possibly an increased rate of coagulation. Since the presence of tannins is widespread in higher plants, this would explain the folk use of so many different plants as 'wound herbs'. An aqueous extract of a tannin-containing herb demonstrated haemostatic activity due to vasoconstriction and the formation of an 'artificial clot' (presumably resulting from a tannin-protein reaction), that tended to produce a mechanical plug to arrest bleeding from small blood vessels.[256] This styptic effect can also be useful for mild internal bleeding.

The topical application of tannins can exert favourable effects on burns, weeping eczema and viral infections. In the early 20th century, tannin sprays were applied to severe burns as preferred therapy. The tannin-protein complex thus formed acted as an artificial semi-permeable membrane known as an eschar.[257] This procedure was abandoned because toxic levels of tannic acid (the hydrolysable tannin used) were sometimes absorbed through the damaged skin. Tannic acid also damaged epithelial stem cells and caused excessive scar formation. However, the procedure is still practised in China using condensed tannins, which are less toxic and kinder to the regenerating epidermis.

One of the notable properties of tannins that has emerged in recent research is their antioxidant effects. Given their polyphenolic nature, this is not surprising. Hamamelitannin (from witchhazel) and gallic acid were more active than ascorbic acid in scavenging reactive oxygen species.[258] Oral administration of geraniin was found to lower the level of lipid peroxide in the serum and liver of rats suffering liver injury.[259] Most of the antioxidant research on tannins and pseudotannins has focused on green tea catechins. As well as impressive in vitro effects, it appears that an antioxidant activity can also be achieved in the human body, presumably brought about by the absorption of decomposition products as well as the catechins (see the Pharmacokinetics section).

A recent review classified the key antioxidant mechanisms of tannins as comprising free radical scavenging, chelation of transition metals and inhibition of pro-oxidative enzymes and lipid peroxidants.[260] Conflicting results have been reported for the antioxidant activity of green tea in clinical studies. The results may have been confounded by how the tea was prepared (e.g. brewing time, concentration) and other dietary and lifestyle factors.[261] A review of trials to 2000 found that antioxidant activity has been demonstrated, although a strong conclusion could not be drawn. In subsequent trials in healthy volunteers, green tea:

- decreased susceptibility of plasma and LDL to oxidation (using lag time of conjugated diene formation). SOD (superoxide dismutase) activity in plasma and serum antioxidant activity remained unchanged[262]
- was associated with a 37.4% reduction in the concentration of oxidised LDL, and a decrease in the levels of antioxidised LDL IgM antibodies[263]
- increased in plasma total antioxidant activity and decreased plasma peroxide levels and DNA oxidative damage in lymphocytes, compared to baseline values.[264]

There are many other clinical benefits demonstrated for green tea catechins.

Good clinical evidence exists for the role of cranberry juice and extracts in the prevention of urinary tract infections.[265] It is believed that consumption of cranberry results in urine that discourages bacterial adherence to the bladder wall. The A-type proanthocyanidins (condensed tannins) are thought to be key here, although they might be too large to be excreted as such in the urine.[266,267] Perhaps their decomposition products are active in urine?

As noted earlier, the pomegranate is a rich source of ellagitannins. Pomegranate extract and juice products standardised for their ellagic acid content are available (presumably the ellagic acid being measured is that contained in the ellagitannins). An initial uncontrolled clinical trial of pomegranate juice in patients with prostate cancer reported a significant prolongation of prostate specific antigen (PSA) doubling time. Anticancer effects in other types of cancers have been observed in vitro and in vivo.[268,269] Pomegranate peel extract also promoted wound healing in rats after topical application, an effect certainly predicted by its tannin content.[270]

As alluded to previously, the many and impressive in vitro effects of tannins may not have clinical relevance because of their poor bioavailability. This is highlighted by a study that postulated hydrolysable tannins were responsible for the anti-prostatic activity of *Epilobium* species via inhibition of 5-alpha-reductase.[271] Sufficient quantities of almost any tannin will non-specifically inhibit almost any enzyme. Other effects of tannins unlikely to have clinical relevance include antiviral activity (except topically and in the gut lumen, see above),[272] inhibition of elastase,[273] cytotoxic effects,[274] reverse transcriptase inhibition,[259] antimutagenic activity,[259] host-mediated antitumour activity[259] and inhibition of lipoxygenase.[259]

The lower than expected rate of coronary artery disease in France has been termed the French paradox. Several reasons have been proposed for this effect, notably the high consumption of red wine rich in OPCs. Independently of this development, a French scientist named Masquelier researched the antioxidant and connective-tissue-stabilising benefits of OPCs over many years. This led to the development of two OPC products (containing predominantly B-type OPCs and their monomers), one from grapeseeds and the other from the bark of the maritime pine (*Pinus pinaster*). These products are prescribed for applications similar to flavonoids and early clinical research supported their use for varicose veins, capillary fragility and chronic venous insufficiency.[275] An impressive array of outcomes from randomised, controlled trials has now accumulated, demonstrating the remarkable clinical diversity of these OPC-rich extracts. For example, a recent review of pine bark extract noted benefits in cardiovascular disorders, type 2 diabetes, cognition, asthma, osteoarthritis and glaucoma, among others.[276] Given the postulated beneficial effects of OPCs in heart disease, it should come as no surprise that hawthorn, the most important herb for the heart in modern phytotherapy, is rich in these substances (for more details on the cardiovascular pharmacology of OPCs, see the hawthorn monograph).

Important tannin-containing herbs not already mentioned include agrimony (*Agrimonia eupatorium*) and bistort (*Polygonum bistorta*). There is also a monograph on witchhazel in Part Three.

Adverse reactions and toxicology

Tannins are found to some extent in many medicinal plants. The following comments about adverse reactions refer only to relatively high doses of herbs containing significant quantities of tannins. It is unlikely that incidental exposure to tannins at low levels has any significant negative impact on health. In fact, condensed tannins are found in several commonly consumed foods. In contrast, hydrolysable tannins are less common in foods (the pomegranate being one exception) and this suggests that the long-term therapeutic intake of this group of tannins should be avoided.

High doses of tannins lead to excessive astringency on mucous membranes, which produces an irritating effect. This probably led to the practice of adding milk to tea whereby the tannins preferentially bind to proteins in the milk rather than the gut wall. However, even adding milk does not prevent the constipation that can result from chronic intake of high levels of tannins. For these reasons, high doses of strongly astringent herbs should be used cautiously in highly inflamed or ulcerated conditions of the gastrointestinal tract and in patients complaining of constipation.

Chronic intake of tannins inhibits digestive enzymes, especially the membrane-bound enzymes on the small intestinal mucosa.[277] Tannins complex metal ions and inhibit their absorption. One study found that as long as tea and iron are consumed separately, iron absorption is not affected.[278] This iron-complexing property of tannins could be exploited in male patients with haemochromatosis, which is now recognised to be a relatively common disorder. (See Appendix C for more information on such potential interactions with tannin-containing herbs.) Tannins can also react with thiamine and decrease its absorption.[279]

Addition of tannic acid, a hydrolysable tannin, to the barium sulphate mixture used in barium enemas increases the yield and accuracy of the examination. The colonic mucosa stands out clearly and tumour visualisation is improved. However, the practice was banned in 1964 by the US FDA (Food and Drug Administration).[280] Several deaths caused by acute hepatotoxicity, the majority in children, were attributed to this practice.[281] In these cases, quantities of tannic acid sufficient to cause massive liver damage were absorbed directly into the bloodstream from the colon. This effect is highly unlikely to follow from use of tannin-containing herbs. Nonetheless, some unexplained cases of herbal hepatotoxicity have been recorded. It is therefore prudent to avoid the use of high doses of highly astringent herbs in patients with very damaged gastrointestinal tracts, other than in the circumstances outlined above. Green tea extract consumption has been linked to rare cases of idiosyncratic hepatotoxicity.[282]

Tannins are carcinogenic when injected subcutaneously[283] and herbal teas containing tannins have been implicated in the possible development of oesophageal cancers.[284,285] While these associations probably have little relevance to phytotherapy, they do suggest caution with the long-term oral and topical use (on damaged skin) of tannin-containing herbs.

Resins

Resins are sticky, water-insoluble substances often exuded by the plant. The term is used in several contexts. When certain plants are damaged, either by incision or naturally due to the action of animals or the environment, they secrete a viscous fluid that soon hardens. This probably serves as protection. The resultant exudate is an amorphous, complex mixture of chemicals that softens on heating. Such resins are often associated with essential oils (oleoresins), with gums (gum resins) or with oil and gum (oleo-gum resins). Their resin components, which mainly comprise diterpenes known as resin acids, resin alcohols and resin phenols, are soluble in alcohol and ether but are insoluble in water and hexane.

In another context, the term 'resin' (or occasionally 'resinoid') means the part of the plant that is soluble in ether or alcohol, as in kava resin, guaiacum resin (also prepared by burning the heartwood) and jalap. These resins are chemically diverse and can contain resin acids, pyrones, lignans, esters and glycosides amongst others. On microscopic examination of the tissues of these plants, secretion cells with resinous contents are sometimes visible.

Myrrh (*Commiphora molmol*) is an oleo-gum resin with astringent and antimicrobial properties. The former quality is probably entirely due to the resin and the latter is a combined effect from the resin and the essential oil. Tincture of myrrh is a potent antiseptic in the mouth and throat. There is a modern tradition that one of its effects is to provoke a local leucocytosis, to effectively stimulate defensive white blood cell responses and so involve the body in eliminating local infections. Clinical experience of long-standing improvement in recurrent throat and gum disease, for example, lends support to this view. In recent times, myrrh has also demonstrated clinical anthelmintic activity, possibly mediated by an effect on immune function. The resin could also play a role here (see the monograph in Part Three for more details).

Resins have also been applied to inflammatory conditions of the upper digestive tract with some benefit. This probably reflects on their astringent property. The oleoresin mastic (*Pistacia lentiscus* var. *chia*) is traditionally used for the relief of dyspepsia and peptic ulcers.[286] Mastic demonstrated a duodenal ulcer healing effect at 1 g/day in a double blind, placebo-controlled clinical trial.[286] Cytoprotective and mild antisecretory effects were demonstrated in a rat model of ulceration, consistent with astringent activity.[287] Its effects on Helicobacter are controversial.[288] Mastic improved dyspepsia symptoms in a randomised, double blind placebo-controlled trial.[289] Boswellia (frankincense) is a resin with considerable anti-inflammatory activity in the digestive tract and elsewhere. (This is reviewed in its monograph in Part Three.)

Important resin-containing herbs not already mentioned include propolis (not actually a herb, but collected by bees from resinous plants), grindelia, calendula, guggul, juniper and the various balsams.

Resins are contact allergens that can cause oral ulceration and contact dermatitis.[290] Myrrh is particularly prone to this effect.

Bitters

Bitters are substances capable of strongly stimulating the bitter receptors in the taste buds at the back of the tongue. The taste stimulus is triggered by an intramolecular bonding with these receptors. Each taste bud contains approximately 20 to 30 sensory cells whose microvilli extend to the bud opening. The taste receptors lie in the membrane of these microvilli and consist of glycoproteins.

Recent research has made considerable advances in our understanding of the bitter taste receptors. A family of approximately 30 such receptors (denoted TAS2R) has been identified in mammals.[291] The TAS2Rs are broadly tuned to each detect multiple bitter substances, explaining how humans can recognise numerous bitter compounds with only a limited set of receptors. The TAS2Rs are expressed in a subset of taste receptor cells that are distinct from those mediating responses to other taste qualities. Cells with these receptors appear to be wired to elicit aversive behaviour, probably because many toxic chemicals are bitter in taste.[291]

One intriguing discovery is that bitter taste receptors are not restricted to the oral cavity.[292] There are numerous reports of TAS2Rs expressed in the gut and in cell lines originating from gastrointestinal tissue, including the stomach. Insulin secretion can be stimulated from clonal pancreatic beta cells in vitro by a bitter molecule (denatonium). Gastric infusion of the same molecule (without it being tasted) delayed gastric emptying in rodents, presumably as a primordial defence against toxicity. There is also evidence of an elevated anion secretion within the large intestines of the rat and human induced by another bitter

compound, 6-n-propyl-thiouracil (presumably against a defensive mechanism). An inactive variant of the TAS2R9 receptor has been associated with altered glucose homeostasis in a human family study.

Although direct humoral effects of bitter compounds in the gastrointestinal tract appear plausible, at least part of the bitter sensing mechanism seems to involve the activation of vagal nerve fibres. It was demonstrated that a mixture of bitter compounds administered intragastrically to mice led to an activation of brainstem neurons, the first relay station of taste information within the brain. This effect was abolished by cutting the vagus nerve, as well as inhibitors of cholecystokinin (CCK) and peptide YY (PYY) receptors. Since vagal nerve fibres contain receptors for these and terminate close to enteroendocrine cells, bitter compounds could stimulate the secretion of these peptide hormones.[292] In other words, bitter taste receptors in the gastrointestinal tract appear to regulate metabolic and digestive functions.

Interesting as this may be, the story becomes even more fascinating with the discovery that TAS2Rs are also expressed on the human respiratory tract.[293] It was demonstrated that bitter taste receptors are located in the nasal respiratory epithelium as well as in ciliated cells of lung epithelium, where they affect respiratory functions in response to noxious stimuli. Moreover, in the epithelium of the lower airways, a cell type of unknown function has been termed 'brush cell' because of an apical tuft of microvilli. Brush cells in the mouse trachea express bitter taste receptors and effect a reduction in respiration when stimulated with a bitter agent.[294] Human airway smooth muscle cells also possess TAS2Rs, and their stimulation with bitter tastants effects a bronchodilation that is 3-fold greater than that elicited by beta-adrenergic receptor agonists.[295] Inhaled bitter tastants decreased airway obstruction in a mouse model of asthma. Perhaps this provides a rational basis for the past use of asthma cigarettes containing bitter herbs?

Given that bitters are defined physiologically based on their interactions with TAS2R, it might be expected that bitter compounds come from a number of different phytochemical classes. This is certainly the case; monoterpenes, sesquiterpenes, diterpenes, flavonoids and triterpenes can all exhibit bitter properties. However, the most notable bitter compounds are the monoterpene secoiridoid glycosides of gentian (particularly amarogentin), centaury and bogbean, and the sesquiterpene lactone dimers (such as absinthin) of wormwood. These compounds are amongst the most bitter substances known.

Absinthin

Amarogentin

The interaction of specific phytochemicals with specific human TAS2Rs (denoted as hTAS2Rs) is now reasonably well documented. For example, andrographolide interacts with hTAS2R50, strychnine with hTAS2R10 and the humulones from hops with hTAS2R10.[296]

Many cultures recognise the value of bitter substances in promoting digestive function and general health. In Holland, older people would celebrate the bitter hour in the early evening when they would partake of bitter food and drink to support their fading digestive powers. In India, it is said that those with liver problems seek bitter-tasting substances. In Africa, the medicinal value of bitter herbs, particularly as digestive stimulants, is commonly recognised in traditional medical systems.[297] Bitter drinks taken before meals are still called aperitifs.

In the early 20th century, it was still widely accepted in medical and scientific circles that bitters promoted digestion. Even Pavlov was said to have acknowledged this connection.[298] However, this was a time when such assumptions were being subjected to scientific scrutiny. In 1915, the American physiologist Carlson and co-workers published a study entitled 'The Supposed Action of the Bitter Tonics on the Secretion of Gastric Juice in Man and Dog'.[298] The group found that bitters either applied to the mouth or directly to the stomach, produced no change in the acidity and pepsin concentration of the gastric juice produced prior to food actually being in contact with the stomach. Despite the fact that this study had a number of methodological flaws, notably that gastric secretions were not tested under the stimulus of actual contact with food, it was largely interpreted as discrediting the concept of bitters as digestive stimulants.

However, work published also in 1915 by Moorhead, a colleague of Carlson, demonstrated a radically different activity profile for bitters.[299] Moorhead found that a tincture of gentian (*Gentiana lutea*) given by mouth or directly into the stomach of cachectic dogs caused a marked increase in appetite. Also, only when gentian was given by mouth (tasted) did

it cause a marked increase in gastric secretion and its acid and pepsin content. This effect only occurred after normal feeding and all the above effects were absent in normal animals.[299]

The conclusions that could be drawn from this early research are several:

- Bitters markedly increase appetite only if a cachectic, malnourished or debilitated state exists in the body.
- Similarly, bitters increase digestive power mainly when it is below optimum, as in a state of cachexia.
- Experiments with bitters should involve actual feeding; that is, the presence of food in the stomach is important for their activity.
- At normal doses, bitters act in the mouth; that is, tasting optimises their activity.

From this research, a key aspect of the mode of action of bitters can be postulated. Bitters applied to the mouth (tasted) before a meal have a priming effect on upper digestive function. This effect is most marked in states where digestion is below optimum, where a positive effect on appetite is also observed. This increase in upper digestive function is probably mediated by a nerve reflex from the bitter taste buds and involves an increase in vagal stimulation (interestingly the very latest research now appears to be supportive of a vagal-mediated mechanism). From physiology, we know that vagal stimulation causes:

- an increase in gastric acid secretion
- a transient rise in gastrin
- an increase in pepsin secretion
- a slight increase in gallbladder motility
- a priming of the pancreas.

Therefore, bitters could have a promoting effect on all components of upper digestive function, namely the stomach, liver and pancreas. Why does this reflex exist? As mentioned above, it probably developed as a protective mechanism, since many poisonous substances taste bitter.

Some more recent research supports this activity profile for bitters. Oral doses of liquid preparations of gentian and wormwood (*Artemisia absinthium*) were tested in human volunteers 5 minutes before a meal.[300] Both bitter tonics stimulated gastric secretion. Gentian also stimulated bile release from the gallbladder and both herbs increased bile production by the liver. Another study found that oral doses of liquid wormwood caused a dramatic increase in the duodenal levels of pancreatic enzymes and bile.[301] Studies have also shown that bitters increase the secretion of saliva. A lemon wedge saturated with Angostura bitters was also found to cure hiccups in 88% of subjects in an open trial.[302]

Some bitter herbs also appear to have a direct effect on the stomach, something that can now be reconciled with the discovery of bitter receptors further down the digestive tract. Wolf and Mack carried out an excellent study on the action of various bitters on the stomach of their famous patient, Tom, who had an occluded oesophagus and a gastric fistula.[303] Bitters were administered by mouth and swallowed into the blind oesophagus; the resulting salivary volume and gastric secretion were compared with direct administration into the stomach. In the 96 experiments conducted, it was found that there was considerable variation in the effects of bitters. Surprisingly, golden seal (*Hydrastis canadensis*) was the most active herb and gentian was virtually inactive at the levels tested. The increase in salivation when the bitter was administered orally was usually comparable with the increase in gastric secretion after direct introduction into the stomach. The alcoholic content of the bitters was shown to evoke no response. It was concluded that bitters exerted a direct effect on the stomach, since no significant effect was observed in Tom's stomach following their oral administration. These results therefore, contrast with the work of Moorhead, but the experimental design did not include a test meal, a common flaw in some of the early research.

A more recent publication also confirms that bitters do indeed exert a direct effect in the stomach.[304] When isolated stomach cells were exposed to different levels of an extract of gentian root, a concentration-dependent rise in gastric acid production was observed. No stimulatory effect was exerted by globe artichoke extract (*Cynara scolymus*). Significant effects for gentian extract were observed at concentrations of 10 to 100 μg/mL. This concentration range can be readily achieved by normal doses of gentian. The author suggested that his results can explain why encapsulated gentian extracts also show therapeutic effects and downplayed the importance of the reflex effect to one of 'supportive importance only'. While this is perhaps an over-extrapolation, the recent discovery of bitter receptors in the stomach makes sense of these findings.

Some support for this concept of direct activity in the stomach also comes from a multicentre, uncontrolled study of gentian capsules involving 205 patients.[305] Patients took on average about five capsules per day, each containing 120 mg of a 5:1 dry extract of gentian root, and achieved rapid and dramatic relief of symptoms, including constipation, flatulence, appetite loss, vomiting, heartburn, abdominal pain and nausea.

Healthy upper digestive function is important for maintaining good health and preventing disease. Low acidity can lead to poor nutrient absorption and abnormal bowel flora. Patients with reduced gastric secretion are more susceptible to bacterial and parasitic enteric infections.[306] The contribution of poor upper digestive function to the chronicity of intestinal dysbiosis is often overlooked by therapists.

Early studies associated low gastric acidity with a number of chronic diseases such as rosacea, gallbladder disease, eczema and asthma, and this has been reflected in writings that are more recent.[307] The experimental method used in these early studies typically measured gastric pH following a test meal. This is now considered an invalid way to investigate a pathological hydrochloric acid deficiency (hypochlorhydria). Instead, a potent gastric cell stimulus such as pentagastrin is currently preferred to establish the diagnosis of hypochlorhydria.

However, the early studies were probably measuring the physiological response of the stomach to food, rather than a pathological absence or deficiency of the secretory apparatus. If this is the case, then the observation is still valid that a poor physiological response to food may be associated with certain chronic diseases. The use of bitters is particularly relevant in this context, since they can act via a vagal reflex, which is the normal physiological way that the upper digestive tract is primed for food.

As early as 1698, Floyer in his Treatise of the Asthma reflected that:

> Some writers, as Sylvius and Etmuller, have observed the hypochondriac symptoms in the stomach, and conclude the asthma is a hypochondriacal flatus, and wants digestives ... It is commonly observed that fulness of diet, and all debauches render the fits most severe, and a temperate diet makes the fits more easy ... This defect of digestion and mucilaginous slime in the stomach are very obvious and observed by writers, and were supposed the immediate cause of the asthma.

A modern study found that allergic asthma was associated with a reduction in histamine-stimulated peak acid output from the gastric mucosa (about 60% of normal). There is therefore a depression of gastric H_2 histamine receptor function in asthma.[308]

Diabetics respond well to bitters, and some herbalists believe they can assist in normalising blood sugar levels in both reactive dysglycaemia and diabetes. A lack of insulin could impair the vagal stimulation of gastric acid secretion[309] and oral doses of a bitter herb lowered blood sugar in healthy rats.[310] Long-standing diabetics may have impaired upper digestive function secondary to vagal neuropathy.[311] The finding that bitter receptors further down the digestive tract appear to be involved will hopefully encourage more research into the role of bitter herbs in insulin resistance.

It has been found that in some cases patients' responses to herbal medicines depend on their upper digestive function.[312] A Japanese study observed that the antioxidant properties of a herbal product could be increased by fermentation. A brewing process degraded high molecular weight polymers to smaller molecules that were more active. The unfermented herbal product was tried on patients with autoimmune diseases. Some responded to the product, others did not. Those who responded had a greater capacity to produce the small antioxidant molecules in their gastric secretions, which was correlated with their acid and pepsin secretion. It was concluded that one of the factors determining the patients' response was the ability of their digestive system to produce low molecular weight compounds from the natural polymers.

Herbalists consider that bitters have a tonic effect on the body and the term 'bitter tonic' is often used. In addition to their use for poor upper digestive function, low appetite and hypochlorhydria and its consequences, bitters are used to treat anaemia. Bitters are valuable for food allergies and intolerances, since poorly digested proteins and other compounds probably contribute to this condition. Herbalists also believe that bitters stimulate immune function and a patient who is pale, lethargic and prone to infections is a prime candidate for bitters. Interestingly, the herb wormwood has been shown to be beneficial for Crohn's disease, an autoimmune disease of the digestive tract, in two clinical trials.[313,314] Whether this is a consequence of interaction with TAS2Rs remains to be investigated.

The famous herbalist Dr Weiss stressed that the action of bitters was most pronounced after continued use (probably because it is a conditioned reflex).[315] He described how a physician in Vienna noted that dyspeptic patients liked wormwood tea and kept asking for it, despite the taste. Another

Viennese paediatrician considered bitters to be an excellent remedy for anorexic children. Weiss claimed that bitters neutralised the negative influence of higher mental functions on digestion, which usually results from chronic stress. He claimed that bitters had a toning effect on the colon when applied over a long period. Interestingly, non-tasters with an inactive hTAS2R38 receptor were found to have an increased risk of colon cancer in one epidemiological study.[316]

Bitters are contraindicated in states of hyperacidity, especially duodenal ulcers. Tasted bitters may actually be beneficial in gastric ulcers, since this condition is often associated with atrophic gastritis. Tasted bitters may also help oesophageal reflux because they could improve the tone of the oesophageal sphincter. However, they should be used with caution here and in relatively mild doses.

The main bitter herbs used in Western herbal medicine are gentian and wormwood. For a reflex effect, bitters do not usually have to be given in high doses. Enough to promote a strong taste of bitterness is usually sufficient. This is typically 5 to 10 drops of the 1:5 tinctures of the above herbs in about 20 mL of water. (Bitters are one exception where drop doses are appropriate.) Since bitters have a priming effect on upper digestive function and work (at least in part) by a visceral reflex (which is slow) they are best taken about 15 minutes before meals. Also, bitters work best if they are sipped slowly, to prolong the stimulation of the reflex. This can be difficult for some people, but will yield optimum results.

In contrast, for a direct effect on the gastric mucosa, higher doses need to be used. About 300 to 600 mg of gentian root before meals would be an appropriate dose. Care should be exercised with such high doses of gentian taken in liquid form, since they might cause nausea in some people.

One question that has vexed herbal clinicians is whether masking the taste of bitters given in liquid form interferes with their reflex activity. This is probably not the case, since masking agents will change the conscious perception of bitterness, but the bitter taste buds will still be stimulated.

A number of papers have been published on the subject of supertasters.[317] Supertasters perceive the greatest bitterness and sweetness from many stimuli, as well as the greatest oral burn from alcohol and capsaicin (from *Capsicum species*). This is an inherited ability produced by a dominant allele. Women are more likely than men to be supertasters. This phenomenon needs to be kept in mind because some patients may be very sensitive to the taste (and possibly effects) of bitter and other strong-tasting herbs. These patients are also more likely to experience nausea if the dose of bitters used is too high.

In epidemiological studies, functional variants in bitter taste receptors have been linked to alcohol dependency,[318] adiposity,[319] eating behaviour disinhibition[320] and body-mass index.[321] Generally, people with lower bitter tasting sensitivity exhibited the poorer health measure.

Pungent constituents

Like bitters, pungency is a physiological classification rather than a phytochemical one. The three most commonly used hot spices are the cayenne pepper (Capsicum), the black pepper and ginger, and while their pungent components (respectively capsaicin, piperine and the gingerols and shogaols) are chemically distinct, it is now known that they act upon a common group of nerve cell receptors: the vanilloid receptors.[322] Capsaicin and piperine are alkaloids based on homovanillic acid (hence vanilloid receptor), whereas the gingerols are substituted alkylphenols.

The transient potential receptor vanilloid 1 (TRPV1) receptor is a non-selective cation channel activated by capsaicin.[323] TRPV1 receptors are predominantly expressed in primary afferent fibres, which are peptidergic sensory neurons, such as the unmyelinated C-fibres. TRPV1 is a pro-inflammatory receptor due to its key role in neuropathic pain, joint inflammation and inflammatory bowel disease. However, it appears to also play a protective role in sepsis and is involved in the physiological regulation of urinary bladder function, thermoregulation, neurogenesis[323] and the cough reflex.[324] Many of these functions are reflected in the traditional uses of cayenne and the modern applications of capsaicin (see below). TRPV1 is also strongly activated by piperine[325] and the gingerols.[326]

Piperine

trans-**Capsaicin**

Gingerols

	n
6-Gingerol	4
8-Gingerol	6
10-Gingerol	8

Since capsaicin-sensitive sensory nerves (rich in TRPV1) are densely distributed in the cardiovascular and gastrointestinal system, activation of TRPV1 either by endogenous ligands or by exogenous agonists has been repeatedly reported to exert hypotensive activity or protective effects against cardiac or gastrointestinal injury. This is via stimulation of the synthesis and release of multiple neurotransmitters such as calcitonin gene-related peptide and substance P.[327] Therefore, TRPV1 is not only a prime target for the pharmacological control of pain, but also a useful target for drug development to treat various diseases including cardiovascular and gastrointestinal diseases. However, considering the contribution of TRPV1 to the development of inflammation in the gastrointestinal tract (as touched on below), the potential side effects of TRPV1 agonists cannot be ignored.

Pharmacodynamics

Capsaicin has been the most commonly studied of the pungent compounds. As mentioned above, the C-fibre sensory neurons, which release inflammatory neuropeptides such as substance P, mediate a wide variety of responses including neurogenic inflammation, thermoregulation and chemical-initiated pain. Capsaicin functions to activate and then, at higher doses and over time, desensitise this class of neurons. This latter response, by a process known as *tachyphylaxis*, provides the basis for the therapeutic interest in capsaicin. Capsaicin stimulates C-fibres by interacting with TRPV1 receptors.[328] The intense sensation of pain and heat which is experienced after eating a hot curry is testimony to this C-fibre activation. But, as experienced curry eaters will testify, they can tolerate hotter and hotter food over time due to tachyphylaxis.

Although the pain and burning from consumption of cayenne or capsaicin can be disturbing, no actual harm results from its consumption. In effect, the specific action on vanilloid receptors creates an illusion of pain and burning. Tissue damage is not concurrent with these sensations. This contrasts strongly with the mustard oils, which are highly corrosive and produce sensations of pain and burning in association with actual tissue damage. On the other hand, capsaicin is a pronounced irritant, as evidenced by the incapacitating effect of capsicum spray. Sometimes ingestion of cayenne does seem to produce lingering sensations of discomfort, and this probably highlights the role of substance P in neurogenic (nervous system-mediated) inflammation. Once the process of neurogenic inflammation has been triggered, it can become self-perpetuating. Neurogenic inflammation has been implicated in a number of chronic functional disorders of uncertain aetiology such as interstitial cystitis and irritable bowel syndrome.

The desensitisation of C-fibres has value for pain relief in a number of chronically painful disorders. Early controlled clinical trials of the topical use of capsaicin cream demonstrated symptom relief in osteoarthritis,[329] neuropathy[330] and postherpetic neuralgia.[331] Topical capsaicin was effective for painful skin disorders such as psoriasis and pruritus and possibly useful for neural dysfunction in the form of cluster headaches and phantom limb pain.[332,333] Vasomotor rhinitis could also be alleviated by topical capsaicin.[334]

However, Cochrane reviews have demonstrated mixed outcomes for the topical application of capsaicin, being negative for pruritus,[335] mildly positive for neuropathic pain[336] and stating insufficient evidence to support intranasal application in allergic rhinitis.[337] Four weeks of a 0.0125% capsaicin gel

was an effective treatment for mild to moderate knee osteoarthritis in a recent placebo-controlled trial involving 100 patients,[338] but its role in this disorder is controversial,[339] despite a positive meta-analysis (yielding moderate evidence of benefit).[340]

The higher fibrinolytic activity observed in Thai people has been attributed to daily intake of cayenne pepper.[341] Cayenne also increases gastric acid output.[342] Since gastric acid is a natural defence against gastrointestinal pathogens, it can be speculated that this could explain the preference for hot, spicy food in tropical countries. In the rat stomach there is clear evidence that capsaicin-sensitive sensory nerves are involved in a local defence mechanism against gastric ulcer. However, excessive capsaicin exposure caused tachyphylaxis and impaired this defensive mechanism.[343] Perhaps the maxim of 'too much of a good thing' applies here.

Like capsaicin, piperine has attracted research interest, but for quite different reasons. Attention has focused on the capacity of piperine to enhance the bioavailability of other agents. These include aflatoxin B1 in rats[344] and propanolol, theophylline,[345] curcumin,[346] vasicine and sparteine in humans.[347] While there is good evidence that piperine inhibits drug metabolism by the intestine and liver,[348] other possibilities include increased permeability of intestinal cells[349] and even complexation with drugs.[350] It strongly inhibits hepatic and intestinal aryl hydrocarbon hydroxylase and UDP-glucuronyl transferase.[351] Hence, piperine also has the potential to induce herb-drug interactions.

In traditional Chinese medicine, a mixture of radish and pepper is used to treat epilepsy. Piperine and some synthetic derivatives have been shown to be anticonvulsant agents that can antagonise convulsions induced by physical and chemical methods.[352] Antiepilepsirine, a derivative of piperine, is used as an antiepileptic drug in China.

Hot spices are used around the world for their general warming effects on the body, in modern terms stimulating circulatory activity. A mechanism for this universal experience is suggested. In a study that compared the effects of various pungent agents, an increase in catecholamine secretion, especially adrenaline, from the adrenal medulla was observed. Capsaicin was most active, but piperine and zingerone (from ginger) also showed activity, although allylisothiocyanate (from mustard) and diallyldisulphide (from garlic) did not have this effect. The effective principles were readily transported from the gut around the body.[353] Capsaicin is known to increase energy expenditure in the body and boost basal metabolic rate, which has implications for its use in weight control.[354]

Epidemiological data reveal that the consumption of foods containing capsaicin is associated with a lower prevalence of obesity. Rural Thai people consume diets containing 0.014% capsaicin.[355] Rodents fed a diet containing 0.014% capsaicin showed no change in caloric intake, but demonstrated a significant 24% reduction in visceral fat weight.

The above findings hark back to the use of cayenne promoted by Samuel Thomson, who regarded it as a life-promoting heating herb and a general metabolic stimulant. The physiomedicalists extended this concept and proposed that cayenne administered in conjunction with another herb would augment the particular stimulatory activity of that herb.

Given what we now know about the bioavailability effects of piperine (and therefore possibly capsaicin), this apparently arcane dictum may have a rational basis.

A discussion of the pharmacology of the gingerols is included in the ginger monograph.

Toxicology

Investigations have been conducted to determine the potential mutagenic and carcinogenic activity of capsaicin and cayenne, but findings are contradictory.[356] Results indicate that capsaicin also demonstrates chemoprotective activity against some chemical carcinogens and mutagens.[357] Piperine appears to lack mutagenic activity.[358] A review of the cayenne and capsaicin toxicity data did not find any reasons for concern.[359]

Saponins

Phytochemistry

Saponins are phytochemicals that produce a foam when dissolved in water. Their name derives from the same root as the word soap (Latin *sapo*=soap). Like soaps or detergents, saponins are large molecules containing a water-loving (*hydrophilic*) part at one end separated from a fat-loving (*lipophilic* or *hydrophobic*) part at the other. In aqueous solution, saponin molecules align themselves vertically on the surface with their hydrophobic ends oriented away from the water. This has the effect of reducing the surface tension of the water, causing it to foam. For this reason, saponins are classified as surface-active agents. Similar to other surface-active agents, saponin molecules can align to form a spherical configuration within the water, creating a micelle. Micelles have a lipophilic centre, and this creation of a fat-loving compartment explains why detergents can dissolve grease and oils.

Saponins are glycosides (the sugar part comprises the hydrophilic end). Two classes are recognised based on the structure of their aglycone or sapogenin: steroidal saponins contain the characteristic four-ringed steroid nucleus, and triterpenoid saponins have a five-ringed structure. Both of these have a glycosidic linkage, usually at carbon 3, and share a common biosynthetic origin via the mevalonic acid pathway. Steroidal saponins are mainly found in the monocotyledons. Triterpenoid saponins are by far the most common. There are some unusual classifications; for example, the ginsenosides in ginseng are grouped with the triterpenoid saponins even though they exhibit a steroidal structure. Steroidal saponins typically contain extra furan and pyran heterocyclic rings, which is not a feature of the ginsenosides. (Furans and pyrans are respectively five- and six-membered rings containing oxygen.)

Saponins are consumed in many common foods and beverages including oats, spinach, asparagus, soya beans and other legumes, peanuts, tea and beer.

Pharmacodynamics

The pharmacological events that result from the ingestion of saponins can be broadly classified into two categories: the general effects from the detergent-like properties of intact saponins, and those specific actions that ensue after a saponin (or more usually the sapogenin) is absorbed into the bloodstream. This discussion will concentrate on the former, but will also provide a context for the specific activities of saponins. Also the anti-inflammatory, tonic, adaptogenic, aldosterone-like and mucoprotective properties (among others) of specific saponins are examined in detail in the monographs on Astragalus, black cohosh, Bupleurum, ginseng, horsechestnut, licorice, poke root, gotu kola and Withania.

Saponins are capable of destroying red blood cells (RBCs) by dissolving their membranes, a process known as *haemolysis*, releasing free haemoglobin into the bloodstream. RBCs are particularly susceptible to this form of chemical attack because they have no nucleus and therefore cannot effect membrane repair. Haemolysis explains why saponins are much more toxic when given by injection than when administered orally. The toxic dose of an injected saponin occurs if sufficient haemoglobin is released to cause renal failure (haemoglobin damages the delicate membranes of the glomerulus). After oral intake, much of the saponin is not absorbed intact. Typically, it is slowly and partially absorbed as the aglycone. The kidneys are thereby spared the sudden influx of haemoglobin. For a long time this feature of saponin toxicity was interpreted by many pharmacologists as an indication that saponins were largely inert after oral doses. While it is true that saponins and even their sapogenins are generally not well absorbed from the gut, there can be no doubt that they can exert significant pharmacological activity after ingestion (for example, the aldosterone-like licorice side effects).

A common misconception is that the haemolytic activity of saponins is related to their detergent-like characteristics. However, as early as the 1960s this was shown to be false. The mechanism of saponin-induced haemolysis was investigated by extracting the active haemolysing factor from ghost cells of saponin-haemolysed blood. The fact that only the corresponding aglycones could be extracted shows that hydrolysis of the glycosidic bond precedes haemolysis (RBC membranes possess a beta-glucosidase). The lack of haemolytic activity of a saponin was either due to the fact that it could not be hydrolysed by the beta-glucosidase or that it could not adsorb onto the RBC membrane.[360] This is further supported by the observation that some sapogenins are also quite haemolytic (for example, glycyrrhetinic acid is actually more haemolytic than glycyrrhizin)[360] and that haemolysis by saponins is inhibited by aldonolactones, which are glycosidase inhibitors.[361]

Saponins are more or less irritant to gastrointestinal mucous membranes (whether this is related to their detergent or haemolytic properties is not understood). This irritant property creates an acrid sensation in the throat when a saponin-containing herb is chewed. One resultant effect, like the emetics, may be by upper gastrointestinal irritation to induce a reflex expectoration. Certainly many of the traditional expectorant herbs such as soapbark, senega, primrose root and ivy leaf are rich in acrid saponins. This reflex expectorant effect, and its relationship to emesis, has been demonstrated in animal models.[362] Presumably, it is mediated via the vagus nerve, as it was abolished when the afferent gastric nerves were cut.

The detergent effect of saponins helps to increase the solubility of lipophilic molecules via micelle formation. One example that illustrates this phenomenon is the kava lactones. These compounds are quite insoluble in water, yet water can readily extract a percentage of lactones from kava root, which also contains a significant amount of saponins. Moreover, the bioavailability of kavain from a kava matrix is much greater than for the pure compound (see the kava monograph), possibly due to the presence of saponins.

However, this phenomenon for kava does not necessarily apply to other herbs. The influence of saponins on the water solubility of compounds having poor aqueous solubility was investigated with the model compounds digitoxin, rutin and aesculin.[363] The saponins that were tested represented the most common structural types. Only slight effects on aqueous solubility were obtained for all the model compounds. These effects include both enhancement and reduction in aqueous solubility, depending on the saponin, the concentration of the saponin solution and the model compound. Hence, saponins generally should not be regarded as solubilisers.

Early research suggested that the incorporation of saponins into the cell membrane probably forms a structure that is more permeable than the original membrane.[364] Saponins readily increase the permeability of the mammalian small intestine in vitro, leading to the increased uptake of otherwise poorly permeable substances and a loss of normal function.[365] The disruptive effect of saponins on the architecture of the enterocyte cell membrane can lead to the impaired absorption of smaller nutrient molecules, which are otherwise rapidly absorbed via specific transporters. This appears to be the case for glucose and ethanol, based on in vitro models.[366,367] Tablets containing an extract of the Ayurvedic herb *Gymnema sylvestre* are sold in Japan as a weight loss agent, which is attributed to reduced glucose absorption rates. Results from one study suggest that the saponin-rich herb *Asparagus racemosus* can act as a transdermal permeation enhancer for larger molecules.[368]

Sapogenins, both steroidal and triterpenoid, resemble cholesterol in their structure and may have a profound effect on cholesterol metabolism in the liver. Diosgenin is well studied in this regard. It interferes with the absorption of cholesterol of both dietary and endogenous origin; such interference is accompanied by increased rates of hepatic and intestinal cholesterol synthesis. Diosgenin also markedly enhanced cholesterol secretion into bile which, in conjunction with the unabsorbed cholesterol, resulted in increased faecal excretion of cholesterol (neutral sterols) without affecting excretion of bile acids.[369] Higher levels of ingestion of saponins or sapogenins lead to cholestasis and jaundice associated with the presence of cholesterol-like crystals in hepatocytes. In grazing animals, this can in turn lead to photosensitivity due to the photosensitising effect of the high plasma levels of chlorophyll metabolites resulting from impaired biliary excretion (see the Tribulus monograph).

It is well established that saponin intake lowers plasma cholesterol levels in animal models.[370] Various mechanisms have been put forward, such as increased faecal excretion of bile salts[370] and loss of cholesterol via exfoliated mucosal cells,[365] but the mechanism suggested by the above research on diosgenin seems most likely.[369] In this context, it is pertinent to note that diosgenin (a sapogenin) inhibits cholesterol absorption, suggesting that the mechanism behind this phenomenon might have more to do with the haemolytic or steroid-like nature of the saponins rather than their detergent properties. As an interesting footnote, it has been suggested that the Masai, who consume 2000 mg of cholesterol per day yet maintain very low blood levels, might achieve this feat by their high consumption of saponins from both foods and medicines.[371] To date this potential for saponin-containing herbs has not really been exploited clinically.

Saponins may have beneficial effects on bowel flora; yucca saponins are added to commercial piggery feeds to suppress ammonia production. As testimony to the fact that a percentage of saponins pass through the digestive tract unabsorbed, the product brochures maintain that the faecal material is easier to hose down because of the detergent action of excreted saponins.

A recent review surveyed research of the effects of saponins on microbial populations and fermentation in ruminants.[372] The primary effect of saponins in the rumen appears to be inhibition of protozoa (defaunation), which might increase the efficiency of microbial protein synthesis and protein flow to the duodenum. Furthermore, saponins may decrease methane production via defaunation and/or directly by decreasing the activities and numbers of methanogens. Saponins may also selectively affect specific rumen bacteria and fungi, which may alter the rumen metabolism. The effects of saponins on rumen fermentation have not been found to be consistent. These discrepancies appear to be related to the chemical structure and dosage of saponins, diet composition, microbial community and adaptation of microbiota to saponins. The clinical effects of saponins on human bowel flora have not yet been adequately explored.

Saponins are very gentle detergents that can be used to wash the hair and skin in conditions such as acne without causing a rebound increase in sebum production. Decoctions of soapwort have been used to wash and restore ancient fabrics in stately homes; modern soaps are too harsh and disintegrate the fabrics.

One of the most interesting effects of saponins (or sapogenins) that follows from their ingestion is their capacity to interact with and influence steroid hormone metabolism. Much of this is covered in the monographs, but some of the principles behind this are worth highlighting here. The role of enzymes that metabolise steroid hormones in the regulation of the activity of these hormones has only been relatively recently appreciated. The most pertinent example for phytotherapy is 11-beta-hydroxysteroid dehydrogenase. This enzyme regulates glucocorticoid action by catalysing the interconversion of hydrocortisone (cortisol) and cortisone, an inactive steroid. In the kidney, hydrocortisone is oxidised to cortisone by the type 2 form of this enzyme, a reaction that prevents circulating hydrocortisone from occupying kidney mineralocorticoid receptors and stimulating a mineralocorticoid response. Aldosterone, being inert to 11-beta-hydroxysteroid dehydrogenase (11beta-HSD), is then available to regulate mineralocorticoid responsive genes in the kidney on its own. Inhibition of 11beta-HSD in the kidney allows

45

hydrocortisone to exert an additional aldosterone-like effect. This is exactly what licorice does.[7]

An important consequence of this mechanism for regulating hormone action is that compounds that inhibit these enzymes will appear to be acting as hormones (or antihormones). Thus the active sapogenin from licorice appears to behave like aldosterone, even though it has no affinity at all for mineralocorticoid receptors. Similar examples need to be better understood. For example, the anti-inflammatory effect of escin from horsechestnut is abolished in the absence of steroid hormones.

The influence of steroidal saponins on oestrogen metabolism may share similar aspects, but perhaps with some noteworthy differences. This is illustrated by research on *Tribulus terrestris*. Saponins from Tribulus appear to increase FSH (follicle-stimulating hormone) in premenopausal women, which in turn increases levels of oestradiol.[373] They may do this by binding with, but only weakly stimulating, hypothalamic oestrogen receptors, which are part of the negative feedback mechanism of oestrogen control. The weak stimulus (as opposed to the strong stimulus of oestrogen) leads the body to interpret that oestrogen levels are lower than they really are. Consequently, the body increases oestrogen production via the negative feedback mechanism. In the postmenopausal woman, herbs such as Tribulus, wild yam (*Dioscorea villosa*) and false unicorn (*Chamaelirium luteum*) appear to alleviate symptoms of oestrogen withdrawal. It is possible that the binding of plant steroids to vacant receptors in the hypothalamus (in this low-oestrogen situation) is sufficient to convince the body that more oestrogen is present in the bloodstream than actually is, and calms the body's response to oestrogen withdrawal.

Claims have arisen in the popular literature that the female body can manufacture progesterone from diosgenin, particularly if a wild yam cream is applied to the skin. This is despite the fact that wild yam contains dioscin and other steroidal saponins, not diosgenin, and there is no information about the dermal absorption of these compounds. Furthermore, no evidence exists for mammalian enzymes that are capable of effecting what is a difficult chemical conversion. The evidence that does exist strongly disputes the possibility of this conversion.[374] Hopefully, the above discussion demonstrates that the interaction of saponins with steroid hormones is far more subtle than this. In fact, diosgenin appears to have oestrogenic properties in mice and lacks progesterogenic effects.[375]

Dioscin (a steroidal saponin)

Diosgenin (a steroidal sapogenin)

Component of quillaia saponin (a triterpenoid saponin)

In addition to this already impressive array of diverse activities for saponins, further effects have been demonstrated using in vitro and in vivo models. However, the results from the former types of studies need to be interpreted with caution, since in the majority of cases saponins will not be absorbed in sufficient quantities to manifest these effects systemically (and the sapogenins do not always share these properties). In vitro findings may have relevance to the topical activity of saponins and effects in the gut lumen, and where the saponin metabolite in the bloodstream has pharmacological properties similar to its parent saponin.

A review of the in vitro and in vivo effects of triterpenoid saponins has documented pharmacological properties such as antiallergic, antiatherosclerotic and antiplatelet, antibacterial, anticomplementary, antidiabetic, contraceptive, antifungal, anti-inflammatory, antileishmanial, antimalarial/antiplasmodial, anti-obesity, anti-proliferative, antipsoriatic, antispasmodic, antisweet, antiviral, cytotoxic/antitumor, gastroprotective, hepatoprotective, immunomodulatory, anti-osteoporotic and insulin-like.[376]

Adverse reactions and toxicology

Saponins are gastrointestinal irritants. In milder examples, this can lead to oesophageal reflux in sensitive or overweight patients, which can be remedied by using enteric-coated preparations or by taking the saponin-containing herbs during a meal. In more severe examples, such as with poke root, this irritation can lead to acute vomiting and diarrhoea. If the irritation is sufficiently prolonged, erosion of the gastrointestinal mucosa can occur, resulting in substantial absorption of saponins into the bloodstream with the expected toxic sequelae. This is probably the mechanism via which acute oral doses of saponins cause death in humans.

Saponins are toxic to fish and other cold-blooded animals and have been used to kill snails that harbour the bilharzia parasite.[377] However, normal intake of the majority of saponins is not toxic to humans, as evidenced by the fact that saponin intake by vegetarians is in the range of 100 to 200/day.[370] Saponins are permitted as food additives in many countries (for example, to give a satisfactory head to beer), although there are inconsistencies in regulations.[378] Long-term feeding of saponins to animals did not demonstrate any signs of toxicity.[378]

As noted previously, grazing animals that consume large amounts of saponins can develop cholestatic liver damage. In South Africa, consumption of Tribulus by sheep contributes to a bilirubin-induced disorder known as geeldikkop (see the Tribulus monograph for a more comprehensive discussion).[379] While it is unlikely that normal human doses would cause cholestasis, this phenomenon should be considered in unexplained cases of this disorder in patients taking herbs. More importantly, saponin-containing herbs are best kept to a moderate level in patients with pre-existing cholestasis.

Cardiac glycosides

Phytochemistry

These compounds, also known as cardioactive glycosides, are steroidal glycosides. They are similar to, but essentially different from, steroidal saponins and constitute a well-defined and highly homogeneous group from both a structural and a pharmacological perspective. They (or the plants that contain them) have been used as conventional medical drugs for over 200 years and are still relatively widely used today, despite their potential toxicity and the controversy over their clinical value. There are two main types, which either have a steroidal aglycone with 23 carbons (the cardenolide glycosides) or 24 carbons (the bufadienolide glycosides). The sugar part usually consists of 2 to 4 sugars joined together (an oligosaccharide).

Hellebrin – a bufadienolide glycoside

The cardenolide aglycone

Pharmacodynamics

The properties of cardiac glycosides are very well documented. They inhibit the sodium-potassium cellular pump leading to a rise in intracellular calcium levels that increases the contractile force and speed of the heart muscle (positive inotropy). In patients with compromised cardiac function, this positive isotropic effect translates into increased cardiac output and associated events that flow from this central effect. Heart rate is decreased (negative chronotropy) via the autonomic nervous system. Digitalis glycosides in particular also cause electrophysiological changes in the heart: conduction velocity at the atrioventricular node is slowed, together with an increase in its refractory period (negative dromotropy). This last feature underlies the use of digitalis glycosides in supraventricular rhythm abnormalities such as atrial fibrillation.

It is beyond the scope of this chapter to discuss the pros and cons of digitalis therapy or the various adverse reactions and toxicity considerations associated with its use. Its medical use certainly appears to be in decline, although there is continued evidence of its frequent clinical utility.[380] Phytotherapists find digitalis to be too powerful for comfort and prefer to see it used, if necessary, under appropriate specialist care (generally the legal restrictions on its use render it available only on a medical prescription).

In some countries, herbalists and physicians practising phytotherapy find value in the use of milder herbs containing cardiac glycosides, in particular lily of the valley (*Convallaria majalis*). Its properties are similar to those of digitalis, but much less cumulative. The principal glycoside is convallatoxin, but the plant contains many minor cardenolides. Convallatoxin is poorly absorbed as a pure compound but the other components in the herb are said to aid its absorption.[381] It is unsuitable for manifest congestive heart failure, but combines well with hawthorn in the management of milder forms of this condition, for digitalis hypersensitivity or for heart failure associated with a low pulse rate.[381] All the usual cautions governing the use of cardiac glycosides should be observed.

Recent reviews have highlighted the novel therapeutic applications of cardiac glycosides, in particular the accumulating in vitro and in vivo studies reporting antitumour activity.[382,383] The first generation of glycoside-based anticancer drugs are in clinical trials.

Anthraquinones

Phytochemistry

Anthraquinones, as the name implies, are phytochemicals based on anthracene (three benzene rings joined together). At each apex of the central ring is a carbonyl group (carbon double-bonded to oxygen), and these provide the quinone part. Not all anthraquinones are strictly quinones; for example, the sennosides are dianthrones consisting of two anthrone units, each bearing only one carbonyl group. Anthraquinones usually occur in plants as glycosides; for example, the sennosides from senna (*Cassia species*) are O-glycosides and the aloins from Aloe are C-glycosides. The cascarosides from cascara (*Rhamnus purshiana*) are unusual molecules in that they are C,O-glycosides, having one glucose linked to a central anthrone via a carbon atom and a second glucose linked via oxygen. If aglycones are present in dried herbs, they are always anthraquinones; anthrones are too unstable in the free state. Dianthrone glycosides such as the sennosides are not

found in the living plant, being formed on harvesting and drying from monomeric anthrone glycosides.

Sennosides A, B (stereoisomers)

Rheinanthrone

Pharmacodynamics

Plants like rhubarb, senna and cascara have been used for their laxative effects since prehistory. Given their widespread contemporary use, it should not be surprising that their pharmacology is relatively well studied. Of particular interest is the pharmacokinetics of the anthraquinone glycosides. This topic will be more extensively discussed in the pharmacokinetics section, but, briefly put, these agents travel to the large bowel where bacterial action forms anthrone aglycones, the true active forms.

The laxative effect on the gut is largely a local one; systemic absorption is limited. Two distinct mechanisms are in force: a modification of intestinal motility and an accumulation of fluid in the intestinal lumen.[384] Experiments in animals and humans have shown that the introduction of anthrones into the colon quickly induces vigorous peristaltic movements.[384] Such a fast response is certainly not a secondary effect resulting from increased faecal water. This effect on motility is at least in part due to the release of prostaglandins, since its action is abolished by indomethacin and other cyclo-oxygenase inhibitors.[385] However, other research shows that inhibition of intestinal tone and segmentation (and therefore reduced colonic transit time) could be the primary motility effect.[384]

Accumulation of fluid in the colonic lumen also leads to a laxative effect. While it has been suggested that this might be due to the inhibitory effect of anthrones on the sodium pump,[384] these agents have instead been shown to stimulate active chloride secretion into the lumen, which is then balanced by an increase in sodium and water flow.[386] Prostaglandins may be involved in this process[387] but not PAF.[388] Alteration of calcium transport may also play a role.[384]

The dual action of anthraquinones highlights an important aspect of their safe and effective usage. In lower laxative doses that produce a normal bowel motion, the effects on motility are dominant. In higher doses, electrolyte secretion and diarrhoea will predominate. Habituation and adverse effects are more likely to result from the excessive electrolyte loss associated with the use of high doses. Chronic abuse of laxatives raises aldosterone levels in response to the electrolyte loss, diminishing their effectiveness. Higher doses also empty a larger portion of the colon. The resulting natural absence of defaecation over the next day or so leads to anthraquinone reuse, perhaps at an even higher dose, and the cycle of laxative need is perpetuated.

Natural anthraquinones in the form of chrysarobin have also been used topically in the treatment of psoriasis. Chrysarobin, a mixture of substances including chrysophanol, is obtained from araroba or goa powder. Araroba is extracted from cavities in the trunk of the South American tree *Andira araroba*.[389] Dithranol (or anthralin), a cheaper synthetic analogue of chrysarobin, has been the focus of the most studies.[390] Chrysarobin is an effective topical agent for psoriasis, as was demonstrated in an open comparative study with coal tar and ultraviolet radiation.[391] However, it has a number of drawbacks: it is only stable in a greasy base and it irritates and stains the skin.

The antiproliferative action of dithranol, and presumably chrysarobin, is thought to be either through effects on DNA, probably mitochondrial DNA, which reduces cell turnover, or through activity on various vital enzyme systems.[392] A possible relationship with reduction-oxidation potential has also been observed.[393] Other research on chrysarobin has been concerned with its tumour-promoting activity.[394] Not surprisingly, this finding has further reduced its use in therapy.

Hypericin and pseudohypericin are dianthrones (structurally related to anthraquinones) with antiviral activity. Several anthraquinone aglycones including rhein, alizarin and emodin have also demonstrated antiviral activity against human cytomegalovirus.[395] This may explain the traditional use of applying the leaves of *Cassia* species to viral skin conditions.[389] It is unlikely that systemic antiviral effects would follow from the ingestion of anthraquinones, due to their low bioavailability.

Rhein

Cascarosides A, B (stereoisomers)

Rhein is an anthraquinone aglycone found in rhubarb that inhibits the activity of cytokines in models of osteoarthritis.[396] This observation led to the development of diacerhein (diacetylrhein), a synthetic derivative with better bioavailability. In early clinical studies, oral diacerhein at 100 mg/day improved symptoms in patients with osteoarthritis.[396] Diarrhoea was a common side effect, as might be expected. A later Cochrane review of seven controlled clinical trials concluded that there is 'gold' level evidence that diacerhein (diacerein) has a small consistent benefit in the improvement of pain in osteoarthritis.[397]

Madder root (*Rubia tinctorum*) contains a characteristic spectrum of intensely coloured anthraquinone glycosides such as glycosides of lucidin and alizarin. As well as being used as a vegetable dye and natural food colouring, madder has traditionally been employed for the prevention and treatment of kidney stones. The anthraquinones in madder can function as chelating agents for some metal ions, such as calcium and magnesium. With oral doses of glycosides and aglycones, a pronounced calcium complexing effect and a significant reduction in the growth rate of kidney stones was observed in an animal model.[389] A therapeutic oral dose of madder root will colour the urine slightly pink, which indicates that significant quantities of anthraquinones are excreted in the urine. Its regular use is said to slowly dissolve kidney stones. Given the concerns (below) over the carcinogenicity of madder, perhaps other anthraquinones sharing this property could be explored for potential value as oral chelation therapy in patients with atherosclerotic lesions.

Adverse reactions and toxicology

Madder has been withdrawn from the German market due to concerns over its mutagenicity and potential carcinogenicity. In particular, rats metabolise alizarin glycosides to alizarin and 1-hydroxyanthraquinone, a known rodent carcinogen.[398] One long-term feeding of madder root to mice failed to produce neoplastic lesions.[399] However, studies that are more recent do tend to confirm carcinogenic activity.[400]

Anthraquinone laxatives may cause mild abdominal complaints such as cramps and abdominal pain and should be used cautiously in patients with these symptoms. Other side effects include discoloration of the urine and haemorrhoid congestion. Overdosage can result in diarrhoea and, coupled with prolonged use, may cause excessive loss of electrolytes, particularly potassium.[384]

Abuse of anthraquinone laxatives has been stated to cause damage to the myenteric plexus. However, results from animal studies and a controlled study in humans have challenged this finding.[401] Habituation can occur with laxative abuse, primarily due to hyperaldosteronism. The evidence is that anthraquinone laxatives used sensibly are unlikely to cause habituation. In fact, in several studies senna has been claimed to have a re-educative function and helped to restore normal bowel function.[402] For example, out of 210 patients in a psychiatric hospital, 44% were taking laxatives at the outset, but 3 months' treatment with senna lowered this to 8%.[403]

Cathartic colon coupled with hypokalaemia (low serum potassium) is a characteristic finding associated with chronic laxative abuse (not just for anthraquinones). The cathartic colon is characterised by the existence of a segment of intestine (typically the ascending colon) that has become largely non-functioning. Cathartic colon presents as chronic diarrhoea resistant to therapy. This is probably a rare disorder and is often associated with psychological abnormalities.[404] Cathartic colon can be reversed; a case was described of a 78-year-old woman with cathartic colon who, after treatment was switched to psyllium, demonstrated complete reversal of the condition after 4 months.[405]

Contraindications for anthraquinone laxatives include ileus from whatever cause. Use in pregnancy and lactation is controversial. In traditional Chinese medicine anthraquinone-containing herbs are contraindicated in pregnancy because they promote a downward movement of energy. Apart from this consideration, they are unlikely to cause adverse effects since their action in the gut is largely topical and systemic absorption is limited (see Pharmacokinetics). Results from several clinical studies on senna indicate that its normal use does not involve any increased risk for the pregnancy or the fetus.[406] Moreover, clinical observations of infants and analytical studies of breast milk both lead to the conclusion that the treatment of lactating mothers with senna does not carry a risk of producing a laxative effect in the infant.[407]

Long-term use of anthraquinone laxatives leads to a condition known as melanosis (or pseudomelanosis) coli. This is a brown discoloration of the intestinal mucosa beginning at the ileocolonic junction and may extend to the rectum. This harmless pigmentation is not due to staining by the anthraquinones, but is instead a lipofuscin-like substance within the macrophages of the colonic mucosa.[384] (Lipofuscin is a pigmented, peroxidised fatty acid residue found in many organs with advancing age.) However, the intrinsic colour of anthraquinones may play some part in the development of this pigment. It is generally accepted that melanosis is a benign, reversible condition.[408,409]

The mutagenicity of isolated anthraquinones has been extensively studied and established in several models, particularly microbial assays such as the Ames test.[410] On the other hand, some studies involving both in vitro and in vivo models found an absence of mutagenicity for senna, sennosides and rhein.[411] The same research group concluded that senna does not represent a genotoxic risk to humans when used periodically at normal therapeutic doses.[412]

Nonetheless, their putative mutagenicity has led to the investigation of carcinogenic effects associated with the use of anthraquinone laxatives. One review examined the relationship between anthraquinone laxatives and colorectal cancer.[413] Danthrone (two studies) and 1-hydroxyanthraquinone (one study) were carcinogenic in rodent models. Three clinical studies did not show an association of colorectal cancer with laxative abuse, but these studies also included bulk laxatives. When melanosis coli was taken as an indicator of anthraquinone laxative use, a retrospective study of 3049 patients undergoing endoscopic diagnosis for suspected colorectal cancer found an association between anthraquinone use and colorectal adenomas.[413] A prospective study by the same research group found that 18.6% of patients with colorectal carcinoma had evidence of anthraquinone use.[413] From their data, they suggested that a relative risk of 3.04 could be calculated for colorectal cancer due to anthraquinone laxative abuse. However, these studies did not differentiate between natural and synthetic (danthrone) laxative use. This is significant, because relatively higher doses of danthrone are required for a laxative effect and, since it is not a glycoside, its systemic absorption is greater. It was later asserted that epidemiological studies do not give conclusive evidence for any association between anthraquinone use and colorectal cancer.[384] Since then, a comprehensive review of the pharmacological and human data concluded that (1) there is no convincing evidence that the chronic use of senna can induce a structural and/or functional alteration of the enteric nerves or the smooth intestinal muscle, (2) there is no relation between long-term administration of a senna extract and the appearance of gastrointestinal tumours (or any other type) in rats, (3) senna is not carcinogenic in rats even after a 2-year daily dose of up to 300 mg/kg/day, and (4) the current evidence does not show that there is a genotoxic risk for patients who take laxatives containing senna extracts or sennosides.[414]

Given the above concerns, whatever their basis in fact, most regulatory authorities now require that anthraquinone laxatives are labelled as a short-term treatment for constipation. Since the goal of the phytotherapist is to effect change (re-educate the bowel) rather than compensate for a deranged physiology, this approach is consistent with good herbal clinical practice.

Coumarins

Phytochemistry

Coumarins owe their name to 'coumarin' which was the common name for the tonka bean (*Dipteryx odorata*), from which the simple compound coumarin was first isolated in 1820. Coumarins are benzo-alpha-pyrones (lactones of *o*-hydroxycinnamic acid) formed via the shikimic acid pathway. Except for a few rare cases, including coumarin itself which is unsubstituted, all plant coumarins contain hydroxy or methoxy groups in position 7. These substituted simple coumarins, such as scopoletin, aesculetin and umbelliferone, are common and widespread in higher plants and often occur as glycosides.

R_1	R_2	R_3	
H	H	H	Coumarin
H	OH	H	Umbelliferone
H	OCH$_3$	H	Herniarin
H	OH	OH	Daphnetin
OH	OH	H	Aesculetin
OCH$_3$	OH	H	Scopoletin

Simple coumarins

Simple coumarin has a pleasant vanilla-like odour. It is probably not present in the intact plant, but is rather formed by enzymatic activity from a glycoside of *o*-hydroxycinnamic acid (such as melilotoside) after harvesting and drying. This accounts for the odour of newly-mown hay, not present in the undamaged plant. Coumarin is used to perfume pipe tobacco and can be sometimes found as an adulterant in commercial vanilla flavouring.[415]

The furanocoumarins are closely related furano derivatives of coumarin (furan is a five-membered heterocyclic ring containing oxygen) commonly found in the Rutaceae (rue family) and Umbelliferae (Apiaceae, celery family). Linear furanocoumarins are often called psoralens and are photosensitising agents (see below).

Linear furanocoumarins

R_1	R_2	
H	H	Psoralen
H	OCH$_3$	Xanthotoxin
H	OH	Xanthotoxol
OCH$_3$	H	Bergapten
OH	H	Bergaptol

The furanochromones such as khellin from *Ammi visnaga* are structural derivatives of benzo-gamma-pyrone (furanobenzo-gamma-pyrones) and therefore are as much related to flavonoids as coumarins. In other words, the carbonyl group is opposite the oxygen rather than adjacent to it. However, they are usually classified as coumarins and will be considered in this section. *Ammi visnaga* also contains visnadin, a pyranocoumarin.

R_1	R_2	
H	CH$_3$	Visnagin
OCH$_3$	CH$_3$	Khellin
H	CH$_2$OH	Khellol

Furanochromones

Visnadin

The widespread nature of coumarins means that they are consumed in the human diet, for example carrots, celery and parsnip.[416] Coumarins are fluorescent compounds and this property is widely utilised in a number of biochemical techniques. Simple substituted coumarins are also used as pigments in sunscreens.

Pharmacodynamics

Dicoumarol is a potent anticoagulant compound formed from coumarin by bacterial action in spoiled sweet clover hay (*Melilotus* species). Its discovery led to the development of modern anticoagulant drugs. Dicoumarol and related anticoagulants are hydroxylated in the 4 position. This is deemed an essential requirement (among others) for powerful anticoagulant activity. All of the common plant coumarins are not substituted at this position and therefore lack significant clinical anticoagulant activity, although many do possess very limited activity when given to animals in high doses.[417] Coumarin has anti-oedema, anti-inflammatory, immune-enhancing and anticancer activities which are more fully described in the Melilotus monograph.

Simple substituted coumarins such as scopoletin and umbelliferone have exhibited a diverse range of pharmacological activities. The spasmolytic activity of scopoletin is probably a major reason for the use of *Viburnum* species such as cramp bark and black haw for hypertension and dysmenorrhoea. Scopoletin and aesculetin were identified in black haw as having significant spasmolytic activity on guinea pig small intestine.[418] Another research team working at the same time also identified scopoletin as a component of the Viburnums that exhibited uterine spasmolytic activity.[419] It has been suggested that the spasmolytic activity of scopoletin might be due to a blockade of autonomic neurotransmitters.[420]

Further studies are required to establish if scopoletin, umbelliferone and related compounds possess clinically relevant anti-inflammatory and analgesic activities, but such activities have been established in animal studies.[421] Inhibition of cyclo-oxygenase and 5-lipoxygenase may play a role.[422] Aesculetin and umbelliferone are also strong xanthine oxidase inhibitors in vitro.[423]

Of eight simple coumarins tested, aesculetin was the most potent at protecting cells in vitro against oxidative damage.[424] The coumarins all inhibited xanthine oxidase in vitro.[424] Aesculetin possessed hypouricaemic activity in rats

(100 mg/kg, ip) and mice (150 mg/kg, ip), but was devoid of xanthine oxidase inhibitory activity at these doses.[425] Scopoletin (50 to 200 mg/kg, ip) was also hypouricaemic after induced elevation of uric acid in mice, but did not affect the serum uric acid level in normal mice.[426] It exhibited both xanthine oxidase inhibition and uricosuric activity. However, the high doses of such phytochemicals given by injection probably have little relevance to phytotherapy.

Like coumarin, substituted coumarins may have a role to play in cancer prevention and treatment. Umbelliferone and scopoletin are antimutagenic[427,428] but were much less protective than coumarin in one model of chemical carcinogenesis.[429] Aesculetin exhibited considerably higher cytotoxic activity than coumarin in vitro on two tumour cell lines, but scopoletin was inactive.[430] Umbelliferone has similar cytotoxic activity to coumarin.[431] Two reviews have outlined the potential of simple natural coumarins in cancer therapy, but most of the data to date are in vitro.[432,433]

Other in vivo properties of simple coumarins include gastroprotective activity for aesculin,[434] and antiasthmatic activity for umbelliferone,[435] all in mice, together with antithyroid activity for scopoletin in hyperthyroid rats[436] and antidiabetic activity for umbelliferone in diabetic rats.[437]

Furanocoumarins have a long history of therapeutic use in humans. More than 3000 years ago, it was recorded in both Egyptian and Ayurvedic medicine that the ingestion of herbs containing psoralens followed by exposure to sunlight could assist in the treatment of vitiligo, a skin condition characterised by a loss of pigmentation.[438] This traditional knowledge was developed into a modern therapy in the 1940s when xanthotoxin (8-methoxypsoralen, 8-MOP) plus sunlight exposure was introduced as a therapy for vitiligo.[439] The treatment was not very successful, mainly due to phototoxic side effects, and it was only when ultraviolet A light sources (UVA) became available that significant advances were made. UVA radiation is less energetic and therefore less damaging than ultraviolet B (UVB) radiation. It was demonstrated that oral 8-MOP and UVA were highly effective in the control of psoriasis and the malignant skin condition mycosis fungoides.[439] The treatment was called PUVA (psoralen plus UVA) and the new field of photochemotherapy was initiated.

Bergapten (5-methoxypsoralen, 5-MOP) is a psoralen with superior therapeutic characteristics in PUVA. Furanocoumarins in conjunction with ultraviolet radiation stimulate melanogenesis (tanning) and cause antiproliferative effects, but they also initiate phototoxic erythema (inflammation). For 8-MOP, the therapeutic dose is similar to the dose that causes erythema. With the use of oral 5-MOP it is possible to obtain melanogenic doses of drug-UVA or drug-sunlight combinations without the development of phototoxicity. This provides a wider margin of safety and permits the induction of a tan (known as a PUVA tan) that is more effective than a normal tan in attenuating the damaging effects of UV exposure. Psoralens are now the basis of yet another new field of therapy: photochemoprotection.[439]

The use of 5-MOP has also provided a more effective treatment for vitiligo and yields fewer side effects in PUVA therapy of psoriasis.[440] As a further development in photochemoprotection, studies have shown that this furanocoumarin, in conjunction with UVB sunscreens, provides a faster

tan (without burning) that is more protective against the harmful effects of ultraviolet radiation[441] and even chemical irritation.[442] It should be noted that certain citrus oils are rich sources of bergapten (5-MOP) and are used in these tanning products in preference to the synthetic chemical.

PUVA therapy is also used for psoriasis,[443] although there are concerns over increased skin cancer risk (see below).[444]

Furanocoumarins in conjunction with UV light kill bacteria and inactivate viruses.[445,446] In addition, they may be responsible for the enhanced bioavailability that grapefruit juice affords to several pharmaceuticals (see the Pharmacokinetics section).

The decoction of the fruits of *Ammi visnaga* has been used since ancient times in Egypt as a spasmolytic for kidney stones and in the treatment of angina pectoris. The pyranocoumarin visnadin was isolated and exhibited positive inotropic and marked coronary vasodilatory activities. Visnadin was developed as a drug treatment for angina, possibly acting as a calcium channel blocker.[447] *Ammi visnaga* also contains the spasmolytic furanochromone khellin, adopted for the treatment of angina and asthma. Its use was discontinued because of side effects such as drowsiness, headache and nausea.

As further evidence that the archetypal plant constituents still provide much of the inspiration for the development of modern drugs, sodium cromoglycate was discovered in an attempt to find a derivative of khellin which was devoid of its side effects. Unlike khellin, the antiasthmatic activity of this drug is believed to result from increased stability of mast cells.[448]

Toxicology

The toxicology of coumarin is reviewed in the Melilotus monograph. It is hepatotoxic in the rat and also less commonly in humans, probably as an idiosyncratic reaction. Coumarins are structurally related to fungal aflatoxins, which are potent hepatotoxins, but it appears that the substituted coumarins do not share this property (see the Melilotus monograph).

Plant coumarins are incorrectly implicated as anticoagulant agents. This is a fundamental misunderstanding of the relevant pharmacology (see Chapter 5 and the Melilotus monograph). Although a case of increased haemorrhagic tendency was attributed to coumarin intake from tonka beans, sweet clover and woodruff, intake was excessive and there were a number of confounding factors.[449]

As noted above, the furanocoumarins are potent photosensitising agents. Chance exposure to these compounds in the field can lead to severe photodermatitis and blistering. The giant hogweed is one example of a plant that consistently causes this problem. Celery pickers can develop photodermatitis after handling celery infected with fungus, which induces celery to produce high levels of psoralens.[450]

Furanocoumarins are powerful mutagens in the presence of UVA and psoralens are light-activated carcinogens.[450] In the presence of UV light, psoralens are capable of binding to and cross-linking DNA, which causes genetic damage and mutations. Only linear furanocoumarins (psoralens) are able to bind two DNA bases to cause cross-links. Non-linear furanocoumarins (isopsoralens) can only bind to one base to form monoadducts. Although concerns were expressed that the development of isopsoralens as photochemotherapeutic agents may increase carcinogenic risk because monoadducts are subject to error-prone DNA repair mechanisms,[450] this does not appear to be the case.[451]

The use of UV filters decreases the photomutagenic and photocarcinogenic effects of psoralens, but the employment of 5-MOP in sun tanning lotions remains controversial.[452,453] Given the advantages of a PUVA tan, it is likely that the benefits will outweigh risks, provided that UV exposure is carefully controlled. This may only occur under clinical supervision.

Use of PUVA therapy in psoriasis is postulated to be associated with an increased risk of skin cancer, particularly squamous cell carcinoma.[454] Risk of developing skin cancer was claimed to be proportional to the number of treatments and the degree of exposure to UVA.[454] However, these associations have been disputed by at least one study, which proposed that prior exposure to arsenic treatments or X-rays largely explained the higher incidence of skin cancer in PUVA-treated psoriasis patients.[455] Significant exposure of the unprotected human eyes to PUVA may accelerate cataract formation, but this is readily alleviated by protective eyeglasses.[454]

Phyto-oestrogens

Phyto-oestrogens are phytochemicals that have oestrogenic activity because they bear some structural similarity to 17-beta-oestradiol. Compounds belonging to several phytochemical classes interact with oestrogen receptors, but research has focused on the isoflavones and lignans. Oestrogenic isoflavones, which include genistein, daidzein and their glycosides, are mainly found in members of the Leguminosae (pea family) such as soya beans and red clover. Linseed (flaxseed) is the richest source of the oestrogenic lignans enterodiol and enterolactone, which are formed by gut bacterial action on the precursor phytochemical secoisolariciresinol diglucoside (SLDG) found in the seed.

Enterolactone

Secoisolariciresinol
R_1 = OH, R_2 = OCH$_3$

Enterodiol
R_1 = H, R_2 = OH

Pharmacodynamics

Interest in the oestrogenic effects of plants first arose in the scientific world when clover disease was identified in Australia in the 1940s. It was observed that infertility developed in sheep after grazing on various species of clover (*Trifolium* species). Research interest at the time focused on understanding the factors that caused clover disease, which were identified as isoflavone glycosides. It was several decades later, when results from epidemiological studies suggested that the dietary consumption of soya products might have a protective role in breast cancer, that interest in the oestrogenic properties of isoflavones was rekindled.[456]

Early studies using various animal tissues demonstrated that, while isoflavones compete strongly with oestradiol at oestrogen receptors, their stimulation of these receptors is much weaker than oestradiol.[457] In other words, they were thought to act as partial oestrogen agonists that could function as oestrogen agonists or antagonists depending on the hormonal milieu. The theory was that in a high-oestrogen environment (such as in the premenopausal woman), their displacement of endogenous oestrogens is postulated to have an antioestrogenic effect. In contrast, in a lower oestrogen environment, as in the postmenopausal woman, they were expected to provide a net oestrogenic effect. While this theory still has some relevance, the situation is now known to be more complex.

There are two isoforms of the oestrogen receptor, ERalpha and ERbeta. Their distribution and density varies, depending on the target tissue. The existence of an oestrogen receptor was first reported in the early 1960s. In 1996, an additional ER was discovered. This receptor was designated ERbeta and consequently the originally discovered receptor was renamed ERalpha.[458] Both ERalpha and ERbeta may coexist in a tissue and relevant proportions often vary. ERalpha is the dominant receptor in the adult uterus. ERbeta is expressed in high levels in prostate, salivary glands, testis, ovary, vascular endothelium, bone, smooth muscle, certain neurons in the central and peripheral nervous system and the immune system.[459] Both isoforms are present in the female breast and reproductive tissue.[460]

Each of the ERs may influence the function of the other. The effects of substances that interact with receptors when both forms are present are complex.[460] It is hypothesised that ERbeta may modulate, or even antagonise, the actions of ERalpha.[461] For example, in the breast ERalpha and ERbeta exhibit opposing functions in cell proliferation: ERalpha promotes epithelial proliferation, whereas ERbeta has a restraining influence.[462] Other studies suggest several possible interactions for the two receptors: antagonistic, synergistic and sequential.[463]

The female sex hormones (the oestrogens) consist of 17beta-oestradiol, oestrone and oestriol. Oestradiol binds to ERalpha and ERbeta with equal affinity.[464] The isoflavone phyto-oestrogen genistein has greater binding affinity for ERbeta than for ERalpha. This preferential binding of genistein to ERbeta indicates such isoflavones probably produce pharmacological and clinical effects quite distinct from oestrogens. In particular, they tend to exhibit antiproliferative activity.[464] Other isoflavone phyto-oestrogens also bind more strongly to ERbeta.[465]

Furthermore, isoflavones bind to ERs with a much lower affinity than oestrogens and therefore produce less potent responses.[466,467] However, they initiate greater gene transcription of ERalpha compared to ERbeta.[467]

As noted above, isoflavones and other phyto-oestrogens are thought to compete with oestradiol for binding and activation of ERs,[460] potentially decreasing the effect of oestradiol in vivo in some circumstances. However, there have been some in vitro results to the contrary.[468] The effect depends on the doses (of both phyto-oestrogens and oestradiol). In a pilot study, a soy protein isolate containing isoflavones (120 mg/day) taken for 6 months did not prevent oestradiol-induced endometrial hyperplasia in postmenopausal women.[469] (But interestingly, there was also no additive effect.)

Research on selective oestrogen receptor modulators (SERMs) such as tamoxifen has provided more insights into how non-steroidal molecules can interact with the oestrogen receptor. A summary of the knowledge thus far is that once a SERM binds to the ER it causes a change in its shape. This allows recruitment of co-activators if it is destined to elicit an oestrogenic response, or co-repressors if its response is anti-oestrogenic. The binding of the coregulatory molecules leads to the activation of the promoter sequence of the oestrogenic responsive gene. Isoflavones have been proposed as natural SERMs.[465]

Studies have found that isoflavones have both agonistic and antagonistic effects, though they are strong ERbeta agonists and weak ERalpha agonists. The presence of a correctly positioned phenolic ring and also the distance between the two opposing phenolic oxygens in the isoflavones structure is similar to that of 17-beta-oestradiol. This similarity allows the isoflavones to bind to the ER, effectively displacing 17-beta-oestradiol. This action may help explain how phyto-oestrogens help protect against breast cancer, because ERbeta inhibits mammary cell growth as well as the stimulatory effects of ERalpha.[465] As with the SERMs, studies have shown that the recruitment of coregulatory molecules may be important in determining the function of phyto-oestrogens. In particular, isoflavones appear to trigger selectively ERbeta transcriptional pathways, especially transcriptional repression.[465]

The in vitro and in vivo studies on phyto-oestrogens can be divided into three general categories: chemoprevention, treatment effects and lifetime exposure studies (in vivo only).[465] This literature is so vast that a thorough review is beyond the scope of this primer. However, one aspect worth emphasising is that isoflavones have been shown to prevent cancer or inhibit cancer cell lines in a variety of models.[470,471] Another is that isoflavones exert favourable effects in vivo and in vitro on parameters relevant to cardiovascular risk including insulin resistance, lipid peroxidation, haemostasis and endothelial function.[472] Probably of greater relevance are the many human studies of the impact of phyto-oestrogens on various health outcomes or parameters. Some of the key findings of these studies are featured below, in a brief outline of the reviews.

A meta-analysis concluded that soya isoflavone consumption was associated with a reduced risk of breast cancer, but this protective effect has only been observed in studies in Asian populations.[473] Soya isoflavone intake was also inversely

associated with the risk of breast cancer recurrence. Moderate consumption of isoflavones in diet does not increase the risk of breast cancer recurrence in Western women who have survived breast cancer, and Asian breast cancer survivors exhibit better prognosis if they continue consuming a soya diet.[474]

Results from Asian epidemiological studies suggest a beneficial impact of isoflavones on bone health.[475] However, clinical trials have yielded conflicting results on bone mineral density and turnover markers that may reflect on differences in study parameters, type and dose of phyto-oestrogen used and the variable metabolism of isoflavones, especially in terms of equol production.[475]

A systematic review and meta-analysis of soya isoflavones versus placebo in the treatment of menopausal vasomotor symptoms concluded that there was a significant tendency in favour of soya.[476] Another meta-analysis found that consumption of 30 mg/day of soya isoflavones (or at least 15 mg genistein) reduced menopausal hot flushes by up to 50%.[477] Individual responses in menopause could be determined by bioavailability and metabolism, especially to equol.[478]

The published effects of isoflavones on the circulating hormones in pre and postmenopausal women were the subject of a systematic review and meta-analysis.[479] In all, 47 studies were included. In premenopausal women, meta-analysis suggested that isoflavone consumption did not affect levels of oestradiol, oestrone or sex hormone binding globulin (SHBG), but did significantly reduce FSH and luteinising hormone (LH) (by about 20%). In postmenopausal women there was no impact of isoflavones on any of these hormones, although there was a 14% non-significant increase in oestradiol.

Epidemiological studies indicate that soya isoflavone consumption is possibly protective against prostate cancer.[480] There is also some suggestion from clinical trials that isoflavones can slow the disease progression.[481]

Isoflavone intake appears to confer cardiovascular benefits that may or may not be related to their phyto-oestrogenic properties. One systematic review identified improvement in arterial stiffness[482] and another used meta-analysis to establish a small reduction in blood pressure.[483] Soya isoflavone intake improved flow-mediated dilation (an indicator of cardiovascular health) based on a meta-analysis of randomised, controlled clinical trials.[484]

Intestinal metabolism of isoflavones to their aglycone form is crucial for ensuring bioavailability and therapeutic activity. In other words, the intestinal microflora is pivotal in the metabolism of oestrogenic isoflavones. Individual differences in intestinal microflora have been proposed as a possible reason why there is some inconsistency in the clinical effects of isoflavones.[485] In particular, daidzein is further metabolised by gut microflora to produce equol, a more active oestrogenic compound. There are large individual variances in the capacity to produce equol and hence possibly a therapeutic effect. Dietary fat consumption is known to reduce this capacity.[486] On the other hand, dietary supplementation with fructo-oligosaccharides such as inulin is known to increase equol.[487]

In contrast to the isoflavones, research on the oestrogenic lignans enterolactone and enterodiol has not been as extensive. Initial interest in these compounds resulted from the observation in the early 1980s that their urinary levels in menstruating women exhibited a cyclic pattern during the menstrual cycle, with maximum excretion in the luteal phase.[488] The relatively high concentrations of these new lignans in urine, their cyclic pattern of excretion and their increased excretion in early pregnancy suggested that they were a new class of human hormone. It transpired what had been found was a plant chemical modified by bacteria in the human digestive tract.[488] Selective antibiotic administration to humans suppressed oestrogenic lignan formation.[488]

Enterolactone, like isoflavones, inhibits oestradiol-stimulated breast cancer cell growth in vitro.[489] Lignan ingestion has been associated with increased concentrations of SHBG, but this was not confirmed in clinical studies.[489–491] Linseed intake by normal premenopausal women was consistently associated with longer luteal phase lengths and higher ratios of luteal phase progesterone to oestradiol.[489] These findings may reflect favourably on breast cancer risk. An earlier animal study found that linseed supplementation reduced early risk markers for breast cancer.[492] Dietary studies and assays of urinary lignans in postmenopausal women have found that lignan excretion is significantly lower in the urine of women with breast cancer,[493] although the situation is not as clear from recent prospective cohort studies.[494]

In more recent times, the health effects of linseed and SLDG supplementation have been investigated in a number of clinical trials. Results of trials involving whole linseed are confounded by its content of mucilage and fixed oil (rich in omega-3 fatty acids), especially the trials investigating its impact on blood lipids or glucose.

The following is obviously not a comprehensive review of the clinical data for linseed and its lignans and focuses on hormonal effects. Linseed (25 g/day) altered oestrogen metabolism more than soya (25 g/day), and significantly shifted oestrogen metabolites to less biologically active forms (2-hydroxyoestrone) in postmenopausal women.[495] This was confirmed in other clinical trials at 10 g/d, in pre- and postmenopausal women.[496,497] At 10 g/day linseed decreased endogenous oestrogen levels and increased prolactin in postmenopausal women.[491] Linseed supplementation does not appear to benefit menopausal symptoms, although more studies are necessary.[498]

Adverse reactions and toxicology

Epidemiological studies have not found adverse effects from the dietary consumption of isoflavones or lignans. However, when quantities well above dietary exposure are used in a therapeutic context, adverse events might well ensue. As noted above, the phyto-oestrogens are partial oestrogen agonists similar to the drug tamoxifen. Research has shown that while tamoxifen has potential for preventing breast cancer and cardiovascular disease, its use increases the risk of developing endometrial cancer. Moreover, concurrent intake of phyto-oestrogens and tamoxifen may reduce the therapeutic effects of the drug in breast cancer. For this reason, and because of the observation that phyto-oestrogens can stimulate the growth of oestrogen-dependent tumours in some circumstances, intake of these phytochemicals should be limited to dietary levels in women with oestrogen-sensitive breast

cancers until clinical studies suggest otherwise. Such data are beginning to emerge (see the discussion on breast cancer risk below).

Controversy has arisen over the possible adverse effects of soya-based infant milk formulas. One earlier study found that infant exposure to isoflavones from these products was relatively much greater than levels shown to alter reproductive hormones in adults.[499] It was suggested that further studies of possible developmental effects are highly desirable.

On the other hand, studies in males have found no indication of adverse effects. For example, a 2010 review found no evidence from rodent studies and nine clinical trials that isoflavone intake impacted oestrogen levels in males. Clinical evidence also indicates no impact on sperm and semen parameters in men.[500] In addition, a meta-analysis that included 15 placebo-controlled clinical trials found that neither soya nor isoflavones altered testosterone parameters in men.[501]

While the epidemiological evidence suggests that a lifetime of moderate to high isoflavone intake is protective against breast cancer incidence in women, the impact of such intake commenced later in life is uncertain. Concerns have been raised that a later intake of high levels of phyto-oestrogens might in fact increase the risk of oestrogen-associated cancers. However, these fears are not supported by the available data.

Mammographic density may be a predictor of breast cancer risk. Women with a high percentage of dense tissue are at 4-fold greater risk of breast cancer. Mammographic parenchymal patterns assess the variation between radiological appearances: fat appears dark and epithelium and stroma appear light. Percentage density is the ratio of dense area to breast area. A meta-analysis of randomised, controlled clinical trials on soya and red clover (*Trifolium pratense*) isoflavones found no impact on mammographic breast density in postmenopausal women.[502] However, isoflavones may cause a small increase in breast density in premenopausal women, which is of uncertain clinical relevance. An epidemiological study in 3315 Chinese women in Singapore found no significant impact of soya intake on breast density, with the suggestion of a possible reduction.[503]

The results of a case-control study involving nearly 800 participants conducted in New Jersey and published in 2009 suggest a reduction in endometrial cancer risk with intake of foods containing isoflavones (but not lignans) in lean women. Four case-control studies prior to this reported conflicting results for the role of dietary phyto-oestrogens in endometrial cancer risk, although there was a suggestion of a reduced risk for soya foods.[504]

A Cochrane meta-analysis of randomised, controlled, clinical trials published to March 2007 investigating relief of menopausal symptoms found no evidence that food or supplements containing phyto-oestrogens caused oestrogenic stimulation of the endometrium when used for up to 2 years. Trials of women who had breast cancer or a history of breast cancer were excluded.[505] The dosage of isoflavones was 50 to 120 mg/day, with many of the soya products containing soya protein.

One concern is that isoflavones may adversely affect thyroid function and interfere with the absorption of synthetic thyroid hormone. A 2006 review evaluated the relevant literature describing the effects of soya on thyroid function.[506] In total, 14 trials (thyroid function was not the primary health outcome in any trial) were identified where the effects of soya foods or isoflavones on at least one measure of thyroid function was assessed in presumably healthy people. Eight involved women only, four involved men, and two both men and women. With only one exception, no effects or only very modest changes, were noted in these trials. Collectively, the findings provide little evidence that soya foods or isoflavones adversely affect thyroid function in euthyroid, iodine-replete individuals. In contrast, some evidence suggests that soya, by inhibiting absorption, may increase the dose of thyroid hormone required by hypothyroid patients. In addition, there remains a theoretical concern based on in vitro and animal data that isoflavone intake by individuals with compromised thyroid function and/or marginal iodine intake may increase their risk of developing clinical hypothyroidism.

Alkaloids

Phytochemistry

Because they are a vast and diverse group of archetypal plant constituents, it is consequently difficult to arrive at a consistent definition of alkaloids. The word derives from the term 'vegetable alkali', referring to the alkaline nature of these compounds, a property that results from the presence of nitrogen. The following definition is concise and descriptive: alkaloids are alkaline (basic) nitrogen-containing heterocyclic compounds derived from higher plants often exhibiting marked pharmacological activity. However, there are several exceptions to this definition. For example, the nitrogen in ephedrine is not part of a ring, so it is not heterocyclic. For this reason, it is sometimes referred to as a protoalkaloid. Berberine is not alkaline and some alkaloids are derived from animals and micro-organisms. Generally, alkaloids are white, but some are highly coloured; for example, berberine is yellow and sanguinarine is red. (By now it should be apparent that names of alkaloids end with the letters -ine.)

Alkaloids were the first chemical drugs to be derived from plants; a mixture of morphine and narcotine was isolated from opium in 1803. They have maintained an important role in conventional drug therapy since then. Names such as codeine, morphine, atropine, quinine, pilocarpine, theophylline, colchicine, pseudoephedrine and vincristine are a familiar part of modern drug medicine. These drugs are potent pharmacological agents and their properties are well described in conventional pharmacology texts. A high risk of adverse reactions ensues from their use. In contrast, while phytotherapists do rely on plants containing alkaloids, their activity is at the milder end of the pharmacological spectrum. Alkaloids as a group are not nearly as important to the phytotherapist as they are to the conventional doctor.

Accordingly, this section will not include a broad and detailed treatment of various classes and subclasses of alkaloids, but will instead focus on a few examples important to phytotherapy. Nevertheless, it is worthwhile to consider the basic structures of the important classes of alkaloids. These are provided in the following diagrams.

Examples of each class named are: pyrrolidine – hygrine; piperidine – lobeline; pyridine – nicotine; indole – strychnine; quinoline – quinine; isoquinoline – morphine; pyrrolizidine – seneciphylline; tropane – hyoscyamine; purine (xanthine) – caffeine; imidazole – pilocarpine; quinolizidine (norlupinane) – sparteine.

Pyrrolidine

Piperidine

Pyridine

Indole

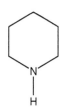

Quinoline

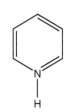

Isoquinoline

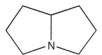

Pyrrolizidine

Tropane

Purine

Imidazole

Quinolizidine

Most alkaloids are synthesised by the plant from amino acids. If they are not, they are called pseudoalkaloids. Most of the known examples of pseudoalkaloids are isoprenoids and are referred to as terpenoid alkaloids. Aconitine from various species of aconite is an example of a diterpene alkaloid and is one of the most toxic substances known. Steroidal alkaloids are also found in plants. Some are combined as glycosides, for example solanine from potato shoots.

Despite being the most important archetypal plant constituents from a conventional perspective, the function of alkaloids in plants is only beginning to be understood. They probably have a defensive or deterrent role, but other theories are still suggested in texts, including they are a by-product of primary metabolism.

Pharmacodynamics

Alkaloids have two key properties that determine much of their pharmacology: an ability to cross the blood-brain barrier and exert depressant or stimulant effects on the central nervous system (CNS), and an ability to interact with various neurotransmitter receptors. Examples include CNS depressants such as morphine and codeine, CNS stimulants such as caffeine and cocaine and sympathetic nervous system stimulants such as ephedrine.

Alkaloids are important to phytotherapy, but their role is less significant than other archetypal plant constituents, as demonstrated by the fact that only three alkaloid-containing herbs are covered by monographs in this text, namely Chelidonium, Berberis and Hydrastis. The research on berberine is now extensive and is comprehensively reviewed in the Berberis and Hydrastis monograph. Some additional examples of important alkaloid-containing herbs and their pharmacodynamic properties are discussed below.

Lobelia (*Lobelia inflata*) and ipecacuanha root (*Cephaelis ipecacuanha*) contain emetic alkaloids (lobeline and emetine, respectively) that act as reflex expectorants at sub-emetic doses (similar to the expectorant saponins). Oral preparations of lobelia are also used as an aid to stop smoking, since lobeline is very similar to nicotine in its pharmacodynamic actions.

Several alkaloid-containing herbs are used as mild analgesics and anxiolytics. California poppy (*Eschscholtzia californica*) is a traditional medicine used by the rural population of California for its analgesic and sedative properties. Animal studies have verified these actions and demonstrated low toxicity.[507] A proprietary formula consisting of 80% California poppy and 20% *Corydalis cava* (both herbs are rich in isoquinoline alkaloids) has been the subject of clinical studies.[508] Results from two clinical trials showed that disturbed sleep behaviour could be normalised by the combination, without evidence of carry-over effects or addiction.[508] In vitro studies suggest that the two herbs co-operate in establishing an advantageous catecholamine status necessary for maintaining sedative and antidepressant effects.[509]

Various species of Ephedra contain the protoalkaloids ephedrine and pseudoephedrine.[510] Ephedra is a commonly used Chinese herb possessing diaphoretic, antipyretic, antiallergic and antiasthmatic properties. It is also favoured in phytotherapy, particularly for the latter two activities. Ephedrine has been used as a conventional treatment for asthma.

Broom tops (*Cytisus scoparius*) contains the alkaloid sparteine and is an important herb for the treatment of cardiac arrhythmias.[511] Sparteine acts as a potassium channel antagonist[512] and delays systolic depolarisation. Normal sinus frequency is slightly reduced, the refractory period is prolonged and the threshold is raised, reducing the risk of fibrillation and extrasystoles. Indications for broom tops include sinus tachycardia, ventricular extrasystoles and arrhythmias following a heart attack.[511] High doses of the herb are necessary to achieve therapeutic levels of sparteine and related alkaloids. Sparteine was once widely used as an oxytocic drug, but it fell out of favour because of the uterine spasm that occurred in women who were unable to metabolise it effectively. About 5% of male and female volunteers studied were unable to metabolise sparteine by N-oxidation[513] and this defect appeared to have a genetic basis.[514]

Pharmacokinetics in herbal medicine

Pharmacokinetics can be defined as the study of the absorption, distribution, metabolism and elimination of pharmacologically active agents in the body. This discussion is not intended to be a primer on the principles of pharmacokinetics (there are appropriate texts for this purpose); however, certain basic issues will be discussed where there is particular relevance to plant chemicals.

One important issue that should underlie much of the study of herbal pharmacokinetics is that herbs are not usually directly introduced into the bloodstream by injection or other means, but rather the traditional oral or topical routes of administration are preferred. This renders the study of bioavailability of paramount importance for active constituents in plants. Bioavailability can be defined as the degree of absorption of active substances into the bloodstream after oral doses. Hence bioavailability is also a factor of the preparation that is used to deliver the dose of active substance. Conventional drugs intended for oral use are designed to have good bioavailability. In contrast, phytochemicals are of natural origin and may exhibit unusual or poor bioavailability that may be further compounded by the choice of dosage preparation.

In this discussion, the issue of the bioavailability of several of the archetypal plant constituents will be emphasised. For pharmacokinetic details related to specific herbs, see the monograph section (Part Three) of this book.

Herbal clinicians and students sometimes question the value of studying herbal pharmacokinetics. The following premises should be considered:

- If it is accepted that medicinal plants act at a chemical level in the body (as well as possibly other levels of activity), then knowledge of how their chemicals behave in the body is vital.
- Given that, with a few exceptions in some countries, oral and topical doses are used for herbal medicines, a better knowledge of bioavailability is critical to meet the challenge of future health problems.

Specifically the information derived from the detailed study of herbal pharmacokinetics can deliver:

- information to further assess the traditional and anecdotal uses of a medicinal plant
- better information on which to base rational dosages
- a better interpretation of scientific information, particularly in vitro research or in vivo studies where the active compounds are administered by injection. There is an abundance of misinformation in the herbal literature related to excessive extrapolation from such studies, with no consideration of bioavailability
- a better appreciation of the safety and toxicity of a plant
- anticipation of potential herb-drug interactions
- supporting evidence for the synergistic nature of herbal medicine

- ways to optimise the bioavailability and hence efficacy of herbal medicines.

The study of herbal pharmacokinetics is a unique and extraordinarily complex field. This is for the following reasons:

- The chemical complexity of plant medicines and the potential interactions between constituents
- The differing bioavailability of different compounds
- Often large polar molecules are involved that might be expected to have poor and unpredictable bioavailability
- The active components are often not known, so the components in the plant that should be studied cannot be identified
- Unlike drugs, herbal medicines are not designed for predictable pharmacokinetic behaviour, and in particular natural compounds are often metabolised in the digestive tract – that is, they are pro-drugs; this key feature is emphasised in this chapter.

But this does not mean to imply that the existing information is without value. On the contrary, many studies now provide a better understanding of this topic and inform clinical practice.

Before particular examples of the pharmacokinetics of plant constituents are discussed, it is worthwhile to examine some of the key issues pertaining to bioavailability. The bioavailability of a molecule depends on several factors that determine how it traverses the barrier of the gastrointestinal tract and survives into the bloodstream. These include:

- the pharmaceutical preparation
- the size of the molecule – very large molecules still have some bioavailability (about 1% or less) which may be due to pinocytosis
- the fat (lipid) solubility of the molecule – the more fat-soluble, the better the bioavailability (see Table 2.2[515] for examples of how fat solubility influences bioavailability for cardioactive glycosides)
- the water solubility of the molecule – if a molecule is both water- and fat-soluble it will exhibit very good bioavailability because it will dissolve in the digestive juices and then cross lipid membranes; otherwise, purely

Table 2.2 Effect of lipid solubility on bioavailability[515]

Cardiac glycoside	P	B%
g-Strophanthin	0.01	6.6
Convallatoxin	0.33	13.6
Digoxin	18.2	26.4
Digitoxin	70	74.9
Oleandrin	338	86.0

B = bioavailability; P = partition between water and octanol, an indication of fat solubility.

water-soluble molecules can be expected to have poor bioavailability; ionisation of a molecule usually denotes poor bioavailability

- specific factors related to crossing the gut wall, such as active transport
- factors within the gut – interaction with food, stability in the gut, gastric emptying
- metabolism in the gut and first-pass metabolism by the liver
- individual factors in the patient, including the influence of genetic and pathological factors.

Food is known to affect the bioavailability of conventional drugs (see Tables 2.3 and 2.4[516] for examples). The presence or absence of food may also influence the absorption and bioavailability of plant constituents. For example, acetyl-11-keto-beta-boswellic acid (AKBA) from *Boswellia serrata* exhibits better bioavailability with a high fat meal,[517] whereas a high fat meal reduces the bioavailability of resveratrol from *Polygonum cuspidatum*.[66]

Grapefruit juice (GFJ) is a plant substance that can exert a marked effect on bioavailability. For example, in early studies it increased the bioavailability of oral 17-beta-oestradiol and its metabolite oestrone.[518] GFJ also substantially increased the bioavailability of the following drugs: felopidine,[519] caffeine,[520] nifedipine and similar drugs,[521] cyclosporine[522] and triazolam[523] and similar drugs. The major interaction seems to be in the gut wall with enzymes belonging to various cytochrome P450 subfamilies.[524] It also appears to inhibit renal 11-beta-hydroxysteroid dehydrogenase in humans and could therefore potentiate the side effects of licorice.[525] Although the flavonoids naringin and naringenin were at first implicated, they are probably not the active components.[526,527] In fact, the furanocoumarin bergamottin and related compounds appear to be largely responsible for this activity.[528] This ability of plant furanocoumarins to inhibit drug-metabolising enzymes was first noted by Korean researchers in 1983.[529] A 2011 review noted that GFJ demonstrated multiple interactions with drugs leading to loss of therapeutic effects or increased side effects.[530] GFJ decreases presystemic metabolism through competitive or mechanism-based inhibition of gut wall CYP3A4 isoenzymes and P-glycoprotein. In addition multidrug resistance protein-2 or organic anion-transporting polypeptide inhibition may play a role. The review confirmed that, although GFJ contains high amounts of flavonoids (such as naringin, naringenin), furanocoumarins (especially 6′,7′-dihydroxybergamottin and bergamottin) are the main phytochemicals involved in the pharmacokinetic interactions. As compounds of GFJ show additive or synergistic effects, all the major furanocoumarins are necessary for the maximal inhibitory effect. Related citrus fruits or other plants containing furanocoumarins may also present pharmacological interactions yet to be discovered.

This phenomenon raises the question of how other plants and their phytochemicals might influence the bioavailability of both drugs and herbal constituents. The example of hyperforin in St John's wort is now well studied in this regard (see the St John's wort monograph).

Bioavailability is also affected by the preparation used to deliver the dose of the medicine. This area of study has been largely neglected for herbal medicines. However, some general statements about aqueous preparations such as infusions and decoctions can be proposed. Infusions and decoctions extract water-soluble compounds from plants. Many of these will have poor bioavailability. One important exception is plants containing essential oils taken by infusion. Here the hot water acts almost as a distillation medium and the oil will collect on the surface of the water. The addition of saponin-containing herbs to the mixture may increase the solubility of compounds not as water-soluble, which may then have better bioavailability. However, this advantage has been disputed (see previously under saponins). This practice is often observed in traditional Chinese medicine, a therapeutic system that relies heavily on aqueous preparations. Changes in water-soluble compounds in the digestive tract, most significantly the conversion of glycosides to aglycones in the caecum and large bowel, will render them more lipid-soluble. They can then be absorbed as the aglycone. In general, however, bioavailability and solubility considerations suggest that infusions and decoctions are inferior preparations for the extraction and delivery of herbal actives. The exception is where

Table 2.3 Drugs with absorption enhanced by food[516]

Drug	Mechanism
Carbamazepine	Increased bile production; enhanced dissolution and absorption
Diazepam	Food enhances enterohepatic recycling; increased dissolution secondary to gastric acid secretion
Griseofulvin	Drug is lipid soluble; enhanced absorption
Metoprolol	Food may reduce first-pass extraction and metabolism
Phenytoin	Delayed gastric emptying and increased bile production improve dissolution and absorption

Table 2.4 Drugs with absorption decreased by food[516]

Drug	Mechanism
Isoniazid	Food raises gastric pH preventing dissolution and absorption; also delayed gastric emptying
Captopril	Mechanism unknown
Chlorpromazine	Drug undergoes first-pass metabolism in gut; delayed gastric emptying affects bioavailability
Tetracyclines	Bind with calcium ions or iron salts forming insoluble chelates

those actives are largely water-soluble anyway, such as some saponins, tannins, polysaccharides and proteins. However, only small quantities of these relatively large molecules will be absorbed as such (see later).

Salicin

A good starting point in the study of herbal pharmacokinetics is those archetypal plant constituents that have been relatively well investigated. The phenolic glycoside salicin and the anthraquinone glycosides are two such examples.

Salicin and its conversion products are illustrated in Figure 2.2 and a schematic diagram of the pharmacokinetics of salicin is provided in Figure 2.3.[531,532] As shown in Figure 2.3, salicin derivatives are first converted into salicin in the stomach or small intestine. The salicin may then be absorbed in the small intestine, but in humans it is mainly carried to the distal ileum or colon where gut flora convert the glycoside into its aglycone, known as salicyl alcohol. The salicyl alcohol is absorbed and oxidised in the blood, tissue and liver to give salicylic acid, the main active form. The excretion of these various products is also outlined in Figure 2.3.

Despite the elaborate route by which salicin (and indeed willow bark) delivers salicylic acid into the bloodstream, the relative bioavailabilities of sodium salicylate and salicin are remarkably similar (Fig. 2.4[531]). The curve for salicin is slightly lower and flatter, indicating a greater half-life. The rapid absorption of salicin as salicylic acid additionally implies

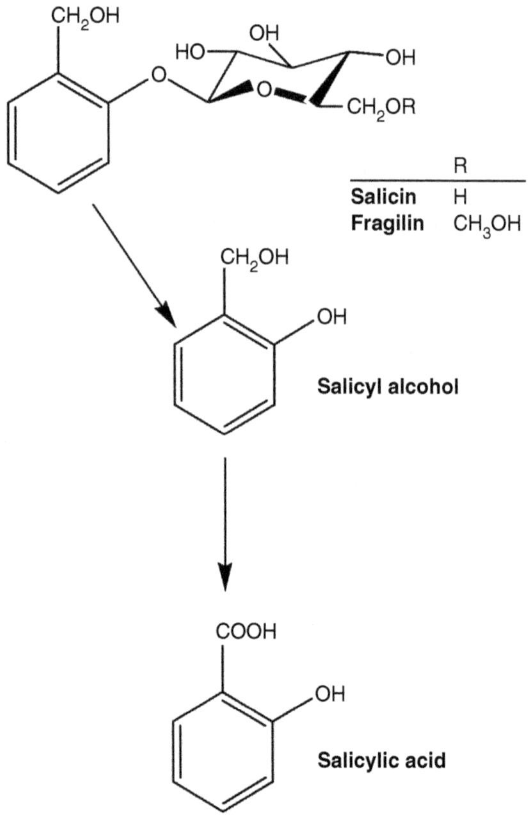

that its conversion is also rapid, suggesting the distal ileum or caecum as the site of conversion rather than the large intestine (orocaecal transit time is typically up to a few hours).

At this point, it is worth reflecting upon the traditional use of willow bark and the history of aspirin. When scientists in the 19th century began to investigate the antipyretic and anti-inflammatory effects of willow bark, salicin was isolated as the active compound. Salicylic acid was more readily synthesised and was adopted into mainstream therapy, but had the drawback of being a strong irritant to the stomach. This led to the development of aspirin, a derivative of salicylic acid, in an attempt to minimise the gastric irritation. (Unfortunately, aspirin was still a gastric irritant, but it was more active than salicylic acid as an analgesic and antiplatelet agent.) Had the early scientists instead preferred salicin, they might have recognised that nature had already designed a derivative of salicylic acid that gave a good yield of bioavailable salicylic acid and was kind to the stomach.

This proposition is supported by an in vivo study.[533] When salicin was administered orally to rats, salicylic acid appeared slowly in the plasma and levels increased gradually, in contrast to the rapid appearance observed after oral administration of sodium salicylate or saligenin. However, oral salicin still significantly reduced yeast-induced fever, producing a normal body temperature. Salicin did not induce gastric lesions, even at a high dose; conversely sodium salicylate and saligenin induced severe gastric lesions in a dose-dependent manner. When given to germ-free rats around 20% of the salicin was recovered intact from the digestive tract and no saligenin was found. These results provided clear evidence that salicin is a pro-drug, as discussed above, that is gradually transported to the lower part of the intestine and hydrolysed to saligenin by intestinal bacteria, producing its therapeutic effects without gastric injury.

Anthraquinone glycosides

Early research on the laxative properties of anthraquinones and their glycosides baffled researchers. When equivalent doses were used, only the glycosides were active orally, not their aglycones. However, when equivalent doses were administered by injection, the reverse situation applied: the aglycones were more active. Equally intriguing were the observations that oral doses of the anthraquinone glycosides took 6 to 8h to exert their laxative effect and the effective dose for laxation often varied dramatically from person to person.

The modern understanding of the pharmacokinetics of anthraquinone glycosides provides a simple explanation for these paradoxical observations. This is illustrated schematically in Figure 2.5.[534]

As anthraquinone glycosides pass through the digestive tract, a significant proportion undergoes polymerisation to inactive polymers. Any remaining glycoside is unchanged and unabsorbed until it reaches the large intestine. There the action of certain bowel flora converts the glycosides into their anthrone aglycones. These active aglycones then exert a laxative action in situ in the colon.[534]

	R
Salicin	H
Fragilin	CH_3OH

Salicyl alcohol

Salicylic acid

Figure 2.2 • Salicin and its conversion products.

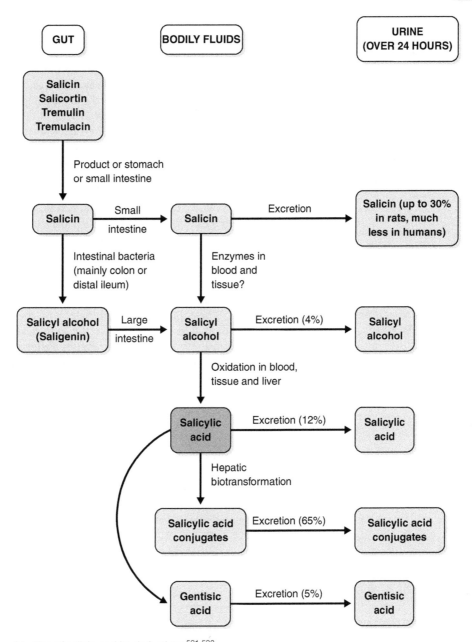

Figure 2.3 • Pharmacokinetics of salicin and its derivatives.[531,532]

Hence, the anthraquinone glycoside given by injection exerts less activity, because this is not the active form. On the other hand, the aglycone given orally also exerts little activity because it is broken down or absorbed before it reaches the colon. (Some modern laxative drugs are anthrone aglycones, but they are administered orally in quite high doses.) The 6 to 8 h lag-time for activity reflects the time it takes for ingested anthraquinone glycosides to reach the appropriate part of the colon for conversion into aglycones.

We can only wonder at this elegant and, when one considers the quantities of liberated anthrone aglycone involved, exquisitely sensitive mechanism designed by nature. One inference from this example is that the composition of an individual's bowel flora is highly relevant to the pharmacokinetic equation and hence to the final pharmacological effect.[534] This is a common theme for several of the archetypal plant constituents and emphasises the herbal clinician's obsession with the health of the gut, not just as the central focus for restoring robust health, but also for delivering effective therapy.

Glycosides and gastric modification

A number of plant glycosides are modified by the action of gastric acid or the alkaline conditions of the duodenum. The following examples and their implications serve to illustrate this phenomenon.

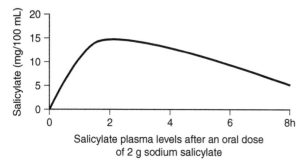

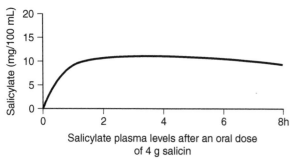

Figure 2.4 • Relative bioavailabilities of salicin and salicylic acid (doses are approximately equivalent).[531]

Harpagoside from devil's claw (*Harpagophytum procumbens*) has oral anti-inflammatory activity (Fig. 2.6). However, when it is incubated with gastric acid, which generates harpagogenin from harpagoside, it tends to lose this activity in oral dose models.[535] While harpagoside may not be the final bioavailable form, this research suggests that the action of gastric acid is detrimental to the anti-inflammatory activity of devil's claw. Preparations of this herb should therefore be enterically coated or at least taken between meals to optimise the bioavailability of anti-inflammatory components. (See the devil's claw monograph for a further discussion of this topic.)

The valepotriates (Fig. 2.7) of valerian have cytotoxic activity when administered by injection, but do not exhibit this effect after oral doses. The former observation initially raised concerns about the safety of valerian, but it is now clear that valepotriates are quite unstable in aqueous solution and are decomposed by gastric acid. The breakdown products of the valepotriates still possess some sedative activity.[536] (See the valerian monograph for more details.)

The following example is not of therapeutic significance but it does illustrate that the empirical basis for the traditional use of plants sometimes reflects an implicit understanding of pharmacokinetic issues. *Salvia divinorum* is a

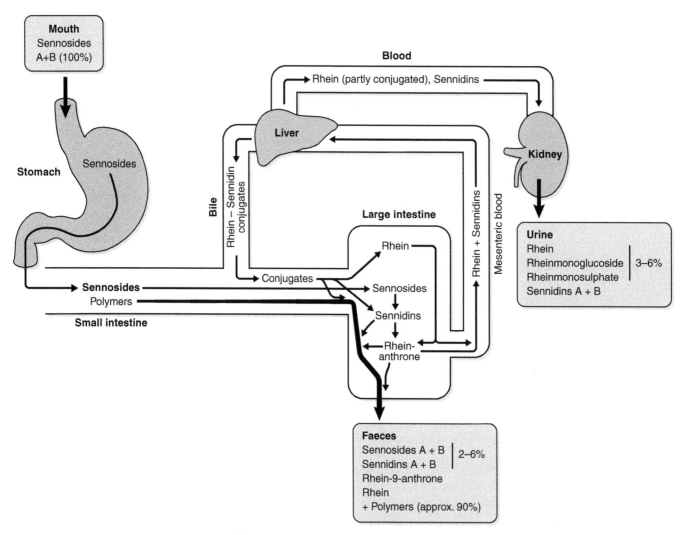

Figure 2.5 • Pharmacokinetics of sennosides.[534]

species of sage with hallucinogenic properties. Traditionally the fresh leaves are chewed for this effect, which led to the belief that the hallucinogenic component(s) were inactivated by drying the herb. Research has revealed that this is not the case. The active hallucinogenic component in *Salvia divinorum* is salvinorin A (Fig. 2.8).[537] This is converted by gastric acid into salvinorin B, which is inactive. Hence the chewing of leaves by the shamans was in fact a delivery mechanism for salvinorin A that bypassed decomposition in the stomach. That the hallucinogenic quantities of salvinorin A can be absorbed through the oral mucosa underlines the potent activity of this compound.

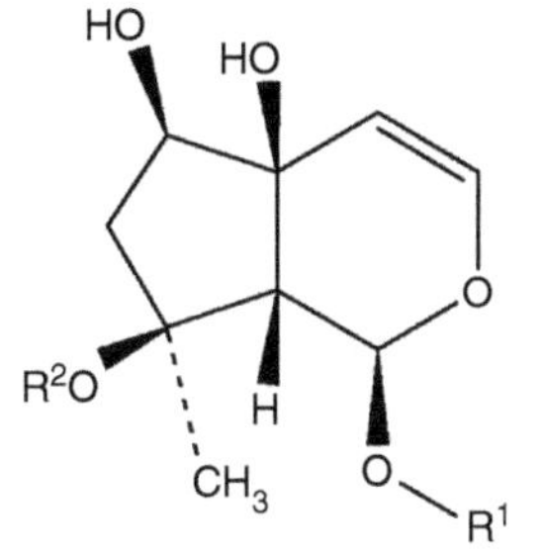

Flavonoid glycosides and enteric modification

Flavonoid glycosides are a common component of many plants and are a significant class of archetypal plant constituents with pharmacological activity. However, in vitro models dominate the pharmacodynamic research on flavonoids and their glycosides. This is of concern because an understanding has existed for some time (and has been repeatedly confirmed) that flavonoids tend to have poor bioavailability as such, because they are largely decomposed by bowel flora.

Studies have shown that flavonoid-O-glycosides are converted into the aglycone by bowel flora. But the decomposition can extend further than this; the aglycones undergo further breakdown by a process known as C-ring fission (the C-ring is the central ring in the flavonoid structure) to give two different phenolic products. An example of C-ring fission is illustrated in Figure 2.9. The ring fission products for several common flavonoids, flavonoid glycosides and related products are summarised in Table 2.5[538] and a general scheme for the pharmacokinetics of many flavonoid glycosides is outlined in Figure 2.10.

Studies have also shown the following:

- Oral doses of flavonoid aglycones are less bioavailable (as the flavonoid) than their glycosides because they are more susceptible to ring fission
- Levels of a flavonoid aglycone in the bloodstream will vary according to:
  - whether it is administered as an aglycone or glycoside
  - if given as a glycoside, the form of the glycosidic pro-drug
  - the nature of the individual bowel flora, which is partly dependent on the individual diet.[539]

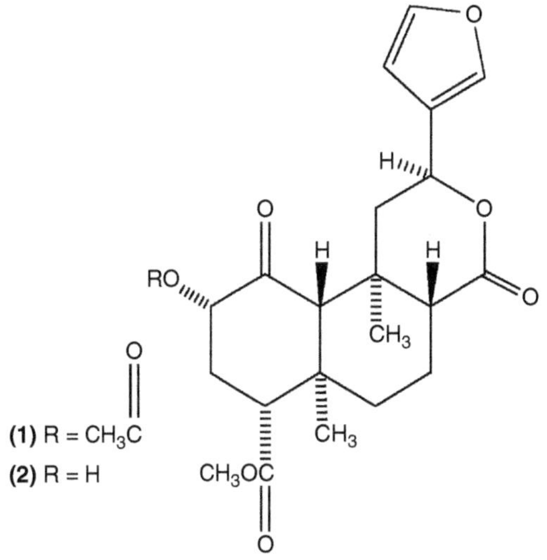

	R¹	R²
Harpagoside	Glucose	*trans*-Cinnamoyl
Harpagide	Glucose	H
Harpagogenin	H	H

Figure 2.6 • Harpagoside from devil's claw.

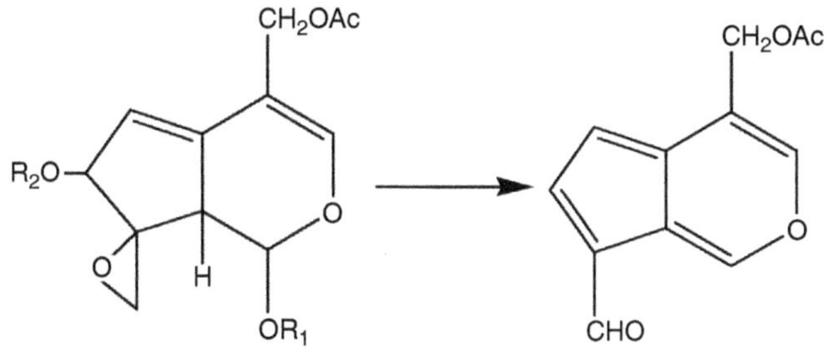

R₁	R₂	
Aiv	Iv	1-Acevaltrate
Iv	Iv	Valtrate

Ac	CH₃CO–	**Acetyl**
Iv		**Isovaleryl**
Aiv		**Acetoxyisovaleryl**

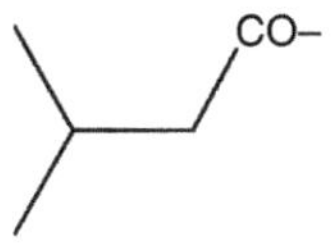

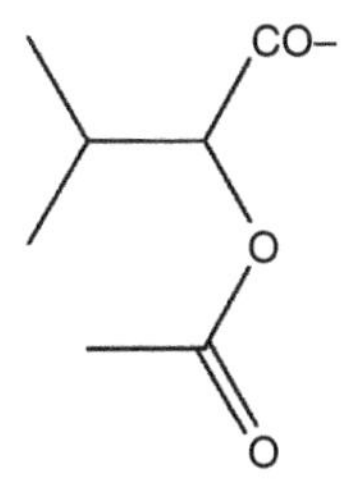

Figure 2.7 • Valepotriates from valerian.

(1) R = CH₃C

(2) R = H

Figure 2.8 • Salvinorins A (1) and B (2) isolated from *S. divinorum*.

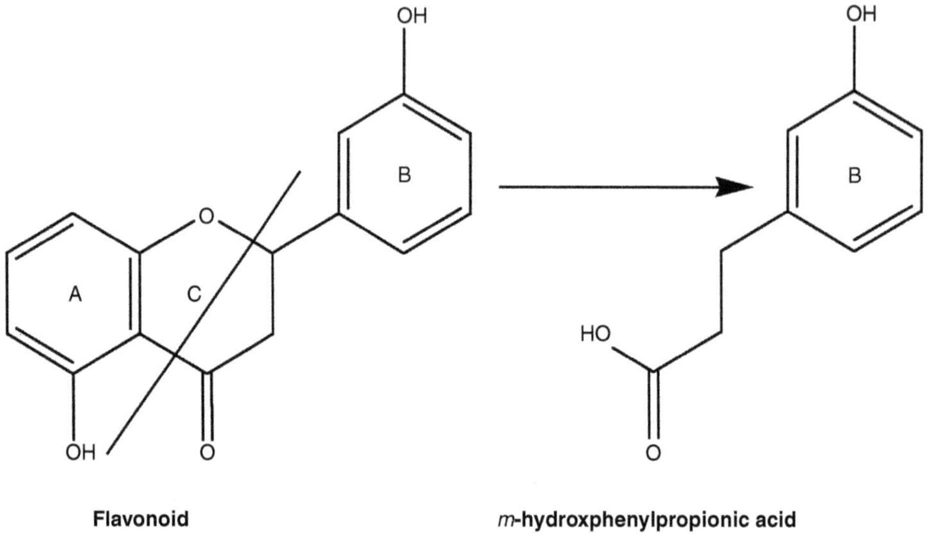

Flavonoid   ***m*-hydroxphenylpropionic acid**

Figure 2.9 • An example of C–ring fission.

This picture of flavonoid pharmacokinetics needs to be modified in one specific area following the work of a German group of scientists early this century. Their study of the bioavailability of quercetin in various forms provided new and important information about the pharmacokinetics of flavonoids.[540–542] The pharmacokinetics of two quercetin glycosides, and plant extracts containing these, were investigated in 12 healthy volunteers in a crossover study.[540,542] This was because prior investigation had indicated that the bioavailability of quercetin may actually be improved by the presence of a sugar on the molecule. That is, certain quercetin glycosides can deliver quercetin more effectively into the bloodstream, presumably via active uptake by enterocytes. (Even this enhanced bioavailability was only about 5% of the amount ingested.)[541]

Each volunteer received an onion extract (containing quercetin-4'-O-glucoside) or pure quercetin-4'-O-glucoside, both equivalent to 100 mg of quercetin; or buckwheat tea (containing quercetin-3-O-rutinoside) or pure quercetin-3-O-rutinoside (rutin), both equivalent to 200 mg of quercetin. Pure quercetin was not detected in the human plasma samples. Instead, four different quercetin glucuronides (QG) were detected. These were presumably formed following uptake by the action of enterocytes.

The form of the flavonoid greatly influenced the rate and extent of QG appearance in the bloodstream. After administration of quercetin-4'-O-glucoside or onions, maximum plasma levels of QG were reached after 0.5 to 1 h. But only 5 to 10 h after administration of rutin or buckwheat tea did QG appear in volunteers' bloodstreams. Despite the fact they were given at half the dose, the levels of QG achieved from onions and quercetin-4'-O-glucoside were about four times those achieved from rutin and buckwheat tea. The plant matrix enhanced the rate and extent of QG appearance, but to a much lesser extent than the form of the flavonoid.

These simple and elegant findings add a new dimension to our understanding of the pharmacokinetics of flavonoids:

- Aglycones (such as quercetin) have poor or even zero bioavailability

Table 2.5 Flavonoid ring fission metabolites[538]

Flavonoid administered	Ring fission products
Quercetin, rutin	3,4-dihydroxphenylacetic acid, 3-methoxy-4-hydroxyphenylacetic acid, *m*-hydroxyphenylacetic acid
Hesperidin, diosmin, eriodictyol, homoeriodictyol	*m*-hydroxyphenylpropionic acid, *m*-coumaric acid (rat), 3-hydroxy-4-methoxyphenyl-hydracrylic acid (human)
(+)-Catechin	delta-(hydroxphenyl)-gamma-valerolactones, *m*-hydroxyphenylpropionic acid, *m*-hydroxybenzoic acid, *m*-hydroxyhippuric acid
Kaempferol	delta-(*p*-hydroxyphenyl)-gamma-valerolactone, *p*-hydroxyphenylacetic acid
Myricetin, myrictrin	3,5-dihydroxyphenylacetic acid
Tricetin, tricin	*m*-hydroxyphenylacetic acid, 3,5-dihydroxyphenylpropionic acid, *m*-hydroxyphenylpropionic acid

- There is an active uptake and metabolism of flavonoid glycosides by enterocytes that is determined by the nature of their sugar (with a preference for glucose)
- Before the flavonoid is taken up by the enterocyte, it is probably hydrolysed to the aglycone by a membrane-bound beta-glucosidase
- Quercetin-4'-O-glucoside is taken up in the small intestine, whereas rutin (which has a glucose and a mannose = rutinoside) is not

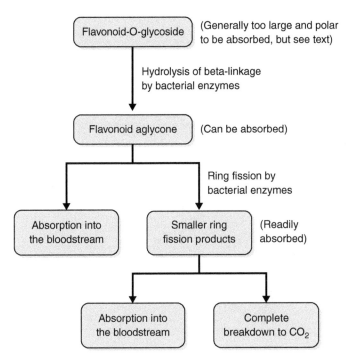

Figure 2.10 • Pharmacokinetics of flavonoid glycosides.

- Presumably rutin travels to the large intestine (hence the lag in QG appearance), where the terminal mannose is removed by bacteria, exposing the glucose which then results in uptake by enterocytes
- Measurement of the renal elimination of flavonoids suggested that at least 6% of the flavonoid dose was absorbed when given as onions.

QG have slightly more antioxidant activity than quercetin, but will not exert much effect in plasma as antioxidants because they are tightly bound to plasma proteins. However, they could well become active at target tissues, especially after removal of the glucuronide group.

The above study could provide no information on the uptake of C-ring fission compounds, since these are also metabolites naturally found in the bloodstream and it was therefore difficult to detect any changes in their levels above the natural background.

A 2011 review supported this perspective, albeit with some subtle modifications.[543] As described above, lactase phlorizin hydrolase (LPH), a membrane-bound beta-glucosidase, is able to liberate aglycones into the intestinal lumen, where they passively diffuse across the small intestinal membrane. However, cytosolic beta-glucosidase may also be involved. As this particular enzyme is located intracellularly in the enterocyte, active transport of the flavonoid glycoside via the sugar transporter SGLT-1 (sodium-dependent glucose transporter) is first required. Flavonoid glycosides that are not substrates of LPH or SGLT-1 will pass to the colon where bacterial hydrolysis will produce the aglycone and C-ring fission products. Of course, the action of LPH or SGLT-1 is not quantitative, with much of the flavonoid glycosides that are

their substrates still passing unchanged to the colon. In other words, the actions of LPH and SGLT-1 only render a small percentage of a flavonoid glycoside bioavailable in the small intestine.

Once absorbed, the flavonoid aglycones are subject to three main types of conjugation: methylation, sulphation and glucuronidation.[543] The extent of conjugation is high and only a small percentage of free flavonoid aglycones is present in the plasma.[543,544] The presence of conjugated metabolites in the portal blood of rats suggests that conjugation first occurs in the enterocytes before further metabolism in the liver.[543,545]

The issue of the bioavailability of the flavonoid aglycone quercetin is controversial. Many nutritional supplement companies market products containing quercetin. The rationale for including quercetin in such products is often largely based on in vitro research or in vivo models following dosage by injection (although there are also clinical trials demonstrating positive effects from high doses - see previous). The consensus of studies is that the bioavailability of quercetin (as quercetin) is poor. This is due to its propensity to undergo C-ring fission. Following the Zutphen Elderly Study and the Netherlands Cohort Study where flavonol and flavone dietary intakes were inversely associated with mortality from coronary heart disease and risk of stroke, Dutch researchers once again studied quercetin bioavailability.[546] Conclusions from their study on ileostomy patients were uncertain because they did not measure quercetin in the bloodstream.[547] It was assumed that, because of the ileostomy, any unrecovered quercetin was absorbed. But significant microbial degradation could also have occurred. This is supported by the minimal level of quercetin (0.5% of original dose) found in subjects' urine. Nonetheless, this study has been misinterpreted by many authors as unequivocally demonstrating a high oral bioavailability for quercetin. More recent studies tend to confirm the relatively low and variable bioavailability of intact quercetin.[230,544] Gut flora metabolism might account for a large part of this variability.

One study of the C-ring fission products of quercetin found that 3,4-dihydroxyphenylacetic acid possessed significant antioxidant activity.[548] In vitro antiplatelet activity is also suggested in another.[549] Pharmacodynamic research on flavonoids should include more studies on their C-ring fission products, which in many instances are probably the main bioavailable and active form of this important group of archetypal plant constituents.[550]

Isoflavones

As noted earlier, the isoflavones are a group of archetypal plant constituents attracting increasing attention because of their affinity for oestrogen receptors. The principal isoflavones are the glycosides genistin and daidzin and their aglycones genistein and daidzein, from the soya plant, and the aglycones formononetin and biochanin A from red clover (see Fig. 2.11). Formononetin can be converted to daidzein, which in turn can be metabolised to equol by bowel flora. This is a significant reaction pathway from a pharmacodynamic perspective, because equol has substantially more oestrogenic activity than

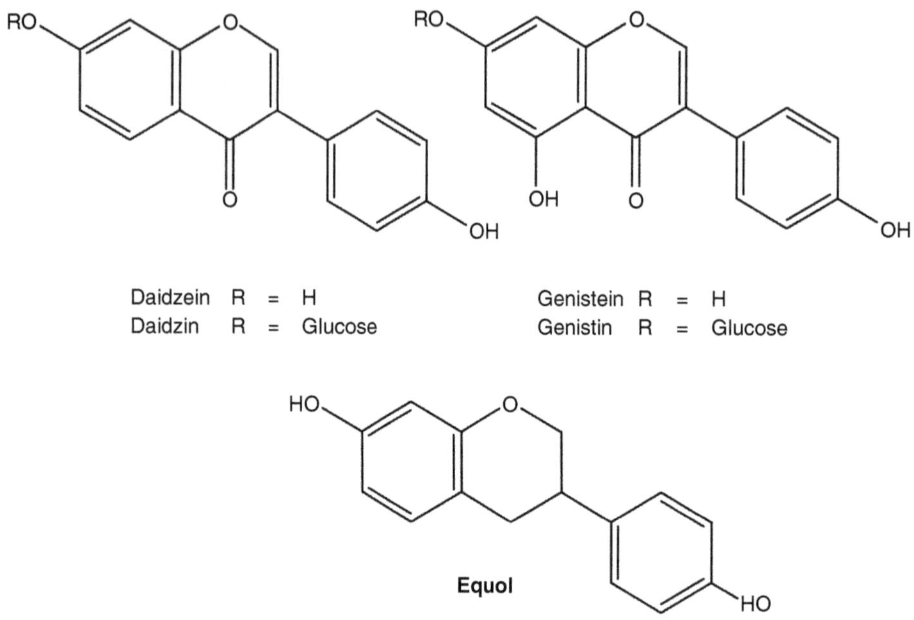

Figure 2.11 • Major isoflavones and equol.

its precursors. However, equol appears to be produced to different degrees in different people. Table 2.6[551] illustrates that individuals can be grouped into high and low equol producers. The high equol producers are likely to experience significantly greater oestrogenic effects from the consumption of soya or red clover.

Early studies also found the following:

- Soya isoflavones are 85% degraded in the intestine[552]
- Differences in faecal flora account for the differing metabolism of soya isoflavones[553]
- Faecal flora could completely degrade genistein and daidzein[553]
- Differences in faecal excretion of isoflavones profoundly altered isoflavone bioavailability: higher faecal excretion was correlated with higher bioavailability. Such people may have fewer bacteria that degrade isoflavones, leaving more intact for absorption.[548] Bioavailability varied from 13% to 35% depending on the individual gut microflora[553]
- Soya protein (containing isoflavone glycosides) increased follicular phase length in women, while miso (containing isoflavone aglycones) did not.[554] This suggests that the glycosidic group delays the degradation of isoflavones, resulting in higher bioavailability of their aglycones or equol.

These earlier studies served to emphasise the importance of bowel flora in determining the bioavailability and hence pharmacodynamic activity of isoflavones.

Recent reviews of the pharmacokinetics of isoflavones have noted similar mechanisms to flavonoids. LPH on the enterocyte cell membrane is thought to play a key role in the removal of sugar from isoflavone glycosides. However, in contrast to the flavonoid glycosides, there is no evidence that isoflavone glycosides are transported by SGLT-1 (or other transmembrane transporters) into the enterocyte cytoplasm.[555] Any glycoside not remaining after passage through the small intestine is converted to the aglycone by colonic bacteria.

Contradictory results have been recorded for the differences in bioavailability between isoflavone aglycones and glycosides.[556] However, a review of 16 human pharmacokinetic studies determined that genistin (the glycoside) was about 60% more bioavailable than genistein (the aglycone). Similarly, daidzin was around 80% more bioavailable than daidzein.[557] These reviewers stated that some comparative studies used different food sources to compare aglycone versus glycoside bioavailability (for example, comparing tempeh with soya bean pieces), yielding contradictory results that were confounded by food matrix effects. Both reviews confirmed that isoflavones possess substantially higher relative bioavailabilities than flavonoids.[556,557]

Equol production was significantly higher after ingestion of daidzin than daidzein, but this has not been confirmed in every study, again possibly because of food matrix effects. Genistin and daidzin exhibit relatively similar bioavailabilities, as do genistein and daidzein. It was thought that the greater urinary excretion of daidzein metabolites reflected its greater bioavailability compared with genistein. However, the explanation for this finding is that a greater fraction of genistein is eliminated via bile.[556,557]

The nature of isoflavone metabolites in plasma is the same after glycoside or aglycone ingestion. Glycosides are not found. Unconjugated aglycones represent about 5% of the total level in plasma, together with their main metabolites the 7-O-glucuronides and 4'-O-glucuronides, with smaller proportions of sulphate esters. Additional metabolites include equol, dihydroequol and dihydrogenistein. Equol itself possesses good bioavailability and is excreted as the glucuronide.[555,556]

Table 2.6 Comparison of the urinary excretion rates of daidzein and two daidzein[551] metabolites in individuals over a 3-day period following soya challenge*

Metabolite	Mean (SD) excretion (μmol) per 3 days	
	<8 μmol equol (n=8)	>25 μmol equol (n=4)
Daidzein	23.05 (12.43)	14.95 (6.69)
Equol	1.53 (2.60)	64.89 (59.23)
O–Dma	21.72 (17.93)	6.97 (6.47)

Note: Equol is substantially more oestrogenic than daidzein or O–Dma.
*Individuals are grouped as either low equol producers (less than 8 μmol in 3 days) or high equol producers (over 25 μmol in 3 days).

Saponins

If a saponin exhibits good fat solubility it can be absorbed unchanged in significant quantities in the small intestine. This is the case for many cardiac glycosides, a related chemical group. If saponins are not absorbed, they will pass to the large intestine where the gut flora will convert them to the sapogenin (aglycone). The sapogenin usually has better lipid solubility and will be absorbed to some extent. Hence, in these cases the saponin acts as a pro-drug. Since the bioactivity of saponins may be due to their aglycone, the extrapolation of in vitro results for saponins is potentially unreliable.

Glycyrrhizin (GL) is a triterpenoid saponin with hepatoprotective activity in vitro and by injection. It also has antiviral activity, even against HIV-1. This has led to suggestions that oral doses of licorice might be used as a systemic antiviral treatment or for hepatoprotective activity. Early pharmacokinetic experiments with licorice or GL demonstrated that the aglycone glycyrrhetinic acid (GA) was the predominant form absorbed into the bloodstream after oral doses.[558,559] GL is converted to GA by human intestinal flora.[560] Some GL may be absorbed, although this could also be recycled GA-glucuronide being misread as GL on chromatograms.[558,561] So licorice may possess antiviral activity after oral doses, but only if the GA-glucuronide or GA itself possesses this activity. GA has been shown to be more hepatoprotective than GL,[562] so licorice may also prove to be a valuable hepatoprotective herb (this awaits clinical confirmation for oral doses). (For a further discussion of the pharmacokinetics of glycyrrhizin, with a focus on the human data, see the licorice monograph.)

Other triterpenoid saponins appear to follow a similar pathway, for example the ginsenosides.[563] The bacterial metabolism and subsequent pharmacokinetics of ginsenosides are complex, because these saponins typically contain several sugars bonded at various positions on the triterpenoid structure. Hence, metabolism by the gut flora usually occurs in several stages as sugars are progressively stripped from the molecule. (For a discussion of the key issues pertaining to the pharmacokinetics of the ginsenosides, see the ginseng monograph.) Some studies on the bioavailability of steroidal saponins have also been published. Ruscus extract (1 g), containing 60 mg degluconeoruscin and other steroidal saponins, was orally administered to three human volunteers.[564] Plasma analysis showed significant absorption: degluconeoruscin concentrations peaked after about 90 minutes. Hence, some steroidal saponins may therefore show good bioavailability (this work does need to be repeated). However, others probably follow the same pattern as glycyrrhizin; the aglycone formed after colonic bacterial metabolism is the absorbed form. This is supported by extensive historical work on cardioactive glycosides showing that some glycosides, such as digitoxin, are quantitatively absorbed (the oral dose of digitoxin is the same as the intravenous dose). In contrast, ouabain (from Strophanthus) exhibited poor and erratic oral absorption and was only given by injection.

Tannins and catechins

Because of their large size, high affinity to bond with proteins and poor lipid solubility, tannins have negligible bioavailability as such. Hence, the activity of tannins (and the herbs that contain them) should be explained in terms of local effects. This poor bioavailability of intact tannins is important, since hydrolysable tannins absorbed into the bloodstream can cause hepatotoxicity. Many common herbs would be poisonous if tannins were highly bioavailable. Also tannins injected subcutaneously cause cancers, so it is also fortunate that they do not penetrate the skin. Breakdown products of tannins produced in the colon by gut flora (and perhaps spontaneously in the small intestine in the case of hydrolysable tannins) are absorbed and probably explain many of the modern uses of tannin and OPC-containing herbs (see previous).

Early in vitro experiments found that ellagic acid was liberated from condensed tannins at pH 7 to 8 (not at pH 2) and also by microflora when in contact with caecum contents (ellagic acid has antioxidant and anticancer properties).[565] About 95% of orally administered tannic acid is decomposed (as assessed by faecal excretion).[566] Tannic acid is a hydrolysable tannin that probably releases gallic acid and other compounds on decomposition. Condensed tannins, OPCs and green tea polyphenols show more complex decomposition patterns, but microflora again produce smaller bioavailable phenolic compounds (see below).[567]

The probable behaviour of tannins as they pass through the digestive tract is summarised in Figure 2.12. Apart from antioxidant activity and other systemic effects from the decomposition products of tannins, all the other possible effects are due to local activity at the designated site. The remote astringency and antihaemorrhagic properties sometimes attributed to oral doses of tannin-containing herbs must be in doubt (in other words, tannins given orally will not, for example, astringe lung tissue or staunch uterine bleeding, unless such effects are due to their smaller breakdown products).

Because of their widespread occurrence in many foods and beverages (for example berries, nuts and wine), the bioavailability and metabolism of ellagitannins has been the subject of several studies and a 2010 review.[568] The review noted the following:

- In vitro digestion studies have shown that in general ellagitannins are stable under stimulated stomach conditions
- Under the physiological conditions of the small intestine (neutral to mild alkaline pH) there is hydrolysis and release of free ellagic acid
- Microbial metabolites of ellagic acid are then formed, mainly urolithins (A to D), which are largely absorbed and glucuronidated by enterocytes and in the liver (in both humans and rodents)
- Low levels of intact ellagitannin and ellagic acid may also be absorbed, although results are inconsistent
- In human studies large interindividual variability has been observed in levels of urolithins (probably related to gut flora variability)
- The urolithins undergo enterohepatic circulation and their conjugates are the main metabolites detected in plasma and urine.

As stated earlier, OPCs are a part of the archetypal group known as condensed tannins. Products high in OPCs, such as pine bark and grapeseed extracts, enjoy enormous popularity as antioxidants and even cure-alls. This popularity was originally based on the work of the French scientist Masquelier, although there is now an impressive body of accumulated clinical data (see previous).

One feature of the early work is the reputed high bioavailability of OPCs, which were even said to cross the blood-brain barrier. Masquelier conducted pharmacokinetic studies on OPCs using radioactively labelled compounds. On the basis of these studies, he concluded that OPCs have good bioavailability and cross the blood-brain barrier. However, the bioavailability of OPCs observed by Masquelier was probably that of their smaller decomposition products, since his study only measured radioactivity, not the chemical entity carrying that radioactivity.

This assertion was certainly supported by a 2005 review[556] which concluded that polymeric procyanidins (condensed tannins) are not absorbed as such and even the absorption of OPC dimers was very minor, about 100-fold lower than the flavonol monomers (catechin and epicatechin).[556] The review pointed out that commercial extracts such as those from grape seed and pine bark contain a substantial percentage of monomers that could be largely responsible for the observed therapeutic effects. In addition, gut flora metabolites of OPCs might also deliver biological effects. Similar to flavonoids, OPCs are degraded by the microflora into various aromatic acids such as m-hydroxyphenylpropionic acid, m-hydroxyphenylacetic acid and their p-hydroxy isomers.

A rat study found that the extent of degradation into aromatic acids decreased as the degree of polymerisation increased. In other words, tannins will tend to resist microbial degradation (presumably because they tend to inactivate the very enzymes that might decompose them).

An in vitro study published since the review found that procyanidin B dimers are metabolised by human gut bacteria to yield 2-(3,4-dihydroxyphenyl) acetic acid and 5-(3,4-dihydroxyphenyl)-gamma-valerolactone (DHPV) as the major metabolites.[569] This finding was corroborated by an investigation in 11 healthy volunteers given a single dose of 300 mg of pine bark extract.[570] Catechin, taxifolin, caffeic acid, ferulic acid and DHPV were the major compounds present in plasma, together with 10 unknown compounds.

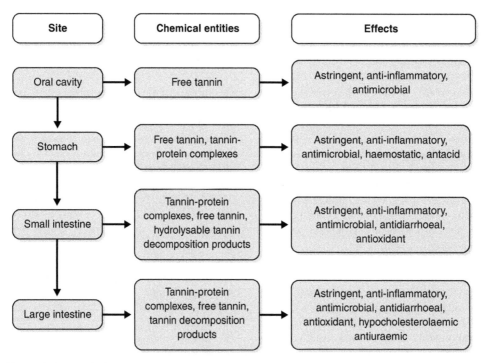

Figure 2.12 • The 'lifecycle' of a tannin through the gut.

Analysis of steady state plasma samples after chronic dosing revealed significant phase II metabolism.

Green tea is rich in polyphenols such as epigallocatechin (EGC) and epigallocatechin gallate (EGCG). Black tea is fermented green tea. During fermentation, the simple polyphenols undergo polymerisation leading to more complex molecules, such as theaflavins and therarubigens (MW 500 to 3000). Green and black tea have marked antioxidant activity in vitro, but green tea is about five times more potent than black. Adding milk has no effect. Early human experiments using oral doses demonstrated that:[571]

* green tea and black tea cause a significant increase in the antioxidant activity of plasma
* green tea is only about 50% stronger than black tea in vivo
* the effect is rapid, peaking at about 30 minutes after consumption for green tea and 50 minutes for black tea
* in contrast to the in vitro study, adding milk completely destroys this effect in people.

One possible explanation is that the tea polyphenols undergo spontaneous decomposition in the gut and the smaller antioxidant molecules are then absorbed. This would explain the similar activities of green and black tea in vivo. Adding milk causes protein binding, which would inhibit this decomposition. This implies that only tea without milk will render significant antioxidant activity in the bloodstream. However, this study did not monitor plasma antioxidant activity after more than a few hours. It is possible that the tannin-protein complexes formed after milk is added are decomposed further down in the gut and bacterial action on the liberated tannins (or just spontaneous breakdown) leads to absorption of antioxidant phenolics from the colon into the bloodstream.

Another possible explanation is that the observed antioxidant effects in plasma were due to absorption of unchanged tea phenolics. Both EGC and EGCG have been detected in the plasma of healthy human volunteers 90 minutes after they consumed capsules containing green tea extract.[572] However, as might be expected for such large polar molecules, levels detected corresponded to only 0.2% to 2.0% of the ingested amount.

The 2005 review quoted above reflected that bioavailability differs markedly among catechins.[556] Galloylation of catechins reduces their absorption. Epigallocatechin (EGC) is methylated on absorption, with 4′-O-methyl-epigallocatechin accounting for 30% to 40% of the total metabolites. EGCG is also methylated, as is catechin itself. EGCG is the only green tea polyphenol present in plasma mainly as the free form, although its overall bioavailability is low (about one-third of catechin and one-tenth of EGC). The other catechins are highly conjugated with glucuronic acid and/or sulphate. Microbial metabolites similar to those found after ingestion of herbal OPC extracts, namely various valerolactone derivatives (mostly in conjugated forms) were identified in the plasma and urine of human volunteers after ingestion of green tea. These metabolites accounted for 6% to 39% of ingested EGC and epicatechin and were 8 to 25 times the levels measured for the unchanged compounds. Galloylated catechins are only eliminated via the bile. These findings were corroborated in a later 3-month study in human volunteers.[573]

Polysaccharides

In some modern herbal literature, great emphasis is placed on the role of polysaccharides as immune-enhancing agents, particularly in the context of herbs such as Echinacea and the medicinal mushrooms. However, the main evidence for this is in vitro research. Polysaccharides are polymers based on sugars and uronic acids. They are found in all plants, especially as a component of the cell wall. However, some plants particularly accumulate polysaccharides. Any herbal extract prepared in 50% ethanol or stronger will not contain significant quantities of polysaccharides because of their insolubility in ethanol. Since they are large water-soluble molecules, which may even carry an ionic charge, polysaccharides will have low (but not zero) bioavailability. Pharmacokinetic considerations therefore dictate that if a herb is to be used as a source of polysaccharides it must be rich in these compounds, be prepared in a way to preserve or extract the polysaccharides and be administered in sufficient doses to compensate for the poor bioavailability. Such considerations will only apply in special cases and probably do not apply for oral doses of any Echinacea preparation (examples might include high doses of aqueous extracts of medicinal mushrooms and Astragalus). Unabsorbed polysaccharides will pass into the large intestine where they are broken down by bowel flora (and may have an effect on flora balance).

Whole-leaf *Aloe vera* preparations appear to be one good source of active polysaccharides, provided they are prepared to contain high levels of acemannan (about 1%). Acemannan is a polysaccharide found under the skin in *Aloe vera* leaves and is often not present in Aloe gel or juice preparations, because the outer leaf is not incorporated or enzymes used during manufacture have destroyed the acemannan. Doses of 50 to 100 mL/day of this concentrate can provide significant doses of acemannan. In a little-known, open, uncontrolled clinical study, 29 AIDS patients received *Aloe vera* whole-leaf juice, essential fatty acids and nutrients.[574] The Aloe dose was the equivalent of 1200 mg/day of acemannan. Karnofsky scores improved in 100% of these patients after 180 days. Although this study had many design flaws, it does suggest that this type of preparation as a source of polysaccharides is worthy of further study.

While medicinal mushroom polysaccharide preparations such as PSK from *Coriolus versicolor* show activity after oral doses,[575] others such as lentinan from *Lentinus edodes* are clinically administered by injection, presumably because of poor oral bioavailability.[576] However, an oral formulation of lentinan (superfine dispersed lentinan) has recently become available.[577]

Optimising efficacy

Hopefully the above discussion demonstrates that knowledge of factors influencing bioavailability can lead to the more effective use of herbal medicines. In particular, the bowel flora characteristics that can optimise the efficacy of many herbal treatments need to be better understood, as highlighted in two recent reviews.[578,579] This factor probably underlines the importance of a wholesome diet and adequate fibre intake, which will lead to healthy bowel flora. Other issues to be considered in the context of optimising efficacy include the following:

- relationship to meals:
  - ○ Polyphenolics should be taken away from meals because of their interaction with protein
  - ○ Components relying on gastric acid hydrolysis should be taken with meals
  - ○ Components damaged by gastric acid should be taken away from meals

- ○ Lipophilic components will probably be better absorbed with a high fat meal and polar (hydrophilic) compounds will probably be better absorbed with a low-fat meal
- saponins can be used to improve absorption
- some foods can be used to inhibit gut biotransformation, for example grapefruit juice
- the frequency of dosage should be based on bioavailability and metabolism.

References

1. Munson PL, Muller RA, Beese GR. *Principles of Pharmacology.* Basic Concepts and Clinical Applications. New York: Chapman and Hall; 1995. pp. 1–5.
2. Currie HA, Perry CC. Chemical evidence for intrinsic 'Si' within Equisetum cell walls. *Phytochemistry* 2009;70(17–18):2089–2095.
3. Vyas S, Collin SM, Bertin E, et al. Leaf concentrate as an alternative to iron and folic acid supplements for anaemic adolescent girls: a randomised controlled trial in India. *Public Health Nutr* 2009;13(3):418–423.
4. Upton R. Classical bontanical pharmacognosy: from Dioscorides to modern herbal medicines. *J Am Herbalists Guild.* 2010;9(2):47–52.
5. Ganora L. *Herbal Constituents: Foundations of Phytochemistry.* Colorado: Herbalchem Press; 2008.
6. Pengelly A. *The Constituents of Medicinal Plants: An Introduction to the Chemistry and Therapeutics of Herbal Medicine,* 2nd ed. Australia: Allen & Unwin; 2004.
7. Baker ME. Endocrine activity of plant-derived compounds: an evolutionary perspective. *Proc Soc Exp Biol Med.* 1995;208:131–138.
8. Croteau R, Kutchan TM, Lewis NG. Natural products (secondary metabolites). In: Buchanan BB, Gruissem W, Jones RL, eds. *Biochemistry and Molecular Biology of Plants.* USA: American Society of Plant Physiologists; 2000.
9. Firn RD, Jones CG. A Darwinian view of metabolism: molecular properties determine fitness. *J Exp Bot.* 2009;60(3):719–726.
10. Macías Galindo JCG, Molinillo JMG, eds. *Allelopathy: Chemistry and Mode of Action of Allelochemicals.* USA: CRC Press; 2004.
11. Efferth T, Koch E. Complex interactions between phytochemicals. The multi-target therapeutic concept of phytotherapy. *Curr Drug Targets.* 2011;12(1):122–132.
12. Laks PE. Wood preservation as trees do it. *Scottish Forestry.* 1991;45(4):275–284.
13. Wink M. Evolution of secondary metabolites from an ecological and molecular phylogenetic perspective. *Phytochemistry.* 2003;64(1):3–19.
14. Castells E, Penuelas J. Towards a global theory of chemical defense: the case of alkaloids (French). *Orsis.* 1997;12:141–161.
15. Oleszek W. Glucosinolates: occurrence and ecological significance (Polish). *Wiad Botaniczne.* 1995;39(1–2):49–58.
16. Zhao J, Davis LC, Verpoorte R. Elicitor signal transduction leading to production of plant secondary metabolites. *Biotechnol Adv.* 2005;23(5):283–333.
17. Bennett RN, Wallsgrove RM. Tansley review no. 72: Secondary metabolites in plant defence mechanisms. *New Phytol.* 1994;127(4):617–633.
18. Dixon RA, Lamb CJ, Masoud S, et al. Metabolic engineering: prospects for crop improvement through the genetic manipulation of phenylpropanoid biosynthesis and defense responses: a review. *Gene.* 1996;179(1):61–71.
19. Inderijt. Plant phenolics in allelopathy. *Bot Rev.* 1996;62(2):186–202.
20. Langenheim HJ. Higher plant terpenoids: a phytocentric overview of their ecological roles. *J Chem Ecol.* 1994;20(6):1223–1280.
21. Macías Galindo JCG, Molinillo JMG, eds. *Allelopathy: Chemistry and Mode of Action of Allelochemicals.* USA: CRC Press; 2004.
22. Callaway R. *Positive Interactions and Interdependence in Plant Communities.* The Netherlands: Springer; 2007.
23. Sharma HM. Phytochemical synergism: beyond the active ingredient model. *Altern Ther Clin Pract.* 1997;4:91–96.
24. Heinrich M, Barnes J, Gibbons S, et al. *Fundamentals of Pharmacognosy and Phytotherapy.* London: Elsevier; 2004. p. 161.
25. Berenbaum MC. What is synergy? *Pharmacol Rev.* 1989;41(2):93–141.
26. Williamson EM. Synergy and other interactions in phytomedicines. *Phytomedicine.* 2001;8(5):401–409.
27. Houghton P. Synergy and polyvalence: paradigms to explain the activity of herbal products. In: Houghton P, Mukherjee PK, eds. *Evaluation of Herbal Medicinal Products. Perspectives on Quality, Safety and Efficacy,* 1st ed. London: Pharmaceutical Press; 2009.
28. Kisa K, Sasaki K, Yamauchi K, et al. Potentiating effect of sennoside C on purgative activity of sennoside A in mice. *Planta Med.* 1981;42(3):302–303.
29. Nho CW, Jeffery E. The synergistic upregulation of phase II detoxification enzymes by glucosinolate breakdown products in cruciferous vegetables. *Toxicol Appl Pharmacol.* 2001;174(2):146–152.
30. Kiuchi F, Goto Y, Sugimoto N, et al. Nematocidal activity of turmeric: synergistic action of curcuminoiods. *Chem Pharm Bull.* 1993;41(9):1640–1643.
31. Onawunmi GO, Yisak W, Ogunlana EO. Antibacterial constituents in the essential oil of Cymbopogon citratus (DC.) Stapf. *J Ethnopharmacol.* 1984;12:279–286.
32. Ye XL, Huang WW, Chen Z, et al. Synergetic effect and structure–activity relationship of 3-hydroxy-3-methylglutaryl coenzyme A reductase inhibitors from Crataegus pinnatifida Bge. *J Agric Food Chem.* 2010;58(5):3132–3138.
33. Gao JL, He TC, Li YB, et al. A traditional Chinese medicine formulation consisting of Rhizoma corydalis and Rhizoma curcumae exerts synergistic anti-tumor activity. *Oncol Rep.* 2009;22(5):1077–1083.
34. Wang XN, Han X, Xu LN, et al. Enhancement of apoptosis of human hepatocellular carcinoma SMMC-7721 cells through synergy of berberine and evodiamine. *Phytomedicine.* 2008;15(12):1062–1068.
35. Wagner H, Ulrich-Merzenich G. Synergy research: approaching a new generation of phytopharmaceuticals. *Phytomedicine.* 2009;16(1):97–110.
36. Savelev SU, Okello EJ, Perry EK. Butyryl- and acetyl-cholinesterase inhibitory activities in essential oils of Salvia species and their constituents. *Phytother Res.* 2004;18(4):315–324.
37. Greay SJ, Carson C, Beilharz et al. Anticancer activity of tea tree oil. *RIRDC Publication No. 10/060* 2010.
38. Eder M, Mehnert W. Bedeutung pflanzlicher Begleitstoffe in Extrakten. *Pharmazie.* 1998;53(5):285–293.
39. Keung W, Lazo O, Kunze L, et al. Potentiation of the bioavailability of daidzin by an extract of Radix puerariae. *Proc Natl Acad Sci USA.* 1996;93:4284–4288.

40. Vinson JA, Bose PB. Comparative bioavailability to humans of ascorbic acid alone or in a citrus extract. *Am J Clin Nutr.* 1988;48:601–604.

41. Vissers MC, Bozonet SM, Pearson JF, et al. Dietary ascorbate intake affects steady state tissue concentrations in vitamin C-deficient mice: tissue deficiency after suboptimal intake and superior bioavailability from a food source (kiwifruit). *Am J Clin Nutr.* 2011;93(2):292–301.

42. Zuo F, Zhou ZM, Zhang Q, et al. Pharmacokinetic study on the multi-constituents of Huangqin–Tang decoction in rats. *Biol Pharm Bull.* 2003;26(7):911–919.

43. Butterweck V, Petereit F, Winterhoff H, et al. Solubilized hypericin and pseudohyerpicin from Hypericum perforatum exert antidepressant activity in the forced swimming test. *Planta Med.* 1998;64(4):291–294.

44. Butterweck V, Jurgenliemk G, Nahrstedt A, et al. Flavonoids from *Hypericum perforatum* show antidepressant activity in the forced swimming test. *Planta Med.* 2000;66(1):3–6.

45. Calapai G, Crupi A, Firenzuoli F, et al. Effects of Hypericum perforatum on levels of 5-hydroxytryptamine, noradrenaline and dopamine in the cortex, diencephalon and brainstem of the rat. *J Pharm Pharmacol.* 1999;51(6):723–728.

46. Butterweck V, Christoffel V, Nahrstedt A, et al. Step by step removal of hyperforin and hypericin: activity profile of different Hypericum preparations in behavioral models. *Life Sci.* 2003;73(5):627–639.

47. Capasso A, Sorrentino L. Pharmacological studies on the sedative and hypnotic effect of *Kava kava* and *Passiflora* extracts combination. *Phytomedicine.* 2005;12(1):39–45.

48. Gertsch J. Botanical drugs, synergy, and network pharmacology: forth and back to intelligent mixtures. *Planta Med.* 2011;77(11):1086–1098.

49. Hopkins AL. Network pharmacology. *Nat Biotechnol.* 2007;25(10):1110–1111.

50. Ulrich–Merzenich G, Panek D, Zeitler H, et al. New perspectives for synergy research with the 'omic'-technologies. *Phytomedicine.* 2009;16(6–7):495–508.

51. Kolodziej H. Fascinating metabolic pools of *Pelargonium sidoides* and *Pelargonium reniforme*, traditional and phytomedicinal sources of the herbal medicine Umckaloabo. *Phytomedicine.* 2007;14(suppl 6):9–17.

52. Agbabiaka TB, Guo R, Ernst E. *Pelargonium sidoides* for acute bronchitis: a systematic review and meta-analysis. *Phytomedicine.* 2008;15(5):378–385.

53. Matthys H, Eisebitt R, Seith B, et al. Efficacy and safety of an extract of *Pelargonium sidoides* (EPs 7630) in adults with acute bronchitis. A randomised, double blind, placebo-controlled trial. *Phytomedicine.* 2003;10(suppl 4):7–17.

54. Patroni C. Aspirin as an antiplatelet drug. *NEJM.* 1994;330(18):1287–1294.

55. Lamaison JL, Petitjean–Freyet C, Carnat A. Lamiacées médicinales à propriétés antioxydantes, sources potentielles d'acide rosmarinique. *Pharma Acta Helv.* 1991;66(7):185–188.

56. Auf'mkolk M, Amir SM, Kubota K, et al. The active principles of plant extracts with antithyrotropic activity: oxidation products of derivatives of 3,4-dihydroxycinnamic acid. *Endocrinology.* 1985;116(5):1677.

57. Chlabicz J, Galasinski W. The components of Melissa officinalis L. that influence protein biosynthesis in-vitro. *J Pharm Pharmacol.* 1986;38(11):791–794.

58. Csiszar A. Anti-inflammatory effects of resveratrol: possible role in prevention of age–related cardiovascular disease. *Ann N Y Acad Sci.* 2011;1215:117–122.

59. Richard T, Pawlus AD, Iglésias ML, et al. Neuroprotective properties of resveratrol and derivatives. *Ann N Y Acad Sci.* 2011;1215:103–108.

60. Szkudelski T, Szkudelska K. Anti-diabetic effects of resveratrol. *Ann N Y Acad Sci.* 2011;1215:34–39.

61. Pezzuto JM. The phenomenon of resveratrol: redefining the virtues of promiscuity. *Ann N Y Acad Sci.* 2011;1215:123–130.

62. Baur JA, Sinclair DA. Therapeutic potential of resveratrol: the in vivo evidence. *Nat Rev Drug Discov.* 2006;5(6):493–506.

63. Shakibaei M, Harikumar KB, Aggarwal BB. Resveratrol addiction: to die or not to die. *Mol Nutr Food Res.* 2009;53(1):115–128.

64. Agarwal B, Baur JA. Resveratrol and life extension. *Ann N Y Acad Sci.* 2011;1215:138–143.

65. Baur JA, Pearson KJ, Price NL, et al. Resveratrol improves health and survival of mice on a high-calorie diet. *Nature.* 2006;444(7117):337–342.

66. la Porte C, Voduc N, Zhang G, et al. Steady-state pharmacokinetics and tolerability of trans-resveratrol 2000 mg twice daily with food, quercetin and alcohol (ethanol) in healthy human subjects. *Clin Pharmacokinet.* 2010;49(7):449–454.

67. Lechtenberg M, Nahrstedt A. Cyanogenic glycosides. In: Ikan R, ed. *Naturally Occurring Glycosides.* UK: John Wiley; 1999. Chapter 5.

68. Miller KW, Anderson JL, Stoewsand GS. Amygdalin metabolism and effect on reproduction of rats fed apricot kernels. *J Toxicol Environ Health.* 1981;7(3–4):457–467.

69. Moertel CG, Ames MM, Kovach JS, et al. A pharmacologic and toxicological study of amygdalin. *JAMA.* 1981;245(6):591–594.

70. Adewusi SR, Oke OL. On the metabolism of amygdalin. 1. The LD50 and biochemical changes in rats. *Can J Physiol Pharmacol.* 1985;63(9):1080–1083.

71. Vetter J. Plant cyanogenic glycoides. *Toxicon.* 2000;38(1):11–36.

72. Fenselau C, Pallante S, Batzinger RP, et al. Mandelonitrile beta-glucuronide: synthesis and characterization. *Science.* 1977;198(4317):625–627.

73. Dorr RT, Paxinos J. The current status of laetrile. *Ann Intern Med.* 1978;89(3):389–397.

74. Hill II GJ, Shine TE, Hill HZ, et al. Failure of amygdalin to arrest B16 melanoma and BW5147 AKR leukemia. *Cancer Res.* 1976;36(6):2102–2107.

75. Moertel CG, Fleming TR, Rubin J, et al. A clinical trial of amygdalin (Laetrile) in the treatment of human cancer. *NEJM.* 1982;306(4):201–206.

76. Hill HZ, Backer R, Hill II GJ. Blood cyanide levels in mice after administration of amygdalin. *Biopharm Drug Dispos.* 1980;1(4):211–220.

77. Syrigos KN, Rowlinson–Busza G, Epenetos AA. In vitro cytotoxicity following specific activation of amygdalin by beta-glucosidase conjugated to a bladder cancer-associated monoclonal antibody. *Int J Cancer.* 1998;78(6):712–719.

78. Cliff J, Muquingue H, Nhassico D, et al. Konzo and continuing cyanide intoxication from cassava in Mozambique. *Food Chem Toxicol.* 2011;49(3):631–635.

79. Elli M, Cattivelli D, Soldi S, et al. Evaluation of prebiotic potential of refined psyllium (*Plantago ovata*) fiber in healthy women. *J Clin Gastroenterol.* 2008;42(suppl 3 Pt 2):S174–S176.

80. Fujimori S, Tatsuguchi A, Gudis K, et al. High dose probiotic and prebiotic cotherapy for remission induction of active Crohn's disease. *J Gastroenterol Hepatol.* 2007;22(8):1199–1204.

81. Rodríguez-Cabezas ME, Gálvez J, Camuesco D, et al. Intestinal anti-inflammatory activity of dietary fiber (Plantago ovata seeds) in HLA-B27 transgenic rats. *Clin Nutr.* 2003;22(5):463–471.

82. Obolentseva GV, Khadzhai YI, Vidyukova AI, et al. Effect of some natural substances on ulceration of the rat stomach caused by acetylsalicylic acid. *Bull Exp Biol Med.* 1974;77:256–257.

83. Rafatullah S, Al-Yahya MA, Al-Said MS, et al. Gastric anti-ulcer and cytoprotective effects of Cyamopsis tetragonolaba ('Guar') in rats. *Int J Pharmacog.* 1994;32(2):163–170.

84. Blackburn NA, Johnson IT. The influence of guar gum on the movements of insulin, glucose and fluid in rat intestine during perfusion in vivo. *Pflügers Archiv.* 1983;397:144–148.

85. Schmidgall J, Schnetz E, Hensel A. Evidence for bioadhesive effects of polysaccharides and polysaccharide-containing herbs in an ex vivo bioadhesion assay on buccal membranes. *Planta Med.* 2000;66(1):48–53.

86. Deters A, Zippel J, Hellenbrand N, et al. Aqueous extracts and polysaccharides from

Marshmallow roots (Althea officinalis L.): cellular internalisation and stimulation of cell physiology of human epithelial cells in vitro. *J Ethnopharmacol.* 2010;127(1):62–69.

87. Morcos SR, El-Baradie AA. Fenugreek mucilage and its relation to the reputed laxative action of this seed. *Egypt J Chem.* 1959;2(1):163–168.

88. Stevens J, Levitsky DA, Van Soest PJ, et al. Effect of psyllium gum and wheat bran on spontaneous energy intake. *Am J Clin Nutr.* 1987;46:812–817.

89. Voinchet O, Mouchet A. Obstruction de l'oesophage par mucilage. *Nouvelle Presse Médicale.* 1974;3(19):1223–1225.

90. [No authors listed]. Health Canada Advises Canadians that Natural Health Products containing Glucomannan May Cause Serious Choking if Used with Insufficient Fluid. Advisory No. 2010–16, January 29, 2010.

91. Nosalova G, Strapkova A, Kardosova A, et al. Antitussive Wirkung des Extraktes und der Polysaccharide aus Eibisch (Althaea officinalis L., var. robusta). *Pharmazie.* 1992;47:224–226.

92. Sutovska M, Nosalova G, Franova S, et al. The antitussive activity of polysaccharides from Althaea officinalis l., var. Robusta, Arctium lappa L., var. Herkules, and Prunus persica L., Batsch. *Bratisl Lek Listy.* 2007;108(2):93–99.

93. Sutovská M, Nosálová G, Sutovský J, et al. Possible mechanisms of dose-dependent cough suppressive effect of Althaea officinalis rhamnogalacturonan in guinea pigs test system. *Int J Biol Macromol.* 2009;45(1):27–32.

94. Smith J, Woodcock A, Houghton L. New developments in reflux-associated cough. *Lung.* 2010;188(suppl 1):S81–S86.

95. Pauwels A, Blondeau K, Dupont L, et al. Cough and gastroesophageal reflux: from the gastroenterologist end. *Pulm Pharmacol Ther.* 2009;22(2):135–138.

96. Thakkar K, Boatright RO, Gilger MA, et al. Gastroesophageal reflux and asthma in children: a systematic review. *Pediatrics.* 2010;125(4):e925–e930.

97. Barberio G, Ruggeri C, Pajno GB, et al. [Gastro-esophageal reflux and asthma. Clinical experience]. *Minerva Pediatr.* 1989;41(7):363–366.

98. Giudicelli R, Dupin B, Surpas P, et al. [Gastroesophageal reflux and respiratory manifestations: diagnostic approach, therapeutic indications and results]. *Ann Chir.* 1990;44(7):552–554.

99. Larrain A, Carrasco E, Galleguillos F, et al. Medical and surgical treatment of nonallergic asthma associated with gastroesophageal reflux. *Chest.* 1991;99(6):1330–1335.

100. Morice AH. Is reflux cough due to gastroesophageal reflux disease or laryngopharyngeal reflux? *Lung.* 2008;186(suppl 1):S103–S106.

101. Avidan B, Sonnenberg A, Schnell TG, et al. Temporal associations between coughing

or wheezing and acid reflux in asthmatics. *Gut.* 2001;49(6):767–772.

102. Kollarik M, Brozmanova M. Cough and gastroesophageal reflux: insights from animal models. *Pulm Pharmacol Ther.* 2009;22(2):130–134.

103. Undem BJ, Carr MJ. Targeting primary afferent nerves for novel antitussive therapy. *Chest.* 2010;137(1):177–184.

104. Roberts DCK, Truswell AS, Bencke A, et al. The cholesterol-lowering effect of a breakfast cereal containing psyllium fibre. *Med J Aust.* 1994;161:660–664.

105. Yu LL, Lutterodt H, Cheng Z. Beneficial health properties of psyllium and approaches to improve its functionalities. *Adv Food Nutr Res.* 2009;55:193–220.

106. Leeds AR. Psyllium – a superior source of soluble dietary fibre. *Food Aust.* 1995;47(suppl 2):S2–S4.

107. Frati-Munari AC, Flores-Garduno MA, Ariza-Andraca R, et al. Effect of different doses of Plantago psyllium mucilage on the glucose tolerance test. *Arch Invest Med (Mexico).* 1989;20(2):147–152.

108. Lis-Balchin M, Deans SG, Eaglesham E. Relationship between bioactivity and chemical composition of commercial essential oils. *Flavour Fragrance J.* 1998;13:98–104.

109. Römmelt H, Zuber A, Dirnagl K, et al. Zur Resorption von Terpenen aus Badezusätzen. *MMW Fortschr Med.* 1974;116(11):537–540.

110. Woronuk G, Demissie Z, Rheault M, et al. Biosynthesis and therapeutic properties of Lavandula essential oil constituents. *Planta Med.* 2011;77(1):7–15.

111. Janssen AM, Scheffer JJC, Baerheim Svendsen A. Antimicrobial activity of essential oils: a 1976–1986 literature review. Aspects of the test methods. *Planta Med.* 1987;53:395–398.

112. Bakkali F, Averbeck S, Averbeck D, et al. Biological effects of essential oils – a review. *Food Chem Toxicol.* 2008;46(2):446–475.

113. Janssen AM, Chin NLJ, Scheffer JJC, et al. Screening for antimicrobial activity of some essential oils by the agar overlay technique. *Pharm Weekbl Sci.* 1986;8:289–292.

114. Baser KH. Biological and pharmacological activities of carvacrol and carvacrol bearing essential oils. *Curr Pharm Des.* 2008;14(29):3106–3119.

115. Soderberg TA, Johansson A, Gref R. Toxic effects of some conifer resin acids and tea tree oil on human epithelial and fibroblast cells. *Toxicology.* 1996;107(2):99–109.

116. Cox SD, Gustafson JE, Mann CM, et al. Tea tree oil causes K$^+$ leakage and inhibits respiration in Escherichia coli. *Lett Appl Microbiol.* 1998;26(5):355–358.

117. Moleyar V, Narasimham P. Antibacterial activity of essential oil components. *Int J Food Microbiol.* 1992;16(4):337–342.

118. Edris AE. Pharmacological and therapeutic potentials of essential oils and their

individual volatile constituents: a review. *Phytother Res.* 2007;21(4):308–323.

119. Pattnaik S, Subramanyam VR, Bapaji M, et al. Antibacterial and antifungal activity of aromatic constituents of essential oils. *Microbios.* 1997;89(358):39–46.

120. Carson CF, Riley TV. Antimicrobial activity of the major components of the essential oil of Melaleuca alternifolia. *J Appl Bacteriol.* 1995;78(3):264–269.

121. Williams LR, Home VN. Factors determining the quality of tea tree oil in formulations for clinical use. *Cosmet Aerosol Toiletries Aust.* 1995;9(2):14–18.

122. Reichling J, Schnitzler P, Suschke U, et al. Essential oils of aromatic plants with antibacterial, antifungal, antiviral, and cytotoxic properties – an overview. *Forsch Komplemented.* 2009;16(2):79–90.

123. Tong MM, Altman PM, Barnetson RS. Tea tree oil in the treatment of tinea pedis. *Aust J Dermatol.* 1992;33(3):145–149.

124. Bassett IB, Pannowitz DL, Barnetson RS. A comparative study of tea-tree oil versus benzoylperoxide in the treatment of acne. *MJA.* 1990;153(8):455–458.

125. Carson CF, Hammer KA, Riley TV. Melaleuca alternifolia (Tea Tree) oil: a review of antimicrobial and other medicinal properties. *Clin Microbiol Rev.* 2006;19(1):50–62.

126. Enshaieh S, Jooya A, Siadat AH, et al. The efficacy of 5% topical tea tree oil gel in mild to moderate acne vulgaris: a randomized, double blind placebo-controlled study. *Indian J Dermatol Venereol Leprol.* 2007;73(1):22–25.

127. Carson CF, Ashton L, Dry L, et al. Melaleuca alternifolia (tea tree) oil gel (6%) for the treatment of recurrent herpes labialis. *J Antimicrob Chemother.* 2001;48(3):450–451.

128. Barker SC, Altman PM. A randomised, assessor blind, parallel group comparative efficacy trial of three products for the treatment of head lice in children – melaleuca oil and lavender oil, pyrethrins and piperonyl butoxide, and a 'suffocation' product. *BMC Dermatol.* 2010;10:6.

129. Heukelbach J, Canyon DV, Oliveira FA, et al. In vitro efficacy of over-the-counter botanical pediculicides against the head louse Pediculus humanus var capitis based on a stringent standard for mortality assessment. *Med Vet Entomol.* 2008;22(3):264–272.

130. Force M, Sparks WS, Ronzio RA. Inhibition of enteric parasites by emulsified oil of oregano in vivo. *Phytother Res.* 2000;14(3):213–214.

131. Kliks MM. Studies on the traditional herbal anthelmintic Chenopodium ambrosioides L.: ethnopharmacological evaluation and clinical field trials. *Soc Sci Med.* 1985;21(8):879–886.

132. Pisseri F, Bertoli A, Pistelli L. Essential oils in medicine: principles of therapy. *Parassitologia.* 2008;50(1–2):89–91.

133. Reiter M, Brandt W. Relaxant effects on tracheal and ileal smooth muscles of the guinea pig. *ArzneimittelForschung.* 1985;35(1A):408–414.

134. Sparks MJ, O'Sullivan P, Herrington AA, et al. Does peppermint oil relieve spasm during barium enema? *Br J Radiol.* 1995;68(812):841–843.

135. Giachetti D, Taddei E, Taddei I. Pharmacological activity of essential oils on Oddi's sphincter. *Planta Med.* 1988;54:389–392.

136. Creamer B. Oesophageal reflux and the action of carminatives. *Lancet.* 1955;1:590–592.

137. Stanic G, Samarzija I, Blazevic N. Time-dependent diuretic response in rats treated with juniper berry preparations. *Phytotherapy Res.* 1998;12:494–497.

138. Schilcher H, Leuschner F. Studies of potential nephrotoxic effects of essential juniper oil (German). *Arzneimittel-Forschung.* 1997;47(7):855–858.

139. Al-Mosawi AJ. Essential oil terpenes: adjunctive role in the management of childhood urolithiasis. *J Med Food.* 2010;13(2):247–250.

140. Dorow P, Weiss TH, Felix R, et al. Effect of a secretolytic and a combination of pinene, limonene and cineole on mucociliary clearance in patients with chronic pulmonary obstruction. *ArzneimittelForschung.* 1987;37(12):1378–1381.

141. Boyd EM. Expectorants and respiratory tract fluid. *Pharma Rev.* 1954;6:521–542.

142. Boyd EM, Pearson GL. On the expectorant action of volatile oils. *Am J Med Sci.* 1946;211:602–610.

143. Boyd EM, Palmer G, Pearson GL. Is there any advantage in combining several expectorant drugs in a compound cough mixture? *Can Med Assoc J.* 1946;54(3):216–220.

144. Sherry E, Warnke PH. Successful use of an inhalational phytochemical to treat pulmonary tuberculosis: a case report. *Phytomedicine.* 2004;11(2–3):95–97.

145. Guillemain J, Rousseau A, Delaveau P. Effets neurodépresseurs de l'huile essentielle de *Lavandula angustifolia* Mill. *Annales de Pharmaceutiques Françaises.* 1989;47(6):337–343.

146. Kasper S, Gastpar M, Müller WE, et al. Efficacy and safety of silexan, a new, orally administered lavender oil preparation, in subthreshold anxiety disorder – evidence from clinical trials. *Wien Med Wochenschr.* 2010;160(21–22):547–556.

147. Kovar KA, Gropper D, Friess D, et al. Blood levels of 1,8-cineole and locomotor activity of mice after inhalation and oral administration of rosemary oil. *Planta Med.* 1987;53:315–318.

148. Haines Jr. DJ. Sassafras tea and diaphoresis. *Postgrad Med.* 1991;90(4):75–76.

149. de Sousa DP. Analgesic-like activity of essential oils constituents. *Molecules.* 2011;16(3):2233–2252.

150. Ghelardini C, Galeotti N, Salvatore G, et al. Local anaesthetic activity of the essential oil of *Lavandula angustifolia.* *Planta Med.* 1999;65(8):700–703.

151. Edris AE. Anti-cancer properties of Nigella spp. essential oils and their major constituents, thymoquinone and beta-elemene. *Curr Clin Pharmacol.* 2009;4(1):43–46.

152. Tisserand R, Balacs T. *Essential Oil Safety: A Guide for Health Care Professionals.* Edinburgh: Churchill Livingstone; 1995.

153. Macht DI. The action of the so-called emmenagogue oils on the isolated uterine strip. *J Pharmacol Exp Ther.* 1912;4:547–552.

154. Arnold WN. Absinthe. *Sci Am.* 1989;260:86–91.

155. Albert-Puleo M. Van Gogh's vision: thujone intoxication. *JAMA.* 1981;246(1):42.

156. Lachenmeier DW. [Absinthe – history of dependence to thujone or to alcohol?] *Fortschr Neurol Psychiatr.* 2007;75(5):306–308.

157. Rutherford T, Nixon R, Tam M, et al. Allergy to tea tree oil: retrospective review of 41 cases with positive patch tests over 4.5 years. *Australas J Dermatol.* 2007;48(2):83–87.

158. Pulverer G. Benzylsenföl: ein Breitbandantibiotikum aus der Kapuzinerkresse. *Dtsch Med Wochenschr.* 1968;93:1642–1649.

159. Sehrawat A, Singh SV. Benzyl isothiocyanate inhibits epithelial-mesenchymal transition in cultured and xenografted human breast cancer cells. *Cancer Prev Res (Phila).* 2011;4(7):1107–1117.

160. Langer P, Stolc V. Goitrogenic activity of allylisothiocyanate – a widespread natural mustard oil. *Endocrinol.* 1965;76:151–155.

161. Higdon JV, Delage B, Williams DE, et al. Cruciferous vegetables and human cancer risk: epidemiologic evidence and mechanistic basis. *Pharmacol Res.* 2007;55(3):224–236.

162. Hayes JD, Kelleher MO, Eggleston IM. The cancer chemopreventive actions of phytochemicals derived from glucosinolates. *Eur J Nutr.* 2008;47(suppl 2):73–88.

163. Herr I, Büchler MW. Dietary constituents of broccoli and other cruciferous vegetables: implications for prevention and therapy of cancer. *Cancer Treat Rev.* 2010;36(5):377–383.

164. Verhoeven DT, Goldbohm RA, van Poppel G, et al. Epidemiological studies on brassica vegetables and cancer risk. *Cancer Epidemiol Biomarkers Prev.* 1996;5(9):733–748.

165. Nestle M. Broccoli sprouts as inducers of carcinogen-detoxifying enzyme systems: clinical, dietary, and policy implications. *Proc Natl Acad Sci USA.* 1997;94(21):11149–11151.

166. Shapiro TA, Fahey JW, Dinkova-Kostova AT, et al. Safety, tolerance, and metabolism of broccoli sprout glucosinolates and isothiocyanates: a clinical phase I study. *Nutr Cancer.* 2006;55(1):53–62.

167. Fahey JW, Zhang Y, Talalay P. Broccoli sprouts: an exceptionally rich source of inducers of enzymes that protect against chemical carcinogens. *Proc Natl Acad Sci USA.* 1997;94(19):10367–10372.

168. Zhang Y, Talalay P, Cho CG, et al. A major inducer of anticarcinogenic protective enzymes from broccoli: isolation and elucidation of structure. *Proc Natl Acad Sci USA.* 1992;89(6):2399–2403.

169. Juge N, Mithen RF, Traka M. Molecular basis for chemoprevention by sulforaphane: a comprehensive review. *Cell Mol Life Sci.* 2007;64(9):1105–1127.

170. Kensler TW, Chen JG, Egner PA, et al. Effects of glucosinolate-rich broccoli sprouts on urinary levels of aflatoxin–DNA adducts and phenanthrene tetraols in a randomized clinical trial in He Zuo township, Qidong, People's Republic of China. *Cancer Epidemiol Biomarkers Prev.* 2005;14(11 Pt 1):2605–2613.

171. Riedl MA, Saxon A, Diaz–Sanchez D. Oral sulforaphane increases Phase II antioxidant enzymes in the human upper airway. *Clin Immunol.* 2009;130(3):244–251.

172. Janssen K, Mensink RP, Cox FJ, et al. Effects of the flavonoids quercetin and apigenin on hemostasis in healthy volunteers: results from an in vitro and a dietary supplement study. *Am J Clin Nutr.* 1998;67(2):255–262.

173. Hughes RE, Wilson HK. Flavonoids: some physiological and nutritional considerations. *Prog Med Chem.* 1977;14:285–301.

174. Amiel M, Barbe R. Study of the pharmacodynamic activity of daflon 500mg. *Ann Cardiol Angiol.* 1998;47(3):185–188.

175. Le Devehat C, Khodabandehlou T, Vimeux M, et al. Evaluation of haemorheological and microcirculatory disturbances in chronic venous insufficiency: activity of Daflon 500mg. *Int J Microcirc Clin Exp.* 1997;17(suppl 1):27–33.

176. Guilhou JJ, Fevrier F, Debure C, et al. Benefit of a 2–month treatment with a micronized, purified flavonoidic fraction on venous ulcer healing. A randomized, double blind, controlled versus placebo trial. *Int J Microcirc Clin Exp.* 1997;17(suppl 1):21–26.

177. Cospite M. Double blind, placebo-controlled evaluation of clinical activity and safety of Daflon 500mg in the treatment of acute hemorrhoids. *Angiology.* 1994;45(6 pt 2):566–573.

178. Gohel MS, Davies AH. Pharmacological treatment in patients with C4, C5 and C6 venous disease. *Phlebology.* 2010;25(suppl 1):35–41.

179. Alonso-Coello P, Zhou Q, Martinez-Zapata MJ, et al. Meta-analysis of flavonoids for the treatment of haemorrhoids. *Br J Surg.* 2006;93(8):909–920.

180. Havsteen BH. The biochemistry and medical significance of the flavonoids. *Pharmacol Ther.* 2002;96(2–3):67–202.

181. Cazarolli LH, Zanatta L, Alberton EH, et al. Flavonoids: prospective drug candidates. *Mini Rev Med Chem.* 2008;8(13):1429–1440.

182. Ferrali M, Signorini C, Caciotti B, et al. Protection against oxidative damage of erythrocyte membrane by the flavonoid quercetin and its relation to iron chelating activity. *FEBS Lett.* 1997;416(2):123–129.

183. Aviram M, Fuhrman B. Polyphenolic flavonoids inhibit macrophage-mediated oxidation of LDL and attenuate atherogenesis. *Atherosclerosis.* 1998;137(suppl):S45–S50.

184. Robak J, Gryglewski RJ. Bioactivity of flavonoids. *Polish J Pharmacol.* 1996;48(6):555–564.

185. Saiija A, Scalese M, Lanza M, et al. Flavonoids as antioxidant agents: importance of their interaction with biomembranes. *Free Radic Biol Med.* 1995;19(4):481–486.

186. Van Acker SA, Tromp MN, Haenen GR, et al. Flavonoids as scavengers of nitric oxide radical. *Biochem Biophys Res Commun.* 1995;214(3):755–759.

187. Hu JP, Calomme M, Lasure A, et al. Structure–activity relationship of flavonoids with superoxide scavenging activity. *Biol Trace Elem Res.* 1995;47(1–3):327–331.

188. Tournaire C, Croux S, Maurette MT, et al. Antioxidant activity of flavonoids: efficiency of singlet oxygen (1 delta g) quenching. *J Photochem Photobiol B Biol.* 1993;19(3):205–215.

189. Cao G, Sofic E, Prior RL. Antioxidant and prooxidant behaviour of flavonoids: structure–activity relationships. *Free Radic Biol Med.* 1997;22(5):749–760.

190. Alcaraz MJ, Ferrandiz ML. Modifications of arachidonic metabolism by flavonoids. *J Ethnopharmacol.* 1987;21:209–229.

191. Okuda J, Miwa I, Inagaki K, et al. Inhibition of aldose reductases from rat and bovine lenses by flavonoids. *Biochem Pharmacol.* 1982;31(23):3807–3822.

192. Chang WS, Lee YJ, Chiang HC. Inhibitory effects of flavonoids on xanthine oxidase. *Anticancer Res.* 1993;13(6A):2165–2170.

193. Ruckstuhl M, Beretz A, Anton R, et al. Flavonoids are selective cyclic GMP phosphodiesterase inhibitors. *Biochem Pharmacol.* 1979;28:535–538.

194. Petkov E, Nikolov N, Uzunov P. Inhibitory effect of some flavonoids and flavonoid mixtures on cyclic AMP phospho diesterase activity of rat heart. *Planta Med.* 1981;43:183–186.

195. Pathak D, Pathak K, Singla AK. Flavonoids as medicinal agents – recent advances. *Fitoterapia.* 1991;62(5):371–389.

196. Pelissero C, Lenczowski MJ, Chinzi D, et al. Effects of flavonoids on aromatase activity, an in vitro study. *J Steroid Biochem Mol Biol.* 1996;57(3–4):215–223.

197. Divi RL, Doerge DR. Inhibition of thyroid peroxidase by dietary flavonoids. *Chem Res Toxicol.* 1996;9(1):16–23.

198. Serafini M, Peluso I, Raguzzini A. Flavonoids as anti-inflammatory agents. *Proc Nutr Soc.* 2010;69(3):273–278.

199. Cushnie TP, Lamb AJ. Antimicrobial activity of flavonoids. *Int J Antimicrob Agents.* 2005;26(5):343–356.

200. Amella M, Bronner C, Briancon F, et al. Inhibition of mast cell histamine release by flavonoids and biflavonoids. *Planta Med.* 1985;51:16–20.

201. Kawai M, Hirano T, Higa S, et al. Flavonoids and related compounds as anti-allergic substances. *Allergol Int.* 2007;56(2):113–123.

202. El Haouari M, Rosado JA. Modulation of platelet function and signaling by flavonoids. *Mini Rev Med Chem.* 2011;11(2):131–142.

203. Hammad HM, Abdalla SS. Pharmacological effects of selected flavonoids on rat isolated ileum: structure–activity relationship. *Gen Pharmacol.* 1997;28(5):767–771.

204. Ko WC, Liu PY, Chen JL, et al. Relaxant effects of flavonoids in isolated guinea pig trachea and their structure–activity relationships. *Planta Med.* 2003;69(12):1086–1090.

205. Kitaoka M, Kadokawa H, Sugano M, et al. Prenylflavonoids: a new class of non-steroidal phytooestrogen (Part 1). Isolation of 8-isopentenylnaringenin and an initial study on its structure–activity relationship. *Planta Med.* 1998;64(6):511–515.

206. Böttner M, Christoffel J, Wuttke W. Effects of long-term treatment with 8-prenylnaringenin and oral estradiol on the GH–IGF-1 axis and lipid metabolism in rats. *J Endocrinol.* 2008;198(2):395–401.

207. Erkkola R, Vervarcke S, Vansteelandt S, et al. A randomized, double blind, placebo-controlled, cross-over pilot study on the use of a standardized hop extract to alleviate menopausal discomforts. *Phytomedicine.* 2010;17(6):389–396.

208. Fremont L, Gozzelino MT, Franchi MP, et al. Dietary flavonoids reduce lipid peroxidation in rats fed polyunsaturated or monounsaturated fat diets. *J Nutr.* 1998;128(9):1495–1502.

209. Mota KS, Dias GE, Pinto ME, et al. Flavonoids with gastroprotective activity. *Molecules.* 2009;14(3):979–1012.

210. Pelzer LE, Guardia T, Osvaldo JA, et al. Acute and chronic anti-inflammatory effects of plant flavonoids. *Farmaco.* 1998;53(6):421–424.

211. Serafini M, Peluso I, Raguzzini A. Flavonoids as anti-inflammatory agents. *Proc Nutr Soc.* 2010;69(3):273–278.

212. Galvez J, Zarzuelo A, Crespo ME, et al. Antidiarrhoeic activity of Euphorbia hirta extract and isolation of an active flavonoid constituent. *Planta Med.* 1993;59:333–336.

213. Elangovan V, Sekar N, Govindasamy S. Chemopreventive potential of dietary bioflavonoids against 20-methylcholanthrene-induced tumorigenesis. *Cancer Lett.* 1994;87:107–113.

214. Yasukawa K, Takido M, Takeuchi M, et al. Inhibitory effects of flavonol glycosides on 12-O-tetradecanoylphorbol-13-acetate-induced tumor promotion. *Chem Pharm Bull (Tokyo).* 1990;38(3):774–776.

215. Prasad S, Phromnoi K, Yadav VR, et al. Targeting inflammatory pathways by flavonoids for prevention and treatment of cancer. *Planta Med.* 2010;76(11):1044–1063.

216. Salgueiro JB, Ardenghi P, Dias M, et al. Anxiolytic natural and synthetic flavonoid ligands of the central benzodiazepine receptor have no effect on memory tasks in rats. *Pharmacol Biochem Behav.* 1997;58(4):887–891.

217. Medina JH, Viola H, Wolfman C, et al. Overview – flavonoids: a new family of benzodiazepine receptor ligands. *Neurochem Res.* 1997;22(4):419–425.

218. Keli SO, Hertog MG, Feskens EJ. Dietary flavonoids, antioxidant vitamins, and incidence of stroke: the Zutphen Study. *Arch Intern Med.* 1996;156(6):637–642.

219. Knekt P, Jarvinen R, Reunanen A, et al. Flavonoid intake and coronary mortality in Finland: a cohort study. *BMJ.* 1996;312(7029):478–481.

220. Rimm EB, Katan MB, Ascherio A, et al. Relation between intake of flavonoids and risk for coronary heart disease in male health professionals. *Ann Intern Med.* 1996;125(5):384–389.

221. Arts IC, Hollman PC, Feskens EJ, et al. Catechin intake might explain the inverse relation between tea consumption and ischemic heart disease: the Zutphen Elderly Study. *Am J Clin Nutr.* 2001;74(2):227–232.

222. Sesso HD, Gaziano JM, Liu S, et al. Flavonoid intake and the risk of cardiovascular disease in women. *Am J Clin Nutr.* 2003;77(6):1400–1408.

223. Song Y, Manson JE, Buring JE, et al. Associations of dietary flavonoids with risk of type 2 diabetes, and markers of insulin resistance and systemic inflammation in women: a prospective study and cross-sectional analysis. *J Am Coll Nutr.* 2005;24(5):376–384.

224. Wang L, Lee IM, Zhang SM, et al. Dietary intake of selected flavonols, flavones, and flavonoid-rich foods and risk of cancer in middle-aged and older women. *Am J Clin Nutr.* 2009;89(3):905–912.

225. Knekt P, Kumpulainen J, Järvinen R, et al. Flavonoid intake and risk of chronic diseases. *Am J Clin Nutr.* 2002;76(3):560–568.

226. Mollace V, Sacco I, Janda E, et al. Hypolipemic and hypoglycaemic activity of bergamot polyphenols: from animal models to human studies. *Fitoterapia.* 2011;82(3):309–316.

227. Levy RM, Khokhlov A, Kopenkin S, et al. Efficacy and safety of flavocoxid, a novel therapeutic, compared with naproxen: a randomized multicenter controlled trial in subjects with osteoarthritis of the knee. *Adv Ther.* 2010;27(10):731–742.

228. Morand C, Dubray C, Milenkovic D, et al. Hesperidin contributes to the vascular protective effects of orange juice: a randomized crossover study in healthy volunteers. *Am J Clin Nutr.* 2011;93(1):73–80.

229. Lin TS, Blum KA, Fischer DB, et al. Flavopiridol, fludarabine, and rituximab in mantle cell lymphoma and indolent B-cell lymphoproliferative disorders. *J Clin Oncol.* 2010;28(3):418–423.

230. Jin F, Nieman DC, Shanely RA, et al. The variable plasma quercetin response to 12-week quercetin supplementation in humans. *Eur J Clin Nutr.* 2010;64(7):692–697.

231. Davis JM, Carlstedt CJ, Chen S, et al. The dietary flavonoid quercetin increases VO(2max) and endurance capacity. *Int J Sport Nutr Exerc Metab.* 2010;20(1):56–62.

232. Abbey EL, Rankin JW. Effect of quercetin supplementation on repeated-sprint performance, xanthine oxidase activity, and inflammation. *Int J Sport Nutr Exerc Metab.* 2011;21(2):91–96.

233. Bigelman KA, Fan EH, Chapman DP, et al. Effects of six weeks of quercetin supplementation on physical performance in ROTC cadets. *Mil Med.* 2010;175(10):791–798.

234. Cureton KJ, Tomporowski PD, Singhal A, et al. Dietary quercetin supplementation is not ergogenic in untrained men. *J Appl Physiol.* 2009;107(4):1095–1104.

235. Egert S, Bosy-Westphal A, Seiberl J, et al. Quercetin reduces systolic blood pressure and plasma oxidised low-density lipoprotein concentrations in overweight subjects with a high-cardiovascular disease risk phenotype: a double blinded, placebo-controlled cross-over study. *Br J Nutr.* 2009;102(7):1065–1074.

236. Nagao M, Naokata M, Yahagi T, et al. Mutagenicities of 61 flavonoids and 11 related compounds. *Environ Mutagen.* 1981;3:401–419.

237. Czeczot H, Tudek B, Kusztelak J, et al. Isolation and studies of the mutagenic activity in the Ames test of flavonoids naturally occurring in medical herbs. *Mutat Res.* 1990;240(3):209–216.

238. Connolly JA, Morgan IM, Jackson ME, et al. The BPV-4 co-carcinogen quercetin induces cell cycle arrest and up-regulates transcription from the LCR of BPV-4. *Oncogene.* 1998;16(21):2739–2746.

239. Barotto NN, Lopez CB, Enyard AR, et al. Quercetin enhances pretumorous lesions in the NMU model of rat pancreatic carcinogenesis. *Cancer Lett.* 1998;129(1):1–6.

240. Chaumontet C, Suschetet M, Honikman-Leban E, et al. Lack of tumor-promoting effects of flavonoids: studies on rat liver preneoplastic foci and on in vivo and in vitro gap junctional intercellular communication. *Nutr Cancer.* 1996;26(3):251–263.

241. Wall ME, Wani MC, Manikumar G, et al. Plant antimutagenic agents, 2. Flavonoids. *J Nat Prod.* 1988;51(6):1084–1091.

242. Duthie SJ, Collins AR, Duthie GG, et al. Quercetin and myricetin protect against hydrogen peroxide-induced DNA damage (strand breaks and oxidised pyrimidines) in human lymphocytes. *Mutat Res.* 1997;393(3):223–231.

243. Zhu BT, Ezell EL, Leihr JG. Catechol-O-methyltransferase-catalyzed rapid O-methylation of mutagenic flavonoids. *J Biol Chem.* 1994;269(1):292–299.

244. Harwood M, Danielewska-Nikiel B, Borzelleca JF, et al. A critical review of the data related to the safety of quercetin and lack of evidence of in vivo toxicity, including lack of genotoxic/carcinogenic properties. *Food Chem Toxicol.* 2007;45(11):2179–2205.

245. Nonaka GI, Sakai R, Nishioka T. Hydrolysable tannins and proanthocyanidins from green tea. *Phytochemistry.* 1984;23(8):1753–1755.

246. Hör M, Rimpler H, Heinrich M. Inhibition of intestinal chloride secretion by proanthocyanidins from Guazuma ulmifolia. *Planta Med.* 1995;61:208–212.

247. Wongsamitkul N, Sirianant L, Muanprasat C, et al. A plant-derived hydrolysable tannin inhibits CFTR chloride channel: a potential treatment of diarrhea. *Pharm Res.* 2010;27(3):490–497.

248. Tomczyk M, Latté KP. Potentilla – a review of its phytochemical and pharmacological profile. *J Ethnopharmacol.* 2009;122(2):184–204.

249. Subbotina MD, Timchenko VN, Vorobyov MM, et al. Effect of oral administration of tormentil root extract (Potentilla tormentilla) on rotavirus diarrhea in children: a randomized, double blind, controlled trial. *Pediatr Infect Dis J.* 2003;22(8):706–711.

250. Maity S, Vedasiromoni JR, Ganguly DK. Anti-ulcer effect of the hot water extract of black tea (Camellia sinensis). *J Ethnopharmacol.* 1995;46:167–174.

251. Ezaki N, Kato M, Takizawa N, et al. Pharmacological studies on Linderae umbellatae Ramus, IV. Effects of condensed tannin related compounds on peptic activity and stress-induced gastric lesions in mice. *Planta Med.* 1985;51(1):34–38.

252. Murakami S, Isobe Y, Kijima H, et al. Inhibition of gastric H+, K+-ATPase and acid secretion by ellagic acid. *Planta Med.* 1991;57:305–308.

253. Alam MS, Alam MA, Ahmad S, et al. Protective effects of Punica granatum in experimentally-induced gastric ulcers. *Toxicol Mech Methods.* 2010;20(9):572–578.

254. Terada A, Hara H, Nakajyo S, et al. Effect of supplements of tea polyphenols on the caecal flora and caecal metabolites of chicks. *Microb Ecol Health Dis.* 1993;6:3–9.

255. Yokozawa T, Fujioka Oura H, et al. Confirmation that tannin-containing crude drugs have a uraemic toxin-decreasing action. *Phytother Res.* 1995;9:1–5.

256. Akah PA. Haemostatic activity of aqueous leaf extract of Ageratum conyzoides L. *Int J Crude Drug Res.* 1988;26(2):97–101.

257. Root-Bernstein RS. Tannic acid, semipermeable membranes and burn treatment. *Lancet.* 1982;2:1168.

258. Haslam E. Natural polyphenols (vegetable tannins) as drugs: possible modes of action. *J Nat Prod.* 1996;9:205–215.

259. Okuda T, Yoshida T, Hatano T. Chemistry and biological activity of tannins in medicinal plants. In: Wagner N, Farnsworth NR, eds. *Economic and Medicinal Plant Research*, vol. 5. London: Academic Press; 1991. pp. 130–165.

260. Koleckar V, Kubikova K, Rehakova Z, et al. Condensed and hydrolysable tannins as antioxidants influencing the health. *Mini Rev Med Chem.* 2008;8(5):436–447.

261. Coimbra S, Castro E, Rocha-Pereira P, et al. The effect of green tea in oxidative stress. *Clin Nutr.* 2006;25(5):790–796.

262. Gomikawa S, Ishikawa Y, Hayase W, et al. Effect of ground green tea drinking for 2 weeks on the susceptibility of plasma and LDL to the oxidation ex vivo in healthy volunteers. *Kobe J Med Sci.* 2008;54(1):E62–E72.

263. Tinahones FJ, Rubio MA, Garrido-Sánchez L, et al. Green tea reduces LDL oxidability and improves vascular function. *J Am Coll Nutr.* 2008;27(2):209–213.

264. Erba D, Riso P, Bordoni A, et al. Effectiveness of moderate green tea consumption on antioxidative status and plasma lipid profile in humans. *J Nutr Biochem.* 2005;16(3):144–149.

265. Rossi R, Porta S, Canovi B. Overview on cranberry and urinary tract infections in females. *J Clin Gastroenterol.* 2010;44(suppl 1):S61–S62.

266. Pappas E, Schaich KM. Phytochemicals of cranberries and cranberry products: characterization, potential health effects, and processing stability. *Crit Rev Food Sci Nutr.* 2009;49(9):741–781.

267. Howell AB, Botto H, Combescure C, et al. Dosage effect on uropathogenic Escherichia coli anti-adhesion activity in urine following consumption of cranberry powder standardized for proanthocyanidin content: a multicentric randomized double blind study. *BMC Infect Dis.* 2010;10:94.

268. Adhami VM, Khan N, Mukhtar H. Cancer chemoprevention by pomegranate: laboratory and clinical evidence. *Nutr Cancer.* 2009;61(6):811–815.

269. Heber D. Multitargeted therapy of cancer by ellagitannins. *Cancer Lett.* 2008;269(2):262–268.

270. Murthy KN, Reddy VK, Veigas JM, et al. Study on wound healing activity of Punica granatum peel. *J Med Food.* 2004;7(2):256–259.

271. Ducrey B, Marston A, Göhring S, et al. Inhibition of 5α-reductase and aromatase by the ellagitannins oenothein A and oenothein B from Epilobium species. *Planta Med.* 1997;63:111–114.

272. Mizuno T, Uchino K, Toukairin T, et al. Inhibitory effect of tannic acid sulfate and related sulfates on infectivity, cytopathic effect, and giant cell formation of human immunodeficiency virus. *Planta Med.* 1992;58:535–539.

273. Lamaison JL, Carnat A, Petitjean-Freytet C. Teneur en tanins et activité inhibitrice de l'élastase chez les Rosaceae. *Ann Pharm Fr.* 1990;48(6):335–340.

274. Kashiwada Y, Nonaka G, Nishioka I, et al. Antitumor agents, 129. Tannins and related compounds as selective cytotoxic agents. *J Nat Prod.* 1992;55(8):1033–1043.

275. Schwitters B, Masquelier J. *OPC in Practice: Bioflavanols and Their Application,* 2nd ed. Rome: Alfa Omega; 1993.

276. Maimoona A, Naeem I, Saddiqe Z, et al. A review on biological, nutraceutical and clinical aspects of French maritime pine bark extract. *J Ethnopharmacol.* 2011;133(2):261–277.

277. Ahmed AE, Smithard R, Ellis M. Activities of enzymes of the pancreas, and the lum-en and mucosa of the small intestine in growing broiler cockerels fed on tannin-containing diets. *B J Nutr.* 1991;65: 189–197.

278. South PK, House WA, Miller DD. Tea consumption does not affect iron absorption in rats unless tea and iron are consumed together. *Nutr Res.* 1997;17(8):1303–1310.

279. Ruenwongsa P, Pattanavibag S. Effect of tea consumption on the levels of alpha-ketoglutarate and pyruvate dehydrogenase in rat brain. *Experientia.* 1982;38: 787–788.

280. Eshchar J, Friedman G. Acute hepatotoxicity of tannic acid added to barium enemas. *Dig Dis.* 1974;19(9): 825–829.

281. Paton A. Tannic acid in barium enemas. *Lancet.* 1964;1:934.

282. Gloro R, Hourmand-Ollivier I, Mosquet B, et al. Fulminant hepatitis during self-medication with hydroalcoholic extract of green tea. *Eur J Gastroenterol Hepatol.* 2005;17(10):1135–1137.

283. Kapadia GJ, Chung EB, Ghosh B, et al. Carcinogenicity of some folk medicinal herbs in rats. *J Natl Cancer Inst.* 1978;60(3):683–686.

284. Morton JF. Further associations of plant tannins and human cancer. *Q J Crude Drug Res.* 1972;12:1829–1841.

285. Chung KT, Wong TY, Wei CI, et al. Tannins and human health: a review. *Crit Rev Food Sci Nutr.* 1998;38(6):421–464.

286. Al-Habbal MJ, Al-Habbal Z, Huwezi FU. A double blind controlled clinical trial of mastic and placebo in the treatment of duodenal ulcer. *Clin Exp Pharmacol Physiol.* 1984;11:541–544.

287. Al-Said MA, Ageel AM, Parmar NS, et al. Evaluation of mastic a crude drug obtained from Pistacia lentiscus for gastric and duodenal anti-ulcer activity. *J Ethnopharmacol.* 1986;15:271–278.

288. Loughlin MF, Ala'Aldeen DA, Jenks PJ. Monotherapy with mastic does not eradicate Helicobacter pylori infection from mice. *J Antimicrob Chemother.* 2003;51(2):367–371.

289. Dabos KJ, Sfika E, Vlatta LJ, et al. Is Chios mastic gum effective in the treatment of functional dyspepsia? A prospective randomised double blind placebo controlled trial. *J Ethnopharmacol.* 2010;127(2):205–209.

290. Lee TY, Lam TH. Allergic contact dermatitis due to a Chinese orthopaedic solution tieh ta yao gin. *Contact Dermatitis.* 1993;28(2):89–90.

291. Meyerhof W. Elucidation of mammalian bitter taste. *Rev Physiol Biochem Pharmacol.* 2005;154:37–72.

292. Behrens M, Meyerhof W. Gustatory and extragustatory functions of mammalian taste receptors. *Physiol Behav.* 2011;105(1):4–13.

293. Behrens M, Meyerhof W. Oral and extraoral bitter taste receptors. *Results Probl Cell Differ.* 2010;52:87–99.

294. Krasteva G, Canning BJ, Hartmann P, et al. Cholinergic chemosensory cells in the trachea regulate breathing. *Proc Natl Acad Sci USA.* 2011;108(23):9478–9483.

295. Deshpande DA, Wang WC, McIlmoyle EL, et al. Bitter taste receptors on airway smooth muscle bronchodilate by localized calcium signaling and reverse obstruction. *Nat Med.* 2010;16(11):1299–1304.

296. Meyerhof W, Born S, Brockhoff A, et al. Molecular biology of mammalian bitter taste receptors. A review. *Flavor Fragrance J.* 2011;26(4):260–268.

297. Ogeto JO, Maitai CK. The scientific basis for the use of Strychnos henningsii (Gilg) plant material to stimulate appetite. *East Afr Med J.* 1983;60:603–607.

298. Carlson AJ, Torchiani B, Hallock R. Contributions to the physiology of the stomach. XXI. The supposed actions of the bitter tonic on the secretion of gastric juice in man and dog. *JAMA.* 1915;64(1):15–17.

299. Moorhead LD. Contributions to the physiology of the stomach. XXVIII. Further studies on the action of the bitter tonic on the secretion of gastric juice. *J Pharmacol Exp Ther.* 1915;7:577–589.

300. Glatzel H, Hackenberg K. [Röntgenologische Untersuchungen der Wirkungen von Bittermitteln auf die Verdauungsorgane.] *Planta Med.* 1967;3:223–232.

301. Baumann IC, Glatzel H, Muth HW. [Untersuchungen der Wirkungen von Wermut (Artemisia absinthium L.) auf die Gallen–und Pankreassaft–Sekretion des Menschen.] *Z Allgemeinmed.* 1975;51(17):784–791.

302. Herman JH, Nolan DS. A bitter cure. *NEJM.* 1981;305:1654.

303. Wolf S, Mack M. Experimental study of the action of bitters on the stomach of a fistulous human subject. *Drug Stand.* 1956;24(3):98–101.

304. Gebhardt R. Stimulation of acid secretion by extracts of Gentiana lutea L. in cultured cells from rat gastric mucosa. *Pharm Pharmacol Lett.* 1997;7(2–3):106–108.

305. Wegener T. [Anwendung eines Trockenextraktes aus Gentianae luteae radix bei dyspeptischem Symptomkomplex.] *Z Phytother.* 1998;19:163–164.

306. Ralph A, Giannella MD, Selwyn A, et al. Influence of gastric acidity on bacterial and parasitic enteric infections. *Ann Intern Med.* 1973;78(2):271–276.

307. Werbach MR. *Nutritional Influences on Illness: A Sourcebook of Clinical Research.* California: Third Line Press; 1987.

308. Gonzalez H, Ahmed T. Suppression of gastric H2-receptor mediated function in patients with bronchial asthma and ragweed allergy. *Chest.* 1986;89(4):491–496.

309. Kemp DR, Herrera F, Isaza J, et al. On the critical nature of blood sugar levels in the vagal stimulation of gastric acid secretion in normal and diabetic dogs. *Surgery.* 1968;64(5):958–966.

310. Mukherjee B, Mukherjee SK. Blood sugar lowering activity of Swertia chirata (Buch–Ham) extract. *Int J Crude Drug Res.* 1987;25(2):97–102.

311. Saltzman MB, McCallum RW. Diabetes and the stomach. *Yale J Biol Med.* 1983;56:179–187.

312. Niwa Y, Miyachi Y, Ishimoto K, et al. Why are natural plant medicinal products effective in some patients and not in others with the same disease? *Planta Med.* 1991;57(4):299–304.

313. Krebs S, Omer TN, Omer B. Wormwood (Artemisia absinthium) suppresses tumour necrosis factor alpha and accelerates healing in patients with Crohn's disease – A controlled clinical trial. *Phytomedicine.* 2010;17(5):305–309.

314. Omer B, Krebs S, Omer H, et al. Steroid-sparing effect of wormwood (Artemisia absinthium) in Crohn's disease: a double blind placebo-controlled study. *Phytomedicine.* 2007;14(2–3):87–95.

315. Weiss RF. Amara in current therapy (German). *Planta Med.* 1966;14(suppl):128–132.

316. Carrai M, Steinke V, Vodicka P, et al. Association between TAS2R38 gene polymorphisms and colorectal cancer risk: a case–control study in two independent populations of Caucasian origin. *PLoS One.* 2011;6(6):e20464.

317. Bartoshuk LM, Duffy VB, Reed D, et al. Supertasting, earaches and head injury: genetics and pathology alter our taste worlds. *Neurosci Behaviour Rev.* 1996;20(1):79–87.

318. Wang JC, Hinrichs AL, Bertelsen S, et al. Functional variants in TAS2R38 and TAS2R16 influence alcohol consumption in high risk families of African–American origin. *Alcohol Clin Exp Res.* 2007;31(2):209–215.

319. Tepper BJ, Koelliker Y, Zhao L, et al. Variation in the bitter-taste receptor

gene TAS2R38, and adiposity in a genetically isolated population in Southern Italy. *Obesity (Silver Spring)*. 2008;16(10):2289–2295.

320. Dotson CD, Shaw HL, Mitchell BD, et al. Variation in the gene TAS2R38 is associated with the eating behavior disinhibition in Old Order Amish women. *Appetite*. 2010;54(1):93–99.

321. Feeney E, O'Brien S, Scannell A, et al. Genetic variation in taste perception: does it have a role in healthy eating? *Proc Nutr Soc*. 2011;70(1):135–143.

322. Papoiu AD, Yosipovitch G. Topical capsaicin. The fire of a 'hot' medicine is reignited. *Expert Opin Pharmacother*. 2010;11(8):1359–1371.

323. Alawi K, Keeble J. The paradoxical role of the transient receptor potential vanilloid 1 receptor in inflammation. *Pharmacol Ther*. 2010;125(2):181–195.

324. Geppetti P, Patacchini R, Nassini R, et al. Cough: the emerging role of the TRPA1 channel. *Lung*. 2010;188(suppl 1):S63–S68.

325. Okumura Y, Narukawa M, Iwasaki Y, et al. Activation of TRPV1 and TRPA1 by black pepper components. *Biosci Biotechnol Biochem*. 2010;74(5):1068–1072.

326. Dedov VN, Tran VH, Duke CC, et al. Gingerols: a novel class of vanilloid receptor (VR1) agonists. *Br J Pharmacol*. 2002;137(6):793–798.

327. Peng J, Li YJ. The vanilloid receptor TRPV1: role in cardiovascular and gastrointestinal protection. *Eur J Pharmacol*. 2010;627(1–3):1–7.

328. Biro T, Acs G, Acs P, et al. Recent advances in understanding of vanilloid receptors: a therapeutic target for treatment of pain and inflammation in skin. *J Invest Dermatol Symp Proc*. 1997;2(1):56–60.

329. Towheen TE, Hochberg MC. A systematic review of randomized controlled trials of pharmacological therapy in osteoarthritis of the knee, with an emphasis on trial methodology. *Semin Arthritis Rheum*. 1997;26(5):755–770.

330. Kingery WS. A critical review of controlled clinical trials for peripheral neuropathic pain and complex regional pain syndromes. *Pain*. 1997;73(2):123–139.

331. Rains C, Bryson HM. Topical capsaicin. A review of its pharmacological properties and therapeutic potential in post-herpetic neuralgia, diabetic neuropathy and osteoarthritis. *Drugs Aging*. 1995;7(4):317–328.

332. Hautkappe M, Roizen MF, Toledano A, et al. Review of the effectiveness of capsaicin for painful cutaneous disorders and neural dysfunction. *Clin J Pain*. 1998;14(2):97–106.

333. Baron R, Wasner G, Lindner V. Optimal treatment of phantom limb pain in the elderly. *Drugs Aging*. 1998;12(5):361–376.

334. Sanico A, Togias A. Noninfectious, nonallergic rhinitis (NINAR): considerations on possible mechanisms. *Am J Rhinol*. 1998;12(1):65–72.

335. Gooding SM, Canter PH, Coelho HF, et al. Systematic review of topical capsaicin in the treatment of pruritus. *Int J Dermatol*. 2010;49(8):858–865.

336. Derry S, Lloyd R, Moore RA, et al. Topical capsaicin for chronic neuropathic pain in adults. *Cochrane Database Syst Rev*. 2009;(4):CD007393.

337. Cheng J, Yang XN, Liu X, et al. Capsaicin for allergic rhinitis in adults. *Cochrane Database Syst Rev*. 2006;(2):CD004460.

338. Kosuwon W, Sirichatiwapee W, Wisanuyotin T, et al. Efficacy of symptomatic control of knee osteoarthritis with 0.0125% of capsaicin versus placebo. *J Med Assoc Thai*. 2010;93(10):1188–1195.

339. Altman R, Barkin RL. Topical therapy for osteoarthritis: clinical and pharmacologic perspectives. *Postgrad Med*. 2009;121(2):139–147.

340. Cameron M, Gagnier JJ, Little CV, et al. Evidence of effectiveness of herbal medicinal products in the treatment of arthritis. Part I: osteoarthritis. *Phytother Res*. 2009;23(11):1497–1515.

341. Visudhiphan S, Poolsuppasit S, Piboonnukarintr O, et al. The relationship between high fibrinolytic activity and daily capsicum ingestion in Thais. *Am J Clin Nutr*. 1982;35:1452–1458.

342. Desai HG, Venugopalan K, Philipose M, et al. Effect of red chilli powder on gastric mucosal barrier and acid secretion. *Indian J Med Res*. 1977;66(3):440–448.

343. Abdel-Salam OM, Szolcsanyi J, Mozsik G. Capsaicin and the stomach. A review of experimental and clinical data. *J Physiol Paris*. 1997;91(3–5):151–171.

344. Allameh A, Sexena M, Biswas G, et al. Piperine, a plant alkaloid of the piper species, enhances the bioavailability of aflatoxin B1 in rat tissues. *Cancer Lett*. 1992;61(3):195–199.

345. Bano G, Raina RK, Zutshi U, et al. Effect of piperine on bioavailability and pharmacokinetics of propranolol and theophylline in healthy volunteers. *Eur J Clin Pharmacol*. 1991;41(6):615–617.

346. Shoba G, Joy D, Joseph T, et al. Influence of piperine on the pharmacokinetics of curcumin in animals and human volunteers. *Planta Med*. 1998;64(4):353–356.

347. Atal CK, Zutshi U, Rao PG. Scientific evidence on the role of Ayurvedic herbals on bioavailability of drugs. *J Ethnopharmacol*. 1981;4(2):229–232.

348. Atal CK, Dubey RK, Singh J. Biochemical basis of enhanced drug bioavailability by piperine: evidence that piperine is a potent inhibitor of drug metabolism. *J Pharmacol Exp Ther*. 1985;232(1):258–262.

349. Johri RK, Thusi N, Khajuria A, et al. Piperine-mediated changes in the permeability of rat intestinal epithelial cells. The status of gamma-glutamyl transpeptidase activity, uptake of amino acids and lipid peroxidation. *Biochem Pharmacol*. 1992;43(7):1401–1407.

350. Khajuria A, Zutshi U, Bendi KL. Permeability characteristics of piperine on oral absorption – an active alkaloid from peppers and a bioavailability enhancer. *Indian J Exp Biol*. 1998;36(1):46–50.

351. Srinivasan K. Black pepper and its pungent principle – piperine: a review of diverse physiological effects. *Crit Rev Food Sci Nutr*. 2007;47(8):735–748.

352. Pei YQ. A review of pharmacology and clinical use of piperine and its derivatives. *Epilepsia*. 1983;24(2):177–182.

353. Kawada T, Sakabe S, Watanabe T, et al. Some pungent principles of spices cause the adrenal medulla to secrete catecholamine in anesthetized rats. *Proc Soc Exp Biol Med*. 1988;188(2):229–233.

354. Doucet E, Tremblay A. Food intake, energy balance and body weight control. *Eur J Clin Nutr*. 1997;51(12):846–855.

355. Leung FW. Capsaicin-sensitive intestinal mucosal afferent mechanism and body fat distribution. *Life Sci*. 2008;83(1–2):1–5.

356. Surh YJ, Lee SS. Capsaicin in hot chili pepper: carcinogen, co-carcinogen or anticarcinogen? *Food Chem Toxicol*. 1996;34(3):313–316.

357. Surh YJ, Lee SS. Capsaicin, a double-edged sword: toxicity, metabolism, and chemopreventive potential. *Life Sci*. 1995;56(22):1845–1855.

358. Karekar VR, Mujumdar AM, Joshi SS, et al. Assessment of genotoxic effect of piperine using Salmonella typhimurium and somatic and germ cells of Swiss albino mice. *ArzneimittelForschung*. 1996;46(10):972–975.

359. [No authors listed]. Final report on the safety assessment of capsicum annuum extract, capsicum annuum fruit extract, capsicum annuum resin, capsicum annuum fruit powder, capsicum frutescens fruit, capsicum frutescens fruit extract, capsicum frutescens resin, and capsaicin. *Int J Toxicol*. 2007;26(suppl 1):3–106.

360. Segal R, Shatkovsky P, Milo-Goldzweig I. On the mechanisms of saponin hemolysis–I. Hydrolysis of the glycosidic bond. *Biochem Pharmacol*. 1974;23:973–981.

361. Segal R, Milo-Goldzweig I. On the mechanism of saponin hemolysis–II. Inhibition of hemolysis by aldonolactones. *Biochem Pharmacol*. 1975;24:77–81.

362. Boyd EM, Palmer ME. The effect of quillaia, senega, squill, grindelia, sanguinaria, chionanthus and dioscorea upon the output of respiratory tract fluid. *Acta Pharmacol*. 1946;2:235–246.

363. Walthelm U, Dittrich K, Gelbrich G, et al. Effects of saponins on the water solubility of different model compounds. *Planta Med*. 2001;67(1):49–54.

364. Bangham AD, Horne RW. Action of saponin on biological cell membranes. *Nature*. 1962;196:952–953.

365. Gee JM, Johnson IT. Interactions between hemolytic saponins, bile salts and small

intestinal mucosa in the rat. *J Nutr.* 1988;118:1391–1397.

366. Yamasaki K. Effect of some saponins on glucose transport system. In: Waller GR, Yamasaki K, eds. *Saponins Used in Traditional and Modern Medicine.* New York: Plenum Press; 1996. pp. 195–206.

367. Yoshikawa M, Yamahara J. Inhibitory effect of oleanene-type triterpene oligoglycosides on ethanol absorption: the structure–activity relationships. In: Waller GR, Yamasaki K, eds. *Saponins Used in Traditional and Modern Medicine.* New York: Plenum Press; 1996. pp. 207–218.

368. Sapra B, Jain S, Tiwary AK. Effect of Asparagus racemosus extract on transdermal delivery of carvedilol: a mechanistic study. *AAPS PharmSciTech.* 2009;10(1):199–210.

369. Cayen MN, Dvornik D. Effect of diosgenin on lipid metabolism in rats. *J Lipid Res.* 1979;20(2):162–174.

370. Oakenfull D, Sidhu GS. Could saponins be a useful treatment for hypercholesterolaemia? *Eur J Clin Nutr.* 1990;44:79–88.

371. Sears C. How to survive the world's worst diet. *New Scientist.* February 10, 1995;18.

372. Patra AK, Saxena J. The effect and mode of action of saponins on the microbial populations and fermentation in the rumen and ruminant production. *Nutr Res Rev.* 2009;22(2):204–219.

373. Milanov S, Maleeva E, Taskov M. Tribestan: effect on the concentration of some hormones in the serum of healthy volunteers. *Medicobiol Info.* 1985;4:27–29.

374. Zava DT, Dollbaum CM, Blen M. Estrogen and progestin bioactivity of foods, herbs and spices. *Proc Soc Exp Biol Med.* 1998;217:369–378.

375. Aradhana Rao AR, Kale RK. Diosgenin – a growth stimulator of mammary gland of ovariectomized mouse. *Ind J Exp Biol.* 1992;30(5):367–370.

376. Dinda B, Debnath S, Mohanta BC, et al. Naturally occurring triterpenoid saponins. *Chem Biodivers.* 2010;7(10):2327–2580.

377. Marston A, Hostettmann K. Plant molluscicides. *Phytochemistry.* 1985;24(4):639–652.

378. Oakenfull D. Saponins in food – a review. *Food Chem.* 1981;6:19–40.

379. Van Tonder EM, Basson PA, Van Rensburg IBJ. Geeldikkop: experimental induction by feeding the plant Tribulus terrestris L (Zygophyllaceae). *J S Afr Vet Assoc.* 1972;43(4):363–375.

380. Weisse AB. A fond farewell to the foxglove? The decline in the use of digitalis. *J Card Fail.* 2010;16(1):45–48.

381. Weiss RF. Herbal Medicine. Beaconsfield: Beaconsfield Publishers; 1988.

382. Prassas I, Diamandis EP. Novel therapeutic applications of cardiac glycosides. *Nat Rev Drug Discov.* 2008;7(11):926–935.

383. Newman RA, Yang P, Pawlus AD, et al. Cardiac glycosides as novel

cancer therapeutic agents. *Mol Interv.* 2008;8(1):36–49.

384. Mascolo N, Capasso R, Capasso F. Senna: a safe and effective drug. *Phytother Res.* 1998;12:S143–S145.

385. Nijs G, De Witte P, Geboes K, et al. In vitro demonstration of a positive effect of rhein anthrone on peristaltic reflex of guinea pig ileum. *Pharmacology.* 1993;47(suppl 1):40–48.

386. Leng–Peschlow E. Sennoside-induced secretion is not caused by changes in mucosal permeability or Na(+), K(+)-ATPase activity. *J Pharm Pharmacol.* 1993;45(11):951–954.

387. Yagi T, Miyawaki Y, Nishikawa A, et al. Suppression of the purgative action of rhein anthrone, the active metabolite of sennosides A and B, by indomethacin in rats. *J Pharm Pharmacol.* 1991;43(5):307–310.

388. Capasso F, Izzo AA, Mascolo N, et al. Effect of senna is not mediated by platelet-activating factor. *Pharmacology.* 1993;47(suppl 1):58–63.

389. Anton R, Haag-Berrurier M. Therapeutic use of natural anthraquinone for other than laxative actions. *Pharmacology.* 1980;20(suppl 1):104–112.

390. van de Kerkhof PC, Vissers WH. The topical treatment of psoriasis. *Skin Pharmacol Appl Skin Physiol.* 2003;16(2):69–83.

391. Rossi–Soffar G. Psoriasis. *Dermatologica.* 1965;130:53–79.

392. Ashton RE, Andre P, Lowe NJ, et al. Anthralin: historical and current perspectives. *J Am Acad Dermatol.* 1983;9(2):173–192.

393. Muller K, Leukel P, Ziereis K, et al. Antipsoriatic anthrones with modulated redox properties. 2. Novel derivatives of chrysarobin and isochrysarobin – antiproliferative activity and 5-lipoxygenase. *J Med Chem.* 1994;37(11):1660–1669.

394. Wang XJ, Warren BS, Rupp T, et al. Loss of mouse epidermal protein kinase C isozyme activities following treatment with phorbol ester and non-phorbol ester tumor promotors. *Carcinogenesis.* 1994;15(12):2795–2803.

395. Barnard DL, Huffman JH, Morris JL, et al. Evaluation of the antiviral activity of anthraquinones, anthrones and anthraquinone derivatives against human cytomegalovirus. *Antiviral Res.* 1992;17(1):63–77.

396. Spencer CM, Wilde MI. Diacerein. *Drugs.* 1997;53(1):98–106.

397. Fidelix TS, Soares BG, Trevisani VF. Diacerein for osteoarthritis. *Cochrane Database Syst Rev.* 2006;(1):CD005117.

398. Blomeke B, Poginsky B, Schmutte C, et al. Formation of genotoxic metabolites from anthraquinone glycosides present in Rubia tinctorum L. *Mutat Res.* 1992;265(2):263–272.

399. Ino N, Tanaka T, Okumura A, et al. Acute and subacute toxicity tests of madder

root, natural colorant extracted from madder (Rubia tinctorum), in (C57BL/6 X C3H)F1 in mice. *Toxicol Ind Health.* 1995;11(4):449–458.

400. Inoue K, Yoshida M, Takahashi M, et al. Induction of kidney and liver cancers by the natural food additive madder color in a two-year rat carcinogenicity study. *Food Chem Toxicol.* 2009;47(1):184–191.

401. Leng-Peschlow E. Senna and its rational use. *Pharmacology.* 1992;44(suppl 1):26–29.

402. Leng-Peschlow E. Senna and its rational use. *Pharmacology.* 1992;44(suppl 1):30–32.

403. Howard LRC, Hughes-Roberts HE. The treatment of constipation in mental hospitals. *Gut.* 1962;3:89–90.

404. Leng-Peschlow E. Senna and its rational use. *Pharmacology.* 1992;44(suppl 1):36–40.

405. Campbell WL. Cathartic colon: reversibility of roentgen changes. *Dis Colon Rectum.* 1983;26:445–448.

406. Leng-Peschlow E. Senna and its rational use. *Pharmacology.* 1992;44(suppl 1):20–22.

407. Leng-Peschlow E. Senna and its rational use. *Pharmacology.* 1992;44(suppl 1):23–25.

408. Leng-Peschlow E. Senna and its rational use. *Pharmacology.* 1992;44(suppl 1):33–35.

409. Harris A, Buchanan GN. Melanosis coli is reversible. *Colorectal Dis.* 2009;11(7):788–789.

410. Brown JP. A review of the genetic effects of naturally occurring flavonoids, anthraquinones and related compounds. *Mutat Res.* 1980;75:243–277.

411. Heidemann A, Miltenburger HG, Mengs U. The genotoxicity status of senna. *Pharmacology.* 1993;47(suppl):178–186.

412. Brusick D, Mengs U. Assessment of the genotoxic risk from laxative senna products. *Environ Mol Mutagen.* 1997;29:1–19.

413. Siegers CP. Anthranoid laxatives and colorectal cancer. *Trends Pharmacol Sci.* 1992;13:229–231.

414. Morales MA, Hernández D, Bustamante S, et al. Is senna laxative use associated to cathartic colon, genotoxicity, or carcinogenicity? *J Toxicol.* 2009; 2009:287247.

415. Marles RJ, Compadre CM, Farnsworth NR. Coumarin in vanilla extracts: its detection and significance. *Econ Bot.* 1987;41(1):41–47.

416. Stohr H, Herrmann K. On the phenolic acids of vegetables. III Hydroxycinnamic acids and hydroxybenzoic acids of root vegetables (German). *Z Lebensmittel Untersuchung Forschung.* 1975;159(4):218–224.

417. Arora RB, Mathur CN. Relationship between structure and anticoagulant activity of coumarin derivatives. *Br J Pharmacol.* 1963;20:29–35.

418. Hörhammer L, Wagner H, Reinhardt H. On new constituents from the barks of Viburnum prunifolium L. (American Snowball) and Virbunum opulus (Common Snowball). *Z Naturforschung.* 1967;22b:768–776.

419. Jarboe CH, Zirvi KA, Nicholson JA, et al. Scopoletin, an antispasmodic component of Viburnum opulus and prunifolium. *J Med Chem*. 1967;10:488–489.

420. Ojewole JAO, Adesina SK. Mechanism of the hypotensive effect of scopoletin isolated from fruit of Tetrapleura tetraptera. *Planta Med*. 1983;49(1):45–50.

421. Chen YF, Tsai HY, Wu TS. Anti-inflammatory and analgesic activities from roots of Angelica pubescens. *Planta Med*. 1995;61(1):2–8.

422. Kimura Y, Okuda H, Arichi S, et al. Inhibition of the formation of 5-hydroxy-6, 8,11,14-eicosatetraenoic acid from arachidonic acid in polymorphonuclear leukocytes by various coumarins. *Biochim Biophys Acta*. 1985;834(2):224–229.

423. Chang WS, Chiang HC. Structure–activity relationship of coumarins in xanthine oxidase inhibition. *Anticancer Res*. 1995;15(5B):1969–1973.

424. Lin HC, Tsai SH, Chen CS, et al. Structure–activity relationship of coumarin derivatives on xanthine oxidase-inhibiting and free radical-scavenging activities. *Biochem Pharmacol*. 2008;75(6):1416–1425.

425. Kong L, Zhou J, Wen Y, et al. Aesculin possesses potent hypouricemic action in rodents but is devoid of xanthine oxidase/dehydrogenase inhibitory activity. *Planta Med*. 2002;68(2):175–178.

426. Ding Z, Dai Y, Wang Z. Hypouricemic action of scopoletin arising from xanthine oxidase inhibition and uricosuric activity. *Planta Med*. 2005;71(2):183–185.

427. Ohta T, Watanabe K, Moriya M, et al. Anti-mutagenic effects of coumarin and umbelliferone on mutagenesis induced by 4-nitroquinoline 1-oxide or UV irradiation in E. coli. *Mutat Res*. 1983;117:135–138.

428. Romert L, Jansson T, Curvall M, et al. Screening for agents inhibiting the mutagenicity of extracts and constituents of tobacco products. *Mutat Res*. 1994;322(2):97–110.

429. Wattenberg LW, Lam LKT, Fladmoe AV. Inhibition of chemical carcinogen-induced neoplasia by coumarins and a-angelicalactone. *Cancer Res*. 1979;39:1651–1654.

430. Kolodziej H, Kayser O, Woerdenbag HJ, et al. Structure–cytotoxicity relationships of a series of natural and semi-synthetic simple coumarins as assessed in two human tumour cell lines. *Z Naturforschung*. 1997;52(3/4):240–244.

431. Weber US, Steffen B, Siegers CP. Antitumor-activities of coumarin, 7-hydroxy-coumarin and its glucuronide in several human tumor cell lines. *Res Commun Mol Pathol Pharmacol*. 1998;99(2):193–206.

432. Lacy A, O'Kennedy R. Studies on coumarins and coumarin-related compounds to determine their therapeutic role in the treatment of cancer. *Curr Pharm Des*. 2004;10(30):3797–3811.

433. Musa MA, Cooperwood JS, Khan MO. A review of coumarin derivatives in pharmacotherapy of breast cancer. *Curr Med Chem*. 2008;15(26):2664–2679.

434. Rios ER, Rocha NF, Venâncio ET, et al. Mechanisms involved in the gastroprotective activity of esculin on acute gastric lesions in mice. *Chem Biol Interact*. 2010;188(1):246–254.

435. Vasconcelos JF, Teixeira MM, Barbosa-Filho JM, et al. Effects of umbelliferone in a murine model of allergic airway inflammation. *Eur J Pharmacol*. 2009;609(1–3):126–131.

436. Panda S, Kar A. Evaluation of the antithyroid, antioxidative and antihyperglycemic activity of scopoletin from Aegle marmelos leaves in hyperthyroid rats. *Phytother Res*. 2006;20(12):1103–1105.

437. Ramesh B, Pugalendi KV. Antihyperglycemic effect of umbelliferone in streptozotocin-diabetic rats. *J Med Food*. 2006;9(4):562–566.

438. Pathak MA, Carbonare MD. Melanogenic potential of various furocoumarins in normal and vitiliginous skin. In: Fitzpatrick TB, Forlot P, Pathak MA, eds. *Psoralens: Past, Present and Future of Photochemoprotection and Other Biological Activities*. Paris: John Libbey Eurotext; 1989. pp. 87–101.

439. Fitzpatrick TB. The psoralen story: photochemotherapy and photochemoprotection. In: Fitzpatrick TB, Forlot P, Pathak MA, eds. *Psoralens: Past, Present and Future of Photochemoprotection and Other Biological Activities*. Paris: John Libbey Eurotext; 1989. pp. 5–10.

440. Kalis B, Sayag S, Forlot P. Photochemotherapy (PUVA) of psoriasis: a double blind comparative study of 5- and 8-methoxypsoralen. In: Fitzpatrick TB, Forlot P, Pathak MA, eds. *Psoralens: Past, Present and Future of Photochemoprotection and Other Biological Activities*. Paris: John Libbey Eurotext; 1989. pp. 277–282.

441. Forlot P. Psoralen induced pigmentation in human skin: overview of clinical evidence, mechanisms of induction and future research. In: Fitzpatrick TB, Forlot P, Pathak MA, eds. *Psoralens: Past, Present and Future of Photochemoprotection and Other Biological Activities*. Paris: John Libbey Eurotext; 1989. pp. 63–71.

442. Kligman AM, Forlot P. Comparative photoprotection in humans by tans induced either by solar stimulating radiation or after a psoralen–containing sunscreen. In: Fitzpatrick TB, Forlot P, Pathak MA, eds. *Psoralens, Past, Present and Future of Photochemoprotection and Other Biological Activities*. Paris: John Libbey Eurotext; 1989. pp. 407–420.

443. Gasparro FP. The role of PUVA in the treatment of psoriasis. Photobiology issues related to skin cancer incidence. *Am J Clin Dermatol*. 2000;1(6):337–348.

444. Matz H. Phototherapy for psoriasis: what to choose and how to use: facts and controversies. *Clin Dermatol*. 2010;28(1):73–80.

445. Musajo L, Rodighiero G, Colombo G, et al. Photosensitizing furocoumarins: interaction with DNA and photoinactivation of DNA containing viruses. *Experientia*. 1965;21:22.

446. Oginsky EL, Green GS, Griffith DG, et al. Lethal photosensitization of bacteria with 8-methoxy-psoralen to long wave length ultra-violet radiation. *J Bacteriol*. 1959;78:821.

447. Rauwald HW, Brehm O, Odenthal KP. The involvement of Ca2+ channel blocking mode of action in the pharmacology of Ammi visnaga fruits. *Planta Med*. 1994;60:101–105.

448. Meyer U. From khellin to sodium cromoglycate – a tribute to the work of Dr. R.E.C. Altounyan (1922–1987). *Pharmazie*. 2002;57(1):62–69.

449. Hogan RP. Hemorrhagic diathesis caused by drinking an herbal tea. *JAMA*. 1983;249(19):2679–2680.

450. Ivie GW. The chemistry of plant furanocoumarins and their medical, toxicological, environmental, and coevolutionary significance. *Rev Latinoam Quim*. 1987;18(1):1–5.

451. Cassier-Chauvat C, Averbeck D. Photomutagenic effects induced by psoralen derivatives in the yeast Saccharomyces cerevisiae. In: Fitzpatrick TB, Forlot P, Pathak MA, eds. *Psoralens: Past, Present and Future of Photochemoprotection and Other Biological Activities*. Paris: John Libbey Eurotext; 1989. pp. 329–335.

452. Marzin D, Olivier P. Study of the protective activity against photomutagenicity of 5-MOP. In: Fitzpatrick TB, Forlot P, Pathak MA, eds. *Psoralens: Past, Present and Future of Photochemoprotection and Other Biological Activities*. Paris: John Libbey Eurotext; 1989. pp. 337–343.

453. Young AR, Walker SL. Experimental photocarcinogenesis of psoralens. In: Fitzpatrick TB, Forlot P, Pathak MA, eds. *Psoralens: Past, Present and Future of Photochemoprotection and Other Biological Activities*. Paris: John Libbey Eurotext; 1989. pp. 357–366.

454. Stern RS. PUVA: its status in the United States, 1988. In: Fitzpatrick TB, Forlot P, Pathak MA, eds. *Psoralens: Past, Present and Future of Photochemoprotection and Other Biological Activities*. Paris: John Libbey Eurotext; 1989. pp. 367–376.

455. Henseler T. Risk of non melanoma skin tumors in patients treated with long–term–photochemotherapy (PUVA). In: Fitzpatrick TB, Forlot P, Pathak MA, eds. *Psoralens: Past, Present and Future of Photochemoprotection and Other Biological Activities*. Paris: John Libbey Eurotext; 1989. pp. 377–386.

456. Messina M. A brief historical overview of the past two decades of soy and isoflavone research. *J Nutr.* 2010;140(7):1350S–1354S.

457. Molteni A, Brizio-Molteni L, Persky V. In vitro hormonal effects of soybean isoflavones. *J Nutr.* 1995;125:751S–756S.

458. Zhao C, Dahlman-Wright K, Gustafsson JA. Estrogen receptor beta: an overview and update. *Nucl Recept Signal.* 2008;6:e003.

459. Koehler KF, Helguero LA, Haldosen LA, et al. Reflections on the discovery and significance of estrogen receptor beta. *Endocr Rev.* 2005;26(3):465–478.

460. Benassayag C, Perrot-Applanat M, Ferre F. Phytoestrogens as modulators of steroid action in target cells. *J Chromatogr B Analyt Technol Biomed Life Sci.* 2002;777(1–2):233–248.

461. Gustafsson JA. ERbeta scientific visions translate to clinical uses. *Climacteric.* 2006;9(3):156–160.

462. McCarty MF. Isoflavones made simple – genistein's agonist activity for the beta-type estrogen receptor mediates their health benefits. *Med Hypotheses.* 2006;66(6):1093–1114.

463. Rissman EF. Roles of oestrogen receptors alpha and beta in behavioural neuroendocrinology: beyond Yin/Yang. *J Neuroendocrinol.* 2008;20(6):873–879.

464. Turner JV, Agatonovic-Kustrin S, Glass BD. Molecular aspects of phytoestrogen selective binding at estrogen receptors. *J Pharm Sci.* 2007;96(8):1879–1885.

465. Oseni T, Patel R, Pyle J, et al. Selective estrogen receptor modulators and phytoestrogens. *Planta Med.* 2008;74(13):1656–1665.

466. Jeng YJ, Kochukov MY, Watson CS. Membrane estrogen receptor-alpha-mediated nongenomic actions of phytoestrogens in GH3/B6/F10 pituitary tumor cells. *J Mol Signal.* 2009;4:2.

467. Wuttke W, Jarry H, Seidlova-Wuttke D. Isoflavones – safe food additives or dangerous drugs? *Ageing Res Rev.* 2007;6(2):150–188.

468. Casanova M, You L, Gaido KW, et al. Developmental effects of dietary phytoestrogens in Sprague–Dawley rats and interactions of genistein and daidzein with rat estrogen receptors alpha and beta in vitro. *Toxicol Sci.* 1999;51(2):236–244.

469. Murray MJ, Meyer WR, Lessey BA, et al. Soy protein isolate with isoflavones does not prevent estradiol-induced endometrial hyperplasia in postmenopausal women: a pilot trial. *Menopause.* 2003;10(5):456–464.

470. Pavese JM, Farmer RL, Bergan RC. Inhibition of cancer cell invasion and metastasis by genistein. *Cancer Metastasis Rev.* 2010;29(3):465–482.

471. Virk-Baker MK, Nagy TR, Barnes S. Role of phytoestrogens in cancer therapy. *Planta Med.* 2010;76(11):1132–1142.

472. Cano A, García-Pérez MA, Tarín JJ. Isoflavones and cardiovascular disease. *Maturitas.* 2010;67(3):219–226.

473. Dong JY, Qin LQ. Soy isoflavones consumption and risk of breast cancer incidence or recurrence: a meta-analysis of prospective studies. *Breast Cancer Res Treat.* 2011;125(2):315–323.

474. Hilakivi-Clarke L, Andrade JE, Helferich W. Is soy consumption good or bad for the breast? *J Nutr.* 2010;140(12):2326S–2334S.

475. Lagari VS, Levis S. Phytoestrogens and bone health. *Curr Opin Endocrinol Diabetes Obes.* 2010;17(6):546–553.

476. Bolaños R, Del Castillo A, Francia J. Soy isoflavones versus placebo in the treatment of climacteric vasomotor symptoms: systematic review and meta-analysis. *Menopause.* 2010;17(3):660–666.

477. Kurzer MS. Soy consumption for reduction of menopausal symptoms. *Inflammopharmacology.* 2008;16(5):227–229.

478. de Cremoux P, This P, Leclercq G, et al. Controversies concerning the use of phytoestrogens in menopause management: bioavailability and metabolism. *Maturitas.* 2010;65(4):334–339.

479. Hooper L, Ryder JJ, Kurzer MS, et al. Effects of soy protein and isoflavones on circulating hormone concentrations in pre- and post-menopausal women: a systematic review and meta-analysis. *Hum Reprod Update.* 2009;15(4):423–440.

480. Kim J. Protective effects of Asian dietary items on cancers – soy and ginseng. *Asian Pac J Cancer Prev.* 2008;9(4):543–548.

481. Van Patten CL, de Boer JG, Tomlinson Guns ES. Diet and dietary supplement intervention trials for the prevention of prostate cancer recurrence: a review of the randomized controlled trial evidence. *J Urol.* 2008;180(6):2314–2321.

482. Pase MP, Grima NA, Sarris J. The effects of dietary and nutrient interventions on arterial stiffness: a systematic review. *Am J Clin Nutr.* 2011;93(2):446–454.

483. Taku K, Lin N, Cai D, et al. Effects of soy isoflavone extract supplements on blood pressure in adult humans: systematic review and meta-analysis of randomized placebo-controlled trials. *J Hypertens.* 2010;28(10):1971–1982.

484. Beavers DP, Beavers KM, Miller M, et al. Exposure to isoflavone-containing soy products and endothelial function: a Bayesian meta-analysis of randomized controlled trials. *Nutr Metab Cardiovasc Dis.* 2012;22(3):182–191.

485. Vatanparast H, Chilibeck PD. Does the effect of soy phytoestrogens on bone in postmenopausal women depend on the equol-producing phenotype? *Nutr Rev.* 2007;65(6):294–299.

486. Rowland IR, Wiseman H, Sanders TAB. Interindividual variations in metabolism of soy isoflavones and lignans: influence of habitual diet on equol production by the gut microflora. *Nutr Cancer.* 2000;36(1):27–32.

487. Tokunaga T. Novel physiological functions of fructooligosaccharides. *Biofactors.* 2004;21(1–4):89–94.

488. Setchell KDR, Lawson AM, Borriello SP, et al. Lignan formation in man – microbial involvement and possible roles in relation to cancer. *Lancet.* 1981;2:4–7.

489. Phipps WR, Martini MC, Lampe JW, et al. Effect of flax seed ingestion on the menstrual cycle. *J Clin Endocrinol Metab.* 1993;77(5):1215–1219.

490. Frische EJ, Hutchins AM, Martini MC, et al. Effect of flaxseed and wheat bran on serum hormones and lignan excretion in premenopausal women. *J Am Coll Nutr.* 2003;22(6):550–554.

491. Hutchins AM, Martini MC, Olson BA, et al. Flaxseed consumption influences endogenous hormone concentrations in postmenopausal women. *Nutr Cancer.* 2001;39(1):58–65.

492. Serraino M, Thompson LU. The effect of flaxseed supplementation on early risk markers for mammary carcinogenesis. *Cancer Lett.* 1991;60:135–142.

493. Adlercreutz H, Fotsis T, Heikkinen R, et al. Excretion of the lignans enterolactone and enterodiol and of equol in omnivorous and vegetarian postmenopausal women and in women with breast cancer. *Lancet.* 1982;2:1295–1299.

494. Sonestedt E, Wirfält E. Enterolactone and breast cancer: methodological issues may contribute to conflicting results in observational studies. *Nutr Res.* 2010;30(10):667–677.

495. Brooks JD, Ward WE, Lewis JE, et al. Supplementation with flaxseed alters estrogen metabolism in postmenopausal women to a greater extent than does supplementation with an equal amount of soy. *Am J Clin Nutr.* 2004;79(2):318–325.

496. Haggans CJ, Travelli EJ, Thomas W, et al. The effect of flaxseed and wheat bran consumption on urinary estrogen metabolites in premenopausal women. *Cancer Epidemiol Biomarkers Prev.* 2000;9(7):719–725.

497. Haggans CJ, Hutchins AM, Olson BA, et al. Effect of flaxseed consumption on urinary estrogen metabolites in postmenopausal women. *Nutr Cancer.* 1999;33(2):188–195.

498. Simbalista RL, Sauerbronn AV, Aldrighi JM, et al. Consumption of a flaxseed-rich food is not more effective than a placebo in alleviating the climacteric symptoms of postmenopausal women. *J Nutr.* 2010;140(2):293–297.

499. Irvine CHG, Fitzpatrick MG, Alexander SL. Phytoestrogens in soy-based infant foods: concentrations, daily intake, and possible biological effects. *Proc Soc Exp Biol Med.* 1998;217:247–253.

500. Messina M. Soybean isoflavone exposure does not have feminizing effects on men: a critical examination of the clinical evidence. *Fertil Steril.* 2010;93(7):2095–2104.

501. Hamilton-Reeves JM, Vazquez G, Duval SJ, et al. Clinical studies show no effects of soy protein or isoflavones on reproductive hormones in men: results of a meta-analysis. *Fertil Steril.* 2010;94(3):997–1007.

502. Hooper L, Madhavan G, Tice JA, et al. Effects of isoflavones on breast density in pre- and post-menopausal women: a systematic review and meta-analysis of randomized controlled trials. *Hum Reprod Update.* 2010;16(6):745–760.

503. Wu AH, Ursin G, Koh WP, et al. Green tea, soy, and mammographic density in Singapore Chinese women. *Cancer Epidemiol Biomarkers Prev.* 2008;17(12):3358–3365.

504. Bandera EV, Williams MG, Sima C, et al. Phytoestrogen consumption and endometrial cancer risk: a population-based case-control study in New Jersey. *Cancer Causes Control.* 2009;20(7):1117–1127.

505. Lethaby AE, Brown J, Marjoribanks J, et al. Phytoestrogens for vasomotor menopausal symptoms. *Cochrane Database Syst Rev.* 2007;(4):CD001395.

506. Messina M, Redmond G. Effects of soy protein and soybean isoflavones on thyroid function in healthy adults and hypothyroid patients: a review of the relevant literature. *Thyroid.* 2006;16(3):249–258.

507. Rolland A, Fleurentin J, Lanahers MC, et al. Behavioural effects of the American traditional plant Eschscholzia californica: sedative and anxiolytic properties. *Planta Med.* 1991;57:212–216.

508. Schäfer HL, Schäfer H, Schneider W, et al. Sedative action of extract combinations of Eschscholtzia californica and Corydalis cava. *ArzneimittelForschung.* 1995;45(1):124–126.

509. Kleber E, Schneider W, Schäfer HL, et al. Modulation of key reactions of the catecholamine metabolism by extracts from Eschscholtzia californica and Corydalis cava. *Arzneimittel-Forschung.* 1995;45(1):127–131.

510. Lui LM, Sheu SJ, Chiou SH, et al. A comparative study on commercial samples of Ephedrae herba. *Planta Med.* 1993;59:376–378.

511. Thies PW. [Spartium und spartein.] *Pharm Unserer Zeit.* 1986;6:172–176.

512. Northover BJ. Effect of pre-treating rat atria with potassium channel blocking drugs on the electrical and mechanical responses to phenylephrine. *Biochem Pharmacol.* 1994;47(12):2163–2169.

513. Eichelbaum M, Spannbrucker N, Steincke B, et al. Defective N-oxidation of sparteine in man: a new pharmacogenetic defect. *Eur J Clin Pharm.* 1979;16:183–187.

514. Vinks A, Inaba T, Otton SV, et al. Sparteine metabolism in Canadian Caucasians. *Clin Pharmacol Ther.* 1982;31(1):23–29.

515. Hempelmann FW, Heinz N, Flasch H. Lipophilicity–protein binding relationship in cardenolides. *Arzneimittel-Forschung.* 1978;28(12):2182–2185.

516. Tschanz C, Stargel WW, Thomas JA. Interactions between drugs and nutrients. *Adv Pharmacol.* 1996;35:1–26.

517. Sterk V, Büchele B, Simmet T. Effect of food intake on the bioavailability of boswellic acids from a herbal preparation in healthy volunteers. *Planta Med.* 2004;70(12):1155–1160.

518. Schubert W, Culberg G, Edgar B, et al. Inhibition of 17 beta-estradiol by grapefruit juice in ovariectomized women. *Maturitas.* 1995;20:155–163.

519. Bailey DG, Arnold JM, Spence JD. Grapefruit juice and drugs. How significant is the interaction? *Clin Pharmacokinet.* 1994;26(2):91–98.

520. Fuhr U, Klittich K, Staib AH. Inhibitory effect of grapefruit juice and its bitter principle, naringenin, on CYP1A2 dependent metabolism of caffeine in man. *Br J Clin Pharmacol.* 1993;35(4):431–436.

521. Miniscalco A, Lundahl J, Regardh CG, et al. Inhibition of dihydropyridine metabolism in rat and human liver microsomes by flavonoids found in grapefruit juice. *J Pharmacol Exp Ther.* 1992;261(3):1195–1199.

522. Min DI, Ku YM, Perry PJ, et al. Effect of grapefruit juice on cyclosporine pharmacokinetics in renal transplant patients. *Transplant.* 1996;62(1):123–125.

523. Hukkinen SK, Varhe A, Olkkola KT, et al. Plasma concentrations of triazolam are increased by concomitant ingestion of grapefruit juice. *Clin Pharmacol Ther.* 1995;58(2):127–131.

524. Lundahl JUE, Regårdh CG, Edgar B, et al. The interaction effect of grapefruit juice is maximal after the first glass. *Eur J Clin Pharm.* 1998;54:75–81.

525. Lee YS, Lorenzo BJ, Koufis T, et al. Grapefruit juice and its flavonoids inhibit 11 beta-hydroxysteroid dehydrogenase. *Clin Pharmacol Ther.* 1996;59(1):62–71.

526. Edwards DJ, Bernier SM. Naringin and naringenin are not the primary CYP3A inhibitors in grapefruit juice. *Life Sci.* 1996;59(13):1025–1030.

527. Runkel M, Bourian M, Tegtmeier M, et al. The character of inhibition of the metabolism of 1,2-benzopyrone (coumarin) by grapefruit juice in humans. *Eur J Clin Pharm.* 1997;53:265–269.

528. He K, Iyer KR, Hayes RN, et al. Inactivation of cytochrome P450 3A4 by bergamottin, a component of grapefruit juice. *Chem Res Toxicol.* 1998;11(4):252–259.

529. Woo WS, Shin KH, Lee CK. Effect of naturally occurring coumarins on the activity of drug metabolizing enzymes. *Biochem Pharmacol.* 1983;32(11):1800–1803.

530. Diaconu CH, Cuciureanu M, Vlase L, et al. Food–drug interactions: grapefruit juice. *Rev Med Chir Soc Med Nat Iasi.* 2011;115(1):245–250.

531. Steinegger E, Hövel H. Analytic and biologic studies on Salicaceae substances, especially on salicin. II. Biological study. *Pharm Acta Helv.* 1972;47:222–234.

532. Fotsch G, Pfeifer S, Bartozsek M, et al. Biotransformation of phenolglycosides leiocarposide and salicin. *Pharmazie.* 1989;44(8):555–558.

533. Akao T, Yoshino T, Kobashi K, et al. Evaluation of salicin as an antipyretic prodrug that does not cause gastric injury. *Planta Med.* 2002;68(8):714–718.

534. Leng-Peschlow E. Senna and its rational use. *Pharmacology.* 1992;44(suppl):10–15.

535. Soulimani R, Younos C, Mortier F, et al. The role of stomachal digestion on the pharmacological activity of plant extracts, using as an example extracts of Harpagophytum procumbens. *Can J Physiol Pharmacol.* 1994;72:1532–1536.

536. Wagner H, Jurcic K, Schaette R. Comparative studies on the sedative action of Valeriana extracts, valepotriates and their degradation products. *Planta Med.* 1980;39:358–365.

537. Valdes III LJ. Salvia divinorum and the unique diterpene hallucinogen Salvinorin (Divinorin) A. *J Psychoactive Drugs.* 1994;26(3):277–283.

538. Griffiths LA, Barlow A. The fate of orally and parenterally administered flavonoids in the mammal. The significance of biliary excretion. *Angiology.* 1972;9(3–6):162–174.

539. Kim DH. Herbal medicines are activated by intestinal microflora. *Nat Prod Sci.* 2002;8(2):35–43.

540. Ishimi Y, Arai N, Wang X, et al. Difference in effective dosage of genistein on bone and uterus in ovariectomized mice. *Biochem Biophys Res Commun.* 2000;274(3):697–701.

541. Pino AM, Valladares LE, Palma MA, et al. Dietary isoflavones affect sex hormone-binding globulin levels in postmenopausal women. *J Clin Endocrinol Metab.* 2000;85(8):2797–2800.

542. Graefe EU, Wittig J, Mueller S, et al. Pharmacokinetics and bioavailability of quercetin glycosides in humans. *J Clin Pharmacol.* 2001;41(5):492–499.

543. Jäger AK, Saaby L. Flavonoids and the CNS. *Molecules.* 2011;16(2):1471–1485.

544. Moon YJ, Wang L, DiCenzo R, et al. Quercetin pharmacokinetics in humans. *Biopharm Drug Dispos.* 2008;29(4):205–217.

545. Zhang L, Zuo Z, Lin G. Intestinal and hepatic glucuronidation of flavonoids. *Mol Pharm.* 2007;4(6):833–845.

546. Hertog MGL, Hollman PCH. Potential health effects of the dietary flavonol quercetin. *Eur J Clin Nutr.* 1996;50(2):63–71.

547. Hollman PC, De Vries JH, Van Leeuwen SD, et al. Absorption of dietary quercetin glycosides and quercetin in healthy ileostomy volunteers. *Am J Clin Nutr.* 1995;62(6):1276–1282.

548. Merfort I, Heilmann J, Weiss M, et al. Radical scavenger activity of three flavonoid metabolites studied by inhibition of chemiluminescence in human PMNs. *Planta Med.* 1996;62(4):289–292.

549. Rechner AR, Kroner C. Anthocyanins and colonic metabolites of dietary polyphenols inhibit platelet function. *Thromb Res.* 2005;116(4):327–334.

550. Rechner AR, Kuhnle G, Bremner P, et al. The metabolic fate of dietary polyphenols in humans. *Free Radic Biol Med.* 2002;33(2):220–235.

551. Kelly GE, Joannou GE, Reeder AY, et al. The variable metabolic response to dietary isoflavones in humans. *Proc Soc Exp Biol Med.* 1995;208(1):40–43.

552. Xu X, Wang HJ, Murphy PA, et al. Daidzein is a more bioavailable soymilk isoflavone than is genistein in adult women. *J Nutr.* 1994;124(6):825–832.

553. Xu X, Harris KS, Wang HJ, et al. Bioavailability of soybean isoflavones depends upon gut microflora in women. *J Nutr.* 1995;125(9):2307–2315.

554. Cassidy A, Bingham S, Setchell K. Biological effects of isoflavones in young women: importance of the chemical composition of soyabean products. *Br J Nutr.* 1995;74(4):587–601.

555. Larkin T, Price WE, Astheimer L. The key importance of soy isoflavone bioavailability to understanding health benefits. *Crit Rev Food Sci Nutr.* 2008;48(6):538–552.

556. Manach C, Williamson G, Morand C, et al. Bioavailability and bioefficacy of polyphenols in humans. I. Review of 97 bioavailability studies. *Am J Clin Nutr.* 2005;81(1 suppl):230S–242S.

557. Nielsen IL, Williamson G. Review of the factors affecting bioavailability of soy isoflavones in humans. *Nutr Cancer.* 2007;57(1):1–10.

558. Wang Z, Kurosaki Y, Nakayama T, et al. Mechanism of gastrointestinal absorption of glycyrrhizin in rats. *Biol Pharm Bull.* 1994;17(10):1399–1403.

559. Krahenbuhl S, Hasler F, Krapf R. Analysis and pharmacokinetics of glycyrrhizic acid and glycyrrhetinic acid in humans and experimental animals. *Steroids.* 1994;59(2):121–126.

560. Hattori M, Sakamoto T, Kobashi K, et al. Metabolism of glycyrrhizin by human intestinal flora. *Planta Med.* 1983;48(1):38–42.

561. Sakiya Y, Akada Y, Kawano S, et al. Rapid estimation of glycyrrhizin and glycyrrhetinic acid in plasma by high-speed liquid chromatography. *Chem Pharm Bull.* 1979;27(5):1125–1129.

562. Nose M, Ito M, Kamimura K, et al. A comparison of the antihepatotoxic activity between glycyrrhizin and glycyrrhetinic acid. *Planta Med.* 1994;60(2):136–139.

563. Hasegawa H, Sung JH, Matsumiya S, et al. Main ginseng saponin metabolites formed by intestinal bacteria. *Planta Med.* 1996;62(5):453–457.

564. Rauwald HW, Grunwild J. Ruscus aculeatus extract: unambiguous proof of the absorption of spirostanol glycosides in human plasma after oral administration. *Planta Med.* 1991;57(suppl 2):A75–A76.

565. Daniel EM, Ratnayake S, Kinstle T, et al. The effects of pH and rat intestinal contents on the liberation of ellagic acid from purified and crude ellagitannins. *J Nat Prod.* 1991;54(4):946–952.

566. Bravo L, Abia R, Eastwood MA, et al. Degradation of polyphenols (catechin and tannic acid) in the rat intestinal tract. Effect on colonic fermentation and faecal output. *Br J Nutr.* 1994;71(6):933–946.

567. Groenewoud G, Hundt HKL. The microbial metabolism of condensed (+)-catechins by rat-caecal microflora. *Xenobiotica.* 1986;16(2):99–107.

568. Larrosa M, García-Conesa MT, Espín JC, et al. Ellagitannins, ellagic acid and vascular health. *Mol Aspects Med.* 2010;31(6):513–539.

569. Appeldoorn MM, Vincken JP, Aura AM, et al. Procyanidin dimers are metabolized by human microbiota with 2-(3,4-dihydroxyphenyl)acetic acid and 5-(3,4-dihydroxyphenyl)-gamma-valerolactone as the major metabolites. *J Agric Food Chem.* 2009;57(3):1084–1092.

570. Grimm T, Skrabala R, Chovanová Z, et al. Single and multiple dose pharmacokinetics of maritime pine bark extract (pycnogenol) after oral administration to healthy volunteers. *BMC Clin Pharmacol.* 2006;6:4.

571. Serafini M, Ghiselli A, Ferro-Luzzi A. In vivo antioxidant effect of green and black tea in man. *Eur J Clin Nutr.* 1996;50(1):28–32.

572. Nakagawa K, Okuda S, Miyazawa T. Dose-dependent incorporation of tea catechins, (–)-epigallocatechin-3-gallate and (–)-epigallocatechin, into human plasma. *Biosci Biotechnol Biochem.* 1997;61(12):1981–1985.

573. Wang JS, Luo H, Wang P, et al. Validation of green tea polyphenol biomarkers in a phase II human intervention trial. *Food Chem Toxicol.* 2008;46(1):232–240.

574. Pulse TL, Uhlig E. A significant improvement in a clinical pilot study utilizing nutritional supplements, essential fatty acids and stabilized aloe vera juice in 29 HIV seropositive ARC and AIDS patients. *J Adv Med.* 1990;3(4):209–230.

575. Sullivan R, Smith JE, Rowan NJ. Medicinal mushrooms and cancer therapy: translating a traditional practice into Western medicine. *Perspect Biol Med.* 2006;49(2):159–170.

576. Yajima Y, Satoh J, Fukuda I, et al. Quantitative assay of lentinan in human blood with the limulus colorimetric test. *Tohoku J Exp Med.* 1989;157(2):145–151.

577. Yoshino S, Watanabe S, Imano M, et al. Improvement of QOL and prognosis by treatment of superfine dispersed lentinan in patients with advanced gastric cancer. *Hepatogastroenterology.* 2010;57(97):172–177.

578. van Duynhoven J, Vaughan EE, Jacobs DM, et al. Metabolic fate of polyphenols in the human superorganism. *Proc Natl Acad Sci USA.* 2011;108(suppl 1):4531–4538.

579. Possemiers S, Bolca S, Verstraete W, et al. The intestinal microbiome: a separate organ inside the body with the metabolic potential to influence the bioactivity of botanicals. *Fitoterapia.* 2011;82(1):53–66.

580. Boyd EM, Sheppard EP. The effect of steam inhalation of volatile oils on the output and composition of respiratory tract fluid. *J Pharmacol Exp Ther.* 1968;163(1):250–256.

581. Boyd EM, Sheppard EP. A bronchomucotropic action in rabbits from inhaled menthol and thymol. *Arch Int Pharmacodyn.* 1969;182(1):206–214.

582. Sheppard EP, Boyd EM. Lemon oil as an expectorant inhalant. *Pharmacol Res Commun.* 1970;2(1):1–16.

583. Boyd EM, Sheppard EP. Nutmeg oil and camphene as inhaled expectorants. *Arch Otolaryngol.* 1970;92(4):372–378.

584. Boyd EM, Sheppard EP. The effect of inhalation of citral and geraniol on the output and composition of respiratory tract fluid. *Arch Int Pharmacodyn.* 1970;188(1):5–13.

Principles of herbal treatment

3

CHAPTER CONTENTS

First principles of traditional herbal treatment

As any review of herbal traditions from around the world will confirm, the use of plants in medicine reflects the enormous diversity of local traditions, with much more variety than consistency. However, more consistent themes emerge in history, most clearly where local folk practices were systematised in the great written traditions, reviewed in Chapter 1.

When these traditions are examined closely, especially when they relate to human experience of illness and medicine, or to recurrent pharmaceutical forms (for example, tannin, resin, laxative, essential oil, acrid or bitter principle formulations rather than the individual remedies) and then translated into modern terminology, it is possible to identify recurrent features. These appear to encapsulate essential characteristics of the material, universal archetypes of the effects plants have on humans. They certainly reflect the therapeutic priorities of earlier ages (and should therefore be adapted before being applied to modern health needs). They are valuable, however, because they probably represent the roots of herbal therapeutics, those characteristics of the remedies that are the most reliable and potent. They also draw stark contrasts with the approaches that have emerged with the development of modern technological medicine. They are antidotes to the modern tendency to view herbs solely as milder versions of modern drugs. In essence, they should underpin any rational phytotherapy.

Note: Therapeutic insights are generally better absorbed from instruction and in practice rather than in the scientific literature and the following information arises from a breadth of sources. Notable among these is the bibliography at the end of the chapter listing authors who mostly were in contact with primary resources or leading teachers. The attempt is to distil rather than list scholastically.

Cleansing: detoxification and elimination

In much traditional practice there was an explicit or implicit assumption that, before healing could take place, noxious influences needed to be removed. In the earliest animistic traditions, pathogens could be literally demons and shamanistic practices emerged to drive them out. However, there was also a consistent, more mundane view of toxins and poisons: these needed to be removed by the body's eliminatory functions. Disease was widely seen as a failure of elimination and the vomiting, diarrhoea, coughing, diaphoresis and diuresis of most acute diseases as evidence that the body was being driven to extraordinary eliminative measures. In Ayurvedic medicine the *doshas* were initially excretions and health their healthy presence; in Chinese medicine the development of chronic disease was a sign that acute eliminatory responses had failed in their primary task of keeping pathogens out and that penetration into the interior had occurred.

The task of the physician was equally clear: to support eliminatory functions as vigorously as possible compatible with the body's vital reserves (eliminatory functions were mostly seen as taxing the body's energies). In practice this meant robust 'heroic' treatments in acute disease, notably involving emetics, purgatives, powerful expectorants and, in fever management, diaphoretics. In chronic and debilitated conditions the aim was to use gentler treatments, peeling away toxic accumulations like the layers of an onion, always making sure that eliminatory measures, laxatives, diuretics, choleretics, expectorants and the more systemic lymphatics and alteratives were supported by adequate sustenance for the vital functions: rest, nourishment and the use of tonic remedies (see below).

DOI: http://dx.doi.org/10.1016/B978-0-443-06992-5.00003-7

Typically in traditional therapeutics, therefore, eliminatory measures were the first stage of treatment, to be followed increasingly by the following more adjustive and sustaining treatments.

Heating: moving the circulation

It was apparent to all humans that heat equated to vitality. The extreme absence of heat was the striking coldness of the corpse. When Samuel Thomson in North America built his therapeutics around the principle that disease was essentially a cold intrusion and that before all else remedies should heat the struggling body, he was only highlighting an almost universal instinct. In every tradition there is frequent use of heating remedies; the hot spices, or 'pungent' remedies, were the strongest for internal use, but there was always a raft of gentler warming remedies as well. Some were applied as aromatic digestives to failing 'cold' digestion, others as warming expectorants or mucolytics in treating the effects of cold and damp on the chest and respiratory system. There were warming tonics (*yang* tonics in traditional Chinese medicine) and a variety of remedies that brought heat to the head, reproductive system or kidneys.

All the above could be used, along with hot packs, hot baths, 'sweat lodges' or hot drinks in fever, which was the major indication for supportive heating. Heating remedies used in fever management are now called 'diaphoretics' as their main effect is to increase perspiration. Sweat was understood not only as a cooling agent but also as the prime eliminatory route in febrile disease; in this context, therefore, heating was an obvious cleansing strategy, as above.

Indications for the use of heating agents apart from fevers were easily understood. If the patient felt cold, as a whole or in the diseased part, or favoured hot food, hot drinks, hot packs or hot baths; if there was diminished vitality; if there was pallor (the nail bed or 'quick' was a particularly sensitive guide) or signs of cumulative cold-damp conditions like mucus or gravity-dependent oedema, then heating remedies were indicated. The fact that a headache or arthritic joint or abdominal swelling was relieved by a hot pack was as important in choosing the course of treatment as determining what pathological factor was involved.

When the focus of cold was clearly demarcated, then extreme heating, in the form of powerful 'counter-irritation', cayenne or mustard plasters, blistering croton oil or formic acid or stinging nettles, might be applied topically, with sometimes dramatic beneficial effects.

Heat in modern terms equates also to circulation: a rationale that includes improved tissue perfusion, oxygenation and metabolite removal can easily be made. A modern phytotherapist might avoid the more drastic topical heating agents and may have less need to manage fevers, but could still consider the role of heating agents in a prescription if these were indicated.

The major caution in modern times is that many patients are also debilitated, at least from the perspective of earlier, more robust times. Heating agents do not heat directly, but instead stimulate increased thermogenesis and circulatory activity. They thus require reserves of energy in the body.

Someone weakened by chronic ill health may suffer if stimulated in this way. An assessment of vital reserves is essential in such treatment.

Cooling: stimulating digestion

Whereas heating was clearly 'on the side of the angels' in traditional healthcare, cooling was altogether a more thoughtful matter. It is, after all, perfectly possible to have hot spicy foods at every mealtime (especially in the tropics where they prompt gastric defences against enteric infections) but, with a few notable exceptions, cooling was confined to therapeutics. Cooling meant reducing vitality. The ultimate cold was death. In their simple restatement of fundamental principles, Samuel Thomson and his followers denied any prospect of cooling in healthcare and even saw something diabolical in it. Nevertheless, more considered views throughout history recognised that one can have too much, or inappropriate, heat. The obvious examples were hyperpyrexia in fevers, inflammatory diseases, hypersensitivity or allergic reactions, nervous agitation and, above all, pain. The respective treatments, febrifuges, anti-inflammatories, antiallergic remedies, sedatives, hypnotics (and narcotics) and analgesics, would all be classified as cooling in these terms. Indeed, some of the eliminatory treatments often applied for these purposes, especially the laxatives and cholagogues, were also seen as cooling. Reference to the Galenic classification (pp. 4–5) will put all this into context.

The classification of sedatives is illuminating. In former times, neurosis and anxiety, irritability and tension were aspects of heat. Children were hotter than adults and there was progressive constitutional cooling with age. Psychological explanations were not prominent and no one was told 'it is all in the mind'. The Cartesian body–mind split had not occurred.

Clearly there was more likely to be care in prescription of cooling remedies. Although many popular treatments existed, it was more likely that professional expertise would be called for, especially in the treatment of severe pains and inflammations. Almost everything now prescribed by modern doctors would have been classified as cooling.

There was one striking exception to the cautions linking cooling to reduced vitality. As referred to in the Galenic classification, the gentlest category of cooling remedy (those 'cold in the first degree') did 'qualify the heat of the stomach and cause digestion'. Digestion was widely seen as a cooling activity, marked of course by a shift of blood flow from the periphery to the core (so that excessive exercise after a big meal can lead to cramps).

The archetypal digestive stimulants were the bitters. Of all the herbal strategies in history, these are probably the most respected (the Chinese even gave them the awesome role in their five-phase classification of tonifying the *Kidneys* – the source of constitutional energies in their system). Bitters are universally used before and after eating as appetite stimulants ('aperitifs') and digestives. They were the first resort in digestive difficulties, especially when associated with heat and hepatobiliary ('damp-heat') disorders (bitters are also the most commonly used choleretics). Critically, they were also favourite febrifuges, apparently lowering body temperature in fever. They appeared to correct an apparent design inconsistency in the febrile response, wherein digestion is shut down, leaving undigested material as a source of new toxicity and even the original source of infection in the case of gastroenteritis. Bitters appeared to switch on digestive defences as well as bring the fever down. In many cultural traditions bitters were seen as primarily cooling (although in northern European traditions especially, some bitter remedies were classified as 'heating' for their stimulant properties – and possibly as a reflection of the prevailing cold environment). Unlike other cooling agents that counteracted vital functions, bitters appeared to transcend these limitations, to convert heat and vitality into nourishment. This was sometimes regarded as magical.

The modern phytotherapist in effect competes in cooling remedies with modern orthodox medicine. Technology has produced the most powerful analgesics, sedatives and anti-inflammatory and antiallergic drugs (although many are still derived from natural sources). Phytotherapy may score in two ways: first, by producing a more gentle and sustained and perhaps even a longer lasting alternative (treating an inflammatory disease with cleansing remedies, for example) and second, by having recourse to the cooling digestives to transform a hot condition in the most constructive way. The phytotherapist might also be sensitive to the risks of excessive cooling; especially when vital reserves are low (there is a well-signed risk of provoking latent kidney inflammations).

Bitters and other cooling herbs and other strategies (such as cooling drinks, baths and cold packs) could be considered by the phytotherapist when the patient, whatever the diagnosis, favours cool applications or is thirsty, abhors heat, has a reddened complexion, is excessively animated or distressed, has a dry and possibly red tongue and/or coloured tongue coating. Any sign of liver difficulties (particularly with fatty food or alcohol) or a history of hepatobiliary problems or digestive troubles strongly indicates bitter remedies. When so appropriate, they are one of the best tactics available.

Tonification: supporting nourishment and repair

So far all the foregoing strategies make demands on the patient's reserves. In more robust times (i.e. when not being robust seriously compromised one's chances of survival) and in the treatment of acute disease, this was not a major issue. However, it quickly becomes one when there is diminished vitality. It can be argued that traditional practitioners would see most modern clinical indications as marked by degrees of debility. The low-grade viral or fungal infections, the persistent catarrhal state, recurrent headaches or migraines, allergies, skin and arthritic disease and other chronic inflammatory diseases, stress problems and anxiety neuroses and cancer are all marked by a failure to cope or adequately to defend. One perspective on this development is that modern medicine has so effectively neutered the acute disease, especially in the too frequent use of antibiotics and anti-inflammatories, that most people in developed countries have never had to muster their defences. Life is also much easier

in these societies and there is generally less rigorous testing of physiological functions.

Whatever the reason, the modern phytotherapist will need to ensure that there are adequate vital supports in their prescriptions. In large part this involves mobilising the principles of convalescence – rest, exercises and diet (see below) – but in herbal terms the remedies to use are the 'tonics'.

Tonics have been poorly defined, with different meanings in different contexts. In this text they are taken to refer to remedies with substantially supportive reputations. Some are also classified as adaptogens, i.e. they appear to encourage the body to better adaptability under stress (so reflecting the concept elaborated by Hans Selye as the general adaptation syndrome, as a marker of health and vitality in the face of stresses). On one hand remedies used as tonics overlap wholly with foods: different parts of the oat, wheat, barley, rye, asparagus and artichoke, for example, have been used as both foods and medicines. In modern times dietary supplements like evening primrose oil and grape seed have further blurred the distinction. Other tonics are more dynamic, notably some of those used in Chinese medicine, particularly the *yang* tonics like Trigonella (fenugreek) and Eucommia and the *qi* tonics like *Panax ginseng* (asiatic ginseng): these move beyond the simply sustaining towards their own contraindications in the very debilitated.

Within this spectrum there is a vast range of remedies which are used in modern phytotherapy because they appear to support some aspect or other of body function: Silybum (St Mary's thistle) and Taraxacum (dandelion root) for the liver and hepatobiliary functions, Crataegus (hawthorn) for the cardiovascular system, *Plantago lanceolata* (ribwort) for the upper respiratory system, Verbascum (mullein) and Inula (elecampane) for the chest, Hypericum (St John's wort), Withania and Turnera (damiana) for nervous with hormonal symptoms, Foeniculum (sweet fennel), Cardamomum (cardamom) for the digestion, Linum (linseed), *Plantago psyllium* (psyllium seed) and Mentha (peppermint) for the bowel, Echinacea, Picrorrhiza and Astragalus for the immune defences, *Vitex agnus-castus* for the female reproductive system, *Serenoa repens* (saw palmetto) for the prostate, and many more in this and other herbal traditions. In earlier times tonification was often the final stage of a course of herbal treatment. The phytotherapist most often has to start a prescription with at least some tonic element.

Approaches to using herbs

Instant treatments: trigger-point phytotherapy

Herbal medicine has developed the reputation in modern times of being an innocuous alternative to conventional drug treatment. It is often thought that if the remedies work at all, it can only be after weeks or months. The French term *médecine douce* sums up a modern European view of herbal medicine; that it is 'soft' and above all safe, free from the side effects of modern chemical drugs.

This is not how herbal medicines were developed. Before ambulances and hospital casualty wards, men and women had to turn to the remedies they had available, sometimes for life-and-death emergencies. Until a few hundred years ago there were few other options than to use plant products. These were often administered in heroic doses and judged on their ability to produce dramatic results. In most people's daily lives there was little room for sentiment or for the modern romantic view of natural medicine maintaining holistic health and balance. The imperative was simple and urgent: 'Will this measure work, and work soon? If not, I do not want to waste time in trying it'.

All this should not be surprising. The notion that people used somehow to be less interested in efficacy or had less wit in seeking out and recommending the best strategies available would be more extraordinary. There is no doubt that the measures actually adopted in the past, often by ordinary people, did work dramatically when needed.

It is of course unlikely that while modern emergency facilities are available anyone would choose to adopt the traditional alternatives, which were often uncomfortable, crude and imprecise. What may be more interesting is to consider the many ways in which these traditional herbal techniques were applied to lesser problems. In having to learn how to survive illnesses, early practitioners appear to have gained considerable insight into the way the body behaves.

One of the tactics adopted was the use of remedies for provocation. The heroic techniques of emesis and catharsis were merely the most dramatic of the approaches used: the bitter digestives and cholagogues, circulatory stimulants, topical rubefacients and expectorants are more gentle examples of remedies that nudge the body towards hopefully useful activity. All these effects are short term, even immediate, as are the measures adopted for symptom relief: the demulcents, carminatives and spasmolytics. These categories of activity link closely to categories of plant constituents (see Chapter 2) and recur again and again in human history. They now may make a persuasive case for modern herbal therapeutics.

Long-term repair

As we have seen, in modern times herbal medicine has come to be seen as gentle, almost innocuous, most suitable for long-term therapy. Patients often expect herbs to take a long time to work. This perspective, however, says more for the conditions being treated than for the herbs themselves. Chronic diseases cannot be corrected quickly. An informal rule of thumb used by some practitioners is to allow 3 months' treatment for a problem of a year's standing and a month for every further year (or a week's treatment for every month in problems of shorter duration). Such formulae can of course only be approximate, but at least they are indicative. They also imply that real correction of chronic disease is possible. This may be unattainable in conditions that are too far established but there are many pleasant surprises in herbal practice and most patients may gain some long-term benefits.

In general, herbal treatment for chronic conditions uses relatively smaller doses, less robust remedies and more tonics.

Other healing strategies

Convalescence

It is ironic that at the very time that healthcare has to deal with so much chronic and debilitating disease it has abandoned the best strategic approach inherited from tradition. In the past it was taken for granted that any illness would require a decent period of recovery after it had passed, a period of recuperation, of convalescence, without which recurrence was possible or likely. For the really debilitating diseases convalescent care was the primary treatment, reaching its apogee in the many European sanatoria for tuberculosis patients.

Convalescence fell out of favour as powerful modern drugs emerged. It appeared that penicillin and the steroid anti-inflammatories produced so dramatic a resolution of the old killer diseases, including tuberculosis, that all the time spent convalescing was no longer necessary. Then, as healthcare provision became generally more effective and public expectations increased, pressure on hospital facilities led to shorter stays, whilst the increasing angst of the modern working rhythm has conspired to ensure that most people now could not consider time off to convalesce after a bout of flu. That this means they are more likely to get another bout the next year is a cruel irony.

A good convalescence is a marvellous thing. It rounds off an illness and gives it meaning; it makes the sufferer stronger for having had the illness. In a way no vaccination could do, it arms and strengthens the immune defences and provides real protection against recurrence, possibly forever. It is probably the only strategy that will allow real recovery from debilitating disease, fatigue syndromes, recurrent infections and states of compromised immunity. It is the therapeutic recognition that healing, like the growth of children, is almost inevitable but that it needs to be allowed to proceed. Convalescence needs time, one of the hardest commodities now to find.

There are four essential features of convalescence, in general agreed through history, though with many cultural embellishments.

Rest

This is by far the most important element. It should include maximum sleep, as physiologically this is the body's time for repair. In the early stages of vigorous convalescence almost constant sleep should be encouraged (as in the former 'sleep clinics'). Thereafter it should be promoted as much as possible. Rest also means less activity: if work has to be done it should be in brief bouts, switching frequently between different activities ('change is as good as a rest'). Patients should be encouraged to pace themselves, to go to bed early, sleep late and not to volunteer for any work that is not absolutely necessary. As much as anything rest becomes a mental priority: all other considerations are secondary. That hour of more sleep is more important than a film on TV, a late-night conversation or night out.

Exercise

This is the flipside and necessary adjunct to rest, the equivalent to 'turning the engine over', to prevent congestion and stagnation. Essentially the body needs to be taken to aerobic exercise (defined for these purposes as any activity producing a pulse rate of between approximately 60–80% of 220 minus one's age, e.g. 108–144 for a 40-year-old) at least briefly each day. Using the pulse rate to set exercise levels has the advantage of being self-adjusting: the very debilitated will reach high pulse rates with minimal activity. Nevertheless, caution is required. The debilitated will have very little stamina and even a minute may be too long. If exercise is followed by more fatigue, it is too much. Rather, one should build up to being able to undertake aerobic activity for up to 15 minutes each day. The main benefit of the aerobic mode is that it quickly dissipates sympathetic-adrenergic effects on the body ('adrenaline'), constantly generated during the day in response to perceived stressors, and the enemy of convalescence. Timing one's exercise for the evening will encourage better sleep that night.

Diet

The principle of the convalescent diet is that it should simply nourish. It should not stimulate or impose demands. Subject to individual dispositions, a convalescent diet is based on vegetables, especially root vegetables, cereals and pulses (if tolerated), fish and eggs, as the most easily assimilated protein sources, and chicken and other fowl if acceptable (chicken stock and soup remain one of the most universal and puzzling convalescent recommendations of history!). There should be no stimulants, caffeine, nicotine, alcohol or sugar, little dairy food and a minimum of convenience foods and food additives. Patients should thus be encouraged to take a simple peasant diet, sharing also with the peasant a simple respect for the food, taking time over it, building their daily rhythm around it.

Medication

It is obviously important to maintain treatment during convalescence: herbal or conventional. However, there is also a key contribution to the measures above in herbal traditions. It was accepted that rest, exercise and diet alone might not be sufficient to bring about recovery. A range of herbal remedies have been directed to facilitating the process, to drive recovery. Many of these are the tonics listed earlier. If recovery is from febrile disease, sustaining warming remedies like Achillea (yarrow), *Angelica archangelica* (common angelica), *Cinnamonum zeylanicum* (Ceylon cinnamon), Cardamomum (cardamom) or Foeniculum (sweet fennel) might be indicated. Recovery from low-grade assault on the immune system, chronic viral or fungal infections, conditions marked by swollen lymph glands, persistent sore throats or catarrhal states would need Echinacea, Picrorrhiza or *Baptisia tinctoria* (wild indigo). Digestion is often in need of support, whether from cooling bitters or warming aromatic digestives. Cleansing should be managed, above all, by gentle eliminatives.

For the phytotherapist convalescence is often the main strategy in making headway in chronic debilitated conditions such as a fatigue syndrome or persistent low-grade infections. Often these problems start with an infection early in life – a glandular fever or infectious mononucleosis, perhaps. The phytotherapist might suggest to the patient that the task is to go back and complete the convalescence from the original illness. The remedies available are probably uniquely appropriate to the job.

Nutrition: helping to convert foods into nourishment

The revival in holistic and traditional healthcare rightly highlights the importance of good diet. It can also be argued that in an age of processed foods and widespread adulteration of the environment, additional foods and food supplements are sometimes essential. Most phytotherapists will attend to these matters as an intrinsic part of their treatment. This text is not the place to rehearse this complex matter but it is the place to explore the phytotherapist's particular perspective on dietary therapy.

One could start with a principle, literally a fundamental principle ('fundament' comes from the Latin for stomach). New-wave dietetics has been associated with the dictum that 'You are what you eat'. This pop simplicity might be derided but it reflects much of what inspires nutritional therapy. A phytotherapist, on the other hand, grounded in the affairs and rude robustness of the digestive tract and liver, might respond: 'No, you are what you assimilate'. To almost every popular dietary measure it is possible to add a functional modifier or a caveat.

Is there any real point giving extra vitamins, minerals or other food supplements if they are not being well absorbed or utilised, or are being excessively metabolised? What is the point of eliminating potential dietary allergens if the gut is in hypersensitivity mode (when one simultaneously reduces vital dietary variety and creates new allergens)? If there is abdominal bloating or flatulence after eating a food, improving digestive performance might be better than removing the food. Correcting bowel environment by attending to biliary or gastric functions may be more useful in containing Candida outbreaks than drastic eliminations of starches and yeasts.

The phytotherapist would want to answer such questions satisfactorily before embarking on extra dietary measures. Referral to the sections on treating digestive, bowel and liver problems and the section on acupharmacology (p. 187) should provide a rich range of tactics to modify digestive performance and modulate dietary measures. Appropriate use of eliminative or heating remedies may provide additional influence on dietary metabolism. Phytotherapy provides unique opportunities to convert food into useful nourishment. It gives dietary therapy much added value.

Bibliography

Brock AR. (trans.) *Galen: On the Natural Faculties*. London: Heinemann; 1952.

Conrad LI, Neve M, Nutton V, et al. *The Western Medical Tradition: 800BC to AD 1800*. Cambridge: Cambridge University Press; 1995.

Cook WH. *The Science and Practice of Medicine*. Cincinnati; 1893.

Dash BV. *Fundamentals of Ayurvedic Medicine*. New Delhi: Konark Publishers; 1987.

Singer PN (trans.). *Galen: Selected Works*. UK: Oxford University Press; 1997.

Lyle TJ. *Physio-Medical Therapeutics, Materia Medica and Pharmacy*. Ohio; 1897.

Nutton V. *Ancient Medicine*. Routledge; 2005.

Porkert M. *The Essentials of Chinese Diagnosis*. Zurich: Acta Medicinae Sinensis; 1983. pp. 39–44.

Porkert M. *The Theoretical Foundations of Chinese Medicine*. Massachusetts: MIT Press; 1978.

Pormann PE, Savage-Smith E. *Medieval Islamic Medicine*. Edinburgh: Edinburgh University Press; 2007.

Thomson S. *New Guide to Health; or the Botanic Family Physician*. Boston; 1835.

Validating herbal therapeutics

4

But do herbs actually work?

Among all the therapies that are called 'complementary', phytotherapy is the one that can draw on the most scientific support. This book is constructed largely on the foundation of published literature. It is clear that there is now a sufficient case to construct a rational therapeutic system from the older traditions. However, in spite of this and the presence in medicinal plants of many pharmacologically active constituents, the most persistent doubt expressed by the medical world is whether whole herbs actually work in practice.

Most published material on phytomedicines is based on laboratory research rather than on observed effects in humans of realistic doses. There is still a relative paucity of top-quality controlled clinical studies of the whole herb. Moreover many good clinical studies show only a modest effect beyond placebo. Critics also point out that pharmacological constituents in most herbs are at relatively low levels in a final therapeutic dose, that the complexity of constituents is at least as likely to reduce as to potentiate activities, and that traditional reputation is often clouded by plagiarism and inappropriate transmission.

On the other hand, most herbal practitioners will attest to consistent therapeutic performance and will also have accounts of dramatic responses from their patients, where genuinely powerful pharmacological effects have followed consumption of herbal prescriptions, often after conventional treatments had failed. They will also point to the essential features of clinical trial data as denying precisely that which they value most about their therapy – the individualisation of treatment and response. As an example, experimental data consistently deny the possibility of appreciable diuretics among plant remedies, yet substantial diuresis in individual patients is one of the most familiar treatment reactions in practice. Such experiences are enough to convince most practitioners that herbal medicine is a serious alternative to conventional drug treatment with few of the adverse effects.

Any move in the stand-off between the sceptics and the believers is, however, likely to include a full discussion of the placebo effect.

The placebo response

Honesty can be painful to all health practitioners: it is likely that most benefits seen in taking any therapy are not produced directly by the treatments themselves. This is the main conclusion reached after taking into account the substantial literature about placebo.

The term 'placebo effect' itself is not wholly appropriate for this discussion. It derived originally from observations in double blind clinical studies where the treatment was compared with a dummy pill made to look as close as possible to the treatment, with neither the patient nor the practitioner aware of which was which. Early observations were that a significant proportion of subjects in such studies who were taking the dummy nevertheless got better. Initial impressions in the 1940s and 1950s, when such rigorous studies became more common, were that figures varied from trial to trial, but it appeared that about a third of subjects were likely to be 'placebo responders'. This behaviour was put down, in the psychosomatic model emerging at the same time, as reflecting a particular suggestibility on the part of that proportion of the population. As a result the placebo response has been seen to be a non-serious event, not something to be confused with real medicine and at worst a confounding nuisance in establishing therapeutic efficacy for treatments.

Many doctors and other practitioners became used to thinking that about a third of their patients would get better whatever they were given and many thought they knew who they were! After discounting this element they were pleased to feel that any further improvement in their patient population was a result of therapeutic efficacy and skill. Herbal practitioners have therefore been able to confirm to themselves that there must be much more to account for the evidence before their eyes.

Both practitioners and sceptics must review their opinion about the placebo effect in the light of overwhelming later evidence. The last 50 years have completely overturned early prejudices. In brief, it is now possible, after analysis of the clinical trial literature, to confirm that:

- placebo benefits can occur in any proportion of a treatment group, from zero to almost 100%,[1] depending on the condition and circumstances[2]
- there are no particular 'placebo responders' as such[3]
- placebos have time–effect curves and peaks, cumulative and carryover effects similar to those of active medications[2]; they can also generate significant levels of interactions with other medications[4] as well as adverse effects[5,6] (see also the discussion of the 'nocebo effect' on p. 109.)
- placebo responses can involve real cures over the long term[7] – they are not, as often thought, transient, imaginary events[8]
- placebo response can lead to long-term benefit even in difficult conditions such as multiple sclerosis,[9] ulcerative colitis,[10] benign prostatic hyperplasia[8] and schizophrenia.[11]

The first real shock to the herbal practitioner is that those 'conditions and circumstances' where placebo responses have been recorded as particularly high include many of those covered by herbal and other complementary treatments. There is support for the cynic's case that the success of herbal tradition over centuries, especially that drawn from close-knit early societies (where placebo responses were likely to be particularly high because of stronger peer pressures and belief systems), could be due to benefits other than the treatment itself.

The shock also applies, however, to conventional medicine and especially surgery, where placebo responses, as evidenced by examining data from non-controlled clinical studies of surgical interventions which were later found to be valueless, are among the highest recorded.[2] The simple instruction from a doctor carries enormous 'placebo' impact.[12] In whole industries, such as those promoting antidepressant drugs, the impact of placebo relative to treatment response has probably been systematically understated.[13]

Among both conventional and complementary healthcare practitioners there is an understandable feeling that cures having nothing to do with the treatment so skilfully provided are something of an embarrassment and even a challenge to one's choice of vocation. Thus the placebo effect is one of the least discussed phenomena in clinical medicine. Yet it is by far the most powerful factor of all.

The way through this potential difficulty is to reconsider what the placebo response means.

Non-specific supports for self-repair: a different therapeutic strategy?

When a moderate cut is sustained, one assumes it will heal itself. A cold or bout of influenza will generally get better on its own. The only treatment for serious trauma like broken bones or operation wounds is to put the tissues back together and leave them for natural healing to occur.

No one doubts that self-repair is a vital phenomenon. Nevertheless, medicine has moved away from the classic principle that all healing is self-healing, that the *vis medicatrix naturae*, the healing power of life, is the only healer and that the physician should do no more than help it on its way. Exasperation at the slow and uncertain pace of natural healing, the realisation that one can save lives and health by stepping in with something direct and powerful, has led to the discovery of healing bullets. The modern success in this venture has allowed medicine to forget the fundamental principle that ultimately no drug or surgery actually heals: its value is in reducing pain and distress, returning an acceptable function and at best enabling spontaneous repair to occur when it had previously been prevented.

There is no problem with the modern strategy in many clinical cases; it is certain that it can save lives and protect health in ways inconceivable to prescientific medicine. Nevertheless, there is another strategy that may be more appropriate in many other clinical conditions, a therapeutic approach with the primary objective of supporting self-repair. This could be most appropriate in facing the challenge of chronic diseases, the broad range of indeterminate syndromes, along with the numerous minor self-limiting symptoms that make up the vast majority of the family practitioner's caseload.

What researchers have labelled as the placebo effect in their clinical trials may be described as an improvement in self-repair. That it was merely the effect of being recruited into the clinical study and being given a dummy treatment (the main feature of most clinical trials is the increased attention that subjects receive for their condition) is surely evidence of how little it can take to mobilise this self-repair. Dismissing placebo healing as just suggestibility is to miss the point; as shown above, placebo healing can occur in any subject when the circumstances are right.

Indeed, some medical practitioners have got the point. There is a long unspoken tradition of non-specific prescribing, with vitamins, laxatives, aspirin and, unfortunately, antibiotics to keep the patient happy (*placebo* means 'I please'), although actual prescription of placebos as such usually breaches ethical and legislative codes.

Many researchers prefer to use the term 'non-specific effects' to describe contributions to improvements in clinical studies that are not caused by the treatment in isolation. As well as the placebo effect itself, they include the natural course of the illness ('getting better anyway' is something 'control groups' of non-treated patients are supposed to quantify in the better organised clinical trials but even here confusion reigns about hidden 'placebo effects'[14]), 'spontaneous remission' (generally used to describe recovery that cannot otherwise be explained), a trend for improvement ('regression to the mean') due to the fact that people tend to get recruited to studies (and come to obtain treatment) when they are at their worst. All these phenomena are aspects of self-repair. A shift in terminology so that the generally prejudicial 'placebo effect' becomes 'non-specific effects' will be welcome.

Herbal remedies and placebos

In reflecting on practice experience with the full impact of the placebo literature in mind, one could easily become dismayed at the difficulty in separating possible herbal treatment effects from non-specific effects. Nevertheless, one is quickly reminded of the peculiar properties of herbal remedies; time and again one sees in practice changes that are characteristic of the remedies, rather than fitting any preconceived notion of a placebo response. Changes in physiological functions, in digestion, bowel performance, expectoration, diuresis, circulation and many others can often be invoked. There is enough evidence to support the view that many herbal remedies have appreciable effects on various organ and tissue functions, much of which is considered throughout this book.

If this is the case and the objectives of treatment are to better mobilise self-repair functions, then herbal remedies could have unique prospects for this job. If non-specific responses are manifestations of such mobilisation then, to put it simply, the role of the herbal practitioner is to improve such responses. No one needs to feel their vocation is challenged if they acknowledge the large contribution of non-specific factors in their professional performance. It may even be possible to develop research questions that test the hypothesis that herbal remedies have unique prospects for mobilising the self-repair functions.

Whatever the argument for or against the benefits of herbal medicine, this has been driven more by prejudice on both sides than by the evidence. It is time to review the status of research so far and pose new, more appropriate methods for the future.

The difficulty of enquiry

Judging by the substantial markets for herbal products in the developed world, let alone the vast use in traditional cultures, a great many people have already found herbal medicines useful. Compared with the experience of most modern drugs, the human use and approval of most herbal remedies is phenomenal. The requirement by the medical and scientific establishment for research to 'prove' that herbs are effective is not found among the population at large. It is apparent that most ordinary people are content to rely on their impressions of the world to get by in it.

Knowledge within traditional medicine has also generally been in the form of received wisdom moulded to the individual needs and prowess of each practitioner. Such means of acquiring healing skills seem temperamentally suited to most practitioners, herbal and conventional, even today. Their interest in inquiry for its own sake, with secure truths up for constant possible refutation, is understandably secondary to their concern to survive in practice. In the case of herbal medicine, adherents understandably tend to give it the benefit of doubt. The view that: 'What worked for our grandparents is good enough for me, and at least it is natural' probably generates a casual approach about research. It is also possible to question the validity of the research forum and only to play it as far as absolutely necessary (so that the rights to supply herbs are not restricted by law).

Moreover, in spite of the public indifference to the evidence base, they do want to be assured that someone is looking after them. They therefore assume the questions are being asked by those who ought to do it. The physician and the regulators are charged with the job of making sure that medicine is safe and effective. There are internal reasons why some practitioners may be willing to submit to the rigours of the research method: a simple pride in the therapy might generate the challenge 'If what you say is so valuable and powerful then it should be able to stand up for itself in any forum'.

There are, however, practical problems in pursuing good clinical research in herbal medicine:

1. To produce results carrying sufficient statistical weight is expensive and laborious (each trial has to be costed in research salaries plus logistical expenses). Herbal medicine in the West can boast no teaching hospitals or research institutes, nor funding by government or a wealthy industrial sector. The necessary infrastructure is lacking. Neither can the costs of undertaking research studies easily be justified commercially. The size of the market for any individual product is not comparable to that for any conventional drug. Commercial investment in clinical trials costing many millions of euros or dollars can only be justified if the manufacturer can recover the investment in the market. A crude herbal is free for anyone to copy and must therefore be transformed into something patentable and different from its natural origins. This leads phytomedicine manufacturers, therefore, to produce new extracts from plants that they can commercially protect. For example there are almost no clinical trial data for Ginkgo leaves as such: on the other hand for proprietary extracts of Ginkgo (EGb761 and other patented extracts[15]) there is a large evidence base.[16] The same is largely true for black cohosh, saw palmetto, St John's wort, horse chestnut and kava. It is difficult for the wider herbal community to claim efficacy for non-standardised products based on these clinical data. The very high and rapidly escalating costs of conducting clinical trials to modern manufacture, ethical standards and regulatory requirements puts off all but the most promising prospects.

2. The indications often claimed for herbal medicines include many without robust outcome measures. Most are destined for the self-medication or over-the-counter (OTC) market so are by definition directed at lesser degrees of morbidity where hard measures are elusive. By contrast most synthetic OTC medicines on the market have 'switched' from prescription status and have acquired their efficacy evidence on harder clinical indications in hospital or clinics. With more variable and lower grade symptoms among the patient population, and with a greater likelihood of self-limiting or other spontaneously changing conditions, clear treatment effects are harder to establish. The result is that it is usually necessary to recruit particularly large patient samples and to devise more artificial exclusion criteria to constrain sample variability. All this places extra logistical demands on those wishing to set up effective clinical trials for these products.

3. Herbs are complex medicines, occupying an unusual position in being medicines with many of the characteristics of foods. Being a complex of pharmacologically active chemicals, the whole package will have different properties from that of any single constituent acting alone. The action of the latter will not predict the effect of the former, particularly if the experimental evidence is based on work done on laboratory animals. It is therefore rare to find the satisfactory preclinical evidence often required by ethics committees for the approval of major clinical studies.

4. There are other unintended consequences of clinical research that can limit their benefits to investors in research. Even the best studies have failed to lead to medicine registrations outside central Europe for example, St John's wort, Ginkgo and hawthorn (Crataegus spp.). In part this is linked to the indications established by such studies. In all three cases the evidence points to uses that are not appropriate for unsupervised self-medication: depression, cardiovascular disease and heart disease respectively. Therefore in countries where the public are more likely to use herbs in self-medication than through a practitioner, there is little incentive for doing such research. Looking ahead there are new reasons for concern. In Europe, where so much of the herbal clinical literature has been generated, there is a new regulatory regime. The 2004 Directive on Traditional Herbal Medicinal Products permits the registration (rather than licensing) as medicines of herbal products on the basis of their traditional use rather than on proven efficacy.[17] Such products still have to comply with pharmaceutical good manufacturing practice and safety monitoring, but there is no longer any incentive to prove their efficacy in clinical trials. In fact, as the Directive does not apply 'where the competent authorities judge that a traditional herbal medicinal product fulfils the criteria for authorisation', any such data may bar a herbal product from the less expensive registration option and lead to a requirement that it be licensed as a full medicine. There is a concern that the new Directive will lead to a progressive devaluing of herbal medicines and a drying up of clinical research activity.[18]

5. The application of herbs and their effect on the body are not always the same as usually understood for conventional medicines. As has been suggested above, herbal medicines may be used more to evoke healing responses in the body than to attack symptoms; this generates a different research question. Clinical trial data will help with, but still not answer, the basic question 'is this remedy going to be good for this patient?' It is also likely that genuinely important benefits for a minority of the population will be overlooked.

6. There are some instances in herbal research where blinding will be difficult. For example, the impact of bitter remedies, potentially mediated by the effects on digestive functions of stimulation of the bitter taste buds, have played important parts in the claims of traditional herbal medicine: this is almost impossible to blind. There will as always be a role for the good single blind study, especially if other elements are rigorously controlled.

Conventional clinical trials

Even with these difficulties, conventional double blind randomised clinical trials can sometimes be completed, although the track record so far is patchy. The controlled trial is a notably flexible instrument and clinical trial data at least involve rigorous observations of human use of plants: of the forms of research available they are by far the most valuable in making clinical judgments. For now there are many hundreds of well-conducted random-assigned, double blind controlled studies, and even systematic reviews of these, at least for the proprietary products on the market. The monographs in this text also include well-conducted clinical trials for products based on valerian, feverfew, ginger, saw palmetto and others. These studies show that the conventional methodology is very powerful and can be suited to understanding herbal remedies in some contexts at least. They also show that even such unremarkable plants, when researched thoroughly, can demonstrate efficacy beyond the placebo.

It is also important to counter some practitioner resistance to clinical trials. Some have decried them as inherently unethical, in denying a proportion of patients the most useful treatment. However, the researcher goes into a controlled clinical study professionally neutral to the outcome: the point is that until the study is complete there is no 'most useful treatment'. Second, no study in a developed country could proceed without painstaking adherence to the principle of informed consent and to other reassurances that the interests of the subject are paramount. The ethics committees that legally review all orthodox study protocols are charged to represent the interests of the subjects (and this includes rejecting studies that are not sufficiently well designed to actually answer the question). Indeed, medical researchers may point out in their terms that administering a remedy that has not been proven by good-quality research is itself unethical. This may not be an argument for herbal practitioners to pursue too far!

Moreover it should be recognised that OTC herbal use far outstrips practitioner prescription, probably by a factor of more than 20:1 even in Europe.[19] For researching OTC label indications for single medicinal products, in which individual responses to remedies are not the critical issue, the double blind controlled clinical trial is clearly the most applicable method. In addition, as the 'patient' is in many cases not being diagnosed professionally and is determining his or her own treatment and prognosis, self-assessment questionnaires are often an appropriate measure of progress. These are not expensive to administer. This is often 'out-patient' medicine. Research costs can be saved as close clinical supervision need not be always be necessary throughout the trial.

Unfortunately clinical research on herbs has often also been of indifferent methodological quality. Modern studies, even those otherwise highly rated, can be undermined because they neglect basic precautions against the very variable quality of herbal products. In a surprising proportion of clinical trial papers the herbal product used is not quantified, stabilised or verified.[20] Other studies may not relate to the herbal remedy as such but to its chemically-defined ingredients.

Perhaps future hopes for a new injection of investment in clinical research lie with the moves towards sustainable economic development in countries around the world. Renewed interest in the potential of indigenous medical traditions, in some cases linked to emerging economies, has increased research activities in a wider range of plants.[21] At best, standards developed for herbal research in Europe can be exported to improve the quality of investigation elsewhere and to new products linked to sustainable 'free trade' arrangements. There is still a hunger for beneficial natural medicines. If there is any substance in the promise, new ways will be found to service that demand. This phenomenon has already begun, as evidenced by the clinical data being generated in India and China, of which this book contains many examples.

So the practical applications of the conventional controlled clinical trial to herbal practice are mixed. It would be helpful to develop other techniques to explore how herbs affect human beings. There have fortunately been some considerable efforts in constructing appropriate methodologies of sufficient weight.[22] These include looking at different outcome measures, applying rigorous observational studies and monitoring individual case studies.

The measurement of transient clinical effects: the functional assay

In the review earlier in this chapter, the tendency to use herbs to support individual self-repair rather than simply to target disturbances was raised as prompting different research questions.

Traditional views of herbal remedies emphasise their primary influence on transient body functions, e.g. they are classed as diaphoretics, expectorants, circulatory stimulants, diuretics, digestive stimulants, laxatives and so on. These effects, contrary to common beliefs about the effect of herbal remedies, can occur very quickly after treatment. The requirement is to devise a process by which such properties can be substantiated.

By working with either healthy individuals or, more appropriately, cohorts of patients, it should be possible to monitor functional changes after administering herbal remedies. Recent advances in electronic biochemical monitors provide the possibility of following changes in liver function and blood levels of various markers very simply. Moreover, monitoring changes

in blood flow to various organs with thermal imaging or cutaneous thermocouples is a most elegant way of pursuing one of the persistent traditional claims for herbal medicines, that they affect the circulation to heat or cool various tissues, organs or functions. With such advances in non-invasive monitoring technologies it is possible to conceive of important trials in human subjects, in both observational and controlled studies.

Rather than pursue isolated effects from isolated chemical entities it may be better to chart several changes within individuals, using such parameters as are relevant, useful and non-invasive. Emphasis would shift to the simultaneous recording of several parameters of change. It is precisely the interdependence of synchronous events that leads to their exclusion from conventional trials as distracting variables. Acceptance of these variables as important data is a key feature of such work and must therefore profoundly change the nature of the information gathered. Instead of trying to eliminate all variables that might cloud the specific issue in question ('Is it drug A that reduces inflammation in this organ or other factors?', for example), the aim of the 'functional assay', as it might be called,* is ideally to define all factors which determine the medicinal substance's influence on the course of disease ('What, in fact, is drug A likely to do in this individual?'). The task would in some ways resemble homeopathic 'proving'; in other ways it might take advantage of modern computerised and multilevel diagnostic techniques known as 'metabolic profiles'.

Any conclusions drawn from such complex information would be qualitative rather than quantitative: relationships may be induced rather than causes analysed. The process will resemble anthropological rather than conventional medical research. It could however augment the collation of exhaustive case stories as described below. The demonstration of transient effects would not always lead to predictable changes in pathologies, representing as these do the somatic accumulation of various, previous functional disorders. However, many clinical presentations are wholly functional (e.g. acute inflammations, asthma, migraine, digestive disorders and the whole range of psychosomatic disorders). Even in the worst case, knowing the functional impact of a herbal remedy would be a most useful guide to its use in clinical practice. (See also later in this chapter under Human phytopharmacological research.)

These latter multiple measurements lead the discussion on to the role of observational studies as a whole in assessing the impact of herbal remedies.

Observational and single-case studies

There are many ways in which rigorous, though uncontrolled, observations can illuminate therapeutic events. Although it is difficult to establish cause and effect in observational or field studies or specifically to separate specific from non-specific treatment effects, there are a number of ways that observational studies could productively be used in herbal research.

Performance and effectiveness of a therapy overall can be measured with various outcome measures, including the whole

---

*After Professor Manfred Porkert at the University of Munich.

range of clinical or biochemical measures, patient question-naires or analysis of records. This information can inform those who are determining health policy or the allocation of resources (a good observational study could demonstrate that herbal medicine was a sufficiently cost-effective strategy in the management of interstitial cystitis, for example, to enable a clinical group to bid for public health funding for treatment of the condition). Of course, only limited evidence of efficacy can be obtained; however, if a herb were to be given to one group of patients with a condition while another group with the same condition was observed as a matching control, then any clear improvement in the first group will suggest follow-up research.

There is another way in which observational studies are a highly appropriate method for herbal medicine. A persistent tradition (see Chapter 1) is that herbal medicines may support self-corrective functions in the body: only by looking globally at the body's responses could this be confirmed. Following the earlier discussion about self-repair and the supportive role of the practitioner of herbal medicine, as well as the review of the self-organisation found in living complex systems in Chapter 1 and the therapeutic principles that arise (p. 15), then it is apparent that different research methodologies are required. These should:

- have regard to global behaviour of the system rather than particular variables in isolation
- aim to measure quantifiable components of health, rather than of morbidity, mortality or other indicators of disease
- involve minimal intervention.

All this suggests observational rather than controlled studies. Non-invasive monitoring of physiological functions, as in the 'functional assay' above, may be applied, perhaps coupled with patient self-rated questionnaires, clinical observations of overall behaviour and epidemiological methods, to establish as far as possible what actually happens to living patients when they do or do not use treatments.

In effect observational studies accrue as sequential single accounts or 'n=1 studies'. The criteria for validity of single case studies have been well reviewed by Reason and Rowan[23] and by Aldridge.[24] A good design can be very rigorous. It includes providing as many points of view on the event as possible, clarifying operational definitions, and recycling observed data around the researchers (including the patient as co-researcher) for checking and possible refutation. As well as applying qualitative research methodologies it is possible to conduct double blind, placebo-controlled studies in a series of such individual case studies with each patient being his or her control. These could allow for a useful database of reliable case histories to be assembled over the years, as both an educational and research exercise.

In an ideal study design, data about a particular treatment could be drawn from:

- the patient, acting as co-researcher and with a uniquely intimate though slanted view of the internal landscape
- the practitioner, with sufficient competence and clinical experience to provide both an informed and empathic account of the encounter
- a third person acting as coordinator and observer.

The account of each participant can be compiled individually and then cross-checked and combined at a case conference so as to produce a final consensus report of the treatment. Each such report can be examined by the coordinating researcher or assistant, applying a form of grounded inquiry similar to that originally proposed by Diesing in the social sciences.[25] In other words, themes of disturbance and incapacity are elicited by formal contents analysis of the original material, and are then used to construct the working case story, both steps being subjected to re-evaluation by all co-researchers. As each case is thus graphically characterised, it can be used for comparative purposes with other cases to see whether a pattern occurs and can be sustained.

Inherent validity in even rigorous consensual research is, of course, no greater than when a number of people agree among themselves that 'all swans are white' (to use Popper's image), but it can still be argued that this is a fair basis on which to base practical predictions and applications (it would be considered very sound intelligence in the business world). It has the advantage that all conclusions are based on real experiences and can more thoroughly be applied to meaningful clinical application.

Such rigorous exercises are best conducted in the environment of a training clinic where there is likely to be a more overt climate of inquiry and debate and extra administrative labour. Routine collection of patient and clinical data at a teaching clinic is feasible, for example, including self-rating questionnaires for general health and target conditions, perhaps combined with a number of other non-invasive observations, compared with general remission rates. Modern database technology and touch-screen inputs facilitate routine data collection and can allow meaningful collation, retrieval and analysis.

The story as evidence

Raising the benefits of using observational, single case studies of pattern recognition rather than reducing events to the single mechanism leads inevitably to one of the oldest and surest currencies in human intercourse: the story or narrative.

Stories have a terrible time in medical research. They are often called anecdotes and studiously ignored. One common truism is: 'the plural of anecdote is not data'. Traditional use evidence for plant medicines, for example (see below), is generally discounted for the purposes of medical research as no more than a series of unconnected anecdotes, not generalisable to the human condition. The story it is argued is only a personal experience, hopelessly tied to the particular circumstance of that person, time and place. Scientific facts need to be removed from the idiosyncratic and are only valuable when they can be applied to a wider population. Medical researchers have generally been the more confident the more they can quantify the probability that what they observe is not due to 'chance'. An individual account remains just that, of little relevance to the rest of us.

However, in clinical medicine there is growing interest in extracting evidence that arises from actual experience of healthcare interventions, the 'narrative evidence base'.

In such an approach each person, patient or research subject is a character living their story, the evidence about each event is obtained by 'living through' rather than 'knowledge about' these characters, the patient's own words and account are the data and the message is in that story.[26] In the narrative evidence base even the derided anecdote has a role. Such evidence can inform clinical and health policy decisions by illuminating the positive and negative consequences of these decisions and the public's eventual compliance with, and outcome of, treatment.

Beyond that, the concept of narrative rather than raw data *as a unit of measure* chimes well with conclusions drawn from observing the behaviour of complex dynamic systems (above and in Chapter 1), especially in the biological and physiological sphere. One can here see life and health as emergent phenomena from systems built on self-similar fractal geometries, where, as described in the field of biosemiotics, organisms extract 'meaning' from the available script, the elements that constitute them.[27] Only a narrative could describe such a phenomenon.

That most human experience of healthcare is ignored is a rebuke to the modern research focus. There is a Sufi story about Nasrudin, who when asked why, when he had lost his key inside his house, he was looking for it in his garden, replied 'because there is more light here'. Perhaps in looking for evidence where there is more light, where the instruments work, the modern scientist is looking for one key in the wrong place. Those most involved in everyday clinical work are perhaps more likely to agree that at the end of the encounter, when the clinical decision is made, it is the individual 'story' that counts most.[28] Human experience is an accretion of billions of stories. Each is meaningful. The challenge is to find rigorous approaches to learn from them.

Using traditional evidence

The value of narrative is finally at its most acute in addressing the great bulk of herbal evidence base. The persistent theme running through any discussion on the efficacy of herbal medicine is that it has been used over centuries and millennia. It is claimed with some justification that at least some value will have been distilled out by this vast store of human bioassay data, especially as there would have been little room for sentiment and idealism in the life-and-death situations that prevailed through most of herbal use.

However, the record of traditional use can appear as little more than a hotchpotch of folk fancies. The review of historical methodologies highlights some limitations, but the power of cultural placebo alone, as discussed above, renders any individual observation almost worthless. What is needed is the identification and extraction of themes, a structure for assessing traditional claims. Fortunately this is possible.

Clinical insight into the traditional record leads to the realisation that, from the very earliest and most primitive accounts of herb use, humans classified the plant material into relatively consistent pharmaceutical categories. The classification was based on subjective properties of taste or appearance and

the immediate impact they made on consumption. These categories, encountered repeatedly in the ethnobotanical records, became the basis of core therapeutic principles in the classic texts of China, India, Graeco-Roman Europe, Islam and almost all other written traditions. The pharmaceutical principles of traditional medicine provide a potentially robust correlation with modern herbal research, provided the latter can be linked to these phytochemical subgroups, as is done in Chapter 2 of this book. In other words, provided both the scientific and the traditional data relate to the same common elements in comparable contexts. By way of example, a recent study compared three independent ethnomedicinal floras.[29] Similarities of usage could be interpreted as independent discoveries, and therefore likely to be an indicator of efficacy. Data from the literature were compiled about the ethnomedicinal floras for three groups of cultures (Nepal, New Zealand and the Cape of South Africa), selected to minimise historical cultural exchange. Ethnomedicinal applications were divided in to 13 categories of use. Regression and binomial analyses were performed at the family level to highlight ethnomedicinal 'hot' families and general and condition-specific analyses were carried out. Several 'hot' families (Anacardiaceae, Asteraceae, Convolvulaceae, Clusiaceae, Cucurbitaceae, Euphorbiaceae, Geraniaceae, Lamiaceae, Malvaceae, Rubiaceae, Sapindaceae, Sapotaceae and Solanaceae) were recovered in common in the general analyses. Several families were also found in common under different categories of use. Although profound differences were found in the three ethnomedicinal floras, common patterns in ethnomedicinal usage were observed in widely disparate areas of the world with substantially different cultural traditions.

Modern ethnopharmacological studies show countless examples where pharmacological activity can be demonstrated in traditional remedies and practices. In effect, the traditional reputation provides the 'human bioassay data', the clinical evidence preceding the preclinical studies, rather than the other way around as is usual in modern pharmaceutical research. This phenomenon has been described as 'reverse pharmacology'.[30] These correspondences may lift the findings of laboratory research into a real clinical context.

If laboratory or preclinical research has a new role in substantiating traditional use, it also has its own rationale that should now be considered.

Preclinical research

Laboratory studies account for the vast majority of published papers on herbal remedies. However, their relevance to human use is clearly often doubtful and the preclinical information provided in the monographs in this book should be viewed from this perspective. They often also include extraction or isolation of 'active principles' and exposure to tissues in forms and at doses very different from what could be seen in human consumption. Nevertheless there are fundamental technical questions raised in building a case for herbal therapeutics that could be usefully addressed. The following reviews highlight areas of preclinical research that really could benefit clinical practice.

Pharmacokinetic issues

Any rationale for herbal medicine is likely to be based on the activity of many plant chemical constituents whose fate in the body is unknown. The following might form the basis of useful pharmacokinetic questions:

- In what ways are plant constituents likely to interact in the gut to affect bioavailability and activity?
- What is known of hepatic action on plant constituents?
- Following from both the above, what plant-derived constituents are likely to reach the systemic circulation?
- How do changes in pharmaceutical formulation affect the bioavailability and activity of plant constituents?

With new biochemical monitoring technology, it is feasible that some of these answers can be obtained non-invasively in healthy human subjects (see Chapter 2 and Part Three). However, such topics have been addressed mainly with animal and organ culture experiments.

Animal experiments

There can be no doubt of the problems of using animals or in vivo research into herbal remedies. Apart from the difficulty of applying findings to the human situation, there are ethical objections from many of those who support the use of herbal medicines, especially in the English-speaking developed world.

Nevertheless, much phytotherapeutic research in Europe and Asia has involved animal experimentation and the findings have entered everyday debate about the action of herbal remedies. It is also possible to devise trials that involve no pain or discomfort to the animals involved, as is the obvious practice in gerontological research (animals live longest when well treated). It is recalled that herbal therapy aims to support vital functions (in China the worth of any therapeutic practice is determined by how successfully its use appears to encourage a long and healthy life). If the intention of a trial was to assess the effects of herbal medication applied in approximately therapeutic doses adjusted for body weight and metabolism, there could be little complaint that the animals would be harmed and they are likely to actually benefit. Advice is that authorities responsible for licensing animal experiments are likely to consider such studies as indistinguishable from keeping animals as pets.

Feasible trials might include monitoring the effects of posited 'adaptogens' on life expectancy, stamina and reproductive capacity, the effects of antimicrobial remedies on normal resistance to disease among large populations and observing changes in digestive and urinary performance (as judged by changes in excretion, appetite and weight). As the common laboratory animal with a metabolism closest to the human being, the humble rat would probably be the creature of choice.

It might also be valuable to have the results of careful observations of the use of herbs in veterinary practice, where many of the limitations attending patient-practitioner interaction can be minimised.

There are examples of how sympathetic animal research can successfully investigate traditional concepts. A team of Chinese scientists decided to tackle the challenge of finding a scientific way to characterise a core hypothesis of Traditional Chinese Medicine (TCM). According to established TCM theory, the hot or cold properties of herbs can be explored by the relationship between environmental temperature and one's perception of it. For example, hot herbs were seen to be able to help the body tolerate a cold environment. The scientists set up a model to study the hot and cold properties of medicinal herbs along these lines, by observing their impact on animal behaviour and function when they were exposed to different environmental temperatures.[31]

Normal male mice were orally administered as a single dose several herbal extracts at doses ranging from 0.38g/kg to 20g/kg, depending on the herb. The experiment was performed on a tri-zone temperature control plate (15, 25 and 40°C). Normal mice given the cold herbs rhubarb (*Rhei spp.*) and Coptis (*Coptis chinensis*, containing bitter alkaloids such as berberine) and the mineral gypsum significantly increased the time that they stayed in the high-temperature zone ($p<0.05$). In contrast, administration of the hot herbs ginger (*Zingiber officinale*), ginseng (*Panax ginseng*) and prepared aconite (processed daughter root of *Aconitum carmichaelii*) resulted in mice dwelling longer in the low-temperature zone ($p<0.05$).

These findings offer a scientific validation of the hot and cold theory of herbs and, being so novel, need to be replicated in other experiments. Should the results and methodology prove to be robust, the technique could provide a useful objective way to better understand the heating or cooling properties of individual herbs. One example is Echinacea root, with opinions varying as to whether it is hot or cold.

Cell, tissue and organ cultures

As part of the modern move to find alternatives to animal experimentation, increasing attention is being paid to techniques for assessing the effects of drugs on cultures of cells, tissues and organs in vitro. Conventional drug research is switching in this direction for preliminary screening in drug discovery programmes and there is a lesser move for at least initial toxicological testing. The advantages are in the opportunity for the direct observation of the action of an agent on target cells, with reduced ethical difficulties (although the sacrifice of animals is often necessary to supply short-lived organ and tissue samples).

The problems are the limited application of such observations to the clinical situation and the need to confirm any in vitro findings anyway. From the point of view of herbal research there is the additional problem that it is impossible at this stage to reproduce that balance of plant constituents that will actually reach internal tissues (after digestion, absorption and the 'first-pass' hepatic effect). Difficulties are increased by the desirability of using tissues most closely mimicking the real situation, i.e. mammalian organ cultures (rather than the easier to culture amphibian tissues or the less sophisticated cell lines).

Nevertheless, in vitro techniques could provide valuable supplementary information to other research, as in the following suggested projects:

- The influence of herbal extracts on epithelial tissue cultures. This represents a point of genuine tissue interaction with herbal remedies and might add much to pharmacokinetic research.

- Observations on the biotransformation of plant constituents using liver cultures.
- Alteration in the migratory behaviour and internal metabolism of macrophages as a result of exposure to herbal extracts.
- The influence of herbal preparations on microbiological cultures.
- Non-specific observations (as in longevity research) on cell migrations, length of interphase, longevity and other pointers to in vitro cell health.
- Observations in vitro of the effects of phytochemicals with proven human bioavailability, for example the alkylamides in Echinacea root.

Human phytopharmacological research

In the face of this uncertainty, and given that most key herbs are already approved for human use, the best possible research model for herbal pharmacological investigation is the human. Listed below are some examples of pharmacological research that has been undertaken on humans.

Such examples include:

- pharmacokinetic and bioavailability studies
- ex vivo research on isolated cells. In this example the volunteer is given the herb and then cells such as blood cells are removed and studied to ascertain if they possess different features to those from someone who did not take the herb (that is, a control)
- use of non-invasive techniques: EEG, ECG, ultrasound, PET (positron emission tomography) scans, polysomnography
- changes in physiological function: hormone levels, urine output and quality, hepatic biotransformation, immune function, gastric acid output and so on
- performance: memory, cognitive function, intelligence, endurance, recovery.

There are many opportunities where herbal research using human volunteers can be creatively devised. Using this kind of research many of the uncertainties are covered off, including extrapolation to the human, bioavailability and dosage (see Part Three for more examples).

Natural product drug discovery

The new reader of the natural product pharmacology literature will find a vast and confusing diversity of research, often into phytochemicals from obscure, exotic and/or toxic plants. This research is largely driven by the desire to find new medical drug leads, rather than to validate or understand traditional herbal medicine. As might be expected, most of this research holds little interest to the herbal clinician.

On the other hand, the use of natural products as therapeutic agents is still an important part of conventional medicine, albeit one that is in decline. Significant drugs discovered from plants in the past few decades include artemisinin (antimalarial), camptothecin and its semisynthetic derivative irinotecan (anticancer), taxol and its semisynthetic derivatives (anticancer) and lovastatin and its statin analogues (hypolipidaemic).[32]

Critically assessing research on herbs

There is now an abundance of preclinical and clinical research on medicinal plants (as evidenced by the content of this book). However, the reader can sometimes mistake the clinical relevance or importance of a published study, or misinterpret its findings. In order to appropriately interpret a herbal scientific study, or the body of work on a particular herb, the following four information filters are proposed:

- The identity filter
- The filter of the relevance to human use
- The filter of the reliability of the data
- The phytoequivalence filter.

If the information passes these filters then it can be assessed as having relevance to the safe and/or effective human use of the plant under investigation.

Questions that might be asked concerning identity are as follows:

- Is it in fact a herbal product?
- Is it from the right species?
- Is it the right variety or chemotype of that species?
- Is it the right part of the plant?
- Was it harvested from the right region and at the right time?

In terms of relevance of the research to normal human use, some of the following questions are relevant:

- Is the information extrapolated from pharmacological studies in animals or test tubes (in vitro)?
- Does the information come from use of a pure phytochemical in vitro, in animals or in humans?
- For animal trials, was the herb or phytochemical administered by injection?
- For all of the above, were the doses or concentrations used well in excess of those that could be realistically achieved from herbal doses or the opposite?

Reliable data are paramount. Poorly designed trials certainly do not inform the efficacy debate for herbal products. Relevant questions include:

- Does the information come from a clinical trial? If so, how good was the trial?
- Was there a control, such as a placebo group?
- Have there been other clinical trials? How do their designs and results compare?
- Has the scientific evidence been comprehensively reviewed and are the conclusions an objective evaluation of all the available information?

Phytoequivalence defines the transferability of herbal data (clinical or traditional) from one herbal product to another. It is a vital concept because clinicians do not use 'herbs' in their clinics, they use herbal *products*. A clinician might seek to reproduce the known clinical properties of a herb (as informed by either tradition or clinical trials), hereby denoted as 'the reference study' with a specific product in his or her practice. Relevant questions to ask include:

- Was the herb extracted under the same conditions as in the reference study?
- Is the proposed dose the same as in the reference study?
- Are the quality markers comparable and relevant, and how were they measured?
- Does the phytochemical profile of the proposed product match that in the reference study?
- Are they similarly formulated?

See also Appendix E on herbal clinical trials and how to read them.

Conclusions and recommendations

There is a substantial evidence base for the use of herbal medicines. However, much of the research data has been generated to find pharmaceutical leads rather than inform clinical decisions. There is scope for integration of the evidence and better research in the future, though only if two conditions are met.

1. **Observations of actual human use, previously marginalised, should become central.** This is accepted when establishing safety but should be acknowledged as the key element in determining benefit as well. Human experience is all that counts in the end. In the case of herbal medicine this experience is already more extensive than in other forms of complementary medicine and it would be unrealistic to ignore it and insist that herbs are only used if proved de novo. Traditional and clinical experience should be rigorously assessed and clearly articulated to make the opening case for efficacy. It can then be refuted or amended by linking that material to research in other areas. Where pharmacological or clinical research supports traditional use, the latter is reinforced. Where modern findings discredit received wisdoms, these should be adjusted or discarded, provided the research is comprehensive and sound. It may also be possible by meta-assessment of the traditional use data to see recurrent patterns of pharmacology or therapeutics that are themselves reinforcing, as touched on previously.[33] It has been shown that much current research does not address clinical questions: a more useful role could be in refuting,

validating or illuminating the issues and answers suggested by human experience.

2. **Herbs need to retain their position as medicines in Europe, Canada and Australia and improve their status elsewhere.** The great part of clinical trial research has been in support of herbal products that are prescribed and dispensed as medicines in central Europe. Although there have been some admirable clinical trials in the USA, these have been in publicly funded research programmes that are generally reactive to public use rather than strategically innovative. The major risk to the future funding of herbal research are regulatory regimes that classify herbs as food supplements or as second-class medicinal products with a status dependent only on traditional use. If manufacturers cannot develop a therapeutic use for a herbal product, they will be unlikely to invest in researching one. If the research funding bodies do not consider herbal remedies as serious contributors to health care, they will not set aside precious resources to develop their potential. Unfortunately the political and market trends are set to diminish the medicinal status of herbs and there is thus a real threat to the future of good herbal research.

Fundamentally, research provides new information and is absolutely necessary in order that the field of phytotherapy evolves to meet the new clinical challenges of the 21st century. But by far the best reason for doing research is that it provides the best education, for herbal students and practitioners alike. Many of the project ideas are feasible for student clinics associated with undergraduate degree training programmes. Being trained to ask questions of their working environment is the best way to produce effective practitioners, able to adapt to different circumstances and avoid formulaic and lazy practice. At its heart research is a process by which it is possible to develop the professional ideal of critical acumen, to select, sort and clarify the information available about a healing technique, to answer the fundamental question: 'Is this treatment likely to make the patient well or is it not?' As Carl Rogers put it:

Scientific methodology needs to be seen for what it truly is: a way of preventing me from deceiving myself in regard to my creatively formed subjective hunches which have developed out of the relationship between me and my material.[34]

Or as Oliver Cromwell is said to have cried: 'By the bowels of Christ, I beseech ye, bethink yourselves that ye may be mistaken'.

References

1. McQuay H, Carroll D, Moore A. Variation in the placebo effect in randomised controlled trials of analgesics: all is as blind as it seems. *Pain.* 1996;64(2):331–335.
2. Turner JA, Deyo RA, Loeser JD, Von Korff M, Fordyce WE. The importance of placebo effects in pain treatment and research. *JAMA.* 1994;271(20):1609–1614.
3. Wilcox CS, Cohn JB, Linden RD, et al. Predictors of placebo response: a retrospective analysis. *Psychopharmacol Bull.* 1992;28(2):157–162.
4. Kleijnen J, De Craen AJM, Van Everdingen J, Krol L. Placebo effect in double blind clinical trials: a review of interactions with medications. *Lancet.* 1994;344:1347–1349.
5. Rosenzweig P, Brochier S, Zipfel A. The placebo effect in healthy volunteers: influence of experimental conditions on the adverse events profile during phase I studies. *Clin Pharmacol Ther.* 1993;54(5):578–583.
6. Barsky AJ, Saintfort R, Rogers MP, Borus JF. Nonspecific medication side effects

and the nocebo phenomenon. *JAMA*. 2002;287(5):622–627.

7. Hansen BJ, Meyhoff HH, Nordling J, et al. Placebo effects in the pharmacological treatment of uncomplicated benign prostatic hyperplasia. *Scand J Urol Nephrol*. 1996;30(5):373–377.

8. Fine PG, Roberts WJ, Gillette RG, et al. Slowly developing placebo responses confound tests of intravenous phentolamine to determine mechanisms underlying idiopathic chronic low back pain. *Pain*. 1994;56(2):235–242.

9. La Mantia L, Eoli M, Salmaggi A, Milanese C. Does a placebo-effect exist in clinical trials on multiple sclerosis? Review of the literature. *Ital J Neurol Sci*. 1996;17(2):135–139.

10. Ilnyckyj A, Shanahan F, Anton PA, et al. Quantification of the placebo response in ulcerative colitis. *Gastroenterology*. 1997;112(6):1854–1858.

11. Lewander T. Placebo response in schizophrenia. *Eur Psychiatry*. 1994;9(3):119–120.

12. Laskin DM, Greene CS. Influence of the doctor–patient relationship on placebo therapy for patients with myofascial pain-dysfunction (MPD) syndrome. *J Am Dent Assoc*. 1972;85(4):892–894.

13. Brown WA. Placebo as a treatment for depression. *Neuropsychopharmacology*. 1994;4:265–269.

14. Hrobjartsson A. The uncontrollable placebo effect. *Eur J Clin Pharmacol*. 1996;50(5):345–348.

15. Kressman S, Muller WE, Blume HH. Pharmaceutical quality of different *Ginkgo biloba* brands. *J Pharm Pharmacol*. 2002;54(5):661–669.

16. The European Scientific Cooperative on Phytotherapy. *The ESCOP Monographs*. Stuttgart and New York: Georg Thieme Verlag; 2003. pp. 178–210.

17. Directive 2004/24/EC of the European Parliament and of the Council. Official Journal of the European Union. L136/86. 30th April 2004; Article 16 (a) 3.

18. Mills S. Herbal research: the good, the bad and the worrying. Editorial. *Complement Ther Med*. 2007;15(1):1–2.

19. IMS/PhytoGold. *Herbals in Europe*. London: IMS Self Medication International; 1998.

20. Wolsko PM, Solondz DK, Phillips RS, et al. Lack of herbal supplement characterization in published randomized controlled trials. *Am J Med*. 2005;118(10):1087–1093.

21. Blumenthal M, Cavaliere C. NCCAM funds new African and Chinese herbal research programs. *Herbalgram*. 2006;71:20–22.

22. Lewith GT, Jonas W, Walach H, eds. *Clinical Research Methodology for Complementary Therapies*. Edinburgh: Elsevier; 2001.

23. Reason P, Rowan J. *Human Inquiry: A Sourcebook of New Paradigm Research*. Chichester: John Wiley; 1981.

24. Aldridge D. Single-case research designs for the clinician. *J R Soc Med*. 1991;84(5):249–252.

25. Diesing P. *Patterns of Discovery in the Social Sciences*. London: Routledge and Kegan Paul; 1972.

26. Greenhalgh T, Hurwitz B, eds. *Narrative Based Medicine: Dialogue and Discourse in Clinical Practice*. London: BMJ Books; 1998.

27. Hoffmeyer J. *Signs of Meaning in the Universe*. Indiana University Press; 1996.

28. Mattingly C. *Healing Dramas and Clinical Plots: The Narrative Structure of Experience*. Cambridge University Press; 1998.

29. Saslis-Lagoudakis CH, Williamson EM, Savolainen V, et al. Cross-cultural comparison of three medicinal floras and implications for bioprospecting strategies. *J Ethnopharmacol*. 2011;135(2):476–487.

30. Gertsch J. Botanical drugs, synergy, and network pharmacology: forth and back to intelligent mixtures. *Planta Med*. 2011;77(11):1086–1098.

31. Zhao YL, Wang JB, Xiao XH, et al. Study on the cold and hot properties of medicinal herbs by thermotropism in mice behavior. *J Ethnopharmacol*. 2011;133(3):980–985.

32. Dev S. Impact of natural products in modern drug development. *Indian J Exp Biol*. 2010;8(3):191–198.

33. See the EXTRACT database project at <www.plant-medicine.com/>.

34. Rogers CR. *On Becoming A Person: A Therapist's View of Psychotherapy*. London: Constable; 1961.

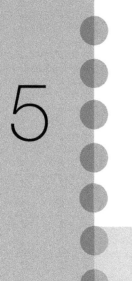

5

Optimising safety

CHAPTER CONTENTS

Introduction

Medical opinion generally has been that it is impossible for any medicine to have effects without side effects, that if herbs are claimed to be free from side effects they are probably not effective either. This is a rational view within its own terms. Any intervention at one site is always likely to lead to reactions at other sites, either because of functional or structural connection or because of similarity in sensitivity.

On the other hand, there is a persistent popular belief that herbs are safe. Probably the main reason why patients first turn to herbs is they assume they are free from side effects, 'not like drugs'. Many herbal clinicians emphasise the same point. They refer to the uninterrupted use of the most established remedies by millions of people since prehistory. They also talk of herbs being used for different reasons than conventional drugs, promoting healing responses rather than targeting pathology or symptoms, of the whole herb being a complex package around the active constituents.

How can these discrepancies be resolved? The answer is not clear or satisfactory. The evidence shows (as abundantly demonstrated in the monographs in this text) that toxic effects of herbal remedies are rarely recorded, although there are a few cases that prompt concern. The main problem is the information vacuum for many herbs into which adherents can project safety and critics hidden dangers. Most significantly, government regulators, in the interests of public safety, can exercise due diligence and reduce access to any herb over which even theoretical doubt may arise. Yet we find that a large diversity of herbal products is available in those countries that observe the most sophisticated regulatory scrutiny for their availability. This certainly must speak to safety, as do the incredibly low insurance premiums enjoyed by herbal clinicians in countries such as the UK, Australia and New Zealand.

Nonetheless, for all concerned, what is needed is more information on safety. This chapter is not intended to be a comprehensive treatise on the issue of herbal safety. There are already a number of textbooks devoted solely to this topic and the monographs in this book provide detailed safety information for each of the 50 herbs covered. The information below is intended more as an introduction to the topic. Texts such as *The Essential Guide to Herbal Safety*[1] and the *Botanical Safety Handbook*[2] are particularly recommended for more information, as they represent a balanced view based on both clinical experience and the published data.

The case for concern

Adverse case reports

There have been a number of cases reported in the medical literature indicating a link between herbal consumption and adverse effects. Many of these are reviewed in the monographs in this book. Most are minor and infrequent in nature. Where serious adverse events are reported, the information is often of poor quality, making a credible link between cause and effect difficult to establish. However, it is worthwhile to note some defining examples of serious adverse events that have occurred in the past few decades. Many of these have resulted from contamination or adulteration, or relate to known toxic herbs.

DOI: DOI: http://dx.doi.org/10.1016/B978-0-443-06992-5.00005-0

During the early 1990s, several patients with renal failure were admitted to hospitals in Brussels with progressive interstitial fibrosis and tubular atrophy that was linked to a herbal slimming preparation. At least 30 individuals were found to have sustained end-stage renal failure from the incident, making it perhaps the single most serious adverse event linked to herbal consumption in modern times. The Chinese herb *Aristolochia fangchi* was found to be an ingredient of the formulation instead of the intended *Stephania tetrandra*. The consequent presence of aristolochic acid, a known toxin, was put forward as a hypothesis for the aetiology of the nephropathies in the literature and the phenomenon became known (perhaps incorrectly) as Chinese herb nephropathy (CHN). However, the case prompted the Association Pharmaceutique Belge at the Service du Contrôle des Médicaments to probe the matter further.[3] They pointed to the idiosyncratic nature of the reactions and the presence of other powerful synthetic drugs in the mixture as suggesting a more complex story. They considered that the cocktail of sometimes powerful preparations adopted by some observing slimming regimes might have significantly lowered the threshold for renal damage. However, aristolochic acid has been known as a nephrotoxin for decades and cases not linked to the concurrent use of drugs have been reported.[4]

In 1997, it was reported that two of the women subsequently developed urothelial cancer caused by the genotoxicity of aristolochic acid.[5] An article published in June 1999 reported further cases of urothelial cancer. Cosyns and co-workers tested 10 patients with CHN.[6] Four (40%) were found to have urothelial carcinoma and abnormal cells were found in all of the 10 patients. Nortier and co-workers[7] (June 2000) concluded that the incidence of urothelial cancer among patients with CHN is high and that the risk was related to the cumulative dose of the herb. They reported treating 105 patients with CHN of whom 43 had been admitted with end-stage renal failure. Thirty-nine of these patients were tested for urothelial carcinoma. Eighteen cases were found, and mild-to-moderate dysplasia was found in a further 19 patients.

Cases of CHN have also been reported in France, Spain, Japan, the UK and Taiwan, where cases of urothelial carcinoma have also been detected.[7] *Aristolochia spp.* can also be used as substitutes for several other Chinese herbs,[8] and Chinese herbal products found to contain aristolochic acid have been recalled in several countries (including Australia[9] and the USA[10]).

This is the first credible, real-world example where the clinical use of a medicinal plant (albeit not the intended one) has resulted in the subsequent development of cancer.

During the early 1990s, liver units in France began to report a number of cases of liver disease possibly linked to the consumption of a slimming herb. The hepatotoxicity of germander (*Teucrium chamaedrys*) was confirmed in isolated rat hepatocytes, particularly a crude fraction containing the diverse furanoditerpenoids. It was concluded that they are activated by cytochrome P450 3A into electrophilic metabolites that deplete glutathione and protein thiols and form plasma membrane blebs.[11] However, these cases were more likely to have been idiosyncratic drug reactions (IDRs) to the germander. Germander was subsequently banned from use in many

countries, although germander-induced hepatotoxicity is probably still occurring, mainly from the fact that certain species of Teucrium are commonly used as a substitute for American skullcap (*Scutellaria lateriflora*).

In fact, so widespread was this adulteration, the macroscopic and microscopic description of skullcap cut herb in the *British Herbal Pharmacopoeia* 1983 was probably for a species of Teucrium. Adulteration of commercial skullcap continued to be an issue in Europe, the UK and the USA into the late 20th century.[12] Idiosyncratic hepatotoxicity was reported for tablets containing skullcap and valerian in 1989[13] and for tablets containing skullcap, mistletoe, kelp, wild lettuce and motherwort in 1981[14] (although the presence of mistletoe was later questioned).[15] The observed hepatotoxicity of these herbal products is probably attributable to a germander species, rather than the herbs mentioned, including skullcap. Case reports of hepatotoxicity caused by germander are not limited to *T. chamaedrys*,[16] other *Teucrium spp.* have caused hepatic failure.[17] One of the reported UK cases of skullcap-related hepatotoxicity was confirmed as being due to *T. canadense* rather than skullcap.[16]

From January 1991 to December 1993, the Medical Toxicology Unit (formerly Poisons Unit) at Guy's and St Thomas's Hospital in London received reports of 11 cases of liver damage following the use of Chinese herbal medicine for skin conditions. There was strong evidence of an association in two cases, as recovery after withdrawal and recurrence of hepatitis after rechallenge were observed. The time-course relationship, recovery after ceasing Chinese herbal medicine and absence of alternative causes of liver damage suggested an association in two further symptomatic cases following a single period of exposure. Herbal material was available for analysis in seven cases. The plant mixtures varied, so no single ingredient could account for liver injury. Effects did not appear dose related and it was concluded they were probably idiosyncratic.[18] Two patients were additionally described who suffered an acute hepatic illness related to taking traditional Chinese herbs for skin disease. Both recovered fully. The mixtures they took included two herbs that were also present in the mixture taken by a previously reported patient who suffered fatal hepatic necrosis.[19] Sporadic cases of IDRs to Chinese herbal formulations resulting in hepatotoxicity have been reported in the literature ever since. A 2009 study from a gastroenterological department in a Chinese hospital concluded that Chinese herbs were a significant factor in idiosyncratic hepatotoxicity, although the liver injury was not severe in most cases.[20] Other studies reviewing patients attending single clinics or hospitals in the UK, Germany and Japan have found a much lower incidence of idiosyncratic hepatitis from the use of Chinese herbal formulations.[21]

Case reports of idiosyncratic hepatotoxicity to Western herbs extend beyond germander. A review of 18 reports of adverse events associated with the ingestion of chaparral reported to the Food and Drug Administration (FDA) between 1992 and 1994 found evidence of hepatotoxicity in 13 cases (causal (10), not followed up (1), probable (2), insufficient data (5)). Of the 13 cases, 10 had ingested chaparral only, with the remainder taking products containing chaparral and other herbs and/or ingredients. Adverse events occurred 3 to 52 weeks after the ingestion of chaparral and resolved 1 to 17 weeks after ceasing intake. The predominant pattern of liver injury was characterised as toxic or drug-induced cholestatic hepatitis. In four individuals there was progression to cirrhosis and in two individuals there was acute fulminant liver failure that required a liver transplant. Of the patients requiring a liver transplant, chaparral was probably not the only factor in one case.[22]

In November 2001 the German Health Authority (BfArM) announced that it was intending to ban the use of kava (*Piper methysticum*) because of reported cases linking kava consumption with hepatotoxicity. Despite submissions from manufacturers, the therapeutic use of kava was banned altogether in Germany in 2002 and several other countries such as Japan, France and Canada followed suit. Late in 2002 it was announced that the Medicines Control Agency (MCA) in the UK would also be banning kava; in February 2003 Swissmedic in Switzerland followed. Like most other herbal hepatotoxicity cases, those linked to kava usage were most likely an immunologically mediated IDR ca rather than a direct toxic effect. Issues associated with this potential IDR to kava are fully explored in the kava monograph.

In 2002 a group of Australian doctors reported suspected hepatotoxicity, presumably an IDR, associated with the ingestion of black cohosh (*Actaea racemosa*).[23] At least 68 more cases have been reported since then, but the association remains a contentious issue. One analysis of the reported cases using the updated Council for International Organisations of Medical Sciences (CIOMS) causality assessment asserted that there was little, if any, evidence for a causal relationship between use of black cohosh and liver damage.[24] For more information on this topic see the black cohosh monograph.

Since its widespread promotion and use in the USA, numerous adverse reactions to the herb Ephedra (*Ephedra sinica*) have been recorded. However, it is difficult to assess meaningfully the majority of these due to insufficient information, the failure to distinguish between its main alkaloid ephedrine and Ephedra as treatments, and the tendency to combine Ephedra with other stimulants in weight loss products (which may potentiate its ability to cause serious side effects).

Nonetheless, the RAND Report undertook a comprehensive analysis of adverse consequences from both clinical trials and case reports submitted to the FDA.[25] Using data from clinical trials, the report concluded that there is sufficient evidence that the use of ephedrine and/or Ephedra or ephedrine plus caffeine is associated with two to three times the risk of nausea, vomiting, psychiatric symptoms such as anxiety and change in mood, autonomic hyperactivity and palpitations. It was not possible to determine the contribution of caffeine to these events. There were no reports of serious adverse events in the controlled trials.[25]

From the adverse events reported by one manufacturer of Ephedra-containing dietary supplements and to the FDA, the RAND Report identified what it termed to be 'sentinel events'. Classification of a sentinel event does not mean to imply a proven cause and effect relationship. These included two deaths, three myocardial infarctions, nine strokes, three seizures and five psychiatric cases associated with prior Ephedra consumption. The report also identified 43 additional

cases as possible sentinel events and noted that about half of all the sentinel events occurred in people aged 30 years or younger.[25] Hepatotoxicity has also been linked to the use of Ephedra both in traditional Chinese formulations and in weight loss supplements.[26-28]

Animal exposure to pyrrolizidine alkaloids (PAs), found in several medicinal plants, has led to a dose-dependent swelling of hepatocytes and haemorrhagic necrosis of perivenular cells of the liver, with concomitant loss of sinusoidal lining cells, with sinusoids filled with cellular debris, hepatocyte organelles and red blood cells. These are all features of veno-occlusive disease.[29] These effects do not represent an IDR, but rather follow from the direct hepatotoxic activity of these alkaloids. The LD_{50} for a pyrrolizidine-rich extract of Senecio was found to be 160 mg/kg.[30] Despite their similarity in structure, PAs differ in their individual LD_{50} values and in the organs in which toxicity is expressed. In one study of four PAs, the proportion of the PA removed by liver cultures varied considerably due to differences in the production of reactive metabolites (dehydroalkaloids), which appear to be largely responsible for the toxicity of PAs, and in their conversion to a safer form (GSDHP).[31] Among pyrrolizidine-containing plants, heliotrope[32] and Senecio[33] have been found to be responsible for veno-occlusive disease in humans. Clinical manifestations of poisoning in humans include abdominal pain, ascites, hepatomegaly and raised serum transaminase levels. Prognosis is often poor with death rates of 20% to 30% being reported.[34] In vivo studies of coltsfoot, containing senkirkine, have shown some evidence of toxicity.[35] However, the key reported case linked to coltsfoot consumption turned out to be a substitution problem. Tea containing peppermint, and what the mother thought was coltsfoot (*Tussilago farfara*), was associated with veno-occlusive liver disease in an 18-month-old boy. Pharmacological analysis of the tea compounds revealed high amounts of PAs, mainly seneciphylline and the corresponding N-oxide. It was calculated that the child had consumed at least 60 mg/kg body weight per day of the toxic pyrrolizidine alkaloid mixture over 15 months. Macroscopic and microscopic analysis of the leaf material indicated that *Adenostyles allariae* had been erroneously gathered by the parents in place of coltsfoot. The child was given conservative treatment only and recovered completely within 2 months.[36]

A review of 18 case reports of pennyroyal ingestion documented moderate to severe toxicity in patients who had been exposed to at least 10 mL of pennyroyal oil. In one fatal case, postmortem examination of a serum sample obtained 72 h after the acute ingestion identified 18 ng/mL of pulegone and 1 ng/mL of menthofuran.[37] In another case of ingestion of 30 mL of pennyroyal oil by a pregnant woman, symptoms included abdominal spasm, nausea, vomiting, alternating lethargy and agitated behaviour. Kidney failure and a solid liver necrosis developed subsequently and death occurred 7 days later. In two similar cases where doses used were 10 mL and 15 mL of oil, vomiting, agitation, fainting, flank pain and dermatitis occurred, but with no lasting toxic symptoms.[38]

Maternal ingestion of blue cohosh (*Caulophyllum thalictroides*) in late pregnancy has been associated with four documented cases of perinatal adverse events. The first case occurred after a normal labour, where a female infant was not able to breathe spontaneously and sustained central nervous system (CNS) hypoxic-ischaemic damage. A midwife had attempted induction of labour using a combination of blue cohosh and black cohosh given orally (dosage undefined) at around 42 weeks' gestation.[39]

In the second case, severe congestive heart failure and myocardial infarction in a newborn male were attributed to maternal consumption of blue cohosh tablets. The woman had been advised to take 1 tablet per day (herb quantity not specified) but she took 3 tablets per day for 3 weeks prior to delivery. Cardiomegaly and mildly reduced left ventricular function were still evident at 2 years of age.[40] The tablets were not analysed for their content. Stroke in an infant was reported as a possible association with a blue cohosh-containing dietary supplement in the FDA's Special Nutritionals Adverse Event Monitoring System database (which listed adverse events but was not subject to preconditions, analysis or peer review).[41] The level of documentation of this case is poor.

Finally, a case report linked stroke in a baby with blue cohosh consumption by the mother.[42] A female infant weighing 3.86 kg was born at just over 40 weeks' gestation to a healthy 24-year-old woman. The obstetrician reportedly had advised the woman to drink a tea made from blue cohosh because induction of labour was a recognised effect of this herb. A caesarean section was performed after a failed attempt at vaginal delivery. The infant had focal motor seizures of the right arm, which began at 26 h of age, and were controlled with phenobarbital and phenytoin. A computed tomographic (CT) scan obtained when the infant was 2 days of age showed an evolving infarct in the distribution of the left middle cerebral artery. There were no other apparent causes for the baby's condition.

In a curious development with this fourth case, urine and meconium were positive for the cocaine metabolite benzoylecgonine, and testing of the mother's bottle of blue cohosh and another brand of the same herb were also positive for this metabolite. Maternal cocaine is a well-known cause of perinatal stroke. Later the authors commented that the finding of a cocaine metabolite in blue cohosh should be interpreted with caution.[43] The finding is most likely due to a false positive reading from the analytical tests used (which did not have a high degree of specificity). In other words, blue cohosh most likely contains a phytochemical which reacts like the cocaine metabolite in terms of the test used, but is not related in any way to cocaine.

Adverse effects have also been documented for a pregnant woman ingesting blue cohosh. Nicotinic toxicity was reported following the attempted use of blue cohosh as an abortifacient.[44] A 21-year-old woman developed tachycardia, sweating, abdominal pain, vomiting and muscle weakness following the ingestion of a blue cohosh tincture. The authors suggested that these symptoms were consistent with nicotinic toxicity and probably resulted from N-methylcytisine, a phytochemical component of blue cohosh. Symptoms resolved over 24 h.

Plants as poisons

Many plants are designated as poisonous, based on toxic effects either after human exposure or following grazing in livestock. Several commonly and safely used medicinal plants are responsible for toxic effects in livestock, notably St John's

wort and Tribulus. However, the issue here is the amount ingested by the animals, which can be several orders of magnitude greater than the human therapeutic dose. Other factors can also influence toxic effects in ruminants. In the case of Tribulus, rumen bacteria apparently metabolise the steroidal saponins into toxic components. This is not relevant to human metabolism. (See the Tribulus monograph for a full discussion of this phenomenon.)

In general, plants have considerably less acute toxicity than many other agents in our modern environment, such as chemicals and drugs. This could be expected since the chemicals in plants are diluted by a large percentage of inert plant material. This assertion is borne out by statistics, for example data from the American Association of Poison Control Centres (AAPCC). In a recent publication, information from the 1983 to 2009 annual reports of the AAPCC was analysed, together with queries of the 2000 to 2009 AAPCC Toxic Exposure Surveillance System and the National Poison Data System databases.[45] During 2000 to 2009, 668 111 plant ingestion exposures were reported, with around 90% of these involving single plants. There was a steady decline in the number of plant exposures, falling from 8.9% of all reported exposures in 1983, to 2.4% in 2009. Young children accounted for more than 80% of plant ingestion exposures. Only 45 fatalities were recorded between 1983 and 2009, with Datura and Cicuta species accounting for about one-third of these. The authors concluded that, while plant ingestion remains a common call for poison information centres, morbidity and mortality associated with these were very low relative to the total number of reported plant exposures.

Given the existence of toxic plants, it is accepted by all involved that not all plants are safe to use as remedies. The incidence of these clearly varies from country to country. Appendix B provides a list of several potentially toxic medicinal herbs. With a few exceptions, their use is best avoided, especially during pregnancy and lactation. The individual herb monographs in this book contain detailed toxicity information, where available.

Adverse reactions

Understanding the key safety issues and demonstrating the safe use of herbal therapy is probably the biggest challenge that faces the future widespread use of medicinal plants. A key issue is that the safety of any given therapy can never be considered in isolation from its efficacy. In every therapeutic task, risks must be weighed against benefits for each particular clinical situation. Therapy is justified only if the possible benefits outweigh the potential risks in an informed risk-benefit analysis. This decision is dependent on an adequate clinical knowledge of the patient and his or her disease, and knowledge of the treatment pertinent to the specific situation.

Although the term 'benefit-risk ratio' is convenient and often used, such an assessment is qualitative not quantitative (in other words, the division of a number for risk by a number for efficacy is rarely actually performed) and hence always involves some element of subjectivity. For a drug that is life-saving, a greater safety risk is acceptable when it is used in that context. This is the reason dangerous therapeutic drugs are tolerated by the regulators.

A major problem in the assessment of many herbs is the lack of hard data supporting their efficacy. Hence, in the eyes of the authorities the benefit is zero, so any risk is unacceptable, as was the case with kava (despite the clinical data). One positive development in this area would be the acceptance of well-established traditional (historical) use as evidence for efficacy. Nonetheless, the fact remains that, in order to preserve the status of herbs, information about efficacy as well as safety is required.

Patients can sometimes experience a mild adverse effect that they attribute to the herbal treatment. Often this is not the case and dechallenge and rechallenge can clarify this. In highly sensitive patients, it can be best to start with a lower dose and build up. The vast majority of clinical trials (see the many examples in the herb monographs) have demonstrated that the side effect profile of a herbal treatment is about the same as placebo.

A number of milder adverse reactions are predictable on the basis of the known phytochemistry of the herb. More details of such side effects are provided in Chapter 2, but a few key examples follow:

- Tannin-containing herbs, such as cranesbill (*Geranium maculatum*) and oak bark (*Quercus robur*), can inhibit trace element and B vitamin absorption. They should therefore not be used in high doses for long periods, or alternatively given away from food and other medications
- Saponins are gastric irritants. Hence, doses of herbs which contain saponins, such as horsechestnut (*Aesculus hippocastanum*) and Gymnema (*Gymnema sylvestre*), can cause reflux and/or vomiting in sensitive individuals. The alternative is to prescribe them in enteric-coated tablets or with meals
- Licorice root (*Glycyrrhiza* spp) can cause sodium and fluid retention and potassium loss. This effect only occurs with extended use at high doses and can be minimised by a high potassium diet. An adult dose equivalent to 3 g/day should not cause this problem
- Korean ginseng (*Panax ginseng*) can cause overstimulation, usually only at higher doses (in excess of 1 g/day)
- Pungent herbs such as capsicum (*Cayenne* spp) and ginger (*Zingiber officinale*) create a burning sensation which patients may find uncomfortable. In the case of herbs that contain mustard oils, such as horseradish (*Armoracia rusticana*), the burning sensation is real and can cause considerable gastric discomfort. High doses of ginger can cause heartburn
- Bitter herbs in high doses may cause some patients to vomit when given in liquid form
- Echinacea and prickly ash (*Zanthoxylum clava-herculis*) in liquid form cause tingling in the mouth and promotion of saliva, which in a few patients can give them a choking sensation and rarely a panic reaction
- Thujone can cause CNS stimulation and possibly epilepsy. Care should be exercised when giving thujone-containing herbs in high doses to epileptics. These herbs include Thuja (*Thuja occidentalis*), sage (*Salvia officinalis*), tansy (*Tanacetum vulgare*), wormwood (*Artemisia absinthium*) and some types of yarrow (*Achillea millefolium*).

Thujone-containing herbs can also cause headaches in high doses

- Garlic can inhibit thyroid function
- Blood root (*Sanguinaria canadensis*) and bryony (*Bryonia alba*) are potent irritants and should only be used in low doses
- Bladderwrack (*Fucus vesiculosus*) and kelp (*Laminaria*) may aggravate or induce hyperthyroidism when given in high doses for prolonged periods
- Laxative herbs can cause abdominal pain. Abuse can lead to electrolyte loss, especially potassium. Chronic use leads to a characteristic pigmentation of the colonic mucosa known as *melanosis coli*. This is harmless and reversible
- Use of kava (*Piper methysticum*) for insomnia can cause a mild lethargy the next morning and chronic use is associated with skin changes
- It is unlikely that St John's wort (*Hypericum perforatum*) causes photosensitivity with normal usage. It may cause an allergic skin rash in some cases, which has been misinterpreted as photosensitivity.

Many other potential side effects have been identified for individual herbs and these are outlined in the monograph section of this text.

Allergic reactions

In general, allergic reactions to herbs are relatively uncommon. A typical allergic reaction, if one occurs, is contact sensitivity. This is acquired only when contact is made with the plant via the skin or mucous membranes. Most herbs have the potential to cause contact sensitivity; however, herbs that contain either resins or sesquiterpene lactones are more likely to have this property. Contact sensitivity can be manifest on the skin either after topical application or in the oral cavity after contact, such as for a gargle or just ingesting a liquid preparation.

Allergic contact dermatitis due to the presence of sesquiterpene lactones (SLs) occurs for many plant species, especially the Asteraceae or daisy family (Compositae). (Note for readers with a chemistry background: in this plant family, the presence of an alpha-methylene on the lactone group is mainly responsible for allergenicity.) It is often observed that individuals who are SL-sensitive tend to develop cross-reactions when encountering other SL-containing species. Commonly used medicinal plants containing SLs include Arnica, feverfew, globe artichoke, elecampane (*Inula helenium*) and dandelion.

Some other herbs which can commonly cause contact sensitivity include myrrh (*Commiphora*), cinnamon (*Cinnamomum spp*), lime flowers (*Tilia*), propolis (not strictly a herb) and balm of Gilead (*Populus candicans*).

Anaphylactic reactions can also occur; however, these are quite rare. The Compositae plants are again often involved and the issues for Echinacea and chamomile are fully discussed in their relevant monographs.

Idiosyncratic reactions

Idiosyncratic reactions are reactions that are peculiar to a single individual or a very small group of people. They are by nature unexpected and unpredictable.

In such cases, unless the herbal formula is rechallenged, it is difficult to be entirely sure that the therapy was the cause. However, when the side effects cause considerable discomfort it may be unethical to rechallenge and in many cases the patient is unwilling to try the same formula again.

We cannot rule out the possibility that many so-called idiosyncratic reactions to herbs could be coincidence or a placebo (or in fact nocebo, which is the opposite of placebo, see later) effect. On the other hand, there are some patients (although they are rare) who appear to react to almost anything. This hyper-reactivity is part of their being unwell and will be revealed during the initial case history taking. For example, if a patient reports a history of 'unusual reactions to drugs' or 'being very sensitive to drugs' it is prudent to take note of this information and make the assumption that, in this particular patient, a reaction to herbal therapy might also occur.

As a general rule, clinicians need to take great care in treating such patients. This is also true for patients who report multiple food sensitivities. When writing a herbal prescription for such patients, it is probably wise to err on the side of caution and use fewer rather than more herbs. This way, if any type of reaction does occur, it may be easier to isolate the cause. In extreme cases, the practitioner may choose to use just one or two herbs initially and add others as the treatment progresses.

Some specific organ toxicities that occasionally seem to occur in herbal therapy may be idiosyncratic reactions. This especially applies in the case of hepatotoxicity (see above). That is, the particular herb does not contain hepatotoxins, but immunologically driven liver destruction is driven by consistent exposure to that herb.

Pregnancy and lactation

It is a general principle that one should refrain from giving medicines to a pregnant woman unless clearly necessary. Although some herbs have been used safely by women when pregnant and may thus be seen to have a degree of positive vetting, they should be prescribed particularly carefully in the crucial first trimester when fetal organ development is underway. Although there are very few accounts that link any pregnancy problems to herb consumption, too little is known for any sweeping recommendation. Particular caution should be exercised for plants with alkaloidal principles, strong volatile constituents (notably including pure essential oils and plants with high levels of thujone) and in cases where there is a history of miscarriage or where low back or abdominal pains occur. Toxic herbs should be avoided; see Appendix B for such a list.

A number of other herbs should be particularly avoided in pregnancy. In many popular herb books, the term 'emmenagogue' is used to refer to a gynaecological remedy. Probably the most frequent indication for such remedies in earlier times was to bring on delayed menstruation; in other words, many 'emmenagogues' were used for birth control, as abortifacients. This was likely to be one of the specialist skills of 'wise women' and, theoretically, remedies affecting the gravid uterus are as likely to harm fetal growth as to abort pregnancy.

The pregnancy safety ratings advocated in *The Essential Guide to Herbal Safety*[1] have been adopted for the monographs in this text. This categorisation is designed to remove

the subjectivity from assessing the safety information for herbs during pregnancy. The ratings are self-explanatory, but a further discussion is provided in Chapter 10 (How to use the monographs). However, some herbal clinicians might prefer a simpler approach of a list of contraindications and cautions, and this is provided in Table 5.1 for more than just the 50 herbs detailed in this book.

In regulatory terms, the caution referred to above in the case of pregnancy is also extended to the stage of lactation. Although critical organ development is not threatened, there remains some doubt in many cases about how secondary plant metabolites, many of which pass easily and even preferentially into breast milk, affect the baby. Practitioners should therefore maintain a degree of caution in attending to clinical problems affecting mother and suckling baby. However, it should be pointed out that documented adverse effects for herbs used during lactation are minimal, other than milk reduction or

Table 5.1 Common herbs under contraindication or caution during pregnancy

Contraindicated

Adhatoda (except at birth)	Jamaica dogwood
Andrographis (first trimester)	Juniper
Baical skullcap (first trimester)	Mugwort
Barberry	Myrrh
Bearberry	Oregon grape
Black cohosh (except to assist with birth)	Pasque flower
Bladderwrack	Pau d'arco
Blue cohosh (except to assist with birth)	Poke root
Cat's claw	Qing hao
Corydalis	Sage
Dan shen	Schisandra (except at birth)
Dong quai (first trimester)	Thuja
Golden seal	Tienchi ginseng
Horseradish (high doses only)	Tylophora
Hyssop	Wormwood

Caution

Aloes resin	Raspberry leaf (best to use in 2nd and 3rd trimesters)
Cascara	Rehmannia
Cinnamon	Rhubarb root
Ginger	Senna pods
Motherwort	Shepherd's purse

Table 5.2 Common herbs under caution or contraindication during breastfeeding

Contraindicated	
Barberry	Pasque flower
Bearberry	Poke root
Bladderwrack	Sage (except to stop milk)
Blue cohosh	Thuja
Golden seal	Tylophora
Mugwort	Willow bark
Oregon grape	Wormwood
Caution	
Aloes resin	Rhubarb root
Cascara	Senna pods
Peppermint	Shepherd's purse

reduced infant feeding. Table 5.2 provides some basic guidelines for commonly used herbs.

Adverse herb-drug interactions

The issue of adverse herb-drug interactions (HDIs) is probably the most contentious problem in the understanding of the safe use of medicinal plants. Many texts carry pages and pages of theoretically possible interactions for each herb, often based on unsupported extrapolations from pharmacological data (typically in vitro studies). Such information is not only needlessly cautious it is potentially alarmist. The reader might experience such difficulty managing the complexity of the provided information that he or she might conclude that the only safe option is never to recommend any herbs in conjunction with conventional drugs. In addition to these hypercautions, there is also considerable misinformation in the field. For a full discussion of these issues, the reader is referred to the relevant chapter in *The Essential Guide to Herbal Safety*.[1]

While adverse HDIs can certainly be theorised, clinically relevant examples that can be predicted on theoretical grounds are probably uncommon. One such example is the combination of licorice (*Glycyrrhiza glabra*, *G. uralensis*) with thiazide diuretics. Prolonged use of both could accelerate potassium depletion. If the patient was also taking digoxin, then a further adverse interaction could occur, since the toxicity of digitalis glycosides is increased by potassium depletion. However, most important adverse HDIs are likely to be unexpected, with case reports representing the best way to discover them.

Adverse HDIs can be either pharmacokinetic or pharmacodynamic in nature. The above example for licorice represents a pharmacodynamic interaction. With a pharmacokinetic interaction, the herb increases or decreases the activity of the drug by altering its absorption, distribution, biotransformation or excretion, or any combination of these. The best-documented example is St John's wort, and this issue is fully discussed in its monograph. Pharmacokinetic HDIs can be investigated via clinical studies in healthy volunteers, where the impact of taking a herb on the pharmacokinetics of one or more probe drugs is explored. This information is substantially more reliable than extrapolation from in vitro studies of the impact of a herb extract on cytochrome P450 enzymes. Such extrapolations should not be given any clinical credibility because of the many uncertainties involved.

Appendix C provides a reference table for HDIs, together with explanatory information. The table is designed to be accurate and responsible and is based on a critical assessment of the clinical relevance of the available information. Entries are mainly drawn from case reports and clinical studies. In addition, the various relevant monographs typically contain a more complete discussion of some of the issues summarised in the appendix.

It must be emphasised that most of the interactions listed are only potential in nature, and the existence of the majority of interactions in the table is not supported by definitive data. However, prudence and good practice suggest that these combinations are considered with caution, the level of which is flagged in the table.

Cases of contention

False alarms?

Over the past two decades, articles have appeared in the media and in journals attributing significant harmful effects to commonly available herbs. In the main, these articles are either imbalanced, misinformed, poorly researched or based on extrapolations from pharmacological studies that have little or no relevance to normal human use. A few examples follow.

In 1999 a team of scientists at Loma Linda University School of Medicine in California undertook studies to analyse the effects of some popular herbs on the fertilisation process and on sperm DNA.[46] They used hamster eggs with their outer coating (zona pellucida) removed, exposed them first to the herbs for 1 h and then to human sperm. In a separate test, human sperm cells were incubated with the herbs for 7 days and then tested for viability and the intactness of their DNA. The coding sequence for an important gene in the sperm was also evaluated as a test for mutagenic activity.

At the lower concentrations tested, there was no effect from the herbs in any of the tests. But at the higher concentrations, St John's wort, *Echinacea purpurea* and Ginkgo prevented human sperm from penetrating the hamster eggs. Exposure of sperm to Echinacea and St John's wort at only the higher concentrations resulted in DNA denaturation, and St John's wort also caused genetic mutation. In contrast, Ginkgo and saw palmetto had no effect.

Despite occasional cautions about the significance of their in vitro (test tube) study, the authors at times appeared to exaggerate the relevance of their findings. For example, they wrote:

> The results of the present study, which demonstrates the effect of high concentrations of St John's wort as a blocker of fertilization, are important for infertile couples who are attempting to conceive and who are taking St John's wort.

The study illustrates several of the pitfalls that can happen in experimental design and interpretation when scientists and clinicians with little training in, or understanding of, herbs attempt research in this field. That the authors of this paper were unfamiliar with herbs is well illustrated by their repeated reference to *Echinacea purpurea* as *Echinacea purpura*. More significantly, the study did not specify whether commercial samples of the plants or their extracts were employed. If extracts were used, these are significantly more concentrated than the original herb, and such an omitted piece of information would reflect markedly on any interpretation of the results. No information is provided about any attempts to verify the authenticity of the herbs used or their quality or phytochemical profile. There is also no information on solvents used to extract the herbs. (Different solvents extract different phytochemicals from herbs, a variability which can substantially influence the outcome of any study.) The exception here was saw palmetto, for which the liposterolic extract was used (see the saw palmetto monograph).

Throughout the paper, it was maintained that each herb was tested at an amount that reflected the normal human dosage. But these amounts were dissolved in only 1 mL of medium instead of the much greater amount of medium required to reflect the normal quantity of human body fluids. As a consequence, the concentrations tested far exceeded typical human exposure to these herbs. The no-effect level was described as representing 'very low' concentrations. In fact, these 'very low' concentrations were equivalent to exposure well above normal human intake (which would suggest that, far from implying harmful effects on fertility, the study found that the herbs were safe). The maximum meaningful concentration for in vitro research on whole herbs is considered to be about 0.1 mg/mL on a dry weight basis. In contrast, the 'low' concentrations used in the study were in fact high at 0.06 to 0.9 mg/mL and the 'high' concentrations (referred to as 'normal' in the text) were excessively high at 0.6 to 9 mg/mL. Furthermore, if these values represent the concentrations of extracts, as opposed to dried herb (as was the case with saw palmetto), then the equivalent dried herb concentrations would be considerably greater still.

But there is an equally important consideration that the authors failed to take into account. Many pharmacological screening programmes using in vitro tests on herbs, such as the programme of the National Cancer Institute in the USA, first remove interfering compounds like tannins. Tannins, which are relatively common in herbs, can bind non-specifically to proteins such as enzymes, effectively producing false positive results. In addition, tannins have very low bioavailability, so any observed non-specific activity on intracellular enzymes is likely to be little more than a scientific curiosity. This consideration was well demonstrated by an elegant but perhaps ultimately futile study published in the *Journal of Ethnopharmacology*.[47] Owen and Johns found that the inhibitory activity of 26 plants on the enzyme xanthine oxidase was positively correlated with their tannin content ($p < 0.001$).

There are many other cautions which govern the extrapolation of in vitro research to living organisms. In the case of herbs, these include the digestive modification, absorption, metabolism and elimination of the many compounds found in plants. To their credit, the authors of the hamster cell study do occasionally acknowledge these cautions. For example, they write: 'The possibility of a lack of a physiological effect in vivo should be considered'.

The international media response to this article was extraordinary, considerably assisted by a press release from the journal in which the editor at the time was quoted as saying: 'This is a very important study that could provide important information to patients suffering from infertility'.

Perhaps the most bizarre episode of a herbal false alarm was the reported occurrence of the toxic alkaloid colchicine in *Ginkgo biloba*. A group of US scientists investigating natural anti-inflammatory substances in pooled placental blood found a compound present that they identified as colchicine.[48] Naturally the scientists were curious as to the origins of this plant chemical, so they decided to examine individual blood samples from 24 pregnant women. Only five of these contained colchicine and the group reported that all of the colchicine-containing blood samples came from women who used herbal supplements. For some undisclosed reason they next tested Ginkgo and Echinacea products from local retail outlets and found that only Ginkgo contained significant levels of colchicine (26 µg per tablet). The authors concluded that due to its potential harmful effects, it would appear that *Ginkgo biloba* should be avoided by women who are pregnant or are trying to conceive.

Colchicine is a drug mainly used to treat acute gout and was originally isolated from the autumn crocus (*Colchicum autumnale*). It is highly toxic and the effective dose is quite close to a toxic dose. Toxic effects include nausea, vomiting and bone marrow suppression.[49] Colchicine inhibits normal cell division (mitosis) and is linked to Down's syndrome. Clearly, it is contraindicated in pregnancy.[50]

Before critiquing the actual scientific merit of the study, some commonsense, logical questions were not answered by the study (and obviously not asked by peer reviewers). These include:

- Were the five women with the colchicine levels taking Ginkgo?
- If not, what herbs were they taking?
- Why would a pregnant woman wish to take Ginkgo?
- Why choose just Echinacea and Ginkgo for analysis?
- How many Ginkgo products were tested?
- Why were not verified Ginkgo leaves tested as well?
- Do the findings match the known safety record of Ginkgo?

Questions about the research from a scientific perspective might include:

- Is it known that Ginkgo contains colchicine?
- Can we expect, from a phytochemical perspective, that Ginkgo should contain colchicine?
- How conclusively was colchicine identified in Ginkgo?
- Could the levels of 'colchicine' in Ginkgo account for the levels found in placental blood?
- Are these levels of 'colchicine' in placental blood toxic? If so, what effects were observed on the mother and child?

In fact colchicine has never before been reported in Ginkgo and a comprehensive literature search by the late Professor

Farnsworth at the University of Chicago found no evidence of colchicine in Ginkgo.[51] According to Professor Farnsworth: 'Based on biogenetic considerations, colchicine should never be found outside of the Monocotyledoneae (Araceae, Liliaceae) and the report of its occurrence in *Saussurea sacra* (Asteraceae) is an anomaly that has not been duplicated by other reports on the chemistry of this species. Thus, colchicine has never been reported as a normal constituent of *Ginkgo biloba* nor would it be expected or predicted to be present'.

Farnsworth also questioned the scientific validity of the study and the editorial process it underwent prior to publication. 'Anyone who thinks that colchicine can be found naturally in Ginkgo is not qualified to be a peer reviewer of this paper,' he said, referring to the editorial process for scientific journals in which papers are reviewed by independent experts to determine their scientific merit and the accuracy of their conclusions prior to publication. Schwabe, the German company that researched and developed Ginkgo extract, tested three separate samples of Ginkgo leaf and failed to find any colchicine. This finding was backed up by industry testing in the USA.[51]

In response to the study, the Australian Therapeutic Goods Administration tested five *Ginkgo biloba* products. Colchicine was not found in any (detection limit $1 \mu g/g$). Interestingly, using a method similar to the study in question, a substance was found in the Ginkgo products which had similar analytical properties to colchicine. Although its identity was not determined, further analysis demonstrated conclusively that it was not colchicine.[52]

Were the levels of colchicine in Ginkgo responsible for those reportedly observed in the pregnant women? The scientists claimed to have found 49 to $763 \mu g/L$ of colchicine in the placental blood of the women allegedly taking herbal supplements.[48] They also claimed to have found $26 \mu g$ of colchicine per Ginkgo tablet. In a multiple dose study of the pharmacokinetics of colchicine, $1 mg/day$ achieved plasma concentrations in human subjects in the range of 0.3 to $2.5 \mu g/L$.[53] Hence to achieve a level of $49 \mu g/L$ of colchicine (the lowest value in the reported range) a person would need to consume around $50 mg$ of colchicine per day. Since each Ginkgo tablet contains only $26 \mu g$, this equates to around 2000 Ginkgo tablet per day. In their defence, the authors claimed that placental tissue is known to concentrate ingredients from the mother's blood. But even assuming a concentration factor of 50, this is still 40 tablets per day to achieve the lowest reported concentration of colchicine, when the normal dose is typically 3 to 4 tablets per day.

Perhaps most astounding of all, the reported levels of colchicine would have been lethal to the unborn children. Several cases involving suicide by the ingestion of colchicine tablets have been reported in the literature. In one case, the plasma level of colchicine 24h after ingestion was $4.5 \mu g/L$,[54] in another the femoral blood level was $62 \mu g/L$.[55] *Colchicum autumnale* is the richest plant source of colchicine. Yet a case report of a man who consumed $17.1 g$ of flowers found that his maximum colchicine level was just $4.34 \mu g/L$, which occurred 13h after ingestion of the flowers.[56] Nonetheless he was hospitalised with nausea, vomiting and abdominal pain.

The authors and the journal involved made sure that their study received due attention by releasing their findings to the press. And despite the many shortcomings of the study the press responded. Press releases and articles ran headings such as:

Ginkgo and Pregnancy Don't Mix

Ginkgo Biloba Compound May Affect Fetus

Magazine Warns Pregnant Women About Herbal Supplement

But perhaps best of all was the quote attributed in London's *Daily Mail* to a UK professor working in the field of complementary medicine who was quoted as saying that the alleged Ginkgo health risk was 'a disaster waiting to happen' and likened it to 'another catastrophe like thalidomide'. Despite criticism from the herbal industry, the scientists and journal editor involved in the publication of the study were reported to be unrepentant.[57]

On April 10, 2003, an Australian newspaper (the Brisbane *Courier-Mail*)[58] ran a brief article relating concerns raised by recent research that the herb black cohosh may increase the toxicity of two chemotherapy drugs. The article went on to say: 'Many women diagnosed with breast cancer use the herb as an alternative to hormone replacement therapy'. Similar alarmist reports of this research were also carried in the US media.

The article was in response to a press release of research findings that were to be presented at the American Association for Cancer Research meeting in Toronto, but the event was cancelled due to concerns over SARS in that city.[59] Notwithstanding the lack of an appropriate forum for the presentation and discussion of their findings, the authors pressed ahead and released their findings via the media.

The first paragraph of the release read: 'Women with breast cancer who are undergoing chemotherapy may want to avoid black cohosh …' The press release then went on to describe that black cohosh extracts appeared to increase the toxicity of the commonly used chemotherapy drugs doxorubicin and docetaxel when tested on cultures of breast cancer cells. Hence, this finding was based on in vitro or test tube research. Black cohosh did not potentiate the toxicity of a third drug tested, cisplatin. No exact details of the experiments were provided. The initial paragraph of the press release seemed to contradict a later statement that: 'Results in laboratory cells may not mimic what happens in the body ….'.

Publication by press release is a growing and controversial trend in scientific circles. But the central problem with this story is that it makes much ado about very little. The reality is that, as already noted, test tube research on herbal extracts is fraught with difficulties and any extrapolations to human use need to be heavily qualified, and certainly do not deserve the type of attention by the media which they typically receive. This case is certainly an example of *in vitro non-veritas*.

Inaccuracies regarding the true risks of HDIs have already been discussed. However, it is worth noting the alarmist issues raised in a recent paper published in the *Journal of the American College of Cardiology*.[60] As one example, concerns over alfalfa and fenugreek interacting with warfarin were expressed; these are not supported by sound science. To phytochemists, the term 'coumarin' means plant chemicals based on the coumarin structure. To pharmacists the term 'coumarin' means anticoagulant drugs derived from or related to coumarin phytochemicals. There is no solid evidence that normal plant coumarins have anticoagulant activity (see Chapter 2).

The article was riddled with other errors, such as confusing *Aloe vera* gel and juice with *Aloe vera* resin. Many of the stated 'commonly used' herbs are not used at all in the US and are known to be toxic, such as oleander, Chinese toad venom, Strophanthus, gossypol and khella. The vast majority of the other potential HDIs described had no clinical data to support them.

The authors claimed green tea interacts with warfarin purely because it is a leafy material (and hence contains vitamin K). Saw palmetto was linked to bleeding and Echinacea to causing arrhythmias, but there is no sound evidence to suggest any such problems with either herb (see the relevant monographs). The irony is that the authors complained about public misinformation about herbs! Despite a detailed and well-credentialled response from the American Botanical Council pointing out the many inaccuracies,[61] the journal was unrepentant.

It appears there is indeed a media bias in the reporting of herbal studies. In late November 2008, a study investigating the print media coverage of clinical trials was published in the open access journal *BMC Medicine*.[62] Public health researchers from Canada investigated the nature and tone of newspaper reporting of clinical trials of herbal medicines compared with reporting of clinical trials of drugs used to treat the same medical conditions. Databases were searched for newspaper articles in the UK and Ireland, the US, Australia/New Zealand and Canada covering the period from January 1995 to June 2005. The clinical trials were identified and sourced. The study was limited to newspaper articles that were directly related to peer-reviewed clinical trials.

The researchers coded 57 trials on herbal medicine mentioned in 352 newspaper articles and 48 drug trials mentioned in 201 newspaper articles. The main comparisons were tone (positive, neutral, negative), quality measures and content between the herbal medicine and drug clinical trials. Newspaper articles on the pharmaceuticals were more likely to be positive or neutral, but those on herbals were likely to be negative (more so than implied by trial results). No report of a pharmaceutical trial was negative, 22% of the herbal reports were. Clearly identified researchers or practitioners expert in herbal therapy were quoted in only 8% of the herbal articles.

It may be easier to publish reports in medical journals on the risks of herbal remedies than it is to prepare a publishable account of their efficacy. In the first case anecdotal evidence is the norm, in the latter case it would be dismissed out of hand. It is therefore incumbent on authors who rely on anecdote (and editors who review the results) to be assiduous in their presentation of the evidence (to get the botanical details correct, for example), to look for other possible factors in the pathogenesis and consistently to insert caveats about their inability to generalise from their evidence.

At the end of the day, risk assessment is more a political than a scientific discipline. The BSE crisis in Europe led to a marked increase in sensitivity to risk, with food policy

measures being made in that case on the basis of risks less than one in many millions. Yet it is inconceivable that truly dangerous activities like driving and smoking would ever be banned, although each may be curtailled to some extent. Unfortunately, for the same reason, herbs as medicines are vulnerable; although political weight is apparent when there have been serious threats to their availability (in Britain, Germany and the US, for example), phytotherapy is less able to muster strong political reasons to save its outlying positions. A question of definition arises in these discussions. What does toxicity actually mean in real life?

Poisonous food

Many ordinary foods naturally contain poisonous constituents:

- Wheat, rye and barley contain the protein gluten (or one that is gluten-like) that is hydrolysed in the digestive system to yield the peptide alpha-gliadin, a well-established and occasionally dangerous intestinal irritant that has caused many thousands of deaths around the world through coeliac disease and sprue.
- Apple seeds and the kernels of apricots, plums and other stone fruits, as well as bitter almonds, contain significant quantities of glycosides that yield cyanide on hydrolysis in the digestive tract.
- The cabbage family contain glucosinolates that yield toxic nitriles and goitrogenic thiocyanates.
- The oil from rapeseed, widely grown in temperate climates as a cheap vegetable oil, can contain erucic acid, which is known to cause heart damage in experimental animals.[63]
- Potatoes are members of the deadly nightshade family; when the tuber turns green under the influence of light it produces the same poisonous alkaloids.
- Many common household pulses, including soya bean, red kidney bean and haricot bean (as in baked beans), contain toxic lectins called phytohaemagglutinins as well as trypsin inhibitors, that can only reliably be neutralised by boiling for at least 30 minutes.

The foods listed above are considered safe to eat, most in unlimited quantities. However, they do demonstrate how difficult it is to predict the toxicity of a plant from the presence of toxic constituents alone. The action of the whole plant and the way in which it is normally consumed clearly in these cases count for more than any individual constituent list. It is at least possible that medicinal plants impugned for their inclusion of toxic constituents are in the same position. In the absence of clear reports of adverse side effects, it can be argued that the burden of proof falls on those who would restrict access to popular remedies.

The nocebo effect

What is much less debated are negative placebo effects. In reports on most double blind clinical trials there are accounts of adverse effects among the placebo group. The symptoms listed cover a wide range and are not necessarily short-term and transient. In one report of studies of 1228 healthy volunteers the overall incidence of adverse events during placebo administration was 19%. Complaints were more frequent after repeated dosing (28%) and in elderly subjects (26%). Overall, the most frequent adverse events were headache (7%), drowsiness (5%) and asthenia (4%), with some variation depending on study design and populations.[64] Pain can certainly be induced by placebo[65] and placebo can also interact negatively with other medications.[66]

The nocebo effect raises an intriguing prospect. It is quite likely that some adverse effects ascribed to a remedy are as non-specific as placebo-induced efficacy. Most of these nocebo effects are likely to be clinically insignificant but there are real possibilities that more serious adverse effects could also have nothing directly to do with the remedy itself.

Unfortunately, placebo-controlled safety studies are not feasible but it will be helpful in assessing overall herbal safety to have some better understanding of the potential of the nocebo effect to confound the picture. For a more extensive discussion of this phenomenon, the reader is referred to *The Essential Guide to Herbal Safety*.[1]

An innocent bystander?

In some cases (perhaps many), an adverse effect attributed to a herb might only represent a coincidental association. One possible example is the hepatotoxic IDRs attributed to black cohosh. Research in several countries has found that one of the most serious causes of liver damage is unknown. Around about one-third of all liver transplants are due to a disorder known as idiopathic or non-A non-B hepatitis.[67,68] The demographics of idiopathic hepatitis (female, late 30s to early 50s) and potential black cohosh use strongly overlap. Hence, there is a distinct possibility that some patients who develop idiopathic hepatitis might also coincidentally be taking black cohosh, given that this herb is now so popular. The herb could then be mistakenly attributed as the cause. Once one mistaken case is described in the literature, however poor its quality, it is likely that others will follow in a process akin to a self-fulfilling prophecy.

A coincidental association is more likely to occur when the quality of reporting a herbal adverse reaction is poor and does not take into account all possible causative factors. (Another problem with most herbal adverse reaction reports is that the identity of the herb purportedly involved is not identified, as is discussed elsewhere in this chapter).

Poor-quality case reports might not only incorrectly attribute a harmful effect to a herb, but they can also hamper the value of case reports as red flags for genuine adverse events. One group recently developed an instrument for assessing the quality of case reports, based on a point-based rating scale incorporating 21 items yielding a total possible score of 42.[69] A review was undertaken of adverse reports for herbal products over three periods, 1986 to 1988, 1996 to 1998 and 2006 to 2008. In total, 137 case reports were included. The percentage of high-quality case reports (scoring 29 or more) rose from 0% in 1986 to 1988, to 27.9% in 1996 to 1998 and 34.2% in 2006 to 2008. This study demonstrates that, while the quality of adverse herbal case reports is improving, there is still a long way to go.

Herbal safety: the arguments

A matter of debate

Given all the above, the issue of herbal safety is indeed a matter of contention. The following are the arguments marshalled by the doubters, particularly those who feel that their duty to public safety is to assume the worst-case scenarios.

The doubts

- Herbal remedies are complex mixtures of chemicals, about whose effects on the body little is known even in their isolated state, let alone when mixed in infinitely variable ways.
- Chemical complexity can work in both directions, buffering against and towards potentiation of adverse effects.
- Traditional use is likely to have spotted only acute and relatively frequent adverse reactions; chronic, delayed or infrequent reactions would probably not have been associated with the herb.
- Traditional reputations are in any case highly unreliable in their transmission.
- It is possible to exceed modern standards of risk, say 1:1000, and still statistically mean that very few working practitioners will see the adverse events in their lifetimes (although this argument does not apply to consumer branded products selling in millions of units per annum).
- There are particularly heavy biases in the way of reporting adverse effects of herbal remedies at the present time (see below); therefore the current state of information is almost certainly understating the risk.

The reassurances

- The remedies used in herbal medicine represent only a tiny proportion of available plant species around the world. It is likely that humans through history moved inexorably to using those plants that were effective with a minimum of toxic or other adverse consequences.
- Even allowing for under-reporting of adverse events, levels in databases are remarkably low and certainly do not compare with the levels of iatrogenic problems in conventional medicine.
- Some benign qualities may arise from the very complexity of the plants, for which they are dismissed by conventional pharmacologists. The existence of tannins, mucilages, saponins or other constituents is likely to buffer or modulate the effect of more active constituents, which are often in any case present in only low levels.
- Most of the serious adverse events reported involve problems of product quality and adulteration (see elsewhere in this chapter). Attendance to pharmaceutical standards of quality assurance and quality control (as is the norm for European herbal medicinal products) and insisting

on minimal training standards for those who prescribe herbal remedies will reduce risk.

- Most importantly, the thrust of treatment in phytotherapy is often different from that of conventional pharmacology. The herbs may better be understood as promoting healing responses in the body rather than directly targeting symptoms or pathology; this allows for a more elliptical, nutritional tilt at the body with consequent reduced negative impact. Certain herbs may be contraindicated in certain cases, not because they can cause side effects or threaten danger, but because they may simply be inappropriate for the job.

Conditional conclusions

None of the arguments presented above are mutually contradictory. An honourable position is possible on either side.

Given the low profile of adverse effects compared with other human activities, however, it could be argued strongly that herbal use should be given the benefit of the several doubts that remain. The burden of proof should lie with the regulator rather than with the herbal sector; that theoretical reasons for impugning safety (such as the presence of constituents with toxic potential in isolation) are not sufficient in themselves for banning herbal remedies. Nevertheless, the herbal sector has a professional responsibility to monitor assiduously and continuously the situation and to react responsibly if genuine concerns arise (see also the discussion of pharmacovigilance later in this chapter).

The impact of quality on safety

Appreciating quality

Medicinal plants are sourced from nature and hence, unlike conventional chemical drugs, will vary from batch to batch. This can be readily understood by comparison with another plant product – wine. In technical terms, wine is the fermented juice of the fruit of *Vitis vinifera*. However, factors such as the grape variety, climatic conditions, soil type, time of harvest and fermentation conditions can all determine whether a batch of wine will be either poor or good quality (which is subsequently reflected in the price of the wine).

In the case of wine, factors such as the texture, colour, aroma and taste determine if the product is of good quality or otherwise. For medicinal plants, the situation is more complex. Most of the chemical components of herbs that are important for therapeutic activity are secondary metabolites. Secondary metabolites are defined as those not likely to be important for normal growth and survival of the plant, although they are sometimes produced in higher levels in response to infection, insect attack and adverse growing conditions. One consequence of this is that, even though they may give an impression of its quality, the appearance and colour of a herb are not necessarily indicators of its therapeutic benefit or safety. Indeed, plants grown under adverse conditions may sometimes have a poor appearance, but higher levels of secondary metabolites. One corollary of this is that

while herb batches that have a good appearance and a pleasant taste might be suitable for a herbal tea, they may not be optimum for use as medicines. Chamomile is a good example. Matricine is considered to be an important active component and varieties of chamomile have been bred that contain higher levels of this phytochemical. Since matricine imparts a bitter taste to the flowers, these high medicinal grade varieties are not suitable for a culinary herbal tea.

Markers of quality?

One approach adopted by the various pharmacopoeias and used by manufacturers is to set minimum levels of marker chemical compounds for a herbal raw material. These are seen to give some indication of activity and hence quality. This approach, although valid, is fraught with difficulties. Even where the marker compound is known to contribute to the therapeutic activity of the herb (and this is not always the case), herbal clinicians stress that the chemical complexity of the plant confers the sum total of its activity. However, until there is better understanding of how individual herbs work in their chemical totality, setting markers is a good beginning. The uncertainties can be lessened by choosing phytochemical classes of marker compounds (flavonoids, essential oil, oligomeric procyanidins and so on) rather than just single chemical constituents. Along these lines, testing for a range of marker compounds (or groups of marker compounds) in the one plant might lead to a better assessment of activity. However, none of this should occur at the expense of the chemical totality of the plant's extractable material.

Pharmaceutical GMP

In a number of countries, including those in Europe as well as Japan and Australia, all herbal medicines must be made according to the code of pharmaceutical GMP (Good Manufacturing Practice). The US now requires compliance with 'GMPs' for dietary supplements, but the standard applied falls short of pharmaceutical GMP in some respects. Pharmaceutical GMP is a fail-safe system of quality assurance and quality control which defines a number of procedures and observances including:

- validation of equipment and processes
- documented standard operating procedures covering every aspect of manufacture
- documented cleaning and calibration logs for equipment
- control of the manufacturing environment, air and water
- quarantining and unique identification and testing of raw materials, labels and packaging
- discrete batch identification
- comprehensive batch record documentation
- reconciliation of raw materials, product, packaging and labels
- quarantining and testing of finished products
- documented release-for-sale procedures
- testing of stability of finished product
- documentation of customer complaints and recall procedures.

Box 5.1

Herbal raw material testing

- Identity and quality with thin layer chromatography
- Microscopic analysis
- Macroscopic analysis and organoleptic assessment
- Pesticide residues
- Microbial levels
- Aflatoxins
- Heavy metals
- Foreign material
- Infestation
- Radiation levels
- Active or marker compounds (quantitative)

Box 5.2

Thin layer chromatography

- An extract of a herb is spotted at the bottom of a thin layer of silica gel on a glass plate
- The plate is dipped in a solvent mixture so that the level of the solvent is below where the herb was applied
- The solvent draws up the layer and carries the phytochemical components in the herb extract different distances
- Sprays and/or ultraviolet light are used to view the components, giving a characteristic pattern of spots
- Each spot corresponds to a phytochemical in the herb
- Different solvent systems draw out different classes of phytochemicals in the herb

Box 5.3

Quality considerations for finished liquid herbal products

- Extraction efficiency
- Identity:
  a. organoleptic assessment
  b. thin layer chromatography or high performance liquid chromatography fingerprint
- Active or marker phytochemicals
- Microbial testing:
  a. total count
  b. pathogens
  c. yeast and mould
- Pesticide residues

Box 5.4

Quality considerations for finished tablet herbal products

- Identity:
  a. organoleptic assessment
  b. thin layer chromatography
- Microbial testing:
  a. total count
  b. pathogens
  c. yeasts and mould
- Hardness and friability
- Disintegration time
- Tablet size
- Weight
- Active or marker phytochemicals

In practice, herbal manufacturing under GMP is more complex than conventional drugs. This is because a herb is biologically rather than chemically defined and:

- may be incorrectly identified
- may vary in chemical content and hence efficacy
- carries with it 'a history', for example it may be contaminated with unwanted substances
- processing of herbs may enhance or impair their safety and efficacy
- stability may be difficult to define and measure.

Nevertheless, all the considerations above point strongly to the importance of herbal product manufacture under appropriate GMP.

As part of GMP, herbal raw materials are subjected to a battery of tests to ensure their quality and purity. These tests are outlined in Box 5.1. A useful guide to the British and European standards in these areas is provided by the *British Herbal Pharmacopoeia* 1996,[70] together with the *current British* and *European Pharmacopoeias* and the *United States Pharmacopeia – National Formulary*.

Thin layer chromatography (TLC) is a particularly useful technique for the identification of plant material. It can also be used to quantify plant constituents. The process of performing TLC is outlined in Box 5.2.

Finished herbal products also need to undergo testing before their release. Boxes 5.3 and 5.4 provide examples of possible testing protocols for finished products.

Microbial contamination

Since plants come from nature, herbal raw materials carry a microbial burden which needs to be reduced during processing. Although microbial contamination of herbs is a potential safety issue, there is relatively little evidence that is a significant issue in practice.

The *European Pharmacopoeia* sets limits for microbial contamination for herbal remedies in Category 4, Section 5.1.4. Microbial Quality of Pharmaceutical Preparations (1997) as follows.

A. Herbal remedies to which boiling water has been added before use:

- Total viable aerobic count. Not more than 10^7 aerobic bacteria and not more than 10^5 fungi per gram or per millilitre
- Not more than 10^2 *Escherichia coli* per gram or per millilitre.

B. Other herbal remedies:

- Total viable aerobic count. Not more than 10^5 aerobic bacteria and not more than 10^4 fungi per gram or per millilitre
- Not more than 10^3 enterobacteria and certain other Gram-negative bacteria per gram or per millilitre
- Absence of *Escherichia coli* (1.0 g or 1.0 mL)
- Absence of salmonella (10.0 g or 10.0 mL).

These levels are incidentally much tighter than those applied to food supply industries where absolute levels are often absent.

Substitution problems in herbal medicine

Substitution of one herbal raw material with another can pose a considerable problem in herbal manufacture. Substitution can occur at several different levels:

- Within a species of a less active chemical race or subspecies
- Of the wrong or less active plant part
- Within a genus of a related plant
- Of a completely different genus.

Many problems associated with herbal quality have been caused by substitution. This particularly threatens remedies that have suddenly become popular so that demand exceeds supply, such as the previous substitution of Echinacea with *Parthenium integrifolium* and the replacement of *Arnica species* with Mexican arnica (*Heterotheca inuloides*). It is particularly serious where safety is compromised, for example the substitution of *Teucrium species* (germander) for *Scutellaria lateriflora* (skullcap), as noted previously.

Some substitution practices may avoid detection at manufacture, even under GMP, and are occasionally detected in over-the-counter products in some countries. However, the knowledge of a specific substitution and the application of an appropriate test method can and does expose such practices. Despite the substitution of Stephania by Aristolochia being implicated in renal disease, apparently this practice still commonly occurs.

Contamination issues in herbal medicine

Herbal products can sometimes be contaminated with other agents and a few isolated instances have raised public health concerns. These include:

- products made in China and India contaminated with heavy metals (sometimes added intentionally) or potentially pathogenic microorganisms
- products made in China contaminated with conventional drugs
- contamination of a safe herb with a toxic herb, for example Digitalis (foxglove leaves) found among *Arctium lappa* (burdock) leaves.

The practice of pharmaceutical GMP in a well-regulated environment should eliminate the possibility of these types of contamination.

As mentioned above, one persistent quality problem that can dramatically impact on safety is the adulteration of herbal products with undeclared conventional drugs. Examples of the adulteration of Chinese herbal medicines with synthetic drugs are provided in two reviews.[71,72] A wide variety of agents including corticosteroids, non-steroidal anti-inflammatory drugs, analgesics, benzodiazepines, anticonvulsants and hypoglycaemic drugs have been found.

Cases of adrenal suppression have been linked to the intake of Chinese herbal products. A Taiwanese study found that 8 of 13 patients with severe illness and low cortisol levels reported using herbal products.[73] Two cases of adrenal suppression were reported in New Zealand and attributed to the intake of the Chinese herbal product Shen Loon.[74] The product was later found to contain the corticosteroid betamethasone, although the authors suggested other factors could be involved as well.

Undeclared codeine was detected in a Chinese antiasthmatic proprietary product.[75] One phenomenon which has fortunately received a high degree of media attention is the adulteration of Chinese weight loss products with banned weight loss drugs such as fenfluramine. This has led to toxic reactions or fatalities in the UK, Singapore, Japan and China.[76–79]

This problem is still current, with the US FDA recently issuing a recall notice on a herbal slimming capsule contaminated with sibutramine, a controlled substance that was withdrawn from the US market in October 2010 for safety reasons.[80]

A particularly cautionary tale is that of PC-SPES. PC-SPES was a herbal formulation specifically targeted at the treatment of prostate cancer (hence PC) developed and patented in the early 1990s by a research chemist.[81] It ostensibly contained seven Chinese herbs and one American herb (saw palmetto: *Serenoa repens*). The product was very successful in the US marketplace and there were consistent anecdotal accounts of its efficacy, especially for controlling PSA (prostate specific antigen) levels. In particular, naturopathic physicians and holistic medical doctors recommended the product to many patients. Being a US-sponsored product they had no reason to believe it was anything other than a herbal product, despite the fact that it was manufactured in China.

PC-SPES soon began to attract the interest of well-respected research scientists including those at Johns Hopkins School of Medicine, Harvard Medical School and the National Center for Complementary and Alternative Medicine.[81] In 2002, three reviews of the use of PC-SPES were published which surveyed the major publications on its pharmacology and clinical activity.[82–84] By early 2002 there were 116 published clinical and laboratory-based studies of PC-SPES.[85]

The reviews highlighted the significant in vitro and in vivo activities of PC-SPES in prostate cancer models and noted the small number of positive but preliminary clinical trials.[82–84] Oestrogenic activity was confirmed for the product, which was consistent with some of the side effects exhibited by patients taking the formulation such as gynaecomastia, loss of libido, decrease in body hair and superficial thrombosis. However, there was also another worrying and paradoxical side effect of PC-SPES: it was linked to severe bleeding in one case[86] and suspected of potentiating the effects of warfarin in another.[87]

Another perspective on PC-SPES began to emerge in 2002 at around the same time the above reviews were published. In early April a group of scientists presented their findings to the 93rd Meeting of the American Association for Cancer Research that PC-SPES samples from 1996 to 2001 contained the oestrogenic drug diethylstilbestrol as well as warfarin and indomethacin.[88] Their comprehensive results were published later that year.[89] Earlier in February 2002, the FDA alerted consumers to stop taking PC-SPES because the California Department of Health Services had detected the presence of warfarin. Another product called SPES from the same corporation had been found to contain the anti-anxiety drug alprazolam.[90] The manufacturer undertook a voluntary recall and PC-SPES was subsequently withdrawn from the market.[81]

Resolving the safety issue: pharmacovigilance initiatives

Postmarketing surveillance

Given that so few herbal extracts have ever been submitted to extensive preclinical studies, the toxicological information about herbal remedies is generally sketchy. In European legislation the principle has been accepted that drugs already widely used in the population need not go back to the laboratory for new toxicological studies. Instead, those supplying such remedies are under increasing burden to establish safety on an ongoing basis; postmarketing surveillance or *pharmacovigilance* are terms generally used to describe this monitoring process. There is an overwhelming mathematical case for systematising observations of adverse reactions. Statisticians have calculated that if, for example, an adverse event occurred in as many as 1 in 1000 cases, one would need to see 3000 cases to have a 95% probability of spotting one.[91] This 'law of three' makes the individual practitioner of little use in identifying even substantial risks.

All modern medicine legislatures have drug monitoring administrations and encourage physicians to report adverse events they encounter. In some countries, reporting to the authority is mandatory and various forms are produced for the purpose. There is thus in most countries a database of adverse drug reactions (ADRs), which contribute to the warnings added to drug labels and datasheets. A very small number of ADRs relate to herbal remedies, but for a number of reasons (see below) these have been poorly evaluated.

In the cases where analysis of the data has been done, reports of adverse effects from human consumption of herbs appear to be relatively infrequent, making up around 1% of spontaneous reporting.[92] There is a widespread concern among the regulatory authorities, however, that these cases represent only a small proportion of such incidents. Spontaneous reporting for even conventional prescribed drugs is an inefficient mechanism, with reporting rates among physicians as low as a few per cent of actual cases.[93] In the case of herbal remedies, so many of which are self-prescribed or are prescribed by non-doctors, there is much less opportunity for doctors to become aware of this factor in adverse events. Reporting mechanisms

---

Box 5.5

Problems affecting the reporting of ADRs involving herbal remedies

There may be fewer adverse drug reactions (ADRs) for herbal remedies due to the following:

- Lethargy (general reporting rates for all drugs are very poor)
- Physicians are usually unaware of natural product consumption
- Physicians do not routinely ask about non-prescribed medications
- Common bias against associating adverse effects with natural medicines
- Ignorance of reporting mechanisms by potential non-physician notifiers
- Users reluctant to talk to professionals if self-prescribed treatment goes wrong
- Potential notifier's reluctance to get involved in 'the system'
- Potential notifier's reluctance to risk losing a favourite remedy
- Uncertainty of connections in multiple ingredient prescriptions

---

Box 5.6

Perceived problems in applying ADRs to assessing the safety of herbal remedies

Adverse drug reaction (ADR) reporting is not sensitive to herbal use. It does not easily:

- detect adverse reactions that are:
  a. subtle
  b. infrequent
  c. delayed
- pick out causative agents from multiple ingredients
- disentangle multiple/multicausal pathologies most often seen in chronic diseases.

There is a wider lack of context in which to place herbal ADRs, in particular concerning:

- market availability/consumption
- pharmacotoxicology
- drug interactions

---

for non-doctors are rarely in place and even pharmacists have only variable opportunities or tradition for notifying adverse events. Even where reporting is possible, there are other reasons why spontaneous notification is likely to be particularly ineffective for herbal remedies (Box 5.5).

On the other hand the herbal sector can claim that uncontrolled observations of adverse events are likely to be misleading for the case of herbal safety, and even the regulators accept that there are particular problems (Box 5.6).

In this context it is an encouraging development that most countries now include herbal adverse reaction reporting in their respective databases, often with a formal requirement on manufacturers to report their knowledge of such events to the relevant statutory authority. Such adverse reaction data from government or WHO databases that have occasionally been drawn on for safety information regarding individual herbs and, where available, in published form, are included in the relevant monograph in Section Three.

In addition, studies are published from time to time that examine the totality of case reports on a specific database. One relatively recent example is from Sweden that drew on adverse reactions submitted to the Swedish Medicinal Products Agency between 1987 and 2006.[94] Among a total of 64 493 reports, 778 concerned 967 suspected adverse reactions related to 175 complementary medicine products. Of these 967 adverse reactions, the most reported substance was *Echinacea purpurea* singly (8.1%) and in combination (7.3%), with *Ginkgo biloba* leaf next at 6.7%. In 221 reports, at least one reaction was categorised as serious, the frequency of these being pulmonary embolism (1.7%), liver reactions (2.8%) and anaphylactic reaction (2%).

For a detailed discussion of the pharmacovigilance of herbal medicines, see Chapter 11 of *The Essential Guide to Herbal Safety*.[1]

Conclusion

There is no absolute safety in life. Every human activity is risky and accidents will happen, even to herbal clinicians.

Some plants are likely to be dangerous when consumed; as material medicines, herbs are bound to interact with the body in ways that are not always convenient. Since little is known about the long-term consequences of herbal intake, it would make good practical sense to discourage patients from taking the same prescriptions for long periods unless there is a clear benefit.

It is surprising, however, how few problems have been laid at the door of medicinal plants. Considering the vast usage around the world of plants as medicines, it is remarkable that there is so little epidemiological or clinical evidence that this is a harmful activity. It is possible even that the safety record for phytotherapy is better than for any other widespread human activity, including eating, drinking, sleeping (a particularly dangerous activity), taking exercise, working or travelling.

The problem for legislators, medical professionals and public guardians is that they inevitably find themselves balancing risk with benefit. If they can see a public benefit as well as a demand for an activity they will feel able to cover themselves against public and media attack if something ever went wrong. Unfortunately, despite the accumulating research, the case for the efficacy of herbal treatments is making relatively slower headway with many legislators and conventional medical practitioners than the case for their safety.

References

1. Mills S, Bone K, eds. *The Essential Guide to Herbal Safety*. St Louis: Elsevier Churchill Livingstone; 2005.
2. Gardner Z, McGuffin M, eds. *The American Herbal Products Association's Botanical Safety Handbook*. Boca Raton, FL: CRC Press; 2012. In press.
3. Violon C. Belgian (Chinese herb) nephropathy: why? *J Pharm Belg*. 1997;52(1):7–27.
4. De Smet PAGM, Keller K, Hansel R, et al. (eds.) *Adverse Effects of Herbal Drugs*, vol 1. Berlin: Springer-Verlag; 1992. p. 79–89.
5. Reginster F, Jadoul M, van Ypersele de Strihou C. Chinese herbs nephropathy presentation, natural history and fate after transplantation. *Nephrol Dial Transplant*. 1997;12(1):81–86.
6. Cosyns JP, Jadoul M, Squifflet JP, et al. Urothelial lesions in Chinese-herb nephropathy. *Am J Kidney Dis*. 1999;33(6):1011–1017.
7. Nortier JL, Martinez MC, Schmeiser HH, et al. Urothelial carcinoma associated with the use of a Chinese herb (*Aristolochia fangchi*). *N Engl J Med*. 2000;342(23):1686–1692.
8. US Food and Drug Administration. Listing of Botanical Ingredients of Concern. US Food and Drug Administration, Center for Food Safety and Applied Nutrition, Office of Nutritional Products, Labeling, and Dietary Supplements. Revised April 9, 2001. Available online. <http://www.fda.gov/Food/DietarySupplements/Alerts/ucm095283.htm> Accessed 15.06.11.
9. Therapeutic Goods Administration. Urgent medicine recall, reference R2001/549, date 6 December 2001. Produced by Therapeutic Goods Administration, 7 December 2001.
10. *Contaminated Chinese Herbs Recalled*. Associated Press; 2001.
11. Lekehal M, Pessayre D, Lereau JM, et al. Hepatotoxicity of the herbal medicine germander: metabolic activation of its furano diterpenoids by cytochrome P450 3A depletes cytoskeleton-associated protein thiols and forms plasma membrane blebs in rat hepatocytes. *Hepatology*. 1996;24(1):212–218.
12. Mills SY. *The A–Z of Modern Herbalism*. London: Thorsons; 1989. pp. 190–191.
13. MacGregor FB, Abernethy VE, Dahabra S, et al. Hepatotoxicity of herbal remedies. *BMJ*. 1989;299(6708):1156–1157.
14. Harvey J, Colin-Jones DG. Mistletoe hepatitis. *Br Med J (Clin Res Ed)*. 1981;282(6259):186–187.
15. De Smet PAGM, Keller K, Hansel R, et al. (eds.) *Adverse Effects of Herbal Drugs*, vol 2. Berlin: Springer-Verlag; 1993. p. 289–296.
16. De Smet PAGM, Keller K, Hansel R, et al. (eds.) *Adverse Effects of Herbal Drugs*, vol 3. Berlin: Springer-Verlag; 1997. p. 137–144.
17. Mattei A, Rucay P, Samuel D, et al. Liver transplantation for severe acute liver failure after herbal medicine (*Teucrium polium*) administration. *J Hepatol*. 1995;22(5):597.
18. Perharic L, Shaw D, Leon C, et al. Possible association of liver damage with the use of Chinese herbal medicine for skin disease. *Vet Hum Toxicol*. 1995;37(6):562–566.
19. Kane JA, Kane SP, Jain S. Hepatitis induced by traditional Chinese herbs; possible toxic components. *Gut*. 1995;36(1):146–147.
20. Wang YP, Shi B, Chen YX, et al. Drug-induced liver disease: an 8-year study of patients from one gastroenterological department. *J Dig Dis*. 2009;10(3):195–200.
21. Shaw D. Toxicological risks of Chinese herbs. *Planta Med*. 2010;76(17):2012–2018.
22. Sheikh NM, Philen RM, Love LA. Chaparral-associated hepatotoxicity. *Arch Intern Med*. 1997;157(8):913–919.
23. Whiting PW, Clouston A, Kerlin P. Black cohosh and other herbal remedies associated with acute hepatitis. *MJA*. 2002;177(8):440–443.
24. Teschke R, Bahre R, Genthner A, et al. Suspected black cohosh hepatotoxicity – challenges and pitfalls of causality assessment. *Maturitas*. 2009;63(4):302–314.
25. Shekelle P, Morton S, Maglione M, et al. Ephedra and ephedrine for weight loss and athletic performance enhancement: clinical efficacy and side effects. Evidence Report/Technology Assessment No. 76 (Prepared by Southern California Evidence–based

Practice Center, RAND, under Contract No. 290–97–0001, Task Order No. 9). AHRQ Publication No. 03–E022. Agency for Healthcare Research and Quality, Rockville, MD; 2003.

26. Borum ML. Fulminant exacerbation of autoimmune hepatitis after the use of ma huang. *Am J Gastroenterol.* 2001;96(5):1654–1655.

27. Nadir A, Agrawal S, King PD, et al. Acute hepatitis associated with the use of a Chinese herbal product, ma-huang. *Am J Gastroenterol.* 1996;91(7):1436–1438.

28. Stolpman DR, Petty J, Ham J, et al. Weight loss supplements and fulminant hepatic failure: a case series. *Hepatology.* 2002;36(4 Pt 2):168A.

29. Yeong ML, Clark SP, Waring JM, et al. The effects of comfrey derived pyrrolizidine alkaloids on rat liver. *Pathology.* 1991;23(1):35–38.

30. White RD, Swick RA, Cheeke PR. Effects of microsomal enzyme induction on the toxicity of pyrrolizidine (senecio) alkaloids. *J Toxicol Environ Health.* 1983;12(4):633–640.

31. Yan CC, Cooper RA, Huxtable RJ. The comparative metabolism of the four pyrrolizidine alkaloids, seneciphylline, retrorsine, monocrotaline, and trichodesmine in the isolated, perfused rat liver. *Toxicol Appl Pharmacol.* 1995;133(2):277–284.

32. Datta DV, Khuroo MS, Mattocks AR, et al. Herbal medicines and veno-occlusive disease in India. *Postgrad Med J.* 1978;54(634):511–515.

33. Ortiz Cansado A, Crespo Valadés E, Morales Blanco P, et al. Veno-occlusive liver disease due to intake of Senecio vulgaris tea. *Gastroenterol Hepatol.* 1995;18(8):413–416.

34. Mokhobo KP. Herb use and necrodegenerative hepatitis. *S Afr Med J.* 1976;50(28):1096–1099.

35. Hirono I, Mori H, Culvenor CC. Carcinogenic activity of coltsfoot, *Tussilago farfara* L. Gann. 1976;67(1):125–129.

36. Sperl W, Stuppner H, Gassner I, et al. Reversible hepatic veno-occlusive disease in an infant after consumption of pyrrolizidine-containing herbal tea. *Eur J Pediatr.* 1995;154(2):112–116.

37. Larrey D. Liver involvement in the course of phytotherapy (editorial). *Presse Med.* 1994;23(15):691–693.

38. Boyd EL. De Smet PAGM, Keller K, Hansel R, et al. (eds.) *Adverse Effects of herbal Drugs,* vol 1. Berlin: Springer-Verlag; 1992. p. 152.

39. Gunn TR, Wright IM. The use of black and blue cohosh in labour. *N Z Med J.* 1996;109(1032):410–411.

40. Jones TK, Lawson BM. Profound neonatal congestive heart failure caused by maternal consumption of blue cohosh herbal medication. *J Pediatr.* 1998;132(3 Pt 1): 550–552.

41. US Food and Drug Administration, Center for Food Safety and Applied Nutrition, Office of Special Nutritionals. The Special Nutritionals Adverse Event Monitoring System.

42. Finkel RS, Zarlengo KM. Blue cohosh and perinatal stroke. *N Engl J Med.* 2004;351(3):302–303.

43. Finkel RS. More on blue cohosh and perinatal stroke/the author's reply. *N Engl J Med.* 2004;351(21):2239–2241.

44. Rao RB, Hoffman RS. Nicotinic toxicity from tincture of blue cohosh (*Caulophyllum thalictroides*) used as an abortifacient. *Vet Hum Toxicol.* 2002;44(4):221–222.

45. Krenzelok EP, Mrvos R. Friends and foes in the plant world: a profile of plant ingestions and fatalities. *Clin Toxicol (Phila).* 2011;49(3):142–149.

46. Ondrizek RR, Chan PJ, Patton WC, et al. An alternative medicine study of herbal effects on the penetration of zona-free hamster oocytes and the integrity of sperm deoxyribonucleic acid. *Fertil Steril.* 1999;71(3):517–522.

47. Owen PL, Johns T. Xanthine oxidase inhibitory activity of northeastern North American plant remedies used for gout. *J Ethnopharmacol.* 1999;64(2):149–160.

48. Petty HR, Fernando M, Kindzelskii AL, et al. Identification of colchicine in placental blood from patients using herbal medicines. *Chem Res Toxicol.* 2001;14(9):1254–1258.

49. Hood RL. Colchicine poisoning. *J Emerg Med.* 1994;12(2):171–177.

50. Levy M, Spino M, Read SE. Colchicine: a state-of-the-art review. *Pharmacotherapy.* 1991;11(3):196–211.

51. American Botanical Council. *Herbal science group debunks research suggesting presence of toxin colchicine in Ginkgo.* News release to national media; 2001.

52. CMEC 29 Complementary Medicines Evaluation Committee. Extracted Ratified Minutes Twenty Ninth Meeting 24 September 2001 Ginkgo and colchicine. <http://www.tga.gov.au/pdf/archive/cmec-minutes-29.pdf>.

53. Chappey O, Scherrmann JM. Colchicine: recent data on pharmacokinetics and clinical pharmacology. *Rev Med Intern.* 1995;16(10):782–789.

54. Dehan B, Chagnon JL, Vinner E, et al. Colchicine poisoning: report of a fatal case with body fluid and post-mortem tissue analysis by high-performance liquid chromatography. *Biomed Chromatogr.* 1999;13(3):235–238.

55. Kintz P, Jamey C, Tracqui A, et al. Colchicine poisoning: report of a fatal case and presentation of an HPLC procedure for body fluid and tissue analyses. *J Anal Toxicol.* 1997;21(1):70–72.

56. Danel VC, Wiart JD, Hardy GA, et al. Self-poisoning with *Colchicum autumnale* L. flowers. *Clin Toxicol.* 2001;39(4):409–411.

57. Borman S. Toxin reported in supplements. *Chem Eng News.* 2001;79(33):33–34.

58. [No author listed] Health risk. *The Courier-Mail* Thursday, 10, 2003; 4.

59. Health – Reuters. Black cohosh may make breast cancer drug more toxic. Yahoo! News, April 7, 2003. Available. <http://www.cancerpage.com/news/article.asp?id=5746> Accessed 15.06.11.

60. Tachjian A, Maria V, Jahangir A. Use of herbal products and potential interactions in patients with cardiovascular diseases. *J Am Coll Cardiol.* 2010;55(6):515–525.

61. Blumenthal M. Cardiology journal refuses to retract error-riddled herb–drug interaction article. *HerbalGram.* 2010;87:8.

62. Bubela T, Boon H, Caulfield T. Herbal remedy clinical trials in the media: a comparison with the coverage of conventional pharmaceuticals. *BMC Med.* 2008;6:35.

63. Rosenzweig P, Brohier S, Zipfel A. The placebo effect in healthy volunteers: influence of experimental conditions on the adverse events profile during phase I studies. *Clin Pharmacol Ther.* 1993;54(5):578–583.

64. Benedetti F, Amanzio M. The neurobiology of placebo analgesia: from endogenous opioids to cholecystokinin. *Prog Neurobiol.* 1997;52(2):109–125.

65. Kleijnen J, De Craen AJM, Van Everdingen J, et al. Placebo effect in double blind clinical trials: a review of interactions with medications. *Lancet.* 1994;344:1347–1349.

66. Atal CK, Zutshi U, Rao PG. Scientific evidence on the role of Ayurvedic herbals on bioavailability of drugs. *J Ethnopharmacol.* 1981;4(2):229–232.

67. Gow PJ, Jones RM, Dobson JL, et al. Etiology and outcome of fulminant hepatic failure managed at an Australian liver transplant unit. *J Gastroenterol Hepatol.* 2004;19(2):154–159.

68. Hoofnagle JH, Carithers Jr RL, Shapiro C, et al. Fulminant hepatic failure: summary of a workshop. *Hepatology.* 1995;21(1):240–252.

69. Hung SK, Hillier S, Ernst E. Case reports of adverse effects of herbal medicinal products (HMPs): a quality assessment. *Phytomedicine.* 2011;19(5):335–343.

70. British Herbal Medicine Association. *British Herbal Pharmacopoeia.* Christchurch: BHMA; 1996. pp. 14–16.

71. Ko RJ. Causes, epidemiology, and clinical evaluation of suspected herbal poisoning. *Clin Toxicol.* 1999;37(6):697–708.

72. Ernst E. Adulteration of Chinese herbal medicines with synthetic drugs: a systematic review. *J Intern Med.* 2002;252(2):107–113.

73. Chang SS, Liaw SJ, Bullard MJ, et al. Adrenal insufficiency in critically ill emergency department patients: a Taiwan preliminary study. *Acad Emerg Med.* 2001;8(7):761–764.

74. Florkowski CM, Elder PA, Lewis JG, et al. Two cases of adrenal suppression following a Chinese herbal remedy: a cause for concern? *NZ Med J.* 2002;115(1153):223–224.

75. Liu SY, Woo SO, Holmes MJ, et al. LC and LC-MS-MS analyses of undeclared

codeine in antiasthmatic Chinese proprietary medicine. *J Pharm Biomed Anal.* 2000;22(3):481–486.

76. Metcalfe K, Corns C, Fahie-Wilson M, et al. Chinese medicines for slimming still cause health problems. *BMJ.* 2002;324(7338):679.

77. Koo E. Chinese medicine appeal outweighs diet pill worry. Reuters August 29, 2002. Available online. <http://www.manilatimes.net/national/2002/aug/29/opinion/20020829opi6.html>.

78. Shimbun Y. Chinese diet aids kill 1, sicken 11. *Daily Yomiuri Online* July 12, 2002. Available online. <http://www.yomirui.co.jp/newse/20020712wo21.htm>.

79. New diet pill blamed for at least 1 death in China. <http://www.voanews.com/english/news/a-13-a-2002-07-15-13-New-67433567.html>. Accessed 15.06.11.

80. US FDA, Public Notification: 'Slim Xtreme Herbal Slimming Capsule' Contains Undeclared Drug Ingredient. <http://www.fda.gov/Drugs/ResourcesForYou/Consumers/BuyingUsingMedicineSafely/MedicationHealthFraud/ucm254905.htm>. Accessed 14.06.11.

81. Ochs R. Going to bat for prostate cancer herbs. *Newsday.com* October 8, 2002. <http://www.newsday.com/going-to-bat-for-prostate-cancer-herbs-1.344309>. Accessed 14.06.11.

82. Oh WK, Small EJ. PC-SPES and prostate cancer. *Urol Clin North Am.* 2002;29(1):59–66.

83. Thomson JO, Dzubak P, Hajduch M. Prostate cancer and the food supplement, PC-SPES. *Neoplasma.* 2002;49(2):69–74.

84. Marks LS, DiPaola RS, Nelson P, et al. PC-SPES: herbal formulation for prostate cancer. *Urology.* 2002;60(3):369–377.

85. Pandha HS, Kirby RS. PC-SPES: phytotherapy for prostate cancer. *Lancet.* 2002;359(9325):2213–2215.

86. Weinrobe MC, Montgomery B. Acquired bleeding diathesis in a patient taking PC-SPE. *N Engl J Med.* 2001;345(16):1213–1214.

87. Davis NB, Nahlik L, Vogelzang NJ. Does PC-SPES interact with warfarin? *J Urol.* 2002;167(4):1793.

88. Arnold K. Tests of three herbal therapies yield disappointing results. *J Natl Cancer Inst.* 2002;94(9):649.

89. Sovak M, Seligson AL, Konas M, et al. Herbal composition PC-SPES for management of prostate cancer: identification of active principles. *J Natl Cancer Inst.* 2002;94(17):1275–1281.

90. Reuters Health. Prostate herbals contain prescription drugs: FDA. February 8, 2002. Available online. <http://abcnews.go.com/wire/Living/reuters20020208_458.html>. Accessed 14.02.02.

91. De Smet PAGM. An introduction to herbal pharmacoepidemiology. *J Ethnopharmacol.* 1993;38:197–208.

92. Report to 9th Meeting of Working Group for International Program on Chemical Safety (IPOS) INTOX Project 2–6th Sept 1996.

93. Leiper JM, Lawson DH. Why do doctors not report adverse drug reactions? *Neth J Med.* 1985;28(12):546–550.

94. Jacobsson I, Jönsson AK, Gerdén B, et al. Spontaneously reported adverse reactions in association with complementary and alternative medicine substances in Sweden. *Pharmacoepidemiol Drug Saf.* 2009;18(11):1039–1047.

PART 2

Practical clinical guides

Introduction

In Part Two, the strategic options in clinical phytotherapy are reviewed. Practical issues of dosage and prescribing are followed by individual chapters on the phytotherapeutic approach to pathological states and to system dysfunctions.

As far as possible the commentary in this section is based on material that is both subjected to modern research and supported by the most persistent therapeutic traditions distilled from the long human battle with illness. If there is a choice between the two sources of information, the text is biased in favour of traditional use; in general, only when there is such use will scientific pointers to plant activity be cited. This is particularly so in the great majority of cases where experimental data are restricted to in vitro or animal or other non-clinical models. Until the modern research effort becomes much more substantial this bias will remain the only appropriate option.

This is not a book on general medicine; not every infirmity encountered in the clinic is covered in depth or even mentioned. Nor is there any attempt to review the wider natural approaches to healthcare; there is little on dietary or other naturopathic strategies. The aim is to highlight the strengths of herbal medicine and to commend the unique approaches to many difficult clinical conditions that are possible. The authors believe that phytotherapy can provide a major resource for future healthcare. The groundwork is set out in these pages.

The evidence base we can use is not complete. The sections vary in substance, size, detail and authority. The support provided by modern research is particularly patchy. In some areas, notably the digestive system, the liver and the urinary system, there is a great deal of underpinning at a theoretical level but modest clinical evidence, although this has grown since the first edition. In most areas, there are some strong therapeutic commendations to make but less pathophysiological or pharmacological rationale or research evidence. Only in the circulatory and nervous systems is there a reasonable mix of theoretical and clinical research support.

In all sections, summary indications and contraindications are included at the beginning. In some sections, summary materia medica for therapeutic group or chemical subgroup is appropriate. A few case histories are included for illumination.

In general, the authors have stayed with the European and North American tradition they practise. Nevertheless, readers who would rather use herbs from other traditions should still find the mechanisms and rationales discussed here appropriate.

Dosage and dosage forms in herbal medicine

6

CHAPTER CONTENTS

The subject of appropriate dose is probably the most controversial aspect of contemporary Western herbal medicine. Among Western herbal practitioners, many different dosage approaches are found from country to country and within countries. Underlying these different approaches are different philosophies about the therapeutic action of medicinal plants.

At one extreme is the assumption that the therapeutic effect relies on a specific dose of the active chemicals contained in each particular plant. At the other extreme, emphasis is placed on the assumption that a herbal medicine, being derived from a living organism, carries a certain energy or vital force. The quality of this energy confers the therapeutic effect and hence the amount of actual herb is not as important, as long as some is present. Others perhaps feel that the active components act as catalysts to restore health and do not need to be present in pharmacological quantities.

The low dosage approach should not be confused with homeopathy, although it has been influenced by this system. One important difference from homeopathy is that the therapeutic indications are not derived from the principle of similars and mainly come from traditional indications. Like homeopathy, this approach probably relies on a high degree of patient susceptibility to the medication.

Both the high and low dosage approaches have their adherents who maintain that their respective systems give good results in the clinic. While it is inappropriate to label one approach as correct and the other incorrect (indeed, even high doses of herbs possibly also act through other unknown interactive factors), it is useful to review and contrast current and historical dosage approaches. By doing this, one can arrive at an appropriate dosage system for modern phytotherapy in that it is consistent with:

* dosage ranges used in other important herbal traditions, e.g. China and India
* dosages used by important historical movements in Western herbal medicine, e.g. the Eclectics
* dosages currently recommended in pharmacopoeias
* dosages established from pharmacological and clinical research.

In any discussion of herbal doses, the influence of dosage form and quality of preparations must also be considered, as should the mechanics of formulation and prescription writing.

Review of dosage approaches

Traditional Chinese medicine

The daily dose for individual non-toxic herbs in traditional Chinese medicine is usually in the range of 3 to 10g, given as a decoction or in pill or powder form.[1] Often higher doses are prescribed by decoction than for pills, as might be expected since not all active components readily dissolve in hot water.[2] (Pills generally consist of the powdered herb incorporated into a suitable base.) Herbs are invariably prescribed in formulations. Doses for such formulations are about 3 to 9g taken three times daily but can be higher in the case of decoctions.

For each individual herb, a wide dosage range is usually given in texts. (This applies for all herbal systems.) One reason for this is that if a herb is used by itself or with just a few other herbs, a larger dose is used than when it is combined with many other herbs.[2] Dose also varies according to the weight and age of patients and the severity or acuteness of their condition.

DOI:http://dx.doi.org/10.1016/B978-0-443-06992-5.00006-2

Recently, a more processed form of dosage has become popular among practitioners of Chinese medicine. This involves the prescription of formulas in a granulated form. The granules are prepared by drying or freeze-drying decoctions, that is aqueous extracts, of herbal formulas. Usually 2 g of granules is prescribed three times daily, which corresponds to about 6 to 10 g of original dried herbs per dose.

Some herbs, or closely related species, are used in both Chinese and Western herbal medicine. Table 6.1[1,3,4] compares dosages for a few of these herbs.

In general, the similarity in the dosage range between the different systems is striking. Discrepancies do exist for Zingiber and Taraxacum, which in the case of Zingiber can be explained by a higher content of the active components in the alcoholic tincture compared to the decoction, and, in the case of Taraxacum may be a reflection on the different species used.

Ayurveda

Ayurveda often involves complex formulations which are prepared over several days and can contain many herbal and mineral components. Consequently, there is more dosage diversity than for Chinese medicine. Dosage ranges for individual non-toxic herbs are generally in the region of 1 to 6 g/day as powders or tinctures, with higher doses often recommended for decoctions.[5]

Eclectic medicine

Eclectic medicine was a largely empirical school of medicine which developed in America during the 19th century.[6] The

movement was most prominent for a brief period from the late 19th to the early 20th centuries, when there were several teaching universities and many eminent scholars in the USA. Although the Eclectics used simple chemical medicines such as phosphoric acid, they mainly prescribed herbal medicines. Their knowledge of materia medica was their greatest contribution to Western herbal medicine; for example, herbs such as Echinacea and golden seal were made popular by them after observation of their use by the Native Americans.

The Eclectics tended to use higher doses than those recommended in current texts and pharmacopoeias, although the ranges tend to overlap. Table 6.2 compares dosages currently used[3,4] with those found in Eclectic texts[7,8] for alcoholic extracts of herbs.

The British Herbal Pharmacopoeia

The *British Herbal Pharmacopoeia* 1983 (BHP) carries extensive dosage information for individual herbs and is generally regarded as an important traditional reference on this subject for Western herbal practitioners. Dosages given in the BHP were derived from earlier texts such as the *British Pharmacopoeia* (BP) and the *British Pharmaceutical Codex* (BPC) but also resulted from a survey of herbal practitioners. More recently, the *British Herbal Compendium* (BHC) has been published in two volumes, with dosage information for the practitioner.[9,10]

The doses given by the BHP 1983 contain some inconsistencies. The main problem is that doses for tinctures often do not correlate to corresponding doses for liquid extracts. For a 1:1 extract and a 1:5 tincture of a particular herb to correlate in terms of dose, the dose range for the tincture should be five times that of the extract, since it is theoretically five times weaker. This problem contrasts with other pharmacopoeias such as the BPC 1934 where the correlation is generally, but

Table 6.1 Comparison of dosages used in Chinese and Western herbal medicine

Herb	Chinese dosage[1] g/day	Western dosage[3,4] g/day
Ephedra sinica	3–9	3–9 (extract)
		3–12 (decoction)
Zingiber officinale	3–9	0.75–3 (decoction)
		0.38–0.75 (tincture)
Taraxacum mongolicum	9–30	6–24 (decoction)
		3–6 (tincture)
Glycyrrhiza uralensis	3–12	3–12 (decoction)
		6–12 (extract)
Rheum palmatum	3–6	2.3–4.5 (decoction)
		1.8–6 (extract)

Note: For dosages of tinctures and extracts given three times daily, the corresponding amount of dried herb per day has been calculated.

Table 6.2 Comparison of dosages used by the Eclectics and modern dosages

Herb	Eclectic dosage[7,8] g/day	Current dosage[3,4] g/day
Euphorbia hirta	1.8–10.8	0.36–0.9
Echinacea angustifolia	0.9–5.4	0.75–3.0
Hydrastis canadensis	0.9–10.8	0.9–3.0
Passiflora incarnata	1.8–10.8	1.5–3.0
Valeriana officinalis	2.1–6.0	0.9–3.0
Rumex crispus	1.8–10.8	6.0–12.0
Viburnum opulus	3.6–10.8	6.0–12.0
Serenoa repens	2.7–10.8	1.8–4.5

Note: The corresponding amount of dried herb per day has been calculated from recommended dosages for fluid extracts.

Table 6.3 Comparison of extract and tincture dosages in the BHP 1983

Herb	Dose range 1:1 extract[3]	Dose range 1:5 tincture[3]	Expected dose range for 1:5 tincture
Agrimonia eupatoria	1–3 mL	2–4 mL	5–15 mL
Achillea millefolium	2–4 mL	2–4 mL	10–20 mL
Eupatorium purpureum	2–4 mL	1–2 mL	10–20 mL
Menyanthes trifoliata	1–2 mL	1–3 mL	5–10 mL

Note: The expected dose range for the 1:5 tincture is calculated by multiplying the dose range for the 1:1 extract by 5.

not exactly, observed. Some examples that highlight this problem are provided in Table 6.3.

The poor correlation demonstrated in Table 6.3, where in the case of *Eupatorium purpureum* the tincture dose is actually *less* than the extract dose, probably arises for two reasons:

1. As stated above, the BHP 1983 doses were in part derived from a survey of herbal practitioners. It is probable that there were different dosage philosophies between practitioners using extracts compared to those using tinctures. Hence, a correlation should not be expected.

2. Tinctures are manufactured using different techniques to 1:1 fluid extracts. This is particularly important. Fluid extracts can be prepared by reconstituting more concentrated extracts, rather than the traditional method of reserved percolation. In either case, the heat or vacuum used in concentration can rob the preparation of important active chemicals. Tinctures better preserve the activity of the whole plant because they are made without heat or a concentration procedure. Fluid extracts were also often manufactured using lower alcohol strengths than tinctures, and important active components may therefore not be extracted from the starting plant material. The result of these factors is that a 1:1 fluid extract can have an activity which is much less than five times that of a 1:5 tincture. This will be dealt with in more detail in the part of this chapter that discusses liquid preparations.

Since tinctures better preserve the chemical profile of the dried herb, more credibility should be given to the tincture doses when using the dosage ranges in the BHP 1983.

Commission E and ESCOP monographs

Under the direction of the German Health Department, the Commission E prepared a series of monographs on commonly used medicinal herbs during the 1980s. The Commission E was an expert committee consisting of doctors, pharmacologists, pharmacognocists and toxicologists from both academia and industry. If a herb did not receive a positive monograph from the Commission E, it could not be readily registered as a medicine in Germany. In the preparation of a monograph, the Commission E took into account relevant traditional use as well as scientific research.

A positive monograph for a herb also included dosage information. Many of the monograph doses are for infusions or decoctions since this reflects the common use of teas in the German marketplace.[11] Such daily doses are usually in the range of 2 to 10 g. Occasionally a monograph will specify a dose for a herb in terms of major active constituents; for example, for Ephedra the daily dose is 45 to 90 mg of alkaloids (about 4 to 8 g of herb) which is similar to the range in Table 6.1. Occasionally, where tincture and extract doses are given by the Commission E, there is not always a good correlation. For example, the single dose for valerian tincture is 1 to 3 mL and yet the single dose for a fluid extract is 2 to 3 mL. The reasons for this may be the same as those discussed above for the BHP 1983.

The Scientific Committee of ESCOP (European Scientific Cooperative of Phytotherapy) has published a series of herbal monographs.[12,13] These were compiled by an international team of expert authors and represent a major contribution to the harmonisation of standards for herbal medicines across the European Union. These monographs contain useful dosage information reflecting the European situation and have been taken into account for the dosage recommendations in this text.

Clinical trials

The clinical trial is arguably the best way to determine the effective dose of either a single herb or a herbal formulation. This will not always be applicable to traditional medicine, however, since prescriptions are usually prepared on an individual basis. Also, a clinical trial does not necessarily determine the optimum dose. However, it does confer a relative certainty to the clinical results. That is, at a given dose of a given preparation a certain percentage of patients are likely to respond; for example, *Ginkgo biloba* standardised extract at 120 mg/day (which corresponds to about 6 g/day of dry leaves), given for 2 months, will improve intermittent claudication in 60% of patients.[14]

Sometimes the clinical trial has used a standardised extract of the herb which can then be correlated to the whole herb; for example, silymarin in liver disorders at 240 mg/day corresponds to 8 to 16 g/day of *Silybum marianum* seeds.[15]

The low dosage approach

Currently in the USA, New Zealand, parts of Europe (especially among homeopaths) and to some extent Australia, there are practitioners who prefer to prescribe drop doses of 1:5 or even more dilute tinctures. It is useful to examine the possible origins of this approach.

In Europe, homeopaths often use combinations of herbal mother tinctures in drop dosage, for example, 'drainage'. This approach is sometimes incorrectly labelled as 'phytotherapy'.

In the USA a more direct influence comes, ironically, from a development of Eclectic medicine. In 1869, the Eclectic physician John Scudder proposed the concept of 'specific medication'.[7] With this concept, medicines were matched specifically to the symptom picture of the patient and then given in the minimum dose required. Although this system may seem similar to homeopathy, there were important differences.[16] Material doses were always used, albeit lower than those prescribed by other Eclectics, and the prescription was not based on the law of similars. However, like classical homeopathy, there was a tendency to use only one medicine at a time.

Scudder initially proposed that 'specific medicines' should be tinctures prepared from the fresh plant.[16] A fresh plant tincture is sometimes still called a 'specific tincture'. Hence, the approach of using drop doses of tinctures, especially fresh plant tinctures, also comes from Scudder.

Although Scudder's system of specific medication was seen as an important development in Eclectic medicine, it was considerably modified by Lloyd.[17] Lloyd felt that drop doses of tinctures were too low and described the preparations proposed by Scudder as 'superficial'. Lloyd proceeded to develop elaborate herbal preparations which were concentrated, semi-purified liquids. He also called these 'specific medicines' and they were widely adopted by Eclectic practitioners. However, in the early 20th century English herbalists aligned themselves with the American physiomedicalists in using simpler formulations, because Lloyd's specific medicines proved too costly to import.

Lloyd sometimes used solvents other than ethanol and water in the preparation of his specific medicines.[17] His methods were kept secret and even today are not widely known. Lloyd writes: 'The aim has been to exclude colouring matters … and inert extractive substances also from these preparations …'. In this sense, he was tending towards the concept of orthodox drugs. However, his preparations were still chemically complex and 'very characteristic' of the original herb.[17] According to Felter, the specific medicines developed by Lloyd were at least eight times stronger than 1:5 tinctures.[7] It is these highly concentrated preparations which were generally used by Eclectic physicians in drop doses, and even then doses could be quite high – up to 60 drops (3 mL) three times daily.[7]

In conclusion, the use of drop doses of tinctures, especially fresh plant tinctures, originated in response to the availability of more concentrated specific medications and was not representative of the general practice of Eclectic medicine, nor initially a challenge to traditional dosages.

The current system in the UK

In the UK in the past herbalists used fluid extracts, usually prepared using heat or from concentrates. However, among newer practitioners in the 1980s there was disenchantment with these preparations because of their inconsistent quality. These practitioners instead adopted the use of 1:5 tinctures. Usually, formulations of tinctures are prescribed at doses of 2.5 to 5 mL three times daily. However, BHP 1983 doses for tinctures can only be achieved by this approach if the formulation contains one to three herbs (see Table 6.3 for

examples). Unfortunately, this restriction is usually not followed and it can be concluded that the move to tinctures has resulted in the use of lower doses.

A rational system for modern phytotherapy

The dosages used by the traditional systems of India and China, by most of the Eclectics and those established by clinical trials or recommended by expert committees or in pharmaceutical texts all tend towards the higher end of the dosage spectrum. Such an agreement should not be ignored if there is to be consistency in modern phytotherapy.

If liquid preparations are to be used, then the BHP 1983 is an appropriate guide. However, as discussed above, more credibility should be given to the tincture doses. The difficulty in using 1:5 tinctures is the large volumes which are required to achieve BHP doses for multi-herb formulations. One way to overcome this problem is to make a more concentrated preparation but without the use of heat or vacuum. Such a preparation would be more akin to a 1:5 tincture than a fluid extract, since it would better reflect the chemical characteristics of the starting herb. The most concentrated preparation which can be achieved from a dried herb without using heat or vacuum concentration, and yet achieving high extraction efficiency, is a 1:2. A process of cold percolation is necessary to achieve a 1:2 extract. Dosages for 1:2 extracts can be calculated as 0.4 of the dose for 1:5 tinctures, since they are 2.5 times stronger.

This approach enables the use of multi-herb formulations consistent with BHP and BHC dosage guidelines. For special preparations, such as herbal extracts standardised for active components, dosages established by clinical trials should be followed.

Oral dosage forms in herbal medicine

It is worth examining the relative advantages and disadvantages of the various oral dosage forms used by practitioners of Western herbal medicine.

Liquids

Liquid preparations have considerable advantages and are widely used. The main advantage is the easy preparation of formulations for each individual patient (extemporaneous dispensing). The other considerable advantage of liquids is that, if properly prepared, they involve minimal processing and truly reflect the chemical characteristics of the herb in a compact, convenient form. They also confer considerable dosage flexibility, which is especially relevant when prescribing low doses for small children. Liquids are readily absorbed and are convenient to take.

Superior bioavailability is also an under-researched advantage of herbal liquids. When a solid dosage preparation is ingested, it must first disintegrate. The plant's phytochemicals need to dissolve in digestive juices (and the water simultaneously imbibed with the tablet or capsule) in order to be absorbed by the body. Research has demonstrated that there is a relationship between the rate and degree of dissolution of the phytochemicals in a solid dosage preparation and their ultimate absorption into the bloodstream. The advantage of herbal liquids is that the all-important phytochemical constituents are already in solution.

The main disadvantage of liquids is taste, although in the case of bitters the taste is an essential part of the therapy. The taste problem is somewhat exaggerated by some patients. Most patients get used to the taste of their mixture and some even grow to like it. If taste becomes a problem, there are flavouring preparations available and these are particularly useful for children.

It is helpful to ask patients before prescribing if they mind taking strong-tasting liquids. This will draw a commitment from those who say it is not a problem and guide the clinician to solid dose alternatives if the answer is otherwise.

The way a herbal liquid is taken can minimise the experience of any unpleasant taste. The most important factors are the contact time of the remedy in the mouth and the intensity of the contact. Some practitioners claim that absorption from the oral cavity is often part of the activity of herbal preparations. So it may in fact be preferable to prolong the contact time. But from the point of view of taste, it should be minimised.

To reduce the intensity of the contact, the herbal liquid must be diluted. However, if it is diluted too much the contact time will be too long. So there is a trade-off between intensity and contact time. It is recommended that a 5 mL dose is diluted with around 10 mL of water or fruit juice. This can easily be swallowed in one go, making the contact time minimal. Another way to reduce further the intensity of the contact is to suck on some ice beforehand. This deadens the taste buds and the olfactory nerve. Chilling the medicine beforehand and adding chilled water is another way to reduce the taste intensity.

Contact time can be further reduced by immediately rinsing the mouth with water or fruit juice. About 50 mL can be quickly consumed immediately after the liquid is taken. To best achieve this, the diluted liquid should be in one hand and the rinse in the other. They are then consumed in a one–two action, as quickly as possible. Using this technique, taste can be dramatically minimised and few patients complain of any problem. For herbs with a lingering aftertaste, eating something afterwards will help.

Another option to avoid the taste of a herbal liquid is to put the liquid (undiluted) into a hard gelatin capsule using a dropper. The capsule will soften slowly over the next hour, so it can be conveniently consumed well before this happens.

Another disadvantage of liquids that applies in a few cases is the alcohol content. This is if the patient is allergic to alcohol or is an ex-alcoholic who does not wish to take alcohol in any form. Also, some strict Muslims will also not take alcohol, even in medicines. Only a very small minority of patients are genuinely sensitive to alcohol. In others, a presumed sensitivity is only an exaggerated reflex response to the medicine. This can usually be alleviated by lower doses at greater frequency, taken with copious water or food. Usually the small quantities of alcohol involved will not affect a mildly damaged liver – a 5 mL dose contains as much alcohol as about one-sixth of a glass of beer or wine. The alcohol content of liquids is not a problem for children since correspondingly lower amounts of liquids, and hence alcohol, are prescribed.

Use of alcohol in herbal liquid preparations is important since it is a good solvent for herbal active components and an excellent preservative. This is discussed in more detail later in this chapter, together with a brief review of the history and context of ethanol use in herbal preparations.

Tablets

Herbal tablets are a convenient dosage form and no problems with taste or alcohol are associated with their use. However, tablets contain fixed formulations which cannot be exactly adapted to the needs of the individual patient. Therefore, it is critical that the herbs contained in a tablet are carefully chosen for the disorder they are intended to treat. Even then, the degree of treatment flexibility is limited.

A major potential problem with tablets is the degree of processing required. Processing is minimal for tablets containing the powdered herb, but the amount of herb which can be incorporated into such tablets is limited (without making them excessively large). Tablets are therefore usually made from extracts, which are more concentrated than the original dried herb. In order to achieve this, the herb is first extracted with a solvent. Often water is used to keep costs down. The resultant liquid is then dried to either a soft or a powdered concentrate using processes such as vacuum concentration or spray drying. Heat-sensitive or volatile components can be damaged or lost by this process. Heat is also sometimes used in the tablet-making process via a granulation step: the tablet mixture may be wetted and then dried in an oven before the final pressing. This risks further damage to the active components. Hence, when manufacturing tablets, quality may be sacrificed for the sake of quantity. One way to compensate for this problem with concentrates is to standardise each herbal ingredient for key active components. However, the components chosen for standardisation must be meaningful in terms of the desired activity of the herb (see later). In other words, they must be meaningful indicators of quality.

Another problem with tablets is that, despite the use of concentrates, they are sometimes formulated to contain low amounts of herbs. Many tablets contain herbs in equivalent dried herb doses of 1 to 50 mg (that is, the herb is there as a concentrate and the equivalent amount of dried herb is calculated from the known strength of the concentrate). It is difficult to see how therapeutic doses can be achieved from such small quantities.

For many patients one liquid formulation may not be enough to treat adequately their complex and varied medical conditions. This is where tablets can be extremely useful. For these patients a herbal formulation can be combined with one or more tablet formulations.

Sometimes only tablets can confer clinically effective doses. Some herbal products have been shown in clinical trials to be only effective at high doses. If these herbs were given in liquid form, the doses of liquid needed would be impractically high. A good example of this is the willow bark tablet that contains around 8 g of willow bark. This means that each tablet is equivalent to 16 mL of a 1:2 liquid extract. The only practical way to give such clinically effective doses of willow bark, based on clinical trials, is to use a herbal tablet.

Boswellia is a highly resinous herb which needs to be extracted in 90% alcohol. Hence, if Boswellia was used as a liquid and administered at clinically effective doses, the amount of alcohol the patient would need to consume would be too high. So the best way to give Boswellia is therefore in tablet form (or as a capsule).

By using herbal tablets, the herbalist does not need to carry an overly large range of herbal liquids in their dispensary. For example, for a condition such as a urinary tract infection, rather than carrying three or four herbs to treat this issue, only one tablet product needs to be stocked. Tablets are also far more easily transported both from the supplier and to patients in remote locations, and for use during travel.

A well-developed tablet formulation, put together by experienced and knowledgeable herbalists, represents a valuable tool, especially for the young and inexperienced practitioner. In a sense, the practitioner who uses such a formulation is drawing on the wealth of clinical experience of the formulators and is more likely to achieve a better clinical result and to learn through that process.

Powders

Sometimes the best way to prescribe a herb is as a powder. This particularly applies to mucilage-containing herbs. When these herbs are mixed with water, the mucilage reacts with the water to form a gel and the wet herb swells to many times its original volume. Mucilage is not very soluble in alcohol-water mixtures, hence it is difficult to use mucilaginous herbs effectively as liquids. In any case, if fluid extracts of, say, slippery elm and marshmallow were properly made, they would be so gelatinous that they could not be poured.

When giving mucilaginous herbs as powders it is best to advise the patient to mix them quickly with water and to take the mixture immediately before it swells. Otherwise, the patient often experiences difficulty negotiating the gelatinous mass which results. A copious amount of water should then be consumed to allow swelling in the stomach. Other herbs given as powders are also best taken slurried with water and rinsed down by additional water.

Tannin-containing herbs for the treatment of colon problems should also be given as powders. This is because the tannins are only slowly dissolved from the herb matrix and, therefore, are still being released in an active form when the powdered herb reaches the colon.

A big advantage of powders is that the total constituents of a herb are presented to the patient's digestive tract, rather than those constituents which only dissolve in alcohol or water. This can also be a disadvantage if the patient has compromised digestion. Where the fat-soluble components are an important part of the activity of a herb, the powder should be followed by a dose of vegetable oil or lecithin to assist absorption.

Capsules

Capsules are a convenient way to give powdered herbs because they conceal unpleasant tastes or textures. A drawback is that even large capsules can only hold 300 to 600 mg of powdered herb, which means that sometimes many capsules need to be taken to achieve adequate doses. Capsules containing herbal formulations are subject to the same limitation of flexibility as tablet formulations. Single herbs in capsules do confer prescription flexibility, since one merely prescribes each of the required herbs in capsule form. The disadvantage is that the patient may need to take a large number of capsules in order to achieve adequate doses for several herbs.

Concentrated extracts can be used in capsules instead of the powdered herb. In this instance, the same advantages and disadvantages discussed above for tablets apply.

Infusions and decoctions

Infusions and decoctions are time-honoured methods for delivering oral doses of herbs. In modern phytotherapy, they are mainly used where the active components of the herb are water soluble, for example, for herbs containing polysaccharides, tannins or mucilage or some glycosides. They also can be advantageous for the treatment of urinary tract problems and for the administration of alterative (depurative) herbs. Diaphoretics should be given hot to maximise their effectiveness, hence they are often administered as infusions or decoctions.

The major disadvantage of infusions or decoctions is that water is not a good solvent for many of the active components in herbs. This problem is compounded by the relatively short extraction time used in their preparation (usually 5 to 10 minutes). In addition, the large volume of hot liquid usually means that exposure to any unpleasant taste is considerably prolonged. The higher doses of herb often used in infusions and decoctions can sometimes compensate for the limitations of hot water as a solvent.

The preparation of liquids

It is useful to consider in detail some of the factors involved in the preparation of herbal liquids.

The strength or ratio

The strength of a liquid preparation is usually expressed as a ratio. For example, 1:5 means that 5 mL of the final preparation is equivalent to 1 g of the dried herb from which the preparation was made. Liquid preparations weaker than 1:2 are usually called 'tinctures' whereas 1:1 and 1:2 preparations are typically called 'extracts'. Tinctures are usually made by a soaking process known as maceration, whereas extracts are best made using percolation. However, tinctures can also be adequately manufactured by a percolation process. These days, 1:1 liquid extracts can be made by reconstituting soft or powdered concentrates (not recommended).

It has been argued that 1:2 extracts are relatively new, are not mentioned in the BHP 1983 or other pharmacopoeias and therefore should not be used. In fact, 1:2 extracts are mentioned in 19th century texts[16,18] and were described in the German Pharmacopoeia (DAB). The seventh edition of the DAB actually defines a liquid extract as a 1:2 extract.[19]

The dominant historical use of 1:1 extracts may not have been the wisest choice because of the extra processing required. In 1953, a Dutch PhD student studied the impact of pharmaceutical processing on some active components of thyme (*Thymus vulgaris*).[20] The components tested were the phenols (thymol and carvacrol), which are responsible for the antiseptic activity of thyme. Thymol and carvacrol are found in the essential (volatile) oil of thyme and could conceivably be lost under conditions of vacuum or heat. The following preparations were made:

1. A 1:1 liquid extract in 50% ethanol by the method of reserved percolation, which is described in most pharmacopoeias
2. A 1:2 liquid extract in 50% ethanol by cold percolation
3. A soft extract (13:1) by evaporating some of the liquid described in (2) under vacuum
4. A powdered extract (16:1) by drying some of the liquid described in (2) in a spray dryer.

The phenol content in all four preparations and in the original herb was measured and the results are summarised in Table 6.4. The table also provides the essential oil content of some of the preparations.

As can be seen from Table 6.4, the 1:2 extract contains only marginally less phenol content than the 1:1. This is presumably because the phenols were largely lost during the heating of the second percolate which occurs in reserved percolation. Hence, on the basis of the active components tested, the 1:2 is almost as strong as the 1:1. It should be noted from Table 6.4 that neither the 1:1 nor the 1:2 quantitatively extracted all the phenols from the dried herb, presumably because these components were not completely soluble at the ethanol percentage chosen. The 1:2 contained 37% of the

original phenol content in the dried herb, compared to 22% for the 1:1.

The results for the soft and powdered extracts are disturbing. For the soft extract, 82% of the phenols were lost in processing, and for the powdered extract the loss was 48%. Compared to spray drying, conditions of vacuum therefore seem more likely to cause the loss of essential oil components, although the losses in both cases are considerable. A Swiss study found that concentration of a chamomile extract under vacuum caused the loss of about half of the essential oil.[21]

The content of essential oil and phenols in the corresponding amount of dried herb are also provided for the various preparations in the right-hand columns of Table 6.4. As can be seen from the table, the soft and powdered extracts only contain a fraction of the essential oil and phenol content of the dried herb. Hence, for this example, the use of these concentrates in the manufacture of liquids, tablets or capsules would clearly represent a substantial sacrifice of quality for the sake of an increase in quantity. If the soft extract was reconstituted to a 1:1 which is a common practice, it would contain about 30% of the phenol content of the 1:2 (0.04% versus 0.11%).

Ethanol-water as the solvent

Ethanol (or alcohol) has been used for hundreds of years to prepare liquid herbal preparations and indeed ethanol-water mixtures do appear to be quite efficient for the extraction of a wide variety of compounds found in medicinal plants. Chemical analyses of organic substances absorbed into pottery jars have recently confirmed the use of medicinal wines in ancient Egypt (about 3150 BC and millennia thereafter) and ancient China (seventh millennium BC). The ancient Egyptian wine contained herbs and tree resins dispensed in wine made from grapes. The jar from ancient China contained a mixed fermented beverage of rice, honey and fruit (hawthorn (*Crataegus spp.*) fruit and/or grape). The medicinal use of wines has been described in ancient documents, and the early Chinese history of fermented beverages is suggested from the shapes and styles of Neolithic pottery vessels.[22,23] Ancient Egyptian papyri describe water, milk, oil (presumably olive oil), honey, beer and wine as carriers for medicinal herbs. Jewish medicine, described in the second-century Talmud, refers to a 'potion of herbs' mixed with beer or wine.[24]

Although the principle of distillation was known to the ancient Greeks, the Arabs adapted the process to produce alcohol, which they then used for medicinal purposes. (The word alcohol, which first appeared in most modern languages in the 16th century, was derived from Arabic (*al-koh'l*).)[25]

The first official British Pharmacopoeia, the *London Pharmacopoeia*, was issued in 1618. It contained a section outlining ethanolic fluid extracts and drew heavily on the classics.[26]

Nicholas Culpeper, the 17th century English herbalist and one of the best-known advocates of Western herbal medicine, described the distillation of one or more herbs in wine, and the maceration of spices in alcohol. Single herbs, such as dried wormwood (*Artemisia absinthium*), rosemary (*Rosmarinus officinalis*) and eyebright (*Euphrasia officinalis*), were steeped in wine and set in the sun for 30–40 days to make a physical wine.[27]

Table 6.4 Essential oil and phenol content of various pharmaceutical preparations of thyme[20]

	Essential oil content %	Phenol content %	Equivalent content in the dried herb	
			Essential oil %	Phenol %
Dried herb	2.81	0.59	2.81	0.59
1:1 extract	–	0.13	–	0.13
1:2 extract	–	0.11	–	0.22
Soft extract (13:1)	0.88	0.51	0.07	0.04
Powdered extract (16:1)	3.54	1.84	0.22	0.12

A number of studies have highlighted the importance of the correct choice of the ethanol percentage in terms of maximising the quality of liquid preparations. The Swiss study mentioned above found that 55% ethanol was the optimum percentage for the extraction of the essential oil from chamomile (*Matricaria chamomilla*).[21] Higher percentages of ethanol did not extract any additional oil and there was a decrease in the solids content of the extract, which indicates that other components were being less efficiently extracted. More recently, Meier found that 40–60% ethanol was the optimum range for achieving the highest extraction efficiency for the active components of a variety of herbs.[28] For example, at 25% ethanol, none of the saponins in ivy leaves (*Hedera helix*) was extracted, but at 60% ethanol they were maximally extracted.

Higher ethanol percentages do not always confer higher activity. French researchers found that *Viburnum prunifolium* bark extracted at 30% ethanol was five times more spasmolytic than a 60% extract.[29]

The basic guidelines for the choice of the ethanol percentage to optimise the activity of the final liquid are as shown in Table 6.5.

Some educators have suggested that herbal liquids are a less desirable dosage form because they are less stable than solid dosage preparations. However, there is little objective evidence to back up this assertion. Some companies now undertake stability studies on their herbal liquids as a requirement of pharmaceutical GMP, and experience in this field is that most liquids maintain their phytochemical profiles within the normal shelf-life requirements of 2 to 3 years.

Provided herbal liquids are purchased through a herbal manufacturer which operates to pharmaceutical GMP standards and has a comprehensive stability programme in place, keeping to within expiry dates is sufficient to ensure retained activity. This is, of course, if the manufacturer's recommended storage conditions are observed. Sunlight is particularly damaging to the phytochemicals in a herbal liquid, so they must be stored in amber glass bottles away from direct sunlight. Temperature is also an important factor. Generally storage below 30°C (86°F) is recommended (temperatures occasionally above 30°C (86°F) will not cause a problem, if the average is below this level). Also a minimum storage temperature of 10°C (50°F) should be maintained. Some herbal liquids such as celery and wild yam will form into a gel if they

become too cold. While gentle reheating will generally make them liquid again, irreversible changes may occur if the cold conditions are prolonged.

Many herbal liquids develop a sediment over time. If the extract has not been heated during its manufacture this is a natural occurrence which generally has only a minor impact on quality. A common question among practitioners is whether this sediment should be rejected or redispersed into the liquid. There are no hard and fast rules here, but a general guide is that if the sediment has tended to aggregate or concrete into a hard mass, then it should be rejected. If, however, the sediment is fine and easily redispersed, then the bottle should be shaken to do this before dispensing. For mixtures of several herbal liquids the sediment should always be redispersed

Glycetracts or glycerites are liquid preparations made using glycerol and water instead of ethanol and water. They are useful preparations where the active components are water-soluble, for example, marshmallow root (*Althaea officinalis*), since they do not contain alcohol and the sweetness of the glycerol gives them a better taste. However, their importance should not be overrated. Glycerol is a poor solvent for many of the active components found in herbs and glycetracts are less stable than alcoholic extracts. Moreover, because of the viscosity of glycerol, concentrated preparations are difficult to make by percolation. The manufacture of 1:1 or 1:2 glycetracts therefore invariably requires the use of a concentration step involving heat or vacuum.

In recent times the use of tinctures made from the fresh plant has become popular among some herbalists. The belief is often that a fresh plant tincture better reflects the plant's 'vitality' or 'energy' and therefore will be a more therapeutic preparation. Other practitioners believe that a fresh plant tincture will better preserve the delicate active components of the plant.

On the other hand, the following observations need to be considered:

- The evidence from phytochemical analysis that fresh plant tinctures contain better levels of active components than dried plant tinctures is generally lacking. In fact, fresh plant tinctures are usually prepared in a low alcohol environment (see below), which means that some less polar (more lipophilic) components may be only poorly extracted. Furthermore, the enzymatic activity of the plant material may not be inhibited in this low alcohol environment, meaning that key phytochemicals may actually be decomposed during the maceration process. This fact was dramatically illustrated by Bauer who found that cichoric acid in fresh plant preparations of *Echinacea purpurea* was largely decomposed by enzymatic activity.[30] So what can be found in the living Echinacea plant was not preserved in the fresh plant tincture.

- Fresh plant tinctures were never official. While fresh plant preparations were included in homeopathic pharmacopoeias (given the energetic considerations in homeopathy this is understandable), they were never listed in conventional pharmacopoeias, other than a few entries for stabilised fresh juices known as succi (singular: succus). Hence, the use of a wide range of fresh plant tinctures is travel into unknown territory.

Table 6.5 Choice of ethanol percentage to optimise the activity of final liquid	
Ethanol (%)	Final liquid
25%	Water-soluble constituents such as mucilage, tannins and some glycosides (including some flavonoids and a few saponins)
45–60%	Essential oils, alkaloids, most saponins and some glycosides
90%	Resins and oleoresins

- Because of the water content of fresh plant tinctures, it is difficult to make preparations which are stronger than a 1:5 on a dry weight basis. This can be readily illustrated by the following example. A leafy, fresh plant material typically contains 80% moisture. Therefore, 100 g of this material represents 20 g of dried herb. To make a 1:5 tincture, this 20 g equivalent of dried herb must be mixed with 100 mL of liquid menstruum. But there is already 80 mL of water from the herb itself. So to preserve the 1:5 ratio only 20 mL of 96% ethanol can be added. This 20 mL of ethanol is not enough to extract the bulky 100 g of fresh plant material. But what is probably just as detrimental is that the effective ethanol percentage is only 20% (20 mL of ethanol and 80 g (or mL) of water from the fresh plant). This is too low to extract lipophilic components and barely enough to preserve the tincture. Some authors suggest the use of multiple macerations to overcome this problem, where the resultant tincture is macerated with a new batch of fresh herb, but this only makes the situation worse, diluting the alcohol to below the level that can stabilise the final tincture.

Quality versus quantity

The issues above arise because herbs are chemically complex biological drugs which need to be processed in some way and losses of activity can occur during this processing. Few of these kinds of problems arise when using pure chemicals.

But even if the problems of processing the herb are ignored, there remains the problem of the quality of the herb itself. A herb is biologically defined and even if this biological definition is adhered to (and sometimes unfortunately it is not), there is an element of chemical uncertainty. The active components of a particular dried herb can vary considerably. This is due to factors such as climate, soil conditions, genetic characteristics, time of harvest, methods of harvest and drying techniques.

One way partially to solve this problem is to use 'organic' and 'wildcrafted' herbs. By definition, these are herbs which not only have been organically grown or harvested from the wild under natural growing conditions, but have also been subjected to maximum care at all stages of harvesting and drying to ensure that quality is optimised.

A more certain way to overcome the problem of the chemical variation of herbs and herbal preparations is to quantify them for indicator or marker chemicals. In other words, the content of a particular component or group of components should always be greater than a minimum level. These components may not be solely responsible for the complete spectrum of the therapeutic effects of the herb, but rather will act as indicators of consistent quality. However, they should be meaningful indicators of quality (see below). Although more research is needed in this direction, many common herbal medicines can now be quantified for active components and the appropriate dosage range can be set accordingly.

Standardised extracts

In the context of herbs, the term 'standardised extract' means different things to different people. To some the concept denotes herbal products which have moved away from a time-honoured traditional basis. To them standardised extracts represent highly concentrated plant extracts (artificially so). Standardised extracts are additionally represented as resulting from processes which have preferentially selected or isolated one phytochemical (or group of phytochemicals) from the herb at the expense of others that might have importance for recognised traditional uses. Or it may be even worse: some herbalists maintain that standardised extracts are frequently adulterated with pure chemicals that are added back to the extract to give it the desired level of 'active constituent'. Moreover, the use of standardised extracts is associated with a limited, reductionist model of herbal therapy where, like conventional drugs, one herb is prescribed for the often-symptomatic treatment of a disorder.

On the other hand, many authorities in the field maintain that standardised extracts represent the future of herbal therapy because they are a way of ensuring consistent activity of a herbal extract from batch to batch. This is particularly important for replicating clinical trials on herbs or extrapolating the results of trials to a clinical setting. Standardised extracts are promoted as being more effective and higher in quality than traditional galenical extracts and the conclusion which the consumer or practitioner might reach is that the latter have no value in modern phytotherapy.

The reality is that there are examples of so-called standardised extracts that reflect all the above positions. Hence, a meaningful understanding of the value and limitations of standardised extracts can only be achieved by reviewing them on a case-by-case basis.

Issues and terminology

Standardised extracts

In the herbal context, a standardised extract is a herbal extract which is made to a consistent standard. This standard can be quite simple, such as the ratio of the starting herbal raw material to the finished extract. Hence, a 4:1 extract, where 4 kg of dried herb is extracted to yield 1 kg of final extract, can technically be called a standardised extract. But generally the term has a more specific meaning: a standardised extract is one that is manufactured to contain a consistent level of one or more phytochemical constituents which are derived from the original starting material.

Extract or concentration ratio

The extract or concentration ratio is the ratio of the starting herbal raw material to the resultant finished concentrated extract. The finished extract is always expressed as the 1 and comes second. Thus, 10:1 means 10 kg of dried herb is used to produce 1 kg of extract.

Galenical extract

A galenical extract is a traditional pharmacopoeial extract of a herb. Guidelines were laid down in the various pharmacopoeias (such as earlier versions of the BPC) which defined the method of preparation, the extracting solvent (which was usually a combination of ethanol and water) and the ratio of the starting material (the herb) to finished product (the extract). Galenical extracts were usually in liquid form, typically tinctures and fluid extracts. However, with the modern trend to solid dosage forms, quite often a galenical extract is dried to its solid residue and incorporated into a tablet or capsule.

Herbalists often regard galenical extracts as 'whole' extracts in that they extract a comprehensive spectrum of the phytochemical content of the plant. While this is generally the case, it should be kept in mind that alcohol-water mixtures are still selective solvents and do not equally extract everything from the plant that is extractable. Something will always be left behind, depending on the percentage of ethanol which is chosen for the solvent.

On the other hand it should be considered that many standardised extracts are merely dried galenical extracts that have been fixed to a consistent level of chosen marker compound(s). Hence they are just as 'whole' as galenical extracts.

Consistent activity

The aim of standardised extracts is to achieve consistent activity of a herbal product from batch to batch. Depending on the circumstances, this is not always the case. If compounds other than the chosen marker compounds (see below for definition) are important for activity and these are not also fixed at consistent levels by the manufacturing process, then a standardised extract will not achieve consistent activity.

Other simpler issues can sabotage the goal of consistent activity. For example, if the analytical method chosen is not very specific towards the desired marker compounds, then this inherent weakness in the yardstick used to measure consistent activity will result in the failure of batch-to-batch consistency. This will be the case even though the certificate of analysis of the extract will provide data to suggest the same 'activity' for each batch.

Although standardised extracts, done well, will ensure consistent activity, they do not necessarily guarantee potency. Potency is a biological term and in this context will relate to some pharmacological or clinical outcome. Only when a particular extract has been shown to be effective in a pharmacological model or (preferably) a clinical trial, can consistent activity be linked to guaranteed potency. Fortunately, many standardised extracts have been shown to be effective in clinical trials, and provided the various caveats above and throughout this article are met, their consistent activity can be linked to guaranteed potency (see also the discussion of phytoequivalence below).

Marker compounds or constituents

Marker compounds are characteristic phytochemicals found in a plant that are chosen to represent the standard for a standardised extract. Hence, in the case of say passionflower (*Passiflora incarnata*), the marker compound is often chosen to be the flavonoid isovitexin and the standardised extract of passionflower is fixed to contain a consistent level of this compound (usually a few per cent). Marker compounds are not necessarily active compounds (see below). However, if well chosen they do serve a useful function in terms of quality, such as the purposes of identification and ensuring appropriate drying, handling and extraction of the herbal starting material.

Usually to achieve a consistent level of a marker compound (or compounds) in a standardised extract, the starting herbal raw material will need to contain a minimum acceptable level. This implies consistent quality practices in terms of harvesting, drying and storage of the herb. Also, the way in which the herb is processed such as extraction conditions and choice of solvent will need to be carefully controlled. Because of this, it is likely that fixing an extract to a consistent level of marker compound(s) will also render the extract more or less consistent in terms of other phytochemical components, at least for that particular manufacturer. This aspect underpins much of the utility of standardised extracts as consistent products.

However, the difficulty arises when another manufacturer then attempts to produce the same standardised extract. Although this 'imitation' extract will obviously be made to contain the same level of marker compound(s), it is not necessarily true that it will be an identical extract to that produced by the original manufacturer (see the concept of phytoequivalence below).

Active compounds or constituents

Active constituents are phytochemicals that are important for a given therapeutic effect of a herbal extract. This is a highly complex issue, but one proposition is simple and clear: marker compounds are not necessarily active compounds. Hence, when *Ginkgo biloba* leaf standardised extract (GBE) was originally manufactured to contain 24% ginkgo flavone glycosides, there was no unequivocal evidence that these compounds conferred the various and exciting therapeutic activities that had been discovered for the extract. Later research suggested that a different group of phytochemicals, the ginkgolides and bilobalide, were more important and GBE is now standardised for these as well. But in terms of say its effects in Alzheimer's disease, the active compounds in GBE are not known. Even if the ginkgolides and bilobalide were found to be important (this could be achieved by a clinical trial comparing two Ginkgo extracts with high and low levels of these compounds which were otherwise identical), it would be unlikely that they were the only compounds important for activity. This observation is also well illustrated by the example of St John's wort where several of its phytochemical components have been shown to have antidepressant activity. (For more details, see the relevant monographs in this book.)

Such a dilemma supports the basic premise of herbalists that the true active component is the herbal extract itself. Nonetheless, it is also likely that an extract low in marker compounds, which from pharmacological experiments have been found to have some relevant activity, will be less likely to confer a therapeutic effect and hence be poorer quality.

This last issue underlies an important point with marker compounds: they should be chosen carefully. Preference must be given to phytochemicals that (on the basis of current knowledge) are likely to have pharmacological activity that is relevant to the proposed use of the extract. On the other hand, if a marker compound is chosen which has no known useful pharmacological activity, it should not be optimised in the extract at the expense of other phytochemicals, for example, selecting for and optimising echinacoside levels in *Echinacea angustifolia* at the expense of alkylamides. Where the marker compound is inactive (on current knowledge), the safest approach to take is to produce a normal galenical extract standardised to the marker.

Sometimes the great body of pharmacological and clinical evidence that we have for a herb relates only to the use of one isolated, purified constituent. Good examples are ephedrine from Ephedra and berberine from *Berberis spp.* Clearly, it makes sense that extracts of these herbs should be standardised to these compounds. On the other hand, the temptation to regard the herbal extracts in question as merely a carrier of this constituent should be resisted. The whole extract will confer matrix effects that might modify the activity of these compounds. Hence, 'standardised extracts' of say Ephedra with greater than 50% ephedrine or of *Berberis spp.* with greater than 50% berberine should be viewed with suspicion. They are chemical medicine, not phytotherapy.

Analytical methodology

One weakness of some standardised extracts on the market is the poor or inappropriate choice of the analytical methodology employed to measure the marker compound(s). A number is only as consistent, reliable or relevant as the technique used to measure it. This is particularly evident for standardised extracts from Ayurvedic or Chinese herbs, but is by no means confined to these.

The following examples will serve to illustrate some aspects of this issue. *Boswellia serrata* extract is standardised to boswellic acids which, because of their anti-inflammatory activity, are important as marker compounds. However, for the majority of extracts on the market the level of boswellic acids is determined by simple acid-base titration. This method will measure the level of any acid in the extract, so an unscrupulous manufacturer could readily add a fruit acid that would result in a false and elevated reading for boswellic acids.

Sometimes gravimetric methods are used to standardise extracts. Here the attempt is to isolate the marker compound from the extract and weigh it. However, the isolation techniques used are generally quite crude and the methodology is consequently prone to much interference. This problem is exemplified by an extract of *Andrographis paniculata* which was supposed to contain 10% andrographolide (determined by a gravimetric technique) but by a more accurate method was found to contain no andrographolide whatsoever. Another example is a *Tribulus terrestris* extract certified to contain 40% saponins (gravimetric), but which contained about 4% when a more accurate analytical technique was applied.

Even the popular St John's wort standardised extract is not free of this problem. The determination of 'total hypericin' is usually based on a method from the DAC (German Pharmaceutical Codex). But there are two methods found in different editions of the DAC. The earlier method will give a number for total hypericin that is about 25% higher than the later, preferred method. However, some manufacturers intentionally base the level of 'total hypericin' in their St John's wort extract on the earlier, outdated method in order to inflate the value. Both these methods give a higher level of total hypericin than that obtained by HPLC (high performance liquid chromatography).

Phytoequivalence

When positive clinical trial data for a standardised extract is made public, because of the fact that patents usually do not protect them, other manufacturers will produce and sell copies of this extract. Certainly, such copies will have the same level of marker compound, but are they really the same as the extract used in the clinical trial? Can the other manufacturers legitimately claim that their extract will produce the same clinical results as the original extract?

In order to answer this question (which is a real regulatory issue in countries such as Germany where prescribed herbal products were rebated under the pharmaceutical benefits scheme) the concept of phytoequivalence has been initiated. So the above questions can be answered in the affirmative only if the two extracts are phytoequivalent.

But what does phytoequivalence mean? Firstly, the second extract should closely match the phytochemical spectrum of the original extract. In other words, not just the level of marker compounds should be the same; all other measurable compounds in the extract should be present at similar levels. Some authorities suggest that a second criterion must also be met: the levels of marker compounds (or their derivatives) achieved in the bloodstream of humans after oral doses of the two products should be similar. This is a much more challenging condition that is often not attempted because of the experimental difficulties involved.

Types of standardised extracts

Based on how they are made, standardised extracts can be classified into three basic types. These are:

1. Galenical-type extracts
2. Highly concentrated extracts
3. Selective phytochemical extracts.

These types of extracts progressively represent a transition from a more traditional herbal product through to more modern types of products, which can be called phytopharmaceuticals. Phytopharmaceuticals are not like conventional drugs, but they are also very different from galenical extracts. Practitioners will wish to choose, based on their philosophical perspective, whether the use of phytopharmaceuticals is acceptable to them. However, as part of this process they should consider that phytopharmaceuticals are often chemically complex (an important criterion for phytotherapy), clinically proven and very safe. Probably, as suggested earlier, the decision is best based on a case-by-case basis.

Galenical-type extracts

Galenical-type standardised extracts have been defined previously. They are not usually highly concentrated. The reason for this is simple: the alcohol-water extractives from a dried herb are typically more than 10% of its weight. Say the alcohol-water extractives from a herb were exactly 10%. When the extract is dried the final weight will be one-tenth of the weight of the starting herb. Therefore, it is a 10:1 extract. In other words, galenical-type extracts are usually less concentrated than 10:1. The concentration ratios typically range from 4:1 to 6:1. Galenical-type standardised extracts represent extracts that are no different from those that have been traditionally used by herbalists for hundreds of years. Examples include standardised extracts of devil's claw, kava, St John's wort and horsechestnut. In fact the majority of standardised extracts are of the galenical type.

Highly concentrated extracts

From the above discussion, it is obvious that highly concentrated extracts (which can be defined for sake of argument as greater than 10:1) are made by processes which are different to galenical-type standardised extracts. These processes usually involve one or more of the following aspects:

- Extraction with solvents different to ethanol-water mixtures such as acetone, chloroform, liquid carbon dioxide or hexane, etc
- Multiple solvent extraction steps (involving ethanol-water mixtures and/or other solvents such as those listed above)
- Standard chemical isolation techniques such as chromatography columns, ion-exchange resins, precipitation and so on.

The drive to produce highly concentrated extracts has several aspects. Fundamentally, it is one of pharmaceutical convenience: the herbal dose can be delivered in a small tablet or capsule. Another aspect of this is the ability to deliver a higher dose: the more concentrated the extract, the greater the temptation to increase the dose (which may or may not be advantageous). Sometimes undesirable components are intentionally removed from the extract as part of this process, for example, the allergenic ginkgolic acids from *Ginkgo biloba* extract. Examples include silymarin and *Ginkgo biloba* extract.

Selective phytochemical extracts

Here one particular phytochemical group is selectively removed from the herb. This could involve any of the processes used to make highly concentrated extracts described above (and these extracts are often, but not always, highly concentrated). Although such extracts might seem removed from herbal therapy (and indeed not herbal products at all), it should be kept in mind that essential oils and evening primrose oil, widely used by natural therapists around the world, are in fact good examples of selective phytochemical extracts. (Essential oils produced either by steam distillation or hexane extraction are more or less identical for many herbs.) Examples include turmeric extract with high levels (90% or more) of curcumin, grapeseed and pine bark extracts.

Closing remarks

Standardised extracts are not a guarantee of quality, as they are often represented. Inappropriate choice of marker compounds, poor design or execution of analytical methods, spiking with pure phytochemicals (which is actually quite rare except for examples where the pure phytochemical is relatively cheap, such as caffeine or rutin) or failure to demonstrate phytoequivalence can mean that the standardised extract is poorer in quality or less effective than a well-made galenical extract. Only those manufacturers who practise good science and have a comprehensive understanding of the many complex issues that impact on herbal quality will be able to produce meaningful standardised extracts.

A mechanism for formulating liquids

There are a number of mechanisms for writing liquid prescriptions but a simple system widely used in the UK is worth describing. This is the system of formulating in terms of weekly doses.

If the dose for a herb is 1 to 2 mL three times daily, then the weekly dose is 21 times this or 21 to 42 mL per week, which is usually rounded down to 20 to 40 mL. Prescriptions for patients are then written in terms of weekly doses.

Assuming the patient is to take 5 mL of a liquid formulation three times daily, this amounts to 105 mL per week which can be rounded down to 100 mL. Hence the weekly dosages of the individual herbs in a formulation should total 100 mL. If the total amount of herbs in a formula is less than 100 mL, water or aqueous ethanol can be added to bring the volume to 100 mL. Using this system the patient then automatically receives the correct amount of each herb in each dose, provided they take 5 mL three times a day (see Table 6.6).

When dispensing for more than 1 week, the weekly doses are simply multiplied by the number of required weeks. This system confers considerable flexibility and ease in prescription writing and dispensing.

Even using 1:1 and 1:2 extracts, formulations based on 100 mL for 1 week should not contain more than about six to seven herbs. Otherwise, therapeutic doses will not be achieved. If more than this number of herbs is required then

Table 6.6 An example prescription for 1 week might be as follows

Sambucus nigra	1:2	20 mL
Echinacea angustifolia	1:2	25 mL
Glycyrrhiza glabra	1:1	20 mL
Mentha piperita	1:2	25 mL
Zingiber officinale	1:2	10 mL
	Total	100 mL

The dosage is 5 mL of the mixture three times daily with water.

the week's formulation should be based on 150 mL. The single dose becomes 7.5 mL (which can be rounded up to 8 mL) three times daily.

Comparing doses

Often it is difficult for practitioners to compare doses between liquid and/or solid preparations made with various types of extracts. The concept of 'dried herb equivalent' is a useful way of comparing doses between different strengths of liquids or between liquids and tablets. Using the product ratio, the dried herb equivalent of a given amount of product can be calculated. The product ratio expresses the weight of original dried herb starting material to the volume or weight of finished product (in that order), e.g. 5:1, 1:4, 1:1, etc. For example, a dried herb equivalent of 1 g might be:

2 mL of a 1:2 liquid
1 mL of 1:1 liquid
250 mg of 4:1 soft extract
200 mg of a 5:1 spray-dried powder.

References

1. Bensky D, Gamble A. *Chinese Herbal Medicine Materia Medica*. Seattle: Eastland Press; 1986.
2. Yanchi L. *The Essential Book of Traditional Chinese Medicine. Volume 2: Clinical practice*. New York: Columbia University Press; 1995.
3. *British Herbal Pharmacopoeia*. Bournemouth: British Herbal Medicine Association; 1983.
4. *British Pharmaceutical Codex*. London: Pharmaceutical Press; 1934.
5. Nadkarni KM, Nadkarni AK. *Indian Materia Medica*. Bombay: Popular Prakashan Private Ltd; 1976.
6. Griggs B. *Green Pharmacy*. London: Jill Norman and Hobhouse; 1981.
7. Felter HW. *The Eclectic Materia Medica, Pharmacology and Therapeutics*. Portland: First published Cincinnati, Ohio, 1922. Reprinted by Eclectic Medical Publications; 1983.
8. Felter HW, Lloyd JU. *King's American Dispensatory*, 18th ed. Portland: Reprinted by Eclectic Medical Publications; 1983.
9. British Herbal Medicine Association. *British Herbal Compendium*. Bournemouth: BHMA. 1992. p. 1.
10. British Herbal Medicine Association. *British Herbal Compendium*. Bournemouth: BHMA; 2006. p. 2.
11. Eberwein E, Vogel G. *Arzneipflanzen in der Phytotherapie*. Bonn: Kooperation Phytopharmaka; 1990.
12. Scientific Committee of ESCOP (European Scientific Cooperative on Phytotherapy). *ESCOP Monographs*, 2nd ed. UK: ESCOP Secretariat; 2003.
13. Scientific Committee of ESCOP (European Scientific Cooperative on Phytotherapy). *ESCOP Monographs*, 2nd ed. Supplement. UK: ESCOP Secretariat; 2009.
14. De Feudis FV. *Ginkgo biloba Extract (EGb 761): Pharmacological Activities and Clinical Applications*. Paris: Elsevier; 1991.
15. Ravanelli OV, Haase W. Zur Wirksamkeit von Silymarin bei Leberkrankheiten. *Z Prakt Anasth Wiederbelebung*. 1976;30(355):1592–1612.
16. Scudder JM. *Specific Medication and Specific Medicines*. Cincinnati: Scudder Bros Co.; 1913.
17. Ellingwood F. *American Materia Medica, Therapeutics and Pharmacognosy*. Portland: Reprinted by Eclectic Medical Publications; 1983.
18. Lyle TJ. *Physio-Medical Therapeutics, Materia Medica and Pharmacy*. London: Originally published Ohio, 1897. Reprinted by The National Association of Medical Herbalists; 1932.
19. *Deutsches Arzneibuch der BRD*, 7 Ausgabe; 1968.
20. Van Es MJ. *Some Applications of the Spray-Dryer in Galenical Pharmacy*. PhD Thesis. Utrecht University; 1953.
21. Munzel K, Huber K. Extraction procedures in the preparation of chamomile fluid extract. *Pharm Acta Helv*. 1961;36:194–204.
22. McGovern PE, Mirzoian A, Hall GR. Ancient Egyptian herbal wines. *Proc Natl Acad Sci USA*. 2009;106(18):7361–7366.
23. McGovern PE, Zhang J, Tang J, et al. Fermented beverages of pre- and proto-historic China. *Proc Natl Acad Sci USA*. 2004;101(51):17593–17598.
24. Bellamy D, Pfister A. *World Medicine: Plants, Patients and People*. Oxford: Blackwell; 1992.
25. Reuben A. Wine hath drowned more men than the sea. *Hepatology*. 2002;36(2):516–518.
26. Brockbank W. Sovereign remedies: a critical depreciation of the 17th-century London pharmacopoeia. *Med Hist*. 1964;8:1–14.
27. Tobyn G. *Culpeper's Medicine: A Practice of Western Holistic Medicine*. Shaftesbury: Element Books; 1997.
28. Meier B. The extraction strength of ethanol/water mixtures commonly used for the processing of herbal drugs. *Planta Med*. 1991;57(suppl 2):A26.
29. Balansard G, Chausse D, Boukef K, et al. Selection criteria for a Viburnum extract, Viburnum prunifolium L., as a function of its veino-tonic and spasmolytic action. *Plantes Med Phytother*. 1983;17(3):123–132.
30. Bauer R, Remiger P, Jurcic K, et al. Beeinflussung der phagozytose-aktivität durch Echinacea-extrakte. *Z Phytother*. 1989;10:43–48.

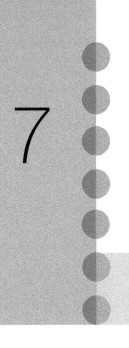

7

A systematic approach to herbal prescribing

CHAPTER CONTENTS

Introduction

In order to appreciate a key element of the approach behind Western herbal therapeutics, we must assume that a normally functioning human body is free from disease and capable of resisting disease. Therefore, a deeper understanding of the cause and treatment of disease should also come from a consideration of physiology, the normal functioning of the body, as well as pathology and pathophysiology. An excessive focus on pathology will lead to a medical system which is interventionist and directed towards compensating for the physiological deficiencies and imbalances that arise in disease (physiological compensation), without seeking a greater understanding of how they arose in the first place. Such a basic strategy will lead to a superficial and short-term approach to treatment. This is increasingly the orthodox medical system we have today. While it is very useful for advanced pathologies and life-threatening states, it is incomplete, and especially inadequate in the treatment of many chronic diseases.

In contrast, most traditional medical systems, which are partially or completely based on herbal medicine, concern themselves more with the underlying physiological imbalances that led to and sustain the disease. As such, they are more focused on physiology than pathology. The treatment is aimed at physiological support or enhancement, rather than just compensating for the chemical deficiencies or excesses resulting from an abnormal physiology. Physiological compensation often requires the constant presence of the medicine to achieve the desired effect, whereas physiological support can, in time, lead to a permanent correction of an abnormal body chemistry.

One group of herbalists in the 19th century recognised these considerations and, in an attempt to translate traditional herbal thinking into more modern concepts, named their discipline 'physiomedicalism'. Obviously, other traditional herbal practitioners did not and could not express their understanding of physiology in terms of modern scientific theories, but this does not detract from the value or elegance of their comprehension of the healthy functioning of the human body.

One example of physiological support versus physiological compensation can be seen in the treatment of bacterial infections. The traditional herbal approach is to support immunity and to fine tune the normal physiological responses to infection such as fever. In contrast, the conventional approach is to suppress the fever and kill the bacteria with antibiotics, thereby compensating for weakened or overloaded bodily defences. The latter approach has life-saving value but will not prevent infections from recurring. The traditional herbal approach may see a higher rate of failure in acute situations, although this is debatable, but could lead to improved immunity and possibly a reduced rate of recurrent infections. Clearly, an important complementary role for traditional herbal medicine can be argued from this and other examples.

Western herbal medicine is also not opposed to employing physiological compensation when needed, although the approach is far less interventionist than that possible with modern drugs. It recognises that a disease process can often create a vicious cycle and that only direct intervention to break that cycle can restore health in some instances. At a pragmatic level, interventionist treatment gives quicker relief of symptoms, which encourages the patient to persist with

DOI: http://dx.doi.org/10.1016/B978-0-443-06992-5.00007-4

the treatment. Sometimes, the very concepts treated might require an interventionist approach because they are orthodox concepts, for example, hypertension and high serum cholesterol. This is not to say that a more traditional herbal approach cannot be of assistance as well.

Therapeutic strategy

The treatment strategy that should inform prescribing in modern Western herbal medicine therefore arises from a consideration of both physiological enhancement and physiological compensation.

Physiological enhancement

General strategy

In general, the goal of physiological enhancement is to create a state of active, robust health. This is more than just the absence of overt disease, although such a positive state of body and mind would be free of disease and capable of resisting disease. It is the optimum state of body chemistry and body energy. The term 'energy' in this context is more than just physical or chemical energy and reflects a subjective quality of good health. All traditional health systems without exception conclude that the obvious extra energy in good health signifies the presence of a vital force that integrates the normal physiological functioning of the body and maintains homeostasis. This controversial concept, 'vitality', represents a fundamental difference between traditional and orthodox medical systems.

The general treatment goals of physiological enhancement can be elaborated as follows:

- Optimise body chemistry by improving nutrition and enhancing detoxification. This applies not just to the body as a whole but to every cell, organ and system within the body.
- Optimise body energy by raising vitality. Improved vitality automatically follows from optimised body chemistry. But it can also be specifically encouraged using tonics, which make more energy available, and adaptogens, which optimise the capacity to cope with stressors of all kinds, thereby helping to conserve vitality.

As noted above, an important general goal of physiological enhancement is the stimulation of detoxification. This is particularly required for problems where toxin overload is significant, as may be the case in chronic fatigue syndrome, autoimmune disease and cancer, for example. Detoxification is traditionally achieved by both stimulating detoxification processes with depuratives, immunostimulants and liver herbs and stimulating elimination with diaphoretics, diuretics, lymphatics, laxatives and expectorants.

Specific strategies

With the exception of 'whole-body' medicines such as the tonics and adaptogens, the general goals of physiological

enhancement are achieved by enhancing the function of individual systems, organs or even tissues and cells. Such enhancement often involves the correction of imbalances. Deficient function in one physiological compartment can lead to overstimulated function in another, which in turn can create a deficiency elsewhere. For this reason the specific treatment is sometimes not aimed at the problem site: for example, in constipation caused by deficient liver function, liver function would be enhanced instead of, or in conjunction with, enhancing bowel function. In another example, an excess of female hormones causing a menstrual problem may again be treated by enhancing liver detoxification processes, since the liver is the organ which breaks down these hormones. Rather than directly manipulating ovarian secretions, it may also be treated by optimising the inputs to the pituitary, which controls ovarian function.

From the brief examples above it becomes apparent that fundamental to the specific strategy of physiological enhancement is the individualisation of the patient. If the concept of a vital force is the first pillar of traditional herbal medicine, the treatment of the patient as an individual is the second. This is in direct contrast to current medical science, since double blind, placebo-controlled clinical trials only examine the effect of a treatment in a group of patients (the more the better, for statistical power) rather than individuals.

Where appropriate, specific physiological enhancement might involve the regulation or boosting of digestive function, immunity, circulation, respiratory function and hormone output. It may also involve the enhancement of specific organs such as the liver, kidneys, ovaries and so on. The focus may be on specific tissues, for example, the exocrine cells of the pancreas. Specific functions of organs may also be supported, for example, the bile secretion from the liver or the detoxification enzyme systems in the liver. In all cases, this must be assessed on an individual basis and periodically reviewed.

Physiological compensation

Sometimes an overstimulated function needs to be directly controlled, or deficiencies need to be compensated, because the pathological process has gone too far. In other cases, a vicious cycle needs to be broken or the patient needs relief from uncomfortable or debilitating symptoms. These are circumstances where physiological compensation is appropriate. Actions which begin with 'anti' usually denote a role in physiological compensation, for example, anti-inflammatory, antiviral, antispasmodic, antiseptic, antiallergic and so on. Sedative and hypnotic actions also involve compensatory mechanisms and there are many other examples. Many of the 'specific' herbs come into this category. Experience has shown that these herbs work well for particular disease states, for example, *Tanacetum parthenium* and migraine, Arnica and bruises, etc. Their mechanism of action is not necessarily known, but probably involves compensatory effects, although mechanisms that are more fundamental might also apply. Knowledge about 'specifics' often originates from folk medicine, where frequently just one herb is used at a time.

Treating the perceived causes

The question which must be asked at the outset and through all stages of treatment is: 'What is the cause of disease in this individual?' Depending on the perceived cause, treatment involving physiological enhancement and/or compensation will be directed at that cause. Using the word 'cause' in any medical discussion can lead ultimately to a metaphysical debate, therefore the adjective 'perceived' becomes an important practical qualification. As the perception and understanding of the patient's problem improve, one gets closer to the 'real' cause. Often there is a chain of causal events. Here the traditional herbal approach is often to treat as many of the links in the chain as are amenable to treatment and active at the time of treatment. Perception of the cause should always be linked to a correct medical diagnosis, although, reflecting the complexity of many clinical conditions and the difficulty that even orthodox medicine has in diagnosing some presentations, a more pragmatic 'assessment' may be at least as useful.

Factors involved in disease causation can be divided into predisposing, excitatory and sustaining causes. A *predisposing* cause is any factor which renders the body more liable to disease. Such predisposing causes include stress, lowered vitality, poor diet, inherited defects and so on. *Excitatory* causes are the direct provoking causes of a disease, such as infection and trauma. *Sustaining* causes usually come into play as a result of the initiation of a disease process and hinder the resolution of the disease. In this context, inflammation can be a sustaining cause. In general, orthodox medical treatment is aimed only at excitatory and sustaining causes, at best.

As much as is possible, predisposing causes should be removed by lifestyle changes, or countered through appropriate physiological enhancement. Neutralisation of excitatory causes often requires both enhancement and compensatory mechanisms. Treatment of sustaining causes usually needs emphasis on physiological compensation to break the sustaining cycle.

An example of treating the links in a causal chain can be illustrated by the following sequence of events:

1. Stress → 2. Insomnia → 3. Lowered vitality →
4. Weakened immunity → 5. Viral infection →
6. Catarrhal state of mucous membranes → 7. Cough

In the context of the above causal sequence, 1–4 are predisposing causes, 5 is the excitatory cause, 6 is a sustaining cause and 7 is the symptomatic expression of the disease.

The treatment approach is set out in Table 7.1.

While not all this may be achievable in one prescription, over time all the links in a chain might be addressed. By choosing herbs which cover several of the required actions, it may be possible to treat many or most links in the one prescription; for example, Hypericum is antiviral and a mild hypnotic, Echinacea is immunostimulant and lymphatic. Other actions might also be required if the body retraces the links in

Table 7.1 Example of a herbal treatment approach for a causal chain

Link in chain	Treatment	Physiological enhancement (E) or compensation (C)
1	Adaptogens	E
2	Sedatives	C
	Hypnotics	C
3	Tonics (choosing those which will not aggravate insomnia)	E
4	Immunostimulants	E
5	Antivirals	C
6	Anticatarrhals	C
7	Expectorants	E
	Antitussives	C

order to resolve the problem; for example, the catarrhal state may be resolved by an acute infection and this would require stimulants (in the herbal sense) and diaphoretics in addition to some of the above. If the catarrhal state were found to be more than just a sustaining cause, then it would require deeper treatment using lymphatic and expectorant herbs.

Sometimes, where there is a good understanding of the main predisposing cause and a very effective treatment, only this cause needs to be treated. For example, Ross River virus infection, which is endemic in Australia, can lead to a chronic condition with joint pain, lethargy and night sweats due to the persistence of the immune imbalance caused by the virus. Treatment with just *Echinacea angustifolia* root (or its combination with *E. purpurea* root) in sufficient doses usually resolves the condition in 6–10 weeks.

Some causes are not treatable by herbal medicine; for example, if insomnia is caused by a traumatic experience, then herbs can compensate but cannot treat or remove the cause. Causes amenable to herbal treatment are listed in Box 7.1.

Some of the causes which cannot be removed but can be compensated for by herbal treatment are listed in Box 7.2.

Often, as part of arriving at an individual treatment framework based on the above considerations, it is necessary to take into account the current medical understanding of the patient's condition. This understanding needs to be carefully interpreted, but nonetheless the current scientific literature is yielding very useful information. For example, potential causative factors identified in autoimmune disease include chronic bacterial and/or viral infections, abnormal bowel flora, dietary allergies and chemical sensitivities. Factors identified in gastric ulceration include bacterial infection, defective sphincter function and poor mucosal resistance.

Box 7.1

Causes amenable to herbal treatment

Lowered vitality
Toxicity
Tumour
Emotional imbalance
Organ malfunction
Organ damage
Inflammation
Hormonal imbalance
Weakened immunity
Allergy
Infection – chronic, subclinical or acute
Stress
Catarrhal state of mucous membranes
Autoimmunity
Unhealthy bowel flora

Box 7.2

Causes which can only be compensated for by herbal treatment

Attitudes to life
Emotional or physical trauma
Heredity
Climate
Age
Lifestyle
Diet

The critical role of case taking

The major aim of case taking is to establish the treatment goals or treatment protocols for that individual. Even for the same medical disorder, this can vary greatly from patient to patient; for example, a patient with eczema with a history of insecticide exposure when young will be treated differently to a patient with eczema which developed after her first child. The following is a basic outline for a consultation which seeks to obtain the information needed to arrive at the treatment framework. Particular emphasis should be given to:

- the historical factors behind the development of the presenting complaint
- factors which modify the presenting complaint
- current and previous medication
- information about the patient's constitution and current condition
- diet
- social history

- past serious disorders or health problems and disorders related to the presenting complaint, as these can lead to information about underlying causes.

The main issue is that the patient should be individualised as much as possible. As part of this process of individualisation, the general morphology and constitution of the patient should also be assessed. All this can be greatly assisted by a symptom checklist. Going through the list may also show up other problems that have a connection to the presenting complaint. A good example is a female patient who complained of regular bouts of thrush. Careful questioning revealed that the thrush always followed a course of antibiotics prescribed for an infected throat. Effective preventative treatment of the infected throat saw that the patient never had a recurrence of thrush. Yet she was never specifically prescribed a treatment for this disorder.

The treatment framework

The treatment framework or protocol sets out the aims or goals of treatment. This is mainly derived from an understanding of the perceived causes of the condition together with an assessment of the need for physiological enhancement or compensation.

Information used to arrive at the treatment framework for a particular disorder is drawn from the following sources:

- The traditional herbal understanding of the disorder
- The clinical experiences of the practitioner in the treatment of the disorder
- A general understanding of the type of the disorder; for example, if it is an infection, what usually leads to this, or if it is an autoimmune disease, the factors that usually precipitate and sustain an autoimmune process
- A scientific understanding of the causes involved in the particular disorder. This information might be derived from clinical and epidemiological studies which have revealed factors which precipitate and sustain the disease process
- A knowledge of scientific studies which have defined the underlying pathological process for that particular disorder
- The individual case history. In a sense, the individual case history acts as a filter for all the above information. An obvious example is lung cancer. Smoking is known to cause lung cancer, but if a patient has never smoked then this consideration is irrelevant to that particular patient. In other words, only those known or suspected causative factors which apply to the particular patient should be incorporated into his or her treatment framework
- The need for symptomatic treatment; again, this relies largely on the individual case history.

For many disorders, development of the treatment framework is a relatively simple process. However, in some instances this process may become quite complex, especially in the case of chronic disorders.

The actions

The concepts that link the treatment goals or treatment framework to the choice of herbs are the actions. These are traditional herbal concepts, but scientific research also yields information about the actions of a herb. The stepwise process in linking treatment goals to choice of herbs for prescription is then suggested as follows:

1. Decide the treatment goals based on traditional herbal concepts, the current medical understanding of the disorder and the patient's case.
2. Ensure that the goals are individualised to the requirements of the individual case.
3. Decide upon the immediate priorities of treatment.
4. On the basis of the immediate treatment goals, decide what actions are required.
5. Choose reliable herbs which have these actions, with as much overlap as possible. For example, if anti-inflammatory and antispasmodic actions are required for the gut, Matricaria can effectively cover both these requirements. Make sure that these herbs are matched to the patient's constitution and general condition according to the considerations outlined in Chapter 3.
6. If a particular action needs to be reinforced, do this by choosing more than one herb with this action or by using a very effective herb in a higher dose.
7. Combine the herbs in a formula with appropriate doses (this is usually done as a mixture of fluid extracts or tinctures). Do not choose too many herbs as this will compromise their individual doses in the formula and may lead to undefined interactions.

To facilitate this process, the practitioner needs a clear understanding of herbs in terms of their reliable, well-established actions. Reference lists of herbs classified under each action and ranked in *order* of priority from the most reliable herb to the least reliable are a useful tool. For example, under the heading of immune stimulants, one might list the following herbs in this order:

Echinacea angustifolia
Echinacea purpurea
Astragalus membranaceus
Andrographis paniculata
Picrorrhiza kurroa
down to *Allium sativum* and *Baptisia tinctoria* which are less proven.

This list could be annotated: for example, *Echinacea spp.*, best at increasing phagocytic activity and early aspects of immune recognition (innate immunity), Andrographis best for acute infections, and Astragalus best in chronic states of impaired immunity and contraindicated in acute infections, and so on. (There will be an element of subjectivity in the compilation of such lists!) The interactive preparation of these lists by a group of practitioners can be a useful learning experience.

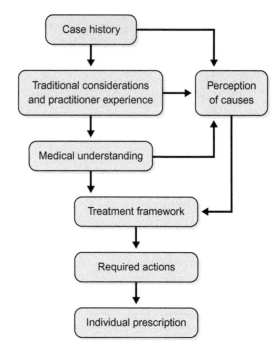

Figure 7.1 • A summary of the event sequence in Western herbal therapeutics.

The event sequence in Western herbal therapeutics is summarised in Figure 7.1.

As part of this process, it can be helpful to draw up a table of treatment goals, corresponding actions and candidate herbs. Depending on the case, this might be quite elaborate, with many treatment goals expanded into even more required actions and yet even more candidate herbs. However, it is also likely that the same herb might appear more than once, indicating that this herb probably (but not necessarily always) needs to be included in the final prescription.

The following brief outline of a case can serve as an illustration of this process. Consider a female patient aged 38 who wants a second child after two miscarriages in the past 4 years. The patient also experiences difficulty conceiving, which makes her miscarriages even more traumatic. Her cycle is long at 36 to 38 days and she experiences marked premenstrual syndrome (PMS) with mastalgia, headaches, emotional lability, anxiety and depression. The patient also suffers from habitual sleep maintenance insomnia. All hormonal tests are normal, save for prolactin, which is elevated.

Table 7.2 provides an example of what might form the key treatment goals, relevant herbal actions and resultant candidate herbs for this patient. Referring to the table it can be seen that a number of herbs appear several times, in particular chaste tree and St John's wort. These are probably the key herbs. Other herbs can be chosen according to their perceived reliability (and associated evidence), the corresponding treatment priorities and the number of times they appear in the table. For this particular case, they would also need to be selected

Table 7.2 Goals, actions and herbs for the case example under discussion (see text)

Treatment goals	Relevant herbal actions	Candidate herbs
Improve sleep (sleep maintenance insomnia)	Melatonin boosting	Chaste tree
	Antidepressant	St John's wort
	Hypnotic	Valerian, passionflower, hops
Alleviate PMS symptoms	Nervine tonic	Skullcap, St John's wort, Schisandra
	Female hormonal balancer	Chaste tree
Reduce prolactin levels	Prolactin inhibitor	Chaste tree
Normalise cycle	Female hormonal balancer	Chaste tree
Stabilise mood and relieve anxiety	Antidepressant	St John's wort
	Anxiolytic	Valerian, passionflower, kava
Promote fertility and ovarian function	Progesterogenic (indirect)	Chaste tree
	Female tonic	Shatavari, dong quai
	Ovarian tonic	False unicorn root, Tribulus
	Oestrogen modulating	False unicorn root, Tribulus, Paeonia, wild yam
Reduce risk of miscarriage (see also actions for promoting fertility and ovarian function above)	Uterine spasmolytic	Black haw, cramp bark, wild yam

according to their suitability in early pregnancy, should the patient successfully conceive. According to these criteria, such herbs might include passionflower, cramp bark, wild yam and false unicorn root. As Tribulus has clinical trial data for promoting fertility, it could be given priority. A case could be argued for a role for adrenal tonic, adaptogen and general tonic herbs for this patient, in which case they could also be included in the table, with stress management as the treatment goal. Patient energetics and relevant herb-drug interactions can also be taken into account to refine further the prescription.

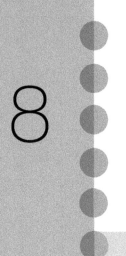

8

Herbal approaches to pathological states

CHAPTER CONTENTS

Topical applications

Scope

Apart from their use to provide non-specific support for recuperation and repair, specific phytotherapeutic strategies include the following.

Treatment of:

- minor wounds and lesions
- sprains and bruises
- seborrhoeic inflammations (such as acne vulgaris)
- cutaneous infections and infestations
- minor inflammations of mouth, throat, anus and nasal and vaginal mucosa
- certain inflammatory conditions affecting the surface of the eye.

Management and relief of:

- pruritic symptoms
- cutaneous eruptions from skin and systemic inflammatory diseases
- inflammations affecting joints, muscles and other subcutaneous tissues
- pain in muscles, joints and subdermal tissues
- varicose ulceration and pressure sores.

Because of its use of secondary plant products, particular caution is necessary in applying topical topical phytotherapy in cases of:

- broken skin
- individuals with certain contact sensitivities.

Orientation

Background

Plants contain many constituents with local physical impact on body tissues. The topical use of herbal remedies is among the first emphases in the earliest and simplest traditions of healthcare. Wound healing was an obvious primal indication for which plant remedies appeared especially suitable.

From a modern perspective, direct effects on tissues are readily testable in research. Most antiseptic, anti-inflammatory and antitumour effects in the research literature relate to in vitro observations, of little direct application to anticipating the effects of oral consumption, but quite relevant to the prediction of topical activity.

Referral to Chapter 2 will provide much of the detail for this review. The following topical properties, however, can be highlighted.

Demulcents and healing agents

Plant material often contains apparently soothing effects on physical contact and plant remedies must have been a very early instinctive application to wounds. Plants with high mucilage content form the basis of poultices and creams. Linum (linseed, flaxseed) is one of the most impressive poultices where the skin (or subdermal tissue in even unbroken skin) is painfully inflamed. *Ulmus rubra* (slippery elm bark) when powdered is one of the most obviously mucilaginous plant materials available for poultices. Stellaria (chickweed) in a cream base provides effective relief for many itchy conditions. Althaea (marshmallow root) and *Trigonella foenum-graecum*

DOI: http://dx.doi.org/10.1016/B978-0-443-06992-5.00008-6

(fenugreek) have notably soothing reputations. The expressed juice of *Aloe vera* also has impressive topical demulcent properties when applied directly to broken or unbroken skin.[1-3]

However, non-mucilaginous herbs like *Alchemilla vulgaris* (lady's mantle) have also demonstrated topical healing effects, in this case on mouth ulcers.[4] The anti-inflammatory remedy Boswellia has been shown topically to heal skin damaged by age and sunlight.[5] The link between anti-inflammatory and healing properties is particularly well illustrated in an ex vivo study on an aqueous extract of *Uncaria tomentosa* (cat's claw). The carboxy alkyl esters, in particular quinic acid esters, easily absorbed across the skin, have been shown to enhance DNA repair and skin resilience to UV damage through anti-inflammatory properties involving the inhibition of nuclear transcription factor kappaB (NF-kappaB).[6]

Perhaps the most thorough healing remedy is Symphytum (comfrey root) cream. When this is applied topically it combines an unparalleled local demulcent action, and tannins (see below) with an active promoter of repair, allantoin, which is known to be very rapidly absorbed into the subdermal tissue.[7] Comfrey has demonstrated healing effects in controlled trials in ankle sprains,[8] and even pain-relieving and anti-inflammatory effects (see below).

Astringents – tannins and OPCs

Tannins and related polyphenols are very common plant constituents with the simple property of curdling protein molecules into which they come in contact. The principle of tanning animal skins to make leather, most often using oak galls or oak bark, follows from this property. Simple washes with strong decoctions of high-tannin preparations (like broadleaved tree bark) are well-established country first-aid treatments for open wounds and third-degree burns and the technique was formally revived among 'barefoot doctors' in China after the Cultural Revolution in the 1960s. The aim here was to produce a sealing *eschar* over the exposed tissues formed from coagulated protein on the surface. In modern clinical application, suspensions of decoctions of high-tannin herbs in gum tragacanth or gum arabic can produce impressive healing effects in open wounds or skin lesions. Plants to be considered for this role include decoctions of Hamamelis (witchhazel bark), *Potentilla tormentilla* (tormentil root), Quercus (oak bark), Krameria (rhatany) and *Geranium maculatum* (American cranesbill root). The antioxidant effects of such preparations have also drawn attention.[9-11] Topically applied tea extracts have been shown to help to restore skin integrity in people with radiation-induced skin damage. On the basis of in vitro cell responses to various tea extracts, these effects are suggested to involve compounds other than the polyphenols.[12] The role of related polyphenols, the oligomeric proanthocyanidins (OPCs), in topical application has been suggested in a clinical study that pointed to a healing effect of combined oral and topical application of an OPC-rich pine bark extract in the treatment of ulcers of diabetic origin.[13]

The usefulness of application of green tea catechins for periodontal disease was investigated in a placebo-controlled trial.[14] Strips containing the catechins as a slow release local delivery system were applied to oral pockets in patients once a week for 8 weeks. The pocket depth and amount of bacteria were markedly decreased in the tannin group, whereas there was no change for the placebo group.

A double blind study investigated the effect of chewing a green tea confectionery on gingival inflammation.[15] A total of 47 volunteers (23 male, 24 female) were randomly assigned to chew either eight green tea or placebo candies per day for 21 days. While there was an improvement in the green tea group, the placebo group deteriorated slightly.

Anti-inflammatories

A number of plant constituents appear to possess topical anti-inflammatory effects, frequently in addition to their demulcent and astringent properties. They might be considered as alternatives to conventional steroidal and other anti-inflammatory prescriptions. For example, herbal Arnica extract compared well with topical non-steroidal anti-inflammatories in the relief of osteoarthritic pain.[16] Calendula (marigold),[17] at least when extracted in high-strength alcohol, and *Matricaria recutita* (German chamomile),[18] both included in creams, have useful benefits in soothing inflamed skin lesions.[19] *Berberis aquifolium*[20] and *Aloe vera*[21] have demonstrated efficacy in the treatment of psoriatic lesions. Echinacea applied topically appears to have local anti-inflammatory effects on minor wounds.[22] Hypericum (St John's wort) extracted in oil as a red pigment is a long-standing remedy for the relief of burns and skin pain, and a hyperforin-rich extract has shown benefit over placebo in relieving atopic dermatitis.[23] Other traditional remedies used topically for anti-inflammatory effects include *Curcuma longa* (turmeric), Juniperus (juniper oil) and *Angelica archangelica* (Angelica oil). Bruising is traditionally treated with external applications of *Aesculus hippocastanum*.[24] The antiseptic properties of tea tree oil (see below) are complemented with an observed topical antihistaminic effect.[25] Many of these applications are fully reviewed in the relevant monographs.

The comfrey ointment referred to above was evaluated for the treatment of knee arthritis.[26] In a large placebo-controlled clinical trial, 220 patients applied 2 g of ointment three times a day for 3 weeks to their painful knee joint. The ointment either contained comfrey or was a matching placebo. In terms of self-rated pain, there was a 55% drop in the comfrey group as opposed to a drop of only 11% in the placebo group. Similar results were also seen for other measures of osteoarthritis symptoms. Overall, pain was reduced, the mobility of the knee improved and quality of life increased.

Comfrey is also good for helping to relieve muscle pain. Two strengths of comfrey cream (10% and 1%) were tested in a double blind study involving 215 people with pain in either the upper or lower back.[27] The stronger cream caused significant improvements in pain on movement, pain at rest and pain on pressure.

A favourite herb for eczema and other forms of inflamed skin (dermatitis) and to promote healing is the Calendula marigold (*Calendula officinalis*). Radiation-induced dermatitis is a common side effect of radiation therapy. For approximately 80% of patients, irradiation induces dermatitis. Apart from the pain and inconvenience associated with the dermatitis, it can lead to interruption of the radiotherapy. There is no standard treatment for the prevention of radiation-induced dermatitis. A survey conducted in 2001 in France indicated that one-third of radiation oncologists prescribed a preventative topical agent for women undergoing irradiation for breast cancer; the most popular choice was the drug trolamine. Hence when French researchers initiated a trial of topical Calendula in patients receiving radiotherapy for breast cancer, they decided to compare its efficacy with that of trolamine.[28]

Between July 1999 and June 2001, 254 patients who had been operated on for breast cancer and who were to receive postoperative radiation therapy were randomly allocated to application of either trolamine (128 patients) or Calendula ointment (126 patients) on the irradiated areas after each session. The occurrence of acute dermatitis of grade 2 or higher was significantly lower (41% versus 63%) with the use of Calendula than with trolamine. Patients receiving Calendula had less frequent interruption of radiotherapy and experienced significantly reduced radiation-induced pain. Calendula ointment was considered to be more difficult to apply, but self-assessed satisfaction was greater.

Antiseptics

The topical effects of herbal remedies can include some antiseptic effects in vitro, although only a few whole preparations have significant clinical prospects. The antimicrobial effects of tea tree oil have been demonstrated in controlled clinical studies in acne vulgaris,[29] dandruff[30] and even methicillin-resistant *Staphylococcus aureus* (MRSA) infections.[31] The oil also has established antifungal properties.[32,33] Another clinical study has demonstrated clinically relevant antifungal effects for a member of the Solanaceae (deadly nightshade) family.[34]

Topical antiviral properties have been demonstrated for the concentrated extract of *Melissa officinalis* (lemon balm) in the relief of herpes infections.[35] One early study found an improved healing rate for 75% of patients, with the time between outbreaks prolonged in 50% of cases.[36] Compared with conventional treatments (at the time), the average healing time of lesions was halved to about 5 days and the time between outbreaks was approximately doubled.[36] In another multicentre study involving 115 patients, treatment of herpes lesions was commenced between 24 and 72h from their outbreak.[37] It was found that lesions in 87% of patients were completely healed within 6 days of treatment. The time between outbreaks was increased for 69% of patients, and this was 2.3 months with lemon balm compared with 1.3 months for conventional drug treatments such as idoxuridine and tromantadine. Minor side effects were observed in only 3% of patients. The delay in new lesions occurring was without any prophylactic application, and it is possible that a preventative application of the cream to normally affected areas would further increase the time between outbreaks. Lemon balm cream can also be used to treat herpes simplex type 2 infection, and probably other similar viral skin infections, including shingles. The cream contained 1% of a concentrated 70:1 extract of lemon balm.

Rhubarb root (*Rheum officinale*) and sage (*Salvia officinalis*) also have activity against viruses, including herpes simplex type 1. In a double blind, controlled trial involving 49 patients, the results for creams containing either 2.3% sage, or 2.3% sage and 2.3% rhubarb, were compared against the conventional antiviral cream containing acyclovir. The average time for the herpes sores to fully heal was 7.6 days with the sage cream, 6.7 days with the rhubarb-sage cream and 6.5 days for acyclovir.[38] Hence, the herbal combination worked as well as the conventional drug.

Many herbs are used as a gargle, lozenge or throat spray to treat a sore throat. These include Calendula, sage, propolis, Echinacea root and golden seal. Acute viral pharyngitis is linked to the common cold and includes symptoms such as sore throat and fever. In a double blind, placebo-controlled clinical trial, the value of a sage throat spray was compared against a placebo spray in almost 300 patients with acute viral pharyngitis.[39] The throat spray was used for seven applications over 3 days, and each application consisted of three sprays. A 15% strength sage spray was found to be much better than placebo for relieving throat pain. Symptomatic relief occurred within 2h of applying the spray.

For a further review of antimicrobial effects of herbal remedies see Chapter 2.

Local anaesthetics and analgesics

As well as the well-known effects on dental pain of topical *Syzygium aromaticum* (clove) oil,[40] and the impact on muscle pain[41] and intractable itching[42] of capsaicin preparations from *Capsicum spp.*, there is now increasing evidence that comfrey (see above) also has pain-relieving properties in arthritis.[43]

Formulations

Many types of topical formulation have evolved for the application of plant materials on body surfaces. A brief summary of their characteristics well reflects the diversity of possible approaches.

Liquids

Liniments (and embrocations)

Semi-liquid preparations prepared in oily or alcoholic solution respectively, with rubefacient or analgesic intentions, are rubbed into unbroken skin. Examples include liniments of mustard and Capsicum, used to stimulate circulation, and liniment of Arnica for healing.

Lotions

These are non-oily liquids applied externally and generally not rubbed in. They are applied to the body surface or any external orifice. Sometimes a lotion will be a herbal tincture used, for example, as a topical treatment for skin or nail fungal infections.

Eardrops

The external ear canal can be treated with oil or alcohol/water-based preparations to help clear obstructions, to treat inflammation or infection of the canal or ear drum or to influence the middle ear by diffusion across the ear drum. Warm olive oil is a popular treatment for waxy obstructions and may be augmented by garlic or Verbascum (mullein flowers) steeped in the oil. However, bacterial contamination of such products is a concern and non-industrially produced preparations are often not to be recommended.

Eyebaths

Aqueous solutions are the usual basis for irrigation of the eye in blepharitis, conjunctival and corneal affections. Bacterial contamination of the eye tissues is particularly hazardous in any home-produced eyebath and these should be discouraged. Great care must be taken to ensure sterility of the fluid which must be boiled for at least 15 minutes in its final container (or added to a sterilised container after boiling). Any water added to the preparation must also be boiled or sterilised. Preparations must be used immediately or stored in sterile frozen blocks. Decoctions of Euphrasia (eyebright), Foeniculum (fennel seed), Agrimonia (agrimony), Glycyrrhiza (licorice root), made at 30 g per 500 mL and then diluted 1:1 with water for application, may be used to reduce inflammatory symptoms.

Gargles

These are preparations in water or alcohol-water solution to be used for throat problems. They may be antiseptic, soothing and/or healing. Herbal gargles may also be swallowed to obtain a secondary, systemic effect. Effective gargles can be made with tinctures of Salvia (sage), Commiphora (myrrh), Calendula and Echinacea, these ideally combined with fluid extract of Glycyrrhiza (licorice) or mucilaginous ingredients. Honey is another effective ingredient.

Inhalants (or vapours)

Volatile components may be inhaled either from a pad applied to the nose and mouth or from liniments or ointments applied to the skin under the nose or on the chest or, most effectively, with steam from hot water. They allow deep and accurate penetration of medicinal agents throughout the whole respiratory system, including the sinuses and middle ear. They will clear catarrhal congestion, soothe irritable mucous membranes and reduce some hypersensitivity reactions. The simplest steaming herb is Matricaria (chamomile) strewn onto the surface of recently boiled water. Recommended oils include pine, aniseed, eucalyptus and, to a limited extent, peppermint.

Baths

Adding herbs or volatile oils to baths has been a traditional technique, with the particular benefit of allowing inhalation of the volatile components in the steam. One common non-volatile application is the mustard bath, used to bathe feet or hands affected by arthritic trouble or as a means of stimulating circulation generally throughout the system. Mustard

powder is added at up to 1% by weight to hand-hot water and the part bathed in it until cool.

Douches

Aqueous solutions may be directed against the body or into a body cavity to cleanse or disinfect. The vaginal douche is the most frequently used: infusions or decoctions of astringent or antiseptic herbs may be prepared and applied deep into the vagina with a bulb syringe or similar applicator whilst the patient is lying supine, for vaginal and cervical infections and inflammations. Douches can also be used for the nasal cavity, although this is rarely done nowadays.

Solids
Creams

These are emulsions of oil in water or water in oil designed to be well absorbed by the skin. They may have various remedies dissolved in either the oil or water fraction. Creams are generally softer than ointments and are more complex in their formulation. For this reason, they were not common in pharmacies of the past but with technical advances are very prominent today, especially in the cosmetics industry. Where available, preparations with Stellaria (chickweed), Calendula, Echinacea and Symphytum (comfrey) are suitable for the treatment of pruritic or inflammatory skin conditions.

Ointments (salves or unguents)

These are semi-solid solutions of various preparations in non-aqueous bases that are not absorbed easily into the skin and are therefore used to provide a protective or remedial film over the skin. Being immiscible with water or skin secretions, ointments effectively form an occlusive layer over the skin, preventing evaporation by transpiration or sweating and allowing the skin to become hydrated. This permits easier absorption of any water-soluble materials in the ointment.

Jellies (or gels)

Suspensions or colloids made from gums, pectin or gelatin allow non-oily applications to be applied to mucous membranes (like the vagina and rectum) and to open or discharging wounds or lesions. They are the most effective way of applying an astringent treatment, especially if gum tragacanth is used as the gelling/suspending agent. Infusions, juices or tinctures may be used for the fluid part. Soothing astringent preparations made, for example, with witchhazel are ideal for irritated wounds, slow-healing leg ulcers or haemorrhoids. Without preservatives, gels should be made and used freshly or from frozen samples.

Plasters

Unlike the modern item, traditional plasters were impregnated dressings applied over the skin where a long-term and concentrated medication was required. The plaster mass was a waxy, rubber, resinous or other base incorporating medical agents, spread on to fabric. It was often designed to convey rubefacient, analgesic or protective effects. Cayenne (capsicum) plasters containing capsaicin are notable applications for arthritic disease.

Poultices

The oldest traditional application was a mass of material soaked in hot water in a fabric bag and applied to the skin while still hot. Poultices have particular ability to draw wounds and infections and to soothe, heal and astringe. Linseed, comfrey, marshmallow and cabbage leaf are frequently used in poultice form in traditional practice.

Suppositories and pessaries

Solid preparations suitable for rectal and vaginal insertion respectively, generally consist of a solution or suspension of active agents in a solid base designed to melt at body temperature (and thus needing to be stored at cool temperatures). Two main types of base are cocoa butter and gelatin-glycerine mixes. The former is most immediately applicable where dry herbal preparations are to be added. Gelatin-glycerine bases are better able to hold fluid; nevertheless, their use may lead to drying of the mucosal membranes and this may provoke inflammation if used frequently.

References

1. Chithra P, Sajithlal GB, Chandrakasan G. Influence of aloe vera on the healing of dermal wounds in diabetic rats. *J Ethnopharmacol*. 1998;59(3):195–201.

2. Strickland FM, Pelley RP, Kripke ML. Prevention of ultraviolet radiation-induced suppression of contact and delayed hypersensitivity by Aloe barbadensis gel extract. *J Invest Dermatol*. 1994;102(2):197–204.

3. Visuthikosol V, Chowchuen B, Sukwanarat Y, et al. Effect of aloe vera gel to healing of burn wound a clinical and histologic study. *J Med Assoc Thai*. 1995;78(8):403–409.

4. Shrivastava R, John GW. Treatment of aphthous stomatitis with topical Alchemilla vulgaris in glycerine. *Clin Drug Invest*. 2006;26(10):567–573.

5. Pedretti A, Capezzera R, Zane C, et al. Effects of topical boswellic acid on photo and age-damaged skin: clinical, biophysical, and echographic evaluations in a double blind, randomized, split-face study. *Planta Med*. 2010;76(6):555–560.

6. Mommone T, Akesson C, Gan D, et al. A water soluble extract from Uncaria tomentosa (cat's claw) is a potent enhancer of DNA repair in primary organ cultures of human skin. *Phytother Res*. 2006;20: 178–183.

7. Sznitowska M, Janicki S. The effect of vehicle on allantoin penetration into human skin from an ointment for improving scar elasticity. *Pharmazie*. 1988;43:218.

8. Koll R, Buhr M, Dieter R, et al. Efficacy and tolerance of a comfrey root extract (Extr. Rad. Symphyti) in the treatment of ankle distortions: results of a multicenter, randomized, placebo-controlled double blind study. *Phytomedicine*. 2004;11: 470–477.

9. Masaki H, Sakaki S, Atsumi T, et al. Active-oxygen scavenging activity of plant extracts. *Biol Pharm Bull*. 1995;18(1):162–166.

10. Sawabe Y, Yamasaki K, Iwagami S, et al. Inhibitory effects of natural medicines on the enzymes related to the skin. *Yakugaku Zasshi*. 1998;118(9):423–429.

11. Mrowietz U, Ternowitz T, Wiedow O. Selective inactivation of human neutrophil elastase by synthetic tannin. *J Invest Dermatol*. 1991;97(3):529–533.

12. Pajonk F, Riedisser A, Henke M, et al. The effects of tea extracts on proinflammatory signaling. *BMC Med*. 2006;4(28):12.

13. Bekcaro G, Cesarone MR, Errichi BM, et al. Diabetic ulcers: microcirculatory improvement and faster healing with Pycnogenol. *Clin Appl Thromb Hemost*. 2006;12(3):318–323.

14. Hirasawa M, Takada K, Makimura M, et al. Improvement of periodontal status by green tea catechin using a local delivery system: a clinical pilot study. *J Periodontal Res*. 2002;37(6):433–438.

15. Krahwinkel T, Willershausen B. The effect of sugar-free green tea chew candies on the degree of inflammation of the gingiva. *Eur J Med Res*. 2000;5(11):463–467.

16. Widrig R, Suter A, Saller R, et al. Choosing between NSAID and arnica for topical treatment of hand osteoarthritis in a randomised, double blind study. *Rheumatol Int*. 2007;27:585–591.

17. Klouchek-Popova E, Popov A, Pavlova N, et al. Influence of the physiological regeneration and epithelialization using fractions isolated from calendula officinalis. *Acta Physiol Pharmacol Bulg*. 1982;8(4): 63–67.

18. Glowania HJ, Raulin C, Swoboda M. Effect of chamomile on wound healing – a clinical double blind study. *Z Hautkr*. 1987;62(17):1262. 1267–1271

19. Shipochliev T, Dimitrov A, Aleksandrova E. Antiinflammatory action of a group of plant extracts. *Vet Med Nauki*. 1981;18(6):87–94.

20. Wiesenauer M, Lüdtke R. Mahonia aquifolium in patients with Psoriasis vulgaris – an intraindividual study. *Phytomedicine*. 1996;3(3):231–235.

21. Choonhakarn C, Busaracome P, Sripanidkulchai B, et al. A prospective, randomized clinical trial comparing topical aloe vera with 0.1% triamcinolone acetonide in mild to moderate plaque psoriasis. *J Eur Acad Dermatol Venereol*. 2010;24(2):168–172.

22. Kinkel JH, Plate M, Töllner HU. Verifiable effect of echinacin ointment on wound healing. *Med Klin*. 1984;79:580–583.

23. Schempp C, Windeck T, Hezel S, et al. Topical treatment of atopic dermatitis with St. John's wort cream – a randomized, placebo controlled double blind half-side comparison. *Phytomedicine*. 2003;10 (suppl IV):31–37.

24. Bombardelli E, Morazzoni P. Aesculus hippocastanum L. *Fitoterapia*. 1996;67(6):483–510.

25. Koh KJ, Pearce AL, Marshman G, et al. Tea tree oil reduces histamine-induced skin inflammation. *Br J Dermatol*. 2002;147:1212–1217.

26. Grube B, Grünwald J, Krug L, et al. Efficacy of a comfrey root (Symphyti offic. radix) extract ointment in the treatment of patients with painful osteoarthritis of the knee: results of a double blind, randomised, bicenter, placebo-controlled trial. *Phytomedicine*. 2007;14(1):2–10.

27. Kucera M, Barna M, Horàcek O, et al. Topical symphytum herb concentrate cream against myalgia: a randomized controlled double blind clinical study. *Adv Ther*. 2005;22(6):681–692.

28. Pommier P, Gomez F, Sunyach MP, et al. Phase III randomized trial of Calendula officinalis compared with trolamine for the prevention of acute dermatitis during irradiation for breast cancer. *J Clin Oncol*. 2004;22(8):1447–1453.

29. Enshaieh S, Jooya A, Siadat AH, et al. The efficacy of 5% topical tea tree oil gel in mild to moderate acne vulgaris: a randomized, double blind placebo-controlled study. *Indian J Dermatol Venereol Leprol*. 2007;73(1):22–25.

30. Satchell AC, Saurajen A, Bell C, et al. Treatment of dandruff with 5% tea tree oil shampoo. *J Am Acad Dermatol*. 2002;47(6):852–855.

31. Dryden M, Dailly S, Crouch M. A randomized, controlled trial of tea tree topical preparations versus a standard topical regimen for the clearance of MRSA colonization. *J Hosp Infect*. 2004;56: 283–286.

32. Buck DS, Nidorf DM, Addino JG. Comparison of two topical preparations for the treatment of onychomycosis: melaleuca

alternifolia (Tea Tree) oil and clotrimazole. *J Fam Prac*. 1994;38(6):601–605.

33. Satchell AC, Saurajen A, Bell C, et al. Treatment of interdigital tinea pedis with 25% and 50% tea tree oil solution: a randomized, placebo-controlled, blinded study. *Australas J Dermatol*. 2002;43(3):175–178.

34. Herrera-Arellano A, Rodriguez-Soberanes A, Martinez-Rivera M, et al. Effectiveness and tolerability of a standardized phytodrug derived from Solanum chrisotrichum on Tinea pedis: a controlled and randomized clinical trial. *Planta Med*. 2003;69:390–395.

35. Koytchev R, Alken RG, Dundarov S. Balm mint extract (Lo-701) for topical treatment of recurring Herpes labialis. *Phytomedicine*. 1999;6(4):225–230.

36. Wölbling RH, Rapprich K. Die Melisse-alte Heilpflanze mit neuem Wirkungsprofil.

Deut Dermatol. 1983;10(31): 1318–1328.

37. Wölbling RH, Milbradt R. Klinik und Therapie des Herpes simplex: Vorstellung eines neuen phytotherapeutischen Wirkstoffes. *Therapiewoche*. 1984;34:1193–1200.

38. Saller R, Buechi S, Meyrat R, et al. Combined herbal preparation for topical treatment of Herpes labialis. *Forsch Komplementarmed Klass Naturheilkd*. 2001;8(6):373–382.

39. Hubbert M, Sievers H, Lehnfeld R, et al. Efficacy and tolerability of a spray with Salvia officinalis in the treatment of acute pharyngitis – a randomised, double blind, placebo-controlled study with adaptive design and interim analysis. *Eur J Med Res*. 2006;11(1):20–26.

40. Alqareer A, Alyahya A, Andersson L. The effect of clove and benzocaine versus

placebo as topical anesthetics. *J Dent*. 2006;34(10):747–750.

41. Gagnier JJ, van Tulder M, Berman B, et al. Herbal medicine for low back pain (review). *Cochrane Database Syst Rev*. 2006;(2):CD004504.

42. Lysy J, Sistiery-Ittah M, Israelit Y, et al. Topical capsaicin – a novel and effective treatment for idiopathic intractable pruritus ani: a randomised, placebo controlled, crossover study. (peri-anal disease). *Gut*. 2003;52(9):1323–1327.

43. Giannetti BM, Staiger C, Bulitta M, et al. Efficacy and safety of a comfrey root extract ointment in the treatment of acute upper or low back pain: results of a double blind, randomised, placebo-controlled, multi-centre trial. *Br J Sports Med*. 2010;44(9):637–641.

Fever

Scope

Apart from their use to provide non-specific support for recuperation and repair, specific phytotherapeutic strategies include the following.

Treatment of:

- uncomplicated and moderate fevers from infectious causes.

Management and relief of:

- febrile symptoms of non-infectious origin.

Particular **caution** is necessary in applying phytotherapy in cases of:

- severe, rampant fever with hyperpyrexia and/or when due to virulent causes.

Orientation

Introduction

Fever is most often associated with viral and bacterial infectious illnesses of varying degrees of severity, such as 'flu', measles, rubella, rheumatic fever, pneumonia, malaria, scarlet fever, polio, tuberculosis and meningitis. It can also accompany a wider range of problems such as cardiovascular and autoimmune diseases, drug reactions and some cancers. Many cases, especially in children, remain mysterious.[1]

It is therefore vital that the onset of any fever is diagnosed as accurately as possible, especially in the very young and elderly, pregnant women, among overseas travellers and those with immune disorders. Conventional drug therapy and even hospitalisation may be essential.

The fever as friend?

Perhaps because of the associations above, the fever process has come to be seen as a problem to be treated in its own

right ('We must bring the fever down'). The serious risks from hyperpyrexia (overheating) are well understood and the accompanying unpleasant symptoms are reason enough to regard fever with suspicion. However, if it is clear that fever is not part of a serious condition there are also good reasons for not suppressing the process unnecessarily. This view is gaining support in conventional medicine,[2,3] particularly in reaction to the fashion for using paracetamol, and previously aspirin, to treat common childhood fevers.[4]

A recent example of such concerns is the New Zealand study that investigated the association between infant and childhood paracetamol use and later atopy and allergic disease.[5] Children given paracetamol before the age of 15 months were 3.6 times more likely to have atopy at age 6 years than infants who had not been given the drug. Paracetamol use between the ages of 5 and 6 years showed dose-dependent associations with wheeze and asthma.

Such modern reassessment of fever treatment echoes the older traditional view that fever was not the disease itself but the body's extraordinary efforts to resist disease. It was therefore something to be supported, or at least managed, rather than unduly suppressed. In this view, a 'good fever', one which went through its natural course satisfactorily, would not only lead to better resolution of the immediate crisis but would actually rearm the body's defences and increase its resistance to future onslaughts. Indeed, it was on this issue above all others that the revivalist practices of Samuel Thomson in the 19th century were based (see p. 11). It was common practice among 'regular' physicians to suppress fevers with mineral drugs based on mercury, arsenic and antimony. Thomson was moved by Indian practices, especially the sweat lodge, to vehemently challenge such principles and insist instead on the view that fever was a sign of healthy defences (the 'natural heat' of the body resisting 'cold' intrusion) and should be supported in its efforts rather than suppressed. To this end, he recommended the use of heating remedies, including cayenne, and other measures to support the body through the episode, managing excesses of the febrile condition along the way. Although

Thomson's message was simple (reflecting the predominance of fevers as the main clinical priority of the times), he identified a fundamental difference between traditional practices and the new direction of orthodox medicine – supporting body defences versus attacking disease processes.

Other traditional approaches to fever management were similar. Because fever was so common, the universal classification of remedies as heating or cooling was made very largely on the basis of their observed effects in this condition. Heating herbs would be used to support a flagging fever and, by promoting perspiration, were additionally seen as aiding elimination through the sweat glands (sweat glands do resemble primitive nephrons and can stand in for kidney function to some extent); cooling remedies would be used to temper excessive pyrexia. Herbs with subtle heating or cooling (such as the Galenic 'hot in the first degree') were seen as exerting a normalising effect, helping to steady body temperature. Other remedies were classified for their ability to reduce the impact of febrile convulsions, diarrhoea, vomiting and distress.

There is modern support for the traditional view.[6] The body's febrile response is accompanied by the arousal of powerful, unpleasant and debilitating defensive measures, the release of inflammatory chemicals, temperature-stimulated activity in the circulation and in various blood cells, including the scavenger white blood cells, and associated alterations in a wide range of other functions.[7,8] In many ways it is like inflammation, for which an analogous traditional view applies (see p. 152): it generally proceeds in defined stages, tends to be self-limiting and is directed to mobilising defensive resources to the rapid elimination of an intrusion into the tissues. Both inflammation and fever are accompanied by what may be regarded as guarding symptoms, in the case of fever often by nausea (leading to reduced eating and unnecessary digestive, eliminative and metabolic burdens), thirst (increasing fluid consumption and compensating for fever-induced dehydration), lassitude and exhaustion (ensuring adequate rest during the process) and photophobia (encouraging withdrawal to a darkened place so as to reduce visual and other stimulation).

In contrast to our forebears, modern practitioners can now accept the far superior diagnostic and treatment prospects that medicine can bring and be grateful that the killer fevers are largely in the past. Nevertheless, there is real value in revisiting some fundamental fever management approaches in the majority of feverish illnesses that do not present a serious threat. There is a real concern that suppressive measures like aspirin and paracetamol and pre-emptive (and often unsuitable) antibiotic treatments are aborting an important natural healing process. Earlier observers predicted that unresolved fevers would lead to recurrent low-grade problems thereafter. The current frequency of chronic catarrhal problems, sore throats, cervical lymphadenopathy (swollen glands), sinusitis, otitis media (glue ear) and atopic allergy, especially among children, reminds many modern practitioners of such a syndrome. Modern studies are beginning to validate these concerns (see above).

It is possible to retrieve some of the early measures as part of a new strategy of fever management, taking advantage of insights and technology unavailable to our forebears.

Practical fever management

Fevers present serious challenges for any practitioner more used to dealing with modern chronic and low-grade conditions. Fevers can be dangerous. **They can change rapidly and initial diagnoses can be wrong. It would be professionally negligent to take responsibility for managing a fever without the necessary personal medical qualifications and experience unless supported by an effective health team. The following suggestions can only be applied in such circumstances.**

After best available medical diagnosis has determined that dangerous disease is unlikely, the phytotherapeutic approach to fever is to see the condition as something to be managed, even nurtured, to allow the body temperature to stay at acceptable febrile levels (usually the range 100–102°F or 37.8–38.9°C) until the fever breaks, then to switch to recuperative measures as required. During the fever the practitioner watches for dangerous symptoms (and ensures ongoing medical supervision as necessary), works with herbal and other measures to prevent body temperature rising too high and provides relief for ancillary symptoms like nausea, vomiting, diarrhoea, coughing, convulsions and general malaise and discomforts.

Many fever-causing bacteria and viruses either produce as metabolites, or present as surface antigens, trigger chemicals, referred to as *exogenous pyrogens*, that stimulate the temperature control mechanism in the hypothalamus – in effect, they 'set the thermostat higher'. The result is a stimulus to the heat-generating and heat-conserving mechanisms of the body so that body temperature can rise to match the new setting in the hypothalamus. Such mechanisms include shutting down the blood flow to the surface (pallor), shivering and seeking warmth. In short, **when the temperature is rising the patient feels cold.**

This is the 'chill' phase of fever. When the body temperature rises to the level set by the hypothalamus, a new stability with balance of heat gain and loss returns. The symptoms of chill recede and a less uncomfortable phase commences.

With the rise in body temperature, blood flow through the tissues and the activity of the phagocytes increase. The body's defences are alerted and mobilised. The intruder's prospects are reduced, as eventually is its production of exogenous pyrogens. The upward stimulus on the hypothalamus is reduced and the thermostat setting falls. The outward sign of this change could be predicted from knowing that the body temperature will now be higher than that set in the thermostat so heat has to be lost. The circulation to the periphery opens up again, the sweat glands operate, clothing and coverings are thrown off. **The temperature falls and for that reason the patient feels hot.** In traditional terms, the fever has 'broken', 'crisis' has been reached and 'lysis' or resolution intervenes. With luck, the infection has been successfully rejected and recovery can commence.

There is a more complex story of course. For example, there are a range of cytokines, such as interleukin (IL)-1 (alpha and beta), IL-6 and tumour necrosis factor-alpha, produced by the body itself and known as *endogenous pyrogens* which, possibly interacting with prostaglandins, can induce relapsing and other complex fever patterns with no clear cause. More recently, it has been shown that inhibitors of cytochrome P450 exacerbate pyrexia and that inducing P450 arachidonic acid metabolism reduces fever.[9–11] There are also endogenous antipyretic mediators including neuroactive substances such as glucocorticoids, vasopressin, IL-10 and melanocortins.[12]

However, the summary account above provides an acceptable basis for a policy of fever management, in which basic principles of nursing can be augmented by herbal remedies.

The first requirement is for some means of monitoring the situation. A clinical thermometer is obviously central but its usefulness is greatly enhanced by knowing how to interpret its findings. Referring to the account of fever above will explain the following points:

1. Feeling cold, with pale cyanosed skin and shivering means that the body temperature is lower than that set in the hypothalamus and is most likely to be *still rising*.

2. Feeling hot, with flushed skin and sweating means that the body temperature is higher than the thermostat setting and is most likely to be *coming down*.

3. Having no dominant feeling of being hot or cold suggests relative equilibrium between thermostat and body temperature.

With these clues and a thermometer, it is generally possible to assess progress through the fever. If, for example, the temperature was 104°F (40°C), its importance would depend on whether the patient was feeling hot or cold. In the former case, one would expect the temperature to fall; in the latter case, some quick treatment would be called for.

Apart from the usual techniques for bringing temperature down, such as cold wet face flannels or tepid baths, there is conventional aspirin.[13] This, however, simply turns the thermostat controls down without attending to any other aspects of the fever; there is the risk of an unresolved problem with symptoms lasting for years.[14]

Its use in children has in any case been discontinued in recent years because of the incidence of serious side effects.[15,16] Paracetamol and ibuprofen[17] are still used for similar purposes; there are reports of adverse effects in the case of paracetamol particularly,[18,19] but a recent systematic review indicates safety of these agents compared with nocebo effects is not a major concern.[20] The wider question is the wisdom of using such agents to bring down the fever, with consequent risks to antibody production and cell repair, when no other risk is present.[21]

Herbal remedies, by contrast, have a number of more complex effects on the body and on the febrile response. There are a number of peripheral antipyretic mechanisms associated with plant remedies,[22–24] including ginger,[25] fennel,[26] boldo[27] and Andrographis.[28] However, it is worth noting in the practical guides to fever management that follow, that the published evidence for efficacy in humans has been undermined by poor methodological quality of the studies.[29]

Herbal treatments during fevers are best provided in the form of aqueous infusions or decoctions (see p. 126), either hot or warm depending on the wider context.

As a steadying influence, the peripheral vasodilators or diaphoretics are appropriate, including remedies such as Achillea (yarrow), Sambucus (elderflower), Matricaria (chamomile),

Tilia (limeflowers), *Nepeta cataria* (catmint) and *Eupatorium perfoliatum* (boneset). Their effect in hot infusion, seen only in a febrile state, is subjectively to reduce chill and encourage cooling perspiration; they also have a variety of other useful benefits for the digestion, mucous membranes and neuromuscular system. They may be combined with peppermint tea for a more accelerated cooling effect.

For gentle but stronger reduction in febrile temperature, the cooling bitters, like Taraxacum (dandelion root), Gentiana (gentian root) and Cichorium (chicory root) and Erythraea (centaury), are favoured. They have the additional advantage of stimulating the otherwise dormant digestive system, thus helping to counter fermentation or infection arising from the gut. Throughout history some plants were particularly favoured for their fever-reducing properties; most were notable bitters as well as having a range of antipathogenic and anti-inflammatory properties. They are, however, inherently more powerful and should be applied with more caution and under closer supervision. They include Cinchona (Peruvian bark that later yielded quinine), various members of the Artemisia or wormwood family, Jateorhiza (calumba), *Berberis vulgaris* (barberry bark) and Hydrastis (golden seal).

Apart from body temperature, there are other symptoms of fever that need to be watched. Many, such as nausea, vomiting, diarrhoea, headaches, coughing, pains and spasms, can usually be controlled by the appropriate herbal remedy, covered elsewhere in this book. Accepting the potential value of the febrile reaction does not mean consigning the patient to unnecessary discomfort. There are of course danger signs as well (a pulse that does not rise with temperature as expected might herald meningitis; convulsions, although common enough in children, can disguise and exacerbate polio; a dry cough of measles can resemble that of pneumonia, which can also be heralded by rapid breathing rates; malaria remains impossible to diagnose without blood tests).[30] The untrained must not attempt to take full responsibility for any such treatment.

Raising fever

In addition to containing excessive body temperature, there may be a need to encourage it to rise. If it is clear that the fever is not adequately materialising and that there is no serious infection or underlying pathology, warming remedies might be chosen. This is a common scenario in affluent societies. Here, fevers are rare after childhood but unresolved low-grade chronic infections are not. In a case of persistent catarrh, for example, it is often useful to take advantage of a partial attempt by the body to raise the stakes, a cold or sore throat perhaps, and set a 'therapeutic fever' in train.

The patient should be advised to prepare properly. Bed rest, a minimal fresh diet and plenty of fluid are basic requirements. It is then possible to take one of the many circulatory stimulants, such as *Cinnamomum zeylanicum* (cinnamon,) *Angelica archangelica* (angelica), Zingiber (ginger), Allium (raw garlic) or even Capsicum (cayenne). A modest febrile process can then be nudged into existence, often to considerable advantage. Echinacea root, being both warming and stimulating to mucosal immune defences, may be particularly useful here.

Aftermath

As important as any other part of the treatment is adequate convalescence (see p. 86) after it is all over. There are a range of remedies traditionally used for post-fever recuperation. These include some of the warming and cooling remedies above, those with additional tonic reputations, like *Inula helenium* (elecampane), Cardamomum (cardamom seed), Echinacea, Taraxacum (dandelion root) and Gentiana (gentian root).

References

1. McCarthy PL, Klig JE, Shapiro ED, et al. Fever without apparent source on clinical examination, lower respiratory infections in children, other infectious diseases, and acute gastroenteritis and diarrhea of infancy and early childhood. *Curr Opin Pediatr.* 1996;8(1):75–93.

2. Kluger MJ, Kozak W, Conn CA, et al. The adaptive value of fever. *Infect Dis Clin North Am.* 1996;10(1):1–20.

3. Klein NC, Cunha BA. Treatment of fever. *Infect Dis Clin North Am.* 1996;10(1):211–216.

4. Adam D, Stankov G. Treatment of fever in childhood. *Eur J Pediatr.* 1994;153(6):394–402.

5. Wickens K, Beasley R, Town I, et al. The effects of early and late paracetamol exposure on asthma and atopy: a birth cohort. *Clin Exp Allergy.* 2011;41(3):399–406.

6. Sullivan JE, Farrar HC. Fever and antipyretic use in children. *Pediatrics.* 2011;127(3):580–587.

7. Norman DC, Castle S, Yamamura RH, et al. Interrelationship of fever, immune response and aging in mice. *Mech Ageing Dev.* 1995;80(1):53–67.

8. Muzyka BC. Host factors affecting disease transmission. *Dent Clin North Am.* 1996;40(2):263–275.

9. Kozak W, Kluger MJ, Tesfaigzi J, et al. Molecular mechanisms of fever and endogenous antipyresis. *Ann NY Acad Sci.* 2000;917:121–134.

10. Sakata T, Kang M, Kurokawa M, et al. Hypothalamic neuronal histamine modulates adaptive behavior and thermogenesis in response to endogenous pyrogen. *Obes Res.* 1995;3(suppl 5):707–712.

11. Derijk RH, Van Kampen M, Van Rooijen N, et al. Hypothermia to endotoxin involves reduced thermogenesis, macrophage-dependent mechanisms, and prostaglandins. *Am J Physiol.* 1994;266(1 Pt 2):1–8.

12. Tatro JB. Endogenous antipyretics. *Clin Infect Dis.* 2000;31(suppl 5):190–201.

13. Bartfai T, Conti B. Fever. *Sci World J.* 2010;10:490–503.

14. Cuddy ML. The effects of drugs on thermoregulation. *AACN Clin Issues.* 2004;15(2):238–253.

15. Chalasani N, Roman J, Jurado RL. Systemic inflammatory response syndrome caused by chronic salicylate intoxication. *South Med J.* 1996;89(5):479–482.

16. Whelton A. Renal effects of over-the-counter analgesics. *J Clin Pharmacol.* 1995;35(5):454–463.

17. Pierce CA, Voss B. Efficacy and safety of ibuprofen and acetaminophen in children and adults: a meta-analysis and qualitative review. *Ann Pharmacother.* 2010;44(3):489–506.

18. Czerwionka-Szaflarska M, Sobkowiak E. Acute gastrointestinal hemorrhage in a 12-month-old child following treatment with panadol. *Pediatr Pol.* 1996;71(5):471–472.

19. Stamm D. Paracetamol and other antipyretic analgesics: optimal doses in pediatrics. *Arch Pediatr.* 1994;1(2):193–201.

20. Perrott DA, Piira T, Goodenough B, et al. Efficacy and safety of acetaminophen vs ibuprofen for treating children's pain or fever: a meta-analysis. *Arch Pediatr Adolesc Med.* 2004;158(6):521–526.

21. Scrase W, Tranter S. Improving evidence-based care for patients with pyrexia. *Nurs Stand.* 2011;25(29):37–41.

22. Lalé A, Herbert JM. Polyunsaturated fatty acids reduce pyrogen-induced tissue factor expression in human monocytes. *Biochem Pharmacol.* 1994;48(2):429–431.

23. Gupta M, Mazumder UK, Kumar RS, et al. Anti-inflammatory, analgesic and antipyretic effects of methanol extract from Bauhinia racemosa stem bark in animal models. *J Ethnopharmacol.* 2005;98(3):267–273.

24. Tsai TH, Lee TF, Chen CF, et al. Thermoregulatory effects of alkaloids isolated from Wu-chu-yu in afebrile and febrile rats. *Pharmacol Biochem Behav.* 1995;50(2):293–298.

25. Chrubasik S, Pittler M, Rougogalis B. Zingerberis rhizoma: a comprehensive review on the ginger effect and efficacy profiles. *Phytomedicine.* 2005;12:684–701.

26. Tanira MOM, Shah AH, Mohsin A, et al. Pharmacological and toxicological investigations on Foeniculum vulgare dried fruit extract in experimental animals. *Phytotherapy Res.* 1996;10:33–36.

27. Backhouse N, Delporte C, Givernau M, et al. Anti-inflammatory and antipyretic effects of boldine. *Agents Actions.* 1994;42(3–4):114–117.

28. Caceres DD, Hancke JL, Burgos RA, et al. Use of visual analogue scale measurements (VAS) to assess the effectiveness of standardized Andrographis paniculata extract SHA-10 in reducing the symptoms of common cold. A randomized double blind-placebo study. *Phytomedicine.* 1999;6(4):217–223.

29. Chen XY, Wu TX, Liu GJ, et al. Chinese medicinal herbs for influenza. *Cochrane Database Syst Rev.* 2007;(4):CD004559.

30. Svenson JE, Gyorkos TW, MacLean JD. Diagnosis of malaria in the febrile traveler. *Am J Trop Med Hyg.* 1995;53(5):518–521.

Infectious diseases

Scope

Apart from their use in providing non-specific support for recuperation and repair, specific phytotherapeutic strategies include the following.

Treatment of:

- minor to moderate acute infections of the respiratory, urinary and gastrointestinal mucosa
- minor to moderate systemic infections especially when accompanied by lymphadenopathy
- topical bacterial and fungal infections
- minor to moderate febrile infections
- minor to moderate chronic viral, bacterial and fungal infections.

Management of:

- refractory cases of chronic viral, bacterial and fungal infections especially accompanied by lowered immune resistance.

Because of its use of secondary plant products, particular **caution** is necessary in applying phytotherapy in cases of infections of the kidney parenchyma.

Note: In most developed countries there are usually legal constraints on non-physicians treating, or claiming to treat, notifiable infections, for example contagious infections, tuberculosis and venereal infections. Severe acute infections, especially involving vital organs, should in general be approached with extreme care and never without full medical supervision unless this is clearly not available.

Orientation

Background

A modern observer might presume that one area where traditional herbal medicine could not be claimed as a useful model is in the area of infections. It is generally accepted that until Pasteur's germ theory of disease and the isolation of effective antimicrobials, humanity had seriously missed the plot. The history of pestilences and plagues, the decimation caused by the killer infections such as smallpox, cholera, typhoid and scarlet fever, the waking medieval nightmares of tuberculosis and syphilis, the Russian roulette that every mother and infant played with perinatal mortality, along with the near universal ignorance of the dangers of living in filth and squalor along with dark mutterings about 'contagions' and 'toxins' in lieu of simple hygienic measures, all looks rather bad for traditional medicine.

Much of this is undeniable. There is no doubt that healthcare shifted beyond recognition with public hygiene measures like clean water and separate sewage systems from the 19th century and the discovery of penicillin in the early decades of the 20th. Herbal practitioners can admit this gracefully and be grateful they no longer have to attempt to thwart life-threatening infectious diseases.

Nevertheless, the herbal cupboard is not entirely bare. Most of the horrors referred to above were features of life in cities and towns, of crowded squalid conditions, far from sources of fresh food (and with no refrigerated delivery) and clean water. The historical and archaeological evidence available suggests that life was more equable in traditional rural communities, that, leaving perinatal mortality aside, average lifespans in the ancient world differed little from those reached until the middle of the 20th century[1-3] and that longevity was not uncommon where land was fertile.[4] In such circumstances, the case against the traditional remedies used by country people is harder to sustain.

Furthermore, if the killer diseases are taken out of the picture and more ordinary everyday infections are considered, the balance shifts in favour of historical treatment. There are a number of traditional remedies that appear to support the body in its battle against infections. From an exhaustive review of traditional cooking practices and recipes and correlation with exposure to infections, it has been concluded that the pungent spices were adopted as flavourings, consciously or unconsciously, at least in part because of their protective effect against enteric infections, with the hottest used where there is greatest exposure.[5] There are other indications that chillies in particular are antimicrobial in moderate doses.[6,7]

As another example of a dietary antimicrobial, various publications indicate that garlic extract also has broad-spectrum antimicrobial activity against many genera of bacteria and fungi. This activity, particularly in respect of Gram-negative bacteria, seems to be stronger than that of other members of the onion family.[8,9] Allicin was the early candidate as the most active constituent in garlic.[10] In terms of the phytochemical world it has been verified as a potent antibacterial agent, but even then its activity is relatively modest compared with conventional antibiotics.[11] Later research has demonstrated that ajoene, the prominent metabolite of allicin, also conveys particular antimicrobial activity, including against such Gram-negative bacteria as *Escherichia coli* and *Klebsiella pneumoniae*. The disulphide bond in ajoene appeared to be necessary for this activity, since reduction by cysteine, which reacts with these bonds, abolished its antimicrobial activity.[12] This activity is, however, significantly exceeded by another metabolite, 10-devinylajoene, marked by substitution of the allyl group in ajoene by a methyl group and sulfinyl group.[13] These findings might explain why a garlic extract was observed to have a more potent anti-staphylococcal activity than an equivalent amount of allicin.[11]

The incidence of stomach cancer is lower in individuals and populations with high allium vegetable intakes. To investigate this further, an aqueous extract of garlic cloves was standardised for its thiosulfinate concentration and tested for its antimicrobial activity on *Helicobacter pylori*. Minimum inhibitory concentration was $40 \mu g/mL$ thiosulfinate. This study may have detected a particular sensitivity of *H. pylori* to garlic constituents as *Staphylococcus aureus* tested under the same conditions was not susceptible to garlic extract up to the maximum thiosulfinate concentration tested ($160 \mu g/mL$).[14] However, clinical trials of the use of garlic in eradicating *H. pylori* have been disappointing, although this might reflect on the form of garlic used.[15,16] Systemic antifungal activity has been supported in a study where commercial garlic extract was given intravenously to two patients with cryptococcal meningitis and three patients with other types of meningitis. Plasma titres of anti-*Cryptococcus neoformans* activity rose two-fold over pre-infusion titres.[17]

The position with other plant constituents is less clear. Essential oils have demonstrated antimicrobial effects in vitro (see, for example references[18-20] and also Chapter 2). In one study, for example, the antimicrobial effects of some essential oils on oral bacteria were surveyed. Tea tree oil, peppermint oil and sage oil proved to be the most potent essential oils, whereas thymol and eugenol were potent essential oil components.[21] Tea tree oil has demonstrated a number of antimicrobial effects, even against MRSA.[22] More studies on tea tree oil are reviewed in Chapter 2. In research on antifungal effects, those of phenolics such as iso-eugenol, cinnamaldehyde, carvacrol, eugenol and thymol were linked to the presence of a free hydroxyl group linked to an alkyl substituent.[23] However, all these studies generally refer to isolated oils rather than to the whole plant and it is difficult to infer from these that traditional treatments had much antimicrobial efficacy.

On the other hand, ethnobotanical reviews of traditional plants (often reported in the excellent *Journal of*

Ethnopharmacology) have shown in vitro efficacy of whole-plant preparations (for example references[24-27]) and in one study a high correlation was demonstrated between traditional use and in vitro antisepsis among plants in North America.[28] It is possible that modest antimicrobial effects may lie in other plant constituents: tannins (especially tannic acid and propyl gallate) have demonstrated such properties. This activity is suggested as being associated with the hydrolysis of ester linkage between gallic acid and polyols, hydrolysed after the ripening of many edible fruits. Tannins in these fruits thus may serve as a natural defence mechanism against microbial infections.[29]

There were other particular remedies, generally at least a few in each tradition, with a role of directly helping the body resist infections. Raw garlic in Europe, Echinacea and Baptisia (wild indigo) in North America, Picrorrhiza in Asia and Andrographis in China were all accorded great respect in their respective cultures. Some were mobilised in managing the fevers that often resulted, others were used to support recovery and the hopefully increased defensive strength of the well-managed convalescence. There is little evidence that any of these are antibiotics in the modern sense: most were understood as supporting some defensive function or other. This list would also contain other supporters of host resistance:

- The powerful bitters – *Artemisia absinthium* (wormwood), Columbo, Marsdenia (condurango), Cinchona (quinine bark), Swertia, *Berberis vulgaris* (barberry bark) and *Hydrastis canadensis* (golden seal root) – that were likely to have been effective protectors against enteric and hepatic infections (see the monograph for the last two herbs)
- The hot pungent spices – *Capsicum spp.* (chillies), Zingiber (ginger) – that complement this role in enteric infections and, with Cinnamomum (cinnamon), that still today provide effective treatments in respiratory infections (see the monograph on ginger)
- Remedies like Juniperus (juniper berries), *Arctostaphylos uva-ursi* (bearberry), *Barosma betulina* (buchu) and *Piper cubeba* (cubeb) in the treatment of urinary infections (see the monographs on bearberry and buchu).

For the many non-serious infections in everyday life, the deathbed recantation attributed to Pasteur is increasingly relevant. No seed can develop without *le terrain*, the soil to nourish it, no infections can establish without the body, by deficit, enabling a sympathetic environment for colonisation to occur. There are very few genuinely aggressive pathogens; there are always some people, usually the majority, unaffected in even the most notorious epidemics. The normal environment, food, air, skin, mouth and gut lining, is full of theoretically pathogenic bacteria (legally allowable counts in many foods are still in the millions of bacteria per milligram). In the absence of supporting immune defences, it is likely that the drive to kill pathogens has gone too far. While antibiotics have changed the prospects for bacterial infections beyond traditional recognition, and antifungals, antiprotozoals and antiviral medicines have played important parts in the management of other infections, it is also clear that infectious diseases remain major clinical problems in even the most modern societies. In particular, there is concern about the increasing resistance of many pathogens to new drugs. Antibiotic resistance is causing particular worries, with

the spectre of 'super-bugs' now occupying the attention of the popular press. In Britain the government instructed doctors in September 1998 to avoid prescribing antibiotics in minor self-limiting infectious conditions such as colds and sore throats or when infections are likely to be viral in origin.

With every new epidemic, be it SARS, bird flu, swine flu or an outbreak of antibiotic-resistant bacteria, it becomes increasingly obvious that the conventional approach to preventing and treating infection is beginning to fail our communities. The hero antibiotics of yesteryear are being rendered next to useless by resistant organisms, with the cost and challenges of developing new antibiotic drugs ensuring that future prospects are relatively bleak. The role for phytotherapy in infectious diseases is likely to increase rather than diminish under these circumstances.

Phytotherapeutics

General approach to infections

It is worthwhile reviewing the considerations for the herbal management of infections. These are as follows:

- Immune-enhancing herbs like *Echinacea angustifolia* or *E. purpurea* root or Baptisia (wild indigo root) are an effective core element in the treatment of any infection acute or chronic (see below for a treatment protocol for Echinacea root). Andrographis is particularly suited to acute infections, with consistent evidence for its clinical efficacy (see the Andrographis monograph).
- Warming circulatory stimulants will act to promote defensive immune activities in many cases of acute infections. Zingiber (ginger) is particularly helpful in these circumstances; Capsicum (cayenne) and Cinnamomum (cinnamon) are respectively stronger and milder substitutes or accompaniments.
- If the infection is located in a particular organ, herbs are often prescribed to support that organ or its defensive functions: strong bitters in the case of enteric infections; Silybum (St Mary's thistle) for liver infections; expectorants for lung infections; Juniperus for the urinary system; Serenoa (saw palmetto) for prostate infections. This is especially the case if these infections are subacute or chronic.
- Hypericum (St John's wort) may be applied in the long-term treatment of infections with enveloped viruses; Thuja (arbor-vitae) more widely for viral infections.
- For topical treatment of accessible surfaces a different range of products can be used. Melaleuca (tea tree oil) can be applied directly to some skin infections and, in suitable carriers, for vaginitis, in the case of either bacterial or fungal origin. Melissa (lemon balm) and Glycyrrhiza (licorice) have topical antiviral activity and can be applied to herpes and similar outbreaks, as can essential oils such as tea tree (provided the virus is enveloped). Thuja and Calendula tinctures and tea tree oil are effective for fungal infections of the skin and nails. For the mouth and throat, mouthwashes and gargles can be made with *Echinacea angustifolia* or *E. purpurea* root, high-strength alcoholic tinctures of Commiphora (myrrh), Calendula, *Populus*

gileadensis (balm of Gilead) or propolis, all best combined with fluid extract of Glycyrrhiza.

Poor immunity and recurrent infections

Patients with poor immunity and/or recurrent infections should receive treatment selected from the following groups:

* Immune-enhancing herbs: Echinacea, Astragalus, Picrorrhiza, Andrographis, Phytolacca. Astragalus should not be prescribed during acute episodes and Picrorrhiza and Andrographis should not be prescribed if the patient is constitutionally cold. Astragalus is particularly indicated for chronically depleted immunity.
* Tonic and adaptogenic herbs: Panax, Eleutherococcus, Withania. It is advisable to hold back on using these during an acute infection.
* Bitter herbs: Gentiana, *Artemisia absinthium* especially where the patient appears anaemic or undernourished. Exercise caution if the patient is also constitutionally

cold; if necessary counter the cooling effect with heating herbs.

Echinacea protocol

Echinacea alone, either the root of *E. angustifolia* or *E. purpurea*, or their combination, has helped countless patients prone to infection in doses equivalent to 2.5 to 7.5 g/day (5 to 15 mL of a 1:2 preparation). The treatment protocol is as follows (equivalent doses in tablet or capsule form can also be used):

1. Take a 5 mL dose each day (2.5 g) as a maintenance dose (take twice this dose for maintenance if immunity is very poor).
2. If infection threatens, double or triple the daily maintenance dose until the threat passes.
3. If infection takes hold, maintain the higher dose until the infection is completely gone and then return to the normal daily dose. Alternatively, or in addition, apply the treatments noted above for acute infections.

See also the Echinacea root monograph.

References

1. Montagu JD. Length of life in the ancient world: a controlled study. *J R Soc Med*. 1994;87(1):25–26.
2. O'Rourke DA. Three score and ten. *MJA*. 1976;131(11):356.
3. Jarcho S. The longevity of the ancient Greeks. *Bull NY Acad Med*. 1967;43(10):941–943.
4. Kottek SS. Old age in Biblical and Talmudic lore. *Isr J Med Sci*. 1996;32(8):702–703.
5. Billing J, Sherman PW. Antimicrobial functions of spices: why some like it hot. *Q Rev Biol*. 1998;73(1):3–49.
6. Cichewicz RH, Thorpe PA. The antimicrobial properties of chile peppers (Capsicum species) and their uses in Mayan medicine. *J Ethnopharmacol*. 1996;52(2):61–70.
7. Caceres A, Alvarez AV, Ovando AE, et al. Plants used in Guatemala for the treatment of respiratory diseases 1. Screening of 68 plants against Gram-positive bacteria. *J Ethnopharmacol*. 1991;31:193–208.
8. Elnima EI, Ahmed SA, Mekkawi AG, et al. The antimicrobial activity of garlic and onion extracts. *Pharmazie*. 1983;38(11):747–748.
9. Dankert J, Tromp TF, De Vries H, et al. Antimicrobial activity of crude juices of Allium ascalonicum, Allium cepa and Allium sativum. *Zentralbl Bakteriol [Orig A]*. 1979;245(1–2):229–239.
10. Adetumbi MA, Lau BH. *Allium sativum* (garlic) – a natural antibiotic. *Med Hypo*. 1983;12(3):227–237.
11. Fujisawa H, Watanabe K, Suma K, et al. Antibacterial potential of garlic-derived allicin and its cancellation by sulfhydryl compounds. *Biosci Biotechnol Biochem*. 2009;73(9):1948–1955.
12. Naganawa R, Iwata N, Ishikawa K, et al. Inhibition of microbial growth by ajoene, a sulfur-containing compound derived from garlic. *Appl Environ Microbiol*. 1996;62(11):4238–4242.
13. Yoshida H, Iwata N, Katsuzaki H, et al. Antimicrobial activity of a compound isolated from an oil-macerated garlic extract. *Biosci Biotechnol Biochem*. 1998;62(5):1014–1017.
14. Sivam GP, Lampe JW, Ulness B, et al. Helicobacter pylori – in vitro susceptibility to garlic (Allium sativum) extract. *Nutr Cancer*. 1997;27(2):118–121.
15. Gail MH, Pfeiffer RM, Brown LM, et al. Garlic, vitamin, and antibiotic treatment for Helicobacter pylori: a randomized factorial controlled trial. *Helicobacter*. 2007;12(5):575–578.
16. Fani A, Fani I, Delavar M, et al. Combined garlic-omeprazole versus standard quadruple therapy for eradication of Helicobacter pylori infection. *Indian J Gastroenterol*. 2007;26(3):145–146.
17. Davis LE, Shen JK, Cai Y. Antifungal activity in human cerebrospinal fluid and plasma after intravenous administration of Allium sativum. *Antimicrob Agents Chemother*. 1990;34(4):651–653.
18. Kartnig T, Still F, Reinthaler F. Antimicrobial activity of the essential oil of young pine shoots (Picea abies L.). *J Ethnopharmacol*. 1991;35(2):155–157.
19. Kalodera Z, Pepeljnjak S, Blaevi N, et al. Chemical composition and antimicrobial activity of Tanacetum parthenium essential oil. *Pharmazie*. 1997;52(11):885–886.
20. Briozzo J, Núñez L, Chirife J, et al. Antimicrobial activity of clove oil dispersed in a concentrated sugar solution. *J Appl Bacteriol*. 1989;66(1):69–75.
21. Shapiro S, Meier A, Guggenheim B. The antimicrobial activity of essential oils and essential oil components towards oral bacteria. *Oral Microbiol Immunol*. 1994;9(4):202–208.
22. Carson CF, Cookson BD, Farrelly HD, et al. Susceptibility of methicillin-resistant Staphylococcus aureus to the essential oil of Melaleuca alternifolia. *J Antimicrob Chemother*. 1995;35(3):421–424.
23. Pauli A, Knobloch K. Inhibitory effects of essential oil components on growth of food-contaminating fungi. *Z Lebensm Unters Forsch*. 1987;185(1):10–13.
24. Ritch-Krc EM, Turner NJ, Towers GH. Carrier herbal medicine: an evaluation of the antimicrobial and anticancer activity in some frequently used remedies. *J Ethnopharmacol*. 1996;52(3):151–156.
25. Cáceres A, Girón LM, Alvarado SR, et al. Screening of antimicrobial activity of plants popularly used in Guatemala for the treatment of dermatomucosal diseases. *J Ethnopharmacol*. 1987;20(3):223–237.
26. Taylor RS, Manandhar NP, Towers GH. Screening of selected medicinal plants of Nepal for antimicrobial activities. *J Ethnopharmacol*. 1995;46(3):153–159.
27. Desta B. Ethiopian traditional herbal drugs. Part II: Antimicrobial activity of 63 medicinal plants. *J Ethnopharmacol*. 1993;39(2):129–139.
28. McCutcheon AR, Towers GHN. *Ethnopharmacology of North American Plants*. Lecture at the 2nd International Congress on Phytomedicine, Munich, Germany, Institute of Pharmaceutical Biology; 1996.
29. Chung KT, Wong TY, Wei CI, et al. Tannins and human health: a review. *Crit Rev Food Sci Nutr*. 1998;38(6):421–464.

Inflammatory and autoimmune diseases

Scope

Phytotherapy includes some unique approaches to influencing inflammatory and immunological mechanisms. Although there is an incomplete evidence base, in some cases there are enough strong themes to influence clinical practice. Phytotherapeutic strategies include the following.

Treatment of:

* acute inflammations of muscles, joints, connective tissues and glandular and gut tissue.

Management of:

* chronic inflammatory diseases of the digestive tract, including gastritis, Crohn's disease and ulcerative colitis
* chronic inflammatory diseases of joints, and other connective tissues, including rheumatoid arthritis (RA) and ankylosing spondylitis (see also Chapter 9)
* psoriasis, scleroderma, other chronic inflammatory skin diseases (dermatitis), including complex and autoimmune conditions such as psoriasis (see also Chapter 9)
* long-term inflammatory processes underlying chronic conditions such as diabetes and atherosclerosis.

Because of the use of secondary plant products, particular **caution** is necessary in applying phytotherapy in cases of:

* inflammatory disease complicated by glomerulonephritis or other kidney disease.

Orientation

Relevant inflammatory mechanisms

The skeletal and connective tissues of the body are primarily designed to cope with wear and tear and have a range of impressive repair mechanisms to reduce consequent problems for the organism, at least until late in life. By far their most frequent problems therefore involve disturbances of the inflammatory and immunological mechanisms. As well as the familiar inflammations of the skin (dermatitis, including eczema and psoriasis) and joints (arthritis), these include those of other connective tissues: arteritis, cellulitis, chondritis, meningitis, osteitis, pericarditis, phlebitis, pleurisy and vasculitis. Chronic inflammatory disturbances also involve glandular tissue: epididymitis, oöphoritis, pancreatitis, prostatitis and thyroiditis, as well as endodermal tissue: Crohn's disease, gastritis and ulcerative colitis. Inflammatory changes in the blood vessel walls have also been shown to be key elements in the chronic deterioration associated with atherosclerosis, and more broadly with several stages in the path through late-onset diabetes, increasing insulin resistance and the later vascular complications of the illness.

In many of these long-term inflammatory conditions, there are also wider disturbances of the immune system, so that mechanisms designed to cope with foreign material begin to attack the body's own tissues. These 'autoimmune' exacerbations in turn provoke their own inflammatory responses. In many chronic inflammatory diseases, there are multiple pathological elements to disentangle. The practitioner rarely has a clear target.

The modern approach to most inflammatory and immunological disturbances is to suppress the manifestations with anti-inflammatory drugs, either steroids or the non-steroidal anti-inflammatories (NSAIDs), or coal-tar products in the case of topical applications to the skin. When steroidal drugs based on cortisone became widely available in the early 1950s, the transformation these made to the prognosis for arthritic, skin and other connective tissue diseases was dramatic. For two decades, any challenge to these drugs would have been derided. However, it then became apparent that both steroids and their non-steroidal counterparts based on aspirin were associated with a range of side effects and diminishing therapeutic returns that now lead physicians to limit their prescription much more than in the past. There is again a demand for other approaches, especially in the case of those sufferers otherwise condemned to a lifetime of powerful and potentially dangerous drugs.

Traditional herbal practice approached these conditions in radically different, although surprisingly consistent, ways. Even though there is very little modern clinical evidence of efficacy, their consistency justifies a rational review, not least because some of the traditional insights concur with the latest findings about the aetiology and mechanisms of inflammatory and immunological diseases. It will be useful to look at some relevant pathophysiological mechanisms.

Chronic low-grade systemic inflammation has come to be defined as a term for a wide variety of conditions marked by a two- to three-fold increase in the systemic concentration of C-reactive protein (CRP) and increased systemic levels of some cytokines. Cytokines are small polypeptides, which were originally discovered to have immunoregulatory roles. The local response to infections or tissue injury involves macrophage activation (often by certain toxins) that causes them to produce cytokines. Some of these facilitate an influx of lymphocytes, neutrophils, monocytes and other cells. The initial cytokines in the cytokine cascade are (in order) tumour necrosis factor (TNF)-alpha, IL-1, IL-6, IL-1 receptor antagonist (IL-1ra) and soluble TNF-alpha receptors. In response to an acute infection or trauma, the cytokines and cytokine inhibitors may increase several-fold and decrease when the infection or trauma is healed.

The key interface in the inflammatory response is the endothelium, the cell lining of the blood vessels, through which the white blood cells that mediate both inflammation and immunity have to pass. Endothelial cells secrete various factors influencing vessel tone, platelet function, coagulation and fibrinolysis and which initiate inflammatory responses. Clinical problems develop when these processes are imbalanced.

In the early stages of the inflammatory response, TNF-alpha and IL-1, among other cytokines, stimulate the endothelial cells to express the cell surface adhesion molecule P-selectin. Within a couple of hours, a second surface adhesion molecule, E-selectin, is produced. Together E- and

P-selectin slow the motion of leukocytes through the bloodstream by causing them to roll along the endothelial surface, allowing other molecules to interact with the slowed leukocytes to stop them and promote their movement into the tissues (described as analogous to throwing a tennis ball at a Velcro surface). Tight adhesion to the rolling leukocyte is performed by two endothelial cell ligands, intercellular adhesion molecule-1 (ICAM-1) and vascular cellular adhesion molecule-1 (VCAM-1), which arrest the motion of the rolling leukocyte.[1] Stopping the leukocyte allows it to enter the tissues by secreting proteases to breach the endothelial basement membrane, a process known as diapedesis.

There are a number of other mediators of endothelium-mediated inflammation. The major cause of the endothelial dysfunction is thought to be decreased availability of nitric oxide (NO), either due to decreased production or enhanced breakdown due to increased oxidative stress.[2] It is the major factor in large arteries mediating endothelial dependent relaxation and inhibits platelet aggregation, cell adhesion and smooth muscle cell proliferation. A number of plant remedies hold promise as promoters of NO activity at the endothelium.[3] The activation of nuclear transcription factor-kappa B (NF-kappaB) has also been linked with a variety of inflammatory diseases. Kappa B kinase catalyses NF-kappaB activation and is implicated in the effects of excessive free fatty acids on the induction of insulin resistance, in atherogenesis, and other inflammatory disorders.

The above are among a number of mechanisms involved in altering endothelial function in the inflammatory response. They therefore represent potential mechanisms in any inflammatory-modulating strategy, and, as will be seen below, there are many plant constituents with this potential.[4] In the case of chronic deteriorations such as increased insulin resistance, diabetes and atherosclerosis, there is the prospect that many dietary plants may have long-term protective effects. The warming spices like ginger,[5] cinnamon[6] and turmeric[7] may share cholinergic 'endothelium-dependent' vasodilator effects mediated by NO and counteracted for example by high glucose levels. Garlic[8] and even daily beverages of tea[9,10] and coffee,[11] have been shown to benefit endothelial markers associated with reduced inflammation in atherosclerosis and diabetes. Among its well-attested benefits on microvascular function,[12] chocolate also reduces inflammatory markers like CRP.[13]

Many commonly consumed herb and spice constituents may inhibit extravasation in the inflammatory response. See Table 8.1.

Others may inhibit migration through inflamed endothelial cells. See Table 8.2.

However, it must be kept in mind that this research is identifying prospects only until such effects are also demonstrated in humans after oral doses. Nonetheless, there can be no harm in increasing the dietary intake of such phytochemicals in cases of chronic inflammation as a background therapy. For a fuller discussion of herbal compounds able to target defined biochemical and molecular mediators of inflammatory, autoimmune arthritis (at least from experimental models), the reader is referred to an excellent recent review.[43]

It is, however, obvious that chronic inflammatory diseases are among the most demanding indications. It is likely that only individual treatments have been truly effective in the past and, apart from the undoubted power of the placebo effect, these are not very amenable to simple recipes or over-the-counter treatments (fish oils in arthritic disease are perhaps the main exception). The required complexity and individualisation of treatments also renders controlled clinical trials near impossible to conduct.

The traditional understanding of inflammatory diseases notably involved ideas of 'toxicity' and, particularly but not exclusively, in Chinese herbal therapeutics, meteorological concepts of 'damp', 'wind', 'heat' and 'cold' (see also p.158). These apparently quaint medieval notions are metaphors for clinical insights into the way the body appears to behave in such illnesses that can indeed inform a modern review. This will now be attempted.

Modern research into the causes of inflammatory diseases has uncovered, in particular, disturbed reactions to infections and significant events in the digestive tract.

Infectious agents

At the turn of the 20th century, the rheumatoid-like condition ankylosing spondylitis was regarded as a venereal disease, though 20 years later the wider association with urinary infection had been made. This, however, was lost by the time steroids transformed the prospects for the condition.

An interesting later brush with ancient notions by modern medical research was seen in an issue of *The British Medical Journal*.[44] It was reported that patients with RA had a significantly higher incidence or history of pulmonary disease than the wider population. It was pointed out that the lungs remain sub-clinically infected, almost indefinitely in many cases, after the incidence of pneumonia, bronchitis and pleurisy, and this persistence is obvious in conditions like emphysema and bronchiectasis. The findings were dramatic and led a linked editorial to speculate, probably reluctantly, that 'toxins' in the infected lung base might provoke the inflammatory changes in the rheumatoid joints.

Modern rheumatology has now taken such notions into orthodoxy, although gratefully abandoning any primitive imagery. Rather than 'toxic' influences, the role of 'immunological cross-reactivity' has emerged as a leading factor in the aetiology of rheumatic diseases. In this view, the autoimmune nature of these diseases is reinforced; it had long been understood that the body's own immune defences were the main cause of many connective tissue inflammations (the term 'collagen diseases' was used to embrace a wide range of such conditions). In immunological cross-reactivity, the immune system is provoked and then confused by the similarity between bacterial, viral or other antigens and those of its own tissues and attacks both. In fact, a survival imperative drives invading organisms to resemble their host, at least at a molecular level, in order to escape immune detection. This phenomenon of 'molecular mimicry' drives immunological cross-reactivity.

Infectious agents are now (controversially) regarded as the major environmental factors that may cause arthritic

Table 8.1 Inhibition of extravasation

Herb or spice constituemt	Properties
Ajoene	Inhibits tumour–endothelial cell adhesion, as well as the in vivo TNF-alpha response to LPS in mouse melanoma cells.[14]
Allicin	Inhibits the spontaneous and TNF-alpha-induced secretion of IL-1beta, IL-8, IP-10 and MIG in a dose-dependent manner from intestinal epithelial cells in vitro, suppresses the expression of IL-8 and IL-1beta mRNA levels.[15]
Allyl isothiocyanate	Significantly inhibits the cellular production of pro-inflammatory mediators such as TNF-alpha and NO.[16]
Anethole	Inhibits NF-kappaB activation induced by TNF, TRAF2 and NIK in vitro, suppresses TNF-induced activation of the transcription factor AP-1, JNK and MAPK in vitro.[17]
Apigenin	Inhibits TNF-alpha in LPS stimulated macrophages resulting in diminished MCP-1 and inhibition of IL-1beta in vitro.[18]
Capsaicin	Blocks the STAT3 activation pathway in multiple myeloma cells in vitro leading to downregulation of cyclin D1, Bcl-2, Bcl-xL, survivin and VEGF.[19]
Carnosol	Decreases LPS-induced iNOS mRNA and protein expression, reduces NF-kappaB subunits translocation and NF-kappaB DNA binding activity in activated macrophages due to inhibition of IKK, inhibits iNOS and NF-kappaB promoter activity.[20]
Caryophyllene	Inhibits the LPS-induced NF-kappaB activation and neutrophil migration in rat paw oedema in vivo.[21]
Cinnamaldehyde	Inhibits age-related NF-kappaB activation and targets inflammatory iNOS and COX-2, inhibits the activation of NF-kappaB via three signal transduction pathways, NIK/IKK, ERK, and p38 MAPK.[22]
Curcumin	Downregulates the constitutive activity of NF-kappaB, decreases expression of NF-kappaB target genes COX-2 and cyclin D1, and induces apoptosis in mouse melanoma cells in vitro.[23] Significantly inhibits the cellular production of proinflammatory mediators such as TNF-alpha and NO.[16]
Diallyl sulphide	Significantly reduces the production of and serum levels of IL-1beta, IL-6, TNF-alpha and GM-CSF in mice with melanoma.[24]
Eugenol	Blocks the release of IL-1beta, TNF-alpha and prostaglandin E2 and suppresses the mRNA expression of IL-1beta, TNF-alpha and COX-2 in LPS-stimulated human macrophages in vitro.[25]
[6]-Gingerol	Inhibits the production of TNF-alpha, IL-1beta and IL-12 in murine peritoneal macrophages exposed to several doses of 6-gingerol in the presence of LPS stimulation.[26]
Humulene	Inhibits the LPS-induced NF-kappaB activation and neutrophil migration in rat paw oedema, prevents the production of TNF-alpha and IL-1beta and the in vivo upregulation of kinin B(1) receptors.[21]
Limonene / myrcene	Inhibits the LPS-induced inflammation including cell migration and production of NO along with significant inhibition of gamma-interferon and IL-4 production in mouse model of pleurisy.[27]
Perillyl alcohol	Reduces NF-kappaB DNA-binding activity.[28]
Phytic acid	Modulates IL-8 and IL-6 release from colonic epithelial cells stimulated with LPS and IL-1beta, suppresses IL-8 basal release, and it dose-dependently reduces IL-8 secretion by colonocytes and downregulates IL-6.[29]
Piperine	Significantly reduces the expression of IL-1beta, IL-6, TNF-alpha, GM-CSF and IL-12p40 genes in melanoma cells.[30]
Quercetin	Attenuates PMACI-induced activation of NF-kappaB,[31] inhibits LPS-induced NO and TNF-alpha production in murine macrophages.[32]
Ursolic acid	Inhibits IKK and p65 phosphorylation leading to the suppression of NF-kappaB activation induced by various carcinogens; this correlates with the downregulation of COX-2, MMP-9 and cyclin D1 in vitro.[33]
Zingerone	Significantly inhibits the cellular production of proinflammatory mediators such as TNF-alpha and NO and inhibits the release of MCP-1 from 3T3-L1 adipocytes.[34]

Table 8.2 Inhibition of invasion

Herb or spice constituemt	Properties
Allicin	Inhibited TNF-alpha induced ICAM-1 expression in human endothelial cells.[35]
Allyl isothiocyanate	Downregulated mRNA level and activity of MMP-2/MMP-9 in human hepatoma SK-Hep1 cells.[36]
Apigenin/kaempferol	Inhibited TNF-alpha induced ICAM-1 expression.[37]
Caffeic acid	Inhibited MMP-9 activity in human hepatocellular carcinoma cell line.[38]
Curcumin	Downregulated MMP-2 expression and activity and expression of integrin receptors, FAK and MT1-MMP in Hep2 cells.[39]
Diallyl disulfide	Inhibited activity of MMP-2 and MMP-9 in human endothelial cells.[24]
[6]-Gingerol	Suppressed expression and enzymatic activity of MMP-2/MMP-9 in human breast cancer cells.[40]
Myricetin	Inhibited expression and activity of MMP-2 in colorectal cancer cells.[41]
Quercetin	Decreased the expressions of MMP-2 and MMP-9 in PC-3 cells.[42]

inflammation in genetically susceptible hosts. Retroviruses, urinary and pulmonary, and especially enteric bacteria are the provocateurs most often discussed.[45–48] *Helicobacter pylori* has been associated with diseases such as autoimmune gastritis, Sjögren's syndrome, atherosclerosis, immune thrombocytopenic purpura, inflammatory bowel diseases and autoimmune pancreatitis, in each of which it seems to play a pathogenic role in some cases. On the other hand, it has also been suggested that it may help to protect against the development of autoimmune gastritis, multiple sclerosis, systemic lupus erythematosus and inflammatory bowel diseases.[49]

Molecular mimicry has been found between a white blood cell protein, HLA-B27, and two molecules, nitrogenase and pullulanase D, in the anaerobic gut bacterium *Klebsiella pneumoniae* among ankylosing spondylitis patients,[50] and between HLA-DR1/DR4 and the haemolysin molecule in another gut anaerobe, *Proteus mirabilis*, among RA patients.[51] Molecular mimicry between HLA-B27 and *K. pneumoniae* molecules in the aetiology of ankylosing spondylitis patients has been extensively studied. It was first proposed by Dr Alan Ebringer in 1976. *K. pneumoniae* was isolated in stool samples more frequently in active phases of the disease and was linked to relapses. High antibody levels in ankylosing spondylitis patients directed against *K. pneumoniae* were found in several studies. Some of these antibodies were shown to cross-react with HLA-B27 as well as spinal collagens. Specific anti-Klebsiella antibodies in ankylosing spondylitis patients have now been reported from 18 different countries. 'B27 disease' is the new terminology proposed by Ebringer.[52]

In another growing association, patients with long-standing active RA have a substantially increased frequency of periodontal disease compared with that among healthy controls. High levels of oral anaerobic bacteria antibodies (such as from *Porphyromonas gingivalis*, *Tannerella forsythensis*, and *Prevotella intermedia*) have been found in the serum and synovial fluid of such patients. Appropriate antibiotics have been shown to be effective against the arthritis[53] (leading to intriguing prospects for herbal oral antiseptics such as gum myrrh). Autoimmunity in RA has been characterised lately

as an antibody response to citrullinated proteins. There is an association with periodontitis that is largely, but not exclusively, caused by *Porphyromonas gingivalis* infection. The citrullination of proteins by *P. gingivalis* and the subsequent generation of autoantigens that drive autoimmunity in RA represent a possible causative molecular mimicry link between these two diseases.[54] As noted above, a further link with the aetiology of RA is with Proteus infection in the urinary tract.[55] Both bacteria can be found as secondary infections elsewhere in the body and prospects for future control of rheumatoid diseases by antibiotic therapy have been raised.[56]

There are some strong indications from archaeology for an infectious trigger for RA. Examinations of skeletal remains from antiquity in Europe do not show signs of RA. In contrast, specimens dating back several thousand years from Native American tribes in North America show clear evidence of the disease. The prevalence of RA in this ethnic group today remains extraordinarily high, with over 5% of individuals affected in some groups. Evidence of RA in Europe first appeared in 17th century art, especially by the Dutch Masters, and the first case report was published in 1676. RA could well be linked to an infectious agent brought from the New World to the Old World.[57]

The site of the trigger for ankylosing spondylitis is not necessarily always the bowel. An association between ankylosing spondylitis and chronic bacterial prostatitis has long been observed. The incidence of chronic prostatitis in male ankylosing spondylitis patients was 83%, compared with 33% in patients with RA.[58] This association was confirmed in a later study.[59] The fact that the prostate may harbour bacteria that contribute to ankylosing spondylitis could explain the higher incidence of this disorder in males. Evidence of Chlamydial urinary tract infection is frequent in female patients with ankylosing spondylitis.[60]

Gut inflammation is a prime candidate for having a bacterial origin (see also below). Johne's disease, which occurs in cattle and other ruminants, is very similar to Crohn's disease and is caused by *Mycobacterium avium* subspecies *paratuberculosis* (MAP). In 1984, Chiodini and co-workers reported the isolation of a strain resembling MAP from the intestinal tissue of three patients with Crohn's disease.[61] This report initiated interest and controversy about a mycobacterial aetiology for Crohn's disease that is still ongoing. MAP has also now been cultured from human milk, faeces, intestinal tissues and peripheral blood of patients with Crohn's disease.[62] Ebringer has also implicated Klebsiella in Crohn's disease and advised a low starch diet (see later).[63] In terms of Crohn's disease, one group of researchers reflected: 'The mycobacterial theory and the autoimmune theory are complementary; the first deals with the aetiology of the disorder, the second deals with its pathogenesis. Combined therapies directed against a mycobacterial aetiology and inflammation may be the optimal treatment …'.[64] The levels of MAP found in Crohn's disease patients is not high, so its presence does not represent a bacterial infection *per se*. Rather it is best viewed as a form of dysbiosis.

Viruses may also be involved in triggering an autoimmune response. For the past 25 years, a potential role of Epstein-Barr virus (EBV) in the pathogenesis of RA has been suspected. The QKRAA amino acid sequence of HLA-DRB1, a tissue marker that carries susceptibility to RA, is found in the EBV envelope. Sera from patients with RA contained higher levels of antibodies to latent and active EBV antigens.[65] RA patients have more EBV-infected B cells than normal controls. Patients with RA have a 10-fold higher EBV load than healthy controls. EBV DNA is detected more frequently in immune cells, synovial fluid and saliva from RA patients than from controls.[65]

In contrast to Crohn's disease, studies over 40 years have associated ulcerative colitis with cytomegalovirus (CMV).[66] A clear association between onset of ulcerative colitis and primary CMV infection was confirmed by viral studies in two patients.[67,68] Higher frequency and amount of antibodies to CMV were found in patients with ulcerative colitis.[66] The simultaneous presence of DNA from several herpes viruses, including CMV, was much greater in ulcerative colitis patients compared to those with Crohn's disease or normal controls.[69] While it is debated that CMV infection may be a causative factor in ulcerative colitis, it is recognised by many clinicians as a complicating event that can increase its severity.[70]

Intestinal wall damage

There is increasing evidence of damage to the gut wall in a range of autoimmune diseases. One category of diseases, classified as spondylarthropathies, involve inflammatory damage of the joints and the skeleton, the eyes, gut, urogenital tract, skin and sometimes the heart.[71,72] Ankylosing spondylitis is the prototype example of this condition; other examples include reactive arthritis, psoriatic arthritis and arthritis in patients with inflammatory bowel disease. In a series of investigations, histological signs of gut inflammation were found in a high proportion of patients with spondylarthropathies.[73] Most of these patients did not present any clinical intestinal manifestations. Remission of the joint inflammation was always connected with a disappearance of the gastrointestinal inflammation. Persistence of locomotor inflammation was mostly associated with the persistence of gastrointestinal inflammation. It was proposed that some patients with a spondylarthropathy had a form of subclinical Crohn's disease in which the locomotor

inflammation was the only clinical expression.[74] Further genomic work substantiates the unique relationship between gut and joint inflammation.[75] These data suggest that spondylarthropathies and Crohn's disease should be scientifically and clinically considered as distinct phenotypes of common immune-mediated inflammatory disease pathways, rather than as separate disease entities.[76]

This hypothesis is supported in prospective long-term studies in which ileocolonoscopied patients were reviewed over periods of up to 9 years. About 6% of spondylarthropathy patients who did not present any sign of Crohn's disease at first investigation (but did show gut inflammation on biopsy) developed full-blown Crohn's disease within 9 years. Electron microscopy of these lesions demonstrated an increase in the number of membranous (M) cells in inflamed mucosa. Necrosis and rupture of these M-cells, with lymphocytes entering the gut lumen, was observed. Such evidence of damage to the gut mucosa could be responsible for an increase in local antigenic stimulation and could readily lead to secondary systemic immunological disorders.[77]

Pathogenic forms of *Escherichia coli* with specific hairs or pilli adhere to the gut mucosa. In 1988, it was first demonstrated that *E. coli* isolated from patients with ulcerative colitis and Crohn's disease showed a significantly greater index of adhesion when compared with normal controls.[78] A new term adherent-invasive *Escherichia coli* (AIEC) was coined to describe this aggressive form. They can replicate intracellularly and survive within macrophages. AIEC strains were found (predominantly in the ileum) in 21.7% of Crohn's disease chronic lesions versus 6.2% of controls.[79] Crohn's disease patients with anti-*E. coli* antibodies were more likely to have internal perforating disease and to require small bowel surgery.[80] Because AIEC can cross and breach the intestinal barrier, move to deep tissues and continually activate macrophages, they can generate persistent inflammation.[81]

As mentioned above, AIEC are found in significant amounts in patients with ulcerative colitis compared with controls.[78] Several workers have shown that isolates of *E. coli* obtained from patients with ulcerative colitis can degrade mucins and produce toxins. Results from one study suggested that connective tissue exposed by bowel ulcerations may result in selection of *E. coli* strains able to bind to them.[82] Compared with healthy people, ulcerative colitis patients have increased levels of IgG directed against their normal flora.[83] There may be an increased number of bowel bacteria in ulcerative colitis, but reduced counts of 'protective' bacteria such as Lactobacilli and Bifidobacteria.[83] Lactobacilli numbers were certainly found to be lower in ulcerative colitis patients during the active phase.[84] This was confirmed in another study that also found the bacterial diversity decreased during a relapse.[85]

In patients with active ulcerative colitis there is an overproduction of hydrogen sulphide, which is toxic to the intestinal mucosa by competing with short-chain fatty acids.[86] This appears to be due to an excess (or greater activity) of sulphate-reducing bacteria (SRB), such as *Desulfovibrio desulfuricans*.[86] In a pilot study, a low sulphur diet for 12 months was associated with a remarkable clinical improvement in four patients with chronic ulcerative colitis.[87] A recent review concluded that there is evidence to implicate SRB in the pathogenesis of ulcerative colitis.[88]

As noted in a *Lancet* review: 'The long-standing assumption that ulcerative colitis is an autoimmune disease has been revised to incorporate evidence suggesting that commensal microflora and their products are autoantigens, and that ulcerative colitis is caused by loss of tolerance towards otherwise harmless components of the normal intestinal flora'.[89]

Hormonal factors

Hormonal factors in rheumatoid disease are well accepted. Risk factors include reduced childbearing and breastfeeding; these apparently contradictory influences are both associated with high prolactin levels.[90]

Several autoimmune diseases have been linked to higher levels of prolactin in the blood, including lupus,[91] RA,[92] Sjögren's syndrome[93] and juvenile arthritis.[94] For systemic lupus erythematosus (SLE), serum prolactin concentrations have been correlated with both clinical activity and remission.[91,95] On the other hand, preeclampsia and breast cancer have a negative association with rheumatic and other autoimmune diseases.[96]

Such links are confusing and even contradictory, but a defective response of the neuroendocrine system to inflammatory stimuli has been proposed as one feature of RA.[97]

Traditional approaches to inflammatory diseases

Anti-inflammatory remedies

The use of willow bark for rheumatism in traditional medicine is a reminder that where remedies clearly provided symptomatic relief, they were used. More recently, there has been a huge research effort to find new anti-inflammatory activities in the plant world. Many chemical subgroups from plants have shown promising experimental activity, including terpenoids and steroids, phenolics and flavonoids, fatty acids, polysaccharides and alkaloids.[98] Most of this work remains on the laboratory bench as interesting markers for the effect of the whole plant; the evidence is more persuasive when demonstrated in clinical trials. For long the potential benefit of sea buckthorn (*Hippophae rhamnoides*) for inflammatory conditions has been assumed on the basis of its high levels of antioxidants but reinforced by clinical trials.[99] Herbal remedies that have shown efficacy in clinical trials for osteoarthritis include *Harpagophytum procumbens* (devil's claw),[100] *Rosa canina* (rosehip),[101] *Uncaria tomentosa* (cats claw)[102] and *Boswellia serrata*. RA has also been relieved by Boswellia.[103] The benefits of *Tripterygium wilfordii* in the same condition were found to be associated with an in vitro suppression of antigen-stimulated T-cell production, immunoglobulin production by B-cells[104] and reduction of IL-2 production and activity.[105] However, while it is a promising intervention in inflammatory disorders, this herb is potentially toxic and has been associated with serious side effects.[106] The effect of the Chinese herbal formulation found effective in London trials in the treatment of atopic eczema has been shown to be associated with changes in a number of immunological functions, such as decreasing the higher levels of circulating IgE complexes and IL-2 receptors and vascular cell adhesion molecules in atopic eczema patients.[107]

Topical anti-inflammatory activity has been observed in clinical studies of *Matricaria recutita* (wild chamomile) in mucositis,[108] and *Melaleuca alternifolia* (tea tree) oil in histamine-induced skin inflammation.[109] (See earlier in this chapter regarding topical anti-inflammatory treatments.)

Counter-irritation

The most common application of counter-irritation was to inflamed arthritic joints and the technique is discussed further in the appropriate chapter (see p. 304). Nevertheless, the approach was also used for other subdermal inflammations, notably in pleurisy and other chest infections, mastitis and other cellulitis conditions. (A traditional treatment of mastitis and pleurisy involved making poultices with cabbage leaves, a relative of mustard.) Heating of inflammations was not always considered appropriate, however. As discussed below, some inflammatory diseases are excessively 'hot' and can react violently to additional heat. Some rheumatic joints can behave in this way.

Diet

One of the persistent dietary notions in European tradition in the case of degenerative diseases, particularly arthritis, has been the distinction between 'acid' and 'alkaline' foods. The view is that as metabolites tend to be acidic, as acid-buffering agents are a major constituent of the body fluids and as eliminatory channels (lungs, kidney, bile and bowel) pass mainly acidic materials, inflammatory diseases may be marked by, and even result from, greater acidosis. Overt metabolic acidosis is well characterised in medicine and may follow excessive alcohol consumption, laxative abuse, excessive vitamin D and NSAIDs (most often prescribed in arthritis) and salicylate use, among other drugs.[110] The case for a more subtle effect is considered further in the section on joint disease in Chapter 9. In addition to the prospects for therapy that could, for example, include diuretic herbal remedies, there are associated dietary observations that reinforce the potential for benefit in some chronic inflammatory diseases. There was, for example, a widespread traditional instinct in many inflammatory diseases to reduce animal protein, although chicken and other fowl were a common exception.

There is modern support for this approach in rheumatic diseases. A combination of fasting and vegetarian diets has been shown to reduce the ability of the urine to support the growth of *Proteus mirabilis* and *Escherichia coli*.[111] A substantial placebo-controlled trial has confirmed that gamma-linolenic acid, (GLA), a component mainly of plant-based foods, has antirheumatic activity.[112] The possibility of cross-reaction between dietary collagen found in animal products and the sufferer's connective tissue has also been postulated.[113,114] The effects of a low-starch diet in reducing the gut levels of anaerobic bacteria such as Klebsiella and serum IgA antibody levels in both normal subjects and those suffering ankylosing spondylitis, and in benefiting symptoms in the latter, have been supported by clinical evidence.[115] Nevertheless, the quality of the research on this issue is too limited to draw firm conclusions on the value of dietary changes on RA.[116]

Phytotherapeutics

The treatment of chronic inflammatory diseases is complex. Traditional strategies rely on the assessment of prevailing conditions within the body and generally incorporate the idea of change and adaptability in ongoing prescription.

In most traditions, inflammatory diseases of the joints, skin and other body tissues were viewed as compounded and deep-seated toxic conditions. It might have been explained that, whereas fevers, acute inflammations and infections were examples of noxious intrusions to which the body mounted a frank and usually successful defence (what modern medicine refers to as the 'self-limiting' condition), chronic problems indicated that the body had not 'repelled boarders' at first attack, had primary defences breached (like the digestive tract, skin and lymphatics: the 'reticuloendothelial' phagocytic wing of the immune response) and had allowed toxic pathogenic influences to penetrate and disturb deeper functions. Treatment often therefore involved characterising the toxicity and constructing the best strategy to help the body better eliminate it. There were many strategies and in the best practice these were tailored to individual circumstances, but certain remedies were more popular for joint and skin diseases than others. These are listed below.

In certain traditions, diagnosis might include assessing the extent of the following characteristics of the disease process; in most cases more than one of which was likely to occur. These are based very much on insights from traditional Chinese medicine and particular Chinese remedies can be readily allocated to each category or blend of categories. Western herbal medicine is less systematised and no such classification of treatments can reliably be made. However, it is most likely that in practice intuitive assessments would resemble what follows.

Damp (the presence of tissue congestion or chronic infection)

Damp was the universal metaphor for toxic congestion, recalling the notions of stagnation, brackishness and mould. As expected, it tended to occur in conditions of poor circulation, most often associated with cold but with a hot 'humid' variant as well. Damp is exacerbated and to some extent caused by external climatic dampness (as the Romans noted, a feature of Britain and the Britons). Associated with cold, it tends to gravitate to the lower regions of the body and can be associated with sluggish digestion and congested abdomen. Associated with heat, it involves the liver, with intolerance to fats, rich food and alcohol and perhaps a history of jaundice/hepatitis. Naturally, it would need treatment with 'drying' remedies: warming aromatics for cold-damp and bitters for hot-damp conditions.

Wind (the degree of fluctuation)

The tendency of rheumatic and some skin problems to fluctuate and move rapidly around the body was obvious. Chinese medicine in particular invoked the universal metaphor of change, wind, to characterise this phenomenon. Wind of course occurs with the juxtaposition of hot and cold and implies that there was similar imbalance within the body. Apart from the fluctuation of symptoms, signs of wind might include, when deep seated (a common occurrence in rheumatic disease) wandering, sudden pains in joints. In Chinese medicine, there were a number of remedies specifically reputed to calm the wind but the deeper view might be that attendance to the underlying imbalances of hot and cold would be the more lasting strategy.

Heat (the violence of the inflammatory reaction and extent of immunological hypersensitivities)

As the obvious vital sign, heat was seen as a mark of vigorous defence (as in fever and inflammation) and in its place was even encouraged. When stuck, however, or marked by destructive symptoms like allergic reactions or eczema, it signified blocked poisons which needed clearing, perhaps with local cooling as well. When coupled with dryness, there would be respiratory symptoms like asthma, allergic rhinitis or hayfever, dry eczema and/or constipation; when coupled with damp, the liver and digestion would be involved as above. It might also be localised to an organ like the lungs or kidneys or to some other part of the body. Heat was often diagnosed on the basis of simple palpation or by the presence of flushing, and a preference for cool drinks, cool weather or cold applications. The tongue might be more red in colour, with less saliva (if associated with dryness) or with a coloured coating (if associated with damp). A range of cooling remedies were used to help clear such hot spots and help with a wider strategy to improve circulation.

Cold (the degree of circulatory, immune and other debility)

Cold is the symptom of diminished vitality and death and marks a condition where the metabolic furnace has faltered, either generally or locally. The patient would prefer heat, in food and drink or as hot applications, abhor cold and might be listless, pale and withdrawn. The tongue might be pale and wet and (if associated with damp) the coating would be white. As long as debility was not too extreme, heating remedies like the spices were indicated either systemically or as hot topical applications.

The modern concepts of immunological diseases as disturbed responses to infection or disrupted gut barriers entirely accord with the intuitive and systematised traditional focus on toxicities. In the particular remedies below, their relevant properties are also listed. Not all plants are ascribed temperaments like warming or drying: some, like diuretics and astringents, were considered to have neutral temperaments; in other cases some Western herbs have no consistent tradition that would allow these qualities to be safely ascribed.

Plants with anti-infective properties

* *Allium sativum* (garlic): heating, disinfectant, especially in lungs and gut
* *Berberis vulgaris* (barberry): cooling and drying
* *Echinacea spp.* (Echinacea): warming and promoting defences, particularly of throat and upper gut wall; this applies specifically to the root

- *Hypericum perforatum* (St John's wort): restorative tonic with potential antiviral support (enveloped viruses only)
- *Lavandula spp.* (lavender): topically warming and antiseptic
- *Thuja occidentalis* (arbor-vitae): warming and stimulating, with potential antiviral support (all viruses)
- *Andrographis paniculata*: cooling and drying, to clear heat and eliminate toxins, especially in respiratory and digestive infections.

Plants with eliminative properties

- *Apium graveolens* (celery): diuretic and eliminating acidic metabolites through the kidneys, particularly used in arthritic disease
- *Arctium lappa* (burdock): general eliminative particularly popular in skin disease
- *Arctostaphylos uva-ursi* (bearberry): diuretic and urinary antiseptic, most likely to be applied in arthritic disease (often to be recommended in ankylosing spondylitis, but more for the latter property)
- *Betula spp.* (birch): diuretic, particularly useful in arthritic disease and where inflammation leads to calcification
- *Berberis aquifolium* (Oregon grape): cooling and drying, cholagogue and popular in treating skin disease
- *Fumaria officinalis* (common fumitory): cholagogue, popular in treating skin disease
- *Galium aparine* (cleavers): diuretic and lymphatic, and used particularly in skin disease
- *Gaultheria procumbens* (wintergreen): topically warming and used over inflammations
- *Inula helenium* (elecampane): warming and aiding elimination (expectoration) from the lungs
- *Juglans nigra* (walnut bark): general alterative and laxative remedy
- *Rumex crispus* (yellow dock): cooling and drying with mild aperient properties for helping bile and bowel elimination
- *Scrophularia nodosa* (figwort): warming and generally eliminative, traditionally for aggressive skin disease
- *Solidago spp.* (goldenrod): traditional diuretic used for skin and sinus conditions, with some anti-inflammatory properties
- *Taraxacum officinale* (dandelion root): cooling and drying with cholagogue and diuretic properties, popularly combined with Apium for arthritic disease and as a remedy in skin disease
- *Trifolium pratense* (red clover): lymphatic and expectorant, used in skin and joint disease
- *Urtica dioica* (nettle leaf): warming and nutritive taken internally, popular in skin and joint disease.

Plants with digestive anti-inflammatory properties

A large number of remedies are effective for intestinal wall problems (see p. 156). The following are immediately obvious options in arthritic, skin and other chronic inflammatory diseases:

- *Aloe vera* (aloe juice): reducing digestive wall inflammation
- *Calendula officinalis* (marigold): lymphatic and reducing inflammation in the throat and stomach

- *Dioscorea villosa* (wild yam): antispasmodic and anti-inflammatory on lower gut wall, possibly steroidal effect systemically
- *Filipendula ulmaria* (meadowsweet): demulcent and astringent effect on stomach wall overwhelming low levels of salicylates
- *Hamamelis virginiana* (witchhazel): astringent throughout the digestive tract
- *Matricaria recutita*: cooling and reducing inflammatory damage in the upper digestive tract, especially bisabolol chemotypes
- *Myrica cerifera* (bayberry): warming and astringent, traditionally used in fever management associated with diarrhoea and dysentery
- *Symphytum officinale* (comfrey leaf): potent healing effects on gut wall, to be used only in the short term
- *Ulmus rubra* (slippery elm): mucilaginous and healing on the upper digestive tract, best used as an early stage of, and preparatory to, wider treatment.

Plants with hormonal properties

Many herbs are rich in stigmasterol and other potentially anti-inflammatory phytosterols, or saponins with anti-inflammatory activity. Some also have reputations for hormone balancing and all those below have a traditional reputation in the treatment of inflammatory diseases:

- *Aesculus hippocastanum* (Horsechestnut seed): particularly useful where inflammation leads to oedema and swelling that interferes with other structures or causes compression syndromes (see monograph)
- *Bupleurum falcatum* (Bupleurum): (see monograph)
- *Cimicifuga racemosa* (black cohosh): has a reputation for arthritis, especially small joint osteoarthritis
- *Pfaffia paniculata* (Brazilian ginseng)
- *Rehmannia glutinosa* (Rehmannia): a useful adrenal tonic and anti-inflammatory in autoimmune diseases (see monograph)
- *Smilax spp.* (sarsaparilla)

Plants with general anti-inflammatory properties

The traditional herbal approach includes anti-inflammatories in the modern medical sense (like NSAIDs). These remedies are, perhaps with a few exceptions, less clinically powerful than modern drugs and are most useful as adjuncts to the therapeutic measures listed above:

- *Boswellia serrata* (Boswellia): a herb that appears to possess a broad range of anti-inflammatory effects (see monograph)
- *Curcuma longa* (turmeric): like Boswellia, a very broad acting anti-inflammatory (see monograph)
- *Fraxinus excelsior* (ash): moderate anti-inflammatory containing coumarins that inhibit T-cells and prostaglandin biosynthesis[117]
- *Guaiacum spp.* (lignum vitae): traditional reputation in arthritic diseases; however, is now an endangered species
- *Harpagophytum procumbens* (devil's claw): mild anti-inflammatory effects (see monograph)

- *Menyanthes trifoliata* (bogbean): a bitter and hepatic remedy applied to rheumatic conditions where such effects are useful
- *Populus spp.* (poplar bark): containing salicylates with established anti-inflammatory properties[117]
- *Salix spp.* (willow bark): the original source of salicylates and with a strong traditional reputation as an antirheumatic, now supported by clinical trials (see monograph)
- *Tanacetum parthenium* (feverfew): potential anti-inflammatory properties (see monograph)
- *Zingiber officinale* (ginger): mild anti-inflammatory effects (see m onograph)

Contraindications for anti-inflammatory remedies

The use of anti-inflammatory herbs is inappropriate when there is already prescription of strong anti-inflammatory medication, unless they are acting by a different mechanism to the drug and/or are aimed to gradually replace the drug.

Traditional therapeutic insights into the use of treatments for inflammatory diseases

Faced with a highly complex condition like a chronic inflammatory disease, the traditional practitioner might of course proceed entirely intuitively to clear the obstacles, using remedies such as the above in their own favoured ways. However, where strategies are systematised, notably in the Chinese tradition, a consistent pattern emerges. There is an almost geological approach. Pathogenic influences are envisaged as penetrating to different strata of the body, becoming more disturbed, disruptive and persistent the deeper they go. In chronic inflammations, by definition, the pathologies are deeply rooted and very intermingled. Looking for a way to disentangle the complexity, the traditional approach was often compared with peeling the layers of an onion, starting from the outside. Any opportunity to use effective 'superficial' eliminative measures would be taken up.

- A cold or fever, provided it could be managed within the patient's often-diminished reserves, could lead to an effective clearing of burdens by mobilising the phagocytic defences. The occurrence of any such event would lead the practitioner to uswitch treatment rapidly and deal with the acute indications intensively until resolved (see also pp. 146–148).

- Primary eliminatory routes would be an early therapeutic focus; diuretics, aperients, depuratives and cholagogues are especially likely to be used, as indicated in the individual's story. These might be step-like interventions, each pursued briefly for particular medium-term goals.
- The gut wall was always a priority zone. Dietary approaches would usually be combined with treatments to enhance the digestive process, like bitters or warming aromatic digestives as required, or remedies with anti-inflammatory or healing effects on the wall itself. For example, one strategy might be to start or rotate a course of treatment with a demulcent remedy like slippery elm.

Chronic inflammatory diseases are often, almost by definition, accompanied by compromised defences and reduced vigour and there may be hot spots of relatively violent inflammations, for example rheumatic joints or skin eruptions. It is thus possible that treatments may be unduly provocative and exacerbations may occur. Contrary to some popular opinion ('Things must get worse before they get better'), these 'healing crises' are rarely a good idea; indeed, they may worsen the condition in the long term. (Therapeutic exacerbations may be justified under carefully controlled conditions to expedite a blocked inflammation or fever but only when the patient is in a sufficiently robust state and the inflammation concerned is relatively simple.) Thus a good practitioner will peel the onion layers with care, only proceeding at a pace the body can stand, avoiding unnecessary exacerbation (for example with remedies that are too heating or cooling or with too strong an eliminative effect) and using remedies that calm and soothe. The practitioner will often take special care to apply strategies that aid recuperation and restoration of a robust and balanced immune system. This may mean, for example, adopting convalescent dietary principles (see p. 87) and combining these with appropriate digestive or hepatic remedies.

Application

Anti-inflammatory remedies are best taken before or, if there is any stomach irritation, after meals.

Long-term therapy with anti-inflammatory remedies is usually acceptable, although this should be kept under review.

Although the conditions involved are sometimes very complex there should still be early endpoints to aim for. The obvious is relief of the symptoms, but there may be stages along the way as well.

References

1. Bevilacqua MP. Endothelial-leukocyte cellular adhesion molecules. *Ann Rev Immunol.* 1993;11:767–804.
2. Panza JA, Quyyumi AA, Brush JE, et al. Abnormal endothelium-dependent vascular relaxation in patients with essential hypertension. *N Engl J Med.* 1990;323:22–27.
3. Achike F, Kwan C. Nitric oxide, human diseases and the herbal products that affect the nitric oxide signalling pathway.

Clin Exp Pharmacol Physiol. 2003;30:605–615.
4. Aggarwal BB, Van Kuiken ME, Iyer LH, et al. Molecular targets of nutraceuticals derived from dietary spices: potential role in suppression of inflammation and tumorigenesis. *Exp Biol Med.* 2009;234(8):825–849.
5. Ghayur MN, Gilani AH, Afridi MB, et al. Cardiovascular effects of ginger aqueous extract and its phenolic constituents are

mediated through multiple pathways. *Vasc Pharmacol.* 2005;43:234–241.
6. Yanaga A, Goto H, Nakagawa T, et al. Cinnamaldehyde induces endothelium-dependent and -independent vasorelaxant action on isolated rat aorta. *Biol Pharm Bull.* 2006;29(12):2415–2418.
7. Goto H, Sasaki Y, Fushimi H, et al. Effect of curcuma herbs on vasomotion and hemorheology in spontaneously

hypertensive rat. *Am J Chin Med.* 2005;33(3):449–457.

8. Williams M, Sutherland W, McCormick M, et al. Aged garlic extract improves endothelial function in men with coronary artery disease. *Phytother Res.* 2005;19:314–319.

9. Pajonk F, Riedisser A, Henke M, et al. The effects of tea extracts on proinflammatory signaling. *BMC Med.* 2006;28:1–12.

10. Steptoe A, Gibson EL, Vuononvirta R, et al. The effects of chronic tea intake on platelet activation and inflammation: a double blind placebo controlled trial. *Atherosclerosis.* 2007;193:262–277.

11. Kempf K, Herder C, Erlund I, et al. Effects of coffee consumption on subclinical inflammation and other risk factors for type 2 diabetes: a clinical trial. *Am J Clin Nutr.* 2010;91:950–957.

12. Grassi D, Necozione S, Lippi C, et al. Cocoa reduces blood pressure and insulin resistance and improves endothelium-dependent vasodilation in hypertensives. *Hypertension.* 2005;46:398–405.

13. di Giuseppe R, Di Castelnuovo A, Centritto F, et al. Regular consumption of dark chocolate is associated with low serum concentrations of C-reactive protein in a healthy Italian population. *J Nutr.* 2008;138:1939–1945.

14. Taylor P, Noriega R, Farah C, et al. Ajoene inhibits both primary tumor growth and metastasis of B16/BL6 melanoma cells in C57BL/6 mice. *Cancer Lett.* 2006;239:298–304.

15. Lang A, Lahav M, Sakhnini E, et al. Allicin inhibits spontaneous and TNF-alpha induced secretion of proinflammatory cytokines and chemokines from intestinal epithelial cells. *Clin Nutr.* 2004;23:1199–1208.

16. Woo HM, Kang JH, Kawada T, et al. Active spice-derived components can inhibit inflammatory responses of adipose tissue in obesity by suppressing inflammatory actions of macrophages and release of monocyte chemoattractant protein-1 from adipocytes. *Life Sci.* 2007;80:926–931.

17. Chainy GB, Manna SK, Chaturvedi MM, et al. Anethole blocks both early and late cellular responses transduced by tumor necrosis factor: effect on NF-kappaB, AP-1, JNK, MAPKK and apoptosis. *Oncogene.* 2000;19:2943–2950.

18. Kowalski J, Samojedny A, Paul M, et al. Effect of apigenin, kaempferol and resveratrol on the expression of interleukin-1beta and tumor necrosis factor-alpha genes in J774.2 macrophages. *Pharmacol Rep.* 2005;57:390–394.

19. Bhutani M, Pathak AK, Nair AS, et al. Capsaicin is a novel blocker of constitutive and interleukin-6-inducible STAT3 activation. *Clin Cancer Res.* 2007;13:3024–3032.

20. Lo AH, Liang YC, Lin-Shiau SY, et al. Carnosol, an antioxidant in rosemary, suppresses inducible nitric oxide synthase through down-regulating nuclear factor-kappaB in mouse macrophages. *Carcinogenesis.* 2002;23:983–991.

21. Medeiros R, Passos GF, Vitor CE, et al. Effect of two active compounds obtained from the essential oil of Cordia verbenacea on the acute inflammatory responses elicited by LPS in the rat paw. *Br J Pharmacol.* 2007;151:618–627.

22. Kim DH, Kim CH, Kim MS, et al. Suppression of age-related inflammatory NF-kappaB activation by cinnamaldehyde. *Biogerontology.* 2007;8:545–554.

23. Marin YE, Wall BA, Wang S, et al. Curcumin downregulates the constitutive activity of NF-kappaB and induces apoptosis in novel mouse melanoma cells. *Melanoma Res.* 2007;17:274–283.

24. Thejass P, Kuttan G. Antiangiogenic activity of iallyl sulfide (DAS). *Int Immunopharmacol.* 2007;7:295–305.

25. Lee YY, Hung SL, Pai SF, et al. Eugenol suppressed the expression of lipopolysaccharide-induced proinflammatory mediators in human macrophages. *J Endod.* 2007;33:698–702.

26. Tripathi S, Maier KG, Bruch D, et al. Effect of 6-gingerol on pro-inflammatory cytokine production and costimulatory molecule expression in murine peritoneal macrophages. *J Surg Res.* 2007;138:209–213.

27. Souza MC, Siani AC, Ramos MF, et al. Evaluation of anti-inflammatory activity of essential oils from two Asteraceae species. *Pharmazie.* 2003;58:582–586.

28. Berchtold CM, Chen KS, Miyamoto S, et al. Perillyl alcohol inhibits a calcium-dependent constitutive nuclear factor-kappaB pathway. *Cancer Res.* 2005;65:8558–8566.

29. Weglarz L, Wawszczyk J, Orchel A, et al. Phytic acid modulates in vitro IL-8 and IL-6 release from colonic epithelial cells stimulated with LPS and IL-1beta. *Dig Dis Sci.* 2007;52:93–102.

30. Pradeep CR, Kuttan G. Piperine is a potent inhibitor of nuclear factor-kappaB (NF-kappaB), c-Fos, CREB, ATF-2 and proinflammatory cytokine gene expression in B16F-10 melanoma cells. *Int Immunopharmacol.* 2004;4:1795–1803.

31. Min YD, Choi CH, Bark H, et al. Quercetin inhibits expression of inflammatory cytokines through attenuation of NF-kappaB and p38 MAPK in HMC-1 human mast cell line. *Inflamm Res.* 2007;56:210–215.

32. Manjeet KR, Ghosh B. Quercetin inhibits LPS-induced nitric oxide and tumor necrosis factor-alpha production in murine macrophages. *Int J Immunopharmacol.* 1999;21:435–443.

33. Shishodia S, Majumdar S, Banerjee S, et al. Ursolic acid inhibits nuclear factor-kappaB activation induced by carcinogenic agents through suppression of IkappaBalpha kinase and p65 phosphorylation: correlation with down-regulation of cyclooxygenase 2, matrix metalloproteinase 9, and cyclin D1. *Cancer Res.* 2003;63:4375–4383.

34. Woo HM, Kang JH, Kawada T, et al. Active spice-derived components can inhibit inflammatory responses of adipose tissue in obesity by suppressing inflammatory actions of macrophages and release of monocyte chemoattractant protein-1 from adipocytes. *Life Sci.* 2007;80:926–931.

35. Mo SJ, Son EW, Rhee DK, et al. Modulation of TNF-alpha-induced ICAM-1 expression, NO and H2O2 production by alginate, allicin and ascorbic acid in human endothelial cells. *Arch Pharm Res.* 2003;26:244–251.

36. Hwang ES, Lee HJ. Allyl isothiocyanate and its N-acetylcysteine conjugate suppress metastasis via inhibition of invasion, migration, and matrix metalloproteinase-2/-9 activities in SK-Hep 1 human hepatoma cells. *Exp Biol Med (Maywood).* 2006;231:421–430.

37. Chen CC, Chow MP, Huang WC, et al. Flavonoids inhibit tumor necrosis factor-alpha-induced up-regulation of intercellular adhesion molecule-1 (ICAM-1) in respiratory epithelial cells through activator protein-1 and nuclear factor-kappaB: structure-activity relationships. *Mol Pharmacol.* 2004;66:683–693.

38. Park WH, Kim SH, Kim CH. A new matrix metalloproteinase-9 inhibitor 3,4-dihydroxycinnamic acid (caffeic acid) from methanol extract of Euonymus alatus: isolation and structure determination. *Toxicology.* 2005;207:383–390.

39. Mitra A, Chakrabarti J, Banerji A, et al. Curcumin, a potential inhibitor of MMP-2 in human laryngeal squamous carcinoma cells HEp2. *J Environ Pathol Toxicol Oncol.* 2006;25:679–690.

40. Lee HS, Seo EY, Kang NE, et al. [6]-Gingerol inhibits metastasis of MDA-MB-231 human breast cancer cells. *J Nutr Biochem.* 2008;19:313–319.

41. Ko CH, Shen SC, Lee TJ, et al. Myricetin inhibits matrix metalloproteinase 2 protein expression and enzyme activity in colorectal carcinoma cells. *Mol Cancer Ther.* 2005;4:281–290.

42. Vijayababu MR, Arunkumar A, Kanagaraj P, et al. Quercetin downregulates matrix metalloproteinases 2 and 9 proteins expression in prostate cancer cells (PC-3). *Mol Cell Biochem.* 2006;287:109–116.

43. Venkatesha SH, Berman BM, Moudgil KD. Herbal medicinal products target defined biochemical and molecular mediators of inflammatory autoimmune arthritis. *Bioorg Med Chem.* 2011;19(1):21–29.

44. Anonymous Respiratory complications of rheumatoid disease [editorial]. *BMJ.* 1978;6125:1437–1438.

45. Krause A, Kamradt T, Burmester GR. Potential infectious agents in the induction of arthritides. *Curr Opin Rheumatol.* 1996;8(3):203–209.

46. Aoki S, Yoshikawa K, Yokoyama T, et al. Role of enteric bacteria in the pathogenesis of rheumatoid arthritis: evidence for antibodies to enterobacterial common antigens in rheumatoid sera and synovial fluids. *Ann Rheum Dis.* 1996;55(6):363–369.

47. Eerola E, Mottonen T, Hannonen P, et al. Intestinal flora in early rheumatoid arthritis. *Br J Rheumatol.* 1994;33(11):1030–1038.

48. Melief MJ, Hoijer MA, Van Paassen HC, et al. Presence of bacterial flora-derived antigen in synovial tissue macrophages and dendritic cells. *Br J Rheumatol.* 1995;34(12):1112–1116.

49. Amital H, Govoni M, Maya R, et al. Role of infectious agents in systemic rheumatic diseases. *Clin Exp Rheumatol.* 2008;26(1 suppl 48):27–32.

50. Rashid T, Ebringer A. Ankylosing spondylitis is linked to Klebsiella – the evidence. *Clin Rheumatol.* 2007;26(6):858–864.

51. Tiwana H, Wilson C, Cunningham P, et al. Antibodies to four gram-negative bacteria in rheumatoid arthritis which share sequences with the rheumatoid arthritis susceptibility motif. *Br J Rheumatol.* 1996;35(6):592–594.

52. Ebringer A, Rashid T. B27 disease is a new autoimmune disease that affects millions of people. *Ann NY Acad Sci.* 2007;1110:112–120.

53. Ogrendik M. Rheumatoid arthritis is linked to oral bacteria: etiological association. *Mod Rheumatol.* 2009;19(5):453–456.

54. Lundberg K, Wegner N, Yucel-Lindberg T, et al. Periodontitis in RA – the citrullinated enolase connection. *Nat Rev Rheumatol.* 2010;6(12):727–730.

55. Ebringer A, Rashid T. Rheumatoid arthritis is an autoimmune disease triggered by Proteus urinary tract infection. *Clin Dev Immunol.* 2006;13(1):41–48.

56. Albani S, Carson DA. A multistep molecular mimicry hypothesis for the pathogenesis of rheumatoid arthritis. *Immunol Today.* 1996;17(10):466–470.

57. Firestein GS. Evolving concepts of rheumatoid arthritis. *Nature.* 2003;423(6927):356–361.

58. Mason RM, Murray RS, Oates JK, et al. Prostatitis and ankylosing spondylitis. *Br Med J.* 1958;1(5073):748–751.

59. Mason RM, Murray RS, Oates JK, et al. Prostatitis and ankylosing spondylitis. *Rheum Phys Med.* 1971;1:78.

60. Lange U, Teichmann J. Ankylosing spondylitis and genitourinary infection. *Eur J Med Res.* 1999;4(1):1–7.

61. Chiodini RJ, Van Kruiningen HJ, Thayer WR, et al. Possible role of mycobacteria in inflammatory bowel disease. I. An unclassified Mycobacterium species isolated from patients with Crohn's disease. *Dig Dis Sci.* 1984;29(12):1073–1079.

62. Greenstein RJ, Collins MT. Emerging pathogens: is Mycobacterium avium subspecies paratuberculosis zoonotic? *Lancet.* 2004;364(9432):396–397.

63. Rashid T, Ebringer A, Tiwana H, et al. Role of Klebsiella and collagens in Crohn's disease: a new prospect in the use of low-starch diet. *Eur J Gastroenterol Hepatol.* 2009;21(8):843–849.

64. Chamberlin W, Graham DY, Hulten K, et al. Review article: mycobacterium avium subsp. paratuberculosis as one cause of Crohn's disease. *Aliment Pharmacol Ther.* 2001;15(3):337–346.

65. Balandraud N, Roudier J, Roudier C. Epstein-Barr virus and rheumatoid arthritis. *Autoimmun Rev.* 2004;3(5):362–367.

66. Farmer GW, Vincent MM, Fuccillo DA, et al. Viral investigations in ulcerative colitis and regional enteritis. *Gastroenterology.* 1973;65(1):8–18.

67. Diepersloot RJ, Kroes AC, Visser W, et al. Acute ulcerative proctocolitis associated with primary cytomegalovirus infection. *Arch Intern Med.* 1990;150(8):1749–1751.

68. Lortholary O, et al. Primary cytomegalovirus infection associated with the onset of ulcerative colitis. *Eur J Clin Microbiol Infect Dis.* 1993;12(7):570–571.

69. Wakefield AJ, Fox JD, Sawyerr AM, et al. Detection of herpesvirus DNA in the large intestine of patients with ulcerative colitis and Crohn's disease using the nested polymerase chain reaction. *J Med Virol.* 1992;38(3):183–190.

70. Hommes DW, Sterringa G, van Deventer SJ, et al. The pathogenicity of cytomegalovirus in inflammatory bowel disease: a systematic review and evidence-based recommendations for future research. *Inflamm Bowel Dis.* 2004;10(3):245–250.

71. Mielants H, Veys EM. Significance of intestinal inflammation in the pathogenesis of spondylarthropathies. *Verh K Acad Geneeskd Belg.* 1996;58(2):93–116.

72. Mielants H, Veys EM, De Vos M, et al. The evolution of spondyloarthropathies in relation to gut histology. I. Clinical aspects. *J Rheumatol.* 1995;22(12):2266–2272.

73. De Keyser F, Mielants H. The gut in ankylosing spondylitis and other spondyloarthropathies: inflammation beneath the surface. *J Rheumatol.* 2003;30(11):2306–2307.

74. Altomonte L, Zoli A, Veneziani A, et al. Clinically silent inflammatory gut lesions in undifferentiated spondyloarthropathies. *Clin Rheumatol.* 1994;13(4):565–570.

75. Jacques P, Mielants H, Coppieters K, et al. The intimate relationship between gut and joint in spondyloarthropathies. *Curr Opin Rheumatol.* 2007;19(4):353–357.

76. Mielants H, De Keyser F, Baeten D, et al. Gut inflammation in the spondyloarthropathies. *Curr Rheumatol Rep.* 2005;7(3):188–194.

77. Nissila M, Lahesmaa R, Leirisalo-Repo M, et al. Antibodies to Klebsiella pneumoniae, Escherichia coli, and Proteus mirabilis in ankylosing spondylitis: effect of sulfasalazine treatment. *J Rheumatol.* 1994;21(11):2082–2087.

78. Burke DA, Axon AT. Adhesive Escherichia coli in inflammatory bowel disease and infective diarrhoea. *BMJ.* 1988;297(6641):102–104.

79. Darfeuille-Michaud A, Boudeau J, Bulois P, et al. High prevalence of adherent-invasive Escherichia coli associated with ileal mucosa in Crohn's disease. *Gastroenterology.* 2004;127(2):412–421.

80. Mow W, Vasiliauskas EA, Lin YC, et al. Association of antibody responses to microbial antigens and complications of small bowel Crohn's disease. *Gastroenterology.* 2004;126(2):414–424.

81. Darfeuille-Michaud A. Adherent-invasive Escherichia coli: a putative new E. coli pathotype associated with Crohn's disease. *Int J Med Microbiol.* 2002;292(3–4):185–193.

82. Olusanya O, Steinrück H, Aleljung P, et al. Surface properties, connective tissue protein binding and Shiga-like toxin production of Escherichia coli isolated from patients with ulcerative colitis. *Zentralbl Bakteriol.* 1992;276(2):254–263.

83. Cummings JH, Macfarlane GT, Macfarlane S. Intestinal bacteria and ulcerative colitis. *Curr Issues Intest Microbiol.* 2003;4(1):9–20.

84. Bullock NR, Booth JC, Gibson GR. Comparative composition of bacteria in the human intestinal microflora during remission and active ulcerative colitis. *Curr Issues Intest Microbiol.* 2004;5(2):59–64.

85. Ott SJ, Plamondon S, Hart A, et al. Dynamics of the mucosa-associated flora in ulcerative colitis patients during remission and clinical relapse. *J Clin Microbiol.* 2008;46(10):3510–3513.

86. Campieri M, Gionchetti P. Bacteria as the cause of ulcerative colitis. *Gut.* 2001;48(1):132–135.

87. Roediger WE. Decreased sulphur aminoacid intake in ulcerative colitis. *Lancet.* 1998;351(9115):1555.

88. Rowan FE, Docherty NG, Coffey JC, et al. Sulphate-reducing bacteria and hydrogen sulphide in the aetiology of ulcerative colitis. *Br J Surg.* 2009;96(2):151–158.

89. Farrell RJ, Peppercorn MA. Ulcerative colitis. *Lancet.* 2002;359(9303):331–340.

90. Fojtíková M, Tomasová Studýnková J, Filková M, et al. Elevated prolactin levels in patients with rheumatoid arthritis: association with disease activity and structural damage. *Clin Exp Rheumatol.* 2010;28(6):849–854.

91. Vera-Lastra O, Mendez C, Jara LJ, et al. Correlation of prolactin serum concentrations with clinical activity and remission in patients with systemic lupus erythematosus. Effect of conventional treatment. *J Rheumatol.* 2003;30(10):2140–2146.

92. Ram S, Blumberg D, Newton P, et al. Raised serum prolactin in rheumatoid arthritis: genuine or laboratory artefact? *Rheumatology (Oxford).* 2004;43(10):1272–1274.

93. El Meidany YM, Ahmed I, Mooustafa H, et al. Hyperprolactinemia in Sjogren's syndrome: a patient subset or a disease manifestation? *Joint Bone Spine*. 2004;71(3):203–208.

94. Picco P, Gattorno M, Buoncompagni A, et al. Interactions between prolactin and the proinflammatory cytokine network in juvenile chronic arthritis. *Ann N Y Acad Sci*. 1999;876:262–265.

95. Pacilio M, Migliaresi S, Meli R, et al. Elevated bioactive prolactin levels in systemic lupus erythematosus – association with disease activity. *J Rheumatol*. 2001;28(10):2216–2221.

96. Polednak AP. Pre-eclampsia, autoimmune disease and breast cancer etiology. *Med Hypotheses*. 1995;44(5):414–418.

97. Panayi GS. Hormonal control of rheumatoid inflammation. *Br Med Bull*. 1995;51(2):462–471.

98. Bingol F, Sener B. A review of terrestrial plants and marine organisms having antiinflammatory activity. *Int J Pharmacog*. 1995;33(2):81–97.

99. Larmo P, Alin J, Salminen E, et al. Effects of sea buckthorn berries on infections and inflammation: a double blind, randomized, placebo-controlled trial. *Eur J Clin Nutr*. 2008;62(9):1123–1130.

100. Grant L, McBean DE, Fyfe L, et al. A review of the biological and potential therapeutic actions of Harpagophytum procumbens. *Phytother Res*. 2007;21(3):199–209.

101. Winther K, Apel K, Thamsborg G. A powder made from seeds and shells of a rose hip subspecies (Rosa canina) reduces symptoms of knee and hip osteoarthritis: a randomized, double blind, placebo-controlled trial. *Scand J Rheumatol*. 2005;34:302–308.

102. Hardin S. Cat's claw: an Amazonian vine decreases inflammation in osteoarthritis. *Complement Ther Clin Pract*. 2007;13:25–28.

103. Etzel R. Special extract of Boswellia serrata (H 15) in the treatment of rheumatoid arthritis. *Phytomedicine*. 1996;3(1):91–94.

104. Tao X, Davis LS, Lipsky PE. Effect of an extract of the Chinese herbal remedy Tripterygium wilfordii Hook F on human immune responsiveness. *Arthritis Rheum*. 1991;34(10):1274–1281.

105. Li XW, Weir MR. Radix Tripterygium wilfordii – a Chinese herbal medicine with potent immunosuppressive properties. *Transplantation*. 1990;50(1):82–86.

106. Cameron M, Gagnier JJ, Chrubasik S. Herbal therapy for treating rheumatoid arthritis. *Cochrane Database Syst Rev*. 2011;2:CD002948.

107. Latchman Y, Banerjee P, Poulter LW, et al. Association of immunological changes with clinical efficacy in atopic eczema patients treated with traditional Chinese herbal therapy (Zemaphyte). *Int Arch Allergy Immunol*. 1996;109(3):243–249.

108. Mazokopakis EE, Vrentzos GE, Papadakis JA, et al. Wild chamomile (Matricaria recutita L.) mouthwashes in methotrexate-induced oral mucositis. *Phytomedicine*. 2005;12:25–27.

109. Koh K, Pearce Marshman G, et al. Tea tree oil reduces histamine-induced skin inflammation. *Br J Dermatol*. 2002;147:1212–1217.

110. Fukuhara Y, Kaneko T, Orita Y. Drug-induced acid-base disorders. *Nippon Rinsho*. 1992;50(9):2231–2236.

111. Kjeldsen-Kragh J, Kvaavik E, Bottolfs M, et al. Inhibition of growth of Proteus mirabilis and Escherichia coli in urine in response to fasting and vegetarian diet. *APMIS*. 1995;103(11):818–822.

112. Zurier RB, Rosetti EW, Jacobsen DM, et al. Gamma-linolenic acid treatment of rheumatoid arthritis: a randomised placebo-controlled trial. *Arthritis Rheum*. 1996;39(11):1808–1817.

113. Terato K, DeArmey DA, Ye XJ, et al. The mechanism of autoantibody formation to cartilage in rheumatoid arthritis: possible cross-reaction of antibodies to dietary collagens with autologous type II collagen. *Clin Immunol Immunopathol*. 1996;79(2):142–154.

114. Mitchison A, Sieper J. Immunological basis of oral tolerance. *Z Rheumatol*. 1994;54(3):141–144.

115. Ebringer A, Wilson C. The use of a low starch diet in the treatment of patients suffering from ankylosing spondylitis. *Clin Rheumatol*. 1996;15(suppl 1):62–66.

116. Hagen KB, Byfuglien MG, Falzon L, et al. Dietary interventions for rheumatoid arthritis. *Cochrane Database Syst Rev*. 2009;21(1):CD006400.

117. Von Kruedener S, Schneider W, Elstner EF. A combination of populus tremula, Solidago virgaurea and Fraxinus excelsior as an anti-inflammatory and antirheumatic drug. A short review. *Arzneimittelforschung*. 1995;45(2):169–171.

Fatigue and debility

Scope

Apart from their use to provide non-specific support for recuperation and repair, specific phytotherapeutic strategies include the following.

Treatment of:

- chronic fatigue syndrome and related conditions such as fibromyalgia
- fatigue and debility after illness, prolonged stress, injury or trauma (convalescence).

Management of:

- fatigue linked to clinical depression
- fatigue due to untreatable or terminal illness.

Because of the use of secondary plant products, **caution** is necessary in applying phytotherapy in cases of:

- severe digestive depletion
- renal or hepatic failure.

Orientation

A debilitating symptom

Phytotherapists increasingly find that a major indication for treatment is a degenerative or debilitating illness. Unlike their forebears, for whom acute diseases were the norm and recuperative support of debility was usually convalescent aftercare, the modern practitioner will be less often involved in first-line treatment. Patients will more often report for help after years of ill health or when conventional medicine has run out of options.

There are many diseases that can lead to such signs of debility as tiredness, inability to rest, weakness, depression, wasting and anorexia. Indeed, any illness of sufficient duration or severity can lead to such symptoms; chronic low-grade infections, especially viral infections, are particular precursors in modern times. In some cases severe or traumatic diseases from the distant past can lead to a legacy of weaknesses of this type. A few are constitutionally enfeebled and are prone to debilitating responses to a range of stressors. A good practitioner will obviously seek to address current problems as far as possible. However, one of the prominent elements of a debilitating condition is that the weakness imposes its own limitations on any treatment. It is often impractical to embark upon the usual treatment strategy while the patient is at a low ebb, as even the gentlest remedies can provoke uncomfortable responses.

Finding a regime of treatment that simply addresses the debility with little consideration of the causes or background factors might be the only strategy feasible if the condition is especially severe. The principles involved in such approaches can best be reviewed for a classic modern syndrome of debility – chronic fatigue syndrome.

Chronic fatigue syndrome

Although the name might be relatively new, chronic fatigue syndrome (CFS) is not a new disorder. While the affliction, described as 'neurasthenia' in Victorian times, does not necessarily represent an early forerunner, the 'bed cases' or 'sofa cases' reported among middle-class women in the period from 1860 to 1910 probably were CFS and, by the time of World War I, a syndrome resembling CFS was a common complaint in Europe and North America.[1] CFS is also known as postviral fatigue syndrome or myalgic encephalomyelitis (ME). Although the medical profession was reluctant at first to recognise CFS as a physical disorder rather than a variant of depression or neurosis, this opinion is changing. Nonetheless, treatment of CFS as a psychiatric problem is still relatively widespread, with a conventional treatment preference for antidepressants. More enlightened thinking is to see the disturbance in biopsychosocial terms, as a complex disruption of a psychoneuroimmunoendocrine information network which, when dysregulated, leads to both psychological and somatic symptoms.[2] The basic principles applied here in the discussion of phytotherapy of CFS will be relevant to the management of patients suffering from most types of fatigue.

CFS was formally defined in 1988 as disabling fatigue of at least 6 months duration of uncertain aetiology. Additional symptoms can include mild fever, sore throat, painful lymph nodes, weight gain, exertional malaise, muscle weakness, muscle and joint pain, headaches, depression, light-headedness, anxiety, visual and cognitive impairment and disturbed sleep patterns. It usually has a relatively definite onset that resembles influenza. Six of these additional symptoms must be present, plus two or more of the following signs: low-grade fever, non-exudative pharyngitis and palpable or tender lymph nodes.[3]

This 1988 definition was amended in 1994 by the United States Centers for Disease Control and Prevention (CDC) to the following:[4]

1. Having severe chronic fatigue for at least 6 months or longer with other known medical conditions (that can cause fatigue) excluded by clinical diagnosis.

2. Concurrently having four or more of the following symptoms:
   ○ post-exertional malaise
   ○ impaired memory or concentration
   ○ unrefreshing sleep
   ○ muscle pain
   ○ multi-joint pain without redness or swelling

   ○ tender cervical or axillary lymph nodes
   ○ sore throat
   ○ headache.

3. The symptoms must have persisted or recurred during 6 or more consecutive months of illness and must not have predated the fatigue.

Currently there is no accepted biochemical test for the condition. Another problem is that the definitions are somewhat restrictive. Many patients with chronic, unexplained fatigue and typical symptoms of CFS may not exactly fulfil the above criteria.

Possible causes of chronic fatigue syndrome
Viruses

The fact that CFS can occur in epidemics has always pointed to an infectious origin. However, despite the fact that various researchers have implicated a number of viruses, a clear association with a single viral infection has not been established. Originally, Epstein-Barr (EBV) virus was thought to be the cause, since CFS can follow glandular fever. Human herpesvirus-6 (HHV-6) is another virus that has been plausibly lined to CFS outbreaks and prevalence.[5]

The link between CFS and some kind of enterovirus, possibly a Coxsackie B virus, is particularly interesting. Coxsackie B viruses are related to the polio virus, which can infect and weaken muscle tissue. There was evidence from British research that enteroviral RNA occurs in the muscle tissue of CFS patients[6] and this may lead to mitochondrial injury.[7] However, a Spanish investigation found only minor changes in muscle tissue, which did not support the hypothesis that viral infection is a cause of muscle fatigue.[8] Also the British research group appears to have abandoned their stance on enteroviruses, concluding it was unlikely that a persistent enterovirus plays a pathogenic role in CFS.[9] Nonetheless, an effect in initiating the disease process should not be excluded,[9] and other groups have certainly pursued the enterovirus connection.[10,11] More recently, the human parvovirus (HPV)-B19 has been the most reported CFS-associated virus,[12] and a new infectious human gamma-retrovirus, xenotropic murine leukaemia virus-related virus, has also been detected at high levels in CFS patients.[13,14]

The only sense which can be made of this research is that:

1. Either a number of viruses are capable of triggering CFS, in which case CFS is not an infection in the strict meaning of the term because there is no single causative agent
   or

2. CFS may involve the reactivation of the immune response to previous viral infections. In other words, the immune system may be fighting the ghosts of past viral infections.

On the latter point it is interesting to note that several investigators have reported increased 2′,5′-oligoadenylate synthetase activity in the mononuclear cells of patients with CFS, with levels correlating with disease severity. This protein is induced by interferons and is an important defence against viral proliferation.[10] It has been suggested that stress-induced EBV reactivation may represent the initial event that leads to a disturbance of immune memory, which in turn leads to a prolongation and accentuation of viral symptoms.

It is worthwhile to examine the implications of CFS epidemics. The Royal Free Hospital epidemic in London was a famous epidemic where a polio-like illness struck down many people. The illness also affected cranial nerves, which is not a feature of CFS. The majority recovered in a matter of weeks to months, but a significant number went on to develop CFS. These susceptible people among the staff at the Royal Free Hospital were left with CFS, and the original epidemic was probably a Coxsackie viral infection.[15] Hence the CFS was probably caused by this viral trigger. The viral infection occurred in an epidemic and created a related epidemic of CFS.[15] It is likely that the same conclusion could be drawn from studying other CFS epidemics.

Other microorganisms

Other microorganisms have also been linked to the incidence of CFS. Polymerase chain reaction (PCR) techniques have established a connection between possible mycoplasmal blood infections and CFS in 50% to 60% of patients.[16–18] However, until these organisms are isolated and cultured from the blood of CFS sufferers, such a link must be regarded as tenuous. Mycoplasmal DNA was not detected in the plasma of 34 sufferers of CFS.[19]

Infection with coagulase negative Staphylococcus has been described as another indirect connection. The pattern of muscle catabolism seen in CFS corresponds to that produced by this organism.[20] Also CFS and fibromyalgia patients treated with staphylococcus toxoid vaccine do show some clinical improvement.[21]

Infection with yeast, possibly *Candida albicans*, has been hypothesised.[22] Since there is a high prevalence in CFS sufferers of non-allergic sinusitis, and this condition is associated with fungal infection and fungal allergy, it was suggested that the upper respiratory tract could harbour a chronic yeast infection in CFS.[23]

Chronic Lyme disease due to past or current infection with *Borrelia burgdorferi* has been described as a possible variant of CFS, although this connection is controversial.[24]

Inflammatory disease and immune abnormalities

Chronically elevated levels of proinflammatory cytokines are associated with inflammatory diseases and psychological symptoms of depression and tiredness. There is now evidence that fatigue correlates closely with inflammatory symptoms (relating to allergy, gastrointestinal upset and to pain) in otherwise healthy populations. It has been suggested that immune dysregulation may explain the existence and covariation of psychological and physical symptoms in the healthy population, including people with medically unexplained symptoms.[25] The immune abnormalities that occur in CFS are, however, inconsistent, perhaps because different viral triggers might cause different malfunctions. One important study found no difference between CFS patients and controls for any white blood cell counts, save the CD8 T-lymphocytes.[26] These cells were activated as in

a viral infection and the cytotoxic cell subset was increased. These differences were significant (p=0.01) in patients with major symptoms of CFS. The study was noteworthy because of the large number of patients involved and also because the degree of these changes corresponded to the severity of the CFS. The authors concluded that immune activation in CFS leads to increased secretion of cytokines causing the observed symptoms. Their findings were consistent with chronic stimulation of the immune system, perhaps by a virus. If this is correct, the feeling of malaise experienced in the early stages of influenza, when cytokine output is increased, is similar to the way CFS sufferers must feel most of the time. Reviews have supported findings that proinflammatory cytokines such as IL-1, IL-6 and TNF-alpha are raised in CFS, with impaired natural killer (NK) cell function as well. Cancer patients treated with the cytokine IL-2 to boost immunity experience side effects remarkably similar to CFS. Serum levels of some cytokines are often raised in CFS. For example, levels of IL-1 alpha,[27] TNF-alpha[10] and TNF-beta[28] were significantly more often increased in CFS patients. A recent review concluded that, despite the heterogeneity in CFS, there is growing evidence that immune dysfunction plays an important role, with cytokine dysregulation a key feature.[10]

Reduced NK cell activity has been reported in several studies. For example, a correlation between low levels of NK cell activity and severity of CFS was found in 20 CFS patients.[29] Also, a marked decrease in NK cell activity was found in almost all patients with CFS, as compared with healthy individuals.[30] However, a Danish study found that NK cell activity in CFS patients was no different from healthy controls.[31] Another relatively common, but inconsistent, finding is the reduced response of lymphocytes to stimulation by mitogens.[32,33]

An increased occurrence of autoantibodies such as rheumatoid factor, thyroid antibodies and antinuclear antibodies (ANA) can be found in CFS patients.[34] This, together with an observed high incidence of circulating immune complexes, led a German research team to conclude that CFS is associated with, or is the beginning of, manifest autoimmune disease.[35] These findings were somewhat supported by a large study on 579 patients from Boston and Seattle that found levels of immune complexes were abnormal in 35% of CFS patients compared with 2% of controls (p=0.0001), and ANA was abnormally high in 15% of CFS patients compared with 0% of controls (p=0.003).[36] The same study found that serum cholesterol and IgG levels were also significantly raised in CFS. Immunodeficiency and disturbed immunological memory have also been explored as contributors to the pathophysiology of CFS.[10]

Gut dysfunction

In any condition marked by immunological disturbances, the digestive system is likely to be implicated. There is increasing evidence of this. CFS is marked by lower levels in the bowel of *Bifidobacteria* and higher levels of aerobic bacteria and higher prevalence and median values for serum IgA against enterobacteria lipopolysaccharides (pointing also to increased leakiness of the gut wall).[37] These findings resonate with clinical experience that symptoms of gut dysbiosis, irritable bowel and food intolerances are widely encountered in chronically fatigued patients.

Circulatory abnormalities

A study of 24 CFS patients who were 50 years or younger found that 100% had slightly abnormal ECG readings, compared with only 22.4% of controls (p<0.01).[38] Mild left ventricular dysfunction was found in 8 of 60 patients with CFS, and gross dysfunction occurred with increasing workloads.[38] Some studies suggest that CFS patients have a low cardiac output due to a small heart[39,40] or perhaps a comorbid hypovolaemic condition.[41] Lower blood pressure and abnormal diurnal blood pressure can be associated with CFS.[42]

A significant breakthrough came with the study by Peckerman and co-workers published in 2003.[43] Impedance cardiography and symptom data were collected from 38 patients with CFS grouped into cases with severe (n=18) and less severe (n=20) illness and compared with those from 27 matched, sedentary control subjects. The patients with severe CFS had significantly lower stroke volume and cardiac output than the controls and less ill patients. Post-exertional fatigue and flu-like symptoms of infection differentiated the patients with severe CFS from those with less severe CFS (88.5% concordance) and were predictive (p<0.0002) of lower cardiac output.

Simpson and co-workers found that subjects complaining of chronic fatigue were more likely to have abnormally shaped (nondiscocytic) red blood cells.[44] They concluded that this association between increased nondiscocytes and impaired muscle function could indicate a cause and effect relationship, which would be in agreement with the physiological concept of fatigue resulting from inadequate oxygen delivery.[44] Simpson advocated the use of evening primrose oil and fish oil to decrease nondiscocytes, and given the favourable influence of *Ginkgo biloba* on red blood cell fragility and blood rheology, it might also be indicated.

Regional cerebral blood flows to the cortex and basal ganglia were significantly reduced in a majority of CFS patients.[45,46] This finding of reduced regional cerebral blood flow in CFS is supported by a study in older patients, which found that the abnormal blood flow in CFS was different to that observed in depression.[47]

Delayed orthostatic hypotension caused by excessive venous pooling (and also linked to a subnormal circulating erythrocyte volume) is a frequent finding in CFS that appears to be linked to fatigue.[48–51] This can be associated with orthostatic hypocapnia.[52]

An autonomic imbalance with a sympathetic dominance expressed as dysregulated cardiac function has been observed in several studies. For example, heart rate during sleep and mean arterial blood pressure were significantly higher in CFS patients,[53] and another study also observed a higher heart rate together with reduced heart rate variability (a sign of sympathetic dominance) during sleep.[54] Reduced heart rate variability also predicts poor sleep quality in CFS[55] and is associated with orthostatic stress in CFS patients.[56]

Brain and cognitive abnormalities

Magnetic resonance imaging (MRI) scans of the brains of CFS sufferers found a high incidence of inflammation (oedema and demyelination) in association with serological evidence of active HHV-6 infection.[57] This controversial finding of brain abnormalities in CFS has been somewhat supported by a study which observed that CFS patients had significantly more abnormal scans than controls: 27% versus 2%.[58] However, the authors felt that this might instead indicate that some patients labelled with CFS could actually be suffering from other medical conditions. Abnormal MRI and single-photon emission computed tomography (SPECT) scans were found with far greater frequency in CFS patients compared to normal controls.[59] SPECT abnormalities were present in 81% of CFS patients versus 21% of control subjects (p<0.01).[59]

The presence of brain abnormalities in CFS, as assessed by MRI, was related to subjective reports of poor physical function[60] and mental fatigue.[61] A strong correlation in CFS between brainstem grey matter volume and pulse pressure suggested impaired cerebrovascular autoregulation.[62] However, abnormal MRI findings have not always been observed in CFS.[63]

It should also be stressed that modern techniques of brain imaging are highly sensitive, and these findings do not necessarily indicate gross organic brain defects. They are probably more indicative of chronic encephalitis, which is possibly either viral or immunological in origin.

A number of objective tests have revealed memory deterioration in CFS patients compared with healthy controls, but findings between studies have not been consistent. Short-term memory,[64] general memory,[65] retrieval from semantic memory[66] and memory requiring cognitive effort[67] have been found to be impaired. Attention can also be impaired.[68] However, other studies have found that memory was not affected,[69] or was only mildly impacted.[70] It has been suggested that impaired information processing, rather than a primary memory dysfunction, may underlie the cognitive problems that afflict so many patients with CFS.[71] A 2010 meta-analysis that included 50 eligible studies concluded that patients with CFS demonstrate moderate to large impairments in simple and complex information processing speed and in tasks requiring working memory over a sustained period of time.[72]

Pituitary and hypothalamic abnormalities

Patients with CFS have a mild central adrenal insufficiency secondary to either a deficiency of corticotropin-releasing hormone or some other central stimulus to the pituitary-adrenal axis.[73] This leads to a decreased response of the adrenal cortex. Abnormalities in the regulation of the hypothalamic-pituitary-adrenal (HPA) axis are also a well-recognised feature of endogenous depression. It has been suggested that, since cytokines potently influence the HPA axis, their activation may underlie many of the features found in CFS and depression.[74]

A comprehensive 2007 review of this topic concluded that there is distinct evidence for a hypofunction of the HPA axis in a proportion of patients with CFS, despite negative studies and methodological difficulties.[75] About half the reviewed studies indicated this finding; the others found no significant changes. The following mechanisms underlying the hypocortisolism were discussed:

- Reduced biosynthesis of releasing factors (CRH, ACTH)
- Downregulation of central receptors
- Increased negative feedback sensitivity to endogenous glucocorticoids
- Decreased availability of free cortisol
- Reduced effects of cortisol on target tissues (relative cortisol resistance).

The above findings suggest that a focus on regulating and restoring normal HPA function in CFS should be a priority for herbal clinicians, one that they are well equipped to deal with. Most patients with CFS were found to have sleep disorders that are likely to contribute to the daytime fatigue and may also be important in the aetiology of the syndrome.[76,77] CFS patients exhibited significant elevations in fatigue, subjective sleep disturbance and objective sleep disorders compared to MS patients and a healthy control group.[78]

A 2008 study confirmed these observations, finding that CFS patients had significant differences in polysomnographic recordings compared with healthy controls and felt sleepier and more fatigued than controls after a night's sleep.[79] CFS patients also had less total sleep time, lower sleep efficiency and less rapid eye movement (REM) sleep than controls.

Biochemical abnormalities

It has been hypothesised that the imbalances in immune function, the HPA axis and the sympathetic nervous system in CFS can be explained by changes in essential fatty acid (EFA) metabolism. Dietary EFA modulation afforded substantial improvement in a majority of cases.[80] A Japanese study did find that serum concentrations of EFAs were depleted in CFS sufferers[81] and controlled clinical trials of evening primrose oil[82] and fish oil demonstrated significant symptom reduction.[83] Japanese scientists have found lower levels of serum acylcarnitine in CFS, which they proposed might explain the fatigue and muscle weakness.[84] Also, the concentration of serum acylcarnitine tended to increase to normal with recovery from fatigue in CFS.[65] However, an open clinical study in 20 CFS patients found no improvement after 3 months of L-carnitine therapy.[8]

Studies on the magnesium status of CFS patients have not resolved this issue. A report on one patient found considerable improvement after 6 weeks of therapy with intravenous magnesium sulphate,[85] but a study of 89 patients with CFS found no evidence of magnesium deficiency in any patient.[86]

When serum folate levels of 60 patients with CFS were assayed it was found that 50% had values below 3.0 μg/L.[87] The authors concluded that some CFS patients are deficient in folic acid.

Clinical trials

There have been a few studies of herbal interventions for CFS or chronic fatigue (not necessarily CFS) in randomised, controlled trials. A randomised, double blind, placebo-controlled clinical study of a standardised *Lycium barbarum* juice product was conducted (by the manufacturer) with 60 older healthy adults (55 to 72 years old). Participants either took 120 mL/day of the juice, equivalent to at least 150 g of fresh fruit, or placebo for 30 days. The Lycium group showed significantly improved measures of fatigue and sleep, and a statistically significant increase in the number of lymphocytes and levels of IL-2 and immunoglobulin G compared to the placebo group. The number of CD4, CD8 and NK cells and levels of IL-4 and immunoglobulin A were not significantly altered.[88]

Consuming high-cocoa liquor/polyphenol-rich chocolate 45 g/day for 8 weeks was beneficial in improving fatigue and residual function in CFS, compared with the consumption of simulated isocaloric low polyphenol chocolate.[89] In a separate study, flavanol-rich cocoa in drinks at 520 mg and 994 mg were compared to matched controls in a randomised, controlled, double blinded, three period crossover trial in 30 healthy adults undergoing the sort of sustained mental demands often leading to fatigue. Various assessments, psychomotor tests and measures of cognitive performance showed the highest dose of cocoa flavanols had the clearest benefit on mood and psychomotor performance in these circumstances.[90] While the mechanisms underlying the effects are unknown, they are thought to be related to known effects of cocoa flavanols on endothelial function and blood flow, a further link between inflammatory processes and the aetiology of fatigue that picks up discussions earlier in this chapter.

A randomised, double blind, controlled trial found that a combination of Astragalus and *Salvia miltiorrhiza* ameliorated chronic fatigue.[91] (See the Astragalus monograph for more details.) There is also the trial assessing Rhodiola in chronic fatigue mentioned later in this chapter.

Phytotherapeutics

Clinical impressions of fatigue

CFS appears to involve a complex interaction between emotional, infectious and environmental stressors leading to subtle immune dysfunction. The extreme debility sometimes encountered has the unfortunate effect of blocking many treatment approaches: rest may be disrupted, exercise may be debilitating and even the simplest foods may seem to be too demanding. Many otherwise useful remedies may be too stimulating or unsettling.

Fatigue may take different forms and arise from different stresses. There may be a deficiency condition, there may be an obstruction to normal functions (such as the effects of clinical depression) or fatigue may follow excessive activity, perhaps marked by anxiety and nervous stress. In other cases it may predispose to recurrent infections, creating a vicious cycle. The therapeutic approach in each case will be different. In the first instance, nutritional and supportive therapies will dominate. In the second, there may be the need to embark upon substantial constitutional and metabolic strategies. Where tension is the predominant factor then repair will be difficult if there is not some relaxant or even sedative relief. If poor immune function is evident, then emphasis needs to be placed here.

The majority of CFS patients were probably devitalised before they contracted the disorder. This might have been due to emotional pressures, work pressures, family pressures, ambition, toxins, pregnancy, or even a bad diet, but the end result is the same. This observation is supported by the finding that stress is a significant predisposing factor in CFS.[92] Any stressor, be it chemical, physical, biological or emotional, then acts to aggravate this condition. This reduced capacity to cope with stress is a key factor in creating the vicious cycle that perpetuates the syndrome.

The devitalisation leads to weakened immunity and finally to an abnormal immune response to a viral infection. A stalemate is reached where the resultant hyperimmune state causes autotoxicity, but is not sufficiently focused to resolve a viral presence, or any other cause, and restore health. It is a curious state where some compartments of the immune system are overactive, but other compartments are deficient.[93] Figure 8.1 summarises the interplay between psychosocial, immune and viral factors in the initiation and perpetuation of CFS.[10]

Sometimes benefits will follow a focus on what could be exacerbating or even causative factors. These might include:

- intestinal dysbiosis, endotoxaemia or similar syndromes, other syndromes involving autotoxicity, chronic inflammation
- allergies or food intolerances
- toxins, e.g. dental amalgam, hair dyes, pesticides
- recurrent fungal, viral or bacterial infection.

Above all else, it is important to ensure that sleep and rest are adequate and much useful treatment effort can be directed to this end as a first priority. Whatever the initiating disturbance, the treatment of fatigue must be marked by extreme gentleness and patience.

Convalescence

With any fatigue syndrome the fundamental principle of treatment is to set up an appropriate recuperative regime. Remedies should be set against a wider programme of convalescence. Convalescence as a strategy is outlined in Chapter 3. Extensive

and appropriate rest is essential and may need to be supported by treatment to help with sleep and relaxation: exercise, even if minimal, will help engage adrenosympathetic disturbances; the diet should be based on the most easily assimilable foods possible. Only when such a regime is in place can herbal treatment have a chance of facilitating further improvements.

Herbal remedies useful in CFS include the following.

Tonic and adaptogenic herbs

Tonics help revitalise the patient and adaptogens improve the response to stress. Tonics were traditionally used to help build strength after illness and trauma and may also build immune function.

Major herbs in this group are:

- *Astragalus membranaceus* (Astragalus): tonic and immune enhancing (see monograph)
- *Eleutherococcus senticosus* (Siberian ginseng): adaptogenic, stimulates T-lymphocyte function (see monograph)
- *Lycium spp.* (goji): a tonic remedy in China with some evidence as an adaptogen
- *Panax ginseng* (Ginseng): tonic, adaptogenic, stimulates hypothalamic output and ACTH and hence adrenal cortex function, increases stamina, spares muscle use of carbohydrate (see monograph)
- *Rhodiola rosea*: a herb with adaptogenic and ergogenic reputations
- *Schisandra chinensis*: a herb with adaptogenic and hepatoprotective reputations[94]
- *Withania somnifera* (Withania): a tonic herb which is not stimulating and facilitates sleep (as its name implies), hence is ideal in situations of sympathetic dominance (see monograph).

Of this group, most interest in recent years has been in Rhodiola, with a wide range of clinical studies reported. These have been unsympathetically reviewed[95] and defended.[96] However, in one case a substantial positive study has been

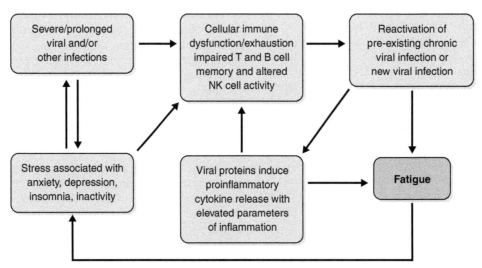

Figure 8.1 • The inter-relationship between psychosocial, immune and viral factors in the initiation and perpetuation of chronic fatigue.[10]
Reproduced from Bansal AS, Bradley AS, Bishop KN, et al. Chronic fatigue syndrome, the immune system and viral infection. *Brain Behav Immun* 2011, with permission from Elsevier.

reported: 60 men and women with stress-related fatigue were randomised into two equal groups, one received four tablets daily of standardised Rhodiola extract (576 mg/day), and the other placebo. After comparing results for various psychomotor and quality of life tests and serum cortisol levels, it was concluded that, compared with placebo, repeated administration of this particular extract exerts an anti-fatigue effect with increased mental performance, ability to concentrate and decreased cortisol response to awakening stress.[97] This probably also has relevance to the use of this herb in CFS. Rhodiola has the additional advantage that its efficacy in depression has been demonstrated in a randomised, placebo-controlled trial and also has considerable pharmacological support.[98]

Adrenal supportive herbs

The main herbs for this purpose are Glycyrrhiza (licorice) and *Rehmannia glutinosa* (see also the relevant monographs). There is one case report of recovery from CFS with the use of licorice that speculates a role in adrenocortical function.[99] Another case report from Japan observed that a chronic fatigue patient went into remission when she developed hyperaldosteronism due to an adrenal tumour. When the adrenal tumour was removed the fatigue returned.[100] Licorice in high doses can cause pseudoaldosteronism due to its aldosterone-like action, but obviously should not be used to this level. A high-potassium, low-sodium diet, as in the Gerson therapy, can also raise plasma aldosterone.

Immune-enhancing herbs

Although these may seem contraindicated, immune-enhancing herbs are often needed to help prevent the recurrent viral infections that can plague patients with CFS. In cases of infection, treatment with tonic herbs may need to be discontinued so that defensive measures can be applied. *Echinacea angustifolia* and *E. purpurea* root are safe to use since, on current knowledge, they mainly enhance innate immunity. This can improve antigen recognition, which leads to better immune responsiveness. *Picrorrhiza kurroa* should be used with caution as it is a potent promoter of all aspects of immune function, but it may be indicated for patients who have frequent viral infections. Andrographis and Astragalus also have a role, especially the latter where there is chronic immune depletion.

Antiviral herbs

Although the viral association is not always clear, these herbs can be useful in many cases. *Hypericum perforatum* (St John's wort) may contribute to antiviral and antidepressant activity. Hypericum is probably active against enveloped viruses such as EBV and HHV-6. *Thuja occidentalis* is also active against enveloped viruses as well as naked viruses, such as the wart virus and enteroviruses.

Immune-depressing and anti-inflammatory herbs

There are a few non-toxic herbs that can depress immune function and may be useful at some stages of treatment. The safest to use is the Indian herb *Hemidesmus indicus* (Indian

sarsaparilla). Rehmannia, Bupleurum and Boswellia can be useful anti-inflammatories and may downregulate cytokine production and responses (see monographs).

Others

Ginkgo biloba, *Salvia miltiorrhiza* and Zanthoxylum (prickly ash) can improve blood flow. Ginkgo decreases erythrocyte fragility and improves blood rheology and short-term memory. Valeriana (valerian), *Passiflora incarnata* (passionflower), *Piper methysticum* (kava) and other such herbs will help the disordered sleep pattern and sympathetic dominance. Crataegus (hawthorn) may help any cardiac and circulatory abnormalities and the sympathetic dominance. Butcher's broom (*Ruscus aculeatus*) and horsechestnut (*Aesculus hippocastanum*), being venous toning, should be considered for orthostatic symptoms (see monographs). EFA therapy with evening primrose oil and fish oil is also recommended.

Notes about treatment

Deep-seated devitalisation is a major part of CFS, so results must be measured in months not weeks. If results are slow to come about the patient should be encouraged, since improvement usually does occur with consistent use of herbs. Patients must be instructed not to overexert themselves when they begin to feel improvement, as this can cause a relapse. They should only partake in mild exercise and not exercise beyond the point of fatigue. Sleep helps to restore the immune system and CFS patients will not improve unless they have adequate sleep, which may be more than they needed previously. They must avoid stress and emotional crises as much as possible. The importance of stress as a cause and sustaining factor of CFS should not be underestimated and appropriate lifestyle measures must be incorporated into the treatment plan.

CASE HISTORY

'William', aged 48, sought treatment for CFS, from which he had suffered for 3 years after exposure to Ross River virus. Symptoms included aches and pains, especially in the first 6 months after the infection, malaise, mild fever, physical weakness, lack of stamina and poor sleep. He worked as a manager at a cemetery and was still able to manage (barely) his job, despite the CFS. He was previously very active. Current medication was salbutamol for asthma and the occasional use of a benzodiazepine to help his sleep

He was placed on the following herbal treatment:

A. Liquid formula:

Echinacea angustifolia and *E. purpurea* (root)	1:2	35 mL
Glycyrrhiza glabra (high in glycyrrhizin)	1:1	15 mL
Astragalus membranaceus	1:2	20 mL
Hypericum perforatum (high in hypericin)	1:2	20 mL
Withania somnifera	1:1	20 mL
	TOTAL	110 mL

Dose: 8 mL with water twice a day.

B. Withania (600 mg) and Korean ginseng (125 mg) tablets 3/day
Eleutherococcus (Siberian ginseng) tablets 1.25 g 3/day
Valeriana edulis (Mexican valerian) tablets 1.0 g 3/day (as required)

There was not much improvement over the first 8 to 12 weeks, but after that he felt the herbs were helping, especially the feeling of malaise and low energy. He then changed to a more stressful job, but was able to cope well with this, relying on the support of the herbal treatment. After another 8 weeks he reported a noticeable improvement all round and was able to undertake a regular programme of exercise.

CASE HISTORY

'Kylie', aged 17, had glandular fever 6 years previously. She had suffered from fatigue ever since, but after beginning Year 12 at school her fatigue was particularly severe. Often catching colds and influenza, her attendance was less than 50%. Even on 'well' days, she often did not have the energy to attend school. Herbal treatment consisted of the following basic formula (written for 1 week):

Astragalus membranaceus	1:2	30 mL
Panax ginseng (standardised extract)	1:2	15 mL
Ginkgo biloba (standardised extract)	2:1	20 mL
Echinacea angustifolia root	1:2	35 mL
	Total:	100 mL

Dose: 5 mL with water three times a day.

In addition, Withania 1:2 5 mL with water once a day was prescribed.

If a cold came on, the above treatment was stopped for 3 to 4 days and the following formula was taken:

Zingiber officinale	1:2	10 mL
Echinacea angustifolia root	1:2	40 mL
Euphrasia officinalis	1:2	20 mL
Achillea millefolium	1:2	30 mL
	Total:	100 mL

Dose: 5 mL with warm water up to five times a day.

Initially, Kylie had difficulty taking the herbal formula because it was too stimulating. So the dose was reduced to half and gradually increased. There was only slight improvement in her condition for 3 months, but then gradual and steady progress was made. While she received herbal treatment from time to time, she was free of CFS for more than 2 years.

CASE HISTORY

'John', was 35 and had not worked for 3 years. By the time he sought herbal treatment he complained that he was getting sicker and sicker. He experienced constant headaches and had suffered from chronic sinusitis for about 10 years. His history showed a previous high exposure to insecticides and years of overwork due to family pressures. His wife could not cope with his not working and his marriage was strained. Various formulas were given but the treatment settled at the following (for 1 week):

Panax ginseng (standardised extract)	1:2	15 mL
Astragalus membranaceus	1:2	30 mL
Crataegus spp. fol.	1:2	20 mL
Ginkgo biloba (standardised extract)		20 mL
Picrorrhiza kurroa	1:2	15 mL
Glycyrrhiza glabra (high in glycyrrhizin)	1:1	20 mL
Scutellaria baicalensis	1:2	30 mL
	Total:	150 mL

Dose: 8 mL with water three times a day.

In addition, *Echinacea angustifolia* root 1:2 5 mL once a day was prescribed from time to time. Also an 'acute formula', similar to the one for 'Kylie', was taken during colds and influenza instead of the basic formula. The Crataegus was for the headaches and circulation and the Baical skullcap for the sinusitis. 'John' actually worsened in the first 3 months of treatment, probably because of the natural progression of the disorder. However, after 5 months he thanked the friend who recommended herbal treatment because it was 'the best thing I could have done'. He gradually improved over a period of several more months.

Tonics

Plant remedies traditionally used as tonics

- *Astragalus membranaceus*
- *Avena sativa* (oatstraw)
- *Glycyrrhiza glabra* (licorice)
- *Hypericum perforatum* (St John's wort)
- *Medicago sativa* (alfalfa)
- *Panax ginseng* (ginseng)
- *Rhodiola rosea*
- *Serenoa repens* (saw palmetto)
- *Swertia chirata* (chiretta)
- *Trigonella foenum-graecum* (fenugreek)
- *Turnera diffusa* (damiana)
- *Verbena officinalis* (vervain)
- *Withania somnifera*.

Indications for tonics

- Convalescence
- Debilitating conditions with or without anorexia
- Chronic fatigue syndrome.

Cautions in the use of tonics

The use of tonic herbs may be difficult in the following circumstances:

- Very severe debility especially if associated with immune or digestive collapse
- Renal or hepatic failure
- Rampant cancer or strong regimes of chemotherapy.

Application

The state of digestion is the main determinant of dosage times. Tonics may be best taken with or after meals if the stomach and digestive system are weakened; in severe cases, they may need to be taken with fluid nourishment. Dosage should be rather more than less frequent: 'little and often' might be a useful axiom. Tonics taken immediately before bed can help when sleep is non-restorative. Withania is ideal for this.

Long-term therapy with tonics is generally indicated and often advisable.

Chinese tonics

In Chinese medicine, tonic remedies are generally divided into four groups, depending on whether they are seen to particularly support *qi*, *yang*, *xue* or *yin*. The first two groups tend to be warming, the last two cooling. They are often more dynamic than the tonics listed above and may thus be more likely to generate adverse reactions. It is more important, therefore, to be careful in their prescription and to take close account of the interpretation of debilitated conditions that Chinese practitioners use. However, they reflect a perspective on debility and its treatment that is not well articulated in the Western traditions. This works both ways: unfortunately methodological limitations have also undermined the evidence for efficacy in the West so far published.[101]

In the following review, Chinese terms will therefore be used. They are briefly introduced in the summary of Chinese herbal medicine in this text (see p. 5) but any practitioner wishing to apply them should be well trained in that tradition. Nevertheless, there is some overlap with Western remedies and some useful insights are possible for a Western phytotherapist.

Qi tonics

These support active energies; they are used for depletion of *qi*, particularly in the *Spleen* and *Lungs*.

In the first case, possibly as a result of prolonged illness or constitutional weakness, debility may affect the functions of assimilation and distribution and be associated with such symptoms as fatigue and depression with depressed digestion, diarrhoea, abdominal pain or tension, visceral prolapse, pale yellow complexion with a tinge of red or purple, pale tongue with white coating and/or languid, frail or indistinct pulses. This may lead in turn to a 'damp' condition developing.

In the second case, extreme or prolonged stress or disease, or chronic pulmonary disease, leads to depletion or cold in the *Lungs*, with easy fatigue and prostration associated with disturbances of regulation, shortness of breath or shallow breathing, rapid, slow or little speech, spontaneous perspiration, pallid complexion, dry skin, pale tongue with thin white coating, weak and depleted pulses.

Plant remedies traditionally used as *Qi* tonics:

- *Astragalus membranaceus* (huang qi)
- *Atractylodes macrocephela* (bai zhu)
- *Codonopsis pilulosa* (dang shen)
- *Glycyrrhiza uralensis* (Chinese liquorice – gan cao)
- *Panax ginseng* (Asiatic ginseng – ren shen)
- *Zizyphus jujuba* (Jujube – da zao).

Yang tonics

These remedies support the active energies, particularly those of the *Kidneys* (but also *Heart* and *Spleen*).

Deficient *Kidney yang* leads to listlessness with a feeling of cold and cold extremities, back and loins; there may be weak legs, poor reproductive function, frequency of micturition, nocturia, diarrhoea (especially early in the morning), pale complexion and submerged weak pulses.

Deficiency affecting the *Heart* involves poor performance and coordination associated with profuse cold sweating, asthmatic states, thoracic or anginal pain on exertion, palpitations and fear attacks, cyanosis, white tongue coating and/or diminished, hesitant or intermittent pulses.

Plant remedies traditionally used as yang tonics:

- *Eucommia ulmoides* (du zhong)
- *Juglans regia* (walnut – hu tao ren)
- *Morinda officinalis* (ba ji)
- *Trigonella foenum-graecum* (fenugreek – hu lu ba).

Xue tonics

These are remedies that support more substantial energies, those manifesting in substantial disturbances or pathologies. By definition, such disturbances are serious and profound and treatment will need to be prolonged. Symptoms of depletion of *xue* may include cyanosis, pallor, vertigo or tinnitus, palpitations, loss of memory, insomnia or menstrual problems.

There is considerable overlap with *yin* tonics.

Plant remedies traditionally used as *xue* tonics:

- *Angelica sinensis* (dang gui)
- *Mori alba* (mulberry fruit – sang shen)
- *Paeonia lactiflora* (paeony root – bai shao)
- *Rehmannia glutinosa* (sheng di huang – fresh, and shu di huang – prepared).

Yin tonics

These are remedies for replenishing the body fluids and essence, supplying condensed energies and nourishment, for the most depleted conditions. Areas in most need of support are the *Kidneys*, *Liver*, *Lungs* and *Stomach*.

Deficient *Kidney yin* often follows very serious debilitating disease or, alternatively, extended sexual or alcohol abuse or overwhelming nervous stress. It may manifest as a deficient Fire condition, marked by a pale complexion with red cheeks, red lips, dry mouth, dry but deeply red tongue, dry throat, hot palms and soles, palpitations, vertigo or tinnitus, pains in the loins, night sweats, nocturnal emissions, nightmares, urinary retention, constipation, accelerated though weak pulses.

Deficient *Liver yin*, usually following the above, is often associated with dry eyes, poor vision and vertigo or tinnitus, deafness, muscle twitching, sleeplessness, hot flushed face with red cheeks, red dry tongue with little coating, diminished, stringy and accelerated pulses.

Deficient *Stomach yin* is marked by anorexia, regurgitation, thirst, abdominal rumbling, red lips and red tongue with no coating.

Deficient *Lung yin*, often following prolonged exposure to dryness or chronic pulmonary disease, is marked by dry cough, haemoptysis, hoarseness and loss of voice, strong thirst and/or restlessness and insomnia.

Plant remedies traditionally used as *yin* tonics:

- *Asparagus cochinchinensis* (tian men dong)
- *Ligustrum lucidum* (nu zhen zi)
- *Lycium chinensis* (gou qi zi)
- *Ophiopogon japonicus* (mai men dong)
- *Panax quinquefolium* (American ginseng)
- *Sesamum indicum* (sesame seeds – hei zhi ma).

References

1. Shorter E. Chronic fatigue in historical perspective. *Ciba Found Symp*. 1993;173:6–16.

2. Hyland ME. Network origins of anxiety and depression. *Behav Brain Sci*. 2010;33(2–3):161–162.

3. Holmes GP, Kaplan JE, Gantz NM, et al. Chronic fatigue syndrome: a working case definition. *Ann Intern Med*. 1988;108(3):387–389.

4. Centers for Disease Control and Prevention. *CFS Case Definition*. <http://www.cdc.gov/cfs/general/case_definition/index.html>. Accessed 28.08.2011.

5. Komaroff AL. Is human herpesvirus-6 a trigger for chronic fatigue syndrome? *J Clin Virol*. 2006;37(suppl 1):S39–S46.

6. Gow JW, Behan WM, Clements GB, et al. Enteroviral RNA sequences detected by polymerase chain reaction in muscle of patients with postviral fatigue syndrome. *BMJ*. 1991;302(6778):692–696.

7. Gow JW, Behan WM. Amplification and identification of enteroviral sequences in the postviral fatigue syndrome. *Br Med Bull*. 1991;47(4):872–885.

8. Grau JM, Casademont J, Pedrol E, et al. Chronic fatigue syndrome: studies on skeletal muscle. *Clin Neuropathol*. 1992;11(6):329–332.

9. Gow JW, Behan WM, Simpson K, et al. Studies on enterovirus in patients with chronic fatigue syndrome. *Clin Infect Dis*. 1994;18(suppl 1):S126–S129.

10. Bansal AS, Bradley AS, Bishop KN, et al. Chronic fatigue syndrome, the immune system and viral infection. *Brain Behav Immun*. 2012;26(1):24–31.

11. Chia JK. The role of enterovirus in chronic fatigue syndrome. *J Clin Pathol*. 2005;58(11):1126–1132.

12. Frémont M, Metzger K, Rady H. Detection of herpes viruses and parvovirus B19 in gastric and intestinal mucosa of chronic fatigue syndrome patients. *In Vivo*. 2009;23(2):209–213.

13. Lombardi VC, Ruscetti FW, Das Gupta J, et al. Detection of an infectious retrovirus, XMRV, in blood cells of patients with chronic fatigue syndrome. *Science*. 2009;326(5952):585–589.

14. Coffin JM, Stoye JP. Virology. A new virus for old diseases? *Science*. 2009;326(5952):530–531.

15. The Medical Staff of the Royal Free Hospital. An outbreak of encephalomyelitis in the Royal Free Hospital group London, in 1955. *BMJ*. 1957;2:895–904.

16. Nasralla M, Haier J, Nicolson GL. Multiple mycoplasmal infections detected in blood of patients with chronic fatigue syndrome and/or fibromyalgia syndrome. *Eur J Clin Microbiol Infect Dis*. 1999;18(12):859–865.

17. Vojdani A, Choppa PC, Tagle C, et al. Detection of mycoplasma genus and Mycoplasma fermentans by PCR in patients with chronic fatigue syndrome. *FEMS Immunol Med Microbiol*. 1998;22(4):355–365.

18. Choppa PC, Vojdani A, Tagle C, et al. Multiplex PCR for the detection of Mycoplasma fermentans, M. hominis and M. penetrans in cell cultures and blood samples of patients with chronic fatigue syndrome. *Mol Cell Probes*. 1998;12(5):301–308.

19. Vernon SD, Shukla SK, Reeves WC. Absence of Mycoplasma species DNA in chronic fatigue syndrome. *J Med Microbiol*. 2003;52(Pt 11):1027–1028.

20. Dunstan RH, McGregor NR, Roberts TK, et al. The development of laboratory-based tests in chronic pain and fatigue: (1) Muscle catabolism and coagulase negative staphylococci which produce membrane damaging toxins. *JCFS*. 2000;7:23–28.

21. Andersson M, Bagby JR, Dyrehag L, et al. Effects of staphylococcus toxoid vaccine on pain and fatigue in patients with fibromyalgia/chronic fatigue syndrome. *Eur J Pain*. 1998;2(2):133–142.

22. Levin AM. Chronic fatigue syndrome: the yeast concept. *JCFS*. 2001;8(2):71–76.

23. Chester AC. Yeast and chronic fatigue syndrome. *JCFS*. 2000;7(3):87–88.

24. Marques A. Chronic Lyme disease: a review. *Infect Dis Clin North Am*. 2008;22(2):341–360.

25. Whalley B, Jacobs PA, Hyland ME. Correlation of psychological and physical symptoms with chronically elevated cytokine levels associated with a common immune dysregulation. *Ann Allergy Asthma Immunol*. 2007;99(4):345–348.

26. Landay AL, Jessop C, Lennette ET, et al. Chronic fatigue syndrome: clinical condition associated with immune activation. *Lancet*. 1991;338(8769):707–712.

27. Linde A, Andersson B, Svenson SB, et al. Serum levels of lymphokines and soluble cellular receptors in primary Epstein-Barr virus infection and in patients with chronic fatigue syndrome. *J Infect Dis*. 1992;165(6):994–1000.

28. Patarca R, Klimas NG, Lugtendorf S, et al. Dysregulated expression of tumor necrosis factor in chronic fatigue syndrome: interrelations with cellular sources and patterns of soluble immune mediator expression. *Clin Infect Dis*. 1994;18(1):147–153.

29. Ojo-Amaize EA, Conley EJ, Peter JB. Decreased natural killer cell activity is associated with severity of chronic fatigue immune dysfunction syndrome. *Clin Infect Dis*. 1994;18(suppl 1):S157–S159.

30. Barker E, Fujimura SF, Fadem MB, et al. Immunologic abnormalities associated with chronic fatigue syndrome. *Clin Infect Dis*. 1994;18(suppl 1):S136–S141.

31. Rasmussen AK, Nielsen H, Andersen V, et al. Chronic fatigue syndrome–a controlled cross sectional study. *J Rheumatol*. 1994;21(8):1527–1531.

32. Straus SE, Fritz S, Dale JK, et al. Lymphocyte phenotype and function in the chronic fatigue syndrome. *J Clin Immunol*. 1993;13(1):30–40.

33. Lloyd A, Hickie I, Hickie C, et al. Cell-mediated immunity in patients with chronic fatigue syndrome, healthy control subjects and patients with major depression. *Clin Exp Immunol*. 1992;87(1):76–79.

34. Hashimoto N, Kuraishi Y, Yokose T, et al. Chronic fatigue syndrome-51 cases in the Jikei University School of Medicine. *Nippon Rinsho*. 1992;50(11):2653–2664.

35. Hilgers A, Frank J. Chronic fatigue syndrome: immune dysfunction, role of pathogens and toxic agents and neurological and cardial changes. *Wien Med Wochenschr*. 1994;144(16):399–406.

36. Bates DW, Buchwald D, Lee J, et al. Clinical laboratory test findings in patients with chronic fatigue syndrome. *Arch Intern Med*. 1995;155(1):97–103.

37. Lakhan SE, Kirchgessner A. Gut inflammation in chronic fatigue syndrome. *Nutr Metab (Lond)*. 2010;7:79.

38. Lerner AM, Lawrie C, Dworkin HS. Repetitively negative changing T waves at 24-h electrocardiographic monitors in patients with the chronic fatigue syndrome. Left ventricular dysfunction in a cohort. *Chest*. 1993;104(5):1417–1421.

39. Miwa K, Fujita M. Cardiovascular dysfunction with low cardiac output due to a small heart in patients with chronic fatigue syndrome. *Intern Med*. 2009;48(21):1849–1854.

40. Miwa K, Fujita M. Cardiac function fluctuates during exacerbation and remission in young adults with chronic fatigue syndrome and 'small heart'. *J Cardiol*. 2009;54(1):29–35.

41. Hurwitz BE, Coryell VT, Parker M, et al. Chronic fatigue syndrome: illness severity, sedentary lifestyle, blood volume and evidence of diminished cardiac function. *Clin Sci (Lond)*. 2009;118(2):125–135.

42. Newton JL, Sheth A, Shin J, et al. Lower ambulatory blood pressure in chronic fatigue syndrome. *Psychosom Med*. 2009;71(3):361–365.

43. Peckerman A, Lamanca JJ, Dahl KA, et al. Abnormal impedance cardiography predicts symptom severity in chronic fatigue syndrome. *Am J Med Sci*. 2003;326(2):55–60.

44. Simpson LO, Murdoch JC, Herbison GP. Red cell shape changes following trigger finger fatigue in subjects with chronic tiredness and healthy controls. *N Z Med J*. 1993;106(952):104–107.

45. Ichise M, Salit IE, Abbey SE, et al. Assessment of regional cerebral perfusion by 99 Tcm–HMPAO SECT in chronic fatigue syndrome. *Nucl Med Commun*. 1992;10:767–772.

46. Biswal B, Kunwar P, Natelson BH. Cerebral blood flow is reduced in chronic fatigue syndrome as assessed by arterial spin labeling. *J Neurol Sci*. 2011;301(1–2): 9–11.

47. Goldstein JA, Mena I, Jouanne E, et al. The assessment of vascular abnormalities in late life chronic fatigue syndrome by brain SPECT: comparison with late life major depressive disorder. *JCFS*. 1995;1(1):55–79.

48. Streeten DH, Thomas D, Bell DS. The roles of orthostatic hypotension, orthostatic tachycardia, and subnormal erythrocyte volume in the pathogenesis of the chronic fatigue syndrome. *Am J Med Sci*. 2000;320(1):1–8.

49. Schondorf R, Freeman R. The importance of orthostatic intolerance in the chronic fatigue syndrome. *Am J Med Sci*. 1999;317(2):117–123.

50. Streeten DH, Anderson Jr GH. The role of delayed orthostatic hypotension in the pathogenesis of chronic fatigue. *Clin Auton Res*. 1998;8(2):119–124.

51. Wilke WS, Fouad-Tarazi FM, Cash JM, et al. The connection between chronic fatigue syndrome and neurally mediated hypotension. *Cleve Clin J Med*. 1998;65(5):261–266.

52. Natelson BH, Intriligator R, Cherniack NS, et al. Hypocapnia is a biological marker for orthostatic intolerance in some patients with chronic fatigue syndrome. *Dyn Med*. 2007;30(6):2.

53. Hurum H, Sulheim D, Thaulow E, et al. Elevated nocturnal blood pressure and heart rate in adolescent chronic fatigue syndrome. *Acta Paediatr*. 2011;100(2):289–292.

54. Boneva RS, Decker MJ, Maloney EM, et al. Higher heart rate and reduced heart rate variability persist during sleep in chronic fatigue syndrome: a population-based study. *Auton Neurosci*. 2007;137 (1–2):94–101.

55. Burton AR, Rahman K, Kadota Y, et al. Reduced heart rate variability predicts poor sleep quality in a case-control study of chronic fatigue syndrome. *Exp Brain Res*. 2010;204(1):71–78.

56. Wyller VB, Barbieri R, Thaulow E, et al. Enhanced vagal withdrawal during mild orthostatic stress in adolescents with chronic fatigue. *Ann Noninvasive Electrocardiol*. 2008;13(1):67–73.

57. Buchwald D, Cheney PR, Peterson DL, et al. A chronic illness characterized by fatigue, neurologic and immunologic disorders, and active human herpesvirus type 6 infection. *Ann Intern Med*. 1992;116(2):103–113.

58. Natelson BH, Cohen JM, Brassloff I, et al. A controlled study of brain magnetic resonance imaging in patients with the chronic fatigue syndrome. *J Neurol Sci*. 1993;120(2):213–217.

59. Schwartz RB, Garada BM, Komaroff AL, et al. Detection of intracranial abnormalities in patients with chronic fatigue syndrome: comparison of MR imaging and SPECT. *Am J Roentgenol*. 1994;162(4):935–941.

60. Cook DB, Lange G, DeLuca J, et al. Relationship of brain MRI abnormalities and physical functional status in chronic fatigue syndrome. *Int J Neurosci*. 2001;107(1–2):1–6.

61. Cook DB, O'Connor PJ, Lange G, et al. Functional neuroimaging correlates of mental fatigue induced by cognition among chronic fatigue syndrome patients and controls. *Neuroimage*. 2007;36(1):108–122.

62. Barnden LR, Crouch B, Kwiatek R, et al. A brain MRI study of chronic fatigue syndrome: evidence of brainstem dysfunction and altered homeostasis. *NMR Biomed*. 2011;24(10):1302–1312.

63. Perrin R, Embleton K, Pentreath VW, et al. Longitudinal MRI shows no cerebral abnormality in chronic fatigue syndrome. *Br J Radiol*. 2010;83(989):419–423.

64. Riccio M, Thompson C, Wilson B, et al. Neuropsychological and psychiatric abnormalities in myalgic encephalomyelitis: a preliminary report. *Br J Clin Psychol*. 1992;31(Part 1): 111–120.

65. Sandman CA, Barron JL, Nackoul K, et al. Memory deficits associated with chronic fatigue immune dysfunction syndrome. *Biol Psychiatry*. 1993;33(8–9):618–623.

66. Smith AP, Behan PO, Bell W, et al. Behavioural problems associated with the chronic fatigue syndrome. *Br J Psychol*. 1993;84(Pt 3):411–423.

67. McDonald E, Cope H, David A. Cognitive impairment in patients with chronic fatigue: a preliminary study. *J Neurol Neurosurg Psychiatry*. 1993;56(7): 812–815.

68. Constant EL, Adam S, Gillain B, et al. Cognitive deficits in patients with chronic fatigue syndrome compared to those with major depressive disorder and healthy controls. *Clin Neurol Neurosurg*. 2011;113(4):295–302.

69. Scheffers MK, Johnson Jr R, Grafman J, et al. Attention and short-term memory in chronic fatigue syndrome patients: an event-related potential analysis. *Neurology*. 1992;42(9):1667–1675.

70. Grafman J, Schwartz V, Dale JK, et al. Analysis of neuropsychological functioning in patients with chronic fatigue syndrome. *J Neurol Neurosurg Psychiatry*. 1993;56(6):684–689.

71. Johnson SK, DeLuca J, Fiedler N, et al. Cognitive functioning of patients with chronic fatigue syndrome. *Clin Infect Dis*. 1994;18(suppl 1):S84–S85.

72. Cockshell SJ, Mathias JL. Cognitive functioning in chronic fatigue syndrome: a meta-analysis. *Psychol Med*. 2010;40(8):1253–1267.

73. Demitrack MA, Dale JK, Straus SE, et al. Evidence for impaired activation of the hypothalamic-pituitary-adrenal axis in patients with chronic fatigue syndrome. *J Clin Endocrinol Metab*. 1991;73(6): 1224–1234.

74. Ur E, White PD, Grossman A. Hypothesis: cytokines may be activated to cause depressive illness and chronic fatigue syndrome. *Eur Arch Psychiatry Clin Neurosci*. 1992;241(5):317–322.

75. Van Den Eede F, Moorkens G, Van Houdenhove B, et al. Hypothalamic-pituitary-adrenal axis function in chronic fatigue syndrome. *Neuropsychobiology*. 2007;55(2):112–120.

76. Morriss R, Sharpe M, Sharpley AL, et al. Abnormalities of sleep in patients with the chronic fatigue syndrome. *BMJ*. 1993;306(6886):1161–1164.

77. McCluskey DR. Pharmacological approaches to the therapy of chronic fatigue syndrome. *Ciba Found Symp*. 1993;173:280–287.

78. Krupp LB, Jandorf L, Coyle PK, et al. Sleep disturbance in chronic fatigue syndrome. *J Psychosom Res*. 1993;37(4): 325–331.

79. Togo F, Natelson BH, Cherniack NS, et al. Sleep structure and sleepiness in chronic fatigue syndrome with or without coexisting fibromyalgia. *Arthritis Res Ther*. 2008;10(3):R56.

80. Gray JB, Martinovic AM, Horrobin D. Eicosanoids and essential fatty acid modulation in chronic disease and the chronic fatigue syndrome. *Med Hypotheses*. 1994;43(1):31–42.

81. Ogawa R, Toyama S, Matsumoto H. Chronic fatigue syndrome – cases in the Kanebo Memorial Hospital. *Nippon Rinsho*. 1992;50(11):2648–2652.

82. Nicolson GL. Lipid replacement as an adjunct to therapy for chronic fatigue, anti-aging and restoration of mitochondrial function. *JANA*. 2003;6(3):22–28.

83. Behan PO, Behan WM, Horrobin D. Effect of high doses of essential fatty acids on the postviral fatigue syndrome. *Acta Neurol Scand*. 1990;82(3):209–216.

84. Kuratsune H, Yamaguti K, Takahashi M, et al. Acylcarnitine deficiency in chronic fatigue syndrome. *Clin Infect Dis*. 1994;18(suppl 1):S62–S67.

85. Takahashi H, Imai K, Katanuma A, et al. A case of chronic fatigue syndrome who showed a beneficial effect by intravenous administration of magnesium sulphate. *Aerugi*. 1992;41(11):1605–1610.

86. Hinds G, Bell NP, McMaster D, et al. Normal red cell magnesium concentrations and magnesium loading tests in patients

with chronic fatigue syndrome. *Ann Clin Biochem.* 1994;31(Pt 5):459–461.

87. Jacobson W, Saich T, Borysiewicz LK, et al. Serum folate and chronic fatigue syndrome. *Neurology.* 1993;43(12): 2645–2647.

88. Amagase H, Sun B, Nance DM. Immunomodulatory effects of a standardized Lycium barbarum fruit juice in Chinese older healthy human subjects. *J Med Food.* 2009;12(5):1159–1165.

89. Sathyapalan T, Beckett S, Rigby AS, et al. High cocoa polyphenol rich chocolate may reduce the burden of the symptoms in chronic fatigue syndrome. *Nutr J.* 2010;9:55.

90. Scholey AB, French SJ, Morris PJ, et al. Consumption of cocoa flavonols results in acute improvements in mood and cognitive performance during sustained mental effort. *J Psychopharmacol.* 2010;24(10):1505–1514.

91. Cho JH, Cho CK, Shin JW, et al. Myelophil, an extract mix of Astragali Radix and Salviae Radix, ameliorates chronic fatigue: a randomised, double blind, controlled pilot study. *Complement Ther Med.* 2009;17(3):141–146.

92. Stricklin A, Sewell M, Austad C. Objective measurement of personality variables in epidemic neuromyasthenia patients. *S Afr Med J.* 1990;77(1):31–34.

93. Patarca-Montero R, Antoni M, Fletcher MA, et al. Cytokine and other immunologic markers in chronic fatigue syndrome and their relation to neuropsychological factors. *Appl Neuropsychol.* 2001;8(1):51–64.

94. Panossian A, Wikman G. Pharmacology of Schisandra chinensis Bail. An overview of Russian research and uses in medicine. *J Ethnopharmacol.* 2008;118(2): 183–212.

95. Blomkvist J, Taube A, Larhammar D. Perspective on roseroot (Rhodiola rosea) studies. *Planta Med.* 2009;75(11):1187–1190.

96. Panossian A, Wikman G, Sarris J. Rosenroot (Rhodiola rosea): traditional use, chemical composition, pharmacology and clinical efficacy. *Phytomedicine.* 2010;17(7):481–493.

97. Olsson EM, von Schéele B, Panossian AG. A randomised, double blind, placebo-controlled, parallel-group study of the standardised extract shr-5 of the roots of Rhodiola rosea in the treatment of subjects with stress-related fatigue. *Planta Med.* 2009;75(2):105–112.

98. Sarris J, Panossian A, Schweitzer I, et al. Herbal medicine for depression, anxiety and insomnia: a review of psychopharmacology and clinical evidence. *Eur Neuropsychopharmacol.* 2011;21(12):841–860.

99. Baschetti R. Chronic fatigue syndrome and licorice. *N Z Med J.* 1995;108(998): 156–157.

100. Kato Y, Kamijima S, Kashiwagi A, et al. Chronic fatigue syndrome, a case of high anti-HHV-6 antibody titer and one associated with primary hyperaldosteronism. *Nippon Rinsho.* 1992;50(11):2673–2678.

101. Adams D, Wu T, Yang X, et al. Traditional Chinese medicinal herbs for the treatment of idiopathic chronic fatigue and chronic fatigue syndrome. *Cochrane Database Syst Rev.* 2009;4:CD006348.

Malignant diseases

Scope

Apart from their use in providing non-specific support for recuperation and repair, specific phytotherapeutic strategies include the following.

Adjunctive treatment of:

* most cancers.

Management of:

* symptoms of cancer treatment, such as nausea/vomiting of chemotherapy
* recuperation from chemotherapy and radiotherapy.

Because of its use of secondary plant products, particular **caution** is necessary in applying phytotherapy in cases of cancers of the stomach, liver and kidneys.

Orientation

Background

Herbal practitioners are often asked to provide treatment for cancer patients. This is most often as a complement to conventional treatments. However, in a few cases they are asked to construct completely alternative treatment strategies. In the latter case especially, the practitioner can be put in a most difficult position. Cancer is undoubtedly one of the most serious and also one of the most complex and diverse diagnoses to receive. Modern oncology has confirmed that finding and attacking malignant targets remains most difficult,

and that different forms of cancer present very different prospects. Modern treatments have, moreover, been powerful, indeed dangerous, assaults on cells that may be more vigorous than their normal neighbours. The efficacy and safety of these treatments depend on being able to focus on their target most selectively. Alternative approaches are usually derided by orthodox authorities because they apparently lack such potency, and reviews tend to reinforce the view that direct efficacy is lacking.[1]

Herbal clinicians respond that they are trying a different approach: mobilising the body's own powerful defences against the proliferation of malignant cells by providing appropriate supportive therapies. They point out that endogenous anticancer defences are formidable in even modest health. It is statistically likely that a tiny fraction of the body's cells (but this could mean thousands of cells) slip out of normal tissue constraints and become malignant each day; through quiet surveillance, the body's defences normally clean up such vagaries without further harm. Against that background, the actual development of a tumour must represent the failure of an impressive protective mechanism. In theory, it may be possible to reactivate these defences, at least in conditions that are not too advanced or debilitating. In practice, there is only modest evidence to guide a practitioner who aims to work in this direction, mainly from in vitro and in vivo studies.

On the positive side, the cases of spontaneous remissions from cancer and unexpected delays in deterioration that all healthcare practitioners encounter are evidence that there are powerful defensive forces to be had. To be set against this, however, is the need for evidence for any strategy towards mobilising these forces. However, there are some pointers, at least to the possibility of improving protection against cancer development before it happens and, by implication (but only by implication), to guide supportive or adjunctive measures to improve the prospects of spontaneous recovery after the event.

Plants and cancer prevention

After a $20 million research campaign over many years and on the basis of in vitro and in vivo studies as well as epidemiological evidence, the American National Cancer Institute (NCI) identified a range of foods with cancer preventive potential in three categories:[2,3]

1. Highest anticancer activity was found in garlic, soya, ginger, licorice and the umbelliferous vegetables (e.g. carrots, celery, parsley and parsnips).

2. Moderate anticancer activity was found in onions, linseed (flaxseed), citrus, turmeric, cruciferous vegetables (e.g. broccoli, Brussels sprouts, cabbage and cauliflower), solanaceous vegetables (tomatoes and peppers), brown rice and whole wheat.

3. Modest anticancer activity has been demonstrated in oats and barley, cucumber and the kitchen herbs such as the mints, rosemary, thyme, oregano, sage and basil.

The chemical groups suggested by the NCI as conveying some of this activity include allyl sulphides in garlic and onions; phytates in grains and legumes; lycopene, limonoids, glucarates and related terpenes; carotenes and flavonoids in citrus; lignans in linseed[4] and soya; isoflavones in soya; saponins in legumes; indoles, isothiocyanates and dithiolthione in cruciferous vegetables;[5] ellagic acid in grapes and other fruit; and phthalides and polyacetylenes in umbelliferous vegetables. Most of these are relatively robust to food preparation and are likely to reach target tissues in the body after oral consumption. Interaction with hormone receptors and other metabolic pathways leading to tumour generation is implicated as a mechanism.

Epidemiological evidence so far supports these findings.[6] For example, a study in Finland, following a cohort of 9959 cancer-free individuals (from a population of 62 440) for 24 years from 1967 found an inverse relationship between the development of lung and other cancers and the consumption of flavonoid-rich fruits and vegetables.[7] In a study in The Netherlands on a randomly selected cohort of 3123 subjects (from a total study size of 120 852), researchers found an inverse relationship between onion consumption and the development of stomach cancers over 3 years.[8] A review of this and other studies concluded that onions, garlic and other allium vegetables were likely to convey protective effects against cancer development, especially in the gastrointestinal tract.[9] There is actually some evidence for similar protective effect on the incidence of breast cancer in women for the use of herbal medicines in general. The Mammary Carcinoma Risk Factor Investigation (MARIE) study, a German population-based case-control study of 10 121 postmenopausal women (3464 with histologically confirmed breast cancer compared to 6657 controls) between 2002 and 2005, included analysis of associations between patterns of herbal preparations use and invasive breast cancer. Accounting for lifestyle and other risk factors, the authors concluded that

those who used herbal preparations – such as black cohosh (*Actaea racemosa*), St John's wort (*Hypericum perforatum*), chaste tree (*Vitex agnus-castus*), pulsatilla (*Pulsatilla pratensis*), rhubarb (*Rheum rhaponticum*) and Asian ginseng (*Panax ginseng*) – to manage their menopausal symptoms reduced their risk of breast cancer by 4% for every year's use of the herbal remedies and up to one-quarter, irrespective of histological type and receptor status.[10]

Some of the most persuasive data on the benefits of plants in at least reducing the incidence of cancer has been in epidemiological studies on the association with tea drinking. In addition to a number of studies demonstrating antitumour effects of extracts of *Camellia sinensis* (green tea) consumption and cancers of the bowel, stomach and breast, there have also been epidemiological studies supporting its protective effect in humans, and there are early studies under way to investigate its benefits in cancer patients.[11]

In the Shanghai Women's Health Study, 69 710 women aged 40 to 70 years were selected for observations over 6 years between 1996 and 2000. Women who reported drinking green tea regularly had around two-thirds of the risk for colorectal cancer compared with non-regular tea drinkers, and there also appeared to be a dose-dependent effect.[12] In a Japanese study, 26 464 men and 38 720 women between the ages of 40 and 80 were studied over 10 years. In all, 37 oral cancer cases were identified in this group. Subjects who consumed 5 or more cups per day had a reduced risk of oral cancer compared with those who consumed less than one cup per day; this was marked mainly in women. Interestingly, the authors proposed that the protective effects of green tea consumption may be through prevention of caries and periodontal disease.[13] Another study also in Japan pooled the results of several studies to indicate that there was a significant decrease in gastric cancer risk in the highest category of green tea consumption (at least five cups per day), but again *only* in women.[14]

Potential benefit in women at least was also suggested in Swedish studies on the links between all tea consumption and epithelial ovarian cancer. In a large study, 61 057 women between the ages of 40 and 76 years (the Swedish Mammography Cohort) were observed over an average of 15 years. After controlling for potential confounders, an inverse association was observed between tea consumption and ovarian cancer, and in a dose-dependent manner.[15]

Although there is criticism of such conclusions being drawn from low incidences of cancer, inadequate descriptions of tea consumption and of confounding factors,[16,17] there is an interesting pointer to the effect of a flavonoid-rich food and the incidence of cancer in women. This picks up on the associations already established with the consumption of flavonoid-rich diets referred to earlier. It also bridges to the interesting debate on the potential of phyto-oestrogen diet sources.

In a large controlled study in China reported in the *British Medical Journal*, data was consistent with the hypothesis that regular intake of soya foods is associated with a reduced risk of endometrial cancer, especially among overweight women.[18] The authors of this report believed that soya foods exert an anti-oestrogenic effect in an oestrogen-rich environment. This view is widely held. It is also postulated as a basis for a protective effect of other plant remedies with oestrogenic properties. However the evidence so far on this point has not been compelling (see also Chapter 2 under Phyto-oestrogens).[19]

On the other hand there seems to be little risk of phyto-oestrogens worsening oestrogen-dependent tumours either. In one study 18861 women were included in a single-blinded observational retrospective cohort study, on survival time from breast cancer and the use of an isopropanolic black cohosh extract. Only about 1000 of these women were taking the black cohosh, but there was no shift in relapse rates in this group compared to controls, even among patients with oestrogen-dependent tumours.[20] In a substantial study conducted in Cambridge, UK, the effect of another phyto-oestrogen source, a red-clover-derived isoflavone extract, on oestrogen-linked mammographic breast density (this is associated with an increased risk for breast cancer) was investigated in 205 women aged 49 to 65 years and without a history of breast cancer. The women received either a placebo or an isoflavone tablet containing 26mg biochanin A, 16mg formononetin, 1mg genistein and 0.5mg daidzein, derived from a proprietary brand of red clover, daily for 1 year. Baseline and 12-month follow-up mammograms were evaluated for density. The supplement did not significantly increase mammographic breast density nor did it have any other effect on hormonal levels. There was no significant effect on menopausal symptoms or hot flushes. The authors conclude that the isoflavone supplement, at the dose given, was acting neither as an oestrogen nor as an anti-oestrogen.[21]

However, this is an area where promising leads rarely translate into firm recommendations: lycopene from tomatoes has inconsistent benefits in human studies,[22] and the disappointing outcomes from the large study on the effects of beta-carotene as a food supplement have acted as a reminder that isolated plant-based solutions may be the wrong targets.[23] There are even data suggesting that some plant beverages, for example maté tea,[24] can have a negative effect on cancer incidence. On the other hand, it is noticeable that reviewers are less dismissive of natural approaches to cancer prevention and even management,[25] with, for example, the role of ginger in treating the side effects of chemotherapy widely appreciated (see below and the ginger monograph).[26] There is even evidence for positive combination effects: 5-fluorouracil is a common chemotherapy that can be limited over time. In one study, an improvement was observed in some patients with combined therapy with standardised Ginkgo biloba (see also later).[27]

There remain future prospects of genuine leads. Anti-inflammatory activity, for example by aspirin and indomethacin, has been shown to have tumour-inhibitory effects in some models (and aspirin consumption has been linked to reduced human colorectal incidence; for example, see the willow bark monograph). Cyclo-oxygenase inhibition by a polyphenol, resveratrol, has been cited as a mechanism for a range of in vitro and in vivo tumour inhibitory effects of red grapeskin products like red wine.[28] There are many other plant mechanisms that may modulate inflammation mentioned in other parts of this text (see, for example, the feverfew and turmeric monographs) and including the flavonoids mentioned earlier. Some

of the key phytochemicals with cancer preventative activity are also discussed in Chapter 2.

Plants and cancer treatment

The potential of plant remedies directly to correct established malignancies is apparently limited. In its intensive programme from 1955, screening plant extracts for anticancer activity, the NCI found less than four extracts in every thousand tested containing compounds that demonstrated efficacy. Of the approximately 114000 extracts studied, 11000 exhibited antitumour activity in the P338 pre-screen, but of these only 500 demonstrated such activity in panel testing and only 26 proceeded to secondary testing. Of the plant isolates that reached this stage, most were alkaloids or terpenoids, with few from plants used in traditional medicine (for example, a triterpene from Withania spp., a diterpene from Brucea spp., a lignan from Podophyllum spp., a quinone from Tabebuia spp., an alcohol from Aristolochia spp. and alkaloids from Camptotheca acuminata, Fagara macrophylla, Ficus spp., Heliotropium indicum, Ochorisia moorei and Zanthoxylum nitidum). Only the diterpene taxol from Taxus brevifolia eventually received marketing approval from the Food and Drug Administration.[29] The anticancer benefits of the alkaloids vinblastine and vincristine from the Madagascar periwinkle, Catharantheus roseus, were identified separately from the NCI programme. The NCI has studied the tamoxifen-like properties of the monoterpene perillyl alcohol, a naturally occurring analogue of limonene in citrus fruits and extracted from oil of lavender.[30]

Other plant isolates from traditional remedies have been identified as having antitumour effects in vitro and in vivo in other research programmes.[31] These include:

- the anthraquinones rhein and emodin from Cassia spp. (the sennas), Rhamnus spp. (cascara sagrada and alder buckthorn) and Rumex crispus (yellow dock)
- the furanocoumarin psoralen from Angelica spp. and other umbelliferous remedies
- the alkaloid berberine from Berberis spp. (barberry and Oregon grape), Hydrastis canadensis (golden seal) and the Chinese remedy Coptis chinensis (see monograph)
- the alkaloids matrine and oxymatrine from the Chinese remedies Sophora spp.
- boswellic acids from Boswellia serrata (see monograph).

There have been a few studies that suggest that plant preparations may have anticancer effects in experimental conditions. An extract of garlic was shown to have effects against bladder cancer in mice.[32] A pectin fraction from citrus demonstrated inhibitory effects on metastasis also in mice,[33] and curcumin has shown consistent laboratory effects (see the turmeric monograph for more details).[34]

Among plant-based treatments for cancer, the fresh plant mistletoe extract marketed as Iscador has been one widely prescribed by physicians in Europe. There is contention in the literature on the strength of the evidence for this. One meta-analysis found broadly in favour of benefit in combination with conventional cancer therapy, although it also called for more rigorous studies.[35] Other reviewers have been more

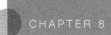

sceptical and deemed the positive studies to be methodologically compromised.[36] It should be noted that this extract is administered by injection.

Phytotherapeutics

Patient expectations

There are several reasons why a patient with cancer might seek herbal treatment. They include:

- As a stand-alone alternative treatment aimed at controlling the tumour and alleviating symptoms. This is often the situation with terminal patients who have no conventional treatment options left: the focus here should be on extending life, improving quality of life (QOL), well-being and palliative care
- As a complementary treatment to enhance survival prospects, reduce side effects and improve QOL and well-being after or in conjunction with surgery and/or chemotherapy and/or radiotherapy
- As a post-conventional treatment to increase survival prospects (prevent recurrence) and improve QOL. In a sense this is tertiary prevention.

An improvement in survival prospects might occur via an enhancement of the effects of conventional therapy, a mitigation of the toxic effects of conventional therapy or a contribution via different pathways, such as promoting the immune response to the tumour.

Surveys tend to back these reasons. For example, an Australian survey of breast cancer patients identified the following key reasons for the use of vitamin and herbal remedies:[37]

- To improve physical well-being (major reason)
- To boost the immune system (major reason)
- To reduce side effects (major reason for herbs only)
- To improve emotional well-being
- To prevent recurrence
- To assist in treating the cancer
- To reduce symptoms.

A US survey across the 10 most common cancers (bladder, colorectal, breast, kidney, lung, lymphoma, ovarian, prostate, melanoma and uterine) assessed dietary supplement use by cancer survivors.[38] Time between diagnosis and participating in the survey averaged 19 months. Over half had localised disease and most (78.22%) did not have recurrence, metastasis or multiple tumours. Almost all (97.3%) underwent conventional treatment and 69.3% had used supplements after diagnosis. Gender (female) and higher education strongly predicted such use. The supplements most commonly used after diagnosis were green tea, multivitamins and protein supplements. The main reasons for use were self-help, to boost immunity and increase energy, and the most common sources for information were doctors (47.3%) and friends or family (37.5%).

In reality the key drivers for patients with cancer seeking herbal treatment can be complex and varied. They might include:

- empowerment, taking control, being an active participant, wanting to do everything possible

- urging of friends and family
- fear of the cancer and the need to find hope and moral support
- fear of failure of conventional treatments
- fear of the side effects of conventional treatments.

Some cancer patients can hold unrealistic expectations about what phytotherapy might have to offer, often encouraged by their encounter with fad cures. Others come in hope or as a last option. In all these difficult circumstances, an evidence-based approach can help to manage expectations on both sides and enable the setting of realistic goals.

Complete eradication of a malignant tumour is not always achieved, even by aggressive mainstream treatments. As already discussed, natural approaches are generally not that active at killing tumour cells or controlling tumour growth. Often they work best in a complementary role in conjunction with the conventional approach. In this context, a highly relevant concept has been suggested by one research group: living with cancer.

Dr Harvey Schipper, Professor of Medicine at the University of Toronto, has proposed this interesting concept.[39] It has profound implications for phytotherapy in the context of cancer. In particular, it challenges the notion that the tumour is the 'disease' in an otherwise healthy body and asserts that cancer is a process, not a specific lump of abnormal tissue. Schipper asserts that for more than 50 years the paradigm underlying cancer research and treatment has been that of irreversibly deranged cells, which would inevitably kill their host unless they were totally eradicated.

Experimentation procedures, evaluation criteria and therapies are all based on cell killing. Yet there is substantial evidence that the kill/cure paradigm has reached its limit, and may be blinding us to other mechanisms. Both old and new data lead to the conclusion that the derangements in cellular function, while profound, are in large measure derivatives of normal mechanisms for organ growth, repair and renewal. Further, these are dynamic processes, potentially capable of reversal.[39]

If cancer is viewed as a community of cells in which signalling and communication is deranged, but functional, it becomes clear that cytotoxic approaches may serve to worsen the very control and communication defects that permit growth, invasion and metastasis. In the new model, the cancer cell is seen as largely normal, but aberrantly regulated. Viewed from this perspective, any 'cures' achieved may not be the result of a total kill, but instead may result from a reassertion of control.

This model leads to an approach aimed at the re-institution of normal regulatory process. In particular, inducing apoptosis, redifferentiation and tumour regulation become specific priorities. In this context the seven strategies proposed by Boik become highly relevant (Box 8.1).[40] However, at the same time the clinician should be guided by clinical outcome evidence and not be blinded by molecular biology theories and purely in vitro evidence.

Phytotherapy

The traditional approach

All the above evidence suggests that in sufferers from cancer it would generally be wise to start supportive treatment with

The seven strategies according to Boik

- Promote genetic stability
- Promote differentiation and apoptosis
- Inhibit abnormal signal transduction
- Promote normal cell-to-cell communication
- Inhibit tumour angiogenesis
- Inhibit tumour invasion and metastasis
- Promote immunity against the tumour

dietary measures to increase fruits, especially citrus fruits and grapes, and vegetables, particularly of the onion, cabbage, umbelliferous and nightshade families and edible fungi. Supplementation with garlic and green tea seems generally to be advisable. Particularly if there is a tendency to constipation (itself a strong naturopathic focus for correction in cancer patients), the use of linseed as a bulking agent for the bowel seems indicated.

So far, so good. However, all generalities are just that, statistical guides for the population as a whole. None of the above can take account of individual differences. Herbal treatment is most consistently predicated on the uniqueness of each patient and his or her story of illness. It is always possible that there will be some for whom the above advice will not be helpful. It is even more difficult to steer more active treatments, especially without rigorous observations for guidance.

Apart from such general supports, therefore, treatment will concentrate in the first place on supporting what are often depleted resources (see the section on Chronic fatigue syndrome, p. 164, for general principles). Only once everything has been done to bolster endogenous defences can gentle active remedies be considered, using only the mildest remedies until or unless the practitioner can be confident that the patient is strong enough to take anything more vigorous. Without any clear clinical evidence for this next step, the practitioner can only be guided by precedent.

The overwhelming instinct through history is to see cancer as an indication for cleansing. Manifestations of this have included strict dietary eliminations (raw food, grain and fruit only, even grape-only diets have been applied). In the nature cure clinics of central Europe, often alpine establishments dedicated originally to the treatment of tuberculosis but switching increasingly to cancer management as the former condition diminished, the emphasis was on strict diets, invigorating hydrotherapy treatments and alterative herbal formulations. The latter might include, depending on other indications:

- *Arctium lappa* (burdock)
- *Calendula officinalis* (marigold)
- *Galium aparine* (cleavers)
- *Phytolacca decandra* (poke root)
- *Rumex acetosella* (sheep's sorrel)
- *Rumex crispus* (yellow dock root)
- *Taraxacum officinale* (dandelion)

- *Thuja occidentalis* (arbor-vitae)
- *Trifolium pratense* (red clover flowers)
- *Urtica dioica* (nettle)
- *Viola odorata* (sweet violet)
- *Viola tricolor* (heartsease).

Laxatives and cholagogues were often applied where indicated. The relatively toxic laxatives *Podophyllum peltatum* (American mandrake) and *P. emodi* from India were specifically used and have been found to have notable cytotoxic constituents that have featured in conventional chemotherapy; however, these are not part of the conservative strategy being discussed here. The full panoply of phytotherapy would additionally be directed at other factors seen to be contributing to the problem. The inclusion of Zingiber (ginger) in cases judged to be in need of circulatory stimulation seems to be supported by its status in the NCI rankings. The use of Glycyrrhiza (licorice) to modulate a prescription is similarly justified. European medicine also features the specific use of mistletoe extract (notably a product Iscador) as a non-toxic stimulant of endogenous defences (see earlier).

There were comparable strategies applied in traditional Chinese medicine, although diagnostic differentiation here is consistently more specific and application of such signs as pulse type and tongue appearance might lead to very individual treatments, particularly in replenishing deficient energies.[41] Nevertheless, cleansing or clearing (of toxins, damp-heat *phlegm* or stagnant *qi*, for example) featured highly. The impression from other cultural traditions is that remedies generally considered as eliminatory are those most often used for cancer.

In a major review of traditional treatments for 'tumours', under the aforementioned NCI programme, researchers at the University of Illinois listed several thousand remedies from around the world.[42–44] Allowing for semantic confusion about what 'tumours' may have meant in early societies (widely encountered 'tumours', for example, are likely to have included faecal impaction, the result of other digestive obstructions or simple lymphadenopathies), it is still notable how many of the remedies listed could be classified as eliminatives.

In North America the theme has been extended into a number of popular approaches to cancer treatment. The controversial Harry Hoxsey treatments (derived from the formulations of a veterinary practitioner), the Essiac formula (based on sheep sorrel and burdock and supported by more commendations and professional and political support than other natural approaches) and many other examples usually emphasise the same or comparable remedies and themes. They usually support their theory with dramatic case reports – encouraging but not entirely persuasive. Whatever the doubts about efficacy, these strategies are at least generally consistent with historical approaches. What is less desirable is the occasional promotion of treatments based on whimsical rationale. The claims for apricot kernels and their constituent 'laetrile' or vitamin B_{17} obscured the fact that this active is a cyanogenic glycoside for which the rationale was in effect a selective toxicity against tumour cells. Apart from the fact that the claim was never adequately tested, it sat uneasily in the alternative culture by competing directly with conventional chemotherapy (see also Chapter 2).

The laetrile incident reminds practitioners that cancer patients are notably vulnerable to marketing hype. Claims for treating cancer are for that reason proscribed for over-the-counter medications in the European Union and have been the subject of proscriptive court judgments. A practitioner faced with a request to help an individual patient through cancer will approach the task with humility and a recognition that, in most cases, the treatment course will be set without a compass or a map. The most responsible practitioner will privately dread the burden.

Combination with conventional treatments

Far safer ground is to use phytotherapy to support the cancer patient undergoing conventional treatments. Phytotherapy may be given prior to conventional treatments to help the patient prepare for them (in order to minimise side effects). They may also be given during conventional treatments to improve treatment outcomes, QOL and reduce side effects. They may be given after conventional treatment for all the above reasons, but also to prevent cancer recurrence and improve survival prospects. This is the most active area of research for phytotherapy in cancer and some relevant clinical studies will be reviewed.

Twenty-five patients with a variety of very advanced cancers of the gastrointestinal tract undergoing palliative radio- or chemotherapy received up to 3g/day of GLA as evening primrose oil (EPO). They were matched to 25 controls.[45] The group receiving EPO exhibited highly statistically significant and clinically relevant survival differences (p=0.0001) and fewer adverse effects were noted from concurrent conventional treatment. Cancer markers also fell in some patients (see monograph).

In a long-term Korean study, the impact of Korean red ginseng (Panax ginseng) therapy on postoperative immunity and survival was investigated in patients with gastric cancer.[46] Forty-nine patients who had undergone gastric resection with lymph node removal by the same surgeon for histologically proven AJCC (American Joint Committee on Cancer) stage III gastric adenocarcinoma were enrolled in the trial. After the application of predefined exclusion criteria, 22 patients were given ginseng (4.5g/day) for the first 6 months after surgery and 20 acted as placebo controls. All patients were also treated with chemotherapy each month for 6 months after surgery. The study demonstrated 5-year disease-free survival and overall survival rates that were significantly higher in patients taking ginseng compared with controls (68.2% versus 33.3% and 76.4% versus 38.5%, respectively; p<0.05). Sun ginseng is a red ginseng extract manufactured under a patented process in Korea. A randomised, placebo-controlled, double blind trial in 53 cancer patients undergoing 'usual medical treatment' found that 12 weeks of 3g/day of sun ginseng significantly improved QOL (p=0.02) and general health (p<0.01).[47] A well-publicised study (n=282) on American ginseng root (Panax quinquefolium) found that 750 to 2000mg/day for 8 weeks significantly reduced cancer-related fatigue.[48]

Nausea is a common side effect of chemotherapy and ginger has been well tested in that context (see the ginger monograph). For example, in a large clinical study funded by the NCI, 644 cancer patients (mostly with breast cancer) were included in a double blind trial[49] and given either a placebo or three different doses of ginger root as 250mg capsules for 6 days, starting 3 days before chemotherapy. On the day of chemotherapy patients were given a standard antiemetic drug. All the tested doses of ginger significantly reduced nausea compared with the placebo, and surprisingly the largest reduction occurred for the lower ginger doses (500mg and 1000mg).

The value of medicinal mushrooms has also been assessed in cancer patients. The results of a randomised, double blind, placebo-controlled trial indicate that reishi (Ganoderma lucidum) extract (equivalent to 90g/day of mushroom) may have an adjunct role in the treatment of patients with advanced lung cancer. After 12 weeks of reishi treatment stable disease occurred in 35% of patients, compared to 22% in the control group.[50] A palliative effect on cancer-related symptoms, and an increase in Karnofsky performance score occurred in a greater number of patients receiving reishi. In uncontrolled trials, reishi extract improved the immune function and stamina of debilitated patients and cancer patients undergoing chemo- and radiotherapies.[51] Oral lentinan from Lentinula edodes has improved immune function in cancer patients, although it is usually given by injection for this application.[52]

PSK is an isolate rich in polysaccharides from the mushroom Coriolus versicolor approved as an adjunctive cancer treatment in Japan. It is usually administered orally at a dose of 3g daily in conjunction with chemotherapy, but also with radiotherapy. Significant improvements in 5-year survival rates in breast, colorectal and gastric cancer have been demonstrated in several controlled clinical trials and in one meta-analysis that included 8009 patients from eight randomised controlled trials.[53] However, differences are often relatively modest.

Chemotherapy and radiotherapy are obviously substantial stressors; hence the stress-adapting role of adaptogens is a strong reason for their consideration. Other compelling reasons for using adaptogens as adjunctive therapy are to help the patient survive the treatment, to support immunity and blood cell counts and to assist with well-being and improve QOL. However, choosing adaptogens that also have some additional benefits on specific cancer mechanisms is a useful parallel strategy. These are best given before conventional therapy for reasons outlined below.

Recently the concept of hormesis has been adopted by biology and medicine as the beneficial adaptive response of cells and organisms to moderate stress. In other words moderate stress promotes health, well-being and mental and physical performance, and increases resistance to toxic influences. There are countless examples: for example, mild 34°C shock protected fruit fly larvae against a long 0°C shock, mild hypoxia can increase lifespan of the roundworm (Caenorhabditis elegans) and induce cross-tolerance to other types of stress.[54]

How can exposure to low levels of toxins or other stressors have beneficial effects? The answer lies in the defence molecules the body calls up in response to threats. Once rallied, these molecules not only deal with the immediate threat, but also increase resistance to other threats. They can even repair existing damage. Examples of these molecular defence agents include heat shock proteins, sirtuin 1, growth factors and cell kinases. Adaptogens are herbs that help the body better adapt to stressors by fine-tuning the stress response. It has recently been shown that the stress-protective effect of adaptogens is not the result of inhibition of the stress response of an organism, but actually comes from the adaptation of the organism to the mild stressful effects of the adaptogen. The repeated administration (adaptation) of adaptogens gives rise to an adaptogenic or stress-protective effect in a manner analogous to repeated physical exercise, leading to a prolonged state of non-specific resistance to stress and increased endurance and stamina under extreme conditions. This is in fact hormesis.[55]

The use of Chinese herbal medicine in conjunction with conventional cancer treatments is widespread in China. There are several books on this topic and a number of systematic reviews and meta-analyses, sometimes by the Cochrane Collaboration. Quite often, individual herbs or formulations are administered by injection. One key adaptogenic and tonic herb that is widely used in China during cancer treatment is Astragalus. A systematic review of Chinese herbs for chemotherapy side effects in colorectal cancer patients found that, while studies were of low quality, results suggest that Astragalus may stimulate immunocompetent cells and decrease side effects.[56] A meta-analysis of randomised trials of Chinese herbal medicine and chemotherapy in the treatment of hepatocellular carcinoma representing 2079 patients found significantly improved survival at 12 months, compared with chemotherapy alone.[57] (Also see the Astragalus monograph.)

Codonopsis is a widely prescribed adaptogen in China, used in conjunction with conventional cancer therapies to reduce side effects and support immunity.[58] It was used as an adjuvant in 76 cancer patients during radiotherapy and reduced its immunosuppressive effect.[59] Pharmacological studies suggest it can help both white and red blood cell production.[60]

A small cohort study following 254 women with ovarian cancer over 3 years found that regular green tea use caused a significant dose-dependent increase in survival rate.[61] Following colorectal adenoma removal, a significant reduction in relapse was observed in a randomised, placebo-controlled trial over 12 months in 125 patients in Japan when green tea consumption was increased (from the equivalent 6 cups/day) to 10 cups/day.[62] Following the report of four cases of remission or regression of chronic lymphocytic leukaemia after green tea consumption,[63] the Mayo clinic undertook a small phase I trial.[64] A proprietary green tea extract was used that was welltolerated. Declines in lymphocyte count and/or lymphadenopathy were observed in the majority of patients.

Several open label trials have shown benefit from Boswellia extract in patients with brain tumours in terms of controlling symptoms by reducing inflammation. Boswellic acids have inhibited growth of various cancer cells in vitro and in vivo at concentrations of the same order of magnitude to those seen in human pharmacokinetic studies (particularly if Boswellia is taken with food). (See the Boswellia monograph for more details.) There is substantial preclinical evidence that curcumin targets multiple factors that sustain tumour development and growth.[53] Curcumin is currently being trialled (albeit in very high doses) in cancer patients with promising findings. It is also being investigated in clinical studies as a cancer preventative. (See the turmeric monograph for more details.)

Despite increasing use by cancer patients, most oncologists recommend avoidance of herbs and supplements throughout most phases of cancer care, especially concurrent use with chemotherapy and radiotherapy.[65] Evidence of harm remains largely theoretical and documented benefit is on the increase. Negative interactions can be either pharmacokinetic or pharmacodynamic, and most evidence for the former exists for extracts of St John's wort (*Hypericum perforatum*), probably those rich in hyperforin (see the monograph). The use of antioxidants with both chemotherapy and radiotherapy is particularly controversial.[65]

A comprehensive two-part review of this topic was published in 2007, which reviewed all published literature from 1965 to 2003.[66,67] Most of the concerns expressed were regarding vitamins, and there was little evidence for any negative interaction with herbs. A 2006 systematic review included 19 randomised, controlled studies in 1554 patients receiving antioxidant supplements (not herbal) concurrent with chemotherapy and concluded that there was no evidence for concern, and perhaps benefit.[68] A 2008 review that included 16 trials of antioxidants with chemotherapy found the same, but suggested the studies were underpowered.[69] The nine radiotherapy studies reviewed suggested less tumour control for vitamin E and beta-carotene. These findings suggest that strongly antioxidant herbs are best avoided within 24 to 48h either side of radiotherapy.

CASE HISTORY

'Robert', aged 57 years, presented with metastatic bladder cancer that had been diagnosed 8 months earlier. The cancer had spread to his local lymph glands and his prostate, and these had been surgically removed. Following diagnosis he was also treated with six 4-week cycles of intravenous chemotherapy using the drugs carboplatin and gemcitabine. This had finished only 1 month prior to his seeking herbal treatment. Despite the chemotherapy, the patient had unfortunately developed extensive secondary tumours throughout his lymphatic system, especially in the supraclavicular fossa. He was about to embark on another six cycles (each over 4 weeks) of a complex intravenous chemotherapy cocktail that included the drugs methotrexate, vinblastine, doxorubicin and cisplatin. Past medical history included testicular cancer 18 years prior that was successfully treated by surgery and chemotherapy. Despite the fact that the patient was attempting another six cycles of chemotherapy, his oncologist expressed the view that he would only be able to tolerate two to three at best, because of the long-term damage to his bone marrow stem cells as a result of past chemotherapy treatments.

He was advised to consume button mushrooms, green tea and vegetable juices in his diet and prescribed the following herbal treatments:

A. Liquid formula:

Withania somnifera	1:1	25 mL
Panax ginseng (standardised extract)	1:2	10 mL
Astragalus membranaceus	1:2	35 mL
Codonopsis pilosula	1:2	40 mL
	TOTAL	110 mL

Dose: 10 mL with water 3 times daily

B. Four tablets/day of the following formulation:*

Polygonum cuspidatum root	8.0 g
Standardised to resveratrol	36 mg
Pinus massoniana bark	5.0 g

Silybum marianum fruit (standardised)	4.2 g
Ginkgo biloba leaf (standardised)	1.5 g
Panax ginseng root (standardised)	250 mg

The patient was able to complete all six rounds of chemotherapy with normal red and white cell counts at the end. He only once needed the treatment reduced due to a low neutrophil count.

* Note added in proof: With the discovery that cancer cells can harness the Nrf2/ARE pathway to enhance their survival during chemotherapy, the use of primers of this pathway such as resveratrol is best avoided within a 48 h window either side of chemotherapy or radiotherapy.

Summary

The validity of using phytotherapy for cancer patients needs to be assessed in terms of risk, benefit, cost, effort and empowerment. More studies are needed to understand risk and benefit, but the most promising area (and least difficult in terms of ethical issues) is the combination with conventional treatments. Antioxidant herbs and supplements are best avoided 24–48 h either side of radiation or chemotherapy, although such caution is largely theoretical and radiotherapy is probably of more concern.

References

1. Weiger W, Smith M, Boon H, et al. Advising patients who seek complementary and alternative medical therapies for cancer. *Ann Intern Med.* 2002;137(11):889–913.

2. Craig WJ. Phytochemicals: guardians of our health. *J Am Diet Assoc.* 1997;97(2): 199–204.

3. Cragg GM. Natural product drug discovery and development at the United States National Cancer Institute. *J Naturopathic Med.* 1996;6(1):38–41.

4. Jenab M, Thompson L. The influence of flaxseed and lignans on colon carcinogenesis and B-glucuronidase activity. *Carcinogenesis.* 1996;17(6):1343–1348.

5. Fowke J, Morrow J, Motley S, et al. Brassica vegetable consumption reduces urinary F2-isoprostane levels independent of micronutrient intake. *Carcinogenesis.* 2006;27(10):2096–2102.

6. Weisburger JH. Practical approaches to chemoprevention of Cancer. *Drug Metab Rev.* 1994;26(1&2):253–260.

7. Knekt P, Järvinen R, Sappänen R, et al. Dietary flavonoids and the risk of lung cancer and other malignant neoplasms. *Am J Epidemiol.* 1997;146(3):223–230.

8. Dorant E, van den Brandt PA, Goldbohm RA, Sturmans F. Consumption of onions and reduced risk of stomach carcinoma. *Gastroenterology.* 1996;110:12–20.

9. Ernst E. Can Allium vegetables prevent cancer? *Phytomedicine.* 1997;4(1):79–83.

10. Obi N, Chang-Claude J, Berger J, et al. The use of herbal preparations to alleviate climacteric disorders and risk of postmenopausal breast cancer in a German case-control study. *Cancer Epidemiol Biomarkers Prev.* 2009;18(8):2207–2213.

11. Muir M. (Green) Tea time: does it help prevent cancer? *Altern Complement Ther.* 1998;4(1):43–47.

12. Yang G, Shu X-O, Li H, et al. Prospective cohort study of green tea consumption and colorectal cancer risk in women. *Cancer Epidemiol Biomarkers Prev.* 2007;16(6):1219–1223.

13. Ide R, Fujino Y, Hoshiyama Y, et al. A prospective study of green tea consumption and oral cancer incidence in Japan. *Ann Epidemiol.* 2007;17(10):821–826.

14. Inoue M, Sasazuki S, Wakai K, et al. Green tea consumption and gastric cancer in Japanese: a pooled analysis of six cohort studies. *Gut.* 2009;58(10):1323–1332.

15. Larsson S, Wolk A. Tea consumption and ovarian cancer risk in a population-based cohort. *Arch Intern Med.* 2005;165: 2683–2686.

16. Liu J, Xing J, Fei Y. Green tea (Camellia sinensis) and cancer prevention: a systematic review of randomized trials and epidemiological studies. *Chin Med.* 2008;3:12.

17. Boehm K, Borrelli F, Ernst E, et al. Green tea (Camellia sinensis) for the prevention of cancer (review). *Cochrane Database Syst Rev.* 2009;3:CD005004.

18. Xu W, Zheng W, Xiang Y, et al. Soya food intake and risk of endometrial cancer among Chinese women in Shanghai: population based case-controlled study. *BMJ.* 2004;10:1285–1290.

19. Magee P, Rowland I. Phyto-oestrogens, their mechanism of action: current evidence for a role in breast and prostate cancer. *Br J Nutr.* 2004;91:513–531.

20. Henneicke-von Zepelin HH, Meden H, Kostev K, et al. Isopropanolic black cohosh extract and recurrence-free survival after breast cancer. *Int J Clin Pharmacol Ther.* 2007;45(3):143–154.

21. Atkinson C, Warren R, Sala E, et al. Red clover-derived isoflavones and mammographic breast density: a double blind, randomized, placebo-controlled trial. *Breast Cancer Res.* 2004;6(3):170–179.

22. Peters U, Leitzmann MF, Chatterjee N, et al. Serum lycopene, other carotenoids, and prostate cancer risk: a nested case-control study in the prostate, lung, colorectal, and ovarian cancer screening trial. *Cancer Epidemiol Biomarkers Prev.* 2007;16(5):962–968.

23. Blumberg JB. Considerations of the scientific substantiation for antioxidant vitamins and beta-carotene in disease prevention. *Am J Clin Nutr.* 1995;62(6 suppl):1521S–1526S.

24. Goldenberg D, Golz A, Joachims H. The beverage mate: a risk factor for cancer of the head and neck. *Head Neck.* 2003;25(7):595–601.

25. White J. The National Cancer Institute's perspective and agenda for promoting awareness and research on alternative therapies for cancer. *J Altern Complement Med.* 2002;8(5):545–550.

26. Boon H, Wong J. Botanical medicine and cancer: a review of the safety and efficacy. *Expert Opin Pharmacother.* 2004;5(12):2485–2501.

27. Hauns B, Haring B, Kohler S, et al. Phase II study of combined 5-fluorouracil/ginkgo biloba extract (GBE 761 ONC) therapy in 5-fluorouracil pretreated patients with advanced colorectal cancer. *Phytother Res.* 2001;15:34–38.

28. Meishiang J, Cai L, Udeani G, et al. Cancer chemopreventative activity of resveratrol, a natural product derived from grapes. *Science.* 1997;275:218–220.

29. Boik J. *Cancer and Natural Medicine: A Textbook of Basic Science and Clinical Research.* USA: Oregon Medical Press; 1995. pp. 110–111.

30. Zeigler J. Raloxifene, retinoids, and lavender: 'Me too' tamoxifen alternatives under study. *J Natl Cancer Inst.* 1996;88(16):1100–1101.

31. Boik J. *Cancer and Natural Medicine: A Textbook of Basic Science and Clinical Research.* USA: Oregon Medical Press; 1995. pp. 112–120.

32. Riggs DR, DeHaven JI, Lamm DL. Allium sativum (garlic) treatment for murine transitional cell carcinoma. *Cancer.* 1997;79(10):1987–1994.

33. Briggs S. Modified citrus pectin may halt metastasis. *Nutr Sci News.* 1997;2(5): 216–218.

34. Shishodia S, Chaturvedi MM, Aggarwal BB. Role of curcumin in cancer therapy. *Curr Probl Cancer.* 2007;31(4):243–305.

35. Ziegler R, Grossarth-Maticek R. Individual patient data meta-analysis of survival and psychosomatic self-regulation from published prospective controlled cohort

studies for long-term therapy of breast cancer patients with a mistletoe preparation (Iscador). *Evid Based Complement Altern Med.* 2010;7(2):157–166.

36. Kleijnen J, Knipschild P. Mistletoe treatment for cancer: review of controlled trials in humans. *Phytomedicine.* 1994;1:255–260.

37. Kremser T, Evans A, Moore A, et al. Use of complementary therapies by Australian women with breast cancer. *Breast.* 2008;17(4):387–394.

38. Ferrucci LM, McCorkle R, Smith T, et al. Factors related to the use of dietary supplements by cancer survivors. *J Altern Complement Med.* 2009;15(6):673–680.

39. Schipper H. Treating cancer: is kill cure? *Ann Acad Med Singapore.* 1994;23(3): 382–386.

40. Boik J. *Natural Compounds in Cancer Therapy.* USA: Oregon Medical Press; 2001.

41. Boik J. *Cancer and Natural Medicine: A Textbook of Basic Science and Clinical Research.* USA: Oregon Medical Press; 1995. pp. 90–104.

42. Hartwell JL. Plants used against cancer. A survey. *Lloydia.* 1970;33(3):288–392.

43. Hartwell JL. Plants used against cancer. A survey. *Lloydia.* 1971;34(1):103–160.

44. Hartwell JL. Plants used against cancer. A survey. *Lloydia.* 1971;34(4):386–425.

45. Manolakis G, van der Merwe CF, Hager ED, et al. The omega-6 metabolite GLA (gamma-linolenic acid) as adjuvant in the management of the very advanced gastrointestinal tract cancer. *Dtsch Z Onkol.* 1995;27(5):124–129.

46. Suh SO, Kroh M, Kim NR, et al. Effects of red ginseng upon postoperative immunity and survival in patients with stage III gastric cancer. *Am J Chin Med.* 2002;30(4): 483–494.

47. Kim JH, Park CY, Lee SJ. Effects of sun ginseng on subjective quality of life in cancer patients: a double blind, placebo-controlled pilot trial. *J Clin Pharm Ther.* 2006;31(4):331–334.

48. Barton DL, Soori GS, Bauer BA, et al. Pilot study of Panax quinquefolius (American ginseng) to improve cancer-related fatigue: a randomized, double blind, dose-finding evaluation: NCCTG trial N03CA. *Support Care Cancer.* 2010;18(2):179–187.

49. Ryan JL, Heckler C, Dakhil SR, et al. Ginger for chemotherapy-related nausea in cancer patients: a URCC CCOP randomized, double blind, placebo-controlled clinical trial of 644 cancer patients. *J Clin Oncol.* 2009;27(suppl 15) Abstract 9511. <http://www.abstract.asco.org/AbstView_65_35351.html>. Accessed 1.08.2011.

50. Gao Y, Dai X, Chen G, et al. A randomized, placebo-controlled, multicenter study of Ganoderma lucidum (W. Curt.: Fr.) Lloyd (Aphylloromycetidae) polysaccharides (Ganopoly R) in patients with advanced lung cancer. *Int J Med Mushrooms.* 2003;5:369–381.

51. McKenna DJ, Jones K, Hughes K, et al. *Botanical Medicines: The Desk Reference for Major Herbal Supplements*, 2nd ed. New York: Haworth Herbal Press; 2002.

52. Morgan M. Immune-enhancing & tonic activity of reishi & shiitake. *Phytotherapist's Perspective.* 2005;64:1–2.

53. Miller S, Stagl J, Wallerstedt DB, et al. Botanicals used in complementary and alternative medicine treatment of cancer: clinical science and future perspectives. *Expert Opin Invest Drugs.* 2008;17(9):1353–1364.

54. Le Bourg E. Hormesis, aging and longevity. *Biochim Biophys Acta.* 2009;1790(10):1030–1039.

55. Panossian A, Wikman G. Evidence-based efficacy of adaptogens in fatigue, and molecular mechanisms related to their stress-protective activity. *Curr Clin Pharmacol.* 2009;4(3):198–219.

56. Taixiang W, Munro AJ, Guanjian L. Chinese medical herbs for chemotherapy side effects in colorectal cancer patients. *Cochrane Database Syst Rev.* 2005(1):CD004540.

57. Shu X, McCulloch M, Xiao H, et al. Chinese herbal medicine and chemotherapy in the treatment of hepatocellular carcinoma: a meta-analysis of randomized controlled trials. *Integr Cancer Ther.* 2005;4(3):219–229.

58. Cao W, Zhao AG. Prescription rules of Chinese herbal medicines in treatment of gastric cancer. *Zhong Xi Yi Jie He Xue Bao.* 2009;7(1):1–8.

59. Zneg XL, Li XA, Zhang BY. Immunological and hematopoietic effect of Codonopsis pilosula on cancer patients during radiotherapy. *Zhongguo Zhong Xi Yi Jie He Za Zhi.* 1992;12(10):607–608. 581

60. Chang H.M. But PP, eds. *Pharmacology and Applications of Chinese Materia Medica*, Vol 2. Singapore: World Scientific; 1987. pp. 975–976.

61. Zhang M, Lee AH, Binns CW, et al. Green tea consumption enhances survival of epithelial ovarian cancer. *Int J Cancer.* 2004;112(3):465–469.

62. Shimizu M, Fukutomi Y, Ninomiya M, et al. Green tea extracts for the prevention of metachronous colorectal adenomas: a pilot study. *Cancer Epidemiol Biomarkers Prev.* 2008;17(11):3020–3025.

63. Shanafelt TD, Lee YK, Call TG, et al. Clinical effects of oral green tea extracts in four patients with low grade B-cell malignancies. *Leuk Res.* 2006;30(6): 707–712.

64. Shanafelt TD, Call TG, Zent CS, et al. Phase I trial of daily oral Polyphenon E in patients with asymptomatic Rai stage 0 to II chronic lymphocytic leukemia. *J Clin Oncol.* 2009;27(23):3808–3814.

65. Hardy ML. Dietary supplement use in cancer care: help or harm. *Hematol Oncol Clin North Am.* 2008;22(4):581–617.

66. Simone II CB, Simone NL, Simone V, et al. Antioxidants and other nutrients do not interfere with chemotherapy or radiation therapy and can increase kill and increase survival, Part 1. *Altern Ther Health Med.* 2007;13(1):22–28.

67. Simone II CB, Simone NL, Simone V, et al. Antioxidants and other nutrients do not interfere with chemotherapy or radiation therapy and can increase kill and increase survival, Part 2. *Altern Ther Health Med.* 2007;13(2):40–46.

68. Block KI, Koch AC, Mead MN, et al. Impact of antioxidant supplementation on chemotherapeutic efficacy: a systematic review of the evidence from randomized controlled trials. *Cancer Treat Rev.* 2007;33(5):407–418.

69. Lawenda BD, Kelly KM, Ladas EJ, et al. Should supplemental antioxidant administration be avoided during chemotherapy and radiation therapy? *J Natl Cancer Inst.* 2008;100(11):773–783.

Herbal approaches to system dysfunctions

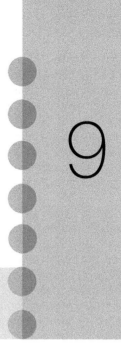

9

CHAPTER CONTENTS

Digestive system and bowel

Scope

Apart from their use to provide non-specific support for recuperation and repair, specific phytotherapeutic strategies include the following.

Treatment of:

- functional disorders such as dyspepsia, gastro-oesophageal reflux, irritable bowel syndrome
- inflammatory conditions of the upper tract, such as aphthous ulcers, oesophagitis, gastritis
- chronic gastrointestinal infections and dysbiosis
- constipation.

Management of:

- digestive deficiency and anorexia
- food intolerances and allergies
- peptic ulceration

- inflammatory diseases of the gut such as Crohn's disease and ulcerative colitis
- diverticulitis.

Modern research provides support for traditional herbal approaches in treating the gastrointestinal tract as **strategic therapy** in cases of:

- allergic conditions and inflammatory diseases of the skin, joints and connective tissues
- oedematous and fluid retention problems
- migraine.

Caution is necessary in applying herbal remedies to:

- severe malabsorption and malnutrition states
- gastric cancer
- biliary obstruction and bile duct cancer.

Orientation

An intelligent self-correcting disassembly line

The gut is a long passage designed to break down and process food, absorb nutrients and reject waste. Like an assembly line in reverse, it will only work efficiently if the delivery of material to the next stage is coordinated closely with the optimum rate of process at that stage. This subtle coordination is achieved by a robust and remarkably reliable network of control systems, orchestrated by a range of neurochemical and endocrine responses reacting to the material in the gut and managed by the complex circuitry and programmes of the enteric nervous system. Smooth muscle cells and the recently reviewed nerve-like interstitial cells of Cajal[1] spontaneously generate electrophysiological slow waves that are then modulated by a network of nerves, ganglia and neurohormones within the abdomen and the intestinal wall that is complex enough to merit the description 'intelligent'. Yet this is a decentralised system, not controlled entirely by the autonomic or higher nervous systems (the gut has approximately 10^8 nerve cells but only thousands of nerve fibres connecting to the central

DOI: http://dx.doi.org/10.1016/B978-0-443-06992-5.00009-8

nervous system, CNS), and most 'decisions' are made at a very local level rather than relying on central controls.[2]

Thus when functions are disturbed, treatments at a local level may have significant impact. Plant constituents have a unique range of topical effects on the gut. The case will be made that, because of the fundamental linkages between gut and other body functions, these effects can account for not only a valuable contribution to the therapeutics of the digestive system, but also for a very wide range of systemic activity as well (see also later).

In phytotherapy there is a traditional emphasis on normalising the functions of the digestive system. This accords well with its dynamics: like other complex dynamic systems in nature, the digestive system is essentially self-correcting. A gentle trigger stimulation of an appropriate reflex response or the temporary dampening of an inappropriate response may be all that is required to prompt or allow the digestive system to revert to normal patterns of behaviour. Plant constituents seem well suited to such tasks. The following text will review some of the areas of the gut where they may work.

Law of the gut: coordinated absorption, secretion and motility

Normal peristalsis is a simple example of the self-correcting and automatous nature of the digestive system. Gut activity is coordinated by a vast complex of nerve fibres, *intrinsic* fibres within the digestive tract linking to networks of *extrinsic* fibres, these in turn linked to *ganglia* within the abdominal cavity. Ascending intrinsic pathways are excitatory on the gut musculature and descending pathways inhibitory, but both are activated by distension. Peristalsis follows the activation by a bolus of food of ascending excitatory pathways proximal to each point along the intestine and the simultaneous inactivation of the descending inhibitory pathways distal to the contraction. The propagation of the circular muscle contraction stops when there is no longer a sufficient distension stimulus ahead.[3] The result of this arrangement is known as the 'law of the gut'. Any bolus of food material in the gut, simply by being there, is normally propelled in one direction, towards the lower bowel;[4] the absence of such a bolus leads to quiescence.

As well as provoking muscular activity, or motility, the presence of food in the gut also stimulates *secretomotor* reflexes via submucous neurons and causes a proportion of water and electrolytes that are absorbed with nutrients such as glucose to be returned to the lumen or instead for more to be lost in diarrhoea.[5] Observations in healthy volunteers point to innate rhythms of absorption, secretion and motility in the small intestine and biliary tract during fasting, these marked by variations in plasma levels of gastrointestinal hormones. Current evidence indicates that this periodicity is generated within the intrinsic innervation,[6] that is probably by local environmental factors, and that disturbances in these rhythms are potent factors in the aetiology of gastrointestinal and hepatic disease.[7] There is a significant correlation between motility and secretory modes, so that they are often coupled as the 'secretomotor' mode. As elaborated below, cholinergic neurons seem to mediate the shift in their direction from the absorptive mode.[8]

Carminative herbal remedies, such as the warming spices, reduce motility[9] (and thus, possibly, secretory activity) and, at least in the case of ginger, increase absorptive activity (see the ginger monograph). Increases in secretory activity and motility may be seen after the prescription of bitters, cholagogues and stimulating laxatives. However, these responses are not always predictable (in the case of bitters and cholagogues they may even be the opposite reaction in some cases) and it is also observed that reactive bowel looseness may follow a much wider variety of treatments. It appears that increases in gut activity are programmed as a response to any potentially perturbing influence, presumably as a simple defence mechanism.

Gut activity and its immune system

If there is gut infection or food intolerance, luminal antigens or bacterial products may be detected by the immune system. This may trigger a cascade of events associated with the release of inflammatory mediators. These mediators lead to increased motility and secretory patterns that are characterised by strong muscular contractions, copious secretion and diarrhoea.[10,11] The close connection between the gut-associated immune responses and the enteric nervous system is confirmed as important in the symptomatology of several functional disorders.[12,13] The enteric nervous system is also increasingly recognised as a regulator of epithelial barrier integrity, especially when the latter is exposed to inflammatory challenge; chronic inflammation has further disabling effects on enteric neuronal function.[14] All this provides further support for an integrated functional model in managing gut and bowel disturbances.

The gut and fluid balance

Diarrhoea is an extreme pattern of fluid and electrolyte loss which, as a consequence of enteric infections and malnutrition, is still the most common immediate cause of death around the world. In developed societies it is rarely as dangerous as it is in impoverished regions, where rehydration with fluids and electrolytes is a critical life-saving measure (as seen in the sugar and salt solution widely used by aid agencies around the world for the purpose). Nevertheless, diarrhoea is relatively common, reflecting a wide variety of events in the gut, from food poisoning and enteric infection through hepatobiliary activity (bile being a prominent potential irritant of the gut wall), food intolerance, to irritable bowel behaviour.[15] Often diarrhoea is of short duration and is not explained. It is even seen as a benign transient cleansing event in some healing strategies ('better out than in').

Any looseness of the bowel involves the loss of considerable amounts of fluid and electrolytes which, with the certainty of the excretion of a wide range of other materials, means that the gut can dwarf the function of the kidneys. Even modest fluctuation in bowel consistency and frequency can have significant impact on fluid balance in the body.

Some herbal traditions use remedies that loosen or bulk the bowel contents to reduce fluid accumulation and retention and even in some circumstances reduce weight. Cathartic remedies were included among those with drastic diuretic effects in the Chinese tradition, and stimulating anthraquinone laxatives clearly lead to fluid and electrolyte loss. In the

French tradition, even bulk laxatives and fibre are used to reduce weight associated with fluid retention.

By contrast, there are also a range of approaches to reducing bowel looseness if this is seen as harmful. These include the temporary use of astringent tannins that reduce reflex irritation of the bowel from the higher reaches of the gut in the case of gastroenteritis, the aromatic digestives and volatile antispasmodics, and the use of demulcent and topically anti-inflammatory remedies such as Althaea (marshmallow), Filipendula (meadowsweet), Glycyrrhiza (licorice), Calendula (marigold) and, for short-term use, Symphytum (comfrey) (see Chapter 2).

Stomach activity

The stomach's functions are closely coordinated with the rest of the digestive tract. It stores masticated food as a hopper, delivering its acidic contents into the alkalinised duodenum only at a rate that can be alkalinised: too fast and it damages the duodenal wall, too slow and it leads to discomfort and inhibits digestion of the following meal.

The stomach is also the first significant point of contact with most herbal remedies. Many have immediate effects on its function, increasing secretions of acid, pepsin and mucus (bitters and pungent constituents), calming activity (mucilaginous, astringent and some aromatic and antispasmodic remedies) or stimulating motility (saponins and emetic alkaloids). It is often highly sensitive to even minor doses of herbal remedies.

Healthy upper digestive function is important for maintaining health and preventing disease. Low acidity can lead to poor nutrient absorption and abnormal bowel flora. Patients with reduced gastric secretion are more susceptible to bacterial and parasitic enteric infections.[16] The contribution of poor upper digestive function to the chronicity of intestinal dysbiosis is often overlooked by therapists: the herbal practitioner has bitters and pungent principles to employ.

The chemical mediators of digestive activity

The coordination of digestive processes is mediated in the first instance by batteries of neurohumoral agents, chemicals that range from familiar endocrine hormones, standard neurotransmitters and chemical mediators, found also in the CNS and other body tissues, to gut-specific chemical agents. Each may be elicited by several receptor types in the gut wall and thus may be sensitive to different secreted, metabolised, dietary or pharmacological agents. These interactions, although highly complex and multilayered, are all integrated into a whole control mechanism for digestive activity.[17] Many constituents of herbal remedies are likely to interact with chemical mediators and this may provide some mechanisms for their effect on gut function. When these interactions are combined with similar examples in the nervous, endocrine, immunological and reproductive systems it appears that herbal medicine might genuinely provide a unique 'psychoneuroimmunological' strategy for the widest body disharmonies, one moreover that is centred on the gut.[18]

One common phytotherapeutic constituent has already established a number of contrasting effects on several neurohumoral mechanisms. Capsaicin, from *Capsicum spp.*, at quite low concentrations blocks the release of calcitonin gene-related peptide, a peptide found in enteric ganglia and known to be elicited directly by local mucosal irritation leading to increased peristaltic and secretomotor activity. Capsaicin thus results in a concentration-dependent decrease in peristaltic activity following mucosal stimulation.[19] Another recent discovery is the reflex release by capsaicin-stimulated nerve fibres of somatostatin, a systemic anti-inflammatory and analgesic with modulating effects on various digestive and pancreatic secretions.[20] Capsaicin also blocks an alternative stimulant to intestinal contraction, vasoactive intestinal peptide (VIP): VIP mediates the effects of noradrenaline and local stressors (such as acute hypoxia in vitro) which both depress cholinergic transmission and stimulate non-cholinergic contractions.[21,22] On the other hand, capsaicin is also known to induce intestinal contractions as a stimulant of sensory substance P-containing neurons,[23] which are also activated by various luminal stimuli such as the presence of food metabolites and simple physical distension to stimulate intestinal contractions. The consumption of hot spices has long been a feature of traditional herbal therapeutics (see also the discussion of 'acupharmacology' below) and the effects of Capsicum on the wider physiology have been confirmed in studies of cutaneous blood flow after ingestion of chillies; variable increases in blood flow have been observed, most consistently in the abdominal area.[24]

One of the most important hormonal regulators of the digestive process is cholecystokinin. This hormone is concentrated in the wall of the upper small intestine and is secreted into the blood on the ingestion of proteins and fats and has also been implicated in the action of bitters. The physiological actions of cholecystokinin include stimulation of pancreatic and gastric acid secretion and gallbladder contraction and regulation of gastric emptying, gastrointestinal motility and satiety, as well as augmenting symptoms of fear and anxiety.[25] (Plants with anxiolytic reputations have been shown to bind to cholecystokinin receptors and one, gotu kola, has been shown to attenuate startle response in human subjects.[26]) It is produced particularly by carbohydrate foods and appears to promote a feeling of fullness.[27] In humans it has been found that foods that lead to high levels of both cholecystokinin and satiety (such as bran) are associated with lower postprandial blood sugar and insulin levels, compared with refined carbohydrate.[28] This may be due to the physical characteristics of the carbohydrate but may also suggest that cholecystokinin helps to suppress hyperinsulinaemia.[29] Cholecystokinin has also been observed to suppress taste when feeding strongly tasting foods to animals.[30] There are suggestions that an increase in cholecystokinin production with age may contribute to the relative anorexia in the elderly.[31]

Gastrin is a polypeptide hormone which is secreted following vagal nerve activity and by the bulk presence of food in the stomach. Some food extractives, including partially digested proteins, alcohol and caffeine have an additional effect and some of the more stimulating plant constituents such as resins, spice ingredients and some saponins are likely to compound this activity.[32] Gastrin stimulates gastric acid and pepsin secretion. It extends and indeed multiplies the short-term effect of vagal stimulation on gastric secretions.

When gastric hydrochloric acid spills over into the intestine it lowers intestinal pH and stimulates the secretion of secretin. This acts to stimulate Brunner's glands and bicarbonate-rich bile and pancreatic secretions so as to alkalinise the intestinal contents. Secretin is also a potential mediator of the antiulcer actions of mucosal protective agents; it appears that secretin inhibits gastric acid secretion via endogenous prostaglandins.[33] Glycyrrhiza (licorice) stimulates the release of secretin in humans.[34]

Serotonin or 5-HT receptors have been shown to mediate the emetic reflex[35] and antagonists of the main receptor concerned, type 5-HT$_3$, have been developed to reduce emesis of cancer chemotherapy. (These are also found to have anxiolytic effects, confirming the overlap in enteric and higher nervous mediators.[36]) There is evidence, referred to in its monograph later in this book, that ginger also acts on this receptor. 5-HT is also a likely mediator in the lower bowel of both sennoside activity and the diarrhoeal response.[37] It is possibly implicated in the action of the emetic plant remedies.

There are a number of herbal constituents shown to have effects on neurosynaptic mediators. These effects are also likely to impinge on gut function, as many mediators have been found common to both. Gamma-aminobutyric acid (GABA), probably affected by a number of plant constituents, is produced in the myenteric plexus in the gut wall and acts via GABA receptors to both stimulate cholinergic and relax VIP motor neurons, contributing to both components of the peristaltic reflex.[38,39] Among many other neuroactive substances and receptor sites now identified as important modulators of gut function, the endocannabinoids[40] and fasting-associated orexins[41] are promising further templates for phytochemical activities. Certain Echinacea alkylamides are cannabinoid 2 receptor agonists (see Echinacea monograph).

Disturbed intestinal permeability

The role of the gut wall is to allow for selective absorption of nutrients while providing vital protection against intrusion into the body tissues of harmful substances from the lumen. Non-steroidal anti-inflammatory drug (NSAID) treatment has adverse effects on enterocyte mitochondria, which may predispose the mucosa to absorption of bacterial and other large molecules that provoke a local inflammatory response. A similar mechanism may operate in patients with untreated Crohn's disease, who show abnormally high permeability. Remission of Crohn's induced by treatment with elemental diets coincides with a reduction in permeability. Significant correlations have been seen between permeability and plasma IgA concentrates in kidney disease and between permeability and the passage of neutrophil chemotactic agents.[42]

It is likely that some plant constituents could reduce excessive intestinal permeability. Tannins are likely to have a limited short-term effect at least in the upper reaches of the tract and healing plants such as *Matricaria recutita* (chamomile), Filipendula (meadowsweet), *Ulmus spp.* (slippery elm),[43] Glycyrrhiza (licorice), Calendula and Symphytum (comfrey) have long been applied with this effect in mind. In theory, local anti-inflammatory activity might effectively reduce some types of increased permeability. However, the most promising effect on intestinal permeability is likely to lie in changing biliary constituents, using hepatics and choleretics (see later in this chapter).

Intestinal flora

The balance of flora populations in the gut is highly complex but, in steady-state health and dietary conditions, probably reasonably stable. In humans, for example, there seems to be a moderately predictable sequence of colonisation after birth and through to adulthood, with fluctuations in the relative numbers of aerobic and anaerobic bacteria in newborns up to a total of 10^{10}/g wet weight, reaching in adulthood between 10^5 and 10^7/g wet weight of aerobic bacteria and between 10^{10} and 10^{11}/g wet weight of anaerobic bacteria.[44]

The benefits of a healthy bacterial population in the gut are clear. Anaerobic bacteria in particular are shown to be responsible for considerable secondary digestion and to decrease intestinal transit time.[45] Normal bacteria like *Escherichia coli*, *Enterococcus faecalis* and *Bacteroides distasonis* have been shown to help protect the gut from pathogenic infiltration and there are a number of other non-specific defences known.[46] Mechanisms are likely to include modification of bile acids, stimulation of peristalsis, induction of immunological responses, competition for substrates and possible elaboration of various bacteriostatic substances.[47] The intestinal flora also contributes to non-specific defences against immunological challenge from dietary antigens by helping to reduce their uptake across the mucosal barrier.[48]

The populations of bacteria and other organisms are, however, obviously dependent on their food supply, the dietary material and its metabolites, reaching the lower intestine. There is a potential for rapid responses to diet: a general reduction in bacteroidetes and increases in firmicutes, clostridia, bacilli and erysipelotrichi are apparent within 1 day of moving the diet from plant based to 'Westernised'.[49] Bowel flora in African populations with a plant-based diet are also found to be much richer in bacteroidetes than Western groups.[50] Probably the most widespread impact on bacterial populations in the gut in modern times, however, is the use of antibiotics. It has long been established that this has an adverse effect on normal gut flora.[51] Antibiotic use can lead to secondary hypersensitivities in the body, presumably through their effects on intestinal flora.[52] For example, they can lead to increased activity of Candida, which has been shown to be a factor in driving allergic responses.[53]

The relationship of bile products with intestinal flora is complex and works in two directions (see also p. 209). Bile salt metabolites variably stimulate growth in bacterial populations,[54] while anaerobic bacteria act on bile products to produce volatile fatty acids that control other pathogenic bacteria.[55] A particularly revealing insight into the relationship is seen in the case of bowel cancer. There are three known endogenous components that affect development of colorectal cancer – colonic bacteria, the mucus layer and bile acids. The major effects of the bacteria are deconjugation and reduction of bile acids, activation of mutagen precursors, fermentation and production of volatile fatty acids, formation of endogenous mutagens and physical adsorption of hydrophobic chemicals. The mucus layer covering the surface acts as a barrier and its composition changes in premalignant and malignant colon tissue. The secretion of protective mucus is elevated by plant cell wall components in the diet. Mucus has some hydrophobic properties and its presence may alter the effect of bile components and bacterial metabolites on the gut wall.

Bowel bacteria have been linked to another cancer. In looking for reasons to explain the epidemiological link between high-fibre diets and lower risks of breast cancer, it was found that both raising fibre content in the diet and suppressing microflora with antibiotics led to reduced intestinal reabsorption of oestrogens and lower levels circulating in the blood. It was concluded that intestinal microflora raise oestrogen levels by deconjugating bound oestrogens that appear in the bile, thereby permitting the free hormones to be reabsorbed.[56] The beneficial levels of a high-fibre diet are likely to be the dominant factor in women susceptible to breast cancer, especially as there is evidence that bacterial flora actually enhance some of its wider benefits.[57]

There are several ways popularly promoted to correct disturbed or damaging bowel flora. Current evidence indicates that varying probiotic strains mediate their effects by a variety of different effects that are dependent on the dosage employed as well as the route and frequency of delivery. Some probiotics act in the lumen of the gut by elaborating antibacterial molecules such as bacteriocins; others enhance the mucosal barrier by increasing the production of innate immune molecules; and other probiotics may mediate their beneficial effects by promoting adaptive immune responses (for example, secretory immunoglobulin A, regulatory T cells, interleukin-10). Some probiotics have the capacity to activate receptors in the enteric nervous system, which could be used to promote pain relief in the setting of visceral hyperalgesia.[58] The value of a high bulk diet with reduced simple sugars intake is, however, more accepted. The phytotherapist might combine the benefits of such dietary moves with attendance to hepatic and biliary function and with bitter or aromatic digestive insurance that food matter is well rendered in the upper digestive tract. The value of direct agents such as *Artemisia absinthium* (wormwood), Marsdenia (condurango) and *Allium sativum* (garlic) on disruptive bowel flora is likely to be upheld (see also later under Intestinal dysbiosis).

Plant fructo-oligosaccharides are associated with 'prebiotic' properties; that is, they selectively stimulate growth and/or activities of health-giving microbial species in the gut.[59] They are a mixture of oligosaccharides typically consisting of glucose linked to fructose units. They are widely distributed in plants such as onions, asparagus and particularly cereals,[60] and in herbal remedies such as Cichorium (chicory) and Taraxacum (dandelion root).[61] They are not hydrolysed by human digestive enzymes but are utilised by intestinal bacteria such as Bifidobacteria, *Bacteroides fragilis* group, Peptostreptococci and Klebsiellae. In clinical studies, improvement of faecal microflora was observed on oral administration of fructo-oligosaccharides at 8 g[62] and 12.5 g[63] per day; the population of bifidobacteria in faeces increased substantially compared with before the administration. Mucilages can also be used to 'feed' healthy bacteria.

Acupharmacology: a pharmacological basis for herbal therapeutics?

Modern insights into the fate of much plant material in the digestive tract support a view that a herbal remedy mostly affects the gut and its immediate surroundings. Adding what is known of the interrelationships between digestive activity and the wider body's physiology allows the modern phytotherapist to develop a rationale for the effect of herbal medicines on the body that is both unique to these remedies and provides potentially very powerful therapeutic strategies.

The body presents two distinct surfaces to the outside world, each of which has its own triggers to initiate reflex responses. The skin is a sensitive template from which it is possible to trigger a wide range of reflex responses elsewhere in the body. When one touches a very hot object, for example, the response is both complex and predictable. More positively the benefits of touch, caressing and massage are increasingly well understood. There are a number of established mechanisms by which cutaneous stimulation can have an impact on both specific internal functions and on general well-being: for example, via dermatomes and spinal afferents, stretch sensor stimulation and somatopsychological connections. These have been used to explain the potential benefits of hands-on therapies.

There are other less well-established mechanisms, possibly involving neurohormonal reflexes, that have been suggested as underpinning acupuncture, acupressure and shiatsu and possibly reflexology – the claim that stimulating particular points on the body surface can effect substantial benefits elsewhere. If stimulation of certain points on the body surface can lead to changes in neurohormones such as enkephalin, then the fact that the stimulant was a steel, stone or gold needle, a warming moxa or finger pressure seems less important than the point that was stimulated. It appears that such reflexes are programmed, even wired, into the system.

If the skin has the potential for mediating complex effects within the body then the second of the body's surfaces has much greater potential. The lining of the gastrointestinal tract has a hundreds of times greater surface than the skin. It is also a dramatically more complex surface structure. Unlike the skin, which has primarily a protective function, the gut surface has a literally intimate engagement with the outer world. It provides by far the largest exposure of the body's immune system and other defences to the outside world.

The main inputs into the decision-making processes involved in digestion are a vast array of receptors and sensory tissues along the gut wall. Each of these provides signals for some effector function elsewhere in the gut or indeed elsewhere in the body. The effects of the following archetypal plant constituents discussed in this chapter and in Chapter 2 can clearly be seen to work primarily on the digestive tract.

There are several general ways by which stimulation along the digestive tract can influence wider body functions, some of which were reviewed earlier.

As a source of enteric reflexes

Through neural links forged during embryonic development, stimulation of neural receptors in the gut wall is theoretically able to effect responses in other areas. Vagal modulation can lead to wider adjustment of autonomic activity in the body and particularly in bronchial muscle activity and cardiovascular control signals originating in the thorax. Pungent principles (hot spices) increase blood flow in other areas after ingestion.[24]

As an endocrine organ

The gut is responsible directly or indirectly for the secretion of insulin, glucagon, somatostatin, gastrin, cholecystokinin and a range of other hormones and transmitters with wide effects on body functions.

Through common neurohormonal mechanisms

The gut wall contains many regulatory neurosecretory cells that produce agents with receptors elsewhere in the body. One obvious example of the neurohormonal and endocrine links is the close relationship between digestive status and emotion.

As the body's largest concentration of immunological activity

The body has by far its greatest exposure to immunological challenge in the digestive system.

As a potential route of access for pathogenic materials

Damage to the digestive defences, the digestive secretions or the intestinal wall can permit the absorption of dangerous materials. As well as the extra strain this may put on the immune system referred to above, there are other potential problems that can arise for which digestive treatments may prove beneficial.

As a determinant of blood sugar levels

The awesome effects on behaviour, on the functions of the CNS, and on the major body hormones of undue fluctuations in levels of blood glucose is a reflection of the importance not only of good carbohydrate intake but of coordinated secretion of enteric hormones such as gastrin and cholecystokinin.

Via the enterohepatic circulation

The absorption of materials from the gut into the portal bloodstream to the liver presents the latter with its main metabolic load. Hepatic processing of this and other circulating material from elsewhere in the body may include excretion of metabolites into the bile. Depending on the extent of secondary breakdown of these metabolites in the gut, particularly with the activity of gut microflora, these products may to varying extents be reabsorbed for recirculation around the body's general circulation. Levels of many physiological and pharmacological agents in the body can therefore be significantly affected by changes in digestive activity.

As the body's major eliminatory organ

The bowel is the obvious outlet not only of digestive residues but also of bowel microflora detritus and bile products.

Any change in eliminatory functions is likely to have significant effects in the body; different traditions around the world have linked catarrhal states, susceptibility to infections, skin and joint diseases, mood disturbances and menstrual problems to disturbed bowel eliminations. The almost universal use in early times of drastic emetics and purgatives, both involving dramatic increase in bile eliminations for the treatment of acute diseases, reflects a widespread human instinct that these eliminatory functions were important.

As the home for the major populations of symbiotic and parasitic organisms in the body

The activity of the gut microflora has an impact on the levels of many nutrients, hormones and drugs in the body.

As the source of all physical and much emotional nourishment and replenishment

The most obvious truism yet provides the phytotherapist with a potent mechanism for effecting better health. Remedies that could be shown to improve digestive performance would be important elements in convalescence and recuperation.

The main advantage of considering herbal therapeutics as acupharmacology is that it provides a basis for rapid responses, a therapeutics based on intervention and review of early results on an iterative process towards recovery. In this approach to treatment, feedback is almost immediate and a muscular strategy of repair can be constructed.

Phytotherapeutic principles

Archetypal digestive remedies

Following Chapter 2, the approach adopted there and in the following section is to look at key chemical groups in plants, the 'archetypal plant constituents', rather than at individual remedies. The fragmentary nature of research support for herbal therapeutics is always a major limitation, but fortunately in the area of the digestive tract there is a more than usually reliable experience of efficacy; the digestive tract is one of the most accessible organs in the body and most traditional treatments relied on immediate clinical effects.

Dosage and other prescription practicalities

Most experience of the impact of herbal remedies on the digestion was associated with the use of heroic doses applied to acute indications. Emetics and cathartics were often the first resort of treatment, and dysentery, life-threatening gastrointestinal infections and hepatitis the most common indications. Even with more robust constitutions, the occasionally dramatic effects of eating unrefrigerated food were very familiar. The remedies outlined above were favoured because they had rapid effect.

The gastrointestinal tract provides a large surface area and the processes of digestion quickly denature and dilute remedies. For most of the effects referred to, therefore, relatively large doses of plant need to be taken (and the preparation needs to contain the relevant constituent – it is no good having a convenient extract of plant without its mucky mucilage, resin or tannin if those are the constituents one needs!). Many modern prescriptions based on quantities measured in drops or milligrams would be unlikely to have much impact on this system. The main exceptions are the bitters and hot spices or other cases where the target receptors are close to the point of entry or the agent is particularly powerful.

It is also likely that for many effects long-term treatment is inappropriate. The cases of tannins and anthraquinones are examples of when this may even be hazardous. In practice, one finds that for most gut-mediated mechanisms the effect is strongest in the earliest days of treatment and often wears off quite quickly.

It is much better to work on short-term prescriptions of relatively strong doses, constantly monitoring for immediate feedback and adjusting accordingly. In any long-term strategy it is generally wise to treat intermittently, maintaining the option of frequent prescription changes according to results.

The following summary of the main phytochemical groups with impact on the digestive system is treatment focused. In each case there is a much more substantial description in Chapter 2 and this should be also referred to before making clinical decisions, particularly for the mucilages (and bulk laxatives), bitters, anthraquinone laxatives and pungent constituents.

Bulk laxatives

Plant materials still provide the primary source of fibre that remains undigested and can swell when hydrated to bulk up the stool contents. The usual reason for consuming these materials is to help reduce constipation. However, an important application for bulk laxatives is constipation-predominant irritable bowel syndrome (IBS). Indeed, this can be the first line of therapy (see below). They are also valuable in correcting disturbed bowel flora as prebiotics, in calming an irritated bowel wall in inflammatory bowel disease, in counteracting potential irritative effects of bile metabolites, and in slowing the absorption of sugars and cholesterol.

Plant remedies traditionally used as bulk laxatives

* Linum (linseed), *Plantago ovata* (ispaghula), *Plantago psyllium* (psyllium seed and husk).

Indications for bulk laxatives

* Constipation
* Inflammatory bowel disease
* Blood sugar disturbances, including the dietary management of diabetes
* Some dyspeptic and gastric inflammatory conditions.

Other traditional indications for bulk laxatives

* Fluid retention
* Obesity.

Contraindications for bulk laxatives

There are few contraindications for the use of fibre and the bulk laxatives. However, their supplementation should be kept under review in cases of:

* iron deficiency anaemia
* osteoporosis
* chronic malnutrition.

Traditional therapeutic insights into the use of bulk laxatives

Some of the bulk laxatives were also used for their obvious mucilaginous properties (see below) in reducing inflammatory problems in the upper sections of the digestive tract.

Application

Bulk laxatives need to be taken whole as powdered material, most conveniently in capsule form, with food.

Long-term therapy with extra supplementation of soluble fibre is not always advisable and both soluble and insoluble fibre intake should be reviewed where absorption of mineral nutrients is a critical issue.

Advanced phytotherapeutics

Bulk laxatives may also be usefully applied in hypercholesterolaemia and in some cases (depending on other factors) of hypertension.

Emetics

Therapeutic vomiting is much less applied than in previous centuries. Even in its usual modern application, it has been demonstrated as an inefficient way to remove ingested poisons, with appreciable amounts being forced into the small bowel.[64] Activated charcoal as a non-emetic treatment for poisoning is likely to be superior,[65] for example in paracetamol poisoning.[66] The main reason to maintain this category is in the use of emetic plant remedies in sub-emetic doses as reflex expectorants – an important pharmacological principle explored in the Respiratory system section of this chapter and in Chapter 2.

Plant remedies traditionally used as emetics

* Cephaelis (ipecacuanha), Urginea (squill).

Traditional indications for emetics

* Any acute toxic and infective condition
* Bronchitis.

Contraindications for emetics

The use of emetics is contraindicated in the following:

* Poisoning associated with coma, convulsions
* Poisoning with petroleum products or corrosive substances
* Any debilitated condition or constitutional weakness.

Traditional therapeutic insights into the use of emetics

Emetics were used as a first line of treatment especially for enteric and bronchitic infections and for any evidence of biliary toxicity. It was always understood that their use was essentially debilitating, so a robust constitution was an essential prerequisite.

Application

For poisoning emergencies use, for example, 15 mL of ipecac syrup for children and adults,[67] repeating the dose in 15 to 30 minutes if necessary. If Ipecac is unavailable, soapy water or detergent with water may be used or manual stimulation of the gag reflex with finger or blunt instrument may be tried.

Mucilages

The demulcent quality of plant mucilages remains one of the most effective short-term reliefs for irritation of the upper digestive tract, notably including reflux into the oesophagus and other effects of acid dyspepsia. The fate of ingested mucilages lower down the tract is not always certain. However, some such as Ulmus (slippery elm) have persistent reputations as remedies for irritation and inflammation lower down the gut; and there may be some mucilaginous effect in some plant materials, where these merge into prebiotic polysaccharide and fibre elements. The authors in one report[68] searched online databases for reports of orally ingested polysaccharides. Fifteen studies were found showing statistically significant effects in humans, although these included open label trials. They involved healthy adults and those with cancer, allergies, or aphthous stomatitis. In healthy human adults, oral arabinogalactans from *Larix occidentalis* (western larch) increased lymphocyte proliferation, CD8+ lymphocytes, and immunoglobulin G response to pneumococcal vaccine in placebo-controlled, randomised, clinical trials. Furanose from American ginseng (*Panax quinquefolius*) reduced incidence and duration of respiratory illness in a trial with healthy older adults. As suggested above, most polysaccharides are partially degraded in the digestive tract. Several are metabolised by gut bacteria and may thereby exert prebiotic effects. Fucoidans and other polysaccharides from seaweeds such as *Fucus vesiculosus* and agar-agar are notably resistant to breakdown and can be included in the bulk laxative category.

As with the emetic category above, there is an important pharmacological principle in the reflex effect of impacts on the upper digestive mucosa onto the function of the respiratory system. Mucilages are consistently used to calm irritating coughs, almost certainly by reflex from their demulcent effect on swallowing.

Plant remedies traditionally used as mucilages

*   Althaea (marshmallow), Ulmus (slippery elm), *Plantago major* (plantain), *Plantago lanceolata* (ribwort), Chondrus (Irish moss), Lobaria (lungwort).

Indications for mucilages

*   Dyspeptic conditions especially with hyperacidity
*   Inflammatory diseases of the digestive tract, e.g. reflux oesophagitis, gastritis, peptic ulceration, enteritis, ileitis and colitis
*   Non-productive, irritable cough
*   Topically: inflamed lesions, pruritus.

Other traditional indications for mucilages

*   Dysuria.

Contraindications for mucilages

The use of mucilages is either contraindicated or at least inappropriate in the following:

*   Congestive bronchial and catarrhal conditions
*   As a substitute for curative treatments where these are available.

Further traditional therapeutic insights into the use of mucilages

Mucilaginous plants were associated in Chinese medicine with a diuretic effect and were also seen as valuable tonics in debilitated conditions, especially with chronic wasting dry lung diseases, such as tuberculosis.

Application

Mucilages should be taken in a formulation that preserves their physical characteristics. Encapsulation is probably the most effective way of administering the whole material (subject to the contents being adequately sterilised) but cold aqueous infusion is the most efficient extraction process, using glycerol later for preservative purposes. Depending on the indication, they may be taken before meals (for digestive problems of the stomach and small intestine), during (for some stomach problems) or after meals (in the case of reflux oesophagitis/hiatus hernia).

Long-term therapy with mucilages presents few problems but, as they are essentially management treatments, such use may disguise the need for more substantial treatments.

Saponins

The detergent properties of this phytochemical group can have a range of mild topical actions on the gut wall. These vary from near emetic activity (for example, with Cephaelis, Senega and Primula species) to a likely effect improving assimilation (as in the saponin content of many vegetables). This group therefore can share some of the properties of both the emetics and mucilages, and in the latter case can add considerably to the demulcent effect (as seen notably with Glycyrrhiza extract and Trigonella).

Plant remedies traditionally used for saponin effects on the gut

*   Primula (cowslip), Glycyrrhiza (licorice), Cephaelis (ipecacuanha), Senega (snakeroot), Trigonella (fenugreek).

Indications for saponin-containing remedies

* Bronchial congestion
* Digestive difficulties.

Other traditional indications for saponin-containing remedies

* As tonics for debilitating conditions
* As hormonal modulators.

Contraindications for saponins

The use of saponins is either contraindicated or at least inappropriate in the following:

* Topically to open wounds
* Coeliac disease, fat malabsorption and vitamins A, D, E, and K deficiency
* In some upper digestive irritations.

Traditional therapeutic insights into the use of saponins

Saponins are common constituents in plants used in Chinese and Asian medicine as tonics and harmonising treatments. Modern pharmacological interest in the effects of ginseng has raised speculation that, as steroidal molecules, some saponins may modulate steroid hormone control mechanisms in the body (see also Chapter 2 and the licorice and ginseng monographs).

Application

Saponin-rich plants may be taken before meals, or if there is a sensitive stomach, immediately after eating.

Long-term therapy with saponin-rich plants should be avoided unless dosage levels are small or clear benefits are apparent which diminish if treatment is stopped. The impact of saponins on digestion and absorption is insufficiently clear.

Tannins

The effects of this phytochemical group have been extensively covered elsewhere in this book. They can provide short-term healing and anti-inflammatory effects on the gut wall, though likely to rapidly reduce with transit through the tract unless in slowly dispersing solid form. Effects on the bowel, for example in diarrhoea, can however be significant if the symptom is a reflex consequence of irritation in the gastric or upper enteric passages (gastroenteritis). The use of tannins is not to be recommended as a long-term solution (see Chapter 2).

Plant remedies traditionally used for tannin constituents

* Hamamelis (witchhazel), *Potentilla tormentilla* (tormentil), Quercus (oak), Agrimonia (agrimony), Geum (avens), Krameria (rhatany), Geranium (cranesbill), *Cnicus benedictus* (blessed thistle), *Acacia catechu* (catechu), Bidens (bur-marigold), Alchemilla (ladies mantle), Polygonum (bistort), Sanguisorba (burnet).

Indications for tannins

* Inflammation of the upper digestive tract
* Diarrhoea following gastrointestinal inflammation
* Topically: open, discharging lesions, wounds, haemorrhoids and third-degree burns.

Contraindications for tannins

The use of tannins is either contraindicated or at least inappropriate in the following:

* Constipation
* Iron deficiency anaemia
* Malnutrition.

Traditional therapeutic insights into the use of tannins

Tannins were used throughout history for forming leather from animal tissues and as effective cauterising agents for burns and other open wounds. The primary traditional indication for the digestive tract was probably diarrhoea.

Application

Tannins should be taken after food in most cases. For some lesions of the upper digestive tract, short-term use between meals or before food is justifiable.

Long-term therapy with high doses of tannins is to be avoided.

Pungent constituents

Spices have long had a central role in digestion and, as discussed elsewhere, have a key role in traditional therapeutics overall. They can both stimulate and calm upper digestive functions, depending on the circumstance and particularly the individual constitution. Usually the patient will know whether these remedies suit them or not and it is always a good question in a consultation.

Plant remedies traditionally used for warming effects

* Capsicum (cayenne), Zingiber (ginger), Armoracea (horseradish).

Indications for pungent constituents

* Congestive dyspepsia
* Gastroparesis (especially ginger)
* Some cases of nausea, emesis, colic, diarrhoea and other hyperperistaltic conditions
* Bronchial congestion
* Poor peripheral circulation
* Topically: for joint and muscle pain, subdermal inflammations.

Other traditional indications for heating remedies

* Any effect of cold on body systems.

Contraindications for pungent constituents

The contraindications for heating remedies are constitutional rather than symptomatic. The same symptoms in two individuals may provide contrasting indications for this group of remedies. The use of hot spices may be contraindicated or inappropriate in the following:

• Concurrently with powerful drug regimes where dosage levels are critical
• Hyperacidity conditions and gastro-oesophageal reflux (unless due to gastroparesis)
• Hepatitis
• Some enteric and bowel inflammatory states with diarrhoea
• Some cases of chronic nephritis.

Traditional therapeutic insights into the use of pungent constituents

Early insights into the impact of 'heating' the body have become very developed in some traditions. Most early physicians would have been familiar with the issues that determined how far to 'heat' or 'cool' a prescription (see p. 4). A quick guide to the applicability would be the presence of white coating on the tongue.

Application

Hot spices can feature in prescriptions taken at various times of the day. When taken primarily for their impact on digestion, they may be taken before meals if there are no local inflammatory conditions in the upper digestive tract, with or after meals if the gut wall proves to be sensitive or there is a tendency to hyperacidity.

Long-term therapy with pungent remedies is acceptable if the individual is comfortable with the regime. It should be discontinued if there are any digestive discomforts.

Aromatics

These can often be regarded as milder version of the pungent constituents above and are often accepted and useful when the stronger spices are not. Consistently they are used in traditional medicine both for digestive and respiratory congestions and as tonic remedies in convalescent recovery from both. They often exert spasmolytic and carminative effects.

Plant remedies traditionally used as aromatics

• Elettaria (cardamom), Angelica, Carum (caraway), Pimpinella (aniseed), Foeniculum (fennel), *Cinnamomum spp.* (cinnamon), Anethum (dill), Alpinia (galangal), Levisticum (lovage), Myristica (nutmeg), Citrus (chen pi).

Indications for aromatics

• Colic and flatulence
• Irritable bowel disease
• Congestive dyspepsia
• Catarrh and bronchial congestion.

Other traditional indications for aromatics

• Sluggish digestion and metabolism
• Congestive chronic infections and inflammatory conditions.

Contraindications for aromatics

The use of aromatics may be contraindicated or inappropriate in gastro-oesophageal reflux, although low doses can sometimes be useful.

Traditional therapeutic insights into the use of aromatics

In Chinese medicine aromatics are used for 'damp' conditions affecting the assimilative functions (represented by the *Spleen* in Chinese medicine). Symptoms include abdominal and thoracic congestion (sometimes associated with cough and breathlessness), loss of appetite and loose stools.

Application

Aromatics are best taken immediately before meals. Their impact on the digestion is often increased if taken in hot aqueous infusions.

Long-term therapy with aromatics is often well tolerated.

Volatile spasmolytics

Volatile essential oils are known to have a range of effects on gut function. Subjectively they are associated in the gut with carminative effects, being helpful in symptoms of colic, flatulence and hyperperistalsis. These benefits tie in with the pharmacologically confirmed spasmolytic and anti-inflammatory effects. There is likely to be an additional contribution from the effects of many of these constituents on the CNS. They are often particularly well suited for children, being both gentle and relatively palatable.

Plant remedies traditionally used as spasmolytics

• Matricaria (chamomile), Mentha (peppermint), Melissa (lemon balm), Achillea (yarrow), *Nepeta cataria* (catmint), Petroselinum (parsley root), *Thymus spp.* (thyme).

Indications for spasmolytics

• Nervous dyspepsia
• Colic and flatulence
• Irritable bowel syndrome
• Gastritis.

Other traditional indications for spasmolytics

• As components of fever management strategies
• General nervous, irritable and anxiety syndromes.

Contraindications for spasmolytics

The use of spasmolytics may be contraindicated or inappropriate in gastric and enteric poisoning incidents.

Traditional therapeutic insights into the use of spasmolytics

These remedies overlap with the aromatics in their effect on the digestive tract but are more appropriate in hot and febrile conditions. However, in many cases predicting efficacy is difficult and patients may be encouraged to try a number of these or aromatic remedies to see which suits best. In all cases effects are very quick.

Application

Spasmolytics are best taken immediately before meals. Their impact on the digestion is often increased if taken in hot aqueous infusions.

Long-term therapy with spasmolytics is often well tolerated.

Resins

The development of glass for chemical investigations has undermined most modern research on these valuable plant constituents, given their well-known impact on glass cleanliness. Thus remedies that were most highly prized in ancient times, such as frankincense and myrrh in biblical times, have been largely lost to modern medicine. High alcoholic extracts of resinous plants will deliver a powerful antiseptic and stimulating effect on the upper digestive mucosa. If delivered in solid form this may be transmitted much lower in the gut passage.

Plant remedies traditionally used as resins

* *Calendula officinalis* (marigold), *Commiphora molmol* (myrrh), *Boswellia serrata*, Ferula (asafoetida), Dorema (ammoniacum), Myrica (bayberry), Pistacia (mastic).

Indications for resin-containing remedies

* Inflammatory conditions of the mouth, throat and upper digestive tract (and in solid form lower regions)
* Lymphadenopathies and recurrent infections.

Application

Resins will only dissolve in alcohol, so resin-rich remedies need to be taken whole or as tinctures with as little water as possible or as the dried extracts made from them (especially if higher doses are required, due to the concurrent ingestion of too much alcohol).

Long-term therapy with resins is inadvisable.

Anthraquinone laxatives

The use of stimulating laxatives should be seen as a short-term measure where no other laxative measures are working. All emphasis should be on finding long-term solutions that progressively reduce the need for these remedies. Phytotherapeutic alternatives to fibre and bulk laxatives include the use of hepatic and biliary remedies and blends of anthraquinone herbs with bulk laxative and volatile spasmolytics, with reducing doses of the former over several months.

Plant remedies traditionally used as anthraquinone laxatives

* Aloe, Cassia (senna), *Rhamnus purshiana* (cascara), *Rhamnus frangula* (frangula), Rheum (rhubarb), *Rumex crispus* (yellow dock).

Indications for anthraquinone laxatives

* Atonic constipation.

Other traditional indications for anthraquinone laxatives

* Fluid retention
* Obesity.

Contraindications for anthraquinone laxatives

The use of anthraquinone laxatives is either contraindicated or at least inappropriate in the following:

* Constipation associated with bowel irritability
* Bowel disease
* Diarrhoea.

Application

Anthraquinones may be taken in laxative doses with the evening meal. Lower doses may be taken with other meals as part of a strategy to increase general bowel activity over the medium term.

Long-term therapy with anthraquinones is formally contraindicated.

Advanced phytotherapeutics

Anthraquinone laxatives may also be usefully applied in some cases (depending on other factors) of detoxifying regimes and reducing kidney stone risk (see Chapter 2).

Bitters

This group is almost entirely focused in their impact on the digestive system, and reference to the Bitters section in Chapter 2 is particularly recommended before incorporating them into a strategic approach. Some listed below are also prominent choleretics and should be further reviewed in that section of this chapter.

Plant remedies traditionally used as bitters

* Gentiana (gentian), Centaurium (centaury), *Artemisia absinthium* (wormwood), Taraxacum (dandelion root), *Hydrastis canadensis* (golden seal), *Berberis vulgaris* (barberry), Aletris (unicorn root), Marsdenia (condurango), Menyanthes (bogbean), Picrasma (quassia), Swertia (chiretta), Veronicastrum (black root).

Indications for bitters

- Poor appetite and digestion
- Liver and bile disturbances (as choleretics)
- Blood sugar disturbances, including the dietary management of diabetes
- Chronic gastritis and gastric ulceration
- Food intolerances and allergies
- Debilitated conditions associated with any of the above.

Other traditional indications for bitters

- Fever management
- Jaundice.

Contraindications for bitters

The use of bitters is either contraindicated or at least inappropriate in the following:

- Duodenal ulceration
- Conditions classed as 'cold-dry' in early medicine, involving for example ready shivering with dry cough and notably including some kidney diseases.

Traditional therapeutic insights into the use of bitters

Bitters were universally classified as cooling in early approaches to medicine (see Chapter 1). This insight is likely to have followed observations that administering bitters helped to contain excesses of temperature in fevers and has been associated in Chinese medicine, for example, with the view that increased digestive activity is intrinsically a cooling phenomenon. In supporting the latter, bitters were seen not only to support nourishment but to reduce the symptoms of excessive heat in some pathologies, including some headaches and migraines, skin and other inflammatory diseases and allergic or hypersensitivity conditions.

Application

Since bitters act by reflex and direct activation of receptors in the upper digestive tract, they do not usually have to be given in high doses. Enough to promote a strong taste of bitterness is usually sufficient. This will typically be seen if 5% to 10% of tinctures are bitters such as Gentiana or *Artemisia absinthium* (wormwood).

Long-term therapy with bitters is possible in those individuals where its effect is beneficial. However, it is always valuable to work to a position where the bitters are taken only when necessary and useful.

Advanced phytotherapeutics

Bitters may also be usefully applied in some cases (depending on other factors) of:

- Headaches and migraines
- Skin and other inflammatory diseases
- Allergic and hypersensitivity conditions.

Phytotherapy for digestive conditions

Recurrent aphthous ulceration (mouth ulcers, canker sores)

Aphthous ulceration is a common recurrent condition characterised by superficial ulcers in the mouth that are round or ovoid and surrounded by inflammatory halos.[69] Ulcers are often multiple and may recur. The cause is unknown, but possible factors include emotional stress, poor innate immunity, imbalanced oral flora, low serum insulin levels, food intolerances and nutrient deficiencies, some medications and dentures.[69] Several of these are controversial. In some women ulcers tend to follow a cyclical pattern and occur premenstrually. The presence of serious diseases such as Crohn's disease, ulcerative colitis, coeliac or Behçet's disease should always be excluded. A multitude of conventional drugs have been attempted as treatments, indicating how poorly understood this condition is.[69]

Treatment

The approach of herbal treatment is to increase mucosal protection, accelerate the healing of the ulcers and to correct any underlying imbalances, especially focusing on immune support. Other aspects of treatment include the minimisation of stress, attention to a wholesome diet with plenty of fruit and vegetables and attention to oral hygiene.

CASE HISTORY

A female patient aged 42 had suffered from mouth ulcers almost continuously for 30 years. All her teeth had been removed when she was 15 because they were 'chalky'. She was a worrier and found it difficult to relax. Initial treatment was as follows (based on 1 week):

Glycyrrhiza glabra (high in glycyrrhizin)	1:1	20 mL
Echinacea angustifolia root	1:2	25 mL
Propolis	1:10	25 mL
Valeriana officinalis	1:2	20 mL
	TOTAL	100 mL

Dose: 5 mL with water three times a day.
The following mixture was to be applied directly to the ulcers:

Propolis	1:10	50 mL
Calendula officinalis	1:2	50 mL
	TOTAL	100 mL

She was also advised to rinse her mouth regularly with a mixture of acidophilus yoghurt and water.
After 4 weeks the patient had only experienced three ulcers, all in the first week of treatment. In the following 4 weeks there was only one ulcer. One year later she was still taking the herbal treatment at a reduced frequency (1 or 2 doses a day) and was relatively free from mouth ulcers.

Topical application of a high alcoholic tincture or extract of Calendula, myrrh, kava or propolis is particularly beneficial. This is because such preparations are quite resinous. When they are painted on to the ulcer the alcohol dries and the resin fixes the active components so that they are not readily washed away by saliva. It is also possible that they promote a local leucocytosis (i.e. attract white blood cells). Topical application of licorice via a dissolving oral patch has been successfully used in clinical trials.[70]

Functional dyspepsia and gastro-oesophageal reflux disease (GORD)

Functional dyspepsia is marked by pain and discomfort, heartburn and epigastric pain, early satiety, bloating and nausea in the upper abdomen, all with no apparent pathological cause (i.e. after gastroscopic and other investigations have proven negative). It is often marked by the production of excess acid in the stomach and is for this reason usually characterised as a stress response. Other symptoms include those of 'diaphragmatic spasm', hyperventilation, shallow breathing, dysphagia and palpitations, and it is tension in this large muscle that probably contributes to the accompanying condition, gastro-oesophageal reflux. The diaphragm in effect is the foundation of the sphincter between oesophagus and stomach: excessive tension in this muscle can lead to a functional hiatus hernia and reflux of stomach acid back into the oesophagus. This condition is initially uncomfortable, then painful ('heartburn') and eventually damaging (erosive oesophagitis).

Early management of this condition is clearly appropriate and important. Useful benefits may be had from simple breathing exercises designed to relax the diaphragm and 'adrenaline reducing' exercise; other stress management tools should be explored. Fortunately the phytotherapist has a range of useful tools to add.

The proprietary preparation Iberogast, used for over 40 years in Germany for the relief of functional dyspepsia, includes a fresh plant extract of *Iberis amara* (bitter candytuft) and extracts of *Angelica archangelica* root, *Silybum marianum* (milk thistle), *Carum carvi* (caraway), *Chelidonium majus* (celandine), *Glycyrrhiza glabra* (licorice), *Matricaria recutita* (German chamomile), *Melissa officinalis* (lemon balm) leaf, and *Mentha × piperita* (peppermint) with 31% ethanol. Four double blind, randomised, clinical trials have demonstrated the therapeutic effects in functional dyspepsia.[71] A previous systematic review including data from the manufacturer allowed analysis of four multicentre, randomised, double blind studies against placebo or reference treatments, with a total of 595 patients; it showed significant reduction in gastrointestinal symptom scores and the conclusion that the combination seems to be an effective phytotherapeutic option without central nervous side effects.[72] Another paper reported a literature search on 350 components of the mixture and found the most common pharmacological activities are motility modulating, anti-inflammatory and antioxidant effects.[73] These constituents happen to overlap considerably the range of phytotherapeutic options below.

In addition to the above discussion, major factors thought to operate in GORD include:[74–77]

- Obesity (especially visceral adiposity) and metabolic syndrome
- Delayed gastric emptying
- Ineffective clearance of reflux from the oesophagus (including deficient saliva production)
- Impaired oesophageal mucosal defence
- Reduced lower oesophageal sphincter (LOS) pressure
- Visceral hypersensitivity, accentuated by psychological stress.

Practical measures in the treatment of GORD include:

- Elevation of the head of the bed by 10 to 15 cm. This improves oesophageal clearance at night
- Regular meal times and not eating on the run
- Avoidance of foods that reduce lower oesophageal sphincter tone. These include chocolate, carminatives (e.g. peppermint and spearmint), fatty foods, coffee, tomato concentrates and onions, but will vary from individual to individual. Spicy foods may also aggravate. Wheat can be a silent factor that seems to predispose to reflux in many patients
- Individual intolerance to certain foods may aggravate reflux, for example dairy products, and these should be avoided. These types of intolerances may not cause immediate reflux, but rather predispose to the condition. Hence an exclusion diet for at least 30 days is the only valid way to assess their role
- Avoidance of drugs which reduce LOS tone such as theophylline, calcium channel blockers and progesterone
- Giving up smoking and excessive alcohol intake (these reduce LOS tone)
- Refraining from overeating
- Avoiding eating at bedtime
- Losing weight if overweight.

For the reasons given, approaches to the herbal treatment of both GORD and functional dyspepsia are similar, although different aspects of treatment are emphasised in each disorder and for individual cases. Main aspects of treatment include the following:

- Improving mucosal resistance with Glycyrrhiza (licorice) and mucilaginous herbs such as Ulmus (slippery elm) and Althaea (marshmallow root) to assist mucoprotection. These are best taken after meals and before bed
- Bitter herbs at low doses can increase LOS tone, improve saliva output and accelerate gastric emptying. However, they also increase gastric acidity and therefore should be used cautiously. Gentiana and Artemisia (wormwood) may be too strong, hence gentler bitters such as Cynara (globe artichoke) or Achillea (yarrow) may be appropriate
- Carminative herbs and essential oils in high doses will aggravate GORD by reducing sphincter tone, but they can be indicated for functional dyspepsia. Also, in lower doses, they can improve gastrointestinal motility
- Treating associated gastroparesis with Zingiber (ginger)
- Anti-inflammatory herbs relieve symptoms and improve healing and include Filipendula (meadowsweet), Stellaria (chickweed) and Matricaria (chamomile), especially those chemotypes of Matricaria rich in bisabolol. Filipendula is also traditionally thought to reduce excess acidity and Matricaria is also spasmolytic. They are indicated in both functional dyspepsia and GORD. An in vivo study found Matricaria also lowered gastric acidity (see monograph)

- GORD and functional dyspepsia may be linked to stress, especially if associated with irritable bowel syndrome. Anxiolytic herbs such as Valeriana, and nervine tonic herbs such as Scutellaria (skullcap), are indicated if this association is evident
- Improving healing with herbs such as Calendula and Centella (gotu kola)
- Gastrointestinal spasmolytics, especially Corydalis, Matricaria and *Viburnum opulus* (cramp bark) may be helpful in GORD because they can exert a regulatory role on lower oesophageal function.

Example liquid formula

Passiflora incarnata	1:2	20 mL
Matricaria recutita (high in bisabolol)	1:2	25 mL
Filipendula ulmaria	1:2	25 mL
Glycyrrhiza glabra (high in glycyrrhizin)	1:1	15 mL
Cynara scolymus	1:2	15 mL
	TOTAL	100 mL

Dose: 5 mL with water three times a day after meals. An extra dose can be taken before retiring in the evening.

For best results combine with Ulmus (slippery elm) powder after meals. Note also that some patients with GORD are aggravated by ethanolic herbal liquids, and tablets or capsules should instead be instituted.

CASE HISTORY

A female patient aged 58 had suffered irregularly from heartburn for 10 to 15 years. Over the years she had learnt to avoid alcohol, smoking, wheat, yeast and rice. She was already taking slippery elm powder and had taken antacids in the past. She sought treatment because she was experiencing frequent attacks of heartburn in the past few months. She hated licorice, so it was not included in her formula.

Treatment consisted of (based on 1 week):

Passiflora incarnata	1:2	25 mL
Matricaria chamomilla	1:2	25 mL
Filipendula ulmaria	1:2	25 mL
Stellaria media (stabilised succus)		25 mL
	TOTAL	100 mL

Dose: 5 mL three times a day.

In the 4 weeks following, the patient experienced only one attack of heartburn and in the following 4 weeks had no problems with heartburn, despite being unwell with influenza.

Poor upper digestive function/anorexia

Poor upper digestive function can be a consequence of prolonged or serious illness or can occur with convalescence. Digestive function can deteriorate with age. Poor digestion is also reflected in children by their failure to thrive, anaemia and susceptibility to infections. Symptoms include anorexia, a prolonged sensation of fullness or stagnation after eating, undigested food in stools, belching or flatulence, intolerance of fatty foods and nausea. However, poor upper digestive function may be largely asymptomatic in itself, but may contribute to other conditions such as food intolerance or allergies, intestinal dysbiosis (abnormal bowel flora), constipation, nutrient deficiencies and migraine headaches. Herbal clinicians believe that many chronic diseases originally begin with poor digestive function and good upper digestive function is a prerequisite for a healthy digestive system.

Herbs that improve upper digestive function can be divided into five major groups:

- Simple bitters such as *Gentiana lutea*, which improve most aspects of upper digestive function
- Aromatic digestives such as *Angelica archangelica*, Cinnamomum (cinnamon) and *Coleus forskohlii* that improve gastric acid secretions. Coleus also improves exocrine pancreatic function
- Pungent herbs such as Zingiber (ginger) and Capsicum (cayenne) that are potent stimulators of gastric acid and other aspects of digestive function (as already noted)
- Choleretic herbs such as *Berberis vulgaris* (barberry), Silybum (St Mary's thistle) and Taraxacum (dandelion root) that improve bile production by the liver
- Cholagogue herbs such *Mentha piperita* (peppermint) that improve gallbladder function.

If there is evidence of liver weakness, including previous pesticide exposure, history of hepatitis or symptoms such as nausea after rich or fatty food, the above treatment might need to strongly focus on the choleretic herbs mentioned above, together with hepatic trophorestoratives. If the patient notices excessive irritability after using any of the above herbs, it is recommended to reduce the dose and/or delete any bitter or choleretic herbs, including Berberis. (See also the above discussion on functional dyspepsia.)

Nausea

Nausea is a symptom rather than a disease state. A number of herbs can be used effectively to give relief. If nausea is traceable to poor liver function, then the treatment approach outlined above should be followed. Other herbs that can provide symptomatic relief in cases of nausea include Zingiber (ginger, very well studied – see monograph), *Mentha piperita* (peppermint), Matricaria (chamomile), *Ballota nigra* (black horehound) and Filipendula (meadowsweet). If herbs are used to prevent motion sickness, they should be taken about 1 h before travel. Ginger is particularly effective for all forms of motion sickness and also for morning sickness. Herbs should not be administered orally to a person who is vomiting.

Peptic ulcer

The herbal approach to the treatment of peptic ulcer disease should take into account all the causative and sustaining factors relevant to the individual patient. Rather than being concerned with inhibiting gastric acid, the herbal clinician stresses the support of factors that protect the mucosa and improve the capacity of the body to heal the ulcer. The prominent shift in attention towards the role of the bacterium *Helicobacter pylori* in causing peptic ulceration has led to many herbal approaches being mooted. These remain largely untested and some research on their role has been negative. For example, in spite of positive in vitro studies indicating an effect on *H. pylori*, consumption of hot spices such as chilli or of raw garlic is not known to offer any benefits in terms of human infection (for example, in Korea where these are consumed in high levels infections are notably high). In a crossover study, of 12 subjects with known *H. pylori* infection were tested with Jalapeno peppers, raw garlic or a bismuth-containing positive control, with clear washouts between different treatments. No benefits as assessed by urea breath test were found.[78]

In vitro evidence exists for an anti-adhesion effect that might reduce the infectivity of *H. pylori* for plant constituents such as proanthocyanidins from *Vaccinium macrocarpon* (cranberry), acidic polysaccharide from *Camellia sinensis* (green tea), carbohydrates from *Panax ginseng* (Korean ginseng), or the false receptors provided by fucoidans and glycosaminoglycans in medicinal algae, including *Fucus vesiculosus* (bladderwrack).[79] All need to be confirmed in human studies (see also pp. 321–322).

With the focus on *H. pylori* and NSAIDs as obvious causes of peptic ulcer disease a number of previously recognised pathogenic factors are now largely overlooked. Only a small percentage of patients positive for *H. pylori* develop peptic ulcer disease. Similarly, not everyone who uses NSAIDs ends up with peptic ulcers. These forgotten factors are likely to be particularly relevant for idiopathic peptic ulcers (an increasingly large patient group), which are by definition not linked to *H. pylori* or NSAIDs.

A review of studies published over 30 years found that soluble fibre from fruit and vegetables was protective and refined sugars a risk factor in peptic ulcers.[80] Alcohol and coffee do not seem to be related to duodenal ulcer, but gastric cancer is linked to diets high in salt and low in fresh fruit.[81] Use of sugar in tea and coffee increases risk, and tea consumption reduces risk of peptic ulcers.[82] Smoking is a strong risk factor.[82,83] Ulcers heal more slowly in smokers and relapse is more likely. Smoking also increases the risk of infection with *H. pylori*[84] and decreases gastric mucosal blood flow.[85] Leisure time physical activity is protective,[82] but skipping breakfast is a risk factor.[86]

As touched on above, the time-honoured role of stress has been neglected recently, but one review concluded:

> The epidemiological, clinical and genetic evidence strongly suggests that host factors, especially the effects of stress (in the broadest psychosocial sense), may be decisive in determining who develops a duodenal ulcer.[87]

As noted above, local defences are an issue in peptic ulcer disease. Gastric mucosal blood flow is considered to be of major importance in maintaining mucosal integrity.[88] Reactive oxygen species and cytokines appear to contribute to the gastric damage.[89] There is an age-related decline in mucosal repair capacity, possibly related to decreased mucosal prostaglandin levels.[90]

Main aspects of phytotherapy include the following:

- Glycyrrhiza (licorice) and mucilaginous herbs such as Ulmus and Althaea to enhance mucoprotection. These are best taken before meals and, in the case of duodenal ulceration, should be taken at least half an hour before eating. Glycyrrhiza also improves pancreatic bicarbonate secretion
- Whilst bitter herbs such as Gentiana are contraindicated in duodenal ulcers, they may be valuable in gastric ulcers because of their trophic effect on the gastric mucous membrane
- *Hydrastis canadensis* (golden seal) is traditionally restorative to mucous membranes and also antibacterial, but would be best avoided in duodenal ulcers
- Immune-enhancing and antiseptic herbs such as Echinacea or high-resin remedies such as *Calendula officinalis* (marigold), *Commiphora molmol* (myrrh) and propolis may help resolve or contain *Helicobacter pylori* presence and improve repair mechanisms. They were traditionally used in peptic ulcer disease long before the importance of *H. pylori* was recognised
- Gently astringent herbs will assist ulcer healing and boost mucoprotection in the vicinity of the ulcer. Good examples are Agrimonia and Filipendula (meadowsweet). Strongly astringent herbs such as *Geranium maculatum* (cranesbill) will aggravate a gastric ulcer, but may be suitable for duodenal ulcer treatment
- Anti-inflammatory herbs such as Stellaria (chickweed) and bisabolol-rich Matricaria (chamomile) and vulneraries such as Calendula and Centella (gotu kola) will help break the vicious cycle of ulceration and accelerate the healing process
- Herbs benefiting the microcirculation, especially in this context Vaccinium (bilberry), Ginkgo and Vitis (grape seed extract), will also assist healing
- Pungent spices have had a common assumption of being contraindicated in peptic ulceration. However, in cultures where these are frequent components of the diet there is a contrary view that they are protective and pharmacological research tends to support this[91]
- Spasmolytic and carminative herbs will improve gastrointestinal motility. Carminative herbs such as Foeniculum (fennel) should be administered only in low doses. Good gastrointestinal spasmolytics include Matricaria and *Viburnum opulus* (cramp bark)
- Herbs that decrease the negative effects of stress can be indicated and include adaptogens, nervine tonics and anxiolytics
- Filipendula is considered by some herbalists to be a normaliser of the acidity of the stomach.[92] It does appear to decrease the negative effects of acid and pepsin on the mucosa, but is probably not a potent antacid. This positive effect on the mucosa is paradoxical since it contains salicylates
- Some patients with peptic ulcer disease may experience irritation from herbal treatment and one approach with more severe or chronic cases is to start with a low dose and gradually increase over several weeks. This can especially apply with liquid preparations, in which case tablets or capsules are more appropriate.

Example liquid formulas

For gastric ulcer

Foeniculum vulgare	1:2	3 mL
Filipendula ulmaria	1:2	25 mL
Glycyrrhiza glabra (high in glycyrrhizin)	1:1	20 mL
Matricaria recutita	1:2	25 mL
Gentiana lutea	1:5	2 mL
Echinacea purpurea/angustifolia root	1:2	25 mL
	TOTAL	100 mL

Dose: 5 mL with water three times a day before meals.

For duodenal ulcer

Filipendula ulmaria	1:2	20 mL
Glycyrrhiza glabra	1:1	20 mL
Matricaria recutita	1:2	20 mL
Vaccinium myrtillus	1:1	20 mL
Echinacea purpurea/angustifolia root	1:2	25 mL
	TOTAL	105 mL

Dose: 5 mL with water three times a day half an hour before meals.

Food intolerance and allergies

Food intolerance can have a number of causes such as enzyme defects (e.g. alactasia), pharmacological activity (e.g. salicylates) and immunological reactions (allergy, coeliac disease). There are also a number of less well-defined and less specific, often idiosyncratic, reactions. Food intolerance can follow hepatitis or gastrointestinal infection. In these instances the reaction to some or many foods can continue long after the actual infection has passed.

In the case of immunological reactions, which represent true food allergy, the best approach to treatment is to avoid the offending foods, if they can be identified and if exclusion is practical. In other instances of food intolerance, herbal treatment may prove beneficial by correcting any physiological defects or deficiencies contributing to the reaction to foods, and by dampening any underlying gastrointestinal inflammation.

Treatable factors that can contribute to a state of food allergy or intolerance include:

- Poor digestion which can lead to chemical fragments from food such as peptides or polypeptides, which are either pharmacologically active or immunogenic
- A leaky gut wall which will allow the passage of unprocessed or partially processed chemicals from food

into surrounding tissue and the portal blood. Factors which can contribute to a leaky gut include alcohol, drugs, intestinal flora dysbiosis, infection and inflammation
- Poor hepatic screening of portal vein contents. Substances absorbed from the gastrointestinal tract are carried by the portal vein to the liver and can be processed by hepatocytes or phagocytosed by the Kupffer cells. In particular Kupffer cells sequester any immunologically active material and thereby dampen any potential immune reaction
- Poor immunity and detoxifying mechanisms in the body, which might lead to an excessive response to a chemical insult.

The herbal approach to the treatment of food intolerance or allergy can include the following:

- Bitter, aromatic, pungent, choleretic and cholagogue herbs to improve upper digestive function
- Hepatotrophorestoratives and stimulants of hepatic metabolism, such as Silybum and Schisandra, to improve hepatic screening and detoxification
- Depurative and lymphatic herbs, such as Arctium (burdock) and Calendula, to assist detoxification mechanisms
- Herbs with healing and protective effects on the gut wall, such as Filipendula (meadowsweet), Calendula, Matricaria (chamomile) and Althaea (marshmallow) root. These can help reduce the impact of a leaky gut
- Immune-enhancing herbs such as Echinacea, which enhances phagocytic activity. Andrographis is both bitter and immune enhancing
- Hydrastis (golden seal) as a restorative to the mucous membranes of the gut wall and a potential modifier of gut flora. Hydrastis is also bitter
- Other treatments to restore normal gut flora. This is covered in detail later in this section
- Antiallergic herbs such as Albizia and *Scutellaria baicalensis* (Baical skullcap) and anti-inflammatory herbs such as Matricaria and turmeric.

Appropriate herbs should be selected from the above treatment approach on the basis of the individual case.

Example liquid formula

Echinacea purpurea/angustifolia root	1:2	30 mL
Andrographis paniculata	1:2	10 mL
Silybum marianum	1:1	20 mL
Matricaria recutita	1:2	20 mL
Filipendula ulmaria	1:2	20 mL
	TOTAL	100 mL

Dose: 5 mL with water three times a day before meals.

CASE HISTORY

A female patient aged 35 had been overseas and developed an acute gastrointestinal infection with pain and diarrhoea. The infection passed but on returning home she experienced bloating and diarrhoea often after eating. Stool culture did not demonstrate the presence of an infection. Symptoms could be controlled by restricting her diet to a very simple one: rice and vegetables.

Treatment consisted of:

Echinacea angustifolia root	1:2	30 mL
Picrorrhiza kurroa	1:2	10 mL
Silybum marianum	1:1	20 mL
Matricaria chamomilla	1:2	20 mL
Filipendula ulmaria	1:2	20 mL
	TOTAL	100 mL

Dose: 5 mL with water three times a day before meals.

Hydrastis tablets 500 mg, one tablet with each meal.

After 4 weeks of treatment, symptoms had improved and she could often be more adventurous with her diet without causing problems. However, symptoms still occurred on many days.

During the next 4 weeks her condition continued to improve with herbal treatment. After another 4 weeks she could eat normally and the herbs were discontinued without adverse effect. **Note** that Andrographis would be a suitable substitute for the Picrorrhiza in the above prescription.

Constipation

Constipation is medically defined as a bowel frequency of less than three times a week or the need to strain more than 25% of the time during defaecation. However, it is probably less than optimum for health to defaecate less than once a day. Phytotherapists certainly believe that regular bowel movements are necessary for the maintenance of good health. Constipation may be associated with diseases such as hypothyroidism and Parkinson's disease and these should always be excluded.

Factors that may cause or contribute to simple constipation include:

- Inadequate fibre and/or fluid intake
- Irritable bowel syndrome
- Psychological factors that can produce constipation through an inhibitory effect on the autonomic innervation of the colon. In some cases this may be related to poor toilet training during youth
- Drugs, excessive tea intake
- Poor liver function (bile is an excellent natural laxative).

Use of the well-known and much maligned anthraquinone-containing herbal laxatives is widespread. On balance, the evidence is that these herbs are safe and effective when used in the short term (see Chapter 2). However, they are best used as a last resort since their effect is only symptomatic. Their tendency to cause wind and griping can aggravate the pain associated with irritable bowel syndrome (IBS) and they are not at all suitable for constipation associated with bowel tension, spasm or irritability (see below). Also, the anthraquinone laxatives may become habit forming. This is for a number of reasons. One simple reason is that in overdose they empty a greater portion of the bowel than normal defaecation does. Hence, it is usual not to have a bowel movement the day following their use while this area of the bowel again fills. But the patient thinks that he or she is constipated again and will repeat the medication, thus perpetuating its use. The way around this is to take sufficient dose to cause a motion of normal consistency. This can vary greatly from person to person. This variability is because bowel flora activate the anthraquinones into their laxative form and bowel flora vary greatly from person to person.

The herbal treatment of constipation can be approached in the following way:

- Improve liver function with choleretic and cholagogue herbs, such as Chionanthus (fringe tree), Taraxacum (dandelion root), Silybum and Cynara
- Increase stool bulk through diet and with bulking herbs such as Ulmus (slippery elm) and *Plantago ovata* (ispaghula)
- Improve motor function with gastrointestinal spasmolytics such as Matricaria (chamomile) and *Viburnum opulus* (cramp bark)
- Improve gastrointestinal lubrication. Linseeds are particularly suitable because of their oil and mucilage content
- Judicious use of laxative herbs, beginning with gentle agents such as *Juglans cinerea* (butternut), Rumex (yellow dock), Glycyrrhiza (licorice) and Rehmannia. Otherwise a minimum quantity of Cassia (senna) or *Rhamnus purshiana* (cascara) can be introduced.

Example liquid formula

Rehmannia glutinosa	1:2	25 mL
Cynara scolymus	1:2	20 mL
Rumex crispus	1:2	20 mL
Taraxacum officinale root	1:2	20 mL
Matricaria recutita	1:2	15 mL
	TOTAL	100 mL

Dose: 8 mL with water twice a day.

Irritable bowel syndrome

Irritable bowel syndrome (IBS) is both a very common condition now attracting new research and a difficult disorder to comprehend and treat. One reason for this is that the diagnosis is only conclusively arrived at after exclusion of other known disorders. There are, however, more positive and integrated approaches available for managing this condition based on a broader psychosocial model,[93] and phytotherapists are likely to find these more attractive. Possible aetiologic factors include hypersensitivity or motor dysfunction in the gut, abnormal response of smooth muscle to CNS signals, visceral and somatic sensory dysfunction and psychosocial distress.[94]

In addition to these 'traditional' factors involved in IBS, much research over the past decade or so has focussed on the pathogenic roles of altered enteric microbiota and inflammation. In addition to gastrointestinal pathogens, recent evidence suggests that patients with IBS have an abnormal composition and higher temporal instability of their intestinal flora.[95] Because this flora is an important determinant of natural gut function and immunity, this instability is probably a contributing factor in IBS and suggests a role for specific management of intestinal dysbiosis in a subset of patients (see below). One specific and typical abnormal gut flora finding in IBS is small intestinal bacterial overgrowth.[96] The fact that gastrointestinal infection or infestation, but not viral gastroenteritis, is a trigger of IBS in 10% of patients speaks to the role of disturbed microbial ecology in this disorder.[97]

On the topic of mucosal inflammation, one recent review of 16 studies found a relationship between mast cell abnormalities and symptom severity and frequency in IBS.[98] The authors suggested that mast cell stabilisers warrant further assessment, suggesting a role for *Albizia lebbek* and *Scutellaria baicalensis*.

After years of inattention, there is a growing body of evidence that dietary components can contribute to IBS.[99] While genuine food allergies are probably rare, food intolerances and especially malabsorption of particular sugars such as fructose (as treated by the so-called low FODMAP diet) do appear to be relevant in many patients. In addition, gluten restriction and sugar/carbohydrate restriction in general have all shown value in individual patients with IBS.[99]

A more definitive approach towards diagnosis and classification in IBS can lead to a better understanding and management. For example, it is unreasonable to assume that IBS characterised by diarrhoea would necessarily respond to the same treatment as IBS for which constipation predominates, yet many clinical trials make no attempt to evaluate therapy in terms of initial symptoms.

IBS is in fact the most common but yet least understood gastrointestinal disorder. There are three basic types:

- Functional diarrhoea with abdominal pain (diarrhoea-predominant IBS)
- Chronic abdominal pain and constipation (spastic colitis, or now termed constipation-predominant IBS)
- Abdominal pain with disturbed and variable bowel habit, typically constipation alternating with diarrhoea.

The dated term 'mucous colitis' refers to the excessive amount of mucus that can be passed with stools. As noted, the exact nature of the herbal treatment should depend on the factors identified in the individual case.

The first line of therapy for IBS is an increase in dietary fibre intake to improve intestinal transit time (especially for constipation-predominant IBS). If this fails, smooth muscle relaxants and/or antispasmodics are conventionally prescribed. A systematic review and meta-analysis to determine the efficacy of fibre intake, antispasmodics and peppermint oil as treatments for IBS identified 615 studies, but concluded that only 35 were eligible for inclusion.[100] The beneficial effect of fibre compared with placebo or no treatment in 12 studies (n=591 patients) was limited to ispaghula (*Plantago ovata*) husk; wheat bran was no more effective than placebo or no treatment. Twelve different antispasmodics were evaluated in 22 studies compared with placebo or no treatment (n=1778 patients). Two antispasmodics (otilonium and hyoscine – an alkaloid from *Hyoscyamus niger* (henbane) and other Solanaceae plants) were deemed to be most efficacious. However, 14% of the patients who took antispasmodics reported adverse events, and more conservative strategies are worth attempting first.

The herbal remedy most researched for IBS is peppermint oil (see the peppermint monograph). Nine clinical trials on peppermint oil and its gastrointestinal effects, including a total of 269 patients, have been reviewed.[101] Most studies of orally administered oil demonstrate a substantial spasmolytic effect on the gut, with slowed motility after prolonged use of doses above 0.2 mL. The authors concluded that an ideal formulation for the treatment of irritable bowel, and prevention of heartburn as a side effect through relaxation of the gastric sphincter, would be enteric coated and have a peak release at about 4 h after ingestion, with a release time of up to 24 h. Of 12 placebo-controlled trials reviewed in a subsequent paper,[102] eight showed a statistically significant positive effect for peppermint oil over the placebo. The conclusion that peppermint oil 'may be the drug of choice in IBS patients with non-serious constipation or diarrhoea to alleviate general symptoms and improve quality of life' is, however, undermined by the wide range of placebo responses reported in the studies reviewed (between 10% and 52%). In a later rigorous study[103] results indicated that 4 weeks of treatment with peppermint oil capsules was superior to a placebo in the treatment of IBS symptoms and its beneficial effect persisted 4 weeks after treatment had ended. This may be due to antibacterial actions of peppermint oil on enteric bacteria, or extended relaxant effects on smooth muscle tissue. Adverse event reports associated with peppermint oil were generally mild and transient and included heartburn and anal discomfort or burning. (See also the peppermint monograph.)

The need for enteric coating to demonstrate an effect for peppermint oil is a caution on the widespread recommendation for the use of other volatile antispasmodic constituents. The aromatic or pungent spices are, however, likely to add additional effects. A partially blinded, randomised, two-dose study on 207 subjects who had self-reported IBS symptoms for at least 3 months provided either 72 mg or 144 mg daily of standardised turmeric extract equivalent to 1800 or 3600 mg of dried root. The report showed overall benefits for both doses, though not clearly differentiated from background trends.[104] Other spices particularly worth trying are *Elettaria cardamomum* (cardamom) and *Foeniculum vulgare* (fennel) and the subjective sensation of relief when taking remedies in this group is often striking.

Another approach is to use remedies with positive benefits on digestion higher up in the system. For example, about one-third of patients with functional dyspepsia also have IBS, and the symptoms of the two disorders overlap considerably: treatment for one might be applicable to the other. A postmarketing surveillance (uncontrolled) German study prospectively collected data over 6 weeks on 279 patients who reported having at least three of five IBS symptoms (abdominal pain, bloating, flatulence, right-sided abdominal cramps and constipation) and who took six capsules daily of a standardised extract of *Cynara scolymus* (artichoke) leaf extract equivalent to 320 mg per capsule. Improvement in their symptoms followed an average of 10 days of treatment (see also further studies in the globe artichoke monograph).[105]

All the above points to the value of trying some of the treatment options below:

- Spasmolytic herbs including Matricaria (chamomile), *Humulus lupulus* (hops), *Viburnum opulus* (cramp bark), *Mentha piperita* (peppermint) and any of the carminative spices
- Corydalis and Zingiber (ginger) may have a role in some patients through a modification of the perception of visceral organ pain
- Sedative and nervine tonic herbs, particularly *Scutellaria lateriflora* (skullcap) and Valeriana (valerian)
- Hepatorestorative and choleretic herbs to improve liver function such as Silybum (St Mary's thistle), Cynara (globe artichoke leaf) and Schisandra
- Mucilage-containing herbs such as Ulmus (slippery elm), especially if there is constipation
- Gastrointestinal antiseptics to restore normal bowel flora such as Hydrastis (golden seal), propolis and oil of oregano. IBS patients may be intolerant of Allium (garlic), but if not it can be useful (see also under Intestinal dysbiosis below)
- The presence of mucus implies irritation, and gastrointestinal anti-inflammatories such as Filipendula (meadowsweet) and Matricaria (chamomile) are indicated
- Constipation should be treated with only gentle herbs such as *Rumex crispus* (yellow dock), *Juglans cinerea* (butternut) and Taraxacum (dandelion root)
- Symptoms of IBS are often confused or conflated with those of premenstrual and other hormonal upsets in women: in this case *Vitex agnus-castus* (chaste berry) and *Trigonella foenum-graecum* (fenugreek) are worth including
- An appropriate controlled exclusion diet should always be conducted to identify food irritants. These should however be done rigorously to avoid unnecessary elimination of nutritious food that has only occasional or apparent effect.

CASE HISTORY

A female patient aged 42 complained of chronic episodes of discomfort and distension in the right lower abdomen. This could be quite sharp at times and was associated with a feeling of malaise. She was intolerant of fatty foods and had what she described as a 'sluggish bowel', although her motions were always 'loose'. Past medical history revealed that she had lived on the Solomon Islands for an extended period during which time she had amoebic dysentery and malaria. A number of recent medical tests, including colonoscopy, could not find any abnormalities. She also had a history of heart damage of undefined origin. For this reason Crataegus (hawthorn) was included in her treatment (the Chinese use Crataegus as a digestive herb).

The following treatment was prescribed:

Crataegus spp. leaves	1:2	20 mL
Filipendula ulmaria	1:2	20 mL
Chionanthus virginicus	1:2	15 mL
Silybum marianum	1:1	15 mL
Matricaria chamomilla	1:2	20 mL
Viburnum opulus	1:2	20 mL
	TOTAL	110 mL

Dose: 5 mL with water three times daily.

Ulmus (slippery elm), one heaped teaspoon with water three times a day, was also recommended. After 4 weeks she reported a stunning transformation. In the whole month the patient had only experienced one bad day. She was feeling very well, eating better and had more energy. The patient will remain on her herbal treatment for some time. This was a patient who had spent many years and thousands of dollars on conventional medical treatment and yet had remained unwell.

Gastrointestinal infections and diarrhoea

The most common causes of acute diarrhoea are infectious agents. Acute diarrhoea may also be caused by drugs or toxins. Chronic diarrhoea is also most likely to be caused by infectious agents. However, other common causes include inflammatory bowel diseases, malabsorption, IBS (idiopathic diarrhoea), medications and food additives. In all cases the source of the diarrhoea should be ascertained and appropriate treatment should then follow.

Acute gastrointestinal diarrhoea with vomiting is generally not suited to herbal therapy. This is because the patient will invariably vomit back the herbal treatment and may consequently develop an aversion to taking herbs.

Acute infectious diarrhoea in the absence of vomiting can be approached in the following way:

- Boost immunity with immune-enhancing herbs, particularly Echinacea and Andrographis
- Control fever with diaphoretic herbs such as *Mentha piperita* (peppermint) and Achillea (yarrow)
- If the infection does not involve a virus, Hydrastis (golden seal) or *Berberis vulgaris* (barberry) is indicated because of the antimicrobial activity of the berberine each contains (see the Berberis monograph). Berberine also inhibits the activity of enterotoxins. Other herbs rich in berberine could also be used such as Phellodendron and Coptis
- Antimicrobial essential oils safe for internal use can also be used to control gut infections. These include oils of anise, thyme and oregano. Allium (garlic) is also a useful, broad-spectrum gut antiseptic (raw crushed cloves or as the allicin-releasing powder)
- If cytotoxins or mucosal invasion are part of the pathogenic process, anti-inflammatory herbs such as Matricaria (chamomile) and mucilage-containing herbs such as *Ulmus rubra* (slippery elm) are indicated
- Tannin-containing herbs, such as *Geranium maculatum* (cranesbill), which act as astringents will also gently control diarrhoea without risk of aggravating the infection by reducing intestinal motility. They also reduce mucosal damage and are particularly indicated if the infection is due to a virus

- Antiprotozoal agents include propolis, *Artemisia annua*, berberine-containing herbs, Euphorbia and essential oil of oregano
- Normal conservative measures such as adequate fluid and electrolyte intake should also be implemented.

Chronic infectious diarrhoea is treated in a similar manner to acute infectious diarrhoea. However, particular emphasis should also be given to factors involved in host resistance:

- Gastrointestinal antiseptics (the essential oils noted above, Hydrastis), especially when used (but not concurrently) with agents that encourage growth of normal flora, will help to restore the protective activity of intestinal flora (see below)
- Herbs to improve gastric acidity to prevent reinfection may also need emphasis. These include Coleus, Angelica, Zingiber (ginger), Capsicum (cayenne) and bitters such as Gentiana.

CASE HISTORY

A female patient aged 35 presented with chronic infection with the protozoan Giardia that had persisted for more than 3 months. She was prescribed the following treatment (based on 1 week):

Echinacea angustifolia root	1:2	35 mL
Picrorrhiza kurroa	1:2	10 mL
Angelica archangelica	1:2	15 mL
Propolis	1:10	20 mL
Zingiber officinale	1:2	5 mL
Matricaria chamomilla	1:2	15 mL
	TOTAL	100 mL

Dose: 5 mL with water three times a day.

Hydrastis (golden seal) 500 mg tablets at 4/day were also prescribed and regular intake of a Lactobacillus culture at separate times was recommended.

After 4 weeks symptoms were about the same. There was even a 1-week period when the patient felt that the herbs were aggravating her condition. After another 4 weeks there was considerable improvement and the condition was resolved by a further 8 weeks' treatment. **Note** that Picrorrhiza in the formula doubled as a bitter to increase gastric acid and as an immune-enhancing agent and could be substituted with Andrographis, which has similar properties.

Diverticular disease

Diverticulosis describes the presence of diverticula or pockets in the wall of the large bowel. Acute diverticulitis is the clinical syndrome that occurs when a diverticulum becomes inflamed and perforates, which is relatively uncommon.

Lack of dietary fibre is probably the main cause of diverticulosis, but other factors that lead to constipation and colonic hypermobility may be involved. (Colonic hypermobility results in excessive mixing activity, which exacerbates constipation and causes areas of raised intraluminal pressure.)

Excessive pressure in the colon associated with age-related weakness and stiffness of the colon wall are probably all involved. If faecal volume is habitually small, pressure may rise to excessive levels during segmenting (mixing) movements. This can result in 'blow outs', which are herniations of the mucosa at naturally weak places in the wall where arteries pass inwards. With age, these can develop into diverticula. Diverticula are potential areas of stagnation in the bowel because they have no muscular wall and, therefore, are less subject to flushing by normal mixing movements.

The main aim of herbal treatment in uncomplicated diverticular disease is to reduce stagnation and further degeneration of the bowel wall. Aspects of treatment include the following:

- Appropriate dietary measures to increase fibre intake (but excluding seeds and nuts) and supplementation with mucilaginous herbs such as Ulmus (slippery elm). This will also help to maintain healthy bowel flora
- Gastrointestinal spasmolytics to decrease intracolonic pressure, including *Viburnum opulus* (cramp bark), Dioscorea (wild yam) and Matricaria (chamomile)
- Herbs to improve connective tissue strength including herbs containing flavonoids and oligomeric procyanidins (OPCs) such as Vitis (grape seed extract) and Crataegus (hawthorn). *Polygonum multiflorum* is also thought to improve connective tissue and is also a gentle laxative
- Gentle treatment of any associated constipation (see above).

Painful or symptomatic diverticular disease can also occur in the absence of diverticulitis. In medical thinking this is considered to be a variant of irritable bowel syndrome. However, it could result from a low-grade 'diverticulosis'. Depending on the assessment of the patient, this problem should either be treated as irritable bowel syndrome or the treatment approach described below to prevent recurrence of acute diverticulitis should otherwise be followed.

Acute diverticulitis usually requires hospitalisation. Herbal treatment is more suited to prevention of its recurrence. As well as incorporating the aspects of treatment of uncomplicated diverticular disease described above, the approach to prevention of acute diverticulitis should additionally include:

- Immune-enhancing herbs such as Echinacea and Andrographis to control pathogenic bacteria
- Gastrointestinal antiseptic herbs (see Gastrointestinal infections above)
- Anti-inflammatory gastrointestinal herbs such as Filipendula (meadowsweet) and Matricaria (chamomile).

CASE HISTORY

A male patient aged 72 suffered an attack of acute diverticulitis and was concerned to prevent another episode.

Treatment consisted of the following prescription (based on 1 week):

Echinacea angustifolia root	1:2	25 mL
Hydrastis canadensis	1:3	20 mL
Viburnum opulus	1:2	20 mL
Matricaria recutita	1:2	20 mL
Propolis	1:10	15 mL
	TOTAL	100 mL

Dose: 5 mL with water three times a day.

Ulmus (slippery elm) powder, one heaped teaspoon with water before each meal, was also prescribed.

The patient was also advised to have more fibre in his diet, particularly more fruit. Fresh crushed garlic, one to two cloves a day, was also recommended for 3 days of every week. After 6 months the herbal treatment was discontinued but the fresh garlic (for 1 to 2 days/week), slippery elm and dietary changes were still observed. Several years later, the patient had not experienced any recurrence of acute diverticulitis.

Intestinal dysbiosis

As well as the obvious involvement of pathogenic gut micro-organisms in acute and chronic gut infections, they are probably contributing factors in the chronicity of disturbances of immune or gut function such as food sensitivity, IBS, asthma, dermatitis, psoriasis and autoimmune diseases such as rheumatoid arthritis, inflammatory bowel disease and ankylosing spondylitis.

The involvement of gut flora in autoimmune disease is exemplified by published studies suggesting the involvement of pathogenic organisms in several autoimmune diseases. Dr Alan Ebringer of King's College Hospital, London, decided to test this association clinically. Patients with ankylosing spondylitis were placed on a low starch diet, because it was postulated that this would reduce the number of Klebsiella organisms in the gut.[106] Most patients on this programme had their disease process halted, but the diet must be adhered to for at least 6 months.

In addition, many people who are chronically unwell but with no specific diagnosis may be suffering from a microbial dysbiosis, which is not sufficiently marked to be classified as an infection. This is well illustrated by the postulated involvement of *Candida albicans* in many such syndromes.

The gastric acid barrier is an important factor in maintaining healthy gut microflora, and other digestive secretions such as bile and pancreatic enzymes also play a role. Immune function, especially secretory IgA, diet and bowel motility can also influence the location and levels of particular microflora.

The assumption made after episodes of gut infection is that recovery is complete. However, several pathogenic microorganisms can take up residence in the gut at low levels following infection. The implication of this can be chronic disease. The role of antibiotics, especially their chronic use, in contributing to gut flora dysbiosis is widely recognised.

The suggested programme below has been adapted from the approach developed by the late Hein Zeylstra (to whom this book is dedicated), for the management of inflammatory bowel disease. It can work well in conjunction with a low starch diet, as per Ebringer above.

Herbal treatment for gut flora dysbiosis is compatible with the use of probiotics and prebiotics. In fact the protocol below relies on the use of a herbal 'prebiotic'. If probiotics are additionally prescribed (either via supplements or diet), then they should not be taken at the same time as antimicrobial herbs:

- The herbal approach is based on the 'weed' and 'feed' hypothesis. In other words, the aim is to manipulate existing microflora to provide a healthier balance and in particular create a predominance of organisms (such as Lactobacilli and Bifidobacteria) that do not imbalance the immune system. By manipulating existing resident microflora, the changes in gut flora are more likely to be permanent

- The 'weed-killer' consists of using broad-spectrum antimicrobial herbs that have activity against bacteria, fungi and protozoa. By using such agents, levels of most microflora are depressed and there is less likelihood of exacerbating the gut flora imbalance. The 'fertiliser' then consists of agents such as marshmallow root glycetract,

aloe vera concentrate or slippery elm powder that selectively encourage healthy microflora, along the same principles as the use of prebiotics

- This process is repeated over weekly cycles. For 2 to 3 days only of each week (preferably the weekend) the antimicrobial herbs are taken throughout the day. Then the 'fertiliser' herbs are used for the rest of the week. The cycle is then repeated for at least 6 weeks, although much longer may be required, especially in the case of chronic diseases such as autoimmune disease

- Key broad-spectrum antimicrobial herbs are garlic, berberine-containing herbs (such as Hydrastis or Phellodendron), essential oils (e.g. oregano) and mild tannin-containing herbs (especially green tea and grape seed extracts). The advantage of tannins is that they are poorly absorbed in the gastrointestinal tract and are carried to the large bowel. Through their capacity to bind proteins, they can inhibit the growth of all microorganisms, but appear to be specifically selective on pathogenic organisms (see below).

For maximum impact:

- The antimicrobial herbs need to be taken in reasonably high doses on the 2 to 3 'weeding' days

- However, the green tea and grape seed extracts are best taken only during the 'feeding' days as they will have minimal impact on healthy flora, but will provide a dampening effect on the regrowth of pathogenic bacteria.

Grape seed oligomeric and polymeric procyanidins demonstrated a beneficial effect on caecal fermentation in rats. Caecal pH decreased, and fermentative activity was stimulated without an increase of deleterious enzymatic activity.[107] A small clinical study in Japan demonstrated that a green tea preparation was able to positively affect intestinal dysbiosis in nursing home patients by raising levels of lactobacilli and bifidobacteria, lowering levels of Enterobacteriaceae, Bacteroidaceae and Eubacteria, and decreasing odorous compounds. Levels of pathogenic bacterial metabolites were also decreased.[108,109] A further study found that supplementation with tea catechins produced favourable improvements in the participant's bowel condition, as evidenced by a reduction in faecal moisture, pH, ammonia, sulphide and oxidation-reduction potential. In both trials the dose was 300 mg/day of tea catechins, which is equivalent to about six cups of green tea.[110]

In summary, on Saturday and Sunday (and perhaps Monday) the patient is advised to take antimicrobial herbs in high doses spread throughout the day. These would include Allium (garlic), oil of oregano and a source of berberine such as Phellodendron. During the rest of the week Ulmus (slippery elm), green tea and grape seed extract are advised. The cycle is then repeated for at least 6 weeks.

Inflammatory bowel disease

The principles of treating chronic inflammatory conditions have been rehearsed in the Inflammatory and autoimmune diseases section in Chapter 8. Inflammatory bowel diseases

(IBDs), like Crohn's disease and ulcerative colitis, however, present local digestive challenges that also deserve separate discussion.

Clearly the main focus in a systematic approach to the digestive role in IBD is to consider diet as a factor. The potential link between Crohn's and wheat consumption has been referred to in Chapter 8 and these and other possibilities are worth rigorously exploring. A low sulphur diet for ulcerative colitis[111] and a dairy- and yeast-free diet for Crohn's disease are also worth trialling.

There is a potential role for topical herbal treatments. Aloe vera gel is widely promoted for the treatment of such digestive disorders. In a randomised, placebo-controlled, blinded study 100 mL of *Aloe barbadensis* (Aloe vera) gel twice daily was shown to have modest benefits in the treatment of mild to moderate ulcerative colitis, though only on subjective symptoms.[112]

IBDs are marked by increased production of pro-inflammatory cytokines such as tumour necrosis factor (TNF)-alpha, interleukin-1 (IL-1) and IL-6. There is the theoretical possibility that reduction in these markers may be obtained by remedies acting primarily on the digestive system. In a randomised, open label, multi-centre trial, 20 patients with active Crohn's receiving standard treatment excluding TNF-alpha inhibitors ingested 250 mg standardised capsules containing wormwood (*Artemisia absinthium*, absinthin at 0.32% to 0.38%) with *Elettaria cardamomum* (cardamom) seeds and *Pistacia lentiscus* (mastic), three times a day. These herbs might all be chosen as treatments for inflammation of the bowel. Blood samples were tested at 3 and 6 weeks to determine TNF-alpha levels compared with baseline and these were significantly lowered in the treatment group compared with placebo.[113]

The important prospect of treating IBD with Boswellia has been commented on in the Boswellia monograph.

It is known that bile can be a co-factor in IBD, particularly following secondary metabolism by bowel flora. Traditional phytotherapeutic approaches have included remedies that are known to have choleretic or hepatic effects and these can be seen as plausible strategies. Disturbed bowel flora may have additional harmful effects and steps to reduce dysbiosis are often justified.

Taking these approaches into account, with the obvious caution of viewing IBD as a systemic disorder as much as a local one, the following measures might be considered. Reference should be made also to the section above on Intestinal dysbiosis for other important therapeutic considerations:

- Immune modulating herbs such as Echinacea root are useful and appear to be able to regulate the inflammation (see the Echinacea monograph for a discussion of its role in autoimmune disease)
- Anti-inflammatory herbs especially Boswellia in solid extract form, as well as *Calendula officinalis* (marigold) and *Curcuma longa* (turmeric) can be helpful (see the Boswellia and turmeric monographs for relevant clinical data)

- As with diverticular disease, increased 'soft' fibre intake and mucilaginous plants and materials, such as aloe gel is likely to be helpful. Mucilaginous gums and prebiotic constituents will also help to maintain healthy bowel flora and counteract negative effects of bile irritation. Those with additional inflammatory-modulating effects such as *Linum usitassimum* (flaxseed) or *Trigonella foenum-graecum* (fenugreek) may be particularly helpful
- Choleretic and hepatic remedies such as *Cynara scolymus* (globe artichoke), *Silybum marianum* (St Mary's thistle), *Hydrastis canadensis* (golden seal) and *Berberis vulgaris* (barberry) are often useful in reducing deleterious effects of the 'wrong sort of bile'.

CASE HISTORY

A 39-year-old woman had suffered from Crohn's disease for 24 years. Lately (the last 2.5 years) it had been out of control. She had a stricture 5 cm from the rectum which made it difficult to control her bowel motions. Her main symptoms were almost continuous diarrhoea. Other symptoms included mouth ulcers, occasional high temperatures and chronically blocked sinuses. Conventional medications were mesalazine 1500 mg/day, oral prednisone (tapering off) and prednisone enemas daily. The following herbal treatments were instituted:

- The intestinal dysbiosis protocol above for 6 weeks and then Hydrastis (golden seal) 1500 mg/day and Ulmus (slippery elm) powder on a regular basis (she could not tolerate garlic)
- Tablets containing *Echinacea angustifolia* root (600 mg) and *Echinacea purpurea* root (675 mg) (3 per day)
- Tablets containing Boswellia (1200 mg), turmeric (2000 mg), celery (1000 mg) and ginger (300 mg) (4 per day)
- A dairy- and yeast-free diet.

After 5 month's treatment there was great symptomatic improvement and the patient commented: 'I no longer view travelling in terms of toilet stops'. She had one relatively normal bowel motion per day, no mouth ulcers and her high temperatures were gone. After 12 months there was no need for the prednisone enemas. After 36 months the patient was completely asymptomatic and on minimal conventional medication. Her lifestyle was transformed!

Haemorrhoids

A haemorrhoid or a pile is a dilation of the internal haemorrhoidal plexus. Internal haemorrhoids are more significant and are covered with mucous membrane. An external pile is really a rupture of a small vein in the perianal region. The exact cause is not known, but is probably associated with a mild partial mucosal prolapse during straining at defaecation.

Haemorrhoids are aggravated by pelvic congestion (constipation and pregnancy) and prostatic enlargement. Some degree of loss of elasticity of the anal sphincter may play a role. Lifting heavy weights may aggravate the condition. Treatment could include the following:

- Increase dietary fibre, both soluble and insoluble
- Mucilage-containing herbs such as Ulmus (slippery elm) and psyllium to keep the stool soft
- Any associated constipation should be treated (see above)
- Oral treatment using herbs to improve venous and connective tissue tone. These include Aesculus (horsechestnut), Ruscus (butcher's broom) and *Polygonum multiflorum*. Flavonoid-containing herbs, such as Crataegus, also have this property. Melilotus (sweet clover) helps to relieve tissue congestion
- Topical treatment with healing and astringent herbs such as Hamamelis (witchhazel), Symphytum (comfrey) and Calendula. Aesculus also works well topically, especially in gel formulations, but should not be applied if the piles are bleeding (see monograph)
- If liver congestion exists, which will exacerbate pelvic congestion, treatment with choleretic and hepatoprotective herbs should be applied.

CASE HISTORY

A male patient aged 35 had suffered from haemorrhoids for 8 years. He had been treated with rubber ligation but was still suffering problems such as irritation and occasional bleeding. He was not experiencing constipation but felt tense in the lower abdomen and was generally an anxious person. Other symptoms included indigestion, abdominal bloating and reflux.

Treatment consisted of (based on 1 week):

Artemisia absinthium	1:5	10 mL
Aesculus hippocastanum	1:2	25 mL
Melilotus officinale	1:2	20 mL
Ruscus aculeatus	1:2	25 mL
Valeriana officinalis	1:2	20 mL
	TOTAL	100 mL

Dose: 5 mL with water three times daily.

Ulmus (slippery elm) powder, one heaped teaspoon twice a day was also prescribed, together with comfrey ointment.

Over the course of the next 16 weeks, the condition improved and he was free of any symptoms related to the haemorrhoids. He also reported feeling more relaxed.

References

1. Du P, O'Grady G, Davidson JB, et al. Multiscale modeling of gastrointestinal electrophysiology and experimental validation. *Crit Rev Biomed Eng*. 2010;38(3):225–254.
2. Altaf MA, Sood MR. The nervous system and gastrointestinal function. *Dev Disabil Res Rev*. 2008;14(2):87–95.
3. Waterman SA, Tonini M, Costa M. The role of ascending excitatory and descending inhibitory pathways in peristalsis in the isolated guinea-pig small intestine. *J Physiol (Lond)*. 1994;481(pt 1):223–232.
4. De Ponti F, Cosentino M, Lecchini S, et al. Physiopharmacology of the peristaltic reflex: an update. *Ital J Gastroenterol*. 1991;23(5):264–269.
5. Wood JD. Enteric nervous system: sensory physiology, diarrhea and constipation. *Curr Opin Gastroenterol*. 2010;26(2):102–108.
6. Wingate DL. The effect of diet on small intestinal and biliary tract function. *Am J Clin Nutr*. 1985;42(5 suppl):1020–1024.
7. Hoogerwerf WA. Role of biological rhythms in gastrointestinal health and disease. *Rev Endocr Metab Disord*. 2009;10(4):293–300.
8. Mellander A, Abrahamsson H, Sjovall H. The migrating motor complex – the motor component of a cholinergic enteric secretomotor programme? *Acta Physiol Scand*. 1995;154(3):329–341.
9. May B, Kuntz H, Kieser M, Koler S. Efficacy of a fixed peppermint oil/caraway oil combination in non-ulcer dyspepsia. *Arzneimittelforschung*. 1996;46(II):1149–1153.
10. De Winter BY, De Man JG. Interplay between inflammation, immune system and neuronal pathways: effect on gastrointestinal motility. *World J Gastroenterol*. 2010;16(44):5523–5535.

11. Cooke HJ. Neuroimmune signaling in regulation of intestinal ion transport. *Am J Physiol*. 1994;266(2 pt 1):167–178.
12. Santos J, Alonso C, Vicario M, et al. Neuropharmacology of stress-induced mucosal inflammation: implications for inflammatory bowel disease and irritable bowel syndrome. *Curr Mol Med*. 2008;8(4):258–273.
13. Wouters MM, Boeckxstaens GE. Neuroimmune mechanisms in functional bowel disorders. *Neth J Med*. 2011;69(2):55–61.
14. Snoek SA, Verstege MI, Boeckxstaens GE. The enteric nervous system as a regulator of intestinal epithelial barrier function in health and disease. *Expert Rev Gastroenterol Hepatol*. 2010;4(5):637–651.
15. Surawicz CM. Mechanisms of diarrhea. *Curr Gastroenterol Rep*. 2010;12(4):236–244.
16. Ralph A, Giannella MD, Selwyn A, et al. Influence of gastric acidity on bacterial and parasitic enteric infections. *Ann Intern Med*. 1973;78(2):271–276.
17. Torsoli A, Severi C. The neuroendocrine control of gastrointestinal motor activity. *J Physiol (Paris)*. 1993;87(6):367–374.
18. Mach T. The brain-gut axis in irritable bowel syndrome – clinical aspects. *Med Sci Monit*. 2004;10(6):125–131.
19. Chen CL, Liu TT, Yi CH, Orr WC. Effects of capsaicin-containing red pepper sauce suspension on esophageal secondary peristalsis in humans. *Neurogastroenterol Motil*. 2010;22(11):1177–1182.
20. Szolcsányi J. Forty years in capsaicin research for sensory pharmacology and physiology. *Neuropeptides*. 2004;38(6):377–384.

21. Serdiuk SE, Komissarov IV, Gmiro VE. The role of the chemosensory systems in the inhibitory regulation of cholinergic transmission in the small intestine. *Fiziol Zh*. 1993;39(1):54–61.
22. Furness JB, Costa M. Projections of intestinal neurons showing immunoreactivity for vasoactive intestinal polypeptide are consistent with these neurons being the enteric inhibitory neurons. *Neurosci Lett*. 1979;15(2–3):199–204.
23. Donnerer J, Bartho L, Holzer P, Lembeck F. Intestinal peristalsis associated with release of immunoreactive substance P. *Neuroscience*. 1984;11(4):913–918.
24. Glatzel H, Rüberg-Schweer M. Regional influence on cutaneous blood flow effected by oral spice intake. *Nutr Dieta Eur Rev Nutr Diet*. 1968;10:194–214.
25. Staljanssens D, Azari EK, Christiaens O. The CCK(-like) receptor in the animal kingdom: functions, evolution and structures. *Peptides*. 2011;32(3):607–619.
26. Bradwejn J, Zhou Y, Koszycki D, Shlik J. A double blind, placebo-controlled study on the effects of Gotu Kola (Centella asiatica) on acoustic startle response in healthy subjects. *J Clin Psychopharmacol*. 2000;20(6):680–684.
27. Eckel LA, Ossenkopp KP. Cholecystokinin reduces sucrose palatability in rats: evidence in support of a satiety effect. *Am J Physiol*. 1994;267(6 pt 2):R1496–1502.
28. Holt S, Brand J, Soveny C, Hansky J. Relationship of satiety to postprandial glycaemic, insulin and cholecystokinin responses. *Appetite*. 1992;18(2):129–141.
29. Hansen JB, Arkhammar PO, Bodvarsdottir TB, Wahl P. Inhibition of insulin secretion

as a new drug target in the treatment of metabolic disorders. *Curr Med Chem.* 2004;11(12):1595–1615.

30. Bartness TJ, Waldbillig RJ. Cholecystokinin-induced suppression of feeding: an evaluation of the generality of gustatory-cholecystokinin interactions. *Physiol Behav.* 1984;32(3):409–415.

31. Morley JE, Silver AJ. Anorexia in the elderly. *Neurobiol Aging.* 1988;9(1):9–16.

32. Khayyal MT, Seif-El-Nasr M, El-Ghazaly MA, et al. Mechanisms involved in the gastro-protective effect of STW 5 (Iberogast) and its components against ulcers and rebound acidity. *Phytomedicine.* 2006;13(suppl 5):56–66.

33. Takeuchi T, Shiratori K, Watanabe S, et al. Secretin as a potential mediator of antiulcer actions of mucosal protective agents. *J Clin Gastroenterol.* 1991;13(suppl):S83–87.

34. Shiratori K, Watanabe S, Takeuchi T. Effect of licorice extract (Fm100) on release of secretin and exocrine pancreatic secretion in humans. *Pancreas.* 1986;1(6):483–487.

35. Minton NA. Volunteer models for predicting antiemetic activity of 5-HT3-receptor antagonists. *Br J Clin Pharmacol.* 1994;37(6):525–530.

36. Costall B, Naylor RJ. Neuropharmacology of emesis in relation to clinical response. *Br J Cancer.* 1992;19:2–7.

37. Beubler E, Schirgi-Degen A. Serotonin antagonists inhibit sennoside-induced fluid secretion and diarrhea. *Pharmacology.* 1993;47(suppl):64–69.

38. Hyland NP, Cryan JF. Gut feeling about GABA: focus on GABA(B) receptors. *Front Pharmacol.* 2010;1:124.

39. Krantis A, Costa M, Furness JB, Orbach J. Gamma-aminobutyric acid stimulates intrinsic inhibitory and excitatory nerves in the guinea-pig intestine. *Eur J Pharmacol.* 1980;67(4):461–468.

40. Izzo AA, Sharkey KA. Cannabinoids and the gut: new developments and emerging concepts. *Pharmacol Ther.* 2010;126(1):21–38.

41. Korczynski W, Ceregrzyn M, Matyjek R, et al. Central and local (enteric) action of orexins. *J Physiol Pharmacol.* 2006;57(suppl 6):17–42.

42. Bjarnason I. Intestinal permeability. *Gut.* 1994;35(suppl 1):18–22.

43. Lee EB, Kim OK, Jung CS, Jung KH. The influence of methanol extract of Ulmus davidiana var. Japonica cortex on gastric erosion and ulcer and paw edema in rats. *Yakhak Hoeji.* 1995;39(6):671–675.

44. Blaut M, Collins MD, Welling GW, et al. Molecular biological methods for studying the gut microbiota: the EU human gut flora project. *Br J Nutr.* 2002;87(suppl 2):203–211.

45. Van Eldere J, Robben J, Caenepeel P, Eyssen H. Influence of a cecal volume-reducing intestinal microflora on the excretion and entero-hepatic circulation of steroids and bile acids. *J Steroid Biochem.* 1988;29(1):33–39.

46. Ozawa A, Ohnishi N, Tazume S, et al. Intestinal bacterial flora and host defense

mechanisms. *Tokai J Exp Clin Med.* 1986;11(suppl):65–79.

47. Rolfe RD. Interactions among microorganisms of the indigenous intestinal flora and their influence on the host. *Rev Infect Dis.* 1984;6(suppl 1):S73–S79.

48. Walker WA, Bloch KJ. Gastrointestinal transport of macromolecules in the pathogenesis of food allergy. *Ann Allergy.* 1983;51(2 pt 2):240–245.

49. Turnbaugh PJ, Ridaura VK, Faith JJ, et al. The effect of diet on the human gut microbiome. *Sci Transl Med.* 2009;1(6):6–14.

50. De Filippo C, Cavalieri D, Di Paola M, et al. Impact of diet in shaping gut microbiota revealed by a comparative study in children from Europe and rural Africa. *Proc Natl Acad Sci USA.* 2010;107:14691–14696.

51. Sullivan A, Edlund C, Nord CE. Effect of antimicrobial agents on the ecological balance of human microflora. *Lancet Infect Dis.* 2001;1:101–114.

52. Wickens K, Pearce N, Crane J, Beasley R. Antibiotic use in early childhood and the development of asthma. *Clin Exp Allergy.* 1999;29:766–771.

53. Noverr MC, Huffnagle GB. Does the microbiota regulate immune responses outside the gut? *Trends Microbiol.* 2004;12:562–568.

54. Parsonnet J. Bacterial infection as a cause of cancer. *Environ Health Perspect.* 1995;103(suppl 8):263–268.

55. Tazume S, Ozawa A, Yamamoto T, et al. Ecological study on the intestinal bacteria flora of patients with diarrhea. *Clin Infect Dis.* 1993;16(suppl 2):77–82.

56. Gorbach SL. Estrogens, breast cancer, and intestinal flora. *Rev Infect Dis.* 1984;6(suppl 1):85–90.

57. Sacquet E, Leprince C, Riottot M, Raibaud P. Dietary fiber and cholesterol and bile acid metabolism in axenic (germfree) and holoxenic (conventional) rats. III. Effect of nonsterilized pectin. *Reprod Nutr Dev.* 1985;25(1A):93–100.

58. Sherman PM, Ossa JC, Johnson-Henry K. Unraveling mechanisms of action of probiotics. *Nutr Clin Pract.* 2009;24(1):10–14.

59. Roberfroid M, Gibson GR, Hoyles L, et al. Prebiotic effects: metabolic and health benefits. *Br J Nutr.* 2010;104(suppl 2):1–63.

60. Broekaert WF, Courtin CM, Verbeke K, et al. Prebiotic and other health-related effects of cereal-derived arabinoxylans, arabinoxylan-oligosaccharides, and xylooligosaccharides. *Crit Rev Food Sci Nutr.* 2011;51(2):178–194.

61. Praznik W, Spies T. Fructo-oligosaccharides from Urginea maritima. *Carbohydr Res.* 1993;243(1):91–97.

62. Mitsuoka T, Hidaka H, Eida T. Effect of fructo-oligosaccharides on intestinal microflora. *Nahrung.* 1987;31(5–6):427–436.

63. Bouhnik Y, Flourié B, Riottot M, et al. Effects of fructooligosaccharides ingestion on fecal bifidobacteria and selected metabolic indexes of colon carcinogenesis

in healthy humans. *Nutr Cancer.* 1996;26(1):21–29.

64. Saetta JP, March S, Gaunt ME, Quinton DN. Gastric emptying procedures in the self-poisoned patients: are we forcing gastric content beyond the pylorus? *J R Soc Med.* 1991;84(5):274–276.

65. Vale JA. Primary decontamination: vomiting, gastric irrigation or only medicinal charcoal? *Ther Umsch.* 1992;49(2):102–106.

66. Underhill TJ, Greene MK, Dove AF. A comparison of the efficacy of gastric lavage, ipecacuanha and activated charcoal in the emergency management of paracetamol overdose. *Arch Emerg Med.* 1990;7(3):148–154.

67. Ilett KF, Gibb SM, Unsworth RW. Syrup of ipecacuanha as an emetic in adults. *Med J Aust.* 1997;2(3):91–93.

68. Ramberg JE, Nelson ED, Sinnott RA. Immunomodulatory dietary polysaccharides: a systematic review of the literature. *Nutr J.* 2010;9:54.

69. Chattopadhyay A, Shetty KV. Recurrent aphthous stomatitis. *Otolaryngol Clin North Am.* 2011;44(1):79–88.

70. Burgess JA, van der Ven PF, Martin M, et al. Review of over-the-counter treatments for aphthous ulceration and results from use of a dissolving oral patch containing Glycyrrhiza complex herbal extract. *J Contemp Dent Pract.* 2008;9(3):88–98.

71. Roesch W, Liebregts T, Gundermann KJ, et al. Phytotherapy for functional dyspepsia: a review of the clinical evidence for the herbal preparation STW 5. *Phytomedicine.* 2006;13(suppl 5):114–121.

72. Milzer J, Iten F, Reichling J, Sallre R. Iberis amara L. and Iberogast – results of a systematic review concerning functional dyspepsia. *J Herbal Pharmacother.* 2004;4(4):51–59.

73. Wegener T, Wagner H. The active components and the pharmacological multi-target principle of STW 5 (Iberogast). *Phytomedicine.* 2006;13(suppl 5):20–35.

74. Rohof WO, Hirsch DP, Boeckxstaens GE. Pathophysiology and management of gastroesophageal reflux disease. *Minerva Gastroenterol Dietol.* 2009;55(3):289–300.

75. Saarela R, Lindroos E, Soini H, et al. Chewing problems and mortality. *J Am Geriatr Soc.* 2011;59(1):181–183.

76. Northridge ME, Nye A, Zhang YV, et al. 'Third places' for healthy aging: online opportunities for health promotion and disease management in adults in Harlem. *J Am Geriatr Soc.* 2011;59(1):175–176.

77. Anand G, Katz PO. Gastroesophageal reflux disease and obesity. *Gastroenterol Clin North Am.* 2010;39(1):39–46.

78. Graham DY, Anderson S, Lang T. Garlic or Jalapeno peppers for treatment of Helicobacter pylori infection. *Am J Gastrol.* 1999;94(5):1200–1202.

79. Yarnell E, Abascal K. Antiadhesion herbs. *Altern Complement Ther.* 2008;14(3):139–144.

80. Misciagna G, Cisternino AM, Freudenheim J. Diet and duodenal ulcer. *Dig Liver Dis.* 2000;32(6):468–472.

81. Calam J, Baron JH. ABC of the upper gastrointestinal tract: pathophysiology of duodenal and gastric ulcer and gastric cancer. *BMJ.* 2001;323(7319):980–982.

82. Suadicani P, Hein HO, Gyntelberg F. Genetic and life-style determinants of peptic ulcer. A study of 3387 men aged 54 to 74 years: The Copenhagen Male Study. *Scand J Gastroenterol.* 1999;34(1):12–17.

83. Rosenstock S, Jørgensen T, Bonnevie O, Andersen L. Risk factors for peptic ulcer disease: a population based prospective cohort study comprising 2416 Danish adults. *Gut.* 2003;52(2):186–193.

84. Parasher G, Eastwood GL. Smoking and peptic ulcer in the Helicobacter pylori era. *Eur J Gastroenterol Hepatol.* 2000;12(8):843–853.

85. Eastwood GL. Is smoking still important in the pathogenesis of peptic ulcer disease? *J Clin Gastroenterol.* 1997;25(suppl 1):S1–S7.

86. Levenstein S. Peptic ulcer at the end of the 20th century: biological and psychological risk factors. *Can J Gastroenterol.* 1999;13(9):753–759.

87. Melmed RN, Gelpin Y. Duodenal ulcer: the helicobacterization of a psychosomatic disease? *Isr J Med Sci.* 1996;32(3–4):211–216.

88. Abdel-Salam OM, Czimmer J, Debreceni A, et al. Gastric mucosal integrity: gastric mucosal blood flow and microcirculation. An overview. *J Physiol (Paris).* 2001; 95(1–6):105–127.

89. Bandyopadhyay D, Biswas K, Bhattacharyya M, et al. Gastric toxicity and mucosal ulceration induced by oxygen-derived reactive species: protection by melatonin. *Curr Mol Med.* 2001;1(4):501–513.

90. Majumdar AP, Fligiel SE, Jaszewski R. Gastric mucosal injury and repair: effect of aging. *Histol Histopathol.* 1997;12(2):491–501.

91. Al Mofleh IA. Spices, herbal xenobiotics and the stomach: friends or foes? *World J Gastroenterol.* 2010;16(22):2710–2719.

92. Roberts F. *Modern Herbalism For Digestive Disorders.* Northamptonshire: Thomsons; 1981.

93. Tanaka Y, Kanazawa M, Fukudo S, Drossman DA. Biopsychosocial model of irritable bowel syndrome. *J Neurogastroenterol Motil.* 2011;17(2):131–139.

94. Hasler WL. Traditional thoughts on the pathophysiology of irritable bowel syndrome. *Gastroenterol Clin North Am.* 2011;40(1):21–43.

95. Bolino CM, Bercik P. Pathogenic factors involved in the development of irritable bowel syndrome: focus on a microbial role. *Infect Dis Clin North Am.* 2010;24(4):961–975.

96. Yamini D, Pimentel M. Irritable bowel syndrome and small intestinal bacterial overgrowth. *J Clin Gastroenterol.* 2010;44(10):672–675.

97. Spiller R, Garsed K. Postinfectious irritable bowel syndrome. *Gastroenterology.* 2009;136(6):1979–1988.

98. Ford AC, Talley NJ. Mucosal inflammation as a potential etiological factor in irritable bowel syndrome: a systematic review. *J Gastroenterol.* 2011;46(4):421–431.

99. Eswaran S, Tack J, Chey WD. Food: the forgotten factor in the irritable bowel syndrome. *Gastroenterol Clin North Am.* 2011;40(1):141–162.

100. Ford AC, Talley NJ, Spiegel BMR, et al. Effect of fibre, antispasmodics, and peppermint oil in the treatment of irritable bowel syndrome: systematic review and meta-analysis. *BMJ.* 2008;337:a2313.

101. Grigoleit HG, Grigoleit P. Gastrointestinal clinical pharmacology of peppermint oil. *Phytomedicine.* 2005;12:607–611.

102. Grigoleit HG, Grigoleit P. Peppermint oil in irritable bowel syndrome. *Phytomedicine.* 2005;12:601–606.

103. Cappello G, Spezzaferro M, Grossi L, et al. Peppermint oil (Mintoil[r]) in the treatment of irritable bowel syndrome: a prospective double blind placebo-controlled randomized trial. *Dig Liver Dis.* 2007;39(6):530–536.

104. Bundy R, Walker A, Middleton R, Booth J. Turmeric extract may reduce irritable bowel syndrome symptomology in otherwise healthy adults: pilot study. *J Altern Complement Med.* 2004;10(6):1015–1018.

105. Walker AF, Middleton RW, Petrowicz O. Artichoke leaf extract reduces symptoms of irritable bowel syndrome in a post-marketing surveillance study. *Phytother Res.* 2001;15:58–61.

106. Ebringer A, Wilson C. The use of a low starch diet in the treatment of patients suffering from ankylosing spondylitis. *Clin Rheumatol.* 1996;15(suppl 1):62–66.

107. Tebib K, Besancon P, Rouanet JM. Effects of dietary grape seed tannins on rat cecal fermentation and colonic bacterial enzymes. *Nutr Res.* 1996;16(1):105–110.

108. Hara Y. Influence of tea catechins on the digestive tract. *J Cell Biochem Suppl.* 1997;27:52–58.

109. Goto K, Kanaya S, Nishikawa T, et al. Green tea catechins improve gut flora. *Ann Long-Term Care.* 1998;6:1–7.

110. Goto K, Kanaya S, Ishigami T, Hara Y. The effects of tea catechins on fecal conditions of elderly residents in a long-term care facility. *J Nutr Sci Vitaminol.* 1999;45(1):135–141.

111. Roediger WE. Decreased sulphur aminoacid intake in ulcerative colitis. *Lancet.* 1998;351(9115):1555.

112. Langmead L, Feakins R, Goldthorpe S, et al. Randomized, double blind, placebo-controlled trial of oral aloe vera gel for active ulcerative colitis. *Aliment Pharmacol Ther.* 2004;19:739–747.

113. Krebs S, Omer B, Omer N. Wormwood (Artemisia absinthium) suppresses tumor necrosis factor alpha and accelerates healing in patients with Crohn's disease – A controlled clinical trial. *Phytomedicine.* 2010;17:305–309.

Biliary system

Scope

Apart from their use to provide non-specific support for recuperation and repair, specific phytotherapeutic strategies include the following.

Treatment of:

- cholecystitis (biliary infection)
- minor or early cholelithiasis (biliary stones)
- conjugated hyperbilirubinaemia.

Management of:

- established cholelithiasis
- chronic and moderate hepatobiliary diseases.

Because of the use of secondary plant products, particular **caution** is necessary in applying phytotherapy to:

- biliary carcinoma
- blocked bile duct
- acute and severe hepatobiliary diseases.

Background

Bile acids/salts and mechanisms of biliary flow

Whereas cholesterol accounts for more than 90% to 95% of the sterols in bile, bile acids and their salts are the most important solutes; they are essential in the management of cholesterol levels and themselves help determine the extent of bile flow. Bile acids are synthesised from cholesterol by the liver. There are three groups. Primary bile acids, in humans mainly cholic and chenodeoxycholic acids and their salts, are produced directly. Secondary bile salts are created by the action of intestinal bacteria on primary bile salts with deoxycholate and lithocholate being formed from cholate and chenodeoxycholate, respectively. Tertiary bile salts are the result of modification of secondary bile salts by intestinal flora or hepatocytes; in humans these include the sulphate ester of lithocholate and ursodeoxycholate and the 7-beta-epimer of chenodeoxycholate.[1]

Bile flow rates and composition are subject to a wide variety of neural, endocrine and paracrine influences. One of the main stimulants of bile flow are bile acids themselves, either in their primary form or reabsorbed as secondary or tertiary forms in the enterohepatic circulation (see below). The cholagogue effects of bile acids have led to their prescription in hepatobiliary disorders. One derivative, ursodeoxycholic acid, has been shown in controlled clinical studies to be a useful agent in the management of patients with primary biliary cirrhosis, autoimmune chronic active hepatitis[2] and cystic fibrosis.[3]

Cholestasis

Infective conditions may lead to cholestasis or reduced bile flow with symptoms including jaundice, pruritus and steatorrhoea. Chronic alcoholics may have hypotonic gallbladder, with increased speed of bile secretion and low biliary levels of cholic acid, cholesterol and bilirubin. Patterns of bile stagnation can occur with increasing severity of alcoholism, especially when associated with cirrhosis.[4] This effect has been attributed to the effects of lipopolysaccharide endotoxins.[5]

The role of inflammatory bowel disease in inducing cholestasis is also well established.[6] In one study serum cholestanol/cholesterol proportions were determined in 79 patients with inflammatory bowel (colonic and ileal) diseases, such as ulcerative colitis and Crohn's disease, and 23 with irritable bowel syndrome as controls. The findings suggested that the increased cholestanol proportion in colonic inflammatory bowel diseases is determined mainly by impaired biliary elimination of this sterol, while in ileal disease the dominating change in sterol balance is activated cholesterol synthesis. Increased serum cholestanol is a novel finding in colonic inflammatory bowel diseases, apparently indicating the presence of subclinical cholestasis in a marked number (20% to 50%) of inflammatory bowel disease patients.[7]

Therapeutic stimulation of bile flow could thus be justified in the management and treatment of any of the above circumstances (see below).

It appears that a substantial amount of urate is also eliminated by the biliary route in humans. Gout and other urate-associated conditions linked to decreased renal urate excretion may therefore benefit from measures that increase biliary urate excretion.[8]

Toxicity of bile acids

Because it is known that high concentrations of bile acids are cytotoxic, it has been speculated that their raised presence in serum and tissues in hepatobiliary diseases contributes to the pathological progression of these disorders. Bile acids are a causative factor in chronic gastritis.[9] Evidence is that oral administration of ursodeoxycholate, being a relatively non-toxic bile acid, can replace more hydrophobic hepatotoxic bile acids in the circulating pool and, by doing so, ameliorate the harmful effects of the latter.[10]

Enterohepatic circulation

An important aspect of bile acid function and toxicity is the constant reabsorption from the intestine into the portal circulation and back to the liver and biliary system – the enterohepatic circulation. Both primary and secondary bile acids are involved in this recycling. In modern medicine a high degree of recycling is assumed. Only 1% of bile acids are lost in the faeces and it was calculated that bile acids are recirculated about 12 times per day.[11] However, it is likely that humans living a more primitive lifestyle with much higher levels of fibre intake had lower reabsorption rates. The implications of enterohepatic circulation are best understood with reference to the kinetics of drugs such as the morphine alkaloids and digoxin, which are largely eliminated from the body through the bile. Increased retention of bile in the enterohepatic circulation is known to increase the half-life of these and other drugs in the body. It is likely, therefore, that the level of bile products (with the formation of tertiary bile acids) and other potentially toxic metabolites may increase, unless the enterohepatic circulation is as low as possible. In practice, this is most likely to follow a relatively fast intestinal transit time, associated with a high-fibre diet.

Bile and cholesterol

Although they are generally cholagogic, the presence of bile acids in the enterohepatic cycle acts to decrease the hepatic production of cholesterol, presumably through a process of negative feedback, and this is likely to control excessive cholesterol secretion in gallstone conditions. As with other hepatic conditions, replacement therapy with bile acids such as chenodeoxycholic and ursodeoxycholic acids is promoted as a treatment, leading even to dissolution of existing gallstones.[12]

Of wider significance is the finding that reduction in the absorption of bile acids from the gut, associated with, for example, diarrhoea, leads to an increase in cholesterol synthesis and cholesterol esterification rate by the liver.[13,14]

Biliary cholesterol excretion is directly linked to two major pathological issues, namely atherosclerotic cardiovascular disease (ACVD) and cholesterol gallstones. In ACVD biliary cholesterol secretion is the final step in the reverse cholesterol transport (RCT) pathway, the transport of peripheral cholesterol back to the liver for excretion.[15] For RCT, enhanced biliary secretion of cholesterol is desirable, although this can lead to biliary cholesterol supersaturation and gallstones. The most relevant source of cholesterol secreted into bile is cholesterol derived from plasma lipoproteins, with HDL (high density lipoprotein) the preferential contributor.[15] However, definitive studies exploring the underlying metabolic pathways are still lacking, although ABC (ATP binding cassette) transporters are known to be involved: specifically ABCB11 for bile acid transport into bile, ABCB4 for phospholipids and ABCG5/G8 for cholesterol.[15]

Effects of bile acids in the intestinal tract

Both primary and secondary bile acids have secretagogue effects on the intestinal mucosa, changing net fluid transport across the villi from absorption to secretion.[16] There is also an atropine-inhibited (i.e. cholinergic) stimulation of intestinal contractions[17] and an increased mucosal vasodilation (blood flow increasing by around 50%), which is not inhibited by atropine.[18] Secondary bile acids in particular are thought to increase permeability at the zonulae occludentes that binds endothelial cells together at their luminal borders, so that normal subepithelial hydrostatic pressure is raised sufficiently to reverse net sodium, chloride and water absorption to net secretion.[19]

Bile has sometimes been referred to as the body's own laxative or 'endolaxative'.[20] Indeed, it is established that bile acids (especially secondary bile acids – see below) can be responsible for bowel looseness and their effects should be borne in mind in cases of unexplained chronic diarrhoea.[21,22]

Bile has a wider range of actions on the intestinal mucosa. Where there is clear reduction in bile levels, there is a reduction in thickness of the mucus blanket, reduced numbers of mucus-associated enterocytes (suggesting a reduced endothelial turnover rate) and lymphocytes and increased populations of bacterial organisms. The implication is that normal bile function is a vital part of the body's gut-related defences.[23] It has also been demonstrated that bacterial endotoxin absorption is increased in the absence of bile salts from the intestine.[24]

Bacterial action on bile acids—consequences and implications

The generally positive functions of primary bile acids become rather more mixed in their effects once bacterial deconjugation and dehydroxylation occur. Secondary bile acids are produced at a very early age – the process is clearly under way even in month-old infants[25] – and are an entirely normal range of metabolites. It is clear that most bacterial deconjugation occurs in the colon[26] but in various less ideal circumstances invasive bacterial populations can lead to secondary bile product formation in the small intestine.

Secondary bile acids have a decidedly irritating effect on the intestinal wall. Exposure of the intestinal wall to deconjugated bile acids stimulates local inflammatory mechanisms, accompanied by the release of prostaglandin E_2 and leukotriene C_4. Such effects are particularly pronounced if there is already latent or active inflammatory disease of the intestinal wall, particularly in small intestinal Crohn's disease.[27] The irritant effect of secondary bile products is especially apparent if their quantities are increased due to stasis in the small intestine. Among a number of ultrastructural alterations to the intestinal mucosa, they increase the numbers of lysosomal vascular structures, fused microvilli and dilated endoplasmic reticulum, which among other implications leads to a reduced absorption of solutes including glucose and other carbohydrates[28,29] and, significantly, fluid absorption:[30] diarrhoea is thus possible. Secondary bile metabolites substantially increase the absorption rates of urea and oxalates from the gut.[31]

There are more insidious potential effects too. Secondary bile acids and their metabolites increase colonic cell proliferation.[32]

The carcinogenic effect is clearly linked to changes in the nature of bacterial populations in the gut, rather than to the nature of the bile acids or indeed other starting materials in the gut.[33] However, there is also little doubt that decreased reabsorption of bile acids (for example, as seen with increasing old age) does increase the likelihood that carcinogenic and other pathogenic bile metabolites will be produced.[34]

Dietary factors are known to affect the balance between intestinal flora and bile metabolism. For example, consumption of sugars was shown in nine volunteers on a crossover basis to significantly prolong transit time through the colon and significantly raise the faecal levels of both primary and secondary bile metabolites.[35] On the other hand, the consumption of 16 g of wheat bran a day on a double blind, 6-month crossover basis by ulcerative colitis sufferers in remission was shown to decrease the faecal concentration of bile acids by almost half. No such effect was observed with psyllium seed.[36]

There are some potential benefits in bacterial action on bile acids. Anaerobic bacteria, for example, can produce volatile fatty acids known to non-specifically inhibit pathogenic bacterial populations.[37]

Bile acids in diseases

Disturbed and pathological states can change the dynamics of bile and other intestinal relationships. In malnutrition, for example, morphological changes in the intestinal wall lead to increased sensitivity to the effects of secondary bile acids, poor absorption of fats and other nutrients, all of which is compounded by changes in intestinal flora.[38]

The impact of inflammatory intestinal diseases like Crohn's is even more pronounced. The damage induced by the disease on the intestinal wall leads to reduced bile acid reabsorption and compensatory increased cholesterol synthesis by the liver,[39] a reaction that probably explains the high level of biliary disease such as gallstones in sufferers from Crohn's.[40,41] The link between inflammatory bowel disease and cholestasis has already been mentioned, and Crohn's disease in particular is linked with disturbed bile metabolism and gallstones.[42] Similar negative impact on enterohepatic circulation follows small intestinal resection, which has been shown to lead to increased synthesis of both bile acids and cholesterol.[43]

The association between biliary and intestinal functions is further highlighted in the condition primary sclerosing cholangitis, a disease characterised by inflammation and obliterative fibrosis of bile ducts. In 70% of cases it is associated with ulcerative colitis. In about two-thirds, there are circulating IgG antibodies to a peptide shared by epithelial cell walls in both bile ducts and colon. Another suggested cause is portal bacteraemia secondary to a diseased bowel wall. The addition of bile acids to the gut has been proposed as a treatment.[44–46]

Phytotherapeutics

Plant constituents, cholesterol and bile function

A useful insight has been made in studies of the metabolism of plant sterols. Plant sterols are structurally similar to cholesterol but, because of poor intestinal absorption, are ordinarily not present in the liver. However, there does appear to be competition in the movement of plant sterols and cholesterol. For example, high plant sterol consumption appears to lower blood cholesterol levels,[47] especially in the short term,[48] and the proportions of plant sterols are significantly lower in cholesterol-rich gallstones than in bile (and stones with low cholesterol content are proportionately richer in plant sterols).[49] One sterol studied, sitostanol, parallels the secretion from and distribution of cholesterol in the liver (for example, both requiring bile salts for secretion in bile) so that it can be used as a physiologic analogue of unesterified cholesterol to trace the transport of sterols through the liver.[50] Such studies, for example, indicate that HDLs are necessary along with bile acids for cholesterol elimination in bile.[51] The use of plant sterols (in this case campesterol and sitosterol) as markers of cholesterol absorption and biliary secretion was also seen in a study referred to above, showing subclinical cholestasis as a feature of inflammatory bowel disease.[52]

When serum concentrations and metabolism of cholesterol were studied in human vegetarians, cholesterol absorption was found to be normal and synthesis was slightly enhanced, though without increase in serum cholesterol precursors. The serum concentrations of total and low-density lipoprotein (LDL)–cholesterol were decreased but, in addition to the obvious lower intake of cholesterol itself, it appeared that the higher intake of plant sterols interfered with cholesterol absorption and thus increased endogenous cholesterol synthesis. Thus, cholesterol saturation and bile acid composition of the bile were not changed. Biliary excretion of plant sterols was apparently relatively inefficient.[53]

Interactions between cholesterol transport and plant constituents extend to another major group. Saponins have been implicated in interference with the absorption of cholesterol, bile acids and fats, leading to reduced animal growth, but also have shown potential in the reduction of blood cholesterol levels.[54] There is evidence of interference with the absorption of vitamins A and E.[55] Their cholesterol-lowering effect may also be linked to their binding of bile salts and increasing their faecal excretion, thus increasing bile salt synthesis from endogenous cholesterol.[56] Further studies to investigate the effects of saponins on bile, cholesterol and lipid metabolism are clearly warranted (see also Chapter 2). One steroidal sapogenin that has been studied, diosgenin, is, like the sterols, also similar enough in structure to cholesterol to interfere with its esterification in the liver.[57] This may contribute to the marked increase observed in biliary cholesterol relative to phospholipids when it was fed for 7 days to rats (see Chapter 2).[58]

Choleretics and cholagogues

There is a traditional differentiation made between cholagogues and choleretics. The former are agents that stimulate the release of bile that has already been formed in the biliary system. Bile acids are the main endogenous cholagogues and fatty foods the most obvious exogenous factors.

Choleretics stimulate bile production by hepatocytes and some have effective cholagogue properties as well. Cholecystokinin, secretin and some of the other humoral agents are involved endogenously. Bitters and some of the botanical agents referred to below are likely to have choleretic activity (see Chapter 2).

There is very little interest in choleretic and cholagogue treatments in conventional medicine, at least in the English-speaking world. Among agents incidentally discovered, NSAIDs, especially aspirin (in one study at a level of 100mg/kg), cause choleresis in animals.[59] Magnesium sulphate (Epsom salts), sometimes used for constipation, has at doses of 500mg been shown to exert a direct effect on the motor activity of the gallbladder in dogs.[60]

Research on herbal choleretics and cholagogues has largely come from Germany and Eastern Europe. It is not comprehensive and most practice in this area is informed by traditional reputation. Given the difficulty in knowing what actually happens in the liver and the potential risks of counterproductive treatments (see below), this is not an ideal situation.

Among the work that has been done, it has been shown that the ethanolic extract of *Chelidonium majus* (greater celandine) in isolated liver culture significantly caused choloresis by increasing bile acid-independent flow,[61] and there is indication of activity in this area in clinical trials (see monograph). A survey of the literature shows that *Cynara scolymus* (artichoke) possesses choleretic, diuretic and hypocholesterolaemic properties (see monograph). The main active components of this plant are mono- and dicaffeoylquinic acids, flavonoids and sesquiterpenes. The most suitable raw material is fresh leaves in the plant's first year of growth.[62] Recent focus has been on the contribution of the claimed choleretic activity to cholesterol reduction. A Cochrane review[63] of three good-quality double blind studies points to a modest effect on total and LDL-cholesterol levels, although not at sufficient levels to recommend to prescribers. In one of the more significant placebo-controlled studies, involving 75 people in the UK, total cholesterol was reduced by 42% in the group receiving 1280mg of standardised artichoke leaf extract per day for 12 weeks, whereas the levels in the placebo group actually rose.[64] The choleretic activity of globe artichoke leaf has also been confirmed in clinical studies (see monograph). Phenolic acids in *Mentha longifolia* were found to possess significant in vivo choleretic and CNS stimulating effects[65] and peppermint leaf is traditionally regarded as a cholagogue. Turmeric (*Curcuma longa*) is also a clinically relevant cholagogue and choleretic herb (see monograph).

Plant remedies traditionally used as choleretics and cholagogues

- *Berberis vulgaris* (barberry), *Berberis aquifolium* (Oregon grape), Chelidonium (greater celandine), Chelone (balmony), Chionanthus (fringe-tree), *Euonymus atropurpureus* (wahoo), Taraxacum (dandelion), Veronicastrum (black root), Peumus (boldo), *Curcuma longa* (turmeric) and Cynara (globe artichoke).

Indications for choleretics and cholagogues

- Non-impacted gallstones
- Moderate cholecystitis (gallbladder infection), in conjunction with immune system support
- Conjugated hyperbilirubinaemia (jaundice due to decreased excretion of conjugated bilirubin through the bile duct).

Other traditional indications for choleretics and cholagogues

- 'Bilious' conditions associated with heaviness in the epigastrium, nausea, intolerance of alcohol and fats, headaches
- 'Toxic' conditions associated with intestinal congestion, especially in skin and autoimmune diseases
- Chronic constipation due to sluggish digestion.

Contraindications for choleretics and cholagogues

The effects of choleretic and cholagogue agents may be different in the diseased liver than the response produced in the normal liver. For example, experimental evidence suggests that the use of choleretic agents where hepatobiliary damage (e.g. cholangitis) is caused by obstructive jaundice might further depress hepatic functions.[66]

The use of choleretics and cholagogues is either contraindicated or at least inappropriate in the following:

- Obstructed bile ducts (due to impacted gallstones, cholangitis or cancer of the bile duct or pancreas)
- Unconjugated hyperbilirubinaemia (jaundice following haemolytic diseases, hereditary disease such as Gilbert's and Crigler-Najjar syndromes)
- Acute or severe hepatocellular disease (for example, following viral hepatitis, cirrhosis, adverse reactions to drugs, such as anaesthetics, steroids, oestrogen, chlorpromazine)
- Septic cholecystitis (where there is a risk of peritonitis)
- Intestinal spasm or ileus
- Hepatic cancer (although hepatoprotective herbs that also have some choleretic activity, such as *Silybum marianum*, can be appropriate, especially for secondary tumours on the liver).

Traditional therapeutic insights into the use of choleretics and cholagogues

Stimulating bile flow has been seen as one of the main eliminative strategies in traditional medicine, reflecting the importance attached by even the most primitive cultures to the role of the liver (the name of the organ was often as evocative as it is in English).

However, bile stimulation was often accompanied by vigorous approaches to eliminating it from the gut as well; the almost universal reliance in folk medicine on emetics and purgatives as first-resort approaches to the treatment of acute disease almost certainly had the effect, intended or otherwise (and in the case of emetics it was often intended), of radically removing bile from the body. It is now easy in modern medicine to dismiss the use of such drastic procedures as useless or dangerous but, unlike the use of bleeding, which was often likely to be counterproductive, emesis and catharsis were almost prehuman measures and established themselves over millennia in the most demanding court of efficacy, the survival from acute disease.

Given what is now known of the retentive qualities of the enterohepatic cycle, the certainty that modern diets and lifestyle have significantly lengthened intestinal transit time compared to that of early humans, thus extending enterohepatic recycling further, it is likely that many modern practitioners might look with some envy at their forebears' ability to get rid of this pool of potentially or actually toxic metabolites. However, emesis and catharsis were seen as an option for the most robust constitutions and, apart from the obvious inappropriateness, they are contraindicated in the more chronic and low-vitality conditions most often seen in the modern clinic.

Modern techniques to eliminate the bile pool generally involve dietary and other measures to decrease intestinal transit time combined with the use of choleretics and cholagogues. Some of the latter actually have laxative effects in any case, either because they contain the appropriate constituents or, more often, because the release of more bile is in itself laxative.

Application

Choleretics and cholagogues are best taken before meals, preferably about 30 minutes, but immediately before will suffice. As many rely at least in part on the effect of bitter constituents, they are best taken in fluid form.

Advanced phytotherapeutics

Choleretics and cholagogues may also be usefully applied in some cases (depending on other factors) of:

- chronic constipation (not due to intestinal spasm nor responding to conventional measures)
- migraine
- acne rosacea
- inflammatory bowel disease
- dysbiotic conditions of the gut
- chronic skin diseases
- autoimmune diseases (especially where associated with any of the above – see relevant sections, especially in Chapter 8).

Phytotherapy

Cholesterol gallstones and biliary pain

Gallstones are formed when cholesterol and other solute levels in bile reach supersaturated concentrations and when the normal glassy-smooth surfaces of the gallbladder are compromised, often by infection. Bile is often supersaturated after a night's metabolism and before breakfast: this could explain the naturopathic practice of recommending lemon juice (a liver and gallbladder stimulant) before breakfast. The concentration of bile also appears to be related to intestinal activity and slow intestinal transit has been linked to gallstone formation in normal-weight women[67] and in other studies.[68]

Certain risk factors for gallstones are inherent: being female, increasing age and ethnicity/family history (genetic traits). Others are modifiable: obesity, metabolic syndrome, hypertriglyceridaemia, rapid weight loss, diet (low in fibre and high in refined carbohydrates and saturated fat) and certain diseases (cirrhosis and Crohn's disease).[69]

Findings largely from in vitro and in vivo studies suggest that infection, inflammation and the response of the immune system can also influence the pathogenesis of cholesterol gallstones.[70] Supersaturated bile can lead to biliary sludge, composed of agglomerated cholesterol crystals. However, human studies have shown that biliary sludge does not necessarily lead to gallstone formation.[70] The missing link could be infection and/or inflammation that seeds stone formation.

Most patients with gallstones have no symptoms and current medical thinking is that there is no distinct advantage in treating asymptomatic gallstones.[71] Small stones are more dangerous than large as they can cause pancreatitis.[72] Oral dissolution therapy with bile salts is still used as a treatment, but is reserved for patients with non-calcified cholesterol gallstones, a patent cystic duct and for those who do not require urgent surgery.[71] These considerations also define the conditions for successful herbal treatment of gallstones. Patients who receive conventional oral therapy usually have a high rate of gallstone recurrence. This underlines the need in herbal therapy for long-term treatment concurrent with appropriate dietary and lifestyle changes.

A key outcome of phytotherapy for cholesterol gallstones is that it can render symptomatic gallstones quiescent. However, its greatest value here will be for stones that are not calcified in a functional gallbladder.

The essential elements of treatment are as follows:

- Bitter herbs to improve digestive and gallbladder function, such as *Artemisia absinthium* (wormwood) or *Gentiana lutea* (gentian)
- Choleretic herbs to improve bile flow, such Chelidonium (greater celandine), Cynara (globe artichoke), *Taraxacum radix* (dandelion root) and Silybum (St Mary's thistle)
- Cholagogue herbs to improve gallbladder motility, such as Chelidonium (greater celandine), Cynara and *Mentha piperita* (peppermint). A proprietary terpene mixture similar to essential oil of peppermint has been shown to dissolve gallstones[73]
- Spasmolytic herbs, selected from *Viburnum opulus* (cramp bark), *Corydalis ambigua*, Matricaria (chamomile) and *Mentha piperita*, can help to relieve gallbladder pain
- Long-term use of herbs containing steroidal saponins such as Dioscorea (wild yam) and Smilax (sarsaparilla) is best avoided, since these herbs may increase cholesterol levels in bile.[74]

A short course of copious olive oil and lemon juice is often recommended to discharge gallstones, although this is controversial.[75,76] However, such a therapy should only be attempted if the gallstones are not calcified, the cystic duct is patent, the gallbladder is functional and herbal therapy to soften the stones has been given for at least 6 months.

The above herbal approach can also be used for functional gallbladder disorder (gallbladder dyskinesia), which is the recurrence of abdominal pain resembling gallbladder pain in the absence of gallstones.[77]

CASE HISTORY

A male patient aged 69 had been experiencing recurrent attacks of biliary pain for several months. A blood test showed the presence of high levels of bilirubin, perhaps due to temporary obstruction caused by the passage of a stone, and tests revealed gallbladder inflammation and gallstones. The patient was offered surgery but wanted to try herbal treatment first.

He was advised to follow a low fat diet and the following formula was prescribed:

Silybum marianum	1:1	25 mL
Cynara scolymus	1:2	25 mL
Taraxacum officinale radix	1:2	20 mL
Picrorrhiza kurroa	1:2	10 mL
Mentha piperita	1:2	20 mL
	TOTAL	100 mL

Dose: 5 mL with water three times a day.

After a few months of treatment all symptoms had abated. The patient continued treatment for another 6 months, during which time he was free of symptoms. Since that time (several years) he has not had any herbal treatment but still remains free of gallbladder symptoms.

CASE HISTORY

An overweight female patient aged 61 years developed recurrent symptoms of nausea, vomiting and upper abdominal pain and was diagnosed as having gallstones. A low fat diet was recommended with avoidance of fried food.

The following herbal formula was prescribed and rapidly ameliorated her symptoms to the point it was no longer required after 6 weeks of use:

Taraxacum officinale radix	1:2	20 mL
Silybum marianum	1:1	20 mL
Cynara scolymus	1:2	25 mL
Matricaria recutita	1:2	20 mL
Corydalis ambigua	1:2	20 mL
		105 mL

Dose: 8 mL with water three times a day initially until symptoms subsided, and then twice a day thereafter.

References

1. Hay DW, Carey MC. Chemical species of lipids in bile. *Hepatology*. 1990;12(3 pt 2): 6–14.
2. Heathcote EJ, Cauch-Dudek K, Walker V, et al. The Canadian multicenter double blind randomized controlled trial of ursodeoxycholic acid in primary biliary cirrhosis. *Hepatology*. 1994;19(5):1149–1156.
3. Van Demeeberg PC, Houwen RHJ, Sinaasappel M, et al. Low-dose versus high-dose in cystic fibrosis-related cholestatic liver disease: results of a randomized study with 1-year follow-up. *Scand J Gastroenterol*. 1997;32(4):369–373.
4. Mikhailovskaya AY, Loranskaya TI, Vasilevskaya LS. Liver bile-secreting function in chronic alcoholics and means of correction of its disorders. *Voprosy Pitaniya*. 1995;5: 34–36.
5. Trauner M, Nathanson MH, Rydberg SA, et al. Endotoxin impairs biliary glutathione and HCO-3-excretion and blocks the choleretic effect of nitric oxide in rat liver. *Hepatology*. 1997;25(5):1184–1191.

6. Huang CS, Lichtenstein DR. Treatment of biliary problems in inflammatory bowel disease. *Curr Treat Options Gastroenterol.* 2005;8(2):117–126.

7. Hakala K, Vuoristo M, Miettinen TA. Serum cholestanol, cholesterol precursors and plant sterols in different inflammatory bowel diseases. *Digestion.* 1996;57(2):83–89.

8. Kountouras J, Magoula I, Tsapas G, Liatsis I. The effect of mannitol and secretin on the biliary transport of urate in humans. *Hepatology.* 1996;23(2):229–233.

9. Kolarski V, Petrova-Shopova K, Vasileva E, et al. Erosive gastritis and gastroduodenitis – clinical, diagnostic and therapeutic studies. *Vutr Boles.* 1987;26(3):56–59.

10. Maillette de Buy Wenniger L, Beuers U. Bile salts and cholestasis. *Dig Liver Dis.* 2010;42(6):409–418.

11. Lester R, Zimniak P. True transport: one or more sodium-dependent bile acid transporters? *Hepatology.* 1993;18(5): 1279–1282.

12. Hofmann AF. Bile acids as drugs: principles, mechanisms of action and formulations. *Ital J Gastroenterol.* 1995;27(2):106–113.

13. Akerlund JE, Reihner E, Angelin B, et al. Hepatic metabolism of cholesterol in Crohn's disease. Effect of partial resection of ileum. *Gastroenterology.* 1991;100(4):1046–1053.

14. Stahlberg D, Reihner E, Angelin B, Einarsson K. Interruption of the enterohepatic circulation of bile acids stimulates the esterification rate of cholesterol in human liver. *J Lipid Res.* 1991;32(9):1409–1415.

15. Dikkers A, Tietge UJ. Biliary cholesterol secretion: more than a simple ABC. *World J Gastroenterol.* 2010;16(47):5936–5945.

16. Gaginella TS, Haddad AC, Go VL, Phillips SF. Cytotoxicity of ricinoleic acid (castor oil) and other intestinal secretagogues on isolated intestinal epithelial cells. *J Pharmacol Exp Ther.* 1977;201(1):259–266.

17. Karlstrom L. Evidence of involvement of the enteric nervous system in the effects of sodium deoxycholate on small-intestinal transepithelial fluid transport and motility. *Scand J Gastroenterol.* 1986;21(3):321–330.

18. Karlstrom L. Mechanisms in bile salt-induced secretion in the small intestine. An experimental study in rats and cats. *Acta Physiol Scand.* 1986;549:1–48.

19. Wanitschke R. Intestinal filtration as a consequence of increased mucosal hydraulic permeability. A new concept for laxative action. *Klin Wochenschr.* 1980;58(6):267–278.

20. Abrahamsson H, Ostlund-Lindqvist AM, Nilsson R, et al. Altered bile acid metabolism in patients with constipation-predominant irritable bowel syndrome and functional constipation. *Scand J Gastroenterol.* 2008;43(12):1483–1488.

21. Kurien M, Evans KE, Leeds JS, et al. Bile acid malabsorption: an under-investigated differential diagnosis in patients presenting with diarrhea predominant irritable bowel syndrome type symptoms. *Scand J Gastroenterol.* 2011;46(7–8):818–822.

22. Ford GA, Preece JD, Davies IH, Wilkinson SP. Use of the SeHCAT test in the investigation of diarrhoea. *Postgrad Med J.* 1992;68(798):272–276.

23. Kalambaheti T, Cooper GN, Jackson GD. Role of bile in non-specific defence mechanisms of the gut. *Gut.* 1994;35(8):1047–1052.

24. Cahill CJ, Pain JA, Bailey ME. Bile salts, endotoxin and renal function in obstructive jaundice. *Surg Gynecol Obstet.* 1987;165(6):519–522.

25. Jonsson G, Midtvedt AC, Norman A, Midtvedt T. Intestinal microbial bile acid transformation in healthy infants. *J Pediatr Gastroenterol Nutr.* 1995;20(4):394–402.

26. Bruwer M, Stern J, Stiehl A, Herfarth C. Changes in fecal bile acid excretion after proctocolectomy. *Z Gastroenterol.* 1996;34(2):105–110.

27. Casellas F, Guarner F, Antolin M, et al. Abnormal leukotriene C4 released by unaffected jejunal mucosa in patients with inactive Crohn's disease. *Gut.* 1994;35(4):517–522.

28. Wehman HJ, Lifshitz F, Teichberg S. Effects of enteric microbial overgrowth on small intestinal ultrastructure in the rat. *Am J Gastroenterol.* 1978;70(3):249–258.

29. Lifshitz F, Wapnir RA, Wehman HJ, et al. The effects of small intestinal colonization by fecal and colonic bacteria on intestinal function in rats. *J Nutr.* 1978;108(12):1913–1923.

30. Fukushima T, Ishiguro N, Tsujinaka Y, et al. Bile acid deconjugation in intestinal obstruction studied by breath test. *Jpn J Surg.* 1977;7(2):73–81.

31. Emmett M, Guirl MJ, Santa Ana CA, et al. Conjugated bile acid replacement therapy reduces urinary oxalate excretion in short bowel syndrome. *Am J Kidney Dis.* 2003;41(1):230–237.

32. Parsonnet J. Bacterial infection as a cause of cancer. *Environ Health Perspect.* 1995;103(suppl 8):263–268.

33. Kanazawa K, Konishi F, Mitsuoka T, et al. Factors influencing the development of sigmoid colon cancer. Bacteriologic and biochemical studies. *Cancer.* 1996; 77(8 suppl):1701–1706.

34. Salemans JM, Nagengast FM, Tangerman A, et al. Effect of ageing on postprandial conjugated and unconjugated serum bile acid levels in healthy subjects. *Eur J Clin Invest.* 1993;23(3):192–198.

35. Kruis W, Forstmaier G, Scheurlen C, Stellaard F. Effect of diets low and high in refined sugars on gut transit, bile acid metabolism, and bacterial fermentation. *Gut.* 1991;32(4):367–371.

36. Ejderhamn J, Hedenborg G, Strandvik B. Long-term double blind study on the influence of dietary fibres on faecal bile acid excretion in juvenile ulcerative colitis. *Scand J Clin Lab Invest.* 1992;52(7):697–706.

37. Tazume S, Ozawa A, Yamamoto T, et al. Ecological study on the intestinal bacteria flora of patients with diarrhea. *Clin Infect Dis.* 1993;16(suppl 2):77–82.

38. Behar M. The role of feeding and nutrition in the pathogeny and prevention of diarrheic processes. *Bull Pan Am Health Organ.* 1975;9(1):1–9.

39. Ejderhamn J, Rafter JJ, Strandvik B. Faecal bile acid excretion in children with inflammatory bowel disease. *Gut.* 1991;32(11):1346–1351.

40. Hutchinson R, Tyrrell PN, Kumar D, et al. Pathogenesis of gall stones in Crohn's disease: an alternative explanation. *Gut.* 1994;35(1):94–97.

41. Murray FE, McNicholas M, Stack W, O'Donoghue DP. Impaired fatty-meal-stimulated gallbladder contractility in patients with Crohn's disease. *Clin Sci (Colch).* 1992;6:689–693.

42. Lapidus A, Akerlund JE, Einarsson C. Gallbladder bile composition in patients with Crohn's disease. *World J Gastroenterol.* 2006;12(1):70–74.

43. Akerlund JE, Bjorkhem I, Angelin B, et al. Apparent selective bile acid malabsorption as a consequence of ileal exclusion: effects on bile acid, cholesterol, and lipoprotein metabolism. *Gut.* 1994;35(8):1116–1120.

44. Stiehl A. Ursodeoxycholic acid in the treatment of primary sclerosing cholangitis. *Ann Med.* 1994;26(5): 345–349.

45. Boberg KM, Lundin KE, Schrumpf E. Etiology and pathogenesis in primary sclerosing cholangitis. *Scand J Gastroenterol.* 1994;204:47–58.

46. Mandal A, Dasgupta A, Jeffers L, et al. Autoantibodies in sclerosing cholangitis against a shared peptide in biliary and colon epithelium. *Gastroenterology.* 1994;106(1):185–192.

47. Deng R. Food and food supplements with hypocholesterolemic effects. *Recent Pat Food Nutr Agric.* 2009;1(1):15–24.

48. Gupta AK, Savopoulos CG, Ahuja J, et al. Role of phytosterols in lipid-lowering: current perspectives. *QJM.* 2011;104(4):301–308.

49. Miettinen TE, Kesaniemi YA, Gylling H, et al. Noncholesterol sterols in bile and stones of patients with cholesterol and pigment stones. *Hepatology.* 1996;23(2):274–280.

50. Robins SJ, Fasulo JM, Pritzker CR, Patton GM. Hepatic transport and secretion of unesterified cholesterol in the rat is traced by the plant sterol, sitostanol. *J Lipid Res.* 1996;37(1):15–21.

51. Robins SJ, Fasulo JM. High density lipoproteins, but not other lipoproteins, provide a vehicle for sterol transport to bile. *J Clin Invest.* 1997;99(3):380–384.

52. Hutchinson R, Tyrrell PN, Kumar D, et al. Pathogenesis of gall stones in Crohn's disease: an alternative explanation. *Gut.* 1994;35(1):94–97.

53. Vuoristo M, Miettinen TA. Absorption, metabolism, and serum concentrations of cholesterol in vegetarians: effects of cholesterol feeding. *Am J Clin Nutr*. 1994;59(6):1325–1331.

54. Francis G, Kerem Z, Makkar HPS, Becker K. The biological action of saponins in animal systems: a review. *Br J Nutr*. 2002;88:587–605.

55. Jenkins KJ, Atwal AS. Effects of dietary saponins on fecal bile acids and neutral sterols, and availability of vitamins A and E in the chick. *J Nutr Biochem*. 1994;5(3):134–137.

56. Oakenfull D, Sidhu GS. Could saponins be a useful treatment for hypercholesterolaemia? *Eur J Clin Nutr*. 1990;44:79–88.

57. Son IS, Kim JH, Sohn HY, et al. Antioxidative and hypolipidemic effects of diosgenin, a steroidal saponin of yam (Dioscorea spp.), on high-cholesterol fed rats. *Biosci Biotechnol Biochem*. 2007;71(12):3063–3071.

58. Roman ID, Thewles A, Coleman R. Fractionation of livers following diosgenin treatment to elevate biliary cholesterol. *Biochim Biophys Acta*. 1995;1255(1):77–81.

59. Nussinovitch M, Zahavi I, Marcus H, et al. The choleretic effect of nonsteroidal anti-inflammatory drugs in total parenteral nutrition-associated cholestasis. *Isr J Med Sci*. 1996;32(12):1262–1264.

60. Sterczer A, Voros K, Karsai F. Effect of cholagogues on the volume of the gallbladder of dogs. *Res Vet Sci*. 1996;60(1):44–47.

61. Táborská E, Bochoráková H, Dostál J, Paulová H. The greater celandine (Chelidonium majus L.) – review of present knowledge. *Ceska Slov Farm*. 1995;44(2):71–75.

62. Dranik LI, Dolganenko LG, Slapke J, Thoma H. Chemical composition and medical usage of Cynara scolymus L. *Rastitel'nye Resursy*. 1996;32(4):98–104.

63. Wider B, Pittler MH, Thompson-Coon J, Ernst E. Artichoke leaf extract for treating hypercholesterolemia. *Cochrane Database Syst Rev*. 2009;(4):CD000335.

64. Bundy R, Walker AF, Middleton RW, et al. Artichoke leaf extract (Cynara scolymus) reduces plasma cholesterol in otherwise healthy hypercholesterolemic adults: a randomized, double blind placebo controlled trial. *Phytomedicine*. 2008;15:668–675.

65. Mimica-Dukic N, Jakovljevic V, Mira P, et al. Pharmacological study of Mentha longifolia phenolic extracts. *Int J Pharmacog*. 1996;34(5):359–364.

66. Ishibashi H, Komori A, Shimoda S, et al. Risk factors and prediction of long-term outcome in primary biliary cirrhosis. *Intern Med*. 2011;50(1):1–10.

67. Heaton KW, Emmett PM, Symes LJ, et al. An explanation for gallstones in normal-weight women: slow intestinal transit. *Lancet*. 1993;341(8836):8–10.

68. Venneman NG, van Erpecum KJ. Pathogenesis of gallstones. *Gastroenterol Clin North Am*. 2010;39(2):171–183.

69. Stinton LM, Myers RP, Shaffer EA. Epidemiology of gallstones. *Gastroenterol Clin North Am*. 2010;39(2):157–169.

70. Maurer KJ, Carey MC, Fox JG. Roles of infection, inflammation, and the immune system in cholesterol gallstone formation. *Gastroenterology*. 2009;136(2):425–440.

71. Portincasa P, Di Ciaula A, Wang HH, et al. Medicinal treatments of cholesterol gallstones: old, current and new perspectives. *Curr Med Chem*. 2009;16(12):1531–1542.

72. Sanders G, Kingsnorth AN. Gallstones. *BMJ*. 2007;335(7614):295–299.

73. Bell GD, Doran J. Gall stone dissolution in man using an essential oil preparation. *BMJ*. 1979;1(6155):24.

74. Thewles A, Parslow RA, Coleman R. Effect of diosgenin on biliary cholesterol transport in the rat. *Biochem J*. 1993;291(3):793–798.

75. Savage AP, O'Brien T, Lamont PM. Adjuvant herbal treatment for gallstones. *Br J Surg*. 1992;79(2):168.

76. Sies CW, Brooker J. Could these be gallstones? *Lancet*. 2005;365(9468):1388.

77. Hansel SL, DiBaise JK. Functional gallbladder disorder: gallbladder dyskinesia. *Gastroenterol Clin North Am*. 2010;39(2):369–379, x.

The liver

Scope

Apart from their use to provide non-specific support for recuperation and repair, specific phytotherapeutic strategies include the following.

Treatment of:

- postpartum symptoms of liver distress, such as after consumption of fatty foods and alcohol
- moderate acute and chronic hepatitis
- poor liver function.

Management of:

- chronic and acute hepatotoxin poisoning
- acute and chronic hepatitis
- cirrhosis.

Because of its use of secondary plant products, particular **caution** is necessary in applying phytotherapy to primary and secondary liver carcinoma.

Orientation

Given its relative lack of attention in most medical books, the liver has an enormous hidden importance. The hub of many of the body's biochemical pathways, and first processor of dietary metabolites, it also has established roles in modulating the immune and endocrine systems (any hormone has two influences on its blood levels, the rate of production and the rate of breakdown in the liver – this is an often varied factor[1]), and cholesterol and blood sugar levels. With its associate Kupffer cells it is a vital defence wall in protecting the body against immunological threat from foodstuffs. In its biliary production it has a key influence on digestion itself and bowel flora and function. All these central roles support the primitive appreciation for the liver as a centre-piece in traditional systems of medicine, and even its name in many languages.

Most obvious is the liver's primary role in detoxification, both of ingested molecules (*xenobiotics*) and internal metabolites and agents such as hormones. There are two phases of hepatic biotransformation involved. During phase I, enzymatic-induced oxidation, reduction or hydrolysis generates a reactive site on the substrate molecule; in phase II a water-soluble (hydrophilic) group is conjugated with this reactive site to make the molecule more polarised (or electrically charged) and thus more able to be excreted by the body.

Phase I by definition creates a potentially toxic reactive oxygen intermediate with free radical activity, for which endogenous antioxidant protection is required. This phase is launched primarily by the cytochrome P450 enzyme family whose role is, like the antibody system, to recognise and initiate the biotransformation of a wide diversity of substrates. Excessive phase I activity can generate more dangerous toxic complications. This might happen, for example, in fasting or other sudden loss of adipose tissue where fat-soluble metabolites are stored. The same challenge may occur if there is a reduction in antioxidant capacity, such as in heavy smoking, exposure to industrial pollutants (which can both induce excessive phase I activity as well) or chronically deficient diets. Its role in oestrogen metabolism is a particularly good example of the liver's significance in health and disease. Unlike other hormones, oestrogen is eliminated by a full phase I and II mechanism, suggesting that the body evolved to see it as a threat (oestrogen is one of the most powerful of the body's major hormones). The rate of phase I detoxification (through cytochromes P450: CYP1A1, CYP1B1, and CYP3A4; see also Chapter 5) is determined by many factors, including individual 'mini-mutations' of P450s known as single nucleotide polymorphisms. As phase I metabolites can have anti-oestrogenic or DNA-damaging effects, then the impact of these variations on the incidence of breast uterine and prostate cancer is known to be substantial.[2] The cancer-protective role of cruciferous vegetables (through glucosinolates) is likely to include a positive effect on these detoxification processes (see also Chapter 2).[3]

Phase II reactions should cut in to neutralise the transformed substrates quickly, to reduce toxic burdens and relieve antioxidant defences. They involve conjugation with glucuronic acid, sulphates, glutathione, glycine or other amino acids, acetylation or methylation. These protective processes are known to be augmented by a diet high in flavonoids, such as fruit and vegetables,[4,5] particularly cruciferous vegetables,[6] onions, red grapes and soy.[7] The onset of diseases, notably cancer, has been often linked to an imbalance between phase I and phase II and the protective benefits of fruit and vegetables against cancer have been put down to this effect. Fundamentally, it is now understood that many of the phytochemicals in fruits and vegetables activate the Nrf2/ARE pathway and thereby induce the production of phase II and antioxidant enzymes. (ARE stands for 'antioxidant response element'.)

Liver remedies may help reduce toxic burdens by shifting the phase I/II balance towards the latter, stimulating cleansing bile flow (see previous section) or by directly protecting the liver tissue itself from oxidant attack. Excessive or phase I or cytochrome P450 activity may lead to mutation, cancer or tissue necrosis, particularly of the liver with its particularly high content of cytochrome P450.[8]

Consequently, the liver is an extremely active organ in the metabolism of ingested materials and it is known to be particularly vulnerable to the effects of agents that are not readily metabolised or excreted. These are known to include many modern drugs, agrochemicals and other modern environmental pollutants. Although severe hepatic damage is not common, constant exposure to new industrial agents, particularly if at relatively high levels and when combined with other well-known burdens on the liver, alcohol and high fat diets, can lead to a modern syndrome of functional liver distress.

Because of the central role of the liver in immunological function and detoxification, there may also be a significant

population of patients, perhaps presenting with other conditions (notably skin and bowel diseases, chronic allergic states, autoimmune disease and other chronic inflammatory disorders), in whom subtle liver damage or dysfunction may already have occurred and can be contributing further to the wider pathology. The increased incidence of viral hepatitis is both the major cause of long-term hepatic disorders and a likely added complication of some of the above adverse changes. The mechanisms of chronic liver damage may include immunological disturbances such as chronic active hepatitis and primary biliary cirrhosis, or may be more subtle with perhaps minor alterations in liver function tests or merely subjective intolerance of fats and alcohol (see Poor liver function below).

As hepatic damage usually starts with classic pathological processes of fatty infiltration, in theory a good liver remedy should have appropriate antioxidant properties. As these need to be focused in liver tissue, they should also be readily absorbed, require little extra liver metabolism and preferably should be retained in the enterohepatic circulation. The best such herbs will contain phytochemicals that activate the Nrf2/ARE pathway, such as curcumin.

Phytotherapeutics

Evidence of beneficial effects on the liver

Many plants contain constituents that have been experimentally shown to have beneficial effects on liver cells, at least under laboratory conditions. Early research investigated the hepatoprotective effects of agents in models of liver toxicity (for example, carbon tetrachloride (CCl_4), D-galactosamine, paracetamol and Amanita mushrooms) and it was such work that identified remedies such as *Silybum marianum* (St Mary's thistle). This and more recent evidence more widely points to benefits on hepatic function of a diet rich in fruit and vegetables (as noted above). The case for traditional herbal practice in its particular focus on the liver as a centrepiece of therapeutics is also supported.

Particularly likely to feature in evidence are flavonoids and related polyphenols. For example, the ubiquitous flavonoid quercetin is one of a number of antioxidants that have been shown to reduce the high level of chromosomal aberrations found in cases of viral hepatitis associated with environmental pollution.[9] Oral administration of the flavonoids daidzin, daidzein and puerarin, from the Chinese herb *Pueraria lobata*, was effective in lowering blood alcohol levels and shortened sleep time induced by alcohol ingestion.[10,11]

Benefits from other notable plant constituents

Glycyrrhizin, a major component of licorice, has been used intravenously for the treatment of chronic hepatitis B in Japan and improves liver function with occasional complete recovery from hepatitis.[12] In vitro studies suggest a hitherto unique mechanism involving intracellular transport across Golgi membranes.[13] In addition, weak binding activity to steroid receptors has been demonstrated.[14] Derivatives of glycyrrhizinic acid promote a decrease in the rate of lipid peroxide oxygenation and in the inhibition of liver enzyme activity (ALT, AST) and also increase choleresis.[15] There is evidence of a choleretic action,[16] also involving glycyrrhizin. (See also the licorice monograph.)

Piperine, an active alkaloidal constituent of the extract obtained from *Piper longum* and *P. nigrum*, was evaluated for its antihepatotoxic potential against CCl_4 and other agents, and was found to have an appreciable benefit, but at levels lower than for silymarin.[17]

The water extract from the root of *Salvia miltiorrhiza* showed a protective effect on cultured rat hepatocytes against CCl_4-induced necrosis. Lithospermate B, a tetramer of caffeic acid, was isolated and found to be an active constituent. Lithospermate B was also found to have a potent hepatoprotective activity, not only in vitro but also for in vivo experimental liver injuries induced by CCl_4 or D-galactosamine-lipopolysaccharide.[18] Various other metabolites of caffeic acid formed in bap are likely to account for many beneficial effects in that organ; these metabolites include cyclolignan derivatives as oxidation products, ferulic and isoferulic acid as methylation products and aesculetin as a cyclisation product.[19]

The Phyllanthus genus has been known to contain a number of biologically active constituents such as an angiotensin-converting enzyme inhibitor and HIV reverse transcriptase inhibitors.[20] *Phyllanthus amarus* has shown antihepatitis B virus activity.[21,22] *P. niruri* from Malaysia contains various constituents with demonstrated effects aginst hepatitis B.[23] *P. ussuriensis*, a Korean native species, has been used to treat several infectious diseases, including hepatitis in folk medicine, and antihepatotoxic effects have been confirmed in vitro.[24] It inhibited hepatitis B virus polymerase activity, decreased episomal hepatitis B virus DNA content and suppressed virus release into culture medium. A number of mechanisms have been elucidated.[25]

Silybum marianum (St Mary's or milk thistle) seed, widely used in Europe for its hepatic reputation, contains the flavonol lignan complex silymarin with antifibrotic activity in diseased liver,[26] and there are other effects observed in diseased liver,[27] including reducing serum transaminases in patients with chronic viral hepatitis.[28] The traditional liver remedy *Schisandra chinensis* contains constituents with antihepatitis activity,[29] and has been shown to reduce circulating monocyte counts (although with no effects on other white blood cell counts) after 2 weeks' treatment of human subjects infected with hepatitis B.[30] (See more in the St Mary's thistle monograph.)

The Chinese remedy *Sophora flavescens* has also been studied experimentally and has shown promising if not conclusive evidence of effectiveness in hepatitis B.[31,32]

Evidence of hepatoprotective effects also arises from studies on other traditional remedies: *Artemisia spp.*,[33,34] *Azadirachta indica* leaf extract,[35] *Picrorrhiza kurroa*,[36] *Osbeckia octandra*,[37] *Gynostemma pentaphyllum*,[38] *Inula britannica* L. subsp. *japonica*,[39] *Salvia plebeia*.[40] Other plant hepatoprotectors have been reviewed.[41–43]

Schisandra has emerged as a key herb for boosting phase I and especially phase II detoxification processes by the liver. As stated previously, phase I and II reactions are involved in the metabolism of mainly xenobiotic substances by the liver. Phase I reactions (which involve cytochrome P450) can result in the production of a more toxic compound (a process called bioactivation). Despite being a postulated powerful inducer of phase I enzymes, Schisandra does not cause harmful bioactivation in

vivo (e.g. after co-administration of paracetamol) and in vitro studies have indicated that constituents of Schisandra decrease the mutagenicity of benzo(alpha)pyrene by influencing hepatic metabolism.[44,45] The probable reason is that Schisandra powerfully induces phase II enzymes as well, which results in the rapid clearance of the potentially toxic metabolite.[46] Other keys herbs in this regard include turmeric (see the turmeric monograph), garlic, green tea, rosemary and broccoli sprouts (all influencing the Nrf2/ARE pathway). St Mary's thistle is unlikely to exert clinically relevant effects on hepatic phase I/II detoxification processes, with its value being more linked to hepatoprotective activity (see below).

Another hitherto little explored hepatic activity may also be a feature of some herbal preparations: extracts of *Thuja occidentalis* and *Echinacea purpurea* have stimulated Kupffer cell phagocytosis in vitro.[47]

Hepatic induction of antitumour effects

The liver has a central role in a wider range of defence mechanisms. For example, the Kupffer cells are a final screen between enteric antigens and the body cavities, various phase II liver enzymes such as glutathione-S-transferase (GST) are important detoxifiers of carcinogens, and the transport of IgA and IgA immune complexes by the liver from serum to bile may provide a host defence against enteric pathogens.[48] These key functions raise the possibility that hepatic remedies might have wider applications.

For example, out of various spices and leafy vegetables screened for their influence on GST in Swiss mice, cumin seeds, poppy seeds, asafoetida, turmeric, neem flowers and basil leaves among other spices increased GST activity high enough in the stomach, liver and oesophagus to be considered as significantly contributing to protection against carcinogenesis.[49] Several naturally occurring flavonoids and other polyphenols, prominently tannic acid, were also shown to exert varying degrees of concentration-dependent inhibition on uncharacterised rat liver GST.[50] Sesquiterpenes such as beta-caryophyllene, beta-caryophyllene oxide, alpha-humulene, alpha-humulene epoxide I and eugenol, all found in cloves, have demonstrated significant activity as inducers of GST in the mouse liver and small intestine,[51] as has myristicin, a major aromatic constituent of parsley.[52] Of course, the most active liver phase II enzyme inducers are the brassica glucosinolates, and their protective properties against experimental carcinogenesis is well described (see Chapter 2). Another key example is turmeric (see the turmeric monograph).

Capsaicin inhibited the formation by liver microsomal fractions of all metabolites of 4-(methylnitrosamino)-1-(3-pyridyl)-1-butanone (NNK), a potent carcinogen in tobacco and tobacco smoke. With other similar results, such findings suggest that it possesses antimutagenic and anticarcinogenic properties through the inhibition of xenobiotic metabolising enzymes.[53]

Hepatoprotectives (or hepatics)

There are few guides to the use of hepatoprotectives (or hepatics) in conventional Western medicine. This is a concept more familiar in mainland Europe and further East, but has become a more popular concept with the marketing of St Mary's thistle (milk thistle) seed.

Hepatoprotectives are remedies claimed to help reduce damage caused to the liver from hepatic stressors and disease. Given what has been said earlier, good hepatoprotectives are most likely to deliver antioxidant activity into liver hepatocytes and induce cellular protective mechanisms.

Plant remedies traditionally used as hepatoprotectives

- *Silybum marianum* (St Mary's thistle), Cynara (artichoke), Bupleurum (chai hu), Schisandra (wu wei zi).

Indications for hepatoprotectives

- Viral and other hepatitis and sequelae
- Adverse effects of alcohol and excess fat consumption
- Exposure to industrial pollutants
- In anticipation of or along with the prescription of powerful medications
- Cirrhosis and other chronic liver diseases.

Other traditional indications for hepatoprotectives

- Many dermatological, enteric and bowel, rheumatic, catarrhal and other chronic inflammatory diseases.

Contraindications for hepatoprotectives

The most widely used hepatoprotectives in European phytomedicine appear to have few contraindications. They are generally mild treatments and, as antioxidants, may have wider benefits. To some extent they may merely extend the known beneficial effect on the liver of plant foods. Nevertheless, some of the remedies mentioned above may have individual characteristics that need consideration, especially in liver carcinoma.

Traditional therapeutic insights into the use of hepatoprotectives

Diseases with early morning symptoms may be associated with liver disturbances on the assumption that the liver has been particularly active overnight during sleep. The occurrence of such signs might in itself be an indication for the use of hepatoprotectives remedies.

Traditional enquiry might also elicit how well a patient handled alcohol and dietary fats. Although difficulties here might rather suggest the use of cholagogues and choleretics, hepatoprotectives would be particularly indicated if symptoms like headaches were associated with such consumption.

Hepatoprotectives are very often employed in the treatment of migraine, often seen traditionally as a liver condition.

Western practitioners are reminded of the ancient Greek humoral concept of 'black bile' (lit: *melancholia*) and the early view of clinical depression as a somatic rather than a psychological phenomenon. Using hepatoprotectives and other treatments for liver and digestive function as part of a fresh approach to the management of depression can be surprisingly productive in some cases.

Application

Hepatoprotectives are best applied before breakfast in the morning and before the last meal of the day, to take account of the extra liver activity during the night. However, they may also be taken before meals throughout the day.

Long-term therapy is quite appropriate for those such as St Mary's thistle and artichoke, which have established their safety from extensive human use.

Advanced phytotherapeutics

Hepatoprotectives may also be usefully applied in some cases (depending on other factors) of:

- migraine
- acne rosacea
- autoimmune diseases (especially where associated with any of the above – see relevant sections)
- fatty liver
- NASH (non-alcoholic steatohepatitis).

There is also a strong case for their use in anticipation of, or association with, the prescription of powerful chemotherapeutic agents in, for example, the treatment of tuberculosis, cancer, psychoses and frequent recourse to general anaesthetics (see also Chapter 8).

For evidence of adverse effects of herbal products on the liver, see Chapter 5.

Phytotherapy for liver conditions

Acute viral hepatitis

The most important causes of acute hepatitis are the hepatitis A, B and C viruses. Other viruses, including Epstein-Barr virus and cytomegalovirus, may also cause acute hepatitis. All these viruses (except A) have a viral envelope and hence may have some susceptibility to *Hypericum perforatum* (St John's wort), which is active against enveloped viruses.

Acute hepatitis can be treated using herbal medicine. In the case of hepatitis A, treatment can lead to rapid recovery and protection against post-hepatitis syndrome. For hepatitis B and C, herbal treatment will mainly help to prevent the disease becoming chronic. The small amounts of alcohol involved from using extracts and tinctures will not be a problem to most patients. However, if there is a difficulty with alcohol then tablets, capsules, glycerol extracts and/or infusions or decoctions can be prescribed. As with other acute infections, oral herbal treatment should not be administered while there is vomiting.

It is hoped that individual strategies will be devised for each patient, taking some of the insights in this and other chapters into account, but essential aspects of treatment are as follows:

- Diaphoretics are indicated in all acute infections accompanied by fever. These include Tilia (lime flowers), Sambucus (elder) and Achillea (yarrow) and are best taken as an infusion. Diaphoretics are assisted by combination with a diffuse stimulant such as Zingiber (ginger)
- Antiviral agents, which for hepatitis include Hypericum, Phyllanthus and Thuja

- Immune-enhancing herbs, especially Echinacea and Andrographis
- Hepatoprotective agents to minimise liver damage such as Silybum, Bupleurum, *Taraxacum radix* (dandelion root), Cynara (globe artichoke) and Andrographis
- Post-hepatitis syndrome should mainly be treated with the hepatoprotectives listed above.

It should be noted that higher doses need to be employed for acute cases (compared to treating chronic conditions).

Chronic viral hepatitis

Chronic viral hepatitis or chronic persistent hepatitis usually results from infection with hepatitis B or C. Especially with hepatitis C, some features of the disease may resemble auto-immune hepatitis. (Frank autoimmune liver disease is known as chronic active hepatitis. A general treatment approach for autoimmune disease is outlined in Chapter 8.)

Treatment

Treatment of chronic viral hepatitis shares many similarities with the treatment of acute viral hepatitis. Essential features of treatment are:

- immune-enhancing agents such as Echinacea, Andrographis and Astragalus for any chronic infection
- hepatoprotective agents as described previously and particularly Schisandra and Silybum in a more concentrated form such as tablets or capsules containing the silymarin extract
- antiviral agents (see above). The use of Phyllanthus may be suitable for chronic viral hepatitis (see previous) as is St John's wort
- herbal antioxidants/cytoprotectives to provide further protection for hepatocytes, such as turmeric and green tea.

CASE HISTORY

A female patient aged 56 years had been diagnosed with chronic hepatitis C 2 years prior. Her genotype (genotype I) was less responsive to interferon therapy, although it had been trialled for 1 year. ALT and AST were moderately elevated at the time of her first consultation (130 and 95 U/L, respectively), although they were severely elevated at the time of diagnosis. Over the 8 years of treatment with phytotherapy her condition has progressively improved. There have been no acute episodes and her ALT and AST readings are nearly normal at 47 and 53 U/L, respectively. This result was achieved with no other additional therapy and the patient remains otherwise well.

Treatment consisted of tablet products delivering the following daily doses:

Astragalus	3.4 g
Echinacea purpurea root	2.6 g
Grape seed extract	100 mg
Turmeric	4 g
Green tea extract	333 mg
Rosemary	2 g
Siberian ginseng	3 g
St John's wort (from standardised extract)	5.4 g
Schisandra	2 g
Silymarin extract (from St Mary's thistle)	630 mg

Cirrhosis of the liver

In cirrhosis, widespread death of liver cells, which can result from many causes but is most commonly due to alcohol abuse, is accompanied and followed by progressive fibrosis and distortion of liver architecture. Since alcohol is forbidden, herbal treatment should be in the form of tablets, capsules, glycerol extracts, infusions and/or decoctions. The main herbal treatment is based around hepatic trophorestoratives, especially concentrated tablets of *Silybum marianum*. Other important herbs in this category include Schisandra, *Taraxacum radix* (dandelion root), Cynara (globe artichoke), Bupleurum and Andrographis. Berberine-containing herbs can also be indicated (see the Berberis monograph). Although cirrhosis is a progressive disease, the rate of progression varies and the outlook is related to many factors. In this context, herbal treatment can make a significant positive contribution.

Antifibrotic activity is another area of herbal activity relevant to cirrhosis that is attracting research interest. The laying down of excessive fibrotic tissue in response to repeated liver damage is the main disruptive pathological change in cirrhosis. *Centella asiatica* (gotu kola) is a herb with potential to reduce an excessive fibrotic response (see gotu kola monograph). *Salvia miltiorrhiza* (dan shen) is also showing promising activity in this regard.[54,55]

Poor liver function and fatty liver

The liver plays a vital role in detoxification and many other metabolic processes in the body. Phytotherapists and naturopaths recognise a condition where liver function is below optimum, although no medically observable liver disease or liver damage may be present. Because of the importance of the liver, a poorly functioning liver can have a wide-ranging impact on health.

Symptoms that may be due to poor liver function include sluggish digestion, fat intolerance, nausea, chronic constipation and chemical, food or drug intolerances. A poorly functioning liver may also contribute to a number of disease states such as psoriasis, autoimmune disease, irritable bowel syndrome, allergies and cancer. Patients might reveal a history of past liver infection, infestation or damage, alcohol or drug abuse, or exposure to medical drugs or environmental pollutants such as pesticides and/or have abdominal obesity. Drug side effects are more likely to occur in patients with poor liver function.

Depending on the symptoms, treatment is based on the following:

- Hepatoprotective and hepatic trophorestorative herbs, especially if there is a history of liver damage or exposure to toxins. Principal herbs include Silybum, Cynara and Taraxacum. Schisandra is particularly useful since it also enhances the detoxifying capacity of the liver (see above). These herbs will assist in cases of nausea and intolerances from any cause
- Choleretic herbs to boost liver function are particularly indicated if digestive symptoms are predominant. They will also boost detoxification via bile and therefore can be valuable in conditions such as psoriasis and cancer. Most of the hepatoprotective herbs listed above have a gentle choleretic activity, but strongly choleretic herbs include

Hydrastis (golden seal), *Berberis vulgaris* (barberry), Chelidonium and bitter herbs. These strongly choleretic herbs tend to cause nausea and irritability in a patient who has some history of liver damage. They should therefore be avoided at first in these circumstances and only introduced after prior treatment with the hepatic trophorestoratives noted above

- Depurative herbs are also indicated in cases where hepatic detoxification may be inadequate. Those which act principally via the liver and digestion include Arctium (burdock), *Rumex crispus* (yellow dock) and Fumaria (fumitory)
- Other herbs (in addition to Schisandra) that specifically boost phase II hepatic detoxification should also be considered, including broccoli sprouts, rosemary, turmeric, garlic and green tea.

CASE HISTORY

A female patient aged 38 wished to take the contraceptive pill. She found that even a low-dose pill still caused symptoms of female hormone excess such as abdominal bloating, weight gain, nausea and depression. She had a past history of liver damage due to hydatid worm cysts during childhood.

Treatment consisted of:

Silybum marianum	1:1	30 mL
Taraxacum officinale radix	1:2	35 mL
Schisandra chinensis	1:2	35 mL
	TOTAL	100 mL

Dose: 5 mL with water twice a day.

The patient found she could take the pill without any adverse effects as long as she also took the herbal treatment.

References

1. Dunning AM. Polymorphisms associated with circulating sex hormone levels in postmenopausal women. *J Natl Cancer Inst.* 2004;96:936–945.

2. Yager JD. Endogenous estrogens as carcinogens through metabolic activation. *J Natl Cancer Inst Monogr.* 2000;27:67–73.

3. Bonnesen C, Stephensen PU, Andersen O, et al. Modulation of cytochrome P-450 and glutathione S-transferase isoform expression in vivo by intact and degraded indolyl glucosinolates. *Nutr Cancer.* 1999;33(2):178–187.

4. Moon YJ, Wang X, Morris ME. Dietary flavonoids: effects on xenobiotic and carcinogen metabolism. *Toxicol In Vitro.* 2006;20(2):187–210.

5. van Breda SG, van Agen E, Engels LG, et al. Altered vegetable intake affects pivotal carcinogenesis pathways in colon mucosa from adenoma patients and controls. *Carcinogenesis.* 2004;25(11):2207–2210.

6. Riedl MA, Saxon A, Diaz-Sanchez D. Oral sulforaphane increases phase II antioxidant enzymes in the human upper airway. *Clin Immunol.* 2009;130(3):244–251.

7. Appelt LC, Reicks MM. Soy feeding induces phase II enzymes in rat tissues. *Nutr Cancer.* 1997;28(3):270–275.

8. Pessayre D. Cytochromes P450 and formation of reactive metabolites. Role in drug induced hepatotoxicity. *Therapie (Paris).* 1993;48(6):537–548.

9. Peresadin NA, Frolov VM, Pinskii LL. Correction with antioxidants of cytogenetic disturbances in viral hepatitis. *Lik Sprava.* 1995;1–2:76–79.

10. Lin RC, Guthrie S, Xie CY, et al. Isoflavonoid compounds extracted from Pueraria lobata suppress alcohol preference in a pharmacogenetic rat model of alcoholism. *Alcohol Clin Exp Res.* 1996;20(4):659–663.

11. Xie CI, Lin RC, Antony V, et al. Daidzin, an antioxidant isoflavonoid, decreases blood alcohol levels and shortens sleep time induced by ethanol intoxication. *Alcohol Clin Exp Res.* 1994;18(6):1443–1447.

12. Sato H, Goto W, Yamamura J, et al. Therapeutic basis of glycyrrhizin on chronic hepatitis B. *Antiviral Res.* 1996;30(2–3):171–177.

13. Takahara T, Watanabe A, Shiraki K. Effects of glycyrrhizin on hepatitis B surface antigen: a biochemical and morphological study. *J Hepatol.* 1994;21(4):601–609.

14. Tamaya T, Sato S, Okada H. Inhibition by plant herb extracts of steroid bindings in uterus, liver and serum of the rabbit. *Acta Obstet Gynecol Scand.* 1986;65(8):839–842.

15. Nasyrov KhM, Chepurina LS, Kireeva RM. Study of hepatoprotective and choleretic activity of glycyrrhizinic acid derivatives. *Eksp Klin Farmakol.* 1995;58(6):60–63.

16. Raggi MA, Bugamelli F, Nobile L, et al. The choleretic effects of licorice: identification and determination of the pharmacologically active components of Glycyrrhiza glabra. *Boll Chim Farm.* 1995;134(11):634–638.

17. Koul IB, Kapil A. Evaluation of the liver protective potential of piperine, an active principle of black and long peppers. *Planta Med.* 1993;59(5):413–417.

18. Hase K, Kasimu R, Basnet P, et al. Preventive effect of lithospermate B from Salvia miltiorhiza on experimental hepatitis induced by carbon tetrachloride or D-galactosamine-lipopolysaccharide. *Planta Med.* 1997;63(1):22–26.

19. Gumbinger HG, Vahlensieck U, Winterhoff H. Metabolism of caffeic acid in the isolated perfused rat liver. *Planta Med.* 1993;59(6):491–493.

20. Munshi A, Mehrotra R, Ramesh R, Panda SK. Evaluation of anti-hepadnavirus activity of Phyllanthus amarus and Phyllanthus maderaspatensis in duck hepatitis B virus carrier Pekin ducks. *J Med Virol.* 1993;41(4):275–281.

21. Liu J, Lin H, McIntosh H. Genus Phyllanthus for chronic hepatitis B virus infection: a systematic review. *J Viral Hepat.* 2001;8(5):358–366.

22. Martin KW, Ernst E. Antiviral agents from plants and herbs: a systematic review. *Antivir Ther.* 2003;8(2):77–90.

23. Bagalkotkar G, Sagineedu SR, Saad MS, Stanslas J. Phytochemicals from Phyllanthus niruri Linn. and their pharmacological properties: a review. *J Pharm Pharmacol.* 2006;58(12):1559–1570.

24. Moon Y-S, Lim WS, Lee MK, et al. Antihepatotoxic effect of callus cultures of the P. ussuriensis. *Seoul Univ J Pharm Sci.* 1995;20:21–31.

25. Lee C-D, Ott M, Thyagarajan SP, et al. Phyllanthus amarus down-regulates hepatitis B virus mRNA transcription and replication. *Eur J Clin Invest.* 1996;26(12):1069–1076.

26. Boigk G, Stroeter L, Waldschmidt J, et al. Silymarin retards collagen accumulation in rat secondary biliary fibrosis. *J Hepatol.* 1995;23(suppl 1):142.

27. Tamayo C, Diamond S. Review of clinical trials evaluating safety and efficacy of milk thistle (Silybum marianum [L.] Gaertn.). *Integr Cancer Ther.* 2007;6(2):146–157.

28. Mayer KE, Myers RP, Lee SS. Silymarin treatment of viral hepatitis: a systematic review. *J Viral Hepat.* 2005;12(6):559–567.

29. Liu GT. Pharmacological actions and clinical use of fructus schizandrae. *Chin Med J (Engl).* 1989;102(10):740–749.

30. Yip AY, Loo WT, Chow LW. Fructus Schisandrae (Wuweizi) containing compound in modulating human lymphatic system – a phase I minimization clinical trial. *Biomed Pharmacother.* 2007;61(9):588–590.

31. Liu J, Zhu M, Shi R, Yang M. Radix Sophorae flavescentis for chronic hepatitis B: a systematic review of randomized trials. *Am J Chin Med.* 2003;31(3):337–354.

32. Long Y, Lin XT, Zeng KL, Zhang L. Efficacy of intramuscular matrine in the treatment of chronic hepatitis B. *Hepatobiliary Pancreat Dis Int.* 2004;3(1):69–72.

33. Janbaz KH, Gilani AH. Evaluation of the protective potential of Artemisia maritima extract on acetaminophen- and CC14-induced liver damage. *J Ethnopharmacol.* 1995;47(1):43–47.

34. Yin J, Wennberg RP, Miller M. Induction of hepatic bilirubin and drug metabolizing enzymes by individual herbs present in the traditional Chinese medicine, yin zhi huang. *Dev Pharmacol Ther.* 1993;20(3–4):186–194.

35. Chattopadhyay RR, Sarkar SK, Ganguly S, et al. Hepatoprotective activity of Azadirachta indica leaves on paracetamol induced hepatic damage in rats. *Indian J Exp Biol.* 1992;8:738–740.

36. Dhawan BN. Picroliv – a new hepatoprotective agent from an Indian medicinal plant, Picrorrhiza kurroa. *Med Chem Res.* 1995;5(8):595–605.

37. Thabrew MI, Hughes RD, Gove CD, et al. Protective effects of Osbeckia octandra against paracetamol-induced liver injury. *Xenobiotica.* 1995;9:1009–1017.

38. Li L, Jiao L, Lau BH. Protective effect of gypenosides against oxidative stress in phagocytes, vascular endothelial cells and liver microsomes. *Cancer Biother.* 1993;8(3):263–272.

39. Iijima K, Kiyohara H, Tanaka M, et al. Preventive effect of taraxasteryl acetate from Inula britannica subsp. Japonica on experimental hepatitis in vivo. *Planta Med.* 1995;61(1):50–53.

40. Lin C-C, Lin J-K, Chang C-H. Evaluation of hepatoprotective effects of 'Chhit-Chan-Than' from Taiwan. *Int J Pharmacog.* 1995;33(2):139–143.

41. Rumyantseva ZhN, Gudivok YS. Search for hepatoprotectors among preparations of plant origin. *Rastitel'nye Resursy.* 1993;29(1):88–97.

42. Rakhmanin YA, Kushnerova NF, Gordeichuk TN, et al. Metabolic responses of the liver exposed to carbon tetrachloride and their correction with plant antioxidants. *Gig Sanit.* 1997;1:30–32.

43. Negi AS, Kumar JK, Luqman S, et al. Recent advances in plant hepatoprotectives: a chemical and biological profile of some important leads. *Med Res Rev.* 2008;28(5):746–772.

44. Liu KT, Cresteil T, Columelli S, et al. Pharmacological properties of dibenzo[a,c]cyclooctene derivatives isolated from Fructus schizandrae chinensis. II. Induction of phenobarbital-like hepatic monooxygenases. *Chem Biol Interact.* 1982;39(3):315–330.

45. Liu KT, Lesca P. Pharmacological properties of dibenzo[a,c]cyclooctene derivatives isolated from Fructus schizandrae chinensis. I. Interaction with rat liver cytochrome P-450 and inhibition of xenobiotic metabolism and mutagenicity. *Chem Biol Interact.* 1982;39(3):301–314.

46. Bone K. Schisandra – the complete liver herb. *Townsend Lett Doctors Patients.* 2003;245:108–112.

47. Vömel T. Effect of a plant immunostimulant on phagocytosis of erythrocytes by the reticulohistiocytary system of isolated perfused rat liver. *Arzneimittel-Forschung.* 1985;35(9):1437–1439.

48. Kleinman RE, Harmatz PR, Walker WA. The liver: an integral part of the enteric mucosal immune system. *Hepatology.* 1982;2(3):379–384.

49. Aruna K, Sivaramakrishnan VM. Plant products as protective agents against cancer. *Indian J Exp Biol.* 1990;11:1008–1011.

50. Zhang K, Das NP. Inhibitory effects of plant polyphenols on rat liver glutathione S-transferases. *Biochem Pharmacol.* 1994;47(11):2063–2068.

51. Zheng GQ, Kenney PM, Lam LK. Sesquiterpenes from clove (Eugenia caryophyllata) as potential anticarcinogenic agents. *J Nat Prod.* 1992;55(7):999–1003.

52. Zheng GQ, Kenney PM, Zhang J, Lam LK. Inhibition of benzo[a]pyrene-induced tumorigenesis by myristicin, a volatile aroma constituent of parsley leaf oil. *Carcinogenesis.* 1992;13(10):1921–1923.

53. Miller CH, Zhang Z, Hamilton SM, Teel RW. Effects of capsaicin on liver microsomal metabolism of the tobacco-specific nitrosamine NNK. *Cancer Lett.* 1993;75(1):45–52.

54. Tao YY, Liu CH. Progress of research on mechanism of Salvia miltiorrhiza and its chemical ingredients against liver fibrosis. *Zhong Xi Yi Jie He Xue Bao.* 2004;2(2):145–148.

55. Stickel F, Brinkhaus B, Krähmer N, et al. Antifibrotic properties of botanicals in chronic liver disease. *Hepatogastroenterology.* 2002;49(46):1102–1108.

Cardiovascular system

Scope

Apart from their use to provide non-specific support for recuperation and repair, specific phytotherapeutic strategies include the following.

Treatment of:

- mild to moderate hypertension
- angina
- palpitations.

Management of:

- chronic, non-severe hypertension
- atheromatous cardiovascular conditions
- recuperation after cardiovascular attacks
- venous insufficiency
- congestive heart failure.

Because of its use of secondary plant products, particular **caution** is necessary in applying phytotherapy in cases of:

- warfarin, heparin and other anticoagulant prescription
- acute cardiovascular incidents
- digitalis glycoside prescription.

Orientation

Old and new perspectives on the circulatory system

A phytotherapeutic perspective on the circulatory system has to take two parts. Most of what modern medicine understands of the system arises from preoccupation with disease states such as hypertension, hypercholesterolaemia, atherosclerosis, clotting disturbances and thrombosis, and coronary diseases that were barely understood in an earlier era and for which traditional physicians cannot have developed therapeutic strategies. There can be no basis therefore for directly applying old treatments to the new conditions. Nevertheless, as this chapter will show, herbal remedies show considerable promise across many of these modern conditions and their use for this purpose, at least in Europe, has been considerably modified compared with their traditional indications. Three of the best-selling herbal products in Europe, Ginkgo, garlic and Crataegus (hawthorn), are traditional remedies highly adapted to new and productive ends.

Nevertheless, to understand more effectively the potential of medicinal plants in affecting circulatory functions, an appreciation of the earlier traditional perspective will be helpful. It is immediately obvious that before modern instruments, human experience of the circulatory system and the effects of treatments upon it were very different. As shall be seen, the insights developed in these early times usefully inform modern prospects.

The circulatory apparatus of William Harvey provided a mechanistic framework for modern advances that was, however, of little application to everyday practice in his time. The common experience was that there was vital movement within the body, as measured by pulse, heartbeat and breathing, and that there was a red fluid whose presence was clearly essential. Even now microscopic film of tissue circulation resonates uncannily with the beats of tribal music! It was relatively easy to link this with the main manifestation of moving blood: the heat of the living body and the variations in that heat in health and disease. In short, blood pulsated and warmed and was generally linked with the common speculation that there must be circulation of energies, fluids and nutrients around the body. Circulation was marked by:

* pulsation
* heat
* blood and reddened complexion and, when in good shape, by a general vital potency.

The heart was obviously associated with all this, but as much as a resonator with the vital pulse as its director. It was the wider pulse itself (reflected in the driving rhythms of early tribal music) that was important in early experience of the circulatory system; it was clearly linked to wider vital events: activity, excitement, emotional stimulation and, in medicine, notably the fever.

Therapeutics in fever focused on dispersing agents to distribute excessive heat and circulation and (as 'diaphoretics') to diffuse the poisons clearly involved through the sweat glands. The detoxifying theme recurred in many traditional concepts of 'blood poisons' as a cause of inflammatory diseases, and the use of 'blood cleansers' or 'blood purifiers', often very vigorously, to treat them.

Also requiring eliminatives (mainly diuretics and laxatives) was oedema, one of the most common indications of poor circulation in the past. As briefly elaborated in Chapter 1, the traditional perspective closely linked circulatory function with elimination.

Traditional views also linked circulation with the assimilation and processing of nutrients. The vital pulse and heat were weakened in debility and exhaustion, conditions associated with coldness and pallor. The main treatments were in effect 'blood tonics', warming nutrients (often since found to be rich in mineral nutrients).

There will be profit in revisiting these perspectives in developing modern strategies for the treatment of circulatory problems using herbal remedies. This is even more justified when the phenomenon of circulation itself is reviewed.

Circulation as currents

Where there has been speculation about the nature of the circulatory system in traditional medicine, it has tended to infer broad currents rather than Harvey's route map. The closest to the latter were the meridians of Chinese medicine, although even these were speculative phenomena not associated with anatomical conduits.[1] The phenomenological perspective of tradition turns out, however, to be closer to the reality than the conventional understanding of arteries, veins and capillaries might suggest.

As far as most tissue cells are concerned, blood flow is not through vessels at all. When plasma filters through the capillary walls to bathe the tissues, it does not diffuse freely. In most tissues, cells are embedded in a gelatinous matrix, formed of complexes of hyaluronic acid which is largely impermeable to aqueous fluids. Movement of plasma is thus confined through clefts and cleavages in the matrix. The interstitial matrix thus both maintains tissue integrity and restricts the free flow of the circulation; oedema is the main symptom of breakdown in this important construct.

The effect of the interstitial matrix on circulatory dynamics is profound. As far as tissues are concerned, circulation is not a Harveyian affair at all, it is more a diffusive process marked by local and wider 'oceanic' currents. Factors that affect tissue circulation are thus different from those that preoccupy modern cardiovascular medicine. Atherosclerosis and thrombosis cause serious local circulatory harm, of course, but they impact on general circulation only when very severe. More important for circulatory health in the tissues are such factors as capillary wall integrity, the local responses to local environmental changes of powerful vasoactive agents such as the kinins and histamine, venous or lymphatic stasis or congestion with subsequent oedema and toxicity.

Antipathogenic benefits of increased tissue perfusion?

A glance at any pathology text will confirm that the cellular processes of disease are remarkably consistent. Pathological deterioration starts with biochemical lesions, then a variety of stages supervene including intracellular lesions, cell hypertrophy and a range of possible degenerative changes, cellular swelling due to water influx into the cell, fatty change or accumulation, atrophy, necrosis, possibly leading to inflammation or calcification. Most detectable disease states in the body are classified by one or more of these processes. Atherosclerosis, for example, involves fatty infiltration and then calcification of the tissues in the arterial walls.

Moreover, the very first initiating trauma is even more consistent. The most likely first step in tissue damage is a relative deficiency of oxygenated blood and fluids. Physical injury is the most likely initiating trauma followed by an accumulation of external or endogenous toxic substances. In both the first and last cases poor tissue perfusion is critical. There are a number of ways in which tissue circulation can be interrupted but there is a clear prima facie case for maintaining tissue perfusion as a core disease-preventing strategy.

One of the most fascinating prospects for the revival of traditional herbal and dietary approaches is in the number of ways in which plant constituents, such as flavonoids, anthocyanins, sesquiterpenes and pungent principles, appear to act beneficially on local circulatory processes.

It is a consistent theme throughout history that the 'heating' remedies were literally life enhancing (see p. 4 and p. 9). The pungent remedies such as cayenne, ginger and raw garlic had reputations that transcended the merely mundane. It is known that they do increase tissue perfusion and blood flow. Everyday subjective experiences of increased body heat after eating spicy food can be confirmed with thermometers. Reference to the ginger monograph reveals a number of studies demonstrating a thermogenic effect, involving such mechanisms as increased catecholamine production and cytokine activity. Supplementing rats' diet with garlic powder increased rectal temperatures, blood noradrenaline levels and mitochondrial activity in brown adipose tissues, an activity that was inhibited by beta-adrenergic blockers.[2]

The prospects for closer investigation are intriguing. It is most probable that the traditional remedies most often used for their tissue warming benefits will show really exciting properties in the treatment of, or prophylaxis against, a range of degenerative diseases that may include atherosclerosis and other cardiovascular diseases. The fact that most are common ingredients of the diet adds even more to this project.

A promise of what may be in store for cayenne, ginger, cinnamon, turmeric and the like is the remarkable story of garlic, now possibly the most intensively studied of all medicinal plants and foods.

Garlic

The chemistry of *Allium sativum* is complex and the multitude of garlic products available in the marketplace reflects this complexity.[3] These types of preparations can be divided into three main groups, to which is added fresh garlic:

1. Carefully dried *garlic powder* that preserves the compound alliin (S-allylcysteine sulphoxide) and the enzyme alliinase. On disintegration of tablets or capsules containing this powder in the digestive tract, alliin comes into contact with alliinase and is converted to allicin. This must take place outside the stomach, as gastric acid inhibits alliinase. Enteric-coating of the tablets or capsules is therefore necessary. (This process mimics the chemical reaction that occurs when a fresh clove of garlic is crushed.) Allicin is unstable and breaks down further into compounds such as diallyl sulphides, ajoene and the vinyl dithiins (the metabolic pathways for allicin in the human body are not fully understood).
2. *Aged garlic extracts* or 'odourless' garlic products that are produced by a fermentation process. These preparations contain modified sulphur compounds such as S-allylcysteine.
3. Steam-distilled preparations of garlic (garlic oil) rich in diallyl sulphides.

Most of the published clinical studies on garlic have used 'garlic powder' preparations, although trials on aged garlic extracts, fresh garlic and garlic oil are also in the literature.

Lipid-lowering effects

Many studies have demonstrated the lipid-lowering effects of garlic and the results of meta-analyses have supported the premise that garlic acts as a lipid-lowering agent. One examined five selected clinical trials on various garlic preparations with a total of 410 patients.[4] The authors concluded that the best available evidence suggests that garlic, in an amount approximating one half to one clove per day, decreased total serum cholesterol levels by about 9%. About a year later a second meta-analysis was published by Silagy and Neil.[5] These scientists included 16 clinical trials with a total of 952 patients. Again, a variety of garlic preparations were included in the meta-analysis. They found that garlic lowered cholesterol levels by 12% and that dried garlic powder preparations also lowered serum levels of triglycerides. In spite of some published negative trials (for example, on garlic[6,7] and on garlic oil[8]), the latest meta-analysis taking 29 clinical trials up to 2007 found garlic significantly reduced total cholesterol and triglycerides, though exhibited no significant effect on LDL or HDL.[9] The results of negative trials are confounded by the observation of Lawson and team that products used in clinical trials where garlic did not lower cholesterol often did not effectively release allicin.[10]

Antiatherogenicity

Perhaps the real value of garlic in the prevention and treatment of cardiovascular disease lies elsewhere. For example, a double blind, placebo-controlled study on 23 patients found that garlic powder tablets reduced the atherogenicity of low-density lipoprotein.[11] In a controlled retrospective study on 202 healthy adults, divided equally between those taking garlic powder and controls, in which measures of the elastic properties of the aorta were used, garlic reduced age-related increases in aortic stiffness.[12]

An important trial looked at the effect of garlic powder intake over 4 years on arterial plaque. The trial was a randomised, double blind, placebo-controlled design involving 152 patients. Plaque volumes in both carotid and femoral arteries were measured by ultrasound. The increase in plaque volume over time was significantly reduced by garlic and in some cases there was a slight regression. The authors were accused of scientific fraud, but subsequently vindicated.[13-15]

Researchers from Germany report that, in test tubes, garlic prevents formation of 'nanoplaques' that can accumulate to cause arteriosclerosis. During a National Institutes of Health workshop on herbs and cardiovascular disease held in Bethesda, MD, in August 2002, Dr Günter Siegel from the Free University of Berlin, described his team's research, which pinpoints exactly how garlic blunts plaque formation.[16] In the presence of calcium, low-density lipoprotein (LDL)-cholesterol binds with molecules secreted from the inner lining of the arteries, forming tiny plaques that can accumulate and harden. HDL-cholesterol inhibits this process by absorbing excess plaque-forming molecules. Siegel's team found that garlic extract works exactly the same way, but more potently. Garlic extract was two and a half times more effective in inhibiting plaque formation than was HDL-cholesterol.[16] This has led to Siegel describing this form of garlic as phyto-HDL, that is a herb acting in the same beneficial way as HDL.

Antihypertensive

A meta-analysis of eight clinical trials (415 patients), all using the same garlic powder preparation, found that garlic caused a modest but significant reduction in both systolic and diastolic blood pressures.[17] However, only three of the trials were specifically conducted in hypertensive patients and many had other methodological shortcomings. A review of aged garlic extract has assigned US National Health and Medical Research Council levels of evidence III-1 ratings on conclusions that 7.2g has been associated with anti-clotting (in vivo studies), as well as modest reductions in blood pressure (an approximate 5.5% decrease in systolic blood pressure).[18] In a recent meta-analysis involving ten trials, garlic reduced systolic blood pressure by 16.3mmHg (95% CI 6.2 to 26.5) and diastolic pressure by 9.3mmHg (95% CI 5.3 to 13.3) compared with placebo, although only in patients with elevated systolic blood pressure.[19] Another contemporary meta-analysis of eleven studies showed a mean decrease of 4.6 ± 2.8mmHg for systolic blood pressure in the garlic groups compared to placebo (n=10; p=0.001), while the mean decrease in the hypertensive subgroup was 8.4 ± 2.8mmHg for systolic (n=4; p<0.001), and 7.3 ± 1.5mmHg for diastolic blood pressure (n=3; p<0.001).[20]

Effects on haemostasis and blood flow

A platelet-inhibiting effect has been described for garlic. In a double blind, placebo-controlled study involving 60 volunteers with elevated cerebrovascular risk factors and increased spontaneous platelet aggregation, it was demonstrated that 800mg/day of garlic powder over 4 weeks led to a significant reduction in platelet aggregation and circulating platelet aggregates.[21] This inhibition of platelet aggregation by garlic powder was confirmed by another research group.[22] However, the confounding issue of the various dosage forms of garlic was highlighted by a study of an oil extract of garlic, which found no significant effect on platelet aggregation.[23] In contrast, consumption of a fresh clove of garlic daily for a period of 16 weeks reduced serum thromboxane by about 80%.[24]

One of the compounds responsible for the antiplatelet effect of garlic powder could be ajoene.[25] This compound inhibits aggregation induced by all known platelet agonists in all species studied and prevents the amplification of platelet responses. Unlike aspirin, it acts by modifying the platelet membrane structure.

A review of published studies found that garlic consistently increased fibrinolytic activity after single or multiple doses. Garlic oil and garlic powder were both active, sometimes after only a single dose. The average increase in the reviewed studies was 58%.[26] A 1991 controlled study using raw garlic demonstrated a significant increase in clotting time and fibrinolytic activity after 2 months in normal volunteers.[27]

In a randomised, placebo-controlled, double blind, crossover study in ten healthy volunteers, a single dose of 600mg of garlic powder significantly reduced haematocrit (p<0.001), plasma viscosity (p<0.05) and plasma fibrinogen (p<0.05).[28] Fibrinolytic activity was also significantly increased (p<0.01). A similar study design also found that a single 900mg dose of garlic powder significantly increased capillary skin perfusion by 55% (p<0.01).[29] Another study found that garlic powder (600mg/day) administered for 7 days increased calf blood flow by approximately 15% (p=0.001).[30]

Garlic and hydrogen sulphide

Two naturally produced gaseous signalling molecules play a key role in the regulation of cardiovascular physiology.[31] These gaseous messengers, nitric oxide (NO) and carbon monoxide (CO), are synthesised by endogenous enzyme systems. Extensive research has shown that agents that improve their production protect the brain and heart against cardiovascular diseases, although this is sometimes controversial.[31]

In an intriguing scientific breakthrough, research on garlic has revealed it is involved in the generation of a significant third gaseous signalling molecule, namely hydrogen sulphide (H_2S).[32] H_2S, also known as rotten egg gas, is toxic in high amounts. But it appears that the small quantities induced by the ingestion of garlic could play a role in its cardiovascular benefits, as well as the characteristic garlic breath. Scientists were able to demonstrate that garlic-derived organic polysulphides, such as diallyl disulphide and diallyl trisulphide, act as H_2S donors.[32] Human red blood cells were able to convert these molecules into H_2S. The authors of the study suggested the major beneficial effects of garlic intake, specifically on cardiovascular disease and more broadly on overall health, are mediated by the biological production of H_2S.[32]

A 2007 review described some of the significant physiological actions of H_2S.[31] It relaxes vascular smooth muscle, induces vasodilation of isolated blood vessels and lowers blood pressure. H_2S is also a potent anti-inflammatory and antioxidant molecule that can increase antioxidant defences. Unlike NO, it does not form a potentially harmful toxic metabolite at the low levels generated in tissue. In addition, H_2S inhibits apoptosis in a number of cell types and promotes the formation of new blood vessels. Several models of cardiovascular disease have demonstrated significant benefit after the administration of H_2S donors. The discovery of this new and novel mechanism of action for garlic adds significant weight to its role in the modification and prevention of cardiovascular disease.

Adverse effects

A number of case reports have reflected these effects of garlic on bleeding parameters. A spontaneous spinal epidural haematoma associated with platelet dysfunction from excessive garlic ingestion was reported.[33] A patient taking garlic prior to cosmetic surgery experienced bleeding complications and had a clotting time of 12.5 minutes. After cessation of garlic, her clotting time dropped to 6 minutes and there were no complications during a second procedure.[34]

Overview

The value of garlic as a prevention and treatment for cardiovascular diseases will best be determined by controlled clinical trials using cardiovascular morbidity or mortality as endpoints. In the meantime, garlic can be prescribed on the basis that it does favourably influence haemorheological parameters (blood flow characteristics) and some cardiovascular risk factors, including modest effect on serum cholesterol and blood pressure. Attention should be paid to the type of garlic preparation used; the strongest published evidence to date is for garlic powder preparations, although other preparations will also be of value. Caution should be exercised when prescribing garlic to patients who are also taking other blood-thinning medications such as aspirin or warfarin and garlic intake should be discontinued 10 days before surgery. However, a clinical trial with healthy volunteers found no adverse effect for garlic powder (enteric-coated standardised tablets, equivalent 4 g/day of fresh garlic) taken with warfarin.[35]

Plant phenolics and the vasculature

When Szent-Gyorgy in the 1930s identified the flavonoid constituents of citrus fruits as a necessary co-factor with ascorbic acid in the prevention of scurvy, he opened an investigation which has actually increased in intensity in recent years. Interest in the flavonols such as rutin and its aglycone quercetin has been augmented by a growing fascination with other phenolic molecules, the oligomeric procyanidins (OPCs) and the polyphenolics linked to the tannins, all very common constituents in dietary fruit and vegetables as well as in herbal remedies.

Flavonoids, a group of phenolic constituents found widely in plants, including most fruits and vegetables, have been found to possess a number of anti-inflammatory effects, including, especially for rutin and others from the flavonol subgroup, effects on the microvasculature[36] (see also the discussion in Chapter 2 under Flavonoids).

Rutin, quercetin-3-rutoside, is a flavonoid glycoside with quercetin as an aglycone and rhamnose and glucose as sugar moieties. It is very widely distributed in the plant kingdom. It is official in many pharmacopoeias and is widely sold as a health supplement, sometimes in association with vitamin C. In experiments it has been shown to increase survival times of rats fed a thrombogenic diet and in other animals to reduce oedema, reduce cholesterol-induced atheroma and inhibit the carcinogenic action of benzo(α)pyrene.[37] Like ascorbic acid, it is an oxygen radical scavenger and has been shown to reduce the mutagenicity of dusts and asbestos[38] and other stressors.[39,40]

Commercial products with a similar structure, hydroxyethylrutosides or oxerutins (containing principally tri-O-(beta-hydroxyethyl)rutoside, as well as a mixture of mono-, di- and tetra-O-(beta-hydroxyethyl)rutosides), are marketed for the treatment of chronic venous insufficiency. There are a number of reports demonstrating positive effects on capillary permeability,[41–43] on venous insufficiency[44] and venous hypertension.[45] Other researchers have reported an improvement in oxygen perfusion of tissues surrounding varicose veins.[46]

The development of synthetic rutosides has followed the finding that natural rutin is poorly absorbed. However, over 95% of all polyphenolic intake passes to the colon and is fermented by the gut microflora into simple phenols. For example, rutin is now known to be rapidly metabolised by bacteria in the intestine, via quercetin, to 3,4-dihydroxyphenylacetic acid, a small phenol with antioxidant properties. Simple phenolic acids derived from cinnamic acid (such as gallic acid, salicylic acid, caffeic acid, vanillic acid and ferulic acid, as their esters including chlorogenic acid and rosmarinic acid), with their derived polyphenols, make significantly larger contributions to dietary phenol, polyphenol and tannin intake

than the flavonols and flavones upon which the vast majority of attention has been focused. It is important to include these in assessments of the total effects of polyphenols.[47] Such degradation products are readily absorbed and are found in urine of animals.[48] Early doubts about the venous efficacy of such flavonoid molecules[49] have therefore not been sustained. (See also the Pharmacokinetics section of Chapter 2.)

There is much in vitro evidence on the effects of flavonoids and other polyphenolics on the microvasculature that can be noted, but which for reasons above need confirmation clinically. For example:

- hawthorn extract[50] and black currant extract[51] have NO-mediated vasodilatory effects on rat arteries
- flavonoids inhibit TNF-alpha induced upregulation of the endothelial adhesion mediator ICAM-1[52]
- phloretin from apples reduces endothelial adhesion molecules and platelet activation.[53]

Compared with the effects of polyphenols in vitro, the effects in vivo are more limited. Several studies, however, show benefits of products in streptozotocin-induced diabetic rats, for example flavonoid-rich citrus fruit extract[54] and rooibos tea (*Aspalathus linearis*).[55] A fundamental point is that in vivo studies are not long enough and rarely consider bioavailability problems. In human studies particularly it is important that studies are long term, to more closely reflect the likely effects of dietary consumption of polyphenols. Two critical and important reviews of the intervention studies for the use of polyphenols have been published[56,57] (see also the relevant section in Chapter 2).

Short-term observations still point to, if not confirm, prospects of vascular changes. In a prospective, placebo-controlled, randomised study, a high rutoside-containing proprietary product (O-(beta-hydroxyethyl rutosides) at 2 g/day for 6 months was tested on patients with diabetic microangiopathy and oedema. Significant decreases in resting flux and rate of ankle swelling were observed in the active treatment groups.[58] In this author's preliminary observations in 1993, 37 patients suffering symptoms of venous insufficiency entered a clinical study to determine the impact on their microcirculation of buckwheat leaf, a popular natural treatment for this condition that contains high levels of plant flavonoids. Using the mild provocation of a suction cup applied to the lower leg and monitoring changes in local circulatory activity with laser Doppler flowmetry, it was possible to identify three characteristics of vascular responses that differentiated sufferers of venous insufficiency from healthy controls: reduced vascular reactivity, flow resolution rate and vasomotor activity. After establishing baseline levels for these characteristics all the subjects took buckwheat leaf for a total of 6 weeks. Twenty-four satisfactorily completed all stages of the study. In this uncontrolled sample it was possible to demonstrate statistically significant changes in vasomotor activity and vascular reactivity. However, flow resolution rate, that might have indicated a beneficial effect on the endothelium, was not changed.

Both short- and long-term improvements in endothelial function have been seen with doses of green tea catechins equivalent to several cups a day.[59] A standardised OPC extract of the bark of the French maritime pine (*Pinus pinaster*) is known to increase capillary resistance. It has been investigated in five clinical trials with a total number of 1289 patients since the late 1960s for treatment and prevention of diabetic retinal microangiopathy, characterised by vascular lesions with exudate deposits and haemorrhages. All of these studies showed that the extract slowed progression of retinopathy and partly recovered visual acuity. It was shown to improve capillary resistance and reduce leakage into the retina. Tolerance was generally very good and side effects were rare, mostly referring to gastric discomfort.[60]

Epidemiological studies suggest that the intake of flavonols and flavones is inversely associated with subsequent coronary heart disease (CHD).[61] There is, however, mixed evidence for a benefit of increased fruit and vegetable intake in vascular health. Improved endothelial function scores and reduced insulin resistance have been observed in a controlled observation of the effects of the Mediterranean diet over 2 years.[62] However, by contrast there was little association found between high fruit and vegetable consumption and the incidence of peripheral arterial disease in a 12-year study of a cohort of 44059 men initially free of cardiovascular disease and diabetes (after adjustment for smoking and other traditional cardiovascular disease risk factors).[63]

Overall, it seems most likely that any benefits of polyphenolic intake will follow long-term and relatively substantial use. However, the prospect for short-term changes in vascular reactivity with relatively high doses of polyphenols needs to be further explored.

The above research highlights that therapeutic herbs can offer value in one aspect of the cardiovascular system that is somewhat neglected in modern drug treatment, namely the health of the small blood vessels or microvasculature. As noted above, flavonoids in general, and specifically OPCs from pine bark or grape seed, possess clinically relevant vasoprotective activity. Other plant agents shown to support the microvasculature with, for example, beneficial clinical effects in microangiopathy include bilberry, gotu kola, Ginkgo and garlic (allicin-releasing preparations). They will have application where structures comprising fine blood vessels are affected, such as the retina (e.g. diabetic retinopathy), neurons (e.g. diabetic neuropathy) and the glomeruli of the kidneys (e.g. diabetic nephropathy).

Phytotherapy for cardiovascular conditions

Congestive heart failure

The original observations by William Withering of the benefits of foxglove in the treatment of dropsy by a country herbalist led to the discovery of the digitalis glycosides that became the primary drug treatment for congestive heart failure. Given its seriousness and the potency of these plant extractives, it has generally been accepted that crude herbal drugs no longer have a place in the rational treatment of the condition.

Nevertheless, there is a consistent tradition for the use of herbs with cardiac glycosides such as *Convallaria majalis* (lily

of the valley) around the world and pharmacological cases have been made for their use as broader spectrum remedies (see Chapter 2). Indeed, the use of crude *Digitalis folium* was favoured by some doctors in Britain over the synthetic isolate until relatively recently. There is also evidence that a wider range of plants may have supportive benefits in the condition. For example, *Terminalia arjuna* 1500 mg/day demonstrated substantial benefits in the treatment of refractory congestive heart failure linked to dilated cardiomyopathy in a placebo-controlled, double blind crossover trial.[64]

There is now substantial clinical evidence for the supportive role of hawthorn (*Crataegus* species) in congestive heart failure, not to supplant conventional medication, but to provide an extra dimension of treatment aimed at supporting the heart muscle itself. (This has been fully reviewed in the hawthorn monograph.)

Other herbs of potential value include *Coleus forskohlii* containing forskolin, a phytochemical with cardiotonic activity,[65] and *Salvia miltiorrhiza* (dan shen).[66] Astragalus also possesses mild cardiotonic activity and can be combined with Korean ginseng for this effect (see the ginseng and Astragalus monographs). Clinical trials from China suggest a clinical benefit from ginseng in patients with congestive heart failure. Mild diuretic herbs may be beneficial for fluid retention, such as dandelion leaves.

CASE HISTORY

A male patient aged 82 with a history of congestive heart failure, stable angina and poor memory (prescribed aspirin and diuretics) was placed on the following formulation:

Ginkgo biloba (standardised extract)	2:1	40 mL
Salvia miltiorrhiza	1:2	30 mL
Panax ginseng	1:2	15 mL
Astragalus membranaceus	1:2	25 mL
	TOTAL	110 mL

Dose: 8 mL twice a day.

In addition, hawthorn leaf and flower extract tablets (containing the equivalent of 1 g of herb) were prescribed at two tablets twice daily.

Over a period of 5 years of this treatment (with some variations) the patient has considerably improved, despite his advancing years. His capacity to exercise is now much greater and he recently repainted his timber house. Relatives of the patient have expressed surprise at his marked improvement.

Essential hypertension

In about 90% of cases with hypertension there is no identifiable cause and the term 'essential hypertension' is used. In the remaining cases a cause can be identified and this is known as 'secondary hypertension'. The main cause is kidney disease; other causes include coarctation of the aorta, endocrine diseases and pregnancy. Generally, the treatment for secondary hypertension is the same as for essential hypertension, but the cause should also be treated if possible. It is important to ensure that patients presenting with essential hypertension do not have a secondary cause. Many patients with hypertension have coexisting cardiovascular risk factors, which should also be addressed.[67]

Although the milder stages of essential hypertension should probably not be considered as a disease, people with hypertension are more likely than those with normal blood pressure to develop a number of cardiovascular diseases. In particular, hypertension is a risk factor for the development of CHD. As such, it is desirable to treat even mild hypertension.

Treatment should aim for gradual reduction in blood pressure. The kidneys will have become adapted to the previously high levels (indeed, an approach to understanding essential hypertension is that it may be a mechanism to ensure adequate kidney function when this is failing). Sudden reduction could lead to other problems. In this sense natural approaches, if effective, can be doubly suitable.

It is apparent to most practitioners that hypertension is an indication for a broad therapeutic strategy, including dietary and lifestyle advice. Some of the features of this advice are therefore outlined below. It is not advisable to attempt to treat severe (greater than 170/110), malignant or accelerated hypertension with only natural approaches; synthetic prescription drugs can be necessary to avoid serious harm in such cases.

Treatment

Diet and lifestyle

Although the physiological mechanisms responsible for the lowering of blood pressure as a result of exercise are still under debate, strong epidemiological and experimental evidence supports a link between the two.[68] Aerobic exercise that uses large muscle groups for 20 to 60 minutes a day for a minimum of 3 days a week is advisable, although there may have to be a gradual build-up to these levels and all stages should be closely monitored.

Obesity and hypertension are strongly linked. There is a continuous linear relationship between excess body fat, blood pressure and the prevalence of hypertension.[69] A cause-and-effect relationship has also been demonstrated. Hence weight loss should always be attempted. The waist:hip ratio is a more accurate predictor of hypertension than either body weight or body mass index.[70] In extreme cases this is now recognised as linked to the condition known as metabolic syndrome.

The role of sodium (salt) restriction in treating hypertension has been controversial, with recent evidence that casts doubt on the conventional view that low sodium intake is always helpful.[71] However, the consensus is that salt reduction does lower high blood pressure readings.[72]

Randomised, controlled trials indicate a specific blood pressure lowering effect of lactovegetarian diets.[73] A non-vegetarian diet rich in fruit and vegetables and low fat dairy products also significantly reduced blood pressure.[74] Although the effects of caffeine on blood pressure are considered to be temporary, many clinicians suggest a reduction in caffeine intake to reduce aggravating factors.[75] Potassium supplementation or the use of a high-potassium, high-magnesium salt has

been shown to reduce blood pressure.[76] Increased calcium intake may also be of value[77] and 6 g/day of fish oil had a mild lowering effect.[78]

Relaxation techniques could be valuable, although their acceptance has been hampered by poorly designed and ambiguous studies.[79] Some self-prescribed non-prescription drugs may cause or exacerbate hypertension. These include ephedrine, pseudoephedrine and other decongestant and weight loss agents.[80]

Herbs

Most of the herbal treatments for hypertension probably act as peripheral vasodilators. They are all slow to exert their activity, except perhaps for Coleus. Important herbs for this condition include the following:

- Crataegus (hawthorn) – as well as reducing high blood pressure this herb has a trophic effect on the heart muscle. This is important because left ventricular heart failure is often caused by prolonged hypertension. The leaves are apparently more potent than the berries for reducing blood pressure (see the hawthorn monograph) and effects are modest.
- *Allium sativum* (garlic) – as well as its mild antihypertensive effects (see previous) this plant also favourably influences other cardiovascular risk factors. Allicin-releasing preparations are most proven in blood pressure management (see previous discussion).
- *Coleus forskohlii* – can have a pronounced lowering effect on high blood pressure. Only varieties containing forskolin should be used. Coleus also has pronounced antiplatelet activity, which may be desirable in some cases.[65]
- *Valeriana* (valerian) – whether this herb acts as a peripheral or central vasodilator or if the activity is due to a general calming effect on the nervous system is not known. It is usually prescribed for stressed patients (see valerian monograph).
- *Olea europaea* (olive leaves) – has been proven to lower high blood pressure in clinical trials, provided the dose is sufficiently high.[81]
- *Viburnum opulus* (cramp bark) – this herb is thought to relax smooth muscle and has been used to augment antihypertensive prescriptions as a vasorelaxant.
- *Achillea millefolium* (yarrow) – is used by some herbalists to specifically lower an elevated diastolic blood pressure.
- *Taraxacum officinale* (dandelion leaves) – has diuretic activity and high levels of potassium and can be useful especially for the treatment of elevated systolic pressure in the elderly.

Other herbs also commonly used to lower high blood pressure include *Tilia* species (lime flowers) and *Viscum album* (mistletoe). The Ayurvedic herb Rauwolfia is a powerful treatment for hypertension, but is usually limited to prescription only.

CASE HISTORY

A female patient aged 48 sought assistance for palpitations, anxiety, angina and mild hypertension. Her ECG did not reveal the presence of a cardiac arrhythmia and her palpitations were less severe in recent times. On examination her blood pressure was 170/95 despite her use of the prescribed drugs labetalol and felodipine.

After treatment over a few months, the following prescription was settled upon:

Ginkgo biloba (standardised extract)	2:1	20 mL
Panax notoginseng	1:2	20 mL
Crataegus folia	1:2	25 mL
Corydalis ambigua	1:2	20 mL
Hypericum perforatum	1:2	25 mL
Passiflora incarnata	1:2	20 mL
Salvia miltiorrhiza	1:2	20 mL
	TOTAL	150 mL

Dose: 7.5 mL with water three times a day.

Over the ensuing months her blood pressure was typically 135/85. She had no problems with palpitations and her anxiety and angina had improved.

The rationale for the herbs chosen was as follows:

* Panax notoginseng, Crataegus and Salvia for her heart and angina
* The above herbs and Ginkgo, Corydalis and Passiflora for palpitations
* Corydalis, Passiflora and Hypericum for anxiety
* Crataegus and the above herbs for anxiety for her hypertension.

CASE HISTORY

A male patient aged 62 with blood pressure as high as 160/100 sought herbal treatment instead of the ACE inhibitor offered by his doctor. He had a high stress job as a property developer and also suffered from benign prostatic hyperplasia.

He was prescribed the following:

Crataeva nurvala	1:2	20 mL
Crataegus folia	1:2	35 mL
Valeriana officinalis	1:2	20 mL
Urtica radix	1:2	15 mL
Zizyphus spinosa	1:2	20 mL
	TOTAL	110 mL

Dose: 8 mL with water twice per day, combined with separate capsules for his prostate containing Serenoa repens.

After 6 months on the treatment his prostate symptoms were considerably reduced and his average blood pressure was 121/76. The patient also followed the lifestyle and dietary advice outlined above.

Angina

Angina pectoris is a manifestation of ischaemia of the heart muscle usually caused by diseased coronary arteries. Stable angina occurs when the frequency, severity, duration, time of appearance and precipitating factors for the angina remain unchanged for 60 days.[82] It is by far the most common form of angina and symptoms typically develop with a defined amount of exercise and abate after a short period of rest. As well as physical activity, stable angina can be precipitated by emotion, eating or cold weather. Angina can also result from an acute reduction in coronary blood flow, and this type of angina can occur at rest. This may result from transient restriction of the flow in the coronary arteries by platelets or a thrombus, or by physiological or pathological vasoconstriction. Vasoconstriction of a normal or minimally diseased coronary artery is referred to as variant or Prinzmetal angina and is now considered to be rare.[83] Unstable angina describes a spectrum of ischaemic events somewhere between stable angina and myocardial infarction (heart attack). An estimated 5% of unstable angina patients die within the first few months of diagnosis.[84]

Stable angina is mostly a distressing rather than dangerous symptom, but there is an increased risk of heart attack and a small proportion will have fatal or serious attacks soon after diagnosis. It is therefore not a condition to be treated casually. Conventional prescription drugs may be necessary, although these most often work well with herbal treatments. Reduction in smoking, hypertension, obesity, any high cholesterol or lipidaemia and a measured increase in exercise is strongly advisable if these measures can be introduced without serious perturbation.

Treatment

The key herb is Crataegus (hawthorn). Preparations from the leaves and flowers and/or berries may be used. As well as being proven in clinical trials to reduce myocardial oxygen demand (see the hawthorn monograph), Crataegus is antioxidant, cardioprotective and a coronary artery vasodilator. Clinical trials have shown that Crataegus is safe to combine with conventional drugs. In patients with ischaemic heart disease, Crataegus decreased the signs of ischaemia as assessed by an exercise ECG test.[85] A related species of Crataegus has been successfully trialled for angina in China in an open label study.[86]

The key Ayurvedic herbs Terminalia arjuna and Inula racemosa (a close relative of elecampane – Inula helenium) have been shown to benefit angina in clinical trials.[87]

Ginkgo (by injection) has improved coronary blood flow in patients with coronary artery disease and favourably affects some cardiovascular risk factors (see Ginkgo monograph).

Salvia miltiorrhiza (dan shen) is a Chinese herb clinically studied for angina and other heart conditions.[88] Its benefits include cardioprotective, vasodilator and antiplatelet activities. Astragalus can also be of potential value (see Astragalus monograph). There is evidence from a clinical trial that Korean red ginseng improved coronary flow reserve in postmyocardial infarction patients.[89]

Antiplatelet herbs such as Coleus forskohlii, Allium sativum (garlic), Zingiber (ginger) and Curcuma longa (turmeric) may have value even if the patient is taking antiplatelet medication, because of their differing mechanisms of action. (They do not appear to decrease prostacyclin production.) They also have other properties that may be beneficial; for example, Coleus is a vasodilator and Curcuma is antioxidant. However, care should be taken to ensure that bleeding time is not excessively prolonged. (See the ginger and turmeric monographs.)

Capsicum spp. (cayenne) has fibrinolytic activity and was traditionally used to improve myocardial blood supply.

Vasodilating and relaxing herbs have been traditionally prescribed for angina and include *Tilia* species (lime flowers) and *Viburnum opulus* (cramp bark). In cases of stable angina they are probably of little value since they would be unlikely to widen a diseased artery restricted by atheroma. However, they might be considered for angina exacerbated by stress and anxiety, together with Valeriana and Corydalis or similar calming herbs.

Example liquid formula

An example formula for stable angina is provided below:

Crataegus folia	1:2	50 mL
Zingiber officinale	1:2	10 mL
Salvia miltiorrhiza	1:2	40 mL
		100 mL

Dose: 8 mL with water twice times daily.

Allicin-releasing garlic tablets (equivalent to about 6 to 12 g/day of fresh garlic and providing at least 12 mg/day alliin).

Hyperlipidaemia and cardiovascular risk factors

Atherogenesis is no longer considered a disorder of lipid accumulation, but a disease process characterised by a dynamic interaction between endothelial (vessel lining) dysfunction, subendothelial inflammation and a 'wound healing' response of the vascular smooth muscle cells. Oxidation of LDL (low-density lipoprotein) triggers the recruitment of macrophages into the arterial wall. They accumulate cholesterol, becoming foam cells.[90,91]

The American Heart Association Prevention Conference in 1999 classified cardiovascular risk factors into three categories. The traditional or conventional risk factors came from the Framingham Heart Study and are thought to have a direct causal role in atherogenesis.[90] Predisposing factors may act through the conventional factors, but may also have independent effects. Conditional risk factors are associated with increased risk of ischaemic heart disease, although their causative and/or independent contributions are still debated. They may further enhance risk if traditional factors are present, hence the term 'conditional'.[90] A fourth category can be added of the emerging risk factors still under preliminary study.

The conventional risk factors comprise cigarette smoking, elevated blood pressure, elevated total or LDL serum cholesterol, low HDL-cholesterol and diabetes mellitus.

Predisposing risk factors are high BMI, visceral adiposity, physical inactivity, male sex, family history of early onset coronary disease, socioeconomic and behavioural factors (e.g. type A personality) and insulin resistance (sometimes regarded as a conditional factor).

Conditional risk factors are currently defined as elevated homocysteine, elevated fibrinogen, elevated lipoprotein(a), small dense LDL particles, elevated C-reactive protein (CRP) and elevated triglycerides.

Emerging risk factors include vascular calcification, infection and periodontal disease, elevated gamma-glutamyltransferase (GGT), low heart rate variability and low red blood cell omega-3 fatty acids (omega-3 index). Some emerging factors are naturally quite controversial.

Hyperlipidaemia may involve hypercholesterolaemia (elevated serum cholesterol) or hypertriglyceridaemia (evaluated serum triglycerides). In adults less than 65 years of age, a total cholesterol concentration greater than 6 mmol/L (240 mg/dL) or a triglyceride concentration greater than 2.8 mmol/L (250 mg/dL) clearly indicates hyperlipidaemia. However, in the presence of other independent risk factors for atherosclerosis, levels lower than these may require treatment (a 'desirable' cholesterol level is less than 5.2 mmol/L). Low HDL-cholesterol, below 0.9 mmol/L (35 mg/dL), is also a risk factor for atherosclerosis, as is a high LDL-cholesterol (with a target often of 2.5 mmol/L or less).

While there is no doubt that hyperlipidaemia, especially hypercholesterolaemia, is associated with increased incidence of premature ischaemic heart disease,[92] intervention with drug therapy, especially in some populations, has been controversial, as for example in healthy women[93] and the elderly (where high cholesterol levels may even be protective of health[94]). However, the benefits of treating raised cholesterol in most patients with CHD after a myocardial infarction (secondary prevention) are clear.[95]

There is certainly a clear consensus in the mainstream literature that LDL-cholesterol is a significant cardiovascular risk factor. However, the predictive value of future cardiovascular events of LDL-cholesterol appears limited.[96] LDL-cholesterol is a more complex issue than previously realised; the subfraction of intermediate density lipoprotein (IDL) cholesterol might be the true atherogenic factor and the number of LDL particles is also important.[96] HDL-cholesterol is a more sensitive predictor of cardiovascular risk and levels are predictive of major cardiovascular events in patients treated with statins, even those with target LDL-cholesterol.[96] Overall, the correlation between HDL-cholesterol and the incidence of CHD is better than for LDL-cholesterol. This holds true for all LDL levels, independent of statin drug treatment.[96] Triglyceride levels are acknowledged by many experts now as an independent risk factor (that is, are not conditional on LDL-cholesterol or HDL-cholesterol levels) and non-fasting levels (VLDL plus chylomicrons) could well be more relevant to predicting risk than fasting triglycerides (VLDL).[97,98]

As one group of cardiologists observed: 'Despite the considerable progress made in cardiovascular disease management in recent decades, there is almost unanimous agreement among epidemiologists and clinicians that coronary risk assessment based exclusively on LDL-cholesterol is not optimal …'.[99]

Despite these considerations, many patients present to herbal clinicians with a clear objective of using phytotherapy to lower elevated cholesterol. In such circumstances, given that herbs are not as powerful as statins, attention to other risk factors is also in the patient's interest. One key herb with a broader activity on cardiovascular risk factors already discussed in the preamble is garlic (especially the allicin-releasing products or the uncooked crushed cloves). Fortunately this broader activity seems to be 'built-in' for many herbs, owing to the molecular promiscuity of their key constituents: turmeric is a good example of this.

As noted earlier, garlic appears to be able to lower plasma fibrinogen. Starting in the 1970s, elevated fibrinogen levels were shown to be a major independent cardiovascular risk factor. Higher fibrinogen levels enhance the CHD risk of patients with hypertension and diabetes and for cigarette smokers. Fibrinogen strongly affects blood rheology and coagulation, platelet aggregation. It is an acute-phase inflammation marker and has direct effects on the vessel wall. The association of fibrinogen with traditional cardiovascular risk factors and its independent contribution suggests it may play a mechanistic role by which the risk factors exert their effect, for example smoking, even LDL-cholesterol. Elevated LDL-cholesterol poses an ominous risk when accompanied by a high fibrinogen level. Reduction of high levels of fibrinogen with drugs reduces cardiovascular morbidity and mortality.[100]

Another interesting risk factor is lipoprotein(a) (Lp(a)). Apolipoprotein(a), a large glycoprotein made by the liver, is linked to an LDL particle to produce Lp(a). Lp(a) has been studied as a cardiovascular risk factor since the 1970s, but interest had declined in the mid-1990s owing to some underpowered epidemiological studies that found no link to cardiovascular disease. Investigation of Lp(a) has also been hampered by inconsistent approaches to its measurement. Several studies, culminating with a large meta-analysis of 126 000 participants published in 2009, have clearly returned Lp(a) to the cardiovascular risk agenda.[101] Linear and independent associations were shown for Lp(a) levels and incidence of CHD and stroke. Two recent genetic studies suggest that this association is causal, at least in people of European ancestry.[102] Ginkgo has been shown to reduce Lp(a) in a small clinical study (see Ginkgo monograph).

Even supporting the immune system and oral health of a patient with or at risk of atheroma might improve their cardiovascular health prospects. A review of the published literature concluded that strong evidence supports an association between acute coronary syndromes and acute respiratory infections.[103] Both peak in winter and acute infections could precede up to a third of events. Large and well-designed retrospective studies consistently find a 2- to 3-fold increase in risk within 1 to 2 weeks after a respiratory infection. It is especially marked in the first few days (nearly a 5-fold increase). Up to half of all deaths during influenza epidemics are attributable to cardiovascular causes. Several, but not all, epidemiological studies have shown that *Chlamydia pneumoniae* antibodies may be related to the development of cardiovascular disease. Additionally Chlamydia seems to be present in atheroma, but not healthy arteries.[104] A meta-analysis of 29 epidemiological studies found the risk of developing cardiovascular disease was a significant 34% higher in people with periodontal disease (7 cohort studies), and the odds ratio was 2.35 from 22 case-control studies.[105]

It should be kept in mind that the process of a heart attack has no direct relationship to cholesterol. Essentially there are three key factors that can lead to a dangerous heart attack. These are the rupture of vulnerable or unstable plaque in a coronary artery wall, the resultant formation of a massive clot or thrombus (thrombosis) that starves the heart of oxygen, and thirdly the dangerous rhythm disturbance that can follow when the heart is shocked in this way. Logically, this process would argue that, through stabilising plaque, making the blood less likely to clot and rendering the heart less prone to dangerous rhythm disturbances, the risk of a dangerous heart attack can be reduced.

Gotu kola could have a role in managing unstable plaque. Other key herbs that might also be useful in this scenario are garlic for blood quality and possibly hawthorn to protect heart rhythm. Vulnerable plaque is one that is at high short-term risk of rupture and plaque rupture is by far the most frequent cause of arterial thrombosis. It is deemed responsible for about 75% of coronary blockages leading to heart attacks and about 90% of carotid artery blockages causing ischaemic stroke. Only plaque with a very thin fibrous cap is at risk of rupture and even just a small area is life-threatening. These plaques are essentially unstable because of a deficiency of connective tissue. Even in the presence of widespread arterial disease, rarely more than a few plaques appear to be at risk of rupture at any given moment.[106] One group of researchers observed: 'It is not clear why some plaques lead to clinical manifestations, whereas many others remain asymptomatic and heal with subsequent fibrosis...'.[107] In a sense, arterial plaque is a type of wound on the blood vessel wall and vulnerable plaque can be seen as either not healing appropriately, or in the early stages of healing (fibrosis).

Gotu kola may help this unstable plaque to heal. In two 12-month placebo-controlled clinical trials, gotu kola stabilised echolucent low density carotid[108] and femoral artery plaque.[109] (See the gotu kola monograph for more details.) Arterial plaque that is echolucent (low echogenicity by ultrasound) has a limited amount of connective tissue and the plaque is weaker and prone to ulceration and rupture. This is not quite the same as vulnerable coronary artery plaque, but shares many similarities. On the basis of these findings, it would be interesting to investigate the impact of the long-term intake of gotu kola on health outcomes in patients with coronary artery disease.

Treatment

Diet and lifestyle

Dietary treatment should be the first-line therapy for hyperlipidaemia, especially in those population groups where the benefit of more aggressive therapy has not been established. All common and most of the rarer types of hyperlipidaemia respond to diet therapy. Saturated fat intake should be reduced. Fibre, especially sticky soluble fibre from fruit, vegetables, legumes, oats and rice, should be increased. Fish consumption, especially of oily fish, should also be increased. There is benefit in the use of monounsaturated vegetable oils such as olive oil, and cholesterol intake should be reduced. Alcohol intake should be moderate and binge drinking avoided.[110]

One interesting protocol that synthesises several aspects of the above recommendations into a systematic approach is known as the 'dietary portfolio'. A Canadian research team headed by David Jenkins has been clinically investigating this strategy for several years, with remarkable results. Their dietary portfolio has been the subject of more than 10 major publications and it is based on the concept of introducing foods that actively reduce cholesterol.[111] In other words, it is a dietary approach based on 'do' rather than 'don't'. The dietary portfolio has four simple aspects:

- Plant sterols (as a supplement or in a functional food) about 2 g/day
- Viscous fibre (oat bran, psyllium, eggplant and so on) about 20 g/day
- Almonds about 30 g/day
- Soya protein about 40 g/day.

The most impressive study using the dietary portfolio was published in *JAMA* in 2003.[111] Here participants were randomised into one of three interventions for 1 month:

- A control diet based on whole wheat cereals and low fat milk which was low in saturated fat
- The above diet plus lovastatin 20 mg/day
- The dietary portfolio.

For the control diet, an average decrease of LDL-cholesterol of 8% was observed. In contrast, those participants receiving the statin or on the dietary portfolio had mean decreases in LDL-cholesterol of 30.9% and 28.6% respectively. In other words, the dietary portfolio achieved a similar cholesterol reduction to a statin drug. Triglycerides were also reduced by 8%.

One key aspect of the dietary portfolio approach is that it incorporates a vegetarian diet, with a large part of the protein coming from soya. This is not acceptable to some patients; hence a partial approach (without the soya) could be adopted, combined with an appropriate selection of the herbal options discussed below.

Herbs

Key herbs to consider are Curcuma (turmeric), *Allium sativum* (garlic), Cynara (globe artichoke) and berberine-containing herbs (in extracts capable of delivering relatively high doses of berberine). Adequate doses of all these herbs need to be prescribed to achieve meaningful clinical results (see previous, and the relevant monographs). There are also some promising in vivo results for hawthorn berries (not the leaves, see the hawthorn monograph).

These herbs can be supported by saponin-containing herbs that are believed to sequester cholesterol in the digestive tract. Gymnema is rich in saponins and has been found to reduce cholesterol in vivo[112] and in a clinical trial in type 2 diabetes.[113] *Medicago sativa* (alfalfa) seed has also been shown to lower cholesterol in a clinical trial.[114] This may be due to both its saponin and mucilage content.

Mucilages are a class of polysaccharide related to soluble fibre. Soluble fibre such as guar gum is thought to lower cholesterol by several possible mechanisms. In particular, bacterial flora in the large bowel metabolise soluble fibre to produce short-chain fatty acids (SCFA). Some of these SCFA are carried by the portal venous system to the liver where they might influence hepatic metabolism to decrease cholesterol biosynthesis. Patients can supplement their soluble fibre intake with mucilages such as Ulmus (slippery elm), Althaea (marshmallow root) and seeds or hulls from *Plantago* species

(psyllium, ispaghula). See also the discussion of mucilages in Chapter 2 for more data on the impact of psyllium on lowering plasma cholesterol in clinical trials.

Green tea consumption has been shown to significantly reduce serum cholesterol and triglycerides and increase HDL.[115]

Example herbal treatment

Cynara scolymus	1:2	45 mL
Gymnema sylvestre	1:1	35 mL
Crataegus laevigata berry	1:2	25 mL
	TOTAL	105 mL

Dose: 8 mL with water two to three times a day.

Together with allicin-releasing garlic tablets (equivalent to about 6 to 12 g/day of fresh garlic) and providing at least 12 mg/day of alliin).

CASE HISTORY

A 74-year-old woman in good overall health was receiving ongoing treatment for emotional and digestive problems. In late 2006 her total serum cholesterol was elevated at 7.0 with LDL-cholesterol at 4.1 (and a high HDL). A powder formulation delivering 4.4 g/day Cynara, 1.85 g/day phytosterols and 4.0 g/day psyllium husks and other aspects of the dietary portfolio were recommended. The patient was able to comply with most of these, but did not like soya, so found taking it difficult. Hence that aspect of the treatment was left out. Around 10 weeks later her total cholesterol tested at 6.0, with an LDL reading of 3.2. Hence, a 22% reduction was achieved, even using the modified dietary portfolio without the soya, but with added Cynara.

Palpitations

Palpitations (undue awareness of the beating of the heart) can be a significant source of anxiety to the sufferer. The awareness is most commonly brought about by a benign change in the rhythm or rate of the heart (rather than the heart being actually damaged), amplified in the resonant chamber of a tense thoracic cavity. However, sinus tachycardia or less benign arrhythmias such as ventricular or atrial tachycardia, heart block or atrial fibrillation may be responsible. These factors should be excluded in diagnosis.

Treatment

Diet and lifestyle

A key element in palpitations is likely to be diaphragmatic spasm, unconscious tension in this large muscle and others in the wall of the chest. Palpitations (along with hyperventilation, some nervous dyspepsia and swallowing difficulties) are therefore an important indication for a coordinated programme of breathing exercises, best initiated under instruction. Patients should avoid excessive nicotine and caffeine intake. Intake of chocolate, cheese and synthetic food preservatives should be reduced. Vasodilator drugs and asthma or nasal treatments containing sympathomimetic (e.g. ephedrine) drugs should be reviewed. Excessive intake of the stimulant herbs Ephedra, Panax and Paulinia (guarana) and Cola should be avoided. Methods to reduce emotional stress should be advised.

Herbs

The combination of benign arrhythmias or ectopic beats with thoracic tension may be treated with *Leonurus cardiaca* (motherwort), Lycopus (bugleweed), Corydalis, Ginkgo, *Salvia miltiorrhiza* (dan shen) and particularly Crataegus (see available monographs).

Lycopus (bugleweed) must be considered if the patient's thyroid is overactive. Emotional and mental tensions can be reduced with the above combined with herbs such as Valeriana, Scutellaria (skullcap), Passiflora, *Piper methysticum* (kava) and Hypericum (St John's wort).

The dyspeptic and reflux conditions often associated with this syndrome should be treated with the appropriate upper digestive relaxants (see the Digestive system section).

Example liquid formula

Corydalis ambigua	1:2	20 mL
Crataegus laevigata leaf	1:2	30 mL
Leonurus cardiaca	1:2	15 mL
Ginkgo biloba (standardised extract)	2:1	20 mL
Scutellaria lateriflora	1:2	20 mL
		105 mL

Dose: 8 mL with water twice a day.

Chronic venous disorders

Varicose veins are a common disorder, with prevalence in the adult population of between 14% for large varices and 59% for small telangiectasias. The term chronic venous insufficiency (CVI) defines functional abnormalities of the venous system producing advanced symptoms including oedema, skin changes and leg ulcers. Both entities, varicose veins and CVI, may be summarised under the term chronic venous disorders, which includes the full spectrum of morphological and functional abnormalities of the venous system. Concerning the aetiology of venous disorders, controversial theories exist leading to different therapeutic concepts. There is probably a vicious circle between structural changes in valves and the venous wall and haemodynamic forces leading to reflux and venous hypertension. Chronic venous insufficiency requires chronic management.[116]

Varicose veins and CVI have long been regarded as disorders of valvular incompetence. However, recent evidence suggests that changes in the vein wall could well precede incompetence. For example, varicosities are often observed below competent valves and can occur before valvular incompetence. Defects in extracellular matrix and collagen composition in the vein wall are thought to be part of this process.[117]

Areas of intimal hyperplasia and smooth muscle cell proliferation are often noted in varicose veins, although regions of atrophy are also present. The total elastin content in varicose veins is reduced compared with non-varicose veins;

changes in overall collagen content are uncertain. Matrix metalloproteinases (MMPs), including MMP-1, MMP-2, MMP-3, MMP-7 and MMP-9, and tissue inhibitor of metalloproteinase (TIMP)-1 and TIMP-3 are upregulated in varicose veins. Activation of the endothelium stimulates the recruitment of leucocytes and release of growth factors, leading to smooth muscle cell proliferation and migration. Dysregulated apoptosis has also been demonstrated in varicose veins.[117]

Although there are few prospects for cosmetically changing established varicosities, herbal treatments stress the need to maintain good venous and connective tissue tone, so as to reduce further trouble and improve venous return from the lower body.

Treatment

Diet and lifestyle

Fruit and vegetable intake should be high to maintain optimum levels of flavonols and other supportive elements. Berries are particularly rich in vasoprotective phytochemicals. Regular walking, and resting or sleeping with the legs elevated, is often to be recommended. Elastic stockings should be useful, especially if applied first thing in the morning. Cold water applied to the legs from the knee to the foot can help to stimulate circulation and tone the area.

Herbs

Aesculus hippocastanum (horsechestnut) and *Ruscus* (butcher's broom), taken internally and also applied topically in a cream, are key aspects of treatment (see monographs). These herbs are proven to increase venous tone. Aesculus should not be applied to broken skin.

Connective tissue stabilising herbs (pine bark and grape seed) and vasoprotective microvascular herbs (bilberry, Ginkgo, grape seed, pine bark and gotu kola) improve connective tissue function. Gotu kola has proven clinical benefits in venous insufficiency and a noted activity for connective tissue regeneration (see monograph).

Improve circulatory function with circulatory herbs, especially Ginkgo, Achillea (yarrow) and rosemary, and antiplatelet herbs such as turmeric.

Melilotus (sweet clover) has anti-oedema activity and improves venous return.

Bilberry's benefits in venous insufficiency are supported by clinical trials and it has the advantage of being safe in early pregnancy (see bilberry monograph).

Herbs beneficial by topical application include Symphytum (comfrey), Arnica, Calendula and Hamamelis (witchhazel).

Example liquid formula

Aesculus hippocastanum	1:2	30 mL
Ruscus aculeatus	1:2	30 mL
Ginkgo biloba (standardised extract)	2:1	20 mL
Centella asiatica (standardised extract)	1:1	30 mL
	TOTAL	110 mL

Dose: 8 mL with water twice a day.

Stasis dermatitis and stasis ulceration

Stasis dermatitis (varicose eczema) develops in the legs as a result of chronic oedema and venous incompetence. It usually begins as a scaling associated with itching over the medial aspect of the ankle and can progress to become stained as a result of extravasation of blood.

Stasis ulceration (varicose ulcer) is a further complication of stasis dermatitis. The ulcers are shallow and can be quite large. They often result from damage such as knocking the leg and can take months or longer to heal. Bacterial infection is present.

Treatment

Treatment is essentially as for varicose veins, but the following additions or modifications are important to prevent further damage and heal any ulcer. Oral doses of Aesculus have demonstrated clinical benefit in varicose ulcers (see Aesculus monograph).

Aesculus or Ruscus should not be applied topically. The best topical treatments consist of Calendula and Echinacea root as a lotion and Calendula cream applied on the good skin around the edge of the ulcer.

Inclusion of Centella (gotu kola) for promotion of healing and Echinacea root for its immune effects in the oral treatment can be beneficial.

CASE HISTORY

A 62-year-old woman had a very bad varicose ulcer, several centimetres in width. She had experienced problems with varicose veins for many years to the point where she could not stand still for any length of time (and had to do her ironing sitting down). Episodes of cellulitis in her legs also occurred from time to time. Her conventional medications were a thiazide diuretic and a cardioselective beta-blocker.

The following treatments were prescribed:

Ginkgo biloba (standardised extract)	2:1	20 mL
Centella asiatica	1:2	35 mL
Ruscus aculeatus	1:2	25 mL
Aesculus hippocastanum	1:2	20 mL
	TOTAL	100 mL

Dose: 5 mL with water three times daily.
Topical treatments consisting of:

- A 50/50 mixture of Calendula 1:2 and *Echinacea angustifolia* root 1:2 diluted one part with five parts of sterile water as a lotion for bathing the ulcer
- Calendula cream and comfrey cream which were to be applied to the good skin **around** the ulcer several times a day.

After about 4 weeks of treatment there was a noticeable improvement in the ulcer. With continued treatment over the next few months the ulcer healed and she could do her ironing standing up. The results of the herbal treatment had far surpassed her expectations.

Deep vein thrombosis

Under certain conditions, a thrombus, composed mainly of platelets and fibrin, can form in a deep vein. In 1856, Virchow described the classic triad of venostasis, hypercoagulability and vascular damage as predisposing factors. These factors underlie the many other risk factors that have been identified, such as surgery, oral contraceptives, air travel, cancer and pregnancy. A patient with a spontaneous deep vein thrombosis (DVT) has one chance in six of having cancer diagnosed within 2 years.

In at least 40% of cases, fragments of thrombus break loose to form a pulmonary embolus. This can be life threatening.

The management of acute DVT and any subsequent pulmonary embolism requires conventional acute medical care. However, phytotherapy does have a role in the prevention of DVT in those at risk, and in the management of the chronic compromised venous return that may subsequently develop (postphlebitic syndrome).

Prevention

Herbs that improve venous tone will decrease the likelihood of venostasis. Aesculus (horsechestnut) has been proven to reduce the risk of DVT in a clinical trial (see monograph). Other herbs listed under chronic venous insufficiency are also relevant.

Integrity of vessel walls can be maintained with OPC-containing herbs including hawthorn, grape seed and pine bark extracts.

Circulation and the quality of the blood can be improved with Ginkgo, dan shen, ginger, garlic and turmeric.

Postphlebitis syndrome

Treatment is similar to above (since recurrences must be prevented) but emphasis is also given to assist venous return and reduce oedema.

Collateral circulation can be promoted with exercise and herbs that improve circulation and the integrity of fine vessels such as Ginkgo, bilberry and grape seed extract.

CASE HISTORY

A male patient aged 39 developed multiple DVTs in one leg and serious pulmonary embolism following a long intercontinental flight. As a result he was left with substantially impaired venous return in one leg, with a tendency to oedema in that limb.

He was prescribed herbal treatments with the aim of improving his venous return by enhancing venous tone and developing collateral circulation. Treatment was superimposed on a regular exercise programme and was as follows:

- Vein tablets (2 tablets/day) each containing:
  Horsechestnut 1.2 g (standardised to contain 40 mg escin)
  Butcher's broom 800 mg (standardised to 20 mg ruscogenin)
  Ginkgo biloba 1.5 g (standardised to contain 7.3 mg flavone glycosides)
  As well as the following:

- Grape seed extract 50 mg tablets. Dose: 2 tablets/day
- Bilberry tablets 6000 mg (fresh weight) standardised to contain 15 mg anthocyanosides. Dose: 4 tablets/day
- Hawthorn leaf tablets (1000 mg). Dose: 2 tablets/day.

Over a period of 3 years there was a considerable improvement in his condition. He can walk and exercise without impairment and is largely free of symptoms.

Hypotension syndrome

Hypotension, or very low blood pressure, can be associated with a number of serious diseases, or can result from drug therapy. Current medical thinking does not associate any health issue with mild hypotension. In fact, mild hypotension (that is, blood pressure in the normal range but significantly lower than average) is considered to be beneficial.

However, herbalists recognise a syndrome associated with mild hypotension that can include depression, lack of energy and episodic dizziness or light-headedness. Some scientific studies now appear to support the existence of this syndrome.[118] Hypotension has been associated with depression in the elderly[119] and in the general population.[120]

The following herbs should be considered:

* Circulatory stimulants such as cayenne and prickly ash
* Ginkgo to improve nourishment of brain tissue and cerebral circulation (see monograph)
* Tonics especially Korean ginseng and adrenal trophorestoratives such as Rehmannia and licorice to help maintain blood pressure and energy
* St John's wort is indicated for any associated depression
* Judicious use of herbs to increase blood pressure such as licorice at higher doses can be considered.

Example liquid formula

Ginkgo biloba (standardised extract)	2:1	20 mL
Zanthoxylum clava-herculis	1:2	15 mL
Hypericum perforatum	1:2	25 mL
Panax ginseng	1:2	15 mL
Glycyrrhiza glabra	1:1	25 mL
	TOTAL	100 mL

Dose: 8 mL with water twice daily.

Cerebral atherosclerosis and peripheral circulation disorders

Cerebral atherosclerosis can lead to vascular dementia, which is the second commonest cause of dementia (after Alzheimer's disease). It can also lead to transient ischaemic attacks.

As with other disorders involving ischaemia, cerebrovascular risk factors should be identified and treated. For example, hypertension may increase the risk of dementia by inducing small vessel disease and white matter lesions (leukoaraiosis).[121,122]

Treatment

* The key herb is Ginkgo, used as the standardised extract in tablet or liquid form. Studies have shown that this extract can compensate for deficits associated with cerebral ischaemia. It may in fact prove to be a specific treatment for white matter disease (see Ginkgo monograph).
* Prickly ash can improve arterial circulation (traditional indication), but should not be used if hypertension is

present. Rosemary and *Salvia miltiorrhiza* (dan shen) should also be considered to improve circulation.

* Garlic, especially in allicin-releasing preparations, improves flow in fine blood vessels and treats cardiovascular risk factors. Other antiplatelet herbs that may be beneficial include turmeric, ginger and Coleus.
* Herbs to boost cognitive function such as Bacopa, sage and Ginkgo should be used to compensate for any reduced cognitive function.
* Antioxidant and vasoprotective herbs such as bilberry and grape seed can be of value to minimise further deterioration.
* The same approach can be applied in peripheral vascular disease, poor circulation and Raynaud's phenomenon.
* In addition, for Raynaud's phenomenon, herbs with peripheral vasodilating properties such as cramp bark, hawthorn and Coleus could be considered.

CASE HISTORY: RAYNAUD'S PHENOMENON

A 60-year-old female patient developed Raynaud's phenomenon in conjunction with scleroderma. On examination she had ischaemic signs on several fingertips in both hands. Her herbal treatment for this problem consisted of the following:

Zingiber officinale	1:2	10 mL
Ginkgo biloba (standardised extract)	2:1	20 mL
Crataegus folia	1:2	20 mL
Zanthoxylum clava-herculis	1:2	15 mL
Echinacea angustifolia root	1:2	35 mL
	TOTAL	100 mL

Dose: 5 mL with water three times a day.

This treatment was able to control her Raynaud's symptoms and prevent the development of gangrene. Echinacea was included in the formula to help prevent infection in the ischaemic fingertips. The treatment did arrest the progression of ischaemic changes and over time improved the health of the fingertips.

Buerger's disease

Buerger's disease is an unusual chronic blood vessel disease.[123,124] In 1908 Leo Buerger from New York first described a pattern of what he termed 'presenile spontaneous gangrene' due to a distinctive disease pattern he called thromboangiitis obliterans (literally the obliteration of blood vessels by inflammatory and clotting processes).[125]

Buerger's disease is indeed an inflammatory, occlusive (blocking) disorder, affecting the small and medium-size arteries and veins.[123] Typical patients are mostly young, male tobacco smokers and the clinical features include ischaemia in the limbs, leg ulcers and even gangrene of the fingers or toes.[123] It is an unusual disorder because the large arteries supplying the heart, brain and abdominal organs are typically spared.[125] The most serious outcome is amputation.

The average age at onset is 34 years and the male to female ratio is 7.5:1.[125] The reported incidence in the US is around

10 cases per 100 000 population, making the total number of cases around 30 000. It has declined in incidence over the past 30 years, possibly because of less smoking. However, the application of a more strict diagnosis is another explanation for this decline.[125] There is a much higher incidence in Eastern Europe, the Mediterranean, India, the Middle East and Japan and Korea.[125] In Japan, Korea and India it can account for up to around half of all cases of peripheral vascular disease.[125]

The cause of Buerger's disease is still unknown, although it has been suggested that it is an autoimmune response triggered when nicotine is present.[126] Certainly, recent observations point to an endothelial dysfunction in arteries not yet involved (particularly impaired vasodilation), and there are elevated levels of antiendothelial cell antibodies.[127] The histological appearance of the inflamed blood vessels does suggest immune involvement, with inflammation of the whole vessel wall and (typically) lymphocytic infiltration.[128] Antiphospholipid antibodies as well as elevated levels of homocysteine have also been implicated,[129] as has excessive exposure to arsenic via tobacco intake.[130]

On the last point, there can be no doubt that tobacco use in some form is crucial to the onset and progression of Buerger's disease.[125] The way the tobacco is ingested appears not to be critical, since the disease has developed in tobacco chewers and snuff users.[125] Ceasing tobacco use favourably impacts the progression and recurrence of active disease and is the best means to avoid limb amputation.[125]

In terms of basic management, all forms of tobacco use and even nicotine patches should be avoided.[131] Intravenous iloprost (a prostaglandin analogue) has shown clinical benefit.[131] Arterial bypass and lumbar sympathectomy are surgical techniques used to avoid amputation, but appear to be of limited application and benefit.[131]

Treatment

There are few clinical data on the use of herbs in the management of Buerger's disease, apart from some studies of traditional Chinese medicines.[132,133] Dong quai (*Angelica sinensis*) has been successfully used to treat Buerger's disease and constrictive aortitis, and is often combined with dan shen (*Salvia miltorrhiza*) in the treatment of peripheral vascular disorders.[134]

Case results for 200 cases of Buerger's disease using a combination of traditional Chinese and conventional medicine were reported.[135] The authors observed three key principles that they believed should be followed in the management of the disease. These were: (1) improve blood circulation and remove blood stasis; (2) control infection in any ischaemic lesions such as leg ulcers; (3) protect the blood flow and promote healing. These principles can also be applied using phytotherapy in the management of Buerger's disease.

Given the above, and the factors and issues identified in the aetiology of Buerger's disease, the following are suggested to be key herbs for managing this disorder:

- Ginkgo (*Ginkgo biloba*), dong quai, ginger (*Zingiber officinale*) and dan shen to improve peripheral circulation and tissue oxygen supply

- Echinacea root (*Echinacea angustifolia* and/or *purpurea*) to support immunity, control infection, promote healing and balance the autoimmune aspects[136]
- Hawthorn leaves (*Crataegus* species) to act as a peripheral vasodilator, support connective tissue and provide antioxidant activity
- Garlic (*Allium sativum*) as the allicin-releasing powdered bulb because of its clinically proven benefits in boosting the microcirculatory blood supply, enhancing fibrinolytic activity, lowering plasma fibrinogen and decreasing platelet aggregation.[137] Garlic is also useful for managing heavy metal toxic exposure
- Gotu kola (*Centella asiatica*) to promote tissue healing and support the venous circulation (see monograph).

CASE HISTORY

A male patient aged 55 presented with a diagnosis of Buerger's disease. He also had cardiomyopathy (undetected at the time of initial presentation), possibly of viral origin, with considerable enlargement of the heart. The Buerger's disease was diagnosed 20 years prior and, despite his having given up smoking for about 15 years (he had smoked for 18 years), was following a progressive course.

Circulation to his legs was severely compromised as assessed by Doppler flow analysis and he was told by his medical specialist to 'get used to the idea of being in a wheelchair'. His walking was impaired, he had pain and his wife stated that his legs 'felt dead' when they brushed against her when they were lying in bed together.

Medical treatment consisted of two lumbar sympathectomies, one half an aspirin a day, enalapril maleate for his raised blood pressure and pentoxifylline. When his cardiomyopathy was discovered (about 1 year into herbal treatment) he was taken off pentoxifylline and placed on nifedipine.

The following herbal formula was prescribed:

Crataegus folia	1:2	30 mL
Salvia miltiorrhiza	1:2	30 mL
Ginkgo biloba (standardised extract)	2:1	20 mL
Echinacea angustifolia root	1:2	30 mL
Zingiber officinale	1:2	10 mL
Angelica sinensis	1:2	30 mL
	TOTAL	150 mL

Dose: 10 mL with water twice a day.

In addition he was prescribed two allicin-releasing garlic tablets (containing 6 mg each of alliin) per day.

Suggested dietary changes were to eat less meat and considerably more fruit and vegetables, especially berries.

Over 3 years of treatment there was a gradual and significant improvement. By his last visit before ceasing herbal therapy he was completely free of symptoms. Towards the end of herbal treatment the patient went on vacation and hiked 20 miles in one day with a pack. He has now taken up hiking over mountains as his hobby and can cover considerable distances for sustained periods, more than the average person.

Circulation had significantly improved in his feet and when he last went for Doppler flow measurements the hospital doctor told him the condition of his legs was so good that he did not require this test. His cardiologist was astounded that his heart had also improved. Ventricular function was now normal and his enlarged heart had reduced to near normal. This was an unexpected but welcome side effect of the herbal treatment.

References

1. Porkert M. *The Theoretical Foundations of Chinese Medicine*. Massachusetts: MIT Press; 1978. pp. 197–212.

2. Oi Y, Okamoto M, Nitta M, et al. Alliin and volatile sulfur-containing compounds in garlic enhance the thermogenesis by increasing norepinephrine secretion in rats. *J Nutr Biochem*. 1998;9(2):60–66.

3. Sendl A. Allium sativum and Allium ursinum: Part 1. Chemistry, analysis, history, botany. *Phytomedicine*. 1995;4:323–339.

4. Warshafsky S, Kamer RS, Sivak SL. Effect of garlic on total serum cholesterol. *Ann Intern Med*. 1993;119:599–605.

5. Silagy C, Neil A. Garlic as a lipid lowering agent – a meta-analysis. *J R Coll Physicians Lond*. 1994;28(1):39–45.

6. Simons LA, Balasubramaniam S, Von Konigsmark M, et al. On the effect of garlic on plasma lipids and lipoproteins in mild hypercholesterolaemia. *Atherosclerosis*. 1995;113:219–225.

7. Isaacsohn JL, Moser M, Stein EA, et al. Garlic powder and plasma lipids and lipoproteins. *Arch Intern Med*. 1998;158:1189–1194.

8. Berthold HK, Sudhop T, Von Bergmann K. Effect of a garlic oil preparation on serum lipoproteins and cholesterol metabolism: a randomized controlled trial. *JAMA*. 1998;279(23):1900–1902.

9. Reinhart KM, Talati R, White CM, Coleman CI. The impact of garlic on lipid parameters: a systematic review and meta-analysis. *Nutr Res Rev*. 2009;22(1):39–48.

10. Lawson LD, Wang ZJ. Low allicin release from garlic supplements: a major problem due to the sensitivities of alliinase activity. *J Agric Food Chem*. 2001;49(5):2592–2599.

11. Orekhov AN, Pivovarova EM, Tertov VV. Garlic powder tablets reduce atherogenicity of low density lipoprotein. A placebo-controlled double blind study. *Nutr Metab Cardiovasc Dis*. 1996;6:21–31.

12. Breithaupt-Grogler K, Ling M, Boudoulas H, et al. Protective effect of chronic garlic intake on elastic properties of aorta in the elderly. *Circulation*. 1997;96(8):2649–2655.

13. Koscielny J, Klüssendorf D, Latza R, et al. The antiatherosclerotic effect of Allium sativum. *Atherosclerosis*. 1999;144(1):237–249.

14. Schiermeier Q. German garlic study under scrutiny. *Nature*. 1999; 401(6754):629.

15. Koscielny J, Schmitt R, Radtke H, et al. Garlic study vindicated by official investigation. *Nature*. 2000;404(6778):542.

16. Vastag B. Garlic prevents plaque. *JAMA*. 2002;288(11):1342.

17. Silagy CA, Neil HAW. A meta-analysis of the effect of garlic on blood pressure. *J Hyperten*. 1994;12(4):463–468.

18. Tapsell LC, Hemphill I, Cobiac L, et al. Health benefits of herbs and spices: the past, the present, the future. *Med J Aust*. 2006;185(4 suppl):S4–S24.

19. Reinhart KM, Coleman CI, Teevan C, et al. Effects of garlic on blood pressure in patients with and without systolic hypertension: a meta-analysis. *Ann Pharmacother*. 2008;42(12):1766–1771.

20. Ried K, Frank OR, Stocks NP, et al. Effect of garlic on blood pressure: a systematic review and meta-analysis. *BMC Cardiovasc Disord*. 2008;8:13.

21. Kiesewetter H, Jung F, Jung EM, et al. Effect of garlic on platelet aggregation in patients with increased risk of juvenile ischaemic attack. *Eur J Clin Pharmacol*. 1993;45:333–336.

22. Legnani C, Frascaro M, Guazzaloca G, et al. Effects of a dried garlic preparation on fibrinolysis and platelet aggregation in healthy subjects. *Arzneimittel-Forschung*. 1993;43(2):119–122.

23. Morris J, Burke V, Mori TA, et al. Effects of garlic extract on platelet aggregation: a randomized placebo-controlled double blind study. *Clin Exp Pharmacol Physiol*. 1995;22:414–417.

24. Ali M, Thomson M. Consumption of a garlic clove a day could be beneficial in preventing thrombosis. *Prostaglandins Leukot Essent Fatty Acids*. 1995;53:211–212.

25. Rendu F. L'ajoene, un antiagrégant efficace et subtil. *Acta Bot Gallica*. 1996;143(2/3):149–154.

26. Reuter HD. Allium sativum and allium ursinum: Part 2. Pharmacology and medicinal application. *Phytomedicine*. 1995;2(1):73–91.

27. Gadkari JV, Joshi VD. Effect of ingestion of raw garlic on serum cholesterol level, clotting time and fibrinolytic activity in normal subjects. *J Postgrad Med*. 1991;37(3):128–131.

28. Kiesewetter H, Jung F, Mrowietz C, et al. Effects of garlic on blood fluidity and fibrinolytic activity: a randomised, placebo-controlled, double blind study. *Br J Clin Pract Symp Suppl*. 1990;69:24–29.

29. Jung EM, Jung F, Mrowietz C, et al. Influence of garlic powder on cutaneous microcirculation. A randomized placebo-controlled double blind cross-over study in apparently healthy subjects. *Arzneimittelforschung*. 1991;41(6):626–630.

30. Anim-Nyame N, Sooranna SR, Johnson MR, et al. Garlic supplementation increases peripheral blood flow: a role for interleukin-6? *J Nutr Biochem*. 2004;15(1):30–36.

31. Lefer DJ. A new gaseous signaling molecule emerges: cardioprotective role of hydrogen sulfide. *Proc Natl Acad Sci USA*. 2007;104(46):17907–17908.

32. Benavides GA, Squadrito GL, Mills RW, et al. Hydrogen sulfide mediates the vasoactivity of garlic. *Proc Natl Acad Sci USA*. 2007;104(46):17977–17982.

33. Rose KD, Croissant PD, Parliament CF, et al. Spontaneous spinal epidural hematoma with associated platelet dysfunction from excessive garlic ingestion: a case report. *Neurosurgery*. 1990;26(5):880–882.

34. Burnham BE. Garlic as a possible risk for postoperative bleeding. *Plast Reconstr Surg*. 1995;95(1):213.

35. Mohammed Abdul MI, Jiang X, Williams KM, et al. Pharmacodynamic interaction of warfarin with cranberry but not with garlic in healthy subjects. *Br J Pharmacol*. 2008;154(8):1691–1700.

36. Lewis DA. *Anti-Inflammatory Drugs from Plant and Marine Sources*. Basel: Birkhäuser Verlag; 1989. pp. 137–164.

37. Leung AY. Rutin. In: Leung AY, ed. *Encyclopedia of Common Natural Ingredients Used in Food, Drugs and Cosmetics*. New York: John Wiley; 1980.

38. Korkina LG, Durnev AD, Suslova TB, et al. Oxygen radical-mediated mutagenic effect of asbestos on human lymphocytes: suppression by oxygen radical scavengers. *Mutat Res*. 1992;265(2):245–253.

39. Negre-Salvayre A, Reaud V, Hariton C, Salvayre R. Protective effect of alpha-tocopherol, ascorbic acid and rutin against peroxidative stress induced by oxidized lipoproteins on lymphoid cell lines. *Biochem Pharmacol*. 1991;42(2):450–453.

40. Teofili L, Pierelli L, Iovino MS, et al. The combination of quercetin and cytosine arabinoside synergistically inhibits leukemic cell growth. *Leuk Res*. 1992;16(5):497–503.

41. Blumberg S, Clough G, Michel C. *Effects of Hydroxyethylrutosides on the Permeability of Frog Mesenteric Capillaries*. Presentation to the AGM of the British Microcirculation Society. London: Department of Physiology, Charing Cross and Westminster Medical School; 1987.

42. Burnand K. *Effect of hydroxyethyl rutosides on transcutaneous PO2 measurements*. Proceedings of the Surgical Research Society, Leeds, 1987.

43. Wismer R. The actions of tri-hydroxyethylrutoside on the permeability of the capillaries in man. *Praxis*. 1963;52:1412.

44. Halborg-Sorenson A, Hansen H. Chronic venous insufficiency treated with hydroxyethylrutosides. *Angiologica*. 1970;7:192.

45. Belcaro G, Rulo A, Candiani C. Evaluation of the microcirculatory effects of Venoruton in patients with chronic venous hypertension by laserdoppler flowmetry, transcutaneous PO2 and PCO2 measurements, leg volumetry and ambulatory venous pressure measurements. *Vasa*. 1989;18(2):146–151.

46. McEwan AJ, McArdle CS. Effort of hydroxyethylrutosides on blood oxygen levels and venous insuffiency symptoms in varicose veins. *BMJ*. 1971;2:138–141.

47. Clifford MN. Diet-derived phenols in plasma and tissues and their implications for health. *Planta Med*. 2004;70(12): 1103–1114.

48. Hollman PC, Katan MB. Bioavailability and health effects of dietary flavonols in man. *Arch Toxicol Suppl*. 1998;20: 237–248.

49. Haeger K. The debatable value of flavonoids in venous insufficiency. *Zbl Phlebol*. 1967;6:23.

50. Chen ZY, Zhang ZS, Kwan KY, et al. Endothelium-dependent relaxation induced by hawthorn extract in rat mesenteric artery. *Life Sci*. 1998;63(22):1983–1991.

51. Nakamura Y, Matsumoto H, Todoki K. Endothelium-dependent vasorelaxation induced by black currant concentrate in rat thoracic aorta. *Jpn J Pharmacol*. 2002;89:29–35.

52. Chen CC, Chow MP, Huang WC, et al. Flavonoids inhibit tumor necrosis factor-alpha-induced up-regulation of intercellular adhesion molecule-1 (ICAM-1) in respiratory epithelial cells through activator protein-1 and nuclear factor-kappaB: structure-activity relationships. *Mol Pharmacol*. 2004;66:683–693.

53. Stangl V, Lorenz M, Ludwig A, et al. The flavonoid phloretin suppresses stimulated expression of endothelial adhesion molecules and reduces activation of human platelets. *J Nutr*. 2005;135(2):172–178.

54. Kamata K, Kobayashi T, Matsumoto T, et al. Effects of chronic administration of fruit extract (Citrus unshiu Marc) on endothelial dysfunction in streptozotocin-induced diabetic rats. *Biol Pharm Bull*. 2005;28(2):267–270.

55. Ulicna O, Vancova O, Bozek P, et al. Rooibos tea (*Aspalathus linearis*) partially prevents oxidative stress in streptozotocin-induced diabetic rats. *Physiol Res*. 2006;55(2): 157–164.

56. Williamson G, Manach C. Bioavailability and bioefficacy of polyphenols in humans. II. Review of 93 intervention studies. *Am J Clin Nutr*. 2005;81(suppl):243–255.

57. Chong MF, Macdonald R, Lovegrove JA. Fruit polyphenols and CVD risk: a review of human intervention studies. *Br J Nutr*. 2010;104(suppl 3):S28–S39.

58. Incandela L, Cesarone MR, DeSanctis MT, et al. Treatment of diabetic microangiopathy and edema with HR (Paroven, Venoruton; O-(beta-hydroxyethyl)-rutosides): a prospective, placebo-controlled, randomized study. *J Cardiovasc Pharmacol Ther*. 2002;7(suppl 1):S11–S15.

59. Oyama J, Maeda T, Sasaki M, et al. Green tea catechins improve human forearm vascular function and have potent anti-inflammatory and anti-apoptotic effects in smokers. *Intern Med*. 2010;49(23): 2553–2559.

60. Schonlau F, Rohdewald P. Pycnogenol for diabetic retinopathy. A review. *Int Ophthalmol*. 2001;24(3):161–171.

61. Hertog MG, Feskens EJ, Hollman PC, et al. Dietary antioxidant flavonoids and risk of coronary heart disease: the Zutphen Elderly Study. *Lancet*. 1993;342(8878):1007–1011.

62. Esposito K, Marfella R, Ciotola M, et al. Effect of a Mediterranean-style diet on endothelial dysfunction and markers of vascular inflammation in the metabolic syndrome: a randomized trial. *JAMA*. 2004; 292(12):1440–1446.

63. Hung HC, Merchant A, Willett W, et al. The association between fruit and vegetable consumption and peripheral arterial disease. *Epidemiology*. 2003;14(6):659–665.

64. Bharani A, Ganguly A, Bhargava KD. Salutary effect of Terminalia Arjuna in patients with severe refractory heart failure. *Int J Cardiol*. 1995;49(3): 191–199.

65. Bone K. *Clinical Applications of Ayurvedic and Chinese Herbs*. Warwick, Australia: Phytotherapy Press; 1996. pp. 103–107.

66. Cheng TO. Cardiovascular effects of Danshen. *Int J Cardiol*. 2007;121(1): 9–22.

67. Erdine S, Ari O, Zanchetti A, et al. ESH-ESC guidelines for the management of hypertension. *Herz*. 2006;31(4): 331–338.

68. Yeater RA, Ullrich IH. Hypertension and exercise; where do we stand? *Postgrad Med*. 1992;91(5):429–434.

69. Beilin L. Epidemiology of hypertension. *Med Int*. 1993;24:351–355.

70. Kochar MS. Hypertension in obese patients. *Postgrad Med*. 1993;93(4):193–200.

71. Stolarz-Skrzypek K, Kuznetsova T, Thijs L, et al. Fatal and nonfatal outcomes, incidence of hypertension, and blood pressure changes in relation to urinary sodium excretion. *JAMA*. 2011;305(17):1777–1785.

72. He FJ, MacGregor GA. Effect of longer-term modest salt reduction on blood pressure. *Cochrane Database Syst Rev*. 2004;(3):CD004937.

73. Berkow SE, Barnard ND. Blood pressure regulation and vegetarian diets. *Nutr Rev*. 2005;63(1):1–8.

74. Appel LJ, Moore TJ, Obarzanek E, et al. A clinical trial of the effects of dietary patterns on blood pressure. *N Engl J Med*. 1997;336(16):1117–1124.

75. Van Horn L, McCoin M, Kris-Etherton PM, et al. The evidence for dietary prevention and treatment of cardiovascular disease. *J Am Diet Assoc*. 2008;108(2):287–331.

76. Geleijnse JM, Witteman JCM, Bak AAA, et al. Reduction in blood pressure with a low sodium, high potassium, high magnesium salt in older subjects with mild to moderate hypertension. *BMJ*. 1994;309:436–440.

77. Blake GH, Beebe DK. Management of hypertension; useful nonpharmacologic measures. *Postgrad Med*. 1991;90(1): 151–158.

78. Bonaa KH, Bjerve KS, Straume B, et al. Effect of eicosapentaenoic and docosahexaenoic acids on blood pressure in hypertension. *N Engl J Med*. 1990;322(12):795–801.

79. Ramsay LE, Yeo WW, Chadwick IG, et al. Non-pharmacological therapy of hypertension. *Br Med Bull*. 1994;50(2):494–508.

80. Bradley JG. Nonprescription drugs and hypertension; which ones affect blood pressure? *Postgrad Med*. 1991;89(6): 195–202.

81. Susalit E, Agus N, Effendi I, et al. Olive (Olea europaea) leaf extract effective in patients with stage-1 hypertension: comparison with Captopril. *Phytomedicine*. 2011;18(4):251–258.

82. Noronha B, Duncan E, Byrne JA. Optimal medical management of angina. *Curr Cardiol Rep*. 2003;5(4): 259–265.

83. Vandergoten P, Benit E, Dendale P. Prinzmetal's variant angina: three case reports and a review of the literature. *Acta Cardiol*. 1999;54(2):71–76.

84. Hung J. Unstable angina: assessment and management. *Mod Med*. 1994;37(10): 18–27.

85. Kandziora J. Crataegutt effect in coronary blood circulation disorders. EEG findings in exercise test. *Munch Med Wochenschr*. 1969;111:295–298.

86. Weng WL, Zhang WQ, Liu FZ, et al. Therapeutic effect of Crataegus pinnatifida on 46 cases of angina pectoris – a double blind study. *J Tradit Chin Med*. 1984;4(4):293–294.

87. Mahmood ZA, Sualeh M, Mahmood SB, Karim MA. Herbal treatment for cardiovascular disease the evidence based therapy. *Pak J Pharm Sci*. 2010;23(1):119–124.

88. Duan X, Zhou L, Wu T, et al. Chinese herbal medicine suxiao jiuxin wan for angina pectoris. *Cochrane Database Syst Rev*. 2008;(1):CD004473.

89. Ahn CM, Hong SJ, Choi SC, et al. Red ginseng extract improves coronary flow reserve and increases absolute numbers of various circulating angiogenic cells in patients with first ST-segment elevation acute myocardial infarction. *Phytother Res*. 2011;25(2):239–249.

90. Kullo IJ, Ballantyne CM. Conditional risk factors for atherosclerosis. *Mayo Clin Proc*. 2005;80(2):219–230.

91. Mahmoudi M, Curzen N, Gallagher PJ. Atherogenesis: the role of inflammation and infection. *Histopathology.* 2007;50(5):535–546.

92. Verschuren WMM, Jacobs DR, Bloemberg BPM, et al. Serum total cholesterol and long-term coronary heart disease mortality in different cultures; twenty-five-year follow-up of the seven countries study. *JAMA.* 1995;274(2):131–136.

93. Walsh JM, Grady D. Treatment of hyperlipidemia in women. *JAMA.* 1995;274(14):1152–1158.

94. Weverling-Rijnsburger AWE, Blauw GJ, Lagaay AM, et al. Total cholesterol and risk of mortality in the oldest old. *Lancet.* 1997;350:1119–1123.

95. Oliver M, Poole-Wilson P, Shepherd J, et al. Lower patients' cholesterol now. *BMJ.* 1995;310:1280–1281.

96. van Wijk DF, Stroes ESG, Kastelein JJP. Lipid measures and cardiovascular disease prediction. *Dis Markers.* 2009;26: 209–216.

97. Morrison A, Hokanson JE. The independent relationship between triglycerides and coronary heart disease. *Vasc Health Risk Manag.* 2009;5(1):89–95.

98. Patel JV, Tracey I, Hughes EA, et al. Omega-3 polyunsaturated fatty acids: a necessity for a comprehensive secondary prevention strategy. *Vasc Health Risk Manag.* 2009;5:801–810.

99. Millán J, Pintó X, Muñoz A, et al. Lipoprotein ratios: physiological significance and clinical usefulness in cardiovascular prevention. *Vasc Health Risk Manag.* 2009;5:757–765.

100. Kannel WB. Overview of hemostatic factors involved in atherosclerotic cardiovascular disease. *Lipids.* 2005;40(12):1215–1220.

101. Danesh J, Erqou S. Lipoprotein(a) and coronary disease – moving closer to causality. *Nat Rev Cardiol.* 2009;6(9):565–567.

102. Clarke R, Peden JF, Hopewell JC, et al. Genetic variants associated with Lp(a) lipoprotein level and coronary disease. *N Engl J Med.* 2009;361(26):2518–2528.

103. Corrales-Medina VF, Madjid M, Musher DM. Role of acute infection in triggering acute coronary syndromes. *Lancet Infect Dis.* 2010;10(2):83–92.

104. Vainas T, Sayed S, Bruggeman CA, et al. Exploring the role of Chlamydia pneumoniae in cardiovascular disease: a narrative review. *Drugs Today (Batrc).* 2009;45(suppl B):165–172.

105. Blaizot A, Vergnes JN, Nuwwareh S, et al. Periodontal diseases and cardiovascular events: meta-analysis of observational studies. *Int Dent J.* 2009;59(4):197–209.

106. Thim T, Hagensen MK, Bentzon JF, et al. From vulnerable plaque to atherothrombosis. *J Intern Med.* 2008;263(5):506–516.

107. Schoenhagen P, Tuzcu EM, Ellis SG. Plaque vulnerability, plaque rupture, and acute coronary syndromes: (multi)-focal manifestation of a systemic disease process. *Circulation.* 2002;106(7): 760–762.

108. Cesarone MR, Belcaro G, Nicolaides AN, et al. Increase in echogenicity of echolucent carotid plaques after treatment with total triterpenic fraction of Centella asiatica: a prospective, placebo-controlled, randomised trial. *Angiology.* 2001; 52(suppl 2):S19–S25.

109. Incandela L, Belcaro G, Nicolaides AN, et al. Modification of the echogenicity of femoral plaques after treatment with total triterpenic fraction of Centella asiatica: a prospective, randomised, placebo-controlled trial. *Angiology.* 2001; 52(suppl 2):S69–S73.

110. Cullum A. The link between diet and CHD. *Practitioner.* 1994;238: 855–857.

111. Jenkins DJ, Kendall CW, Marchie A, et al. Effects of a dietary portfolio of cholesterol-lowering foods vs lovastatin on serum lipids and C-reactive protein. *JAMA.* 2003;290(4):502–510.

112. Shigematsu N, Asano R, Shimosaka M, Okazaki M. Effect of administration with the extract of Gymnema sylvestre R. Br leaves on lipid metabolism in rats. *Biol Pharm Bull.* 2001;24(6): 713–717.

113. Baskaran K, Kizar Ahamath B, Radha Shanmugasundaram K, et al. Antidiabetic effect of a leaf extract from Gymnema sylvestre in non-insulin-dependent diabetes mellitus patients. *J Ethnopharmacol.* 1990;30(3):295–300.

114. Mölgaard J, von Schenck H, Olsson AG. Alfalfa seeds lower low density lipoprotein cholesterol and apolipoprotein B concentrations in patients with type II hyperlipoproteinemia. *Atherosclerosis.* 1987;65(1–2):173–179.

115. Imai K, Nakachi K. Cross sectional study of effects of drinking green tea on cardiovascular and liver diseases. *BMJ.* 1995;310:693–696.

116. Partsch H. Varicose veins and chronic venous insufficiency. *Vasa.* 2009;38(4):293–301.

117. Lim CS, Davies AH. Pathogenesis of primary varicose veins. *Br J Surg.* 2009;96(11):1231–1242.

118. Pilgrim JA, Stansfeld S, Marmot M. Low blood pressure, low mood? *BMJ.* 1992;304(6819):75–78.

119. Kim BS, Bae JN, Cho MJ. Depressive symptoms in elderly adults with hypotension: different associations with positive and negative affect. *J Affect Disord.* 2010;127(1–3):359–364.

120. Licht CM, de Geus EJ, Seldenrijk A, et al. Depression is associated with decreased blood pressure, but antidepressant use increases the risk for hypertension. *Hypertension.* 2009;53(4):631–638.

121. Kalaria RN. Vascular basis for brain degeneration: faltering controls and risk factors for dementia. *Nutr Rev.* 2010;68(suppl 2):S74–S87.

122. Brown WR, Thore CR. Review: cerebral microvascular pathology in ageing and neurodegeneration. *Neuropathol Appl Neurobiol.* 2011;37(1):56–74.

123. Lazarides MK, Georgiadis GS, Papas TT, et al. Diagnostic criteria and treatment of Buerger's disease: a review. *Int J Low Extrem Wounds.* 2006;5(2):89–95.

124. Frost-Rude JA, Nunnelee JD, Spaner S. Buerger's disease. *J Vasc Nurs.* 2000;18(4):128–130.

125. Mills JL, Sr. Buerger's disease in the 21st century: diagnosis, clinical features, and therapy. *Semin Vasc Surg.* 2003;16(3):179–189.

126. Lazarides MK, Georgiadis GS, Papas TT, et al. Diagnostic criteria and treatment of Buerger's disease: a review. *Int J Low Extrem Wounds.* 2006;5(2):89–95.

127. Olin JW, Shih A. Thromboangiitis obliterans (Buerger's disease). *Curr Opin Rheumatol.* 2006;18(1):18–24.

128. Frost-Rude JA, Nunnelee JD, Spaner S. Buerger's disease. *J Vasc Nurs.* 2000;18(4):128–130.

129. Adar R, Papa MZ, Schneiderman J. Thromboangiitis obliterans: an old disease in need of a new look. *Int J Cardiol.* 2000;75:S167–S170.

130. Noël B. Thromboangiitis obliterans a new look for an old disease. *Int J Cardiol.* 2001;78(2):199.

131. Olin JW. Thromboangiitis obliterans Buerger's disease. *N Engl J Med.* 2000;343(12):864–869.

132. Men J, Men J. TCM treatment of thromboangiitis obliterans – a report of 64 cases. *J Tradit Chin Med.* 2005;25(1):34–36.

133. Yang BH, Zhang SG. Study of thromboangiitis obliterans treated with 'vascular no. 3' using Doppler ultrasound. *Zhong Xi Yi Jie He Za Zhi.* 1989;9(10):596–598.

134. Bone K. *Clinical Applications of Ayurvedic and Chinese Herbs.* Warwick: Phytotherapy Press; 1996. p. 5.

135. Zhao XD, Jin X. Clinical analysis of 200 cases of necrotic thromboangiitis obliterans. *Zhong Xi Yi Jie He Za Zhi.* 1990;10(12):729–731.

136. Bone KM. Autoimmune disease: a phytotherapeutic perspective. *Townsend Lett Doctors Patients.* 1999;193/194: 94–98.

137. Bone KM. Cardiovascular activity of garlic powder products. *Townsend Lett Doctors Patients.* 2002;229/230:46–48.

Respiratory system

Scope

Apart from their use to provide non-specific support for recuperation and repair, specific phytotherapeutic strategies include the following.

Treatment of:

- inflammatory catarrhal conditions of the upper respiratory mucosa (e.g. common cold, rhinitis, sinusitis, otitis media)
- acute bronchial and tracheal infections
- allergic rhinitis
- nervous coughing patterns.

Management of:

- chronic obstructive pulmonary diseases (chronic bronchitis, bronchiectasis, emphysema, silicosis)
- asthma
- chronic tracheitis
- coughing due to persistent local irritation.

Because of its use of secondary plant products, particular **caution** is necessary in applying phytotherapy in cases of known allergic reactions to specific medicinal plant products.

Rationale and orientation

To the Chinese, the lungs were the internal organs most in contact with the exterior. So as well as ascribing to them the source of the body's rhythm and the site of the catalysis of vital energies, they were seen to be the organs in charge of defences. In earlier times the role of the respiratory system was obvious in all cultures; the first cry was generally taken to be the first sign of life, the bronchial gasp on the deathbed the last, and a consistent fear throughout history was the hacking, bloody cough of consumption or tuberculosis, the disease that once cast its baleful influence over the popular imagination like cancer and AIDS now do, the constant reminder of how fatal debility followed weakening of the lungs. It was obvious that the lungs, even more than the stomach, were susceptible to contagion, the conceptual medieval precursor to viruses and bacteria. In this imagery, the key to resistance lay not in attacking alien invaders but in strengthening innate resources. Traditional strategies for treating respiratory disease were notably founded on supportive and tonifying remedies. Given that the modern virus remains as elusive as it ever was, an emphasis on supporting defences may seem appropriate again.

Modern interpretations of respiratory illness have shifted in recent years to identifying underlying inflammatory processes, involving leukotrienes and cytokines. Given that most pathologies have a strong inflammatory element, this is a promising avenue of further research for phytotherapy.[1]

This is, however, the one area where the divide between traditional and modern approaches is not very wide. Elsewhere, there are very few modern endorsements of early treatment strategies.[2] Modern medical science, which at first embraced such agents in the earlier part of this century, now sees no role for their use. For example, modern editions of

Martindale's Extra Pharmacopoeia claim that: 'There is little evidence to show that expectorants are effective'. Some modern drugs may have expectorant activity, such as bromhexine, but they are usually referred to as 'mucolytic'. The impact of traditional remedies on the respiratory system is relatively poorly researched. Reliable external measures of change in mucosal function are elusive; many respiratory diseases are either self-limiting or are among some of the most persistent conditions in the clinic. Even in asthma, where peak flow rates provide a simple measure of benefit, the complexity of the condition and the usual presence of confounding and violent influences make easy characterisation of the condition, and the measurement of all but the most powerful across-the-board remedies, unreliable.

A sense that traditional approaches should be relegated to history is possibly reinforced in the medical psyche by the knowledge that one of the most dramatic advances of modern drugs was in controlling at last the old scourge of tuberculosis. However, this dismissal is not as conclusive as once thought. Tuberculosis is making a serious come-back on the world stage, attacking first the very impoverished and malnourished as it always did. As modern drugs struggle with this new manifestation, there may once again be value in looking at the lessons from the past, that treatment should be based on supportive remedies in a regime of convalescence. With the luxury of choice, with the option of taking modern drugs where these are necessary, but also being able to select more supportive strategies at other times, there is real value in reviewing the treatments forged out of desperate but not always unsuccessful battles with disease in earlier times. These lessons are fortunately quite well learnt.

The dominant feature of respiratory conditions is how readily changes in their behaviour are appreciated subjectively. The often immediate effects of eating and drinking different foods and drinks, of temperature and humidity changes and of the various treatments used through history have been the main guide in determining therapeutic strategy. From such experience has come the view of the respiratory mucosa and musculature as being particularly sensitive to reflex responses, notably from the upper digestive tract, from the pharynx to the stomach. There is a persistent tradition in many cultures that respiratory problems are extensions of digestive dysfunctions. Embryology supports such links, with the bronchial tree originating as a diverticulum of the pharyngeal zone of the alimentary duct and sharing common vagal innervation, and the association, for example, between asthma and histamine H_2 receptors in the stomach[3] add further support to such connections.

Phytotherapeutics

Part of the problem with expectorants probably arises from confusion over their definition. Another stems from the difficulties involved with measuring their efficacy.

Overview of expectorants

- An expectorant is a substance that enhances those physiological mechanisms by which respiratory tract secretions are cleared from the lungs. In the course of doing this they often render the consistency of respiratory tract secretions more fluid and/or more demulcent. They do not necessarily increase the quantity of coughed-up phlegm, nor are they necessarily antitussive (see below).

- Since reflex and warming expectorants act by different mechanisms, and on different parts of the lung tissue, an effective herbal prescription can combine these two types of expectorants, but depending on the patient's condition as noted above.
- The effect and mechanism of action of reflex expectorants have been demonstrated by scientific experiments. However, since their effect seems to involve vagal stimulation of secretory glands, there may also be vagal stimulation of smooth muscle tissue in the lungs. Hence they should be used with caution in asthma, and combined with bronchiolar spasmolytics (but not anticholinergics that can dry respiratory secretions).
- Many lower respiratory tract disorders will benefit from the action of expectorants, but particularly those where mucus is tenacious and difficult to cough up. However, it depends on the cause of a cough whether an expectorant action is also antitussive.

The four definitions of expectorants given below highlight the difficulties. The dictionary meaning is only concerned with the actual oral production of phlegm or sputum. Since the majority of mucus produced from the lungs is swallowed, this definition is clearly unsatisfactory. Definitions from the pharmacologists Boyd and Lewis are more useful, but probably the best definition comes from Brunton, a 19th century pharmacologist. Brunton's functional definition best explains the various ways in which medicinal plants can act as expectorants.

Definitions of expectorants

- *Oxford Dictionary* – 'Promoting the ejection of phlegm by coughing or spitting.'
- Boyd (1954) – 'An expectorant may be pharmacologically defined as a substance which increases the output of demulcent respiratory tract fluid.'
- Lewis (1960) – 'Expectorants increase the secretions of the respiratory tract and so reduce the viscosity of the mucus which can then act as a demulcent. By virtue of the presence of increased quantities of fluid mucus, expectorants produce a "productive cough" which is less exhausting and less painful to the patient.'
- Brunton (1885) – 'Remedies which facilitate the removal of secretions from the air passages. The secretion may be rendered easier of removal by an alteration in its character or by increased activity of the expulsive mechanism.'

Why expectorants?

Many respiratory conditions are characterised by abnormal mucus (catarrh) that can narrow airways. This abnormal mucus may be thick and tenacious and hence very difficult to clear from the airways.

If expectorants can render this catarrh more fluid and/or assist in its expulsion, then a clinical benefit should be achieved.

Expectorants can help to relieve debilitating cough. The presence of an irritation in the airways (such as tenacious abnormal mucus) invokes the cough reflex. (The cough reflex is most sensitive in the trachea and larger airways. The sensitivity progressively decreases in the finer airways and in the very fine airways there is no reflex at all. So in alveolitis, there is little stimulation of the cough reflex, whereas for tracheitis the stimulus is strong.) By clearing abnormal mucus or by changing its character and making it more demulcent, expectorants can allay cough and are therefore antitussive.

In spite of the incomplete scientific case and lack of a consensus orthodox view, traditional approaches to expectoration are strong and consistent across cultures and history. They include mechanisms that are rational and usually immediately apparent.

The following are categories of herbal remedies acting on the respiratory tract.

Stimulating (reflex) expectorants

These are remedies that provoke increased mucociliary activity by reflex stimulation of the upper digestive wall. The classic examples were originally used as emetics. It was noted that this drastic action was accompanied by a noticeable expectoration. In fact, traditional practitioners in Britain used emesis as a technique to clear the lungs in asthma and chronic bronchitis until quite recent times. Application of these remedies in sub-emetic doses was thus a consistent feature in all major herbal traditions. Herbs such as ipecacuanha, squills and Lobelia have been standards in Western medicine. There is some limited modern investigation of mechanisms involved. For example, ipecac-induced emesis is thought to be mediated through both peripheral and central 5-HT_3 receptors.[4] Other plants have been used as stimulating expectorants, although not used as emetics; members of the Primula, Bellis, Saponaria and Polygala genera are often included in this category in Western traditions. High saponin levels seem to be a common feature of this group and saponins are certainly nauseating in high doses.

Plant remedies traditionally used as stimulating (reflex) expectorants

- Cephaelis (ipecacuanha), *Lobelia inflata* (Lobelia), Urginea (squills), *Primula veris* (cowslip), Bellis (daisy), Saponaria (soapwort), *Polygala senega* (snakeroot).

Indications for stimulating expectorants

- Cough linked to bronchial congestion, especially where mucus is thick and tenacious or where there is unproductive cough
- Bronchitis, emphysema.

Other traditional indications for stimulating expectorants

- In some cases as emetics in higher doses.

Contraindications for stimulating expectorants

Although there is no firm evidence of unsuitability, as gastric irritants they can transiently upset some individuals (immediately relieved by withdrawing or changing the remedy). In addition, the use of stimulating expectorants should be kept under review in cases of:

- dry and irritable conditions of the lungs
- asthma
- young children
- dyspeptic conditions.

Application

Stimulating expectorants are best taken in hot infusions or as tinctures or fluid extracts, before food.

Long-term therapy with stimulating expectorants is appropriate in the management of chronic bronchial conditions as long as digestive functions are not affected.

Advanced phytotherapeutics

Stimulating expectorants may also be usefully applied in some cases (depending on other factors) of rheumatic and connective tissue diseases.

Warming expectorants (mucolytics)

Many of the spices were highly prized in the cold damp climates of northern Europe for their apparent ability to counteract associated chest problems. In particular, ginger had an almost mythical reputation; where this or imported cinnamon and cloves were not available, Europeans resorted to fennel, aniseed, garlic, mustard and horseradish for the same ends. Later cayenne or chilli peppers were used for this purpose, although generally taken to be too drying in most cases. The effect of the pungent spices probably includes increased blood flow to the respiratory mucosa, a reflex irritation of the upper digestive mucosa (as with the stimulating expectorants) and, especially in the sulphur-containing garlic and mustard family, a decrease in the thickness of mucus by altering the structure of its mucopolysaccharide constituents; the sensation usually is of a clearing of catarrh and the shifting of congestion up from the lungs.[5] A simple infusion of fresh ginger and cinnamon remains one of the most effective home treatments for the common cold.

Essential oils from various herbs (either administered as essential oils or contained in herbal extracts or tinctures) are the most important agents that directly influence goblet cells to secrete more respiratory tract fluid and mucus. Boyd studied the effects of several essential oils in various experimental models (see Chapter 2). The most pronounced increase of respiratory tract fluid was seen after ingestion of oil of anise. Interestingly ingestion of oil of eucalyptus had a moderate effect that was not eliminated by cutting afferent gastric nerves. This finding supports the premise that essential oils do not generally act as reflex expectorants.

Plant remedies traditionally used as warming expectorants

- *Pimpinella anisum* (aniseed), *Cinnamomum zeylanicum* (cinnamon), Foeniculum (fennel), Zingiber (ginger), *Allium sativum* (garlic), *Angelica archangelica* (angelica).

Indications for warming expectorants

- Productive cough associated with cold
- Bronchitis, emphysema
- Profuse catarrhal conditions
- Dry cough, as per Boyd.

Other traditional indications for warming expectorants

- As aromatic digestives
- Congestive chronic infections and inflammatory conditions.

Contraindications for warming expectorants

The use of warming expectorants may be contraindicated or inappropriate in gastro-oesophageal reflux.

Traditional therapeutic insights into the use of warming expectorants

There is a close association in traditional medicine between catarrhal congestion and the digestive/assimilative functions. The warming remedies were seen to act seamlessly across both respiratory and digestive functions treating disturbances in either or both together. Symptoms most often found with catarrhal conditions might include abdominal distension, loss of appetite and loose stools.

Applications

Warming expectorants are best taken immediately before meals. They are particularly effective taken in hot aqueous infusions.

Long-term therapy with warming expectorants is usually acceptable.

Respiratory demulcents

These herbs contain mucilage and have a soothing and anti-inflammatory action on the lower respiratory tract. Although the mechanism is not clear, an opposite effect to that of the stimulating expectorants has been postulated; that is the effect is a reflex one from the demulcent effect on the pharynx and upper digestive tract, again involving common embryonic origins and vagal innervation.

The major respiratory demulcent herbs are *Althaea officinalis* (marshmallow root or leaves) and other members of the Malvaceae (mallows), *Ulmus spp.* (slippery elm), members of the Plantago genus, *Cetraria islandica* (Iceland moss) and *Chondrus crispus* (Irish moss). Tussilago (coltsfoot) and Symphytum (comfrey) were very widely popular before concerns about pyrrolizidine alkaloids constrained their sale.

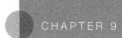

Pronounced antitussive activity has been demonstrated experimentally with oral doses of 1000 mg/kg body weight of extract of *Althaea officinalis* (marshmallow), with comparable effects at 50 mg/kg of the isolated polysaccharides.[6] These animal studies might suggest enormous doses necessary for clinical effect but if, as implied, the effect is a mechanical one, it is likely that only marginal increases in dose would be necessary to have similar impact in larger animals like humans (see also Chapter 2 under Mucilages).

Respiratory demulcents were popular for children's cough and generally for dry, irritable and ticklish coughing. They were seen as intrinsically contraindicated in wet, damp chest problems, although they can sometimes be quite well suited to these if there is an irritable element.

Plant remedies traditionally used as respiratory demulcents

- Althaea (marshmallow), *Plantago spp.* (ribwort and plantain), Verbascum (mullein, especially leaf), Chondrus (Irish moss), Cetraria (Iceland moss), Glycyrrhiza (licorice).

Indications for respiratory demulcents

- Dry, non-productive, irritable cough
- Coughing in children
- Asthmatic wheezing and tightness.

Other traditional indications for respiratory demulcents

- As mucilaginous digestive remedies
- The effects of dryness on the respiratory system.

Contraindications for respiratory demulcents

The use of respiratory demulcents may be inappropriate in profuse catarrhal or congestive conditions of the mucosa (but see above).

Traditional therapeutic insights into the use of respiratory demulcents

As with other respiratory remedies, there is a close association between effects here and on the digestive tract. Respiratory demulcents are at their most appropriate if there are parallel indications in the gut: dry inflamed conditions such as gastritis and oesophagitis associated with hyperacidity, dry constipation and its various associated problems.

Application

Respiratory demulcents are best taken before meals. They are particularly effective taken in cold aqueous infusions. However, if gastro-oesophageal reflux is contributing to the pathology, as can be the case in asthma, they should be taken after meals.

Long-term therapy with respiratory demulcents is usually well tolerated.

Respiratory spasmolytics

Respiratory spasmolytics relax the bronchioles of the lungs. Traditionally they included the solanaceous plants (the nightshade family) with powerful atropine-related antiparasympathetic constituents: Datura, Atropa and Solanum were the prominent antiasthmatics of early history. As could now be explained pharmacologically, these remedies tended also to dry up the mucosa and had other less desirable effects, so less powerful remedies were also popular. *Ephedra sinica* (ma huang) from Asia was popular when it reached Europe and works through a sympathomimetic action. Other gentle remedies include culinary herbs such as hyssop and especially thyme, horehound, the North American gumplant, *Grindelia camporum* and elecampane (*Inula helenium*).

Plant remedies traditionally used as respiratory spasmolytics

- Ephedra (ma huang), *Datura stramonium* (jimson weed), *Atropa belladonna* (deadly nightshade), *Solanum dulcamara* (bittersweet), Hyssopus (hyssop), *Thymus vulgaris* (thyme), *Lobelia inflata* (lobelia), *Marrubium vulgare* (horehound), *Grindelia camporum* (gumplant), *Euphorbia hirta* (pill-bearing spurge), *Coleus forskohlii*, Glycyrrhiza (licorice), Inula (elecampane).

Indications for respiratory spasmolytics

- Tight, breathless, non-productive coughing
- Wheezing and other asthmatic symptoms.

Other traditional indications for respiratory spasmolytics

- Many of the gentler remedies were used as relaxants
- The solanaceous plants have potent neuroactive properties.

Contraindications for respiratory spasmolytics

The use of respiratory spasmolytics may be contraindicated or inappropriate in the following:

- In the case of solanaceous plants: glaucoma, urinary retention, paralytic ileus, intestinal atony and obstruction
- In the case of Ephedra: appetite disorders, glaucoma, prescription of monoamine oxidase (MAO) inhibitors.

Application

Respiratory spasmolytics may be taken at any time of the day as required for immediate effect.

Long-term therapy with respiratory spasmolytics is acceptable in the case of the gentler examples, but not for the solanaceous plants or Ephedra, and in all cases there should be attention to treatment of underlying causes rather than relying on symptomatic relief.

Anticatarrhals

There are a range of popular herbal treatments for a range of respiratory mucosal conditions whose action still remains mysterious. Indications for their use range from catarrhal congestion to some types of mucosal hypersensitivity such as hay-fever and allergic rhinitis.

Plant remedies traditionally used as anticatarrhals

- *Euphrasia spp.* (eyebright), *Plantago lanceolata* (ribwort), *Sambucus nigra* flowers (elder), *Mentha piperita* (peppermint), *Nepeta hederacea* (ground ivy), *Solidago virgaurea* (goldenrod), *Verbascum thapsus* (mullein flowers) and *Hydrastis canadensis* (golden seal). Ephedra also has pronounced anticatarrhal activity.

Anticatarrhal herbs for the upper respiratory tract include eyebright, ribwort, Ephedra, elder, peppermint, ground ivy and golden seal. Golden seal is particularly indicated where there is copious yellow to green discharge of a chronic nature. Golden rod may also fit into this category. Anticatarrhal herbs for the lower respiratory tract include mullein, Ephedra and ribwort.

Sage has a general drying effect on bodily secretions including the mucous membranes and may be indicated where secretions are particularly copious and watery.

Indications for anticatarrhals

- Catarrhal conditions of the upper and lower respiratory tract
- Sinusitis, otitis media
- Allergic rhinitis, asthma and other hypersensitivity conditions.

Contraindications for anticatarrhals

Anticatarrhals are generally regarded as gentle and safe.

Application

Anticatarrhals are best taken before meals. Long-term therapy with anticatarrhals is usually well tolerated.

Herbs modulating inflammation and allergy

The inflammatory basis of many respiratory conditions has been clearer in recent years, with the role of dietary approaches, for example increasing the consumption of omega-3 fatty acids, being increasingly justified.[7] The role of plant flavonoids and phenolics (such as the proprietary remedy Pycnogenol derived from the *Pinus pinaster* – maritime pine) as at least an adjunct for inflammatory respiratory conditions such as allergic rhinitis[8] and childhood asthma[9] has been supported in double blind, controlled clinical trials against placebo. Traditional remedies such as Ephedra and *Scutellaria baicalensis* (Baical skullcap) have been refocused on the management of mild asthmatic conditions.

A number of herbs in recent years have accumulated a reasonable evidence base of efficacy in dealing with upper respiratory disease and in asthmatic symptoms. In the first instance,

research has been driven by products in the over-the-counter (OTC) industry, given that 'cough-cold' is the largest single OTC sector, especially in winter. Generally these remedies have in common preclinical research pointing to various anti-inflammatory activities, but there is little suggestion that they have antiviral or other wider asthmatic properties. The remedies most researched in this area include *Petasites hybridus* (butterbur) and the South African *Pelargonium sidoides* (umckaloabo).

Petasites is a traditional European remedy that has been used less in recent years since its pyrrolizidine alkaloid (PA) content was confirmed. Two pyrrolizidine alkaloid reduced proprietary extracts, one from the root and one from the leaf, have come on the market with claims to treat allergic rhinitis and migraine. Preclinical studies have shown that the sesquiterpenes isopetasin, oxopetasin and petasin are active constituents. They have demonstrated smooth muscle relaxant activity and in addition their esters inhibited the in vitro synthesis of leukotrienes, COX-2 and PGE_2.[10] Clinical trials of the efficacy of Petasites in allergic rhinitis have included a significant study showing comparability with a conventional antihistamine[11] and one showing reduced reaction to the inflammatory agonist adenosine monophosphate (AMP).[12] Other trials have been smaller or less rigorous,[13] though add to the case for this new discovery.

Pelargonium is known in Germany for a range of respiratory conditions including acute bronchitis and has been marketed more widely as an OTC remedy for the common cold. In the former indication the clinical evidence, drawn from six randomised controlled trials, was judged as 'encouraging' in a recent meta-analysis.[14] In relation to the common cold, a Cochrane review was tentatively positive in its conclusions, albeit from limited evidence (see also Chapter 2).[15]

There is less evidence for a proprietary preparation based on *Sambucus nigra* (elderberry), which as well as showing some promise clinically in the treatment of colds, has stimulated anti-inflammatory cytokines in human monocytes ex vivo.[16]

Plant remedies traditionally used as anti-inflammatory or antiallergy remedies

- Ephedra, *Albizia lebbek* and *Scutellaria baicalensis* (Baical skullcap), *Tylophora indica* et *cordifolia* (Indian ipecac),[17] *Picrorhiza kurroa*, *Coleus forskohlii*, Urtica (nettle leaf) *Boswellia serrata* (frankincense)[18] and *Hedera helix* (ivy).[19]

Indications for anti-inflammatory or antiallergy remedies

- Mild and chronic asthmatic symptoms, including reactive wheeziness even without diagnosis of asthma
- Allergic rhinitis and other hypersensitivity conditions.

Contraindications for anti-inflammatory or antiallergy remedies

Any remedy that might modulate anti-inflammatory activity in the body needs to be applied with caution in autoimmune disease, although actual interactions with such conditions has not been widely reported.

Application

Most of the remedies in this category are appropriate for relatively long-term use and may need some weeks to demonstrate benefits.

Antitussives

Antitussives are remedies that allay coughing. Some may work through soothing irritability (respiratory demulcents); others are claimed to relieve coughs at source, by removing congestive mucus or other mobile provocations (expectorants).

However, the term 'antitussive' is often used specifically to refer to remedies that depress the cough reflex and, in particular in herbal terms, to those with appreciable levels of cyanogenic glycosides. The notable example in the Western tradition is *Prunus serotina* (wild cherry). Another tradition was to use opiates, and the gentle version of that strategy, Lactuca (wild lettuce), is still applied to the problem in some traditions. Hops (*Humulus lupulus*) were also used for the same reason. Such cough suppressants are not ideal treatments and could even be counterproductive if they reduce cleansing of the lungs. However, there are many cases where they provide helpful relief and they may be the only solution for coughing not due to movable irritants (for example, nervous cough on the one hand, tumours on the other).

Plant remedies traditionally used as antitussives

* *Prunus serotina* (wild cherry bark), Lactuca (wild lettuce), Glycyrrhiza (licorice), Bupuleurum.

Indications for antitussives

* Non-productive, severe or persistent cough refractory to expectorants
* Nervous cough
* Cough due to external irritation or obstruction (e.g. tumour).

Contraindications for antitussives

Antitussives should be used only as needed and limited as soon as practical.

Application

Antitussives are best taken before meals.

Long-term therapy with antitussives is not advisable, except for palliative care.

Topical agents

Throat applications

The surfaces at the back of the mouth and pharynx are the first point of contact for ingested or inhaled pathogens and irritants; the dense masses of lymphatic tissue in the region confirm their important role in defence. The use of gargles, lozenges and cough drops to mobilise local defences can be an effective way to encourage the body's response to a wide range of respiratory infections. In the case of sore throats, demulcent remedies such as licorice and marshmallow,[20] and astringents such as sage (*Salvia* species) and Hamamelis (witchhazel) could at least reduce irritation, and there are a range of remedies with more substantial reputations as topical anti-inflammatories. These can be used as levers to improve resistance and recovery in rhinitis, sinusitis and otitis as well as treating more local inflammations. Rather than attempting local antisepsis, resinous tinctures such as Calendula and myrrh, balm of Gilead, propolis and Tolu balsam appear to mobilise activity in the surrounding lymphatic tissues through the mildly provocative effect of their resins and essential oils. Other essential oil herbs can provide a mild antiseptic activity, for example thyme (*Thymus vulgaris*).

Plant remedies traditionally used as throat applications

* *Calendula officinalis* (marigold), *Commiphora molmol* (myrrh), *Populus gileadensis* (Balm of Gilead) – all in 90% alcohol extraction and most effectively combined with 1:1 or 1:2 extracts of *Glycyrrhiza glabra* (licorice); *Salvia officinalis* (sage), *Thymus vulgaris* (thyme); (for more soothing action) tannin- or mucilage-containing herbs such as *Althaea officinalis* (marshmallow), *Rubus nigra* (blackberry leaf), *Hamamelis virginiana* (witchhazel) and *Ulmus fulva* (slippery elm).

Indications for throat applications

* Sore and inflamed throats
* Persistent or recurrent upper respiratory infections, sinusitis, otitis media
* Gum disease and dental caries.

Contraindications for throat applications

Occasionally a very inflamed throat with enlarged lymphatic tissues (e.g. tonsillitis) may make the throat tissues too sensitive; this can usually be rectified with more licorice or other mucilaginous or tannic content.

Application

Throat applications are best taken between meals and at least 10 minutes before eating or drinking.

Inhalations

The obvious topical applications for the respiratory mucosa, traditional approaches to inhalations included smoking (Datura for asthma, for example, a high-risk treatment not recommended today), inhaling steam from herbal infusions to relieve congestion, and simple humidification. When the technology for extracting essential oils was developed these were frequent applications. Most apparent activity is found with the oils from mints (especially menthol), Eucalyptus, camphor, the Melaleuca family (tea tree – *M. alternifolia*, cajuput – *M. leucadendron*, niaouli – *M. viridiflora*), the Artemisia family (especially the aromatic *A. abrotanum* or southernwood[21]) and the pine family (turpentine – *Pinus palustris, P. sylvestris, P. excelsa*). These were widely used for symptomatic relief of respiratory congestion, although in the case of menthol there are doubts as to the real benefits (see peppermint monograph).[22] It is possible that some volatile principles could exert anti-inflammatory effects[23] (steam inhaled from chamomile flower infusions in some allergic rhinitis and pine oils in bronchitis, for example). Small doses of volatile oils may have a complex combination of activities, either reducing or stimulating ciliary activity[24] or mucosal secretions.[25] (See also Essential oils in Chapter 2.)

Multipurpose remedies

As can be seen from the above, some herbs may fall into several categories. This is because they contain either several active components or a group of active components acting in several different ways. For example, Verbascum (mullein) contains saponins that are expectorant, mucilage that is demulcent and iridoids that are anticatarrhal. Lobelia, although an emetic and stimulating expectorant, was used primarily as a relaxant remedy in 19th century North America; it thus has a broad spectrum of effects on the respiratory system. Probably the broadest acting remedy in common use, however, is Glycyrrhiza (licorice) which combines a saponin stimulant effect, a soothing effect and appreciable anti-inflammatory properties.

Phytotherapy for respiratory conditions

Allergic and non-allergic rhinitis

Rhinitis is an inflammation of the lining of the nose characterised by one or more of the following symptoms: nasal congestion, nasal discharge, sneezing and itching. Acute infectious rhinitis (and sinusitis) is usually due to the common cold and the appropriate treatment is described later in this chapter. Chronic infectious rhinitis is treated using the same approach as described later under chronic sinusitis. Allergic rhinitis is triggered by inhaled allergens and may be perennial or seasonal (hayfever). Non-allergic or vasomotor rhinitis has no identified medical cause, although in naturopathic traditions it is understood as being caused or exacerbated by diet. Rhinitis may also be drug-induced, rhinitis medicamentosus, by overuse of nasal sprays containing decongestants.

In phytotherapy for rhinitis, it is important to identify whether or not inhaled allergens are involved, since this determines the approach to treatment. Allergic rhinitis is usually characterised by sneezing, itching, nasal discharge, conjunctivitis and nasal congestion. There will usually be a family history of allergy and secretions are often copious, clear and thin. Diagnosis is confirmed by positive skin prick test or radioallergosorbent test (RAST) to aeroallergens. In contrast, non-allergic rhinitis is mainly characterised by chronic nasal congestion with a scant, thin, whitish discharge. Skin prick tests and RAST are negative, and it usually has an adult onset.

The acute allergic response in rhinitis results from the interaction of an inhaled allergen with a specific IgE antibody on the surface of mast cells and basophils. This leads to the release of histamine and other factors that cause the acute symptoms. In chronic, persistent rhinitis, T cells recruit eosinophils (in a process quite similar to asthma) and this leads to chronic symptoms such as nasal blockage, loss of smell and nasal hyper-reactivity.

Allergens involved in seasonal allergic rhinitis are usually grass pollens, but pollens from other plants including trees may be implicated. In perennial allergic rhinitis, house dust mite, molds, cockroaches and cats are common sources of allergen.

Treatment

The approach suggested for the herbal treatment of rhinitis is to control symptoms and remove causes. Avoidance measures to reduce exposure to aeroallergens should be part of this treatment, such as the standard procedures to reduce levels of dust mite allergens. Staying at high altitudes or by the sea can substantially reduce pollen exposure (sea breezes are low in pollen).

Dietary exclusions should be trialled for both allergic and non-allergic rhinitis. Herbalists believe that diet can create a state of hypersensitivity and catarrh of the mucous membranes that predisposes to rhinitis. The dietary components that contribute to this process do not necessarily give a positive reaction on the RAST or skin prick test. They include dairy products, wheat, salt and refined carbohydrates. Excessive consumption of these should be avoided by sufferers of rhinitis and complete exclusion of one component (e.g. dairy products) should be tried for at least 2 months, or prior to and during the allergy season.

In order for an allergic reaction to occur, an allergen must penetrate deep into the nasal lining. If the mucous membranes are healthy and intact, the allergen will never reach the mast cells to trigger an allergic reaction. This is why traditional herbalists have stressed the importance of healthy upper respiratory mucous membranes in the management of allergic rhinitis and rely on upper respiratory anticatarrhal herbs (which is really just another way of saying herbs that promote a healthy condition of the mucous membranes) as their mainstay of treatment.

Eyebright is often misunderstood in mass-market products and popular literature. Because of the common name it is often promoted to help vision. But this has never been the case. Because of its favourable effect on upper respiratory mucous membranes, the conjunctiva acquires a healthy sheen, hence the 'eye is bright'. The herb will have this effect if taken orally or applied topically.

Essential aspects of treatment are as follows

- Immune-enhancing herbs such as Echinacea root and Astragalus. This is especially the case for allergic rhinitis
- Antiallergic herbs only in the case of allergic rhinitis, including Albizia, Baical skullcap and Nigella
- Upper respiratory anticatarrhal herbs for both types of rhinitis, including Euphrasia, Hydrastis and *Plantago lanceolata*
- When treating seasonal allergic rhinitis, treatment must be commenced 6 weeks before the season starts

and continued through the season. Any helpful dietary exclusions should also follow this time pattern
- Stress can exacerbate rhinitis and should be treated if it is considered to be a factor with tonic herbs, nervine tonics, sedative herbs and adaptogens as appropriate
- Treatment of rhinitis at a deeper level may involve the use of depuratives (e.g. Galium – clivers), lymphatics (e.g. Phytolacca – poke root) and choleretics and other liver herbs.

CASE HISTORY

A 30-year-old female patient with chronic persistent rhinitis. Symptoms were worse in the morning with clear nasal discharge and irritated eyes. She was sensitive to house dust mite and had suffered tonsillitis, adenoids and otitis media as a child. She regularly took antihistamines.

Treatment consisted of a dairy-free diet, protective measures against house dust mite and the following herbs:

Echinacea angustifolia root	1:2	30 mL
Picrorrhiza kurroa	1:2	5 mL
Zingiber officinale	1:2	5 mL
Euphrasia officinalis	1:2	25 mL
Scutellaria baicalensis	1:2	20 mL
Albizia lebbek	1:2	20 mL
	TOTAL	105 mL

Dose: 8 mL with water twice a day.

Hydrastis 500 mg tablets, one tablet three times a day. After 3 months of herbs, her antihistamine use was greatly reduced and symptoms were very much improved. Note that Picrorrhiza can be replaced by Andrographis if it is not available.

Common cold and influenza

The common cold (acute rhinitis) is a benign viral infection of the upper respiratory tract that usually occurs in the winter months. Viruses commonly involved are rhinovirus, adenovirus, influenza virus and parainfluenza virus. It usually begins with a sore throat, nasal congestion, sneezing with clear discharge and mild fever. After a few days, a mucopurulent discharge occurs due to secondary bacterial infection. A few days of bed rest may be necessary and full recovery usually occurs 7 to 10 days after onset. Complications or sequelae include acute sinusitis, sore throat, tonsillitis and otitis media (covered in this chapter).

In contrast, influenza is often a more severe respiratory infection which can result in loss of life. The main viruses that cause influenza are enveloped viruses known as influenza A and B. These viruses are capable of mutating and new strains constantly appear. Sometimes influenza A virus can exchange a segment of its genetic material with another virus. This produces a new strain of influenza A to which no-one is immune, leading to a worldwide outbreak or pandemic. These have occurred in 1918, 1957, 1968 and 2009. Influenza is also mainly a winter disease. The influenza virus can produce a range of disease, from a mild common cold to fatal pneumonia (especially in the elderly or severely debilitated). True influenza is usually differentiated from other 'flu-like' illnesses by its marked systemic illness with high fever, malaise and muscle pain. Bed rest is usually always required.

(For prevention of respiratory infections, see Chapter 8.)

Treatment

The basic treatment approaches for the common cold and influenza are similar. However, in the case of more severe forms of influenza, treatment is more vigorous (e.g. higher or more repeated doses), and the use of St John's wort (*Hypericum perforatum*) and garlic (*Allium sativum*) as putative antiviral agents is included.

Essential aspects of treatment are as follows:

- Diaphoretics and heating remedies to manage and improve febrile responses. For the most direct agents, circulatory stimulants Zingiber (ginger, especially fresh grated) and cinnamon taken in hot water can dramatically improve mucosal symptoms and fend off the sensation of cold. For more gentle but sustained effects, especially in children, hot teas of *Mentha piperita* (peppermint), *Eupatorium perfoliatum* (boneset), *Nepeta cataria* (catmint), Achillea (yarrow), Tilia (lime flowers) and Sambucus (elderflower) are well-established diaphoretic approaches, which in the context of a cold can exert surprisingly different effects than when consumed at other times. *Asclepias tuberosa* (pleurisy root) is indicated if there are pulmonary or bronchial complications. *Allium sativum* (garlic, taken raw) may also be useful as a general and warming defensive agent
- Immune-enhancing herbs such as Echinacea root and Andrographis to help support the body's fight against the virus. Andrographis is particularly suited to acute respiratory infections, whereas the data for Echinacea root is mixed. Note that Astragalus and tonics such as *Panax ginseng* are contraindicated in the acute stage of infection. *Pelargonium sidoides* and elderberry also have positive clinical data and may support immunity and have other relevant activities
- Anticatarrhal herbs for upper respiratory catarrh, especially Euphrasia (eyebright), Sambucus (elderflower) and Hydrastis (golden seal). Traditionally, Hydrastis was said to be contraindicated in the acute stage of infection, so its use may be best in the later stages of the secondary bacterial infection
- Hypericum (St John's wort) as an antiviral treatment for influenza.

Since these are acute disorders, dosages should be high and often.

CASE HISTORIES

The following case history demonstrates the value of immune-enhancing therapy as an early intervention. John aged 42 was about to fly from Brisbane to London (24 h) and had just caught a cold. He was concerned about the adverse effect of flying on his condition. He was prescribed *Echinacea angustifolia* root tablets 500 mg and was advised to take two tablets every hour, if possible. By the time John arrived in London his cold was almost gone. He continued to take two Echinacea root tablets every few hours the next day and the cold did not reappear.

The next case history illustrates a more complete approach to treating the common cold. Anne, aged 38, presented with the early stages of a cold including a clear discharge and fever. She was treated with the following formula and recovered quickly with only mild symptoms:

Echinacea angustifolia root	1:2	40 mL
Picrorrhiza kurroa	1:2	10 mL
Zingiber officinale	1:2	5 mL
Achillea millefolium	1:2	25 mL
Sambucus nigra flower	1:2	20 mL
	TOTAL	100 mL

Dose: 5 mL with 40 mL hot water five to six times daily.

Treatment was also supplemented with regular intake of peppermint infusions and up to six allicin-releasing garlic (*Allium sativum*) tablets (5000 mg fresh weight equivalent) a day. Rest was also advised.

Note: for the treatment of influenza the above regime could be followed but the elderflower could be replaced by a high hypericin extract of St John's wort which has antiviral activity. Where Picrorrhiza is referred to it can be replaced with appropriate doses of Andrographis.

Acute and chronic bacterial sinusitis

With sinusitis, drainage of the sinuses is partially blocked, usually by congestion and mucosal oedema. This results in stasis that allows a bacterial infection to take hold. Pain is caused by either negative pressure (due to absorption of gases by the vasculature) or the positive pressure of mucosal congestion.

Factors involved in the aetiology of chronic sinusitis include pollution, occupational dust exposure, tobacco smoke, adenoids, allergy (especially in children), rhinitis, cold and damp weather, dental problems, trauma and flying. A deviated nasal septum or other structural causes may be present. Phytotherapists also believe that dietary factors can cause excessive mucus discharge, which may cause and sustain the disease. Particularly implicated are dairy products, salt and wheat. Stasis and congestion may be aggravated if the patient has inadequate fluid intake.

Treatment

The treatment approaches for acute and chronic bacterial sinusitis are similar. For acute sinusitis the dose should be higher and given more frequently and treatment may need to be supplemented with diaphoretics etc., as for acute rhinitis, if fever is present. Key aspects are:

- supporting the immune system in its fight against the bacteria involved using immune-enhancing herbs such as Echinacea and Andrographis
- anticatarrhal herbs (e.g. Euphrasia) to help clear the stasis
- mucolytic herbs to help clear the stasis, such as *Allium sativum* (garlic) and Armoracia (horseradish)
- particularly indicated is Hydrastis (golden seal), which has antimicrobial and anticatarrhal properties and is a mucous membrane trophorestorative. Regularly chewing a Hydrastis tablet can be very beneficial, but they are exceedingly bitter
- A steam inhalation containing antimicrobial and anti-inflammatory essential oils, such as tea tree, pine or aniseed oils, or chamomile flowers, may be useful.

For chronic sinusitis only

- Patients with chronic sinusitis should avoid antihistamines and steroid-based decongestant drugs as these will weaken immunity in the region further.
- Chronic sinusitis may represent a vicarious elimination and this can be additionally treated with depuratives such as Galium (cleavers), and lymphatics such as Phytolacca (poke root)
- Exposure to the environmental factors listed above should be reduced and a dairy-free, low-salt diet should be trialled for at least 3 months. Antiallergic herbs may also be relevant
- The sinuses are relatively inaccessible regions of the body and once a chronic infection has taken hold it can be difficult to eradicate.

The following topical treatment can be beneficial:

Capsicum annuum	1:3	20 mL
Lobelia inflata	1:8	20 mL
Hydrastis canadensis	1:3	20 mL
Commiphora molmol	1:5	20 mL
Myrica cerifera	1:2	20 mL
	TOTAL	100 mL

Work over the affected sinuses for 10 minutes once to twice a day. Keep away from the eyes. Use a glove or wash hands after using.

The Capsicum and Myrica act as decongestants, the myrrh is antiseptic and Lobelia assists penetration. The properties of Hydrastis are given above. If Lobelia is unavailable, substitute with a saponin-containing herb such as Bupleurum or Aesculus (horsechestnut).

CASE HISTORY

A male patient aged 36 presented with chronic sinusitis that followed a bout of the common cold. There was a history of allergic rhinitis with chronic use of antihistamines and nasal steroids. Antibiotics had failed to resolve the condition, which had been present for 4 years. The patient had a high dairy intake and had been a cigarette smoker. Treatment consisted of the following:

Echinacea angustifolia root	1:2	40 mL
Euphrasia officinalis	1:2	30 mL
Hydrastis canadensis	1:3	25 mL
Phytolacca decandra	1:5	5 mL
	TOTAL	100 mL

Dose: 5 mL with water three times daily

In addition, allicin-releasing garlic (*Allium sativum*) tablets (5000 mg fresh weight equivalent) three per day and Picrorrhiza 500 mg tablets, two per day, were prescribed. The patient was placed on a dairy-free and low-salt diet and advised not to use antihistamines and steroid decongestant drugs. The above sinus rub was also prescribed.

After a period of 6 months of treatment, symptoms were considerably improved.

Note that the Picrorrhiza can be substituted by Andrographis and the *E. angustifolia* root by a mixture of *E. purpurea* and *E. angustifolia* roots.

Chronic tonsillitis and chronic sore throat

Chronic sore throat may be a symptom of other disorders, such as sinusitis. However, it may exist in its own right as a chronic bacterial infection in a patient with or without tonsils. The organism usually responsible is a group A Streptococcus.

The approaches to the herbal treatment of chronic tonsillitis and chronic sore throat are similar. The main aspects of treatment are as follows:

- Immune-enhancing herbs. Being a chronic condition, Astragalus may be used as well as Echinacea root and Andrographis. Echinacea root is best taken as a liquid to obtain a local effect on the throat
- Lymphatic and depurative herbs are particularly indicated in tonsillitis and include Phytolacca, Echinacea root, Galium and *Arctium lappa* (burdock)
- Anticatarrhal herbs, particularly eyebright and golden seal
- A local treatment such as a throat spray or lozenge using herbs such as:
  - Glycyrrhiza (licorice) – soothing, anti-inflammatory, topically antiviral
  - Salvia (sage) – astringent and antiseptic to the mucous membranes
  - Propolis – antiseptic, healing and anaesthetic
  - Kava – local anaesthetic to provide a soothing effect (or clove essential oil)
  - Echinacea root – immune-enhancing, anti-inflammatory
  - Capsicum – stimulant, antiseptic
  - Hydrastis (golden seal) – antiseptic, mucous membrane trophorestorative
  - Althaea (marshmallow root) – demulcent
  - Myrrh – vulnerary and antiseptic, induces local leucocytosis
- A dairy-free diet rich in fruit and vegetables should be observed.

Example liquid formula

Echinacea purpurea/angustifolia root	1:2	40 mL
Euphrasia officinalis	1:2	25 mL
Phytolacca decandra	1:5	5 mL
Salvia fructicosa	1:2	15 mL
Hydrastis canadensis	1:3	25 mL
	TOTAL	110 mL

Dose: 8 mL with water twice a day. Ideally gargle medicine briefly before swallowing.

CASE HISTORY

A male patient aged 65 complained of a chronic sore throat that had been present for years. Other conditions were also being treated, but for the sore throat he was prescribed:

Echinacea angustifolia root	1:2	5 mL once a day with water

A gargle consisting of:

Echinacea angustifolia root	1:2	40 mL
Propolis	1:5	30 mL
Salvia officinalis	1:2	30 mL
	TOTAL	100 mL

Dose: 2 mL in 10 mL water as a gargle on the affected area of the throat twice a day. Swallow after use.

After 8 weeks the sore throat was considerably improved and with continuing treatment it became a minor trouble.

Otitis media

Inflammation of the middle ear, or otitis media, can be divided into suppurative or acute otitis media (AOM), and inflammation accompanied by effusion, termed non-suppurative or secretory otitis media or otitis media with effusion (OME). Viral upper respiratory tract infection is most commonly associated with the onset of AOM, although the major infection present is bacterial. Symptoms can include pain, purulent discharge from the ear, hearing loss, vertigo, tinnitus and fever. Examination will demonstrate a red, dull and bulging or perforated ear drum.

Recurrent AOM is common, affecting between 10% and 20% of children up to 12 months of age.[26] Young children have immature immunity and short and poorly functional Eustachian tubes (the latter results in poor middle ear ventilation). Chronic otitis media with discharge from the ear can result from ineffectively treated acute or recurrent otitis media. The infection is clearly bacterial.

OME is an enigmatic disorder that also usually occurs in children. Examination of the ear drum shows that it is retracted ('sucked in') and there is fluid in the middle ear cavity that can lead to conductive hearing loss. Allergy, nasal infection and chronic sinus infection may be involved and it is associated with increased frequency of respiratory infections. Medical treatment can involve the use of grommets to drain the middle ear cavity. The overuse of antibiotics is probably ill advised, although bacterial infection may play a role in some patients with this disorder.

Treatment

The treatments of acute and chronic otitis media are similar to the treatments of acute and chronic sinusitis respectively (with the exclusion of the topical treatment).

OME should be regarded as an allergic disorder, as well as possibly a vicarious elimination. A dairy-free, low-salt diet should be tried or otherwise a full elimination diet. However, the presence of microorganisms that contribute to the inflammation or the malfunction of the Eustachian tube should also be considered. If adenoids are implicated, then the OME should be treated similarly to tonsillitis. The following herbs are emphasised during OME treatment:

- Antiallergic and decongestant herbs such as Albizia, *Scutellaria baicalensis* and Nigella
- Upper respiratory anticatarrhal herbs such as Euphrasia, Solidago, Hydrastis, *Plantago lanceolata* and *Glechoma hederacea*

- Depurative and lymphatic herbs such as Galium (clivers) and Phytolacca
- Immune-enhancing herbs, particularly Echinacea root and Astragalus, to correct the presence of allergy and possibly infection
- Chewing on a Hydrastis tablet (difficult for children because of its bitterness) will accentuate its mucous membrane trophorestorative and antibacterial effects on the upper respiratory tract.

Example liquid formula for AOM

Echinacea purpurea/angustifolia root	1:2	35 mL
Sambucus nigra flower	1:2	25 mL
Pelargonium sidoides	1:5	20 mL
Euphrasia officinalis	1:2	25 mL
	Total	105 mL

Adult dose is 5 mL with warm water five to six times a day for acute AOM and 5 mL three times a day as a preventative for recurrent AOM. Children's doses should be calculated from the application of an appropriate dosage rule.

Acute bronchitis

Acute bronchitis is an acute inflammation of the trachea and bronchi. It commonly follows the common cold, influenza, measles or whooping cough. Patients with chronic bronchitis are particularly prone to develop episodes of acute bacterial bronchitis (where their sputum turns from grey or white to yellow or green). Other factors that can predispose to this kind of bacterial infection include cold, damp, dust and cigarette smoking.

Initially there is an irritating, unproductive cough that eventually progresses over a few days to copious, mucopurulent sputum. Infection usually starts in the trachea and progresses to the bronchi and with this spread there is a general febrile disturbance with temperatures of 38°C to 39°C. Gradual recovery should occur over the next 4 to 8 days. However, it may progress to bronchiolitis or bronchopneumonia.

Treatment

Being an acute disorder, it is important to give frequent doses of herbs and, if possible, to follow the progression of the infection, adapting the treatment to the various stages:

- Antiseptic herbs such as *Inula helenium*, *Thymus vulgaris* and *Allium sativum* (garlic) should be prescribed throughout the course of the infection and preferably should be continued for 1 week into recovery to prevent relapse
- During the dry, unproductive cough phase, demulcents such as Althaea glycetract should be prescribed. This combines well with a small quantity of Glycyrrhiza (licorice) (see under Chronic obstructive pulmonary disease below)
- Diaphoretic herbs are indicated during the febrile phase, particularly *Asclepias tuberosa* (pleurisy root), which

is almost a specific for acute lower respiratory tract infections. It is often combined with Zingiber (ginger) to enhance its effectiveness. Other diaphoretics such as Tilia and Achillea can also be prescribed
- Expectorant herbs, which include *Inula helenium*, *Thymus vulgaris*, Polygala and other saponin-containing herbs, Foeniculum (fennel), Pimpinella (aniseed) and Marrubium (white horehound) can be prescribed throughout the course of the disorder
- Anticatarrhal herbs, especially Verbascum, *Plantago lanceolata* and Hydrastis, may be indicated when the sputum is particularly copious or if the productive cough lingers beyond the acute stage
- Antitussive herbs should be used to help the cough, especially at night, and *Prunus serotina* (wild cherry) is particularly indicated if tracheitis predominates.

Example liquid formula

Echinacea purpurea/angustifolia root	1:2	25 mL
Asclepias tuberosa	1:2	20 mL
Zingiber officinale	1:2	5 mL
Inula helenium	1:2	20 mL
Glycyrrhiza glabra	1:1	15 mL
Foeniculum vulgare	1:2	20 mL
	Total	105 mL

Dose: 5 mL with 40 mL warm water five to six times a day.

Whooping cough

Whooping cough or pertussis is a highly infectious disease caused by *Bordetella pertussis*. About 90% of cases occur in children under 5 years.

The first stage consists of respiratory infection lasting about 1 week during which conjunctivitis, rhinitis and an unproductive cough are present. Diagnosis is difficult at this stage, since it resembles other respiratory infections.

The coughing stage follows and is characterised by severe bouts of coughing. Each paroxysm consists of many short sharp coughs, gathering in speed and duration and ending in a deep inspiration when the characteristic whoop may be heard. The paroxysms can end with vomiting. This stage can last from one to several weeks. The sputum is particularly tenacious and difficult to expectorate.

Treatment

The treatment approach is similar to acute bronchitis but different aspects of the treatment are emphasised:

- Immune-enhancing herbs such as Echinacea and Andrographis and respiratory antiseptic herbs such as *Inula helenium*, *Thymus vulgaris* and *Allium sativum* (garlic) should be prescribed throughout to treat the infection and prevent complications

- In the coughing stage, expectorant herbs such as *Inula helenium*, *Thymus vulgaris*, Polygala, Glycyrrhiza (licorice) and other saponin-containing herbs, Foeniculum (fennel), Pimpinella (aniseed) and Marrubium (white horehound) should be emphasised to loosen the tenacious sputum
- Also, antitussive and demulcent herbs are required to dampen and soothe the cough reflex. If vomiting is occurring, these should be extended by gastrointestinal spasmolytics such as *Viburnum opulus*. (See also the marshmallow-licorice formulation below under Chronic obstructive pulmonary disease)
- Respiratory spasmolytics with expectorant activity, such as Grindelia and *Inula helenium*, should also be emphasised in the coughing stage. A combination of Inula, Glycyrrhiza and Lobelia is worth trying for the most severe symptoms
- Mucolytic herbs such as *Allium sativum* and Armoracia may also be required to help loosen the tenacious sputum.

Chronic obstructive pulmonary disease (COPD)

Although chronic bronchitis and pulmonary emphysema are distinct disorders, they often coexist in the patient and it can be difficult to determine the relative importance of each condition in the individual case. The term 'COPD' often applies to a combination of the two. In emphysema, the fine architecture of the alveoli is damaged, leading to impairment of ventilatory capacity. There is probably little that can be done to reverse this destruction (although some clinicians feel that bioavailable silica and herbs rich in this mineral, such as Equisetum and Urtica can help restore lung architecture).

In contrast, chronic bronchitis is a syndrome that can develop in response to long-term exposure to various types of irritants to the bronchial mucous membranes. These include cigarette smoke, dust and automobile or industrial air pollution, especially in conjunction with a damp climate. Acute infection is usually a precipitating or aggravating factor and chronic infection is usually present, with regular acute episodes. Hence, there are many factors in chronic bronchitis that are treatable, and long-term herbal treatment can dramatically alter the course of chronic bronchitis.

In chronic bronchitis, ventilatory capacity is reasonably preserved but hypoxia, pulmonary hypertension and right ventricular failure occur early – 'the blue bloater'. In emphysema, the impairment of ventilatory capacity and exertional dyspnoea lead to the sufferer being labelled a 'pink puffer'. A mixed syndrome is most common and all patients should be treated along the following lines, regardless of their clinical label. The treatment outcome will, however, depend on how much the changes in their lungs can be reversed.

Treatment

In chronic bronchitis there is overactivity of the mucus-secreting glands and goblet cells. The vast excess of mucus coats the bronchial walls and clogs the bronchioles. Exacerbating this, many ciliated columnar cells are replaced by goblet cells in response to the chronic irritation. Therefore the excessive mucus is also less able to be cleared from the lungs. Hence, the use of expectorants is emphasised in the treatment of chronic bronchitis, despite the fact that an easily productive cough can be a feature of this disease. (In some patients sputum may be scanty and tenacious, which also requires treatment with expectorants.)

- Bronchial irritation must be avoided. Giving up smoking and a change in occupation or climate may be necessary. Mucus-producing foods such as dairy products and bananas should be reduced
- Any chronic infection should be treated and acute infections prevented by immune-enhancing herbs, especially Echinacea root and Astragalus (discontinue Astragalus during acute febrile infections). The role here of *Panax ginseng* has been supported in at least one clinical trial.[27] Many chronic bronchitis patients are constitutionally cold, so the cold herbs Picrorrhiza and Andrographis are best avoided. Heating herbs such as cinnamon may be helpful and could possibly be used in conjunction with these cold herbs
- Expectorant herbs, such as *Inula helenium*, *Thymus vulgaris*, Polygala and other saponin-containing herbs, Foeniculum (fennel), Pimpinella (aniseed) and Marrubium (white horehound) can be prescribed throughout the course of the disorder. The diffusive stimulant properties of Zingiber will potentiate the activity of expectorants
- Respiratory antiseptic herbs that also have expectorant or mucolytic properties are particularly indicated, such as *Inula helenium*, *Thymus vulgaris* and *Allium sativum*
- Since the goblet cells are oversecreting, anticatarrhal herbs such as Verbascum, *Plantago lanceolata* and Hydrastis can help to reduce this excessive secretion
- If there is an unproductive cough at night, a separate formula containing demulcents such as Althaea glycetract and Glycyrrhiza, and antitussives such as Glycyrrhiza and Bupleurum, may be prescribed (see below)
- Inhalation of peppermint and eucalyptus oils combined can help loosen mucus and dilate airways to make breathing easier
- Bronchodilating herbs such as Coleus and Lobelia may be helpful. Ephedra should probably be avoided. Those with expectorant activity such as Grindelia can also be selected
- Since chronic inflammation is present, anti-inflammatory herbs such as Glycyrrhiza, Bupleurum and Rehmannia will be of value, as well as omega-3 fatty acids
- Support for the heart and general circulation with Crataegus and Ginkgo may be required.

Demulcent/antitussive formula

The following demulcent formula can also be used to relieve an irritable cough:

Althaea officinalis glycetract	1:5	80 mL
Glycyrrhiza glabra (high in glycyrrhizin)	1:1	20 mL
	Total	100 mL

Dose: 4 mL sipped undiluted (that is no water is added) as required up to 6 times a day.

A male patient, 66 years, has received herbal treatment for chronic bronchitis for 7 years. During this time there has been considerable improvement in the patient's condition and friends often now comment on how well he looks. The frequency of acute episodes has substantially reduced and his lung function parameters have improved. Although treatment varied over this time period, a representative herbal treatment is as follows.

Immune formula (mainly):

Echinacea angustifolia/purpurea root	1:2	45 mL
Arctium lappa	1:2	15 mL
Achillea millefolium	1:2	20 mL
Withania somnifera	1:2	20 mL
	TOTAL	100 mL

Dose: 5 mL with water three times a day.

Lung formula:

Glycyrrhiza glabra	1:1	15 mL
Inula helenium	1:2	20 mL
Zingiber officinale	1:2	10 mL
Foeniculum vulgare	1:2	15 mL
Thymus vulgaris	1:2	20 mL
Grindelia camporum	1:2	20 mL
	TOTAL	100 mL

Dose: 5 mL with water three times a day.

Bronchiectasis

'Bronchiectasis' describes an abnormal dilatation of the bronchi that becomes a focus for chronic infection. In most cases it develops as a complication of a severe bacterial infection and then follows a chronic course. Clinical features include chronic cough, often with copious purulent sputum, and febrile episodes with malaise and night sweats that can last from a few days to weeks, and sometimes haemoptysis. The disorder can be debilitating. Although continual use of antibiotics is inadvisable, patients can often receive this regime.

Treatment

Essential aspects of the treatment of bronchiectasis are as follows:

- Immune-enhancing herbs such as Echinacea root, Andrographis and Astragalus
- Respiratory antiseptic herbs such as *Inula helenium*, *Thymus vulgaris* and *Allium sativum*
- Diaphoretics such as *Asclepias tuberosa* (pleurisy root) during the febrile episodes
- Tonics such as Panax, Rhodiola, Eleutherococcus and/or Withania if debility is present
- Anticatarrhal herbs, including Verbascum, *Plantago lanceolata* and Hydrastis
- Expectorant herbs such as *Inula helenium*, *Thymus vulgaris*, Polygala and other saponin-containing herbs, Foeniculum (fennel), Pimpinella (aniseed) and Marrubium (white horehound)
- Note that Astragalus, Panax and Eleutherococcus should be discontinued during any acute febrile phases.

Example liquid formula

Echinacea purpurea/angustifolia root	1:2	40 mL
Inula helenium	1:2	25 mL
Glycyrrhiza glabra (high in glycyrrhizin)	1:1	15 mL
Hydrastis canadensis	1:3	30 mL
	TOTAL	110 mL

Dose: 8 mL with water twice daily.

A male patient, 59 years, with bronchiectasis. He was initially coughing up an egg cup of sputum every morning and experiencing occasional febrile episodes and acute viral infections. This patient has now been maintained on phytotherapy for more than 15 years. Apart from the occasional winter respiratory infection he remains well. His sputum production is minimal and he freely claims that herbs have 'kept me alive'.

- Herbal treatment consisted of the following: *Echinacea purpurea/ angustifolia* root tablets (1.275 g), two tablets one to two times daily. The Echinacea liquid disagreed with this patient, hence the tablets. The higher dose is taken during febrile episodes and acute infections.

The following liquid formula:

Aesculus hippocastanum	1:2	15 mL
Foeniculum vulgare	1:2	10 mL
Thymus vulgaris	1:2	30 mL
Astragalus membranaceus	1:2	25 mL
Inula helenium	1:2	20 mL
	TOTAL	100 mL

Dose: 8 mL twice a day.

The Aesculus was mainly for circulatory problems but it also has expectorant properties due to its saponin content.

- Garlic, 1 to 2 fresh crushed cloves per day
- A dairy-free diet was followed.

Asthma

In terms of phytotherapy, asthma is probably the most complex of the respiratory disorders. The successful management of asthma hence embodies most of the principles already discussed. Asthma can be defined as the occurrence of dyspnoeic bronchospasmodic crises linked to an airways hyper-responsiveness (AHR). Like autoimmune disease it is a chronic disturbance of immunological function that can be controlled to some extent, but not eradicated by modern drug therapy. In other words asthma is not just the attacks (crises); it is a chronic disturbance of the immune system with the attacks being the 'tip of the iceberg'. Hence any treatment aimed only at relaxing airways and relieving symptoms, be it orthodox or herbal, is superficial and will not change the chronicity of the disease.

Recent research has identified many factors that contribute to the aetiology and morbidity of asthma. Traditional herbal medicine also recognises the role of inefficient digestion, poor immunity, stress, diet and unhealthy mucous membranes in the development of the disease. In order to treat asthma more effectively with phytotherapy, it is necessary to have an understanding of the causative and sustaining factors contributing to the condition. For each individual it is likely that the disease process has been precipitated by a unique and complex interaction of contributive events. A multi-factorial model that allows the individualisation of the patient, yet at the same time incorporates the most likely factors operating in asthma, is discussed below. This in turn requires the synthesis of traditional herbal understanding with the latest research findings, which is fundamental to the practice of modern phytotherapy.

Asthma can be classified as extrinsic (allergic asthma) or intrinsic asthma. Although there has been some confusion with the terms, and some medical scientists feel that the classification is meaningless,[28] the differentiation is quite clear. Patients with extrinsic asthma comprise the majority of cases and exhibit a positive skin test to common aeroallergens and foods. Serum IgE levels are usually raised. However, extrinsic asthmatics can still be exacerbated by non-specific stimuli such as cold air and exercise. Intrinsic asthmatics have negative skin tests, and chronic infection and other factors are thought to play a role in the disease process. Intrinsic asthma is usually later in onset and more severe.[29] Aspirin-sensitive asthma (ASA) is a form of intrinsic asthma. Both types of asthma show an increased family occurrence.[30]

Pathophysiology

Asthmatic lungs are characterised by epithelial cell loss, goblet cell hyperplasia, increased collagen deposition, mast cell degranulation and inflammatory cell infiltration.[31] Asthma is now primarily classified as an inflammatory disorder. The desquamation allows allergens to penetrate more easily and exposes irritant receptors.

There has been an increased understanding over the past two decades that asthma is a chronic, immunologically mediated condition with a disturbance of the normal airway repair mechanism, which results in inflammatory changes and airway remodelling.[32] The airway inflammation and remodelling together likely explain the clinical manifestations of asthma. The mechanisms by which the external environmental cues, together with the complex genetic actions, propagate the inflammatory process that characterise asthma are beginning to be understood. There is also an evolving awareness of the active participation of structural elements, such as the airway epithelium, airway smooth muscle and endothelium in this process. In tandem with this has come the realisation that inflammatory cells respond in a coordinated, albeit dysfunctional, manner via an array of complex signalling pathways that facilitate communication between these cells; these structural elements within the lung and the bone marrow

serve as reservoirs for and the source of inflammatory cells and their precursors. Although often viewed as separate mechanistic entities, innate and acquired immunity often overlap in the propagation of the asthmatic response.[32]

Classically, asthma, specifically allergic asthma, has been attributed to a hyperactive Th2 cell immune response. However, the Th2 cell-mediated inflammation model has failed to adequately explain many of the clinical and molecular aspects of asthma.[33] In addition, the outcomes of Th2-targeted therapeutic trials have been disappointing. Thus, asthma is now believed to be a complex and heterogeneous disorder, with several molecular mechanisms underlying the airway inflammation and AHR that is associated with it. The original classification of Th1 and Th2 pathways has recently been expanded to include additional effector Th cell subsets. These include Th17, Th9 and Treg cells. Emerging data highlight the involvement of these new T helper cell subsets in the initiation and augmentation of airway inflammation and asthmatic responses.[33]

That regulatory T cells (Tregs) have a crucial role in controlling allergic diseases such as asthma is now undisputed. The cytokines most commonly implicated in Treg-mediated suppression of allergic asthma are transforming growth factor-beta (TGF-beta) and interleukin (IL)-10. In addition to naturally occurring Tregs, adaptive Tregs, induced in response to foreign antigens, have been shown in recent studies. The concept of inducible/adaptive Tregs (iTregs) has considerable significance in preventing asthma, if such cells are generated early enough in life.[34]

Other inflammatory cells implicated in asthma include natural killer T cells, although their role is controversial,[35,36] mast cells, neutrophils and eosinophils.[37] Platelets and endothelial cells also play a role.

As touched on above, some experts are arguing for a re-evaluation of the therapeutic implications informed by a pathophysiological understanding of asthma. A case is made that asthma has its origins in the airways themselves, involving defective structural and functional behaviour of the epithelium in relation to environmental insults, with wall thickening.[38] Specifically, a defect in barrier function and an impaired innate immune response to viral infection may provide the substrate upon which allergic sensitisation takes place. Once sensitised, the repeated allergen exposure will lead to disease persistence. These mechanisms could also be used to explain the observed airway wall remodelling and the susceptibility of the asthmatic lung to exacerbations provoked by respiratory viruses, air pollution episodes and exposure to biologically active allergens. It seems that the problem lies in placing allergy at the centre of disease pathogenesis, when in practice other environmental factors may be equally if not more important in the induction and then progression of asthma. Instead a defect of epithelial barrier function exists that, as in atopic dermatitis, allows greater access of environmental allergens, microorganisms, and toxicants to the airway tissue. Evidence indeed indicates that both the physical and functional barrier of the airway epithelium is defective in asthma with disrupted tight junctions, reduced antioxidant activity, and impaired innate immunity. Viewing asthma primarily as an epithelial disease, with the conceptual adoption of a chronic wound scenario, also provides a route to understand the observed airway wall remodelling and the varying asthma phenotypes over its life course.[39]

A host of inflammatory mediators have been identified in the pathophysiology of asthma. However some mediators may be more involved in triggering the inflammatory process than others. In this context, important mediators are the Th2 cytokines and probably histamine, platelet activating factor (PAF), major basic protein, leukotrienes especially (leukotriene B4)[40] and to a lesser extent prostaglandins.[37] Patients with ASA have increased PAF responsiveness, reduced prostaglandin levels and increased leukotrienes compared with normal controls.[41,42] TGF-beta is a key player in airway remodelling.

The host of inflammatory cells and mediators involved in the pathogenic process means that treatment directed at a single mediator or cell is unlikely to be successful. A multifaceted approach to treatment is required. This is compatible with herbal therapy, which has traditionally used combinations of plants to treat diseases.

The above considerations also explain the current preference in conventional medicine for steroid use in asthma. These drugs have a broad suppressing effect on many inflammatory mechanisms. In this context the 'magic bullet' is more like an ordinary shotgun.

Factors associated with asthma

Differentiation should be made between the causes that initiate or sustain the underlying condition, which are probably factors that result in injury to the lining of the lungs, and the triggers that precipitate the asthmatic attack. While avoidance of the latter group is of course important, it is only attention to the former that will reduce the progression of the disease. There is no better illustration of this issue than the subject of dairy products. Traditional knowledge suggests that consumption of dairy products can lead to a state of unhealthy mucous membranes in sensitive patients. However, these patients may not give a positive skin test to dairy products, and these products may not provoke an acute asthmatic attack. In the classical sense there is no allergy to dairy products. Yet the avoidance of this food group will, in time, give appropriate patients considerable relief from their asthmatic condition. Key factors amenable to treatment are reviewed below.

Allergens

The most significant allergen in the long-term development of asthma is now considered to be the house dust mite. However, this does not necessarily mean that the degree of house dust mite exposure will correlate with the day-to-day severity of asthma. This is because sensitivity to the house dust mite feeds the underlying pathological process. Unfortunately, chemical and physical methods aimed at reducing exposure to house dust mite allergens have yielded disappointing results.[43]

Other common factors involved in asthma development may include cats, cockroaches, grass pollens and molds, but the situation is complex, as for dust mite.[44] Association with severe asthma in children was seen between non-feather

bedding, especially foam pillows and the current ownership of furry pets, or ownership at birth.[45] A Finnish study of school children aged 7 to 13 found that moisture and mold problems in the school building were linked to respiratory infections and asthma.[46]

Of course, all the above allergens can trigger an asthma attack, as can many foods, especially dairy products, eggs and nuts. Dust mite contamination of wheat flour caused anaphylactic reactions and cooking had no effect. It was suggested that flour be stored in the refrigerator.[47] Royal jelly should be used cautiously as it is now a well-known trigger of asthma attacks.

Air quality

Maternal or parental smoking has been linked to asthma incidence and severity.[48] Air pollution parameters such as NO_2, ozone and particulates have also been associated with the incidence of asthma.[49]

Exposure to dust, irritants and allergens at the workplace can also cause asthma. Usually withdrawal from the irritant or allergen results in remission, but in some cases where exposure is prolonged the asthma becomes self-sustaining despite such withdrawal.

Sinusitis

Sinusitis has been associated with asthma in several studies,[50,51] although this has received less attention recently. This is not considered to be due to aspiration of sinus contents.[52] In one study 79% of asthma cases had chronic rhinitis or rhinosinusitis.[53] In 69% of cases the nasal symptoms coincided with or preceded the onset of asthma. In 59% of associated cases, nasal symptoms coincided with acute asthmatic episodes. Treatment of the nasal condition improved the asthma. The link between sinusitis and asthma is strongest in patients with intrinsic asthma. Evidence supports the concept that rhinosinusitis and asthma may be the expression of an inflammatory process that appears in different sites of the respiratory tract at different times.[54]

Poor digestion

A number of researchers in the 1930s found a high incidence of hypochlorhydria in asthmatic patients.[55] In these studies the test meal method was used. This method is now considered inappropriate for the assessment of histological hypochlorhydria. However it does assess for functional hypochlorhydria, that is a deficiency of vagal stimulation of acid production. Hydrochloric acid therapy improved the asthma.[55] Since this kind of gastric deficiency is due to deficient vagal output, the use of bitter herbs that act through a vagal reflex to increase gastric digestion is indicated (see Chapter 2).

Gastro-oesophageal reflux (GOR) has been linked to asthma in several studies. In fact there is evidence that GOR is an important aetiological factor for some asthmatics. Monitoring of oesophageal pH revealed GOR in seven out of nine patients with persistent asthma.[56] In another study 61% of patients with intrinsic asthma exhibited GOR.[57] From studies on children it was concluded that asthma symptoms were more often elicited by exposure of the distal oesophagus to gastric acid, possibly by a vagal reflex, than by aspiration of gastric juice.[58] However, other studies have implicated the importance of aspiration.[59,60] In support of the reflex hypothesis, subjects with GOR (but not asthma) showed a significantly greater bronchial reactivity to histamine than normal matched controls.[61]

Treatment of GOR by surgery or drugs can result in improvement or cure of asthma, although results are mixed and suggest that targetting of individual patients is necessary.[62] (Also see Chapter 2, under Mucilages.)

Diet

Particular foods are well-known causes of asthma attacks. However, the contribution of diet to the underlying pathophysiological processes of asthma is not well studied. It has been postulated that dietary changes may have contributed to the rise in asthma mortality.[63] In particular, increased consumption of polyunsaturated fatty acids has resulted in the doubling from 8% to 15% of the linoleic content of body fat.[63] Such a change could be regarded as pro-inflammatory.

Coffee consumption was found to be inversely correlated to the prevalence of bronchial asthma in an Italian study.[64] Epidemiological studies found that consumption of oily fish may protect against asthma in childhood[65] and adults,[66] and a connection between low magnesium intake and increased asthma risk has also been suggested.[67] Consumption of apples (five per week) was found to improve lung function.[68] This benefit was attributed to the flavonoids found in apples.

A systematic review and meta-analysis found weak but supportive protective evidence with respect to dietary vitamins A, D and E, zinc, fruits and vegetables and a Mediterranean diet.[69]

Infection and infestation

Viral infections are known to exacerbate asthma. Viral infection in the upper airways frequently triggers deterioration in airways hyperreactivity in asthmatics.[70] Most hospital admissions for asthma occur over the winter months and soon after the start of school terms.[70] Viral infections also worsen asthma in adults.[71,72]

There is also some evidence to suggest that viral infections may also contribute to the development of asthma, especially in children. About 92% of children hospitalised with respiratory syncytial virus (RSV) bronchiolitis in the first year of life subsequently developed symptoms suggestive of asthma within 5 years.[73] Of this group, 71% had clinical evidence of asthma.[73] Recurrent upper respiratory tract infections are associated with asthma risk in children[74] and 37% of children with viral lower respiratory tract infections in infancy subsequently developed asthma.[75] With the development of molecular diagnostics, human rhinovirus wheezing illnesses have been recognised more recently as a stronger predictor of school-age asthma than RSV.[76]

In contrast, bacterial infection has been linked to adult-onset asthma. The first study linking repeated or prolonged exposure to *Chlamydia pneumoniae* with wheezing, asthmatic bronchitis and asthma was published in 1991.[77] Patients with evidence of *C. pneumoniae* exposure comprised 81%

of 26 patients with asthmatic bronchitis, 100% of asthmatic bronchitics 40 years and older, and 8 out of 10 patients with asthma. However, findings from later studies have been inconsistent.[78] Associations between *Mycoplasma* species and chronic asthma are relatively well-established.[78]

A group of 12 adult patients with asthma and chronic fungal skin infection were found to have hypersensitivity to *Trichophyton spp.*[79] Several patients had many of the features of late-onset intrinsic asthma. A Russian study in children with bronchial asthma living near a microbiological factory found that most were hypersensitive to Candida.[80] Asthma has also been associated with parasitic infestation with *Strongyloides stercoralis.*[81]

Salt intake and dehydration

Regional sales of table salt in England and Wales are strongly correlated with deaths from asthma in men and children.[82] A study of 138 men found a close relation between AHR and 24h urinary sodium excretion.[83] Other studies have yielded conflicting results. A large randomised controlled trial of slow sodium supplementation showed an increase in AHR in men, but not women,[84] and a low salt intake was correlated with improved asthma in men.[85] Several mechanisms for this association have been postulated, such as an increase in circulating Na,K-ATPase inhibitors or a decrease in catecholamine concentration.[86] Data supporting dietary salt restriction for reducing AHR in asthmatics are encouraging.[87]

Exercise-induced asthma may be related to dehydration of the intrathoracic airways during hyperpnoea.[88] A high salt intake may interfere with rehydration of the airways. Mouth breathing as a result of sinusitis may also cause airway dehydration.

Hormonal factors

Glucocorticoid insufficiency related to various adrenal and extra-adrenal mechanisms has been associated with asthma in a Russian study.[89] Reduced nocturnal catecholamine and cortisol levels, which are a natural part of circadian rhythm, may be linked to the nocturnal exacerbation commonly associated with asthma.[90] Stress-induced corticosteroid resistance or insensitivity in asthma is receiving research attention,[91] as is hyporesponsiveness of the HPA (hypothalamic-pituitary-adrenal) axis (see also below).[92]

It was postulated that an increase in brain norepinephrine can reflect depression of the HPA axis.[93] In asthmatic children such an increase was found compared with controls.[93]

Premenstrual asthma has been observed, which was improved by progesterone injection.[94] Dynamic changes in hormone concentrations during the perimenstrual period are thought to be responsible for the rise in emergency admissions of asthmatic women at this time. Hormonal variation may prove to be a significant and independent risk factor for acute exacerbations of asthma.[95] Although the observed 4-fold increase in emergency admissions suggested that hormonal variation may influence the timing of an asthma attack, the severity of symptoms was no worse than that among women who presented at any other time in their menstrual cycle.

Stress

Low-income patients were more likely to report exacerbation of asthma when upset or anxious.[96] Parents of children who developed asthma were more likely to have problems in coping and parenting.[97]

Stress and associated muscular tension might influence lung function. One study suggested that an intrinsic impairment of the ability of inspiration to stretch airway smooth muscle is a major feature of asthma.[98] In other words, defective deep breathing could be a factor in airway narrowing. This would suggest a role for relaxation and breathing techniques in asthma.

Antioxidant status

The role of oxidative stress in asthma is gaining increasing research attention.[99] Activation of the Nrf2/ARE pathway could prove to be of therapeutic benefit.[100] Patients with acute asthma had decreased antiperoxide plasma activity compared with normal controls.[101] Moreover the severity of the asthma was inversely associated with the above parameter. In patients with steroid-dependent asthma the free radical process was more intensive.[101] Low selenium concentrations in whole blood have been correlated to increased asthma risk in New Zealand.[102]

Traditional factors associated with asthma

Poor digestion

Floyer in his *Treatize of the Asthma* published in 1698 wrote:

> Some writers ... have observed the hypochondriac symptoms in the stomach and conclude the asthma ... wants digestives .... It is commonly observed that fullness of diet, and all debauches render the fits most severe, and a temperate diet makes the fits more easy .... The defect of digestion and mucilaginous slime in the stomach are very obvious and observed by writers ....

Salter in 1868 stated that:

> ... the precursory symptoms are connected with the stomach and consist of loss of appetite, flatulence, costiveness and certain peculiar uneasy sensations in the epigastrium; but here I think we have something more than mere premonitory signs; I think the relation of these symptoms to the spasm which follows is often that of cause and effect.

Unhealthy mucous membranes and diet

Mucus secreted by mucous membranes (MM) is normal and has many important physiological functions. When MM become unhealthy, the nature and the quantity of the mucus changes. This can be referred to as a catarrhal condition. The degree of catarrhal congestion of the lungs can vary in asthma, and is best assessed by auscultation and case history. The association of chronic sinusitis with asthma is indicative of unhealthy MM. Despite the excessive mucus, catarrhal MM are thought to provide less protection than healthy MM, and in the case of asthma render the lungs more prone to damaging environmental factors such as allergens and pathogens. This traditional concept ties in well with the newer understanding of asthma as primarily a defect of airway epithelium, as described above.

Diet is a significant factor in causing a catarrhal state of the respiratory MM. Excessive protein, refined carbohydrate or salt consumption can lead to excessive and unhealthy mucus production. In some individuals, particular food groups especially dairy and/or wheat can also contribute to this process.

Catarrhal MM can also be regarded as a vicarious elimination due to inefficient detoxification and elimination in the body. Hence in traditional terms the detoxifying and eliminative processes need to be supported and stimulated.

Stress

Traditionally asthma has been regarded as imbalance in the autonomic nervous system. Stress and nervous anxiety contribute to this imbalance which may also cause muscular tension in the diaphragm and disturb the rhythmic nature of the breathing apparatus.It has been postulated that asthma results from a disturbance of the rhythmic activity of the respiratory centre in the brain.[103] This disorder is then reflected in the airways and the respiratory muscles through their respective innervations to cause a subclinical template of asthma. This rhythmic disturbance is reflected in the EEG of asthmatic patients, which generally contain certain abnormalities.[103]

Treatment

Treatment goals will obviously vary according to the needs of the individual case at the particular time of treatment. However, based on the above considerations they can be divided into two main categories: symptomatic treatment and treatment of the underlying issues (Table 9.1). The required actions related to the specific treatment goals and relevant herbs are also provided. Some treatment goals, such as resolving sinusitis, are complete therapeutic subjects in themselves and are covered elsewhere in this chapter.

This approach is informed by modern research and contrasts with the traditional approach that merely focussed on bronchodilator and expectorant activities (Table 9.2).

Some key herbs in asthma

Some plants have specialised effects on the inflammatory or allergic mechanisms known to occur in asthma. Since some of these effects have only recently been discovered or studied, a discussion of the research findings follows.

Cepaenes and thiosulfinates from *Allium cepa* (onion) are dual inhibitors of arachidonic acid metabolism, as are the gingerols from *Zingiber officinale* (ginger). See also the monograph on turmeric regarding its relevant anti-inflammatory and antiasthmatic activities. Boswellia has been successfully trialled in asthma on the basis of its anti-inflammatory activity (see monograph).

Isothiocyanates, cepaenes and thiosulfinates from *Allium cepa* have demonstrated an asthma-protective effect in animal models. The thiosulfinates counter platelet activating factor (PAF) and histamine-induced bronchoconstriction. In a human experiment, allergen-induced asthma attacks were almost completely inhibited by an *Allium cepa* extract.[104]

In vitro studies in the late 1980s discovered that the ginkgolides from the *Ginkgo biloba* leaf are potent and specific PAF antagonists (see monograph). In vivo animal studies (oral and injected routes) confirmed this activity.[105] Ginkgo and ginkgolides have also shown some beneficial clinical activity in asthma (see monograph).

Table 9.1 Asthma: symptomatic treatment and treating the underlying issues

Goal	Required actions	Herbs
Symptoms		
Control the allergic response	Antiallergic	Baical skullcap, Albizia, Nigella
Control acute respiratory infection	Diaphoretic, immune-enhancing, etc.	Echinacea, Andrographis, ginger, yarrow, etc.
Reduce inflammation	Anti-inflammatory, reflex demulcent	Ginkgo, Bupleurum, turmeric, marshmallow root, Boswellia, Sophora
Clear the airways	Expectorant	Adhatoda, Elecampane, fennel
Relax bronchial smooth muscle	Bronchospasmolytic	Adhatoda, Elecampane, Grindelia, Coleus
Allay debilitating cough	Expectorant, demulcent, antitussive	Elecampane, marshmallow root, Bupleurum, licorice
Underlying issues		
Control the allergic response	Antiallergic	Baical skullcap, Albizia, Nigella
Treat sinusitis	Anticatarrhal, antiallergic, immune-enhancing, etc.	Eyebright, Andrographis, golden seal, golden rod
Increase gastric acid	Bitter tonic, digestive	Gentian, Andrographis
Control reflux	Antispasmodic, demulcent, antacid, mucoprotective	Meadowsweet, marshmallow root, licorice
Eliminate infection	Immune-enhancing, antiviral, antibacterial	Echinacea root, Andrographis, Hypericum
Reduce the physical effects of stress	Adaptogen	Astragalus, Siberian ginseng
Reduce anxiety and tension	Sedative and nervine tonic	Valerian, St John's wort, Passiflora
Boost the hypothalamic-pituitary-adrenal axis	Tonic, adrenal tonic	Withania, Rehmannia, licorice
Balance immunity	Immune modifying, immune depressant	Echinacea root, Hemidesmus, Tylophora
Improve antioxidant status	Antioxidant, prime Nrf2/ARE	Ginkgo, rosemary, turmeric, grape seed, green tea
Improve the health of mucous membranes	Anticatarrhal, mucous membrane trophorestorative, lymphatic, depurative	Eyebright, golden seal, Verbascum

Table 9.2 Major herbs for asthma according to the *British Herbal Pharmacopoeia 1983*

Herb	Action
Datura	Spasmolytic
Drosera	Bronchodilator, expectorant
Ephedra	Bronchodilator (antiallergic)
Euphorbia	Spasmolytic, expectorant
Grindelia	Antispasmodic, expectorant
Lobelia	Spasmolytic, expectorant

Tylophora indica (*Tylophora asthmatica*) is a potent anti-asthmatic herb that depresses cell-mediated immunity.[106] It also stimulates the adrenal cortex, increasing plasma steroid levels and antagonising steroid-induced suppression of adrenal activity.[107] Several poorly designed clinical trials using Tylophora have shown benefits.[108]

Flavonoids from *Scutellaria baicalensis* have marked antiallergic activity. Baicalin and baicalein demonstrated antiallergic and antiasthmatic activity in several animal models.[109] For example oral administration of baicalin to egg-white-sensitised guinea pigs protected them against allergic reaction from re-inspiration of the antigen. Both compounds suppressed cutaneous allergy in guinea pigs.[109] A soluble derivative of baicalein was antiallergic after oral administration[110] and demonstrated more extensive antiallergic activity than sodium cromoglycate in vitro.[111] Other flavonoids from Baical skullcap were active in inhibiting the histamine release from rat peritoneal mast cells in vitro,[112] and baicalein inhibited basophil histamine content and growth in vitro.[113]

Saiboku-To (TJ-96) is a Kampo medicine comprising 10 herbs including Baical skullcap. It has been used in Japan for glucocorticoid-dependent asthmatic patients with the aim of reducing the dose of administered glucocorticoids. The antiallergic action of Saiboku-To is based on the suppression of type I and IV allergic reaction, which has been confirmed in animal studies.[114]

Albizia lebbek has mast cell stabilising activity.[115] Its antiallergic effects may also be mediated by suppression of lymphocyte function.[116]

Adhatoda vasica is a small evergreen, subherbaceous bush that grows on the plains of India, in the lower Himalayan ranges and in Sri Lanka, Burma and Malaysia. Adhatoda leaf has been used extensively in the Ayurvedic system for over 2000 years.[117] It has antiasthmatic, bronchodilating and expectorant activities and is traditionally used for the treatment of asthma, bronchitis cough and common cold.[118] In the World Health Organization publication *The Use of Traditional Medicine in Primary Health Care: A Manual for Health Workers in South-East Asia*, Adhatoda was said to facilitate breathing and to make sputum more fluid, thereby facilitating its removal. Adhatoda preparations are recommended for long-term use in adults and children.[119] However, it is contraindicated during pregnancy.

Key constituents of Adhatoda leaf are the quinazoline alkaloids (0.5% to 2%). The major alkaloid is vasicine present at levels of 45% to 95%. Minor alkaloids include vasicinine, vasicinone, oxyvasicinine, deoxyvasicine, deoxyvasicinone and vasicinol.[120,121] The drug bromhexine was developed from vasicine in Europe prior to the 1960s and is still used as an aid to expectoration by reducing the viscosity of secretions.[122] Oral administration of a mixture of vasicine and vasicinone (25 mg, three times per day) showed good bronchodilating activity in asthma patients. Seventy per cent demonstrated clinical improvement and improvement in spirometry.[123]

Uncontrolled clinical trials conducted in India as early as 1925 suggested that Adhatoda had an expectorant action. In acute bronchitis Adhatoda provided relief, especially where the sputum was thick and tenacious. In patients with chronic bronchitis cough was relieved and the sputum thinned, which facilitated removal. Mild relief was achieved for asthma.[118]

There are approximately 40 to 60 species of Grindelia native to temperate, mostly arid and semi-arid regions of North and South America. Species of Grindelia (commonly called gumweeds or gumplant) are not well differentiated and the taxonomy of the genus is still poorly understood. The resins produced by Grindelia consist mostly of labdane-type diterpenoid resin acids, similar in chemistry and physical properties to those obtained from pine trees. Resins from various species of Grindelia have been patented for use in adhesives, rubber, coatings and textiles.[124]

Several species of Grindelia are used in phytotherapy including *Grindelia camporum*, *G. robusta*, *G. squarrosa* and *G. humilis*. Constituents of the medicinal *Grindelia spp.* include the resin together with phenolic acids, flavonoids, an essential oil and small amounts of saponins.[125]

Grindelia is an expectorant herb with bronchospasmolytic activity. It is traditionally recommended for the treatment of spasmodic respiratory conditions such as asthma and bronchitis. The *British Herbal Pharmacopoeia 1983* lists the specific indication as bronchial asthma with tachycardia.[126] Eclectic physicians also utilised Grindelia for asthma.[127]

The Chinese herb *Sophora flavescens*, both on its own and in a formulation, has yielded promising results in asthma management. Its pharmacological properties include diuretic, antiviral, antitumour, sedative and anti-inflammatory activities. The main active components are matrine-type alkaloids, particularly matrine and oxymatrine.[128] It has been suggested that the Sophora alkaloids can act as modulators of cell membrane excitability. This is based on its CNS effects, anti-arrhythmic activity and inhibition of glutamate-induced responses.[128] On the hypothesis that an excitatory modulator (especially in the context of glutamate responses) may be beneficial in asthma, an open trial of Sophora in refractory asthma was initiated.[128]

From February 1997 to December 2005, 14 patients with moderate to severe asthma (six men and eight women) aged 22 to 70 years were treated. These patients had been diagnosed with asthma by their allergists and had been receiving medication for asthma for 3 to 6 years. Despite years of moderate to high doses of inhaled corticosteroids and beta-2 agonists, they still suffered episodes of dyspnoea, expectoration,

coughing, wheezing or chest tightness more than two times a week and waking up at night with asthma symptoms more than two times a week.[128] The patients were given a dried powder of a hot water extract of *S. flavescens* root, which contained a high content of matrine and oxymatrine (1.8% to 3.2%). The extract was provided in capsules, with a dose equal to 4 g of dried root, three times daily for 3 months and two times daily for 6 months and once daily for 27 months thereafter. Since the study was open, non-randomised and selective, the results below are summarised based on the records of the diary card of symptoms, PEF (peak expiratory flow), medication use and quality of life.[128]

After 4 weeks, the daytime asthma symptoms were reduced by 78%, and the night-time symptoms by 75%. Beta-2 agonist dose was reduced by 72% and the dose of corticosteroid inhaler reduced by 45%. The mean PEF rate improved by 12%. Two patients had remarkable improvements of eczema symptoms. No side effects were observed.[128] At 1 year, the daytime symptoms of asthma reduced by 94% and night-time symptoms by 95%. Beta-2 agonist use was reduced by 95%; corticosteroid inhaler was reduced by 92%. The mean PEF had increased by 18%. After 3 years, the daytime symptoms of asthma were reduced by 97%, night-time symptoms by 98%. The dose of beta-2 agonist was reduced by 97% and no patients inhaled corticosteroids. The mean PEF had increased by 21%. At 3 years, nine of the patients had achieved a symptom-free, medication-free and also an asthma-free condition, meaning they did not develop asthma symptoms when they were exposed to the previous triggers of their asthma attacks. Two of the patients with functional and radiological evidence of emphysema achieved an improvement in both breathing capacity and airway fibrosis (emphysema) to the extent that they were no longer considered to have emphysema. Two patients had complete remission of their eczema.[128]

Despite these striking results, they must be viewed with caution since this was an open label trial and there was no placebo group. Hence, it is encouraging to learn that Sophora in conjunction with two other traditional Chinese herbs (*Glycyrrhiza uralensis* (licorice) and *Ganoderma lucidum*) was found to be active in a controlled trial.[129] The efficacy and tolerability of this formula was investigated in 91 patients with moderate to severe asthma in a double blind, randomised trial. The herbal treatment was compared with oral prednisone therapy.[129]

Patients in the herbal group received oral capsules (3.6 g/ day of the mixture) and placebo tablets similar in appearance to prednisone. Those in the prednisone group received oral prednisone tablets (20 mg/day in the morning) and 'herbal placebo capsules', for 4 weeks. Treatment was administered daily over a period of 4 weeks. No medications other than rescue beta-2 agonists were allowed. This study found that post-treatment lung function (FEV_1 and PEF values) was significantly improved in both groups. The improvement was slightly but significantly greater in the prednisone group ($p < 0.05$). There was a significant and a similar degree of reduction in clinical symptom scores in both treated groups.[129]

Of interest, the Th2 cytokines IL-5 and IL-13 were significantly reduced in both treated groups ($p < 0.001$ for each).

Strikingly, serum interferon (IFN)-gamma and cortisol levels were significantly decreased in the prednisone group (p<0.001), but significantly increased in the herbal group (p<0.001). In addition, the herbal treatment had no significant effect on body weight (increases in body weight post-therapy, 2.8 kg in the prednisone group versus 0.8 kg in the herbal group). No significant side effects were observed.

Prescription construction

Asthma is a deep-seated protracted condition that requires herbal treatment in pharmacological doses. Hence a high dosage protocol is proposed. Based on the treatment goals outlined above it is suggested that two formulations, each of four to six herbs, are developed for the individual patient, or otherwise one formulation and a herbal tablet or capsule.

One should be a long-term treatment aimed at treating the underlying factors behind the asthmatic condition. The second can be aimed at the symptoms and sustaining causes. (A third formula could be developed which is only to be taken to alleviate acute attacks, but these days most patients will resort to a bronchodilating drug in these circumstances.)

The herbs in the two formulations should be chosen so that there is as much overlap of the required actions as possible. This reduces the number of herbs needed to give a broad range of required actions (as informed by Table 9.1). For example:

- Ginger has expectorant, digestive-stimulant and anti-inflammatory activities.
- Adhatoda is expectorant and bronchodilating.

The adult patient is then prescribed an 8 mL dose of each formula two to three times a day. Dosages are adjusted for children based on their body weight.

The treatment should be varied over time depending on the patient's response. Also not every factor can necessarily be treated at the one time, so particular treatment goals may need to be changed from time to time. This should be a dynamic and interactive approach. The following case histories illustrate some aspects of this strategy.

CASE HISTORY

The patient, 16-year-old teenage girl, had had asthma since the age of 6. She had been hospitalised several times, including recently. She had marked upper respiratory allergy and 'had a constant cold all last year'. Medication was inhaled bronchodilators and steroids. The patient was advised to eliminate all dairy products from her diet.

The following herbal tablets were prescribed:

- A tablet containing *Echinacea angustifolia* root 500 mg, *Ocimum tenuiflorum* 500 mg, *Andrographis paniculata* 1000 mg and *Ocimum tenuiflorum* leaf essential oil 10 mg. Dose 4/day
- A tablet containing *Boswellia serrata* 1.9 g, *Apium graveolens* 1000 mg, *Zingiber officinale* 300 mg and *Curcuma longa* 2 g. Dose 2/day
- A tablet containing *Echinacea angustifolia* root 600 mg and *Echinacea purpurea* root 675 mg. Dose 1/day
- A tablet containing *Scutellaria baicalensis* 800 mg, *Albizia lebbek* 800 mg and *Tanacetum parthenium* 50 mg. Dose 2/day.

Over a 6-month treatment period the patient's condition improved dramatically. The need for inhaled conventional drugs was reduced to almost zero, her sinuses cleared and there was a considerable enhancement of general well-being.

The following case illustrates how herbal tablets can be effectively used to manage asthma in patients who have difficulty negotiating tinctures and liquid extracts. Here the tablets were largely aimed at controlling inflammation and allergy, and supporting immune function.

CASE HISTORY

A 75-year-old female patient developed late onset asthma following a bout of lower respiratory infections and was prescribed prednisone by her medical doctor (now stopped). She also had pronounced sinus congestion and was under stress because of selling and moving house.

The following herbal treatments were instituted:

Euphrasia officinalis	1:2	25 mL
Ginkgo biloba (standardised extract)	2:1	25 mL
Echinacea angustifolia/purpurea root	1:2	25 mL
Eleutherococcus senticosus	1:2	25 mL
	TOTAL	100 mL

Dose: 8 mL with water twice a day

Three herbal tablets per day containing: *Scutellaria baicalensis* 500 mg, *Adhatoda vasica* 750 mg, *Grindelia camporum* 300 mg, *Curcuma longa* 1000 mg, *Ginkgo biloba* leaf 1000 mg and *Foeniculum vulgare* essential oil 5 mg.

After 4 weeks, the patient reported that her asthma had substantially improved. This improvement was also sustained by the next consultation 4 weeks later. The patient was then subsequently maintained with just the herbal tablets, which according to her reports provided substantial relief for her asthma on an ongoing basis.

References

1. Chen S. Natural products triggering biological targets – a review of the anti-inflammatory phytochemicals targeting the arachidonic acid pathway in allergy asthma and rheumatoid arthritis. *Curr Drug Targets*. 2011;12(3):288–301.
2. Passalacqua G, Bousquet PJ, Carlsen KH, et al. ARIA update: 1. Systematic review of complementary and alternative medicine for rhinitis and asthma. *J Allergy Clin Immunol*. 2006;117:1054–1062.
3. Gonzalez H, Ahmed T. Suppression of gastric H2-receptor mediated function in patients with bronchial asthma and ragweed allergy. *Chest*. 1986;89(4):491–496.
4. Minton NA. Volunteer models for predicting antiemetic activity of 5-HT3-receptor antagonists. *Br J Clin Pharmacol*. 1994;37(6):525–530.
5. Muller-Limmroth W, Frohlich HH. Effect of various phytotherapeutic expectorants on mucociliary transport. *Fortsch Med*. 1980;98(3):95–101.
6. Nosál'ova G, Strapková A, Kardosová A, et al. Antitussive action of extracts and polysaccharides of marsh mallow (Althea officinalis L., var. robusta). *Pharmazie*. 1992;47(3):224–226.
7. Horwitz R. Controlling asthma: the role of nutrition. *Explore*. 2005;1(5):393–395.

8. Wilson D, Evans M, Guthrie N, et al. A randomized, double blind, placebo-controlled exploratory study to evaluate the potential of Pycnogenol® for improving allergic rhinitis symptoms. *Phytother Res.* 2010;24(8):1115–1119.

9. Lau B, Riesen S, Truong K, et al. Pycnogenol as an adjunct in the management of childhood asthma. *J Asthma.* 2004;41(8):825–832.

10. Giles M, Ulbricht C, Khalsa KPS, et al. Butterbur: an evidence-based systematic review by the Natural Standard Research Collaborative. *J Herbal Pharmacother.* 2005;5(3):119–143.

11. Schapowal A. Treating intermittent allergic rhinitis: a prospective, randomized, placebo and antihistamine-controlled study of butterbur extract Ze 339. *Phytother Res.* 2005;19:530–537.

12. Lee K, Carstairs I, Haggart K, et al. Butterbur, a herbal remedy, attenuates adenosine monophosphate induced nasal responsiveness in seasonal allergic rhinitis. *Clin Exp Allergy.* 2003;33:882–886.

13. Danesch U. Petasites hybridus (butterbur root) extract in the treatment of asthma – an open trial. *Altern Med Rev.* 2004;9(1):54–62.

14. Agbabiaka TB, Guo R, Ernst E. Pelargonium sidoides for acute bronchitis: A systematic review and meta-analysis. *Phytomedicine.* 2008;15:378–385.

15. Timmer A, Günther J, Rücker G, et al. Pelargonium sidoides extract for acute respiratory tract infections. *Cochrane Database Syst Rev.* 2008;(3):CD006323.

16. Barak V, Berkenfeld S, Halperin T, Kalickman I. The effect of herbal remedies on the production of human inflammatory and anti-inflammatory cytokines. *Isr Med Assoc J.* 2002;4:919–921.

17. Guo R, Pittler MH, Ernst E. Herbal medicines for the treatment of allergic rhinitis: a systematic review. *Ann Allergy Asthma Immunol.* 2007;99(6):483–495.

18. Ernst E. Frankincense: systematic review. *Br Med J.* 2008;337 a2813.

19. Hofmann D, Hecker M, Volp A. Efficacy of dry extract of ivy leaves in children with bronchial asthma – a review of randomized controlled trials. *Phytomedicine.* 2003;10:213–220.

20. Kurz H. *Antitussiva und Expektoranzien.* Stuttgart: Wissenschaftliche Verlagsgesellschaft; 1989.

21. Remberg P, Bjork L, Hedner T, Sterner O. Characteristics, clinical effect profile and tolerability of a nasal spray preparation of Artemisia abrotanum L for allergic rhinitis. *Phytomedicine.* 2004;11(1):36–42.

22. Eccles R, Morris S, Tolley NS. The effects of nasal anesthesia upon nasal sensation of airflow. *Acta Otolaryngol (Stockholm).* 1988;106:152–155.

23. Hedayat KM. Essential oil diffusion for the treatment of persistent oxygen dependence in a three-year-old child with restrictive lung disease with respiratory syncytial virus pneumonia. *Explore.* 2008;4(4):264–266.

24. Dorow P. Welchen Einfluss hat Cineol auf die mukoziliare Clearance? *Therapiewoche.* 1989;39:2652–2654.

25. Lorenz J, Ferlinz R. Expektoranzien: pathophysiologie und therapie der mukostase. *Arzneimitteltherapie.* 1985;3:22–27.

26. Kleigman RM, Behrman RE, Jenson HB, et al. *Nelson Textbook of Pediatrics,* 18th ed. Philadelphia: Saunders Elsevier; 2007.

27. Scaglione K, Weiser M. Effects of the standardised Ginseng extract G115 in patients with chronic bronchitis. *Clin Drug Invest.* 2001;21(1):41–45.

28. Burrows B, Martinez FD, Halonen M, et al. Association of asthma with serum IgE levels and skin-test reactivity to allergens. *N Engl J Med.* 1989;320(5):271–277.

29. Ulrik CS, Backer V, Dirksen A. Mortality and decline in lung function in 213 adults with bronchial asthma: a ten-year follow up. *J Asthma.* 1992;29(1):29–38.

30. Pirson F, Charpin D, Sansonetti M, et al. Is intrinsic asthma a hereditary disease? *Allergy.* 1991;46(5):367–371.

31. Beasley R, Roche W, Holgate ST. Inflammatory processes in bronchial asthma. *Drugs.* 1989;37(suppl 1):117–122.

32. Murphy DM, O'Byrne PM. Recent advances in the pathophysiology of asthma. *Chest.* 2010;137(6):1417–1426.

33. Durrant DM, Metzger DW. Emerging roles of T helper subsets in the pathogenesis of asthma. *Immunol Invest.* 2010;39(4–5):526–549.

34. Ray A, Khare A, Krishnamoorthy N, et al. Regulatory T cells in many flavors control asthma. *Mucosal Immunol.* 2010;3(3):216–229.

35. Umetsu DT, Dekruyff RH. Natural killer T cells are important in the pathogenesis of asthma: the many pathways to asthma. *J Allergy Clin Immunol.* 2010;125(5):975–979.

36. Thomas SY, Chyung YH, Luster AD. Natural killer T cells are not the predominant T cell in asthma and likely modulate, not cause, asthma. *J Allergy Clin Immunol.* 2010;125(5):980–984.

37. Murdoch JR, Lloyd CM. Chronic inflammation and asthma. *Mutat Res.* 2010;690(1–2):24–39.

38. Holgate ST, Arshad HS, Roberts GC, et al. A new look at the pathogenesis of asthma. *Clin Sci (Lond).* 2009;118(7):439–450.

39. Holgate ST, Roberts G, Arshad HS, et al. The role of the airway epithelium and its interaction with environmental factors in asthma pathogenesis. *Proc Am Thorac Soc.* 2009;6(8):655–659.

40. Hallstrand TS, Henderson Jr WR. An update on the role of leukotrienes in asthma. *Curr Opin Allergy Clin Immunol.* 2010;10(1):60–66.

41. Taylor ML, Stewart GA, Thompson PJ. The differential effect of aspirin on human platelet activation in aspirin-sensitive asthmatics and normal subjects. *Br J Clin Pharmacol.* 1993;35(3):227–234.

42. Yamashita T, Tsuji H, Maeda N, et al. Etiology of nasal polyps associated with aspirin-sensitive asthma. *Rhinology Suppl.* 1989;8:15–24.

43. Gøtzsche PC, Johansen HK. House dust mite control measures for asthma: systematic review. *Allergy.* 2008;63(6):646–659.

44. Arshad SH. Does exposure to indoor allergens contribute to the development of asthma and allergy? *Curr Allergy Asthma Rep.* 2010;10(1):49–55.

45. Strachan DP, Carey IM. Home environment and severe asthma in adolescence: a population based case-control study. *BMJ.* 1995;311:1053–1056.

46. Taskinen T, Hyvarinen A, Meklin T, et al. Asthma and respiratory infections in school children with special reference to moisture and mold problems in the school. *Acta Paediatr.* 1999;88:1373–1379.

47. Carpi J. Mite-contaminated foods linked to anaphylaxis. *Fam Pract News.* May 1996;1:19.

48. Bakirtas A. Acute effects of passive smoking on asthma in childhood. *Inflamm Allergy Drug Targets.* 2009;8(5):353–358.

49. Sarnat JA, Holguin F. Asthma and air quality. *Curr Opin Pulm Med.* 2007;13(1):63–66.

50. Brugman SM, Larsen GL, Henson PM, et al. Increased lower airways responsiveness associated with sinusitis in a rabbit model. *Am Rev Respir Dis.* 1993;147(2):314–320.

51. Friday Jr GA, Fireman P. Sinusitis and asthma: clinical and pathogenetic relationships. *Clin Chest Med.* 1988;9(4):557–565.

52. Bardin PG, Van Heerden BB, Joubert JR. Absence of pulmonary aspiration of sinus contents in patients with asthma and sinusitis. *J Allergy Clin Immunol.* 1990;86(1):82–88.

53. Jarikre LN, Ogisi FO. Nasal symptoms in bronchial asthma. *East Afr Med J.* 1990;67(1):9–12.

54. de Benedictis FM, del Giudice MM, Severini S, Bonifazi F. Rhinitis, sinusitis and asthma: one linked airway disease. *Paediatr Respir Rev.* 2001;2(4):358–364.

55. Bray GW. The hypochlorhydria of asthma of childhood. *Q J Med.* 1931;24:181–197.

56. Barberio G, Ruggeri C, Pajno GB, et al. Gastro-esophageal reflux and asthma. Clinical experience. *Minerva Pediatr.* 1989;41(7):363–366.

57. Giudicelli R, Dupin B, Surpas P, et al. Gastroesophageal reflux and respiratory manifestations: diagnostic approach, therapeutic indications and results. *Ann Chir.* 1990;44(7):552–554.

58. Gustafsson PM, Kjellman NI, Tibbling L. Bronchial asthma and acid reflux into the distal and proximal oesophagus. *Arch Dis Child.* 1990;65(1):1255–1258.

59. Geller LI, Glinskaia TP, Nikolaeva LI, Petrenko VF. Gastroesophageal reflux and bronchial asthma. *Ter Arkh.* 1990;62(2):69–72.

60. Donnelly RJ, Berrisford RG, Jack CI, et al. Simultaneous tracheal and esophageal pH monitoring: investigating reflux-associated asthma. *Ann Thorac Med*. 1993;56(5):1029–1033.

61. Agarwal A, Rishi JP, Gupta AN, Bhandari VM. Histamine bronchoprovocation tests in subjects with gastro-oesophageal reflux disease. *J Assoc Physicians India*. 1990;38(2):159–161.

62. McCallister JW, Parsons JP, Mastronarde JG. The relationship between gastroesophageal reflux and asthma: an update. *Ther Adv Respir Dis*. 2011;5(2):143–150.

63. Chang CC, Phinney SD, Halpern GM, Gershwin ME. Asthma mortality: another opinion – is it a matter of life and … bread? *J Asthma*. 1993;30(2):93–103.

64. Pagano R, Negri E, Decarli A, La Vecchia C. Coffee drinking and prevalence of bronchial asthma. *Chest*. 1988;94(2):386–389.

65. Hodge J, Salome CM, Peat JK, et al. Consumption of oily fish and childhood asthma risk. *MJA*. 1996;164:137–140.

66. Laerum BN, Wentzel-Larsen T, Gulsvik A, et al. Relationship of fish and cod oil intake with adult asthma. *Clin Exp Allergy*. 2007;37(11):1616–1623.

67. Britton J, Pavord I, Richards K, et al. Dietary magnesium, lung function, wheezing, and airway hyperreactivity in a random adult population sample. *Lancet*. 1994;344(8919):357–362.

68. Stuttaford T. Medical Briefing: Apple of the doctor's eye. *The Times*. February 2000;3:15.

69. Nurmatov U, Devereux G, Sheikh A. Nutrients and foods for the primary prevention of asthma and allergy: systematic review and meta-analysis. *J Allergy Clin Immunol*. 2011;127(3):724–733. e1–e30.

70. Bardin PG, Johnston SL, Pattemore PK. Viruses as precipitants of asthma symptoms. II. Physiology and mechanisms. *Clin Exper Allergy*. 1992;22(9):809–822.

71. Beasley R, Coleman ED, Hermon Y, et al. Viral respiratory tract infection and exacerbations of asthma in adult patients. *Thorax*. 1988;43(9):679–683.

72. Kloepfer KM, Gern JE. Virus/allergen interactions and exacerbations of asthma. *Immunol Allergy Clin North Am*. 2010;30(4):553–563.

73. Sly PD, Hibbert ME. Childhood asthma following hospitalization with acute viral bronchiolitis in infancy. *Pediatr Pulmonol*. 1989;7(3):153–158.

74. Rylander E, Pershagen G, Eriksson M, Nordvall L. Parental smoking and other risk factors for wheezing bronchitis in children. *Eur J Epidemiol*. 1993;9(5):517–526.

75. Liu WJ, Lo WS, Hsieh HJ, et al. Increased incidence of asthma and pulmonary dysfunction after severe lower respiratory tract infection in infancy. *Zhonghua Min Guo Xiao Er Ke Yi Xue Hui Za Zhi [Acta Paediatr Sin]*. 1991;32(6):348–357.

76. Jackson DJ, Lemanske Jr RF. The role of respiratory virus infections in childhood asthma inception. *Immunol Allergy Clin North Am*. 2010;30(4):513–522.

77. Hahn DL, Dodge RW, Golubjatnikov R. Association of Chlamydia pneumoniae (strain TWAR) infection with wheezing, asthmatic bronchitis, and adult-onset asthma. *JAMA*. 1991;266(2):225–230.

78. Guilbert TW, Denlinger LC. Role of infection in the development and exacerbation of asthma. *Expert Rev Respir Med*. 2010;4(1):71–83.

79. Ward Jr GW, Karlsson G, Rose G, Platts-Mills TA. Trichophyton asthma: sensitisation of bronchi and upper airways to dermatophyte antigen. *Lancet*. 1989;1(8643):859–862.

80. Pronina EV, Karaev ZO, Alferov VP. Increased sensitivity to Candida in patients with bronchial asthma. *Pediatria*. 1990;5:14–18.

81. Strazzella WD, Safirstein BH. Asthma due to parasitic infestation. *N J Med*. 1989;86(12):947–949.

82. Burney P. A diet rich in sodium may potentiate asthma. Epidemiologic evidence for a new hypothesis. *Chest*. 1991;91(6 suppl):143S–148S.

83. Burney PGJ, Britton JR, Chinn S, et al. Response to inhaled histamine and 24 hour sodium excretion. *BMJ*. 1986;292:1483–1486.

84. Burney PGJ, Neild JE, Twort CH, et al. Effect of changing dietary sodium on the airway response to histamine. *Thorax*. 1989;44(1):36–41.

85. Carey OJ, Locke C, Cookson JB. Effect of alterations of dietary sodium on the severity of asthma in men. *Thorax*. 1993;48(7):714–718.

86. Knox AJ. Salt and asthma. *BMJ*. 1993;307:1159–1160.

87. Mickleborough TD. Salt intake, asthma, and exercise-induced bronchoconstriction: a review. *Phys Sportsmed*. 2010;38(1):118–131.

88. Daviskas E, Gonda I, Anderson SD. Local airway heat and water vapour losses. *Respir Physiol*. 1991;84(1):115–132.

89. Fedoseev GB, Trofimov VI, Sinitsina TM, et al. [Current views on the role of disorders of hormonal regulation in the development of altered sensitivity and reactivity of the bronchi]. *Vestn Akad Med Nauk SSSR*. 1989;2:29–33.

90. van Aalderen WM, Meijer GG, Oosterhoff Y, Bron AO. Epidemiology and the concept of underlying mechanisms of nocturnal asthma. *Respir Med*. 1993;87(suppl B):S37–S39.

91. Haczku A, Panettieri Jr. RA. Social stress and asthma: the role of corticosteroid insensitivity. *J Allergy Clin Immunol*. 2010;125(3):550–558.

92. Di Marco F, Santus P, Centanni S. Anxiety and depression in asthma. *Curr Opin Pulmon Med*. 2011;17(1):39–44.

93. Scanlon TR, Chang S. Brain norepinephrine: a possible role in bronchial asthma. *Ann Allergy*. 1988;60(4):333–338.

94. Beynon HL, Garbett ND, Barnes PJ. Severe premenstrual exacerbations of asthma: effect of intramuscular progesterone. *Lancet*. 1988;2:370–372.

95. Skobeloff EM, Spivey WH, Silverman R, et al. The effect of the menstrual cycle on asthma presentations in the emergency department. *Arch Intern Med*. 1996;156(16):1837–1840.

96. Rumbak MJ, Kelso TM, Arheart KL, Self TH. Perception of anxiety as a contributing factor of asthma: indigent versus nonindigent. *J Asthma*. 1993;30(3):165–169.

97. Mrazek DA, Klinnert MD, Mrazek P, Macey T. Early asthma onset: consideration of parenting issues. *J Am Acad Child Psychiatry*. 1991;30(2):277–282.

98. Skloot G, Permutt S, Togias A. Airway hyperresponsiveness in asthma: a problem of limited smooth muscle relaxation with inspiration. *J Clin Invest*. 1995;96(5):2393–2403.

99. Dozor AJ. The role of oxidative stress in the pathogenesis and treatment of asthma. *Ann N Y Acad Sci*. 2010;1203:133–137.

100. Riedl MA, Nel AE. Importance of oxidative stress in the pathogenesis and treatment of asthma. *Curr Opin Allergy Clin Immunol*. 2008;8(1):49–56.

101. Boljevic S, Daniljak IG, Kogan AH. Changes in free radicals and possibility of their correction in patients with bronchial asthma. *Vojnosanit Pregl*. 1993;50(1):3–18.

102. Flatt A, Pearce N, Thomson CD, et al. Reduced selenium in asthmatic subjects in New Zealand. *Thorax*. 1990;45(2):95–99.

103. Kashalikar SJ. A common denominator in the pathogenesis of asthma. *Med Hypotheses*. 1988;27(4):255–259.

104. Dorsch W, Adam O, Weber J. Antiallergic and antiasthmatic effects of onion extracts. *Folia Allergol Immunol Clin*. 1983;30(suppl 4):17.

105. Braquet P. Proofs of involvement of PAF-acether in various immune disorders using BN 52021 (ginkgolide B): a powerful PAF-acether antagonist isolated from Ginkgo biloba L. *Adv Prostaglandin Thromboxane Leukot Res*. 1986;16:179–198.

106. Atal CK, Sharma A, Kaul A, Khajuria A. Immunomodulating agents of plant origin. I: Preliminary screening. *J Ethnopharmacol*. 1986;18(2):133–141.

107. Udupa AL, Udupa SL, Guruswamy MN. The possible site of anti-asthmatic action of Tylophora asthmatica on pituitary-adrenal axis in albino rats. *Planta Med*. 1991;57(5):409–413.

108. Bone K. *Clinical Applications of Ayurvedic and Chinese Herbs*. Warwick, Australia: Phytotherapy Press; 1996. pp. 134–136.

109. Chang HM, But PP. *Pharmacology and Applications of Chinese Materia Medica*. Singapore: World Scientific; 1987.

110. Nagai H, Osuga K, Koda A. Inhibition of hypersensitivity reactions by soluble derivatives of baicalein. *Jpn J Pharmacol*. 1975;25:763.

111. Amella M, Bronner C, Briancon F, et al. Inhibition of mast cell histamine release by flavonoids and bioflavonoids. *Planta Med*. 1985;1:16–20.

112. Kubo M, Matsuda H, Tanaka M, et al. Studies on Scutellariae radix. VII. Anti-arthritic and anti-inflammatory actions of methanolic extract and flavonoid components from Scutellariae radix. *Chem Pharm Bull (Tokyo)*. 1984;32(7):2724–2729.

113. Tanno Y, Shindoh Y, Takishima T. Modulation of human basophil growth in vitro by xiao-qing-long-tang (syo-seiryu-to), chai-pu-tang (saiboku-to), qing-fei-tang (seihai-to), baicalein and ketotifen. *Am J Chin Med*. 1989;17(1–2):45–50.

114. Taniguchi C, Homma M, Takano O, et al. Pharmacological effects of urinary products obtained after treatment with saiboku-to, a herbal medicine for bronchial asthma, on type IV allergic reaction. *Planta Med*. 2000;66(7):607–611.

115. Tripathi RM, Sen PC, Das PK. Studies on the mechanism of action of Albizzia lebbeck, an Indian indigenous drug used in the treatment of atopic allergy. *J Ethnopharmacol*. 1979;1(4):385–396.

116. Tripathi RM, Sen PC, Das PK. Further studies on the mechanism of the anti-anaphylactic action of Albizzia lebbeck, an Indian indigenous drug. *J Ethnopharmacol*. 1979;1(4):397–400.

117. Atal CK. *Chemistry and Pharmacology of Vasicine: A New Oxytocic and Abortifacient*. Jammu-Tawi: Regional Research Laboratory; 1980.

118. Chopra RN, et al. *Chopra's Indigenous Drugs of India*, 2nd ed. Calcutta: Academic Publishers; 1982.

119. World Health Organization. *The Use of Traditional Medicine in Primary Health Care: A Manual for Health Workers in South-East Asia*. New Delhi: WHO Regional Office for South-East Asia; 1990.

120. Wagner H, Bladt S. *Plant Drug Analysis: A Thin Layer Chromatography Atlas*, 2nd ed. Berlin: Springer-Verlag; 1996.

121. Rastogi RP, et al. *1990–1994 Compendium of Indian Medicinal Plants*, vol 5. Lucknow and New Delhi: Central Drug Research Institute and National Institute of Science Communication; 1998.

122. Bruce RA, Kumar V. The effect of a derivative of vasicine on bronchial mucus. *Br J Clin Pract*. 1968;22(7):289–292.

123. Aulakh GS, Mahadevan G. Herbal drugs for asthma – a review of clinical evaluation of anti-asthmatic drugs. *Indian Drugs*. 1989;26(11):593–599.

124. McLaughlin SP. *Grindelia New Crop Factsheet*. University of Arizona: Office of Arid Lands Studies; 1995.

125. Mills S, Bone K. *The Essential Guide to Herbal Safety*. USA: Churchill Livingstone; 2005. pp. 457–458.

126. British Herbal Medicine Association. *British Herbal Pharmacopoeia*. Bournemouth: BHMA; 1983.

127. Felter HW, Lloyd JU. *King's American Dispensatory*, 18th ed., rev 3, vol II. First published, Portland, 1905; reprinted Sandy, Oregon, Eclectic Medical Publications, 1983.

128. Hoang BX, Shaw DG, Levine S, et al. New approach in asthma treatment using excitatory modulator. *Phytother Res*. 2007;21:554–557.

129. Li X-M. Traditional Chinese herbal remedies for asthma and food allergy. *J Allergy Clin Immunol*. 2007;120:25–31.

Urinary system

Scope

Apart from their use to provide non-specific support for recuperation and repair, specific phytotherapeutic strategies include the following.

Treatment of:

- acute and recurrent urinary infections
- functional disturbances of micturition.

Management of:

- interstitial cystitis
- urinary stones
- oedema with renal involvement
- moderate autoimmune kidney disease
- bedwetting.

Because of its use of secondary plant products, **extreme caution** is necessary in applying phytotherapy in cases of:

- renal failure
- urinary obstruction
- severe glomerulonephritis
- acute pyelonephritis.

Orientation

Herbal diuretics

Plants have been used as diuretic remedies throughout history (Pliny the Elder mentions that many plants have diuretic properties in his *Naturalis Historia*[1]). However, the early indications for such use were often different: urinary stones, nephritis, cystitis, strangury, urinary retention and incontinence.[2] The excruciating pain of urinary stones would of course be well known and would have driven many urgent treatments. Because of the severity of such conditions, diuretic remedies would have been more drastic than nowadays. Remedies would have been given in much higher doses, for shorter duration, and stronger agents were used. The diuretic effects of purgatives, for example, were well understood and these may well have been used in desperate attempts to relieve the symptoms of ascites in advanced liver failure – a not uncommon condition given the frequency of hepatitis. (This reputation of laxatives, although easily experienced, remains unsupported in clinical research, although it has been found in vivo that anthraquinone derivatives induce experimental diuresis associated with the inhibition of ATPases in the kidney medulla.[3]) Another drastic treatment of dropsy forms the basis of one of medicine's best historical stories. When William Withering found that the active principle of one effective remedy for dropsy was the cardioactive foxglove he initiated a whole new medical tradition as well as confirming that dropsy was a symptom of heart failure rather than of the kidneys (see also Chapter 2).

Inducing appreciable consistent diuresis generally involves drastic pharmacological activity and modern diuretic drugs are powerful agents. Examples of plants with direct diuretic effects producing consistent activity in controlled conditions in the literature are rare, and there are some studies that specifically show a negative effect in these circumstances.[4–7] There is, for example, the suggestion that essential oils may prove to have direct effects on tubular function: a paper on the effects of aqueous parsley seed extract has implicated tubular inhibition of the sodium/potassium pump, albeit with relatively large doses in rats, that would lead to a reduction in sodium and potassium reabsorption and an osmotic water flow into the urinary lumen.[8] Other examples where a diuretic effect has been observed experimentally include a study showing significant increase in 24-hour urine volume, urine and serum sodium levels in nine mild hypertensives administered a whole-plant preparation of *Phyllanthus amarus*.[9] In another study, *Aerua lanata* flowers at doses of 10g induced significant diuresis in 70% of subjects in uncontrolled clinical conditions.[10] A study on a product based on asparagus and parsley root has also shown limited diuretic effect in the management of congestive heart failure.[11] The benefits of the Indian remedy *Terminalia arjuna* bark extract at 500mg every 8 hours, as adjuvant therapy to conventional medications, have been attested in a double blind, crossover trial on 12 patients with chronic congestive heart failure (although this is most likely a cardiac rather than a renal effect).[12]

There is some evidence of diuretic effects of various popular diuretics in experimental animals, but often at very high doses (40mL/kg[13] and 1g/kg[14,15]), levels outside any therapeutic range. Other plants with experimental diuretic effects in animals that have been observed at various dosages include Taraxacum (dandelion),[16] members of the Equisetum family,[17] Orthosiphon leaf[18] and Orthosiphon seeds,[19] various *Solidago* species,[20,21] *Agrimonia eupatoria* (agrimony),[22] *Lactuca virosa* (wild lettuce)[23] and Parietaria (pellitory).[24] Diuretic activity (including renal vasodilation and urinary sodium excretion) has been observed in experimental studies on *Clerodendron trichotomum*,[25] and *Rehmannia radix*.[26] However, studies on *Alpinia speciosa*[27] and *Polygonum punctatum*[28] showed no diuretic properties in spite of other pronounced pharmacological activities, and the main effect in rats of administering oral doses of *Opuntia ficus-indica* infusions was a marked loss of potassium, with only modest diuresis and sodium loss at lower concentrations.[29]

In more recent pharmacological studies, several common herbs have exhibited interesting diuretic activity that might prove clinically relevant, including fennel (see fennel monograph). Others have been the subject of an extensive 2007 review.[30] A few clinical trials have also been undertaken. Powdered cherry stalk (*Cerasus avium*) at 2g caused a mild increase in urine volume in 13 healthy volunteers in an open label trial.[31] In another open label, pilot study, three 8mL doses in 1 day of a hydroethanolic extract of fresh dandelion leaf given to 17 healthy volunteers caused a significant (p<0.05) increase in the frequency of urination in the 5-hour period after the first dose.[32] There was also a significant (p<0.001) increase in the excretion ratio in the 5-hour period after the second dose of extract. The third dose failed to change any of the measured parameters. The herb *Eclipta alba* leaf powder 3g/day caused a remarkable increase in urine volume (34%) and urine sodium (24%) in a placebo-controlled 60-day trial involving 60 mildly hypertensive patients.[33]

The modest research evidence apart, the experience of even mild herbal prescriptions having sometimes dramatic diuretic effects is well known to practitioners and this is one of the most common reactions to treatment that patients report. One conclusion that can be drawn is that diuretic responses are variable, perhaps reflecting other indeterminate susceptibilities in the individual patient.

Aquaretics and diuretic depuratives

Two variations on the diuretic theme have emerged from earlier Western traditions. In German practice, the concept of 'aquaretic' has been used to describe diuretic agents that excrete water from the body, most probably associated with potassium, but not other electrolyte, excretion.[34] They may exert their effect due to increased blood flow to the kidney. Most herbal diuretics in tradition are likely to be of this class. They are thus not easily comparable with modern diuretics that interfere with resorption at the distal tubule of the nephron, leading to wider electrolyte elimination, and thus may be less effective in treating hypertension and oedematous conditions. They are speculated to act on the glomerulus, increasing fluid loss from the body in a physiological manner by increasing the formation of primary urine.[35]

In the case of hypertension, the main benefit of herbal aquaretics may be in replacing the potassium lost through the use of modern diuretic prescriptions. High potassium levels relative to sodium have been shown to be a feature of herbal drugs with traditional diuretic activity.[36] Compared to a ratio in the average diet of 2:1, herbal remedies such as Urtica (nettle tops), Equisetum (horsetail), Betula (birch), Sambucus (elder), Agrimonia (agrimony), *Phaseolus vulgaris* (bean pods), Matricaria (chamomile) and tilia (lime flowers) had ratios greater than 150:1 potassium to sodium, especially in decoction form. It is difficult with current information to link high potassium levels to any aquaretic or diuretic effect, but given that diuresis is almost by definition accompanied by potassium loss, to have an effective potassium supplement seems convenient.

The herb combination that has been most studied in the context of aquaretic activity is asparagus root (*Asparagus officinalis*) with parsley herb (*Petroselinum crispum*).[11] In uncontrolled trials, this combination caused significant weight loss in overweight patients and significantly lowered blood pressure in patients with hypertension, without changing other biochemical parameters.[11]

In the case of oedema, phytotherapeutic strategies should emphasise activity on other body functions (see below) rather than any diuretic impact.

A second concept of 'diuretic depurative' is more compatible with the general meaning of diuretics in Western herbal tradition; it implies that the remedy removes metabolites and waste products as well as water, that is as an aid to excretion.

There is one very gentle diuretic mechanism that may underlie the effect of several plants.

Osmotic diuresis

The principle of osmotic diuresis has been established since the end of the 19th century when Ustimowitsch, Falck and Richet stressed the influence of urinary solutes on urine flow, although over a century earlier Segalas and Wohler observed that an extra load of urea, or any other substance that is excreted by the kidney, causes a diuresis.[37]

The osmotic plant-based diuretic mannitol is used, by intravenous injection, in acute oliguric renal failure.[38] Mannitol is found in some plants, including the popular diuretic *Elymus repens* (couch grass); however, its absorption from the gut wall is limited and it is unlikely to play a significant role in the effect of couch grass. Nevertheless, a number of similar sugar molecules may account for a gentle diuretic effect of many herbal remedies, as well as, more generally, fruits and vegetables. For example, the plant starch inulin is used in commercial preparations to measure glomerular filtration rate and in experiments of kidney microperfusion as a marker of tubular water reabsorption. A number of plant extracts of inulin have been shown to have a comparable effect.[39]

The kidneys and oedema

Although clearly active in the elimination of water from the body and the control of fluid levels within the tissues, the impact of the kidneys in oedema is not always obvious, compared with a failing heart, a cirrhotic liver or lymphatic or venous insufficiency in their relevant syndromes. Nevertheless, in all such cases prescription of conventional diuretic drugs is commonplace and it is widely assumed that the kidney is centrally involved in most cases.

This assumption has mixed support in the scientific literature. For example, renal complications of liver cirrhosis are certainly implicated in the development of ascites. These complications include inadequate renal prostaglandin production and the negative effect on the kidney of raised nitric oxide production. Such complications may actually reduce the effect of diuretics, but they remain indicated in the treatment of ascites as long as they are effective.[40] In phytotherapy, however, the main effort now would be on using hepatics and other treatments for the liver.

Although undoubtedly effective symptomatically, the value of diuretics used alone for congestive heart failure in the long term has been challenged, because of their possible excitation of the renin-angiotensin system. Concomitant prescription of ACE inhibitors has been proposed and positively evaluated, because they suppress this excitation.[41] As seen below, herbal diuretics are unlikely to raise the same concerns but may be only second-tier treatments compared to the cardioactive glycosides.

The localised oedema of lymphatic and venous insufficiency is treated in phytotherapy with particular remedies said to act on the vessel walls. These may have incidental diuretic effects.

In phytotherapy, there are few traditional strategies that are likely to bear directly on the kidney cortex itself, with emphasis placed instead on activity lower down the urinary system. Nevertheless, little is known about the full impact of plant constituents on this organ and, although there are very few cases where actual nephrotoxicity occurs, a general caution in using herbal treatments is advisable where the kidneys are already damaged.[42]

Beneficial effects of plant remedies on the kidney

Kidney disease such as glomerulonephritis and cystic disease presents awesome and possibly overwhelming odds for the phytotherapist. By definition the kidney in such cases, especially where the basement membrane is involved, is vulnerable to further damage with any new active metabolite and the practitioner needs to proceed with extreme caution. Nevertheless, there is experimental and case report evidence, mainly from China and Japan, suggesting that some herbal remedies might have beneficial effects in such cases, including such conditions as nephrotic syndrome (Chinese herbs Astragalus and Angelica

(see monographs),[43] diabetic nephropathy (*Abemoschus manihot*[44]) and other kidney diseases.[45-49] *Andrographis paniculata* has shown experimental ability to reduce pyuria and haematuria as complications of urinary stone destruction (see Andrographis monograph)[50] and magnesium lithospermate B, a component of *Lycopus* and *Lithospermum* species, has shown potential as a therapeutic agent for inhibiting the progression of renal dysfunction.[51] The use of various Chinese bitter ('cooling and drying') herbs has been shown to improve biochemical markers associated with free radical damage in patients with chronic glomerulonephritis compared with matched controls.[52]

Other plant materials have shown apparent antinephrotoxic activity and may provide the basis for strategies following the adverse effects of heavy metals, antibiotics, analgesic and other prescription drugs, Amanita mushroom and aflatoxins and industrial agents. Protective effects of *Arctostaphlos uva-ursi*, *Orthosiphon stamineus* and *Polygonum aviculare* have been noted against the nephrotoxic effects of mercuric chloride,[53] and beneficial effects against the nephrotoxin aminoglycoside in elderly patients have also been noted in controlled studies for *Cordyceps sinensis*.[54] Aqueous rhubarb extract (at 150 mg/day) reduced proteinurea and glomerulosclerosis in rats exposed to experimental chronic renal fibrosis in controlled models.[55] More recently curcumin and Withania have demonstrated nephroprotective activity in vivo (see monographs) and there have been some interesting reviews of this topic.[56-59]

Phytotherapeutics: diuretics (aquaretics and diuretic depuratives)

Terminology

As noted above, most plants used primarily for their effects on the urinary system are collectively referred to as 'diuretics' in many texts. Nevertheless, this covers a broad range of traditional activities and probably very variable actual diuretic effects so the terms 'aquaretics' and 'diuretic depuratives' (see above) may be more accurate. However, the conventional terminology will be used here, as demarcation between the two categories is currently inadequate.

Plant remedies traditionally used as diuretics

- *Eupatorium purpureum* (gravel root), *Elymus repens* (couch grass), *Eryngium maritimum* (sea holly), *Zea mays* (corn silk), *Aphanes arvensis* (parsley piert), *Daucus carota* (wild carrot), *Parietaria diffusa* (pellitory), *Taraxacum officinale* (dandelion), *Apium graveolens* (celery).

Indications for diuretics

- Dysuria and oliguria linked to urinary infections or stones (although simply increasing fluid intake can achieve the same flushing effect)
- Heart failure (as an adjunct to cardioactive glycosides)
- Ascites (combined with hepatic remedies)
- Nocturnal enuresis and other functional disturbances of micturition
- Urinary stones.

Other traditional indications for diuretics

- Haematuria
- Arthritis and skin disorders.

Contraindications in the use of diuretics

The use of diuretic herbs may be inappropriate and possibly even contraindicated in the following:

- Renal failure
- Diabetes.

Other traditional therapeutic insights into the use of diuretics

The traditional treatment of arthritic disease often involved using herbs that were otherwise considered diuretics. There is a more modern tradition that suggests these diuretics act to increase the elimination of metabolic acid wastes (e.g. uric acid), factors popularly associated with arthritic disease. The precise explanation for the apparent efficacy of remedies such as birch, celery seed and nettle leaf in arthritic diseases may be more complex.

This tradition is a reminder of the wider assumption that diuretics were among the eliminative strategies applied to a range of toxic conditions associated especially with inflammatory diseases and persistent or recurrent infections (see p. 149). Any hint of fluid retention accompanying such conditions would be a traditional indication for diuretics.

Application

Diuretics, when prescribed overtly as such, are best taken in relatively high quantities at any time relative to eating. However, dramatic diuresis in some cases may follow quite small doses of many herbs, perhaps directed to other ends.

Phased treatments may be appropriate, for example, early morning and lunchtime dosages as part of a strategy for treating nocturnal enuresis.

Long-term therapy with many diuretics is quite acceptable.

Advanced phytotherapeutics

Diuretics may also be usefully applied in some cases (depending on other factors) of:

- osteoarthritis
- dermatitis
- other chronic inflammatory diseases accompanied by fluid retention
- premenstrual syndrome.

Urinary antiseptics

Plant remedies traditionally used as urinary antiseptics

- *Arctostaphylos uva-ursi* (bearberry, see monograph), *Vaccinium macrocarpon* (cranberry), *Barosma betulina* (buchu, see monograph), *Juniperus communis* (juniper), *Berberis vulgaris* (barberry, see monograph), *Chimaphila umbellata* (pipsissewa), *Hydrastis canadensis* (golden seal), *Piper cubeba* (cubeb).

The main role of cranberry appears to be in the prevention of urinary tract infections; possibly by reducing bacterial adherence to the bladder wall.[60] The accumulated evidence for its role in this regard is relatively good, especially in terms of managing recurrent infections.[61,62]

Indications for urinary antiseptics

- Urinary infections or stones
- Prostatitis
- Interstitial cystitis (possibly).

Contraindications in the use of urinary antiseptics

The use of urinary antiseptic herbs may be inappropriate and possibly even contraindicated in the following:
- Kidney disease
- Renal failure
- Pregnancy.

Application

Urinary antiseptics may be taken before or with meals. It may be found that taking whole ground preparations in capsule form may be more effective than tinctures, but this is not a critical matter. Long-term therapy with many urinary antiseptics is not advisable.

Other relevant agents

Urinary tract demulcents

These agents will exert a soothing effect on the lining of the urinary tract and are indicated for inflammation and infections such as urethritis and cystitis. They may also be of value for inflammation higher up the urinary tract and the irritation of kidney stones. Some urinary tract demulcents such as marshmallow leaf act by a reflex effect (reflex demulcents). Others, specifically couch grass and corn silk probably have a direct effect.

Antilithics

These herbs decrease the likelihood of urinary stone formation and may also act to weaken and slowly dissolve existing stones. Antilithic herbs include Crataeva, horsetail, gravel root (*Eupatorium purpureum*), parsley piert (*Aphanes arvensis*) and pellitory of the wall (*Parietaria* species). Gravel root may act particularly against uric acid stones, whereas the other herbs act on mineral stones. Some antilithics such as Crataeva[63] can help the expulsion of small stones.

Bladder tonics

These herbs have a toning effect on the smooth muscle of the bladder. They are therefore useful in the treatment of hypotonic bladder, as can occur with the urinary outlet obstruction caused by benign prostatic hyperplasia, and other neurological conditions of the bladder. During bladder infection, bacteria may remain with the residual urine that is left in the bladder after each voiding. Bladder tonics decrease this residual volume and therefore assist greatly with the flushing of the bladder. In this context they can be particularly valuable in the resolution of recurrent cystitis. The best established bladder tonic is Crataeva bark.[63]

Kidney tonics

In Western herbal terminology kidney tonics are herbs which tonify the function of the kidneys and may be useful in poor kidney function in conjunction with diuretic depuratives. They may also help protect the kidney during diseases such as glomerulonephritis. Unfortunately there is little reliable information about herbs that might have this role. In the European tradition, Solidago virgaurea (golden rod) stands out[64] and there could also be a role for horsetail in this context.

In traditional Chinese medicine the term 'kidney tonic' is also used, but it has no relationship with the anatomical kidney. The 'kidney tonics' of Chinese medicine are typically adrenal cortex tonics. It is important that they are not confused with the above.

Phytotherapy for urinary conditions

Recurrent urinary stones

A theme that emerges from the research is the complexity of mineral and electrolyte disturbance, involving other body systems, which can underlie urinary stone formation. For example, the pathogenesis of renal calculi may involve relative changes in concentrations of other urinary trace elements, notably copper and phosphorus,[65] that clearly reflect wider metabolic changes.

In industrialised countries, about 80% of stones that form in the kidneys are composed of calcium salts and usually occur as calcium oxalate and less commonly calcium phosphate.[66,67] The remaining 20% of stones are largely composed of uric acid, struvite or cystine.

Because urine is supersaturated with calcium, crystal formation occurs readily if urine calcium rises, as when there is fluid depletion or increased calcium excretion. Calcium is also less soluble as the urine becomes more alkaline. Factors in urine that inhibit crystallisation processes include:[68]

- magnesium, which complexes oxalate
- citrate, which complexes calcium
- pyrophosphate, which impairs crystallisation of calcium oxalate.

About 50% of patients with calcium stones have excessive calcium in their urine. The most common cause of this is a genetically determined increased calcium absorption in the intestine. Excessive urinary calcium can also be caused by a diet rich in sodium or animal protein. Low levels of citrate in the urine is another factor, which affects between 20% and 60% of patients.[66] Factors involved here can include urinary tract infection, a high sodium intake, chronic diarrhoea, potassium loss, excessive physical exercise and an excessively acid-forming diet (rich in high protein foods). High excretion of oxalate in the urine is largely of dietary or genetic origin. Ironically, the dietary factor most often responsible for oxalate stones is a low calcium intake. However, reducing the intake of oxalates is probably a safer option than increasing dietary calcium beyond normal levels,[68] although calcium supplementation has been shown to be beneficial in stone prevention.[69]

High protein consumption may be a factor in stone formation, since the resultant sulphates formed generate an acid load in the urine that is buffered by bone.[67] Animal protein also has a high purine content, which will increase uric acid excretion. An inverse relationship occurs between renal potassium and calcium excretion, which brings attention to the role of potassium-rich fruits and vegetables as preventatives.[67] Obesity and insulin resistance are linked to both calcium and uric acid stones.[67,70]

Recurrent oxalate stone formers are significantly less likely to be colonised with the gut-dwelling bacterium Oxalobacter formigenes.[71] This organism is able to degrade dietary oxalate. Probiotic use of lactic acid bacteria that metabolise oxalate might also provide a valid alternative to this organism.

Lifestyle and diet are best aimed at preventing stone formation, and, since the recurrence rate of stones is 75% over 20 years, the following guidelines could be followed by all patients with a history of kidney stones.[66]

Regular weight-bearing exercise will help store calcium in bones, which would otherwise be excreted in the urine. However, exercise should not be excessive since this increases dehydration and can cause lactic acidosis, both factors in stone formation. Fluid intake should be adequate, especially in warm climates, but commercial drinks are to be avoided (these are sometimes loaded with phosphate and sugar).

The diet should be based on fruit, vegetables and unrefined carbohydrates. Animal protein (including cheese) intake should not be excessive and dietary salt should be restricted.[72] Fruit, which is rich in potassium and citrate, should be emphasised, together with foods rich in magnesium such as fermented soya products, legumes, nuts and green leafy vegetables. Calcium intake, specifically dairy foods, should be moderate, but should also not be restricted unless there are other reasons for this, such as dairy protein allergy. Restriction of calcium can lead to excessive oxalate absorption.[73] If there is a history of oxalate stones, then foods rich in oxalate are best avoided. These include rhubarb, spinach, strawberries, ginger, almonds, cashews and beetroot. A probiotic supplement may be relevant here as well.

There is substantial evidence of interaction between urinary urates and oxalates, so that higher urinary levels of the former, following disturbances of purine metabolism including gout, can lead to 'salting out' of calcium oxalate stones; drugs such as allopurinol, which reduce urinary urate, also reduce oxalate stones.[74] This calls into question the use, in the case of incipient or actual oxalate calculi (for example, in cases of severe small intestinal disease as above), of some plants such as the fruits of Apium graveolens (celery) and Petroselinum crispum (parsley), Eupatorium purpureum (gravel root), Betula spp. (birch) and Urtica dioica (nettle leaf), that are considered to increase urinary excretion of urates.

Other studies suggest that urate stones themselves may be linked to low blood urate levels following enhanced tubular secretion of urate within the kidney. In such cases, agents increasing urate excretion would be clearly contraindicated and alkalinisation of urine may be the most effective treatment,[75] since overly acidic urine is the key feature of these types of stones. It may be the factor that connects the disorder with metabolic syndrome.[76,77]

In pregnancy, hyperuricuria and hypercalciuria, changes in metabolic inhibitors of lithiasis formation, urinary stasis, relative dehydration and the presence of infection all increase the likelihood of stone formation.[78]

Herbal remedies and urinary stones

In seven plants (*Verbena officinalis*, *Lithospermum officinale*, *Taraxacum officinale*, *Equisetum arvense*, *Arctostaphylos uva-ursi*, *Arctium lappa* and *Silene saxifraga*) studied for their effects on experimental risk factors for urinary stones (citraturia, calciuria, phosphaturia, pH and diuresis), moderate solvent action on uric stones was linked to the alkalinising capacity of the herb infusion and to a possible urinary antiseptic activity.[79]

Other Asiatic herbal products have been shown to reduce experimental renal stone formation.[80–82] In Ayurveda, *Crataeva nurvala* is highly acclaimed for its use in the management of urinary tract disorders, especially kidney stones. Research has demonstrated a range of activity on urinary structures, including improved performance in clinical studies of benign prostatic hyperplasia[83] and with urinary stones[84,85] and in reducing oxalate stone formation,[86] with the steroid lupeol being a possible active constituent.[87] A pharmacological study found that Crataeva influenced small intestinal Na,K-ATPase, which in turn influenced the transport of minerals.[88] This is a reminder that oxalate problems may well originate from the digestive tract (see above).

Herbal teas in general have been recommended as alternatives to the usual black tea consumption because of the latter's association with increased risk of formation of calcium oxalate stones, but this is unlikely to reflect a general benefit of plant extractives as such.[89]

Herbal treatment can augment the above dietary and lifestyle measures designed to prevent kidney stones and can also be used to treat existing stones. The regime is largely the same for these two treatment scenarios. In the case of managing existing stones, therapy is aimed at passing small stones and/or gradually weakening or dissolving larger stones:

- A key herb is Crataeva, which research has shown can assist the passage of small stones and prevent the formation of new stones (see the detailed information above). Other antilithic herbs such as horsetail and golden rod are indicated, as are aquaretics which will render the urine more dilute (as will copious fluid intake). Dandelion leaf is also useful, given that it is rich in potassium.
- Anthraquinone-containing herbs such as cascara and yellow dock can help by binding calcium in the urine and making it less likely to precipitate. The herb madder (*Rubia tinctorum*) was particularly used for this effect in Europe, but has now been banned due to concerns over carcinogenicity.
- Infection can provide a focus for stone formation; hence the treatment strategies for cystitis should also be followed if infection is thought to play a role. This includes immune supporting herbs such as Echinacea root and antibacterial herbs such as cranberry and buchu. However, there is some clinical evidence to suggest that cranberry may slightly increase the risk of oxalate stone formation.[90]

- If a stone is lodged and causing pain then urinary tract demulcents and spasmolytic herbs such as cramp bark and wild yam are additionally indicated. The prescription-only spasmolytic *Ammi visnaga* was traditionally used in Egypt to aid the passage of urinary stones. While stones are causing damage to the urinary tract mucosa, immune-enhancing herbs and urinary tract antiseptics will lower the risk of infection. A species of oak *Quercus salicina* (*Q. stenophylla*) has been used to treat urinary stones in Japan since 1969. Clinical trials have demonstrated efficacy in assisting the passage of both renal and ureteral stones.[91,92]

Example liquid formula

Taraxacum officinale leaf	1:1	25 mL
Equisetum arvense	1:2	25 mL
Viburnum opulus	1:2	20 mL
Solidago virgaurea	1:2	20 mL
Rumex crispus	1:2	20 mL
	TOTAL	110 mL

Dose: 8 mL with water twice a day (if Crataeva 1:2 liquid is available it can be used instead of the dandelion leaf in the above formulation).

Urinary infections

Urinary infections are very common, affecting for example up to 20% of women at some time in their lives. Practitioner experience is that herbal remedies can be effective treatments for conditions such as urethritis, cystitis, ureteritis and even pyelonephritis (especially if chronic). Infections of the prostate gland (i.e. prostatitis) are also potentially amenable, although two general caveats are raised here. There are usually legal and ethical issues in the way of tackling urinary infections of venereal origin without referral to conventional sexually transmitted disease clinics. From a clinical point of view also, a urinary infection that has progressed beyond the walls of the tubules, as in pyelitis and prostatitis, can present other treatment challenges. That being said, the judicious use of the urinary antiseptics described below is often productive and there are many cases of recurrent cystitis that have been permanently corrected with phytotherapy.

Several plant constituents have at least theoretical antiseptic effects when eliminated in the urinary tract and a number of plants have firm clinical reputations for long-term efficacy in uncomplicated urethritis and cystitis, especially when caused by Gram-negative bacteria such as *Escherichia coli* (accounting for 80% of adult cases), *Staphyloccocus saprophyticus*, Klebsiella and Proteus.

When urinary tract infections are complicated by pregnancy, diabetes, immunosuppression or other abnormalities, prudence will determine that these are considered before simple urinary antiseptics are applied. Except in pregnancy and severe kidney disease, however, the treatments are rarely contraindicated. They may also show effectiveness in urinary tract conditions linked to fungal (e.g. Candida) and parasitic infections (for example, following malaria, leishmaniasis, trichomoniasis and bilharziasis) and for those without obvious infective cause. In the last case at least alkalinisation of the urine is a helpful accompaniment, conventionally with half a teaspoon of sodium bicarbonate in water every 3 to 4 hours but also with increased consumption of fruit juice (and vegetable juice especially).

Urinary infection probably requires adhesion of the bacteria to the otherwise glassy surface of the urinary tract and those usually responsible have mechanisms to do this. Constituents of berries of the heather family, notably *Vaccinium macrocarpon* (cranberry) and *V. myrtillus* (blueberry, bilberry), appear at least in vitro to interfere with this adhesion mechanism,[93] especially in the case of *Escherichia coli* (responsible for 80% of such infections). This may be due to the D-mannose in the berries preferentially adhering to the bacterial surface, or to proanthocyanins. There have been a number of clinical trials pursuing this effect and recently an updated Cochrane report chose 10 that were of methodologically good quality for systematic review and four for meta-analysis. The conclusion from the latter was that cranberry juice products can be effective in reducing urinary tract infections, although perhaps favouring women and having less impact in the elderly.[62] They pointed to more work being needed, particularly in establishing effective dosage and other elements of treatment regime.

The benefits of cranberry may be pointers to the clinical benefits seen with its relative, *Arctostaphylos uva-ursi* (bearberry), although in this case it is the leaves that are used and it is the conversion of the glycoside arbutin into the antiseptic hydroquinone in the urinary tract that is seen as the likely mechanism.[94] Another traditional urinary antiseptic *Chimaphila umbellata* (pipsissewa) also contains arbutin.[95] (Also see the bearberry monograph.)

Another plant constituent with clinical antiadhesive properties, at least in the gut and in synthetic form, is berberine from the Berberis genus including *Berberis aquifolium* (Oregon grape) and *Hydrastis canadensis* (golden seal), both used traditionally for cystitis.[96] These also have separate activity against *E. coli, Klebsiella spp.* and other urinary pathogens (see berberis monograph).

It is also possible that herbs may help in the condition known as interstitial cystitis. This difficult condition, marked by inflammatory infiltration in the bladder wall but no obvious infection, is generally thought to be an autoimmune disorder. However, an infective cause has not been ruled out,[97] and in spite of its name, it appears that there is no increased bladder permeability.[98] There do appear to be changes in neurotransmitter sensitivity (increasing resistance to atropine and histamine and a switch towards purinergic transmission in parasympathetic nerve terminals)[99] and impairment of bladder perfusion in patients has also been observed, especially when the bladder was full.[100] It is for these reasons that in herbal treatments urinary antiseptics can be combined with other agents with an apparent benefit on the bladder wall (e.g. Equisetum, Zea, *Crataeva nurvula* and Althaea).

A major and debilitating problem is recurrent acute bacterial cystitis (otherwise known as recurrent cystitis), where the woman suffers repeated acute infections, often close to one another. As already noted the bacteria that cause cystitis can cling to and invade the cells lining the bladder wall and there they can

remain dormant and resistant to antibiotic attack. Their activation leads to the next infection. Up to 20% of young women with cystitis develop recurrent infections of the urinary tract.[101]

Recurrent cystitis responds positively to herbal treatment, which is recommended on a continuing basis to prevent the acute attacks. After freedom from acute infections for 3 to 4 months, the herbal treatment can be reduced and eventually discontinued if the response is still favourable. Dietary measures (especially cranberry intake) should then continue, including reduced refined carbohydrate intake and dairy products. Adequate fluid intake should be ensured. Also, during acute cystitis any use of herbs needs to be combined with copious intake of fluid to flush the bladder. Cystitis is an infection, so it is always a good idea to support the immune system. For this either Echinacea root or the Ayurvedic herb *Andrographis paniculata* can be used. In a clinical trial Andrographis prevented the typical development of urinary tract infections in patients undergoing shock wave therapy for kidney stones (see andrographis monograph). Andrographis is appropriate at around 6g/day during acute cystitis and about 3g/day of Echinacea root can be used to prevent recurrent cystitis.

Other herbs to consider in cystitis include urinary tract demulcents such as couch grass and corn silk and licorice (*Glycyrrhiza glabra*), which may reduce bacterial adherence to the bladder wall (see licorice monograph).

Example liquid formula: acute cystitis

Echinacea purpurea/angustifolia root	1:2	35 mL
Barosma betulina	1:2	20 mL
Glycyrrhiza glabra (high in glycyrrhizin)	1:1	15 mL
Zea mays	1:1	30 mL
	TOTAL	100 mL

Dose: 8 mL with water 3–4 times daily.

CASE HISTORY

A 26-year-old woman presented with recurrent bouts of cystitis. She had been experiencing these attacks for about 7 years, but they had increased in frequency since she became sexually active. In the past 18 months the frequency of her cystitis had been particularly high, and she had tried many courses of antibiotics, some very powerful. Her cystitis symptoms were almost continuous by her first herbal consultation, but in frustration she had ceased all antibiotics about 6 weeks prior.

Results of all investigations were normal and a procedure during which the trigone area of the bladder had been scraped had failed to change the frequency or morbidity of her cystitis.

The patient was advised to drink 100 mL/day cranberry juice and prescribed the following formulation:

Echinacea angustifolia/purpurea root	1:2	50 mL
Barosma betulina	1:2	30 mL
Glycyrrhiza glabra	1:1	25 mL
Crataeva nurvala	1:2	45 mL
	TOTAL	150 mL

Dose: 8 mL with water three times daily.

After 5 weeks of herbal treatment the patient reported no cystitis, only two mornings of mild burning which passed without developing further. Following another 6 weeks of treatment, the report was the same. Her dose was then adjusted to 8 mL twice a day without adverse consequences.

The rationale for the herbal treatment was as follows (see also above):

- Echinacea improves immunity and thereby decreases the tendency to infections.
- Buchu is a urinary tract antiseptic.
- Licorice contains compounds that decrease bacterial adherence to the bladder wall.
- Crataeva improves bladder tone and reduces residual volume in the bladder, which decreases residual bacteria in the bladder.

Nocturnal enuresis (bedwetting)

Childhood sleep (nocturnal) enuresis (bedwetting) is the inappropriate voiding of urine by a child who has reached the age at which satisfactory control is expected. Since a large proportion of young children wet their beds, it is inappropriate to use the term enuresis until at least 5 years of age. At least 90% of children with nocturnal enuresis are reliably dry during the day.[102]

More than 80% of children with nocturnal enuresis have never been dry at night for a prolonged period, but nearly all will have had an occasional dry night. This can be referred to as intermittent enuresis. True primary enuresis, in which the child has never had a single dry night, is very rare. Secondary (or acquired) enuresis is less prevalent than intermittent enuresis, and is where enuresis develops after the age of 5 years in a child who has previously been reliably dry at night for at least 1 year.[102]

Nocturnal enuresis is more common in boys, first-born children, lower social classes and in children who have experienced stress in early life.[102] Given the association with families, genetic factors may be involved with this disorder. Disorders such as diabetes, renal failure, urological abnormalities and epilepsy are rarely the cause, but should be excluded.

Stress is probably a factor, especially in relapses. Obviously the condition itself can be stressful. A child with nocturnal enuresis may have a smaller functional bladder capacity (that is, the child has the habit of emptying the bladder when it contains a relatively small volume of urine).[103] Urinary tract infection is not common, but should be tested for. Constipation can be an unrecognised factor and should be attended to.[104] Food allergies may be present (especially dairy, wheat or yeast) and soft drinks, tea and coffee should be avoided. Sleep apnoea should be considered and appropriate measures taken if relevant (including herbal treatment for adenoids and sinus conditions).

It is now generally agreed that nocturnal polyuria, detrusor overactivity and high arousal thresholds are, in various combinations, central to enuresis pathogenesis.[105]

In addition to the measures described above, the following considerations can be useful. If the child shows symptoms consistent with food allergies or intolerances, then a relevant exclusion diet should be tested. Intake of refined carbohydrates should be reduced and a natural whole food diet followed as much as possible.

Restriction of fluid intake is not helpful. In fact increasing fluid intake during the day to generate higher urine flow rates increases the awareness of bladder filling and, by encouraging urine holding, achieves an increase in functional bladder size.[106]

Many research projects have confirmed the merits of conditioning using alarms. Body-worn alarms are usually preferred.[106,107] Rewarding dry nights can reinforce behaviour. It might be particularly valuable to reward dry nights without making an obvious connection, so that a subconscious impression is encouraged.

Key herbs to consider are as follows:

- The bladder-toning effect of Crataeva is helpful, particularly in conjunction with increased diurnal fluid intake. Horsetail has been traditionally prescribed for nocturnal enuresis and may have a similar function to Crataeva.
- St John's wort is another traditional treatment and its nervine tonic and mild antidepressant activities will alleviate the vicious cycle of stress. Other nervine tonics such as skullcap can be considered.
- Chamomile is another nervous system herb that is particularly relevant for children. Stronger calming herbs such as valerian should not be excluded if the need arises.
- Urinary tract demulcents such as corn silk will alleviate any irritation of the urinary tract; ribwort is traditionally used.
- Allergies may need to be treated with herbs such as Albizia and Baical skullcap.

Example liquid formula
The following formula is an example treatment for an 8-year-old child:

Hypericum perforatum	1:2	25 mL
Crataeva nurvala	1:2	35 mL
Zea mays	1:1	20 mL
Equisetum arvense	1:2	20 mL
		100 mL

Dose: 4 mL with water twice a day (morning and afternoon).

CASE HISTORY

A mother came with her 8-year-old son seeking treatment for his nocturnal enuresis. He had always had the problem. While his enuresis improved during school holidays, on average he was only dry for a maximum of two to three consecutive nights. During the school term he would wet the bed almost every night. He was a highly strung boy, suffered nightmares, was easily agitated, prone to respiratory allergies and a very fussy eater. He found school stressful and difficult.

The following formulation was prescribed:

Hypericum perforatum	1:2	20 mL
Zizyphus spinosa	1:2	20 mL
Passiflora incarnata	1:2	15 mL
Crataeva nurvala	1:2	30 mL
Plantago lanceolata	1:2	25 mL
	TOTAL	110 mL

Dose: 5 mL with water twice a day.

For the first 2 weeks he experienced dry nights, the first time ever in his life. However, this was followed by wetting every night for the next 2 weeks. Over the ensuing 6 months of treatment there was a gradual improvement, to the point that wetting the bed was a rare event. The mixture was reduced to one dose a day. Over the ensuing 2 years the bedwetting would return from time to time when he was stressed, but reinstitution of the mixture at the full dose quickly restored the dry nights.

References

1. Melillo L. Diuretic plants in the paintings of Pompeii. *Am J Nephrol*. 1994;14(4–6): 423–425.

2. Aliotta G, Capasso G, Pollio A, et al. Joseph Jacob Plenck (1735–1807). *Am J Nephrol*. 1994;14(4–6):377–382.

3. Zhou XM, Chen QH. Biochemical study of Chinese rhubarb. XXII. Inhibitory effect of anthraquinone derivatives on Na+-K+-ATPase of the rabbit renal medulla and their diuretic action. *Yao Hsueh Hsueh Pao*. 1988;23(1):17–20.

4. Doan DD, Nguyen NH, Doan HK, et al. Studies on the individual and combined diuretic effects of four Vietnamese traditional herbal remedies (Zea mays, Imperata cylindrica, Plantago major and Orthosiphon stamineus). *J Ethnopharmacol*. 1992;36(3):225–231.

5. Goonaratna C, Thabrew I, Wijewardena K. Does Aerua lanata have diuretic properties? *Indian J Physiol Pharmacol*. 1993;37(2):135–137.

6. Black HR, Ming S, Poll DS, et al. A comparison of the treatment of hypertension with Chinese herbal and Western medication. *J Clin Hypertens*. 1986;2(4):371–378.

7. Laranja SM, Bergamaschi CM, Schor N. Evaluation of three plants with potential diuretic effect. *Rev Assoc Med Bras*. 1992;38(1):13–16.

8. Kreydiyyeh SI, Usta J. Diuretic effect and mechanism of action of parsley. *J Ethnopharmacol*. 2002;79(3):353–357.

9. Srividya N, Periwal S. Diuretic, hypotensive and hypoglycaemic effect of Phyllanthus amarus. *Indian J Exp Biol*. 1995;33(11):861–864.

10. Udupihille M, Jiffry MT. Diuretic effect of Aerua lanata with water, normal saline and coriander as controls. *Indian J Physiol Pharmacol*. 1986;30(1):91–97.

11. Von Beitz G, Hippe SK, Schremmer D. Asparagus-P, das pflanzliche Diuretikum in der Herz-Kreislauf-Therapie. *Naturheilpraxis*. 1996;2:247–252.

12. Bharani A, Ganguly A, Bhargava KD. Salutary effect of Terminalia arjuna in patients with severe refractory heart failure. *Int J Cardiol*. 1995;49(3):191–199.

13. De Ribeiro RA, De Barros F, De Melo MM, et al. Acute diuretic effects in conscious rats produced by some medicinal plants used in the state of Sao Paulo, Brasil. *J Ethnopharmacol*. 1988;24(1):19–29.

14. Cáceres A, Girón LM, Martínez AM. Diuretic activity of plants used for the treatment of urinary ailments in Guatemala. *J Ethnopharmacol*. 1987;19(3):233–245.

15. Cáceres A, Saravia A, Rizzo S, et al. Pharmacologic properties of Moringa oleifera. 2: Screening for antispasmodic, antiinflammatory and diuretic activity. *J Ethnopharmacol*. 1992;36(3):233–237.

16. Racz-Kotilla E, Racz G, Solomon A. The action of Taraxacum officinale extracts on the body weight and diuresis of laboratory animals. *Planta Med*. 1974;26:212–217.

17. Pérez Gutiérrez RM, Laguna GY, Walkowski A. Diuretic activity of Mexican equisetum. *J Ethnopharmacol*. 1985;14(2–3):269–272.

18. Englert J, Harnischfeger G. Diuretic action of aqueous Orthosiphon extract in rats. *Planta Med*. 1992;58(3):237–238.

19. Casadebaig-Lafon J, Jacob M, Cassanas G, et al. Adsorbed plant extracts, use of extracts of dried seeds of Orthosiphon stamineus benth. *Pharm Acta Helv*. 1989;64(8):220–224.

20. Leuschner J. Anti-inflammatory, spasmolytic and diuretic effects of a commercially available Solidago gigantea herb extract. *Arzneimittelforschung*. 1995;45(2):165–168.

21. Chodera A, Dabrowska K, Sloderbach A, et al. Effect of flavonoid fractions of Solidago virgaurea L on diuresis and levels of electrolytes. *Acta Pol Pharm*. 1991;48(5–6):35–37.

22. Giachetti D, Taddei E, Taddei I. Diuretic and uricosuric activity of Agrimonia eupatoria L. *Boll Soc Ital Biol Sper*. 1986;62(6):705–711.

23. Gu WZ, Deng LJ. Studies on the chemical constituents of the essential oil in the seed of Lactuca setiva L. and its diuretic action. *Chung Yao Tung Pao*. 1987;11(33–35):63.

24. Giachetti D, Taddei E, Taddei I. Diuretic and uricosuric activity of Parietaria judaica L. *Boll Soc Ital Biol Sper*. 1986;62(2):197–202.

25. Lu GW, Miura K, Yukimura T, Yamamoto K. Effects of extract from Clerodendron trichotomum on blood pressure and renal function in rats and dogs. *J Ethnopharmacol*. 1994;42(2):77–82.

26. Lee HS, Kim ST, Cho DK. Effects of rehmanniae radix water extract on renal function and renin secretion rate in unanesthetized rabbits. *Am J Chin Med*. 1993;21(2):179–186.

27. Mendonca VL, Oliveira CL, Craveiro AA, et al. Pharmacological and toxicological evaluation of Alpinia speciosa. *Mem Inst Oswaldo Cruz*. 1991;86(suppl 2):93–97.

28. Simões CM, Ribeiro-do-Vale RM, Poli A, et al. The pharmacologic action of extracts of Polygonum punctatum Elliot (= P. acre HBK). *J Pharm Belg*. 1989;44(4):275–284.

29. Perfumi M, Tacconi R. Effect of Opuntia ficus-indica flower infusion on urinary and electrolyte excretion in rats. *Fitoterapia*. 1996;67(5):459–464.

30. Wright CI, Van-Buren L, Kroner CI, Koning MM. Herbal medicines as diuretics: a review of the scientific evidence. *J Ethnopharmacol*. 2007;114(1):1–31.

31. Hooman N, Mojab F, Nickavar B, Pouryousefi-Kermani P. Diuretic effect of powdered Cerasus avium (cherry) tails on healthy volunteers. *Pak J Pharm Sci*. 2009;22(4):381–383.

32. Clare BA, Conroy RS, Spelman K. The diuretic effect in human subjects of an extract of Taraxacum officinale folium over a single day. *J Altern Complement Med*. 2009;15(8):929–934.

33. Rangineni V, Sharada D, Saxena S. Diuretic, hypotensive, and hypocholesterolemic effects of Eclipta alba in mild hypertensive subjects: a pilot study. *J Med Food*. 2007;10(1):143–148.

34. Schilcher H, Emmrich D. Pflanzliche Urologika zur Durchspülungstherapie. Deutsche Apotheker Zeitung 1992;132(47):2549–2555. In: Awang DVD (ed). Tyler's Herbs of Choice: The Therapeutic Use of Phytochemicals. 3rd ed, USA: CRC Press; 2009, p. 59.

35. Werk W. Wasser ausleiten: elektrolytneutral. *Erfahrungsheilkunde*. 1994;11:712–714.

36. Szentmihályi K, Kéry A, Then M, et al. Potassium-sodium ratio for the characterisation of medicinal plant extracts with diuretic activity. *Phytother Res*. 1998;12:163–166.

37. Richet GC. Osmotic diuresis before Homer W. Smith: a winding path to renal physiology. *Kidney Int*. 1994;45(4):1241–1252.

38. Archer DP, Freymond D, Ravussin P. Use of mannitol in neuroanesthesia and neurointensive care. *Ann Fr Anesth Reanim*. 1995;14(1):77–82.

39. Dias-Tagliacozzo GM, Dietrich SMC, Mello-Aires M. Measurement of glomerular filtration rate using inulin prepared from Vernonia herbacea, a Brazilian native species. *Braz J Med Biol Res*. 1996;29(10):1393–1396.

40. Roberts LR, Kamath PS. Ascites and hepatorenal syndrome: pathophysiology and management. *Mayo Clinic Proc*. 1996;71(9):874–881.

41. Taylor SH. Refocus on diuretics in the treatment of heart failure. *Eur Heart J*. 1995;16(suppl):7–15.

42. Markell MS. Herbal therapies and the patient with kidney disease. *Q Rev Nat Med*. 1997 Fall:189–200.

43. Li L, Wang H, Zhu S. Hepatic albumin's mRNA in nephrotic syndrome rats treated with Chinese herbs. *Chung Hua I Hsueh Tsa Chih*. 1995;75(5):276–279.

44. Yu JY, Xiong NN, Guo HF. Clinical observation on diabetic nephropathy treated with alcohol of Abelmoschus manihot. *Chung Kuo Chung Hsi I Chieh Ho Tsa Chih*. 1995;15(5):263–265.

45. Li P, Fujio S. Effects of chai ling tang on proteinuria in rat models. *J Tradit Chin Med*. 1995;15(1):48–52.

46. Zheng JF, Chen SY. Observations on therapeutic effects of huangdan decoction and Tripterygium wilfordii compound tablet on membranous glomerulonephritis in rats. *J Tongji Med Univ*. 1995;15(1): 31–34.

47. Shida K, Imamura K, Katayama T, et al. Clinical efficacy of sairei-to in various

urinary tract diseases centering on fibrosis. *Hinyokika Kiyo.* 1994;40(11):1049–1057.

48. Kawachi H, Takashima N, Orikasa M, et al. Effect of traditional Chinese medicine (sairei-to) on monoclonal antibody-induced proteinuria in rats. *Pathol Int.* 1994;44(5):339–344.

49. Ren G, Chang F, Lu S, et al. Pharmacological studies of Polygonum capitatum Buch Ham. ex D. Don. *Chung Kuo Chung Yao Tsa Chih.* 1995;20(2):107–109, 128.

50. Muangman V, Viseshsindh V, Ratana-Olarn K, Buadilok S. The usage of Andrographis paniculata following extracorporeal shock wave lithotripsy (ESWL). *J Med Assoc Thai.* 1995;78(6):310–313.

51. Yokozawa T, Zhou JJ, Hattori M, et al. Effects of a Dan Shen component, magnesium lithospermate B, in nephrectomized rats. *Nippon Jinzo Gakkai Shi.* 1995;37(2):105–111.

52. Yu EK. Anti-free radical damage of chronic glomerulonephritis with febrifugal and diuretic medicinal herbs. *Chung Kuo Chung Hsi I Chieh Ho Tsa Chih.* 1993;13(8):464–466, 452.

53. Shantanova LN, Mondodoev AG, Lonshakova KS, Nikolaev SM. Pharmacotherapeutic effectivity of plant nephrophyte polyextractions in cases of mercuric chloride necronephrosis. *Rastitel'nye Resursy.* 1996;32(1–2):110–117.

54. Bao ZD, Wu ZG, Zheng F. Amelioration of aminoglycoside nephrotoxicity by Cordyceps sinensis in old patients. *Chung Kuo Chung Hsi I Chieh Ho Tsa Chih.* 1994;14(5):271–273, 259.

55. Zhang G, El Nahas AM. The effect of rhubarb extract on experimental renal fibrosis. *Nephrol Dial Transplant.* 1996;11(1):186–190.

56. Wojcikowski K, Johnson DW, Gobé G. Medicinal herbal extracts – renal friend or foe? Part two: herbal extracts with potential renal benefits. *Nephrology (Carlton).* 2004;9(6):400–405.

57. Wojcikowski K, Johnson DW, Gobe G. Herbs or natural substances as complementary therapies for chronic kidney disease: ideas for future studies. *J Lab Clin Med.* 2006;147(4):160–166.

58. Li X, Wang H. Chinese herbal medicine in the treatment of chronic kidney disease. *Adv Chronic Kidney Dis.* 2005;12(3):276–281.

59. Jha V. Herbal medicines and chronic kidney disease. *Nephrology (Carlton).* 2010;15(suppl 2):10–17.

60. Côté J, Caillet S, Doyon G, et al. Bioactive compounds in cranberries and their biological properties. *Crit Rev Food Sci Nutr.* 2010;50(7):666–679.

61. Rossi R, Porta S, Canovi B. Overview on cranberry and urinary tract infections in females. *J Clin Gastroenterol.* 2010;44(suppl 1):S61–S62.

62. Jepson RG, Craig JC. Cranberries for preventing urinary tract infections. *Cochrane Database Syst Rev.* 2008;(1):CD001321.

63. Bone K. *Clinical Applications of Ayurvedic and Chinese Herbs.* Warwick: Phytotherapy Press; 1996. pp. 112–114.

64. Melzig MF. Goldenrod – a classical exponent in the urological phytotherapy. *Wien Med Wochenschr.* 2004;154(21–22):523–527.

65. Rodgers AL, Barbour LJ, Pougnet BM, et al. Re-evaluation of the 'week-end effect' data: possible role of urinary copper and phosphorus in the pathogenesis of renal calculi. *J Trace Elem Med Biol.* 1995;9(3):150–155.

66. Pak CYC. Kidney stones. *Lancet.* 1998;351:1797–1801.

67. López M, Hoppe B. History, epidemiology and regional diversities of urolithiasis. *Pediatr Nephrol.* 2010;25(1):49–59.

68. Whitfield HN, Mallick NP. Renal calculi. *Medicine.* 1995:199–204.

69. Goldfarb DS. Prospects for dietary therapy of recurrent nephrolithiasis. *Adv Chronic Kidney Dis.* 2009;16(1):21–29.

70. Sakhaee K, Maalouf NM. Metabolic syndrome and uric acid nephrolithiasis. *Semin Nephrol.* 2008;28(2):174–180.

71. Siva S, Barrack ER, Reddy GP, et al. A critical analysis of the role of gut Oxalobacter formigenes in oxalate stone disease. *BJU Int.* 2009;103(1):18–21.

72. Burtis WJ, Gay L, Insogna KL, et al. Dietary hypercalciuria in patients with calcium oxalate kidney stones. *Am J Clin Nutr.* 1994;60:424–429.

73. Curhan GC, Willet WC, Rim EB, Stampfer MJ. A prospective study of dietary calcium and other nutrients and the risk of symptomatic kidney stones. *N Engl J Med.* 1993;328:833–838.

74. Grover PK, Ryall RL. Urate and calcium oxalate stones: from repute to rhetoric to reality. *Miner Electrolyte Metab.* 1994;20(6):361–370.

75. Hisatome I, Tanaka Y, Kotake H, et al. Renal hypouricemia due to enhanced tubular secretion of urate associated with urolithiasis: successful treatment of urolithiasis by alkalization of urine K+, Na(+)-citrate. *Nephron.* 1993;65(4):578–582.

76. Maalouf NM. Metabolic syndrome and the genesis of uric acid stones. *J Ren Nutr.* 2011;21(1):128–131.

77. Cicerello E, Merlo F, Maccatrozzo L. Urinary alkalization for the treatment of uric acid nephrolithiasis. *Arch Ital Urol Androl.* 2010;82(3):145–148.

78. Swanson SK, Heilman RL, Eversman WG. Urinary tract stones in pregnancy. *Surg Clin North Am.* 1995;75(1):123–142.

79. Grases F, Melero G, Costa-Bauza A, et al. Urolithiasis and phytotherapy. *Int Urol Nephrol.* 1994;26(5):507–511.

80. Yamaguchi S, Jihong L, Utsunomiya M, et al. The effect of takusha and kagosou on calcium oxalate renal stones in rats. *Hinyokika Kiyo.* 1995;41(6):427–431.

81. Hirayama H, Wang Z, Nishi K, et al. Effect of Desmodium styracifolium-triterpenoid on calcium oxalate renal stones. *Br J Urol.* 1993;71(2):143–147.

82. Kawamura K, Moriyama M, Nakajima C, et al. The inhibitory effects of Takusha on the formation, growth and aggregation of calcium oxalate crystals in vitro. *Hinyokika Kiyo.* 1993;39(8):695–700.

83. Deshpande PJ, Sahu M, Kumar P. Crataeva nurvala Hook and Forst (Varuna) – the Ayurvedic drug of choice in urinary disorders. *Indian J Med Res.* 1982;76(suppl):46–53.

84. Prabhakar YS, Kumar DS. The Varuna tree, Crataeva nurvala, a promising plant in the treatment of urinary stones. A review. *Fitoterapia.* 1990;61(2):99–111.

85. Varalakshmi P, Shamila Y, Latha E. Effect of Crataeva nurvala in experimental urolithiasis. *J Ethnopharmacol.* 1990;28(3):313–321.

86. Anand R, Patnaik GK, Kulshreshtha DK, et al. Antiurolithiatic activity of Crataeva nurvala ethanolic extract on rats. *Fitoterapia.* 1993;64(4):345–350.

87. Anand R, Patnaik GK, Kulshreshtha DK, et al. *Antiurolithiatic and diuretic activity of lupeol, the active constituent isolated from Crataeva nurvala (Buch. Ham).* Proceedings of the 24th Indian Pharmacological Society Conference, Ahmedabad, Gujarat, India, A10, 1991.

88. Varalakshmi P, Latha E, Shamila Y, et al. Effect of Crataeva nurvala on the biochemistry of the small intestinal tract of normal and stone-forming rats. *J Ethnopharmacol.* 1991;31(1):67–73.

89. McKay DW, Seviour JP, Comerford A, et al. Herbal tea: an alternative to regular tea for those who form calcium oxalate stones. *J Am Diet Assoc.* 1995;95(3):360–361.

90. Gettman MT, Ogan K, Brinkley LJ, et al. Effect of cranberry juice consumption on urinary stone risk factors. *J Urol.* 2005;174(2):590–594.

91. Higashi Y, Yamada H, Kobori G, et al. Clinical equivalence trial of UROCALUN miniaturized tablet in patients with upper urinary tract stone disease. *Hinyokika Kiyo.* 2005;51(3):215–223.

92. Watanabe K, Yuri K. [A clinical study on spontaneous passage of ureteral stone – effect of urocalun and jumping exercise to ureteral stone]. *Hinyokika Kiyo.* 1989;35(5):769–773.

93. Ofek I, Goldhar J, Zafiri D, et al. Anti-Escherischia adhesin activity of cranberry and blueberry juice. *N Engl J Med.* 1991;324:1559.

94. Schindler G, Patzak U, Brinkhaus B, et al. Urinary excretion and metabolism of arbutin after oral administration of Arctostaphylos uvae ursi extract as film-coated tablets and aqueous solution in healthy humans. *J Clin Pharmacol.* 2002;42(8):920–927.

95. Galván IJ, Mir-Rashed N, Jessulat M, et al. Antifungal and antioxidant activities of the phytomedicine pipsissewa, Chimaphila umbellata. *Phytochemistry.* 2008;69(3):738–746.

96. Rabbani GH, Butler T, Knight J, et al. Randomised controlled trial of berberine

sulfate therapy for diarrhea due to enterotoxigenic Escherichia coli and Vibrio cholerae. *J Infect Dis.* 1987;155:979–984.

97. Warren JW. Interstitial cystitis as an infectious disease. *Urol Clin North Am.* 1994;21(1):31–39.

98. Ruggieri MR, Chelsky MJ, Rosen SI, et al. Current findings and future research avenues in the study of interstitial cystitis. *Urol Clin North Am.* 1994;21(1):163–176.

99. Paella S, Artibani W, Ostardo E, et al. Evidence for purinergic neurotransmission in human urinary bladder affected by interstitial cystitis. *J Urol.* 1993;150(6):2007–2012.

100. Irwin P, Galloway NT. Impaired bladder perfusion in interstitial cystitis: a study of blood supply using laser Doppler flowmetry. *J Urol.* 1993;149(4):890–892.

101. Williams DH, Schaeffer AJ. Current concepts in urinary tract infections. *Minerva Urol Nefrol.* 2004;56:15–31.

102. Meadow R. Childhood enuresis. *Medicine.* 1995:211–214.

103. Yeung CK. Nocturnal enuresis (bedwetting). *Curr Opin Urol.* 2003;13(4):337–343.

104. Robson WL. Current management of nocturnal enuresis. *Curr Opin Urol.* 2008;18(4):425–430.

105. Nevéus T. Diagnosis and management of nocturnal enuresis. *Curr Opin Pediatr.* 2009;21(2):199–202.

106. Knapp M. How to treat enuresis. *Australian Doctor*1994;(August suppl): i–vii.

107. Mathew JL. Evidence-based management of nocturnal enuresis: an overview of systematic reviews. *Indian Pediatr.* 2010;47(9):777–780.

Nervous system

Scope

Apart from their use to provide non-specific support for recuperation and repair, specific phytotherapeutic strategies include the following.

Treatment in some circumstances of:

- stress symptoms
- psychosomatic conditions
- anxiety states, panic attacks
- neuralgia
- nervous exhaustion
- insomnia
- visceral spasm.

Management of:

- moderate visceral pain
- mild to moderate depressive conditions
- nervous debility
- dose reduction for prescription hypnotics and sedatives.

As with any pharmacological agent, particular **caution** is necessary in applying phytotherapy in cases of:

- severe psychosis or depression
- prescription of powerful antipsychotics, antiepileptics, anaesthetics
- addictive personality.

Orientation

Receptor activity

Although herbal remedies are not exactly comparable to conventional drugs in terms of directness of action, it is most likely that the primary effect of plant constituents on the nervous system is similar in terms of the synaptic junctions between nerve and nerve and nerve and muscle or other tissue. The receptor sites involved, whether on the presynaptic or postsynaptic membranes, are the communication junctions in the nervous system where its modulation is generally effected. The transmitter chemicals involved are among the most powerful molecules in the body and play a major part in the functions of other body systems; as seen in the relevant chapters of this book, plant constituents have been widely shown to engage with receptors in the hormonal, immunological and other control systems in the body. These systems form a whole, whose study, psychoneuroimmunology, has attracted the attention of the more imaginative medical researchers since the 1960s. The ability of plant constituents to engage cell receptors is also a particular feature of activity within the digestive system, which in clinical reality for herbal remedies is probably the most accessible interface in the chemical control of the nervous system.

There are ample opportunities for herbal constituents to interact with synaptic function in the nervous system. Various herbal extracts have been shown in vitro to act on adrenergic and cholinergic,[1] muscarinic, $5\text{-}HT_{1A}$ and $5\text{-}HT_2$ receptors, dopamine (D_1 and D_2), the benzodiazepine and the gamma-aminobutyric acid (GABA) binding sites.[2,3] Notable examples of such activity follow; the literature cited reflects the fact that much published research in this area emanates from China and Japan. While these experimental examples might not always reflect real clinical effects, some are given here to reflect the wide spectrum of possible activities of herbal remedies.

Calcium channel activity

A modification of the movement of calcium ions through channels in the cell wall is a common factor in many receptor mechanisms. As well as the calcium channel-blocking effect of opioid alkaloids like protopine and tetrandine[4] (and see the Analgesic section below), this has also been observed in vascular tissues for ginseng saponins.[5,6] A coumarin, scoparone, from Capillaris also inhibits calcium influx.[7] From the Chinese remedy *Dictamnus dasycarpus*, calcium channel block was found with fraxinellone and dictamine, two constituents with vasorelaxant effect.[8]

Adrenergic effects

The adrenergic effects of alkaloids of Ephedra, ephedrine and pseudoephedrine, have been understood for many years. Beta-2-adrenergic receptor stimulation has also been mooted to explain the effect of *Angelica sinensis* in reducing experimental pulmonary hypertension.[9] The nociceptive effect of processed aconite was demonstrated as involving adrenergic rather than opioid receptors[10] and hypaconitine appears to be the most active of the alkaloids.[11] The bronchorelaxant (antiasthmatic) effect of coumarins in the fruit of *Cnidium monnieri* is mediated by a beta-2 receptor and blocked by propranolol.[12]

Acetylcholine receptors

Plant remedies with anticholinergic effects (i.e. blocking acetylcholine receptors) are important in traditional medicine. Acetylcholine-sensitive or 'cholinergic' receptors are divided into many types, depending on their other sensitivities. 'Nicotinic' receptors are also sensitive to the alkaloid from *Nicotiana tabacum* (tobacco). 'Muscarinic' receptors are also sensitive to muscarine from the fly agaric mushroom. The atropine-like alkaloids in plants of the Solanaceae (such as deadly nightshade, henbane and jimson weed) block muscarinic receptors in the parasympathetic nervous system. As well as these well-known alkaloidal cholinergic blockers, there are likely to be other plants with more modest, though significant, positive effects on these receptors. For example, the effect of dried orange peel on digestive activity was blocked by atropine, suggesting activity on the muscarinic receptors.[13] More modern interest in this category has focused on a potential role of herbal products in the management of Alzheimer's disease.[14]

GABA and benzodiazepine receptors

The benzodiazepine drug valium was named in recognition of recent research that had established valerian as manifesting some tranquillising properties. Although there are no chemical similarities between valerian constituents and benzodiazepines, some pharmacological similarities have emerged, with evidence that, like the benzodiazepines, valerian acts in part through an effect on the receptors on inhibitory neurons sensitive to GABA (see also the valerian monograph). GABA-A and benzodiazepine receptor binding has been shown as a feature of a number of herbal remedies.[15,16] For example, *Salvia miltiorrhiza* (dan shen), much researched in Beijing as a postulated treatment for ischaemic damage after strokes,[17] and in the repair of other nerve tissue damage,[18] has effects which apparently include stimulating GABA release[19,20] and blocking calcium input.[21]

Dopaminergic receptors

The main pharmacological interest in dopaminergic activity is in Parkinsonism research and a number of plants have shown some promise in pharmacological research, though not yet clinically.[22] The Ayurvedic herb *Mucuna pruriens* is a natural source of L-DOPA also showing promise in the management of Parkinson's disease.[23] Tetrahydrocolumbamine from *Polygala tenuifolia* inhibits dopamine receptors, in part competitively,[24] as does tetrahydropalmatine from Corydalis (and see below). (In the monograph on chaste tree other evidence for dopaminergic receptor activity is outlined.)

Analgesic activity

Analgesics present a major challenge to the modern phytotherapist. Painkillers are by definition relatively powerful agents. Natural analgesics are likely to have been identified early in human history for their immediate benefits in pain relief and/or for their psychoactive properties. Obvious examples are the opium poppy (morphine alkaloids), the nightshade family (atropine alkaloids), willow (see monograph), poplar and birch barks among other sources of salicylates and phenols, as well as the many psychoactive plants (coca, cannabis, psilocybin, mescaline, etc.). Most are now only legally prescribed by doctors, if at all, and it would appear that there is little scope for relatively gentle remedies to compete with the improved targeting of synthetic analgesics.

There are, however, a number of traditional remedies with general and specific analgesic reputations that have been less well exploited in modern times and which are relatively well tolerated in clinical use. Although not as powerful as some of the modern synthetic analgesics, they do show sufficient activity to be taken seriously and are particularly likely to be helpful in pain linked to inflammation and to visceral and vascular spasm. The research papers cited in the following examples demonstrate that even in the demanding area of analgesia there is ample evidence to support useful clinical intervention by the phytotherapist. None of the following remedies are safe for widespread use by the public; their use is to be confined to the experienced clinician who can take account of all factors, including the increased likelihood of adverse effects.

Eschscholtzia californica (California poppy)

A traditional medicinal plant of the Indians, this herb is now used mainly by the rural population of western USA for its mild analgesic and sedative properties (and as the state flower of California). In studies on a prescription herbal formulation in Germany containing *E. californica* and *Corydalis cava* (see below) at 4:1 relative concentration, investigators identified interactions with opioid receptors,[25] as well as other neurotransmitter activity.[26] Aqueous alcoholic extracts from *E. californica* also were shown to inhibit the enzymatic degradation of catecholamines as well as the synthesis of adrenaline, dopamine beta-hydroxylase and monoamine oxidase (MAO-B).[27] A clinical trial of a mixture of Eschscholtzia, Crataegus (hawthorn) and magnesium showed significant benefits compared with placebo in reducing the symptoms of anxiety.[28]

A key alkaloidal constituent, chelerythrine, is a well-known protein kinase C inhibitor with antitumour activity (see also the Chelidonium monograph).[29] Activation of protein kinase C in spinal cord dorsal horn neurons contributes to persistent pain following noxious thermal[30] and chemical stimulation; chelerythrine produced significant reductions of nociceptive responses in one study.[31] Another Canadian study suggests that chelerythrine can attenuate the development of morphine dependence.[32] It also demonstrates a range of potent anti-inflammatory activities.[33,34]

Chelerythrine and another alkaloidal constituent, sanguinarine, exhibited affinity for rat liver vasopressin V1 receptors and are competitive inhibitors of [³H]-vasopressin binding. These alkaloids represent two of the first non-peptidic structures providing original chemical leads for the design of synthetic vasopressin compounds.[35]

Corydalis cava et spp. (yan hu suo)

This remedy has been widely used in China and the East for pain, especially of dysmenorrhoea and the abdomen. In the studies referred to above on its combination with *E. californica*, *Corydalis cava* was generally the stronger of the two ingredients.

Whole Corydalis extract demonstrated antispasmodic activity in acetylcholine-induced contractions at around half that seen for papaverine,[36] and its isoquinoline constituents including familiar alkaloids such as protopine, berberine and palmatine have exhibited anticholinesterase activity.[37] Consistently with the pharmacological profiles of this group, isocoryne produced an inhibitory effect on GABA-activated currents.[38] Isocorypalmine has close affinity for the D1 dopamine receptor.[39] Dehydrocorydaline appears to block noradrenaline release and an experimental antiulcerative action is posited.[40] Corydalis also has powerful anti-inflammatory effects.[41,42]

Traditional vinegar-processed preparations of the fresh Corydalis tuber have been shown to have stronger analgesic effects in vivo than those of the dried preparation.[43] There appeared to be higher concentrations of total alkaloids in the fresh specimen.[44]

Evodia rutaecarpa (wu zhu yu)

This remedy was traditionally used for pain, especially arising from abdominal and digestive causes with headaches and abdominal pain, including dysmenorrhoea.

At least some of the effectiveness of Evodia has been linked to the fraction containing evodiamine and rutaecarpine.[45] A cholinergic mechanism has been implicated in this activity.[46,47] On the other hand, in the case of Evodia's vasodilatory activity, an alpha-adrenoceptor blocking and 5-HT antagonising action are suggested,[48] including for a recent isolate, synephrine,[49] as well as for the powerful cardiotonic and uterotonic evodiamine[50,51] and for the vasorelaxant and hypotensive dehydroevodiamine.[52,53] Direct action on muscarinic receptors has been linked to its antidiarrhoeal action.[54]

Among a number of plants tested, Evodia showed a strong inhibitory effect on acetylcholinesterase in vitro[55] and an antiscopolamine effect in vivo. This antiamnesic effect was more potent than that of tacrine, an older drug for Alzheimer's disease approved by the FDA.[56] The active component was identified as dehydroevodiamine hydrochloride.

Anxiolytic activity

Modern research is investigating a number of medicinal plants for anxiolytic activity. The key anxiolytic herbs covered by monographs in this text are *Piper methysticum* (kava) and *Valeriana officinalis* (valerian). Withania (*Withania somnifera*), hawthorn (*Crataegus* species) and Ginkgo (*Ginkgo biloba*) have also demonstrated clinical anxiolytic effects, and these trials have been included in their respective monographs.

Another anxiolytic herb with a growing body of evidence is passionflower (*Passiflora incarnata*). The unusual common name is not a reference to earthly passions. It comes instead from the Christian symbolism (Christ's Passion) seen in the flower by the Spanish conquistadores when they first encountered the vine growing in South America. This was later elaborated by the scholarly monk Jacomo Bosio, who maintained that the flowers contained a profound symbolism of Christ's final days on earth.[57] For example, the five stamens were the number of wounds, the three pistil stigmas represented nails and the 72 filaments were the number of thorns in the crown given to Jesus.

Despite this focus on the flower, the part of the plant used medicinally is the aerial part or the vine. Phytochemicals found here that contribute to the anxiolytic activity are not fully understood, but they include flavonoids, maltol and flavonoid-related molecules such as benzoflavone.[58]

There are now several clinical trials providing evidence to support the value of passionflower for anxiety symptoms. In a pilot, randomised, double blind, controlled trial, passionflower extract was as efficacious as oxazepam for the management of generalised anxiety disorder. However, herbal treatment resulted in a lower incidence of impairment of job performance. The daily dosage of the undefined passionflower extract was 45 drops.[59] A passionflower and valerian combination improved symptoms of insomnia in uncontrolled trials.[60,61] The side effects characteristic of benzodiazepine tranquilisers were not observed.[61] In a controlled trial with comparison against chlorpromazine (an antipsychotic drug), electroencephalographic (EEG) recordings showed a sedative activity after 6 weeks' treatment with the herbal combination.[60] In a randomised, double blind, placebo-controlled study, a single dose of passionflower extract (equivalent to about 7 g of dried herb) demonstrated a calming effect in healthy female volunteers, as assessed by a self-rating scale for alertness.[62]

Passionflower has also been used to help drug withdrawal symptoms. A randomised, double blind, controlled, 14-day trial compared clonidine plus passionflower extract against clonidine plus placebo in the outpatient detoxification of opiate addicts. Both treatments were equally effective at treating the physical symptoms of withdrawal, but the group receiving passionflower showed superiority over clonidine alone in terms of the management of mental symptoms.[63]

Many patients suffer from anxiety before surgery, but any premedication must be sufficiently strong without causing undue sedation or interacting with general anaesthesia. A recent clinical study found that a single dose of passionflower prior to outpatient surgery reduced anxiety without increasing sedation.[64] In a double blind, randomised, placebo-controlled trial, 60 patients received either 500 mg of passionflower herb as a tablet or a matching placebo as a premedication 90 minutes before surgery. The passion flower tablet was standardised to contain 1.01 mg of benzoflavone. A numerical rating scale of 1 to 10, with 10 being the worst possible anxiety, was used to assess anxiety and sedation before and 10, 30, 60 and 90 minutes after premedication. Psychomotor function was assessed at arrival in the operating theatre and 30 and 90 minutes after tracheal extubation. Anxiety scores were similar for both groups at baseline, being 4.6 ± 1.7 for the passionflower group and 5.1 ± 2.0 for the placebo control group. After 90 minutes these had changed to 0.97 for the herbal treatment versus 3.88 for control treatment (p<0.001). There were no significant differences between the groups in the level of sedation before surgery and the recovery of function after surgery. Discharge times were also similar and no side effects were observed.

A clinical study presented as a poster at the European College of Neuropsychopharmacology Congress held in Vienna during October 2007 found that a combination of St John's wort (*Hypericum perforatum*) and passionflower was helpful for the symptoms of depression with anxiety.[65] Each tablet in the combination contained 450mg of St John's wort extract (about 2.7g of herb) and 350mg of passionflower extract (about 1.4g of herb) and it was given at a dose of 2 per day. In the trial, 162 patients received either the herbal tablets or a matching placebo for 8 weeks using a randomised, double blind design. Herbal treatment resulted in a highly significant reduction in the Hamilton depression score in the mildly depressed patients (15.64 ± 0.93 to 8.05 ± 1.69) versus an increase for placebo. Results were similar for anxiety scores, indicating that the anxiety that often accompanies mild depression also responded to the herbal combination, no doubt due largely to the passionflower.

Preliminary findings from a clinical trial suggest passionflower improves subjective sleep quality, a result entirely consistent with its traditional reputation as a mild hypnotic. A double blind, placebo-controlled trial conducted in Australia investigated the efficacy of passionflower on sleep.[66] Forty-one healthy volunteers (18 to 35 years) without extreme sleep problems received passionflower or placebo for 1 week, then after a 1-week washout they received the other treatment for 1 week. They drank a cup of tea 1 hour before bedtime. The tea was prepared from 2g passionflower or placebo (parsley, *Petroselinum crispum*; 2g) in 250mL of boiling water, infused for 10 minutes. There was a significant improvement in sleep quality when taking passionflower (5.2% mean increase relative to placebo; $p<0.01$). No significant effects were found for other parameters, although the participants had initially low levels of anxiety.

Antidepressant activity

Herbs with antidepressant activity form part of the herbal category known as the nervine tonics (or nervous system trophorestoratives). The best known example is St John's wort (*Hypericum perforatum*), which is the subject of a lengthy monograph in this book.

In addition, there is some encouraging research that has highlighted some unlikely herbal candidates for antidepressant activity, namely lavender (*Lavandula officinalis*) and saffron (*Crocus sativa*). Also, perhaps not unexpectedly, the tonic herb Rhodiola now has some reasonable evidence for a supporting role in depression.

Lavender has a strong reputation as a herb for the nervous system. In aromatherapy it has been used to calm anxiety and boost mood for some time. The use of lavender oil in depression is also supported by evidence from clinical studies.[67] A small double blind clinical trial was conducted to compare the oral use of 60 drops/day of a lavender 1:5 tincture with the drug imipramine.[68] A third group of patients also took both treatments. While the lavender tincture showed some benefit, it was not as effective as the imipramine for depression.

Perhaps a higher dose of lavender might have yielded better results, as the dose used in the trial was quite low. But the interesting finding was that the combination of lavender with imipramine worked better than imipramine alone, without any accentuation of the drug's side effects.

The evidence for saffron is more extensive, with a number of clinical trials showing promising results, although again these are all small, involving around 40 patients each. Trials tested its efficacy against a placebo and against conventional antidepressants, both a tricyclic (imipramine) and a selective serotonin re-uptake inhibitor (fluoxetine).

Two double blind placebo-controlled trials found that saffron extract at a dose of just 30mg/day was significantly better ($p<0.001$) than placebo in improving the mood of patients with mild to moderate depression.[69,70] There were no more side effects in the saffron group than in the placebo. There was a dramatic drop in the Hamilton depression rating scale for the patients taking the saffron that was evident at 2 weeks and continued to fall until the end of the trial at 6 weeks. In all, it fell from around 23 to 9 in the group taking saffron, versus a fall of only around 23 to 18 in the placebo group.

In the comparative clinical trials, saffron was found to be as effective as the conventional drugs tested. In the trial comparing saffron with imipramine, patients taking the drug experienced the typical side effects of a dry mouth and excessive sedation.[71] No such side effects occurred for saffron. Saffron was compared with fluoxetine in two published trials[72,73] and found to have a similar remission rate for depression to the drug, of around 25%. There were no significant differences between the two patient groups in terms of side effects.

Saffron is a very expensive spice and dye commonly used in Indian and Middle Eastern cuisine. The reason why it is expensive is that just a small part (the stigma) of each flower of this attractive Crocus is harvested by hand.

Research from Sweden has supported the role of *Rhodiola rosea* in depression.[74] In an experimental model of depression Rhodiola performed as well as St John's wort and the antidepressant drug imipramine. The activity was dose dependent and several key phytochemicals in Rhodiola including rosavin were shown to be active.

This research led to a clinical trial of Rhodiola extract in mild and moderate depression. In a randomised, double blind, placebo-controlled design, male and female patients aged 18 to 70 years with Hamilton Rating Scale for Depression (HAMD) scores of 21 to 31 were divided into three groups.[75] Over 6 weeks Group A (31 patients) received 340mg/day of Rhodiola extract, Group B (29 patients) received 680mg/day of extract and Group C (29 patients) were assigned a matching placebo. Both the Hamilton and the Beck Depression Inventory (BDI) were used to assess treatment outcomes at 6 weeks. The BDI is a series of questions developed to measure the intensity, severity and depth of depression.

In terms of overall depression, there were highly significant reductions ($p<0.0001$) in both the HAMD and BDI scores 6 weeks after Rhodiola treatment that was not evident in the placebo group. The average HAMD score in Groups A and B fell from around 25 to around 18 for both groups, indicating that a dose-response effect was not seen for this outcome. In contrast, a dose-response relationship was observed for the

BDI scale, with values falling from around 11 to 8 in Group A and from about 11 to 5 in Group B. In terms of the HAMD subgroup scores, significant reductions were seen for insomnia, emotional instability and somatisation (physical symptoms caused by mental or emotional factors), but not for self-esteem (except in the high dose Group B). No serious side effects were seen.

In discussing a mechanism of action for Rhodiola, the authors emphasised its adaptogenic and antistress activities.[74] In depression it is theorised that stress hormones such as cortisol and indeed the HPA (hypothalamic-pituitary-adrenal) axis are overactivated and do not switch off appropriately via the normal negative feedback (see later in this section). The influence of certain stress chemicals released by cells (stress kinases) is thought to play a key role in this overactivity. In particular, they inhibit the sensitivity of receptors in the brain to cortisol. In an experimental model, Rhodiola extract decreased the release of stress kinases and cortisone in response to stress. This suggests that Rhodiola inhibits the stress-induced activation of stress kinases in depressed patients and so restores the impaired sensitivity of their brain receptors to cortisol. This 'resistance' of the cortisol receptors is a noted feature in many patients with major depression (see also p. 338).

Phytotherapeutics

Analgesics

Plant remedies traditionally used as analgesics

- *Corydalis spp.* (yan hu suo), *Eschscholtzia californica* (California poppy), *Evodia rutaecarpa* (wu zhu yu), *Gelsemium sempervirens* (yellow jasmine), *Paederia scandens* (ji shi teng), *Piscidia erythrina* (Jamaica dogwood). Topically: *Bryonia alba* (white bryony), *Piper methysticum* (kava), *Syzygium aromaticum* (clove bud).

Indications for herbal analgesics

- Pain associated with inflammation (e.g. arthritis, chondritis, tendinitis, myalgia)
- Pain associated with visceral spasm (e.g. gallbladder, urinary and intestinal colic)
- Pain associated with vascular spasm (e.g. migraine, spasmodic dysmenorrhoea)
- Neuralgic pain (in limited cases).

Other traditional indications for analgesics

- Primitive anaesthesia.

Contraindications for herbal analgesics

As powerful agents, herbal analgesics should be restricted in their application to experienced and well-trained practitioners only. There is a theoretically increased risk of neurotoxicity and other adverse effects (although little known incidence) and there is always the possibility that individual examples could be withdrawn from use by regulatory authorities; this

is most likely after cases of irresponsible use. The following cases should be approached with particular caution:

- Concurrent prescription of powerful analgesics
- Pain in children
- Neurological disease
- Depression and psychosis
- Liver and kidney disease
- History of allergic or anaphylactic reactions.

Application

Herbal analgesics may be taken as required or before food. There is likely to be a longer delay compared with synthetic analgesics and the temptation to dose excessively must be resisted.

Long-term therapy with analgesics is not advisable, except in palliative care.

Advanced phytotherapeutics

Herbal analgesics may also be usefully applied in some cases (depending on other factors) of inflammatory disease.

Herbal sedatives and hypnotics

In conventional pharmacological terms, sedatives reduce nervous activity and hypnotics promote sleep. There is obviously overlap in practice between the two categories, and both imply a degree of depression of nervous activity and consequent dangers (as seen most obviously in the barbiturates). There is a third category of calming agent that was postulated as an ideal anxiolytic strategy: the tranquilliser. This was originally defined as a treatment whose effect was confined to the reticular activating system that determined the level of arousal in the central nervous system (CNS), and did not otherwise sedate. Although the benzodiazepines were hailed as tranquillisers on their discovery, this ideal has been clearly compromised and these remedies are now seen to have appreciable sedative and hypnotic effects as well.

Many traditional herbal remedies have various degrees of sedative and tranquillising activity, and some have had this effect supported in experimental and clinical studies. However, it is probably misleading to apply the strict pharmacological definitions to them; their effects are much broader in clinical experience, with strong sedation rare. For the purposes of this text, therefore, the terms 'herbal sedatives and hypnotics' will be used to describe remedies that are actually relaxing, with little evidence of depressive activity.

Plant remedies traditionally used as sedatives and hypnotics

- *Corydalis spp.* (yan hu suo), *Humulus lupulus* (hops), *Lactuca virosa* (wild lettuce), *Passiflora incarnata* (passionflower), *Piper methysticum* (kava), *Piscidia erythrina* (Jamaican dogwood), *Scutellaria laterifolia* (skullcap), *Zizyphus spinosa*.[76,77]

Indications for herbal sedatives and hypnotics

- Moderate tension and anxiety syndromes (short-term or intermittent use)
- Insomnia (difficulty in getting off to sleep first thing at night)
- Weaning off conventional sedative prescriptions.

Other traditional indications for sedative and hypnotics

- Restlessness disturbing convalescence.

Contraindications for herbal sedatives and hypnotics

As generally milder than prescribed sedatives, herbal equivalents should not be seen as immediate substitutes in the more serious indications. It would be unwise and even dangerous to drop the use of strong sedative medication without careful planning, preferably with the cooperation of the prescribing physician:

- Depression
- Insomnia marked by increasing restlessness during the early hours of the morning.

Traditional therapeutic insights into the use of sedatives and hypnotics

In what were usually harsher and more robust times, the need for sedatives was often urgent, and opium extracts were the most favoured. The main tradition of use of moderate herbal sedatives was as short-term components of convalescent management, particularly to help with sleep. There was apparently little use of sedatives for wider lifestyle management.

Application

Herbal sedatives and hypnotics may be taken as required, at bedtime or before food.

Advanced phytotherapeutics

Herbal sedatives and hypnotics may also be usefully applied in some cases (depending on other factors) of inflammatory disease.

Spasmolytics and relaxants (anxiolytics)

Most medical preoccupation has been with the nervous system as an entity in itself, with the goal of better analgesics, sedatives, tranquillisers and antipsychotics. Traditional interest in such areas was of course also strong and many plants were favoured for their powerful psychoactive properties. However, probably the most widespread use of neuroactive plants, or nervines, nowadays is for their effects on innervated structures rather than on nervous tissue alone.

The spasmolytic is a modern descriptor of the effect of an agent on visceral muscle in vitro, often the isolated guinea pig ileum. The technique is widely used as a model to indicate muscarinic or related receptor activity as above, but is a property with little therapeutic application. By contrast, herbal spasmolytics or relaxants are remedies used to reduce the symptoms of tension in the body. Pre-Cartesian insights into the human condition had no separation between body and mind and this particular holistic view is a constant feature of Asian medicine still. Apart from the obvious psychoactives, remedies were not seen to be acting on the nervous system as such; rather there were many remedies that treated various manifestations of turbulence in the body linked to what nowadays would be described as 'stress-related' conditions.

Even though using other terms, early texts described such conditions as classic hypertension ('Liver qi rising'), nervous headaches, palpitations, breathless attacks and hyperventilation ('constriction of the chest'), nervous dyspepsia, dysphagia, irritable bowel and urinary frequency.

The remedies selected for these conditions were seen as somatic in emphasis. The markers for application and effectiveness were physical symptoms. Nowadays modern phytotherapists refer to many of them as antispasmodics or spasmolytics or, more recently, 'visceral relaxants'. They are offered to the modern stressed patient as a welcome antidote to the culture of tranquillisers and sedatives, treatments working from the 'neck down' to reduce the physical effects of tension without befuddling the brain or impugning their sanity. Western remedies such as those listed later have all developed reputations as useful management measures in helping patients handle and even overcome psychosomatic disorders, perhaps combined with appropriate breathing exercises and adrenaline-reducing aerobic activity. Some Chinese remedies such as *Uncaria rhynchophylla* were targeted at such conditions and hold out the promise of modern applications.

Plant remedies traditionally used as spasmolytics and relaxants (anxiolytics)

- *Corydalis spp.*, *Dioscorea spp.* (wild yam), *Leonurus cardiaca* (motherwort), *Lobelia inflata* (lobelia), *Matricaria recutita* (chamomile), *Melissa officinalis* (lemon balm), *Passiflora incarnata* (passionflower), *Piper methysticum* (kava), *Scutellaria lateriflora* (skullcap), *Tilia spp.* (lime flowers), *Valeriana officinalis* (valerian), *Viburnum opulus* (cramp bark).

Indications for spasmolytics and relaxants (anxiolytics)

- Anxiety, irritability and restlessness, including in children
- Sleeplessness due to anxiety and irritability
- Nervous dyspepsia
- Irritable bowel and intestinal colic
- Tension headaches and migraines
- Spasmodic dysmenorrhoea.

Contraindications for spasmolytics and relaxants (anxiolytics)

As a group these remedies are generally safe and well tolerated.

Traditional therapeutic insights into the use of spasmolytics and relaxants

Early use of spasmolytics also appears to have been dominated by their emergency indications, notably urinary and biliary colic. The use of milder relaxant treatments was mainly as tisanes for children and in the largely unrecorded but vast realm of family care. As expected, systematic classifications of medicine throughout history are generally silent on this area of popular healthcare.

Relaxants were obviously indicated for functional overactivities; indications such as dyspeptic and colicky conditions were probably the most common (and carminatives such as the spices the most frequent tisanes). Headaches, teething and restlessness in children and menstrual pains were likely to make up most of the remaining indications. These were usually treated within the home by local remedies with recipes handed down through the family.

Some remedies are more sedative than others in this class (see above). These might be added to a relaxant prescription to increase its impact. However, sedation may be depleting: the more a remedy is chosen for its sedative effects, the shorter the treatment should be and the more tonifying remedies should be added (see following section). The latter should also be a major element in prescriptions for the increasing proportion of tension conditions linked with fatigue, debility, depression and exhaustion.

Application

Spasmolytics and relaxants (and also those aromatics and volatile spasmolytics used for this purpose) may be best taken as hot infusions, though the ordinary teabag may not be sufficiently strong compared with the traditional brew, and in acute cases traditional doses were very high indeed. However, the following herbs probably work better in aqueous ethanolic extracts: *Dioscorea spp.*, *Lobelia inflata*, *Passiflora incarnata*, *Piper methysticum*, *Valeriana officinalis*, and *Viburnum opulus*.

Long-term therapy is generally well tolerated and may be appropriate, although the use of more sedative remedies should be reduced.

Nervine tonics (nervous trophorestoratives)

Herbal medicine has had to adapt significantly from its traditional roots. There is evidence that in many earlier cultures there were different perspectives on anxiety and depression syndromes. Whether there was genuinely less opportunity for the modern diagnosis in highly structured communities living on the edge of survival or whether such symptoms were not recognised as such is arguable. There is, however, less emphasis on treatments to relieve stress and mood conditions in most traditional texts.

There were also no powerful synthetic agents that relieved pain and distress. It is thus an entirely modern notion that herbs could provide gentle back-up for sufferers with nervous or mental problems.

In the West, where such adjustments have been made over many decades, the group of remedies that has emerged to meet modern needs is sometimes referred to as 'nervines'. In recognition of the common observation that many conditions of tension are linked with fatigue, debility and depression, there is also a category of remedies that were seen to restore energies and build up strength. These have sometimes been referred to as 'trophorestoratives'. It was a general principle that some tonifying element be included in most nervine prescriptions, so as to aim for lasting value rather than just short-term alleviation.

Plant remedies traditionally used as nervous system trophorestoratives

- *Avena sativa* (oatstraw), *Centella asiatica* (gotu kola), *Hypericum perforatum* (St John's wort), *Schisandra chinensis*, *Scutellaria lateriflora* (skullcap), *Turnera diffusa* (damiana), *Verbena officinalis* (vervain), *Withania somnifera* (Indian ginseng).

Indications for nervous system trophorestoratives

(See also Tonics in Chapter 8.)
- Nervous exhaustion
- Neuralgia, herpes infections
- Depressive states
- Insomnia (waking up in the small hours after getting off to sleep easily).

Other traditional indications for nervous system trophorestoratives

- Convalescence
- Neurasthenia.

Contraindications for nervous system trophorestoratives

True trophorestoratives are almost nutritional in their effects, with few risks of adverse effects except in those patients with extremely debilitated constitutions (see also the discussion on tonics).

Traditional therapeutic insights into the use of nervous system trophorestoratives

Neurasthenia encompassed a wider range of disorders than nervous exhaustion. In days before psychoanalysis and neurology, it included symptoms where the nervous tissues were seen to be affected such as neuralgia and neuritis, depression, anxiety states and neurosis. The trophorestoratives were thus often combined with other tonics and convalescent foods such as molasses, yeast and malt extract (now known as rich sources of the B vitamins), oatmeal and other cereals.

Application

Nervous system trophorestoratives may be taken as required or before food.

Long-term therapy with trophorestoratives is generally the norm.

Phytotherapy for nervous system conditions

Anxiety

There are several types of anxiety defined in the various diagnostic manuals including panic disorder, phobias, social anxiety disorder, obsessive-compulsive disorder, separation anxiety and post-traumatic stress disorder. However, the condition classified as generalised anxiety disorder (GAD) is probably the most common form suffered by patients seeking phytotherapy. This is with good reason, since this often milder form of anxiety is more amenable to subtle treatments.

The DSM-IV (American Psychiatric Association 2000) defines GAD as troublesome excessive anxiety and worry (apprehensive expectation) occurring more days than not for at least 6 months and not associated with any other condition.[78] Three or more of the following will be present: restlessness or feeling on edge, being easily fatigued, difficulty in concentration, irritability, muscle tension and sleep disturbances.

One interesting discussion suggests that several factors have led contemporary psychiatry away from neuroses and anxiety disorders and towards depression as a social paradigm of distress.[79] These included a perception that anxiety disorders have less relevance, the downfall of the benzodiazepines and the failure to replace them with better anxiolytics, and the development of newer antidepressants. The article suggests that having promoted cognitive-behavioural therapy as the treatment for anxiety disorders, these conditions have become more the domain of clinical psychologists.

The discussion does touch on an important consideration: that patients suffering from anxiety must be viewed as a whole. Aspects of lifestyle and diet should be considered and extremes corrected where possible, for example excessive use of alcohol, recreational drugs or sexual indulgence, imbalanced diet, excessive tea and coffee intake, and cigarette smoking. Such corrections will need to be carefully considered, since often these factors can be used by the patient to allay anxiety and their abrupt withdrawal could exacerbate symptoms. Appropriate professional guidance and counselling, with the introduction of simple techniques for relaxation, can be beneficial.

Aspects of herbal treatment to be considered for the patient with GAD are as follows:

- Dampening symptoms of anxiety with anxiolytic and sedative herbs such as kava, valerian and passionflower. Other herbs in these categories can provide valuable assistance and include lavender, California poppy, Zizyphus seed, Corydalis, Magnolia and Bacopa
- The nervine tonic herbs also have a role (these herbs are calming, but also lift mood) in the treatment of anxiety. They include St John's wort, Schisandra, lemon balm, skullcap, oats and damiana
- Spasmolytic herbs to alleviate spasm. Cramp bark and chamomile may be useful for any visceral symptoms associated with the anxiety, and hawthorn berry can be prescribed where there are cardiac symptoms. Motherwort is also useful for palpitations

- Anxious patients stress their bodies and deplete their adrenal reserves. This can create a vicious cycle. Hence adrenal restorative, adaptogenic and tonic herbs may be required. The herb of choice in this context is Withania, since it has calming properties, supported by Rehmannia and licorice (Glycyrrhiza)
- Patients who have access to a bath can be advised to add a few drops of lavender oil to the bath for its calming effect
- Any associated sleep disturbance should be treated with a separate formula at night (see Insomnia in this section)
- Anxiolytic herbs can be used to aid the withdrawal of benzodiazepine drugs. The herbs should be taken for a few weeks before the drugs are gradually withdrawn. Additive effects to the benzodiazepines are minimal.

Anxiolytic herbs should not in general make the patient drowsy or affect their capacity to drive or use machinery. However, some sensitive patients may complain of this. These are usually people who are sleep-deprived or 'living on their nerves' and the herbs are probably only making them aware of how tired their bodies are. Due attention to rest and sleep usually eliminates this effect over a few weeks.

Note: Terminology to describe the classification of medicines is often applied loosely and inconsistently in modern usage. Sedatives (according to the *Oxford Dictionary*) soothe the nervous system. Implied in the term, however, is a resultant state of sedation. In contrast, anxiolytics allay anxiety, without necessarily inducing a state of sedation. In modern parlance, sedatives are often used to describe substances that induce sleep. But the correct term for this is hypnotic. That said, it is obvious that most sedatives will assist someone with disturbed sleep (but probably work better as such when taken throughout the day, rather than just before bed).

Example liquid formula

Valeriana officinalis	1:2	20 mL
Passiflora incarnata	1:2	20 mL
Withania somnifera	1:2	35 mL
Hypericum perforatum	1:2	25 mL
	TOTAL	100 mL

Dose: 8 mL with water twice a day.

CASE HISTORY

A female patient aged 45 was suffering from anxiety and depression and had been diagnosed as having bipolar disorder and prescribed lithium and dothiepin hydrochloride. Three years ago she experienced a nervous breakdown. She had recently left a difficult and unstable husband, whom she felt had persecuted her. The dothiepin caused side effects so the patient had recently discontinued it.

The patient was prescribed the following herbs:

Hypericum perforatum	1:2	20 mL
Piper methysticum	1:2	25 mL
Scutellaria lateriflora	1:2	15 mL
Valeriana officinalis	1:2	20 mL
Bacopa monniera	1:2	20 mL
	TOTAL	100 mL

Dose: 5 mL with water three times a day.

Also, to help with sleep, valerian tablets 500 mg, three before bed were suggested. After taking the herbs for 4 weeks she reported that she felt better in herself and was coping well and her sleep had improved. She continued on the herbs for another 6 months with good results. (The patient was also recommended to consult a clinical psychologist skilled in counselling, which she did.)

Note: Bacopa was included in the formula because of its use in India for extreme mental states. Kava might be substituted with tablets or capsules if a liquid is not available. Alternatively other herbs such as Corydalis could have been used instead of the kava.

Depression

Unipolar depressive disorders (depression without a manic or hypomanic phase) not associated with medical illness are typically classified as follows in various diagnostic manuals:

* Major depression characterised by sadness, apathy, irritability, disturbed sleep, disturbed appetite, weight loss, fatigue, poor concentration, guilt and thoughts of death
* Dysthymic disorder, which consists of a pattern of chronic, ongoing mild depressive symptoms that are less severe than major depression
* Seasonal affective disorder (SAD), which is more common in women and related to seasonal changes. The prevalence increases with increasing latitude and it can be treated by light therapy. Symptoms include lack of energy, weight gain and carbohydrate craving.

The DSM-IV defines major depressive disorder (MDD) as a clinical depressive episode that lasts longer than 2 weeks and is uncomplicated by recent grief, substance abuse or a medical disorder.[78] Various theories about the cause of MDD have been proposed, and include the monoamine-deficiency hypothesis (that underlies modern drug therapy) and a dysfunction in the hypothalamic-pituitary-adrenal (HPA) axis with an abnormal stress response.[80] Elevated cortisol is consistently present in depressed patients. This overactivity of the HPA axis may be related to a conditioned response to traumatic events in childhood.

MDD has various degrees of expression, and phytotherapy is most appropriate for its mild to moderate manifestations. Patients experiencing severe MDD with acute suicidal thoughts or exhibiting other forms of self-endangerment should be referred to appropriate care. Impaired circulation to the brain, especially in elderly patients, is another cause of depression. Low systolic blood pressure was also associated with a poor perception of well-being in 50-year-old men[81] and depression in men aged 60 to 89 years.[82]

The general considerations outlined in the treatment of anxiety also apply here. Patients suffering from depression should be treated as a whole with due attention to lifestyle, diet, drug use and mental hygiene (productive attitudes for coping with life events). Professional guidance and counselling is often appropriate, rather than the relegation of depression to just a biochemical imbalance to be corrected with pharmacological agents.

As noted above, phytotherapy is most appropriate for mild to moderate episodes of MDD, dysthymic disorder and SAD. Episodes of severe depression may require the more strident therapy offered by conventional drugs, although herbs can

have a supportive role, especially in terms of boosting vitality. Herbs can also be relevant when the patient has improved and wishes to discontinue drug therapy.

Key elements of herbal treatment are as follows:

* The nervine tonic herbs are the mainstay of treatment, especially St John's wort, which is a well-proven treatment for mild to moderate depression (see monograph). Other important herbs in this category include damiana, skullcap, Schisandra and Bacopa.
* Patients who are also anxious should be prescribed anxiolytic herbs. Valerian, passionflower and Zizyphus are also useful, but hops is traditionally contraindicated.
* Depressed patients are low in vitality, so adrenal restorative (licorice and Rehmannia), tonic and adaptogenic herbs are often indicated. Ginseng may have antidepressant activity, but it should be used cautiously if anxiety is present. Rhodiola, Withania and Siberian ginseng are better choices in these cases. Licorice and Schisandra also have exhibited some antidepressant activity in animal models. These herbs will also help correct the adverse long-term effects of stress on the physiology of the stress response.
* If required, herbs that improve circulation to the brain should be prescribed, especially Ginkgo.
* Recent research supports the value of lavender, Rhodiola and saffron (see above).

Example liquid formula

Valeriana officinalis	1:2	20 mL
Hypericum perforatum	1:2	25 mL
Rhodiola rosea	2:1	20 mL
Schisandra chinensis	1:2	20 mL
Glycyrrhiza glabra	1:1	15 mL
	TOTAL	100 mL

Dose: 5 mL with water three times a day.

CASE HISTORY

A male patient, aged 72, came seeking help for depression following the death of his daughter from cancer about 6 months ago. He did not want to take conventional medication. He was prescribed St John's wort extract 300 mg in tablets, 3 per day. Each tablet was standardised to 0.9 mg total hypericin and equivalent to 1500 to 1800 mg of flowering tops. There was a steady improvement in his mood over 6 to 8 weeks and he felt much better and more positive about life. The patient was maintained at 2 tablets per day with continued benefit.

Insomnia

Generally patients seek phytotherapy for insomnia that has become a chronic problem. The DSM-IV additionally requires that with chronic primary insomnia the patient's sleep disturbance disrupts his or her daily performance and quality of life.[78] It can be difficult in practice to differentiate primary insomnia from possible secondary causes such as alcohol and medical problems. Hence, it is more practical to address all the issues that might be contributing to the insomnia, while prescribing herbs as if it was primary insomnia. This approach therefore requires a detailed and careful case history and appropriate counselling of the patient.

Insomnia, or inadequate sleep, can be categorised for phytotherapy according to the difficulties experienced by the patient. These include difficulty falling asleep (sleep-onset insomnia), awakening during the night with difficulty falling back to sleep (sleep-maintenance insomnia), early morning awakening (sleep-offset insomnia) and a sense of not having enough sleep (non-restorative sleep). Patients can report a combination of these.

Major causes of sleep-onset insomnia include anxiety, pain or discomfort, caffeine and alcohol. Sleep-maintenance insomnia can be linked to depression, sleep apnoea, fibromyalgia syndrome, nocturnal hypoglycaemia, pain or discomfort and alcohol. If restless legs syndrome is a cause of insomnia, this should be addressed separately (see later in this section). Any obvious causes of the insomnia (such as pain) should also be treated separately.

It is important to ensure that the patient sleeps in a darkened, noise-free environment in a comfortable bed. The use of stimulants should be reduced, especially coffee, tea, guarana and cola drinks. Alcohol intake should also be reduced. Unwinding at night can be important and a few drops of lavender oil added to an evening bath can help this process. Where the insomnia has been precipitated by anxiety or other psychological problems, appropriate counselling or phytotherapy should be recommended. The key herbs for insomnia to be considered will depend on the pattern of the insomnia:

- Anxiolytic and hypnotic herbs are the mainstay of treatment. These can be taken throughout the day to prevent a build-up of tension or mental excitability that might result in insomnia. An additional dose is then recommended around 1 hour before bed. If the insomnia is not severe, then the herbs can be taken as a single dose before bed. Key herbs include valerian, kava, Zizyphus, hops, lemon balm, Magnolia, lavender, passionflower, California poppy and chamomile. Best results with valerian come from continuous use for at least 2 weeks (see monograph).
- Antidepressant and nervine tonic herbs are indicated, especially if the insomnia is associated with fibromyalgia or is sleep-maintenance insomnia. These include St John's wort, saffron, skullcap, damiana, Rhodiola and Schisandra.
- If the patient is debilitated and suffers from sleep-maintenance insomnia, then adrenal restorative herbs such as licorice or Rehmannia are also indicated. These herbs will additionally help to maintain blood sugar levels during the night.
- Tonic and adaptogenic herbs used throughout the day can help to break the vicious cycle of non-restorative sleep in stressed patients. The safest and best herb to use in this context is Withania, although a small amount of ginseng will not be too stimulating for most patients. Also use of those herbs taken just before bed can tonify (and thereby improve) the sleep of patients experiencing non-restorative sleep.
- If pain interferes with sleep then analgesic herbs for pain management are indicated. For example, willow bark is useful for pain associated with inflammation, whereas Corydalis, cramp bark, kava and wild yam will help to alleviate pain associated with smooth muscle cramping. (See also the treatments for restless legs syndrome and nocturnal myoclonus.)

Recent research with Vitex (chaste tree) and melatonin represents a promising new development in the herbal treatment of maintenance insomnia (see monograph).

Example liquid formulas

Sleep-onset insomnia

Valeriana officinalis	1:2	30 mL
Passiflora incarnata	1:2	25 mL
Zizyphus spinosa	1:2	25 mL
Withania somnifera	1:1	20 mL
	TOTAL	100 mL

Dose: 5 mL with water three times a day. Take the last dose 1 hour before bed.

Sleep-maintenance or sleep-offset insomnia

Valeriana officinalis	1:2	25 mL
Hypericum perforatum	1:2	30 mL
Vitex agnus-castus	1:2	20 mL
Scutellaria lateriflora	1:2	25 mL
	TOTAL	100 mL

Dose: 5 mL with water three times a day. Take the last dose 1 hour before bed.

CASE HISTORY

A male patient aged 47 complained of difficulty falling asleep some nights. He was prescribed kava tablets, 2 to 3 about 50 minutes before bed. Each tablet contained 200 mg of extract standardised to 60 mg of kava lactones and equivalent to about 1800 to 2000 mg of root. He found the tablets very effective, but did find that they caused early morning drowsiness on some, but not all, mornings after he used them.

CASE HISTORY

A female patient, aged 59, suffered from fibromyalgia (which was treated with a herbal mixture taken during the day). However, a significant problem (typically associated with fibromyalgia) was her terrible insomnia. She claimed that some nights she only slept for about 1 hour. Valerian tablets and kava tablets were tried to no effect.

She was prescribed the following formula:

Zizyphus spinosa	1:2	30 mL
Scutellaria lateriflora	1:2	25 mL
Lavandula officinalis	1:2	20 mL
Corydalis ambigua	1:2	25 mL
	TOTAL	100 mL

Dose: 8 mL with water about 30 minutes before bed. Repeat a few hours later if still awake.

The above sleep mixture helped tremendously and, with the sleep improvement, her fibromyalgia also improved more rapidly.

Restless legs syndrome (and nocturnal myoclonus)

Restless legs syndrome (RLS) has been described as 'the most common disorder you've never heard of'.[83] It is an unusual sensation (paraesthesia) in the legs that typically occurs at bedtime and is a common cause of insomnia. The cause of RLS is not known. It is known to be associated with a number of medical conditions including iron deficiency, pregnancy and dialysis.

RLS is surprisingly common and plagues the sleep of many sufferers. Various estimates have ranged from 2% to 15% of the adult population, with the real number likely to be about 6%. It is more common in women.[84] The older the person, the more likely he or she will suffer from restless legs. It is rare in young children, but for those older than 65 years around 10% to 28% are affected.

Lower iron levels in the brain affect dopamine metabolism, specifically inhibition of tyrosine hydroxylase needed for the synthesis of dopamine and requiring iron as a cofactor.[85] In one study, 75% of patients with RLS had decreased iron stores. Iron concentrations in the blood drop by 50% to 60% at night. Ferritin concentrations of <50 ng/mL have been correlated with decreased sleep efficiency and increased leg movements in sleep in RLS. Oral supplementation of iron has resulted in significant clinical improvement in RLS. Some patients with RLS improve with folate supplementation, which is also involved in tyrosine hydroxylase production.[84]

Magnesium therapy (12.4 mmol/day=301 mg/day) has been shown to be beneficial.[86] A placebo-controlled trial found that 800 mg/day Valerian root for 8 weeks improved RLS symptoms and daytime sleepiness.[87] A recent pilot trial with Vitex (chaste tree) was also promising (see monograph). A number of lifestyle factors have been associated with RLS. These include heavy smoking, advanced age, obesity, hypertension, loud snoring, use of antidepressant drugs,[83] diabetes and lack of exercise.[88]

Conventional medical treatment for RLS focuses on drugs for the nervous system, especially dopaminergic agents. Many of these drugs are quite powerful and dangerous and should be reserved for more severe cases.[82] A study found that RLS was very common in people with varicose veins (22% incidence).[89] After treatment for superficial varicose veins (sclerotherapy or vein stripping), 98% reported an immediate improvement in their restless legs.

When the blood is not circulating properly, the walls of the deeper veins can stretch, resulting in unpleasant sensations in the legs. The sluggish circulation can cause red blood cell aggregation that can further add to the paraesthesia and restless legs. Consistent with this, the condition is much more common during pregnancy.[82] One survey of 500 women found that 19% reported RLS during pregnancy, that 7% described their symptoms as 'severe' and that the condition abated in 96% of affected women within 1 month of giving birth.[82]

Key herbs to consider for RLS are:

- anxiolytic and hypnotic herbs such as valerian, kava (especially), skullcap and passionflower to alleviate the nervous system imbalance that is part of RLS
- many of the factors involved in RLS (smoking, pregnancy, obesity, age, diabetes) all point to an involvement of the circulation. Hence venotonic herbs such as horsechestnut and butcher's broom and herbs that enhance circulation such as Ginkgo have a key (but often neglected) role to play
- chaste tree and other herbs for insomnia may be of value.

CASE HISTORY

A female patient aged 61 complained of sleep-onset insomnia and sleep latency largely brought about by restless legs at night. There was a history of anxiety and poor venous circulation. She was prescribed tablets (2 per day) containing *Aesculus hippocastanum* (horsechestnut) 1.2 g, *Ginkgo biloba* (Ginkgo) 1.5 g and *Ruscus aculeatus* (butcher's broom) 800 mg and a magnesium supplement. Kava tablets (providing 120 to 180 mg kava lactones per day) were also to be taken as required.

This patient was successfully treated for about 2 years as above and then found that the treatment could be stopped for many months without problem. The treatment was started again if symptoms returned. This on and off approach was followed for 3 years.

Chronic tension headache

Chronic tension-type headache (TTH) is a neurological disorder characterised by frequent attacks of mild to moderate headache with few other symptoms.[90] The headaches are typically bilateral, have a pressing (non-pulsatile) quality and are not aggravated by routine physical activity. They are not characterised by nausea or vomiting and no other causes are found. TTH affects up to 78% of the general population and 3% suffer from the chronic form.[91]

Peripheral factors are implicated in episodic TTH, whereas central factors probably underlie chronic TTH. Activation of hyperexcitable peripheral afferent neurons from head and neck muscles is the most likely explanation for infrequent headaches.[90] Muscle and psychological tension are associated with and can aggravate TTH, but are not believed to be the cause. Abnormalities in central pain processing and a generalised increase in pain sensitivity are present in some patients with chronic TTH.[90,92]

The treatment of a single episode of tension headache is rarely an issue for a consultation for herbal treatment. The commonly encountered clinical situation is recurrent or chronic TTH, hence the approach to treatment described below is more aimed at the prevention of headaches, but many of the herbs below will also alleviate tension headache pain. Herbs with mild analgesic properties still have a role in this context because they generally also possess some relaxing or anxiolytic activity.

Aspects of herbal treatment that should be considered:

- If the headaches are related to trigger foods, or there are signs of problems with digestion, then bitter herbs to improve upper digestive and choleretic herbs to improve liver function should be included.
- Anxiolytic and nervine tonic herbs should be prescribed if appropriate, especially those which have some analgesic activity such as Corydalis and kava.
- Spasmolytic herbs, particularly those with an effect on the circulation can help to prevent tension headaches. These include wild yam, hawthorn, cramp bark and chamomile.
- Analgesic herbs include willow bark, California poppy and Corydalis. As well as its role in migraine, feverfew is a useful anti-inflammatory herb in TTH.
- If the headaches have a relationship with the menstrual cycle, then hormonal regulating herbs may be valuable, for example chaste tree if the headaches occur premenstrually.
- If eye strain is a factor then higher doses of bilberry (equivalent to at least 80 mg of anthocyanins per day) are indicated.
- In elderly people, cerebral ischaemia may contribute to headaches and can be treated with Ginkgo if there is evidence of its presence.
- Topical application of peppermint oil to the temples has been shown to relieve headache pain in clinical trials (see monograph).
- If the above approach does not give results then localised traction or compression of veins or nerves may be a cause, and anti-inflammatory and antioedema herbs such as horsechestnut and butcher's broom should be tried in conjunction with St John's wort (similar to the approach described next for trigeminal neuralgia).
- For headaches due to sinusitis, treatment should focus on this condition. An analgesic herb such as willow bark could also be recommended.

Example liquid formula

Corydalis ambigua	1:2	25 mL
Viburnum opulus	1:2	25 mL
Crataegus monogyna leaf	1:2	30 mL
Matricaria recutita (high in bisabolol)	1:2	20 mL
	TOTAL	100 mL

Dose: 8 mL with water twice a day.

CASE HISTORY

A male patient, aged 74, complained of headaches and fatigue. He had experienced about one headache per week on and off for years. He had some sinus problems, with post-nasal drip at night and his nose could be blocked at times. He used to have migraines and his headaches were worse with stress. He worked long hours and was anxious and worried.

He was prescribed the following herbs:

Euphrasia officinalis	1:2	20 mL
Viburnum opulus	1:2	15 mL
Tanacetum parthenium	1:5	10 mL
Matricaria recutita	1:2	15 mL
Corydalis ambigua	1:2	20 mL
Crataegus monogyna leaf	1:2	20 mL
	TOTAL	100 mL

Dose: 5 mL with water three times a day.

For the fatigue he was also prescribed 2 tablets per day, each containing Withania root 600 mg and ginseng main root 125 mg. The eyebright was included in the treatment because of the possible association of the headaches with his sinus condition. After 8 weeks on the herbal treatment he was relatively free from headaches.

Trigeminal neuralgia

Trigeminal neuralgia, also known as tic douloureux, is a frequent cause of facial pain that involves the trigeminal nerve and occurs almost exclusively in middle-aged or elderly people. The pain is severe and fleeting and may be so severe that the patient winces (hence the term *tic*). Pain attacks tend to occur in clusters that can go on for several weeks.[93]

The pathogenesis of trigeminal neuralgia is speculated to be an ephaptic conduction caused by segmental demyelination and artificial synapse formation (in other words the trigeminal nerve becomes cross-wired due to demyelination). The cause of the demyelination might be multiple sclerosis, vascular degeneration or ageing. However, one recent review suggested that the most common aetiology is vascular compression of the trigeminal nerve root entry zone that leads to a focal demyelination.[94] The blood vessels involved are said to be aberrant or tortuous.[92] Studies have demonstrated proximity of the nerve root to such vessels, usually the superior cerebellar artery.

Under a relatively new classification from the International Headache Society, for the diagnosis of classical trigeminal neuralgia no cause of symptoms other than vascular compression can be found. In contrast, symptomatic trigeminal neuralgia has the same clinical picture, but an underlying cause such as multiple sclerosis, amyloid filtration, small brain infarcts or bony compression is identified.[92]

Relevant herbs to consider include the following:

- A key herb is St John's wort, which is traditionally prescribed for any neuralgia related to nerve irritation or compression.
- The health of large blood vessels and the microcirculation can be improved with grape seed and pine bark extracts and bilberry, Ginkgo, garlic, gotu kola and hawthorn.
- Any compression caused by oedema associated with inflammation or tortuous vessels can be treated with horsechestnut. The venous-toning effect of this herb may also be of value.

- Anti-inflammatory herbs could be tried, such as Boswellia and turmeric.
- Analgesic herbs such as Corydalis or willow bark can be prescribed for the painful episodes.
- Effects from demyelination can be somewhat improved by ensuring adequate intake of essential fatty acids (for example evening primrose oil, which is also anti-inflammatory) and improving the microvasculature (see above).
- A published case history described the successful use of consumption of 30 to 60 mL/day of Aloe vera juice for 3 months. The patient's pain diminished significantly within 2 weeks of initiating therapy. When she stopped the Aloe juice her pain returned and it went within a few days of starting it again.[95]

CASE HISTORY

A male patient, aged 77, presented with trigeminal neuralgia on the right side of his face. He had had the condition for about 9 years and it was first diagnosed as a dental problem. His episodes of attacks numbered 2 to 3 per year and each episode lasted 3 weeks to 3 months. While he was experiencing attacks he found it difficult to shave or wash his face. He was told by a specialist that a blood vessel was impinging on the trigeminal nerve (he had a history of atherosclerosis of the carotid arteries and angina pectoris). He was prescribed carbamazepine for the trigeminal neuralgia, but was concerned that this medication made him feel sluggish. His case history revealed that he suffered from hayfever with bouts of sneezing and he drank an enormous amount of tea each day (which he was advised to reduce).

He was prescribed the following herbal treatments:

- Grape seed extract tablets 100 mg/day
- Tablets (3 per day) containing the following herbs:
  - horsechestnut extract equivalent to dry seed 1.2 g containing escin 40 mg
  - butcher's broom extract equivalent to dry root and rhizome 800 mg
  - Ginkgo extract 30 mg equivalent to dry leaf 1.5 g containing Ginkgo flavone glycosides 7.3 mg
- Liquid formulation:

Scutellaria baicalensis	1:2	30 mL
Hypericum perforatum	1:2	30 mL
Crataegus monogyna leaf	1:2	30 mL
Ginkgo biloba (standardised extract)	2:1	10 mL
	TOTAL	100 mL

Dose: 5 mL with water twice a day.

(The Ginkgo in the liquid supplemented the amount in the tablets containing horsechestnut and butcher's broom.) Over the ensuing months the intensity and frequency of the neuralgia abated and after 6 months he was free of pain and not taking carbamazepine. Continued treatment maintained the freedom from neuralgia. He was also sneezing less.

RATIONALE

Given the association with circulation, grape seed extract and Ginkgo were prescribed to boost the integrity of the microvascular circulation, hawthorn for the arteries and horsechestnut and butcher's broom for any pressure on the nerve associated with oedema or venous congestion.

Baical skullcap and grape seed were to help reduce the sneezing and St John's wort was given for the irritated trigeminal nerve.

Migraine

Results from the American Migraine Prevalence and Prevention Study indicate that the cumulative lifetime incidence of migraine in the USA is 43% for women and 18% for men. This frequency is likely to be reflected in most Western countries and, given that the diagnostic criteria used were relatively stringent, the incidence may be even greater.[96]

A migraine is a complex brain event that can produce a wide array of neurological and systemic symptoms. Although the term migraine is derived from the word *hemicrania*, meaning one side of the head, the pain is not necessarily one-sided. Symptoms include extreme and prolonged head pain, photophobia, nausea and vomiting. Sometimes the migraine is preceded by sensory (especially visual) or motor symptoms (the aura). More commonly there is no aura.

The vascular theory of migraine was proposed by Wolff and others in the 1930s. It attributes migraine to an initial intracranial vasoconstriction (which accounts for the aura) followed by an extracranial vasodilation (the headache). However, this theory was not consistent with later experimental observations.

There has been further movement away from the concept of migraine as a primarily vascular disorder.[96] Although intracranial vasodilation is an appealingly simple explanation for migraine pain, this hypothesis has never been capable of explaining the wide range of symptoms that may precede, accompany, or follow the pain. Multiple imaging studies have now confirmed that vasodilation is not required for migraine headache. In fact cortical hypoperfusion during the headache is more characteristic.

A corollary of the vascular hypothesis of migraine is the concept that vasoconstriction is a primary mechanism by which caffeine, ergotamines and triptans exert their therapeutic effect. But experimental studies do not support this understanding and suggest that the mode of action of each drug class is complex and distinct.[96] However, the vascular hypothesis still has its supporters as well as detractors.[97]

Migraine is currently hypothesised by some researchers as an episodic disorder of brain excitability, akin to epilepsy and episodic movement disorders. Waves of altered brain function, such as cortical spreading depression could be responsible for translating changes in cellular excitability into a migraine attack.[96] This suggests a role for sedative and antiepileptic herbs.

Another suggestion is that migraine is an episode of local sterile meningeal inflammation and the subsequent activation of trigeminal neurons that supply the intracranial meninges and related large blood vessels.[98] Meningeal mast cells could be involved here as triggers, suggesting a role of *Scutellaria baicalensis*, given the neurological and mast cell activities of its flavonoids.

Epidemiological studies suggest that migraine is associated with disorders of the cerebral, coronary, retinal, dermal and peripheral vasculature. There is evidence that migraine is associated with vascular endothelial dysfunction and impaired vascular reactivity, both as a cause and a consequence.[99] This suggests a role for microvascular herbs and could explain the role of feverfew in migraine, including this herb's possible effects on platelet function (see the feverfew monograph).

Migraine is a potentially progressive disorder, and progression of episodic migraine to chronic migraine (migraine chronification) is associated with a range of co-morbidities and risk factors, that could represent either cause or effect. Hypertension is one such co-morbidity,[100] others include obesity, excessive use of medications, caffeine overuse, stressful life events, depression, sleep disorders, cutaneous allodynia,[101] temporomandibular disorders,[102] white matter lesions in the brain,[103] cardiac and vascular problems, psychiatric disorders,[104] head injury, pro-inflammatory states and prothrombotic states.[105]

The higher frequency of migraine in women has already been noted, and menstrual migraine, which occurs before or during menstruation, is believed to be associated with the fall of oestrogen.[106] In other women, oral contraceptive use can trigger migraines.[105] At menopause, migraine can regress, worsen or remain unchanged.[105]

Other factors linked to migraine development or migraine attacks include prolonged stress,[107,108] and trigger foods such as cheese, coffee, chocolate or citrus fruits. Alcohol drinks, especially red wine, can also act as a trigger. About 40% of migraine sufferers tested positive for *Helicobacter pylori*, and eradicating this organism resulted in a significant clinical improvement.[109]

As well as trigger foods it has been suggested that other food allergies could also be a factor in migraine headaches. Commonly implicated foods include cow's milk products, wheat and eggs.[110] Poor body alignment and the benefits of spinal manipulation are particularly relevant to this condition.

In general, patients seeking phytotherapy for migraine will be sufferers of chronic migraine. Hence therapy is best aimed at preventing attacks, although a separate formula to abort attacks if taken early can be prescribed. This abortive treatment could include herbs such as feverfew, willow bark, ginger and Corydalis, all in relatively high doses.

Considerations for preventative herbal treatment include selection from the following:

- Anxiolytic and nervine tonic herbs are used for the effects of stress, especially those having some analgesic activity such as Corydalis. St John's wort may be particularly valuable, as will herbs with some antiepileptic properties such as kava, Bacopa, Withania and valerian.
- Feverfew works well as a migraine prophylactic, but it must contain good levels of parthenolide. It takes about 4 to 6 months to fully work (see feverfew monograph). Since its primary effect may be on platelets, its role may be supported by antiplatelet herbs such as ginger and turmeric.
- If the migraines are related to trigger foods or there are signs of problems with digestion, then herbs to improve upper digestive and liver function should be included. Phytotherapy places an emphasis on the relationship between migraine headaches and liver function. It is good practice to include a liver herb in a migraine preventative formula, be it a choleretic herb such as globe artichoke or ones that aid hepatic detoxification such as turmeric or Schisandra. In France, this liver connection is acknowledged by phytotherapists, as evidenced by a study of migraine treated by the liver herb *Fumaria officinalis* (fumitory).[111] *Helicobacter pylori* can be treated with bitters, garlic, sage, thyme, Nigella and golden seal (see also pp. 321–322).
- Menstrual migraine should be treated with herbs with oestrogenic effects such as shatavari, wild yam and Tribulus. Premenstrual migraine may be alleviated by prescribing chaste tree.
- Ginkgo should be included in a preventative formula, given that cortical hypoperfusion is associated with migraine. The anti-PAF activity of Ginkgo (PAF is platelet activating factor) may also be an advantage.
- Spasmolytic herbs, particularly those with an effect on the circulation, can help to prevent a migraine. These include hawthorn, cramp bark and chamomile. The spasmolytic herb butterbur is used in Europe for migraine prophylaxis. (Caution: butterbur contains toxic pyrrolizidine alkaloids, but these compounds have been removed from products permitted for sale in Europe.)
- Given that a pro-inflammatory cascade might be involved in the aetiology of migraine, anti-inflammatory herbs such as Boswellia, turmeric and ginger could be of value as preventive agents.
- Herbs for microvasculature and promoting endothelial health could be of value. These include garlic, bilberry, pine bark and grape seed extracts, Ginkgo, green tea, turmeric, and *Polygonum cuspidatum* (as a source of resveratrol).

Example liquid formula

Tanacetum parthenium	1:5	20 mL
Hypericum perforatum or *Bacopa monniera*	1:2	30 mL
Schisandra chinensis	1:2	25 mL
Zingiber officinale	1:2	10 mL
Viburnum opulus	1:2	20 mL
	TOTAL	105 mL

Dose: 8 mL with water twice a day.

CASE HISTORY

A female patient aged 43 suffered from about two severe migraines a month. There did not appear to be any association with trigger foods and they tended to occur premenstrually. She was prescribed the following treatments:

- Feverfew tablets 150 mg standardised to contain 900 μg parthenolide, 2 tablets per day
- Three tablets per day of an anti-inflammatory formula containing Boswellia extract 200 mg equivalent to dry gum resin 2400 mg containing boswellic acids 135 mg, celery seed oil equivalent to dry seed 3000 mg, and ginger rhizome 300 mg
- Chaste tree 500 mg tablets, 2 tablets on rising.

Over a period of about 4 to 6 months the migraines reduced substantially in frequency and severity. She found that conventional analgesics such as aspirin could better abort or allay an attack than previously (this is a common finding with feverfew therapy).

Enhancing cognition

Although not a health issue, there is considerable interest in herbs that may be able to effect cognition enhancement, for example among students studying for exams or older people whose memories are weakening. In addition, these herbs form a central part of the treatment of more serious conditions such as Alzheimer's disease.

On current evidence, Ginkgo has been shown to improve cognitive function, although there have been some negative findings (see Ginkgo monograph). In particular, the combination of Ginkgo and ginseng seems to be particularly powerful at improving cognition in both acute and long-term studies (see the ginseng monograph).

The Ayurvedic herb *Bacopa monniera*, also known as brahmi in India, has a strong traditional reputation for improving cognitive function and intelligence.[112] Several clinical trials have found that various Bacopa extracts (typically at around 300 mg/day) improved cognitive function in healthy volunteers, usually when given over 90 days.[113–115] Features of some of these trials included effects being maximal at 90 days and Bacopa decreasing the rate of forgetting of new information. A short-term trial (2 hours) on Bacopa showed no benefit.[113]

In a 12-week randomised, double blind trial conducted in the USA, the effect of 300 mg/day of Bacopa on cognitive function was investigated in healthy elderly volunteers. The main outcome was measured by the delayed recall score from the AVLT (Auditory Verbal Learning Test) word memory task. Also measured was the Stroop Task which assesses the ability to ignore irrelevant information. The following results were obtained:[116]

- Bacopa significantly enhanced AVLT delayed word recall memory scores
- Stroop results were similarly significant, with the Bacopa group improving and the placebo group unchanged
- Depression and anxiety scores and heart rate significantly decreased over time for the Bacopa group, compared to an increase in the placebo group
- No effects were found on the DAT (Divided Attention Task).

A team of British and Australian scientists, including Professor Andrew Scholey now at Swinburne University, have undertaken a series of investigations on sage (*Salvia officinalis*) because of its traditional reputation as a tonic for the nervous system and memory. For example, the 16th century English herbalist John Gerard wrote about sage: 'It is singularly good for the head and brain and quickeneth the nerves and memory'. The investigators used a randomised, placebo-controlled, double blind, crossover design to investigate the effects of a single dose of sage in healthy older volunteers over a 6-hour period.[117] Compared with the placebo phase (which generally exhibited the characteristic decline in performance over the 6-hour test period), the 333 mg extract dose of sage caused a highly significant enhancement of secondary memory at all testing times. Secondary memory is longer term memory where, in this case, recently supplied information is

processed. There were also significant improvements in accuracy of attention following this dose, but not for the other doses. The extract used in the study was also shown to inhibit cholinesterase in test tube experiments. The authors concluded that the overall pattern of results was consistent with a benefit to pathways involved in efficient processing of information and/or consolidation of memory, rather than enhanced efficiencies in retrieval or working memory. The optimum sage dosage of 333 mg (about 2.5 g of herb) improved secondary memory by about 30 units. The decline with age for the healthy group tested (compared to healthy 18 to 25 year olds) was around 40 units. Hence the benefits seen in the present study reflect a substantial temporary reversal of the deterioration in secondary memory that typically occurs with about 50 years of normal ageing.

Other herbs demonstrated to improve cognitive function include gotu kola (see monograph), Schisandra and Rhodiola. In two sets of experiments, young (21 to 24 year old) telegraph-operators were asked to transmit Morse code at maximum speed for a period of 5 minutes.[118,119] Following treatment with a single dose of Schisandra extract (3 g herb) the test was repeated. The error frequency was within the range 84% to 103%, whilst that of the control group (treated with a placebo of glucose or 70% ethanol) was 130%. It was concluded that Schisandra prevented or reduced exhaustion-related errors. By using a test method involving the correction of texts in which fatigue affected the accuracy but not the speed of work[120] it was demonstrated that 38 (65%) of a group of 59 students treated with Schisandra showed an improvement in performance. Of these, seven presented an increase in the amount of work performed, 14 exhibited an enhancement in the quality of correction, and 17 showed improvements with respect to both of these.

A combination of Rhodiola, Siberian ginseng and Schisandra, used either in single or repeated doses, significantly increased the mental working capacity of healthy volunteers (computer operators on night duty).[121] A relatively low dose of Rhodiola extract at 170 mg/day for 2 weeks improved five different tests of cognitive function in a double blind, placebo-controlled trial in 56 young, healthy doctors on night duty.[122]

Cognition-enhancing herbs can also be of value in children, including those suffering attention deficit hyperactivity disorder (ADHD), and Bacopa is a good example of this. BR-16A is an Ayurvedic herbal formulation containing Bacopa as the main ingredient. It was evaluated for its efficacy in an open label trial in 25 children aged between 4 and 14 years having hyperkinetic behavioural problems. The duration of the problem ranged from 6 months to 3 years. Fifteen children were mentally disadvantaged and amongst them 10 had a history of brain damage. The herbal syrup brought about 'marked improvement' in five children as judged by both parents and doctors. No side effects were noted.[123]

In terms of controlled trials in ADHD, two have been conducted: one with BR-16A and the other using Bacopa alone. A randomised, double blind, placebo-controlled trial was undertaken to evaluate the efficacy of BR-16A in school-going children with ADHD. A total of 195 children were screened, out of which 60 satisfied the medical criteria for ADHD. Among those enrolled in the study, 30 received herbal treatment and 30 received placebo. An assessment of academic functioning along with psychological tests was done before and after the treatment. Statistical analysis was carried out in only 50 children and showed improvement in these tests in the herbal group compared with the placebo group. However, none of these differences achieved statistical significance because of the low number of trial participants.[124]

The study of Bacopa in ADHD was a small pilot study only published in abstract form. In this trial, a double blind, randomised, placebo-controlled design was employed. A total of 36 children were involved. Of these, 19 received Bacopa extract 100 mg/day for 12 weeks and 17 were given placebo. The active herbal treatment was followed by a 4-week placebo administration, making the total duration of the trial 16 weeks in both groups. One child in the Bacopa group and six in the placebo group dropped out. The mean ages were 8.3 years and 9.3 years in the Bacopa and placebo groups respectively. The children were evaluated on a battery of tests including mental control, sentence repetition, logical memory and word recall. Evaluation was undertaken before, during and at the end of the study. Data analysis revealed a significant improvement with sentence repetition, logical memory and learning following 12 weeks' administration of Bacopa. This improvement was maintained at 16 weeks. During the clinical trial Bacopa exhibited excellent tolerability and no treatment-related adverse effects were reported.[125]

Pycnogenol, a proprietary, standardised extract of French maritime pine bark (Pinus pinaster) has shown promising results in ADHD and the clinical trial data in children is more robust than for Bacopa. Initial positive case reports stimulated the interest to study this extract further.[126–128] However, a double blind, placebo-controlled comparative study in adults with ADHD failed to yield significant results.[129] No significant differences were found between placebo, the drug methylphenidate and pine bark extract. However, the sensitivity of this study can be questioned since it also found no activity for the reference drug.

A pilot study found a significant improvement in ADHD for the pine bark extract in children at 1 mg/kg/day.[130] This then led to a double blind, placebo-controlled study in 61 children, using the same dose over 4 weeks.[131] Patients were examined at start of trial, 1 month after treatment and 1 month after the end of treatment period by standard questionnaires: CAP (Child Attention Problems) Teacher Rating Scale, Conner's Teacher Rating Scale (CTRS), the Conner's Parent Rating Scale (CPRS) and a modified Wechsler Intelligence Scale for children. Results showed that 1 month of the pine bark extract caused a significant reduction of hyperactivity and improved the attention, coordination and concentration of children with ADHD. No positive effects were found in the placebo group. A relapse of symptoms was noted 1 month after termination of treatment.

Example liquid formulas

For stress-associated memory impairment:

Glycyrrhiza glabra	1:1	20 mL
Rhodiola rosea (standardised extract)	2:1	25 mL
Ginkgo biloba (standardised extract)	2:1	40 mL
Panax ginseng (standardised extract)	1:2	20 mL
	TOTAL	105 mL

Dose: 8 mL with water twice a day.

For acutely improving short-term memory and cognitive function (the student or speaker's friend):

Ginkgo biloba (standardised extract)	2:1	60 mL
Panax ginseng (standardised extract)	1:2	40 mL
	TOTAL	100 mL

Dose: 8 mL twice within a 1 hour period about 1 to 2 hours before an exam or lecture.

For age-associated cognitive decline:

Ginkgo biloba (standardised extract)	2:1	35 mL
Salvia fruticosa	1:2	30 mL
Panax ginseng (standardised extract)	1:2	15 mL
Rhodiola rosea (standardised extract)	2:1	25 mL
	TOTAL	105 mL

Dose: 8 mL with water twice a day.

Combine with tablets containing an extract of Bacopa capable of providing the equivalent of at least 10 g of herb per day (100 mg bacosides).

CASE HISTORY

A student studying for university exams requested a formula to improve performance in the exam and concentration and memory while studying. She was prescribed the following formula:

Ginkgo biloba (standardised extract)	2:1	20 mL
Eleutherococcus senticosus	1:2	30 mL
Schisandra chinensis	1:2	25 mL
Bacopa monniera	1:2	25 mL
	TOTAL	100 mL

Dose: 8 mL with water twice a day. (Note: The Siberian ginseng was prescribed for the stressful effects of studying as well as its effects on performance.)

The student reported improved concentration and memory and less fatigue while studying. She passed her exams.

References

1. Hsieh MT, Peng WH, Wu CR, et al. Review on experimental research of herbal medicines with anti-amnesic activity. *Planta Med.* 2010;76(3):203–217.

2. Leung JW, Xue H. GABAergic functions and depression: from classical therapies to herbal medicine. *Curr Drug Targets CNS Neurol Disord.* 2003;2(6):363–374.

3. Johnston GA. GABA(A) receptor channel pharmacology. *Curr Pharm Des.* 2005;11(15):1867–1885.

4. Ko FN, Wu TS, Lu ST, et al. Ca(2+)-channel blockade in rat thoracic aorta by protopine isolated from Corydalis tubers. *Jpn J Pharmacol.* 1992;58(1):1–9.

5. Low AM, Berdik M, Sormaz L, et al. Plant alkaloids, tetrandrine and hernandezine, inhibit calcium-depletion stimulated calcium entry in human and bovine endothelial cells. *Life Sci.* 1996;58(25):2327–2335.

6. Kwan CY. Vascular effects of selected antihypertensive drugs derived from traditional medicinal herbs. *Clin Exp Pharmacol Physiol.* 1995;22(suppl 1):S297–S299.

7. Yamahara J, Kobayashi G, Matsuda H, et al. Vascular dilatory action of the Chinese crude drug. II. Effects of scoparone on calcium mobilization. *Chem Pharm Bull (Tokyo).* 1989;37(2):485–489.

8. Yu SM, Ko FN, Su MJ, et al. Vasorelaxing effect in rat thoracic aorta caused by fraxinellone and dictamine isolated from the Chinese herb Dictamnus dasycarpus Turcz: comparison with cromakalim and Ca2+ channel blockers. *Naunyn Schmiedebergs Arch Pharmacol.* 1992;345(3):349–355.

9. Sun RY, Yan YZ, Zhang H, Li CC. Role of beta-receptor in the radix Angelicae sinensis attenuated hypoxic pulmonary hypertension in rats. *Chin Med J (Engl).* 1989;102(1):1–6.

10. Isono T, Oyama T, Asami A, et al. The analgesic mechanism of processed Aconiti tuber: the involvement of descending inhibitory system. *Am J Chin Med.* 1994;22(1):83–94.

11. Kimura M, Muroi M, Kimura I, et al. Hypaconitine, the dominant constituent responsible for the neuromuscular blocking action of the Japanese–sino medicine 'bushi' (aconite root). *Jpn J Pharmacol.* 1988;48(2):290–293.

12. Chen Z, Duan X. Mechanism of the antiasthmatic effect of total coumarins in the fruit of Cnidium monnieri (L.) Cuss. *Chung Kuo Chung Yao Tsa Chih.* 1990;15(5):304–305, 320.

13. Huang ZH, Yang DZ, Wei YQ. Effect of atropine on the enhancing action of Fructus aurantii immaturus on the myoelectric activity of small intestine in dogs. *Chung Kuo Chung Hsi I Chieh Ho Tsa Chih.* 1996;16(5):292–294.

14. Anekonda TS, Reddy PH. Can herbs provide a new generation of drugs for treating Alzheimer's disease? *Brain Res Rev.* 2005;50(2):361–376.

15. Yamada K, Hayashi T, Hasegawa T, et al. Effects of Kamikihito, a traditional Chinese medicine, on neurotransmitter receptor binding in the aged rat brain determined by in vitro autoradiography (2): Changes in GABAA and benzodiazepine receptor binding. *Jpn J Pharmacol.* 1994;66(1):53–58.

16. Sugiyama K, Kano T, Muteki T. Intravenous anesthetics, acting on the gamma-amino butyric acid (GABA) A receptor, potentiate the herbal medicine 'saiko-keishi-to'-induced chloride current. *Masui.* 1997;46(9):1197–1203.

17. Kuang P, Wu W, Zhu K. Evidence for amelioration of cellular damage in ischemic rat brain by radix salviae miltiorrhizae treatment – immunocytochemistry and histopathology studies. *J Tradit Chin Med.* 1993;13(1):38–41.

18. Hu Y, Ge Y, Zhang Y, et al. Treatment of 100 cases of nerve deafness with injectio radix salviae miltiorrhizae. *J Tradit Chin Med.* 1992;12(4):256–258.

19. Chang HM, Chui KY, Tan FW, et al. Structure–activity relationship of miltirone, an active central benzodiazepine receptor ligand isolated from Salvia miltiorrhiza Bunge (Danshen). *J Med Chem.* 1991;34(5):1675–1692.

20. Kuang P, Xiang J. Effect of radix salviae miltiorrhizae on EAA and IAA during cerebral ischemia in gerbils: a microdialysis study. *J Tradit Chin Med.* 1994;14(1):45–50.

21. Tao Y, Kuang P, Zuo P. Inhibitory effect of 764-3 on Ca2+ uptake in rat brain synaptosomes. *J Tradit Chin Med.* 1996;16(4):288–292.

22. Chen LW, Wang YQ, Wei LC, et al. Chinese herbs and herbal extracts for neuroprotection of dopaminergic neurons and potential therapeutic treatment of Parkinson's disease. *CNS Neurol Disord Drug Targets.* 2007;6(4):273–281.

23. Kasture S, Pontis S, Pinna A, et al. Assessment of symptomatic and neuroprotective efficacy of Mucuna pruriens seed extract in rodent model of Parkinson's disease. *Neurotox Res.* 2009;15(2):111–122.

24. Shen XL, Witt MR, Dekermendjian K, Nielsen M. Isolation and identification of tetrahydrocolumbamine as a dopamine receptor ligand from Polygala tenuifolia Willd. *Yao Hsueh Hsueh Pao.* 1994;29(12):887–890.

25. Reimeier C, Schneider I, Schneider W, Schäfer HL, Elstner EF. Effects of ethanolic extracts from Eschscholtzia californica and Corydalis cava on dimerization and oxidation of enkephalins. *Arzneimittelforschung.* 1995;45(2):132–136.

26. Schäfer HL, Schäfer H, Schneider W, Elstner EF. Sedative action of extract combinations of Eschscholtzia californica and Corydalis cava. *Arzneimittelforschung.* 1995;45(2):124–126.

27. Kleber E, Schneider W, Schäfer HL, Elstner EF. Modulation of key reactions of the catecholamine metabolism by extracts from Eschscholtzia californica and Corydalis cava. *Arzneimittelforschung.* 1995;45(2):127–131.

28. Hanus M, Lafon J, Mathieu M. Double blind, randomised, placebo-controlled study to evaluate the efficacy and safety of a fixed combination containing two plant extracts (Crataegus oxyacantha and Eschscholtzia californica) and magnesium in mild-to-moderate anxiety disorders. *Curr Med Res Opin.* 2004;20(1):63–71.

29. Herbert JM, Augereau JM, Gleye J, Maffrand JP. Chelerythrine is a potent and specific inhibitor of protein kinase C. *Biochem Biophys Res Commun.* 1990;172(3):993–999.

30. Meller ST, Dykstra C, Gebhart GF. Acute thermal hyperalgesia in the rat is produced by activation of N-methyl-D-aspartate receptors and protein kinase C and production of nitric oxide. *Neuroscience.* 1996;71(2):327–335.

31. Yashpal K, Pitcher GM, Parent A, et al. Noxious thermal and chemical stimulation induce increases in 3H-phorbol 12,13-dibutyrate binding in spinal cord dorsal horn as well as persistent pain and hyperalgesia, which is reduced by inhibition of protein kinase C. *J Neurosci.* 1995;15(5 Pt 1):3263–3272.

32. Fundytus ME, Coderre TJ. Chronic inhibition of intracellular Ca2+ release or protein kinase C activation significantly reduces the development of morphine dependence. *Eur J Pharmacol.* 1996;300(3):173–181.

33. Shah BH, Shamim G, Khan S, Saeed SA. Protein kinase C inhibitor, chelerythrine, potentiates the adrenaline-mediated aggregation of human platelets through calcium influx. *Biochem Mol Biol Int.* 1996;38(6):1135–1141.

34. Pavlakovic G, Eyer CL, Isom GE. Neuroprotective effects of PKC inhibition against chemical hypoxia. *Brain Res.* 1995;676(1):205–211.

35. Granger I, Serradeil-le Gal C, Augereau JM, Gleye J. Benzophenanthridine alkaloids isolated from Eschscholtzia californica cell suspension cultures interact with vasopressin (V1) receptors. *Planta Med.* 1992;58(1):35–38.

36. Boegge SC, Kesper S, Verspohl EJ, Nahrstedt A. Reduction of ACh-induced contraction of rat isolated ileum by coptisine, (+)–caffeoylmalic acid, Chelidonium majus, and Corydalis lutea extracts. *Planta Med.* 1996;62(2):173–174.

37. Kim DK, Lee KT, Baek NI, et al. Acetylcholinesterase inhibitors from the aerial parts of Corydalis speciosa. *Arch Pharm Res.* 2004;27(11):1127–1131.

38. Chernevaskaja NI, Krishtal OA, Valeyev AY. Inhibitions of the GABA-induced currents of rat neurons by the alkaloid isocoryne from the plant Corydalis pseudoadunca. *Toxicon*. 1990;28(6):727–730.

39. Ma ZZ, Xu W, Jensen NH, et al. Isoquinoline alkaloids isolated from Corydalis yanhusuo and their binding affinities at the dopamine D1 receptor. *Molecules*. 2008;13(9):2303–2312.

40. Kurahashi K, Fujiwara M. Adrenergic neuron blocking action of dehydrocorydaline isolated from Corydalis bulbosa. *Can J Physiol Pharmacol*. 1976;54(3):287–293.

41. Matsuda H, Tokuoka K, Wu J, Shiomoto H, Kubo M. Anti-inflammatory activities of dehydrocorydaline isolated from Corydalis Tuber. *Nat Med*. 1997;51(4):293–297.

42. Matsuda H, Tokuoka K, Wu J, Shiomoto H, Kubo M. Inhibitory effects of dehydrocorydaline isolated from corydalis tuber against type I-IV allergic models. *Biol Pharm Bull*. 1997;20(4):431–434.

43. Liu L, Li G, Zhu Y, et al. Comparison of analgesic effect between locally vinegar-processed preparation of fresh rhizoma Corydalis and traditionally vinegar-processed rhizoma Corydalis. *Chung Kuo Chung Yao Tsa Chih*. 1990;15(11):666–667, 702.

44. Wang Y, Zhu F, Zhang J, et al. Chemical evaluation of vinegar-processing method for fresh rhizoma Corydalis. *Chung Kuo Chung Yao Tsa Chih*. 1990;15(9):526–528.

45. Yamahara J, Yamada T, Kitani T, Naitoh Y, Fujimura H. Antianoxic action and active constituents of evodiae fructus. *Chem Pharm Bull (Tokyo)*. 1989;37(7):1820–1822.

46. Yamahara J, Yamada T, Kitani T, Naitoh Y, Fujimura H. Antianoxic action of evodiamine, an alkaloid in Evodia rutaecarpa fruit. *J Ethnopharmacol*. 1989;27(1–2):185–192.

47. Yu LL, Liao JF, Chen CF. Effect of the crude extract of Evodiae fructus on the intestinal transit in mice. *Planta Med*. 1994;60(4):308–312.

48. Chiou WF, Liao JF, Chen CF. Comparative study of the vasodilatory effects of three quinazoline alkaloids isolated from Evodia rutaecarpa. *J Nat Prod*. 1996;59(4):374–378.

49. Hibino T, Yuzurihara M, Kase Y, Takeda A. Synephrine, a component of Evodiae Fructus, constricts isolated rat aorta via adrenergic and serotonergic receptors. *J Pharmacol Sci*. 2009;111(1):73–81.

50. Shoji N, Umeyama A, Takemoto T, Kajiwara A, Ohizumi Y. Isolation of evodiamine, a powerful cardiotonic principle, from Evodia rutaecarpa Bentham (Rutaceae). *J Pharm Sci*. 1986;75(6):612–613.

51. King CL, Kong YC, Wong NS, et al. Uterotonic effect of Evodia rutaecarpa alkaloids. *J Nat Prod*. 1980;43(5):577–582.

52. Chiou WF, Liao JF, Shum AY, Chen CF. Mechanisms of vasorelaxant effect of dehydroevodiamine: a bioactive isoquinazolinocarboline alkaloid of plant origin. *J Cardiovas Pharmacol*. 1996;27(6):845–853.

53. Yang MC, Wu SL, Kuo JS, Chen CF. The hypotensive and negative chronotropic effects of dehydroevodiamine. *Eur J Pharmacol*. 1990;182(3):537–542.

54. Yu LL, Liao JF, Chen CF. Effect of the crude extract of the Evodiae Fructus on the intestinal transit in mice. *Planta Med*. 1994;60(4):308–312.

55. Kim HJ, Jang YP, Kim YC. A constituent from Evodiae fructus having inhibitory effect on acetylcholinesterase. *Seoul Univ J Pharm Sci*. 1995;20:1–11.

56. Park CH, Kim SH, Choi W, et al. Novel anticholinesterase and antiamnesic activities of dehydroevodiamine, a constituent of Evodia rutaecarpa. *Planta Med*. 1996;62(5):405–409.

57. The Symbolism of the Passion Flower. <http://www.paghat.com/passiflorasymbolism.html>. accessed 9.09.2011.

58. Bone K. *Clinical Guide to Blending Liquid Herbs Herbal Formulations for the Individual Patient*. USA: Churchill Livingstone; 2003. pp. 362–365.

59. Akhondzadeh S, Naghavi HR, Vazirian M, et al. Passionflower in the treatment of generalized anxiety: a pilot double blind randomized controlled trial with oxazepam. *J Clin Pharm Ther*. 2001;26(5):363–367.

60. Kammerer E, Wegener T. Schlafstörungen und deren Behandlung: stellenwert hochdosierter pflanzlicher Kombinationen. *Nat Med*. 1995;10(2):1–8.

61. Mollenhauer C. Anwendung eines hochdosierten Schlafsaftes aus Passionsblumenkraut and Baldrianwurzelextrakt (Dormo-Sern®) in der ambulanten Praxis bei Patienten mit Ein- und Durchschlafstörungen (EDS). *Z Phytother Abstractband*. 1995:22.

62. Schulz H, Jobert M, Hubner WD. The quantitative EEG as a screening instrument to identify sedative effects of single doses of plant extracts in comparison with diazepam. *Phytomedicine*. 1998;5(6):449–458.

63. Akhondzadeh S, Kashani L, Mobaseri M, et al. Passionflower in the treatment of opiates withdrawal: a double blind randomized controlled trial. *J Clin Pharm Ther*. 2001;26(5):369–373.

64. Movafegh A, Alizadeh R, Hajimohamadi F, et al. Preoperative oral passiflora incarnata reduces anxiety in ambulatory surgery patients: a double blind, placebo-controlled study. *Anesth Analg*. 2008;106(6):1728–1732.

65. Chaudhry HR, Taj R, Saeed N, et al. Effectiveness of a combination of Hypericum and Passiflora for the treatment of depression with concomitant anxiety. *Eur Neuropsychopharmacol*. 2007;17(suppl 4):S394.

66. Ngan A. Conduit R. A double blind, placebo-controlled investigation of the effects of Passiflora incarnata (Passionflower) herbal tea on subjective sleep. *Phytother Res*. 2011;25(8):1153–1159.

67. Lee IS, Lee GJ. Effects of lavender aromatherapy on insomnia and depression in women college students. *Taehan Kanho Hakhoe Chi*. 2006;36(1):136–143. (Article in Korean).

68. Akhondzadeh S, Kashani L, Fotouhi A, et al. Comparison of Lavandula angustfolia Mill. tincture and imipramine in the treatment of mild to moderate depression: a double blind, randomized trial. *Prog Neuropsychopharmacol Biol Psychiatry*. 2003;27(1):123–127.

69. Akhondzadeh S, Tahmacebi-Pour N, Noorbala AA, et al. Crocus sativus L. in the treatment of mild to moderate depression: a double–blind, randomized and placebo-controlled trial. *Phytother Res*. 2005;19(2):148–151.

70. Moshiri E, Basti AA, Noorbala AA, et al. Crocus sativus L. (petal) in the treatment of mild-to-moderate depression: a double blind, randomized and placebo-controlled trial. *Phytomedicine*. 2006;13(9–10):607–611.

71. Akhondzadeh S, Fallah-Pour H, Afkham K, et al. Comparison of Crocus sativus L and imipramine in the treatment of mild to moderate depression: a pilot double blind randomized trial [ISRCTN45683816]. *BMC Complement Altern Med*. 2004;4:12.

72. Noorbala AA, Akhondzadeh S, Tahmacebi-Pour N, et al. Hydro-alcoholic extract of Crocus sativus L versus fluoxetine in the treatment of mild to moderate depression: a double blind, randomized pilot trial. *J Ethnopharmacol*. 2005;97(2):281–284.

73. Akhondzadeh Basti A, Moshiri E, Noorbala AA, et al. Comparison of petal of Crocus sativus L and fluoxetine in the treatment of depressed outpatients: a pilot double blind randomized trial. *Prog Neuropsychopharmacol Biol Psychiatry*. 2007;31(2):439–442.

74. Darbinyan V, Aslanyan G, Aroyan E, et al. Rhodiola SHR-5 extract and the treatment of depression. *Planta Med*. 2007;73:813–814.

75. Darbinyan V, Aslanyan G, Amroyan E, et al. Clinical trial of Rhodiola rosea L. extract SHR-5 in the treatment of mild to moderate depression. *Nord J Psychiatry*. 2007;61(5):343–348.

76. Della Loggia R, Tubaro A, Redaelli C. Evaluation of the activity on the mouse CNS of several plant extracts and a combination of them. *Riv Neurol*. 1981;51(5):297–310.

77. PellaLoggia R, Zilli C, Del Negro P, et al. Isoflavones as spasmolytic principles of Piscidia erythrina. *Prog Clin Biol Res*. 1988;280:365–368.

78. American Psychiatric Association. *Diagnostic and Statistical Manual of Mental Disorders*, 4th ed. Arlington: American Psychiatric Association; 2000.

79. Starcevic V. Have anxiety disorders been disowned by psychiatrists? *Aust Psychiatry*. 2011;19(1):12–16.

80. Belmaker RH, Agam G. Major depressive disorder. *N Engl J Med*. 2008;358(1):55–68.

81. Rosengren A, Tibblin G, Wilhelmsen L. Low systolic blood pressure and self

perceived wellbeing in middle aged men. *BMJ.* 1993;306(6872):243–246.

82. Barrett-Connor E, Palinkas LA. Low blood pressure and depression in older men: a population based study. *BMJ.* 1994;308(6926):446–449.

83. Clark MM. Restless legs syndrome. *J Am Board Fam Pract.* 2001;14(5):368–374.

84. Ohayon MM, Roth T. Prevalence of restless legs syndrome and periodic limb movement disorder in the general population. *J Psychosom Res.* 2002;53(1):547–554.

85. Patrick L. Restless legs syndrome: pathophysiology and the role of iron and folate. *Altern Med Rev.* 2007;12(2):101–112.

86. Hornyak M, Voderholzer U, Hohagen F, et al. Magnesium therapy for periodic leg movements-related insomnia and restless legs syndrome: an open pilot study. *Sleep.* 1998;21(5):501–505.

87. Cuellar NG, Ratcliff SJ. Does valerian improve sleepiness and symptom severity in people with restless legs syndrome? *Altern Ther Health Med.* 2008;15(2):22–28.

88. Phillips B, Young T, Finn L, et al. Epidemiology of restless legs symptoms in adults. *Arch Intern Med.* 2000;160(14):2137–2141.

89. Kanter AH. The effect of sclerotherapy on restless legs syndrome. *Dermatol Surg.* 1995;21(4):328–332.

90. Loder E, Rizzoli P. Tension-type headache. *BMJ.* 2008;336(7635):88–92.

91. Bendtsen L, Jensen R. Tension-type headache. *Neurol Clin.* 2009;27(2):525–535.

92. Cathcart S, Winefield AH, Lushington K, Rolan P. Stress and tension-type headache mechanisms. *Cephalalgia.* 2010;30(10):1250–1267.

93. Krafft RM. Trigeminal neuralgia. *Am Fam Physician.* 2008;77(9):1291–1296.

94. Cheshire WP. Trigeminal neuralgia: for one nerve a multitude of treatments. *Expert Rev Neurother.* 2007;7(11):1565–1579.

95. Hayes SM. Tic douloureux: report of successful treatment. *Gen Den.* 1984;32(5):441–442.

96. Charles A. Advances in the basic and clinical science of migraine. *Ann Neurol.* 2009;65(5):491–498.

97. Panconesi A, Bartolozzi ML, Guidi L. Migraine pain: reflections against vasodilatation. *J Headache Pain.* 2009;10(5):317–325.

98. Levy D. Migraine pain, meningeal inflammation, and mast cells. *Curr Pain Headache Rep.* 2009;13(3):237–240.

99. Tietjen GE. Migraine as a systemic vasculopathy. *Cephalalgia.* 2009;29(9):987–996.

100. Barbanti P, Aurilia C, Egeo G, Fofi L. Hypertension as a risk factor for migraine chronification. *Neurol Sci.* 2010;31 (suppl 1):S41–S43.

101. Aguggia M, Saracco MG. Pathophysiology of migraine chronification. *Neurol Sci.* 2010;31(suppl 1):S15–S17.

102. Bevilaqua Grossi D, Lipton RB, Bigal ME. Temporomandibular disorders and migraine chronification. *Curr Pain Headache Rep.* 2009;13(4):314–318.

103. Kruit MC, van Buchem MA, Launer LJ, et al. Migraine is associated with an increased risk of deep white matter lesions, subclinical posterior circulation infarcts and brain iron accumulation: the population-based MRI CAMERA study. *Cephalalgia.* 2010;30(2):129–136.

104. Negro A, D'Alonzo L, Martelletti P. Chronic migraine: comorbidities, risk factors, and rehabilitation. *Intern Emerg Med.* 2010;5(suppl 1):S13–S19.

105. Bigal M. Migraine chronification – concept and risk factors. *Discov Med.* 2009;8(42):145–150.

106. Silberstein SD. Migraine and women. *Postgrad Med.* 1995;97(4):147–153.

107. Klingler D, Bauchinger B. Migraine – summary of diagnostic and therapeutic strategies. *Wien Med Wochenschr.* 1994;144(5–6):117–120.

108. Sauro KM, Becker WJ. The stress and migraine interaction. *Headache.* 2009;49(9):1378–1386.

109. Gasbarrini A, De Luca A, Fiore G, et al. Beneficial effects of Helicobacter pylori eradication on migraine. *Hepatogastroenterology.* 1998;45:765–770.

110. Pizzorno Jr JE, Murray MT, Joiner-Bey H. Chapter 55: Migraine headache. In: *The Clinician's Handbook of Natural Medicine.* 2nd ed. Edinburgh: Churchill Livingstone; 2008. pp. 502–520.

111. Barre Y. Migraine and Fumaria officinalis. *Sem Ther.* 1967;43(5):307–308.

112. Bone K. *Clinical Applications of Ayurvedic and Chinese Herbs.* Warwick: Phytotherapy Press; 1996. pp. 101–102.

113. Stough C, Lloyd J, Clarke J, et al. The chronic effects of an extract of Bacopa monniera (Brahmi) on cognitive function in healthy human subjects. *Psychopharmacology (Berl).* 2001;156(4):481–484.

114. Roodenrys S, Booth D, Bulzomi S, et al. Chronic effects of Brahmi (Bacopa monnieri) on human memory. *Neuropsychopharmacology.* 2002;27(2):279–281.

115. Stough C, Downey LA, Lloyd J, et al. Examining the nootropic effects of a special extract of Bacopa monniera on human cognitive functioning: 90 day double blind placebo-controlled randomized trial. *Phytother Res.* 2008;22(12):1629–1634.

116. Calabrese C, Gregory WL, Leo MJ, et al. Effects of a standardized Bacopa monnieri extract on cognitive performance, anxiety, and depression in the elderly: a randomized, double blind, placebo-controlled trial. *Altern Complement Med.* 2008;14(6):707–713.

117. Scholey AB, Tildesley NTJ, Ballard CG, et al. An extract of Salvia (sage) with anticholinesterase properties improves memory and attention in healthy older volunteers. *Psychopharmacology (Berl).* 2008;198:127–139.

118. Lebedev AA. On the pharmacology of Schizandra. In: Lazarev NV, ed. *Materials for the Study of Ginseng and Schizandra.* Moscow: Far East Branch of USSR Academy of Science; 1955. pp. 178–188.

119. Lebedev AA. Schizandrin – a new stimulant from Schizandra chinensis fruits. Dissertation for a Degree in Medicine. Tashkent, Tashkent University, 1967. p. 16.

120. Kochmareva LI. The effect of *Schizandra chinesis* and Ginseng on processes of concentration. In: Lazarev NV. (ed). *Materials for the Study of Ginseng and Schizandra.* Leningrad: Far East Branch of USSR Academy of Science; 1958. pp. 12–17.

121. Vezirishvili MO, Roslyakova NA, Wikman G. The experience in developing an up-to-date biologically active supplement. *Med Altera.* 1999:44–46.

122. Darbinyan V, Kteyan A, Panossian A, et al. Rhodiola rosea in stress induced fatigue – a double blind cross-over study of a standardized extract SHR-5 with a repeated low-dose regimen on the mental performance of healthy physicians during night duty. *Phytomedicine.* 2000;7(5):365–371.

123. Shah LP, Seth GS. An open clinical trial of mentat in hyperkinetic children. *Probe.* 1992;31(2):125–129.

124. Kalra V, Hina Z, Pandey RM, Kulkarni KS. A randomized double blind placebo-controlled drug trial with Mentat in children with attention deficit hyperactivity disorder. *Neurosci Today.* 2002;6(4):223–227.

125. Negi KS, Singh YD, Kushwaha KP, et al. Clinical evaluation of memory enhancing properties of memory plus in children with attention deficit hyperactivity disorder. *Indian J Psychiatry.* 2000;42(suppl 2).

126. Hanley JL. *Attention Deficit Disorder.* Green Bay: Impact Communication Inc.; 1999.

127. Passwater RA. *All about Pycnogenol®.* New York: Average Publishing Group; 1998.

128. Masao H. *Pycnogenol®'s therapeutic effect in improving ADHD symptoms in children.* Mainichi Shimbun (Japan). 2000.

129. Tenenbaum S, Paull JC, Sparrow EC, et al. An experimental comparison of Pycnogenol® and methylphenidate in adults with attention-deficit/hyperactivity disorder (ADHD). *J Atten Disord.* 2002;6:49–60.

130. Trebaticka J, Skodacek I, Suba J, et al. Treatment success of ADHD by Pycnogenol®. In: Hoikkala A, Soidinsal O, Wahala K, eds. *XXII International Conference on Polyphenols Polyphenols 2004.* Finland, Jyvaskyla: Gummerus Printing; 2004. pp. 179–180.

131. Trebaticka J, Kopasova S, Hradecna Z, et al. Treatment of ADHD with French maritime pine bark extract, Pycnogenol®. *Eur Child Adolesc Psychiatry.* 2006;15(6):329–335.

Female reproductive system

Scope

Apart from their use to provide non-specific support for recuperation and repair, specific phytotherapeutic strategies include the following.

Treatment of:

- irregular menstruation and dysmenorrhoea (painful periods)
- some cases of menorrhagia (heavy menstrual bleeding)
- premenstrual syndromes
- menopausal syndrome
- impaired lactation
- postnatal syndromes
- some cases of infertility
- functional ovarian cysts
- some cases of vaginitis, cervicitis, vulvitis.

Management of:

- fibroids and endometrial polyps
- endometriosis and pelvic inflammatory diseases
- polycystic ovary syndrome.

Because of its use of secondary plant products and for ethical and legal reasons, particular **caution** is necessary in applying phytotherapy in cases of:

- delayed menstruation
- pregnancy and lactation
- venereal disease
- ovarian cancers
- hormone antagonist treatment for cancer (e.g. tamoxifen).

Orientation

Introduction

The female reproductive system provides perhaps the most substantial challenge to modern medical procedures and at the same time potentially the richest prospects for an inspired phytotherapy. Modern medicine finds disorders of the system difficult to treat conservatively. The reproductive structures themselves are the most dramatic examples of structure following function and, indeed, a function that is notably rhythmic. Beyond this is the historical and social reality: the experience of women has been neglected in medical science and their illnesses poorly charted. On the other hand women have often been the health care practitioners in society, they have necessarily had to focus a great deal on matters of their own reproductive health, fertility and, as midwives, childbirth and child-rearing. They have mastered the skills of intuitive diagnosis and treatment of functions that are notably difficult to isolate and measure and have developed some non-medical approaches to them. Nowadays they may feel particularly aggrieved about the medicalisation of their reproductive functions and are receptive to a new appreciation of their own insights.

The medical challenge

It has proven difficult to devise modern treatments for disorders of the female reproductive system that are genuinely appropriate to the task. It has always been hard to get a true measure of the job in the first place. Many problems start with dysfunctions in menstrual cycles or with hormonal disruptions, for which treatment outcome measures are not agreed and where subjective distress is not matched by technological monitoring. Even pathologies are more variable than consistent. Endometriosis and fibroids remain largely inexplicable; there are more categories of ovarian cysts and tumours than can easily be grasped; pelvic inflammatory conditions are almost defined by their unchartability.

Treatments therefore tend to bluntness. The primary recourse is to hormones, hormone analogues or hormone antagonists. These often have a crude effect on reproductive tissues that can be beneficial. However, they cannot interact comfortably with the astonishing choreography of multiple hormonal interactions that shape normal reproductive functions. They work by blocking this complexity, changing the force of negative feedback from subtle rhythm generation to the dictator of an artificial regime. As with almost everything else in this area, clear indicators of the wider impact of such treatments are hard to obtain but many women do not feel happy with them. Other conventional treatments are even more intrusive. Surgery is probably used for gynaecological and obstetric problems more extensively than for any other area of medicine. Although the days of routine hysterectomies, ovariectomies and mastectomies may be passing, it is still the case that surgery is undertaken too quickly for many sufferers, simply for want of any alternatives. Other measures – antibiotics for pelvic inflammatory disease, short-wave diathermy, dilation and curettage and laser ablation – appear often to be used without a clear treatment strategy and without an evidence base of efficacy.

One only needs to review the social history of obstetrics in the modern world, the move by women in many countries to reclaim home births, the move to less medicalised labour wards in hospitals, the increasing restoration of the midwife as arbiter of labour management and the exceptionally high professional liability insurance premiums required of obstetricians, to see that medicine has not always served women's needs well. There appears to be a case for a different approach to their healthcare, one ideally that involves them better.

Structures and functions

Neither reproductive functions nor structures are fixed through life. In the case of the female, there is additional variability due to the need to ensure ideal conditions for pregnancy. In most mammals ovulation, and the associated transformation of the reproductive system, only occurs in certain situations and at certain times of the year (early hunter nomad women also probably ovulated only when food and circumstances were acceptable). Nevertheless, there is in the human female the mechanism for constant menstrual cycles that switches on in adolescence and, circumstances permitting (adequate food is still important), is maintained to the sixth decade of life. The menstrual cycle is a transformative cycle, generated by the interplay of secretory sites, the hypothalamus, the anterior pituitary and the ovaries, and of the hormones they produce. It leads to real changes in reproductive structures so that the relevant anatomy actually changes through the month. The hormone secretions appear to be the outcome of a rhythmic pulse.[1] The anatomical changes in the ovarian hormone secretors, the development and ripening of the follicle to ovulation and the formation of the new secretory apparatus, the corpus luteum, out of the remnants of the follicle are rate-limiting elements in the equation and, with the functional pulsation, can be seen to provide the structural mechanism for the 'ovarian clock'. If pregnancy occurs the corpus luteum is enabled to increase its activity, so priming the whole body towards the major shifts in both structure and function required to support a developing embryo and eventually give birth.

The main characteristic of the female reproductive system, therefore, is its mobility and changeability. Many disorders of it are thus functional disorders and most start that way. Dysfunctions are medical challenges in their own right. There is by definition no physical damage or pathological change to observe, as functional measures (for example biochemical markers such as metabolite and hormone levels) are notoriously unreliable in complex systems. There is a more subjective impression than objective monitoring. For example, relative dominance of oestrogen or progesterone is as much determined by symptoms as by blood tests. Oestrogen dominance may be implicated by sore breasts, heavier periods, increased fat distribution in hips and thighs, and presence of fibrocystic changes in the breast, fibroids and endometriosis. Progesterone lack may be seen in spotting between periods, increased premenstrual symptoms and early premenopause.

Treatments that aim to correct such dysfunctions can do so in two ways: suspend normal activity, in this case often with hormonally active agents – the contraceptive pill or hormone replacement therapy, for example, or hormonal antagonists; or, secondly, engage the causes of dysfunction at source. In this case treatments should be interactive, should support rather than interfere with normal checks and balances and should in part be guided by the woman herself. Even when treating actual pathologies, a strategy that also supported the return to underlying functional rhythms could be commended. In modern times exposure to oestrogens in the diet and environment has added a significant new factor to reproductive health in both women and men.

The herbal strategy: prompts to self-organisation

As there is a particular paucity of hard scientific data for the herbal treatment of female reproductive problems, practitioners have to be guided by case evidence. In treating menstrual disorders, this can be striking. Typically, a woman suffering dysmenorrhoea, irregular menstruation, premenstrual syndrome or menorrhagia will be given a mixture of traditional women's remedies. For 1 or 2 months there are likely to be unfamiliar changes in the menstrual cycle, occasionally even

a worsening of the original problem. Then from the third or fourth cycle there is often a real sense that a normal rhythm is emerging. It is as if the original software programme has been rebooted: the disturbance is diminished or even disappears. Most importantly, it is often possible to stop the medication soon after this point without relapse.

Such cases, and there are many in practice, are very illuminating. Whatever mechanisms are involved, and these can only be speculative, there appears to be a strong self-corrective tendency to the menstrual cycle. It is of course very robust and consistent among women all over the world and in all sorts of circumstances. A tendency to self-organisation would be consistent with the behaviour of other complex dynamic systems in biology. It is also highly reassuring. It suggests that to return to normal, menstrual function requires only the lightest nudge, even a placebo nudge (see p. 91). (It is also striking, however, how often women through the ages spontaneously chose plants with high levels of steroidal molecules for this work.)

The herbal nudge to self-correction is a feature of other gynaecological treatment strategies. Menopausal disturbances are another example. A typical scenario might involve a woman in her late 40s with increasing menstrual difficulties, premenstrual syndrome, congestive dysmenorrhoea and/or emotional turbulence. She thinks they may be signs of impending menopause but of course cannot be sure. A herbal treatment that might include *Vitex agnus-castus* (chaste berry) and Hypericum (St John's wort) could be given, with one of two possible endpoints. Either periods stop and a smooth menopause, with hopefully few symptoms, could be underway in a few months or normal menstrual cycles could be resumed over the same time frame. The treatment seems to prompt the body to revert to its programme, whatever that might be. Again, there is the assumption of self-organisation, extended in this context to the view that menopause is programmed to be a smooth transition, that menopausal syndrome is an aberration (this could be argued if even one woman had a quiet and positive menopause; in fact a good proportion of women do).

Similar assumptions underpin the traditional herbal treatment of infertility, difficulties after childbirth and with lactation, and even of more overtly pathological states, functional ovarian cysts, some cases of endometriosis and the management of fibroids and pelvic inflammatory disease. Even when faced with more serious pathologies where conventional medical treatment is already underway, such as breast and cervical cancers, polycystic ovaries or the aftermath of hysterectomies, provided that there is some prospect of returning normal ovarian-pituitary dialogue and rhythms, then herbal prompts to this end are plausible and attractive strategies towards improved health.

Emmenagogues and abortifacients

Women in earlier times lived very different lives with radically different aspirations compared with their descendants in modern societies. Childbirth and child-rearing were generally more central to their lives. Infertility was one of the worst social problems a woman could suffer, often seriously threatening her position in the community. In all cultures considerable effort was put into treatments to improve fertility. These might well have worked to the principles set out above. Nevertheless, childbirth needed to be paced. For those who were normally fertile the priority became birth control. The absence at the due time of a period was not always welcome and there would be a regular demand in most communities for remedies that could prompt menstruation when delayed: emmenagogues. These would clearly need to be uterine stimulants and might need to be taken in heroic dosages. In modern times they might be classified as abortifacients.

Many herbs passed down as 'women's remedies' were probably for this purpose, although the term 'emmenagogue' has come in popular books to refer to menstrual regulators in general and is no longer a reliable pointer to such an effect. In reviewing the modern application of traditional women's remedies, it will be useful to keep this category of remedies in mind, however. Although generally taken in small doses in modern times, they may be contraindicated in pregnancy or where pregnancy is being sought and may be more stimulating than the menstrual modulators described earlier. In the Anglo-American tradition, emmenogogues could include Caulophyllum (blue cohosh), *Actaea racemosa* (black cohosh), *Mitchella repens* (squaw vine), *Ruta graveolens* (rue), *Thuja occidentalis* (arbor-vitae), *Mentha pulegium* (pennyroyal), *Gossypium herbaceum* (cotton root), *Artemisia spp.* (the wormwoods) as well as the stimulating laxatives and cathartic remedies. Uterostimulant action has also been shown for Chinese herbs *Carthamus tinctorius*, *Angelica sinensis* and *Leonurus sibiricus* with H_1 and alpha-adrenergic receptors as postulated mediators.[2] Some traditional effects on reproductive structures and functions have been linked with herbal activities on various prostaglandin receptors and functions that may also constitute stimulation of this type.[3]

The use of emmenagogues as abortifacients cannot be recommended in this text. Ethicolegal issues aside, getting the dose and timing right to terminate an early pregnancy was undoubtedly either a skilled or a messy affair and the possibility of embryo-damaging mistakes is high.

Phytotherapy in gynaecological and obstetric conditions

Note: The first edition of this book often cited the remedy *Chamaelirium luteum* (helonias or false unicorn root) as a major remedy in 'rebooting' normal menstrual cycles. This plant with its steroidal saponins was one of the more dramatic legacies of indigenous women's medicine in North America. However it has not fared well in recent decades and is now in danger in the wild. There are programmes to grow the plant commercially and a few reliable sources of supply are available, but at the time of writing these are in the minority and the majority of stock on the market is likely to arise from wild harvesting. One possible substitute is shatavari (*Asparagus racemosus*) from the Ayurvedic tradition. Hence on the few occasions where false unicorn is mentioned in the following

sections, it should be read in the context that it is only being recommended if sustainable sources are available.

Premenstrual syndrome

Premenstrual syndrome (PMS) is a variety of psychological, behavioural and physical symptoms which occur in the luteal phase of the menstrual cycle. Up to 85% of menstruating women report having one or more premenstrual symptoms, and 2% to 10% report these as disabling. More than 200 symptoms have been associated with PMS, but irritability, tension and dysphoria are the most prominent and consistently described. Of a number of potential causes that have been considered, evidence points to two being particularly significant:[4]

1. Enhanced sensitivity to progesterone in women with underlying serotonin deficiency
2. An inability to convert linoleic acid to prostaglandin precursors.

In anovulatory cycles, symptom cyclicity (PMS) disappears, and there exists a consensus that the cyclical changes are provoked by factors from the corpus luteum.[5] The nature of the provoking factor, however, is unknown; but the ovarian steroids, 17beta-oestradiol and progesterone, are suspected.[6,7] The response systems within the brain known to be involved in PMS symptoms are the serotonin (as noted above) and GABA systems. Progesterone metabolites, especially allopregnanolone, are neuroactive, acting via the GABA system in the brain. Allopregnanolone has similar effects to benzodiazepines, barbiturates and alcohol.[6,7]

The symptoms experienced vary from woman to woman and Abraham has created five distinct subgroups (Table 9.3).[8] This classification is relevant since a pilot clinical trial conducted in England found that the herb *Vitex agnus-castus* (chaste berry) gave good results for PMS-A, PMS-D and PMS-H. A second larger clinical trial with Vitex found no statistical significance over placebo, although there was a tendency to improvement for breast tenderness and symptoms of fluid retention (see also the chaste tree monograph).[9]

Table 9.3 Abraham's five PMS subgroups and symptoms

PMS-A	PMS-C	PMS-D	PMS-H	PMS-P
Nervous tension	Increased appetite	Depression	Fluid retention	Aches and pains
Irritability	Headaches	Forgetfulness	Weight gain	Reduced pain threshold
Mood changes	Fatigue	Crying	Swelling of extremities	
Anxiety	Dizziness	Confusion	Breast tenderness	
	Heart pounding	Insomnia	Abdominal bloating	

Since then the evidence for chaste tree has improved. A systematic review of herbal treatments for PMS found that chaste tree was the most investigated treatment and, after excluding trials because of poor quality or unsuitable diagnostic criteria, identified four eligible trials involving 500 women.[10] The review concluded that chaste tree was useful for PMS. Several other trials showing benefit in premenstrual mastalgia have also been published, including one that demonstrated that it lowered prolactin levels, another possible factor implicated in PMS (see chaste tree monograph).

The aims of herbal treatment in PMS are as follows:

* Correct any hormonal imbalance. Vitex is often prescribed throughout the cycle on a long-term basis. (See monograph for dosage recommendations and discussion.) Actaea (black cohosh) and Paeonia (white peony) can also have a role here

* Correct essential fatty acid status, especially with evening primrose oil at doses of 3000 to 4000 mg/day. According to Abraham it is particularly indicated in PMS-C, which is associated with a prostaglandin deficiency

* Treat the main physical symptoms as they occur, for example treat fluid retention with diuretics such as Taraxacum leaves (dandelion), aches and pains with herbal analgesics such as Salix (willow bark) and sweats with Salvia (sage). Ginkgo throughout the cycle was found to be useful for breast symptoms. Sometimes symptomatic treatment will not be necessary if the other aims are addressed. Ruscus (butcher's broom) has also shown benefits for the congestive symptoms in a clinical trial (see butcher's broom monograph)

* Treat the emotional disturbances. This can often be the most important part of the therapy. Treatment is usually throughout the cycle. Nervine tonics such as Hypericum (St John's wort) have been shown in double blind controlled trials directly to reduce symptoms of PMS, even after excluding non-luteal depression,[11] and sedatives such as Valeriana (valerian) for anxiety or insomnia are also valuable

* Compensate for the adverse effects of stress on the body using adaptogenic herbs such as Schisandra, Eleutherococcus (Siberian ginseng) and Withania. Sources of stress should be examined and dealt with if possible and diet should be balanced and mainly consist of unprocessed foods

* Treat the liver if signs of sluggishness are apparent, for example difficulty digesting fats, tendency to constipation, history of liver disease, tendency to nausea, preference for light or no breakfasts, etc. The liver is the site of the breakdown of female hormones and a sluggish liver may contribute to hormonal imbalance. Herbs to use include Taraxacum root and Silybum (St Mary's thistle), but especially those that promote hepatic detoxification such as Schisandra and Curcuma (turmeric)

* In some cases oestrogen-modulating herbs such as Asparagus (shatavari) and Dioscorea (wild yam) can be beneficial (especially for PMS-D).

CASE HISTORY

A woman, aged 34, with one child, aged 3, experienced severe depression, irritability, anxiety, fluid retention and breast tenderness that began about 7 days before the onset of menstruation and persisted until the first day of bleeding. Questioning revealed a history of viral hepatitis and increased levels of stress and devitalisation caused by caring for a young child. Initial treatment consisted of the following:

Valeriana officinalis	1:2	20 mL
Hypericum perforatum	1:2	30 mL
Silybum marianum	1:1	30 mL
Withania somnifera	1:1	25 mL
	TOTAL	105 mL

Dose: 5 mL with water three times a day

Tablets containing 500 mg Vitex agnus-castus extract were prescribed at 2 per day.

After 4 weeks there was a mild improvement. After another 3 months of treatment there was a substantial improvement. The breast and fluid symptoms were gone and her emotional symptoms and energy levels were considerably better. Treatment was continued. After some time of consistent benefit the patient continued on chaste tree only (as above) and remained virtually symptom-free.

Dysmenorrhoea

There are two types of dysmenorrhoea (painful menstruation) recognised:

1. Spasmodic or primary dysmenorrhoea in which the pain is directly related to the onset of menstruation and is uterine in origin. A widely prevalent and common complaint among young women, estimated to be present in 40% to 50%, with severe forms giving rise to work or school absenteeism in 15%. Prevalence is highest in the early 20s and decreases progressively thereafter. It only occurs in ovulatory cycles. Advances in the last three decades suggest that in primary dysmenorrhea there is abnormal and increased secretion of proinflammatory prostaglandins, thromboxane A_2, prostacyclin and leukotrienes, which in turn induce abnormal uterine contractions similar to the way they induce contractions in labour. The contractions reduce uterine blood flow, leading to uterine hypoxia and pain, analagous to that of angina in the heart.[12] Unlike endometriosis, primary dysmenorrhoea can be relieved by non-steroidal inflammatory drugs and usually the contraceptive pill.

2. Secondary or congestive dysmenorrhoea, which occurs before or late in menstruation and may arise in the uterus or in some other organ.

Since primary dysmenorrhea usually only causes problems for 1 to 2 days each month, it makes sense to use herbs that can help to control the pain at these times. Treatment throughout the whole menstrual cycle is best reserved for severe cases only.

Short-term treatment consists of uterine spasmolytics, analgesics, sedatives and herbs that decrease prostaglandin production. They can be given at around the onset of menstruation. However, these remedies are usually more effective for severe pain when given prior to the onset of menstruation by a few days. High doses need to be recommended to control acute symptoms.

Overall treatment focusses on the following herbs:

- Since Vitex (chaste berry) might enhance progesterone production, it could aggravate spasmodic dysmenorrhoea and should not be used. However, if a woman with spasmodic dysmenorrhoea also suffers from PMS with congestive symptoms (e.g. breast tenderness), Vitex can help both disorders when used as a long-term treatment.
- Herbs that support oestrogen function in the body (they may not be intrinsically oestrogenic themselves) can be indicated and include Asparagus (shatavari) and Dioscorea (wild yam). These herbs will help long term.
- Lamium (white dead nettle) is a specific that may decrease the condition when given long term.
- Short-term treatment consists of uterine spasmolytics and herbs that decrease prostaglandin production. The former include *Angelica sinensis* (dong quai), Dioscorea, Rubus (raspberry leaves) and *Viburnum* species (cramp bark or black haw). Achillea (yarrow) is spasmolytic and will check excessive bleeding if taken long term. Fennel has shown value in a clinical trial (see monograph). The latter include Zingiber (ginger), Curcuma (turmeric) and Salix (willow bark). Ginger at 1g daily dose has been shown in early controlled trials to be particularly effective here.[13] Actaea (black cohosh) is an anti-inflammatory and hormonal herb that can also be indicated and Corydalis and Eschscholtzia (California poppy) are useful analgesics.
- Aromatherapy with herbal oils of lavender, clary sage and rose has been shown to be an effective option in managing dysmenorrhoea symptoms.[14]
- For congestive dysmenorrhoea, herbs that help reduce localised oedema are indicated, including Aesculus (horsechestnut) and butcher's broom.

Example liquid formulas

Spasmodic dysmenorrhoea About 3 to 4 days before the period is due, start the following herbal formula:

Corydalis ambigua	1:2	25 mL
Dioscorea villosa	1:2	30 mL
Viburnum opulus	1:2	35 mL
Zingiber officinale	1:2	10 mL
	TOTAL	100 mL

Dose: 5mL with water twice a day. Then just before menstruation, increase to 5mL with water six times a day and stop treatment when pain has gone.

Not all women experience dysmenorrhoea. Hence it is not an inevitable consequence of menstruation. If the patient desires to treat the underlying condition an additional long-term hormonal-balancing formula can be tried. In more severe cases of spasmodic dysmenorrhoea, this hormonal-balancing treatment throughout the cycle is an essential requirement. An example is as follows:

Cimicifuga racemosa	1:2	10 mL
Zingiber officinale	1:2	15 mL
Angelica sinensis	1:2	40 mL
Dioscorea villosa	1:2	35 mL
	TOTAL	100 mL

Dose: 5mL with water two times a day. Symptomatic treatment should also be used as above, but taken just prior to menstruation.

Chaste tree 1:2 liquid (1 to 2mL with water on rising) so long as PMS or congestive symptoms are also present.

Congestive dysmenorrhoea

Vitex agnus-castus	1:2	20 mL
Aesculus hippocastanum	1:2	25 mL
Dioscorea villosa	1:2	30 mL
Angelica sinensis	1:2	25 mL
	TOTAL	100 mL

Dose: 8mL with water twice a day.

Abnormal uterine bleeding

Excessive or abnormal bleeding from the uterus is a symptom, not a disease. The pattern of bleeding can vary, as can the cause. Metrorrhagia, where the bleeding is irregular in amount, acyclical in nature and often prolonged in duration, is usually due to a pathological condition of the uterus. A number of conditions, largely dysfunctional in nature, can respond to herbal treatment and are described below. Where abnormal bleeding is due to an organic cause, treatment should be directed at that cause. Such problems may be beyond the scope of herbal treatment.

A key herb for dysfunctional uterine bleeding is shepherd's purse (*Capsella bursa-pastoris*). This is antihaemorrhagic and astringent, traditionally used to treat chronic menorrhagia and uterine haemorrhage.[15,16] European herbalists regarded shepherd's purse as useful for heavy bleeding associated with fibroids.[17,18] In the late 19th century, and during World War I in Europe, shepherd's purse was commonly used as a substitute for ergot in uterine bleeding.[19–21] (Ergot is the product of a fungus (*Claviceps purpurea*) that grows on grain, especially rye. By the end of the 19th century, ergot was a standard drug used to induce contractions during labour. It was also used to treat postpartum haemorrhage.[22]) Ethanolic extracts of shepherd's purse were also found to have a haemostatic action in a clinical setting in Japan.[23,24]

Menorrhagia

This is excessively profuse or prolonged bleeding occurring with a normal cycle. The iron status of women with menorrhagia should always be checked. Fibroids (see below) are the most likely cause, but other underlying causes must be investigated. In severe cases herbs can be taken throughout the cycle with doses increased to acute levels just prior to menstruation. In milder cases herbs can be commenced at acute doses just prior to menstruation only and continued until it has ceased.

Treatment may include Vitex (chaste berry), Paeonia (white peony) and antihaemorrhagic herbs, for example Achillea (yarrow), *Panax notoginseng* (Tienchi ginseng) and Equisetum (horsetail) and uterine antihaemorrhagics such as Capsella (shepherd's purse) and Trillium (beth root).

Functional secondary amenorrhoea

This is the absence of menses for 6 months or for longer than three of the patient's normal menstrual cycles. First exclude pregnancy, lactation, drugs, premature menopause, polycystic ovary syndrome (PCOS), poor diet or excessive exercise as causes. Other organic causes should also be excluded.

Herbal treatment of amenorrhoea is aimed at:

- correcting hypothalamic malfunction and the resultant hormonal imbalance using herbs such as Vitex (chaste berry), *Asparagus racemosus* (shatavari) and Caulophyllum (blue cohosh)
- treating the effects of any co-morbid depression with nervine tonics such as Hypericum (St John's wort)
- treating the effects of stress with adaptogens, nervine tonics and sedative herbs
- treating debility with tonic herbs such as Withania and *Panax ginseng*; *Angelica sinensis* (dong quai) is specifically indicated where amenorrhoea follows menorrhagia or is associated with anaemia.

Difficulty with conception

This has a number of causes, many of which are not treatable by herbs. It should first be established if the problem truly exists with the woman. If this is the case, then the cause or causes should be isolated, if possible. Endometriosis and PCOS are common causes that will be treated as separate subjects below.

Some categories of difficult conception are listed below with the corresponding herbal approach to treatment:

- With anovulatory cycles, first establish the cause. Obesity or being underweight and overall health may determine whether ovulation occurs or not. Serious liver or kidney disease and other metabolic disorders all affect ovulation. Thyroid disease, even when mild, is a common problem affecting fertility. Lifestyle factors such as stress, excessive or too little exercise, diet, tea, coffee, alcohol, smoking and drugs should all be investigated. Treat the underlying cause and additionally give Vitex (chaste tree). Nervine tonics are frequently called for. Actaea (black cohosh, at higher doses) and *Angelica sinensis* (dong quai) may also be tried to establish ovulation. Tribulus and other saponin-containing oestrogen-modulating herbs are often appropriate and can either be given during the follicular phase of the menstrual cycle or for the whole cycle. Paeonia (white peony) can normalise folliculogenesis.
- Defective luteal function may be the problem, possibly associated with latent or frank hyperprolactinaemia. Treat mainly with Vitex and oestrogen-modulating herbs such as Tribulus. Paeonia may alternatively be of value.

- Cervical mucus may be too viscous. Cervical mucus may be 'hostile' for reasons other than hormonal. If this is suspected, recommend an alkaline diet (low protein, high fruit and vegetables). Lifestyle factors should be addressed (see below) and alkalinising herbs such as Apium (celery seed) prescribed together with oestrogen-promoting herbs (Dioscorea, Tribulus, and Asparagus) which will help to stabilise vaginal flora.
- Immunological rejection of sperm can occur. Sperm carries foreign proteins and a woman will often mount an immunological reaction against the sperm of her partner. With a consistent partner, this reaction usually abates but sometimes it does not. Treat with immune-regulating herbs such as Echinacea. Also attend to any factors which may be causing immune system dysregulation (see Chapter 8 under Autoimmunity).
- After investigation of difficulty with conception, no known factor can be identified in 20% to 30% of cases. Emotions can affect hypothalamic-pituitary hormone secretion and release. Stress and other emotional stimuli are known to increase prolactin release, which may affect reproductive function. Emotional factors may be involved in producing oviductal spasm which is sometimes observed in diagnostic tests. Obesity or being underweight and overall health may determine whether conception occurs or not. Lifestyle factors such as excessive or too little exercise, diet, tea, coffee, alcohol, smoking and drugs should be investigated. Treatment should be based on the above considerations and could include Vitex, Caulophyllum (blue cohosh), Actaea (higher doses) Tribulus and Asparagus for the hormonal side, *Viburnum opulus* for oviductal spasm and tonics, adaptogens, nervine tonics and sedatives as appropriate.

Example liquid formula

Chaste tree 1:2, 1 to 2 mL with water on rising each day and the following:

Asparagus racemosus	1:2	30 mL
Dioscorea villosa	1:2	30 mL
Cimicifuga racemosa	1:2	10 mL
Angelica sinensis	1:2	30 mL
	TOTAL	100 mL

Dose: 8 mL with water twice a day.

Pelvic inflammatory disease

Pelvic inflammatory disease is infection of the uterus, fallopian tubes and adjacent pelvic structures not associated with surgery or pregnancy. It is also known as chronic salpingitis. The most common organisms involved are *Chlamydia trachomatis* and *Neisseria gonorrhoeae*. There may be an original or current venereal origin, which if possible should be elicited. Misdiagnosis by the woman or by the practitioner of vaginal infections, with symptoms including discharge, irritation, dyspareunia, urinary complaints, and malodour may lead to secondary infections or pelvic inflammatory disease. Three likely causes, bacterial vaginosis, vulvovaginal candidiasis and trichomoniasis, should be distinguished and appropriate treatment instituted.[25]

Any vaginal infection provides a possible topical treatment route to a pelvic infection. The healthy vagina is an impressive barrier to infection and first steps should be to maintain its healthy microenvironment of lactic-acid-producing commensal bacteria (whose activity is maintained by moderate levels of oestrogen). Excessive douching, common among some women, is a known factor in bacterial vaginitis and should be discouraged.

For pelvic inflammatory conditions uncomplicated by vaginal infection the following systemic approaches can be tried:

- Immune-enhancing herbs such as Echinacea, Andrographis and Astragalus
- Dioscorea and Asparagus to support the female organs
- Hydrastis (golden seal) is a mucous membrane tonic useful for chronic infections of the oviducts
- Corydalis may assist to relieve the pain.

The above approach to treatment is compatible with and will actually assist conventional antibiotic treatment.

Uterine myoma (fibroids)

Uterine fibroids are benign, slow-growing smooth muscle tumours. They are probably the most common neoplasm in women. They are made up of myometrial cells that, under various hormonal and unknown stimuli, express increased aromatase activity and thus increase local oestrogen production; this further increases local tissue growth. Medically they are treated by gonadotrophin releasing hormone (GnRH) agonists or by surgery or ablation. The most common problem they cause is menorrhagia, but this disorder may be suspected in any combination of symptoms of lower abdominal congestion such as bloating, urinary frequency, painful intercourse, as well as infertility and complications of pregnancy.

A significant inverse association between risk of fibroids and age at menarche was reported. Compared with women who were 12 years of age at menarche, those who were ≤10 years of age at menarche were at increased risk (relative risk, RR, 1.24), whereas women who were age ≥16 years of age at menarche were at lower risk (RR 0.68).[26,27]

Several studies have shown an inverse relationship between the number of pregnancies and the risk of fibroids.[26] One explanation is that pregnancy reduces the time of exposure to unopposed oestrogens. The reduced risk of fibroids requiring surgery in postmenopausal patients is probably due to tumour shrinkage in the reduced oestrogen environment following menopause.[26]

The role of the use of oral contraceptives is controversial and may depend on the actual components of the pill used.[26] A significantly elevated risk of fibroids has been reported among women who first used oral contraceptives in their early teenage years (13 to 16 years of age) compared with those who had never used them.[26,27] In contrast, hormone replacement therapy may not only prevent the shrinkage of fibroids after menopause, it may even stimulate their growth (or at least the growth of some of the tumours in women with multiple tumours).[26] While tamoxifen is anti-oestrogenic, in breast tissue it probably exerts oestrogenic effects on the uterus. Hence it has been linked to promoting fibroid growth in a percentage of women in several clinical studies.[26]

Several studies have found a marked association between obesity and an increased incidence of fibroids.[26] This may be related to hormonal factors, especially excess oestrogen. In obese premenopausal women, decreased metabolism of oestradiol by the 2-hydroxylation route reduces the conversion of oestradiol to inactive metabolites, which could result in a relatively hyperoestrogenic state.[26,28] (See the studies cited later on how linseed may help to correct this effect.) A prospective study from the UK found that the risk of fibroids increased approximately 21% for each 10 kg increase in body weight.[29] A large US study found a correlation between BMI and fibroid risk.[30]

One study has addressed the question of dietary influences on the prevalence of fibroids. In an Italian population, 843 women with fibroids were compared with 1557 women without. A diet weighted toward green vegetables was protective (RR 0.5), whereas a higher intake of meat was associated with a greater incidence of fibroids (RR 1.7).[31,32] It is known that vegetarians have lower plasma oestrogen levels compared with non-vegetarians, so this fact could explain this observation. Also low fat diets are known to reduce oestrogen levels.[26]

Several studies have shown a reduced risk of fibroids associated with current smoking, but not past smoking.[26] Again this has been attributed to the reputed anti-oestrogenic effect of cigarette smoking. One study found no change in risk for caffeine consumption and an increased risk for more than seven drinks of beer per week.[33]

A case-control study of 318 women found, after adjustment for other known risk factors, that the incidence of uterine fibroids was positively correlated with a history of pelvic infection.[31,34] A history of three separate episodes of pelvic inflammatory disease conferred a relative risk of 3.7. Similarly a history of infection with Chlamydia gave a relative risk of 3.2.

High blood pressure is known to damage the smooth muscle lining of the arteries, and atherosclerosis is in part a proliferative condition of blood vessel walls. A prospective study of hypertension and risk of uterine fibroids found that diastolic blood pressure was an independent risk factor.[31,35] Hypertensive women were 24% more likely to report fibroids, and for every 10 mgHg increase in diastolic blood pressure the risk for fibroids increased 8% to 10%.

It is widely accepted that oestrogen and the interaction with oestrogen receptors in the nucleus of the smooth muscle cell influence the growth of uterine fibroids. At menopause, fibroids begin to shrink in most patients; hence ovarian hormones are thought to play a key role in fibroid growth.[36] While there are a considerable amount of both experimental results and clinical findings to support this connection, not the least being the use of GnRH agonists as treatments for fibroids, the mechanism remains poorly understood.[36] Oestrogen may directly increase proliferation of leiomyoma cells or might indirectly increase growth by augmenting the effects of progesterone.[36]

As noted above, the enzyme aromatase is present in fibroids. This enzyme governs the conversion of androstenedione into oestrone and testosterone into oestradiol. Also 17beta-hydroxysteroid dehydrogenase (17beta-HSD), which converts oestrone into oestradiol (the active form of oestrogen), is overexpressed.[37]

The growth promoting effects of oestrogen and progesterone on the uterine smooth muscle cells is probably mediated by various locally produced growth factors.[26] In particular, TGF-beta appears to be the only factor overexpressed in fibroid cells that is hormonally regulated.[38] Other growth factors have also been extensively investigated, but their role remains unclear.[26]

One interesting observation is the connection with prolactin.[26] Prolactin is produced by uterine tissues as well as the pituitary gland, and is a known growth promoter for vascular smooth muscle.[26] While this is speculative at this stage, it does provide further support for the use of Vitex (chaste tree), which has been shown to decrease circulating prolactin levels in clinical trials.[39]

Treatment

The aim of herbal treatment for uterine fibroids is to minimise any further growth of the tumours and to manage any associated symptoms, especially the menorrhagia. It is unlikely that herbal treatments will substantially shrink fibroids (although see the study cited below). Treatment needs to be trialled for at least 3 months and combined with attention to those lifestyle issues identified by the risk factors listed above. In particular, attention should be given to achieving a healthy body weight and diet.

One review observed that no controlled trials of complementary treatments for uterine fibroids could be found in the literature.[40] However, a traditional Chinese herbal formula also used in Kampo was found by Japanese medical scientists to shrink uterine myomas.[41] The formula, known in Japanese as Keishibukuryo-gan (KBG) and in Mandarin as Kuei-chih-fui-ling-wan, contains *Cinnamomum cassia*, *Paeonia lactiflora*, *Prunus persica* seeds, *Poria cocos* and *Paeonia suffruticosa*. In English it is known as cinnamon and hoelen combination. This formula is frequently used in gynaecological disorders such as pelvic inflammatory disease, menopausal symptoms, and menorrhagia and dysmenorrhoea related to venous congestion of the pelvic region.

In an open study, 110 premenopausal women, average age 43.2 years (ranging from 27 to 52 years) were treated with the equivalent of 22.5 g/day of the dried herb formula administered as a freeze-dried decoction (1.5 g) for 12 weeks or more. These women had symptomatic uterine myomas all less than 10 cm in diameter. Clinical symptoms of menorrhagia and dysmenorrhoea were improved in more than 90% of cases, with shrinkage of the fibroids in about 60% of patients.

There is evidence to suggest that linseed supplementation causes a change in oestrogen metabolism that may be favourable for inhibition of uterine fibroids. Oestradiol is the biologically active oestrogen that drives the tumour growth. It is metabolised in the liver by the CYP450 enzymes 2-hydroxylase and 16alpha-hydroxylase into 2-hydroxyoestrone and 16alpha-hydroxyoestrone, respectively. The latter is still potently oestrogenic, with uterotropic activity similar to oestradiol. Hence excessive formation of 16alpha-hydroxyoestrone contributes to oestrogen excess. Controlled clinical studies have shown that supplementation with linseed (10 to 25 g/day) significantly reduced the relative formation of 16alpha-hydroxyoestrone in both pre- and postmenopausal women.[42,43]

The most enlightened approach to controlling fibroid growth would be to reduce oestrogen levels and especially aromatase activity. Factors that stimulate aromatase include excessive adipose tissue, high insulin levels (associated with insulin resistance), and levels of the proinflammatory prostaglandin PGE_2. Obesity includes all these negative factors (adipose tissue also produces many proinflammatory cytokines). A number of herbs and herbal constituents are considered to have aromatase inhibitory properties, including Serenoa (saw palmetto) and Linum (linseed or flax seed) and flavonoids in general.[44] However, much of this represents in vitro data and clinical research is needed. Other approaches may include reducing exposure to dietary oestrogenic sources by choosing organic diets. To modify the effects of oestrogen, the intake of (oestrogen-blocking) phyto-oestrogens and oestrogenic lignans (e.g. from soya and linseed) should be increased (see above).

Vitex (chaste tree) is a major part of herbal treatment and can be given in high doses (e.g. 5 mL twice a day) if the fibroids are severe. Paeonia can potentially exert anti-oestrogenic and other favourable hormonal effects. Liver herbs, especially Schisandra, may help the breakdown and elimination of excessive oestrogen. Antihaemorrhagic and uterine antihaemorrhagic herbs are indicated for the menorrhagia (see above). Herbs that have been traditionally used to control benign growths include Echinacea, Thuja (arbor-vitae) and Chelidonium (greater celandine). *Ginkgo biloba* standardised extract can relieve pain associated with fibroids. Other immune herbs may also be beneficial. Oestrogen-promoting herbs such as Dioscorea and Tribulus are best avoided.

Example liquid formula

Capsella bursa-pastoris	1:2	20 mL
Equisetum arvense	1:2	20 mL
Echinacea purpurea/angustifolia root	1:2	20 mL
Panax notoginseng	1:2	20 mL
Paeonia lactiflora	1:2	20 mL
	TOTAL	100 mL

Dose: 8 mL with water twice a day.
And chaste tree 1:2, 4 to 6 mL with water once a day.

CASE HISTORY

A patient aged 43 presented with uterine fibroids characterised by menorrhagia and pain, especially with menstruation. She did not want surgery and asked for herbs to control her symptoms.

Treatment was as follows (based on 1 week):

Capsella bursa-pastoris	1:2	20 mL
Achillea millefolium	1:2	25 mL
Thuja occidentalis	1:5	20 mL
Echinacea angustifolia root	1:2	20 mL
Panax notoginseng	1:2	15 mL
	TOTAL	100 mL

Dose: 5 mL with water 3 times a day.

She was also prescribed Vitex 1:2, 2.5 mL with water twice a day, with the first dose on rising in the morning. *Ginkgo biloba* 50:1 standardised extract, 40 mg per tablet, 2 tablets per day, was also prescribed.

After 10 weeks of treatment there was considerable improvement in the menorrhagia and pain. Herbal treatment was maintained for continued symptom control.

A female patient aged 41 presented with multiple uterine fibroids and heavy bleeding. A few of the tumours were quite large (>8cm). She was placed on the following treatment:

Astragalus membranaceus	1:2	20 mL
Paeonia lactiflora	1:2	30 mL
Hypericum perforatum	1:2	25 mL
Withania somnifera	1:2	35 mL
	TOTAL	110 mL

Dose: 5 mL with water twice a day.

Chaste tree 1:2 liquid. Dose: 4 mL with water on rising.

This patient also regularly took Echinacea root 1:2 liquid at 5 mL per day.

The Hypericum and Withania were for the stress the patient was experiencing due to other issues. Over the ensuing 5 years of treatment her fibroids grew slightly (but not rapidly) but she now experiences normal uterine bleeding. Her gynaecologist cannot understand why this is so. Note that, unlike the previous case, this patient received no uterine antihaemorrhagic herbs.

Endometriosis

Endometriosis is the presence of functioning endometrial tissue in an abnormal location. This may occur between the muscle fibres of the myometrium (uterine endometriosis) or in various locations in the pelvic cavity. The ectopic endometrium forms a cyst that can often rupture, resulting in inflammation and formation of multiple adhesions. Unlike normal endometrial tissue, the ectopic cells contain aromatase and are thus able to generate and be further stimulated by oestrogen (like cells that make up fibroids). The prostaglandin PGE_2 is a potent stimulant of aromatase in endometriosis, emphasising the inflammatory factors in the origin of this condition.

Treatment

The most important herb for the treat of endometriosis is *Vitex agnus-castus* (chaste tree). Higher doses may be necessary, similar to those recommended for uterine fibroids (see chaste tree monograph).

Because of the prostaglandin abnormalities, evening primrose oil can also be indicated. Other herbs indicated for the symptoms include:

- *Viburnum opulus* (cramp bark), Corydalis, *Angelica sinensis* (dong quai), *Rubus idaeus* (raspberry leaf) and Zingiber (ginger) for dysmenorrhoea and chronic pelvic pain
- Pulsatilla for ovarian and ovulation pain
- *Centella asiatica* (gotu kola) and *Saliva miltiorrhiza* (dan shen) to reduce formation of adhesions
- antihaemorrhagic and uterine antihaemorrhagic herbs for the menorrhagia
- sedative, nervine tonic and adaptogenic herbs for the exacerbating effects of stress
- anti-inflammatory herbs such as Zingiber (ginger), Curcuma (turmeric), Boswellia, Bupleurum, Vitis (grape seed extract), Pinus (pine bark extract), Glycyrrhiza (licorice) and Rehmannia.

Herbs that may influence the underlying pathology include:

- Vitex, because of its regulating effect on ovarian function
- liver herbs, especially Schisandra to accelerate the breakdown of oestrogen, supported by hepatotrophorestoratives such as Silybum (St Mary's thistle)
- immune-enhancing herbs to help prevent and resolve endometrial cysts (e.g. Echinacea, Astragalus and Phytolacca (poke root))
- herbs to control benign growths (e.g. Thuja (arbor-vitae) and Echinacea).

To modify the effects of oestrogen, the intake of phyto-oestrogens and oestrogenic lignans should be increased.

Polycystic ovary syndrome

Full recognition and understanding of this most common cause of infertility has been slow, with international conferences in 1990 and 2003 marking landmarks in definition and clinical approach. PCOS affects up to 7% of young women with a combination of intermittent or absent ovulation, hyperandrogenism and very often insulin resistance and hyperinsulinaemia. This last connection is significant as 60% of sufferers are obese, half of even normal weight PCOS sufferers also have insulin resistance, and there is also an increased risk of type 2 diabetes and associated cardiovascular conditions among PCOS sufferers later in life. Insulin-sensitising drugs like metformin are now common treatments to stabilise cycles. Anovulatory cycles and relatively excessive androgen and luteinising hormone (LH) production are normal features of puberty for young girls, a product of spurts in growth hormone. Early weight gain is now regarded as a potent factor in the development of fully fledged PCOS from this normal stage of development.[45]

The most common symptoms of PCOS are hirsutism and other signs of hyperandrogenism, such as oily skin and acne.

The evidence of a link between PCOS and insulin resistance, although not universal, now dominates clinical approaches. Any moves that can reduce adipose tissue levels and other causes of hyperinsulinaemia appear to be merited. Other hormonal interventions are less clear (the use of the contraceptive pill disguises rather than prevents PCOS in adolescence).

Key biochemical features of PCOS are as follows:

- Increased serum androgen (testosterone, androstenedione, dehydroepiandrosterone sulphate (DHEAS))[46] with or without hyperinsulinaemia
- Decreased SHBG (sex hormone binding globulin) levels[46]
- Increased LH levels and serum LH:FSH (follicle stimulating hormone) ratio >2[46]
- Increased prolactin levels in some cases[46]
- Increased oestrone levels. Oestradiol can be increased, but is typically low or normal[47]
- Increased fasting insulin or fasting glucose.[46]

Due to long-standing unopposed oestrogen stimulation, there is increased risk for endometrial carcinoma.[48] Women with PCOS also have many abnormalities in lipid profiles, and are at increased risk of cardiovascular disease.[48]

A combination of white peony (*Paeonia lactiflora*) and licorice roots has been used in Chinese and Japanese traditional medicine and has the following names: Shaoyao Ganchao Tang (Chinese),

Shakuyaku-Kanzo-To (SKT, Japanese) and TJ-68 (a Japanese proprietary product). In these combinations *Glycyrrhiza uralensis* is used, but *Glycyrrhiza glabra* would also be suitable, since in traditional Chinese medicine *G. uralensis*, *G. glabra* and *G. inflata* are medicinally interchangeable species.[49] The combination has also been evaluated in uncontrolled clinical trials in PCOS.

SKT significantly decreased serum testosterone in women with defined PCOS, and in those described as infertile, oligomenorrhoeic or amenorrhoeic. All women had high serum testosterone levels. The dosage of extract was 5 to 7.5g/day (equivalent to 4 to 6g of dried white peony root and 4 to 6g of dried licorice root), and given for periods ranging from 2 to 8 weeks up to 24 weeks. The extent of the reduction in mean testosterone is illustrated by the before and after values in two trials: 137 to 85ng/dL (p<0.001) and 94ng/dL dropping to below 70% of this value at 4 and 6 weeks (p<0.005). In some cases regular ovulation was established and some women conceived. Several trials documented that no side effects were observed.[50–52] SKT (7.5g/day, equivalent to 6g of dried white peony root and 6g of dried licorice root, and taken for 12 weeks) also significantly decreased serum free testosterone compared to baseline values in women with acne vulgaris. The herbal treatment significantly decreased the number of comedomes. No difference was observed for the other hormones measured: total testosterone, dihydrotestosterone, DHEAS and SHBG.[53] The white peony and licorice combination may also be of benefit in lowering raised prolactin levels. A rapid decrease in prolactin levels was observed in 10 anovulatory women with elevated serum prolactin after administration of SKT (7.5g/day). The decrease reached significance 2 weeks after the start of treatment.[54] In case observation studies SKT (7g/day) successfully treated drug-induced hyperprolactinaemia in men and a woman.[55,56]

Herbal treatment is centred on the following strategy:

- If appropriate, address central obesity as the driver of insulin resistance with Coleus and licorice
- If appropriate, address insulin resistance with St Mary's thistle, Gymnema, ginseng, pine bark, Korean ginseng, Polygonum and berberine-containing herbs
- Chaste tree for hormonal regulation, doses depending on androgen and especially prolactin levels (see monograph)
- Licorice and white peony are clinically proven in PCOS and especially help to restart ovulation
- Tribulus and shatavari will improve fertility if that is a goal
- Support adrenal function with licorice and Rehmannia.

Example liquid formula

Vitex agnus-castus	1:2	20 mL
Glycyrrhiza glabra	1:1	15 mL
Paeonia lactiflora	1:2	30 mL
Gymnema sylvestre	1:1	25 mL
Schisandra chinensis	1:2	20 mL
	TOTAL	110 mL

Dose: 8mL with water two to three times daily.

When a cycle has been initiated, add Tribulus concentrated extract, equivalent to furostanol saponins (as protodioscin) 300 to 400mg/day on days 5 to 14 of the cycle to ensure cyclic regularity and fertility.

CASE HISTORY

'Karen' was 27 years old and was diagnosed with PCOS when she was 18. Her periods were very irregular, usually between 60 and 90 day cycles, she had no hirsutism and was of normal weight.

Prior to her period she developed severe sugar cravings, depression, became very anxious and did not sleep well. Her diet was poor ('Karen' described herself as a vegetarian, but mostly ate junk food, chocolate and fruit) containing very low levels of vegetables, protein and complex carbohydrate.

She was placed on a 'grazing' diet to improve possible glucose tolerance: small, frequent meals, no refined carbohydrates and emphasis on a better balance of food groups.

Herbal formula

Paeonia lactiflora	1:2	40 mL
Glycyrrhiza glabra	1:1	30 mL
Taraxacum officinale root	1:2	30 mL
	TOTAL	100 mL

Dose: 5mL three times daily.

After 3 months she had experienced three menstrual cycles at 27 day intervals and was feeling very well with no PMS. Her herbal formula was continued for another two cycles.

Benign breast disorders

Many terms have been used in the past to describe benign breast disorders. These include such descriptions as benign mammary dysplasia, cystic mastopathy, chronic cystic mastitis and cystic epithelial hyperplasia. Often they were grouped under the term 'fibrocystic breast disease' but this nomenclature is considered to be inappropriate and benign breast disease can be more appropriately categorised as the following:

- Fibroadenoma (FA)
- Cystic disease of the breast (fibrocystic changes, breast cysts).

One novel concept has been proposed to describe benign breast disorders. They are seen as aberrations of normal breast development and involution (ANDI). This is based on the fact that most benign breast disorders are not neoplastic growths, but rather arise on the basis of normal changes occurring in the breast throughout the various stages of reproductive life. They are no more benign neoplasms than is endometriosis.[57]

FA is a common, usually single lesion, typically seen in patients between ages 20 and 40. This lesion may enlarge during pregnancy, but usually becomes smaller as patients age. Clinically, FAs are usually sharply demarcated, with well-circumscribed smooth borders.[58]

Fibrocystic changes are commonly seen in the breast.[58] The term describes pathological changes seen under the microscope and should not be used to describe clinical findings. The histological changes include varying amounts of fibrosis and cyst sizes. If predominantly fibrosis is present, the lesion may be referred to as fibrous mastopathy. Calcification may be seen in association with fibrocystic changes.

FA is classified in most surgical texts as a neoplasm. However, evidence supports the fact that FAs come under the category of ANDI.[57] The natural history of FA is unlike that of benign tumours. The average FA grows to a diameter of 1 to 1.5 cm and then remains static. It regresses at menopause. FA are more hormonally responsive than most benign tumours, they lactate during pregnancy. FA-like lesions occur in most women's breasts. In fact, histologically there is a complete spectrum from normal lobules to large lobules, to subclinical FA, to clinical FA. Moreover, a FA develops from a single lobule, not a single cell.

FA accounts for about 12% of all palpable symptomatic breast masses. They are quite common in women under 25 years and rare in women over 40. As noted, FA is probably an aberration of normal lobule development, a process which begins in the early stages of reproductive life. They can be removed surgically, usually after a period of observation.

Mechanisms controlling FA development and growth are poorly understood. In addition to the role of oestrogen and progesterone receptors expressed by epithelial cells, recent studies describe a possible role for growth factors and their receptors in the pathogenesis and growth FA, suggesting that multiple receptor signalling pathways could be involved in the growth and differentiation of benign breast lesions.[59] However, concerning the risk of development of subsequent breast cancer, one large retrospective study has concluded that there is no increased risk for a woman with a simple FA and no family history of breast cancer.

Discrete palpable breast cysts are most common in the 40 to 50 year age group and are uncommon below 30 and over 54. A breast cyst is probably an aberration of lobular involution, a process that begins in the later stages of reproductive life.[59] Some studies have looked at breast cancer risk in patients with palpable breast cysts.[60] There may be an increased risk of between 2 to 4 times average, but this finding may be exaggerated.[60] Patients with macrocysts do appear to have a higher risk of later developing breast cancer,[61] although terminology and classifications have confused the issue.[59]

Elimination of caffeine and other methylxanthines from the diet (tea, coffee, chocolate and cola) can result in considerable clinical improvement in women with benign breast disorders.[62] Some women may also respond to a diet low in tyramine (i.e. remove aged cheese, wine, mushrooms, bananas and aged and processed meats).[62] Nicotine also contributes to the disorder.[62] The common biochemical link between these observations is the enhancement of catecholamine release and increase of circulating catecholamines (epinephrine and norepinephrine).[62] This also underlines the role of physical and emotional stress. Women with benign breast disease had a significantly higher level of urinary catecholamines than women without breast disease.[63]

Treatment for fibroadenoma

Vitex is the main treatment, because of its regulating effect on ovarian function. Herbs for growths such as Thuja (arbor-vitae) and Echinacea are also indicated. Oestrogen-promoting herbs such as Asparagus (shatavari) and Paeonia may be beneficial because an FA is an aberration of normal lobule development. Any stress aspects should also be addressed by prescribing nervine tonics, sedatives or tonics as the case history dictates.

CASE HISTORY

'Jenny' was 31 and had a breast lump which was diagnosed as an FA. Her GP recommended 3 months' observation but the surgeon wanted the lump removed. Being concerned at the prospect of surgery, she decided to try herbal treatment during the observation period.
Treatment was as follows (based on 1 week):

Echinacea angustifolia root	1:2	30 mL
Scutellaria lateriflora	1:2	30 mL
Paeonia lactiflora	1:2	25 mL
Thuja occidentalis	1:5	15 mL
	TOTAL	100 mL

Dose: 5 mL with water three times a day.
Vitex 1:2, 2 mL with water on rising, was also prescribed.
Treatment was continued for 3 months. When she returned to the surgeon, he could find no trace of the FA.

Treatment for breast cysts

The herbal treatment of breast cysts is similar to the approach used for FA, except that oestrogen-promoting herbs are best avoided. Vitex is the most important herb and the alleviation of the negative physiological effects of stress should also be emphasised. Abstinence from stimulants, as described above, should also be observed. To modify the effects of oestrogen, intake of phyto-oestrogens and oestrogenic lignans should be increased. This could also reduce any risk of breast cancer. Ginkgo could help control mastalgia symptoms (see Ginkgo monograph).

Menopause

The climacteric or menopause is a period of waning ovarian function that marks the end of the reproductive lifespan. As such, it is a normal event in the life of a woman and should not be regarded as a disease. Menopause is a retrospective diagnosis usually made after 12 months of amenorrhea.[64] The average age for the menopause is around 51 years and has changed little in the last century. The average age of onset of the perimenopause is about 46 to 47 years and it lasts about 4 years.

The aim of herbal treatment is to assist the adjustment to this important change and provide symptomatic alleviation of the effects of oestrogen withdrawal. It is not intended that herbal treatment for the menopausal change should be prescribed indefinitely, although it may be required for several years until the body has adapted to the new hormonal levels. The principle form of circulating oestrogen in postmenopausal women is oestrone, synthesised by the peripheral conversion of androstenedione (mainly from the adrenals, with a small amount from the postmenopausal ovary) in the liver and adipose tissue.

Many symptoms are associated with menopause, but the two that are the most distressing are hot flushes (which often cause insomnia) and vaginal dryness. These are experienced by over 70% of women and are directly related to the drop in oestrogen.[64] Hot flushes typically last for 6 months to 5 years, but may persist for as long as 15 years.[64] Other physical symptoms include night sweats, headaches, bone and joint pain, tiredness and breast tenderness. Psychological symptoms associated with the menopause include depression, poor memory, irritability and loss of confidence. Whether these are directly related to the fall in oestrogen is controversial.

Hot flushes tend to persist longer and are more severe in women who have had a surgically induced menopause.[64] They occur most often in the first year after the final period. Symptoms consist of sweating on the face, neck and chest as well as peripheral vasodilation. There is a rise in skin temperature of several degrees Celcius and a transient increase in heart rate. The body's core temperature falls slightly. Symptoms last for 4 to 5 minutes each time.

The aetiology of the hot flush is unknown.[65,66] Probably the rate of change of plasma oestrogen influences the thermoregulatory system via the hypothalamus. Neurotransmitter activity, especially in the serotonergic and noradrenergic pathways, is altered. Hot flushes occur in conjunction with the pulsatile release of LH. There is a suggestion that women who experience more extreme hot flushes may have a less healthy cardiovascular system.[67]

An emerging conclusion from clinical practice is that the extent of distress in menopause is directly associated with conditions and circumstances that would imply adrenal exhaustion. One could suggest that during reproductive life the woman has two steroid-producing pairs of glands working in tandem (and overlapping considerably). With menopause the loss of one pair is felt considerably harder. Strategies that support adrenal function and relieve stress burdens on the body are well justified.

Treatment

There are many remedies sold in the open market for the treatment of menopause. However, the results of rigorous clinical trials have so far not been overly encouraging for the most popular such as Actaea (black cohosh)[68] and *Trifolium pratense* (red clover).[69] A positive result for a Hypericum and Actaea combination[70] has been limited by lack of controls and other methodological defects (see the black cohosh monograph). However, recent results of a placebo-controlled study for St John's wort point to a benefit.[71] In fact, phytotherapists often rely on different herbs to these for the management of the menopausal transition.

The main aims of herbal assistance with the menopausal change are as follows:

- To assist the body to adapt to the new hormonal levels by reducing the effects of oestrogen withdrawal. This is achieved by prescribing saponin-containing herbs such as Tribulus, *Chamaelirium luteum* (helonias root), Asparagus (shatavari), Dioscorea (wild yam) and Actaea (black cohosh) (see Chapter 2). *Alchemilla vulgaris* (ladies mantle) is also indicated in this context and can be a useful backup when other herbs fail to deliver the expected result. Some recent clinical studies with hops (*Humulus*

lupulus) are encouraging. Panax (ginseng) is a tonic saponin-containing herb with some disputed evidence for oestrogenic activity; however, it may aggravate irritability and insomnia and should be used cautiously

- To provide support for the nervous system and adrenal function using tonic and nervine tonic herbs with adaptogens and adrenal restoratives. Hypericum (St John's wort) is almost a specific for menopausal depression. Avena (oats) is also popular. Rehmannia, Panax (ginseng), Eleutherococcus (Siberian ginseng), Glycyrrhiza (licorice) and Withania are all potentially indicated
- To abate the intensity of the hot flushes or sweating. The important herb here is Salvia (sage), although cardiovascular herbs such as Crataegus (hawthorn) and Leonurus (motherwort) also can be useful
- Vitex has a role to play for the perimenopausal woman with PMS-like symptoms (which may or may not be premenstrual due to menstrual irregularity). Some herbalists are of the opinion that Vitex also helps allay other menopausal symptoms such as flushes (see Vitex monograph). Its influence on pituitary function might be the key here
- Phyto-oestrogen intake should be increased through soya products, linseeds and herbal teas, but it should not be excessive as this may interfere with the main herbal treatment.

Despite its popularity, there is little traditional or clinical evidence to support the claim that *Angelica sinensis* (dong quai) has a specific role in menopause, although it has been helpful in combination (see dong quai monograph). Its tonic effect will also be of some value. Evening primrose oil appears to have no place in a therapeutic regime for the menopause.

The above approach will reduce the severity of menopausal symptoms in a majority of cases. Many women will find that, although hot flushes still occur, their intensity and frequency are so reduced as not to be a problem. A small percentage of women cannot be helped by the above approach, presumably because their levels of oestrogen are too low or have dropped too rapidly. Often these are women who have received extensive hormone replacement therapy in the past. After menopause, oestrogen is manufactured in fat and muscle tissue from adrenal hormones. Such unresponsive cases may eventually respond to adrenal support.

CASE HISTORY

A woman 47 years old presented with hot flushes, sweating, depression and interrupted sleep caused by the hot flushes. She was irritable, low in energy and under stress at work. The hot flushes had started 18 months ago.

The following formula was prescribed (based on 1 week):

Hypericum perforatum	1:2	20 mL
Chamaelirium luteum	1:2	20 mL
Dioscorea villosa	1:2	20 mL
Crataegus oxyacantha (fruit)	1:2	15 mL
Withania somnifera	1:2	25 mL
	TOTAL	100 mL

Dose: 5 mL with water three times a day.

After 1 month of treatment there was little change, but by the end of the second month there were considerable reductions in the frequency and severity of the hot flushes. She was less irritable and depressed. After 1 year of treatment the herbs were stopped and no return of menopausal symptoms occurred.

CASE HISTORY

A 49-year-old woman was experiencing hot flushes. It had been 8 months since her last period. She was waking up one to two times a night and having five or six flushes a day, including with sweating. Herbal tablets containing *Dioscorea villosa* (wild yam) 400mg, *Asparagus racemosus* (shatavari) 400mg, *Actaea racemosa* (black cohosh) 100mg, *Hypericum perforatum* (St John's wort) 600mg, *Salvia fruticosa* (sage) 290mg and *Panax ginseng* 75mg were prescribed at 3 tablets per day.

After 5 weeks she reported a lower severity and frequency of flushes; that outcome was maintained through the following months.

Therapy during pregnancy

After taking into account the professional reluctance to prescribe herbs in pregnancy, there are nevertheless a number of herbs invaluable for the treatment of some common problems of pregnancy.

Morning sickness

In the first trimester, Zingiber (ginger) can provide effective relief in mild to moderate cases of morning sickness (see monograph). About 10 drops (approx 0.3mL) of a 1:2 extract with water can rapidly relieve nausea. This can be repeated up to nine times more in a day if required. More severe cases may require liver herbs such as Silybum (St Mary's thistle) and Taraxacum (dandelion root). *Mentha piperita* (peppermint), Filipendula (meadowsweet), Gentiana and Ballota (black horehound) are also useful herbs. For morning sickness and nausea that extends into the second trimester, Rubus (raspberry leaf) is usually an effective treatment.

Threatened miscarriage

Vitex (chaste berry) is indicated for threatened miscarriage if progesterone levels are relatively low (at the lower dosage end). Other herbs usually indicated include Dioscorea (wild yam), *Viburnum opulus* or *prunifolium* for cramping or bearing down sensations and Capsella (shepherd's purse) for bleeding.

Varicose veins

Varicose veins are more likely to develop during pregnancy, probably because of the weakening effect on connective tissue of higher levels of female hormones. The main basis of treatment is therefore to maintain connective tissue; safe herbs which do this include Vaccinium (bilberry) and Crataegus (hawthorn). A cream containing Aesculus and Hamamelis (witchhazel) can be applied to problem areas.

Preparation for childbirth

To help the mother prepare for birth, *Rubus idaeus* (raspberry leaf) and Mitchella (squaw vine) can be taken continuously after the first trimester. It is not known how these herbs act, but Rubus probably builds up the strength of the myometrium (uterine muscle), which leads to an easy birth. The value of Rubus in pregnancy has been proven in many cases and there is no evidence for any deleterious effect. During labour, Rubus should be taken with increased frequency, up to six 5mL doses in a day. *Viburnum opulus* (cramp bark) may also be prescribed if there is a problem with dilation of the cervix, as can Mitchella and Actaea.

Therapy following pregnancy
Herbs and breastfeeding

Herbs that promote milk include: Galega (goats rue), Asparagus (shatavari), *Silybum marianum*, Foeniculum (fennel), Trigonella (fenugreek), Verbena (vervain), Urtica (nettles) and *Euphorbia pilulifera*. The role of chaste tree is controversial and only low doses should be used.

Herbs that decrease milk include Salvia (sage), *Mentha piperita* (peppermint) and Lycopus (gypsywort or bugleweed).

Some herbal components may be passed in the milk. A breastfed baby can sometimes be effectively treated by medicating the mother, especially if there is infant colic.

Postnatal depression

Postnatal depression is caused by a combination of female hormonal effects with the adrenal depletion that can follow pregnancy and childbirth. Treatment is based around Vitex, tonics and nervine tonics.

A typical treatment is as follows (based on 1 week):

Panax ginseng	1:2	10mL
Hypericum perforatum	1:2	25mL
Glycyrrhiza glabra (high in glycyrrhizin)	1:1	15mL
Withania somnifera	1:2	30mL
Rhodiola rosea	2:1	20mL
	TOTAL	100mL

Dose: 5mL with water three times a day.

Also Vitex 1:2, 1 to 2mL with water once a day on rising.

References

1. Filicori M, Tabarelli C, Casadio P, et al. Interaction between menstrual cyclicity and gonadotrophin pulsatility. *Horm Res.* 1998;49(3–4):169–172.

2. Shi M, Chang L, He G. Stimulating action of Carthamus tinctorius L., Angelica sinensis (Oliv.) Diels and Leonurus sibiricus L. on the uterus. *Chung Kuo Chung Yao Tsa Chih.* 1995;20(3):173–175. 192.

3. Li W, Zhou CH, Lu QL. Effects of Chinese materia medica in activating blood and stimulating menstrual flow on the endocrine function of ovary-uterus and its mechanisms. *Chung Kuo Chung Hsi I Chieh Ho Tsa Chih.* 1992;12(3):165–168. 134.

4. Dickerson LM, Mazyck PJ, Hunt MH. Premenstrual syndrome. *Am Fam Physician.* 2003;67(8):1743–1752.

5. Freeman EW, Sammel MD, Rinaudo PJ, et al. Premenstrual syndrome as a predictor of menopausal symptoms. *Obstet Gynecol.* 2004;103(5 pt 1):960–966.

6. Seippel L, Backstrom T. Luteal-phase estradiol relates to symptom severity in patients with premenstrual syndrome. *J Clin Endocrinol Metab.* 1998;83(6):1988–1992.

7. Backstrom T, Andreen L, Birzniece V, et al. The role of hormones and hormonal treatments in premenstrual syndrome. *CNS Drugs.* 2003;17(5):325–342.

8. Abraham GE. Nutritional factors in the etiology of the premenstrual tension syndromes. *J Reprod Med.* 1983;28(7):446–464.

9. Mills S, Turner S. A double blind clinical trial on a herbal remedy for premenstrual syndrome: a case study. *Comp Ther Med.* 1993;1(2):73–77.

10. Dante G, Facchinetti F. Herbal treatments for alleviating premenstrual symptoms: a systematic review. *J Psychosom Obstet Gynaecol.* 2011;32(1):42–51.

11. Canning S, Waterman M, Orsi N, et al. The efficacy of Hypericum perforatum (St. John's wort) for the treatment of premenstrual syndrome: a randomized, double blind, placebo-controlled trial. *CNS Drugs.* 2010;24(3):207–225.

12. Dawood MY. Primary dysmenorrhea: advances in pathogenesis and management. *Obstet Gynecol.* 2006;108(2):428–441.

13. Ozgoli G, Goli M, Moattar F. Comparison of effects of ginger, mefenamic acid, and ibuprofen on pain in women with primary dysmenorrhea. *J Altern Complement Med.* 2009;15(2):129–132.

14. Han S, Hur M, Buckle J, et al. Effect of aromatherapy on symptoms of dysmenorrhea in college students: a randomized placebo-controlled trial. *J Altern Complement Med.* 2006;12(6):535–541.

15. British Herbal Medicine Association. *British Herbal Pharmacopoeia.* Bournmouth: BHMA; 1983.

16. Felter HW, Lloyd JU. *King's American Dispensatory*, 18th ed., rev 3. Portland: First published 1905. Reprinted Eclectic Medical Publications: 1983.

17. Leclerc H. *Précis de Phytothérapie*, 5th ed. Paris: Masson; 1983.

18. Weiss RF. *Herbal Medicine*, translated by AR Meuss from the 6th German edn of *Lehrbuch der Phytotherapie*. Sweden: Gothenburg, AB Arcanum; 1988.

19. Bisset NG, ed. *Herbal Drugs and Phytopharmaceuticals: a Handbook for Practice on a Scientific Basis.* Stuttgart: Medpharm Scientific Publishers; 1994.

20. Grieve M. *A Modern Herbal.* New York: Dover Publications; 1971.

21. Maisch JM. Notes on some old remedies. *Am J. Pharm.* 1888;60(7):4.

22. De Costa St C. Anthony's fire and living ligatures: a short history of ergometrine. *Lancet.* 2002;359(9319):1768–1770.

23. Kuroda K, Kaku T. Pharmacological and chemical studies on the alcohol extract of Capsella bursa-pastoris. *Life Sci.* 1969;8(3):151–155.

24. Kuroda K, Takagi K. Studies on Capsella bursa-pastoris. I. General pharmacology of ethanol extract of the herb. *Arch Int Pharmacodyn.* 1969;178(2):382–391.

25. Mashburn J. Etiology, diagnosis, and management of vaginitis. *J Midwifery Womens Health.* 2006;51(6):423–430.

26. Flake GP, Andersen J, Dixon D. Etiology and pathogenesis of uterine leiomyomas: a review. *Environ Health Perspect.* 2003;111(8):1037–1054.

27. Marshall LM, Spiegelman D, Goldman MB, et al. A prospective study of reproductive factors and oral contraceptive use in relation to the risk of uterine leiomyomata. *Fertil Steril.* 1998;70:432–439.

28. Schneider J, Bradlow HL, Strain G, et al. Effects of obesity on estradiol metabolism: decreased formation of nonuterotropic metabolites. *J Clin Endocrinol Metab.* 1983;56(5):973–978.

29. Ross RK, Pike MC, Vessey MP, et al. Risk factors for uterine fibroids: reduced risk associated with oral contraceptives. *Br Med J (Clin Res Ed).* 1986;293:359–362.

30. Marshall LM, Spiegelman D, Manson JE, et al. Risk of uterine leiomyomata among premenopausal women in relation to body size and cigarette smoking. *Epidemiology.* 1998;9:511–517.

31. Payson M, Leppert P, Segars J. Epidemiology of myomas. *Obstet Gynecol Clin North Am.* 2006;33(1):1–11.

32. Chiaffarino F, Parazzini F, Vecchia C, et al. Diet and uterine myomas. *Obstet Gynecol.* 1999;94:395–398.

33. Wise L, Palmer J, Harlow B, et al. Risk of uterine leiomyomata in relation to tobacco, alcohol, and caffeine consumption in the Black Women's Health Study. *Hum Reprod.* 2004;19:1746–1754.

34. Stewart E, Nowak R. New concepts in the treatment of uterine leiomyomas. *Obstet Gynecol.* 1998;92:624–627.

35. Boynton-Jarrett R, Rich-Edwards J, Malspeis S, et al. A prospective study of hypertension and risk of uterine leiomyomata. *Am J Epidemiol.* 2005;161:628–638.

36. Marsh EE, Bulun SE. Steroid hormones and leiomyomas. *Obstet Gynecol Clin North Am.* 2006;33(1):59–67.

37. Shozu M, Murakami K, Inoue M. Aromatase and leiomyoma of the uterus. *Semin Reprod Med.* 2004;22(1):51–60.

38. Sozen I, Arici A. Interactions of cytokines, growth factors, and the extracellular matrix in the cellular biology of uterine leiomyomata. *Fertil Steril.* 2002;78(1):1–12.

39. Bone K. *Clinical Guide to Blending Liquid Herbs: Herbal Formulations for the Individual Patient.* USA: Churchill Livingstone; 2003. pp. 142–146.

40. Fugh-Berman A, Kronenberg F. Complementary and alternative medicine (CAM) in reproductive-age women: a review of randomized controlled trials. *Reprod Toxicol.* 2003;17(2):137–152.

41. Sakamoto S, Yoshino H, Shirahata Y, et al. Pharmacotherapeutic effects of huei-chih-fu-ling-wan (keishi-bukuryo-gan) on human uterine myomas. *Am J Chin Med.* 1992;20(3-4):313–317.

42. Brooks JDS, Ward WE, Lewis JE, et al. Supplementation with flaxseed alters estrogen metabolism in postmenopausal women to a greater extent than does supplementation with an equal amount of soy. *Am J Clin Nutr.* 2004;79(2):318–325.

43. Haggans CJ, Travelli EJ, Thomas W, et al. The effect of flaxseed and wheat bran consumption on urinary estrogen metabolites in premenopausal women. *Cancer Epidemiol Biomarkers Prev.* 2000;9(7):719–725.

44. Wang C, Makela T, Hase T, et al. Lignans and flavonoids inhibit aromatase enzymes in human preadipocytes. *J Steroid Biochem Mol Biol.* 1994;50(3-4):205–212.

45. Pasquali R, Gambineri A. Polycystic ovary syndrome: a multifaceted disease from adolescence to adult age. *Ann NY Acad Sci.* 2006;1092:158–174.

46. Harwood K, Vuguin P, DiMartino-Nardi J. Current approaches to the diagnosis and treatment of polycystic ovarian syndrome in youth. *Horm Res.* 2007;68(5):209–217.

47. Vignesh JP, Mohan V. Polycystic ovary syndrome: a component of metabolic syndrome? *J Postgrad Med.* 2007;53(2):128–134.

48. Lobo RA, Carmina E. The importance of diagnosing the polycystic ovary syndrome. *Ann Intern Med.* 2000;132(12):989–983.

49. Pharmacopoeia Commission of the People's Republic of China. *Pharmacopoeia of the People's Republic of China*, English ed. Beijing: Chemical Industry Press; 1997.

50. Takahashi K, Kitao M. Effect of TJ-68 (shakuyaku-kanzo-to) on polycystic ovarian disease. *Int J Fertil Menopausal Stud*. 1994;39(2):69–76.

51. Takahashi K, Yoshino K, Shirai T, et al. Effect of a traditional herbal medicine (shakuyaku-kanzo-to) on testosterone secretion in patients with polycystic ovary syndrome detected by ultrasound. *Nihon Sanka Fujinka Gakkai Zasshi*. 1988;40(6):789–792.

52. Yaginuma T, Izumi R, Yasui H, et al. Effect of traditional herbal medicine on serum testosterone levels and its induction of regular ovulation in hyperandrogenic and oligomenorrheic women (author's transl). *Nihon Sanka Fujinka Gakkai Zasshi*. 1982;34(7):939–944.

53. Aizawa H, Niimura M. Serum androgen levels in women with acne vulgaris. The effects of shakuyaku-kanzo-to (SK). *Skin Res*. 1996;38:37–41.

54. Hosoya E, Yamamura Y, eds. *Recent Advances in the Pharmacology of Kampo (Japanese Herbal) Medicines*. Amsterdam: Excerpta Medica; 1988.

55. Yamada K, Kanba S, Yagi G, Asai M. Herbal medicine (Shakuyaku-kanzo-to) in the treatment of risperidone-induced amenorrhea. *J Clin Psychopharmacol*. 1999;19(4):380–381.

56. Yamada K, Kanba S, Yagi G, Asai M. Effectiveness of herbal medicine (shakuyaku-kanzo-to) for neuroleptic-induced hyperprolactinemia. *J Clin Psychopharmacol*. 1997;17(3):234–235.

57. Hughes LE. Benign breast disorders: the clinician's view. *Cancer Detect Prev*. 1992;16(1):1–5.

58. Miltenburg DM, Speights Jr. VO. Benign breast disease. *Obstet Gynecol Clin North Am*. 2008;35(2):285–300.

59. Courtillot C, Plu-Bureau G, Binart N, et al. Benign breast diseases. *J Mammary Gland Biol Neoplasia*. 2005;10(4):325–335.

60. Dixon JM. Cystic disease and fibroadenoma of the breast: natural history and relation to breast cancer risk. *Br Med Bull*. 1991;47(2):258–271.

61. Angeli A, Dogliotti L, Naldoni C, et al. Steroid biochemistry and categorization of breast cyst fluid: relation to breast cancer risk. *Steroid Biochem Mol Biol*. 1994;49(4–6):333–339.

62. Minton JP, Abou-Issa H. Nonendocrine theories of the etiology of benign breast disease. *World J Surg*. 1989;13(6):680–684.

63. Dogliotti L, Orlandi F, Angeli A. The endocrine basis of benign breast disorders. *World J Surg*. 1989;13(6):674–679.

64. Bruce D, Rymer J. Symptoms of the menopause. *Best Pract Res Clin Obstet Gynaecol*. 2009;23(1):25–32.

65. Andrikoula M, Prelevic G. Menopausal hot flushes revisited. *Climacteric*. 2009;12(1):3–15.

66. Rossmanith WG, Ruebberdt W. What causes hot flushes? The neuroendocrine origin of vasomotor symptoms in the menopause. *Gynecol Endocrinol*. 2009;25(5):303–314.

67. Andrikoula M, Hardiman P, Prelevic G. Menopausal hot flush: is it only a nuisance or also a marker of cardiovascular disease risk? *Gynecol Endocrinol*. 2009;25(7):450–454.

68. Borrelli F, Ernst E. Black cohosh (Cimicifuga racemosa) for menopausal symptoms: a systematic review of its efficacy. *Pharmacol Res*. 2008;58(1):8–14.

69. Booth N, Piersen C, Banuvar S, et al. Clinical studies of red clover (Trifolium pratense) dietary supplements in menopause: a literature review. *Menopause*. 2006;13(2):251–264.

70. Briese V, Stammwitz U, Friede M, et al. Black cohosh with or without St. John's wort for symptom-specific climacteric treatment – results of a large-scale, controlled, observational study. *Maturitas*. 2007;57(4):405–414.

71. Abdali K, Khajehei M, Tabatabaee HR. Effect of St John's wort on severity, frequency, and duration of hot flashes in premenopausal, perimenopausal and postmenopausal women: a randomized, double blind, placebo-controlled trial. *Menopause*. 2010;17(2):326–331.

Joint diseases

Scope

Apart from their use to provide non-specific support for recuperation and repair, specific phytotherapeutic strategies include the following.

Treatment of:

- early and transient joint inflammation
- gout
- repetitive strain injury.

Management of:

- long-standing joint disease with joint damage
- low back pain
- fibromyalgia.

Because of its use of secondary plant products, particular **caution** is necessary in applying phytotherapy in cases of:

- very aggressive joint inflammations.

Orientation

Background

Degeneration of one or more joints in the body affects almost all persons from the fifth decade of life and there are equally universal clinical signs by the age of 70 years. There is evidence of the problem occurring in the bone records from the distant past as well, and it is a condition found in almost all vertebrates, even dinosaurs, whales, fish and birds. It is probable that the joint structures reach the limit of their regenerative capacity earlier than other body tissues. They certainly operate at the limit of engineering tolerance and circulatory renewal at the best of times. A number of environmental conditions, life circumstances, traumatic events, infections and other diseases and genetic factors might reduce the regenerative capacity even further.

In fact, there is still much uncertainty over the aetiology of osteoarthritis (OA). Wear and tear is a factor in prolonged overuse of a certain joint, but use is generally better than inactivity (long-distance runners have no worse incidence of the disease but even moderate forced inactivity can accelerate the condition). The immediate event is a disturbance in the behaviour of the chondrocyte, normally a very quiescent and isolated cell responsible for maintaining the cartilage of the joint, leading to its mitosis, then an interactive stimulation of neighbouring osteoblasts to produce the bony overgrowth. Whatever provokes the chondroblasts, it is fair, in the absence of hard evidence, to look at the widest systemic evidence for disturbance around the body and the interpretations of such events by earlier observers.

In looking at the wider picture to understand localised OA, one is taking a similar path to that for the more overtly inflammatory arthritic conditions, the diffuse connective tissue diseases: rheumatoid arthritis, Sjögren's and Behçet's syndromes, polymyalgia rheumatica, the lupus erythematoses, polymyositis and the like, as well as the spondylitic diseases, ankylosing spondylitis, Reiter's syndrome and psoriatic arthropathy. These all share a substantial immunological component and their treatment is best taken along with other diseases of this type (see Chapter 8). Nevertheless, even these diseases, inasmuch as the joints are involved, can be approached with some of the following points in mind.

As with skin diseases (see p. 315), the verdict of the ancients on joint diseases was unanimous. Arthritis represented a toxic accumulation at the site. There was probably an appreciation that joints were uniquely vulnerable structures, fairly obvious 'bottlenecks' in the circulatory flow; the notion of a 'toxic log jam' at such sites seems commonplace, evidenced in part by the topical treatments usually applied.

Phytotherapeutics

Counter-irritation

There was, of course, an immediate imperative in joint pain in the past. It quickly affected mobility and threatened survival. It was also easily focused upon. If the problem represented a local toxic accumulation then local measures to improve circulation were the obvious treatment. Applying heat to the joint would most often reduce pain. Applying stronger heating measures could often have a longer term benefit. Thus throughout the world drastic heating measures were applied to affected joints. At the least, hot poultices or baths with mustard, pepper or cayenne would be used as rubefacients (a milder effect can be had with proprietary liniments and embrocations). Indeed there is currently evidence that ginger applied topically[1] or internally[2] can benefit OA (see also the ginger monograph). For more dramatic effects stronger remedies were used, those in Galenic terms that would be classified as 'hot in the fourth degree', that 'corrode and cause blisters if outwardly applied' (see Chapter 1).

Blistering in arthritis was a common technique. A very strong mustard or cayenne application might do it and flaying with stinging nettles (see nettle monograph for relevant clinical trials) was favoured in ancient Europe (even birds and some animals will expose themselves to ant bites in certain circumstances), but more corrosive substances such as croton oil and formic acid (found in ant bites and stinging nettle) became favoured as they were isolated. Blistering was used, for example, among the new industrial working classes of 19th century Britain who still favoured their rural herbal traditions and would visit the recently urbanised herbalist because in this way, and without effective social security or system of disability payments, they would be able to get back to work more quickly (they often did not pay until such results were achieved either!). The application could produce a large blister in minutes; lancing this could yield an impressive quantity of fluid. The fact that pain could be instantly reduced and mobility often at least temporarily improved led to the obvious supposition that the blister

fluids carried toxins away and that the associated and obvious heating brought in more healing circulation to do the rest. In modern central Europe, blistering applications have sometimes been replaced with precision-depth epidermal puncture devices followed by irritant applications; fluids pass through the puncture holes without blisters having to form. Similar simple devices are also used in traditional Chinese medicine.

Counter-irritation is often in modern accounts explained as resulting from some form of stimulation of nerve receptors leading to reflex analgesia. This does not do justice to the technique or to its therapeutic context; indeed, both rubefacients and blistering agents, expertly applied, are intrinsically comforting sensations. A better speculation might be that counter-irritation is a proinflammatory technique; the increased vasoactivity and stimulation of other inflammatory mediators can be seen as constituting a therapeutic inflammation, doing painlessly what the body itself does with pain, swelling and disability. It is a principle espoused by Samuel Thomson in 19th-century North America (see Chapter 1), that fever and its local counterpart, inflammation, are not the disease themselves but the body's defence against disease. Like Thomson's cayenne and Galen's heating remedies generally, the topical counter-irritations, whether simply warming liniments and embrocations or blistering heating packs, were recognition that the best therapy was to improve upon nature's defences and even extend them.

In modern practice blistering is rarely acceptable. However, good results can often be had with heating poultices, footbaths or handbaths, using an agent such as powdered mustard. For a poultice, a slurry made with the yellow powder sold to make English mustard can be smeared on a gauze and held over the affected joint under a hot wet flannel pad. Occasional glimpses of the area under the dressing should warn if blistering is impending, but the most common reaction is a mild erythema only. Fifteen to 20 minutes should be enough application. For a hand- or footbath a dessertspoonful of mustard powder is put into a bowl of hot water just large enough to immerse the affected limb; this in turn is best placed in a larger bowl of hot water better to maintain the temperature for up to 20 minutes. It is still possible to obtain cayenne plasters from specialist suppliers, rubber material impregnated with cayenne, and it may be possible to make one's own substitute. Russian ointment includes cayenne for a particularly robust liniment. Otherwise strong muscle rubs or the Asian product 'Tiger Balm' will provide moderate relief for arthritic joints. Most accessibly, many embrocations and liniments are available in pharmacies and elsewhere, mostly based on mentholated ointments with various rubefacient constituents (e.g. eucalyptus and wintergreen oils) added, although these are likely to have only mild benefits.

The above approaches are mostly indicated for the low level of inflammatory activity associated with OA. They may also be indicated in more volatile inflammations of rheumatic disease, but are sometimes not. Gout is another joint condition that is usually contraindicated. If the joint is too inflamed and hot already, these techniques may be aggravatory. Sensitivity to liniments or heat may be a good guide not to proceed further.

Internal treatments

As indicated earlier, a consistent theme in traditional medicine was to remove toxic accumulations from the affected joints. Equally consistent was the view that this was particularly a burden on the kidneys. Many traditional treatments for arthritis were also diuretic (or diuretic depurative) remedies, perceived as helping the body remove toxic waste through the urine. In European medicine herbs such as Apium (celery), Betula (birch), Taraxacum (dandelion) and Filipendula (meadowsweet) were widely used diuretics in the treatment of arthritic disease.

The juxtaposition of kidney function and joint disease was elaborated in the European naturopathic and North American Eclectic traditions in their focus on acid/alkali balance (the kidneys of course are dedicated largely to maintaining electrolyte equilibrium in the body fluids). The concept has permeated folk culture: acids are bad for joints, alkalis good.

It is widely understood that the body has to eliminate acid metabolites and that joint problems are a classic outcome of failure to do this. Under such circumstances it makes sense to reduce acidic foods from the diet; not (and this is one detail causing much confusion) foods that taste acidic such as citrus and other fruits, but foods that leave an acidic residue after digestion, due to a preponderance of sulphates and phosphates. Proteins are the major example of the latter. One guide is to test the acidity of ash after combustion of the food, given that digestion is enzymatically an analogous process; in this test lemons leave an alkaline ash, and cheese, meat and eggs leave an acidic ash.

However, estimates based on the acid or alkaline nature of the mineral ash of the food do not take into account the incomplete intestinal absorption of various nutrients. A useful paper has reviewed the clinical impact of the potential renal acid loads (PRAL) of various foods and elaborated on clinical strategies for the treatment of chronic inflammatory diseases.[3]

The PRAL of various foods is calculated from their sodium, potassium, calcium, magnesium, phosphorus, chloride and sulphur content, taking into account the known percentage absorption rates for protein (in the case of sulphur) and minerals.[4] It is expressed as milli-equivalents (mEq) per 100 g. The PRAL content averages for various food groups are shown in Box 9.1.[4] A positive value means that the food is acidic and a negative value indicates alkalinity.

The most acidic food was parmesan cheese (PRAL 34.2) and the most alkaline food was raisins (PRAL −21.0).[4] Plant-based beverages such as wine, tea and coffee are generally alkaline if taken without milk. However, some beers and cola drinks were acidic. Mineral water could be quite alkaline (PRAL −1.8) depending on its origin. The most alkaline fruit was the banana (PRAL −5.5), closely followed by apricots (PRAL −4.8). The most alkaline vegetable was spinach (PRAL −14.0), mainly due to its very high calcium content. The least alkaline vegetables were cucumber and asparagus. Processed meats were the most acidic form of meat or fish consumption and lentils and peas were also mildly acidic. Nuts were variable: hazelnuts were alkaline and peanuts and walnuts were acidic. Egg yolks were highly acidic (PRAL 23.4) and chocolate and cake were moderately so.

In the 1930s William Howard Hay, an American doctor, published his theories on health and disease (for example

---

Box 9.1

PRAL of certain food groups and combined foods

Food group	PRAL (mEq/100 g)
Fats and oils	0
Fish	7.9
Fruits and fruit juices	−3.1
Grain products	
Bread	3.5
Flour	7.0
Noodles	6.7
Meat and meat products	9.5
Milk and dairy products	
Milk and non-cheese products	1.0
Cheese with lower protein content*	8.0
Cheeses with higher protein content**	23.6
Vegetables	−2.8

*Less than 15 g protein per 100 g.
**More than 15 g protein per 100 g.

Hay WH. *A New Health Era*. London: George G Harrap and Co. Ltd; 1935). His system of health became known as the Hay Diet or the Hay System and for a time was very popular. Its influence on naturopathic thinking is still in evidence. Hay realised that foods were either acid or alkaline in nature and that this was not based on their pH before consumption. Instead, in a predecessor to PRAL values, Hay proposed that, since foods are combusted in the body to give energy, it is the pH of the residue of a food after combustion (or ashing) that will indicate its acidity or alkalinity in the body (as noted above). Hay realised that acid foods are those which are rich in protein, since the sulphur content of the protein creates acidity after combustion. In contrast, the alkaline foods are those rich in potassium, sodium and calcium, since these combust to give an alkaline ash.

Although the Hay System was very similar to naturopathy, the original contribution made by Hay was that the modern diet was too acidic and that many modern diseases resulted from this. Hay also developed the concept of food combining, where high protein foods were separated in the diet from high carbohydrate foods. He also proposed that one day of the week should be 'alkaline', when only alkaline foods were to be consumed. As noted above, Hay's classification of alkaline or acidic foods correlates very closely with the PRAL values developed by Remer and Manz.[4]

Using the work of Remer and Manz,[4] the Hay System can be put on a modern scientific basis. Moreover, excessively acidic foods can be identified and largely avoided and replaced by highly alkaline foods. According to Hay, this will not only result in benefits for OA and other rheumatic conditions, but also many other chronic disorders. Urine pH can be used to measure progress with the diet and adjustments made accordingly. Recent studies indicate that rendering the urine more alkaline will have a sparing effect on calcium excretion. This implies that an alkaline diet may help to prevent osteoporosis, although a recent study suggests this is not the case, except in older men.[5]

A number of other points about the paper of Remer and Manz are worth noting.[4] Since the body excretes organic acids in proportion to body weight, the more overweight a person is the more acidic their system becomes. If this excess acidity is linked to some of the negative health aspects associated with obesity, then a more alkaline diet could help to counter these negative influences. The fact that the body excretes organic acids also means that the diet needs to be quite alkaline before the urine pH rises above 7.0 into alkalinity. One flaw in the proposed PRAL values is that some organic acids can be consumed in the diet, for example oxalic and tartaric acids, which are not metabolised by the body. These could influence the PRAL values of certain foods (e.g. oranges, grapes and spinach).

The herbal diuretics mentioned above can be understood as usefully complementing a high-alkali diet based on vegetables and fruits in reducing the rate of joint deterioration in many sufferers from OA.

Diuretic herbs may be augmented by inflammatory modulators traditionally used in arthritic disease. There are a number of treatments that have been subjected to systematic review and found to be promising, including gamma-linolenic acid products such as *Borago officinalis* (borage seed oil), *Oenothera biennis* (evening primrose oil) and *Ribes nigrum* (blackcurrant seed oil), capsaicin from *Capsicum annuum* (cayenne), curcumin from *Curcuma longa* (turmeric), *Tanacetum parthenium* (feverfew), *Linum usitatissimum* (linseed or flaxseed oil) and *Boswellia serrata*.[6] Given the wide disparity of treatments and relatively low number of good studies there was understandably a request for confirmatory trials in each case,[6] some of which have since been conducted. (See also Chapter 2 and the respective monographs.)

Salix (willow) and Populus (poplar) have appreciable levels of anti-inflammatory salicylates. The review referred to above included a double blind trial that one of the authors of this book conducted on a product that contains a mixture of the two. It showed moderate but significant benefit in the relief of chronic arthritic pain in a placebo-controlled study on 82 patients.[7] In an open prospective cohort study, researchers examined the effect of a standardised aqueous ethanolic willow bark extract on knee and hip symptoms due to gonarthrosis (chronic wear of the cartilage in the knee joint) and coxarthrosis (non-inflammatory degenerative disease of the hip joint). Eighty-eight patients received the equivalent of 120 to 240 mg/day salicin, 40 patients a standard drug treatment as a reference for 6 weeks. As the study progressed there was a trend towards greater improvement in the willow bark group with better tolerability than for the conventional treatment.[8] A recent systematic review of other studies on Salix concluded that there was moderate evidence of efficacy for the use of ethanolic willow bark extract in low back pain at doses equivalent to 240 mg/day of salicin (see willow bark monograph).[9]

Other traditional anti-inflammatories have also been investigated in modern times: in a recent double blind, placebo-controlled trial, a standardised *Boswellia serrata* (frankincense) extract was investigated for the treatment of OA of the knee. Seventy-five patients with mild to moderate symptoms were randomised into three equal groups: placebo, low-dose and high-dose extract. Both doses of Boswellia conferred clinically

and statistically significant improvements in pain scores and physical ability scores throughout the 90 days of treatment (see also Boswellia monograph).[10] In two randomised controlled clinical trials, a traditional European remedy, comfrey (applied topically), has been found helpful in reducing ankle swelling.[11,12] Harpagophytum (devil's claw) is a remedy that has attracted a considerable research effort, generally positive though with some poor-quality studies (see devil's claw monograph).[13,14] A number of alterative remedies are used non-specifically for arthritis. Notable in European tradition is Urtica (nettle), for which there is now some pilot evidence of efficacy available (see also nettle monograph).[15]

A Cochrane review of clinical trials for low back pain, usually with arthritic elements, found that there was positive evidence for *Harpagophytum procumbens*, *Salix alba* and *Capsicum spp.* although there were methodological shortcomings in each case.[16]

A more recent contender for an arthritic treatment has been standardised preparations of *Rosa canina* (rosehip). In one double blind, controlled study among 100 patients with OA of the knee or hip, a modest benefit over placebo was detected over 4 months.[17] In another double blind, placebo-controlled crossover trial in 94 patients with the same condition, researchers found that the effect was minimal, but included some reduction of stiffness and symptoms, and reduced use of back-up analgesics.[18] Others are less obvious in their rationale and rely on traditional reputation to support their use; *Actaea racemosa* (black cohosh), *Curcuma longa* (turmeric) and Juniperus (juniper) may feature. However, there are now positive results for curcumin from turmeric, especially in high dose or enhanced bioavailability preparations (see turmeric monograph). The efficacy of some of the above together has been established in a double blind controlled clinical trial and evidence for similar combinations exists elsewhere.[19] Zanthoxylum (prickly ash) might be added in cases where cold and poor circulation are identified as factors.

Phytotherapy

Osteoarthritis

The diarthrodial joint functions to enable smooth articulation of the two adjoining bone ends, at the same time providing both strength and resilience.[20] The joint capsule is stiff fibrous tissue to offer structural support, often reinforced by other structures such as collateral ligaments. The inner lining of the joint capsule is the synovial membrane, consisting of an inner thin (1 to 3 cells thick) layer, supported by an outer innervated and vascularised stromal layer. Synovial fluid fills the joint cavity and acts as the lubricant. It is an ultrafiltrate of blood plasma made viscous with hyaluronic acid. The hyaline cartilage covers the articular surfaces and is a highly specialised connective tissue adapted to load bearing and shock absorption. A sparse population of chondrocytes is distributed through the cartilage extracellular matrix, which is mainly type II collagen, proteoglycans (aggrecans), glycoproteins and water.[20]

Osteoarthritis (OA) has been defined as the failed repair of damage caused by excessive mechanical stress on joint tissues.[20] All joint structures are affected, but the major hallmarks are the destruction of articular cartilage and changes in the subchondral bone. Historically OA was called 'osteoathrosis', a term implying the absence of inflammation. However, high-sensitive assays (such as for C-reactive protein, CRP) demonstrate that low-grade inflammation is present and that synovial tissue is also involved in the pathology.[21]

OA is the most common joint disorder and the leading cause of disability in the elderly. Among adults 60 years or older the prevalence in the US of symptomatic knee OA is 10% in men and 13% in women.[22] Total hip replacements are estimated to increase by seven times from 2005 to 2030.[20] Clinically diagnosed OA occurs in more than 50% of adults older than 65 years and in more than 30% aged 45 to 64 years.[23] Widely accepted risk factors are age, obesity, joint injury, genetics (39% to 65% in twin studies), gender, joint misalignment and metabolic disorders.[24–27] However, the robustness of many of these is still debated.

A Canadian study examined the link between primary OA and occupation.[28] Agricultural workers showed a significant excess prevalence of OA, with an observed to expected (O/E) ratio of 1.7 in women and 2.3 in men. Linear trends in prevalences between white collar, 'mixed' collar and blue collar workers were also significant, with O/E ratios respectively of 1.0, 2.9, and 2.6 in women and 1.0, 1.2, and 1.7 in men. Specific excess prevalence was found in women among housekeepers (O/E 4.4), and in men among unskilled labour workers (O/E 10.3) and truck drivers (O/E 6.7).[28]

OA results from a complex interaction of mechanical, biochemical, molecular and enzymatic feedback loops.[29] The final common pathway is joint tissue destruction resulting from the failure of cells to maintain the homeostatic balance between matrix synthesis and degradation. As OA advances, the dominant catabolic processes lead to progressive joint tissue lesions. The articular cartilage, subchondral bone, synovial membrane and synovial fluid are all affected.

The precise mechanisms behind cartilage degradation are still unclear. Early on there is an increase of water and a decrease of proteoglycans (aggrecans) and type II collagen.[30] The predominant enzymes responsible for cartilage matrix degradation in OA are the matrix metalloproteinases (MMPs) and aggrecanases. Aggrecan is a large aggregating proteoglycan that contains chondroitin sulphate and keratan sulphate and is important for the weight-bearing properties of cartilage. A subclass of MMPs known as ADAMTS appears to be activated in OA and break down aggrecan.[30] Later, cartilage mineralisation (predominantly calcium pyrophosphate and phosphate) occurs and can accelerate the inflammation.

Synovial inflammation (synovitis) occurs in early OA but can be subclinical. It is possibly induced by cartilage matrix degradation[29] and becomes more extensive as OA progresses, with synovial hypertrophy and hyperplasia occurring.[31] There are increased numbers of immune cells, such as activated B cells and T lymphocytes. In turn, the synovitis may contribute to progression of the cartilage degradation.

The degeneration and erosion of cartilage has recently been challenged as the primary pathological event in OA.[29] Subchondral bone is suggested to play a key role: after all the disease was originally called *osteo*arthritis because of the prominence of the bone reaction. The subchondral bone plate is in direct contact with the cartilage and could influence its degradation. Evidence from humans and animal models has shown that subchondral bone alterations may precede cartilage degeneration. The nutrition of the articular cartilage is provided in part by the vascular bed of the subchondral bone. Early microvascular damage affecting the venous circulation in subchondral bone is found in OA. There is also increasing evidence that bone marrow lesions (BMLs) and bone cysts have an important role in the pathogenesis of knee OA.[32] BMLs are strongly associated with radiological progression of knee OA and BML enlargement predicts increased cartilage loss and the reverse.

The common observation that chronic OA patients can experience flare-ups speaks to it being an inflammatory disease. Inflammation seems to be a very early event in OA, perhaps elicited by the initial traumatic injury. Elevated levels of CRP can be observed well before clinical disease.[21] Inflammation and its triggers directly affect synovial cells (fibroblasts and macrophages), as well as cartilage chondrocytes, causing them to produce cytokines, particularly interleukin (IL)-1beta and later tumour necrosis factor (TNF)-alpha. (The macrophage is a key inflammatory cell in OA.)[21] OA cartilage produces a large amount of nitric oxide (NO) and reactive oxygen species. This is attributable to increased expression of inducible NO synthase (iNOS). NO reduces the major anabolic processes and increases the catabolic processes.

Eicosanoids, namely leukotrienes (LT) and prostaglandins (PG) are involved, particularly PGE_2 produced from arachidonic acid by cyclo-oxygenase (COX)-2, followed by PG synthase.[29] The use of non-steroidal anti-inflammatory drugs (NSAIDs) and COX-2 selective inhibitors has shown that PGE_2 inhibition does not alter the course of progressive OA.[33] LTs produced by 5-lipoxygenase (5-LOX) could be the reason for this, as COX inhibitors might shunt more arachidonic acid into the 5-LOX pathway, paradoxically worsening the progression of OA. LTB_4 potently increases IL-1beta and TFN-alpha from the synovium. Hence dual inhibitors of eicosanoids, acting on both COX and 5-LOX, are desirable.[33] Upstream activation of nuclear factor-kappaB is stimulated by cytokines, excessive mechanical stress and matrix degradation products, and in turn regulates the expression of cytokines, inflammatory mediators (including COX-2) and several matrix degrading enzymes. It may cause chondrocytes to malfunction.[34]

While the OA definition links it to mechanical stress, predisposition to such stress could be more important. One study found that OA is more widespread in the body than is apparent from clinical studies.[35] This is consistent with other data suggesting that OA is a disease that is primarily dependent on systemic predisposition to a particular type of bone response to mechanical stress. Generalised OA is a strong predictor of disease progression.[27] One factor in operation here could be advanced glycation endproducts (AGEs). Increased severity of OA correlates with higher cartilage AGE levels.[36] AGEs in cartilage trigger AGE receptors (RAGE) on chondrocytes and fibroblast-like synoviocytes causing increased catabolic activity, for example production of cytokines and matrix degrading enzymes, which degrade and breakdown cartilage.[37]

The source of pain in OA remains enigmatic, especially at the level of the individual patient. Cartilage is aneural; hence it cannot be the tissue that directly generates pain.[20] In contrast, subchondral bone, synovium, marginal periosteum, ligaments and the joint capsule are all richly innervated, but rarely can the precise tissue origin of pain be identified in the individual patient. Imaging studies at the knee joint have shown a correlation between pain and both synovitis and subchondral bone changes. The relatively immediate reduction in pain following total knee replacement could be due to the excision of the subchondral plate in this procedure. Grosser pathological changes such as subchondral bone exposure, osteophytes and oedema probably cause pain in highly advanced disease. In addition, alterations of CNS pathways associated with chronic pain states (central sensitisation or 'wind-up') have also been identified in OA patients; the neurotransmitter substance P might be involved here.[23] While PGE_2 is generally acknowledged as a major pain mediator, there are indications that leukotrienes can also play a role in pain.[38]

Growing evidence from epidemiological studies suggests that OA is also linked to primary cardiovascular disease.[39] High prevalences of cardiovascular risk factors and vascular co-morbidity have been described in OA. Factors strongly associated include hyperlipidaemia and hypertension. A higher risk of cardiovascular death is associated with widespread OA and one large study found that men with OA in any finger joint were 40% more likely to die from cardiovascular disease.[40] One study found that the same risk factors that predict for cardiovascular disease, especially those related to coagulation, thrombosis and blood rheology, predict for OA, but with a lower threshold.[41] The study concluded: 'that there is a hypercoagulable and prothrombotic condition in osteoarthritis, with hypofibrinolysis and indirect evidence of increased fibrin generation'.

One recent review suggested there is mounting evidence that microvascular pathology plays a key role in the initiation and/or progression of OA.[42] Disruption of microvascular blood flow in subchondral bone may reduce nutrient diffusion to articular cartilage in OA. Ischaemia in subchondral bone due to microthrombi may produce osteocyte death, bone resorption and articular damage in OA. Another slightly earlier review suggested that vascular disease in subchondral bone may accelerate the OA process.[40] This is either by reducing cartilage nutrition or via direct ischaemic effects on bone, depending if cartilage damage is a primary or secondary inflammatory event. As further evidence, BML formation could be secondary to vascular events. Regardless of what initiates OA (which is more relevant for prevention), vascular disease is suggested to be highly relevant to the progression of OA.

Based on the above information, any rational therapy in OA must recognise the following issues:

- OA is not simply mechanical wear and tear
- Neither is OA a solely PGE_2-mediated inflammatory disease
- The source of pain in OA can be enigmatic
- OA is an active and complex biological process of matrix degradation mediated by cells within and adjacent to the joint, involving a range of inflammatory factors and pathological processes

- Underlying issues such as vascular and microvascular health and insulin resistance should be addressed
- Therapy for OA should target the processes driving matrix degradation and the true sources of pain and inflammation.

The herb *Boswellia serrata* is a key agent in the rational therapy of OA. A 2010 review noted the following anti-inflammatory effects of Boswellia or boswellic acids from in vitro and in vivo experiments[43]: inhibition of 5-LOX, but only minor activity on PGE production, downregulation of TNF-alpha by inhibition of NF-kappaB, inhibition of IL-1beta production and inhibition of C3-convertase of the complement system. Particularly active are 11-keto-beta-boswellic acid (KBA) and acetyl-11-keto-beta-boswellic acid (AKBA). The clinical evidence for Boswellia in OA is good. In particular, there are suggestions from some trials that Boswellia treatment might be disease-modifying, rather than just providing symptom control (see Boswellia monograph). This disease-modifying effect should be no surprise given the range of its anti-inflammatory effects relevant to OA.

Another key rational treatment is the proprietary pine bark extract known as Pycnogenol. A double blind, placebo-controlled trial involving 38 knee OA sufferers found 150mg/day of the proprietary pine bark OPCs (PBO) for 3 months reduced pain and stiffness and improved physical function.[44] Differences were quite significant clinically, with a 49% reduction in the WOMAC score and a significant drop in conventional painkiller use. A similar design trial, but with 156 patients and PBO at 100mg/day again showed a 50% reduction in the WOMAC score and a significant drop in oedema.[45] A follow-up study of this trial found CRP was lowered by 71% by PBO, and fibrinogen by 37%.[46] Another similar trial in 100 patients receiving 150mg/day found reduced stiffness and use of other painkillers.[47] PBO has beneficial effects on the microvasculature, which, in addition to anti-inflammatory activity, could explain its benefits in OA.

The above discussion proposes that microcirculatory and cardiovascular factors may predispose to OA. This was supported by a UK study in female twins that found a strong protective effect on radiographic hip OA for 'Allium' consumption (odds ratio 0.70).[48] Non-citrus fruit was also protective (OR 0.56). Of course, a major Allium species is garlic, well known for its vascular and microvascular effects.

It is hoped that individual strategies will be devised for each patient with OA, taking some of the insights in this and other chapters into account, but essential elements of herbal treatment are as follows:

- Phytotherapy regards OA not as a focal joint disease, but a systemic disorder, with emphasis placed on an alkaline-forming diet
- Herbs that make the body more alkaline are a key part of support in OA; the main herb in this category is Apium (celery seed). This herb is considered to increase the excretion of acidic metabolites in the urine. It probably also has anti-inflammatory activity. Another herb used for OA in this category is dandelion leaves
- Depuratives (alteratives), which are believed to aid in the clearance of metabolic waste from the body, are often recommended. These include Burdock and yellow dock, but the key herb is nettle leaf, which has been found to also have anti-inflammatory activity in arthritis (see nettle monograph)

- Bladderwrack is used for obese patients with arthritis because of its thyroid-stimulating activity, but may also have other effects
- St John's wort can be used where nerve entrapment is present. Because of its positive effect on the nervous system, particularly in cases of depression, it can also help to compensate for negative psychosocial factors and improve sleep quality
- Anti-inflammatory herbs are indicated and these include Boswellia, ginger and turmeric. Herbs which may modify cytokines and other inflammatory processes, for example Rehmannia, Bupleurum and Boswellia, and those working on NF-kappaB activation, such as feverfew, should be considered
- Willow bark is the key analgesic herb (see monograph)
- The importance of improving the circulation to affected joints has long been recognised and traditional support such as prickly ash can be supplemented with modern support from garlic, Ginkgo and celery seed
- Herbs to benefit the microcirculation are also relevant, such as grape seed and pine bark extracts (sources of OPCs), bilberry, gotu kola and Ginkgo
- Gotu kola should be considered as part of a long-term management to improve viability of chondrocytes.

Example liquid formula

Apium graveolens	1:2	35 mL
Urtica dioica	1:2	35 mL
Zingiber officinale	1:2	10 mL
Curcuma longa	1:1	30 mL
	TOTAL	110 mL

Dose: 8 mL with water twice per day.

CASE HISTORY

A 66-year-old male had been diagnosed with spinal stenosis, with a tendency to calcification in his body (e.g. the lower aorta). He was experiencing pain in the left side (referred pain) and also pain in his left hip (OA of the hip was confirmed by X-ray diagnosis). He was taking NSAID drugs and was previously a long-term smoker.

He was prescribed the following:

Ginkgo biloba (standardised extract)	2:1	20 mL
Hypericum perforatum	1:2	25 mL
Apium graveolens	1:2	35 mL
Taraxacum officinale leaf	1:1	20 mL
	TOTAL	100 mL

Dose: 8 mL with water twice a day.

Also nettle and birch leaf decoction, one to two heaped teaspoons per dose twice a day was recommended. After 7 months of treatment he was no longer experiencing any symptoms and was not taking the NSAID. He continued with the treatment at half the above doses.

The nettle and birch were prescribed for the arthritis and calcification tendency. Ginkgo was to improve microcirculation to joints and nerves (history of smoking) and St John's wort was for nerve entrapment pain.

CASE HISTORY

Small joint OA can be difficult to treat and is quite stubborn, presumably because of its hereditary aspect. A 58-year-old female patient had quite advanced disease with large deformities on all of her fingers, marked stiffness and moderate pain.

The patient was initially prescribed the following liquid formula:

Zingiber officinale	1:2	15 mL
Apium graveolens	1:2	50 mL
Urtica dioica	1:2	35 mL
	TOTAL	100 mL

Dose: 8 mL with water twice per day.

Tablets containing 1.9 g *Boswellia serrata*, 2.0 g *Curcuma longa*, 1.0 g *Apium graveolens* and 300 mg *Zingiber officinale* at 2 per day were also included.

Progress was initially steady but not dramatic. In the following 6 months tablets containing 8 g of *Salix purpurea* at 2 per day were added and the patient reported a big improvement in her pain and stiffness, despite being more active than usual.

Gout

Gout is a common arthritis caused by deposition of mono-sodium urate (MSU) crystals within joints following chronic hyperuricaemia.[49] It affects 1% to 2% of adults in developed countries where it is the most common inflammatory arthritis in men. Epidemiological studies suggest its incidence is rising. Diet, lifestyle and genetic defects in renal transporters of urate seem to be the main causative factors in primary gout. Gout and hyperuricaemia are associated with hypertension, type 2 diabetes, metabolic syndrome and renal and cardiovascular diseases.[49] In fact, gout appears to be a risk factor for all cause mortality and cardiovascular mortality and morbidity that is additional to the risk conferred by its association with traditional cardiovascular risk factors.[50] These co-morbidities can be either a cause or effect of gout. For example, elevated uric acid contributes to the development of essential hypertension.[51]

A 2011 review of the risk factors for gout identified 53 relevant studies.[52] Alcohol consumption, especially beer and spirits, increased the risk of incident gout. Several dietary factors are also implicated, including meat, seafood, sugar sweetened soft drinks and consumption of foods high in fructose (in keeping with gout's links to metabolic syndrome). Dairy, folate and coffee intake were each associated with a lower incidence of gout.

Many patients with gout present with an acute attack (flare) of gouty arthritis.[53] About 20% of patients have urinary tract stones and can develop an interstitial urate nephropathy. When the serum urate levels persistently exceed 6.8 mg/dL (0.4 mmol/L), extracellular fluids become saturated and hyperuricaemia occurs, with an increased risk of MSU precipitation. Although any joint can be affected, the metatarsophalangeal joint of the big toe is the first joint involved in half of all cases.

MSU crystals are potent inducers of inflammation. Within the joint they trigger a local inflammatory reaction, neutrophil recruitment and the production of proinflammatory cytokines.[54] Uptake of MSU crystals by monocytes involves interaction with components of the innate immune system, including Toll-like receptors (TLRs) and the NALP-3 (NLRP 3) inflammasome complex that drives production of interleukin(IL)-1beta. The inflammatory effects of MSU are IL-1-dependent.

Arthritic disease caused by accumulation of urate crystals at joints provides a particular indication for herbal remedies. There are a number which are claimed to increase elimination of urate from the kidneys, notably Apium (celery), Urtica (nettle) and Betula (birch). There is no doubt that prescriptions based on such herbs appear to ease the symptoms and even help to prevent recurrence. They thus provide a simple and probably safe treatment, especially when combined with a low purine diet (reduced red meat, offal, oily fish, red wine and port), so that urate metabolites are as reduced as far as possible.

Recent research has further informed the dietary and lifestyle advice for patients. Specifically, moderate intake of purine-rich vegetables (asparagus, mushrooms, peas and so on) or protein is not associated with an increased risk of gout.[55] Hence, these foods can be consumed in moderation. However, the above advice regarding avoidance or reduction of meat, seafood and alcohol has been soundly confirmed.[55,56] Low fat dairy products can be increased, as these appear to be protective,[57] and there are some promising preliminary studies supporting the time-honoured association of cherries with lowering serum uric acid.[58,59] Weight reduction with daily exercise and a low glycaemic index diet are also important considerations.[60]

The essentials of herbal treatment are as follows:

- Herbs containing significant levels of salicylates such as willow bark and meadowsweet are probably best avoided, since they may inhibit uric acid excretion (salicylates certainly block the action of uricosuric drugs).
- As noted above, the key herb is celery seed, which is believed to act as a uricosuric agent. Relatively high doses are necessary, and its activity can be improved by combination with dandelion leaves. Gravel root has been traditionally used for uric acid kidney stones and may contain components that inhibit xanthine oxidase. Nettle and birch leaves are also said to have the property of assisting uric acid removal.
- Depurative herbs, especially sarsaparilla, are also considered to be a key part of treatment.
- Anti-inflammatory herbs (perhaps except for willow bark) can be used for acute symptoms. (These are fully listed under Osteoarthritis in this section of the chapter.) Given the involvement of cytokines, Boswellia is probably a key choice.
- Uric acid is also excreted via the liver, and choleretic herbs such as dandelion root and globe artichoke can be indicated in a patient who exhibits symptoms of poor bile production.

- The beneficial effect of cherries may be due to the anthocyanins they contain. Hence bilberry may also have similar activity.

Example liquid formula

Apium graveolens	1:2	40 mL
Taraxacum officinale leaf	1:1	30 mL
Smilax ornata	1:2	30 mL
	TOTAL	100 mL

Dose: 8 mL with water twice a day.

CASE HISTORY

A male patient aged 56 years presented with severe gouty tophi in several fingers. He had been suffering gout for several years and had only recently commenced conventional medical treatment with allopurinol. He basically sought help with the reduction of the size and degree of inflammation of the tophi, otherwise his doctor wanted to remove part of two fingers. His serum uric acid was currently normal. Treatment consisted of the following:

Apium graveolens	1:2	70 mL
Smilax ornata	1:2	30 mL
	TOTAL	100 mL

Dose: 5 mL with water twice a day.

Topical treatment of the affected fingers, by bathing in a strong Epsom salts solution (once a day) and in a lotion of half Echinacea angustifolia root 1:2 and half Calendula 1:2, diluted 1 in 10 with water (twice a day), was instituted.

After several weeks of treatment, his fingers were much less painful and the swelling had reduced in size. After 6 months the appearance of his fingers was almost normal.

Repetitive strain injury/carpal tunnel syndrome

According to a 2007 review in The Lancet, repetitive strain injury (RSI) remains a controversial topic.[61] The label is applied to a wide range of specific disorders affecting the upper limbs or neck. The best known is carpal tunnel syndrome (CTS). Others include cubital tunnel syndrome, tendonitis of the wrist or hand, trigger finger, tennis elbow and so on. As the name implies, RSI results from repetitive movements, awkward postures, sustained force and other factors that impact on the normal use of a joint or group of joints. Other descriptive names for the problem include cumulative trauma disorder and occupational overuse syndrome.[61]

RSI is relatively common in adults of working age. The overall prevalence is conservatively thought to be between 5% and 10% of adults, but depending on the occupation this can go up to 40%.[61] Statistics show that industrial workers performing repetitive, monotonous movements are at a high risk, but athletes and musicians are also at risk. Long hours at a computer keyboard or using a mouse also can be factors.

The occurrence of CTS is quite high, with estimates ranging up to 14% of adults.[62] RSI is said to cost US industry about $6.5 billion every year.[61]

Given the high cost of RSI, it is surprising to learn that, relatively speaking, not much is known about its causes. Stresses at work and psychological distress seem to be contributive factors.[61] However, the factor common to all cases of RSI is overuse of muscle tendon units, causing a reactive inflammation that leads to pain and swelling (oedema) in the local tissues. This can lead to impairment or entrapment of nerves, which adds to the pain and causes other sensations such as parasthesia.[61] In the case of CTS, pressure at the carpal tunnel in the wrist is the most important factor, and being overweight can add to this.[62] In fact, some experts suggest that CTS is not really a sub-category of RSI, because overuse of the hands is not thought to play a significant role.[62]

Conventional medical treatment for RSI basically comprises the use of anti-inflammatory drugs, including cortisone injections.[61] For CTS, surgery is often used as a final resort. For non-specific, work-related RSI, immobilisation followed by exercise and manual therapy is often suggested. From the herbal perspective, published clinical studies in RSI are lacking, but clinical experience suggests there is much that can be done.

Herbs for RSI can be recommended on the basis of the known problems associated with the condition, such as inflammation, restricted blood flow, local oedema and nerve entrapment. There are many relevant anti-inflammatory herbs. These include devil's claw (*Harpagophytum procumbens*), cat's claw (*Uncaria tomentosa*), Boswellia (*Boswellia serrata*), celery seed (*Apium graveolens*), turmeric (*Curcuma longa*), ginger (*Zingiber officinale*) and willow bark (*Salix* species). Anti-inflammatory herbs also work well applied topically; the best ones for this purpose are Arnica (*Arnica montana*) and comfrey (*Symphytum* species). (See the relevant monographs for more details.)

Other key aspects of herbal treatment for RSI are as follows:

- St John's wort for the nerve entrapment
- Ginkgo for any ischaemic aspects associated with the nerve entrapment or restricted blood flow
- Horsechestnut and butcher's broom as anti-oedema agents to ameliorate local pressure.

Example liquid formula

Aesculus hippocastanum	1:2	25 mL
Hypericum perforatum	1:2	30 mL
Ginkgo biloba (standardised extract)	2:1	20 mL
Zingiber officinale	1:2	10 mL
Zanthoxylum clava-herculis	1:2	15 mL
	TOTAL	100 mL

Dose: 8 mL with water twice a day.

CASE HISTORY

Carpal tunnel syndrome

A 43-year-old woman had been diagnosed with carpal tunnel syndrome, with symptoms of pins and needles in both her hands. She also had periodical nosebleeds, although her blood pressure was normal, as were all other tests. She was prescribed the following formula:

Achillea millefolium	1:2	20 mL
Crataegus monogyna	1:2	20 mL
Panax notoginseng	1:2	20 mL
Aesculus hippocastanum	1:2	15 mL
Ginkgo biloba (standardised extract)	2:1	15 mL
Zanthoxylum clava-herculis	1:2	10 mL
	TOTAL	100 mL

Dose: 5 mL with water three times daily.

The yarrow (Achillea) and Tienchi ginseng were for the nosebleeds. After about 4 months of treatment, she commented that her hands were the best they had been for years and she had very few problems with her nose bleeding. Note that the treatment for the carpal tunnel syndrome in this case was largely circulatory.

Fibromyalgia syndrome

Fibromyalgia syndrome (FMS) is a disorder of unknown cause characterised by chronic widespread musculoskeletal pain and symptoms such as fatigue, sleep disturbances, gastrointestinal complaints and psychological problems.[63] One key diagnostic condition was the presence of multiple tender points on the body (11 of 18 tender points should be present, as defined by the American College of Rheumatology). However, not all patients meet this diagnostic hurdle. This has led to other diagnostic approaches. One such approach uses a widespread pain index in conjunction with a symptom severity scale.[64] Subclassification of FMS has also been proposed to better inform treatment approaches.[65]

Some clinicians now consider FMS is part of the spectrum of central sensitivity syndrome (CSS).[64] Clinical entities included under CSS include chronic fatigue syndrome (CFS), irritable bowel syndrome, temporomandibular disorder, idiopathic low back pain, multiple chemical sensitivity (MCS) and interstitial cystitis. Augmented pain and sensory processing in the CNS is suggested as the most reproducible pathogenic feature of these illnesses. This could be due to deficiencies in serotonergic and noradrenergic, but not opioidergic, transmission in the CNS, together with increases in pronociceptive neurotransmitters such as glutamate and substance P.[66]

As alluded to above, there is considerable co-morbidity between FMS, CFS and MCS. For example, a study of a cohort of CFS sufferers found 40.6% met the criteria for MCS and 15.6% met the criteria for fibromyalgia.[67] Another study found that 70% of tested CFS patients met the criteria for fibromyalgia.[68] The reverse association is also strong: 58% of a female group with fibromyalgia met the full criteria for CFS compared to 26.1% of a control group; for males the rates were even higher, 80.0% versus 22.2% for controls.[69] In fact, it has been suggested that FMS and CFS are possibly the same condition.[70]

However, while the literature does support the concept that there is much overlap between CFS and FMS, there are also studies that have been able to clearly differentiate the two conditions (see below). Since CFS and FMS have radically different clinical definitions that form the basis of their respective diagnoses, the possibility exists that they could represent the same underlying condition, but with different aspects of clinical expression. The analogy is somewhat akin to the proverb of the seven blind wise men who sought to explain the nature of the elephant. One felt the trunk of the elephant and concluded it was like a snake, another felt the tail and concluded it was like a rope, and so on.

In this context, an interesting US study examined 646 patients with CFS and/or FMS in terms of the presence or absence of a set of 32 common symptoms.[71] A technique known as latent class analysis demonstrated that essentially patients could be assigned, on the basis of their symptoms, into one of four classes. The mean symptom counts in Classes 1 to 4 were 26±2.0, 20±2.5, 16±2.8 and 11±2.9 respectively. Hence, each class was reasonably discrete from the others. It was found that the presence of CFS was lowest in the more severe class (Class 1) and highest in Class 4. FMS showed the reverse trend. Severity of fatigue was highest in Class 1 and lowest in Class 4. Hence, FMS could represent a more severe form of CFS:

> If our interpretation of our results is correct, what are the implications for understanding the clinical heterogeneity of chronic fatigue syndrome and fibromyalgia? In particular, it is notable that latent class analysis did not yield classes corresponding to chronic fatigue syndrome alone, fibromyalgia alone and comorbid chronic fatigue syndrome/fibromyalgia. These analyses would suggest that the clinical definitions of chronic fatigue syndrome and fibromyalgia are not particularly distinctive and that these syndromes are characterized by greater similarities than differences... . If the notion is correct – that the distinction between chronic fatigue syndrome and fibromyalgia is very fuzzy rather than sharp – rigid application of the existing case definitions of chronic fatigue syndrome and fibromyalgia may be more likely to lead to confusion than to clarity.

> There may be a clinical implication of our findings. It may prove to be the case that classifying patients according to a severity-related construct is more important or useful than (other) classification.

Despite the considerable evidence of the co-morbidity between CFS and FMS reviewed above, and the suggestion that they are not distinct clinical entities, a number of studies have found distinctive differences between them. A well-proven case in point is the observation that only patients fulfilling the definition of FMS (and not those with CFS) have elevated levels of substance P in their cerebrospinal fluid.[72,73] Substance P is a neurotransmitter involved in pain modulation. Higher levels in cerebrospinal fluid may promote peripheral nerve growth and abnormal pain perception. This suggests that more emphasis must be placed on pain management in the treatment of FMS.

Other differences noted in clinical studies include higher nocturnal levels of melatonin in FMS patients compared with CFS and healthy controls,[74] elevated levels of plasma endothelin-1 in FMS whereas levels in CFS are normal,[75] and differing protein profiles in cerebrospinal fluid[76] and urinary electrophoretic profiles between the two disorders.[77]

Some cardiovascular parameters differ between CFS and FMS. For example, haemodynamic instability using a tilt test demonstrated abnormalities for CFS in two studies. Values for FMS patients did not differ from healthy controls.[78,79] The results suggest that more emphasis must be placed on the cardiovascular system in the management of CFS. Patients with FMS often have marked sleep disturbances. In the opinion of one group, sleep disturbances are more marked in FMS than CFS. For CFS patients often the main complaint about sleep is that it is excessive and non-restorative. In contrast, FMS patients almost invariably suffer from less than average time asleep.[80]

There also appear to be marked differences in the neuroendocrine response between CFS and FMS. In particular, with CFS there may be a deficiency of corticotropin releasing 'hormone (CRH) production, while in FMS there may be excess. Patients with CFS have a mild central adrenal insufficiency, secondary to either a deficiency of CRH or some other central stimulus to the pituitary-adrenal axis.[81] In contrast, a review on hormonal perturbations in FMS asserted:[82]

> Recent studies of the entire endocrine profile of FM patients following a simultaneous challenge of the hypophysis with corticotropin-releasing hormone (CRH), thyrotropin-releasing hormone, growth hormone-releasing hormone, and luteinizing hormone-releasing hormone support the hypothesis that an elevated activity of CRH neurons determines not only many symptoms of FM but may also cause the deviations observed in the other hormonal axes.

These findings and the work of others suggest that an adrenal hyporesponsive state (adrenal depletion) is a distinctly characteristic feature of FMS.

In addition, there appears to be a state of autonomic dysfunction (dysautonomia) in FMS, with sympathetic nervous system hyperactivity.[83] Growth hormone levels may be abnormal in FMS and not in CFS.[73,79] Adult growth hormone deficiency is a well-described syndrome with many features reminiscent of fibromyalgia.[84] It has been postulated that thyroid hormone resistance is also a factor in FMS.[85] Patients with FMS were less responsive to injections of thyrotropin-releasing hormone in terms of thyrotropin and thyroid hormone production.[86] However, this could be the result of hypothalamic malfunction.

Like CFS, FMS can have an infectious trigger.[87] But also like CFS a wide variety of viruses have been associated with the disorder. Viral induced changes in cytokines have been suggested to play a role in fibromyalgia,[88,89] and one study found abnormal cytokine levels,[90] but not another.[91]

Given the similarities between CFS and FMS discussed above, the recommended herbs for FMS are similar to those for CFS outlined in Chapter 8. Specifically, these include:

- nervine tonic herbs such as *Hypericum perforatum* (St John's wort), which boosted growth hormone in a small uncontrolled trial,[92] Bacopa and *Scutellaria lateriflora*
- tonic, adaptogenic herbs and adrenal supportive herbs including Astragalus, Eleutherococcus, Rhodiola, *Panax ginseng*, Withania, Glycyrrhiza and Rehmannia
- immune-modulating herbs such as Echinacea root and Hemidesmus
- herbs supporting cognition such as Ginkgo and Bacopa.

In addition, issues that are more unique to FMS also require specific attention. Suggested herbal strategies include:

- anxiolytic and hypnotic herbs to reduce sympathetic overactivity and improve sleep quality such as *Piper methysticum* (kava), Valeriana, Passiflora, Vitex, *Zizyphus spinosa*, *Magnolia officinalis* and Crataegus
- anti-inflammatory and analgesic herbs to help address the disorder of central afferent processing and for pain management including Rehmannia, Apium, Boswellia, Curcuma, Salix, Bupleurum and OPCs from Vitis and Pinus
- antidepressant herbs such as Rhodiola, Hypericum and Lavandula
- a particular emphasis on the adrenal restorative herbs Glycyrrhiza and Rehmannia.

CASE HISTORY

A male patient aged 50 sought treatment for chronic fibromyalgia (considerably worse in the last 18 months). Fibromyalgia diagnosis was verified by a rheumatologist. Symptoms started around 10 years ago after a bout of Ross River virus.

Current problems, symptoms, issues included:

- persistent urinary tract infection, coughing bouts, postnasal drip
- lightheaded, blurred vision, poor memory and concentration
- anxious, disturbed sleep
- agonising muscular pain and a burning sensation in his feet

- frequent use of antibiotics and conventional NSAIDs
- fatigue and poor energy reserves
- constant nausea (which developed in prominence after the first consultation)
- sweet craving and a high carbohydrate diet.

The treatment approach settled on:

Ginkgo biloba (standardised extract)	2:1	20 mL
Hypericum perforatum (high hypericin)	1:2	20 mL
Echinacea purpurea/angustifolia root	1:2	30 mL
Euphrasia officinalis	1:2	20 mL
Cynara scolymus	1:2	20 mL
	TOTAL	110 mL

Dose: 8 mL with water twice daily.

Tablets containing 350 mg *Rehmannia glutinosa*, 700 mg *Bupleurum falcatum*, 500 mg *Hemidesmus indicus* and 165 mg *Tanacetum parthenium* at four tablets per day and also tablets containing 950 mg *Withania somnifera*, 750 mg *Glycyrrhiza glabra*, 470 mg *Scutellaria lateriflora* and 100 mg *Panax ginseng* at three per day.

Progress was very slow, but there were promising signs with some symptoms reducing after 2 to 3 months. Only after 5 months was an all-round improvement acknowledged when the patient reported:

- aches and pains generally much better
- last few weeks felt terrific, but overdid it
- nausea gone, energy levels good
- use of NSAIDs only needed when overdoes things
- sleep improved but still wakes up in the early hours.

Globe artichoke was replaced by chaste tree in the liquid formula to improve sleep quality, specifically to address his sleep maintenance insomnia.

References

1. Yip BY, Tam ACY. An experimental study on the effectiveness of massage with aromatic ginger and orange essential oil for moderate-to-severe knee pain among the elderly in Hong Kong. *Complement Ther Med.* 2008;16:131–138.

2. Altman RD, Marcussen KC. Effects of a ginger extract on knee pain in patients with osteoarthritis. *Arthritis Rheum.* 2001;44(11):2531–2538.

3. Minich DM, Jeffrey S, Bland JS. Acid-alkaline balance: role in chronic disease and detoxification. *Altern Ther Health Med.* 2007;13(4):62–65.

4. Remer T, Manz F. Potential renal acid load of foods and its influence on urine pH. *J Am Diet Assoc.* 1995;95(7):791–797.

5. McLean RR, Qiao N, Broe KE, et al. Dietary acid load is not associated with lower bone mineral density except in older men. *J Nutr.* 2011;141(4):588–594.

6. Soeken K, Miller S, Ernst E. Herbal medicines for the treatment of rheumatoid arthritis: a systematic review. *Rheumatology.* 2003;42:652–659.

7. Mills SY, Jacoby RK, Chacksfield M, Willoughby M. Effect of a proprietary herbal medicine on the relief of chronic arthritic pain: a double blind study. *Br J Rheumatol.* 1996;35:874–878.

8. Beer AM, Wegener T. Willow bark extract (Salicis cortex) for gonarthrosis and coxarthrosis – results of a cohort study with a control group. *Phytomedicine.* 2008;15:907–913.

9. Vlachojannis JE, Cameron M, Chrubasik S. A systematic review on the effectiveness of willow bark for musculoskeletal pain. *Phytotherapy Res.* 2009;23(7):897–900.

10. Sengupta K, Alluri KV, Satish AR, et al. A double blind, randomized, placebo controlled study of the efficacy and safety of 5-Loxin® for treatment of osteoarthritis of the knee. *Arthritis Res Ther.* 2008;10(4):85.

11. Kucera M, Barna M, Horacek O, et al. Efficacy and safety of topically applied Symphytum herb extract cream in the treatment of ankle distortion: results of a randomized controlled clinical double blind study. *Wien Med Wochenschr.* 2004;154:498–507.

12. Predel H, Giannetti B, Koll R, et al. Efficacy of a comfrey root extract ointment in comparison to a Diclofenac gel in the treatment of ankle distortions: results of an observer-blinded, randomized, multicenter study. *Phytomedicine.* 2005;12:707–714.

13. Brien S, Lewith GT, McGregor G. Devil's claw (Harpagophytum procumbens) as a treatment for osteoarthritis: a review of efficacy and safety. *J Altern Complement Med.* 2006;12(10):981–993.

14. Chrubasik S, Conradt C, Roufogalis BD. Effectiveness of Harpagophytum extracts and clinical efficacy. *Phytother Res.* 2004;18(2):187–189.

15. Chrubasik S, Enderlein W, Bauer R, Grabner W. Evidence for antirheumatic effectiveness of Herba Urticae dioicae in acute arthritis: a pilot study. *Phytomedicine.* 1997;4(2):105–108.

16. Gagnier JJ, van Tulder M, Berman B, Bombardier C. Herbal medicine for low back pain. *Cochrane Database Syst Rev.* 2006;(2):CD004504.

17. Warholm O, Skaar S, Hedman E, et al. The effects of a standardized herbal remedy made from a subtype of Rosa canina in patients with osteoarthritis: a double blind, randomized, placebo-controlled clinical trial. *Curr Ther Res Clin Exp.* 2003;64(1):21–31.

18. Winther K, Apel K, Thamsborg G. A powder made from seeds and shells of a rose hip subspecies (Rosa canina) reduces symptoms of knee and hip osteoarthritis:

a randomized, double blind, placebo-controlled trial. *Scand J Rheumatol.* 2005;34:302–308.

19. Von Kruedener S, Schneider W, Elstner EF. A combination of populus tremula, solidago virgaurea and fraxinus excelsior as an anti-inflammatory and antirheumatic drug. *Arzneimittelforschung.* 1995;45(2):169–171.

20. Van Weeren PR, de Grauw JC. Pain in osteoarthritis. *Vet Clin North Am Equine Pract.* 2010;26(3):619–642.

21. Heinegård D, Saxne T. The role of the cartilage matrix in osteoarthritis. *Nat Rev Rheumatol.* 2011;7(1):50–56.

22. Zhang Y, Jordan JM. Epidemiology of osteoarthritis. *Clin Geriatr Med.* 2010;26(3):355–369.

23. Valdes AM, Spector TD. The clinical relevance of genetic susceptibility to osteoarthritis. *Best Pract Res Clin Rheumatol.* 2010;24(1):3–14.

24. Felson DT. An update on the pathogenesis and epidemiology of osteoarthritis. *Radiol Clin North Am.* 2004;42(1):1–9.

25. Lohmander LS, Felson D. Can we identify a 'high risk' patient profile to determine who will experience rapid progression of osteoarthritis? *Osteoarthritis Cartilage.* 2004;12(suppl A):S49–S52.

26. Dawson J, Juszczak E, Thorogood M, et al. An investigation of risk factors for symptomatic osteoarthritis of the knee in women using a life course approach. *J Epidemiol Community Health.* 2003;57(10):823–830.

27. Cheung PP, Gossec L, Dougados M. What are the best markers for disease progression in osteoarthritis (OA)? *Best Pract Res Clin Rheumatol.* 2010;24(1):81–92.

28. Rossignol M, Leclerc A, Hilliquin P, et al. Primary osteoarthritis and occupations: a national cross sectional survey of 10 412 symptomatic patients. *Occup Environ Med.* 2003;60(11):882–886.

29. Martel-Pelletier J, Pelletier JP. Is osteoarthritis a disease involving only cartilage or other articular tissues? *Eklem Hastalik Cerrahisi.* 2010;21(1):2–14.

30. Umlauf D, Frank S, Pap T, et al. Cartilage biology, pathology, and repair. *Cell Mol Life Sci.* 2010;67(24):4197–4211.

31. Attur M, Samuels J, Krasnokutsky S, et al. Targeting the synovial tissue for treating osteoarthritis (OA): where is the evidence? *Best Pract Res Clin Rheumatol.* 2010;24(1):71–79.

32. Kwan Tat S, Lajeunesse D, Pelletier JP, et al. Targeting subchondral bone for treating osteoarthritis: what is the evidence? *Best Pract Res Clin Rheumatol.* 2010;24(1):51–70.

33. Bondeson J. Activated synovial macrophages as targets for osteoarthritis drug therapy. *Curr Drug Targets.* 2010;11(5):576–585.

34. Marcu KB, Otero M, Olivotto E, et al. NF-kappaB signaling: multiple angles to target OA. *Curr Drug Targets.* 2010;11(5):599–613.

35. Rogers J, Shepstone L, Dieppe P. Is osteoarthritis a systemic disorder of bone? *Arthritis Rheum.* 2004;50(2):452–457.

36. DeGroot J, Verzijl N, Wenting-van Wijk MJ, et al. Accumulation of advanced glycation end products as a molecular mechanism for aging as a risk factor in osteoarthritis. *Arthritis Rheum.* 2004;50(4):1207–1215.

37. Steenvoorden MM, Huizinga TWJ, Verzijl N, et al. Activation of receptor for advanced glycation end products in osteoarthritis leads to increased stimulation of chondrocytes and synoviocytes. *Arthritis Rheum.* 2006;54(1):253–263.

38. Ogino S, Sasho T, Nakagawa K, et al. Detection of pain-related molecules in the subchondral bone of osteoarthritic knees. *Clin Rheumatol.* 2009;28(12):1395–1402.

39. Kornaat PR, Sharma R, van der Geest RJ, et al. Positive association between increased popliteal artery vessel wall thickness and generalized osteoarthritis: is OA also part of the metabolic syndrome? *Skeletal Radiol.* 2009;38(12):1147–1151.

40. Conaghan PG, Vanharanta H, Dieppe PA. Is progressive osteoarthritis an atheromatous vascular disease? *Ann Rheum Dis.* 2005;64(11):1539–1541.

41. Cheras PA, Whitaker AN, Blackwell EA, et al. Hypercoagulability and hypofibrinolysis in primary osteoarthritis. *Clin Orthop Relat Res.* 1997;334:57–67.

42. Findlay DM. Vascular pathology and osteoarthritis. *Rheumatology.* 2007;46(12):1763–1768.

43. Ammon HP. Modulation of the immune system by Boswellia serrata extracts and boswellic acids. *Phytomedicine.* 2010;17(11):862–867.

44. Farid R, Mirfeizi Z, Mirheidari M, et al. Pycnogenol supplementation reduces pain and stiffness and improves physical function in adults with knee osteoarthritis. *Nutr Res.* 2007;27(11):692–697.

45. Belcaro G, Cesarone MR, Errichi S, et al. Treatment of osteoarthritis with Pycnogenol. The SVOS (San Valentino Osteo-arthrosis Study). Evaluation of signs, symptoms, physical performance and vascular aspects. *Phytother Res.* 2008;22(4):518–523.

46. Belcaro G, Cesarone MR, Errichi S, et al. Variations in C-reactive protein, plasma free radicals and fibrinogen values in patients with osteoarthritis treated with Pycnogenol. *Redox Rep.* 2008;13(6):271–276.

47. Cisár P, Jány R, Waczulíková I, et al. Effect of pine bark extract (Pycnogenol) on symptoms of knee osteoarthritis. *Phytother Res.* 2008;22(8):1087–1092.

48. Williams FM, Skinner J, Spector TD, et al. Dietary garlic and hip osteoarthritis: evidence of a protective effect and putative mechanism of action. *BMC Musculoskelet Disord.* 2010;11:280.

49. Richette P, Bardin T. Gout. *Lancet.* 2010;375(9711):318–328.

50. Roddy E, Doherty M. Epidemiology of gout. *Arthritis Res Ther.* 2010;12(6):223.

51. Mazzali M, Kanbay M, Segal MS, et al. Uric acid and hypertension: cause or effect? *Curr Rheumatol Rep.* 2010;12(2):108–117.

52. Singh JA, Reddy SG, Kundukulam J. Risk factors for gout and prevention: a systematic review of the literature. *Curr Opin Rheumatol.* 2011;23(2):192–202.

53. Becker MA, Ruoff GE. What do I need to know about gout? *J Fam Pract.* 2010;59(suppl 6):S1–S8.

54. So A. Developments in the scientific and clinical understanding of gout. *Arthritis Res Ther.* 2008;10(5):221.

55. Choi HK, Atkinson K, Karlson EW, et al. Purine-rich foods, dairy and protein intake, and the risk of gout in men. *N Engl J Med.* 2004;350(11):1093–1103.

56. Schlesinger N. Dietary factors and hyperuricaemia. *Curr Pharm Des.* 2005;11(32):4133–4138.

57. Choi HK, Liu S, Curhan G. Intake of purine-rich foods, protein, and dairy products and relationship to serum levels of uric acid: the third national health and nutrition examination survey. *Arthritis Rheum.* 2005;52(1):283–289.

58. Jacob RA, Spinozzi GM, Simon VA, et al. Consumption of cherries lowers plasma urate in healthy women. *J Nutr.* 2003;133(6):1826–1829.

59. Howatson G, McHugh MP, Hill JA, et al. Influence of tart cherry juice on indices of recovery following marathon running. *Scand J Med Sci Sports.* 2010;20(6):843–852.

60. Choi HK. A prescription for lifestyle change in patients with hyperuricemia and gout. *Curr Opin Rheumatol.* 2010;22(2):165–172.

61. van Tulder M, Malmivaara A, Koes B. Repetitive strain injury. *Lancet.* 2007;369(9575):1815–1822.

62. Bland JDP. Carpal tunnel syndrome. *BMJ.* 2007;335:343–346.

63. Adler GK, Manfredsdottir VF, Creskoff KW. Neuroendocrine abnormalities in fibromyalgia. *Curr Pain Headache Rep.* 2002;6(4):289–298.

64. Smith HS, Harris R, Clauw D. Fibromyalgia: an afferent processing disorder leading to a complex pain generalized syndrome. *Pain Physician.* 2011;14(2):E217–E245.

65. de Miquel CA, Campayo JG, Flórez MT, et al. Interdisciplinary consensus document for the treatment of fibromyalgia. *Actas Esp Psiquiatr.* 2010;38(2):108–120.

66. Clauw DJ. Fibromyalgia: an overview. *Am J Med.* 2009;122(suppl 12):S3–S13.

67. Jason LA, Taylor RR, Kennedy CL. Chronic fatigue syndrome, fibromyalgia, and multiple chemical sensitivities in a community-based sample of persons with chronic fatigue syndrome-like symptoms. *Psychosom Med.* 2000;62(5):655–663.

68. Goldenberg DL, Simms RW, Geiger A, Komaroff AL. High frequency of fibromyalgia in patients with chronic fatigue seen in a primary care practice. *Arthritis Rheum.* 1990;33(3):381–387.

69. White KP, Speechley M, Harth M, Ostbye T. Co-existence of chronic fatigue syndrome with fibromyalgia syndrome in the general population. A controlled study. *Scand J Rheumatol*. 2000;29(1): 44–51.

70. McKay PG, Duffy T, Martin CR. Are chronic fatigue syndrome and fibromyalgia the same? Implications for the provision of appropriate mental health intervention. *J Psychiatr Ment Health Nurs*. 2009;16(10):884–894.

71. Sullivan PF, Smith W, Buchwald D. Latent class analysis of symptoms associated with chronic fatigue syndrome and fibromyalgia. *Psychol Med*. 2002;32(5): 881–888.

72. Evengard B, Nilsson CG, Lindh G, et al. Chronic fatigue syndrome differs from fibromyalgia. No evidence for elevated substance P levels in cerebrospinal fluid of patients with chronic fatigue syndrome. *Pain*. 1998;78(2):153–155.

73. Nampiaparampil DE, Shmerling RH. A review of fibromyalgia. *Am J Manag Care*. 2004;10(11 Pt 1):794–800.

74. Korszun A, Sackett-Lundeen L, Papadopoulos E, et al. Melatonin levels in women with fibromyalgia and chronic fatigue syndrome. *J Rheumatol*. 1999;26(12):2675–2680.

75. Kennedy G, Spence V, Khan F, et al. Plasma endothelin-1 levels in chronic fatigue syndrome. *Rheumatology (Oxford)*. 2004;43(2):252–253.

76. Baraniuk JN, Casado B, Maibach H, et al. A chronic fatigue syndrome – related proteome in human cerebrospinal fluid. *BMC Neurol*. 2005;5:22.

77. Casado B, Zanone C, Annovazzi L, et al. Urinary electrophoretic profiles from chronic fatigue syndrome and chronic fatigue syndrome/fibromyalgia patients: a pilot study for achieving their normalization. *J Chromatogr B Analyt Technol Biomed Life Sci*. 2005;814(1):43–51.

78. Naschitz JE, Sabo E, Naschitz S, et al. Hemodynamic instability in chronic fatigue syndrome: indices and diagnostic significance. *Semin Arthritis Rheum*. 2001;31(3):199–208.

79. Parker AJ, Wessely S, Cleare AJ. The neuroendocrinology of chronic fatigue syndrome and fibromyalgia. *Psychol Med*. 2001;31(8):1331–1345.

80. Schaefer KM. Sleep disturbances linked to fibromyalgia. *Holist Nurs Pract*. 2003;17(3):120–127.

81. Demitrack MA, Dale JK, Straus SE, et al. Evidence for impaired activation of the hypothalamic-pituitary-adrenal axis in patients with chronic fatigue syndrome. *J Clin Endocrinol Metab*. 1991;73(6): 1224–1234.

82. Neeck G, Riedel W. Hormonal pertubations in fibromyalgia syndrome. *Ann N Y Acad Sci*. 1999;876:325–338.

83. Martinez-Lavin M. Biology and therapy of fibromyalgia. Stress, the stress response system, and fibromyalgia. *Arthritis Res Ther*. 2007;9(4):216.

84. Bennett RM. Adult growth hormone deficiency in patients with fibromyalgia. *Curr Rheumatol Rep*. 2002;4(4):306–312.

85. Garrison RL, Breeding PC. A metabolic basis for fibromyalgia and its related disorders: the possible role of resistance to thyroid hormone. *Med Hypotheses*. 2003;61(2):182–189.

86. Neeck G, Riedel W. Thyroid function in patients with fibromyalgia syndrome. *J Rheumatol*. 1992;19(7):1120–1122.

87. Buskila D, Atzeni F, Sarzi-Puttini P. Etiology of fibromyalgia: the possible role of infection and vaccination. *Autoimmun Rev*. 2008;8(1):41–43.

88. Thompson ME, Barkhuizen A. Fibromyalgia hepatitis C infection, and the cytokine connection. *Curr Pain Headache Rep*. 2003;7(5):342–347.

89. Rea T, Russo J, Katon W, et al. A prospective study of tender points and fibromyalgia during and after an acute viral infection. *Arch Intern Med*. 1999;159(8):865–870.

90. Wallace DJ, Linker-Israeli M, Hallegua D, et al. Cytokines play an aetiopathogenetic role in fibromyalgia: a hypothesis and pilot study. *Rheumatology (Oxford)*. 2001;40(7):743–749.

91. Amel Kashipaz MR, Swinden D, Todd I, et al. Normal production of inflammatory cytokines in chronic fatigue and fibromyalgia syndromes determined by intracellular cytokine staining in short-term cultured blood mononuclear cells. *Clin Exp Immunol*. 2003;132(2):360–365.

92. Franklin M, Chi J, McGavin C, et al. Neuroendocrine evidence for dopaminergic actions of hypericum extract (LI 160) in healthy volunteers. *Biol Psychiatry*. 1999;46(4):581–584.

Skin diseases

Scope

Apart from their use to provide non-specific support for recuperation and repair, specific phytotherapeutic strategies include the following.

Treatment of:

- eczema (atopic dermatitis)
- some cases of psoriasis and immunological skin diseases
- contact and other allergic skin disease
- superficial fungal infections
- acne and furunculosis
- viral infections.

Management of:

- chronic psoriatic disease
- rosacea.

Because of its use of secondary plant products, **caution** is necessary in applying phytotherapy topically over some:

- broken skin
- mucosal surfaces.

Note: contact sensitivity reactions are possible to almost any ingredient in the vehicles (e.g. creams and ointments) for topical applications to skin disease.

Orientation

Internal and external applications

Phytotherapy provides two unique approaches to the treatment of skin inflammations. Firstly, there are particular physical and pharmacological properties in plant constituents that possess topical and cosmetic benefits directly on external application,[1,2] and which are discussed further in Chapter 8 and below. Secondly, there are developed medicinal strategies for treating skin problems as manifestations of internal disease, such that most herbal prescriptions are taken orally.[3] For both reasons, and in spite of a relative lack of clinical research data, phytotherapy can be recommended as a dermatological strategy. Nevertheless, skin diseases are among the most complex and inconsistent categories in medicine. There are many (including malignant tumours, bullous diseases, alopecia areata and pigmentary disorders) that are probably beyond conservative treatment, others (such as pityriasis rosea and lichen planus) that usually do not need treatment at all and some that are wholly unpredictable. It is unrealistic to claim consistent performance for phytotherapy either. What is offered below is a number of pragmatic options, productively to be considered along with conventional prescription, as well as other complementary approaches, dietary and psychotherapeutic treatments.

A signpost to an enigma?

There are few clear guides to understanding skin diseases. The origin of a proportion can be traced to simple sources, bacterial, viral or fungal infections for example (although a good practitioner would still aim to investigate ultimate causes for these too) or toxic exposures, but the great majority are largely mysterious. Even attempts to distinguish external (exogenous) and endogenous disease are not very helpful. It may look a simple matter that someone has a contact dermatitis to this, that or the other, or that eliminating milk products apparently resolves eczema, but the internal reasons for such sensitivity are left unaddressed. For most skin disease, it is almost impossible to pick out substantive causative factors. Although dermatology is an impressive discipline in terms of differential diagnosis (distinguishing plantar psoriasis from tinea pedis or sarcoidosis from granuloma anulare), there is remarkably little to say about the causes of most skin diseases and the specialty is remarkably bereft of curative strategies. Topical and systemic corticosteroids largely replaced coal-tar products in the 1950s, but these remain the pillars of dermatological treatment, although palliative only.

It is clear that much skin disease is very complex. Notable are those linked to immunological disorders. Psoriasis is specifically an immunological skin disease, but there are many others with greater or lesser association with internal autoimmune disorders: discoid lupus erythematosus, scleroderma, and dermatomyositis. Already in some such cases links have been made between the skin symptoms and events deep in the body (see also Chapter 8). These conditions are also the most inconsistent and refractory; remission may be possible in some individuals but relapses are at least as common and neither change is likely to show much pattern. Clinical experience is that each individual case history is unlike any other and that the landmarks of deterioration, used by practitioners as clues to the construction of a therapeutic strategy, show few common themes.

Although the various skin inflammations diagnosed as eczema are more likely to be considered as local defects (a dermatitis only), it is also certain that these can reflect a wide variety of environmental, dietary and psychological/emotional influences. Again it is hard to avoid the conclusion that the skin manifests deeper disorders; that treatment seems more appropriate directed from the inside out.

Traditional observers of skin disease were almost unanimous in seeing it as a wider disturbance within. Given the paucity of treatment options in conventional dermatology, it may be time to reconsider some of the older strategies.

A suitable case for cleansing

An almost universal view of skin diseases in the past was that they were signals of inner toxicities, accumulations of irritants

that the normal eliminatory functions had failed to remove. The variety of possible problems reflected a great variety of toxicities and most developed traditions had a wide range of diagnoses and treatments. The metaphors used were those found elsewhere in these humoral systems. In the meteorological analogies used, toxicity was often equated with 'damp', which in turn reflected disorders of the digestive system and liver. The fluctuation in some skin problems was seen to reflect the influence of 'wind', the consequence of disturbances in metabolic balance, in the balance of heating and cooling. Those that currently would be classified as allergic eczemas might have been considered 'dry' in earlier times, with reference to the gut and respiratory system. Skin disease could also be predominantly 'hot' or 'cold'. In other words, treatments might extend across the whole range of traditional materia medica, depending on details of the indication, mostly through applying remedies that were also seen to be eliminative.

Folk traditions were generally less sophisticated, but the concept of skin disease as a toxicity symptom was consistent. In European traditions, for example, skin problems were treated with 'blood cleansers' and 'blood purifiers' and the terms 'depurative' and 'dyscratic' are also derived from this perspective. In China, some remedies were seen as simply good at eliminating poison and were often used as folk treatments for skin diseases. The more acute and severe the skin inflammations, the more robust the remedy used.

Unfortunately there is a gaping lack of modern clinical research for the traditional internal strategies for skin disease. The one notable exception is, however, encouraging.

Two double blind, controlled, clinical trials published by a London team of dermatologists and immunologists in 1992 showed significant efficacy of a herb formulation taken internally. In one study, 40 adult patients with chronic, refractory, widespread atopic dermatitis in crossover between active treatment and placebo herbs showed that substantial benefits followed the use of the Chinese herbs.[4] In a second, 47 children with a chronic extensive morbilliform variant of non-exudative atopic eczema were given Chinese herbs and placebo herbs in random order, each for 8 weeks, with an intervening 4-week washout period. In 37 who completed the study, the difference in benefits was clear.[5] Follow-up studies in both cases were also positive. One year after the trial, all subjects on treatment in the first study showed significant benefit; although none were able to discontinue permanently, most had reduced dosage. By contrast, mean scores for untreated individuals showed deterioration.[6] A 1-year follow-up on the children trial showed that over 50% of patients showed significant lasting benefit and 20% were able to stop treatment with complete remission.[7]

Inevitable safety issues were raised, not least by the authors of the papers themselves (who recommend routine monitoring of liver function tests and tight exclusion criteria for treatment). For example, two cases of acute hepatic illness have been associated with the use of Chinese herbs for eczema[8] and one case of severe cardiomyopathy was reported after a 2-week course of such treatment.[9] Nevertheless, actual reports in the clinical trials were not alarming. In the follow-up of the children trial after a year of continuous treatment, two patients taking treatment had raised asymptomatic AST (aspartate aminotransferase) levels, but there were no abnormalities in either full blood counts or biochemical parameters in any adult patient on continued treatment after a year.

The implications of such work have been lost on wider medical thinking, and follow-up attempts to develop a less complex marketable formula foundered. However, it demonstrates that it is possible to design appropriate studies applying traditional diagnoses as inclusion criteria and it is fervently to be hoped that more studies will be forthcoming. One case where internal approaches have been tested is a study on the effects of orally consumed cocoa flavanols on photosensitivity (as measured by skin sensitivity, cutaneous blood flow, transepidermal water loss, and skin structure, texture and hydration after UV irradiation). In a controlled study comparing high and low flavanol cocoa in 24 healthy women over 12 weeks, those consuming the high flavanol version had significantly reduced skin sensitivity to UV.[10] This study reinforces similar protective properties reported for carotenoids and lycopene products. Similar studies exist for the internal use of *Centella asiatica* (see the gotu kola monograph).

Topical treatments

Chapter 2 will lead the reader to many plant constituents with appreciable direct action on body tissues. There is a wide range of herbal applications to skin lesions, where the skin barrier is damaged. The section on topical applications in Chapter 8 should also be consulted. In summary, the following characteristics of herbal remedies are relevant.

Demulcents

These are helpful in reducing pruritus (itching) and inflammatory pain due to skin disease. In some cases, longer-term healing can result.

Lipids

Plant lipids can slow moisture loss from and smooth rough, scaly skin. *Ricinus communis* (castor bean) oil is a common basis for ointment, sometimes combined with zinc. Oils of *Oenothera biennis* (evening primrose), *Borago officinalis* (borage, starflower), *Cannabis sativa* (hemp) and *Ribes nigrum* (black currant) seeds have high gamma-linolenic acid and are also widely applied.

Astringents

These can sometimes be dramatically helpful where the skin is broken and discharging. As well as providing temporary relief, a strong astringent application can reduce discharge, reduce sepsis and promote healing.

Antiseptics

On a basic level, these are used for containing fungal conditions (like tinea and candida) and bacterial infections (erysipelas, furunculosis). The oil of *Melaleuca alternifolia* (tea tree) has been shown to be modestly effective in cases of the fungal skin infection tinea pedis after 4 weeks' application of two doses in a blinded, placebo-controlled clinical trial with 158 patients (see also Chapters 2 and 8).[11]

Topical anti-inflammatories

In addition to immediate, often physical, properties, a number of plants have demonstrated useful anti-inflammatory properties in skin conditions in clinical trials (see also Chapter 8). The known systemic effects of the boswellic acids were tested topically in a double blind placebo-controlled study on the effects of photo-aging on the faces of 15 women, each acting as her own control. The cream containing boswellic acids comparatively reduced measures of photo-ageing skin damage, such as transepidermal water loss and skin thinning over 30 days, sustained after 2 months of followup.[12] It was considered that this benefit involved improved keratinisation and repair in the damaged skin. In another study that claimed to be blinded, 86 patients diagnosed with alopecia areata were divided into treatment and control groups. The treatment group performed a daily scalp massage with the essential oils *Thymus vulgaris* (thyme), *Lavandula angustifolia* (lavender), *Rosmarinus officinalis* (rosemary) and *Cedrus atlantica* (cedar) in a carrier oil blend of jojoba and grapeseed. They then wrapped a warm towel around the head to aid absorption of the oils. The control group performed the same procedure with only a moderately perfumed carrier oil combination. On a blind double-marking of standardised photographs, 44% of the treatment group showed significant improvement compared with 15% of the control group.[13]

Curcumin from turmeric also has pronounced anti-inflammatory action on the skin. An open label study found that phosphorylase kinase was highly elevated in 10 untreated psoriasis patients and was substantially and significantly reduced to near normal in 10 patients using a topical curcumin (as a 1% gel preparation).[14] A small uncontrolled trial in 12 patients with psoriasis given curcuminoids (4.5g/day) for 12 weeks found that two of the eight patients who completed the trial had responded to treatment.[15] A larger placebo-controlled trial is necessary, as suggested by the authors. A US dermatologist described the successful outcomes of a number of cases treated with topical curcumin in the same gel preparation referred to above (see turmeric monograph for more details).[16]

Phytotherapeutics

A strategic approach

A good clinician will have no set treatments for skin diseases. It is of course helpful to have a good diagnosis, so that treatment can be better directed. However, even then one reverts quickly to first principles. How are the fundamental body functions? In particular, is there evidence of difficulties in digestive, hepatobiliary and bowel or other eliminatory functions? If there is an immunological component, as in autoimmune or allergic conditions, then events at the gut wall or lumen are even more likely to be factors; they should be tracked down assiduously, with techniques such as rigorous experimental dietary eliminations to elucidate particular difficulties. The priority of treatment is to work at such 'primary lesions'. It may then be helpful to apply a humoral classification; is there evidence of patterns that might once have been classified as damp, dryness, cold, heat and/or wind? Remedies that dry, moisten, cool, heat or balance respectively could then feature in the prescription. More widely, skin disorders can be considered as inflammatory conditions and approached strategically using insights developed in the relevant sections in Chapter 8.

The treatment of acne and furunculosis may particularly suggest bowel treatments: rosacea and allergic drug eruptions, heptobiliary and bowel remedies. Particularly in such cases one would understandably revert to traditional alterative depurative remedies (see below), especially if their role overlapped with what had been determined as primary problems.

Healing crises?

Skin disease is particularly prone to exacerbations during treatment. It can take very little to provoke this adverse result and 'healing crises' are common in homeopathic and dietary treatments of skin disease (for example, in fasting). Some proponents of the latter disciplines claim these are a good thing, a sign that 'toxins are coming out'. An immersion in pathophysiological mechanisms of skin inflammation would discourage this view and it is not even internally consistent as a notion. Skin inflammation is by definition an extraordinary event, involving a range of traumata in the dermal tissues that have little intrinsic value. If in traditional terms skin diseases suggest inadequacies in the ordinary eliminatory and processing functions, then having even more toxins coming out of the skin, even briefly, does not recommend itself.

There is only one exception to the inadequacy of the healing crisis as a technique in treating skin disease. In cases of low-grade chronic skin trouble, where lack of activity is a characteristic of the condition, promoting subacute or acute crises has been a traditional manoeuvre to render the condition a little more vulnerable to treatment. In most other cases, clinical experience suggests exacerbations beyond a few initial days rarely lead to benefits in the long term; indeed, the opposite is normally true.

A good herbal practitioner will therefore aim for the minimum exacerbation, promoting the defective functions so as to diffuse the pathology. Given the readiness with which exacerbation does occur, a treatment strategy that led to progressive relief without a healing crisis would be something of a triumph.

Plant remedies traditionally used as alteratives/depuratives

- *Arctium lappa* (burdock root), *Berberis aquifolium* (Oregon grape root),[17] *Fumaria officinalis* (fumitory), *Galium aparine* (cleavers), *Iris versicolor* (blue flag), *Juglans regia* (walnut), *Rumex crispus* (yellow dock root), *Scrophularia nodosa* (figwort), *Trifolium pratense* (red clover flowers), *Urtica dioica* (nettle), *Viola tricolor* (heartsease).

Indications for alteratives/depuratives

- Skin disease traditionally associated with toxaemia or septicaemia (e.g. furunculosis, some cases of acne)
- Many cases of eczema
- Some cases of urticaria
- Most other skin diseases (as components of wider acting prescriptions).

Other traditional indications for alteratives/depuratives

- Joint diseases
- Connective tissue diseases
- Any wider detoxification regime (e.g. spring fasts).

Contraindications for alteratives/depuratives

Depuratives can in many cases be provocative to skin disease. Care needs to be taken to reduce the prospects for major exacerbations (see Healing crises? above).

Traditional therapeutic insights into the use of alteratives/depuratives

Depuratives were seen primarily to detoxify, to help eliminatory and processing functions reduce the metabolic waste products accumulating. It was seen to be better to stimulate elimination than processing or at least to conduct therapy in that order. Increased processing, without elimination would be exacerbatory. Similarly, any remedy that led to increased constipation or other elimination would often be accompanied by exacerbation. Arctium (burdock) is notable for its potential for exacerbation; it should be used carefully, well combined with, or preceded by, more eliminatory remedies.

Application

Long-term therapy with depuratives is often appropriate and is usually safe.

Phytotherapy

Atopic dermatitis (eczema)

Eczema, or dermatitis, is a pruritic inflammatory skin reaction that manifests with variable clinical and histological pictures. Atopic dermatitis (AD) is a dermatitis linked to the atopic state. The patient is troubled by itching skin and there is a history of chronic or chronically relapsing dermatitis, worse on the flexures, and a family or personal history of atopy (asthma, hayfever and urticaria). The incidence of AD is increasing worldwide. Patients with AD are at a higher risk for progressing in the atopic march to asthma.[18]

AD can be categorised into extrinsic and intrinsic types.[19] Extrinsic or allergic AD shows high total serum IgE levels and the presence of specific IgE for environmental and food allergens, whereas patients with intrinsic or non-allergic AD exhibit normal total IgE values and the absence of specific IgE. While extrinsic AD is the classical type with a high prevalence, the incidence of intrinsic AD is approximately 20%, with a female predominance. Clinical features of intrinsic AD include relatively late onset, milder severity and Dennie-Morgan folds, but no ichthyosis vulgaris or palmar hyperlinearity. The skin barrier is perturbed in the extrinsic, but not the intrinsic, type. Filaggrin gene mutations are also not a feature of intrinsic AD (see below). The intrinsic type is immunologically characterised by the lower expression of interleukin (IL)-4, IL-5 and IL-13, and the higher expression of IFN-gamma. It is suggested that intrinsic AD patients are not sensitised with protein allergens, which induce Th2 responses, but with other antigens, and metals might be one of the candidates for such antigens.[19]

As touched on above, specific genetic defects in the epidermal barrier occur in a significant percentage of AD sufferers. The loss-of-function mutations in the structural protein filaggrin, with resultant enhanced transepidermal water loss, are consistent with a unifying hypothesis that offers a mechanistic understanding of AD pathogenesis.[20] A diminished epidermal defence to allergens and microbes is followed by polarised Th2 lymphocyte responses with resultant chronic inflammation, including autoimmune mechanisms.

There is a longstanding controversy as to whether allergy is a major pathogenic factor in AD. Several studies have associated food allergy, inhalant allergens and skin contact with airborne allergens with AD.[21] Even in the absence of a specific IgE for house dust mites, infants with AD have proliferative T cell responses to these antigens. The role of restricting food allergens in the treatment of AD remains controversial in the mainstream literature,[22] although one review suggested that egg-exclusion diets could be of value.[23] Another review proposed that, while food allergy is an important provoking cause of AD, elimination diets are only relevant in about 35% of affected individuals.[24] Milk, eggs, wheat, soya and peanuts account for 75% of the cases of food-induced AD. Other clinicians do advocate elimination diets over a period of 4 to 6 weeks in AD sufferers with a high serum IgE and positive skin prick tests.[25]

Other allergens implicated in AD include those from microorganisms and aeroallergens such as pollen, mold and dust mite.[25] Dust mite sensitivity appears to be particularly important.[26] One clinic with experience of more than 18 000 AD patients also suggested a role for pseudoallergic mechanisms through toxic environmental agents (pollutants, solvents, pesticides and so on).[27] A double blind, controlled trial found that house dust mite avoidance measures greatly reduced the activity of AD, especially in children.[28] Responses to this therapy varied considerably, despite the fact that allergic reactivity to house dust mite antigens can be established by prick-test challenge in virtually all patients with AD.

These observations highlight a potential misconception concerning allergen exposure in this disorder: a positive skin-prick test (which tests for an IgE-based response) does not necessarily identify those allergens that might be contributing to the underlying immunological disturbance. Some patients with a positive skin reaction to dust mite do not respond to reduced exposure. A corollary is that food allergens are not necessarily identified by a prick-test challenge, although the study described below illustrates that it can be a useful, but not infallible, guide.

Twenty-six children with AD and markedly elevated serum IgE concentrations were evaluated for clinical evidence of hypersensitivity to foods with double blind, placebo-controlled food challenges. Selection of foods for challenges was based on positive skin prick tests (>3 mm wheal) or a convincing history. At least one positive skin test to a food antigen was found in 24/26 patients. A total of 111 double blind, placebo-controlled challenges were performed in these children after suspect foods were eliminated from their diets for 10 to 14 days. There were 23 positive challenges in 15 children, 21 of which manifested as cutaneous symptoms, primarily pruritus and an erythematous macular and/or maculopapular rash involving 5% (or greater) of the body surface. In all, 14 children (54%) developed cutaneous symptoms after food challenges. All symptoms occurred within 10 minutes to 2 hours of challenge; nasal symptoms, mild wheezing and gastrointestinal symptoms were seen in some children. No symptoms occurred in 104 placebo challenges. There were 86/111 clinically insignificant positive skin tests (77%) and three false-negative skin tests. These studies demonstrate that, in some children with AD, immediate food hypersensitivity can provoke cutaneous pruritus and erythema, which leads to scratching and subsequent eczematous lesions. Foods that commonly elicited symptoms on challenge were milk, wheat, eggs, soya and peanuts.[29] (This study highlights that replacing cow's milk with soya milk is not advisable in some patients.) In a follow-up study, elevated plasma histamine levels were found in the group of subjects who had positive reactions to food challenges.[30] Other studies have found that chocolate, seafood, oranges, celery and yeast can also commonly provoke symptoms in patients with AD.[31,32]

Many types of inflammatory cells are present in AD skin lesions, but the major abnormality is thought to involve hyperstimulatory T cells.[21] Much interest has focused on the shift in T-helper-cell activity towards a Th2 type response. Both Th1 and Th2 cells can induce B cells to produce immunoglobulins, but only Th2 cells induce IgE.[21] Regulatory mechanisms are also relevant, with an important role for T regulatory cells.[33]

Innate immune responses are also defective in AD, leading to increased susceptibility to viral, bacterial and fungal infections.[34] An example of this is the almost 90% rate of colonisation of the skin with *Staphylococcus aureus* in AD patients, compared with only 5% colonisation in healthy people. Circulating NK cells are significantly reduced in AD patients and are functionally defective, as noted by the reduced release of IFN-gamma. A striking finding in lesional biopsies from AD patients is the absence of neutrophils.[35]

Although the Th1/Th2 paradigm, with Th2 responses predominating in AD, has been helpful, the actual processes involved are more complex. Patients appear to develop a biphasic helper T-cell pattern, with Th2 cytokine predominance seen early in the acute stage, but then a switch to a more Th1-like profile, with higher levels of IFN-gamma in the chronic stage.[34]

As noted, the cutaneous microbial flora of atopic dermatitis patients shows striking differences in terms of the presence of *Staph. aureus*. The relative rarity of colonisation on normal skin is in sharp contrast to the high rate found in patients with AD, ranging from 76% on unaffected areas up to 100% on acute, weeping lesions.[36] *Staph. aureus* can induce inflammatory reactions via a range of activities, including toxin and protein secretion. Among these are the superantigens, which have potent inflammatory and immunological effects.[36] (Superantigens bind directly to macrophages without antigen processing. This can have profound pathological effects due to the release of cytokines by these cells or via the subsequent activation of T-cells.[37,38]) The superantigen *Staph. aureus* enterotoxin B induces the expansion of Th2 cells, leading to increased IgE synthesis.[36]

An interesting prospective study comparing, 110 AD patients and 30 healthy volunteers (age 11 to 45 years) demonstrated a high colonisation density of skin lesions and nasal, pharyngeal and vaginal mucosa with *Staph. aureus* in 102 cases, with streptococci in 53 cases and with Candida, Aspergillus or *Penicillium* sp. in 36 cases. Quantitative investigations of faecal and duodenal aspirate microflora in the same AD group revealed significantly increased counts of haemolytic coliforms, Candida/Geotrichum and pathogenic Clostridia, generally associated with dramatically reduced counts of lactic acid producing bacteria. By contrast, positive skin cultures with *Staph. aureus* were isolated in only two controls and increased Candida counts in faeces were found in another three. Specific IgE antibodies against *Candida albicans*, *Aspergillus fumigatus* and *Saccharomyces cerevisiae* were evident in 61, 32 and 56 cases, respectively, suggesting an increased infectious susceptibility and sensitivity to fungal antigens in the disease group. Thirty-one of 58 tested AD sera showed obviously decreased gamma-globulin levels (IgG and IgM, p<0.005) and in 24 of 35 patients tested for delayed cutaneous hypersensitivity reactions, a severe depression of the cellular immune response was recorded. The authors suggested that their experience shows that correction of the intestinal and dermal dysbiosis, along with appropriate nutritional support and immune modulating therapy, are essential steps in the management of AD.[39] However, a Cochrane review failed to find evidence that conventional therapy against *S. aureus* was clinically helpful in people with AD that is not clinically infected.[40]

Some early studies (for example, Ayers in 1929 and Brown and co-workers in 1935) found a low gastric production of hydrochloric acid was correlated with incidence of AD. Therapy with hydrochloric acid resulted in a dramatic improvement in some cases.[41] A Russian study found markedly reduced activity of membrane-bound small-intestinal enzymes in 346 patients with AD. Correction of this dysfunction resulted in improvements in both digestion and skin.[42] A related study found a similar problem in infants with AD and reduction of disaccharide intake (e.g. lactose, sucrose and maltose) was instituted.[43]

A meta-analysis of 21 studies found that current intestinal parasite infection was protective against allergic sensitisation.[44] This supports the 'old friends' hypothesis, a modification of the hygiene hypothesis, where exposure to certain relatively harmless microorganisms (including helminths) supports immunological regulation via gut-associated T regulatory and regulatory dendritic cells.[45] A less diverse gut microbiota, with high counts of Bacteroides, Clostridium,

Enterobacteriaceae and Staphylococcus early in life has been associated with an increased risk for AD.[46]

Based on the above discussion, the following lifestyle and dietary changes can be recommended. Measures to eliminate exposure to house dust mite antigen should be instituted. Simple or multiple exclusion diets should be considered, based on the clinical information. Elimination of cow's milk (and related dairy products) is recommended as the starting diet if a simple exclusion diet is chosen. Care should be taken to substitute protein and calcium in young children. If there is no symptom improvement in about 4 to 6 weeks, different foods in turn could be tried such as eggs, peanuts or seafood.[47] Various multiple exclusion diets are available.[47] These typically involve avoidance of dairy products, eggs, nuts, pork, bacon, shellfish, yeast and fruit. Such diets can be severe and should not be instituted as a first resort. The diet should otherwise be well balanced and should not contain excessive amounts of junk food, sugar and refined carbohydrate.

It is hoped that individual strategies will be devised for each patient with AD, taking some of the insights in this and other chapters into account, but essential elements of herbal treatment are as follows:

- Echinacea root will help to balance the immune response. Experience shows that it does not aggravate AD (and may even help shift responses away from Th2 type to Th1). Boosting the innate immune response with Echinacea, Andrographis and other immune herbs may help to control *Staph. aureus* infection.
- Antiallergic herbs (such as Albizia, Baical skullcap and nettles) and anti-inflammatory herbs (such as licorice and Bupleurum) can help to control symptoms.
- Bitter herbs and ginger will improve digestion (if indicated).
- Long-term treatment with depuratives such as burdock, figwort, clivers, yellow dock and sarsaparilla. *Solanum dulcamara* (bittersweet) is a depurative herb that also possesses anti-inflammatory properties.[48] Heartsease is specifically used for infantile eczema.
- Evening primrose oil as a source of gamma-linolenic acid can correct an essential fatty acid imbalance, confer anti-inflammatory effects and support the epidermal barrier.
- Topical treatment with anti-inflammatory and antiseptic herbs. The antiseptic herbs will help to control skin microflora imbalance and infection with *Staph. aureus*. Calendula has both antiseptic and anti-inflammatory properties. Myrrh and tea tree oil have antiseptic properties and topical treatment with myrrh and Echinacea could improve the cutaneous immune response (watch for contact dermatitis with myrrh). Witchhazel with its tannins has antimicrobial activity and other components in the herb confer anti-inflammatory effects. Golden seal contains antimicrobial alkaloids (hence it should not be combined with tannins). Licorice, chamomile and St John's wort oil have topical anti-inflammatory activity (see monographs).
- Hemidesmus and Rehmannia can be used to modulate the Th2 response.
- Therapeutic baths can be of value in AD. A bag of oatmeal suspended in a coarse cloth (run the bath water out of the

tap through the bag and then suspend the bag in the bath) will soothe irritated and inflamed skin. Antiseptic essential oils in a bath will help to correct skin microflora imbalance.

- Gut dysbiosis should be addressed, if appropriate (see p. 203).

CASE HISTORY

An 8-year-old girl had eczema that started about 4 years ago. It was worse each summer, perhaps as a result of swimming in the local pool. The mother had tried removing dairy products from her diet, with not much success. The girl seemed to be eating quite a few sweet biscuits and so it was suggested that these be reduced. Her doctor had prescribed a topical steroid. On examination the lesions on her face showed signs of a secondary infection. The following formula and dosage was prescribed (based on her weight of 25 kg):

Echinacea angustifolia root	1:2	50 mL
Scutellaria baicalensis	1:2	25 mL
Urtica dioica	1:2	25 mL
	TOTAL	100 mL

Dose: 3 mL with water twice a day.

Topical application of a chickweed cream was also recommended for the lesions and one 500 mg capsule of evening primrose oil was to be broken and taken internally or applied topically (on the abdomen where the skin is thin for dermal absorption) twice a day.

On review after 4 weeks the rash had improved substantially and her face was clear. Use of the local swimming pool did not seem to aggravate the condition as it did previously. Treatment was continued for several months and improvement was maintained.

CASE HISTORY

A woman aged 23 years presented with severe AD. It was itchy and infected and affected her hands, legs, scalp, face (around the lips) and chest. The condition started about 6 years ago and was currently being treated with topical steroids. It was worse premenstrually and she had a family history of atopy and suffered from asthma. She was prescribed the following formula (feverfew for antiallergic effects):

Astragalus membranaceus	1:2	25 mL
Echinacea angustifolia root	1:2	25 mL
Centella asiatica	1:1	20 mL
Tanacetum parthenium	1:5	10 mL
Bupleurum falcatum	1:2	20 mL
	TOTAL	100 mL

Dose: 5 mL with water three times daily.

In addition she was advised to avoid all dairy products, take chaste tree 1:5 2.5 mL with water on rising each morning and three 1000 mg evening primrose capsules per day. A chickweed cream was prescribed for topical application.

Four weeks later her condition was about the same. She had made a decision (without seeking advice) to completely stop her steroid cream and her rash grew much worse (a characteristic rebound effect). Since then it had stabilised, but not improved. Treatment was continued.

After another 8 weeks of treatment there was a significant improvement in her skin condition. Treatment was continued over several more months, after which her AD had more or less subsided.

Chronic urticaria

Chronic urticaria can be defined as the occurrence of transient wheals lasting more than 6 weeks in duration. In many cases a specific cause is not identified and this is classified as chronic idiopathic urticaria. A physical trigger (heat, cold, exercise, etc.), vasculitis or systemic disease (mainly autoimmunity, especially thyroid disease) can act as a cause.[49] Associations with *Helicobacter pylori*, candida infection, malignancy and food intolerances have been reported. An elimination diet focusing on salicylate and amine sensitivities should be considered on a trial basis.

A subset of patients with chronic idiopathic urticaria has autoantibodies to the high affinity IgE receptor, or, rarely, anti-IgE antibodies. Autologous serum skin testing for these autoantibodies can be performed.[49] These autoantibodies have been shown to activate blood basophils and skin mast cells in vitro. Activation of basophils or mast cells causing histamine release is quite specific for chronic urticaria and defines the autoimmune subgroup.[50] New research suggests that in some patients the activation of the extrinsic coagulation pathway with thrombin generation might play an important role.[51]

It is hoped that individual strategies will be devised for each patient with chronic urticaria, taking some of the insights in this and other chapters into account, but essential elements of herbal treatment are as follows:

- Depuratives are an important aspect of treatment, especially the stinging nettle leaf. Perhaps some principle of homeopathy applies here, since the stinging nettle produces urticarial lesions on contact with the skin. Other depurative herbs include yellow dock, Oregon grape and burdock.
- Antiallergic herbs, especially Albizia and Baical skullcap, will help to control symptoms created by mast cell activation and prevent recurrence of urticaria.
- Echinacea will help to balance the immune response and resolve any relevant infection. If infection is suspected to be the cause, other immune-enhancing herbs should also be prescribed, and St John's wort for antiviral activity if appropriate.
- Rehmannia has been shown to benefit urticaria in uncontrolled clinical trials conducted in China. Hemidesmus may also be of value.
- Digestive function should be improved using bitters, ginger and choleretic herbs if food allergies are suspected.
- A clinical study found that 21 of 30 patients suffering from chronic urticaria which had lasted from 3 months to 5 years had proven *Helicobacter pylori* infection.[52] After therapy for Helicobacter, all 21 became free of urticaria.
- Herbs that can help to control Helicobacter if the patient tests positive include garlic, thyme, turmeric, cranberry, sage, Nigella, barberry and other berberine-containing herbs (such as golden seal) and herbs containing tannins (note that tannins are incompatible with alkaloids such as berberine and should be taken at different times). Berberine-containing herbs are particularly active.

Echinacea should also form part of the treatment and garlic will work best as a fresh, crushed clove.

- Factors involved in autoimmunity should be addressed if appropriate (see Chapter 8).

Example liquid formula

Echinacea purpurea/angustifolia root	1:2	35 mL
Scutellaria baicalensis	1:2	20 mL
Urtica dioica	1:2	20 mL
Rehmannia glutinosa	1:2	30 mL
	TOTAL	105 mL

Dose: 8 mL with water two times a day.

CASE HISTORY

A girl aged 14 years presented with recurrent urticaria. Her first episode occurred about 4 to 5 years ago, when she experienced urticaria every day for about a month. Her hands and feet were affected first, but sometimes the itchy rash would cover most of her body. Despite the fact that she was now avoiding certain foods and triggers such as contact with couch grass, she was currently experiencing an attack every 2 to 3 days. There was no history of hayfever, asthma or eczema.

Given that she might react to certain herbs, her prescription was three herbs, dispensed separately. The herbs were:

Echinacea angustifolia root	1:2	4 mL/day
Scutellaria baicalensis	1:2	4 mL/day
Urtica dioica	1:2	4 mL/day

Her instructions were to take the first herb only for 3 days, followed by the second and the third, each for 3 days. If none of the herbs aggravated her condition (which was the case), she was then to commence all three herbs each day at the above doses.

After taking the herbs for about 8 weeks the bouts of urticaria had ceased. She stopped the herbal treatment and 3 years later the urticaria had not returned.

Herpes simplex and shingles

Herpes simplex skin outbreaks are characteristic mucocutaneous lesions which are caused by new infection with herpes simplex virus 1 (HSV-1) or 2 (HSV-2), or by reactivation of latent virus residing in the nervous system. Typically HSV-1 affects the face, lips or mouth and HSV-2 affects the genitals, although either virus can infect either location.

HSV is a double-stranded DNA, enveloped virus. HSV infection of some neuronal cells does not result in cell death. Instead, viral genomes are maintained by the cell in a repressed state compatible with survival and normal activities of the cell, a condition known as latency. Immune competency is of primary importance in preventing and dealing with outbreaks caused by latent virus.

The treatment approach for shingles is basically the same as for herpes simplex infection.

Phytotherapy should be centred on the following:

- Immune-enhancing herbs will assist the fight against the virus in acute outbreaks and prevent reactivation of latent virus. Key herbs include Echinacea root, Andrographis and Astragalus. Astragalus should not be used in acute outbreaks.
- Internal treatment with St John's wort preparations high in hypericin appears to exert a significant activity against HSV-1 and -2 (see monograph).
- Debilitated patients suffering from recurrent outbreaks may benefit from adrenal tonics, tonics, adaptogenic herbs and nervine tonics between outbreaks. Key herbs in these categories include Rehmannia, licorice, Withania, Siberian ginseng and St John's wort.
- Topical treatment of lesions includes Calendula extract (applied neat to the lesions) and lemon balm, licorice and/or tea tree in ointment or cream form (see Chapter 8). Clinical studies have shown that use of lemon balm ointment on lesions helps to prevent future outbreaks of herpes simplex (see Chapter 8).
- Post-herpetic neuralgia is treated with St John's wort and analgesic herbs for the neuralgia, together with adaptogens, tonics and immune-enhancing agents. Peppermint oil can be applied topically (see monograph).
- Clinical trials have demonstrated that cream containing capsaicin (or cayenne extract) might also have value for post-herpetic neuralgia (see Chapter 2).

Example liquid formula

For acute outbreaks the following formula has helped several patients in conjunction with topical application of Calendula extract for both herpes simplex and shingles:

Echinacea purpurea/angustifolia root	1:2	70 mL
Hypericum perforatum (high hypericin)	1:2	30 mL
	TOTAL	100 mL

Dose: 5 mL with water four to five times a day until the lesions heal.

CASE HISTORY

A 27-year-old woman was suffering from recurrent cold sores. She had been experiencing an outbreak at least every month and the sores were large and painful. This had been happening for many years. Treatment prescribed was:

Echinacea angustifolia root	1:2	70 mL
Hypericum perforatum (high hypericin)	1:2	30 mL
	TOTAL	100 mL

Dose: 5 mL with water three times a day.

Picrorrhiza tablets 500 mg at two per day and topical application of Calendula 1:2 extract was also prescribed.

After 4 weeks there was a noticeable improvement. She still had an outbreak but it was not as severe and healed more quickly. During the next 4 weeks she was free from outbreaks of cold sores. Treatment was continued for another 8 weeks, again with no outbreaks. For the following 4 months she remained free of lesions without herbal treatment and has been more or less free of lesions for several years after.

CASE HISTORY

A 25-year-old woman had a large, painful lesion on her face which had been diagnosed as shingles (herpes zoster) by her doctor. She was concerned and depressed because she had been told that the sore could possibly leave a scar. The following treatment for this acute condition was prescribed:

Echinacea angustifolia root	1:2	70 mL
Hypericum perforatum (high hypericin)	1:2	30 mL
	TOTAL	100 mL

Dose: 5 mL with water five to six times a day.

Picrorrhiza 500 mg tablets at three per day were also prescribed, and she was advised to apply Calendula 1:2 extract (90% alcohol) to the sore, followed by Calendula cream when it started to heal. (Caution with Picrorrhiza at this dose as it may induce abdominal pain and diarrhoea due to the cucurbitacins it contains.)

After 5 days she rang to report that the lesion was healing well and that the pain had abated on the first dose of herbal mixture. After only 10 days the lesion had completely healed without a trace of a scar and she was free from any pain or other symptoms. Note regarding these cases: Andrographis at 3 to 4 g/day is a suitable clinical alternative to the Picrorrhiza.

Warts

Warts are a common skin condition, especially before the age of 20. They result from infection with the DNA human papillomavirus, of which there are numerous subtypes. Transmission is by contact with the virus either in live or shed skin.

Most warts eventually resolve spontaneously in healthy people. In immunocompromised patients they can persist and spread (this highlights the importance of immune function). The spontaneous resolution probably results when the immune system 'discovers' the virus.

The general approach to treating infections has been provided in Chapter 8. Treatment for warts centres on:

- immune-enhancing herbs, particularly Echinacea root but also other herbs with this property will be of value
- internal and topical treatment with Thuja
- topical treatment with other antiviral agents such as tannin-rich herbs (abrade the surface of the wart to allow access), Calendula and the fresh, yellow latex of greater celandine
- other topical treatments include comfrey (the crushed fresh leaves are preferred by some) and the white latex of the petty spurge (Euphorbia peplus). These treatments may also exert some antiviral activity.

CASE HISTORY

A male patient aged 23 had been treated for a wart on his knee by conventional cryotherapy. Instead of being free of warts, his whole knee became covered with them. Being reluctant to use cryotherapy again, he sought herbal treatment. He was prescribed the following formula:

Echinacea angustifolia root	1:2	80 mL
Thuja occidentalis	1:5	20 mL
	TOTAL	100 mL

Dose: 5 mL with water three times a day.

After 4 weeks there was no change and he received a repeat prescription. About 2 weeks after this he rang to say that he woke up that morning to find that all his warts were gone.

Tinea pedis

Tinea pedis or athlete's foot is the most common type of human fungal infection. It appears to be spread through sharing of bathing facilities and via swimming pools. Occlusive footwear and infrequent washing of socks can lead to chronicity and relapses. The most common organisms involved include Trichophyton rubrum and T. mentagrophytes.

Phytotherapy is centred on:

- improving immune function with immune-enhancing herbs to fight the infection
- topical treatment with herbal antifungal agents such as Calendula, tea tree oil, orange or lemon essential oil, greater celandine and thyme or thyme essential oil. Be careful that the topical agents do not excessively irritate the skin.

If the toe nails are involved, tea tree oil application to the quick of the nail (eponychium) is particularly useful, but in chronic cases may need to be applied for up to 3 months.

CASE HISTORY

A male patient aged 53 presented with severe, chronic tinea in the right foot. The tinea caused the skin to crack which resulted in secondary bacterial infection. Sometimes this was complicated by cellulitis and localised oedema in the lower leg (he had to wear a compression stocking on the lower right leg when the oedema was bad).

At the time of presentation he was experiencing acute bacterial infection and cellulitis and had been prescribed antibiotics. Griseofulvin had been prescribed some time ago for the fungal infection and he maintained this treatment throughout.

The immediate aim of initial treatment was to control the bacterial infection. Being an ex-alcoholic, he requested that tablets be prescribed. He was placed on:

- A tablet containing Echinacea angustifolia root 600 mg and Echinacea purpurea root 675 mg per tablet. Dose: four tablets/day.
- A tablet containing Echinacea angustifolia root 500 mg, holy basil 500 mg and essential oil 10 mg, and Andrographis 1.0 g per tablet. Dose: four tablets/day.
- A tablet containing horsechestnut 1.2 g, butcher's broom 800 mg and Ginkgo 1.5 g per tablet. Dose: three tablets/day.

The treatment rationale was as follows. The first two tablets were prescribed to boost immune function against the bacteria and fungus. The other tablet was for the localised oedema and stasis. In addition the patient was given a lotion containing equal parts of Calendula 1:2 and Echinacea angustifolia root 1:2 to use diluted with water to bathe the infected foot. Afterwards a comfrey cream was to be applied to the unbroken skin of this foot.

Two weeks later the foot had settled down, but another week later the cellulitis flared up again. He was maintained on the same treatment to prevent the cellulitis and to work on the fungal infection. Over the next 6 months the condition settled, the bouts of cellulitis ceased and the skin on the foot healed over. However, the fungal infection remained and he was prescribed topical tea tree oil in addition. As long as the patient maintained the treatment his condition was stable and the fungal infection was kept under control, with no outbreaks of cellulitis.

Acne

Acne is the most common disease of the skin.[53] It affects 85% of teenagers, 42.5% of men, and 50.9% of women between the ages of 20 and 30 years. The role of hormones, particularly as a trigger of sebum production and sebaceous growth and differentiation, is well known. Excess production of hormones, specifically androgens, growth hormone, IGF-1 (insulin-like growth factor 1), insulin, CRH, and glucocorticoids, is associated with increased rates of acne development. Acne may be a feature in many endocrine disorders, including polycystic ovary disease, Cushing syndrome, androgen-secreting tumours and acromegaly. Other non-endocrine diseases associated with acne include Apert syndrome, SAPHO syndrome, Behçet syndrome and PAPA syndrome. Acne medicamentosa is the development of acne vulgaris or an acneiform eruption with the use of certain medications. These medications include testosterone, progesterone, steroids, lithium, phenytoin, isoniazid, vitamins B2, B6 and B12, halogens and epidermal growth factor inhibitors. Management of acne medicamentosa includes standard acne therapy. Discontinuation of the offending drug may be necessary in recalcitrant cases.

Basic medical interventions for acne include topical therapy, systemic antibiotics, hormonal agents, isotretinoin and physical treatments. Generally, the severity of acne lesions determines the type of acne regimen necessary. The emergence of drug-resistant *Propionibacterium acnes* and adverse side effects are current limitations to effective acne management.[53]

Acne is a disorder of the sebaceous follicles (sebaceous glands associated with hair follicles), which are located on the face, chest and back. Several factors play a pivotal role in the pathogenesis of acne:

- Androgen dependence
- Excessive sebum production (lipogenesis)
- Abnormal follicular differentiation (retention hyperkeratosis)
- Increased colonisation with *Propionibacterium acnes*
- Inflammatory processes.

Sebum is the fatty secretion produced by sebaceous glands. Patients with acne have higher rates of sebum production than unaffected individuals and severity of acne can be correlated to sebum production.[54] Enlargement of the sebaceous glands and increased production of sebum is stimulated by the increase in adrenal and gonadal androgens that precedes the onset of puberty. The first signs of acne commonly occur at this time.

High (but within normal range) serum concentrations of the testosterone precursor dehydroepiandrosterone sulphate (DHEAS) correlate with the presence of acne in prepubertal children and in some adults.[55] In particular, some women with acne do have raised serum concentrations of testosterone and DHEAS, but in men the situation is less consistent.

Increased local metabolism of DHEAS in sebaceous glands to more potent androgens such as dihydrotestosterone may take place under the influence of androgen-metabolising enzymes such as type I 5alpha-reductase.[55] Low levels of SHBG in the plasma may act in concert with this process.[56] This, in addition to a possible role of growth factors, may influence sebum production and hence acne.[55]

Desquamated cornified cells of the upper canal of the sebaceous follicle become abnormally adherent. Instead of undergoing the normal process of shedding, they instead form a microscopic plug (the microcomedo) in the follicular canal.[55] The mechanism of this process, known as comedogenesis, is not known, but a local deficiency of linoleic acid may be involved.[57] These lower levels of linoleic acid in sebum may result from accelerated sebum production.[57]

Progressive enlargement of microcomedones gives rise to clinically visible comedones, the non-inflammatory lesions of acne. The follicular canal becomes blocked, but sebum production continues with the resultant proliferation of *P. acnes*, a normal resident of the sebaceous follicle.[56] Sebaceous follicles containing microcomedones provide an anaerobic, lipid-rich environment in which these bacteria flourish. Glycerol is a nutritional requirement of *P. acnes* and is obtained through lipolysis of triglycerides in the sebum, with the release of free fatty acids as a byproduct.

The free fatty acids have proinflammatory and comedogenic properties. *P. acnes* also releases chemotactic factors, which attract neutrophils to the follicular lumen, resulting in further inflammatory damage.[58] *P. acnes* further contributes to the inflammatory process through complement activation and release of other hydrolytic enzymes such as proteases. Follicular rupture and extension of the inflammatory process into the surrounding skin results in the formation of the inflammatory lesions of acne – papules, pustules and nodules. Abnormalities in neutrophil chemotaxis and phagocytosis of *P. acnes* and activation of macrophages contribute to the chronic, haphazard nature of inflammation in severe acne.[59,60]

Interest in sebaceous gland physiology and its diseases is rapidly increasing. Exploration of sebaceous gland biology, hormonal factors, hyperkeratinisation, role of bacteria, sebum, nutrition, cytokines and TLRs is receiving research attention. Sebaceous glands play an important role as active participants in the innate immunity of the skin. They produce neuropeptides, excrete antimicrobial peptides and exhibit characteristics of stem cells. Androgens affect sebocytes and infundibular keratinocytes in a complex manner influencing cellular differentiation, proliferation, lipogenesis and comedogenesis. Retention hyperkeratosis in closed comedones and inflammatory papules is attributable to a disorder of terminal keratinocyte differentiation. *P. acnes*, by acting on TLR-2, may stimulate the secretion of cytokines, such as IL-6 and IL-8 by follicular keratinocytes and IL-8 and IL-12 in macrophages, giving rise to inflammation. Certain *P. acnes* strains may induce an immunological reaction by stimulating the production of sebocyte and keratinocyte antimicrobial peptides, which play an important role in the innate immunity of the follicle. Qualitative changes of sebum lipids induce alteration of keratinocyte differentiation and induce IL-1 secretion, contributing to the development of follicular hyperkeratosis. High glycaemic load food and milk may induce increased tissue levels of 5alpha-dihydrotestosterone. These new aspects of acne pathogenesis lead to the considerations of possible customised therapeutic regimens.[61]

One interesting hypothesis offers a solution for the pathogenesis of acne and explains all major pathogenic factors at the genomic level: this theory is a relative deficiency of the nuclear transcription factor forkhead box-containing transcription factor (Fox)O1.[62] This poorly understood transcription factor modulates energy homeostasis at both the cellular and whole-body levels. Nuclear FoxO1 suppresses androgen receptor, other important nuclear receptors and key genes of cell proliferation, lipid biosynthesis and inflammatory cytokines. Elevated growth factors during puberty and persistent growth factor signals due to Western lifestyle stimulate the export of FoxO1 out of the nucleus into the cytoplasm via activation of the phosphoinositide-3-kinase (PI3K)/Akt pathway. By this mechanism, genes and nuclear receptors involved in acne are derepressed, leading to increased androgen receptor-mediated signal transduction, increased cell proliferation of androgen-dependent cells, induction of sebaceous lipogenesis and upregulation of TLR-2-dependent inflammatory cytokines. All known acne-inducing factors exert their action by reduction of nuclear FoxO1 levels. In contrast, retinoids, antibiotics and dietary intervention can increase the nuclear content of FoxO1, thereby normalising increased transcription of genes involved in acne.

As touched on above, despite the popular conventional view that diet is not related to acne, several experts in the field are encouraging a reassessment of this position, partly because the data refuting any association are weak.[63] For example, one review pointed out that acne is virtually unknown in traditional hunter-gatherers.[64] The review goes on to suggest an association between dairy products (from the protein, not the fat) and dietary fat (especially in terms of increased sebum production). The severe methodological shortcomings of the negative trials involving chocolate were stressed. Such trials have been used to refute any connection between diet and acne.

Recent evidence has demonstrated that the hormonal cascade triggered by diet-induced hyperinsulinaemia elicits an endocrine response that simultaneously promotes unregulated tissue growth and enhances androgen synthesis.[65] This former aspect is regulated by IGF-1, a potent mitogen, required for keratinocyte proliferation. Another review considered that there was compelling evidence that high glycaemic load diets may exacerbate acne.[66]

The view is growing that acne can be regarded as an indicator disease of the exaggerated insulinotropic effects of modern Western diets.[67] Especially milk- and whey protein-based products contribute to elevations of postprandial insulin and basal IGF-1 plasma levels. This is a key aspect of mammalian milk designed to promote growth in the neonate. Increased insulin/IGF-1 signalling reduces nuclear FoxO1.[67] IGF-1 stimulates 5alpha-reductase, adrenal and gonadal androgen synthesis, androgen receptor signal transduction, sebocyte proliferation and lipogenesis.[68]

The use of strong soaps and shampoos that strip sebum from the skin and hair and initiate a rebound increase in sebum production should be avoided. Herbal extracts such as licorice, which are rich in saponins, can act as a gentle skin wash which will not cause a rebound in sebum production.

Appropriate dietary strategies for acne, as supported by the above evidence, stress the avoidance of high glycaemic index foods and dairy products. The diet should also not contain excessive levels of fat.

It is hoped that individual strategies will be devised for each patient with acne, taking some of the insights in this and other chapters into account, but essential elements of herbal treatment are as follows:

- Depurative herbs are again the mainstay of treatment. In particular Calendula and burdock may reduce excess sebum production, but other important depuratives for acne include yellow dock, poke root and Oregon grape.
- A more effective immune response will help to control levels of *P. acnes*. Echinacea has been traditionally used in acne, possibly for this reason. Andrographis is another candidate.
- Chaste tree given to men and women has shown benefit in acne in early clinical trials, possibly due to its hormonal effects (see chaste tree monograph). Linseeds contain lignans that may raise SHBG (see Chapter 2). Studies have found that consumption of licorice can lower testosterone levels, but high doses may be necessary (see licorice monograph).
- Other internal herbs used to treat acne include garlic and golden seal. On the surface it might appear that these herbs are selected because of their antimicrobial properties. However, their oral use for acne could be explained by depurative and immune-regulating effects.
- Gugulipid, an extract of *Commiphora mukul* standardised for guggulsterones, produced a similar improvement to tetracycline in a controlled clinical trial in 20 patients.[69] Patients with oily skin responded better to gugulipid. This herb is thought to act by improving thyroid function; bladderwrack can also be used in this context.
- Topical treatments can be of benefit, especially as resistance is growing to antibiotics used in acne.[70] A single blind clinical trial found that topical treatment with fresh basil juice (*Ocimum basilicum*) was as effective as conventional treatment.[71] Topical tea tree oil was found to be effective (see Chapter 2). Calendula and comfrey are also popular topical treatments.
- Topical treatments with herbs can also have value in lowering sebum production and assisting exfoliation. For example, in vitro lipogenesis in guinea pig sebaceous glands was suppressed by wogonin, a component of Baical skullcap.[72]
- Case observations and even clinical studies have shown that insulin and antidiabetic drugs appear to cause clinical improvement in acne.[73] It has even been suggested that acne is 'skin diabetes'. Hence it is conceivable that the oral use of herbs used to treat diabetes may have a similar beneficial effect, particularly Gymnema, and this is supported by the involvement of insulin/IGF-1 in the modern understanding of the pathogenesis of acne.

Example liquid formula

Vitex agnus-castus	1:2	15 mL
Calendula officinalis	1:2	20 mL
Arctium lappa	1:2	20 mL
Scutellaria baicalensis	1:2	20 mL
Phytolacca decandra	1:5	5 mL
Echinacea purpurea/angustifolia root	1:2	30 mL
	TOTAL	110 mL

Dose: 8 mL with water twice a day.

CASE HISTORY

A female patient of 33 years was a flight attendant. Her onset of acne was at 21 years and the use of the oral contraceptive pill (OCP) had kept her condition under control. She had recently ceased the OCP and was now experiencing a major worsening on her back, chest and jaw line. The patient also had difficulties in preventing weight gain. The following was prescribed:

Calendula officinalis	1:2	15 mL
Vitex angus-castus	1:2	15 mL
Echinacea purpurea/angustifolia root	1:2	25 mL
Rehmannia glutinosa	1:2	25 mL
Bupleurum falcatum	1:2	20 mL
	TOTAL	100 mL

Dose: 5 mL with water three times a day
   Also the following were recommended:

- A tablet containing Gymnema extract 4.0 g. Dose: one tablet before meals three times a day
- Topical wash of 5% Calendula 1:2 in water two times per day
- Diet: low glycaemic index diet, no grains or dairy products.

   Within 5 days the lesions began to clear; however, it took a period of 12 weeks to totally clear. The patient remained free of acne thereafter. (Case history kindly provided by Rob Santich, Sydney.)

Assisting healing and repair

The basic response of all living organisms to damage or loss of body tissues is to initiate repair and regenerate the damaged part. So while surgeons may claim that they save the lives of their patients (and they often do), without this capacity of the body to heal itself surgery would in fact be a death sentence.

There are three basic processes involved in wound healing:[74]

- Regeneration of damaged tissue (such as skin)
- Regeneration of damaged connective tissue (connective tissue is the building block of the body, providing the structural matrix for the functional tissues)
- The replacement by fibrous tissue of dead cells that cannot regenerate.

When part of the body is wounded the essential sequence of events is as follows. The damaged tissue and the bleeding around it stimulate the body's inflammatory response. White blood cells (particularly macrophages and neutrophils) invade the damaged tissue in large numbers and begin engulfing (by phagocytosis) and processing the large amounts of debris. This usually takes several days. During this process fine and delicate new blood vessels begin to form by the process known as angiogenesis. These new blood vessels provide nutrition to support the next stage of healing, which is the regeneration of connective tissue. During this time other necessary tissues such as nerve cells and lymph vessels begin to form.

Fibroblasts are the cells that synthesise the non-cellular constituents of connective tissue, namely collagen and glycosaminoglycans, the jelly-like ground substance into which the collagen is embedded.

With the passage of time there is organisation and remodelling of the new connective tissue, which becomes progressively denser. The zone of new dense connective tissue is known as a scar. The fibroblasts contract, pulling the margins of the wound together. Scar remodelling continues for months or years after the wound has healed,[74] and this suggests a long-term role for herbs such as gotu kola to minimise the scar.

Regeneration of connective tissue is half of wound healing; the other half is restoration of the cells that line the surfaces of tissue (known as epithelium). Skin cells are a form of epithelium and the skin cells around the margin of a wound begin to multiply and cover the gap created by the wound.

Other tissues (apart from skin) regenerate by a similar process (if they are capable of doing so). For example, bone heals in a very similar way, except that osteoblasts are involved. Hence the approach suggested below should also assist bones to heal.

If the scavenging phase of the macrophages is disturbed, say by infection, healing will be slow. Also, a good blood supply to the general area is essential for efficient healing. Excess movement of the wound edges can also impair healing; this is the main reason why broken limbs are placed in a cast.

Hence the key steps in healing are:

- cleaning up of debris by immune cells, infection can slow this down
- establishment of new blood vessels
- regeneration of the connective tissue elements
- regeneration of epithelial cells.

The following herbs can assist these steps:

- *Echinacea purpurea* or *E. angustifolia* root (or their combination) will not only enhance the activity of the phagocytic cells, but will also help to prevent any complicating infection.
- Ginkgo will ensure that the wounded area receives adequate oxygen and blood supply, and will also help maintain the integrity of the newly formed blood vessels (see Ginkgo monograph).
- Bilberry is a key herb for the microcirculation (as evidenced by its positive effects on damage to the retina of the eye) so it will additionally assist the role of the Ginkgo in supporting the new blood supply (see monograph). Grape seed extract not only supports microcirculation,[75] it also helps to maintain the strength of connective tissue[76] and provides valuable antioxidant activity.
- Gotu kola stimulates the activity of both the fibroblasts (or osteoblasts) and epithelial cells to ensure efficient regeneration and repair (see gotu kola monograph).
- Topical use of healing (vulnerary) herbs such as Calendula will also assist the regeneration of epithelial cells.

Example liquid formula

Echinacea purpurea/angustifolia root	1:2	40 mL
Centella asiatica (standardised extract)	1:1	40 mL
Ginkgo biloba (standardised extract)	2:1	30 mL
	TOTAL	110 mL

Dose: 8 mL with water twice a day.

References

1. Aburjai T, Natsheth FM. Plants used in cosmetics. *Phytother Res.* 2003;17:987–1000.

2. Ahshawat M, Saraf S, Saraf S. Preparation and characterization of herbal creams for improvement of skin viscoelastic properties. *Int J Cosmet Sci.* 2008;30:183–193.

3. Dweck AC. The internal and external use of medicinal plants. *Clin Dermatol.* 2009;27:148–158.

4. Sheehan MP, Rustin MHA, Atherton DJ, et al. Efficacy of traditional Chinese herbal therapy in adult atopic dermatitis. *Lancet.* 1992;340:13–17. (ii)

5. Sheehan MP, Atherton DJ. A controlled trial of traditional Chinese medicinal plants in widespread non-exudative atopic eczema. *Br J Dermatol.* 1992;126(2):179–184.

6. Sheehan MP, Stevens H, Ostlere LS, et al. Follow-up of adult patients with atopic eczema treated with Chinese herbal therapy for 1 year. *Clin Exp Dermatol.* 1995;20(2):136–140.

7. Sheehan MP, Atherton DJ. One-year follow up of children treated with Chinese medicinal herbs for atopic eczema. *Br J Dermatol.* 1994;130(4):488–493.

8. Kane JA, Kane SP, Jain S. Hepatitis induced by traditional Chinese herbs; possible toxic components. *Gut.* 1995;36(1):146–147.

9. Ferguson JE, Chalmers RJ, Rowlands DJ. Reversible dilated cardiomyopathy following treatment of atopic eczema with Chinese herbal medicine. *Br J Dermatol.* 1997;136(4):592–593.

10. Heinrich U, Neukan K, Tronnier H, et al. Long-term ingestion of high flavanol cocoa provides photoprotection against UV-induced erythema and improves skin condition in women. *J Nutr.* 2006;136:1565–1569.

11. Satchell AC, Sauragen A, Bell C, Barnetson RS. Treatment of interdigital tinea pedis with 25% and 50% tea tree oil solution: a randomized, placebo-controlled, blinded study. *Australas J Dermatol.* 2002;43(3):175–178.

12. Calzavara-Pinton P, Zane C, Facchinetti E, et al. Topical boswellic acids for treatment of photoaged skin. *Dermatol Ther.* 2010;23(suppl 1):S28–S32.

13. Hay IC, Jamieson M, Ormerod AD. Randomized trial of aromatherapy: successful treatment for alopecia areata. *Arch Dermatol.* 1998;134(11): 1349–1352.

14. Heng MC, Song MK, Harker J, et al. Drug-induced suppression of phosphorylase kinase activity correlates with resolution of psoriasis as assessed by clinical, histological and immunohistochemical parameters. *Br J Dermatol.* 2000;143(5):937–949.

15. Kurd SK, Smith N, VanVoorhees A, et al. Oral curcumin in the treatment of moderate to severe psoriasis vulgaris: A prospective clinical trial. *J Am Acad Dermatol.* 2008;58(4):625–631.

16. Heng MC. Curcumin targeted signaling pathways: basis for anti-photoaging and anti-carcinogenic therapy. *Int J Dermatol.* 2010;49(6):608–622.

17. Donsky H, Clarke D, Reliéva A. Mahonia aquifolium extract for the treatment of adult patients with atopic dermatitis. *Am J Ther.* 2007;14:442–446.

18. Spergel JM. Epidemiology of atopic dermatitis and atopic march in children. *Immunol Allergy Clin North Am.* 2010;30(3):269–280.

19. Tokura Y. Extrinsic and intrinsic types of atopic dermatitis. *J Dermatol Sci.* 2010;58(1):1–7.

20. O'Regan GM, Sandilands A, McLean WH, Irvine AD. Filaggrin in atopic dermatitis. *J Allergy Clin Immunol.* 2009;124(3 suppl 2):R2–R6.

21. Rudikoff D, Lebwohl M. Atopic dermatitis. *Lancet.* 1998;351:1715–1721.

22. Bath-Hextall F, Delamere FM, Williams HC. Dietary exclusions for established atopic eczema. *Cochrane Database Syst Rev.* 2008;1:CD005203.

23. Finch J, Munhutu MN, Whitaker-Worth DL. Atopic dermatitis and nutrition. *Clin Dermatol.* 2010;28(6):605–614.

24. Greenhawt M. The role of food allergy in atopic dermatitis. *Allergy Asthma Proc.* 2010;31(5):392–397.

25. Caubet JC, Eigenmann PA. Allergic triggers in atopic dermatitis. *Immunol Allergy Clin North Am.* 2010;30(3):289–307.

26. Schäfer T. The impact of allergy on atopic eczema from data from epidemiological studies. *Curr Opin Allergy Clin Immunol.* 2008;8(5):418–422.

27. Ionescu JG. New insights in the pathogenesis of atopic disease. *J Med Life.* 2009;2(2):146–154.

28. Tan BB, Weald D, Strickland I, Friedmann PS. Double blind controlled trial of effect of housedust-mite allergen avoidance on atopic dermatitis. *Lancet.* 1996;347:15–18.

29. Sampson HA. Role of immediate food hypersensitivity in the pathogenesis of atopic dermatitis. *J Allergy Clin Immunol.* 1983;71:473–480.

30. Sampson HA, Joliei PL. Increased plasma histamine concentrations after food challenges in children with atopic dermatitis. *N Engl J Med.* 1984;311:372–376.

31. Molkhou P, Waguet J-C. Food allergy and atopic dermatitis in children: treatment with oral sodium cromoglycate. *Ann Allergy.* 1981;47:173–175.

32. André C, André F, Colin L. Effect of allergen ingestion challenge with and without cromoglycate cover on intestinal permeability in atopic dermatitis, urticaria and other symptoms of food allergy. *Allergy.* 1989;44:47–51.

33. Pucci S, Incorvaia C. Allergy as an organ and a systemic disease. *Clin Exp Immunol.* 2008;153(suppl 1):1–2.

34. Dokmeci E, Herrick CA. The immune system and atopic dermatitis. *Semin Cutan Med Surg.* 2008;27(2):138–143.

35. De Benedetto A, Agnihothri R, McGirt LY, et al. Atopic dermatitis: a disease caused by innate immune defects? *J Invest Dermatol.* 2009;129(1):14–30.

36. Abeck D, Mempel M. *Staphylococcus aureus* colonization in atopic dermatitis and its therapeutic implications. *Br J Dermatol.* 1998;139:13–16.

37. Leung DYM, Hauk P, Strickland I, et al. The role of superantigens in human diseases: therapeutic implications for the treatment of skin diseases. *Br J Dermatol.* 1998;139:17–29.

38. Ong PY, Leung DY. The infectious aspects of atopic dermatitis. *Immunol Allergy Clin North Am.* 2010;30(3):309–321.

39. Ionescu G, Kiehl R, Wichmann-Kunz F, Leimbeck R. Immunobiological significance of fungal and bacterial infections in atopic eczema. *J Adv Med.* 1990;3(1):47–58.

40. Bath-Hextall FJ, Birnie AJ, Ravenscroft JC, Williams HC. Interventions to reduce Staphylococcus aureus in the management of atopic eczema: an updated Cochrane review. *Br J Dermatol.* 2010;163(1):12–26.

41. Ayers S. Gastric secretion in psoriasis, eczema and dermatitis herpetiformis. *Arch Derm Syphilol.* 1929;20:854–859.

42. Nikitina LS, Shinsky GE, Trusov VV. Contribution of the membranous digestion and the small intestine absorption to the pathogenesis of eczema. *Vestn Dermatol Venerol.* 1989;2:4–7.

43. Vasiliev YV. Digestive activity of intestinal disaccharidases in infants suffering from eczema. *Vestn Dermatol Venerol.* 1984;10:16–20.

44. Feary J, Britton J, Leonardi-Bee J. Atopy and current intestinal parasite infection: a systematic review and meta-analysis. *Allergy.* 2011;66(4):569–578.

45. Rook GA, Brunet LR. Microbes, immunoregulation, and the gut. *Gut.* 2005;54(3):317–320.

46. Vael C, Desager K. The importance of the development of the intestinal microbiota in infancy. *Curr Opin Pediatr.* 2009;21(6):794–800.

47. Ursell A. Dietary manipulation in eczema. *Practitioner.* 1994;238:284–288.

48. Niedner R. Solanum dulcamara L. – a "plant cortisone"? *Med Monatsschr Pharm.* 1996;19(11):339–340.

49. Fernando S, Broadfoot A. Chronic urticaria—assessment and treatment. *Aust Fam Physician.* 2010;39(3): 135–138.

50. Kaplan AP, Greaves M. Pathogenesis of chronic urticaria. *Clin Exp Allergy.* 2009;39(6):777–787.

51. Boguniewicz M. The autoimmune nature of chronic urticaria. *Allergy Asthma Proc.* 2008;29(5):433–438.

52. Kolibášová K, Cervenková D, Hegyi E, et al. Helicobacter pylori – a possible etiologic factor of chronic urticaria. *Dermatosen*. 1994;42(6):235–236.

53. Lolis MS, Bowe WP, Shalita AR. Acne and systemic disease. *Med Clin North Am*. 2009;93(6):1161–1181.

54. Janiczek-Dolphin N, Cook J, Thiboutot D, et al. Can sebum reduction predict acne outcome? *Br J Dermatol*. 2010;163(4): 683–688.

55. Thiboutot DM. Acne: an overview of clinical research findings. *Dermatol Clin*. 1997;15(1):97–109.

56. Baur DA, Butler RCD. Current concepts in the pathogenesis and treatment of acne. *J Oral Maxillofac Surg*. 1998;56: 651–655.

57. Leyden JJ. New understandings of the pathogenesis of acne. *J Am Acad Dermatol*. 1995;32(5 Pt3):S15–S25.

58. Brown SK, Shalita AR. Acne vulgaris. *Lancet*. 1998;351:1871–1876.

59. Grange PA, Weill B, Dupin N, Batteux F. Does inflammatory acne result from imbalance in the keratinocyte innate immune response? *Microbes Infect*. 2010;12(14–15):1085–1090.

60. Dessinioti C, Katsambas AD. The role of Propionibacterium acnes in acne pathogenesis: facts and controversies. *Clin Dermatol*. 2010;28(1):2–7.

61. Kurokawa I, Danby FW, Ju Q, et al. New developments in our understanding of acne pathogenesis and treatment. *Exp Dermatol*. 2009;18(10):821–832.

62. Melnik BC. FoxO1 – the key for the pathogenesis and therapy of acne? *J Dtsch Dermatol Ges*. 2010;8(2):105–114.

63. Costa A, Lage D, Moisés TA. Acne and diet: truth or myth? *An Bras Dermatol*. 2010;85(3):346–353.

64. Davidovici BB, Wolf R. The role of diet in acne: facts and controversies. *Clin Dermatol*. 2010;28(1):12–16.

65. Berra B, Rizzo AM. Glycemic index, glycemic load: new evidence for a link with acne. *J Am Coll Nutr*. 2009;28(suppl):450S–454S.

66. Bowe WP, Joshi SS, Shalita AR. Diet and acne. *J Am Acad Dermatol*. 2010;63(1):124–141.

67. Melnik BC. Evidence for acne-promoting effects of milk and other insulinotropic dairy products. *Nestle Nutr Workshop Ser Pediatr Program*. 2011;67:131–145.

68. Melnik BC, Schmitz G. Role of insulin, insulin-like growth factor-1, hyperglycaemic food and milk consumption in the pathogenesis of acne vulgaris. *Exp Dermatol*. 2009;18(10):833–841.

69. Thappa DM, Dogra J. Nodulocystic acne: oral gugulipid versus tetracycline. *J Dermatol*. 1994;21(10):729–731.

70. Smith EV, Grindlay DJ, Williams HC. What's new in acne? An analysis of systematic reviews published in 2009–2010. *Clin Exp Dermatol*. 2011;36(2):119–122.

71. Balambal R, Thiruvengadam KV, Kameswarant L, et al. Ocimum basilicum in acne vulgaris – a controlled comparison with a standard regime. *J Assoc Physicians India*. 1985;33(8):507–508.

72. Seki T, Morohashi M. Effect of some alkaloids, flavonoids and triterpenoids, contents of Japanese-Chinese traditional herbal medicines, on the lipogenesis of sebaceous glands. *Skin Pharmacol*. 1993;6(1):56–60.

73. McCarty M. High-chromium yeast for acne? *Med Hypotheses*. 1984;14: 307–310.

74. Park JE, Barbul A. Understanding the role of immune regulation in wound healing. *Am J Surg*. 2004;187(5A):11S–16S.

75. Dartenuc JY, Marache P, Choussat H. Resistance capillaire en geriatrie etude d'un microangioprotecteur – Endotelon. *Bord Med*. 1980;13:903–907.

76. Tixier JM, Godeau G, Robert AM, Hornebeck W. Evidence by in vivo and in vitro studies that binding of pycnogenols to elastin affects its rate of degradation by elastases. *Biochem Pharmacol*. 1984;33:3933–3939.

Male reproductive system

Scope

Apart from their use to provide non-specific support for recuperation and repair, specific phytotherapeutic strategies include the following.

Treatment of:

- erectile dysfunction
- some cases of low fertility.

Management of:

- andropause and associated low libido
- benign prostatic hyperplasia with lower urinary tract symptoms
- acute and chronic prostatitis
- early stages of prostate cancer.

Orientation

The key to good health in a man is no secret. Men are more prone to poor health habits and over time this can lead to the expected chronic diseases. Epidemiological studies support this proposition. For example, a US study followed nearly 6000 American men of Japanese descent for 40 years and looked at whether or not they survived to 85 years.[1] Overall 42% survived, but only 11% were healthy. The healthy men avoided six particular risk factors: being overweight, high blood sugar, hypertension, high blood fats, smoking and excessive alcohol. All save the last two are linked to insulin resistance. A more recent study in men >90 years confirmed these findings and noted the beneficial effects of healthy exercise.[2]

However, it is not just the killer diseases that are particularly related to lifestyle choices by men. Many of the common male disorders, that were once thought to be accidents or the consequence of ageing, are now known to heavily feature dietary and lifestyle factors in their aetiology. In fact, reduced testosterone, erectile dysfunction, prostate cancer (PC) and benign prostatic hyperplasia show a strong pattern of co-morbidity, reflecting on common causes. The key causes featured in the literature are focused on factors that lead to insulin resistance and 'inflammaging'. Hence appropriate dietary and lifestyle changes are particularly relevant in the comprehensive management of most male disorders.

Phytotherapy

Andropause

In contrast to women, men do not experience a sudden cessation of gonadal function comparable to menopause. However, there is a progressive reduction in male hypothalamic-pituitary-gonadal axis function. Testosterone levels decline through both central (pituitary) and peripheral (testicular) mechanisms and there is loss of the circadian rhythm of testosterone secretion.

Overall, at least 25% of men over age 70 meet laboratory criteria for hypogonadism (testosterone deficiency). This has been termed andropause or PADAM (partial androgen deficiency of ageing men) or popularly 'male menopause'. It is thought to be responsible for a variety of symptoms in ageing men, including reduced muscle and bone mass, fatigue and erectile dysfunction.[3] However, its diagnosis and the subsequent use of testosterone therapy are still controversial.[4]

Numerous cross-sectional and longitudinal studies indicate that testosterone declines with age (1% per year from 40 years). There is an even greater decline in free or bioavailable (free + albumin bound) testosterone, partly because of the 1.2% per year increase in SHBG (sex hormone-binding globulin).[5] Despite the large body of evidence that testifies to a decline in testosterone with age, it is by no means universal. Numerous studies have demonstrated that fit and healthy men in their 70s could achieve testosterone levels within the range expected for young men, provided they took regular exercise, were non-smokers, were not overweight and in general good health.[6]

The ADAM (androgen deficiency of ageing men) questionnaire forms a validated test for screening for symptoms related to a low testosterone level. In addition, the questions are informative themselves in defining the changes in a man associated with declining testosterone. In particular, they highlight that testosterone very much functions as a coping hormone in men. The questions are:

1. Do you have a decrease in libido?
2. Do you have a lack of energy?
3. Do you have a decrease in strength and/or endurance?
4. Have you lost height?
5. Have you noticed a decreased 'enjoyment of life'?
6. Are you sad and/or grumpy?
7. Are your erections less strong?
8. Have you noted a recent deterioration in your ability to play sports?
9. Are you falling asleep after dinner?
10. Has there been a recent deterioration in your work performance?

A recent study found that questions 1 and 7 were the most diagnostic of low testosterone (especially if three other questions were positive).[7]

A number of epidemiological studies have identified key factors associated with PADAM. For example, obesity and metabolic syndrome have been linked to accelerated testosterone decline.[8] Alcohol use and stress are also implicated.[9,10] In turn, low testosterone predicts an increased risk of Alzheimer's disease,[11] cognitive decline,[12] insulin resistance and type 2 diabetes.[13] Low testosterone is associated with increased mortality in men and a higher risk of cardiovascular disease.[14]

A key herb in the management of PADAM is *Tribulus terrestris*. This herb possibly acts on the central regulation of testosterone production, at the level of the pituitary and hypothalamus. Clinical and in vivo studies have demonstrated increased testosterone, libido and sexual activity (see Tribulus monograph). *Withania somnifera* also improved testosterone levels in infertile men and boosted DHEAS (dehydroepiandrosterone sulphate) levels in stressed patients (see Withania monograph). Another traditional male tonic that will certainly help the stress and insulin resistance aspects linked to PADAM is *Panax ginseng* (see monograph). *Serenoa repens* is traditionally regarded as a herb for atrophy of the sexual tissues in both men and women and can be included in formulations to address the peripheral (testicular) decline in testosterone output (see monograph).

Example liquid formula

Withania somnifera	2:1	20 mL
Panax ginseng	1:2	10 mL
Tribulus terrestris	2:1	50 mL
Serenoa repens	1:2	30 mL
	TOTAL	110 mL

Dose: 8 mL with water twice a day.

Low male fertility

About 15% of all couples are sub-fertile and the man is responsible in 30% of these cases. In another 20% abnormalities are detected in both partners.[15] Ejaculation volume may be reduced, sperm count may be low or sperm may be abnormal. The cause in the male is usually unknown, although prescribed or recreational drugs can be identified in some cases. Excessive exposure to heat, as from hot tubs, can decrease sperm production, as can tight underwear. A percentage of men with varicoceles are sub-fertile because of them. Varicoceles can be treated with vascular herbs such as horsechestnut, gotu kola, butcher's broom and the circulatory herbs listed below.

Treatment should attend to all lifestyle factors, since sperm are a reflection of the overall health of the male. Any major health problems and weaknesses, such as poor immunity, effects of stress, anxiety and so on, should be specifically addressed. A healthy diet rich in fruit and vegetables and low in refined carbohydrate should be observed.

Specific herbal guidelines for low fertility in the male are:

- male hormone and fertility promoting herbs: Korean ginseng, saw palmetto, Tribulus and Withania
- tonic and adaptogenic herbs: Korean ginseng, Withania and Siberian ginseng
- prostate herbs if prostatic secretions are abnormal (usually there will be a history of prostatitis): saw palmetto and nettle root
- antioxidant and circulatory herbs to improve microcirculation: grape seed, green tea, bilberry and Ginkgo.

Example liquid formula

Panax ginseng (standardised extract)	1:2	35 mL
Serenoa repens	1:2	25 mL
Ginkgo biloba (standardised extract)	2:1	20 mL
Withania somnifera (standardised extract)	2:1	20 mL
	TOTAL	100 mL

Dose: 8 mL with water twice a day.

A couple were participating in an IVF programme. Sperm count and motility in the man were below normal. He took 4 mL of Korean ginseng 1:2 with water each day for 8 weeks. At the end of the 8 week period his sperm count was the highest recorded that month at the clinic.

A 42-year-old male had very low sperm count, 38% abnormal forms and poor motility. No pregnancy with unprotected sex (same partner) for last 7 years. Therapy was Tribulus one tablet twice a day. His wife was pregnant before the 3 months when planned repeat of his semen analysis was due. This tablet contained *Tribulus terrestris* herb, standardised for 100 mg steroidal saponins calculated as protodioscin. (Case history kindly provided by Dr Therese Lovell, Sydney.)

Erectile dysfunction

Obviously the development of drugs such as sildenafil has revolutionised the medical management of erectile dysfunction (ED). These drugs act as inhibitors of phosphodiesterase-5 (PDE-5) and increase cyclic GMP (cGMP). Maximal erectile function results from the relaxation of the smooth muscle of the penile arterial vessels through the activation of neuronal nitric oxide synthase (NOS), together with relaxation of the smooth muscle around the sinusoids of the corpora cavernosa through release of endothelial NO. The smooth muscle relaxation brought about by NO is mediated by cGMP release, and PDE acts to break down this cGMP. However, in most men with ED, poor lifestyle choices and resulting endothelial dysfunction and vascular disease result in insufficient NO and cGMP functions for the PDE-5 inhibitors to achieve their full potential.

ED in an otherwise healthy man is in fact a warning sign of endothelial dysfunction and impending vascular disease. In terms of risk factors, obesity is strongly associated with ED and the disorder is three times more common in diabetic men. In fact, one study found 12% of men with ED had unrecognised diabetes. Insulin resistance and metabolic syndrome are also risk factors for ED. In another study in men without diabetes, ED was strongly correlated with waist:hip ratio and was significantly improved by weight loss and exercise (with improved endothelial NO production). Smoking doubles the risk of ED, but limited alcohol intake is not a problem. ED is commonly co-morbid with hypertension, low testosterone, diabetes, obesity and benign prostatic hyperplasia and lower urinary tract symptoms (LUTS).[16,17]

Some studies have delved deeper into the link between insulin resistance and ED. For example, a strong association was established between metabolic syndrome, insulin resistance and the incidence of ED. A fasting blood glucose >6.1 mmol/L was found to be positively correlated to increasing severity of ED.[18]

A systematic review and meta-analysis identified seven randomised controlled trials of Korean red ginseng in the treatment of ED.[19] Six of the trials compared the effect of ginseng against placebo, enabling a meta-analysis. This demonstrated a highly significant and clinical relevant effect of ginseng on ED (p<0.00001). However, the authors cautioned that the low methodological quality and small sample size precluded

absolute conclusions. Doses used in the trials were relatively high at typically 2 to 3 g/day (see monograph).

Specific herbal guidelines for ED are as follows:

- Treat any stress and anxiety with anxiolytic herbs such as valerian. Nervine tonics are often required, particularly damiana, skullcap and St John's wort.
- Devitalisation is often a factor that can be alleviated by tonic and adaptogenic herbs such as Korean ginseng, Withania and Rhodiola. Adrenal tonics can be required such as Rehmannia.
- Male hormone levels can be improved with male tonics: saw palmetto, Withania and particularly Tribulus as previously described.
- Improving circulation will provide a benefit to maintain erection, and circulatory herbs, particularly ginger, Ginkgo and prickly ash, can assist.
- Address insulin resistance and cardiovascular/endothelial health with appropriate herbs.

Example liquid formula

Ginkgo biloba (standardised)	2:1	20 mL
Panax ginseng (standardised)	1:2	30 mL
Serenoa repens	1:2	20 mL
Turnera diffusa	1:2	20 mL
Withania somnifera	2:1	20 mL
	TOTAL	110 mL

Dose: 8 mL with water twice a day.

Combine with Tribulus leaf tablets (three per day) providing 300 mg/day steroidal saponins calculated as protodioscin for low testosterone and/or libido.

A male patient aged 46 presented with ED. He was relatively healthy but his blood pressure was slightly elevated at 125/95 mmHg. Otherwise no circulatory issues were apparent. On questioning he was regularly drinking a licorice and fennel tea – both herbs are potentially oestrogenic in high doses. He had tried a PDE-5 inhibitor but was not overly impressed and did not like using it. He was advised to substantially reduce the tea, drink green tea instead (hence supporting endothelial function) and do regular exercise. After two visits his prescription settled on the following:

Withania somnifera (standardised extract)	2:1	20 mL
Turnera diffusa	1:2	30 mL
Ginkgo biloba (standardised extract)	2:1	30 mL
Passiflora incarnata	1:2	30 mL
	TOTAL	110 mL

Dose: 5 mL with water twice a day.

In addition, energy tonic tablets containing 600 mg *Rhodiola rosea* dry root, standardised to contain salidroside 1.5 mg, and 500 mg *Panax ginseng* dry root, standardised to contain ginsenosides calculated as Rg and Rb 8 mg, were prescribed at two tablets twice a day.

On review 3 months after his initial visit his blood pressure was normal (drinking much less licorice/fennel tea as advised), he reported having more energy and that the herbs were 'working'.

The following case history of a successful, simple treatment is kindly provided by Dr Therese Lovell, Sydney. A 72-year-old male presented with a loss of ability to get the penile head (distal half) to harden during intercourse. This had been occurring for about 12 months and he now had great difficulty in achieving any penetration for his partner of many years. He had no other symptoms or signs of neurovascular compromise outside the presenting complaint. He did have excess trunkal fat, which was suggested would only serve to increase his overall metabolic risks and would intensify his erectile dysfunction.

He had been using Ginkgo extract tablets (60 mg) at a dose of one twice daily for some years for general vascular support. Tribulus leaf 9 g tablets (each containing 100 mg protodioscin) were introduced on a trial basis for 3 months. Dose was one twice daily. The patient returned after 3 months and reported a 95% improvement in his ED. He was keen to continue the Tribulus tablets at the same dose and was absolutely delighted with the results.

Benign prostatic hyperplasia

BPH is a progressive, benign growth of the prostate gland that gradually narrows the urethra.[20] The clamping effect eventually obstructs the flow of urine. As a result, the bladder fails to empty completely. Urine remaining in the bladder stagnates, leaving the patient vulnerable to infections, bladder stones and kidney damage. The poor bladder capacity can cause frequent urination especially at night. Associated with BPH is therefore a set of LUTS. However, there is not always an exact correlation between the size of the prostate and the degree of LUTS, suggesting that other urodynamic factors are also involved.

The exact cause of BPH is not known and there have been various theories proposed.[21] The recent understanding downplays androgens, both testosterone and dihydrotestosterone; their role is said now to be permissive. A higher oestrogen/testosterone ratio could be a causative hormonal factor. Increased peripheral conversion of testosterone to oestradiol by aromatase could be at play here.[21] Chronic inflammation is also a common finding and one theory has proposed that BPH is an immune-mediated inflammatory disease caused by either infection or autoimmunity (more likely the latter).[22] There is a strong link between chronic prostatitis and BPH.[23] Another theory proposes that higher circulating insulin stimulates prostate growth, and hence links BPH to insulin resistance.[24,25]

Indeed, multiple experimental, clinical and epidemiological studies have demonstrated the link between either hyperinsulinaemia, elevated fasting blood glucose or type 2 diabetes and prostate enlargement and LUTS.[24] An association with obesity has also been observed.[26] The sympathetic overactivity linked to obesity, metabolic syndrome and hypertension may specifically increase the risk of manifesting LUTS.[27,28] LUTS and metabolic syndrome have been shown to be co-morbid, as has LUTS and ED. Improving testosterone can help symptoms of LUTS[29] and inflammation may also play a role in LUTS (insulin resistance is a pro-inflammatory condition); elevated serum C-reactive protein (CRP) correlates well with severity of LUTS.[30]

Increased levels of physical activity have been associated with a decreased risk of BPH and LUTS in several large studies.[31]

A low fat, low animal protein diet appears to be protective, as does alcohol consumption against BPH, but it might increase LUTS.[32] High glycaemic load foods appear to contribute to risk,[31,33] whereas consumption of fruit and vegetables appears protective.[34] A recent review of 14 studies confirmed the beneficial effect of exercise and proposed that decreased sympathetic tone, lower insulin resistance and reduced oxidative damage to the prostate could be the mechanisms involved.[35]

Herbal remedies have a long history in the management of BPH/LUTS. The early association of the symptoms of prostatic enlargement (urinary frequency, retention and diminished flow) with ageing in men led to the inevitable association of remedies that reduced these symptoms with rejuvenating male tonics and promoters of male potency. Given the eternal demand for such agents, it is not surprising that they feature in most traditions. In some it is difficult to distinguish the stimulant aphrodisiac from the prostatic remedy; whereas cola (kola nuts) and *Pausinystalia yohimbe* (yohimbe), used in male virility ceremonies in west Africa, are obvious stimulants (the former a high caffeine source once briefly combined with the cocaine-containing coca leaves in the stimulant tonic drink of that name), it is less easy to distinguish the modest euphoric effects of high doses of the central American plant *Turnera diffusa* (damiana) from its reputation in aiding at least some of the problems of older men. *Panax ginseng* (Korean ginseng) was used particularly for elderly men in traditional Asian culture and is still favoured for prostatic enlargement symptoms – it has potential hormonal activity as a rationale. The most notable remedy from the southern USA is *Serenoa repens* (saw palmetto), initially used as a male tonic (as noted previously) but with increasing evidence of benefits in BPH. However, the consensus view appears to be shifting against its efficacy. Positive 1998 and 2002 Cochrane reviews[36] have been supplanted by a negative 2009 revision, which suggested that in a total of 26 studies there was no benefit above placebo.[37] (See the monograph for a discussion of these issues.) Saw palmetto is widely prescribed by urologists in Germany for early symptoms of benign prostatic hyperplasia, along with *Urtica dioica* (nettle root) and *Curcurbita pepo* (pumpkin seed).[38] There is consistent evidence for benefit in the case of *Urtica* in double blind, controlled studies (see monograph).[39] In the case of pumpkin seed, evidence is disappointing: one large multi-centre, placebo-controlled, double blind study on 542 early stage BPH patients looked at the effect of 500 mg standardised pumpkin seed extract or placebo twice daily for 12 months and found no difference in the two groups on subjective and laboratory measures.[40] The African remedy *Pygeum africanum* has been beneficial in clinical trials and is popular in France. However, it has been classified as an endangered species, with bleak prospects for its sustainability.[41] *Crataeva nurvala* improves bladder tone and decreases bladder emptying and is a useful symptomatic treatment for urinary obstruction, including that linked to prostatic enlargement (see the Urinary system in this chapter).

Specific herbal guidelines for BPH/LUTS are:

* improve prostate function with antiprostatic herbs that act by various mechanisms and include saw palmetto and nettle root (with clinical evidence for the benefit of this combination)

- improve compromised bladder function with the bladder tonic Crataeva
- control infection with Echinacea and Andrographis and urinary antiseptic herbs such as buchu and cranberry
- alleviate excess sympathetic tone/LUTS with spasmolytic herbs especially cramp bark, Corydalis, wild yam, valerian and kava.

Example liquid formula

Serenoa repens	1:2	40 mL
Urtica dioica	1:2	30 mL
Crataeva nurvala	1:2	40 mL
	TOTAL	110 mL

Dose: 8 mL with water twice per day.

CASE HISTORY

A male patient aged 69 complained of urinary problems, especially frequency. He was needing to go more frequently during the day and was getting up three to four times each night. It was assumed he had BPH/LUTS. Saw palmetto and nettle root were prescribed, but after 3 months of treatment there was no improvement. Enquiry to his doctor revealed that his prostate was not enlarged and his PSA (prostate specific antigen) was very low. A trial of relaxing herbs, plus Crataeva to improve bladder function was instituted to treat what might be excess sympathetic tone causing LUTS. He noted steady improvement over the next 5 months to the point where he was only needing to get up once during the night.

The new treatment consisted of:

Zizyphus spinosa	1:2	20 mL
Scutellaria lateriflora	1:2	20 mL
Viburnum opulus	1:2	20 mL
Crataeva nurvala	1:2	40 mL
	TOTAL	100 mL

Dose: 8 mL with water twice per day.

Chronic prostatitis

Prostatitis literally means inflammation of the prostate gland. It can be caused by a bacterial infection, in which case it is usually acute and short-lived. More common, however, is chronic prostatitis (also known as chronic prostatitis/chronic pelvic pain syndrome, CP/CPPS), for which the cause is basically unknown (bacteria are rarely involved). This painful and debilitating disorder can affect up to 15% of men at some stage in their lives and between 2% and 10% of adult men suffer from prostatitis at any given time.[42] There is evidence suggesting that CP may be associated with an increased risk of prostate cancer (PC) as well as enlargement of the prostate (BPH).[42]

The main symptoms of CP/CPPS are, as the name implies, chronic genitourinary pain or discomfort, with or without difficulties on urination. There is no known effective conventional treatment. Doctors often prescribe antibiotics, but they are rarely effective. Even if bacteria are involved (and they are mostly not), the prostate gland is notoriously difficult for antibiotics to gain effective access.

The exact cause of CP is unknown, but many relevant factors have been identified that probably all contribute to the problem. Feedback from patients is that prolonged sitting or riding a pushbike can make the condition worse, which suggests that poor circulation to the prostate is a probable factor. Many also complain that their pain flares up when they drink alcohol, so if this is the case it should be avoided.

From the published research, chronic inflammation possibly due to an autoimmune reaction is identified as an important factor. Men with CP have signs of significant inflammation in biopsy tissue taken from their prostates, with T cells apparently driving this reaction.[43] Another factor is stress. A study in Finland found that psychological stress is common in men with CP/CPPS.[44]

One of the key herbs for CP/CPPS is saw palmetto, because of the thinking that it improves the overall health of the prostate gland. One clinical trial found a liposterolic extract of saw palmetto did not improve CP/CPPS,[45] but it can work well in combination, especially as the galenical. Another key herb is Echinacea, indicated to balance the immune system and also to help the body resolve any low level bacterial presence that might be driving the autoimmune response (also a case for urinary antiseptics such as buchu). Other relevant herbs include nettle root (which is again another herb to support the prostate), cramp bark and chamomile for pain and spasm. The Ayurvedic herb Crataeva is useful where bladder symptoms are also involved, since it is the best herb to support bladder function. Sometimes other immune herbs such as the mushrooms Ganoderma and shiitake can be valuable in stubborn cases.

In addition, herbs for chronic immune weakness such as Astragalus and tonic and adaptogenic herbs should be considered, as should mucous membrane tonic and anticatarrhal herbs such as golden seal and ribwort. Anti-inflammatory herbs may be appropriate, such as Bupleurum, Rehmannia and even Boswellia.

Example liquid formula

Echinacea purpurea/angustifolia root	1:2	25 mL
Serenoa repens	1:2	30 mL
Glycyrrhiza glabra (high in glycyrrhizin)	1:1	15 mL
Barosma betulina	1:2	20 mL
Zea mays	1:1	20 mL
	TOTAL	110 mL

Dose: 8 mL with water twice a day.

CASE HISTORY

A male patient aged 53 years presented with chronic prostatitis of 20 years' duration. He experienced episodes of pain and cramping and sexual intercourse was painful (meaning it did not happen very often). Semen had been bloody at times, which supported the diagnosis of chronic prostatitis. Antibiotics had been prescribed over long periods but had been of no help. Occasionally there was a clear discharge.

The following formula was prescribed:

Echinacea purpurea/angustifolia root	1:2	25 mL
Barosma betulina	1:2	25 mL
Urtica dioica	1:2	20 mL
Crataeva nurvala	1:2	30 mL
	TOTAL	100 mL

Dose: 8 mL with water twice a day.

In addition, immune-enhancing tablets containing 400 mg *Echinacea angustifolia* root powder, 1000 mg *Andrographis paniculata* herb standardised to contain 8 mg andrographolide, 500 mg *Ocimum tenuiflorum* herb and 10 mg *Ocimum tenuiflorum* leaf essential oil were prescribed at four tablets per day, together with 320 mg/day of the liposterolic extract of saw palmetto.

After 4 weeks there was considerable improvement. On intercourse there was no sharp pain, but still a burning sensation. The patient described himself as 'the best I have been for a long time'. Over the ensuing months the treatment was continued, and the patient became symptom-free on maintenance doses that are half those given above.

Prostate cancer

Older men are at increased risk of prostate cancer (PC), especially those with a family history and/or with a higher prostate specific antigen (PSA) level.[46] Autopsy results reveal that a man's percentage risk of harbouring PC is about the same as his age in years. African Americans have a much higher risk. The risk is low in Asia, but when Japanese men move to the US their risk increases.[47] Infection and inflammation (prostatitis) also appear to be causative factors. Many men with PC also have prostatitis on biopsy and regular use of anti-inflammatory drugs lowers risk of developing PC. The role of androgens is unclear and controversial; 5alpha-reductase inhibitors may prevent the condition, but their value in studies might result from improved screening (more reliable PSA and biopsies).[48]

PSA is a protease enzyme produced by the prostate to keep the semen liquid. The use of serum PSA to screen for prostate cancer is highly controversial. Some medical experts have likened it to 'tossing a coin'. Around 75% of men with an elevated PSA reading do not have active PC and around 20% of men with PC will have a normal PSA. This is largely because elevated PSA is also associated with prostatitis and BPH.[46,49]

A high-grade prostatic intraepithelial neoplasia (HGPIN or just PIN) may be found on biopsy. This is a pre-cancerous state, like carcinoma in situ, that can regress or progress.[50,51]

The phenomenon of 'watchful waiting' (active surveillance) for men with intermediate PSA and/or Gleason score (GS) readings provides an opportunity for herbal management of men with low-grade PC. This is also the case for the pre-cancerous state HGPIN.

Key aspects of a plausible phytotherapeutic strategy are as follows:

- Address inflammation and downregulate inflammatory pathways
- Supplement with phyto-oestrogens

- Improve immune regulation
- Exploit specific pathways of cancer cell regulation (as per Boik, see pp. 177–178) using multifunctioning herbs[52]
- Dietary recommendations.

In terms of downregulating inflammatory pathways in PC, herbs that can reduce NF-kappaB transcription should be emphasised.[53] A complex protocol mainly involving an anti-inflammatory herbal formula (rosemary, turmeric, ginger, holy basil, green tea, Polygonum, Coptis, barberry, oregano and Baical skullcap) was evaluated over 18 months in 23 men with HGPIN in an open label trial. The mean starting PSA was 6.13 ± 3.56 ng/mL and by the end of the trial 48% of the men demonstrated a 25% to 50% reduction. Of the 15 participants who had the 18-month biopsy, 60% had reverted to benign, 27% still had HGPIN and 13% progressed to PC (GS 6). Serum CRP and NF-kappaB (in prostate tissue) were significantly reduced.[54]

Baical skullcap flavonoids are being actively researched for antitumour properties, including PC models. Attenuation of NF-kappaB activity is a large part of this activity.[55] Curcumin has demonstrated apoptosis and a radiosensitising effect in prostate cancer cell lines (see also monograph).[56,57] Boswellia is anti-inflammatory and a boswellic acid (AKBA) induced apoptosis in PC cell lines and at 10 mg/kg suppressed PC tumour growth in mice and inhibited angiogenesis.[58,59] Red wine, but not alcohol, has been linked to a significantly lower risk of PC.[60] Resveratrol and OPCs are anti-inflammatory components found in wine. Grape seed extract inhibited advanced human prostate tumour growth and angiogenesis in mice at 100 mg/kg/day.[61] Resveratrol at about 12.5 mg/kg suppressed PC growth in rats[62] and inhibited NF-kappaB-regulated gene expression in PC cells.[63] In vitro and in vivo studies suggest that a key tumour-inhibiting mechanism for cat's claw is suppression of NF-kappaB. Cat's claw has also demonstrated clinical anti-inflammatory activity in a trial in rheumatoid arthritis patients.[64] Feverfew also has profound effects on NF-kappaB, but there are problems with bioavailability and hence an effective dose (see monograph).

In terms of phyto-oestrogens, there is promising research on linseed and isoflavones. Linseeds (30 g/day) for an average of 30 days prior to surgery significantly reduced cellular proliferation rates in a controlled trial involving 161 men with PC.[65] There were no changes in testosterone or PSA. Metabolites of the linseed lignans (such as enterolactone) inhibit PC cell growth in vitro.[66]

There is good evidence from a recent meta-analysis of 14 epidemiological studies that soya foods will lower the risk of PC by around 26%.[67] Non-fermented sources of soya such as tofu or soya milk showed a higher degree of protection than fermented soya products such as miso. There is also good evidence that soy isoflavone supplementation can help patients with PC. Yet extraordinarily in 2007 the Cancer Council NSW, Australia, issued a press release warning patients with PC not to take soya foods 'because they can accelerate the growth of tumours'.[68] Clinical studies with soya in healthy men have found favourable alterations in sex hormone levels and metabolism.[69,70] Prostatic fluid concentrations of isoflavones in soya consumers are sufficient to inhibit PC cell growth in vitro[71] and isoflavones have been detected in prostate tissue after supplementation.[72] In fact, prostatic levels exceeded serum levels.[73] Healthy men receiving 100 mg/day of soya isoflavones were protected from TNF-alpha-induced NF-kappaB activation (assessed in lymphocytes).[74] Four clinical studies have shown reductions in PSA or PSA velocity or other favourable effects in men with various stages of PC after intake of soya isoflavones or soya drinks. Typical isoflavone doses were 100 to 200 mg/day.[75–78] In a controlled trial 50 g/day of soya grits significantly reduced PSA and increased free PSA compared with a control wheat diet in men with PC scheduled for a radical prostatectomy.[79] Isoflavone intake is best increased via both diet and supplements.[80]

The effect of an isoflavonoid-rich extract of red clover (60 mg/day isoflavones) on 20 men with elevated PSA levels (mean 10.16 ng/mL) but negative prostate biopsy was investigated over 1 year in an uncontrolled study. Mean PSA fell to 7.15 ng/mL (p<0.019).[81] Randomised controlled trials are needed in biopsy-positive men.

In terms of immune regulation, investigations of medicinal mushrooms have mainly been undertaken. Activated hemicellulose compound is an extract of shiitake mushroom mycelia. It acts by enhancing cellular immune responses.[82,83] Modest benefits were observed in patients with advanced PC[83] and a dramatic remission was published for a patient with metastatic castration-resistant PC (GS 9).[84] Similar modest trial results were seen for a soya product combined with Ganoderma mycelia polysaccharides (5 g daily of the mushroom extract and also delivering around 900 mg/day isoflavones) in patients with PC.[85] However, another dramatic remission was published of a patient with confirmed PC (GS 6) who received a low dose of the product for 6 weeks.[86] PSA fell from 19.7 to 4.2 and no PC was found after prostatectomy. Cases such as these are a clear validation of applying the living with cancer principles in early stage cancers (see Chapter 8).

Green tea could prove to be a key herb in PC cell regulation, but promising results with silymarin from St Mary's thistle are hampered by its poor access to the prostate. Preclinical (in vivo and in vitro) studies suggest that green tea and epigallocatechin gallate possess multi-targeted activity in PC.[87,88] Induction of apoptosis and reduction in NF-kappaB activity appear to be important in vitro mechanisms. Tea polyphenols were present in human and mouse prostate tissue after green tea consumption.[89]

Early clinical studies with green tea were not promising, but both trials were in advanced, hormone-refractory PC patients.[90,91] A subsequent double blind, placebo-controlled study of 60 men with HGPIN over 1 year found that 60 mg/day of green tea catechins reduced LUTS and reduced the incidence of PC development (one case with green tea versus nine in placebo).[92] A follow-up study of around half the men 2 years later (after no further treatment) found two more PC cases in the placebo group and one in the green tea group, establishing that the benefits were maintained.[93] Twenty-six men with positive biopsies took 1.3 g/day green tea catechins until surgery.[94] PSA was decreased, as were growth factors in prostatic tissue.

Silymarin has demonstrated multiple mechanisms of activity against PC in vitro and in vivo.[95,96] Silymarin also synergises with chemotherapeutic drugs in vitro.[97] One mechanism involves inhibition of multi-drug resistance pumps. However, after oral dosing of high amounts in men only very low levels were found in prostatic tissue.[98]

The use of the PSA biomarker has provided for some interesting studies in prostate cancer. An uncontrolled study of pomegranate juice (8 oz daily containing 570 mg of polyphenolics) in men with rising PSA after surgery or radiotherapy was conducted in 48 patients with PSA 0.2 to <5.0 ng/mL and GS≤7. Mean PSA doubling time significantly increased from 15 months at baseline to 54 months post-treatment (p<0.001).[99]

The research team of Dr Dean Ornish in the US has looked at the impact of diet in PC patients under watchful waiting. In the first study, a very low-fat vegan diet (12% dietary fat) plus supplements (soya, vitamin E, fish oil, selenium and vitamin C), exercise and stress management was compared to controls. PSA declined 4% over 12 months versus a 6% rise in the control arm. At follow-up 2 years later, 13 men in the control group had progressed to PC treatment versus just two in the intervention group. A second study with similar intervention examined prostate biopsies after 3 months. Gene expression changes in tissue consistent with lower tumourigenesis were observed. A low glycaemic index, moderate fat diet in four men for 6 weeks found favourable gene expression changes after radical prostatectomy compared with controls.[100,101]

Example treatments
Watchful waiting and post-treatment The following liquid formulation:

Panax ginseng	1:2	15 mL
Echinacea purpurea/angustifolia root	1:2	35 mL
Uncaria tomentosa	1:2	30 mL
Scutellaria baicalensis	1:2	30 mL
	TOTAL	110 mL

Dose: 8 mL with water twice a day.
In addition, select from the following:
- 60 to 120 mg/day resveratrol from Polygonum
- Medicinal mushrooms (dose depends on species, etc.)
- Soy or red clover isoflavones 100 to 200 mg/day (if appropriate)
- Boswellia extract 2 g/day
- Ideally a low fat, low GI, organic, vegan diet with soya products
- 30 g of linseeds daily
- Green tea (as much as possible)
- Organic carrot (two thirds) and beetroot (one third) juice, 200 to 400 mL daily
- A good consumption of brassica vegetables
- Tomato paste (40 g daily, containing about 20 to 30 mg lycopene) and turmeric powder (5 g daily)
- Orange juice (including the peel – best if organic) 300 to 600 mL daily.

CASE HISTORY

A male patient aged 54 presented with a diagnosis of PC with a rising PSA of 6.1 and a biopsy with three positive cores, GS 9. He had been booked for a radical prostatectomy the following month and was advised to go ahead. A few months later the patient returned to report the surgery was successful in controlling his PC (PSA <0.01) but unfortunately left him without the control of his bladder and he was suffering infections. No follow-up radiotherapy or hormone therapy had been offered.

The following liquid formulation was prescribed:

Panax ginseng	1:2	10 mL
Barosma betulina	1:2	20 mL

Echinacea purpurea/angustifolia root	1:2	30 mL
Glycyrrhiza glabra (high in glycyrrhizin)	1:1	15 mL
Crataeva nurvala	1:2	35 mL
	TOTAL	110 mL

Dose: 8 mL with water two to three times daily.

In addition, the patient was recommended a tea formulation (containing *Rumex acetosella*, *Arctium lappa*, *Ulmus rubra* and *Rheum palmatum*) and tablets providing 6 g/day POA-type cat's claw. After 6 years, the patient has no urinary infections and is currently maintained on Astragalus, Echinacea and the herbal tea formulation, all in tablet form, together with many of the dietary recommendations noted above. His PSA is still low.

References

1. Willcox BJ, He Q, Chen R, et al. Midlife risk factors and healthy survival in men. *JAMA*. 2006;296(19):2343–2350.

2. Yates LB, Djoussé L, Kurth T, et al. Exceptional longevity in men: modifiable factors associated with survival and function to age 90 years. *Arch Intern Med*. 2008;168(3):284–290.

3. Clapauch R, Braga DJ, Marinheiro LP, et al. Risk of late-onset hypogonadism (andropause) in Brazilian men over 50 years of age with osteoporosis: usefulness of screening questionnaires. *Arq Bras Endocrinol Metabol*. 2008;52(9):1439–1447.

4. [No authors listed] Testosterone for 'late-onset hypogonadism' in men? *Drug Ther Bull*. 2010;48(6):69–72.

5. Morley JE. Hormones and the aging process. *J Am Geriatr Soc*. 2003;51(7 suppl):S333–S337.

6. Diver MJ, Imtiaz KE, Ahmad AM, et al. Diurnal rhythms of serum total, free and bioavailable testosterone and of SHBG in middle-aged men compared with those in young men. *Clin Endocrinol (Oxf)*. 2003;58(6):710–717.

7. Blümel JE, Cedraui P, Gili SA, et al. Is the Androgen Deficiency of Aging Men (ADAM) questionnaire useful for the screening of partial androgenic deficiency of aging men? *Maturitas*. 2009;63(4):365–368.

8. Rodriguez A, Muller DC, Metter EJ, et al. Aging, androgens, and the metabolic syndrome in a longitudinal study of aging. *J Clin Endocrinol Metab*. 2007;92(9):3568–3572.

9. Hafez B, Hafez ESE. Stress/aging: endocrine profiles/reproductive dysfunction in men. *Arch Androl*. 2004;50(4):207–238.

10. Emanuele MA, Emanuele N. Alcohol and the male reproductive system. *Alcohol Res Health*. 2001;25(4):282–287.

11. Moffat SD, Zonderman AB, Metter EJ, et al. Free testosterone and risk for Alzheimer disease in older men. *Neurology*. 2004;62(2):188–193.

12. Moffat SD, Zonderman AB, Metter EJ, et al. Longitudinal assessment of serum free testosterone concentration predicts memory performance and cognitive status in elderly men. *J Clin Endocrinol Metab*. 2002;87(11):5001–5007.

13. Saad F. The role of testosterone in type 2 diabetes and metabolic syndrome in men. *Arq Bras Endocrinol Metabol*. 2009;53(8):901–907.

14. Jones TH. Testosterone deficiency: a risk factor for cardiovascular disease? *Trends Endocrinol Metab*. 2010;21(8):496–503.

15. Howards SS. Treatment of male infertility. *N Engl J Med*. 1995;332(5):312–317.

16. Berookhim BM, Bar-Chama N. Medical implications of erectile dysfunction. *Med Clin North Am*. 2011;95(1):213–221.

17. Meldrum DR, Gambone JC, Morris MA, et al. A multifaceted approach to maximize erectile function and vascular health. *Fertil Steril*. 2010;94(7):2514–2520.

18. Bansal TC, Guay AT, Jacobson J, et al. Incidence of metabolic syndrome and insulin resistance in a population with organic erectile dysfunction. *J Sex Med*. 2005;2(1):96–103.

19. Jang DJ, Lee MS, Shin BC, et al. Red ginseng for treating erectile dysfunction: a systematic review. *Br J Clin Pharmacol*. 2008;66(4):444–450.

20. Wiygul J, Babayan RK. Watchful waiting in benign prostatic hyperplasia. *Curr Opin Urol*. 2009;19(1):3–6.

21. Roehrbornb CG. Pathology of benign prostatic hyperplasia. *Int J Impot Res*. 2008;20(suppl 3):S11–S18.

22. Kramer G, Mitteregger D, Marberger M. Is benign prostatic hyperplasia (BPH) an immune inflammatory disease? *Eur Urol*. 2007;51(5):1202–1216.

23. Sciarra A, Mariotti G, Salciccia S, et al. Prostate growth and inflammation. *J Steroid Biochem Mol Biol*. 2008;108(3–5):254–260.

24. Vikram A, Jena G, Ramarao P. Insulin-resistance and benign prostatic hyperplasia: the connection. *Eur J Pharmacol*. 2010;641(2–3):75–81.

25. Bushman W. Etiology, epidemiology, and natural history of benign prostatic hyperplasia. *Urol Clin North Am*. 2009;36(4):403–415.

26. Parsons JK, Sarma AV, McVary K, et al. Obesity and benign prostatic hyperplasia: clinical connections, emerging etiological paradigms and future directions. *J Urol*. 2009;182(6 suppl):S27–S31.

27. Moul S, McVary KT. Lower urinary tract symptoms, obesity and the metabolic syndrome. *Curr Opin Urol*. 2010;20(1):7–12.

28. Sarma AV, Parsons JK, McVary K, et al. Diabetes and benign prostatic hyperplasia/lower urinary tract symptoms-what do we know? *J Urol*. 2009;182(6 suppl):S32–S37.

29. Yassin AA, El-Sakka AI, Saad F, et al. Lower urinary-tract symptoms and testosterone in elderly men. *World J Urol*. 2008;26(4):359–364.

30. Sarma AV, Kellogg Parsons J. Diabetes and benign prostatic hyperplasia: emerging clinical connections. *Curr Urol Rep*. 2009;10(4):267–275.

31. Parsons JK. Modifiable risk factors for benign prostatic hyperplasia and lower urinary tract symptoms: new approaches to old problems. *J Urol*. 2007;178(2):395–401.

32. Parsons JK, Im R. Alcohol consumption is associated with a decreased risk of benign prostatic hyperplasia. *J Urol*. 2009;182(4):1463–1468.

33. Ranjan P, Dalela D, Sankhwar SN. Diet and benign prostatic hyperplasia: implications for prevention. *Urology*. 2006;68(3):470–476.

34. Barnard RJ, Aronson WJ. Benign prostatic hyperplasia: does lifestyle play a role? *Phys Sportsmed*. 2009;37(4):141–146.

35. Sea J, Poon KS, McVary KT. Review of exercise and the risk of benign prostatic hyperplasia. *Phys Sportsmed*. 2009;37(4):75–83.

36. Wilt T, Ishani A, MacDonald R. Serenoa repens for benign prostatic hyperplasia. *Cochrane Database Syst Rev*. 2002;(3):CD001423.

37. Tacklind J, MacDonald R, Rutks I, Wilt TJ. Serenoa repens for benign prostatic

hyperplasia. *Cochrane Database Syst Rev.* 2009;(2):CD001423.

38. Bombardelli E, Morazzoni P. Cucurbita pepo L. *Fitoterapia.* 1997;68(4):291–302.

39. Safarinejad MR. Urtica dioica for treatment of benign prostatic hyperplasia: a prospective, randomized, double blind, placebo-controlled, crossover study. *J Herbal Pharmacother.* 2005;5(4):1–11.

40. Bach D. Placebo-controlled, long-term therapeutic study of a pumpkin seed extract product in patients with micturition complaints from benign prostatic hyperplasia. *Urology.* 2000;40:437–443.

41. Stewart KM. The African cherry (Prunus africana): can lessons be learned from an over-exploited medicinal tree? *J Ethnopharmacol.* 2003;89(1):3–13.

42. Krieger JN. Classification, epidemiology and implications of chronic prostatitis in North America, Europe and Asia. *Minerva Urol Nefrol.* 2004;56(2):99–107.

43. John H, Barghorn A, Funke G, et al. Noninflammatory chronic pelvic pain syndrome: immunological study in blood, ejaculate and prostate tissue. *Eur Urol.* 2001;39(1):72–78.

44. Mehik A, Hellstrom P, Sarpola A, et al. Fears, sexual disturbances and personality features in men with prostatitis: a population-based cross-sectional study in Finland. *BJU Int.* 2001;88(1):35–38.

45. Kaplan SA, Volpe MA, Te AE. A prospective, 1-year trial using saw palmetto versus finasteride in the treatment of category III prostatitis/chronic pelvic pain syndrome. *J Urol.* 2004;171(1): 284–288.

46. Kell JS. Prostate-specific antigen tests and prostate cancer screening: an update for primary care physicians. *Can J Urol.* 2010;17(suppl 1):18–25.

47. Patel AR, Klein EA. Risk factors for prostate cancer. *Nat Clin Pract Urol.* 2009;6(2):87–95.

48. Jacobs EJ, Rodriguez C, Mondul AM, et al. A large cohort study of aspirin and other nonsteroidal anti-inflammatory drugs and prostate cancer incidence. *J Natl Cancer Inst.* 2005;97(13):975–980.

49. Thanigasalam R, Mancuso P, Tsao K, et al. Prostate-specific antigen velocity (PSAV): a practical role for PSA? *Aust N Z J Surg.* 2009;79(10):703–706.

50. Epstein JI. An update of the Gleason grading system. *J Urol.* 2010;183(2): 433–440.

51. Punnen S, Nam RK. Indications and timing for prostate biopsy, diagnosis of early stage prostate cancer and its definitive treatment: a clinical conundrum in the PSA era. *Surg Oncol.* 2009;18(3):192–199.

52. Boik J. *Cancer and Natural Medicine: A Textbook of Basic Science and Clinical Research.* USA: Oregon Medical Press; 1995. pp. 110–111.

53. Aggarwal BB. Nuclear factor-kappaB: the enemy within. *Cancer Cell.* 2004;6(3):203–208.

54. Capodice JL, Gorroochurn P, Cammack S, et al. Zyflamend in men with high-grade prostatic intraepithelial neoplasia: results of a phase I clinical trial. *J Soc Integr Oncol.* 2009;7(2):43–51.

55. Li-Weber M. New therapeutic aspects of flavones: the anticancer properties of Scutellaria and its main active constituents Wogonin, Baicalein and Baicalin. *Cancer Treat Rev.* 2009;35(1):57–68.

56. Hilchie AL, Furlong SJ, Sutton K, et al. Curcumin-induced apoptosis in PC3 prostate carcinoma cells is caspase-independent and involves cellular ceramide accumulation and damage to mitochondria. *Nutr Cancer.* 2010;62(3):379–389.

57. Chendil D, Ranga RS, Meigooni D, et al. Curcumin confers radiosensitizing effect in prostate cancer cell line PC-3. *Oncogene.* 2004;23(8):1599–1607.

58. Lu M, Xia L, Hua H, et al. Acetyl-keto-beta-boswellic acid induces apoptosis through a death receptor 5-mediated pathway in prostate cancer cells. *Cancer Res.* 2008;68(4):1180–1186.

59. Pang X, Yi Z, Zhang X, et al. Acetyl-11-keto-beta-boswellic acid inhibits prostate tumor growth by suppressing vascular endothelial growth factor receptor 2-mediated angiogenesis. *Cancer Res.* 2009;69(14):5893–5900.

60. Schoonen WM, Salinas CA, Kiemeney LALM, et al. Alcohol consumption and risk of prostate cancer in middle-aged men. *Int J Cancer.* 2005;113(1):133–140.

61. Singh RP, Tyagi AK, Dhanalakshmi S, et al. Grape seed extract inhibits advanced human prostate tumor growth and angiogenesis and upregulates insulin-like growth factor binding protein-3. *Int J Cancer.* 2004;108(5):733–740.

62. Harper CE, Cook LM, Patel BB, et al. Genistein and resveratrol, alone and in combination, suppress prostate cancer in SV-40 tag rats. *Prostate.* 2009;69(15): 1668–1682.

63. Benitez DA, Hermoso MA, Pozo-Guisado E, et al. Regulation of cell survival by resveratrol involves inhibition of NF kappa B-regulated gene expression in prostate cancer cells. *Prostate.* 2009;69(10): 1045–1054.

64. Morgan M. Major Therapeutic activity of cat's claw. *Phytotherapist's Perspective.* 10:2010. Available from <www.mediherb. com.au>.

65. Demark-Wahnefried W, Polascik TJ, George SL, et al. Flaxseed supplementation (not dietary fat restriction) reduces prostate cancer proliferation rates in men presurgery. *Cancer Epidemiol Biomarkers Prev.* 2008;17(12):3577–3587.

66. McCann MJ, Gill CI, Linton T, et al. Enterolactone restricts the proliferation of the LNCaP human prostate cancer cell line in vitro. *Mol Nutr Food Res.* 2008;52(5):567–580.

67. Yan L, Spitznagel EL. Soy consumption and prostate cancer risk in men: a revisit of a meta-analysis. *Am J Clin Nutr.* 2009;89(4):1155–1163.

68. Weaver C. Cancer warning on soy foods. 2007. <http://www.news.com.au/features/ cancer-patients-warned-off-soy-rich-foods/ story-e6frfl49-1111112828191>. Accessed 17 August 2011.

69. Hamilton-Reeves JM, Rebello SA, Thomas W, et al. Soy protein isolate increases urinary estrogens and the ratio of 2:16alpha-hydroxyestrone in men at high risk of prostate cancer. *J Nutr.* 2007;137(10):2258–2263.

70. van Veldhuizen PJ, Thrasher JB, Ray G, et al. Dose effect of soy supplementation in prostate cancer: a pilot study. *Oncol Rep.* 2006;16(6):1221–1224.

71. Hedlund TE, van Bokhoven A, Johannes WU, et al. Prostatic fluid concentrations of isoflavonoids in soy consumers are sufficient to inhibit growth of benign and malignant prostatic epithelial cells in vitro. *Prostate.* 2006;66(5):557–566.

72. Guy L, Vedrine N, Urpi-Sarda M, et al. Orally administered isoflavones are present as glucuronides in the human prostate. *Nutr Cancer.* 2008;60(4):461–468.

73. Gardner CD, Oelrich B, Liu JP, et al. Prostatic soy isoflavone concentrations exceed serum levels after dietary supplementation. *Prostate.* 2009;69(7): 719–726.

74. Davis JN, Kucuk O, Djuric Z, et al. Soy isoflavone supplementation in healthy men prevents NF-kappa B activation by TNF-alpha in blood lymphocytes. *Free Radic Biol Med.* 2001;30(11):1293–1302.

75. Kwan W, Duncan G, Van Patten C, et al. A phase II trial of a soy beverage for subjects without clinical disease with rising prostate-specific antigen after radical radiation for prostate cancer. *Nutr Cancer.* 2010;62(2):198–207.

76. Pendleton JM, Tan WW, Anai S, et al. Phase II trial of isoflavone in prostate-specific antigen recurrent prostate cancer after previous local therapy. *BMC Cancer.* 2008;8:132.

77. Hamilton-Reeves JM, Rebello SA, Thomas W, et al. Effects of soy protein isolate consumption on prostate cancer biomarkers in men with HGPIN, ASAP, and low-grade prostate cancer. *Nutr Cancer.* 2008;60(1):7–13.

78. Hussain M, Banerjee M, Sarkar FH, et al. Soy isoflavones in the treatment of prostate cancer. *Nutr Cancer.* 2003;47(2):111–117.

79. Dalais FS, Meliala A, Wattanapenpaiboon N, et al. Effects of a diet rich in phytoestrogens on prostate-specific antigen and sex hormones in men diagnosed with prostate cancer. *Urology.* 2004;64(3):510–515.

80. Gardner CD, Chatterjee LM, Franke AA. Effects of isoflavone supplements vs. soy foods on blood concentrations of genistein and daidzein in adults. *J Nutr Biochem.* 2009;20(3):227–234.

81. Engelhardt PF, Riedl CR. Effects of one-year treatment with isoflavone extract from red

clover on prostate, liver function, sexual function, and quality of life in men with elevated PSA levels and negative prostate biopsy findings. *Urology*. 2008;71(2): 185–190.

82. deVere White RW, Hackman RM, Soares SE, et al. Effects of a mushroom mycelium extract on the treatment of prostate cancer. *Urology*. 2002;60(4):640–644.

83. Terakawa N, Matsui Y, Satoi S, et al. Immunological effect of active hexose correlated compound (AHCC) in healthy volunteers: a double blind, placebo-controlled trial. *Nutr Cancer*. 2008;60(5):643–651.

84. Turner J, Chaudhary U. Dramatic prostate-specific antigen response with activated hemicellulose compound in metastatic castration-resistant prostate cancer. *Anticancer Drugs*. 2009;20(3):215–216.

85. deVere White RW, Hackman RM, Soares SE, et al. Effects of a genistein-rich extract on PSA levels in men with a history of prostate cancer. *Urology*. 2004;63(2):259–263.

86. Ghafar MA, Golliday E, Bingham J, et al. Regression of prostate cancer following administration of Genistein Combined Polysaccharide (GCP), a nutritional supplement: a case report. *J Altern Complement Med*. 2002;8(4):493–497.

87. Stuart EC, Scandlyn MJ, Rosengren RJ. Role of epigallocatechin gallate (EGCG) in the treatment of breast and prostate cancer. *Life Sci*. 2006;79(25):2329–2336.

88. Khan N, Adhami VM, Mukhtar H. Review: green tea polyphenols in chemoprevention of prostate cancer: preclinical and clinical studies. *Nutr Cancer*. 2009;61(6): 836–841.

89. Henning SM, Aronson W, Niu Y, et al. Tea polyphenols and theaflavins are present in prostate tissue of humans and mice after green and black tea consumption. *J Nutr*. 2006;136(7):1839–1843.

90. Choan E, Segal R, Jonker D, et al. A prospective clinical trial of green tea for hormone refractory prostate cancer: an evaluation of the complementary/ alternative therapy approach. *Urol Oncol*. 2005;23(2):108–113.

91. Jatoi A, Ellison N, Burch PA, et al. A phase II trial of green tea in the treatment of patients with androgen independent metastatic prostate carcinoma. *Cancer*. 2003;97(6):1442–1446.

92. Bettuzzi S, Brausi M, Rizzi F, et al. Chemoprevention of human prostate cancer by oral administration of green tea catechins in volunteers with high-grade prostate intraepithelial neoplasia: a preliminary report from a one-year proof-of-principle study. *Cancer Res*. 2006;66(2):1234–1240.

93. Brausi M, Rizzi F, Bettuzzi S. Chemoprevention of human prostate cancer by green tea catechins: two years later. A follow-up update. *Eur Urol*. 2008;54(2):472–473.

94. McLarty J, Bigelow RL, Smith M, et al. Tea polyphenols decrease serum levels of prostate-specific antigen, hepatocyte growth factor, and vascular endothelial growth factor in prostate cancer patients and inhibit production of hepatocyte growth factor and vascular endothelial growth factor in vitro. *Cancer Prev Res (Phila)*. 2009;2(7): 673–682.

95. Cheung CW, Gibbons N, Johnson DW, et al. Silibinin – a promising new treatment for cancer. *Anticancer Agents Med Chem*. 2010;10(3):186–195.

96. Singh RP, Raina K, Sharma G, et al. Silibinin inhibits established prostate tumor growth, progression, invasion, and metastasis and suppresses tumor angiogenesis and epithelial-mesenchymal transition in transgenic adenocarcinoma of the mouse prostate model mice. *Clin Cancer Res*. 2008;14(23):7773–7780.

97. Colombo V, Lupi M, Falcetta F, et al. Chemotherapeutic activity of silymarin combined with doxorubicin or paclitaxel in sensitive and multidrug-resistant colon cancer cells. *Cancer Chemother Pharmacol*. 2011;67(2):369–379.

98. Flaig TW, Glode M, Gustafson D, et al. A study of high-dose oral silybin-phytosome followed by prostatectomy in patients with localized prostate cancer. *Prostate*. 2010;70(8):848–855.

99. Pantuck AJ, Leppert JT, Zomorodian N, et al. Phase II study of pomegranate juice for men with rising prostate-specific antigen following surgery or radiation for prostate cancer. *Clin Cancer Res*. 2006;12(13):4018–4026.

100. Freedland SJ, Aronson WJ. Dietary intervention strategies to modulate prostate cancer risk and prognosis. *Curr Opin Urol*. 2009;19(3):263–267.

101. Van Patten CL, de Boer JG, Tomlinson Guns ES. Diet and dietary supplement intervention trials for the prevention of prostate cancer recurrence: a review of the randomized controlled trial evidence. *J Urol*. 2008;180(6):2314–2322.

Endocrine disorders

Scope

Apart from their use to provide non-specific support for recuperation and repair, specific phytotherapeutic strategies include the following:

Treatment of:

- adrenal depletion
- reactive dysglycaemia
- functional endocrine deficiencies.

Management of:

- metabolic syndrome
- type 2 diabetes
- hyper- and hypothyroidism.

Particular **caution** is necessary in applying phytotherapy in cases of:

- brittle type 1 diabetes.

Orientation

Hormone resistance

Declining endocrine function is one key manifestation of ageing. However, it appears to have been exacerbated in modern times by the phenomenon of functional hormone resistance, with insulin resistance being the least controversial, significant and most prevalent example.

Functional hormone resistance occurs when the endocrine gland produces adequate amounts of a given hormone, but the target cells are unable to utilise that hormone properly. The consequences are that either the effect of this hormone is reduced, or the body responds by producing more of the hormone to compensate. Both outcomes can lead to chronic health problems.

Insulin resistance is a curse of modern lifestyle that can lead to metabolic syndrome and type 2 diabetes. It has also been linked to a wide variety of other diseases such as breast and prostate cancer, PCOS (polycystic ovary syndrome), Alzheimer's disease, gout and NASH (non-alcoholic steatorrhoeic hepatitis). Abdominal or central obesity (visceral adiposity) is probably the most significant issue in metabolic syndrome[1,2] and underlies the key metabolic change, which is insulin resistance.[1] 'Insulin resistance syndrome' is in fact an alternative name preferred by some scientists.

Many patients show clinical evidence of low thyroid function (especially low body temperature) but have normal laboratory tests for TSH (thyroid stimulating hormone), T3 and T4. It has been recently and controversially proposed that this phenomenon is due to thyroid hormone resistance (THR), similar to insulin resistance.[3] This is not to be confused with subclinical hypothyroidism, which is medically defined as normal T3 and T4 with mildly elevated TSH (less than 10.0 MIU/L, normal range typically given as 0.3 to 5.5),[4] although the two issues could occur together.

Subclinical hypothyroidism is usually associated with antithyroid antibodies but THR is not.[4] Attributed causes of THR include mitochondrial dysfunction and environmental toxins including heavy metals, dioxins and pesticides acting as endocrine disrupters.[3] Adrenal and thyroid function are connected, and elevated cortisol can interfere with thyroid function and possibly also lead to THR.[5] It has also been proposed that chronic infection, chronic inflammation and hypercoagulation can cause THR.[6]

The most reliable method of diagnosis of THR is the symptom picture coupled with a positive Barnes Basal Temperature test. Temperatures below 36.6°C indicate hypothyroid function and possible THR if thyroid hormone tests are normal. A favourable response to thyroid treatment (phytotherapeutic or medical) confirms the diagnosis. Signs to look for include puffy face and lips, thinning hair and outer eyebrows, swollen skin, lack of alertness, cold extremities, weight gain and tendency to chronic infections. However, low thyroid function is the 'great imitator' that can mimic a vast number of medical conditions.

Functional cortisol resistance is probably even more controversial. The best example of chronic hyperactivation of the stress system (both the HPA axis and the noradrenergic system), probably due to a functional cortisol resistance, is melancholic depression.[7] Hypersecretion of CRH from the hypothalamus has been shown in depression, with associated increases in ACTH and plasma cortisol. This hypersecretion of CRH is thought to be due to an impaired sensitivity of glucocorticoid receptors in the cerebral cortex, hypothalamus and pituitary, which impedes the normal negative feedback effect of cortisol. The higher amount of cortisol in melancholic depression has damaging effects leading to osteoporosis, metabolic syndrome, chronic infections and cancers.[7] When not treated, these patients have a reduced life expectancy of 15 to 20 years, after excluding suicide. Other conditions possibly associated with functional cortisol resistance include anorexia nervosa, obsessive compulsive disorder, metabolic syndrome, chronic alcoholism and overtraining syndrome. In contrast, for fibromyalgia syndrome the resistance is probably to ACTH, rather than cortisol, due to poorly functioning adrenal glands.

The antidepressant activity of *Rhodiola rosea* is interesting in this context. Stress-activated protein kinase (SAPK, also known as JNK) inhibits the sensitivity of glucocorticoid receptors to cortisol. In an experimental model, both Rhodiola extract and salidroside decreased the release of SAPK/JNK and cortisone in response to stress. Hence the authors postulated that Rhodiola inhibits the stress-induced activation of SAPK/JNK in depressed patients and thereby restores the impaired sensitivity of glucocorticoid receptors to cortisol. Rhodiola also lowered awakening cortisol levels in patients with chronic stress and fatigue.[8]

The three key hormones discussed above exhibit functional relationships with each other. For example, exercise and weight loss-induced improvements in insulin resistance were blunted by poor thyroid status (subclinical hypothyroidism).[9] The relationship between excess cortisol and insulin resistance or impaired thyroid function has already been discussed.

As touched on above, modern exposure to endocrine disrupters could play a significant role in endocrine disorders, including functional hormone resistance, metabolic syndrome, type 2 diabetes and hypothyroidism. One particularly relevant class of potent endocrine disruptors comprises the persistent organic pollutants (POPs).

These are mainly the organochlorines, which largely comprise the PCBs and DDT and metabolites. They have been banned from use in Western countries for several decades, but are incredibly stable in the environment and accumulate in fat tissue. Consumption of animal products means humans are particularly prone to POP accumulation. Some examples of their potential chronic effects on the body follow.

Serum levels of PCBs correlate with blood pressure, which is independent of BMI or age.[10] In utero exposure to PCBs in concentrations slightly higher than average impacts on intellectual function.[11] PCB exposure from a waste incinerator was found to adversely impact thyroid function in children.[12] POPs including PCBs have been linked to increased incidences of oestrogen receptor-positive breast cancer[13] and breast cancer in general.[14]

A major metabolite of DDT is DDE.[15] The body's DDE level is a risk factor for liver cancer, but associations with other cancers are controversial. Elevated DDE levels have been linked to CFS. DDT/DDE has been associated with female infertility, male infertility and miscarriages.

Gamma-glutamyltransferase (GGT) is the main predictor among serum liver enzymes for type 2 diabetes incidence.[16] Relatively recently it has been linked to increased incidences of metabolic syndrome[17] and insulin resistance.[18] Even values at the high end of the normal range are predictive of a marked increase in risk. It has been shown that an increase in GGT predicts new onset of metabolic syndrome, incident (as opposed to silent) cardiovascular disease and death, suggesting that GGT is a marker of metabolic and cardiovascular risk.[19]

Various theories have been proposed, for example that GGT indicates the development of fatty liver disease[16] or is a measure of inflammation and oxidative stress.[20] However, one compelling suggestion is that POPs are acting as endocrine disruptors, with GGT representing a measure of this exposure. After adjustment for all other known factors, including BMI and waist circumference, diabetes prevalence was strongly positively associated with POPs.[21] In two studies, POPs (mainly as organochlorine pesticides) have been positively linked to insulin resistance[22] and metabolic syndrome.[23]

In humans BMI and fat mass are positively correlated with plasma POPs.[24] Lipolysis is associated with an increase in POP release, leading to a hyperconcentration of these pollutants in plasma and tissues during body weight and fat loss. This release of POPs during weight loss has been associated with decreased energy expenditure, such as resting metabolic rate. It accounts for around half of the adaptive drop in thermogenesis that occurs with weight loss. It is partly explained by a drop in T4 and T3, indicating significant endocrine disruption. POPs have even been described as environmental obesogens.[24]

Such information regarding POPs highlights the need to support the body's detoxification mechanisms where functional hormone resistance is evident. Enhancing phase I and especially phase II clearance by the liver is critical to reduce the burden of endocrine disruption, as is eating organic foods, especially animal products. Nutrients supporting the liver and providing the substrates of phase II clearance such as glutamine, glycine, taurine, cysteine, methionine and choline are important. Key herbs for boosting detoxification include Schisandra, rosemary (Rosmarinus), garlic (*Allium sativum*), green tea (Camellia), turmeric (*Curcuma longa*) and the Brassica species. Choleretic herbs also have a role since the phase II products will be largely excreted in the bile. During weight loss, supporting the hepatic metabolism of POPs becomes critical, as does additional thyroid support.

Arresting hormone decline

As mentioned above, the function of most endocrine glands declines with age, so it is relevant here to consider whether therapeutic plants can play a role in arresting endocrine ageing.

The industrialised world is facing a major challenge. The anticipated almost exponential increase in the number of older people will have dramatic and potentially disastrous consequences for public health, healthcare financing and delivery, informal caregiving and pension systems.[25] Take the US as a key example. In the US the proportion of the population aged 65 years or older is projected to increase from 12.4% in 2000 to 19.6% in 2030, being 71 million citizens. The number of people aged 80 years or older will more than double from 9.3 million to 19.5 million. By 2025 the proportion of Florida's population aged 65 years or older is projected to be 26%. This demographic transition, which is due to the ageing of the baby boomers and increased life expectancy, represents a huge social challenge. About 80% of people aged greater than 65 years will have at least one chronic health condition, and 50% at least two. For example, about 10% of all adults aged 65 years or more will suffer from Alzheimer's disease.[25]

> My relationship with death remains the same. I am very strongly against it.... There's no advantage in getting older. I'm 74 now. You don't get any wiser, you don't get more mellow.... Nothing good happens. Your back hurts more. You get more indigestion. Your eyesight isn't as good. You need a hearing aid. It's a bad business getting older, and I would advise you not to do it.
>
> Woody Allen, 2010

Should getting older be just about 'nothing good happens'? Are we really meant to only become sicker and frailer as we age, with declining adrenal, thyroid and pancreatic function? The above quote from Woody Allen touches on a key issue here: that successful ageing is not just about living longer; it

is about maintaining optimal mental, social and physical well-being and function.[26] In other words, healthspan is as important as lifespan, in fact even more so. Preserving endocrine function into old age is a key part of this.

The famous ageing researcher Leonard Hayflick once observed that ageing is 'an increase in molecular disorder'.[27] One recently proposed theory that builds on this basic concept, and ties many ageing concepts together into one model, has been dubbed the 'green theory' of ageing. This model proposes that ageing is the result of damage to large key molecules, especially proteins, that has accumulated as a result of toxic metabolic byproducts (including damage caused by oxidation). A primary determinant of healthspan is therefore the efficiencies of either the protection against toxic products, the removal of these toxic products, including phase I/II detoxification by the liver, or the repair of this large molecule damage.[28,29] Protect, detoxify and repair is the catch-cry of preserving cellular health into old age.

The body has many pathways for detoxification, protection and repair:[30,31]

- Multiple pathways of repair of nuclear and mitochondrial DNA
- Processes for sensing and responding to intra- and extracellular stressors
- Pathways for protein repair, including chaperones
- Pathways for the removal and turnover of defective proteins (involving protease enzymes)
- Antioxidative and enzymic defences against oxygen free radicals
- Processes for the detoxification of harmful chemicals in the diet and from the environment (phase I/II)
- Immune responses against pathogens and parasites
- Processes of wound healing and tissue regeneration
- Maintenance of optimum blood glucose levels to minimise the damage glucose does to proteins (the damaged proteins are known as advanced glycation endproducts or AGEs)
- Pathways for the normal programmed death (apoptosis) of irreversibly damaged cells.

According to the green theory, as long as these detoxification, protection and repair pathways are operating at their optimum efficiency, healthy ageing and preserved endocrine function should be a given. These themes sound remarkably like those in an old-fashioned naturopathy book. A key secret in achieving this goal is embedded in the concept of hormesis.

The term 'hormesis' was originally developed by toxicologists. In the recent context it conveys a simple message: what does not kill you makes you stronger. Medical and biological scientists now use the word hormesis to describe a key, fundamental concept of life: that moderate stress is not only healthy, it actually actively promotes optimum health. Hormesis therefore describes the beneficial adaptive response to moderate, healthy stress. It possibly represents the universal tonic and perhaps the one true fountain of youth.

Examples of hormesis in the research are many. For example, moderate levels of exercise promote excellent health, whereas excessive levels are debilitating and can lead to overtraining syndrome. There are countless examples from experimental models. For example, mild heat shock protected fruit fly larvae against a freezing shock that would normally kill them. Mild hypoxia stress can increase the lifespan of the roundworm (*Caenorhabditis elegans*) and can induce cross-tolerance to other types of stress.

The beneficial effects of mild to moderate stress (or hormetic effects) on ageing and longevity have been studied for several years, but especially in the last decade. In summary, mild to moderate stress has been found to increase longevity, delay behavioural ageing and increase resistance to other stresses in many animal models.[32-35]

How can exposure to low levels of toxins or other stressors have beneficial effects? The answer lies in the defence molecules the body calls up in response to threats. Once rallied, these molecules not only deal with the immediate threat, but also increase resistance to other threats. They can even repair pre-existing damage, as per the green theory. Examples of these molecular defence agents include heat shock proteins (HSPs), sirtuin1, and the various beneficial growth factors and cell kinases. HSPs are produced when cells are exposed to high temperatures, toxins or inflammation. Their role is to protect (chaperone) other key proteins from damage by binding to them and shielding them from attack. Another 'bodyguard', sirtuin1 (or SIRT1), senses cellular stress and activates multiple genes that code for protective proteins such as antioxidants and cell-membrane stabilisers.[36]

At this point it is worth mentioning the first class of herbs that can induce or mimic hormetic effects in the body: these are the adaptogens and they include ginseng (*Panax ginseng*), Rhodiola, Eleutherococcus and Withania. Recent research suggests that Echinacea root could be an adaptogen (see monograph). The basic theory of adaptogens was that they helped the body cope with stress by fine-tuning (and hence conserving) the stress response. They were also thought to support immune responses. However, current research has shed new light on how adaptogens might confer these benefits, and this is via hormesis.

It has recently been shown that the stress-protective effect of adaptogens is not the result of an inhibition of the stress response, but actually the result of the adaptation of the organism to the mild stress-mimicking effect of the adaptogen. In other words adaptogens mimic healthy stress in the body and turn on protective hormetic-response molecules, such as HSPs, thereby extending healthspan.[37,38]

Another key antiageing concept that ties in well with the green theory and hormesis is the value of calorie restriction (CR). All ageing researchers universally acknowledge that dietary restriction or CR by 20% to 40% is proven to extend lifespan by up to 50%. No other known intervention has such a consistent and profound effect: experiments on single yeast cells up to primates have verified this outcome. But the key story here is not the extension of lifespan; it is the significant compression of morbidity (or extension of healthspan and normal endocrine function) that also takes place. At advanced ages CR animals are more youthful-looking, display inquisitive behaviour and are highly active, just like much younger animals. The exact way that CR works to extend youthfulness and lifespan is not fully understood, but several researchers have proposed that it is due to hormesis, with CR acting as a moderate healthy stressor.[39-41]

A strong advocate of the hormesis hypothesis for CR is Dr David Sinclair, an Australian scientist working at Harvard on ageing research. He argues that the hormesis hypothesis links so many of the diverse observations about CR from experimental models. The pathways involved are a hardwired survival mechanism to enhance the chance of survival during stress and reduced food availability – a defensive response to a survival threat. Sinclair proposes that this very basic survival mechanism should be and is regulated by a few genes and their corresponding proteins. These genes have been identified as *SIRT1* to 7. *SIRT1* is particularly important. The sirtuin proteins are increased in CR and regulate a multitude of beneficial metabolic effects, as noted above.

Since phytochemicals can cause hormetic responses and may act as environmental signals to shift into survival mode ahead of an environmental decline, Sinclair's team investigated whether simple phytochemicals might increase the SIRT1 protein. Resveratrol, found in grapes and several other foods and herbs, was identified to be the most active natural agent at activating SIRT1.[42] *Polygonum cuspidatum*, the giant knotweed from Chinese traditional medicine, is a rich phytotherapeutic source of resveratrol. This plant is a common weed in many countries.

CR in practice can be difficult. The mental and physical stress of being hungry in conjunction with a modern life might provide more stress than is beneficial for a hormetic effect. Depression- and anxiety-like symptoms have been observed in CR rats. Diminished libido is a common side effect in humans and animals. CR might also reduce resistance to infection.[39,40]

A more compelling strategy to practising actual CR is to find herbs and other supplements that can mimic its effects in the body, in the same way that adaptogens might directly mimic hormesis. The best example of how to do this to date is resveratrol (see above). In yeast cells, resveratrol was found to mimic CR by stimulating Sir2 (the yeast equivalent of SIRT1), and as a result increasing DNA stability and extending lifespan.[42] Resveratrol significantly increased the survival of mice fed a high calorie diet and caused favourable physiological changes similar to CR.[43] While the intense focus has been on resveratrol, other phytochemicals have been shown to activate SIRT1 or the SIRT1 pathway in various in vitro models. For example components of silymarin from Silybum (St Mary's or milk thistle) are active.[44,45]

In addition to resveratrol, there are other ways to mimic CR effects in the body. Three key biochemical changes are observed in CR primate experiments: reductions in body temperature (by around 0.5°C), and plasma insulin, and a prevention of the decline in DHEAS. When men in the Baltimore Longitudinal Study on Ageing were divided into upper and lower halves for each of these values, there was a clear survival benefit observed.[46] The most marked survival benefit was observed for a higher level of DHEAS, followed by a lower level of insulin. A lower body temperature might reflect the benefits of slower metabolism, better oxidative control and reduced workload for the thyroid. Lower insulin probably results in lower AGEs and other favourable metabolic effects, and a higher DHEAS possibly reflects the sparing of the adrenal glands. On the insulin resistance front, metformin (a diabetes drug that promotes insulin sensitivity) prolonged lifespan in rodents and additionally seems to cause biochemical changes similar to CR.[47] Insulin resistance is known to contribute to the risk of developing many chronic diseases (see above and elsewhere in this chapter).

Hence, the beneficial consequences of CR can be simulated by improving insulin sensitivity (lowering insulin resistance) and better preserving DHEA. Perhaps not surprisingly, the adaptogens can help to improve DHEA levels. After oral administration of 6g of Korean red ginseng for 30 days to postmenopausal women, DHEAS was increased by around 13%. Withania (*Withania somnifera*) significantly increased DHEAS by 30% in a placebo-controlled clinical trial (p<0.001).[48,49]

Research has found that many herbs can improve insulin sensitivity. But two herbs are key in a healthy ageing context. A placebo-controlled clinical trial found that a St Mary's thistle extract (delivering 600mg/day of silymarin) for 4 months exerted a beneficial effect on glycaemic profile in relatively well-controlled patients with type 2 diabetes (on medication). There were also significant reductions in HbA_{1c} (13%), fasting blood glucose (15%), total cholesterol (12%), LDL-cholesterol (11%) and triglycerides (25%).[50] In well-controlled type 2 diabetic patients, ginseng caused no change in HbA_{1c} or fasting plasma glucose in a placebo-controlled clinical trial. However, fasting plasma insulin was significantly reduced by the ginseng (by 34%), whereas it increased in the placebo group (by 10%). In other words the ginseng lowered insulin resistance.[51]

In summary, the phytotherapeutic approach to healthy endocrine ageing should:

- maintain healthspan as well as lifespan and help to compress morbidity
- address several of the key insights associated with ageing (based on 'state of the art' information)
- act consistently with current theories of slowing ageing, such as the green theory
- specifically mimic the beneficial effects of CR by activating sirtuin-mediated pathways (SIRT1 especially)
- provide hormetic challenge, support detoxification pathways, help maintain insulin sensitivity and protect the adrenal glands.

Four key herbs discussed above meet many of these targets, being *Polygonum cuspidatum* (with resveratrol), St Mary's thistle (with silymarin), ginseng and Withania.

Phytotherapeutics

Some herbs have a long history of use for endocrine problems, but probably few can match the time-honoured use of *Gymnema sylvestre*. Nature sometimes has an intriguing way of revealing the therapeutic properties of plants. For example, the resemblance of the yellow sap oozing from the broken end of a greater celandine plant (*Chelidonium majus*) to bile has led some herbalists to conclude that this herb is beneficial to the liver and gallbladder. Modern clinical research has supported this traditional insight.

The association between the physical characteristics of a plant and its potential to heal is known as the Doctrine of Signatures. Another cited example is the modern use of mistletoe injections in Europe for the treatment of cancer. The mistletoe is a plant that grows, like a tumour, on other plants.

The Doctrine of Signatures should never be assumed as an absolute rule and it is typically not that useful in describing the potential uses for a herb. However, in the case of the Ayurvedic herb Gymnema or gurmar (which in Hindi means sugar destroyer), the association between one of its physical properties and its use for diabetes is striking.

Gymnema when applied to the mouth (by chewing the leaf or tablet or dropping a liquid extract on the tongue) has the remarkable property of anaesthetising the sweet taste buds. This effect wears off after an hour or two. Hence, the herb, which has been used for over 2000 years for the treatment of diabetes (ancient texts describe its use for when the urine is sweet), makes its 'sugar-destroying' actions known by its effect on the sweet taste buds one of the most dramatic and profound examples of the Doctrine of Signatures.

Gymnema sylvestre is a liana or climbing plant with stems up to 8m in length. It grows in open woods and bush land at an altitude of 300 to 3000 feet in India, China, Indonesia, Japan, Malaysia, Sri Lanka, Vietnam and South Africa. The sweet taste suppressant property of Gymnema was revealed to a British officer by the inhabitants of a northern Indian village in the mid-19th century. As stated previously, the herb is traditionally used for the treatment of diabetes, but Gymnema extracts are also sold in Japan for the control of obesity.

Gymnema contains a group of compounds known as gymnemic acids that appear not only to be largely responsible for its sweet-abolishing properties, but also contribute substantially to its antidiabetic activity. Many in vivo studies have verified the antidiabetic properties of Gymnema, but one study in particular made a remarkable finding, which if verified in time could substantially expand our understanding of the value of this herb for diabetes. Gymnema extracts returned fasting blood glucose levels to normal after 20 to 60 days of oral administration to diabetic rats. Surprisingly, there was a rise in insulin levels towards normal values and the number of beta cells in the pancreas increased.[52] This suggests that Gymnema might actually restore damaged pancreatic tissue, provided the damage has not gone too far. The possibility is supported, to some extent, by the clinical trials on Gymnema (see below).

A controlled study in patients with type 1 diabetes found that a water-soluble Gymnema extract (400mg/day) reduced insulin requirements (by about 50%). Over the duration of treatment Gymnema lowered fasting blood glucose (by about 35%) and glycosylated haemoglobin levels. Cholesterol was also significantly reduced and brought to near normal levels, as were triglycerides. The treatment period ranged from 6 to 30 months. The significant decrease in glycosylated haemoglobin occurred after 6 to 8 months, but this parameter remained significantly higher than normal values. None of these reductions was observed in control patients on insulin therapy alone, who were studied over a period of 10 to 12 months. The authors suggested that Gymnema enhanced insulin production, even from the damaged pancreatic tissue of type 1 diabetic patients, possibly by pancreatic regeneration. As proof of this they found that levels of C-peptide, a byproduct of the conversion of proinsulin to insulin, were apparently raised.[53]

A second study by the same research group found that the same Gymnema preparation (400 mg/day) produced similar results in type 2 diabetics. Fasting blood glucose and glycosylated haemoglobin were significantly reduced compared with baseline values after 18 to 20 months of treatment. None of these reductions was observed in patients receiving conventional therapy alone, who were studied over a period of 10 to 12 months. By the end of the treatment period cholesterol and triglycerides were also significantly reduced in those receiving Gymnema. Fasting and post-meal serum insulin levels were significantly increased in the Gymnema group compared with the patients taking only conventional drugs. Twenty-one of the 22 patients were able to reduce their medication; five of these discontinued it entirely and maintained their blood glucose with Gymnema extract alone. The authors' suggestion of beta cell regeneration or repair facilitated by Gymnema was supported by the higher insulin levels in the serum of patients after Gymnema supplementation.[54]

Despite the long time period for the clinical trials, clinical experience suggests Gymnema can work quickly to control blood sugar levels. Used on its own it will not drop blood sugar to the point of causing hypoglycaemia. However, as the trials demonstrated, its real value probably only follows after prolonged use, in the order of months or years. The doses used in the trials corresponded to about 12 g of herb/day.

Another key endocrine herb is *Coleus forskohlii*, also from the Indian subcontinent. This herb is a significant and recent development in phytotherapy. The root has been used for centuries in Ayurvedic medicine for cardiovascular disorders, abdominal pain and constipation.[55,56] Modern Ayurvedic uses include hypothyroidism.[57]

The plant is a small member of the mint family (Lamiaceae or Labiatae).[58] It grows as a perennial on the Indian plains and lower Himalayas. Coleus is also cultivated as a garden ornamental and is now grown commercially as a medicinal plant. The root contains a distinctive essential volatile oil and various diterpenes, especially 0.2% to 0.3% forskolin. No other species of Coleus contains forskolin and not even all varieties of C. forskohlii. In 1981 it was first demonstrated that forskolin possessed a special property: it could activate in a unique way the enzyme involved in the production of cyclic AMP (cAMP, adenylate cyclase).[58]

cAMP was first discovered in 1956.[57] A large number of hormones and neurotransmitters use cAMP to transfer their effects deep within a cell. In other words, the hormones or neurotransmitters do not enter the cell but instead activate a receptor on the cell surface that is part of the adenylate cyclase enzyme complex. This activation results in the production of cAMP. The cAMP then activates cAMP-dependent protein kinase, which results in changes in the cell's function. Given this, cAMP is often referred to as the 'second messenger'.

The physiological and biochemical effects of raised intracellular cAMP are many. They include inhibition of platelet activation, increased force of contraction of the heart muscle and relaxation of smooth muscle. Metabolic effects include increased insulin secretion, increased ACTH from the pituitary, increased thyroid function and increased fat breakdown in fat cells.

Because of the fundamental effects of cAMP, the pharmacology of forskolin is very broad. Basically forskolin acts synergistically with the wide range of hormones and neurotransmitters that activate adenylate cyclase. Effects have been noted in most bodily systems including the circulatory, respiratory, endocrine, gastrointestinal and nervous systems.[58]

In terms of its endocrine and metabolic effects, forskolin increases thyroid hormone production (and acts similarly to TSH).[58] It acts synergistically with calcitonin in inhibiting osteoclast function. In fat cells forskolin stimulates fat breakdown and inhibits glucose uptake. It potentiates the secretagogue effects of glucose and stimulates the release of glucagon.

Given the role of central adiposity in insulin resistance, the recent clinical discovery that Coleus encourages fat loss has a high relevance to endocrine health. In an open trial (8 weeks), Coleus extract (50 mg/day of forskolin) to six overweight women (BMI >25) resulted in significant reduction of body weight and fat content. Lean body mass was significantly increased. In an open, 12-week trial conducted in Japan, involving 13 overweight volunteers (13 women, one man; BMI 29.9), there was a significant decrease in body weight, BMI and body fat from Coleus extract (25 mg/day of forskolin).[59] In the US, a randomised, double blind, 12-week trial observed that, although there was no difference in food intake, overweight female volunteers taking Coleus extract (50 mg/day of forskolin) experienced weight loss (mean: 0.7 kg) while the placebo group gained weight (mean: 1 kg). Volunteers taking Coleus experienced significantly less hunger and greater fullness. No clinically significant side effects were observed.[60]

A trial of similar design conducted in India with obese men and women (BMI: 28 to 40 and/or body fat >30% (males), >40% (females)) found that the difference in body weight between the groups was significant. Coleus-treated patients lost an average of 4% of total body weight (1.73 kg), compared to a gain of 0.3% (0.25 kg) in the placebo group.[59] Also statistically significant was the effect on body fat and lean body mass. The loss of body fat in the Coleus-treated group was replaced with lean body mass, while those on placebo gained body fat and experienced a decrease in lean body mass. Serum HDL-cholesterol significantly increased in those receiving Coleus (compared to baseline values and compared to placebo).

In a double blind clinical trial conducted in the USA, 30 overweight/obese male volunteers (BMI >25) were randomised to receive Coleus extract (containing 50 mg/day of forskolin) or placebo for a period of 12 weeks.[61] Administration of Coleus resulted in a significant decrease in fat mass and body fat. The reduction in fat mass from baseline to after treatment with Coleus was 4.5 kg. There was also a trend toward a significant increase for lean body mass in the Coleus group compared with the placebo group. The average change in weight for those treated with Coleus was a loss of 0.07 kg, in contrast to an average gain of 1.57 kg for the placebo group. This extensive trial also found that treatment with Coleus significantly increased bone mass.[61]

In addition to its well-described effects on adrenal function, licorice (*Glycyrrhiza glabra*) may also have a role in encouraging fat loss. The enzyme 11beta-hydroxysteroid dehydrogenase (11beta-HSD) exists as two types in the body. Type 1 activates cortisol and type 2 inactivates it, and they are expressed in different tissues. Adipose tissue 11beta-HSD type 1 is increased in obesity. Increased cortisol in adipose tissue may contribute to the development of metabolic syndrome.[62,63]

Licorice is well documented to inhibit the activity of 11beta-HSD type 2. This is responsible for its aldosterone-like side effects. A group of Italian scientists found that licorice for 2 months reduced body fat mass in 15 healthy volunteers without any change in calorie intake. BMI did not change.[64] The authors attributed this effect to inhibition of 11beta-HSD type 1 at adipocytes and later showed that topical application of glycyrrhetinic acid for 1 month reduced the thickness of subcutaneous thigh fat (placebo-controlled trial).[65]

The number of herbs in various traditions attributed with a capacity for glycaemic control is probably testimony to the constant challenge that diabetes has posed in the past 100 or so years. In fact, the first major diabetic drug, metformin (still a mainstay in type 2 diabetes today), was developed from a medicinal plant. A key constituent of the herb goat's rue (*Galega officinalis*) is the guanidine alkaloid galegine. In 1927 it was found that galegine possessed hypoglycaemic properties, leading to the development of biguanide drugs such as metformin that potentiate the activity of insulin.[66] The structures of galegine and metformin are closely related.

Both fenugreek leaf and seed (*Trigonella foenum-graecum*) have demonstrated hypoglycaemic activity in experimental models, with mucilage and the free amino acid 4-hydroxyisoleucine likely candidates for such activity. Clinical trials using either whole or defatted fenugreek seed (5g/day and more) have led to improved blood sugar levels in patients with type 2 diabetes.[67]

More recently, research attention has shifted to the common spice cinnamon (*Cinnamomum verum*), with most of the focus on cassia cinnamon (*Cinnamomum cassia*). Initial clinical trials were promising,[68,69] although results were not always positive.[70] A 2009 review of eight clinical trials concluded the herb does possess the potential to lower postprandial blood glucose levels.[71]

Berberine has shown significant blood-sugar lowering activity in clinical trials in type 2 diabetes (albeit in high doses). This suggests a role for berberine-containing herbs in this context (see the monograph for Berberis).

Phytotherapy

Adrenal depletion

Adrenal depletion can be defined as a reduced capacity to cope with stress. It usually arises from the chronic effects of continued stress brought about by the pace and demands of modern living. In a sense it represents a precursor state to chronic fatigue and fibromyalgia syndromes. Although not recognised as a medical condition, this syndrome is very common and often underlies why patients seek herbal treatment for fatigue. Typical signs and symptoms of adrenal depletion include constant fatigue and need for extra sleep, inability to cope with stress, irritability and anxiety, reduced libido, sighing and yawning, low back pain in the adrenal area, recurrent and often prolonged colds or influenza, sweet craving and reactive dysglycaemia, sensitive to cold and heat and low core temperature. Pigmentation in skin creases and loss of body hair may be

evident, as can poor digestion and assimilation, postural hypotension (Raglan's sign) and unstable pupillary reflex.[72]

Treatment for adrenal depletion includes the following objectives:

- Support adrenal gland function with adrenal restorative herbs such as Glycyrrhiza (licorice) and Rehmannia
- Decrease the detrimental effects of stress on the adrenal glands with adaptogens such as Eleutherococcus, Withania and Panax (ginseng)
- Enhance adrenal function with tonics such as ginseng and Withania
- Minimise the effects of stress on the nervous system with nervine tonics such as Hypericum (St John's wort) and *Scutellaria lateriflora* (skullcap)
- Support immune function with Echinacea, Astragalus and Andrographis if required.

Example liquid formula

Glycyrrhiza glabra	1:1	10mL
Rehmannia glutinosa	1:2	20mL
Withania somnifera	1:1	30mL
Hypericum perforatum	1:2	20mL
Eleutherococcus senticosus	1:2	20mL
	TOTAL	100mL

Dose: 8mL with water twice a day.

CASE HISTORY

A female patient aged 36 complained of low energy, mouth ulcers, poor concentration, difficulty in staying awake in the evenings, low libido and stress at work. She was concerned that she would not be able to cope with a new job plus help her husband at night with his business.

Herbal treatment was aimed at supporting her immunity, energy and concentration and helping her to better cope with the stressful demands of her life. The patient was treated with herbs over several years and was able to function well with good energy levels overall. As much as possible she changed her lifestyle to ensure adequate rest and holidays, but still needed to often work long hours. Herbal treatment was largely based on the following:

Withania 2:1, 2mL with water on rising, together with:

Glycyrrhiza glabra	1:1	15mL
Echinacea angustifolia/purpurea root	1:2	25mL
Ginkgo biloba (standardised extract)	2:1	20mL
Hypericum perforatum (high in hypericin)	1:2	20mL
Eleutherococcus senticosus	1:2	20mL
	TOTAL	100mL

Dose: 8mL with water twice a day.

Idiopathic reactive hypoglycaemia

Reactive hypoglycaemia (RH) is a postprandial hypoglycaemic state occurring 2 to 5 hours after food intake. While it can occur in association with diabetes, gastrointestinal dysfunction and hormone deficiency states, a large patient group is characterised as having idiopathic RH.[73] The definition of idiopathic RH is controversial. Patients with idiopathic RH are proposed to have a delayed discharge of insulin that occurs inappropriately with falling levels of plasma glucose. It might also result from an exaggerated insulin response or a high insulin sensitivity.[73] It has been suggested that RH can occur in lean young women with polycystic ovary syndrome (PCOS), where it could be predictive of future diabetes.[73] RH is generally more common in people with low body weight.[74]

Postprandial RH is characterised by sympathetic and neuroglucopenic symptoms developing concurrently with a lower blood sugar.[74] These include anxiety, trembling, sweating, hunger, dizziness, poor concentration and headaches. Being postprandial, symptoms typically occur mid-to-late mornings and afternoons.

People with RH are probably more sensitive to a drop in blood sugar, possibly due to excessive caffeine intake, stress and/or poor cerebral blood flow.[75] Diet is an important issue. Generally there is excessive consumption of refined carbohydrates and a low protein intake (especially at breakfast). Adrenal depletion can mean that counter-regulatory mechanisms of blood sugar control are not adequate.

Basic dietary advice is as follows:

- Refined carbohydrates should be avoided and the diet should have a low glycaemic load
- Intake of caffeine is best avoided
- Protein intake at each meal is encouraged (protein stimulates gluconeogenesis resulting in a consistent output of glucose by the liver).

Herbal treatment includes the following objectives:

- Support of adrenal gland function with adrenal restorative herbs such as licorice and Rehmannia. Use only Rehmannia if the patient has high blood pressure
- Decrease the detrimental effects of stress on the adrenal glands with adaptogens such as Withania, ginseng and Eleutherococcus
- Boost adrenal function with tonics such as ginseng
- Improve cerebral circulation with *Rosmarinus officinalis* (rosemary) and Ginkgo
- Lower doses of Gymnema in liquid preparations (for example 10 mL of 1:1 extract per 100 mL formula) can help to control reactive hypoglycaemia and sugar craving, as can bitter herbs such as Gentiana
- Support liver function with Schisandra and *Silybum marianum* (St Mary's thistle), since the liver also has a role in regulating blood sugar.

Example liquid formula

Rehmannia glutinosa	1:2	30 mL
Glycyrrhiza glabra	1:1	15 mL
Gymnema sylvestre	1:1	10 mL
Ginkgo biloba (standardised extract)	2:1	25 mL
Eleutherococcus senticosus	1:2	25 mL
	TOTAL	105 mL

Dose: 5 mL with water three times a day before meals.

Metabolic syndrome

As noted above, metabolic syndrome is an insulin-resistant state and as such is a precursor to type 2 diabetes. It is characterised by a cluster of cardiovascular risk factors and was first proposed in 1988, although alluded to in earlier literature.[76] These include various combinations of abdominal obesity, glucose intolerance, hypertension and atherogenic dyslipidaemia. The dyslipidaemia includes elevated triglycerides, low HDL-cholesterol, elevated apolipoprotein B and small LDL particles.

There are three main definitions of metabolic syndrome.[77] The first was developed by the WHO in 1998 with hyperglycaemia and insulin resistance as a central feature, associated with two or more related metabolic abnormalities (hypertension, dyslipidaemia, abdominal obesity or micro-albuminuria). Up until this consensus definition, metabolic syndrome was not widely accepted as a medical entity and it is still controversial. The US National Cholesterol Education Program (NCEP) definition requires three or more of: abdominal obesity, elevated triglycerides (>1.7 mmol/L), low HDL-cholesterol (<1.0 mmol/L men, <1.3 women), hypertension (>130/85 mmHg) or elevated fasting glucose.[77] In 2005 the International Diabetes Federation (IDF) proposed a definition similar to the NCEP, but elevated abdominal obesity as a necessary requirement.

The prevalence of metabolic syndrome has reached alarming proportions.[77] Depending on the definition, the incidence in US adults aged 20 years or more is between 35% and 39%. For Australia the estimated prevalence is between 24% and 26%. Metabolic syndrome is more prevalent with increasing age, affecting about 50% of adults aged 60 years and over. It is also more common in men. Despite the current high incidence, the prevalence of metabolic syndrome is increasing. For the first time in decades, medical scientists are proposing that the average life expectancy might *fall* in industrialised countries.

The key aspects of management of metabolic syndrome are:

- lifestyle: especially exercise and managing stress loads
- dietary: a calorie-restricted low glycaemic load (GL) or low carbohydrate diet with good fibre levels and the optional use of a protein-based meal replacement supplement
- herbs and nutrients: to address the triad of central weight loss, improving insulin sensitivity and managing the metabolic disturbances.

It is acknowledged by all consensus groups that metabolic syndrome is linked to lack of physical activity.[78] Physical activity not only assists weight loss, it also improves insulin sensitivity. The current recommendation of the US American Heart Association for metabolic syndrome is at least 60 minutes of continuous or intermittent aerobic activity a day. Resistance training is also recommended.

A 2007 study compared a low GL diet against a low fat diet in obese (BMI >30) young adults.[79] For those with insulin resistance, the low GL diet produced a greater decrease in weight (−5.8 versus −1.2 kg, p=0.004) and body fat percentage (−2.6% versus −0.9%, p=0.03) than the low fat diet at 18 months. There was no significant difference for these measures between diet groups for those with a normal insulin response. In the full cohort, HDL-cholesterol increased and triglycerides decreased more on the low GL diet, whereas LDL-cholesterol decreased more on the low fat diet.

Key herbs and their rationale in the management of metabolic syndrome are as follows:

- Coleus and licorice – for weight loss/fat loss (see above)
- Gymnema, St Mary's thistle, ginseng and fenugreek for better glycaemic control
- Gymnema, St Mary's thistle, giant knotweed (as a source of resveratrol) and ginseng for decreasing insulin resistance
- Gymnema, grape seed and pine extracts and green tea for reducing the glycaemic index of food intake (taken just before meals, see Chapter 2).
- St Mary's thistle for excessive iron stores and fatty liver and elevated GGT (see monograph)
- Hawthorn, Coleus, garlic, green tea, grape seed extract and psyllium for any cardiovascular metabolic disturbances
- Globe artichoke for weight loss and cardiovascular metabolic disturbances (see monograph)
- Grape seed, green tea, rosemary, St Mary's thistle, turmeric for the pro-oxidant, pro-inflammatory metabolic disturbances
- Schisandra, rosemary, green tea, turmeric, broccoli sprout extract for improving xenobiotic clearance
- Ginseng, licorice, Rehmannia, Withania, Rhodiola and Eleutherococcus, as appropriate, for managing the negative metabolic effects of stress.

Being a highly complex disorder, the treatment strategy for metabolic syndrome will vary depending on the specific issues for the patient. Lifestyle and dietary changes and a reduction in central adiposity must be set as the primary objectives in the initial stages of treatment. Herbs for the insulin resistance and to improve glycaemic control should also be a priority.

Be guided by the case: for example, if there is a fatty liver and high ferritin then Silybum is the herb of choice (as the silymarin concentrate). If there are sugar cravings and borderline diabetes, preference should be given to Gymnema. If there is hypertension then hawthorn could be included. Stress management and attention to the cardiovascular and other metabolic disturbances, as indicated by the case, can be prioritised as appropriate.

Type 2 diabetes

In a 2008 editorial of the *Medical Journal of Australia*, the growing epidemic of type 2 diabetes in Australia was described as a 'juggernaut'.[80] In an older population (Blue Mountains Eye Study) the overall incidence was 9.3%, with impaired fasting glucose in another 15.8% of participants.[81] A 2003 study found that the prevalence of type 2 diabetes has doubled in the past 20 years to represent >7% of Australian adults.[82] The incidence is also rising rapidly in children and adolescents.[83] These findings would also be typical of most Western countries.

The primary aim in type 2 diabetes is to achieve better glycaemic control through herbs, nutritional supplements, diet and exercise. However, type 2 diabetes is a chronic progressive disease which attacks the eyes, kidneys, nerves and blood vessels. Hence therapies aimed to treat and prevent these complications may also be necessary.

In terms of the diabetic complications, three major metabolic issues appear to be involved.[84,85] These are glycosylation of proteins, disturbances of the polyol pathway and inflammation and oxidative stress.

Glycosylation of proteins is directly related to glucose levels in the blood. Later stages are represented by the formation of irreversible advanced glycation endproducts (AGEs). These are a direct product of glucose concentration, time and oxidant stress. AGEs are potentially pathogenic; they accelerate atherogenesis, enhance protein deposition and cross-linking, derange normal physiology and create oxidative damage and inflammation.[84]

Not all tissues require insulin for glucose transport, for example nerves, the lens, kidneys, blood vessels and endothelium.[86] Hyperglycaemia leads to an increase in intracellular glucose in these tissues, which is subsequently metabolised by aldose reductase (AR) into sorbitol, a polyol, and eventually fructose. This causes cellular damage. Increased activity of the hexosamine pathway can also lead to disturbed cell function via increased fructose production.

Hyperglycaemia increases oxidative stress through several pathways, including the interaction of glycosylated proteins with receptors (RAGEs) as noted above.[85] A major mechanism appears to be the overproduction of the superoxide anion by the mitochondrial electron transport chain. Hyperglycaemia also promotes inflammation via increased cytokine induction.

Flavonoids and related compounds show strong inhibitory activity on aldose reductase (AR) in vitro. Licorice and baicalein from Baical skullcap (*Scutellaria baicalensis*) have shown significant AR inhibitory activity in an animal model and could prove to be useful in preventing some of the long-term complications of diabetes.[87] Treatment with silybin (231 mg/day for 4 weeks) in 14 type 2 patients resulted in significant reduction of red blood cell sorbitol levels (suggestive of AR inhibitory activity, see monograph).

A link between ferritin, iron stores and type 2 diabetes has been proposed.[88] Frequent blood donations improve insulin sensitivity and glycaemic control in normal people and diabetics. Iron stores may contribute to diabetic complications, and being a frequent blood donor appears to confer some protection against developing type 2 diabetes. A correlation between serum ferritin and diabetic retinopathy has been observed.[89] Silybum (St Mary's thistle) as the concentrated extract has been shown to lower serum ferritin in a clinical study (see St Mary's thistle monograph).

The glycaemic index is an assessment of the rate of glucose elevation in the bloodstream following the intake of a particular food. Any herb which delays gastric emptying will reduce the glycaemic index. These include mucilage herbs and other sticky fibre foods. Tannins (e.g. grape seed) also interfere with digestive processes, and saponins (e.g. Gymnema) can disrupt glucose transport (see also Chapter 2).

Key herbs to consider on the basis of the individual case in type 2 diabetes include:

- hypoglycaemic herbs such as Gymnema, Silybum (as silymarin), pine bark, ginseng, berberine-containing herbs and cassia cinnamon to maintain better glycaemic control
- antioxidant and microvascular-stabilising herbs such as bilberry, Ginkgo, grape seed and pine bark extracts to

prevent and treat complications involving fine blood vessels such as diabetic retinopathy, nephropathy and neuropathy

- Gotu kola, which has demonstrated benefits in diabetic microangiopathy in clinical trials, as have Ginkgo and bilberry (see respective monographs)
- herbs with meals to lower the GI of diet (Gymnema, green tea and grape seed and pine bark extracts)
- potential AR inhibitors such as licorice, Baical skullcap and Silybum to prevent the long-term complications of diabetes attributed to activation of the polyol pathway
- St Mary's thistle (as the silymarin extract) for insulin resistance, AR inhibitory activity and reducing iron.

Treatment

A comprehensive protocol for type 2 diabetes patients might include the following:

- St Mary's thistle standardised extract (70% to 80% silymarin) capsules/tablets 150 to 200 mg of extract, one with each meal
- High potency Gymnema tablets/capsules to match the clinical trial doses, one before each meal
- An antioxidant, vasoprotective herbal tablet (see above for ingredient candidates)
- Green tea, one cup with each meal
- Mucilage, either psyllium hulls or slippery elm, 2 to 5 g before each meal
- * And the following formula:

Glycyrrhiza glabra	1:1	15 mL
Scutellaria baicalensis	1:2	30 mL
Galega officinalis	1:2	40 mL
Panax ginseng	1:2	20 mL
	TOTAL	105 mL

Dose: 8 mL with water twice a day.

CASE HISTORY

A male patient aged 55 years presented with boils (furuncles) and a partially rejected corneal graft with eye irritation. He received a liquid combination of Echinacea root 1:2 and Euphrasia (eyebright) 1:2 (8 mL twice a day) and a healing tablet formula containing gotu kola, grape seed extract and Ginkgo. His cornea and boils improved, but when the boils did not resolve completely and examination showed some muscle wasting in the legs and buttocks, he was sent for a blood sugar test. His fasting blood sugar was around 17 mmol/L and HbA$_{1c}$ around 12%. His doctor wanted to prescribe insulin, despite the diagnosis being type 2 diabetes. Instead he started the drug metformin and his herbal treatment eventually settled at:

- Tablets containing Gymnema sylvestre (Gymnema) 4 g (one before each meal)

- Tablets containing Polygonum cuspidatum (giant knotweed) root 8.0 g, Pinus massoniana (Masson pine) bark 5.0 g, Silybum marianum (St Mary's thistle) fruit 4.2 g, Ginkgo biloba (Ginkgo) leaf 1.5 g and Panax ginseng (Korean ginseng) root 250 mg (one before each meal)
- Tablets containing Vitis vinifera (grape seed) extract 6.0 g, Curcuma longa (turmeric) extract 2.0 g, Camellia sinensis (green tea) extract 4.17 g and Rosmarinus officinalis (rosemary) extract 1.0 g (one before two main meals).

The patient's fasting blood sugar now ranges at 6 to 7 mmol/L and his HbA$_{1c}$ is stable at around 7%.

Clinical and subclinical hypothyroidism

An underactive thyroid is a common condition that may often go undiagnosed. Because of the difficulty in detecting an underactive thyroid from symptoms, clinicians now rely heavily on laboratory tests. These thyroid function tests usually measure thyroid stimulating hormone (TSH, produced by the pituitary gland) and thyroid hormone output (T3 and T4). Also if it is suspected that a disease is causing the poor thyroid function, such as a disturbance of the immune system as in Hashimoto's disease, then other tests such as antibody tests may be conducted.

If TSH is raised and T4 is low (that is, the stimulus to the thyroid is higher than normal, but its output is lower than normal), this is diagnostic of an underactive thyroid. Sometimes TSH is raised, but T4 is normal. This is termed sub-clinical hyperthyroidism. But how accurately do the blood tests reflect ideal thyroid function? Thyroid hormones regulate many key functions of the body and levels in the blood do not always reflect what is happening in the tissues.

This point was underlined by the case history of a 12-year-old boy who had many of the characteristic signs and symptoms of an underactive thyroid, such as increased body weight, lethargy, no appetite, puffy face, poor initiative and relatively slow pulse. Yet his thyroid function tests were normal. He had previously suffered from an overactive thyroid that had been treated with the standard drugs. Whether the drugs overcorrected, or whether his thyroid just naturally went underactive, could not be known for certain. But the important observation was that his tests were normal when his guardians were claiming he was a very different boy to when he was normal. See also p. 338 on THR.

It has been suggested that the diagnosis of hypothyroidism on the basis of thyroid function tests is flawed.[90] A better way to assess thyroid function is to measure basal metabolic rate (BMR), but this is seldom used. Some time ago Barnes suggested that many people have subtle thyroid dysfunction that the blood tests fail to detect, and controversially advocated the use of basal body temperature (BBT) to assess BMR.[91] BBT is measured using a thermometer placed under the armpit on waking for 5 consecutive days. (For menstruating women measurement should start on day 2 or 3 of the cycle.) Readings less than 36.6°C (97.8°F) can indicate underactivity.

The key plant used to boost thyroid function is bladderwrack (*Fucus vesiculosis*). Bladderwrack is a shore-dwelling seaweed containing fluid-filled bladders that allow it to float as the tide comes in, hence its name. The part used is the whole seaweed plant, known as the thallus. The common understanding of this herb is often confused. It is not the same as kelp (although many people call it this). Kelp is a large, deep-sea seaweed harvested in significant quantities from ocean-going ships. In contrast, bladderwrack is collected by hand from inter-tidal regions. Although both kelp and bladderwrack, like all seaweeds, are rich sources of iodine, herbalists believe that bladderwrack additionally contains organic-bound iodine, which stimulates thyroid function in a way that simple iodine supplementation cannot.

Experiments as early as 1910 indicated that oral doses of bladderwrack had a stimulatory action on the thyroid gland.[92] In a controlled clinical trial, overweight participants taking bladderwrack extract in addition to a controlled diet achieved a significantly greater average weight loss than those on the diet alone.[93]

Caution does need to be exercised when taking bladderwrack, especially long term. Kelp and bladderwrack can cause overactive thyroid in the short term, and if taken in excess quantities over a long period can even induce a compensatory phenomenon that results in an underactive thyroid.[94,95] However, on the other hand, to be effective at stimulating thyroid function at least 3 to 4g/day of bladderwrack is needed, or its equivalent in extract form.

Another herb with a mild stimulatory effect on the thyroid is the root of *Withania somnifera*.[96,97] Withania is widely regarded as a tonic (see monograph). Its stimulatory effect on thyroid output was shown in an in vivo model, especially on T4 output (which indicates a direct effect on the thyroid).[96,97] How it works is not known, but this herb favourably influences the function of several endocrine glands, as does another herb from India *Coleus forskohlii*. Coleus makes thyroid-hormone producing cells in the thyroid more sensitive to the effects of TSH (see p. 342).

If thyroid autoantibodies are above normal, then active thyroid destruction is occurring and these autoimmune manifestations should be taken into account during treatment (see Chapter 8). Issues pertaining to endocrine disruption should also be investigated (as discussed above) and antithyroid dietary components:[98]

- Some plants are characterised as goitrogens, and although they can cause goitre formation in some instances, the mode of action can differ greatly.
- Plants containing cyanogenic glycosides can reduce thyroid function by inhibiting iodine uptake, (e.g. linseeds – not the oil).
- Brassica species (e.g. cabbage, cauliflower) and garlic contain sulphur compounds that interfere with thyroid hormone synthesis.
- In contrast walnuts and soya beans cause increased faecal clearance of thyroxin by somehow interfering with enterohepatic cycling.

- They increase iodine uptake but this is insufficient to compensate for the thyroxin loss.
- Excessive soya intake, especially in children, might depress thyroid function.

Example liquid formula

Fucus vesiculosis	1:1	40 mL
Coleus forskohlii	1:1	35 mL
Withania somnifera	2:1	25 mL
	TOTAL	100 mL

Dose: 8 mL with water twice a day.

Hyperthyroidism (Grave's disease)

Symptoms of an overactive thyroid include weight loss with increased appetite, tremor, racing heart, increased sweating, soft nails and hair, diarrhoea, palpitations, restlessness, irritability and raised blood pressure. Also with Grave's disease there can be bulging of the eyes known as exophthalmos.

Herbs can be used to regulate an overactive thyroid, and there are two key plants, both members of the mint family, that have been used by herbalists for many generations to calm an overactive thyroid. They are Lycopus (bugleweed) and Leonurus (motherwort). The recent evidence suggests that they mainly counter the cardiovascular symptoms (see the bugleweed monograph).

In addition, the following therapeutic goals related to the autoimmune aspects could be considered:

- Balance immune system function with immune-modifying herbs such as Echinacea root and immune-depressing herbs such as Hemidesmus
- Reduce inflammation with anti-inflammatory herbs such as Rehmannia and Bupleurum
- Treat any suspected viral aetiology with antiviral herbs such as St John's wort (active only against enveloped viruses).

Antithyroid dietary components should be encouraged (see previous).

Example liquid formula

Lycopus spp.	1:2	20 mL
Leonurus cardiaca	1:2	20 mL
Echinacea purpurea/angustifolia root	1:2	20 mL
Bupleurum falcatum	1:2	25 mL
Hypericum perforatum (high hypericin)	1:2	20 mL
	TOTAL	105 mL

Dose: 5 to 8 mL with water three times a day.

CASE HISTORY

A female patient aged 42 presented with thyrotoxicosis. Her main symptoms were palpitations, tachycardia, weight loss and nervous agitation. Some exophthalmia was present. It was apparently precipitated by a bad bout of influenza the previous winter. Since then she had frequent colds and was highly stressed. The patient was on the highest recommended dose of the antithyroid drug carbimazole (six tablets per day). Her TSH was very low and thyroid hormones were considerably elevated. She was given basic dietary advice (a more healthy diet) and it was suggested that she reduce her tea and coffee intake. The following herbs were prescribed:

- Tablets containing *Andrographis paniculata* (Andrographis) extract 2.0 g, *Ocimum tenuiflorum* (holy basil) extract 500 mg, *Echinacea purpurea/angustifolia* root 500 mg and *Ocimum tenuiflorum* (holy basil) essential oil 10 mg (three per day).
- Tablets containing *Hypericum perforatum* (St John's wort) extract 1.8 g (three per day)
- Tylophora 1:5, 10 to 30 drops for the first 10 days of each month.

Echinacea purpurea/angustifolia root	1:2	20 mL
Lycopus spp.	1:2	35 mL
Rehmannia glutinosa	1:2	20 mL
Eleutherococcus senticosus	1:2	25 mL
	TOTAL	100 mL

Dose: 8 mL with water twice a day.

The rationale for the treatment:

- Andrographis and Echinacea root to balance immunity
- St John's wort: antiviral, nervine tonic
- Tylophora: downregulate immune response
- Rehmannia: anti-inflammatory, inhibits cytokines
- Bugleweed: antithyroid
- Siberian Ginseng: adaptogen.

Progress (herbal treatment maintained throughout):

- Only minor improvement in the first 3 months (which her doctor attributed to her drug)
- One month later, thyroid function nearly normal so drug reduced to three tablets per day
- One month later, thyroid normal, only very mild symptoms
- Six months later, off drug, thyroid test normal
- One year later: in remission, receiving no treatments.

In treating autoimmune disease it is important to identify the underlying issues that feed the pathological process. Herbs to balance immunity, remove pathogenic agents, balance bowel flora and control inflammation should be emphasised in the treatment plan.

References

1. Fulop T, Tessier D, Carpentier A. The metabolic syndrome. *Pathol Biol (Paris)*. 2006;54(7):375–386.

2. Shen W, Punyanitya M, Chen J, et al. Waist circumference correlates with metabolic syndrome indicators better than percentage fat. *Obesity (Silver Spring)*. 2006;14(4): 727–736.

3. Sylver N. Hypothyroidism type 2: a new way of looking at an old problem. *Townsend Letter for Doctors and Patients*. 2008;305:66–73.

4. Fatourechi V. Subclinical hypothyroidism: an update for primary care physicians. *Mayo Clin Proc*. 2009;84(1):65–71.

5. Andrews C, Morgan M. Nutritional and herbal support for healthy thyroid and adrenal function. *Nutritional Perspective* 2006;25:1–4.

6. Garrison RL, Breeding PC. A metabolic basis for fibromyalgia and its related disorders: the possible role of resistance to thyroid hormone. *Med Hypotheses*. 2003;61(2):182–189.

7. Tsigos C, Chrousos GP. Hypothalamic-pituitary-adrenal axis, neuroendocrine factors and stress. *J Psychosom Res*. 2002;53(4):865–871.

8. Olsson EM, von Schéele B, Panossian AG. A randomised, double blind, placebo-controlled, parallel-group study of the standardised extract shr-5 of the roots of Rhodiola rosea in the treatment of subjects with stress-related fatigue. *Planta Med*. 2009;75(2):105–112.

9. Amati F, Dubé JJ, Stefanovic-Racic M, et al. Improvements in insulin sensitivity are blunted by subclinical hypothyroidism. *Med Sci Sports Exerc*. 2009;41(2):265–269.

10. Kreiss K, Zack MM, Kimbrough RD, et al. Association of blood pressure and polychlorinated biphenyl levels. *JAMA*. 1981;245(24):2505–2509.

11. Jacobson JL, Jacobson SW. Intellectual impairment in children exposed to polychlorinated biphenyls in utero. *N Engl J Med*. 1996;335(11):783–789.

12. Osius N, Karmaus W, Kruse H, et al. Exposure to polychlorinated biphenyls and levels of thyroid hormones in children. *Environ Health Perspect*. 1999;107(10):843–849.

13. Dewailly E, Dodin S, Verreault R, et al. High organochlorine body burden in women with estrogen receptor-positive breast cancer. *J Natl Cancer Inst*. 1994;86(3): 232–234.

14. Høyer AP, Grandjean P, Jørgensen T, et al. Organochlorine exposure and risk of breast cancer. *Lancet*. 1998;352(9143):1816–1820.

15. Crinnion WJ. Environmental medicine, part 4: pesticides – biologically persistent and ubiquitous toxins. *Altern Med Rev*. 2000;5(5):432–447.

16. Lim J-S, Lee D-H, Park J-Y, et al. A strong interaction between serum gamma-glutamyltransferase and obesity on the risk of prevalent type 2 diabetes: results from the Third National Health and Nutrition Examination Survey. *Clin Chem*. 2007;53(6):1092–1098.

17. André P, Balkau B, Vol S, et al. Gamma-glutamyltransferase activity and development of the metabolic syndrome (International Diabetes Federation Definition) in middle-aged men and women: Data from the Epidemiological Study on the Insulin Resistance Syndrome (DESIR) cohort. *Diabetes Care*. 2007;30(9):2355–2361.

18. Kang YH, Min HK, Son SM, et al. The association of serum gamma glutamyltransferase with components of the metabolic syndrome in the Korean adults. *Diabetes Res Clin Pract*. 2007;77(2):306–313.

19. Lee DS, Evans JC, Robins SJ, et al. Gamma glutamyl transferase and metabolic syndrome, cardiovascular disease, and mortality risk: the Framingham Heart Study. *Arterioscler Thromb Vasc Biol*. 2007;27(1):127–133.

20. Yamada J, Tomiyama H, Yambe M, et al. Elevated serum levels of alanine aminotransferase and gamma glutamyltransferase are markers of inflammation and oxidative stress independent of the metabolic syndrome. *Atherosclerosis*. 2006;189(1):198–205.

21. Lee DH, Lee IK, Song K, et al. A strong dose–response relation between serum concentrations of persistent organic pollutants and diabetes: results from the National Health and Examination Survey 1999–2002. *Diabetes Care*. 2006;29(7): 1638–1644.

22. Lee DH, Lee IK, Jin SH, et al. Association between serum concentrations of persistent organic pollutants and insulin resistance among nondiabetic adults: results from the National Health and Nutrition Examination

Survey 1999–2002. *Diabetes Care.* 2007;30(3):622–628.

23. Lee DH, Lee IK, Porta M, et al. Relationship between serum concentrations of persistent organic pollutants and the prevalence of metabolic syndrome among non-diabetic adults: results from the National Health and Nutrition Examination Survey 1999–2002. *Diabetologia.* 2007;50(9):1841–1851.

24. Major GC, Doucet E, Trayhurn P, et al. Clinical significance of adaptive thermogenesis. *Int J Obes.* 2007;31:204–212.

25. Goulding MR, Rogers ME, Smith SM. *Public Health and Aging: Trends in Aging-United States and Worldwide.* <http://www.cdc.gov/mmwr/preview/mmwrhtml/mm5206a2.htm>. Accessed 13.09.11.

26. *Creating Healthy Communities for an Aging Population Work Group,* 2006. <http://www.health.state.mn.us/divs/orhpc/pubs/healthyaging/healthyagingsumm.pdf>. Accessed 13.09.11.

27. Hayflick L. Biological aging is no longer an unsolved problem. *Ann NY Acad Sci.* 2007;1100:1–13.

28. Faragher RGA, Sheerin AN, Ostler EL. Can we intervene in human ageing. *Expert Rev Mol Med.* 2009;11:e27.

29. Gems D, McElwee JJ. Broad spectrum detoxification: the major longevity assurance process regulated by insulin/IGF-1 signaling? *Mech Ageing Dev.* 2005;126(3):381–387.

30. Holliday R. Aging is no longer an unsolved problem in biology. *Ann NY Acad Sci.* 2006;1067:1–9.

31. Rattan SIS. Theories of biological aging: genes, proteins, and free radicals. *Free Radic Res.* 2006;40(12):1230–1238.

32. Son TG, Camandola SN, Mattson MP. Hormetic dietary phytochemicals. *Neuromol Med.* 2008;10(4):236–246.

33. Hayes DP. Nutritional hormesis. *Eur J Clin Nutr.* 2007;61(2):147–159.

34. Radak Z, Chung HY, Koltai E, et al. Exercise, oxidative stress and hormesis. *Ageing Res Rev.* 2008;7(1):34–42.

35. Le Bourg E. Hormesis, aging and longevity. *Biochim Biophys Acta.* 2009;1790(10):1030–1039.

36. Mattson M, Calabrese E. Best in small doses. *New Scientist.* 2008;199(2668):36–39.

37. Panossian A, Wikman G. Evidence-based efficacy of adaptogens in fatigue, and molecular mechanism related to their stress-protective activity. *Curr Clin Pharmacol.* 2009;4(3):198–219.

38. Panossian A, Wikman G. *Molecular Mechanisms of Stress Protective Effect of Adaptogens.* UNE International Conference: Evidence-Based Complementary Medicine. Armidale, Australia, 2009.

39. Hayes DP. Nutritional hormesis. *Eur J Clin Nutr.* 2007;61(2):147–159.

40. de Magalhães JP. *Integrative Genomics of Ageing Group. Caloric Restriction.* <http://www.senescence.info/calories.html>. Accessed 13.09.11.

41. Sinclair DA. Toward a unified theory of caloric restriction and longevity regulation. *Mech Ageing Dev.* 2005;126(9):987–1002.

42. Howitz KT, Bitterman KJ, Sinclair DA, et al. Small molecule activators of sirtuins extend Saccharomyces cerevisiae lifespan. *Nature.* 2003;425:191–196.

43. Baur JA, Pearson KJ, Price NL, et al. Resveratrol improves health and survival of mice on a high-calorie diet. *Nature.* 2006;444(7117):337–342.

44. Li LH, Wu LJ, Tashiro SI, et al. Activation of the SIRT1 pathway and modulation of the cell cycle were involved in silymarin's protection against UV-induced A375-S2 cell apoptosis. *J Asian Nat Prod Res.* 2007;9(3–5):245–252.

45. Zhou B, Wu LJ, Li LH, et al. Silibinin protects against isoproterenol-induced rat cardiac myocyte injury through mitochondrial pathway after up-regulation of SIRT1. *J Pharmacol Sci.* 2006;102(4):387–395.

46. Roth GS. Caloric restriction and caloric restriction mimetics: current status and promise for the future. *J Am Geriatr Soc.* 2005;53(9 suppl):S280–S283.

47. Anisimov VN, Berstein LM, Egormin PA, et al. Metformin slows down aging and extends life span of female SHR mice. *Cell Cycle.* 2008;7(17):2769–2773.

48. Tode T, Kikuchi Y, Hirata J, et al. Effect of Korean red ginseng on psychological functions in patients with severe climacteric syndromes. *Int J Gynaecol Obstet.* 1999;67(3):169–174.

49. Auddy B, Hazra J, Mitra A, et al. A standardized *Withania somnifera* extract significantly reduces stress-related parameters in chronically stressed humans: a double blind, randomized, placebo-controlled study. *J Am Nutr Assoc.* 2008;11(1):50–56.

50. Huseini H, Larijani B, Heshmat R, et al. The efficacy of Silybum marianum (L.) Gaertn. (silymarin) in the treatment of type II diabetes: a randomized, double blind, placebo-controlled, clinical trial. *Phytother Res.* 2006;20(12):1036–1039.

51. Vuksan V, Sung MK, Sievenpiper JL, et al. Korean red ginseng (Panax ginseng) improves glucose and insulin regulation in well-controlled, type 2 diabetes: results of a randomized, double blind, placebo-controlled study of efficacy and safety. *Nutr Metab Cardiovasc Dis.* 2008;18(1):46–56.

52. Shanmugasundaram ER, Gopinath KL, Radha Shanmugasundaram K, et al. Possible regeneration of the islets of Langerhans in streptozotocin-diabetic rats given Gymnema sylvestre leaf extracts. *J Ethnopharmacol.* 1990;30(3):265–279.

53. Shanmugasundaram ER, Rajeswari G, Baskaran K, et al. Use of Gymnema sylvestre leaf extract in the control of blood glucose in insulin-dependent diabetes mellitus. *J Ethnopharmacol.* 1990;30(3):281–294.

54. Baskaran K, Kizar Ahamath B, Shanmugasundaram KR, et al. Antidiabetic effect of a leaf extract from Gymnema sylvestre in non-insulin-dependent diabetes mellitus patients. *J Ethnopharmacol.* 1990;30(3):295–300.

55. Srivastava SK, Mehrotra S, Srivastave GK, Chauhan DK. Folk uses of herbs from Mahabaleshwar Region of Sahyadri Hills. *J Econ Taxon Bot.* 2003;27(4):857–863.

56. Varma N, Srivastava V, Tandon JS, et al. Effect of Coleus forskohlii against caecal amoebiasis of rats. *Int J Crude Drug Res.* 1990;28(1):1–3.

57. Ding X, Staudinger JL. Induction of drug metabolism by forskolin: the role of the pregnane X receptor and the protein kinase a signal transduction pathway. *J Pharmacol Exp Ther.* 2005;312(2):849–856.

58. Bone K. *Clinical Applications of Ayurvedic and Chinese Herbs.* Warwick: Phytotherapy Press; 1996. pp. 103–107.

59. Sabinsa Corporation. *ForsLean® Product Information.* Available from <www.forslean.com>. Accessed 12.09.11.

60. Henderson S, Magu B, Rasmussen C, et al. Effects of coleus forskohlii supplementation on body composition and hematological profiles in mildly overweight women. *J Int Soc Sports Nutr.* 2005;2(2):54–62.

61. Godard MP, Johnson BA, Richmond SR. Body composition and hormonal adaptations associated with forskolin consumption in overweight and obese men. *Obes Res.* 2005;13(8):1335–1343.

62. Engeli S, Böhnke J, Feldpausch M, et al. Regulation of 11beta-HSD genes in human adipose tissue: influence of central obesity and weight loss. *Obes Res.* 2004;12(1):9–17.

63. Desbriere R, Vuaroqueaux V, Achard V, et al. 11beta-hydroxysteroid dehydrogenase type 1 mRNA is increased in both visceral and subcutaneous adipose tissue of obese patients. *Obesity (Silver Spring).* 2006;14(5):794–798.

64. Armanini D, De Palo CB, Mattarello MJ, et al. Effect of licorice on the reduction of body fat mass in healthy subjects. *J Endocrinol Invest.* 2003;26(7):646–650.

65. Armanini D, Nacamulli D, Francini-Pesenti F, et al. Glycyrrhetinic acid, the active principle of licorice, can reduce the thickness of subcutaneous thigh fat through topical application. *Steroids.* 2005;70(8):538–542.

66. Bone K. *Clinical Guide to Blending Liquid Herbs. Herbal Formulations for the Individual Patient.* USA: Churchill Livingstone; 2003. pp. 243–245.

67. Bone K. *Clinical Guide to Blending Liquid Herbs. Herbal Formulations for the Individual Patient.* USA: Churchill Livingstone; 2003. pp. 210–218.

68. Khan A, Safdar M, Ali Khan MM, Khattak KN, Anderson RA. Cinnamon improves glucose and lipids of people with type 2 diabetes. *Diabetes Care.* 2003;26(12):3215–3218.

69. Mang B, Wolters M, Schmitt B, et al. Effects of a cinnamon extract on plasma glucose, HbA, and serum lipids in diabetes mellitus type 2. *Eur J Clin Invest.* 2006;36(5):340–344.

70. Vanschoonbeek K, Thomassen BJ, Senden JM, et al. Cinnamon supplementation does not improve glycemic control in postmenopausal type 2 diabetes patients. *J Nutr.* 2006;136(4):977–980.

71. Kirkham S, Akilen R, Sharma S, Tsiami A. The potential of cinnamon to reduce blood glucose levels in patients with type 2 diabetes and insulin resistance. *Diabetes Obes Metab.* 2009;11(12):1100–1113.

72. Durrant-Peatfield B. *Your Thyroid and How to Keep It Healthy.* London: Hammersmith Press; 2007.

73. Altuntas Y, Bilir M, Ucak S, Gundogdu S. Reactive hypoglycemia in lean young women with PCOS and correlations with insulin sensitivity and with beta cell function. *Eur J Obstet Gynecol Reprod Biol.* 2005;119(2):198–205.

74. Brun JF, Fedou C, Mercier J. Postprandial reactive hypoglycemia. *Diabetes Metab.* 2000;26(5):337–351.

75. Debrah K, Sherwin RS, Murphy J, Kerr D. Effect of caffeine on recognition of and physiological responses to hypoglycaemia in insulin-dependent diabetes. *Lancet.* 1996;347(8993):19–24.

76. Johnson LW, Weinstock RS. The metabolic syndrome: concepts and controversy. *Mayo Clin Proc.* 2006;81(12):1615–1620.

77. Chew GT, Gan SK, Watts GF. Revisiting the metabolic syndrome. *Med J Aust.* 2006;185(8):445–449.

78. Grundy SM, Cleeman JI, Daniels SR, et al. Diagnosis and management of the metabolic syndrome: an American Heart Association/ National Heart, Lung, and Blood Institute Scientific Statement. *Circulation.* 2005;112:2735–2752.

79. Ebbeling C, Leidig MM, Feldman HA, et al. Effects of a low-glycemic load vs low-fat diet in obese young adults: a randomized trial. *JAMA.* 2007;297(19):2092–2102.

80. Zimmet PZ, James WPT. The unstoppable Australian obesity and diabetes juggernaut. What should politicians do? *Med J Aust.* 2008;185(4):187–188.

81. Cugati S, Wang JJ, Rochtchina E, Mitchell P. Ten-year incidence of diabetes in older Australians: the Blue Mountains Eye Study. *Med J Aust.* 2007;186(3):131–135.

82. Shaw JE, Chisholm DJ. Epidemiology and prevention of type 2 diabetes and the metabolic syndrome. *Med J Aust.* 2003;179(7):379–383.

83. McMahon SK, Haynes A, Ratnam N, et al. Increase in type 2 diabetes in children and adolescents in Western Australia. *Med J Aust.* 2004;180(9):459–461.

84. Fauci AS, Braunwald E, Isselbacher KJ, et al. *Harrison's Principles of Internal Medicine.* New York: McGraw-Hill; 1998. pp. 2071–2077.

85. Aronson D. Hyperglycemia and the pathobiology of diabetic complications. *Adv Cardiol.* 2008;45:1–16.

86. Aronson D, Rayfield EJ. How hyperglycemia promotes atherosclerosis: molecular mechanisms. *Cardiovasc Diabetol.* 2002; 1:1.

87. Zhou YP, Zhang JQ. Oral baicalin and liquid extract of licorice reduce sorbitol levels in red blood cell of diabetic rats. *Chin Med J (Engl).* 1989;102(3):203–206.

88. Fernández-Real JM, López-Bermejo A, Ricart W. Cross-talk between iron metabolism and diabetes. *Diabetes.* 2002;51(8):2348–2354.

89. Canturk Z, Cetinarslan B, Tarkun I, Canturk NZ. Serum ferritin levels in poorly- and well-controlled diabetes mellitus. *Endocr Res.* 2003;29(3):299–306.

90. Skinner GR, Thomas R, Taylor M, et al. Thyroxine should be tried in clinically hypothyroid but biochemically euthyroid patients. *BMJ.* 1997;314(7096):1764.

91. Barnes B, Galton L. *Hypothyroidism: The Unsuspected Illness.* New York: Harper Row; 1976.

92. Hunt R, Seidell A. Thyrotropic iodine compounds. *J Pharmacol Exp Ther.* 1910;2:15–47.

93. Curro F, Amadeo A. L'Estratto di Fucus vesiculosus L. nel trattamento medico dell'obesità e delle alterazioni metaboliche connesse. *Arch Med Intern.* 1976;28:19–32.

94. Eliason BC. Transient hyperthyroidism in a patient taking dietary supplements containing kelp. *J Am Board Fam Pract.* 1998;11(6):478–480.

95. Shilo S, Hirsch HJ. Iodine-induced hyperthyroidism in a patient with a normal thyroid gland. *Postgrad Med J.* 1986;62(729):661–662.

96. Panda S, Kar A. Changes in thyroid hormone concentrations after administration of ashwagandha root extract to adult male mice. *J Pharm Pharmacol.* 1998;50(9):1065–1068.

97. Panda S, Kar A. Withania somnifera and Bauhinia purpurea in the regulation of circulating thyroid hormone concentrations in female mice. *J Ethnopharmacol.* 1999;67(2):233–239.

98. Bone K. ed. Antithyroid plants reviewed. *MediHerb Prof Monit.* 1992;(3):3–4.

PART 3

Materia medica

How to use the monographs

10

General considerations

In this book, the monographs on individual herbs are designed to be as user-friendly as possible and hence are divided into two sections:

- A summary monograph which provides at a glance a definition, background material and clinically relevant information.
- A technical data section which extensively reviews the botany, pharmacology, clinical trial data, safety data and regulatory status in selected countries.

If the reader requires only information about the clinical applications of a particular herb, and the general sources from which this information is derived, he or she needs only to refer to the summary monograph. On the other hand, if more detailed technical information is required, this is available in the technical data section. The review of the technical material has been conducted as widely and as comprehensively as possible at the time of writing. However, due to limits on space, for certain herbs such as Ginkgo, St John's wort, turmeric and ginseng it was not possible to review all of the published studies known to the authors. In these instances, a selection was made of what were considered the most important publications.

Common and botanical names

The monographs are headed and ordered according to the English common name of each herb. This is followed by the currently accepted botanical name of the plant from which the herb is derived.

Linnaeus' system of nomenclature for all living things was first published in 1735 and is the classification system in current use. Nomenclature (naming) and taxonomy (classification) are continually changing scientific disciplines, so the botanical name (and its ranking) may change over time.

For example, the *Echinacea* species are currently being revised. A potential change includes *E. angustifolia→E. pallida* var. *angustifolia*.[1] Changes which have been proposed, but will not be enacted due to possible detriment to the pharmaceutical, herbal and agricultural industries, include:[2]

E. purpurea→E. serotina

E. laevigata→E. purpurea

With the use of gene-sequencing techniques, changes may increase in the future as a greater understanding of taxonomy at a genetic level develops. Of an estimated 5 million species (of living things), only about 1.5 million are documented at present and they are constantly being renamed and moved in the 20 or so categories of the Linnaean classification system. A new approach (phylogenetic nomenclature), which names groups of organisms that descend from a common ancestor is gaining popularity.[3]

Information about the botanical name and family has been sourced from the following (in order of preference):

- Mabberley DJ. *The Plant Book*, 2nd Edn. Cambridge University Press, Cambridge, 1997. In the preparation of this book the authors followed the system of Cronquist (1981) as modified by Kubitzki (1990) (pp. ix-xiii)
- PLANTS database, United States Department of Agriculture, USDA
- GRIN Taxonomy database, Agricultural Research Service, USDA
- Global Plant Checklist, International Organisation for Plant Information

The *Flora of China* database provides additional information for certain plants not covered by the above sources.

The botanical name is usually a Latin binomial consisting of a generic name, which comes first and then the specific epithet. Both components of the name are italicised. The generic name, which is capitalised, defines the genus to which the plant belongs. The authority that follows the specific epithet further defines the species. It indicates the taxonomist credited with naming the species (and hence the

DOI: http://dx.doi.org/10.1016/B978-0-443-06992-5.00010-4

author of the name) and is often abbreviated (e.g. 'Linnaeus' becomes 'L'). The authority has been included in the initial identifying information in these monographs and if necessary in the Adulteration section, but is not retained throughout the remainder of the monograph.

Arnica montana L.

Generic name	Arnica
Specific epithet	montana
Plant species	Arnica montana
Authority	L. (short for Linnaeus)

A botanical name may contain three Latin names when the species is further divided into subspecies or varieties: for example, *Arnica chamissonis* subsp. *foliosa*, *Viburnum opulus* var. *americanum*. In the name *Mentha* × *piperita*, the × indicates that this is a hybrid.

After the first appearance in the text, the first Latin name may be abbreviated to its initial letter (e.g. *E. purpurea*).

Synonyms

Other English common names, alternative botanical names and common names in several other languages are listed.

What is it?

This section includes historical and background information about the herb, the plant parts commonly used and other relevant details.

Effects

This section describes how the herb acts in simple language.

Traditional view

The traditional view reviews the traditional uses of the herb. As recounted elsewhere in this book, traditional use data are more than just anecdotal information and can often provide valuable insights into the therapeutic potential of a particular plant. This section is referenced so that the sources of this traditional use information are transparent.

Summary actions

The actions are important because they encompass the traditional pharmacology of herbal medicine and link the therapeutic requirements of the patient to the choice of herbs (see the

Chapter 7). Only those actions which are considered to be well supported are listed.

Can be used for

This section is divided into two parts. The part headed 'Indications supported by clinical trials' summarises those indications for which it is felt that there is good justification from clinical trial data.

The part headed 'Traditional therapeutic uses' is not just a repetition of the 'Traditional view' section. Rather these traditional uses have been selected as being those most relevant and supported by contemporary practice.

This section effectively covers the clinical uses that can be recommended in practice.

May also be used for

Again, this section is often divided into two parts. The part headed 'Extrapolations from pharmacological studies' lists clinical indications that might be reasonably expected to follow from sound pharmacological data. Unfortunately, such extrapolations are often made in herbal writings, but not stated to be such. This can leave the reader confused as to what recommended indications come from sound clinical or traditional data and what are merely speculative.

The second part headed 'Other applications' lists applications of interest which may not strictly involve medical conditions (e.g. cosmetic applications), or potential medical applications that derive from the extrapolation of limited clinical, folk or traditional information.

The information in this section should be read in the spirit that it is speculative, but may provide a useful solution to a particular therapeutic problem.

Preparations

The various preparations of the herb that can be used in therapy are described.

Dosage

Typical adult dosages are usually given for a range of dosage forms. The information is obtained from authoritative traditional texts and authorities and reflects typical modern use. Doses above these levels might increase the risk of adverse reactions or toxicity (see the section on Overdosage).

The authoritative texts used mainly comprise the following:

- British Herbal Medicine Association's Scientific Committee. *British Herbal Pharmacopoeia*. BHMA, Bournemouth, 1983
- British Herbal Medicine Association's Scientific Committee. *British Herbal Pharmacopoeia*, 4th Edn. BHMA, Bournemouth, 1996

- Pharmacopoeia Commission of the People's Republic of China. *Pharmacopoeia of the People's Republic of China*, English Edn. Chemical Industry Press, Beijing, 1997
- Bensky D, Gamble A. *Chinese Herbal Medicine Materia Medica*. Eastland Press, Seattle, 1986
- Scientific Committee of ESCOP (European Scientific Cooperative on Phytotherapy). *ESCOP Monographs*. European Scientific Cooperative on Phytotherapy, ESCOP Secretariat, UK, March 1996–October 1999
- Blumenthal M, et al (eds). *The Complete German Commission E Monographs: Therapeutic Guide to Herbal Medicines*. American Botanical Council, Austin, 1998.
- Kapoor LD. *CRC Handbook of Ayurvedic Medicinal Plants*. CRC Press, Boca Raton, 1990
- Regional Research Laboratory and Indian Drug Manufacturers' Association. *Indian Herbal Pharmacopoeia*. Indian Drug Manufacturers' Association, Mumbai and Regional Research Laboratory, Jammu-Tawi, 1998

In addition, dosages used in clinical trials were also taken into account.

Duration of use

This section provides information about the duration of safe use of the herb.

Summary assessment of safety

This section summarises the safety data detailed in the Technical data section.

Technical data

Botany

A brief description of the plant is provided.

Adulteration

Correct botanical species identification is both a quality and a potential safety issue. Administration of an incorrect species may lower the efficacy of the herb, but in some cases may cause an adverse reaction due to substitution with a toxic herb. This section also includes information regarding endangerment. Practitioners need to act to avert the potential loss of therapeutic plants, but this information is also relevant to safety also because scarcity increases the cost of the herb and the potential for adverse reactions through substitution or adulteration.

CITES (the Convention on International Trade in Endangered Species of Wild Fauna and Flora) currently provides the only international instrument for the listing of species considered to be sufficiently endangered to the extent that commercial trade must be either monitored and controlled or prohibited.[4]

Key constituents

The main phytochemical content of the plant is summarised, and levels of particular constituents are provided where available. Chemical diagrams of some key constituents are included.

Pharmacodynamics

This section reviews pharmacodynamic studies of various extracts of the herb (using different solvents) and of isolated key constituents. Sometimes the powdered herb is given instead of an extract. This information is grouped under relevant headings. In general, in vitro studies are provided first, followed by animal studies. It should be kept in mind that, because of their chemical complexity and uncertain pharmacokinetics, in vitro studies of herbal extracts do not necessarily provide clinically relevant information. In particular, some in vitro studies (and also animal studies) use excessive concentrations or doses, which are difficult to relate to normal therapeutic regimes. The reader is cautioned to refer to the original publication, taking these and other relevant factors into account, before drawing conclusions about use in humans.

When extrapolating from animal studies a common misconception is that the dose used in the animal (mg/kg) directly relates to the human dose on a body weight basis. In other words, the mg/kg dose in the animal is to be multiplied by the average human weight of 70 kg to give the corresponding human dose in mg. Such considerations are important in toxicology and new drug development (where an effective human dose needs to be worked out from prior animal studies). But animals have much faster metabolism, so a correction factor needs to be applied. One publication has defined the scale-up factors for common animal models. This is around 6 for the mouse and 11 for the rat.[5] In other words if a rat study used 100 mg/kg of extract, the corresponding human dose (for 70 kg) is 1.135 g, not 7.0 g. This can only apply if oral doses were used in the animal model. Other assumptions are that the model is relevant to the human disease and the animal metabolises the agent in the same way as humans.

The pharmacodynamic section also includes healthy volunteer studies that were seeking to establish information about the human pharmacodynamics of the herb in question.

Pharmacokinetics

The known pharmacokinetics of key constituents is reviewed, giving emphasis to human studies.

Clinical trials

Emphasis is given to randomised, controlled, double blind clinical trials. However, open (not blinded) and uncontrolled (no control group) trials are also briefly summarised. Where a number of clinical trials have been subjected to meta-analysis, or systematic review, this publication is primarily reviewed rather than those individual trials included in the meta-analysis or review, although important individual studies may also be highlighted. Also see Appendix E.

- In vitro: no relevance
- In vivo, herb given by injection: no relevance unless known active components have established bioavailability, even then of limited value
- In vivo, herb given orally: some relevance, depending on dose and validity of the animal model
- Clinical study: highly relevant, but depending on the design of the trial and being able to reproduce the treatment used.

Toxicology and other safety data

Toxicology

This section provides the reader with information about the acute and chronic toxicology (including the lethal dose), mutagenicity and carcinogenicity for the herb and/or key herbal constituents. The route of administration is reported for both the toxicological and teratogenicity data, since it effects the extrapolation to human use of the herb.

Abbreviations used throughout this section:

ig*	intragastric
im	intramuscular
ip	intraperitoneal
iv	intravenous
LD$_{50}$	lethal dose for 50% of the tested population
LOAEL	lowest observed adverse effects level
MLD	minimum lethal dose
	The least amount of a chemical that can produce death
MOAEL	minimum observed adverse effect level
MTD	maximum tolerated dose
NOAEL	no observed adverse effect level
	The highest dosage administered that does not produce toxic effects
Sc	subcutaneous
TLV	threshold limit value
TTL	threshold toxic limit

*In some cases 'oral' has been used for 'gavage' and 'ig' administration.

LD$_{50}$ test

The LD$_{50}$ test was introduced in 1927 for the biological standardisation of drugs.[6] With the mean lethal dose (LD$_{50}$) test, groups of experimental animals are treated with graduated doses of a test substance with the aim of obtaining a 50% or even higher mortality at the highest doses. The scientific significance of the classical LD$_{50}$ test has been questioned on the basis of the relatively broad variability of the test results (more than 2-fold and up to 11-fold differences) and for animal welfare reasons.[7] Three recently developed alternative animal tests that significantly improve animal welfare – the fixed dose procedure, the acute toxic class method, and the up and down procedure – can now be used within a strategy of acute toxicity testing for all types of test substances and for regulatory and in-house purposes. In vitro cytotoxicity tests could be used as adjuncts to these alternative animal tests to improve dose level selection and reduce (at least modestly) the number of animals used. However, the total replacement of animal tests requires a considerable amount of further development[8] and such modern data are not yet currently available for most herbs.

The LD$_{50}$ values can be grouped into toxicity levels,[9] as outlined in the following table with examples.

Lethal dose	Toxicity level	Example(s)
<1 mg/kg	Dangerously toxic	Dioxin – 0.045 mg/kg (oral, rat (female))
1–50 mg/kg	Extremely toxic	Indomethacin – 12.6 mg/kg (oral, rat)
		Dieldrin – 46 mg/kg (oral, rat)
50–500 mg/kg	Very toxic	Aristolochic acid – 55.9 mg/kg (oral, mouse (male))
		Curare – 270 mg/kg (oral, rabbit)
		Paracetamol – 338 mg/kg (oral, mouse)
		Caffeine – 355 mg/kg (oral, rat (male))
500–5000 mg/kg	Moderately toxic	Atropine – 622 mg/kg (oral, rat)
		Aspirin – 1500 mg/kg (oral, rat)
		Baking soda – 4220 mg/kg (oral, rat)
5000–15 000 mg/kg	Slightly toxic	Sodium cyanide – 6444 mg/kg (oral, rat)
		Monosodium succinate (food additive) –>8 g/kg (oral, rat)
>15000 mg/kg	Practically non-toxic	Propylene glycol (cosmetics) – 20 000 mg/kg (oral, rat)

In terms of categorising the acute toxicity of different herbs, assessments were based on dried herb equivalent quantities. In other words, a LD$_{50}$ of 2000 mg/kg for a 5:1 extract would give a dried herb equivalent dosage of 10 000 mg/kg, indicating slight toxicity.

To calculate an approximate human toxic dose from an animal dose, see the discussion on dosage extrapolation in the Pharmacodynamics section of this chapter.

Ames salmonella/microsome mutagenicity assay (Salmonella test, Ames test)

This is a short-term bacterial reverse mutation assay specifically designed to detect a wide range of chemical substances producing genetic damage leading to gene mutations.[10] The test was developed by Ames and colleagues in the mid-1970s and became the most used test because of its initial promise of high qualitative (yes/no) predictivity for cancer in rodents and, by extension, in humans. The relationship between mutagenic potency prediction and quantitative carcinogenicity, however, is now known to be weak,[11] despite the fact that early studies with this assay indicated that greater than 90% of the known carcinogens tested were mutagenic and that 90% of the non-carcinogens tested were non-mutagenic. The power of this assay was derived from the use of a liver microsome fraction (S9 mix) containing the mixed function oxidase (cytochrome P450) enzymes required to activate the test substance into precarcinogens (as might occur in the body after phase I metabolism by the liver). As the basis of the selection of chemicals for mutagenicity testing shifted to relative environmental importance, the sensitivity of the Salmonella assay for detecting carcinogens decreased. A negative result does not imply that the chemical will be non-carcinogenic. There are a large number of false-negatives produced (i.e. non-genotoxic carcinogens).[12] Some plant components such as flavonoids give a false positive on this test.

Micronucleus test

This is the induction and quantitative measurement of chromosomal damage leading to the formation of micronuclei in cells that have been exposed to genotoxic agents or ionising radiation.

SOS chromotest

The SOS chromotest is a simple bacterial colorimetric assay for genotoxicity that may be used as a primary screening tool or as part of a battery of short-term tests for carcinogens.

Contraindications

The information presented here is a critical review of traditional references, clinical trials and the modern understanding based on clinical practice. Often contraindications are described for herbs in popular literature and medical articles that have little realistic basis for recommendation. Contraindications listed in this section are advised with a definite rationale and, where disagreement exists with other recognised references, the rationale is provided.

Special warnings and precautions

Appropriate warnings and cautions are provided. These may arise from the consideration of material such as contraindications, clinical studies, case reports, the phytochemicals in the herb (if they are present in significant quantities) and its traditional uses.

Interactions

Herb–drug interactions are presented from reliable case reports, clinical studies and the opinion of expert committees such as the German Commission E (see Regulatory status for explanation). In general, a herb–drug interaction causing a possible beneficial effect such as the herb increasing the effectiveness of an administered drug is not included, particularly where it involves a known major action of the herb. A clinician prescribing a herbal treatment to a patient concurrently taking a drug with a similar activity would be alert to such a possibility and should monitor the patient. However, the exception is where a positive reinforcement of the action of a drug by a herb might lead to harmful effects, such as with hypoglycaemic drugs and insulin. Concerns of this kind have been included.

In general, information about potential interactions between herbs and drugs derived from in vitro studies are not featured, due to the unknown relevance of this work to oral administration in humans. However, they may be included as part of a comprehensive review. Studies using experimental models (in vivo animal studies) are typically included since they may provide a basis for a possible interaction in humans.

Use in pregnancy and lactation

The pregnancy category descriptions outlined in the following table are assigned on the basis of the available and relevant traditional and scientific information. Generally, traditional information about herbs with an emmenagogue action (bringing on menstruation) and in vitro studies demonstrating contraction of isolated uterine tissue are not emphasised in the assessment. Information that is more reliable is instead included, such as traditional pregnancy contraindications, animal models of the use of the herb or its constituents during pregnancy as well as in vivo teratogenicity studies. It must be stressed that this categorisation is driven by the data and is designed to, as much as possible, remove the subjective element from assessing the safety of herbs in pregnancy. Therefore, to some readers there may be surprises in how the various herbs have been assigned.

(The pregnancy categories are adapted from the Australian publication *Medicines in Pregnancy*, 4th Edn, 1999.)

Category A	No proven increase in the frequency of malformation or other harmful effects on the fetus despite consumption by a large number of women.
Category B1	No increase in frequency of malformation or other harmful effects on the fetus from limited use in women. No evidence of increased fetal damage in animal studies.
Category B2	No increase in frequency of malformation or other harmful effects on the fetus from limited use in women. Animal studies are lacking.
Category B3	No increase in frequency of malformation or other harmful effects on the fetus from limited use in women. Evidence of increased fetal damage in animal studies exists, although the relevance to humans is unknown.
Category C	Has caused or is associated with a substantial risk of causing harmful effects on the fetus or neonate without causing malformations.
Category D	Has caused or is associated with a substantial risk of causing fetal malformation or irreversible damage.
Category X	High risk of damage to the fetus.

Category A has been usually assigned where the use of the herb in pregnancy is known to be widespread and there is at least one published study of its safe use in pregnancy. However, in some cases where the herb is widely used as a food, for example bilberry (*Vaccinium myrtillus*), the requirement for a published study was not enforced.

Although the A to X classification provides a general guide to increasing safety concerns, it must be stressed again that these categories are assigned according to the data. Hence there are many herbs assigned to the category B2. It is likely that the vast majority of these herbs are safe during pregnancy and in terms of risk deserve a category A. However without documented studies of safe use during pregnancy, the category A cannot be assigned to such herbs.

As stated earlier this categorisation is designed to remove the subjectivity from assessing the safety information for herbs during pregnancy. The subjective element comes in when the reader interprets this information to guide the advice they give to their patients. For example, a highly cautious approach might be to only use or advise herbs in category A. It is up to each practitioner to use this data to conduct a risk–benefit analysis for each individual case, also taking into account the confidence and experience of the therapist in recommending herbs during pregnancy.

Use in lactation

Information is provided based on the existing evidence of safety or otherwise. In several cases this is not known, and hence is stated as such.

Effects on ability to drive and use machines

In most cases there is very little pharmacological and clinical research to make a definite recommendation. In these instances, the recommendation is presented on the basis of knowledge of the herb, its constituents and traditional information. Where clinical trial information is available, it is referred to.

Side effects

This section includes adverse reactions documented in traditional texts, regulatory information, clinical trials and case reports. Reactions caused by both topical and systemic administration are included.

Contentious side effects are often discussed in greater detail. The listing of side effects does not automatically imply causality. In the majority of published cases there is a deficiency of information, including identification of the plant material ingested (correct species, plant part) and dosage. There is rarely any verification that the product was not contaminated. Due consideration of concomitant drug ingestion is often not undertaken.

Overdosage

Poisoning and adverse reactions resulting from overdosage (mostly in humans) is listed. Poisoning by parts of the plant other than the used part is sometimes included for clarification, since some texts can assign such information to the herb without elaborating which plant part was involved.

Safety in children

Little specific scientific information about the safety of herbs in children exists. Recommendations are usually based on the knowledge of the herb, its constituents and traditional evidence of safe use in children.

Regulatory status in selected countries

The regulatory status of the herb in Australia, China, Germany, the UK and the USA is presented.

Australia

Part 4 of Schedule 4 of the Therapeutic Goods Regulations specifies herbs which cannot be contained in any products listed on the Australian Register of Therapeutic Goods (ARTG), or which can only be present in minute doses or if other specified conditions are met. In other words, herbs in Part 4 of Schedule 4 are considered to be more toxic and cannot be included in over-the-counter herbal products without further safety evaluations (see below).

Herbs on this list may be supplied as raw materials to practitioners provided they are not included in retail products. Products containing herbs on this list can be registered on the ARTG after first passing evaluation for quality, safety and efficacy by a Therapeutic Goods Administration committee.

UK and Europe

The General Sale List indicates the substances that can, with reasonable safety, be sold or otherwise supplied by or under the supervision of a pharmacist. Generally, such products may be sold in retail outlets. The GSL records substances often without a definitive common name or with a genus name only, and generally this convention is followed here. Maximum dose means the maximum quantity of the substance that can be delivered in a single dose (denoted as 'maximum single dose' in the monographs). Maximum daily dose means the maximum quantity of the substance recommended in any period of 24 hours.

As of April 2011, all manufactured herbal medicines in the UK are required to have either a traditional herbal registration or a product licence. Under the Framework of the European Union Directive on Traditional Herbal Medicinal Products, the Traditional Herbal Medicines Registration Scheme began on 30 October 2005 in the UK. Products are required to meet specific standards of safety and quality and be accompanied by agreed indications, based on traditional usage. Herbal products sold as raw materials for practitioner compounding and dispensing are exempt from these requirements, as are products commissioned by appropriately registered healthcare providers.

The German Commission E was an expert committee of the German Federal Health Department set up in 1978. The committee reviewed the available scientific data and traditional information to assess the safety and efficacy of selected herbs. They published their findings as concise and unreferenced monographs – the supporting reference material is stored at the German Health Department. The Commission was discontinued in the early 1990s, but much of the information remains largely valid. A positive Commission E monograph means that the indications are officially recognised by the German government, primarily for non-prescription and clinical applications. A negative Commission E monograph means that the German government does not advocate the use of the herb, either because of a lack of adequate scientific evidence for current or historical usage and/or because of potential or documented risks associated with its use.

USA

GRAS (Part 582, US Code of Federal Regulations Title 21 – Food and Drugs) is a listing of substances generally recognised as safe for their intended use, for example, for inclusion in food.

The DSHEA legislation (Dietary Supplement Health and Education Act of 1994) has defined dietary supplements as 'safe within a broad range of intake, and safety problems within the supplements are relatively rare'. The intent of this legislation was to meet the concerns of consumers and manufacturers to help ensure that safe and appropriately labelled products remain available to consumers. The provisions of DSHEA define dietary supplements and dietary ingredients, establish a new framework for assuring safety, outline guidelines for literature displayed where supplements are sold, provide for use of claims and nutritional support statements, regulate ingredient and nutrition labelling and grant the FDA (Food and Drug Administration) the authority to establish good manufacturing practice regulations.

The references listed at the end of each monograph alert the reader to the primary source of the information presented. In order to save space, references are provided in abbreviated form, as demonstrated below for the references for this chapter.

References

1. Binns SE, Baum BR, Arnason JT. *Syst Bot*. 2002;27(3):610–632.
2. Binns SE, Baum BR, Arnason JT. *Taxon*. 2001;50(4):1199–1200.
3. Milius S. *Sci News*. 1999;156(17):268–270.
4. Lewington A.. *Traffic Int*. 1993:31–32.
5. Reagan-Shaw S, Nihal M, Ahmad N. *FASEB J*. 2008;22(3):659–661.
6. DePass LR. *Toxicol Lett*. 1989;49(2-3):159–170.
7. Schlede E, Mischke U, Roll R, et al. *Arch Toxicol*. 1992;66:455–470.
8. Botham PA. *ILAR J*. 2002;43(suppl):S27–S30.
9. Munson PL, Mueller RA, Breese GR, eds. *Principles of Pharmacology: Basic Concepts and Clinical Applications*. New York: Chapman & Hall; 1995.
10. Mortelmans K, Zeiger E. *Mutat Res*. 2000;455(2):29–60.
11. Fetterman BA, Kim BS, Margolin BH, et al. *Environ Mol Mutagen*. 1997;29(3):312–322.
12. Munson PL, Mueller RA, Breese GR, eds. *Principles of Pharmacology: Basic Concepts and Clinical Applications*. New York: Chapman & Hall; 1995. pp. 1602–1603.

Andrographis

(*Andrographis paniculata* (Burm. f.) Nees)

Synonyms

Chiretta, King of bitters (Engl), kalmegh (Bengali, Hindi), kirata (Sanskrit), chuan xin lian (Chin), senshinren (Jap).

What is it?

Andrographis, commonly known as kalmegh (meaning 'king of bitters'), is grown in hedgerows and gardens in India where it is highly valued by the local people as a medicine. It has often been used as a substitute for the bitter herb *Swertia chirata*, and as such also has the Indian common name of chirayta. At one point, Andrographis was advertised in England as a substitute for quinine (possibly due to its bitterness). However, this was discontinued due to a lack of antimalarial activity (although new research studies demonstrate there is such activity in experimental models). The whole herb, including the root, has been used for medicinal purposes in India, but use of the leaf or aerial parts is more common. As well as in Ayurveda, Andrographis is found in the materia medica of other traditional medical systems, particularly those of China and south-east Asia.

Effects

Enhances immune system function; stimulates bile production and flow; protects the liver from toxins; counters the damaging effects of free radicals; helps to normalise blood sugar.

Traditional view

In Ayurvedic medicine, the herb is used for its bitter tonic, stomachic, antipyretic and laxative properties. It is said to increase appetite, strengthen digestion and diminish flatulence, hyperacidity and biliousness.[1] The herb is also utilised for treatment of many other conditions, including diabetes, debility and hepatitis.[2] The roots and leaves have a reputation for being depurative and anthelmintic.[3] In traditional Chinese medicine, Andrographis is bitter and 'cold', and is used to clear *Heat* from the *Blood* (especially in the lungs, throat and urinary tract) and to detoxify *Fire Poison* (manifesting as skin sores and carbuncles). In addition to gastrointestinal complaints, it is prescribed for throat infections, cough with thick sputum and snake bites.[4,5] Since Andrographis is regarded as a 'cold' herb, it is ideally suited to treating acute infections, which are 'hot' conditions.

Summary of actions

Bitter tonic, choleretic, immunostimulant, hepatoprotective, antipyretic, anti-inflammatory, antiplatelet, antioxidant.

Can be used for

Indications supported by clinical trials

Bacterial and viral respiratory infections including the common cold, acute sinusitis and pharyngotonsillitis (good evidence), enteric infections (low-level evidence); prevention of urinary tract infections; prophylaxis of the common cold; familial Mediterranean fever (in combination); ulcerative colitis.

Traditional therapeutic uses

Loss of appetite, atonic dyspepsia, flatulence, diarrhoea, dysentery, gastroenteritis, bowel complaints of children, sluggish liver, diabetes, general debility and for convalescence after fevers; respiratory and skin infections.

May also be used for

Extrapolations from pharmacological studies

To boost immune function in bacterial and viral infections, for protection against hepatotoxicity; to enhance the detoxifying capacity of the liver; to alleviate inflammation. May be a useful adjunctive treatment in cancer and diabetes, especially to provide immune support.

Preparations

Dried or fresh herb as a decoction, infusion and fluid extract for internal use. Dry extracts standardised to andrographolides have been used in tablet or capsule form in clinical trials. The leaf juice is also used in traditional Ayurveda.

Dosage

Being very bitter, some people may find Andrographis difficult to take in liquid preparations. Whichever way it is taken, the daily preventative dose for an adult is about 2 to 3 g or its equivalent (for example, 4 to 6 mL/day of a 1:2 fluid extract). During infection, the effective dose is nearer to 6 g/day (up to 12 mL/day of the 1:2). Standardisation for andrographolides is preferable.

Since Andrographis is energetically 'cold', it is preferably taken in combination with 'warm' herbs when used during winter as a preventative treatment, especially if the user has a 'cold' constitution. Warming herbs include ginger, Astragalus and tulsi (*Ocimum sanctum*).

Duration of use

May be taken long term.

Summary assessment of safety

No significant adverse effects from ingestion of Andrographis are expected, although high doses may cause gastric discomfort. Andrographis is best avoided during early pregnancy.

Technical data

Botany

Andrographis paniculata is an annual shrub belonging to the Acanthaceae family. It grows to a height of 1 metre with branches that are sharply quadrangular, often narrowly winged towards the apical region. The leaves are lanceolate (5 to 8 cm long), and the flowers are small, solitary in panicles, with a corolla ranging from white to rose pink in colour and hairy externally. The fruit is approximately 2 cm long, linear-oblong in shape and acute at both ends. The seeds are numerous, yellowish-brown and glabrous.[6] It grows wild as an undershrub in tropical moist deciduous forests[6] and is also cultivated as a rainy season crop.[2]

Key constituents

- Diterpenoid lactones, collectively referred to as andrographolides, and consisting of aglycones (such as andrographolide) and glucosides (such as neoandrographolide and andrographiside)[7,8]
- Diterpene dimers,[7] flavonoids[9]
- Xanthones in the roots.[10]

Many of the diterpenoid lactones (such as andrographolide) are bitter; however, neoandrographolide is not.[8]

Adulteration

Andrographis echioides is an adulterant of *A. paniculata*.[11] Purchased extracts of *Andrographis paniculata* are sometimes devoid of any andrographolide content, despite claims to the contrary on product specifications.[12]

Andrographolide

Pharmacodynamics

Anti-infective and immunomodulating activity

Although Andrographis is widely used in infections and infestations, the most likely opinion is that its value here is mainly as an immune-enhancing treatment. Early reports in China attributed an antibacterial activity to the plant that was not supported in a later review.[5] No direct antibacterial activity could be demonstrated for an aqueous extract of Andrographis against Salmonella, Shigella, *Escherichia coli*, group A streptococci and *Staphylococcus aureus* in vitro. Animal studies using orally administered Andrographis (0.12 to 0.24 g/kg) for 6 months failed to demonstrate bactericidal activity.[13] Serum taken from 10 healthy volunteers after a single oral dose of Andrographis (ranging from 1 g to 6 g) showed no bactericidal activity against a number of organisms.[13]

However, an alcoholic extract of Andrographis did show significant activity against an *E. coli* enterotoxin-induced secretory response (that causes diarrhoea) in vivo,[14] and in another study effected in vitro inhibition of adherence of *Streptococcus mutans*.[15] Andrographolide potentiated the sensitivity of two strains of *Pseudomonas aeruginosa* to several antibiotic drugs in vitro.[16] Significant growth inhibition (compared to five other herbs) was recently demonstrated for an Andrographis aqueous extract in vitro against *Streptococcus agalactiae*.[17] Feeding Nile tilapia fish (*Oreochromis niloticus*) with Andrographis reduced mortality following infection with this species of Streptococcus (although such an outcome could also reflect enhanced immunity).

Liquid extract of Andrographis root demonstrated strong in vitro anthelmintic activity against human *Ascaris lumbricoides*.[18] Subcutaneous administration of a decoction of Andrographis leaves to infected dogs reduced nematode larvae in the blood by 85%.[19]

Early uses as a substitute for quinine in malaria have been supported by recent research. An in vitro study revealed that xanthones from Andrographis root bearing a hydroxyl group at position 2 demonstrated the most potent antimalarial activity, while xanthones with a hydroxyl group at position 1, 4 or 8 possessed very low activity. Further, in vivo antimalarial testing of the most active xanthone on Swiss Albino mice with *Plasmodium berghei* infection demonstrated a substantial reduction (62%) in parasitaemia after treatment with 30 mg/kg.[10] However, more relevant to current herbal use are studies on Andrographis leaf or whole plant. An earlier study showed that a chloroform extract of the whole plant demonstrated complete parasite growth inhibition within a 24 hour incubation period in vitro at concentrations as low as 0.05 mg/mL. There was significant reduction in mortality rates in mice administered Andrographis whole plant extract (5 mg/kg/day, ip for 4 days) just after malarial infection.[20] Methanolic extracts of Andrographis leaves[21] and aerial parts[22] were active in vitro against both chloroquine resistant and sensitive strains of *Plasmodium falciparum*.

Dehydroandrographolide succinic acid monoester (DASM), a drug derived from andrographolide, has been found to inhibit HIV in vitro. This effect was observed on several HIV strains and DASM was non-toxic to other cells in the concentration range. However, the diterpenoid lactones of Andrographis (dehydroandrographolide and andrographolide) were devoid of anti-HIV activity.[23] Moreover, in vitro studies with aqueous extracts of Andrographis showed little or no inhibition of HIV-1. Modes of inhibition studied comprised inhibition of HIV-1 protease,[24] inhibition of the interaction between HIV-1 gp 120 and immobilised CD4 receptor, inhibition of HIV-1 reverse transcriptase and inhibition of glycohydrolase enzymes.[25]

Andrographolides showed in vitro activity against herpes simplex virus 1 in vitro[26] and both Andrographis ethanolic extract (25 μg/mL) and andrographolide (5 μg/mL) inhibited the expression of Epstein-Barr virus lytic proteins in vitro, thereby inhibiting viral maturation.[27] Andrographolide showed significant activity against influenza A viruses in vitro, including the H5N1 strain.[28] Administration of andrographolide (100 to 200 mg/kg/day, oral) to mice infected with avian influenza A strains H9N2 and H5N1 and the human strain H1N1 significantly reduced death rate, prolonged life, inhibited lung consolidation and reduced viral titres in the lung.[28] However, such in vivo activity might also be the consequence of immune effects.

Early research suggested an immunostimulant action for Andrographis. Enhanced phagocytosis was demonstrated in vitro for a decoction of the herb and in vivo after injection of the soluble derivatives.[5] Isolated andrographolide (4 mg/kg/day, ip for 2 days) and an ethanolic Andrographis extract (25 mg/kg/day, oral for 7 days) significantly stimulated both antigen-specific and innate immune responses in mice. The whole extract produced stronger immunostimulation.[29] Prolonged survival in animals after snakebite was observed after pretreatment with extracts of Andrographis.[30]

Four later studies (three from the same research group) have demonstrated a downregulation of immune response by andrographolide using both in vitro and in vivo models. In vitro, andrographolide reduced T cell activation in splenocytes,[31] reduced IL-2 production in stimulated Jurkat T cells by interfering with nuclear factor of activated T cells (NFAT) and mitogen-activated protein kinases (MAPK),[32] reduced IL-2 and interferon-gamma in stimulated murine T cells,[33] and downregulated macrophage immune responses

and cytokine expression.[34] In vivo, andrographolide (4 mg/kg/day, ip) reduced T cell function and significantly reduced the severity of experimental autoimmune encephalomyelitis in mice, including antimyelin T cell and antibody responses.[31] Andrographolide (1 mg/kg/day for 7 days, ip) also reduced antibody production and the number of IL-4-producing splenocytes in mice after antigen challenge.[34]

However, several other later publications have observed an enhanced immune response from andrographolide or Andrographis extract, most notably the in vivo studies summarised in the Antitumour activity section that follows. In addition, andrographolide and a combination of Andrographis and Siberian ginseng extracts (Kan Jang) demonstrated lymphocyte proliferation and stimulation of some cytokines in vitro in a whole blood cell culture.[35] Andrographis extract (25 or 50 mg/kg/day, oral for 14 or 28 days) and andrographolide (1 or 4 mg/kg/day, oral for 14 or 28 days) enhanced specific antibody and cell-mediated immune responses in mice inoculated with an inactivated Salmonella vaccine.[36] A mixture of andrographolides (1.0, 1.5 and 2.5 mg/kg, oral) potentiated delayed-type hypersensitivity (DTH) in mice inoculated with sheep red blood cells, but also countered the increase in DTH after cyclophosphamide treatment.[37] This suggests an immunomodulatory activity. Further experimentation at the same doses revealed that the andrographolide mixture significantly stimulated phagocytic activity, white blood cell counts and spleen and thymus weights in mice.

Antitumour activity

A methanol extract of Andrographis showed potent cell differentiation-inducing activity on mouse leukaemia cells in vitro. Some of the isolated diterpenes also demonstrated this activity.[7,38] Andrographolide was shown to inhibit the in vitro proliferation of more than 30 tumour cell lines representing various types of cancers, specifically breast, CNS, colon, lung, melanoma, ovarian, prostate, renal and leukaemia. The compound was found to exert direct anticancer activity on cancer cells by cell-cycle arrest via induction of p27 and decreased expression of cyclin-dependent kinase 4 (CDK4). It also enhanced tumour necrosis factor-alpha (TNF-alpha) in lymphocytes, and possibly via this mechanism increased their cytotoxic activity against cancer cells in vitro.[39] Andrographolide (100 and 200 mg/kg/day for 10 days, oral) significantly inhibited the growth of B16 melanoma and HT-29 colon tumours in mice.[39]

Since these publications there has been a considerable number of in vitro investigations of the antineoplastic activity of andrographolide against a wide variety of cancer cell lines. An extensive review of material up to 2008 by Varma and co-workers identified the key mechanisms involved.[40] These included induction of cell-cycle arrest (possibly due to increased levels of p21) and apoptosis (via a variety of mechanisms involving caspase-3, caspase-8, BcL-2 and TNF-alpha-related apoptosis inducing ligand). Other mechanisms have been proposed from recent research, including a downregulation of epidermal growth factor receptors,[41] a decrease of cell-cycle related proteins,[42] changes in the intracellular redox system[43] and a novel cell differentiating activity.[44] Other andrographolides have also been shown to induce cell-cycle arrest in vitro.[45]

Neoandrographolide sensitised the cytotoxic action of etopiside against a leukaemia cell line[46] and andrographolide was found to sensitise cancer cells (such as colorectal, cervical and hepatic) to doxorubicin.[47]

Other researchers have investigated inhibition of angiogenesis as an anticancer prospect for Andrographis extract and andrographolide. Intraperitoneal administration of both in angiogenesis-induced mice led to substantial reductions in elevated proinflammatory cytokines such as IL-1beta, IL-6, TNF-alpha and granulocyte-macrophage colony-stimulating factor (GM-CSF) and the most potent angiogenic factor, vascular endothelial growth factor (VEGF). Antiangiogenic factors such as tissue inhibitor of metalloproteinase 1 (TIMP-1) and IL-2 levels were elevated after treatment.[48] The inhibitory effect on VEGF production was supported by a later in vitro study.[49]

Andrographolide inhibited the adhesion of gastric cancer cells to endothelial cells in vitro by blocking E-selectin expression in the latter.[50] Taiwanese scientists have found inhibition of migration and invasion of cancer cell lines in vitro via the downregulation of matrix metalloproteinase-7 (MMP-7)[51,52] and MMP-2.[53]

There have also been additional in vivo anticancer studies on andrographolide and Andrographis extract (both administered intraperitoneally). A 70% ethanolic extract of Andrographis (10 mg/animal for 10 days, ip) substantially reduced tumour growth, helped maintain total white cell count, improved IL-2 and GM-CSF levels and reduced TNF-alpha in mice inoculated with Dalton's lymphoma ascites cells.[54] These effects were maintained for 11 to 20 days after the final herb dose and were also observed for animals concurrently treated with a combination of cyclophosphamide, radiation and whole body hyperthermia. The same authors also observed that both Andrographis extract (10 mg/animal for 10 days, ip) and andrographolide (0.5 mg/animal for 10 days, ip) substantially prolonged the survival times of mice inoculated with EL4 thymoma cells.[55] IL-2 and interferon-gamma levels were increased and the authors concluded, based on this and a series of complex experiments, that the two treatments increased cytotoxic T lymphocyte activity. In general, the Andrographis extract was more active than andrographolide. The same research group using similar models and treatments has also demonstrated enhanced natural killer cell activity and antibody-dependent cytotoxicity in normal and tumour-bearing (Ehrlich ascites carcinoma) mice.[56]

Hepatoprotective and choleretic activity

Andrographolide showed protective activity against chemically induced toxicity in rat hepatocytes in vitro. The observed hepatoprotective effect was greater than silymarin.[57] Intraperitoneal administration of andrographolide, andrographiside and neoandrographolide (100 mg/kg) to mice protected against hepatotoxic damage caused by carbon tetrachloride and tert-butylhydroperoxide. Andrographiside and neoandrographolide had the greatest effect on reducing lipid peroxidation and were comparable to silymarin.[58] Similar studies suggest that andrographolide is the major active antihepatotoxic principle in Andrographis.[59] Intraperitoneal administration of three diterpene constituents of Andrographis showed protective effects on hepatotoxicity induced in mice by various chemicals. The protective effect of andrographiside and neoandrographolide was as strong as silymarin, and could be due to the glucoside groups acting as strong antioxidants.[60] Andrographolide exhibited hepatoprotective activity after oral or intraperitoneal administration to rats with chemically induced acute hepatitis. Treatment with the herb led to complete normalisation of five biochemical parameters and improved histopathological changes in the liver.[61]

Intraperitoneal pretreatment of mice with different doses of andrographolide or arabinogalactan proteins from Andrographis for 7 days was followed by intraperitoneal injection of ethanol (7.5 g/kg of body weight). At 500 mg/kg and 125 mg/kg, respectively, the protective activity of these two preparations against hepatic and renal alcohol toxicity was comparable to silymarin.[62]

Oral administration of Andrographis extract and andrographolide to rats demonstrated a protective action against carbon tetrachloride-induced hepatotoxicity. The leaf extract showed stronger activity than andrographolide.[63] Pre- and post-treatment with oral doses of Andrographis (0.5 g/kg/day) normalised alcohol-induced increases in serum transaminase activity in rats. The researchers concluded that Andrographis has a protective as well as a curative effect on alcohol-induced toxic liver damage.[64]

Andrographolide (5, 7 and 10 mg/kg, oral) improved levels of antioxidant parameters such as glutathione, superoxide dismutase and catalase in mice treated with the liver carcinogen hexachlorocyclohexane (BHC).[65] It also reduced parameters of liver damage and the development of liver tumours in BHC-treated mice at the same doses.[66]

Significant hepatoprotective activity was demonstrated for an alcohol extract of Andrographis and two of its diterpenes – andrographolide and neoandrographolide – against the hepatotoxicity caused by *Plasmodium berghei* infection in animals. The protective effect of Andrographis was thought to be partially due to reactivation of superoxide dismutase, which in turn counteracted peroxidative damage caused by the infection. Andrographis may also induce drug metabolising systems that detoxify hepatotoxins.[67] Administration of Andrographis (0.5 g/kg/day) or andrographolide (5.0 mg/kg/day) to rats for 7 to 30 consecutive days induced the liver microsomal drug-metabolising enzymes aniline hydroxylase, N-demethylase and O-demethylase.[68]

Andrographolide produced a dose-dependent choleretic effect (increased bile flow, bile salt and bile acids) in rats and guinea pigs after oral administration[69] and by intraperitoneal injection in rats.[70] The effect was stronger than silymarin.[69] Aqueous extract of Andrographis orally administered to rats at 3.75 mL/kg increased bile flow and liver weight. A maximal increase in flow and weight was reached after 2 days.[71]

Cardiovascular activity

An early study investigating an aqueous extract by intravenous administration suggested that Andrographis may limit the expansion of the ischaemic focus, may exert a marked protective effect on the reversible ischaemic myocardium and could demonstrate a weak fibrinolytic action.[72] Andrographis alleviated myocardial ischaemia-reperfusion injury in vivo.[73] It upregulated cellular reduced glutathione and protected cardiomyocytes against hypoxia/reoxygenation injury in vitro.[74] The mechanism was probably via a decrease in the harmful effect of oxygen free radicals.[75] A study using rabbits found Andrographis alleviated atherosclerotic arterial stenosis induced by both de-endothelialisation and a high cholesterol diet. In addition, it lowered the restenosis rate after experimental angioplasty.[76] Andrographolide (5 mg/kg, presumably ip) suppressed the hyperplasia of arterial neointima (about a 60% reduction) in a murine model of arterial restenosis. This was via the downregulation of NF-kappaB target genes that are critical in thrombosis and inflammation.[77]

An aqueous extract of Andrographis given by intraperitoneal infusion to rats exhibited a dose-dependent reduction in systolic blood pressure in spontaneously hypertensive rats and normotensive controls.[78] A crude water extract of Andrographis, and two semi-purified n-butanol and aqueous fractions, significantly reduced mean arterial blood pressure in anaesthetised rats without decreasing heart rate after ip administration. The hypotensive substance in the crude water extract appeared to be concentrated in the butanol fraction.[79]

Following the observation that some patients exhibited a hypotensive response while taking Andrographis, the in vitro and in vivo actions of the herb and three of its diterpenoids were investigated.[80] The diterpenoid 14-deoxy-11,12-didehydroandrographolide (DIAP) was most active at reducing the chronotropic response of isolated rat atria and exerting spasmolytic activity in rat aortic rings. An Andrographis aqueous extract with the highest levels of DIAP (delivering 19 mg/kg of this compound, oral doses for 7 days) was the most potent (compared to two other extracts with lower levels of DIAP) at reducing systolic blood pressure in rats. Mechanistic studies suggested that vascular smooth muscle was the major site of the hypotensive effect.

Andrographolide inhibited PAF-induced human platelet aggregation[81] and deoxyandrographolide antagonised PAF-mediated processes in neutrophils,[82] as did andrographolide,[83] all in vitro.

Anti-inflammatory, antipyretic, antiallergic and analgesic activity

Several early in vivo studies found antipyretic and anti-inflammatory effects for andrographolides (after oral administration or injection). The anti-inflammatory activity of the andrographolides may be due to the promotion of ACTH (adrenocorticotrophic hormone) and consequent enhancement of adrenocortical function.[5] Andrographolide administered orally (30, 100 and 300 mg/kg) significantly reduced inflammation in a number of animal models including adjuvant-induced arthritis.[84] The addition of andrographolide to an endothelial cell culture together with TNF-alpha caused a concentration-dependent reduction of the enhancement of endothelial monocyte adhesion, which is part of the inflammatory process.[85] Another in vitro study found that andrographolide inhibited NF-kappaB binding to DNA, thereby reducing the expression of pro-inflammatory proteins such as COX-2 in neutrophils.[83] Andrographolide prevented oxygen radical production by human neutrophils in vitro.[86]

As well as demonstrating antioxidant activity in vitro and in vivo, a 70% methanolic extract of Andrographis (10 mg/animal for 5 days, ip) completely inhibited carrageenan-induced paw oedema in mice.[87] Oral administration of neoandrographolide (150 mg/kg) also demonstrated anti-inflammatory activity in mice as well as in vitro, using several experimental models.[88]

In a murine model of asthma, andrographolides (30 mg/kg, ip) inhibited the elevation of bronchoalveolar fluid (BAF) levels of TNF-alpha and GM-CSF, and almost abolished the accumulation in BAF of lymphocytes and eosinophils.[89] In a similar model, andrographolide (0.1, 0.5 and 1 mg/kg, ip) dose-dependently inhibited increases in total cell count, eosinophil count and IL-4, IL-5 and IL-13 levels in BAF.[90] It also attenuated IgE responses, eosinophilia and airway mucus production and hyper-responsiveness. Examination of lung tissue specimens and further in vitro investigations suggested that andrographolide might act by inhibiting the NF-kappaB pathway. An anti-inflammatory mechanism mediated by reduced NF-kappaB expression was also observed for andrographolide (2 mg/kg/day for 7 days, ip) in another study in mice, using a similar experimental model of asthma.[91]

Oral doses of andrographolide at 300 mg/kg demonstrated analgesic activity; at 100 and 300 mg/kg significant antipyretic effects were also observed after 3 h. In addition, this dose exhibited significant protective activity against aspirin-induced ulceration in rats.[92] An aqueous extract of Andrographis (40 and 100 mg/kg, oral) and andrographolide (25, 50 and 100 mg/kg, oral), but not a 95% ethanolic extract (100 and 200 mg/kg, oral), demonstrated significant analgesic activity in mice.[93] The aqueous extract and andrographolide were also active at oral doses of 100 mg/kg in reducing carrageenan-induced rat paw oedema. A similar activity profile (analgesic and antioedema) was demonstrated for subcutaneous injection of andrographolide (10, 25 and 50 mg/kg).[94] Analgesia was probably mediated via non-opioid pathways, since naloxone failed to antagonise the activity of andrographolide. A methanolic extract of Andrographis (100 to 300 mg/kg, ip) slightly lowered body temperature, increased pentobarbitone sleeping time, demonstrated analgesic activity, reduced exploratory behaviour and curiosity, and exhibited some muscle-relaxing activity in mice.[95] The same doses in rats also reduced exploratory behaviour in the Y-maze test.

Hypoglycaemic activity

An aqueous extract of Andrographis (10 mg/kg) was found to prevent glucose-induced hyperglycaemia in rabbits, but failed to prevent glucose absorption from the gut.[96] In a screening of several traditional remedies, only Andrographis (as aqueous extract, and especially freeze-dried extract, administered at 50 mg/kg and 6.25 mg/kg body weight) significantly lowered blood glucose levels in streptozotocin-induced hyperglycaemic rats.[97] In a further study Andrographis decoction was orally administered to alloxan-induced diabetic rats, with a significant reduction in blood glucose levels observed compared with controls.[98]

In a study comparing normal and streptozotocin-induced diabetic rats, an ethanolic extract of Andrographis not only demonstrated hypoglycaemic effects, but also reduced oxidative stress in the diabetic rats. Normal and diabetic rats were randomly divided into groups and treated orally with distilled water, metformin (500 mg/kg) or Andrographis (400 mg/kg) twice daily for 14 days. Both Andrographis and metformin significantly increased body weight and reduced fasting serum glucose in the diabetic rats, but had no such effects in the normal rats. Both treatments also significantly increased the activity of the antioxidant enzymes superoxide dismutase (SOD) and catalase in the diabetic rats, but again not in the normal rats.[99] In another study, Andrographis extract (400 mg/kg, oral) decreased blood glucose and increase activities of the antioxidant enzymes SOD and catalase in streptozotocin-induced diabetic rats.[100]

Inhibition of the digestive enzymes alpha-glucosidase and alpha-amylase can significantly decrease the postprandial increase in blood glucose. In vitro testing demonstrated that a 20% ethanolic extract of Andrographis possessed an appreciable alpha-glucosidase inhibitory effect, but demonstrated only weak inhibition of alpha-amylase.[101] Supporting this observation, a single oral dose of Andrographis extract (250, 500 or 1000 mg) dose-dependently and significantly reduced blood glucose in streptozotocin-induced diabetic rats challenged with starch and sucrose, but not after a glucose challenge.[101] In contrast, andrographolide (0.5 to 1.5 mg/kg, oral) dose-dependently decreased plasma glucose in streptozotocin-induced diabetic rats, and at 1.5 mg/kg (oral) significantly attenuated plasma glucose after glucose challenge in normal rats.[102]

As a possible contradiction of the above results for sucrose, oral administration of Andrographis extract and andrographolide produced a dose- and time-dependent activation of brush-border membrane-bound hydrolases (lactase, maltase, sucrase) in rats, suggesting it accelerated the intestinal digestion and absorption of disaccharides.[103]

Other activity

An aqueous extract of Andrographis (200 mg/kg, oral) largely countered the nephrotoxic impact of gentamicin in rats, in terms of tending to normalise serum creatinine and urea, blood urea nitrogen and urine volume.[104] Whether this effect was due to antioxidant activity or represented a specific renoprotective activity is not clear.

Three studies cited above attest to significant in vivo and in vitro antioxidant activity for the herb,[87,93,100] as do some of the hepatoprotection studies. Oral administration of an aqueous extract of Andrographis (10, 20 and 30 mg per mouse) caused a significant elevation of catalase, SOD and glutathione-S-transferase activities in lymphoma-bearing mice, as well as exhibiting some antitumour activity.[105]

Other studies have demonstrated protection against toxins, in some cases linked to antioxidant activity. Andrographolide and an aqueous extract of Andrographis (250 mg/kg/day for 7 days, ip) protected against nicotine-induced neurotoxicity in rats by reducing oxidative stress.[106] A similar protective activity against nicotine-induced oxidative stress was demonstrated in vitro for lymphocytes.[107]

A 70% ethanolic extract of Andrographis (10 mg/animal/day for 10 days, ip) was also shown to protect against cyclophosphamide toxicity in mice in two separate but similar studies conducted by the same research group.[108,109] The

elevation of TNF-alpha induced by the drug was lowered by Andrographis treatment. Andrographolide was also active.[109]

Topical application of Andrographis extract (10%) improved wound healing in rats.[110] Wounds dressed with Andrographis showed markedly less scar width, higher fibroblast proliferation, more collagen, less angiogenesis and an absence of inflammatory cells.

Pharmacokinetics

An early study found that oral doses of radiolabelled andrographolide given to mice were rapidly absorbed and distributed to organs, especially gallbladder, kidney, ovary and lung. Andrographolide levels appeared to be low in spleen, heart and brain. Approximately 90% was excreted in the urine and faeces after 24 h, and 94% after 48 h. At 48 h, radiolabelled andrographolide only accounted for approximately 11% of urine and liver fractions, the remainder consisted of metabolites.[111]

Using isolated rat small intestine it was observed that P-glycoprotein (P-gp) was involved in the intestinal transport and absorption of andrographolide.[112] One recent study using in vitro models and rats calculated that andrographolide had low absolute bioavailability (2.67%) because of its rapid biotransformation and efflux by P-gp.[113] Metabolites of andrographolide found in rats included sulphates[114] and an unusual sulphonic acid derivative (in urine).[115]

Studies in human volunteers have identified sulphate[116] and glucuronide[117] conjugates in urine after ingestion of andrographolide. Administration of a single 200 mg dose of andrographolide to each of 20 healthy volunteers revealed mean values of Tmax and Cmax of 1.6 h (range 1.5 to 2.0 h) and 58.6 ng/mL (range 29.3 to 81.2 ng/mL), respectively.[118] The elimination half-life of andrographolide was 10.5±2.1 h. These results are consistent with a relatively low bioavailability for andrographolide.

Andrographolides might exhibit better bioavailability from Andrographis extracts. After oral administration of 1 g/kg of an extract (containing 4.52% andrographolide and 2.95% 14-deoxy-11,12-didehydroandrographolide (DIAP)) to rats, the respective Cmax and Tmax values observed were 1.42±0.09 μg/mL and 3.0±0.12 h for andrographolide and 1.31±0.05 μg/mL and 3.0±0.15 h for DIAP.[119] Similarly in rabbits, 2 mL/kg of a liquid extract of Andrographis (containing 35.2 mg andrographolide and 20.7 mg DIAP) resulted in respective Cmax and Tmax values of 2.28 μg/mL and 1.0 h for andrographolide and 1.33 μg/mL and 0.75 h for DIAP.[120]

The amount of andrographolide was determined in the blood plasma of rats and 15 human volunteers following the oral administration of a 60% ethanolic Andrographis extract to rats and its combination with Siberian ginseng to humans (Kan Jang).[121] In rats it was found that andrographolide is rapidly and almost totally (91%) absorbed after oral administration of 20 mg/kg of the Andrographis extract. Less than 10% was found in the urine, presumably because of extensive metabolism. The pharmacokinetics of andrographolide was found to be highly variable in humans after the single oral administration of 20 mg via Kan Jang, although it was reasonably rapidly absorbed (Tmax 1.37 h). The calculated steady-state plasma concentration after the normal multiple doses of the herbal combination was around 0.66 μg/mL, with a Cmax after each dose of about 1.34 μg/mL.

Clinical trials

Respiratory infections

A recent systematic review of two systematic reviews and eight clinical trials concluded that there was evidence that Andrographis was useful in the treatment of upper respiratory tract infections, but expressed concerns about publication bias and particularly the fact that most of the trials had been conducted in association with product manufacturers.[122] The authors called for more independent clinical trials.

The two systematic reviews included in the above were as follows. In one, seven double blind, controlled trials (n=896) that met inclusion criteria for evaluation of efficacy were considered. All trials scored at least three (out of a maximum of five) for methodological quality on the Jadad scale. Collectively, the data suggested that Andrographis was superior to placebo in alleviating the subjective symptoms of uncomplicated upper respiratory tract infection. There was also preliminary evidence of a preventative effect. Adverse events reported following the herb administration were generally mild and infrequent.[123] In the second review, 433 patients from three trials were included in the meta-analysis. Andrographis either alone or in combination with Siberian ginseng was more effective than placebo in the treatment of uncomplicated acute upper respiratory tract infection.[124]

In a general review of the literature for evidence of the efficacy and safety of complementary and alternative medicine for the prevention and treatment of upper respiratory tract infection in children, the authors concluded that Andrographis decreased nasal secretions (p<0.01), but not other symptoms.[125]

The subjects of these reviews as well as other studies follow.

Uncontrolled early Chinese clinical studies in patients with bacterial and viral respiratory infections suggested beneficial effects after oral administration of Andrographis or andrographolides, implying an immune enhancing action.[5] Investigations from the Sichuan Traditional Medicine Research Institution found Andrographis exerted a beneficial effect in the treatment of infectious diseases associated with cold symptoms. The major finding was the lowered body temperature within 48h after treatment with Andrographis. Of 84 cases of common cold, 70 achieved normal body temperature within 48h.[126]

A randomised double blind study of 152 patients with pharyngotonsillitis found Andrographis (6g/day) for 1 week to be as effective as paracetamol (acetaminophen) in relieving fever and sore throat. For both groups the difference between baseline symptoms and final evaluation was significant (p<0.0001). Lower doses of Andrographis were not as effective.[127]

Tablets containing a total of 1200 mg Andrographis extract (standardised to 4% andrographolides) or placebo were given to 61 patients suffering symptoms of common cold in a double blind, placebo-controlled clinical trial. After 4 days of treatment, measured symptoms were significantly reduced in the Andrographis-treated group compared to placebo: strength of disease (p=0.0001), tiredness (p=0.0001), sweating/shivering (p=0.001), sore throat (p=0.0001) and muscular ache (p=0.0001). In terms of clinical signs (rhinitis, sinus pains and headaches, lymphatic swellings), there was no significant difference between the treated and placebo groups at day 4. However, when the groups were compared over time (specifically day 0 versus day 4), there was a significant decrease in the intensity of these signs only for the Andrographis group (p<0.05). The overall reduction in the symptom score over time was also significant (p<0.01). The authors concluded that, based on their findings, Andrographis can significantly reduce the symptoms and duration of the common cold.[128]

In a randomised, double blind, placebo-controlled clinical trial, 107 healthy children received either Andrographis extract tablets (200mg/day of extract, standardised to 11.2mg andrographolide) or placebo for 3 months during the winter season. This dose corresponds to about 1g of original herb. Analysis after the first month indicated no significant change for Andrographis treatment. However, by the third month there was a significant decrease in the incidence of colds compared with placebo (30% versus 62%; p<0.01). The relative risk of catching a cold was 2.1 times lower for the Andrographis group.[129] The same research team conducted a further randomised, placebo-controlled, double blind study of an Andrographis extract at 1200mg/day over 5 days in 158 adult patients. Visual analogue scale evaluations of the intensity of headache, tiredness, earache, sleeplessness, sore throat, nasal secretion, phlegm and frequency and intensity of cough were performed by the patients at days 0, 2 and 4 of the treatment. Using a logistic regression model of assessment, there was a significant decrease in the intensity of the symptoms of tiredness, sleeplessness, sore throat and nasal secretion in the Andrographis group at day 2, as compared with the placebo group. By day 4, a significant decrease in the intensity of all symptoms was observed for the Andrographis group. No adverse effects were observed or reported.[130]

In another randomised, double blind, placebo-controlled pilot study, 50 outpatients with symptoms of common cold were treated with tablets containing Andrographis extract (1020mg/day, about 6g of herb). The patients were advised to make their first clinic visit not later than 3 days after the occurrence of cold symptoms. After 5 days of therapy, subjective evaluation demonstrated a significantly reduced number of sick leave days (p<0.03), improved symptoms (p<0.025) and hastened recovery (p<0.05). Side effects were very few and mild.[131]

Recently, a randomised, double blind, placebo-controlled clinical trial observed that treatment with a standardised extract of Andrographis reduced the symptoms of uncomplicated upper respiratory tract infection.[132] A total of 223 patients received either 200mg/day of an Andrographis extract (about 2.5g of herb, containing 60mg of andrographolides) or a matching placebo for 5 days after experiencing the typical symptoms of a common cold. Nine self-evaluated symptoms were used to assess the efficacy of the herbal treatment: cough, expectoration, nasal discharge, headache, fever, sore throat, earache, malaise/fatigue and sleep disturbance. Both groups showed improvement in these scores from days 1 to 3. However, from days 3 to 5 most of the symptoms in the placebo group were unchanged, whereas symptom improvement continued for the Andrographis group. The difference in the overall symptom score between the two groups was significant at day 5 (p<0.05). For individual symptoms on day 5, all were significantly improved for the Andrographis group versus placebo (p<0.05), except for earache. The overall efficacy of Andrographis was a significant 2.1 times higher than placebo (p<0.05), and the herbal treatment was well tolerated. One weakness of the trial design was that patients were not treated for longer than 5 days. Hence the impact of Andrographis on shortening the duration of the common cold could not be assessed.

In two randomised, parallel-group clinical studies, a standardised extract of Andrographis (as the combination Kan Jang) was compared with amantadine in the treatment of diagnosed viral influenza infection.[133] Each tablet comprised 85 mg of Andrographis extract (containing 5 mg andrographolides) and 10 mg of Siberian ginseng extract (from 120 mg root). The typical acute dose was four tablets three times daily. In the first pilot study, 71 Kan Jang-treated patients were compared with 469 patients on amantadine; in the second phase 66 patients were enrolled. Duration of sick leave and frequency of post-influenza complications were used as outcome measures and indicated that the herbal combination contributed to a quicker recovery. It reduced the risk of post-influenza complications and was also well tolerated.

A three-arm study compared the efficacy of standard treatment, Kan Jang and a preparation containing *Echinacea purpurea* extract in patients with uncomplicated common colds.[134] Of the 130 children aged between 4 and 11 years studied over a period of 10 days, 39 patients received only standard treatment, 53 were treated with the Andrographis combination plus standard treatment and 41 were treated with Echinacea plus standard treatment. It was found that adjuvant treatment with the Andrographis combination was significantly more effective than the Echinacea preparation when started at an early stage of uncomplicated common colds. The effect was particularly pronounced in terms of the amount of nasal secretion and congestion. It also accelerated the recovery time compared to other treatments. The need for standard medication was significantly less in the Andrographis combination group compared with the others and it was well tolerated, with no adverse reactions reported.

The same Andrographis combination was also tested in a phase III randomised, double blind, placebo-controlled parallel group clinical trial in the treatment of uncomplicated upperrespiratory tract infections. After an initial pilot trial involving 46 patients over 3 to 8 days, 179 patients completed the 3-day study according to protocol. Both the total symptom score (from patients' evaluation) and the total diagnosis score (from physicians' evaluation) showed highly significant improvements (p<0.0006 and p=0.003, respectively), as compared with placebo. Throat signs and symptoms demonstrated the most significant improvement.[135]

A double blind, placebo-controlled clinical study evaluated the impact of Kan Jang treatment for 5 days in the management of acute upper respiratory symptoms (including sinusitis) in 185 patients. At the end of the treatment, significant differences compared with placebo were in evidence for total symptoms in the group as a whole (p<0.001) and in the acute and recurrent sinusitis subgroups. In terms of individual symptoms in the whole group, significant differences against placebo (p<0.001) were observed for sore throat, headache, malaise and catarrh.[136]

Enteric infections

Many early Chinese studies used oral administration of Andrographis or andrographolides in acute bacillary dysentery and enteritis and observed a marked benefit.[5] Patients with acute diarrhoea were treated with powdered leaves and stems of Andrographis. The Andrographis was more effective in reducing the number of *Shigella*, but was less effective for cholera compared with tetracycline. Oral administration of 1 g every 12 h for 2 days was more effective than giving a dose of 500 mg every 6 h for 2 days.[137]

Inflammatory disorders

Familial Mediterranean fever (FMF) is a recessively inherited inflammatory disorder characterised by recurrent attacks of fever and serositis (inflammation of the serous tissues such as pleura, pericardium and peritoneum). A combination of Andrographis extract 600 mg/day (containing 48 mg andrographolide), Siberian ginseng extract 120 mg/day (standardised to >9.6 mg eleutheroside E), *Schisandra chinensis* extract 600 mg/day (standardised to >9.6 mg schisandrins) and licorice extract 120 mg/day (standardised to >7.2 mg glycyrrhizin) was assessed over 30 days in a pilot study involving 24 children with FMF.[138] Using a double blind, placebo-controlled design, it was found that duration, frequency and severity of attacks were all significantly less compared with placebo following the herbal treatment (p=0.0003). A separate publication investigated the impact of the herbal combination on plasma nitric oxide (NO) levels during the trial.[139] Additional control groups were used, consisting of healthy volunteers and FMF patients treated with colchicine. Basal levels of NO in FMF patients during attack-free periods over the 30-day trial were found to be no different to the healthy controls. Surprisingly, NO levels fell during attacks. The herbal formulation with Andrographis was found to normalise blood levels of NO and decrease IL-6 in FMF patients during attacks.

A 14-week randomised, double blind, placebo-controlled clinical trial in 60 patients examined the impact of a 75% ethanolic extract of Andrographis (300 mg/day corresponding to 3 g of herb and containing 90 mg of andrographolides) in active rheumatoid arthritis.[140] All trial patients were given methotrexate and were allowed to take prednisone or chloroquine in stable doses if already prescribed. Compared with baseline there were significant improvements observed in the Andrographis group by week 14 for tender joints (p=0.001), number of swollen joints (p=0.02), severity of swollen joints (p=0.01), severity of tender joints (p=0.002), levels of rheumatoid factor (p=0.01) and quality of life measures (p<0.001). However, compared with the placebo group these changes were not statistically significant. Perhaps a larger trial with a higher dose might have yielded results that were more definite.

A randomised, double blind trial was conducted at five centres in Shanghai to compare a standardised extract of Andrographis with the non-steroidal anti-inflammatory drug mesalazine (4.5 g/day, in slow release form) in patients with mildly to moderately active ulcerative colitis (confirmed by colonoscopy).[141] One hundred and eight patients completed the trial. The aqueous-ethanolic extract provided about 108 mg/day of andrographolide. Treatment with Andrographis extract demonstrated similar efficacy to mesalazine. Scores for clinical symptoms (fever, stool frequency, stool consistency, stool blood, abdominal pain, mucous stool, tenesmus (straining) and abdominal tension) were assessed throughout treatment. Symptom scores decreased over time in both groups. Clinical efficacy was also assessed by the percentage of patients attaining remission, partial remission or improvement in symptoms. Mucosal healing was evaluated by colonoscopy and, in the 34 patients with biopsies available, histopathology was evaluated. Such outcomes were significantly better (p<0.001) for both groups compared with baseline, and there was no significant difference between the two treatment groups. Thirteen per cent of patients in the Andrographis group and 27% of patients in the mesalazine group had at least one adverse event. Most adverse events appeared to be related to the underlying disease.

Other conditions

In a phase I clinical trial, 13 HIV positive patients and 5 healthy volunteers took 5 mg/kg andrographolide for 3 weeks, escalating to 10 mg/kg for 3 weeks, which was then intended to rise to 20 mg/kg for a final 3 weeks. However, the trial was interrupted at 6 weeks due to adverse events, including an anaphylactic reaction in one patient. All adverse events had resolved by the end of observation. A significant rise in the mean CD4+ lymphocyte level in HIV patients occurred after administration of 10 mg/kg andrographolide (from 405 to 501 cells/mm^3, p=0.002). There were no statistically significant changes in mean plasma HIV-1 RNA levels throughout the trial.[142]

An open study in Thailand compared parameters of urinary tract infection in patients undergoing shock wave dissolution of kidney stones (lithotripsy). The study found that 1 g of Andrographis was as effective as the antibiotics co-trimoxazole and norfloxacin in reducing pyuria and haematuria.[143]

A phase I clinical study of Kan Jang in healthy men revealed a slightly positive benefit on sperm count, sperm activity and other indices of fertility when it was taken at three times the normal dose.[144]

Sixty-three patients with cardiac and cerebrovascular diseases were observed at 3 h and/or 1 week after taking Andrographis extract. Results showed that platelet aggregation induced by ADP was significantly inhibited (p<0.001). The aggregation rate was lower at 1 week. In other volunteers taking Andrographis, serotonin release from platelets was decreased (p<0.01), but plasma serotonin levels remained unchanged. A rise in platelet cAMP levels might be the mechanism behind the antiplatelet activity of Andrographis.[145]

A majority of 20 patients with infective hepatitis showed marked improvement in symptoms after approximately 24 days of treatment with an Andrographis decoction (equivalent to 40 g of herb per day). Significant decreases in various liver function tests were also observed. Overall, 80% of cases were 'cured' and 20% were relieved.[146]

Toxicology and other safety data

Toxicology

The following LD$_{50}$ data have been recorded for Andrographis extract and its constituents:

Substance	Route, model	LD$_{50}$ value	Reference
Andrographis methanol-aqueous (1:1) extract of whole plant	ip, mice	>1.0 g/kg	147
Andrographis alcohol extract (part not specified)	oral, mice	>15 g/kg	148
Andrographis alcohol extract (part not specified)	ip, mice	14.98 g/kg	148
Andrographis alcohol extract (part not specified)	sc, mice	>15 g/kg	148
total lactones	oral, mice	13.4 g/kg	5
andrographolide	oral, mice	>40 g/kg	5
andrographolide sulphonate	iv, mice	2.47 to 2.94 g/kg	5
deoxyandrographolide	oral, mice	>20 g/kg	5
neoandrographolide	oral, mice	>20 g/kg	5

In acute toxicity studies, no toxic effects were observed in mice after oral administration of a suspension of Andrographis leaf powder (2 g/kg), a suspension of leaf alcohol extract (2.4 g/kg) or andrographolide (3 g/kg).[149] Similarly, subcutaneous administration of Andrographis leaf decoction (0.33 g/kg) to rabbits did not exhibit toxic effects.[19] Female rats treated for 14 days with an oral dose of 5 g/kg of a methanolic Andrographis extract also demonstrated no adverse effects.[150]

No toxic effects were observed in subacute oral toxicity tests when either a leaf powder suspension (200 and 400 mg/kg) or straight leaf powder (50 to 150 mg/kg) was administered on alternate days for 4 weeks to mice or for 14 weeks to rats, respectively.[149] Also andrographolide (1 g/kg/day) administered to rats and rabbits for 7 days did not cause toxic effects.[5] Rats administered Andrographis powder (part and route not specified) at dosages of 0.12, 1.2

and 2.4 g/kg/day for 6 months exhibited no abnormalities in growth rate, food consumption, clinical signs, serum biochemical parameters or histology.[148]

Oral administration of andrographolide (2 g/day) for 4 days caused a transient elevation of the liver enzyme ALT in healthy volunteers. Levels normalised upon discontinuation of the andrographolide. Hepatic and renal functions were not impaired after doses of 0.9 g/day for 5 days.[5]

Effects of Androgrphis on male fertility show conflicting results, but there is probably no cause for concern based on the more recent studies. Reduced fertility and prolongation of gestation were observed in mice when the male was fed Androgrphis stem powder (0.75% of diet) prior to mating. As mating rates were not confirmed, these effects may have been due to a reduction in libido. Treated females mated with untreated males showed no appreciable change in fertility or gestational period.[151] In contrast, antifertility effects were not observed in mice fed the powdered leaf or root (1% of diet; approximately 2 g/kg/day) for 2 weeks prior to mating and for 3 weeks during mating.[151,152]

Oral administration of Androgrphis leaf powder (50 and 100 mg/kg/day) for 24 to 60 days to male rats resulted in the cessation of spermatogenesis and biochemical and degenerative changes in the testes and male accessory organs.[153,154] Decreased sperm counts, spermatozoa abnormalities, histopathological changes in the testes and lack of fertility were observed after oral administration of high doses of andrographolide (25 and 50 mg/kg) for 48 days.[155] However, no significant differences were observed in reproductive organ weights, testicular histology or serum testosterone levels after oral administration of an Androgrphis dried herb (5:1) ethanol extract (containing 5.6% andrographolide) at dosages of 20, 200 and 1000 mg/kg/day for 60 days. The authors concluded that the above variation in results might be due to differences in the preparation of the plant material used.[156]

Recently Androgrphis extract (20, 200 and 1000 mg/kg/day orally for 65 days)[157] and andrographolide (50 mg/kg/day for 2 to 8 weeks)[158] demonstrated no significant effects on sperm morphology, motility and counts and were without significant adverse effects. There is also the phase I clinical study in men cited earlier.[144]

After nitrosation with nitrite under acidic conditions, an ethanol extract of Androgrphis became mutagenic to strains TA 98 and TA 100 (Salmonella/microsome test) tested either in the presence or absence of S-9 mix.[159] A methanolic extract of Androgrphis was devoid of significant genotoxic effects in three different in vitro models.[150]

Contraindications

Androgrphis should not be used during pregnancy without professional advice, especially in early pregnancy. Bitters are contraindicated in states of hyperacidity, especially duodenal ulcers. Bitters should be used with caution in oesophageal reflux.

Special warnings and precautions

Caution in early pregnancy.

Interactions

Antiplatelet activity was demonstrated ex vivo in the blood from patients with cardiac and cerebrovascular diseases taking Androgrphis extract.[145] This could possibly lead to an adverse interaction with antiplatelet and anticoagulant drugs. However, oral doses of Androgrphis with Siberian ginseng exhibited no interaction with warfarin in rats.[160]

Androgrphis should not be prescribed long-term with immunosuppressant medication as it may decrease the effectiveness of the drug. This is a theoretical concern based on the immune-enhancing activity of Androgrphis. No case report of such an interaction has been published.

There have been several studies examining the in vitro or in vivo impact of either Androgrphis extract or andrographolide on drug metabolising enzymes. However, the clinical relevance of these findings remains uncertain. In vitro, andrographolide induced the expression of cytochrome P450 superfamily 1 members CYP1A1 and CYP1A2, but not CYP1B1, in a concentration-dependent manner in murine hepatocytes.[161,162] In isolated human and rat liver microsomes Androgrphis extract and andrographolide inhibited CYP3A4 and 2C9 activity.[163] Androgrphis extracts and andrographolide significantly induced glutathione-S-transferase activity in rat primary hepatocytes.[164,165]

Of more relevance are the in vivo studies. An aqueous or an ethanolic extract of Androgrphis (equivalent to 5 mg/kg/day andrographolide orally for 14 to 30 days) induced CYP1A1 and CYP2B in mice.[166] Similar doses of Androgrphis extract and andrographolide given orally to rats decreased CYP2C11 activity.[167] Andrographolide (5 mg/kg/day, sc) enhanced CYP1A1 expression only in polycyclic aromatic hydrocarbon responsive mice, and only in males (probably via an interaction with testosterone).[168]

Theophylline is a typical substrate of CYP1A2 in rats. Oral Androgrphis extract (1 or 2 g/day) or andrographolide (154 mg/kg/day) pretreatment for 3 days in rats increased the clearance of subsequently administered theophylline, confirming results from in vitro studies.[169] The doses used were relatively high and do not reflect typical human doses.

Use in pregnancy and lactation

Category B3 – no increase in frequency of malformation or other harmful effects on the fetus from limited use in women. Evidence of increased fetal damage in animal studies exists, although the relevance to humans is unknown.

However, Androgrphis is best avoided during early pregnancy until more information is available regarding its antifertility activity. A product containing standardised extract of Androgrphis leaf has been used to treat the common cold in Scandinavia for over 20 years and no cases of pregnancy termination have been reported.[170] Results from experiments regarding possible antifertility effects in female animals are conflicting (see below).[151,152,170–173]

Oral administration of an Androgrphis extract (200, 600 and 2000 mg/kg) for the first 19 days of pregnancy did not impact progesterone levels in pregnant rats.[170] Female mice fed high doses of Androgrphis powder (2 g/kg/day) for

6 weeks failed to conceive when mated with males of proven fertility in a controlled experiment.[171] Intraperitoneal injection of Andrographis whole plant decoction prevented implantation in mice and caused abortion at different stages of gestation in mice and rabbits. The decoction also terminated early pregnancy when administered by oral, intravenous, subcutaneous, intramuscular and intrauterine routes in mice.[172] However, oral administration of Andrographis extract to rats at doses less than 2 g/kg during the first 9 days of pregnancy failed to interrupt pregnancy, induce fetal resorption or alter the number of live offspring.[173] Andrographis stem powder (0.75% of diet) had no appreciable effect on fertility when fed to female mice for up to 4 weeks prior to mating.[151] Antifertility effects were not observed in mice fed the powdered leaf or root (1% of diet; approximately 2 g/kg/day) for 2 weeks prior to mating and for 3 weeks during mating.[151,152]

No teratogenic or toxic effects were observed when a suspension of Andrographis leaf powder (200 and 400 mg/kg) was orally administered on alternate days for 4 weeks to mice in a controlled experiment.[149]

In vitro tests, which are of uncertain relevance to normal human use, have shown the following effects. Andrographis chloroform extract and andrographolide sodium succinate suppressed hormonal secretion and had a cytotoxic effect on cultured human placental chorionic trophoblastic tissue (aged between 6 to 8 weeks of pregnancy) in vitro.[174] Andrographis extract demonstrated uterine relaxant activity in vitro.[175]

There are no data available on the use of Andrographis during lactation.

Effects on ability to drive and use machines

No adverse effects expected.

Side effects

In general, Andrographis has been well tolerated in clinical trials. One of 90 patients receiving Andrographis extract reported unpleasant sensations in the chest and intensified headache,[131] and 2 of 50 patients reported urticaria,[135] in randomised, double blind, placebo-controlled trials investigating respiratory infections. Andrographis extract was administered

for 3 to 5 days at a dose of 1020 mg/day (containing 63 mg andrographolide and deoxyandrographolide).

A high incidence of adverse effects, including headache, fatigue, pruritus/rash, metallic/decreased taste and diarrhoea, was reported in a trial of pure andrographolide in HIV patients. One patient experienced an anaphylactic reaction.[142] The oral dose of andrographolide, 15 mg/kg/day for 3 weeks followed by 30 mg/kg/day for a further 3 weeks, was very high compared with normal therapeutic dosages of Andrographis extract. Cases of anaphylactic shock after injection of Andrographis extract have been reported in China.[5]

Overdosage

No incidents found in published literature. High doses may cause gastric discomfort, anorexia and vomiting.[5]

Safety in children

Adverse events were not reported in a randomised, double blind, placebo-controlled trial investigating the prevention of the common cold in which healthy children were orally administered Andrographis extract (200 mg/day), 5 days per week for 3 months.[129]

Regulatory status in selected countries

Andrographis is official in the *Pharmacopoeia of the People's Republic of China* (English Edition 1997). The usual adult dosage, usually administered in the form of a decoction, is listed as 6 to 9 g.

Andrographis is not on the UK General Sale List and is not covered by a Commission E monograph.

Andrographis does not have GRAS status. However, it is freely available as a 'dietary supplement' in the USA under DSHEA legislation (Dietary Supplement Health and Education Act of 1994).

Andrographis is not included in Part 4 of Schedule 4 of the Therapeutic Goods Act Regulations of Australia and is freely available for sale.

References

1. A Panel of Vaidyas. *Clinical Application of Ayurvedic Remedies*. Indian Medical Science Series No. 3, 4th ed. Delhi: Sri Satguru Publications; 1998. p. 100.
2. Kapoor LD. *CRC Handbook of Ayurvedic Medicinal Plants*. Boca Raton: CRC Press; 1990. p. 39.
3. Chopra RN, Chopra IC, Handa KL, et al. *Chopra's Indigenous Drugs of India*. Reprint, 2nd ed. Calcutta: Academic Publishers; 1982. p. 278.
4. Bensky D, Gamble A. *Chinese Herbal Medicine Materia Medica*. Seattle: Eastland Press; 1986. p. 136.

5. Chang H, But P. *Pharmacology and Applications of Chinese Materia Medica*, 2. Singapore: World Scientific; 1987. pp. 918–928.
6. Thakur RS, Puri HS, Husain A. *Major Medicinal Plants of India*. Central Institute of Medicinal and Aromatic Plants: Lucknow; 1989. p. 61.
7. Matsuda T, Kuroyanagi M, Sugiyama S, et al. *Chem Pharm Bull*. 1994;42(6):1216–1225.
8. Tang W, Eisenbrand G. *Chin Drugs of Plant Origin*. Berlin: Springer Verlag; 1992. pp. 97–103.

9. Zhu PY, Liu GQ. *Chin Trad Herb Drugs*. 1984;15:373–376.
10. Dua VK, Ojha VP, Roy R, et al. *J Ethnopharmacol*. 2004;95(2–3):247–251.
11. Regional Research Laboratory and Indian Drug Manufacturers' Association. *Indian Herbal Pharmacopoeia*. Jammu-Tawi: Indian Drug Manufacturers' Association, Mumbai and Regional Research Laboratory; 1998. pp. 18–29.
12. Lehmann R, Penman K. *Information on File*. St Lucia, Queensland, Australia: MediHerb Research Laboratory, University of Queensland; 2001.

13. Leelarasamee A, Trakulsomboon S, Sittisomwong N. *J Med Assoc Thai.* 1990;73(6):299–304.

14. Gupta S, Chaudhry MA, Yadava JNS. *Int J Crude Drug Res.* 1990;28(4):273–283.

15. Limsong J, Benjavongkulchai E, Kuvatanasuchati J. *J Ethnopharmacol.* 2004;92(2–3):281–289.

16. Wu CM, Cao JL, Zheng MH, et al. *J Int Med Res.* 2008;36(1):178–186.

17. Rattanachaikunsopon P, Phumkhachorn P. *J Biosci Bioeng.* 2009;107(5):579–582.

18. Raj RK. *Ind J Physiol Pharmacol.* 1975;19(1):47–49.

19. Dutta A, Sukul NC. *J Helminthol.* 1982;56(2):81–84.

20. Najib Nik ARN, Furuta T, Kojima S, et al. *J Ethnopharmacol.* 1999;64(3):249–254.

21. Siti Najila MJ, Noor Rain A, Mohamad Kamel AG, et al. *J Ethnopharmacol.* 2002;82(2–3):239–242.

22. Mishra K, Dash AP, Swain BK, et al. *Malar J.* 2009;8:26.

23. Chang RS, Ding L, Chen GQ, et al. *Proc Soc Exp Biol Med.* 1991;197(1):59–66.

24. Xu H, Wan M, Loh B, et al. *Phytother Res.* 1996;10:207–210.

25. Collins RA, Ng TB, Fong WP, et al. *Life Sci.* 1997;60(23):345–351.

26. Wiart C, Kumar K, Yusof MY, et al. *Phytother Res.* 2005;19(12):1069–1070.

27. Lin TP, Chen SY, Duh PD, et al. *Biol Pharm Bull.* 2008;31(11):2018–2023.

28. Chen JX, Xue HJ, Ye WC, et al. *Biol Pharm Bull.* 2009;32(8):1385–1391.

29. Puri A, Saxena R, Saxena RP, et al. *J Nat Prod.* 1993;56(7):995–999.

30. Martz W. *Toxicon.* 1992;30(10):1131–1142.

31. Iruretagoyena MI, Tobar JA, González PA, et al. *J Pharmacol Exp Ther.* 2005;312(1):366–372.

32. Carretta MD, Alarcón P, Jara E, et al. *Eur J Pharmacol.* 2009;602(2–3):413–421.

33. Burgos RA, Seguel K, Perez M, et al. *Planta Med.* 2005;71(5):429–434.

34. Wang W, Wang J, Dong SF, et al. *Acta Pharmacol Sin.* 2010;31(2):191–201.

35. Panossian A, Davtyan T, Gukassyan N, et al. *Phytomedicine.* 2002;9(7):598–605.

36. Xu Y, Chen A, Fry S, et al. *Int Immunopharmacol.* 2007;7(4):515–523.

37. Naik SR, Hole A. *Planta Med.* 2009;75(8):785–791.

38. Kumar RA, Sridevi K, Kumar NV, et al. *J Ethnopharmacol.* 2004;92(2–3):291–295.

39. Rajagopal S, Kumar RA, Deevi DS, et al. *J Exp Ther Oncol.* 2003;3(3):147–158.

40. Varma A, Padh H, Shrivastava N. *eCAM.* 2009;9.

41. Tan Y, Chiow KH, Huang D, et al. *Br J Pharmacol.* 2010;159(7):1497–1510.

42. Shen KK, Liu TY, Xu C, et al. *Yao Xue Xue Bao.* 2009;44(9):973–979.

43. Ji L, Shen K, Liu J, et al. *Redox Rep.* 2009;14(4):176–184.

44. Manikam SD, Stanslas J. *J Pharm Pharmacol.* 2009;61(1):69–78.

45. Geethangili M, Rao YK, Fang SH, et al. *Phytother Res.* 2008;22(10):1336–1341.

46. Pfisterer PH, Rollinger JM, Schyschka L, et al. *Planta Med.* 2010;76(15):1698–1700.

47. Zhou J, Ong CN, Hur GM, et al. *Biochem Pharmacol.* 2010;79(9):1242–1250.

48. Sheeja K, Guruvayoorappan C, Kuttan G. *Int Immunopharmacol.* 2007;7(2):211–221.

49. Zhao F, He EQ, Wang L, et al. *J Asian Nat Prod Res.* 2008;10(5–6):467–473.

50. Jiang CG, Li JB, Liu FR, et al. *Anticancer Res.* 2007;27(4B):2439–2447.

51. Lee YC, Lin HH, Hsu CH, et al. *Eur J Pharmacol.* 2010;632(1–3):23–32.

52. Shi MD, Lin HH, Chiang TA, et al. *Chem Biol Interact.* 2009;180(3):344–352.

53. Chao HP, Kuo CD, Chiu JH, et al. *Planta Med.* 2010;76(16):1827–1833.

54. Sheeja K, Kuttan G. *Immunopharmacol Immunotoxicol.* 2008;30(1):181–194.

55. Sheeja K, Kuttan G. *Immunopharmacol Immunotoxicol.* 2007;29(1):81–93.

56. Sheeja K, Kuttan G. *Integr Cancer Ther.* 2007;6(1):66–73.

57. Visen PK, Shukla B, Patnaik GK, et al. *J Ethnopharmacol.* 1993;40(2):131–136.

58. Kapil A, Koul IB. Hepatoprotective agents from Indian traditional plants. In: Pushpangadan P, ed. *Glimpses of Indian Ethnopharmacology (Proceedings of the First National Conference on Ethnopharmacology).* India: Tropical Botanic Garden and Research Institute; 1995. pp. 283–297.

59. Handa SS, Sharma A. *Indian J Med Res.* 1990;92:276–283.

60. Kapil A, Koul IB, Banerjee SK, et al. *Biochem Pharmacol.* 1993;46(1):182–185.

61. Handa SS, Sharma A. *Indian J Med Res.* 1990;92:284–292.

62. Singha PK, Roy S, Dey S. *J Ethnopharmacol.* 2007;111(1):13–21.

63. Choudhury BR, Poddar MK. *Methods Find Exp Clin Pharmacol.* 1984;6(9):481–485.

64. Choudhury BR, Poddar MK. *Methods Find Exp Clin Pharmacol.* 1983;5(10):727–730.

65. Trivedi NP, Rawal UM, Patel BP. *Integr Cancer Ther.* 2007;6(3):271–280.

66. Trivedi NP, Rawal UM, Patel BP. *Integr Cancer Ther.* 2009;8(2):177–189.

67. Chander R, Srivastava V, Tandon JS. *Int J Pharmacog.* 1995;33(2):135–138.

68. Choudhury BR, Haque SJ, Poddar MK. *Planta Med.* 1987;53(2):135–140.

69. Shukla B, Visen PKS, Patnaik GK, et al. *Planta Med.* 1992;58(2):146–149.

70. Tripathi GS, Tripathi YB. *Phytother Res.* 1991;5:176–178.

71. Chaudhuri SK. *Indian J Exp Biol.* 1978;16:830–832.

72. Zhao HY, Fang WY. *J Tongji Med Univ.* 1990;10(4):212–217.

73. Guo ZL, Zhao HY, Zheng XH. *J Tongji Med Univ.* 1994;14(1):49–51.

74. Woo AY, Waye MM, Tsui SK, et al. *J Pharmacol Exp Ther.* 2008;325(1):226–235.

75. Guo ZL, Zhao HY, Zheng XH. *J Tongji Med Univ.* 1995;15(4):205–208.

76. Wang DW, Zhao HY. *Chin Med J.* 1994;107(6):464–470.

77. Wang YJ, Wang JT, Fan QX, et al. *Cell Res.* 2007;17(11):933–941.

78. Zhang CY, Tan BK. *Clin Exp Pharmacol Physiol.* 1996;23(8):675–678.

79. Zhang CY, Tan BK. *J Ethnopharmacol.* 1997;56(2):97–101.

80. Yoopan N, Thisoda P, Rangkadilok N, et al. *Planta Med.* 2007;73(6):503–511.

81. Amroyan E, Gabrielian E, Panossian A, et al. *Phytomedicine.* 1999;6(1):27–31.

82. Burgos RA, Hidalgo MA, Monsalve J, et al. *Planta Med.* 2005;71(7):604–608.

83. Hidalgo MA, Romero A, Figueroa J, et al. *Br J Pharmacol.* 2005;144(5):680–686.

84. Madav S, Tandan SK, Lal J. *Fitoterapia.* 1996;67(5):452–458.

85. Habtemariam S. *Phytother Res.* 1998;12:37–40.

86. Shen YC, Chen CF, Chiou WF. *Br J Pharmacol.* 2002;135(2):399–406.

87. Sheeja K, Shihab PK, Kuttan G. *Immunopharmacol Immunotoxicol.* 2006;28(1):129–140.

88. Liu J, Wang ZT, Ji LL. *Am J Chin Med.* 2007;35(2):317–328.

89. Abu-Ghefreh AA, Canatan H, Ezeamuzie CI. *Int Immunopharmacol.* 2009;9(3):313–318.

90. Bao Z, Guan S, Cheng C, et al. *Am J Respir Crit Care Med.* 2009;179(8):657–665.

91. Li J, Luo L, Wang X, et al. *Cell Mol Immunol.* 2009;6(5):381–385.

92. Madav S, Tripathi HC. Tandan. *Ind J Pharm Sci.* 1995;57(3):121–125.

93. Lin FL, Wu SJ, Lee SC, et al. *Phytother Res.* 2009;23(7):958–964.

94. Sulaiman MR, Zakaria ZA, Abdul RA, et al. *Biol Res Nurs.* 2010;11(3):293–301.

95. Mandal SC, Dhara AK, Maiti BC. *Phytother Res.* 2001;15(3):253–256.

96. Borhanuddin M, Shamsuzzoha M, Hussain AH. *Bangladesh Med Res Counc Bull.* 1994;20(1):24–26.

97. Husen R, Pihie AH, Nallappan M. *J Ethnopharmacol.* 2004;95(2–3):205–208.

98. Reyes BA, Bautista ND, Tanquilut NC, et al. *J Ethnopharmacol.* 2006;105(1–2):196–200.

99. Zhang XF, Tan BK. *Clin Exp Pharmacol Physiol.* 2000;27(5–6):358–363.

100. Dandu AM, Inamdar NM. *Pak J Pharm Sci.* 2009;22(1):49–52.

101. Subramanian R, Asmawi MZ, Sadikun A. *Acta Biochim Pol.* 2008;55(2):391–398.

102. Yu BC, Hung CR, Chen WC, et al. *Planta Med.* 2003;69(12):1075–1079.

103. Choudhury BR, Poddar MK. *Methods Find Exp Clin Pharmacol.* 1985;7(12):617–621.

104. Singh P, Srivastava MM, Khemani LD. *Ups J Med Sci*. 2009;114(3):136–139.

105. Verma N, Vinayak M. *Mol Biol Rep*. 2008;35(4):535–540.

106. Das S, Gautam N, Dey SK, et al. *Appl Physiol Nutr Metab*. 2009;34(2): 124–135.

107. Das S, Neogy S, Gautam N, et al. *Toxicol In Vitro*. 2009;23(1):90–98.

108. Sheeja K, Kuttan G. *Asian Pac J Cancer Prev*. 2006;7(4):609–614.

109. Sheeja K, Kuttan G. *Integr Cancer Ther*. 2006;5(3):244–251.

110. Al-Bayaty FH, Abdulla MA, Hassan MI, et al. *Nat Prod Res*. 2011:1–7 [Epub ahead of print].

111. Zheng ZY, Wan YD, He GX. *Chin Trad Herb Drugs*. 1982;13:417–420.

112. Daodee S, Wangboonskul J, Jarukamjorn K, et al. *Pak J Biol Sci*. 2007;10(12): 2078–2085.

113. Ye L, Wang T, Tang L, et al. *J Pharm Sci*. 2011 [Epub ahead of print].

114. He X, Li J, Gao H, et al. *Chem Pharm Bull (Tokyo)*. 2003;51(5):586–589.

115. He X, Li J, Gao H, et al. *Drug Metab Dispos*. 2003;31(8):983–985.

116. Cui L, Qiu F, Wang N, Yao X. *Chem Pharm Bull (Tokyo)*. 2004;52(6): 772–775.

117. Cui L, Qiu F, Yao X. *Drug Metab Dispos*. 2005;33(4):555–562.

118. Xu L, Xiao DW, Lou S, et al. *J Chromatogr B Analyt Technol Biomed Life Sci*. 2009;877(5–6):502–506.

119. Akowuah GA, Zhari I, Mariam A, et al. *Food Chem Toxicol*. 2009;47(9): 2321–2326.

120. Chen L, Yu A, Zhuang X, et al. *Talanta*. 2007;74(1):146–152.

121. Panossian A, Hovhannisyan A, Mamikonyan G, et al. *Phytomedicine*. 2000;7(5):351–364.

122. Kligler B, Ulbricht C, Basch E, et al. *Explore (NY)*. 2006;2(1):25–29.

123. Coon JT, Ernst E. *Planta Med*. 2004;70(4):293–298.

124. Poolsup N, Suthisisang C, Prathanturarug S, et al. *J Clin Pharm Ther*. 2004;29(1):37–45.

125. Carr RR, Nahata MC. *Am J Health Syst Pharm*. 2006;63(1):33–39.

126. Pharmacology Department, Sichan, 1975. Cited in Melchior J, Palm S, Wikman G. *Phytomedicine* 1996/7;3(4):315–318.

127. Thamlikitkul V, Dechatiwongse T, Theerapong S, et al. *J Med Assoc Thai*. 1991;74(10):437–442.

128. Hancke J, Burgos R, Caceres D. *Phytother Res*. 1995;9:559–562.

129. Caceres DD, Hancke JL, Burgos RZ, et al. *Phytomedicine*. 1997;4(2):101–104.

130. Caceres DD, Hancke JL, Burgos RA, et al. *Phytomedicine*. 1999;6(4):217–223.

131. Melchior J, Palm S, Wikman G. *Phytomedicine*. 1996/7;3(4):315–318.

132. Saxena RC, Singh R, Kumar P, et al. *Phytomedicine*. 2010;17(3–4):178–185.

133. Kulichenko LL, Kireyeva LV, Malyshkina EN, et al. *J Herb Pharmacother*. 2003;3(1):77–93.

134. Spasov AA, Ostrovskij OV, Chernikov MV, et al. *Phytother Res*. 2004;18(1):47–53.

135. Melchior J, Spasov AA, Ostrovskij OV, et al. *Phytomedicine*. 2000;7(5):341–350.

136. Gabrielian ES, Shukarian AK, Goukasova GI, et al. *Phytomedicine*. 2002;9(7): 589–597.

137. Chaicharntipyuth C, Thanangkul P. The Eighth Conference, Thailand, Faculty of Pharmacy, Chulalongkorn University, 1989.

138. Amaryan G, Astvatsatryan V, Gabrielyan E, et al. *Phytomedicine*. 2003;10(4): 271–285.

139. Panossian A, Hambartsumyan M, Panosyan L, et al. *Nitric Oxide*. 2003;9(2):103–110.

140. Burgos RA, Hancke JL, Bertoglio JC, et al. *Clin Rheumatol*. 2009;28(8):931–946.

141. Tang T, Targan SR, Li ZS, et al. *Aliment Pharmacol Ther*. 2011;33(2):194–202.

142. Calabrese C, Berman SH, Babish JG, et al. *Phytother Res*. 2000;14(5):333–338.

143. Muangman V, Viseshsindh V, Ratana-Olarn K, et al. *J Med Assoc Thai*. 1995;78(6):310–313.

144. Mkrtchyan A, Panosyan V, Panossian A, et al. *Phytomedicine*. 2005;12(6–7):403–409.

145. Zhang YZ, Tang JZ, Zhang YJ. *Zhongguo Zhong Xi Yi Jie He Za Zhi*. 1994;14(1): 28–30, 24, 35.

146. Chaturvedi GN, Tomar GS, Tiwari SK, et al. *Ancient Sci Life*. 1982;2:208–215.

147. Nakannishi K, Sasaki SI, Kiang AK, et al. *Chem Pharm Bull*. 1965;13:822.

148. Sithisomwongse N, Pengchata J, Cheewapatana S, et al. *Thai J Pharm Sci*. 1989;14(2):109–117.

149. Dhammaupakorn P, Chaichantipyuth C. 8th Symposium, Thailand, Faculty of Pharmacy, Chulalongkorn University, 1989.

150. Chandrasekaran CV, Thiyagarajan P, Sundarajan K, et al. *Food Chem Toxicol*. 2009;47(8):1892–1902.

151. Shamsuzzoha M, Rahman MS, Ahmed MM. *Bangladesh Med Res Conc Bull*. 1979;5(1):14–18.

152. Shamsuzzoha M, Shamsur RM, Mohiuddin AM, et al. *Lancet*. 1978;2(8095):900.

153. Akbarsha MA, Manivannan B, Hamid KS, et al. *Indian J Exp Biol*. 1990;28(5): 421–426.

154. Akbarsha MA, Manivannan B. *Indian J Comp Animal Physiol*. 1993;11(2):103–108.

155. Akbarsha MA, Murugaian P. *Phytother Res*. 2000;14(6):432–435.

156. Burgos RA, Caballero EE, Sanchez NS, et al. *J Ethnopharmacol*. 1997;58(3): 219–224.

157. Allan JJ, Pore MP, Deepak M, et al. *Int J Toxicol*. 2009;28(4):308–317.

158. Sattayasai J, Srisuwan S, Arkaravichien T, et al. *Food Chem Toxicol*. 2010;48(7):1934–1938.

159. Ieamworapong C, Kangsadalumpai K, Rojanapo W. *Environ Mol Mutagen*. 1989;14(suppl 15):93.

160. Hovhannisyan AS, Abrahamyan H, Gabrielyan ES, et al. *Phytomedicine*. 2006;13(5):318–323.

161. Jaruchotikamol A, Jarukamjorn K, Sirisangtrakul W, et al. *Toxicol Appl Pharmacol*. 2007;224(2):156–162.

162. Chatuphonprasert W, Jarukamjorn K, Kondo S, et al. *Chem Biol Interact*. 2009;182(2–3):233–238.

163. Pekthong D, Martin H, Abadie C, et al. *J Ethnopharmacol*. 2008;115(3):432–440.

164. Chang KT, Lii CK, Tsai CW, et al. *Food Chem Toxicol*. 2008;46(3):1079–1088.

165. Yang AJ, Li CC, Lu CY, et al. *J Agric Food Chem*. 2010;58(3):1993–2000.

166. Jarukamjorn K, Don-in K, Makejaruskul C, et al. *J Ethnopharmacol*. 2006;105(3): 464–467.

167. Pekthong D, Blanchard N, Abadie C, et al. *Chem Biol Interact*. 2009;179(2–3): 247–255.

168. Jarukamjorn K, Kondo S, Chatuphonprasert W, et al. *Eur J Pharm Sci*. 2010;39(5):394–401.

169. Chien CF, Wu YT, Lee WC, et al. *Chem Biol Interact*. 2010;184(3):458–465.

170. Panossian A, Kochikian A, Gabrielian E, et al. *Phytomedicine*. 1999;6(3):157–162.

171. Zoha MS, Hussain AH, Choudhury SA. *Bangladesh Med Res Counc Bull*. 1989;15(1):34–37.

172. But PPH. *Abstr Chin Med*. 1988;2(2): 247–269.

173. Hancke J. 1997. Cited in Panossian A, Kochikian A, Gabrielian E et al. *Phytomedicine* 1999;6(3):157–162.

174. Zhang X, Zhuang L, Li S, et al. *Acta Zool Sin*. 1985;31(1):52–58.

175. Burgos RA, Aguila MJ, Santiesteban ET, et al. *Phytother Res*. 2001;15(3): 235–239.

Arnica flowers

(*Arnica montana* L.)

Synonyms

Leopard's or wolf's bane, Mountain tobacco (Engl), Arnicae flos (Lat), Arnikablüten, Berwohlverleih (Ger), Fleurs d'arnica (Fr), Polmonaria di montagna (Ital), Guldblomme (Dan).

What is it?

Arnica flowers have been traditionally used for the external treatment of sprains and bruises, typically as the tincture. Homeopathic preparations are also used internally and externally, but are not covered in this monograph. A macerated oil from Arnica flowers known as 'Arnica oil' can be applied topically as well. The attractive bright yellow flowers of Arnica are native to the mountain pastures in central Europe. The plant is pleasantly aromatic. *Arnica montana* is a protected species in Germany and its declining occurrence in Europe may be related to soil quality. For this reason, another closely related species (*A. chamissonis* ssp. *foliosa*) is also used there. Products adulterated with Mexican Arnica (*Heterotheca inuloides*), a common substitute, should be avoided.

Effects

Arnica stimulates the peripheral blood supply and has anti-inflammatory activity in external use for bruising, sprains, swellings, muscle pain, symptoms of varicose veins and haemorrhoids.

Traditional view

Traditionally Arnica has been a popular remedy used externally for sprains, bruises, painful swellings, injuries and wounds. However, topical application was avoided in cases of tender or broken skin. It was often applied diluted and the surface deliberately not covered with bandages. Arnica was also used internally as a stimulant and diuretic, but to a much lesser extent due to its allergenic and irritant effects.[1-3]

Summary actions

Anti-inflammatory, anti-ecchymotic (against bruises), analgesic, antiseptic.

Can be used for

Indications supported by clinical trials

Topically for chronic venous insufficiency, muscle ache and osteoarthritis.

Traditional therapeutic uses

Externally for bruises, sprains, swellings, unbroken chilblains, haematomas, inflammation, dislocations, oedema associated with fractures; haemorrhoids; rheumatic, muscle and joint complaints; inflamed insect bites; surface phlebitis and symptoms of varicose veins.[2,3]

May also be used for

Extrapolations from pharmacological studies

Topical use for antimicrobial activity, although the effect is likely to be mild.

Other applications

External use for alopecia neurotica,[4] in hair preparations to prevent dandruff and to stimulate circulation in the scalp.[5]

Preparations

To prepare a poultice, 2 to 3 g of Arnica flowers are covered with approximately 150 mL of hot water and strained after 10 minutes. Bandages, gauze or cotton is soaked in the infusion and then placed on the affected area of the body.

'Arnica oil' is obtained by macerating 1 part Arnica flowers in 5 parts vegetable oil.

Arnica tincture (1:5, 45% ethanol) is also used topically as a lotion or incorporated into creams or ointments. Recently a supercritical carbon dioxide extract with a high sesquiterpene lactone content has been introduced to the market.[6]

Dosage

Lotion: dilute a 1:5 tincture five times with water. Apply two to three times per day.

Ointment typically contains 10% to 25% tincture or about 15% 'Arnica oil'. Apply two to three times per day.

Duration of use

Not for prolonged application.

Summary assessment of safety

Arnica is potentially toxic if taken internally. Contact dermatitis can occur, but is probably relatively rare. Arnica preparations should not be applied to open wounds or near the eyes and mouth.

Technical data

Botany

Arnica, a member of the Compositae or Asteraceae (daisy) family, is a perennial herb with a horizontally growing rhizome. It grows to 30 to 60 cm, the lower leaves are up to 17 cm long, elliptical in shape, 5-veined and form a rosette at the base of the stem. The flower heads number 1 to 3, and are up to 8 cm wide. They consist of peripheral, ligulate flowers, which are yellow-orange and central flowers which are tubular.[7,8]

Adulteration

Since *Arnica montana* is a protected species in many countries, it is liable to adulteration with various yellow flowering Compositae plants.[2,9–11] Arnica flower does not contain rutin and can therefore be easily distinguished from the most commonly occurring adulterant *Heterotheca inuloides* (Mexican Arnica).[9,10] In addition to this species, the *European Pharmacopoeia* regards *Calendula officinalis* as an adulterant.

Shortage of *A. montana* has led to a more widespread use of related species including *A. chamissonis, A. alpina, A. cordifolia, A. sororia, A. fulgens, A. longifolia* and *A. sachalinensis*. The latter three are particularly used for tinctures.[12,13] However, only *A. montana* is listed as official in the *British Herbal Pharmacopoeia, British Pharmacopoeia* and *European Pharmacopoeia*.[4,14,15] *A. chamissonis* subsp. *foliosa* is accepted by the German Commission E.[16]

Key constituents

- Sesquiterpene lactones (SLs) of the pseudoguaianolide type (0.2% to 1.5%), including helenalin and 11alpha, 13-dihydrohelenalin and their ester derivatives[17,18]
- Triterpenes, including arnidiol[19]
- Flavonoids (0.4% to 0.6%)[17] including quercitin 3-O-glucuronic acid[20]
- Lignans including pinoresinol[21]

- Coumarins, carotenoids[10]
- Non-toxic pyrrolizidine alkaloids (tussilagine and isotussilagine)[22]
- Polyacetylenes[19]
- Essential oil (0.23% to 0.35%) containing sesquiterpenes, thymol derivatives and other monoterpenes[19]
- Caffeoylquinic acids (phenolic acids) including 3,5- and 1,5-dicaffeoylquinic acids.[23]

One study found that the mean total SL levels were higher in the disk florets of Arnica (0.87%) than in the ray florets (0.71%), lower in the flower receptacles (0.35%) and lowest in the stems (0.03%).[24] The total SL content increased progressively as the flowers matured, from 0.51% in buds to 0.94% in withered flowers. An investigation of the SL content of Arnica tincture stored for 3 years at 4, 25 and 30°C found a decrease in content of 13%, 32% and 37% respectively.[25]

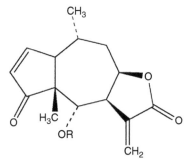

Helenalin (R = H) and its ester derivatives (R = acyl)

Pharmacodynamics

Arnica and its key constituents have demonstrated a range of pharmacological activities in experimental models. However, it should be noted that some of the effects below would be mainly relevant to the ingestion of the herb, which is not recommended. Most relevant to the topical use of Arnica are the anti-inflammatory and antimicrobial activities.

Anti-inflammatory and immune regulatory activity

Like parthenolide from feverfew, helenalin and certain other SLs in Arnica exert potent anti-inflammatory activity in vitro by inhibiting the activation of the transcription factor nuclear factor (NF)-kappaB. This was first demonstrated in 1997 and found to be quite selective, as the activity of four other transcription factors was not affected.[26] Follow-up research indicated that helenalin acts by selectively alkylating the p65 subunit of NF-kappaB, rather than by inhibiting the degradation of IkappaB.[27] (NF-kappaB, composed of a p50 and a p65 subunit, is retained in an inactive cytoplasmic complex by binding to a third (inhibitory) subunit IkappaB. Degradation of IkappaB results in its activation.)

Inhibition of NF-kappaB has also been demonstrated in vitro for various extracts of *Arnica* species, including Arnica tincture.[28–30] Consistent with inhibition of NF-kappaB activation, an Arnica extract inhibited nitric oxide production and cyclooxygenase (COX)-2 activity in activated murine macrophages.[31]

Other related anti-inflammatory activity has been found for the SLs in Arnica. The transcription factor nuclear factor of activated T cells (NFAT) is also inhibited in vitro by Arnica extract.[30] Suppression of matrix metalloproteinase (MMP)-1 and MMP-13 mRNA levels in bovine and human articular chondrocytes was also observed.[32] This latter effect may be due to inhibition of activation of the transcription factors activator protein (AP)-1 and NF-kappaB, and implies possible activity in osteoarthritis.

Arnica SLs have also demonstrated additional anti-inflammatory mechanisms in vitro. Two derivatives of 11alpha, 13-dihydrohelenalin inhibited the stimulated release of the pro-inflammatory enzyme neutrophil elastase from human neutrophils.[33] Helenalin provoked irreversible inhibition of leukotriene C4 (LTC4) synthase in human platelets and inhibited both 5-lipoxygenase and LTC4 synthase in human granulocytes.[34] Polymorphonuclear neutrophil chemotaxis was inhibited at low concentrations, whereas prostaglandin synthetase activity was inhibited at a higher concentration by a series of sesquiterpene lactones, including helenalin and dihydrohelenalin.[35]

Helenalin also appears to modulate immune activity in vitro. It induced apoptosis in activated CD4+ T cells by triggering the mitochondrial pathway of apoptosis, or otherwise inhibiting their proliferation.[36] As previously demonstrated, activation of NFAT (specifically NFATc2) was also found.

Additional results from in vitro studies suggest that the mechanism of the anti-inflammatory activity of Arnica and its constituents also possibly occurs at several other sites:[35]

* Uncoupling of oxidative phosphorylation in polymorphonuclear neutrophils
* Elevation of cAMP in neutrophils and liver cells
* Inhibition of lysosomal enzymatic activity in neutrophils and liver cells.

Several sesquiterpene lactones, including those from Arnica, have demonstrated anti-inflammatory activity by intraperitoneal injection (2.5 mg/kg/day) in animal models such as carrageenan-induced paw oedema and chronic adjuvant arthritis. The alpha-methylene-gamma-lactone structure was required for inhibitory activity in both models and the 6-hydroxy group of helenalin was required for potency in the former model. Inhibition of writhing reflex (an indication of analgesic activity) was also demonstrated.[37]

Topical Arnica was shown to be an effective anti-inflammatory in a rat model of acute muscle damage.[38] The Arnica gel (containing 200 mg/g of an unspecified Arnica tincture) was either applied by massage or ultrasound, with the latter failing to exert an anti-inflammatory effect above the control group.

Antimicrobial activity

Components of the essential oil of Arnica have demonstrated potent activity against Gram-positive and Gram-negative bacteria and against *Candida spp.* in vitro.[39] Helenalin and helenalin acetate were also active in vitro against Gram-positive bacteria and *Proteus vulgaris*.[40] The polyacetylenes have shown broad-range antimicrobial activity against pathogenic fungi (*Trichophyton spp., Microsporum gypseum,*

Epidermophyton spp.) and bacteria (*Staphylococcus aureus, Pseudomonas aeruginosa, Escherichia coli*) in vitro.[41] However, compared with propolis, an Arnica extract showed little antibacterial activity against oral pathogens.[42] Some modest activity for Arnica was demonstrated against periodontal bacteria.[43] SLs including helenalin were also quite active against *Leishmania mexicana* with IC50 values of 2 to 4 μM.[44]

Helenalin and related sesquiterpene lactones have antitrypanosomal activity (with an IC50 as low as 0.05 μM for helenalin)[45] and the pseudoguaianolide SLs show high activity against asexual blood forms of *Plasmodium falciparum*.[46]

Staph. aureus is a major udder pathogen causing bovine mastitis. Some pro-inflammatory cytokines, including tumour necrosis factor (TNF)-alpha, enhance its growth. Helenalin markedly reduced the growth of *Staph. aureus* in the presence of TNF-alpha in bovine mammary epithelial cells.[47] Helenalin also reduced *Staph. aureus* infection and associated inflammation in a murine model of mastitis following ip administration (20 mg/kg).

Antitumour activity

Like parthenolide from feverfew, helenalin has exhibited antitumour activity in vitro, although it has been less extensively studied. In a screening of 21 flavonoids and five SLs from *Arnica* species, helenalin demonstrated the strongest cytotoxic activity of the SLs when tested on lung carcinoma cells. The flavonoids showed moderate to low cytotoxicity compared with the reference compound.[48]

Helenalin strongly induced apoptosis in leukaemia Jurkat T cells,[49] even if they lacked the CD95 death receptor or over-expressed antiapoptotic proteins.[50] It probably acts by inducing a mitochondria-dependent pathway. The cytotoxicity of helenalin against KB tumour cells was decreased by cysteine, but the cytotoxicity of 11alpha,13-dihydrohelenalin was not affected.[51]

The effect of flavones and flavonols from *Arnica spp.* on the cytotoxicity of helenalin was investigated in the human lung carcinoma cell line. At non-toxic concentrations, all flavonoids (except kaempferol) significantly reduced helenalin-induced cytotoxicity.[52]

Arnica SLs inhibited Walker 26 carcinosarcoma and Ehrlich ascites tumour growth in vivo (2.5 mg/kg day for rats and 25 mg/kg/day for mice, both ip).[53]

Other activity

The stabilisation of the lysosomal membrane in liver cells by SLs was dependent on the alpha-methylene-gamma-lactone structure.[35]

Helenalin and 11alpha,13-dihydrohelenalin in vitro have inhibited human platelet function via thiol-dependent pathways. The reduction in platelet sulphydryl groups is probably associated with reduced phospholipase A_2 activity.[54]

Helenalin, dihydrohelenalin and epoxyhelenalin (20 mg/kg/day in mice) produced a lowering of serum cholesterol (30%) and serum triglycerides (25%). Thiol-bearing enzymes of lipid synthesis were inhibited by these compounds in vitro, suggesting they alkylate thiol nucleophiles by a Michael-type addition.[55]

Pharmacokinetics

In vitro studies using pig skin stratum corneum investigated the penetration kinetics of different preparations of Arnica. It was observed that SLs penetrate the skin in amounts sufficient to confer an anti-inflammatory effect.[56] SLs in tinctures penetrated better than isolated SLs. A later study by the same group using a similar model suggested that the degree of total penetration depended more on the type of the formulation (ointment being superior to gel) and its SL content, rather than the SL composition or extraction method used.[57]

Oleic acid and dimethylsulphoxide acted as skin permeation enhancers of SLs from a supercritical carbon dioxide extract of Arnica, as assessed using human stratum corneum and epidermis as an in vitro membrane.[58] Using a similar model, 11,13-dihydrohelenalin derivatives were found to exhibit the most permeation from an Arnica tincture.[59] A study using an in vitro pig skin membrane observed that a micro-emulsion was a good vehicle for the permeation of helenalin.[60]

Clinical trials

A 6-week, open, multicentre trial involving 26 men and 53 women with mild to moderate osteoarthritis of the knee concluded that an Arnica gel (containing 50g/100g of a 1:20 fresh plant tincture) applied mornings and evenings was an effective treatment, as assessed using the WOMAC scale.[61] The overall local adverse event rate of 7.6% included only one allergic reaction.

In a randomised, double blind study over 3 weeks, 204 patients with active osteoarthritis of interphalangeal joints of hands were treated topically with gel preparations of either ibuprofen (5%) or Arnica (50g/100g of 1:20 fresh plant tincture). There were no differences between the two groups in terms of pain and hand function improvements, or for any secondary endpoints evaluated. Adverse events reports were comparable and rare.[62] The study was planned and performed according to strict international guidelines for studies of multiple sites of osteoarthritis of the fingers: OARSI (Osteoarthritis Research Society International), EMEA (European Agency for the Evaluation of Medicinal Products) guidelines for controlled studies and their statistical evaluation as well as according to good clinical practice rules. This was the very first herbal study looking at this condition to be performed according to these strict guidelines.

A double blind, randomised, controlled trial was conducted in healthy volunteers with laser-induced bruises who were given either a 20% Arnica ointment, a 5% vitamin K preparation, a 1% vitamin K/0.3% retinol mix or white petrolatum (as a placebo) twice a day under occlusion for 2 weeks. Independent assessments of bruise resolution observed that the Arnica ointment was comparable to vitamin K and significantly more effective than the petrolatum (p=0.003) or vitamin K/retinol mix (p=0.01).[63]

In a double blind study, 570 patients with acute ankle joint distortion were randomised to four treatment groups: Arnica tincture (diluted 10g tincture/100mL solution), hydroxyethyl salicylate (HES, 3%), their combination, and a placebo.[64] The medication was applied four to five times daily (0.5mL each time) as a spray. Efficacy was assessed on days 3 to 4 by evaluating pain on motion using a visual analogue scale (VAS). The base preparation for all four treatments contained essential oils and camphor, ensuring that the different study preparations were not discernible by their organoleptic properties. Pain improvement for the combination was highly significant compared with all other groups, and approximately corresponded to the cumulative effect of the single constituents. According to the VAS assessment, the Arnica tincture contributed about one-third to the treatment effect of the combination. Interestingly, no adverse local reaction occurred in the group using the Arnica spray (unlike any other treatment group). The same research group conducted an earlier preliminary clinical study that demonstrated an additive analgesic effect of Arnica and HES. This was a single blind trial involving healthy volunteers following the creation of pain by transcutaneous electrostimulation.[65]

A placebo-controlled, double blind, randomised clinical study involving 89 patients with pronounced symptoms of chronic venous insufficiency tested the efficacy of an Arnica gel (containing 20% Arnica tincture). After 3 weeks, the symptom of feeling heaviness in the legs (which is strongly associated with peripheral oedema), together with objective measurements of oedema and venous tone, were assessed. The 'heavy leg' feeling improved significantly more in the Arnica group compared with placebo. In addition, venous tone and oedema were improved. This efficacy of Arnica for the treatment of symptoms associated with varicose veins is believed to be due to a protective effect against oedema.[66]

Twelve male volunteers externally applied preparations for muscle ache. Arnica gel was more effective than placebo gel.[67]

A randomised, double blinded, placebo-controlled study showed no difference between an Arnica gel and its vehicle on post laser treatment burns, with 19 patients acting as their own controls.[68]

Toxicology and other safety issues

Toxicology

The following LD_{50} data have been recorded for Arnica extract and its constituents:

Substance	Route, model	LD_{50} value	Reference
A. montana extract	oral, mice	123 mg/kg	69
A. montana extract	oral, rats	>5 g/kg	69
A. montana extract	ip, mice	31 mg/kg	69

Substance	Route, model	LD$_{50}$ value	Reference
Sesquiterpene lactone enriched extract of *A. Montana*	ip, mice	280 mg/kg	11
helenalin	oral, mice	150 mg/kg	70
helenalin	oral, rats	125 mg/kg	70
helenalin	oral, hamsters	85 mg/kg	70
helenalin	oral, rabbits	90 mg/kg	70
helenalin	oral, sheep	100 to 125 mg/kg	70
helenalin	ip, mice	43 mg/kg	71
helenalin	ip, mice	9.86 mg/kg	72

An aqueous-ethanolic extract of Arnica did not demonstrate irritating, sensitising or phototoxic activity after topical application to the skin of rabbits or guinea pigs. Minimal irritant activity was observed when the 50% extract was instilled in the eyes of rabbits.[69] In contrast, a short chain ether extract of Arnica demonstrated strong dermal sensitising activity in guinea pigs.[73]

Arnica absolute is an alcohol extract of Arnica concrete, which is obtained from the fresh flowers by an organic solvent extraction process. Arnica absolute (5% to 100%) induced slight patchy to moderate erythema in guinea pigs upon topical application. However, 75% absolute was neither irritating nor phototoxic to the skin of mice. Also, 4% absolute was neither irritating nor sensitising to human volunteers in a maximisation study. The absolute did not induce dermal sensitisation in guinea pigs.[69]

Arnica tincture was weakly mutagenic in the Ames test in vitro. The mutagenic activity was thought to be due to the flavonoid content and was found to vary, depending on plant origin and method of preparation.[74] Helenalin was inactive in this test.[75]

In male mice, a single injection of helenalin (25 mg/kg) increased serum alanine aminotransferase, lactate dehydrogenase, urea nitrogen and sorbitol dehydrogenase within 6 h. Intraperitoneal injection of helenalin (25 mg/kg/day) increased differential polymorphonuclear leukocyte counts and decreased lymphocyte counts and liver, thymus and spleen weights. Histological evaluation revealed substantial effects on lymphocytes in the thymus, spleen and mesenteric lymph nodes. Multiple helenalin exposure (25 mg/kg/day) also inhibited hepatic microsomal enzyme activities and decreased cytochrome P450 and cytochrome B5 contents.[71] Helenalin and helenalin acetate demonstrated dermal sensitising activity in guinea pigs at concentrations of 0.1% to 1.0%.[76]

The activity of helenalin has been attributed to its ability to alkylate sulphydryl groups.[19] In vitro and in vivo studies suggest that the cytotoxicity of helenalin is strongly dependent on hepatic glutathione levels, which can be rapidly depleted by even low concentrations of helenalin.[77,78] Helenalin demonstrated chromosome-damaging activity in vitro in Chinese hamster ovarian cells.[11] The relevance of this result to the in vivo activity of Arnica has not been established.

A recent review on the safety of *Arnica montana* and its extract concluded that there are insufficient data to support their safe use in cosmetic formulations.[69]

Contraindications

Not to be taken internally. Do not apply to broken skin or near the eyes or mouth. Withdraw use on the first sign of dermatitis. Contraindicated in those with known allergy to Arnica.

Special warnings and precautions

Not for prolonged external application. Individuals with known sensitivity to other members of the Asteraceae family (such as ragweed, daisies and chrysanthemums), or to plants from other families with SLs, chemically related to Arnica (such as the Lauraceae), should use Arnica cautiously.[79]

Interactions

None currently known.

Use in pregnancy and lactation

Category X – high risk of damage to the fetus when taken internally. No adverse effects are expected with topical use.

Miscarriage has been reported after overdose of ingested Arnica tincture or infusion[11,80] (see Overdosage). Constituents of Arnica have been shown to increase uterine tone and contraction, but Arnica tincture has not demonstrated these actions. Arnifolin (1 to 5 mg/kg) increased the tone and strengthened periodical contractions of the rabbit uterus in situ and 6-O-acetyl-11,13-dihydrohelenalin contracted isolated rat uterus.[11,81] Arnica tincture did not increase tone or contraction of isolated pregnant rabbit uteri.[11] Similar negative results were demonstrated in the cat after intravenous administration of 0.3 mL of fresh Arnica extract.[82]

Internal use of Arnica is contraindicated in breastfeeding. Do not apply near the nipple.

Effects on ability to drive and use machines

No adverse effects expected for topical use.

Side effects

Cases of allergic or irritant contact dermatitis caused by topical application of Arnica were first reported in 1844.[83]

A review of the literature up to 1980 found more than 100 cases of contact dermatitis due to sensitisation with Arnica. Most cases were induced by self-treatment with Arnica tincture.[13] Reactions have also been reported after the use of other Arnica preparations, including ointments, creams, soaps, lotions and shampoos.[79] Arnica ointments and plasters are considered to pose a much lower risk of reaction than other types of applications.[12,84] Several case reports of allergic contact dermatitis from the topical use of Arnica, proven by patch testing, have been published since the 1980 review.[85–87]

Arnica-sensitive individuals are known to cross-react with other Compositae and Lauraceae species.[79] SL and epoxy-thymol-diester constituents of the plant have been proven to be both sensitising agents and to act as allergens.[13,88] It is likely that other constituents of Arnica also contribute to the acquired hypersensitivity.[89] SL-sensitive individuals tend to develop cross-reactions to chemically related SLs in other species.[90] The presence of an alpha-methylene-gamma-lactone group has been shown to be important for cross-reactivity between SLs.[12]

A 1992 review reported that Arnica contact allergy was recognised in 11% to 75% of patients at dermatology clinics.[79] However, several studies published since this review have reported much lower percentages, only up to 1.14%.[84,89,91,92] Further to this, a survey of 38 physicians provided data for 18830 patients who received 42378 Asteraceae-containing products.[93] Adverse reactions to the topical use of Arnica were rare and not serious.

A relatively recent study investigated eight patients with a recent history of Arnica allergy.[94] Although all eight had previously exhibited a positive reaction to an Arnica test preparation, this could only be reproduced in five. Moreover, the majority of the patients were not sensitive to Arnica SLs. This demonstrates that the issues governing contact sensitivity to Arnica are complex. One experimental study suggested that the anti-inflammatory and immune modulating properties of Arnica SLs (see above under Pharmacodynamics) reduce their potential for contact sensitisation.[95] As examples of this, contact hypersensitivity to Arnica could not be induced in a standard murine model and Arnica tinctures suppressed contact hypersensitivity to the strong sensitiser trinitrochlorobenzene.[95]

The Commission E advises that prolonged treatment of damaged skin with Arnica can cause oedematous dermatitis with the formation of pustules. Extended use may cause eczema. In treatment involving higher concentrations, primary toxic skin reactions with the formation of vesicles or even necrosis may occur.[16] Extensive oral mucosal ulceration was reported in a 48-year-old woman who misused a mouthwash containing 70% ethanol, Arnica tincture and oil of peppermint.[96] The preparation should be diluted five times with water, but was instead used neat.

A case of leukaemia-related Sweet's syndrome, reportedly triggered by topical application of a cream containing 1.5% Arnica, has been published. Pathergy (skin hyper-reactivity) to Arnica was suspected.[97]

Overdosage

The symptoms of overdose after oral ingestion of Arnica include nausea, vomiting, diarrhoea, dizziness, trembling, increased heart rate, cardiac rhythm disturbances, difficulty with breathing and collapse.[98] Arnica poisoning has been observed to cause death due to circulatory paralysis with secondary respiratory arrest.[98]

A 19-year-old male mistakenly consumed an unknown amount of tea made from the leaves and flowers of Arnica. Two hours later he experienced myalgia, headache and shaking chills. He developed hyperthermia, tachycardia, hypotension and raised serum levels of creatinine, aspartate aminotransferase and alanine aminotransferase. After treatment with fluid and dopamine, he was discharged 6 days later when his symptoms had improved.[99] A man experienced stomach cramping and died within 36h of consuming 70g of Arnica tincture.[11]

Miscarriage has been reported after overdose with ingested Arnica tincture or infusion.[11,80] A woman in the second month of pregnancy miscarried after a few days when she ingested an infusion of 20g Arnica flower. Ingestion of three tablespoons of a self-prepared tincture of Arnica flowers led to miscarriage within 24h.[11] Multisystem failure has been reported following the ingestion of Arnica with abortive intent.[100]

Safety in children

For topical use only.

Regulatory status in selected countries

Atrogel, an external application, has a Traditional Herbal Medicinal Product Registration in the UK with the following claims: 'traditionally used for the symptomatic relief of muscular aches and pains, stiffness, sprains, bruises and swelling after contusions'.

Arnica is official in the European Pharmacopoeia (2011).

Arnica for external use is covered by a positive Commission E monograph and has the following applications: injuries and accidents, for example for haematomas, dislocations, sprains, bruising, oedema associated with fractures, in rheumatic muscle and joint complaints, inflammation of the mucous membranes of the mouth and throat, furuncles, inflamed insect bites and surface phlebitis.

Arnica does not have GRAS status. It is available as a 'dietary supplement' in the USA under DSHEA legislation (1994 Dietary Supplement Health and Education Act). However, topical preparations are not technically covered by the DSHEA legislation.

Arnica for internal use is included in Part 4 of Schedule 4 of the Therapeutic Goods Act Regulations of Australia and hence is restricted, except for homeopathic products. External use of Arnica is unrestricted, provided products with a therapeutic claim are listed with the Therapeutic Goods Administration.

References

1. Grieve M. *A Modern Herbal*, Vol 1. New York: Dover Publications; 1971. p. 55.
2. Felter HW, Lloyd JU. *King's American Dispensatory*, 18th ed, rev 3, vol 1, 1905. Reprinted Portland: Eclectic Medical Publications; 1983. pp. 278–281.
3. Felter H. *The Eclectic Materia Medica, Pharmacology and Therapeutics*, 1922. Reprinted Portland: Eclectic Medical Publications; 1983. pp. 206–207.
4. British Herbal Medicine Association's Scientific Committee. *British Herbal Pharmacopoeia*. West York: BHMA; 1983. pp. 30–31.
5. Sanderson L. *How to Make Your Own Herbal Cosmetics*. New Canaan: Keats Publishing Inc; 1977. p. 51.
6. Bilia AR, Mc Bergonzi, Mazzi G, et al. *J Pharm Biomed Anal*. 2006;41(2):449–454.
7. Chiej R. *The Macdonald Encyclopedia of Medicinal Plants*. London: Macdonald; 1984. Entry No. 40.
8. Launert EL. *The Hamlyn Guide to Edible and Medicinal Plants of Britain and Northern Europe*. London: Hamlyn Publishing; 1981. p. 210.
9. Wagner H, Bladt S. *Plant Drug Analysis: A Thin Layer Chromatography Atlas*, 2nd ed. Berlin: Springer-Verlag; 1996. pp. 197, 214–215.
10. Bisset NG, ed. *Herbal Drugs and Phytopharmaceuticals*. (Wichtl, M. (ed), German edition). Stuttgart: Medpharm Scientific Publishers; 1994. pp. 83–87.
11. Blaschek W, Ebel S, Hackenthal E, et al. *HagerROM 2002: Hagers Handbuch der Drogen und Arzneistoffe*. Heidelberg: Springer; 2002.
12. Hausen BM, Herrmann HD, Willuhn G. *Contact Dermatitis*. 1978;4(1):3–10.
13. Hausen BM. *Hautarzt*. 1980;31(1):10–17.
14. *British Pharmacopoeia* 2002. CD–ROM. Crown Copyright, 2002.
15. *European Pharmacopoeia*, 4th ed. Strasbourg: Council of Europe; 2002;(suppl 4.3):672–674.
16. Blumenthal M, ed. *The Complete German Commission E Monographs: Therapeutic Guide to Herbal Medicines*. Austin: American Botanical Council; 1998. pp. 83–84.
17. Wagner H, Bladt S. *Plant Drug Analysis: A Thin Layer Chromatography Atlas*, 2nd ed. Berlin: Springer-Verlag; 1996. p. 197.
18. Staneva J, Denkova P, Todorova M, et al. *J Pharm Biomed Anal*. 2011;54(1):94–99.
19. Willuhn G. Chapter 10: *Arnica* flowers: pharmacology, toxicology, and analysis of the sesquiterpene lactones – their main active substances. In: Lawson LD, Bauer R, eds. *Phytomedicines of Europe. Chemistry & Biological Activity*. Washington: American Chemical Society; 1998. pp. 118–132.
20. Ganzera M, Egger C, Zidorn C, et al. *Anal Chim Acta*. 2008;614(2):196–200.
21. Schmidt TJ, Stausberg S, Raison JV, et al. *Nat Prod Res*. 2006;20(5):443–453.
22. de Smet PAGM, editor. *Adverse Effects of Herbal Drugs*, Vol 1. Berlin: Springer-Verlag; 1992. pp. 194, 238.
23. Lin LZ, Harnly JM. *J Agric Food Chem*. 2008;56(21):10105–10114.
24. Douglas JA, Smallfield BM, Burgess EJ, et al. *Planta Med*. 2004;70(2):166–170.
25. Schmidt TJ, Matthiesen U, Willuhn G. *Planta Med*. 2000;66(7):678–681.
26. Lyss G, Schmidt TJ, Merfort I, et al. *Biol Chem*. 1997;378(9):951–961.
27. Schaffner W. *Biol Chem*. 1997;378(9):935.
28. Lyss G, Schmidt TJ, Pahl HL, et al. *Pharm Pharmacol Lett*. 1999;9(1):5–8.
29. Ekenäs C, Zebrowska A, Schuler B, et al. *Planta Med*. 2008;74(15):1789–1794.
30. Klaas CA, Wagner G, Laufer S, et al. *Planta Med*. 2002;68(5):385–391.
31. Verma N, Tripathi SK, Sahu D, et al. *Mol Cell Biochem*. 2010;336(1–2):127–135.
32. Jäger C, Hrenn A, Zwingmann J, et al. *Planta Med*. 2009;75(12):1319–1325.
33. Siedle B, Gustavsson L, Johansson S, et al. *Biochem Pharmacol*. 2003;65(5):897–903.
34. Tornhamre S, Schmidt TJ, Näsman–Glaser B, et al. *Biochem Pharmacol*. 2001;62(7):903–911.
35. Hall IH, Starnes CO, Lee KH, et al. *J Pharm Sci*. 1980;69(5):537–543.
36. Berges C, Fuchs D, Opelz G, et al. *Mol Immunol*. 2009;46(15):2892–2901.
37. Hall IH, Lee KH, Starnes CO, et al. *J Pharm Sci*. 1979;68(5):537–542.
38. Alfredo PP, Anaruma CA, Pião AC, et al. *Ultrasonics*. 2009;49(4–5):466–471.
39. Kellner W, Kober W. *Arzneimittelforschung*. 1955;5:224.
40. Willuhn G, Rottger PM, Quack W. *Pharm Ztg*. 1982;127:2183–2185.
41. Reisch J, et al. *Arzneimittelforschung*. 1967;17:816.
42. Koo H, Gomes BP, Rosalen PL, et al. *Arch Oral Biol*. 2000;45(2):141–148.
43. Iauk L, Lo Bue AM, Milazzo I, et al. *Phytother Res*. 2003;17(6):599–604.
44. Barrera PA, Jimenez–Ortiz V, Tonn C, et al. *J Parasitol*. 2008;94(5):1143–1149.
45. Schmidt TJ, Brun R, Willuhn G, et al. *Planta Med*. 2002;68(8):750–751.
46. Grancois G, Passreiter CM. *Phytotherapy Res*. 2004;18(2):184–186.
47. Boulanger D, Brouillette E, Jaspar F, et al. *Vet Microbiol*. 2007;119(2–4):330–338.
48. Woerdenbag HJ, Merfort I, Passreiter CM, et al. *Planta Med*. 1994;60(5):434–437.
49. Gertsch J, Sticher O, Schmidt T, et al. *Biochem Pharmacol*. 2003;66(11):2141–2153.
50. Dirsch VM, Stuppner H, Vollmar AM. *Cancer Res*. 2001;61(15):5817–5823.
51. Heilmann J, Wasescha MR, Schmidt TJ. *Bioorg Med Chem*. 2001;9(8):2189–2194.
52. Woerdenbag HJ, Merfort I, Schmidt TJ, et al. *Phytomedicine*. 1995;2(2):127–132.
53. Hall IH, Lee KH, Starnes CO, et al. *J Pharm Sci*. 1978;67(9):1235–1239.
54. Schroder H, Losche W, Strobach H, et al. *Thromb Res*. 1990;57(6):839–845.
55. Hall IH, Lee KH, Starnes CO, et al. *J Pharm Sci*. 1980;69(6):694–697.
56. Wagner S, Suter A, Merfort I. *Planta Med*. 2004;70(10):897–903.
57. Wagner S, Merfort I. *J Pharm Biomed Anal*. 2007;43(1):2–38. 3
58. Bergonzi MC, Bilia AR, Casiraghi A, et al. *Pharmazie*. 2005;60(1):36–38.
59. Tekko IA, Bonner MC, bowen RD, et al. *J Pharm Pharmacol*. 2006;58(9):1167–1176.
60. Bergamante V, Ceschel GC, Marazzita S, et al. *Drug Deliv*. 2007;14(7):427–432.
61. Knuesel O, Weber M, Suter A. *Adv Ther*. 2002;19(5):209–218.
62. Widrig R, Suter A, Saller R, et al. *Rheumatol Int*. 2007;27(6):585–591.
63. Leu S, Havey J, White LE, et al. *Br J Dermatol*. 2010;163(3):557–563.
64. Ku era M, Kolar P, Barna M, et al. *Pain Res Treat*. 2011;7. Article ID 365625.
65. Ku era M, Horácek O, Kálal J, et al. *Arzneimittelforschung*. 2003;53(12):850–856.
66. Quartz P, Landgrebe N, Wöbling D, et al. Paper presented at the 6th Phytotherapy Congress. Berlin; 1995.
67. Moog-Schulze JB. *Tijdschr Integr Geneeskunde*. 1993;9:105–112.
68. Alonso D, Lazarus MC, Baumann L. *Dermatol Surg*. 2002;28(8):686–688.
69. [No authors listed] Final report on the safety assessment of Arnica montana extract and Arnica montana. *Int J Toxicol*. 2001;20(suppl 2):1–11.
70. Witzel DA, Ivie GW, Dollahite JW. *Am J Vet Res*. 1976;37(7):859–861.
71. Chapman DE, Roberts GB, Reynolds DJ, et al. *Fundam Appl Toxicol*. 1988;10(2):302–312.
72. Kim HL. *Res Commun Chem Pathol Pharmacol*. 1980;28(1):189–192.
73. Hausen BM. *Contact Dermatitis*. 1978;4(5):308.
74. Goggelmann W, Schimmer O. *Prog Clin Biol Res*. 1986;206:63–72.
75. MacGregor JT. *Food Cosmet Toxicol*. 1977;15(3):225–228.
76. Herrmann HD, Willuhn G, Hausen BM. *Planta Med*. 1978;34(3):299–304.
77. Merrill J, Kim HL, Safe S. *Adv Exp Med Biol*. 1986;197:891–896.
78. Merrill JC, Kim HL, Safe S, et al. *J Toxicol Environ Health*. 1988;23(2):159–169.

79. Hausen BM, De Smet PAGM. Keller K, Hansel R, eds. *Adverse Effects of Herbal Drugs*, Vol 1. Berlin: Springer-Verlag; 1992. pp. 237–242.

80. Merdinger O. *MMW*. 1938;85: 1469–1470.

81. Rybalko KS, Trutneva EA, Kibal'chich PN. *Aptetschnoje Delo*. 1965;14:32–33.

82. Kreitmair H. *Mercks Jahresber*. 1936;50:106–107.

83. Ochsenheimer J. *Osterr Med Wschr*. 1844:226–227.

84. Bruynzeel DP, van Ketel WG, Young E, et al. *Contact Dermatitis*. 1992;27(4): 278–279.

85. Hormann HP, Korting HC. *Occup Environ Dermatoses*. 1994;42(6):246–249.

86. Hormann HP, Korting HC. *Phytomedicine*. 1995;4:315–317.

87. Pirker C, Moslinger T, Koller DY, et al. *Contact Dermatitis*. 1992;26(4):217–219.

88. Passreiter CM, Florack M, Willuhn G, et al. *Derm Ber Umwelt*. 1988;36(3):79–82.

89. Hausen BM, *Am J Contact Dermatitis*. 1996;7(2):94–99.

90. Hausen BM, De Smet PAGM, Keller K, Hansel R, eds. *Adverse Effects of Herbal Drugs*, Vol 1. Berlin: Springer-Verlag; 1992. pp. 227–236.

91. Paulsen E, Andersen KE, Hausen BM. *Contact Dermatitis*. 1993;29(1):6–10.

92. Reider N, Komericki P, Hausen BM, et al. *Contact Dermatitis*. 2001;45(5): 269–272.

93. Jeschke E, Ostermann T, Lüke C, et al. *Drug Saf*. 2009;32(8):691–706.

94. Jocher A, Nist G, Weiss JM, et al. *Contact Dermatitis*. 2009;61(5):304–306.

95. Lass C, Vocanson M, Wagner S, et al. *Exp Dermatol*. 2008;17(10):849–857.

96. Moghadam BK, Gier R, Thurlow T. *Cutis*. 1999;64(2):131–134.

97. Delmonte S, Brusati C, Parodi A, et al. *Dermatology*. 1998;197(2):195–196.

98. Hänsel R, Haas H. *Therapie mit Phytopharmaka*. Berlin: Springer-Verlag; 1983. p. 272.

99. Topliff A, Grande G. *J Toxicol Clin Toxicol*. 2000;38(5):518.

100. Ciganda C, Laborde A. *J Toxicol Clin Toxicol*. 2000;39(3):318–319.

Astragalus

(*Astragalus membranaceus* (Fisch.) Bge.)

Synonyms

Membranous milk-vetch root (Engl), Astragali Radix (Lat), huang qi (Chin), ogi (Jap), hwanggi (Kor), astragel (Dan).

What is it?

The root of *Astragalus membranaceus* has been used for many hundreds of years in traditional Chinese medicine. The *Pharmacopoeia of the People's Republic of China* defines *A. membranaceus* and *A. membranaceus* var. *mongholicus* (synonym: *A. mongholicus*) as the medicine Radix Astragali. Another species of the Astragalus genus that grows in the mountainous districts of Iran and Iraq yields tragacanth gum from its thorny stems. Although many species are used as forage for livestock and wild animals, some (including the locoweeds) are known to cause intoxication in livestock, which can be passed to humans through milk and meat. *Astragalus membranaceus* is not one of these species. In Western herbal medicine Astragalus is largely viewed as an immune tonic.

Effects

Restores, strengthens and balances the body's immune response; increases vitality; strengthens cardiac function.

Traditional view

In traditional Chinese medicine Astragalus is classified as a herb that tonifies the *Qi* (energy) and *Blood* (nutrition), hence it is used for postpartum fever and recovery from severe loss of blood. It tonifies the *Spleen* (being used for fatigue linked to decreased appetite), raises the *Yang Qi* of the *Spleen* and *Stomach* (used for organ prolapse and uterine bleeding) and promotes urination, tissue healing and the discharge of pus. Its properties are sweet and slightly warm.[1] Traditionally, Astragalus is taken as the powdered dried root or decoction. This is reflected in the body of pharmacological research on the properties of the Astragalus polysaccharides, which would occur in these dosage forms.

Summary actions

Immune-enhancing, tonic, adaptogenic, cardiotonic, diuretic, hypotensive, antioxidant, immune-regulating.

Can be used for

Indications supported by clinical trials

Impaired immunity, especially if associated with leucopenia; adjunct in the treatment of cancer; viral infections including the common cold, cervical erosion associated with herpes simplex virus infection and viral myocarditis; allergic rhinitis, fatigue and heart conditions (usually in combination).

Traditional therapeutic uses

Postpartum fever and recovery from severe loss of blood; fatigue; decreased appetite; organ prolapse, uterine bleeding; to raise vitality[1]; palpitation with shortness of breath; spontaneous sweating; prostration; chronic diarrhoea.[2]

May also be used for

Extrapolations from pharmacological studies

General prevention of infection; autoimmune diseases; conditions resulting in immune suppression, such as for patients receiving chemotherapy; viral infections (for example infection with Japanese encephalitis, coxsackie B2 and B3, parainfluenza virus type I and viral myocarditis); general debility; hypertension.

Other applications

Skin care, cosmetics and hair tonics for its healing, nourishing and vasodilating properties.[3]

Preparations

Dried root for decoction; liquid extract, tablets and capsules; powdered root.

Dosage

* 10 to 30 g/day of the dried root by decoction. Larger doses are used in traditional Chinese medicine as required, for example to treat paralysis[1]
* 4 to 8 mL/day of the 1:2 liquid extract or equivalent doses of the dried extract in tablet or capsule form.

Duration of use

May be taken long term for most applications but is contraindicated during acute infection.

Summary assessment of safety

No adverse effects are expected if used as recommended. Astragalus might aggravate acute infection.

Technical data

Botany

Astragalus is a member of the Leguminosae (pea) family, the Papilionoideae subfamily, and grouped in the same tribe as the licorice genus.[4] *Astragalus mongholicus* is a perennial herb growing 60 to 150 cm high. The leaves are pinnate, with 25 to 37 leaflets, and elliptic. The racemes are axillary, the calyx is 5 mm long and tubular. The root is flexible, long and covered with a tough, wrinkled, yellowish-brown epidermis. The woody interior is of a yellowish-white colour.[5]

Adulteration

Astragalus propinquus, A. lepsensis, A. aksuensis, A. hoantchy, A. hoantchy subsp. *dshimensis, A. lehmannianus, A. sieversianus* and *A. austrosibiricus* have all been identified as adulterants of *Astragalus membranaceus*, whilst *Hedysarum polybotrys* is a substitute. Astragaloside IV is normally used as a marker for quality control. In the *Japanese Pharmacopoeia* 1996, substitutes including *A. chrysopterus, A. floridus* and *A. tongolensis* are officially permitted, but these are not accepted in China.[6] More recently *Glycyrrhiza pallidiflora* has been suggested as a common adulterant.[7]

Key constituents

- Triterpenoid saponins (including astragalosides I to VIII), isoflavonoids (including formononetin), polysaccharides[8]
- Phytosterols, flavonoids, essential oil, amino acids (gamma-aminobutyric acid, canavanine).[9]

The important biologically active constituents in Astragalus are the polysaccharides and saponins.[8] Depending on the method of preparation, their levels will vary in extracts. Polysaccharides are mainly present in aqueous extracts such as a decoction, and can be isolated from these. Hot water extracts will also contain saponins. Ethanolic extracts will contain only low levels of polysaccharides, with the solubility of Astragalus saponins more or less increasing with the ethanol content used (for an extract made at room temperature).

Several pharmacological studies have investigated 'Astragalus polysaccharides'. However, the purity and composition of such isolates are likely to vary considerably. One recent Chinese study described isolation by sequential decoction with subsequent removal of proteins and colour.[10] Another described the preparation of a decoction of the defatted root, followed by protein removal and preliminary isolation using ethanol precipitation. This crude polysaccharide extract was then further purified by ionexchange, followed by gel filtration.[11] As a result, two polysaccharides (APS-I and APS-II) were isolated (consisting of arabinose and glucose, or rhamnose, arabinose and glucose, respectively).

The chemical composition of Astragalus was found to vary with the region of cultivation.[12] Moreover, the content of astragalosides in the root bark is up to 74 times that in the xylem, hence thin roots contain higher levels than thick roots.[12]

	R[1]	R[2]	R[3]
Astragaloside I	COCH$_3$	COCH$_3$	H
Astragaloside II	COCH$_3$	H	H
Astragaloside IV	H	H	H

Astragalosides

Pharmacodynamics

As touched on above, various preparations of Astragalus have been studied in pharmacological models, including Astragalus polysaccharides, individual or complex saponin isolates, crude aqueous or ethanol extracts, and a commercial preparation known as 'Astragalus injection' (which ironically was administered orally in some pharmacological studies).

Since polysaccharides are very large molecules with relatively low oral bioavailability, the relevance of any in vitro outcomes is questionable, especially to the oral use of an Astragalus decoction. This also applies for in vivo models where the polysaccharides were administered by injection. Hence, this research is mainly noted in passing and emphasis has been placed on the in vivo studies where the polysaccharides were administered orally. Also it should be kept in mind that the oral polysaccharide research is only relevant to the use of Astragalus as a decoction.

Saponins do have reasonable oral bioavailability, but they are generally changed by gut flora before systemic absorption (see Chapter 2). Hence, the relevance of the saponin in vitro research is also uncertain, but probably higher than for the polysaccharides. Again emphasis has been placed on in vivo studies where the saponins were given orally.

Astragalus injection is used clinically in China, hence it is logical that its pharmacological properties would also be studied. However, the relevance of this research to the oral use of Astragalus is low, so again such studies are briefly mentioned in this monograph without much detail, or even omitted from this review.

Of course, the relevance of any pharmacological research to human use needs to be interpreted with caution, especially in the case of medicinal plants (given their chemical complexity).

One limitation of this review is that several of the studies referred to are published in Mandarin. In these cases information was only available as the English abstract, rather than the full paper. This sometimes rendered interpretation difficult, especially when such critical issues as dose and route of administration were omitted from the abstract.

Astragalus can be combined with dong quai in the formulation known as DBT. Research on this combination can be found in the dong quai monograph.

Immune function

Astragalus markedly enhanced the cytotoxicity of natural killer cells,[13] potentiated interleukin-2-generated LAK (lymphokine-activated killer) cell cytotoxicity manifested by tumour cell lysis[14] and reversed tumour-associated macrophage suppression in urological tumours,[15] all in vitro. Using an in vitro local graft-versus-host reaction as a test assay for T-cell function, Astragalus extract restored the reaction in cells taken from 9 of 10 cancer patients.[16] Saponins from Astragalus stimulated the natural killer (NK) cell activity of human peripheral blood lymphocytes and restored steroid-inhibited NK cell activity, both in vitro.[17] Astragalus saponins reduced nicotinic acetylcholine receptor antibodies in blood cell cultures from myasthenia gravis patients.[18]

More recently, Astragalus was found in vitro to correct the immunological dysfunction in peripheral dendritic cells taken from children with Henoch–Schönlein purpura[19] and modified responses from lipopolysaccharide-stimulated macrophages, reducing cytokines in a dose-dependent manner.[20] Astragalosides significantly increased phagocytic activity against *Mycobacterium tuberculosis* in vitro.[21] Peripheral blood mononuclear cells (PBMCs) from 27 children with recurrent tonsillitis were stimulated and cultured with Astragalus in vitro for 48 hours.[22] Astragalus improved interferon-gamma output. Similar results were seen for Astragalus in PBMCs from 15 asthma patients, suggesting a reversal of Th2 predominant status.[23]

Oral doses of Astragalus in mice (200 mg/kg) enhanced several aspects of immunity, including increased thymus weight, potentiation of phagocytic function, superoxide anion production by peritoneal macrophages and proliferation of splenocytes.[24] Protective effects on immune suppression in mice were observed after co-administration of Astragalus with a carcinogen. Macrophage numbers and white cell function

were raised to the same as or greater than normal levels.[25] Co-administration of Astragalus with an antitumour agent resulted in protection against the immunosuppression induced by the antitumour agent.[26] Oral administration of Astragalus (5 g/kg/day for 7 days) increased phagocytic activity[27] and significantly increased the lymphocyte transformation rate in a suppressed cellular immunity model.[28] Astragalus promoted interleukin-2 production in splenic lymphocytes of blood-deficient mice.[29] A protective effect of Astragalus extract after oral administration against Japanese encephalitis virus infection in mice was demonstrated. The authors proposed that the protective effect of Astragalus is based on a non-specific mechanism during the early stage of infection, before shifting to antibody production, and that macrophages play an important role by inducing the production of active oxygen.[30]

Astragaloside IV (50 mg/kg/day, iv) mitigated the development of the characteristic features of ovalbumin-induced chronic experimental asthma in mice.[31] Astragalus saponins (400 mg/kg, oral) exerted a protective effect against microbial sepsis in mice.[32] An ethanolic extract of Astragalus modified Th1/Th2 cytokine secretion patterns in vitro and in vivo (1.25 g/kg/day, oral for 7 days), favouring Th2 responses.[33] In contrast, oral doses of Astragalus attenuated the expression of IgA nephropathy in rats, possibly by diminishing Th2 cytokine responses.[34] Astragalus improved the phagocytic activity of peritoneal macrophages in mice.[35] The effect of ip injection was higher than for oral doses, but the difference was not significant. The immune response of carp (including phagocytic activity) was enhanced after including Astragalus at 0.5% of diet.[36]

Astragalus injection (at the equivalent of 6 g/kg/day of root by oral gavage) protected against cyclophosphamide-induced thymus injury in mice.[37] In other experiments, injection of Astragalus protected the immune organs of rats with obstructive jaundice,[38] and improved haematopoiesis in myelosuppressed mice.[39,40] Astragalus extract by injection demonstrated potential as a vaccine adjuvant[41] (this is a common property of saponins, including those in Astragalus).[42] The injection of an Astragalus decoction (10 g/kg) prevented airway hyper-reactivity in the ovalbumin mouse model of chronic asthma by inhibiting Th2 cytokine release.[43]

High oral doses of Astragalus decoction given to healthy subjects (15.6 g/day for 20 days) significantly increased serum IgM, IgE and cAMP.[44] Two months of oral treatment in people susceptible to the common cold greatly increased levels of IgA and IgG in nasal secretions, and administration for 2 weeks or 2 months enhanced the induction of interferon by peripheral white blood cells.[45] Healthy human volunteers treated with Astragalus fresh root tincture (15 mL/day, equivalent to 1.23 g of root for 7 days) demonstrated significant increases in white blood cell CD69 expression (a marker for lymphocyte activation) after 1 and 7 days compared with placebo in a small, double blind trial.[46] Patients receiving chronic haemodialysis treated with intravenous Astragalus injection (30 mL two to three times a week for 2 months) exhibited significantly greater levels of interleukin-2 than patients in the control group in a small trial involving 31 people, suggesting a favourable effect on immune function.[47] The expression of CD25 on T cells was also significantly increased in a similar clinical study using the same doses after 24 hours (p<0.02), but not after 7 days.[48]

There is a substantial number of in vitro studies on the immune effects of Astragalus polysaccharides of varying composition. Astragalus polysaccharides in vitro potentiated the immune-mediated antitumour activity of interleukin-2[49] and the activity of monocytes.[50] Astragalus polysaccharides improved the in vitro responses of lymphocytes taken from normal volunteers and cancer patients[51] and enhanced the NK cell activity in vitro of blood samples from normal volunteers and systemic lupus erythematosus (SLE) patients.[52] The polysaccharide fraction F3 potentiated the lymphokine-activated killer cell-inducing activity of interleukin-2 in blood taken from cancer and AIDS patients.[53] Other studies have shown that Astragalus polysaccharides in vitro activated and exerted mitogenic activity on B cells,[54,55] promoted neutrophil adhesion to vascular endothelial cells,[56] activated macrophages[55,57] and dendritic cells,[58,59] improved the innate immune response of bladder epithelial cells,[60] and induced differentiation of splenic dendritic cells, followed by the shifting of Th2 to Th1 balance, with enhancement of T cell function.[61]

Injection of Astragalus polysaccharides downregulated the immune response in rats with glomerulonephritis[62] and mice with type 1 diabetes,[63] augmented antibody responses[54] and restored the lymphocyte blastogenic response in older mice.[54] Astragalus polysaccharides (2 g/kg/day, oral) also prevented the development of type 1 diabetes in NOD mice by correcting the Th1/Th2 cytokine imbalance.[64] Oral doses of Astragalus polysaccharides (2 mg per chick) improved immune responses in chickens vaccinated against Newcastle disease[65] and at 220 mg/kg of feed acted synergistically with probiotic bacteria in modulating chick immune responses.[66] The innate immune response (phagocytic activity) was enhanced in sea cucumbers fed Astragalus polysaccharides (0.3% of feed) and superfine root powder (3.0% of feed).[67]

A comparison of oral doses of the whole extracts of *Astragalus membranaceus*, *A. membranaceus* var. *mongholicus* and *Hedysarum polybotrys* (all at 560 mg/kg) and their various chemical fractions (all at 560 mg/kg) demonstrated that the polysaccharide fractions of all three herbs were the most active fractions and exerted similar levels of immune enhancement in two separate assays in mice.[68] Another study found that the polysaccharides from four Chinese herbs, including Astragalus, were all active at inducing serum antibodies and promoting T cell proliferation following ip injection in chickens.[69] These studies highlight a key paradox of the research into the contribution of polysaccharides to the immune activity of herbs, namely that the polysaccharide fraction from any plant is likely to have immune-enhancing activity. A key question is: why has a particular herb, such as Astragalus, developed a strong traditional reputation as an immune-enhancing herb if such activity is solely due to similarly acting components common to most other plants?

Antiviral activity

The antiviral activity of Astragalus is most likely to be due to increased immunity and possibly enhanced interferon production.[2] In support of this, Astragalus demonstrated slight inhibitory activity against adenovirus type 7 in vitro. Natural and recombinant interferon enhanced the inhibitory activity of Astragalus.[70] It also promoted the production of interferon by mouse lung against parainfluenza virus type I and Newcastle disease virus in vitro.[71] Astragalus exhibited potent hepatitis B surface antigen-inactivating activity in vitro,[72] inhibited the activity of murine retroviral reverse transcriptase and human DNA polymerases[73] and had a protective effect on cultured beating heart cells infected with coxsackie B2 virus.[74]

Astragalus extract exhibited activity against herpes simplex virus type 1 in vitro[75] and countered the growth-inhibitory effect of cytomegalovirus infection on human cord blood progenitor cells.[76] Calycosin-7-O-beta-glucopyranoside, a major isoflavonoid in Astragalus, inhibited coxsackie virus B3 (CVB3) in vitro and was also active (24 mg/kg, oral) in an acute myocarditis model in mice.[77]

Oral or intranasal administration of Astragalus decoction protected mice from infection with parainfluenza virus type I.[24,45,78] Results from a series of in vivo experiments indicated that the effect of Astragalus resembled that of both bronchitis vaccine and the interferon mediator tilorone.[45] Astragalus polysaccharides had a weak inhibitory effect on hepatitis B virus in mice,[79] but astragaloside IV was quite active against the virus in vitro.[80]

Astragalus increased the survival rate and improved some abnormal electrophysiological parameters in acute CVB3 viral myocarditis in vivo.[81] In vitro and in vivo studies indicate Astragalus may act by decreasing the secondary damage caused by calcium ion influx, thereby improving abnormal myocardial electric activity, as well as inhibiting the replication of CVB3 virus RNA in the myocardium.[82,83]

Astragalus feeding (2.2 mg/kg/day) increased survival rate, alleviated pathological changes and reduced markers of cardiac damage in mice with CVB3 myocarditis.[84] In contrast to other work, an inhibitory effect on virus RNA replication in vivo was not correlated with the induction of beta-interferon,[85] but was greater than a calcium channel blocker (verapamil) and a steroidal anti-inflammatory drug (dexamethasone) in vitro.[86] Routine therapy combined with oral administration of Astragalus to viral myocarditis patients significantly enhanced immune parameters when compared with patients receiving routine therapy alone.[87]

Adaptogenic and tonic activity

Addition of Astragalus enhanced growth, metabolism and longevity in cell cultures.[2] It lowered oxygen consumption in mitochondria, enhanced tolerance to stress and prolonged the life of human embryonic kidney cells in culture.[88] Two isomers of the molecule HDTIC extracted from Astragalus extended the lifespan of human fetal lung diploid fibroblasts in vitro by slowing telomere shortening, reducing DNA damage and improving DNA repair.[89] They also delayed replicative senescence in the same model.[90] The telomerase activator cycloastragenol (TA-65, found at low levels in Astragalus) elongated short telomeres in mouse embryonic fibroblasts and improved some healthspan indicators in adult/old mice without increasing cancer incidence.[91] Such observations have been interpreted by some as suggestive that Astragalus or these components will promote human longevity, but this is clearly premature on current limited evidence.

Administration of Astragalus over 2 weeks to mice markedly increased plasma cAMP.[92] Astragalus decoction improved learning performance in animal maze tests[93] and improved memory in two models (50 g/kg/day for 7 days, oral).[94] Administration over 15 days inhibited field search behaviour, decreased spontaneous activity and increased sleep time.[93] Decoction of Astragalus improved endurance in mice and increased weight gain compared with controls.[1] A mixture of ginseng and Astragalus demonstrated antifatigue activity in mice. This activity was partly due to an improvement of energy metabolism.[95] Astragalus extract (400 mg/kg/day) countered the adverse effects of repeated restraint stress in rats, improving spatial learning and memory and reducing anxiety.[96] Oral administration of Astragalus increased the turnover of proteins in serum and liver in animals treated daily for 10 days.[97] Astragalus lowered collagen content in the aorta and lung of old rats to near levels found in young animals[98] and improved the density of M-cholinergic brain receptors.[99] In early research, oral administration of Astragalus increased plasma cAMP in healthy subjects.[100]

Cardiovascular and haemorheological activity

Astragalus saponins demonstrated a positive inotropic action on isolated heart and decreased the resting potential of cultured myocardial cells, suggesting an inotropic effect exerted through modulation of Na^+,K^+-ATPase.[101] Astragalosides reduced intracellular calcium overload in rat cardiomyocytes and enhanced free radical removal, both suggestive of a protective effect against myocardial injury.[102] Astragaloside IV improved post-ischaemic heart function and ameliorated reperfusion arrhythmias in rat hearts in vitro,[103] and improved intracellular calcium handling in hypoxia-reoxygenated cardiomyocytes.[34] Astragalus extract prevented daunorubicin-induced apoptosis of cultured cardiomyocytes by decreasing free radical release[104] and demonstrated a cardiotonic effect in isolated beating rabbit atria.[105] Astragaloside IV improved homocysteine-induced endothelial dysfunction in rat aortic rings via antioxidant activity.[106]

Oral administration of aqueous extract of Astragalus countered the rise in blood pressure and plasma renin activity in a hypertensive model.[107] Intragastric administration of Astragalus produced a hypotensive effect in another experimental model.[108] Gamma-aminobutyric acid was isolated as a potential hypotensive constituent.[109] Oral Astragalus improved impaired endothelial-dependent vasodilation in obese rats.[110,111] Astragaloside IV has exhibited vasodilatory effects in vivo,[112,113] as has the whole extract.[114]

Improvement of cardiac function has been demonstrated for Astragalus or its isolates in a number of in vivo models. In several such studies Astragalus or Astragalus components were given by injection. Examples of oral dose studies include the inhibitory effect of Astragalus (5, 10 and 20 g/kg/day) on left ventricular hypertrophy induced by pressure overload in rats.[115] Astragalus (20 g/kg, oral) also counted abnormal cardiac function in rats with pressure overload-induced heart failure, and at oral doses of 3.3 or 10 g/kg/day improved cardiac function in doxorubicin-injured rat hearts.[116] All these doses are rather high. Astragalosides have also demonstrated

cardioprotective activity in vivo following administration by injection,[103,117] as has Astragalus injection.[118]

Cardiac output increased in 20 patients with angina pectoris after 2 weeks of treatment with Astragalus.[119] Astragalus strengthened left ventricular function and had an anti-OFR (oxygen free radical) effect in acute myocardial infarction patients compared with controls. The decrease in the pre-ejection period:left ventricular ejection time ratio was closely correlated with the increase in superoxide dismutase activity of red blood cells and the decrease in lipid peroxidation of plasma. This anti-OFR activity of Astragalus may be one of the mechanisms behind its cardiotonic activity.[120]

Astragalus extract demonstrated a protective effect on erythrocyte deformability in vitro for blood taken from normal subjects and patients with SLE.[121] Astragalus significantly enriched the blood, as measured by improvement in haemorheological indices,[122] and, in a 'blood stagnation' experimental model, decreased whole-blood specific viscosity and increased plasma specific viscosity.[123]

Hepatoprotective activity

Astragalus saponins were protective against chemically induced liver injury in vitro and in vivo.[124] Oral doses of Astragalus polysaccharides (200 mg/kg/day) also demonstrated hepatoprotective activity in rats.[125] Astragalus extracts exhibited hepatoprotective activity and increased the activity of hepatic lysozymes, tissue dehydrogenase and liver glycogen.[126–128] Oral doses of an extract combination of Astragalus and *Paeonia lactiflora* (60, 120 and 240 mg/day) protected against immunological liver injury in mice.[129] The total flavonoids of Astragalus (100 mg/kg, oral) protected against paracetamol liver damage in mice.[130,131]

Some studies suggest that Astragalus in combination might protect against the hepatic fibrosis associated with chronic liver damage. Oral doses of the Astragalus and Paeonia combination mentioned above (80 and 160 mg/kg/day) reduced liver damage and fibrosis in rats with carbon tetrachloride-induced liver injury and decreased the elevation of tumour growth factor (TGF)-beta1.[132] Oral doses of a combination of Astragalus and *Salvia miltiorrhiza* (60, 120 and 240 mg/kg/day) also demonstrated antifibrotic activity in a similar model.[133]

Renal activity

A 2009 systematic review examined the published in vivo studies for Astragalus in early diabetic nephropathy in rats.[134] Of 41 articles identified, 13 reports that fulfilled the inclusion criteria were reviewed. Meta-analysis revealed that Astragalus extract (orally or by injection depending on the study, but mainly the former) significantly reduced fasting blood glucose, glomerular filtration rate, urinary albumin excretion and thickness of the glomerular basement membrane (p values ranging from <0.00001 to 0.03).

Several other in vivo studies have demonstrated protective effects on renal function in a variety of models, including IgA nephropathy.[135–140] Doses used were often relatively high and the route of administration was not always specified.

See also the Clinical trials section for diuretic activity in a human study.

Antidiabetic activity

In addition to the studies included in the meta-analysis above, the effects of Astragalus or its components have also been examined in several diabetic models. For example, oral doses of Astragalus polysaccharides (400 to 2000 mg/day) alleviated glucose toxicity and restored glucose homeostasis,[141] lowered blood glucose and reduced insulin resistance[142–144] and reduced cardiomyopathy[145] in various diabetic models. Other components have also been shown to have antidiabetic activity, including the isoflavonoids[146] and astragaloside IV, which protected against diabetic neuropathy in rats (3, 6 and 12 mg/kg twice a day, oral).[147]

Anticancer activity

Astragalus saponins,[148–150] Astragalus injection[151,152] and an Astragalus extract[153] have all shown growth inhibitory activity against a variety of tumour cell lines in vitro. Mechanisms included promotion of apoptosis,[148,149,153] growth inhibition[150] and downregulation of Akt phosphorylation.[151]

Astragalus saponins (100 and 200 mg/kg/day for 20 days, oral) reduced tumour volume in a mice xenograft model of colon cancer, demonstrating activity comparable to 5-fluorouracil.[150] Various fractions of Astragalus polysaccharides (prepared by decoction followed by stepwise ethanol precipitation) demonstrated weak cytotoxic activity in vitro, but promoted immune response in a mouse cancer model after ip injection.[154] Astragalus extracts demonstrated chemopreventative activity in mice (10, 20 and 40 mg/kg/day, oral)[155] and rats (90 and 180 mg/kg/day, oral).[156]

Antioxidant and anti-inflammatory activities

Astragalus flavonoids demonstrated a protective effect on mammalian cell damage caused by the hydroxyl radical, inhibited lipid peroxides and increased superoxide dismutase activity in vitro.[157] Three Astragalus saponins demonstrated superoxide anion scavenging activity in vitro.[158] Astragalus extract reduced free radical-mediated injury to renal tubules in rabbits (2.4 g/kg, iv).[159] Astragalus injection reduced measures of oxidative stress and inflammation in a controlled trial involving 60 haemodialysis patients.[160]

An aqueous extract of Astragalus demonstrated a broad anti-inflammatory effect on human amnion cells in vitro.[161] Astragalosides inhibited the formation of advanced glycation endproducts during the incubation of bovine serum albumin with ribose.[162]

Astragalus polysaccharides (250, 500 and 1000 mg/kg/day, oral) were anti-inflammatory in rats with adjuvant arthritis[163] and the 8:1 dried aqueous extract of Astragalus (30 and 100 mg/kg/day, oral) reduced the expression of various inflammatory mediators in zymosan air-pouch mice.[164] Astragalus decoction (100 mg/kg/day, oral) also inhibited the development of experimental atopic dermatitis in mice.[165] High oral doses of an aqueous extract of Astragalus either before (2 and 4 g/kg/day) or after (4 and 8 g/kg/day) hapten provocation reduced experimental colitis in rats.[166] Oral (4 and 8 g/kg/day) or intracolonic (200 and 800 mg/kg/day) doses of this Astragalus extract also demonstrated similar therapeutic activity in the same colitis model, but by modulation of different colonic cytokines, depending on the mode of administration.[167]

Neurological activity

Astragalus extract,[168] astragaloside IV[169] and Astragalus isoflavones[170] exhibited neuroprotective activity in various in vitro models. Peripheral nerve regeneration was demonstrated in vitro and in vivo (in rats via local administration) for an Astragalus extract.[171] An Astragalus extract (150 and 300 mg/kg, oral) also protected against pentylenetetrazole-induced seizures in mice.[172]

Other activity

Astragalus inhibited aldose reductase,[173] promoted the replication of hepatic DNA,[174] inhibited mitochondrial oxygen consumption caused by lipid peroxidation[175] and stimulated the motility of human sperm,[176] all in vitro. Incubating sperm from infertile men with Astragalus decoction significantly enhanced motility.[177,178] Intraperitoneal injection of Astragalus extract into rats made infertile by cadmium resulted in significant increases in sperm counts and reduced sperm malformation, compared with untreated controls.[179]

A methanolic extract of Astragalus inhibited the growth of the human intestinal bacterium *Clostridium perfringens* in vitro.[180] Oral administration of Astragalus normalised the imbalance in intestinal flora in an experimental model of senility.[181]

Oral administration of a concentrated solution of Astragalus strengthened small intestine movement and muscle tonus, especially in the jejunum.[182] This activity supports its traditional use in organ prolapse.

Astragaloside IV (3, 10 and 30 mg/kg/day, oral) exerted gastroprotective effects in rats with ethanol-induced gastric mucosal damage.[183]

Pharmacokinetics

A pharmacokinetic investigation of astragaloside IV administered by intravenous injection to rats and dogs found highest concentrations in the lung and liver.[184] The compound was relatively quickly eliminated and does not appear to cross the blood-brain barrier.

The bioavailabilities of the flavonoids in Astragalus decoction were examined using various models, namely a computational chemistry prediction method, a Caco-2 cell monolayer and an improved rat everted gut sac model.[185] The computational model suggested that 26 compounds in Astragalus, including 12 flavonoids, were potentially bioavailable. The two in vitro models found that 21 compounds were absorbed, including flavonoid and isoflavonoid aglycones and some of their glycosides and metabolites. Following a multiple-dose study in a healthy male volunteer who ingested 60 g of the crude herb via decoction twice a day for 5 days, several of the same compounds were also detected in his urine, but mainly the metabolites (as might be expected for urine).

Clinical trials

Immune function

In an open, randomised clinical trial, 115 patients with leucopenia received a high dose of a concentrated Astragalus preparation (equivalent to 30 g/day of Astragalus) or a low dose (equivalent to 10 g/day) over a period of 8 weeks. There was a significant rise of average white blood cell (WBC) counts in both groups after treatment (p<0.001). The average WBC count for the high-dose group was significantly higher than for the low-dose group (p<0.05). On the basis of these findings, the author suggested that Astragalus is an effective treatment for leucopenia and increasing the dosage could enhance its effectiveness.[186] In an open study, 1000 volunteers received Astragalus either orally, as a nasal spray or in a compound formula. A prophylactic effect for the common cold was observed, as evidenced by decreased incidence and shortened duration of infection.[45]

A combination of Astragalus (320mg/day of an 18:1 extract containing 40% polysaccharides) and calcium-aluminium silicate as a mineral carrier and possible synergist was investigated in a 6-week double blind, placebo-controlled clinical trial involving 48 patients with seasonal allergic rhinitis.[187] Both the attending physicians and the patients judged the active treatment as more efficacious than placebo (p=0.003 and p=0.026, respectively). However, no statistically significant differences were detected between the groups for serum IgE, IgG and nasal eosinophils, although there was a trend to lower IgG for Astragalus plus minerals (p=0.18). In a post hoc analysis of 21 patients with weed pollen allergy, Astragalus plus minerals significantly improved total symptom score (p=0.022) and quality of life (p<0.001) compared with placebo. All adverse events were mild and not considered to be connected to the active treatment.

Astragalus in combination with other herbs has also been investigated for clinical effects on immune function. In a double blind, placebo-controlled trial, 85 children aged 7 to 15 years with asthma were randomly assigned to receive either an oral herbal formula (0.619 g/day, comprising equal weights of dried aqueous extracts from Astragalus, Cordyceps, Stemona, Fritillaria and Scutellaria baicalensis), or placebo for 6 months.[188] There was no significant difference recorded for any of the trial endpoints between the active treatment and placebo groups. The impact of Compound Astragalus Recipe was investigated in 60 patients with myasthenia gravis in a controlled trial.[189] While clinical outcomes were similar in the herbal and control groups, the herbal treatment significantly lowered the CD4+/CD8+ ratio (p<0.05).

Astragalus injection has demonstrated a range of effects on immune function in open label clinical trials. For example, it improved cellular immunity in patients with serious abdominal trauma,[190] promoted recovery of haematopoietic function in patients with chronic aplastic anaemia,[191] improved immune function in patients with congestive heart failure[192] and enhanced the efficacy of conventional treatment for SLE.[193]

Antiviral activity

Administration of Astragalus to a large number of patients with chronic viral hepatitis resulted in a success rate of 70% in an open trial. In most cases, elevated serum ALT levels returned to normal after 1 to 2 months.[194]

In a double blind clinical trial, 235 patients with typical chronic cervicitis (associated with viral infection) received one of the following treatments applied locally by gauze: recombinant interferon-alpha1 (at 5 or 10 mg), combined interferon (5 mg) and Astragalus (0.5 mL of a 1:1 extract), or Astragalus alone (0.5 mL of a 1:1 extract). These treatments were applied twice per week for 3 weeks. The Astragalus plus interferon group showed a similar improvement to the higher dose interferon group, with approximately 60% of patients demonstrating complete resolution or marked improvement. Only 8% of patients treated with Astragalus alone exhibited marked improvement and no patients were completely cured. These results suggest that Astragalus acted synergistically with interferon therapy.[195] An earlier double blind trial showed a similar result for 164 patients with cervical erosion associated with herpes simplex virus infection.[196] In 106 patients with herpes simplex keratitis, those randomly assigned to Astragalus treatment (dose and route not specified in the English abstract) exhibited significant improvement in the rebalancing of Th1/Th2 cytokines, an effect not observed in the comparative control group receiving ribavirin.[197]

An infused formulation of six herbs with Astragalus as the main component was significantly better than a control treatment (including silymarin) in terms of clinical improvement and greater negative seroconversions in an open label trial involving 208 patients with chronic viral hepatitis B.[198]

A formulation containing extracts of Astragalus combined with Glycyrrhiza glabra, Artemisia capillaris, Morus alba and Carthamus tinctorius was investigated in HIV positive patients in Thailand. In an open label study, 28 HIV-1 infected adults (CD4 count >200 cells/mm^3 and HIV-1 RNA >20000 copies/mL) received 5g/day of the combination plus sulfamethozaxole and trimethoprim for 12 weeks.[199] Up to 36% of patients demonstrated a reduction in plasma HIV-1 RNA of more than 0.5 log during the trial, but CD4 counts were unchanged. In a subsequent randomised, double blind, 24-week clinical trial, the efficacy of the herbal combination (7.5 g/day) given with zidovudine and zalcitabine was compared against the two drugs plus a herbal placebo in 60 HIV-1 positive patients.[200] The decline in HIV RNA was significantly greater in the group receiving the herbal combination (p<0.001) and CD4 cell counts were higher compared with baseline (p<0.05), versus no change in the control group. Serious adverse events were not observed.

A 2004 Cochrane review of herbal medicines for viral myocarditis found 40 randomised trials involving 3448 patients.[201] Twenty-five different herbal treatments were tested in the included trials. Astragalus was given as a single treatment in 10 trials (oral doses in three, by injection in seven) and as part of a herbal combination in another 13 trials (all doses oral). Analysis of the 10 Astragalus-only trials (plus one where the formulation was mainly Astragalus) found Astragalus significantly improved premature beat, cardiac output, ejection fraction and some levels of myocardial enzymes (indicating cardiac damage). Overall the authors stressed the low methodological quality, but suggested some herbal medicines such as Astragalus deserve further examination in this context in rigorous trials.

Cardiovascular conditions (other than viral myocarditis)

In a comparative trial, 92 patients suffering from ischaemic heart disease were treated with Astragalus, Salvia miltiorrhiza or the anti-anginal drug nifedipine. Results were superior for the Astragalus-treated group, as demonstrated by marked relief from angina pectoris and improvement in several objective clinical parameters. Treatment of ischaemic heart disease by Astragalus was significantly more effective compared with the control group (p<0.05).[202] In an open label trial in 20 patients with angina pectoris, Astragalus (60g/day, presumably by decoction) significantly improved cardiac output by 16.9% after 2 weeks (p<0.01), with no improvement of left ventricular diastolic function.[203] Unlike digitalis, the herb did not inhibit ATP activity.

Forty-five patients with chronic heart failure (defined in TCM (traditional Chinese medicine) terms by Xin-qi or Xin-yang deficiency) were randomised to receive conventional medicine or conventional medicine plus 4.5g/day (oral) of an Astragalus granule containing only Astragalus.[204] While improvements from baseline in TNF-alpha, left ventricular ejection fraction (LVEF) and walking distance were observed in both groups, they were all significantly higher in the group receiving Astragalus (p<0.05).

Ninety chronic heart failure patients (TCM diagnosis as above) were randomly assigned to receive perindopril (4mg/day) and one of three different doses of Astragalus granule (15, 9 or 4.5g/day).[205] Clinical improvements, including for LVEF, walking distance and quality of life, were greatest in the highest dose group (p<0.01).

Ninety-four patients with vascular disease secondary to type 2 diabetes mellitus were randomly assigned to either Astragalus with saponins from *Panax notoginseng*, or simvastatin, in an open label trial. Blood cholesterol and triglyceride levels and a measure of vascular inflammation (MMP-9) improved similarly in the two groups.[206]

Astragalus injection has demonstrated a range of effects in cardiac patients in clinical trials. For example, it improved cardiac function and haemodynamics in children with tetralogy of Fallot,[207] improved heart function parameters in patients with congestive heart failure[208,209] and acute myocardial infarction,[210] and decreased inflammatory cytokine production in patients undergoing heart valve replacement.[211] Injected doses typically contained high levels of the crude herb (up to 80g).

Kidney disease

A randomised, double blind, placebo-controlled crossover study in 12 healthy men assessed the impact of a single oral dose of Astragalus (0.3g/kg of a dried 4:1 aqueous extract) on diuresis.[212] Compared with placebo, Astragalus markedly increased urinary sodium excretion, fractional sodium excretion and urinary excretion of chloride during the first 4 hours. The authors concluded that Astragalus induces marked natriuresis in healthy men and attributed this to enhanced renal responses to endogenous ANP (atrial natriuretic peptide).

A US group of doctors described two separate cases (published 3 years apart) of remission of idiopathic membranous nephropathy (IMN, probably autoimmune in origin) after therapy with Astragalus. The first case described a 77-year-old woman with nephrotic syndrome secondary to IMN who was largely unresponsive to conventional treatments.[213] After beginning Astragalus (15g/day as part of the formulation Shen-Yan Siwei Pian) there was a marked decrease in proteinuria. Nephrotic syndrome recurred after a temporary cessation of the formulation, with complete remission after its reintroduction. Remission persisted even after stopping the herbal treatment. The second case was a 63-year-old man with nephrotic syndrome due to IMN.[214] In addition to conventional treatments (which had not resolved his proteinuria) he took Astragalus (15g/day herb equivalent of a 4:1 extract – presumably aqueous) for around 12 months, after which he experienced complete remission of nephrotic syndrome.

In an open clinical trial, a combination of *Arctium lappa* fruit and tincture of Astragalus orally for 3 months with losartan was compared with losartan alone in 54 patients with diabetic nephropathy. The herbal combination reduced hyperlipidaemia, proteinuria and postprandial hyperglycaemia significantly compared with losartan alone.[215] Patients with diabetic nephropathy were randomly assigned to take simvastatin or a combination of Astragalus and Panax saponins. Both treatments reduced hyperlipidaemia and various markers of renal damage.[206] In an open label trial, 21 patients with type 2 diabetes and microalbuminuria received 150mL four times a day of an unspecified Astragalus and Ligusticum decoction for 6 months.[216] The herbal combination improved both urinary albumin excretion and endothelial dysfunction.

Astragalus injection improved renal tubular function in patients with IgA nephropathy[217] and primary nephrotic syndrome.[218]

Cancer therapy

A meta-analysis of 34 randomised clinical trials involving patients with non-small-cell lung cancer treated with platinum-based chemotherapy and Astragalus-based Chinese herbs suggested a benefit from the combination.[219] Most trials involved formulas featuring Astragalus, but two were of Astragalus alone. The herbs were administered by injection in around one-third of the trials. Twelve trials measuring such outcomes reported significantly lower mortality rates after 12 months when Astragalus was combined with chemotherapy (risk ratio 0.67). Nine studies reported significantly lower mortality rates after 24 months when Astragalus was combined with chemotherapy (risk ratio 0.73). Most of the studies included were of low methodological quality. A Cochrane review indentified four relevant trials where a decoction of Astragalus and a formulation featuring Astragalus was combined with chemotherapy regimens in patients with colorectal cancer.[220] Chemotherapy-induced nausea, vomiting and leucopenia were all decreased by concomitant administration of Astragalus decoction, and immune function was improved. The trials were of low quality, suggesting larger, more rigorous trials are needed to confirm these results.

A systematic review and meta-analysis of Chinese herbs in the treatment of hepatocellular carcinoma found that formulations containing Astragalus had a larger treatment effect than the pooled broad estimate (odds ratio 1.35, p=0.048).[221] Products containing Astragalus significantly improved 12-month survival rates (odds ratio 1.28, p<0.0001). While there were questions over trial design, the authors considered this to be compelling evidence that needs to be evaluated in high-quality clinical trials. The herbal treatments were often administered by injection.

In an open label trial, 20 children with acute leukaemia in remission received Astragalus (90 g/day, mode of administration not specified in the English abstract) plus chemotherapy for 1 month, while another 24 in the control group received chemotherapy alone.[222] The herbal treatment increased dendritic cell induction of peripheral mononuclear cells and enhanced antigen-presenting ability.

Other conditions

In a double blind, placebo-controlled clinical trial involving 507 elderly people, oral administration of Astragalus in combination with *Polygonum multiflorum* and *Salvia miltiorrhiza* demonstrated significant antiageing effects. Improvements were noted in vigour, strength, vision, cellular immunity and serum lipofuscin levels. The total effective rate was 76.6% compared with 34.5% for placebo (p<0.001).[223]

Eighty-four patients with liver cirrhosis and portal hypertension were randomly assigned to receive either conventional treatment or a combination of Astragalus and *Salvia miltiorrhiza* (dan shen) for 3 months in an open label trial.[224] There were significant improvements in haemodynamic measures and indices of liver fibrosis in the group treated with the herbal combination compared with the control group.

A 4-week randomised, double blind, placebo-controlled clinical trial was conducted with 36 adults with chronic fatigue (but not necessarily chronic fatigue syndrome).[225] The trial participants were divided into a control group (receiving a 'placebo' Chinese herbal formulation known as Hyangsapyunweesan (in Korean), 3 g/day) or 3 or 6 g/day of a 3.3:1 concentrated aqueous extract from equal parts of Astragalus and dan shen. This combination significantly decreased subjective fatigue severity scores compared with the control group (p<0.05).

Toxicology and other safety data

Toxicology

No adverse effects were observed within 48 hours after oral administration of Astragalus at doses of 75 and 100 g/kg. The ip LD_{50} of Astragalus has been reported to be 40 g/kg in mice. However, ip injection of 50 g/kg elicited no significant toxic reactions in mice in another study.[2] A 3-month subchronic toxicity evaluation of Astragalus given by injection found no distinct toxicity at doses up to 39.9 g/kg in rats and 19.95 g/kg in dogs.[226]

The aqueous extract of Astragalus (1.25 mg/mL) modestly increased the incidence (16%) of aberrant cells in the Ames test in vitro.[227] In contrast, aqueous-methanolic extract of Astragalus showed no mutagenic effects[228] and an aqueous extract demonstrated antimutagenic activity in vitro.[229] A Chinese herbal formula (Man-Shen-Ling) that contains Astragalus did not exhibit toxic, mutagenic, teratogenic or carcinogenic effects in acute and chronic toxicity tests in animal models.[230]

Contraindications

Based on traditional considerations, it is not advisable to prescribe Astragalus in acute infections.

Special warnings and precautions

None required.

Interactions

In vivo studies suggest that Astragalus may reduce the efficacy of cyclophosphamide (an immunosuppressive agent).[231,232] However, the clinical relevance of this is uncertain. In principle, immune-enhancing herbs should not be given long-term to transplant recipients receiving immune-suppressing drugs.

Use in pregnancy and lactation

Category B1 – no increase in frequency of malformation or other harmful effects on the fetus from limited use in women. No evidence of increased fetal damage in animal studies for oral doses.

Some species of Astragalus are known to induce locoism (a condition that can cause reproductive alterations), abortion and occasional skeletal deformities in livestock.[233,234] *A. membranaceus* has not been identified as one of these species and swainsonine, the indolizidine alkaloid responsible for locoism,[235] has not been detected in *A. membranaceus*. It is unlikely that the Astragalus species used medicinally are teratogenic, since those species that induce teratogenic effects are also known to be toxic. Moreover, a Chinese herbal formula (Man-Shen-Ling) that contains Astragalus did not demonstrate teratogenic activity in animal models.[236] Intravenous astragaloside IV was maternally toxic at 1.0 mg/kg in rats and fetotoxic at a dose higher than 0.5 mg/kg, but was devoid of teratogenic effects in rats and rabbits.[237]

There are no data available concerning the safety of Astragalus in breastfeeding.

Effects on ability to drive and use machines

No adverse effects expected.

Side effects

Controlled clinical studies suggest a low incidence of significant side effects.

Overdosage

No incidents found in published literature.

Safety in children

Limited information available, but adverse effects are not expected.

Regulatory status in selected countries

Astragalus is official in the *Pharmacopoeia of the Republic of China* (English edition, 1997) and the *Japanese Pharmacopoeia* (15th edition, English version 2006).

Astragalus is not covered by a Commission E monograph and is not on the UK General Sale List.

Astragalus does not have GRAS status. However, it is freely available as a 'dietary supplement' in the USA under DSHEA legislation (1994 Dietary Supplement Health and Education Act).

Astragalus is not included in Part 4 of Schedule 4 of the Therapeutic Goods Act Regulations of Australia and is freely available for sale.

References

1. Bensky D, Gamble A. *Chinese Herbal Medicine Materia Medica*. Seattle: Eastland Press; 1986. pp. 457–459.
2. Chang H, But P. *Pharmacology and Applications of Chinese Materia Medica*, vol 2. Singapore: World Scientific; 1987. pp. 1041–1046.
3. Leung AY, Foster S. *Encyclopedia of Common Natural Ingredients Used in Food, Drugs and Cosmetics*, 2nd ed. New York: John Wiley; 1996. p. 52.
4. Mabberley DJ, ed. *The Plant Book*, 2nd ed. Cambridge: Cambridge University Press; 1997. 64, pp. 396–398.
5. World Health Organization. *Medicinal Plants in China*. Manila: World Health Organization, Regional Office for the Western Pacific; 1989. p. 47.
6. Ma XQ, Shi Q, Duan JA, et al. *J Agric Food Chem*. 2002;50(17):4861–4866.
7. Huang DL, Sun SQ, Xu YQ, et al. *Guang Pu Xue Yu Guang Pu Fen Xi*. 2009; 29(9):2396–2400. [Article in Chinese].
8. Tang W, Eisenbrand G. *Chinese Drugs of Plant Origin*. Berlin: Springer Verlag; 1992. pp. 191–197.
9. Katsura E, Katoh Y, Yamagishi T. *Hokkaidoritsu Eisei Kenkyushoho*. 1983;33:136–137.
10. Mu LX, Zhu L, Zhao AH, et al. *Zhong Yao Cai*. 2009;32(11):1741–1745. [Article in Chinese].
11. Xu DJ, Xia Q, Wang JJ, et al. *Molecules*. 2008;13(10):2408–2415.
12. Song JZ, Yiu HH, Qiao CF, et al. *J Pharm Biomed Anal*. 2008;47(2):399–406.
13. Jing JP, Lin WF. *Chin J Microbiol Immunol*. 1983;3:293–296.
14. Wang Y, Qian XJ, Hadley HR, et al. *Mol Biother*. 1992;4(3):143–146.
15. Rittenhouse JR, Lui PD, Lau BHS, et al. *J Urol (Paris)*. 1991;146(2):486–490.
16. Sun Y, Hersh EM, Talpaz M, et al. *Cancer*. 1983;52(1):70–73.
17. You L, Zhou Y, Zhang Y, et al. *Zhongguo Mianyixue Zazhi*. 1990;6(1):60–63.
18. Tu LH, Huang DR, Zhang RQ, et al. *Chin Med J (Engl)*. 1994;107(4):300–303.
19. Wang J, Zhang QY, Chen YX. *Zhongguo Zhong Xi Yi Jie He Za Zhi*. 2009;29(9):794–797. [Article in Chinese].
20. Clement-Kruzel S, Hwang SA, Kruzel MC, et al. *J Med Food*. 2008;11(3):493–498.
21. Xu HD, You CG, Zhang RL, et al. *J Int Med Res*. 2007;35(1):84–90.
22. Yang Y, Wang LD, Chen ZB. *Zhongguo Dang Dai Er Ke Za Zhi*. 2006;8(5):376–378.
23. Wang G, Liu CT, Wang ZL, et al. *Chin J Integr Med*. 2006;12(4):262–267.
24. Sugiura H, Nishida H, Inaba R, et al. *Nippon Eiseigaku Zasshi*. 1993;47(6):1021–1031.
25. Jin R, Mitsuishi T, Akuzawa Y, et al. *Kitakanto Med J*. 1994;44(2):125–133.
26. Jin R, Wan LL, Mitsuishi T. *Chung Kuo Chung Hsi I Chieh Ho Tsa Chih*. 1995;15(2):101–103.
27. Isotopes laboratory, Beijing institute of tuberculosis. *Xinyiyaexue Zazhi* 1974;8:12.
28. Wang JY, Zhong JX, Zhou ZH, et al. *Chin J Integr Trad West Med*. 1987;7(9):543.
29. Chen YC. *Chung Kuo Chung Yao Tsa Chih*. 1994;19(2):739–741.
30. Kajimura K, Takagi Y, Ueba N, et al. *Biol Pharm Bull*. 1996;19(9):1166–1169.
31. Du Q, Chen Z, Zhou LF, et al. *Can J Physiol Pharmacol*. 2008;86(7):449–457.
32. Gao XH, Xu XX, Pan R, et al. *J Nat Med*. 2009;63(4):421–429.
33. Kang H, Ahn KS, Cho C, et al. *Biol Pharm Bull*. 2004;27(12):1946–1950.
34. Xu XL, Chen XJ, Ji H, et al. *Pharmacology*. 2008;81(4):325–332.
35. Ning KJ, Ruan XC, Lu JF, et al. *Zhongguo Zhong Yao Za Zhi*. 2005;30(21): 1670–1672. [Article in Chinese]
36. Yin G, Ardó L, Thompson KD, et al. *Fish Shellfish Immunol*. 2009;26(1):140–145.
37. Wei X, Zhang J, Li J, et al. *Am J Chin Med*. 2004;32(5):669–680.
38. Zhang RP, Zhang XP, Ruan YF, et al. *World J Gastroenterol*. 2009;15(23):2862–2869.
39. Zhu XL, Zhu BD. *Phytother Res*. 2007;21(7):663–667.
40. Lv Y, Feng X, Zhu B. *Zhong Yao Cai*. 2005;28(9):791–793. [Article in Chinese].
41. Yang X, Huang S, Chen J, et al. *Vaccine*. 2010;28(3):737–743.
42. Yang ZG, Sun HX, Fang WH. *Vaccine*. 2005;23(44):5196–5203.
43. Shen HH, Wang K, Li W, et al. *J Ethnopharmacol*. 2008;116(2):363–369.
44. Institute of Basic Medical Sciences, Chinese Academy of Medical Sciences. *Chung Hua I Hsueh Tsa Chih* 1979;59:31–34.
45. Institute of Epidemic Prevention, Chinese Academy of Medical Sciences. *Med Commun* 1978;4:4.
46. Brush J, Mendenhall E, Guggenheim A, et al. *Phytother Res*. 2006;20(8):687–695.
47. Qun L, Luo Q, Zhang ZY, et al. *Clin Nephrol*. 1999;52(5):333–334.
48. Zwickey H, Brush J, Iacullo CM, et al. *Phytother Res*. 2007;21(11):1109–1112.
49. Chu D, Sun Y, Lin J, et al. *Chung Hsi I Chieh Ho Tsa Chih*. 1990;10(1):34–36.
50. Chu DT, Sun Y, Lin JR. *Chung Hsi I Chieh Ho Tsa Chih*. 1989;9(6):351–354.
51. Wang DC. *Chung Hua Chung Liu Tsa Chih*. 1989;11(3):180–183.
52. Zhao XZ. *Chung Kuo Chung Hsi I Chieh Ho Tsa Chih*. 1992;12:669–671. 645
53. Chu DT, Lin JR, Wong W. *Chung Hua Chung Liu Tsa Chih*. 1994;16(3):167–171.
54. Cho WC, Leung KN. *J Ethnopharmacol*. 2007;113(1):132–141.
55. Shao BM, Xu W, Dai H, et al. *Biochem Biophys Res Commun*. 2004;320(4):1103–1111.
56. Hao Y, Qiu QY, Wu J. *Zhongguo Zhong Xi Yi Jie He Za Zhi*. 2004;24(5):427–430.
57. Lee KY, Jeon YJ. *Int Immunopharmacol*. 2005;5(7–8):1225–1233.
58. Shao P, Zhao LH, Zhi-Chen *Int Immunopharmacol*. 2006;6(7): 1161–1166.
59. Chen CJ, Li ZL, Fu Q, et al. *Nan Fang Yi Ke Da Xue Xue Bao*. 2009;29(6): 1192–1194. [Article in Chinese].
60. Yin X, Chen L, Liu Y, et al. *Biochem Biophys Res Commun*. 2010;397(2):232–238.
61. Liu QY, Yao YM, Zhang SW, et al. *J Ethnopharmacol*. 2010. [Epub ahead of print].
62. Li S, Zhang Y, Zhao J. *Int Immunopharmacol*. 2007;7(1):23–28.
63. Li RJ, Qiu SD, Chen HX, et al. *Biol Pharm Bull*. 2007;30(3):470–476.
64. Chen W, Li YM, Yu MH. *Exp Clin Endocrinol Diabetes*. 2008;116(8):468–474.
65. Chen Y, Wang D, Hu Y, et al. *Int J Biol Macromol*. 2010;46(4):425–428.
66. Li SP, Zhao XJ, Wang JY. *Poult Sci*. 2009;88(3):519–525.

67. Wang T, Sun Y, Jin L, et al. *Fish Shellfish Immunol.* 2009;27(6):757–762.

68. Liu J, Hu X, Yang Q, et al. *J Biomed Biotechnol.* 2010:12. Article ID 479426.

69. Qiu Y, Hu YL, Cui BA, et al. *Poult Sci.* 2007;86(12):2530–2535.

70. Peng J, Wu SH, Zhang LL, et al. *Zhongguo Yixue Kexueyuan Xuebao.* 1984;6(2): 116–119.

71. Institute of Epidemic Prevention, Chinese Academy of Medical Sciences. *Stud on Epidemic Prev* 1976;3:204.

72. Zheng MS, et al. *Chin Trad Herbal Drugs.* 1987;18(10):459–461.

73. Ono K, Nakane H, Meng ZK, et al. *Chem Pharm Bull (Tokyo).* 1989;37(7):1810–1812.

74. Yuan WL, Chen HZ, Yang YZ, et al. *Chin Med J (Engl).* 1990;103(3):177–182.

75. Sun Y, Yang J. *Di Yi Jun Yi Da Xue Xue Bao.* 2004;24(1):57–58. [Article in Chinese].

76. Liu WJ, Liu B, Guo QL, et al. *Zhonghua Er Ke Za Zhi.* 2004;42(7):490–494.

77. Zhu H, Zhang Y, Ye G, et al. *Biol Pharm Bull.* 2009;32(1):68–73.

78. Institute of Epidemic Prevention, Chinese Academy of Medical Sciences. *Stud Epidemic Prev* 1976;2:124.

79. Dang SS, Jia XL, Song P, et al. *World J Gastroenterol.* 2009;15(45):5669–5673.

80. Wang S, Li J, Huang H, et al. *Biol Pharm Bull.* 2009;32(1):132–135.

81. Rui T, Yang YZ, Zhou TS. *Chung Kuo Chung Hsi I Chieh Ho Tsa Chih.* 1994;14(5):292–294. 262

82. Peng TQ, Yang YZ, Kandolf R. *Chung Kuo Chung Hsi I Chieh Ho Tsa Chih.* 1994;14(11):664–666.

83. Guo Q, Peng TQ, Yang YZ. *Chung Kuo Chung Hsi I Chieh Ho Tsa Chih.* 1995;15(8):483–485.

84. Chen XJ, Bian ZP, Lu S, et al. *Am J Chin Med.* 2006;34(3):493–502.

85. Peng T, Yang Y, Riesemann H, et al. *Chin Med Sci J.* 1995;10(3):146–150.

86. Guo Q, Peng T, Yang Y, et al. *Virol Sin.* 1996;11(1):40–44.

87. Huang ZQ, Qin NP, Ye W. *Chung Kuo Chung Hsi I Chieh Ho Tsa Chih.* 1995;15(6):328–330.

88. Xiong ZY. *Zhejiang J Trad Chin Med.* 1983;18(5):235–238.

89. Wang P, Zhang Z, Sun Y, et al. *DNA Cell Biol.* 2010;29(1):33–39.

90. Wang P, Zhang Z, Ma X, et al. *Mech Ageing Dev.* 2003;124(10–12):1025–1034.

91. De Jesus BB, Schneeberger K, Vera E, et al. *Aging Cell.* 2011;10(4):604–621.

92. Isotopes Section of the Pharmacology Department, Basic Sciences Research Unit, Capital Hospital of the Chinese Academy of Medical Sciences, et al. *Med Res Commun.* 1977;10:27.

93. Pan SY, Hou JY, Jiang MY, et al. *Chung Yao Tung Pao.* 1986;11(9):559–561.

94. Hong GX, Qin WC, Huang LS. *Chung Kuo Chung Yao Tsa Chih.* 1994;19(11):687–688, 704.

95. Nagai K, Hanazuka M, Hizume S, et al. *Jpn Pharmacol Therapeut.* 1992;20(9):47–53.

96. Park HJ, Kim HY, Yoon KH, et al. *Korean J Physiol Pharmacol.* 2009;13(4):315–319.

97. Liu J, et al. *Chin Trad Herbal Drugs.* 1981;12(6):264–265.

98. Xu P, Jin G, Shen X. *Chung Kuo Chung Yao Tsa Chih.* 1991;16(1):49–50.

99. Shi r, He L, Hu Y, et al. *J Tradit Chin Med.* 2001;21(3):232–235.

100. Institute of Basic Medical Sciences, Chinese Academy of Medical Sciences. *Zhonghua Yixue Zazhi* 1979;1:23.

101. Wang Q. *Chung Kuo Chung Yao Tsa Chih.* 1992;17(9):557–559.

102. Meng D, Chen XJ, Bian YY, et al. *Am J Chin Med.* 2005;33(1):11–20.

103. Zhang WD, Chen H, Zhang C, et al. *Planta Med.* 2006;72(1):4–8.

104. Luo Z, Zhong L, Han X, et al. *Phytother Res.* 2009;23(6):761–767.

105. Liu Y, Hua SD, He YG, et al. *Zhongguo Zhong Yao Za Zhi.* 2008;33(19):2226–2229.

106. Qiu LH, Xie XJ, Zhang BQ. *Biol Pharm Bull.* 2010;33(4):641–646.

107. Song DJ, Gu DG, Mao SY, et al. *Chin Trad Herbal Drugs.* 1989;20(8):361–364.

108. Chengdu Institute for Drug Control. Chengdu Medical and Health Information 1971;1:90.

109. Hikino H, Funayama S, Endo K. *Planta Med.* 1976;30(4):297–302.

110. Li MR, Yu YR, Deng G. *Nan Fang Yi Ke Da Xue Xue Bao.* 2010;30(1):7–10. [Article in Chinese].

111. Deng G, Yu YR. *Sichuan Da Xue Xue Bao Yi Xue Ban.* 2009;40(4):608–611. [Article in Chinese].

112. Zhang C, Wang XH, Zhong MF, et al. *Clin Exp Pharmacol Physiol.* 2007; 34(5–6):387–392.

113. Zhang WD, Zhang C, Wang XH, et al. *Planta Med.* 2006;72(7):621–626.

114. Zhang BQ, Hu SJ, Qiu LH, et al. *Biol Pharm Bull.* 2005;28(8):1450–1454.

115. Su D, Xu B, Shi HL, et al. *Zhongguo Zhong Yao Za Zhi.* 2008;33(14):1724–1727. [Article in Chinese].

116. Su D, Li HY, Yan HR, et al. *Am J Chin Med.* 2009;37(3):519–529.

117. Chen XJ, Meng D, Feng L, et al. *Am J Chin Med.* 2006;34(6):1015–1025.

118. Ma L, Guan ZZ. *Zhongguo Zhong Xi Yi Jie He Za Zhi.* 2005;25(7):646–649. [Article in Chinese].

119. Lei ZY, Qin H, Liao JZ. *Zhongguo Zhong Xi Yi Jie He Za Zhi.* 1994;14(4):199–202. [Article in Chinese].

120. Chen LX, Liao JZ, Guo WQ. *Zhongguo Zhong Xi Yi Jie He Za Zhi.* 1995;15(3):141–143. [Article in Chinese].

121. Dai JH, Liang ZJ, Qin WZ, et al. *Guizhou Med J.* 1987;11(1):23–24.

122. Xue JX, Jiang Y, Yan YQ. *Chung Kuo Chung Yao Tsa Chih.* 1993;18(10): 621–630, 640.

123. Xue JX, Yan YQ, Jiang Y. *Chung Kuo Chung Yao Tsa Chih.* 1994;19(2):108–110, 128.

124. Zhang YD, Shen JP, Zhu SH, et al. *Yao Hsueh Hsueh Pao.* 1992;27(6):401–406.

125. Dang SS, Zhang X, Jia XL, et al. *Chin Med J (Engl).* 2008;121(11):1010–1014.

126. Han DW, Xu RL, Yeung SCS. *Abstr Chin Med.* 1988;2(1):114–115.

127. Zhang ZL, Wen QZ, Liu CX, et al. *J Ethnopharmacol.* 1990;30(2):145–150.

128. Yan XW, et al. *Symposium of the Chinese Pharmaceutical Association.* 1962; 332.

129. Sun WY, Wei W, Gui SY, et al. *Basic Clin Pharmacol Toxicol.* 2008;103(2):143–149.

130. Wang DQ, Critchley JA, Ding BG, et al. *Zhongguo Zhong Yao Za Zhi.* 2001;26(9):617–620. [Article in Chinese].

131. Wang DQ, Ding BG, Ma YQ, et al. *Zhongguo Zhong Yao Za Zhi.* 2001;26(7):483–486. [Article in Chinese].

132. Sun WY, Wei W, Wu L, et al. *J Ethnopharmacol.* 2007;112(3):514–523.

133. Yang Y, Yang S, Chen M, et al. *J Ethnopharmacol.* 2008;118(2):264–270.

134. Zhang J, Xie X, Li C, et al. *J Ethnopharmacol.* 2009;126(2):189–196.

135. Zuo C, Xie X, Deng Y, et al. *Zhongguo Zhong Yao Za Zhi.* 2009;34(2):193–198. [Article in Chinese].

136. Zuo C, Xie X, Deng Y, et al. *Wei Sheng Yan Jiu.* 2008;37(5):566–570. [Article in Chinese].

137. Zhang GZ, Wu XC, Peng XJ, et al. *Zhongguo Dang Dai Er Ke Za Zhi.* 2008;10(2):173–178. [Article in Chinese].

138. Huang LM, Shi XQ, Liang H. *Zhongguo Zhong Yao Za Zhi.* 2007;32(13):1324–1328. [Article in Chinese].

139. Zuo C, Xie XS, Qiu HY, et al. *J Zhejiang Univ Sci B.* 2009;10(5):389–390.

140. Li X, He DL, Cheng XF, et al. *Zhongguo Zhong Yao Za Zhi.* 2005;30(20): 1606–1609. [Article in Chinese].

141. Zou F, Xq Mao, Wang N, et al. *Acta Pharmacol Sin.* 2009;30(12):1607–1615.

142. Mao XQ, Yu F, Wang N, et al. *Phytomedicine.* 2009;16(5):416–425.

143. Liu M, Wu K, Mao X, et al. *J Ethnopharmacol.* 2010;127(1):32–37.

144. Wu Y, Ou-Yang JP, Wu K, et al. *Acta Pharmacol Sin.* 2005;26(3):345–352.

145. Chen W, Yu MH, Li YM, et al. *Acta Diabetol.* 2010;47(suppl 1):35–46.

146. Ma W, Nomura M, Takahashi-Nishioka T, et al. *Biol Pharm Bull.* 2007;30(11): 2079–2083.

147. Yu J, Zhang Y, Sun S, et al. *Can J Physiol Pharmacol.* 2006;84(6):579–587.

148. Auyeung KK, Mok NL, Wong CM, et al. *Int J Mol Med.* 2010;26(3):341–349.

149. Auyeung KK, Law PC, Ko JK. *Int J Mol Med.* 2009;23(2):189–196.

150. Tin MM, Cho CH, Chan K, et al. *Carcinogenesis.* 2007;28(6):1347–1355.

151. Deng Y, Chen HF. *Zhong Xi Yi Jie He Xue Bao.* 2009;7(12):1174–1180. [Article in Chinese].

152. Ye MN, Chen HF. *Zhong Xi Yi Jie He Xue Bao*. 2008;6(4):399–404. [Article in Chinese].

153. Cheng XD, Hou CH, Zhang XJ, et al. *Acta Biochim Biophys Sin (Shanghai)*. 2004;36(3):211–217.

154. Cho WC, Leung KN. *Cancer Lett*. 2007;252(1):43–54.

155. Kurashige S, Akuzawa Y, Endo F. *Cancer Invest*. 1999;17(1):30–35.

156. Cui R, He J, Wang B, et al. *Cancer Chemother Pharmacol*. 2003;51(1): 75–80.

157. Wang D, Shen W, Tian Y, et al. *Chung Kuo Chung Yao Tsa Chih*. 1995;20(4):240–242. 254

158. Liu XJ, Jiang M, Yu Z, et al. *Tianran Chanwu Yanjiu Yu Kaifa*. 1991;3(4): 1–6.

159. Sheng BW, Chen XF, Zhao J, et al. *Chin Med J (Engl)*. 2005;118(1):43–49.

160. Qu XL, Dai Q, Qi YH, et al. *Zhong Xi Yi Jie He Xue Bao*. 2008;6(5):468–472. [Article in Chinese].

161. Shon YH, Nam KS. *Phytother Res*. 2003;17(9):1016–1020.

162. Motomura K, Fujiwara Y, Kiyota N, et al. *J Agric Food Chem*. 2009;57(17): 7666–7672.

163. Li HQ, Qiu JD, Yang LH. *Yao Xue Xue Bao*. 2009;44(7):731–736. [Article in Chinese].

164. Ryu M, Kim EH, Chun M, et al. *J Ethnopharmacol*. 2008;115(2):184–193.

165. Lee SJ, Oh SG, Seo SW, et al. *Biol Pharm Bull*. 2007;30(8):1468–1471.

166. Ko JK, Lam FY, Cheung AP. *World J Gastroenterol*. 2005;11(37):5787–5794.

167. Ko JK, Chik CW. *Cytokine*. 2009;47(2):85–90.

168. Her X, Li C, Yu S. *J Tongji Med Univ*. 2000;20(2):126–127.

169. Chan WS, Durairajan SS, Lu JH, et al. *Neurochem Int*. 2009;55(6):414–422.

170. Yu D, Duan Y, Bao Y, et al. *J Ethnopharmacol*. 2005;98(1–2):89–94.

171. Lu MC, Yao CH, Wang SH, et al. *J Trauma*. 2010;68(2):434–440.

172. Aldarmaa J, Liu Z, Long J, et al. *Neurochem Res*. 2010;35(1):33–41.

173. Zhang JQ, Zhou YP. *China J Chin Materia Medica*. 1989;14(9):557–559.

174. Mu DW. *Yixueyanjiu Tongxun*. 1985;10:289–290.

175. Hong CY, Lo YC, Tan FC, et al. *Am J Chin Med*. 1994;22(1):63–70.

176. Hong CY, Ku J, Wu P. *Am J Chin Med*. 1992;20(3–4):289–294.

177. Liu J, Liang P, Yin C, et al. *Andrologia*. 2004;36(2):78–83.

178. Hong CY, Ku J, Wu P. *Am J Chin Med*. 1992;20(3–4):289–294.

179. Liang P, Li H, Peng X, et al. *Zhonghua Nan Ke Xue*. 2004;10(1):42–45. 48, [Article in Chinese].

180. Ahn YJ, Kwon JH, Chae SH, et al. *Micro Ecol Health Dis*. 1994;7(5):257–261.

181. Yan M, Song H, Xie N, et al. *Chung Kuo Chung Yao Tsa Chih*. 1995;20(10): 624–626.

182. Yang DZ. *Zhongguo Zhong Xi Yi Jie He Za Zhi*. 1993;13(10):616–617. 582, [Article in Chinese].

183. Navarrete A, Arrieta J, Terrones L, et al. *J Pharm Pharmacol*. 2005;57(8): 1059–1064.

184. Zhang WD, Zhang C, Liu RH, et al. *Life Sci*. 2006;79(8):808–815.

185. Xu F, Zhang Y, Xiao S, et al. *Drug Metab Dispos*. 2006;34(6):913–924.

186. Weng XS. *Chung Kuo Chung Hsi I Chieh Ho Tsa Chih*. 1995;15(8):462–464.

187. Matkovic Z, Zivkovic V, Korica M, et al. *Phytother Res*. 2010;24(2):175–181.

188. Wong EL, Sung RY, Leung TF, et al. *J Altern Complement Med*. 2009;15(10):1091–1097.

189. Niu GH, sun X, Zhang CM. *Zhongguo Zhong Xi Yi Jie He Za Zhi*. 2009;29(4):305–308. [Article in Chinese].

190. Wu J, Wang YX, Su WL, et al. *Chin J Integr Med*. 2006;12(1):29–31.

191. Wang MS, Li J, Di HX, et al. *Chin J Integr Med*. 2007;13(2):98–102.

192. Liu ZG, Xiong ZM, Yu XY. *Zhongguo Zhong Xi Jie He Za Zhi*. 2003;23(5): 351–353. [Article in Chinese].

193. Cao XY, Xu YL, Lin XJ. *Zhongguo Zhong XI Yi Jie He Za Zhi*. 2006;26(5):443–445. [Article in Chinese].

194. Zhou QJ. *Advances in Chinese Medicinal Materials Research*. Singapore: World Scientific; 1985. p. 216.

195. Qian ZW, Mao SJ, Cai XC, et al. *Chin Med J*. 1990;103(8):647–651.

196. Qian ZW, Mao SJ, Cai XC, et al. *Chin J Integr Trad West Med*. 1987;7(5):268–269, 287.

197. Mao SP, Cheng KL, Zhou YF. *Zhongguo Zhong Xi Yi Jie He Za Zhi*. 2004;24(2):121–123. [Article in Chinese].

198. Tang LL, Sheng JF, Xu CH, et al. *J Int Med Res*. 2009;37(3):662–667.

199. Kusum M, Klinbuayaem V, Bunjob M, et al. *J Med Assoc Thai*. 2004;87(9): 1065–1070.

200. Sangkitporn S, Shide L, Klinbuayaem V, et al. *Southeast Asian J Trop Med Public Health*. 2005;36(3):704–708.

201. Liu J, Yang M, Du X. *Cochrane Database Syst Rev*. 2004(3): CD003711.

202. Li SQ, Yuan RX, Gao H. *Chung Kuo Chung Hsi I Chieh Ho Tsa Chih*. 1995;15(2):77–80.

203. Lei ZY, Qin H, Liao JZ. *Zhongguo Zhong Xi Yi Jie He Za Zhi*. 1994;14(4):199–202. 195, [Article in Chinese].

204. Yang QY, Lu S, Sun HR. *Zhongguo Zhong Xi Yi Jie He Za Zhi*. 2010;30(7):699–701.

205. Yang QY, Lu S, Sun HR. *Chin J Integr Med*. 2011;17(2):146–149.

206. Liu KZ, Li JB, Lu HL, et al. *Zhongguo Zhong Yao Za Zhi*. 2004;29(3):264–266. [Article in Chinese].

207. Li ZP, Cao Q, Xing QS. *Zhongguo Zhong Xi Yi Jie He Za Zhi*. 2003;23(12):891–894. [Article in Chinese].

208. Zhang JG, Yang N, He H. *Zhongguo Zhong Xi Yi Jie He Za Zhi*. 2005;25(5):400–403. [Article in Chinese].

209. Zhou ZL, Yu P, Lin D. *Zhongguo Zhong Xi Yi Jie He Za Zhi*. 2001;21(10):747–749. [Article in Chinese].

210. Zhang JG, Gao DS, Wei GH. *Zhongguo Zhong Xi Yi Jie He Za Zhi*. 2002;22(5):346–348. [Article in Chinese].

211. Wang F, Xiao MD, Liao B, et al. *Zhongguo Zhong Xi Yi Jie He Za Zhi*. 2008;28(6):495–498. [Article in Chinese].

212. Ai P, Yong G, Dingkun G, et al. *J Ethnopharmacol*. 2008;116(3):413–421.

213. Ahmed MS, Hou SH, Battaglia MC, et al. *Am J Kidney Dis*. 2007;50(6):1028–1032.

214. Leehey DJ, Casini T, Massey D. *Am J Kidney Dis*. 2010;55(4):772.

215. Wang HY, Chen YP. *Zhongguo Zhong Xi Yi Jie He Za Zhi*. 2004;24(7):589–592. [Article in Chinese].

216. Lu ZM, Yu YR, Tang H, et al. *Sichuan Da Xue Xue Bao Yi Xue Ban*. 2005;36(4):529–532.

217. Li SM, Yan JX, Yang L. *Zhongguo Zhong Xi Yi Jie He Za Zhi*. 2006;26(6):504–507.

218. Chen LP, Zhou QL, Yang JH. *Zhong Nan Da Xue Xue Bao Yi Xue Ban*. 2004;29(2):152–153.

219. McCulloch M, See C, Shu XJ, et al. *J Clin Oncol*. 2006;24(3):419–430.

220. Taixiang W, Munro AJ, Guanjian L. *Cochrane Database Syst Rev*. 2005(1):CD004540.

221. Wu P, Dugoua JJ, Eyawo O, et al. *J Exp Clin Cancer Res*. 2009;28:112.

222. Dong J, Gu HL, Ma CT, et al. *Zhongguo Zhong Xi Yi Jie He Za Zhi*. 2005;25(10): 872–875. [Article in Chinese].

223. Du X, Zhang ZL. *Chung Hsi I Chieh Ho Tsa Chih*. 1986;6(5) 258–259, 271–274.

224. Tan YW, Yin YM, Yu XJ. *Zhongguo Zhong Xi Yi Jie He Za Zhi*. 2001;21(5):351–353.

225. Cho JH, Cho CK, Shin JW, et al. *Complement Ther Med*. 2009;17(3):141–146.

226. Yu SY, Ouyang HT, Yang JY, et al. *J Ethnopharmacol*. 2007;110(2):352–355.

227. Tadaki S, Yamada S, Miyazawa N, et al. *Jap J Toxicol Environ Health*. 1995;41(6): 463–469.

228. Yamamoto H, Mizutani T, Nomura H. *Yakugaku Zasshi*. 1982;102(6):596–601.

229. Wong BY, Lau BH, Tadi PP, et al. *Mutat Res*. 1992;279(3):209–215.

230. Su ZZ, He YY, Chen G. *Zhongguo Zhong Xi Yi Jie He Za Zhi*. 1993;13(5) 259–260, 269–272.

231. Chu DT, Wong WL, Mavligit GM. *J Clin Lab Immunol*. 1988;25(3):125–129.

232. Chu DT, Sun Y, Lin JR. *Zhong Xi Yi Jie He Za Zhi*. 1989;9(6):351–354, 326.

233. James LF, Shupe JL, Binns W, et al. *Am J Vet Res*. 1967;28(126):1379–1388.

234. James LF, Keeler RF, Binns W. *Am J Vet Res*. 1969;30(3):377–380.

235. Molyneux RJ, James LF. *Science*. 1982;216(4542):190–191.

236. Su ZZ, He YY, Chen G. *Zhongguo Zhong Xi Yi Jie He Za Zhi*. 1993;13(5):259–260, 269–272.

237. Jiangbo Z, Xuying W, Yuping Z, et al. *J Appl Toxicol*. 2009;29(5):381–385.

Bearberry

(*Arctostaphylos uva ursi* (L.) Spreng.)

Synonyms

Arctostaphylos officinalis Wimm., *Arbutus uva ursi* L. (botanical synonyms), mountain cranberry, green manzanita, uva ursi (Engl), Uvae ursi folium (Lat), Bärentraube (Ger), busserole, raisin d'ours (Fr), uva d'orso, uva ursina (Ital), melbær (Dan).

What is it?

The Arctostaphylos genus contains 50 species indigenous to western North America; *A. uva ursi* has circumpolar distribution and is found in central and northern Europe, as well as in North America.[1,2] Bearberry leaves have been used as a urinary antiseptic in the UK since the 13th century.[1] It is also a traditional herb of the Native Americans, who used the leaves for ceremonial smoking. However, their main use was in the form of a tea to treat venereal disease and inflammation of the genitourinary tract.[3] The berries of *Arctostaphylos* species have provided food, not only for wildlife such as birds and bears but also for humans. *Arctostaphylos* species suppress the growth of neighbouring plants due to the hydroquinone formed from the arbutin in their leaves, bark and roots.[3]

Effects

Antibacterial, astringent and anti-inflammatory effects in the genitourinary tract.

Traditional view

Bearberry was traditionally used for its astringent property and was considered of great value in diseases of the bladder and kidneys, strengthening and imparting tone to the urinary passages and alleviating inflammation of the urinary tract.[4] Uses by the Eclectic physicians included chronic irritation of the bladder, enuresis, excessive mucus and bloody discharges in the urine, chronic diarrhoea, dysentery, menorrhagia, leucorrhoea, diabetes, chronic gonorrhoea and strangury.[5]

Summary actions

Urinary antiseptic, astringent, anti-inflammatory.

Can be used for

Indications supported by clinical trials

Cystitis, recurrent cystitis (in conjunction with other herbs).

Traditional therapeutic uses

Urinary infections such as cystitis, urethritis, prostatitis, pyelitis, lithuria, diarrhoea and intestinal irritations, and any condition requiring an astringent action including chronic diarrhoea. The specific indication listed in the *British Herbal Pharmacopoeia* 1983 is acute catarrhal cystitis with dysuria and highly acid urine.[6]

May also be used for

Extrapolations from pharmacological studies

Internally and externally as adjuvant treatment of inflammatory conditions such as contact dermatitis, inflammatory oedema and arthritis.

Other applications

As a whitening agent for the skin and may assist in the control of hyperpigmentary disorders.[7]

Preparations

Dried leaves as a cold infusion or liquid extract for internal or external use. Cold water extraction of powdered leaves results in better levels of arbutin and lower levels of tannins compared to hot water extraction.[8]

Dosage

- 3 to 12 g dried leaf per day (the latter equivalent to at least 700 mg arbutin) prepared as an infusion or cold macerate
- 4.5 to 8.5 mL of 1:2 liquid extract per day, 11 to 22 mL of 1:5 tincture per day or the equivalent in tablet or capsule form.

Some studies have found that the antimicrobial effect of bearberry is optimal when the urine has an alkaline pH.

However, the majority of urinary tract infections produce acid urine. Alkalinisation of the urine may therefore be beneficial in conjunction with herbal therapy using bearberry (although the need for this has been questioned in a recent study). This can be achieved, at least in the short term, by concurrent administration of bicarbonate or a proprietary urinary alkalinising product. An alkaline-forming diet high in fruit and vegetables could also be consumed during treatment. Consumption of plenty of water during treatment is also advised.

Duration of use

Due to its high tannin content, bearberry is not suitable for prolonged internal use at higher doses.

Summary assessment of safety

There is a very low risk associated with the short-term administration of bearberry, but its use should be avoided during pregnancy and lactation.

Technical data

Botany

Arctostaphylos uva ursi is a small, evergreen, prostrate, mat-forming shrub belonging to the Ericaceae (heath) family. The leathery leaves are alternate, obovate from a wedge-shaped base, 1 to 2 cm long, dark green on the upper surface and pale green underneath. The small pink flowers with a bell-shaped corolla are arranged in drooping clusters. The fruit is shiny, small, round and scarlet-red.[4,9]

Adulteration

Substitution with other species of Ericaceae is relatively common in commerce. *Vaccinium vitis idaea* L., *V. uliginosum* L., *V. myrtillus* L. (bilberry), *Gaultheria procumbens* L. (wintergreen), *Arctostaphylos alpinus* (L.), *Buxus sempervirens* L. (box) have all been detected in batches of 'bearberry leaves'.[10] According to the *German Pharmacopoeia*, samples containing less than 6% arbutin should be considered as adulterated.

Arctostaphylos uva ursi is protected and/or has restrictions for wildcrafting in several areas of Europe.[11]

Key constituents

- Hydroquinone glycosides (normally between 6.3% and 9.2% – higher in autumn crops)[12] including arbutin and methylarbutin[13]
- Polyphenols (predominantly gallotannins); phenolic acids, flavonoids, triterpenes.[13]

Interestingly, arbutin is found at high concentrations in some plants capable of surviving extreme and sustained dehydration.[14]

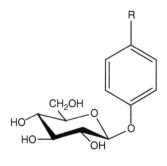

	R
Arbutin	OH
Methylarbutin	OCH$_3$

Hydroquinone derivatives

Pharmacodynamics

Antimicrobial activity

There is some debate as to whether the antimicrobial effect of bearberry is due to hydroquinone esters such as arbutin or to free hydroquinone.[13] The antimicrobial activities of arbutin and an aqueous extract of bearberry were tested in vitro against bacterial strains implicated in urinary tract infections. The antibacterial activity of arbutin was directly correlated with the beta-glucosidase activity of the bacteria. (This enzyme converts arbutin into free hydroquinone.) The highest enzyme activity was found in Streptococcus, Klebsiella and Enterobacter, the lowest in *Escherichia coli*.[15] Arbutin (128 µg/L) inhibited three of eight clinical isolates of *Pseudomonas aeruginosa* tested in vitro.[16] Arbutin and hydroquinone inhibited the growth of *Ureaplasma urealyticum* and *Mycoplasma hominis* in vitro.[17] These bacteria are associated with non-gonococcal urethritis.

Piceoside, a glucoside isolated from bearberry, did not demonstrate antibacterial activity in vitro, but its aglycone p-hydroxyacetophenone showed activity against *Proteus vulgaris*, *Enterobacter aerogenes* and *Bacillus subtilis*.[18] Another study found antimicrobial activity for bearberry extracts in vitro against *E. coli*, *Proteus vulgaris*, *Enterobacter aerogenes*, *Streptococcus faecalis*, *Staphylococcus aureus*, *Salmonella typhi* and *Candida albicans*.[19] The summer and autumn leaves were more potent than the winter leaves.[20]

The antibacterial activity of various agents was tested in vitro using 74 different strains of bacteria isolated from the urinary tract including *E. coli*, *Proteus mirabilis*, *Pseudomonas aeruginosa*, *Staphylococcus aureus* and species of Enterobacter, Citrobacter and Klebsiella. Urine was collected from healthy volunteers 3 h after oral administration of 0.1 g or 1.0 g of arbutin; several synthetic antibiotics were also tested. Of all test substances, only gentamicin, nalidixic acid and urine collected after intake of 1.0 g of arbutin and adjusted to pH 8 were active against every strain used.[21]

A hydroethanolic extract of bearberry was amongst the most active of 14 traditional Canadian medicinal plants tested against a wide variety of strains of *Neisseria gonorrhoeae*, including isolates resistant to antibiotics.[22] A minimum inhibiting concentration of 32 µg/mL was demonstrated in vitro.

A study of the dry leaf extract of bearberry on the course of acute bacterial pyelonephritis (caused by *E. coli*) in white rats showed that bearberry extract (25 mg/kg) had a marked antibacterial and nephroprotective effect.[23]

Samples of both normal urine and urine collected from healthy subjects after consuming bearberry tea were compared for resistance to bacterial contamination. Urine from the bearberry tea drinkers was more bacteriostatic than normal urine samples. However, the addition of arbutin to normal urine did not result in the same bacteriostatic activity. A series of solutions were then tested for their inhibition of the growth of strains of *Staph. aureus* and *E. coli* in vitro. The solutions included hydroquinone, methylhydroquinone and arbutin, normal urine and urine from bearberry tea drinkers. They were tested at normal pH and at pH elevated to 8.0 by the addition of potassium hydroxide. Only the hydroquinone and methylhydroquinone solutions inhibited bacterial growth at normal pH. However, incubation of bacteria with bearberry tea drinkers' urine adjusted to pH 8 also resulted in inhibition of bacterial growth. This inhibitory effect was also seen for urine adjusted to pH 8 from subjects given pure arbutin.[24] The authors suggested that antibacterial activity would only occur when the excretion products of arbutin (hydroquinone paired with glucuronate and sulphate) appear in sufficiently high concentrations in an alkaline urine. It was hypothesised that at an alkaline pH these excretion products of arbutin released small amounts of free hydroquinone in the presence of bacteria, thereby conferring antibacterial activity to the urine. The maximum antibacterial effect from the hydroquinone glucuronides and sulphates formed from arbutin was obtained about 3 to 4h after taking the herb.[25] Free hydroquinone is only excreted in trace amounts, which is desirable given the toxic potential of this agent.

A recent paper has expressed a contradictory view. In this study, urine was collected from four healthy individuals after ingestion of 420 mg of arbutin.[26] The samples were added to an *E. coli* suspension and it was noted that the concentration of hydroquinone in bacteria was 20-fold higher than a control. The authors commented that the pH of urine is unlikely to be important, as the intracellular pH of *E. coli* is not affected by urine alkalinisation. They concluded that deconjugating enzymes such as beta-glucuronidases found in the bacteria enrich and deconjugate hydroquinone glucuronides and/or sulphates regardless of pH. The pH of the test urine was not stated, but in the study design attempts to increase it to more than 6.5 via a vegetarian diet were instituted.

Urine produced by a healthy person consuming a meat and fish diet is typically in the pH range 4.5 to 6.0; a vegetarian diet will make urine more alkaline. A urine of pH >7 during a urinary tract infection indicates infection by a micro-organism capable of splitting urea, with the release of ammonia.[27] Urea-splitting organisms include *Proteus spp.*, *Klebsiella spp.*, some *Citrobacter spp.*, some *Haemophilus spp.*, *Bilophila wadsworthia*, the yeast *Cryptococcus neoformans* and several other bacteria and fungi.[28] Infection with these organisms should be particularly susceptible to treatment with bearberry if alkaline urine does enhance its activity. Alkalinisation of the urine with

buffering agents (for example containing sodium bicarbonate, sodium citrate, citric acid and tartaric acid) in conjunction with bearberry intake may prove to be clinically effective for the treatment of cystitis caused by non-urea-splitting bacteria, but given the conflicting findings noted above, this requires further research.

The antibacterial effect of bearberry may also be useful in the gastrointestinal tract. An aqueous extract of bearberry was found to modulate cell surface hydrophobicity and demonstrated antibacterial effects on ten strains of *Helicobacter pylori* in vitro.[29] The research team concluded that the hydrolysable tannins were largely responsible, as pure tannic acid produced comparable results.

Anti-inflammatory and antiallergic activities

Co-administration of arbutin (50 mg/kg, oral) and indomethacin (subcutaneous) showed an inhibitory effect on swelling in a delayed-type hypersensitivity model, which was stronger than that of indomethacin alone.[30] In the same model, arbutin (10 and 50 mg/kg, oral) plus prednisolone or dexamethasone showed stronger effects than each of the anti-inflammatory drugs alone.[31] Arbutin may therefore have a synergistic anti-inflammatory activity on type IV allergic reaction-induced inflammation. In the same model, oral administration of a bearberry methanolic extract (100 mg/kg) demonstrated an inhibitory effect on swelling. When administered simultaneously with subcutaneous prednisolone, the inhibitory effect was more potent than that of prednisolone alone.[32]

Although ointments containing 1% and 2% aqueous extract of bearberry did not inhibit the ear swelling caused by experimentally induced contact dermatitis or carrageenan-induced paw oedema in rats and mice, they did increase the anti-inflammatory effect of a steroid ointment (dexamethasone). Co-administration of bearberry did not increase the side effects of dexamethasone.[33] Topical doses of bearberry might also increase the anti-inflammatory effects of other steroid-like compounds, such as plant-derived saponins.

Effect on melanin synthesis

Arbutin at a concentration of 5×10^{-5} M decreased melanin content to approximately 39% when compared to untreated melanoma cells in vitro, without affecting cell growth. Tyrosinase activity also dropped significantly in the arbutin-treated cells. (This enzyme is involved in melanin synthesis.) Arbutin was not hydrolysed to hydroquinone, suggesting that the observed inhibitory effect was for arbutin itself, not hydroquinone.[34] Further studies have revealed that the depigmenting mechanism of arbutin in humans involves inhibition of melanosomal tyrosinase activity, rather than the suppression of expression and synthesis of tyrosinase.[35]

A 50% methanolic extract of bearberry inhibited melanin synthesis in vitro. Both the bearberry extract and arbutin had an inhibitory effect on tyrosinase activity and inhibited the production of melanin by both tyrosinase and autoxidation.[7] Bearberry extract could have a bleaching effect on freckles and may assist in the control of hyperpigmentary disorders.

Other activity

Oral doses of arbutin (50 mg/kg) suppressed experimentally induced cough reflex. The effect of arbutin was stronger than that of the non-narcotic antitussive dropropizine and comparable to that of codeine.[36]

Oral administration of a bearberry infusion (3 g/L in drinking water) to healthy rats fed a standard diet containing calcium (8 g/kg) and magnesium (2 g/kg) did not induce significant diuresis, nor affect calcium or citrate concentration levels.[37]

Aqueous and methanolic extracts of bearberry have demonstrated in vitro molluscicidal activity against the freshwater snail *Biomphalaria glabrata* (the intermediate host of schistosomiasis). The methanol extract was active at a concentration of 50 ppm.[38]

A methanol extract of bearberry showed algicidal activity when tested in ponds. It is believed the tannins precipitated the algal proteins.[39]

Pharmacokinetics

Urinary excretion of phenolic metabolites after the oral administration of either bearberry leaf tea or arbutin occurs within 1 to 2h and reaches a maximum 4h after administration. In healthy subjects given bearberry tea, 70% to 75% of the administered dose was excreted within 24h. Arbutin is altered after its passage through the body; it only occurs in trace amounts in urine when high doses are given. Free hydroquinone is only excreted in trace amounts, if at all.

It has been suggested that there are two possible processes for the absorption and metabolism of arbutin.[40] The major process involves the absorption of intact arbutin by small intestinal enterocytes via the sodium-glucose pump. On first-pass metabolism in the liver, arbutin is deconjugated to hydroquinone and then reconjugated to sulphate and glucuronide phase II derivatives, which are then excreted via the urine. The minor process involves the conversion to free hydroquinone of arbutin in the colon by the action of bacterial beta-glucosidase. The hydroquinone is then converted by colonic enterocytes into sulphate and glucuronide derivatives which are absorbed into the bloodstream and passed into the urine.

In a crossover study involving six healthy volunteers, enteric-coated bearberry tablets demonstrated the same bioavailability within a 24-h period as an equivalent bearberry extract. The release of arbutin metabolites was retarded by at least 3h with the tablets. In a pilot study conducted prior to this main study, no free hydroquinone was found in the urine of volunteers, although the above hydroquinone derivatives were found.[41] This study was designed to compare the bioavailability of enterically coated tablets containing bearberry extract with uncoated tablets, but it does also add some support to the above metabolic pathways. Additionally, a small, randomised crossover trial in sixteen adults evaluated the bioavailability of an aqueous solution of bearberry as compared to film-coated tablets.[42] The maximum mean urinary concentration of hydroquinone equivalents was marginally higher and peaked a little earlier in the tea group, although this was not statistically significant. The authors concluded there were no significant differences between the two groups in terms of metabolites or total amounts of hydroquinone equivalents excreted.

Some other studies investigating the elimination of arbutin in rats have arrived at different conclusions, which cast doubt on their relevance to humans. In these studies, orally administered arbutin was excreted unchanged in urine[43] and oral administration of bearberry tea resulted in the excretion of six unidentified phenolic compounds, but no hydroquinone. No degradation products were observed after the perfusion of isolated rat liver with arbutin, thus leading to the conclusion that it was hydrolysed in the kidneys.[44] As noted above, the results of these studies are not supported by the human studies. Moreover, in the case of the orally administered arbutin, the authors may have actually measured arbutin metabolites and mistakenly assigned them as arbutin.

Clinical trials

Urinary disorders

In a double blind, placebo-controlled, randomised clinical trial, 57 women who had experienced at least three episodes of cystitis during the preceding year received either herbal medicine or placebo. The herbal medicine consisted of bearberry extract (standardised for arbutin and methylarbutin content) and extract of dandelion root and leaf (dose of individual herbs not specified). Treatment for 1 month significantly reduced the recurrence of cystitis during the 1-year follow-up period, with no incidence of cystitis in the herbal group and a 23% occurrence in the placebo group (p<0.05). No side effects were reported.[45]

Toxicology and other safety data

Toxicology

Hydroquinone is a recognised toxic compound. However, arbutin and bearberry extracts are considerably less toxic than hydroquinone, as somewhat evidenced by the studies cited below.

The oral LD_{50} of hydroquinone as a 2% aqueous solution has been reported as between 320 and 550 mg/kg in various laboratory animals.[46] Hydroquinone is non-mutagenic in the Ames test but induces chromosome aberrations and karyotypic effects in eukaryotic cells.[47] In contrast, arbutin did not induce mutations in concentrations up to 10^{-2} M in a gene mutation assay. An increase in mutation frequency was observed with concentrations of 10^{-3} M and higher when arbutin was preincubated with beta-glucosidase. Hydroquinone, used as a positive control, also exhibited clear effects. In vivo, hydroquinone administered by intraperitoneal injection induced elevated micronucleus incidences. However, there was no induction of micronuclei in bone marrow when arbutin was administered orally (0.5 to 2.0 g/kg). This research suggests that arbutin itself is not mutagenic, but any generated hydroquinone could exert a mutagenic potential.[48]

Contraindications

According to the *British Herbal Compendium*, bearberry is contraindicated in kidney disorders[13] but there is no evidence to support this, and the contraindication probably arose out of a theoretical caution.

According to the Commission E, bearberry is contraindicated in pregnancy and lactation and for children less than 12 years of age.[49]

Special warnings and precautions

Bearberry is not suitable for prolonged use. Use cautiously in highly inflamed or ulcerated conditions of the gastrointestinal tract.[50]

In principle, the prolonged use of herbs with high levels of tannins is inappropriate in constipation, iron deficiency anaemia and malnutrition.[51]

Interactions

Concomitant acidification of the urine (for instance by medication) may result in a reduction of efficacy,[24] although this is hypothetical and of uncertain relevance to the urinary antiseptic mechanism of bearberry.

Oral or topical use of bearberry or arbutin has been observed to augment the anti-inflammatory effects of indomethacin,[30] prednisolone,[31,32] and dexamethasone[31,33] in experimental models. The clinical relevance of these findings is uncertain.

Bearberry extract markedly potentiated the action of beta-lactam antibiotics against methicillin-resistant *Staph. aureus* in vitro. The constituent corilagin (a polyphenol) was responsible for the activity.[52] However, whether this leads to a clinical interaction is uncertain.

The high tannin levels will cause interference with the absorption of various nutrients and drugs, especially metal ions, thiamine and alkaloids. Bearberry should be consumed at least 2 h away from oral thiamine, mineral supplements such as iron and alkaloid-containing drugs.[51]

Use in pregnancy and lactation

Pregnancy category C – has caused or is associated with a substantial risk of causing harmful effects on the foetus or neonate without causing malformations.[10]

There is a minor theoretical risk to fetal development due to the uterotonic properties of arbutin in vivo.[53,54] However, arbutin also occurs in food: wheat products (1 to 10 ppm), pears (4 to 15 ppm), and coffee and tea (0.1 ppm).[55]

The transfer of arbutin or hydroquinone to breast milk is not advisable, and therefore the herb should be avoided in lactation.

Effects on ability to drive and use machines

No adverse effects expected.

Side effects

Hydroquinone depigmenting creams may cause exogenous ochronosis (hyperpigmentation)[56] and/or allergic contact dermatitis.[57] However, these side effects have not been reported for cosmetic creams containing bearberry.[56]

A case of bilateral bull's-eye maculopathy has been reported in a 56-year-old woman after ingestion of bearberry tea for 3 years, dose unknown.[58] While it is generally acknowledged that bearberry inhibits melanin production, which is present in ocular tissue, therapeutic doses for short periods of time are routinely considered safe.

Due to the high tannin content, internal use of high doses of bearberry may cause cramping, nausea, vomiting and constipation.

Overdosage

Inflammation of the urinary mucosa and haematuria have been claimed as a consequence of high doses,[59] and there is a stated risk of liver damage.[60] Long-term use of high doses is to be avoided.

Safety in children

Treatment is not recommended for children under the age of 6 years.

Regulatory status in selected countries

Bearberry is official in the *European Pharmacopoeia* (2006).

Bearberry is covered by a positive Commission E Monograph and has the following application: inflammatory disorders of the lower urinary tract.

Bearberry is on the UK General Sale List and in France the herb is accepted for the internal treatment of benign urinary infections and to promote the renal elimination of water.

Bearberry does not have GRAS status. However, it is freely available as a 'dietary supplement' in the USA under DSHEA legislation (1994 Dietary Supplement Health and Education Act). Bearberry has been present in the following over-the-counter (OTC) drug products: weight control drug products and orally administered menstrual drug products. The FDA, however, advises: 'that based on evidence currently available, there is inadequate data to establish general recognition of the safety and effectiveness of these ingredients for the specified uses'.

Bearberry is not included in Part 4 of Schedule 4 of the Therapeutic Goods Act Regulations of Australia and is freely available for sale.

References

1. Mabberley DJ. *The Plant Book*, 2nd ed. Cambridge: Cambridge University Press; 1997. p. 53.

2. Evans WC. *Trease and Evans' Pharmacognosy*, 14th ed. London: WB Saunders; 1996. p. 223.

3. Brinker FJ. *Eclectic Dispensatory of Botanical Therapeutics*, vol 2, *Section 1: Native Healing Gifts*. Sandy: Eclectic Medical Publications; 1995. pp. 19–23.

4. Grieve MI. *A Modern Herbal*, vol 1. New York: Dover; 1971. pp. 89–90.

5. Felter HW, Lloyd JU. *King's American Dispensatory*, 18th ed., 3rd rev, vol 2, 1905. Reprinted by Eclectic Medical Publications; 1983. pp. 2038–2040.

6. British Herbal Medicine Association's Scientific Committee. *British Herbal Pharmacopoeia*. West York: BHMA; 1983. pp. 29–30.

7. Matsuda H, Nakamura S, Shiomoto H, et al. *Yakugaku Zasshi*. 1992;112(4): 276–282.

8. Frohne D. *Pharm Ztg*. 1980;125: 2582–2583.

9. Launert EL. *The Hamlyn Guide to Edible and Medicinal Plants of Britain and Northern Europe*. London: Hamlyn; 1981. p. 128.

10. Mills S, Bone K. *The Essential Guide to Herbal Safety*. St Louis: Elsevier; 2005. p. 259.

11. Lange D. *Europe's Medicinal and Aromatic Plants: Their Use, Trade and Conservation*. Traffic International; 1998. p. III.

12. Parejo I, Viladomat F, Bastida J, et al. *Phytochem Anal*. 2001;12(5):336–339.

13. British Herbal Medicine Association British Herbal Compendium, vol 1. Bournemouth: BHMA; 1992. pp. 211–213.

14. Oliver AE, Crowe LM, De Araujo PS, et al. *Biochim Biophys Acta*. 1996;1302(1):69–78.

15. Jahodar L, Jilek P, Patkova M, et al. *Cesk Farm*. 1985;34(5):174–178.

16. Ng TB, Ling JM, Wang ZT, et al. *Gen Pharmacol*. 1996;27(7):1237–1240.

17. Robertson JA, Howard LA. *J Clin Microbiol*. 1987;25(1):160–161.

18. Jahodar L, Kolb I. *Pharmazie*. 1990;45(6):446.

19. Holopainen M, Jabodar L, Seppanen-Laakso T, et al. *Acta Pharm Fenn*. 1988;97(4): 197–202.

20. Skvortsov SS, Khan-Fimina VA. *Fitontsidy Mater Soveshch*. 1969;6:207–209.

21. Kedzia B, Wrocinski T, Mrugasiewicz K, et al. *Med Dosw Mikrobiol*. 1975;27: 305–314.

22. Cybulska P, Thakur SD, Foster BC, et al. *Sex Trans Dis*. 2011;38(12):1–5.

23. Nikolaev SM, Shantanova LN, Mondodoev AG, et al. *Rastitel'Nye Resursy*. 1996;32(3):118–123.

24. Frohne D. *Planta Med*. 1970;18:1–25.

25. German Federal Minister of Justice. German Commission E for Human Medicine Monograph, Bundes-Anzeiger (German Federal Gazette) no. 228, dated 05.12.84 and no. 109, dated 15.06.1994.

26. Siegers C, Bodinet C, Ali SS, et al. *Phytomedicine*. 2003;10(suppl 4):58–60.

27. Bouchier IAD, Morris JS, eds. *Clinical Skills – A System of Clinical Examination*, 2nd ed. London: WB Saunders; 1982. p. 243.

28. Baron EJ, Peterson LR, Finegold SM. *Bailey and Scott's Diagnostic Microbiology*, 9th ed. St Louis: Mosby Year Book; 1994. p. 106.

29. Annuk H, Hirmo S, Turi E, et al. *FEMS Microbiol Lett*. 1999;172(1):41–45.

30. Matsuda H, Tanaka T, Kubo M. *Yakugaku Zasshi*. 1991;111(4–5):253–258.

31. Matsuda H, Nakata H, Tanaka T, et al. *Yakugaku Zasshi*. 1990;110(1):68–76.

32. Kubo M, Ito M, Nakata H, et al. *Yakugaku Zasshi*. 1990;110(1):59–67.

33. Matsuda H, Nakamura S, Tanaka T, et al. *Yakugaku Zasshi*. 1992;112(9):673–677.

34. Akiu S, Suzuki Y, Asahara T, et al. *Nippon Hifuka Gakkai Zasshi*. 1991;101(6): 609–613.

35. Maeda K, Fukuda M. *J Pharmacol Exp Ther*. 1996;276(2):765–769.

36. Strapkova A, Jahodar L, Nosalova G. *Pharmazie*. 1991;46(8):611–612.

37. Grases F, Melero G, Costa-Bauza R, et al. *Int Urol Nephrol*. 1994;26(5):507–511.

38. Schaufelberger D, Hostettmann K. *Planta Med*. 1983;48(2):105–107.

39. Ayoub SMH, Yankov LK, Hussein-Ayoub SM. *Fitoterapia*. 1985;6(4):227–229.

40. Garcia de Arriba S, Stammwitz U, Pickartz S, et al. *Z Phytother*. 2010;31(2):95–97.

41. Paper DH, Koehler J, Franz G. *Pharm Pharmacol Lett*. 1993;3:63–66.

42. Schindler G, Patzak U, Brinkhaus B, et al. *J Clin Pharmacol*. 2002;42(8):920–927.

43. Jahodar L, Leifertova I, Lisa M. *Pharmazie*. 1983;38(11):780–781.

44. Leifertova I, Lisa M, Jahodar L, et al. *Rozvoj Farm Ramci Ved-Tech Revoluce, Sb Prednasck Sjezdu Cesk Farm Spol*, 7th ed. Prague: University of Karlova; 1979. Meeting date 1977; pp. 41–43.

45. Larsson B, Jonasson A, Fianu S. *Curr Ther Res Clin Exp*. 1993;53(4):441–443.

46. Woodard G, Hagan CE, Radomski JL. *Fed Proc*. 1949;8:348.

47. Devillers J, Boule P, Vasseur P, et al. *Ecotoxicol Environ Saf*. 1990;19(3): 327–354.

48. Mueller L, Kasper P. *Mutat Res*. 1996;360(3):291–292.

49. German Federal Minister of Justice. *German Commission E for Human Medicine Monograph*, Bundes-Anzeiger (German Federal Gazette) no. 109, dated 15.06.94; no. 19, dated 28.01.1994.

50. Blumenthal M, Busse WR, Goldberg A, et al. *The Complete German Commission E Monographs*. Texas: American Botanical Council; 2000. pp. 224–225.

51. Mills S, Bone K. *The Essential Guide to Herbal Safety*. St Louis: Elsevier; 2005. p. 260.

52. Shimizu M, Shiota S, Mizushima T, et al. *Antimicrob Agents Chemother*. 2001;45(11):3198–3201.

53. Shipochliev T. *Vet Med Nauki*. 1981;18(4):94–98.

54. Itabashi M, Aihara H, Inoue T, et al. *Iyakuhin Kenkyu*. 1988;19:282–297.

55. Deisinger PJ, Hill TS, English JC. *J Toxicol Environ Health*. 1996;47(1):31–46.

56. Howard KL, Ferner BB. *Cutis*. 1990;45(3):180–182.

57. Engasser PG, Maibach HI. *J Am Acad Dermatol*. 1981;5(2):143–147.

58. Wang L, Del Priore LV. *Am J Ophthalmol*. 2004;137(6):1135–1137.

59. Stübler M, Krug E. *Leesers Lehrbuch der Homöopathie, Pflanzliche Arzneistoffe II*. Heidelberg: Haug-Verlag; 1988. pp. 403–406.

60. Standardzulassung für Fertigarzneimittel. *Pharmazeutischer Verlag, Deutscher Apotheker*, Frankfurt/Main, 1987/89, Verlag.

Synonyms

Berberis vulgaris: barberry (Engl), Berberidis cortex (Lat), Berberitze, Sauerdorn (Ger), epinevinette, vinettier (Fr), berberi (Ital), almindelig Berberis (Dan). *Hydrastis canadensis*: golden seal (Engl), Hydrastidis rhizoma (Lat), Goldsiegel, Kanadische Gelbwurzel (Ger), guldsegl (Dan).

What is it?

There are more than 500 species of the Berberis genus. *Berberis vulgaris*, the common or European barberry, is indigenous to Europe and naturalised in Britain. Many parts of the plant have been utilised: the fine wood for turning, the root and stems providing dyestuff for fabrics, leather and wood (also formerly a hair dye) and the fruit for jams.[1] The root and stem bark are used medicinally.

Hydrastis canadensis was known to the Cherokee nation long before the settlement of America by Europeans. They employed its underground portion for dyeing and as an internal remedy, and acquainted the early settlers with most of its properties.[2] Hydrastis became a very prominent herb in the Eclectic tradition. The plant is indigenous to central and eastern North America, but its population is now much reduced through overexploitation.[3,4] Hence, it is preferable to use cultivated sources of Hydrastis because of its endangered status. The high price commanded by the root and rhizome means that Hydrastis is susceptible to adulteration.

The activities of Berberis and Hydrastis are thought to be mainly due to their isoquinoline alkaloids, in particular berberine and hydrastine (the latter occurs only in Hydrastis). Other plants also contain berberine, but will generally not be examined in this monograph unless they provide some relevant insights regarding this phytochemical. However, most of the research cited here for berberine will be relevant to its other herbal sources such as *Coptis chinensis* and *Phellodendron amurense*.

Effects

Berberis vulgaris: controls gastrointestinal infections; improves the flow of bile.

Hydrastis canadensis: in addition to the above, restores the integrity of mucous membranes of the respiratory and digestive tract, and promotes gastric digestive processes.

Traditional view

Berberis vulgaris has had a long history of use in Western herbalism. A decoction was taken in the spring months as a blood purifier and used externally as a mouth and eyewash. The Eclectics regarded Berberis primarily as a tonic, but it was also used for conditions affecting the liver and gallbladder, and for diarrhoea, dysentery and parasitic infestations including malaria.[5,6]

Hydrastis canadensis was specifically indicated for catarrhal states of the mucous membranes when unaccompanied by acute inflammation (except in the case of acute purulent otitis media, where it was considered to work better than in the chronic condition). Muscular debility was another key traditional indication. As a bitter stomachic, it was used to sharpen appetite and aid digestion, and was considered valuable for disordered states of the digestive apparatus, especially when functional in character. Hydrastis was considered a valuable local agent in affections of the nose and throat. It was also used in cutaneous diseases, especially when dependent upon gastric difficulties; concurrent internal and external use was said to hasten the cure.[7] In addition, Hydrastis was recommended for submucosal myoma, haemorrhagic endometriosis and heavy menstrual bleeding.[8]

Summary actions

Berberis vulgaris: antimicrobial, cholagogue, choleretic, antiemetic, mild laxative, bitter.

Hydrastis canadensis: stomachic, reputed oxytocic, antihaemorrhagic, anticatarrhal, trophorestorative for mucous membranes, antimicrobial, bitter, anti-inflammatory, depurative, vulnerary, choleretic.

Can be used for

Indications supported by clinical trials

From clinical trials on berberine: acute infectious diarrhoea; trachoma (as eyedrops); giardiasis; hypertyraminaemia; type 2 diabetes mellitus; elevated blood lipids; protection from radiation injury; cutaneous leishmaniasis (topically).

Traditional therapeutic uses

Berberis vulgaris: jaundice (when there is no obstruction of the bile ducts); biliousness, cholecystitis, gallstones; functional derangement of the liver; digestive stimulant, diarrhoea; in larger doses for constipation.[5,6,9]

Hydrastis canadensis: catarrhal states of the mucous membranes when unaccompanied by acute inflammation (except in acute purulent otitis media); disordered states of the gastrointestinal tract (particularly gastritis, gastric ulcer, diarrhoea) including conditions with hepatic symptoms; as a tonic during convalescence; haemorrhagic conditions of the uterus and pelvis (but it was considered too slow for active postpartum haemorrhage); internally and externally for skin disorders including eczema and acne, especially with gastrointestinal involvement; discharges from the genitourinary tract (e.g. leucorrhoea, gonorrhoea); disorders of the ear, nose, mouth, throat; externally for superficial disorders of the eye (but has no suggested value in intraocular infection).[7]

May also be used for

Extrapolations from pharmacological studies

Berberine-containing herbs may also be used for bacterial and fungal infections, protozoal infections (cutaneous and visceral leishmaniasis, amoebic dysentery, malaria, giardiasis, trichomoniasis), tapeworm infestation; possibly as an adjunct in treatment of congestive heart failure, arrhythmia; possibly in prevention of cancer; thrombocytopenia.

Hydrastis: the above indications plus anorexia and conditions requiring increased flow of gastric juices; conditions of visceral and/or smooth muscle spasm.

Other applications

Hydrastis was used as a component of eyewashes, and both Hydrastis and Berberis are used in bitter tonic preparations. Berberine salts are used in ophthalmic products, usually in eyedrops and eyewashes.[10] Despite the traditional contraindication for Hydrastis in acute respiratory infections such as the common cold, it is often used in this way, particularly in modern practice in the USA. Notwithstanding some popular use, Hydrastis has no value in masking drug-screening tests.

Preparations

Dried or fresh stem bark or root bark (Berberis) or rhizome and rootlets (Hydrastis) for decoction, liquid extract, tincture, tablets and capsules for internal or external use.

Dosage

*   *Berberis vulgaris*: 1.5 to 3 g/day of the dried root or stem bark or 3 to 6 mL/day of the 1:2 liquid extract; 7 to 14 mL/day of the 1:5 tincture
*   *Hydrastis canadensis*: 0.7 to 2 g/day of the dried rhizome/root or 2 to 5 mL/day of the 1:3 tincture; 3.5 to 8.0 mL/day of the 1:5 tincture.

Equivalent herb doses can also be taken in tablet or capsule form.

Higher doses of both herbs are necessary in acute conditions and to achieve the clinical effects for berberine noted in most of the clinical trials.

Duration of use

Both herbs may be taken long term within the recommended dosage.

Summary assessment of safety

No adverse effects from ingestion of either Berberis or Hydrastis are expected when used within the recommended dosage. Berberine-containing plants are not recommended for use during pregnancy, although there is a view that this concern is overstated. High doses of berberine increase the bioavailability of cyclosporin.

Technical data

Botany

Berberis vulgaris, a member of the Berberidaceae family, is a deciduous shrub 0.75 to 1.75 m tall with thick, creeping roots and a much-branched, greyish stem. The leaves are arranged in clusters on short axillary shoots, obovate to oblong-obovate, up to 4 cm long with spiny-toothed margins and short petioles. Its yellow flowers are six-sepalled and six-petalled, falling in loose clusters. The edible berries are red, oblong and about 1 cm in size.[11,12]

Hydrastis canadensis, a member of the Ranunculaceae (buttercup) family, is a small perennial. The stems are purplish and hairy above ground, but below the soil the root hairs and rhizome are yellow. The yellow rhizome is characteristically marked with depressions caused by the falling away of the annual stems (hence golden seal, as in the impression in wax once used to seal letters). The rhizome is about 5 cm in length, producing a profusion of yellow roots at its sides, 30 cm or more in length. The stems bear two or three large, slightly hairy five part leaves. The small solitary, greenish white or rose-coloured flower develops into a berry-like fruiting head, bright red in colour when fully ripe, resembling a raspberry and containing 10 to 30 black seeds.[13]

The Ranunculaceae and Berberidaceae are part of the same order (Ranunculales).

Adulteration

Due to the price of genuine Hydrastis, commercial products have been found not to contain the authentic plant material.[14,15] Hydrastis was listed on Appendix II of the Convention on International Trade in Endangered Species (CITES) as of 18 September 1997[16] and is currently listed. It is preferable to use cultivated sources (rather than wildcrafted sources) of Hydrastis because of its endangered status.

A 1933 source indicated that *Berberis aristata* was often confused with other *Berberis spp.* (such as *B. lycium*, and *B. vulgaris*) in India.[17] Commercially available barberry root bark may contain branch and stem bark. *Berberis vulgaris* is a protected species in one or more regions of France.[18]

Key constituents

Berberis vulgaris (root bark):

- Alkaloids (up to 13%), including those of the isoquinoline group: protoberberines (berberine (up to 6%), jatrorrhizine, palmatine) and bisbenzylisoquinolines (total <5%, including oxyacanthine).[19] Levels are much lower in the stem bark.

Hydrastis canadensis:

- Alkaloids (2.5% to 6%), including those of the isoquinoline group, the protoberberines: berberine (2% to 4.5%), canadine (0.5% to 1%), hydrastine (2.2% to 4%).[14,20]

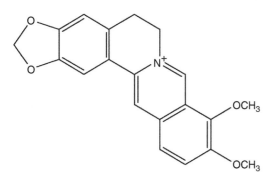

Berberine

Hydrastine

Pharmacodynamics of key constituents

The activities of Berberis and Hydrastis are thought to be largely due to the presence of their isoquinoline alkaloids. An earlier pharmacological review indicated that berberine has the following activities:[21]

- Antimicrobial, antifungal, antiparasitic
- Antidiarrhoeal, intestinal antisecretory, inhibits enterotoxins, cholera toxin antagonist
- Antiarrhythmic, positive inotropic (cardiotonic)
- Cytotoxic, antimitotic, antitumoral, increases the action of antitumoral agents, inhibits the action of carcinogens
- Cholagogue, choleretic, increases bilirubin excretion
- Mydriatic (dilates the pupil), increases lacrimal secretion
- Anticariogenic
- Inhibits acetylcholinesterase
- Hypoglycaemic.

More recently discovered properties (see below) include hypolipidaemic, antidepressant and anticonvulsant activities.

Hydrastine has the following activities:[22]

- Choleretic
- Sedative
- Antibacterial
- Vasoconstrictive.

Antimicrobial and antiparasitic activity

Berberine possesses extensive antimicrobial activity and does appear, in general, to be more active against Gram-positive bacteria (see Table 1). However, most of the research has been published before 2000, with relatively few studies conducted since.

Berberine sulphate blocked the adhesion of a uropathogenic strain of *E. scherichia coli*, in vitro. The reduction in adherence is related to the loss of the synthesis and expression of fimbriae (hairlike appendages) on the surface of the berberine-treated bacteria. Inhibition of microbial adherence results in termination of infection and may explain the anti-infectious activity of berberine in *E. coli* urinary tract infections, since the direct antimicrobial activity of berberine against *E. coli* is relatively low (see Table 1).[23] Berberine reduces FtsZ (a protein involved in bacterial cell division) in *E. coli*, thereby inhibiting the replication of this organism.[24]

Berberine has also demonstrated antibacterial activity against methicillin-resistant *Staphylococcus aureus* (MRSA) in vitro.[25] It was effective against all strains of MRSA, with 90% growth inhibition obtained at concentrations of 64 µg/mL or less. Berberine also restored the efficacy of antibiotics commonly used for MRSA. It was found to have an additive effect when combined with ampicillin, and a synergistic activity with oxacillin. Another study found that berberine chloride exhibited antimicrobial activity against all 43 tested strains of *Staph. aureus*.[26] Biofilm formed by *Staphylococcus epidermidis* is a common cause of infection in orthopaedic joint prostheses. Berberine was found to inhibit *Staph. epidermidis* adhesion to titanium alloy at a concentration of 45 µg/mL and prevented biofilm formation.[27,28]

Berberine sulphate has demonstrated antimycotic activity against several fungal species (see Table 1). Relatively high concentrations of 10 to 25 mg/mL inhibited the growth of Alternaria, *Aspergillus flavus*, *Asp. fumigatus*, *Candida albicans*, Curvularia, Drechslera, Fusarium, Mucor, Penicillium, *Rhizopus oryzae* and Scopulariopsis. The growth of Syncephalastrum was inhibited by a concentration of 50 mg/mL.[29] The minimum inhibitory concentration (MIC) of the antifungal drug fluconazole against *Candida albicans* was 1.9 µg/mL. However, this decreased to 0.48 µg/mL in the presence of just 1.9 µg/mL berberine.[30]

Berberine and protoberberine derivatives exhibited a potency comparable to that of quinine in vitro against two clones of human malaria: *Plasmodium berghei* and *P. falciparum*. None of the compounds, however, were active

Table 1 In vitro sensitivity of micro-organisms to berberine[33,44–46]

Test organism	Causative agent for the following conditions in humans	Inhibitory concentration (µg/mL)*
Bacteria		
Bacillus cereus	Food poisoning	25.0
B. pumilus	As for B. subtilis	25.0
B. subtilis	Food poisoning and various infections including septicaemia	25.0
Clostridium tetani	Tetanus	50
Corynebacterium diphtheriae	Diphtheria	6.2
Enterobacter aerogenes	Opportunistic infections	2500
Escherichia coli	Toxic strains can cause enteritis, peritonitis, infections of the urinary tract	600
Klebsiella spp.	Infections of the respiratory tract	>100.0
K. pneumoniae	Responsible for severe pneumonitis	25.0
Proteus spp.	Infant diarrhoea, urinary tract infection, suppurative lesions	>100.0
Pseudomonas pyocyanea	Various suppurative (pus-forming) infections	>100.0
Salmonella paratyphi	Enteric fever	>100.0
S. schottmuelleri	Enteric fever	>100.0
S. typhimurium	Gastroenteritis, food poisoning in Western countries	>100.0
S. typhi	Typhoid fever	>100.0
Shigella boydii	Bacillary dysentery	12.5
Staphylococcus aureus	Abscesses, endocarditis, pneumonia, osteomyelitis, septicaemia	6.2–50.0
S. albus	Occasionally endocarditis and infection of central nervous system	50.0
Streptococcus pyogenes	Variety of suppurative diseases including acute pharyngitis, impetigo and non-suppurative diseases including rheumatic fever	12.5
Vibrio cholerae	Cholera	25–50.0
Fungi		
Candida albicans	Thrush and candidiasis, and infection involving various parts of the body	12.5
C. utilis	As for C. albicans	12.5
C. tropicalis	As for C. albicans	3.1
Cryptococcus neoformans	Cryptococcosis (an infection involving lungs, bones or skin but often the CNS (meningitis))	150**
Microsporum gypseum	Tinea	50**
Saccharomyces cerevisiae	Associated with endocarditis and occasionally pulmonary infection	100**
Sporothrix schenkli	Sporotrichosis (a granulomatous disease of the skin, occasionally of internal organs and bones)	6.2
Trichophyton mentagrophytes	Attacks skin, hair and nails including dermatophytosis (a skin eruption)	100**

Table 1 In vitro sensitivity of micro-organisms to berberine[33,44–46]

Test organism	Causative agent for the following conditions in humans	Inhibitory concentration (μg/mL)*
Other		
Entamoeba histolytica	Protozoa responsible for amoebiasis	200
Erwinia carotovora	A plant pathogen	100
Leishmania donovani	Visceral leishmaniasis	5.0
Mycobacterium tuberculosis	Tuberculosis	200**
Xanthomonas citri	A plant pathogen	3.1

*Minimum concentration that totally inhibits growth in a liquid medium at pH 8.0. Maximum concentration tested was 100 μg/mL, unless otherwise noted.
**Tested in a solid medium, which typically required 4 to 10 times greater concentration for the same level of inhibition.

in *P. berghei*-parasitised mice.[31] Berberine sulphate inhibited the growth of *Entamoeba histolytica*, *Giardia lamblia* and *Trichomonas vaginalis* in vitro and induced morphological changes in the parasites.[32] Berberine chloride (1 μg/mL) significantly inhibited the growth of *Leishmania donovani* promastigotes by approximately 50%, in vitro. A concentration of 5 μg/mL resulted in complete inhibition of growth. *L. donovani* causes visceral leishmaniasis.[33] A recent study confirmed a half maximal inhibitory concentration (IC^{50}) for berberine chloride of 2.6 μg/mL against *L. donovani* promastigotes.[34] The mechanism involved was apoptosis following enhanced oxidative damage.

In vivo berberine demonstrated significant activity (greater than 50% suppression of lesion size) against *Leishmania braziliensis panamensis* in golden hamsters.[35] In both the 8-day and long-term models of *L. donovani* infection in hamsters, berberine markedly diminished the parasitic load, rapidly improved the haematological picture and was less toxic than pentamidine. Berberine sulphate administered into the lesion (1% four times per week) was found to be highly effective against cutaneous leishmaniasis in dogs. Cutaneous leishmaniasis (oriental sore) is caused by the protozoan *Leishmania tropica*.[36]

Berberine hydrochloride demonstrated a high degree of activity against *E. histolytica* in vitro with a minimum amoebicidal concentration of 10 μg/mL. Oral administration of berberine (100 mg/kg) to rats with experimental amoebiasis (protozoal infection) reduced the infection by 83%. Berberine also reduced the level of infection to 20% in infected hamsters.[37]

Studies have shown that certain antimicrobial agents can block the adherence of micro-organisms to host cells at doses much lower than those needed to kill cells or inhibit cell growth. At concentrations below the MIC, berberine caused an increase in release of lipoteichoic acid (LTA) from streptococci. LTA is the major ligand responsible for the adherence

of the bacteria to host cells, including host cell receptors (fibronectin). Release of LTA from the streptococcal cells means a reduction in the capacity of the bacteria to adhere to the host. Berberine also interfered with bacterial adherence by directly preventing the complexing of LTA with fibronectin or by dissolving the complexes once they were formed.[38] (See also the berberine research above regarding biofilms.)

Antimicrobial research on hydrastine is more limited. It exhibited relatively weaker killing activity than berberine against *Staph. aureus* and *Streptococcus sanguis*.[39] An MIC^{50} of 100 μg/mL was demonstrated against *Helicobacter pylori* (see also later under Pharmacodynamics of the herbs).[40] The effect of hydrastine on the protoscolices (larvae) of the tapeworm *Echinococcus granulosus* was measured in vitro and in vivo. Hydrastine at 0.3% concentration produced 70% mortality of the larvae in both experiments.[41]

Berberine demonstrated in vitro antiviral activity against herpes simplex virus types 1 and 2 with an IC^{50} of 82 and 90 μg/mL, respectively.[42] The in vitro antiviral activity (IC^{50}) of berberine chloride against human cytomegalovirus using the plaque assay was 0.68 μM (0.25 μg/mL), which was similar to the drug ganciclovir.[43]

Antidiarrhoeal activity

Oral doses of berberine (>25 mg/kg) and Geranium extract (a source of tannins) showed significant inhibition of diarrhoea in mice, and both substances inhibited spontaneous peristalsis in rat intestine. Comparison with atropine and papaverine indicated that the antidiarrhoeal activity of berberine differs from that of Geranium extract.[47] Intragastric administration of berberine sulphate reduced the purging effect of castor oil or *Cassia angustifolia* (senna) leaf in mice. It did not affect the gastrointestinal transport of Chinese ink in normal mice.[48]

A goal of therapy for diarrhoeal diseases is to decrease stool water. This can be done in two ways: by increasing the absorption of water and electrolytes or decreasing the stimulated secretion of fluid. Berberine probably does the latter.[49] It did not significantly alter normal ileal water and electrolyte transport as measured in vivo[50] and in vitro.[51] However, it inhibited secretion caused by *Vibrio. cholerae* and *E. coli* heat-labile enterotoxins, even when administered after the enterotoxin had bound to intestinal mucosa. The antisecretory effect was therefore not dependent on the type of enterotoxin.[52] In contrast, while simultaneous oral administration of berberine (0.1 mg/rat) and *E. coli* enterotoxin resulted in a significant reduction in fluid accumulation (p<0.01), treatment with berberine prior to or after the enterotoxin was ineffective.[53] Two studies are contradictory as to whether berberine alters cholera toxin-induced stimulation of the adenylate cyclase–cAMP system.[44,54] Hence, the exact mechanism of action of berberine is not certain, but its site of action appears to be distal to second messenger production and may be at a level common to all stimuli of colonic chloride secretion.[55]

A more recent investigation of the antidiarrhoeal activity of berberine used a model of thyroid hormone-induced diarrhoea in rats and measured gastrointestinal peptides.[56] While both plasma motilin and gastrin were elevated by thyroxine, they were normalised by the berberine (60 mg/kg/day for 7 days, oral). As a result, berberine also normalised increases in the number and volume of intestinal goblet cells.

Cardiovascular activity

A review concluded that berberine possesses a range of cardiovascular properties, including positive inotropic, negative chronotropic, antiarrhythmic and vasodilatory activities.[57] An in vitro study indicated that berberine inhibits voltage-dependent and ATP-sensitive potassium channels, hence the hypoglycaemic and antiarrhythmic activity of berberine might be due to its potassium channel-blocking effect.[58] Intravenous administration of berberine (1 mg/kg) decreased the amplitude of delayed after-depolarisations and blocked arrhythmias in rabbit ventricular muscles. The mechanism of antiarrhythmic activity of berberine might therefore instead be due to suppression of delayed after-depolarisations caused by a decrease in sodium influx.[59]

Berberine prevented the development of pressure-overload-induced left ventricular hypertrophy in vivo after aortic banding.[60] Oral administration of 10 mg/kg decreased left ventricular and diastolic pressures, and whole heart and left ventricular weights were lower after 8 weeks of treatment. A follow-up study was conducted to investigate the effects of berberine on catecholamine levels in a similar experimental model.[61] Plasma and left ventricular levels of adrenaline and noradrenaline were decreased after treatment with berberine. Berberine (5 to 10 mg/kg) improved cardiac contractility and inhibited left ventricular remodelling (especially myocardial fibrosis) in a rat model of hypertension.[62] Such effects might be partially associated with increased nitric oxide (NO) and cAMP in left ventricular tissue.

Administration of berberine sulphate increased the number of thrombocytes, decreased the activity of factor XIII and promoted blood coagulation in intact and gamma-irradiated rats and mice.[63] Berberine inhibited platelet aggregation and platelet adhesiveness in rats with reversible middle cerebral artery occlusion. Thromboxane B_2 levels after treatment with berberine were lower than levels in untreated ischaemic controls. The decline of platelet aggregation and decrease of thromboxane B_2 may be one of the important factors behind the anti-ischaemic activity of berberine.[64] Berberine also markedly inhibited clot retraction in vitro, which may be due to direct inhibition of calcium ion influx.[65]

Recent research has also focused on the cholesterol-lowering activity of berberine and its mechanism of action. The compound upregulates hepatic LDL (low density lipoprotein) receptor expression in vitro via post-transcriptional mRNA stabilisation.[66] This appears to be mediated by the extracellular signal-regulated kinase signalling pathway. Canadine, along with two other constituents of Hydrastis, have also demonstrated the same ability.[67] While berberine and the whole root preparation of Hydrastis both upregulated the expression of LDL receptors in a human liver cell line (HepG2 cells), the latter preparation was more effective (see also later in this monograph). Berberine was also found to inhibit cholesterol and triglyceride synthesis in HepG2 cells by increasing AMP-activated protein kinase (AMPK).[68]

Oral administration of berberine (50 and 100 mg/kg/day) to hyperlipidaemic hamsters for 10 days resulted in 26% and 42% decreases in total cholesterol and LDL-cholesterol, respectively. A 3.5-fold increase in hepatic LDL receptor mRNA and a 2.6-fold increase in LDL protein was seen in hamsters taking the higher dose.[69] LDL receptors in the liver increase the uptake and clearance of cholesterol from the bloodstream. The same researchers found that a combination of berberine (90 mg/kg/day, oral) and simvastatin (6 mg/kg/day, oral) in food-induced hyperlipidaemic rats was more effective than either agent alone at reducing serum LDL-cholesterol (p<0.01). A more effective reduction of serum triglyceride levels was also demonstrated.[70] The combination also upregulated LDL receptor mRNA in the rat livers to a level 1.6 times higher than either monotherapy, with a corresponding reduction of liver fat storage and improvement in hepatic histology.

A different research group investigated the effect of berberine and plant stanols (inhibitors of cholesterol absorption from the diet) on plasma cholesterol levels in rats with diet-induced hyperlipidaemia. Berberine (100 mg/kg/day, oral) slightly, but not significantly, lowered plasma total cholesterol, while the plant stanols (1% in diet) showed a borderline significant reduction (18%, p=0.067).[71] However, the combination markedly and significantly lowered plasma total cholesterol (41%, p=0.0002). Follow-up research by the same investigators sought to understand the mechanisms involved. Diet-induced hyperlipidaemic hamsters were chosen as the experimental model, since these animals are regarded as a good correlate for human cholesterol metabolism.[72] Using the same doses as above, it was again demonstrated that total plasma cholesterol was most reduced by the combination (43%, p=0.0001).[73] Neither berberine nor the plant stanols affected plasma triglyceride levels, whereas their combination resulted in a significant 37% reduction (p<0.001). As to the possible sites of action of berberine, a series of tests suggested that it interfered with intestinal cholesterol absorption in a different manner to the stanols, possibly by interfering with micelle formation. In addition bile acid synthesis was increased, which can increase cholesterol clearance via the digestive tract. In contrast, cholesterol synthesis by the liver was also increased (this is a known property of other cholesterol absorption inhibitors), but not by enough to counter the cholesterol-lowering mechanisms. Contrary to research cited above, the authors found that berberine did not affect hepatic LDL receptor mRNA expression.

Tissue factor (TF) plays an essential role in coagulation by binding factor VII, which activates factor X. TF is expressed in cells within the atherosclerotic vessel wall, is induced by inflammatory mediators and enhances plaque thrombogenicity. Human aortic endothelial cells treated with berberine (1 to 30 μM) exhibited enhanced TF expression following inflammatory stimulants.[74] This was via stabilisation of TF mRNA. Also berberine countered the inhibitory effects of statins on endothelial TF in vitro. Berberine also enhanced TF and inhibited TFPI (tissue factor pathway inhibitor), a TF antagonist, in *ApoE*$^{-/-}$ mice after oral doses of 100 mg/kg/day. The authors suggested that this prothrombotic effect of berberine indicates it should be considered with caution as a cholesterol-lowering agent and that large-scale clinical trials are needed to prove its safety in this regard. In addition, berberine might promote atherosclerosis and foam cell formation by inducing scavenger receptor-A expression in macrophages (which mediates LDL uptake), as determined by in vitro and in vivo (mice, 5 mg/kg/day, ip) experiments.[75]

On the other hand, berberine might reduce the incidence or pathogenesis of arterial disease by other mechanisms: in vitro berberine inhibited lysophosphatidylcholine-induced vascular smooth muscle cell (VSMC) proliferation and migration via inhibition of intracellular reactive oxygen species, suggesting potential in the prevention of atherosclerosis.[76] Berberine also inhibited the in vitro growth and migration of VSMC induced by platelet-derived growth factor.[77] LDL oxidation and LDL-induced cytotoxic effects on human endothelial cells were also reduced by berberine in vitro.[78] Atherosclerotic plaque rupture is usually the initiating event in a heart attack. Overproduction of MMPs (matrix metalloproteinases) by macrophages can lead to plaque rupture by degrading the extracellular matrix. Berberine reduced MMP-9 expression in activated macrophages in vitro.[79]

Berberine might benefit vascular endothelial cell integrity and function by improving protective mechanisms, such as increasing the production of NO and enhancing resistance to hyperglycaemic-induced injury. This was observed in blood vessels and vascular endothelial cells taken from mice and rats.[80] In human studies, 1.2 g/day (oral) of berberine for 30 days mobilised circulating endothelial progenitor cells (improving small artery elasticity),[81] augmented their function (a result of enhanced plasma NO levels)[82] and reduced circulating endothelial microparticles in parallel with improved flow-mediated vasodilation.[83] This suggests berberine has beneficial effects on human vascular endothelial health.

Anticancer activity

There have been numerous investigations into the anticancer properties of berberine, mainly via in vitro studies using human and animal cancer cell lines. A 2009 systematic review cited more than 100 studies, with most published since the year 2000.[84] Antiproliferative activity at concentrations typically up to 100 μM (about 34 μg/mL) has been demonstrated in vitro for a range of tumour cell lines including liver, lung, breast, uterus, melanoma, prostate and leukaemia. According to the review, the antiproliferative effect of berberine is relatively slow and gentle, requiring exposure times of at least 24 h for significant effects. Various mechanisms underlying this antiproliferative/cytotoxic activity of berberine have been proposed, but the most widely investigated mechanism is its role in cell cycle arrest (with sometimes conflicting results). Induction of apoptosis is another possible key mechanism, via regulation of reactive oxygen species production, mitochondrial transmembrane potential and NF-kappaB activation. Other possible anticancer mechanisms according to the review include transcriptional regulation of some oncogene and carcinogenesis-related gene expression, interaction with DNA and RNA, and inhibition of key enzymes such as DNA topoisomerase.

The review also notes studies, relatively few in number, where berberine has inhibited metastasis, invasion and angiogenesis in vitro, especially via MMP inhibition. Despite earlier studies suggesting that berberine might be relatively inactive against cancer in vivo, later studies have demonstrated significant effects. The review cites studies for Dalton's lymphoma ascites tumour cells in mice (ip treatment was more effective than oral) and human tongue squamous carcinoma, also in mice (berberine 10 mg/kg, ip). Berberine has also prevented cancer development in models of chemical carcinogenesis.

Another 2009 review of the antineoplastic activity of berberine noted many of the same studies and came to similar conclusions regarding mechanisms of action.[85] The review also included additional positive in vivo studies for berberine including inhibition of leukaemia cells and lung tumours inoculated into mice (berberine dose 100 mg/kg, oral). Berberine also strongly suppressed the growth of human prostate cancer xenografts in mice. This review did caution that antagonistic activity of berberine on chemotherapeutic drugs has been observed in vitro, due to the upregulation of multidrug resistance pumps in cancer cells. Hence there is a risk that co-administered berberine might compromise cancer chemotherapy. However, in vivo research is needed to clarify this issue.

Anti-inflammatory activity

Berberine was shown to inhibit COX-2 transcription in human colon cancer cells (at >0.3 μM)[86] and reduce COX-2 protein (but not enzyme activity) in an oral cancer cell line in vitro (1, 10 and 100 μM).[87] Activator protein 1 (AP-1) activity was also decreased in human hepatoma cells[88] and oral cancer cells treated with berberine.[87] AP-1 is a pro-inflammatory transcription factor also involved in carcinogenesis.

Berberine inhibited cellular proliferation of human peripheral lymphocytes in vitro. Some effects of berberine, especially its anti-inflammatory activity, may arise in part from the inhibition of DNA synthesis in activated lymphocytes.[89] The phytochemical also suppressed pro-inflammatory responses via AMPK activation in macrophages in vitro.[90] Berberine suppressed the induction of the interleukin IL-1beta and tumour necrosis factor (TNF)-alpha by inflammatory agents in human lung cells in vitro.[91]

The alkaloid berbamine demonstrated suppressive effects via ip administration on delayed hypersensitivity and mixed lymphocyte reactions and significantly prolonged allograft survival, compared with untreated transplanted mice.[92] In an early study berberine significantly inhibited the proliferative response of spleen cells to mitogens in vitro and reduced the amount of haemolytic plaque-forming cells. The ratio of CD4+ to CD8+ cells was decreased, which may be one of the mechanisms of action.[93]

An ethanol extract of Berberis, three alkaloidal fractions and isolated alkaloids (berberine and oxyacanthine) were applied by the ip route in acute inflammation models. The ethanol extract demonstrated the highest anti-inflammatory activity. It also demonstrated activity in chronic inflammation (adjuvant arthritis). The two fractions containing only protoberberines and berberine suppressed the delayed-type hypersensitivity reaction. The other fraction (containing protoberberines and bisbenzylisoquinoline alkaloids) and berberine reduced the antibody response against sheep red blood cells in vivo.[94]

Researchers assessed the effect of berberine in a colitis model in rats.[95] Oral berberine (15 mg/kg/day for 7 days) reduced histological lesions, tissue damage and myeloperoxidase activity. IL-8 was also reduced in vitro when berberine was added to inflamed rectal mucosa tissue.[95]

The isoquinoline alkaloids berberine, berbamine, palmatine, oxyacanthine, magnoflorine and columbamine were isolated from the root bark of a Turkish Berberis plant (*B. crataegina*) and investigated for their anti-inflammatory and antinociceptive effects in various in vivo models.[96] Berberine, berbamine and palmatine were found to be effective in a dose-dependent manner in mice at oral doses of 100 and/or 200 mg/kg. The antipyretic activity of the three alkaloids in mice was particularly marked, with doses of 25 to 50 mg/kg proving active.

Berberine pretreatment (5 and 10 mg/kg, ip) inhibited the production of exudate and the prostaglandin PGE_2 in carrageenan-induced inflammation in rats.[90] The acute inflammatory response induced by lipopolysaccharide (LPS) in broiler chickens was largely mitigated by berberine (15 mg/kg, oral).[97] Berberine also attenuated LPS-induced acute lung injury by inhibiting TNF-alpha production and expression and activation of phospholipase A_2 in mice (50 mg/kg, oral).[98]

Neurological activity

A recent review examined the neurological potential of berberine.[99] The authors noted that, like many alkaloids, it readily crosses the blood-brain barrier and has exhibited neuroprotective, antidepressant and anxiolytic activities in various test models. The alkaloid is reported to modulate neurotransmitters and their receptor systems in the brain in vitro and in vivo, exhibiting D2 dopamine antagonist activity and noradrenaline, serotonin and dopamine transporter inhibition. In one study berberine (50 mg/kg, oral) significantly reversed

amyloid-beta memory damage in rats[100] and in another it exhibited antidepressant activity in mice (5 to 20 mg/kg, ip).[101] Oral doses of berberine (mice, 20 mg/kg) potentiated the effect of antidepressant drugs in a depression model and increased noradrenaline and serotonin levels in the hippocampus and frontal cortex.[102] Berberine (100 and 500 mg/kg, oral) displayed anxiolytic activity in mice, with effects comparable to diazepam (1 mg/kg) and buspirone (2 mg/kg).[103]

Anticonvulsant activity has also been demonstrated in various models in mice (10 and 20 mg/kg, ip).[104] This was attributed to a modulation of neurotransmitter systems. Berberine also significantly improved scopolamine-induced amnesia in rats. This anti-amnesic effect of berberine may be related to an increase in activity in the peripheral and central cholinergic neuronal systems.[105]

Antidiabetic activity

Much recent research has focused on the antidiabetic properties of berberine. One in vitro mechanistic study compared the glucose-lowering effects of berberine with metformin and troglitazone.[106] Similar to metformin, berberine reduced the uptake of glucose by hepatocytes in an insulin-independent manner. Another in vitro study found that it increased glucose uptake by adipocytes via an insulin-independent mechanism that may involve AMPK.[107] Further to this berberine and dihydroberberine were found to inhibit mitochondrial respiratory complex I in vitro, thereby activating AMPK and improving insulin action.[108] Results from another in vitro study suggested that inhibition of DPP IV (human dipeptidyl peptidase IV) is another possible hypoglycaemic mechanism of berberine.[109]

In vitro models of insulin resistance have provided further information. Berberine reversed free-fatty-acid (FFA) induced insulin resistance in adipocytes.[110] It also reduced insulin resistance through protein kinase C-dependent upregulation of the insulin receptor in cultured human liver cells[111] and improved FFA-induced insulin resistance in muscle cells by inhibiting fatty acid uptake.[112] Berberine also modulated insulin signalling transduction in insulin-resistant muscle cells.[113]

In cultured rat glomerular mesangial cells exposed to high glucose, incubation with berberine significantly decreased cell proliferation and aldose reductase activity.[114] Aldose reductase facilitates the conversion of excess cellular glucose into toxic metabolites, which probably facilitates the development of diabetic nephropathy. In the same model, berberine also inhibited fibronectin and collagen accumulation, suggesting a renoprotective effect.[115]

The hypoglycaemic activity of berberine has been demonstrated in a number of in vivo studies. One in vivo study investigated the activity of berberine in streptozotocin-induced diabetic rats and found that oral doses (187.5 and 562.5 mg/kg) significantly reduced fasting blood glucose, triglycerides, total cholesterol, FFAs and apolipoprotein B, and increased HDL-cholesterol and apolipoprotein AI in a dose-dependent manner.[116] A follow-up in vivo experiment in normal mice found that berberine increased serum insulin and decreased blood glucose after oral doses of 93.75, 187.5 and 562.5 mg/kg.[116]

One study examined the metabolic effects of berberine in models of diabetes and insulin resistance in vivo, and in insulin-responsive cell lines in vitro.[117] In a diabetic mouse model, berberine (5 mg/kg/day, ip) reduced body weight and significantly improved glucose tolerance. Similarly, berberine (380 mg/kg/day, oral) reduced body weight and plasma triglycerides and improved the activity of insulin in Wistar rats fed a high fat diet. Berberine also reduced lipogenesis by downregulating the genes involved, and was found to upregulate those involved in energy expenditure in both muscle and adipose tissue. The in vitro arm of the study showed once again that berberine increased AMPK activity. It also increased GLUT4 (glucose transporter type 4) translocation and reduced lipid accumulation in adipocytes. Another study explored the impact of berberine on diabetes induced by alloxan and a high fat and cholesterol diet in rats.[118] Oral administration of berberine (100 and 200 mg/kg) significantly decreased fasting blood glucose levels, total cholesterol, LDL-cholesterol and triglycerides, whilst increasing HDL-cholesterol, NO, superoxide dismutase and glutathione peroxidase. Histopathological results demonstrated that berberine was able to restore damaged pancreatic tissue,[118] which was also found in another study.[119] Similar favourable effects on lowering insulin and plasma glucose and on metabolism (including lipid levels) have been demonstrated in other in vivo studies.[111,119,120–123]

As touched on above, berberine has also demonstrated favourable effects in animal models of insulin resistance, suggesting a possible role in the management of metabolic syndrome. In dietary obese rats, berberine (250 mg/kg/day, oral for 5 weeks) markedly increased insulin sensitivity.[124] Associated in vitro experiments suggested that it stimulates glycolysis, and the observed increase in AMPK activation is a consequence of the associated mitochondrial inhibition.[124] In high-fat-diet rats, berberine (150 mg/kg/day, oral for 6 weeks) significantly decreased plasma glucose and insulin levels, along with a reduction in body weight and improvement of blood lipid profiles.[125] In rats with fructose-induced insulin resistance, berberine (187.5 mg/kg/day, oral for 4 weeks) reduced plasma insulin, insulin resistance and triglyceride levels, but did not change plasma glucose.[126]

One possible antidiabetic mechanism of berberine could be via the inhibition of intestinal disaccharidases, thereby retarding postprandial sugar absorption. Berberine (100 mg/kg/day, oral) attenuated intestinal disaccharidase activities in streptozotocin-induced diabetic rats,[127] a finding that was also observed in vitro.[128] These results were supported in another investigation that found berberine significantly lowered postprandial blood glucose (PBG) following sucrose or maltose loading in normal rats.[129]

Berberine also inhibits aldose reductase activity in vivo. It ameliorated renal injury in streptozotocin-induced diabetic rats at 200 mg/kg/day (oral) by suppressing both oxidative stress and aldose reductase activity, as well as lowering blood glucose.[114,130] The alkaloid also demonstrated some protective activity against retinal pathology in a diabetic rat model.[131]

Other activity

Berberine reduced the tonic contraction induced by carbachol in isolated longitudinal muscle of gastric fundus. It mainly acted by inhibiting extracellular calcium entry induced by both carbachol and potassium chloride.[132] Comparative examinations were made of the relative activity of various isoquinoline alkaloids on isolated mouse intestine and uterus. Berberine, palmatine, jatrorrhizine, dihydroberberine and dihydropalmatine caused marked contraction of uterus. Only tetrahydroberberine, tetrahydropalmatine and tetrahydrojatrorrhizine showed strong papaverine-like spasmolytic activity on intestine.[133] Berberine was also found to inhibit the influx of extracellular calcium and calcium-release from intracellular stores in smooth muscle cells of guinea pig colon in a dose-dependent manner.[134]

Acute doses of berberine (2.5 mg/rat, oral) significantly increased the secretion of bilirubin in experimental hyperbilirubinaemia ($p < 0.05$), without affecting the functional capacity of the liver. Chronic administration of 5 mg/day for 8 days abolished the effect, resulting in normal biliary bilirubin excretion.[135]

An in vitro study conducted on the sebaceous glands of the hamster ear found that lipogenesis was suppressed 63% by 100 μM berberine ($p < 0.01$). Lipogenesis was also suppressed by wogonin, a flavonoid in Scutellaria baicalensis. Herbal medicines containing berberine and/or wogonin may therefore be useful in the treatment of acne vulgaris, especially topically. It is likely that berberine inhibits lipogenesis at the level of synthesis of triglyceride from FFA.[136]

Intragastric administration of berberine sulphate significantly inhibited the increased vascular permeability induced by intraperitoneal acetic acid in mice. Subcutaneous administration markedly inhibited the increased vascular permeability in rats and inhibited mouse ear swelling.[37]

Berberine inhibited osteoclast formation and survival in vitro[137] and promoted osteoblast differentiation.[138] In another in vitro study it inhibited osteoclast formation, differentiation and bone resorption.[139]

Berberine (3 mg/kg/day, ip for 36 days) reduced weight gain and food intake, inhibited adipogenesis and lowered serum glucose, triglycerides and total cholesterol in high-fat-diet-induced obese mice.[140] It improved lipid dysregulation in obese mice at 5 mg/kg/day ip by controlling central and peripheral AMPK activity.[141]

Berberine has an antiurolithic effect that is mediated through multiple pathways. In Wistar rats, berberine (5 to 20 mg/kg, ip) increased urine output accompanied by increased pH and sodium and potassium excretion and decreased calcium excretion, similar to the diuretic drug hydrochlorothiazide.[142] At 10 mg/kg (ip) it also prevented and eliminated chemically induced calcium oxalate crystal deposition in renal tubules and protected against the deleterious effects of lithogenic treatment, including weight loss and oxidative stress.

Pharmacodynamics of the herbs

Antimicrobial activity

A more efficient inhibition of growth was observed for a 1:4 tincture of Berberis compared with 0.2% berberine chloride solution against a variety of microorganisms in vitro. This effect of the Berberis tincture was the result of a higher concentration of berberine (0.31%) and the presence of other active components, including alkaloids.[143]

A 70% alcohol–water extract of Hydrastis and the major isolated alkaloids berberine, hydrastine, canadine and canadaline all demonstrated antibacterial activity against *Staph. aureus*, *E. coli*, *Streptococcus sanguis* and *Pseudomonas aeruginosa* in vitro.[39] The whole extract was as active or more than pure berberine in terms of MIC values, despite the lower content of alkaloids. However, its killing activity was weaker than berberine. The crude methanolic extract of Hydrastis was found to inhibit *Helicobacter pylori* in vitro, with an MIC^{50} of 12.5 µg/mL.[40] Berberine and beta-hydrastine were considered to be the most active constituents with MIC^{50} values of 12.5 and 100 µg/mL, respectively.

Hydrastis was among the most potent of 21 herbal extracts screened for in vitro activity against *Helicobacter pylori*, but sage (*Salvia officinalis*) was more active.[144] The Hydrastis extract exhibited only relatively modest activity against *Campylobacter jejuni*.

Effect on smooth muscle

Berberine caused a slow diminution of tone, amplitude, rate and response to acetylcholine in rat uterus. Hydrastine increased the rate of uterine contraction, with slowly decreasing tone and amplitude. Berberine and hydrastine together produced a rapid decrease in tone and amplitude, similar to that produced by Hydrastis extract.[145] The author commented that, although commonly regarded as a uterine stimulant, Hydrastis was in fact a uterine sedative in this model. Hydrastis extract and the total crude alkaloids of Hydrastis demonstrated spasmolytic activity on isolated mouse intestine and uterus.[146]

In contrast, an alcohol extract of Hydrastis exerted a vasoconstrictive activity in rabbit aorta. It also inhibited the contraction of rabbit aorta induced by adrenaline, serotonin and histamine in vitro. However, berberine and hydrastine did not show this vasoconstrictive effect. Berberine demonstrated some inhibitory activity on aortic contraction induced by adrenaline, but hydrastine was inactive.[147] The observed vasoconstrictive activity of Hydrastis extract may be due to the presence of hydrastinine, a decomposition product of hydrastine.

The four major alkaloids of Hydrastis (berberine, hydrastine, canadine and canadaline) were tested on rabbit aorta strips for adrenolytic activity (inhibition of adrenaline-induced contraction). The total extract had a lower adrenolytic potency than the alkaloid mixture. The authors suggested that berberine, canadine and canadaline acted synergistically and the presence of other compounds (in particular hydrastine) probably counteracted their activity.[148]

Another study by the same research group found that the major alkaloids of Hydrastis evoked contractile activity in isolated guinea pig ileum through an indirect cholinergic mechanism, acting on acetylcholine release from nerve endings. They demonstrated differing contractile potencies for the alkaloids, depending on chemical structure.[149]

In confirmation of earlier research, an ethanolic extract of Hydrastis exhibited reversible relaxant activity on spontaneous contractions in non-pregnant rat uterus and also on contractions induced by serotonin, oxytocin and acetylcholine.[150] The extract also relaxed carbachol precontracted guinea pig trachea. An ethanolic extract of Hydrastis induced strong relaxation in rabbit bladder detrusor muscle, but the four major individual alkaloids were inactive.[151]

Other activity

Berberis tincture increased contractions in isolated rabbit intestine and demonstrated cholagogue activity in guinea pigs and cholekinetic activity in rats.[152]

An extract of *Berberis aristata* root inhibited the PAF-induced aggregation of rabbit platelets in a dose-dependent manner in vitro. It also inhibited the binding of radiolabelled PAF to rabbit platelets in a competitive manner.[153]

Conflicting results have been recorded for Berberis in pyresis. An early study demonstrated an antipyretic effect for Berberis decoction in rabbits with fever.[154] However, in a later study water, chloroform and hexane extracts showed no activity.[155]

A study of the action of bitters was conducted in 1956 on the stomach of a man named Tom, who had an occluded oesophagus and a gastric fistula.[2] Bitters were administered by mouth and swallowed into the blind oesophagus; the resulting salivary volume and gastric secretion were compared with direct administration into the stomach. In the 96 experiments conducted it was found that there was considerable variation in effects of the bitters. Hydrastis was the most active herb and gentian was virtually inactive at the levels tested (see also Chapter 2).[156]

Hydrastis tincture (0.06 mL/mouse) showed some anticarcinogenic and hepatoprotective activity in p-dimethylaminoazobenzene-induced hepatocarcinogenesis in mice.[157]

Hypercholesterolaemic hamsters received either berberine (15 mg/kg/day, ip) or Hydrastis extract (containing berberine 7.5 mg/kg/day, ip).[67] The Hydrastis significantly lowered plasma total cholesterol, LDL-cholesterol, triglycerides and FFAs, and to the same extent as the berberine. It also significantly reduced liver fat storage, and hepatic LDL receptor mRNA was increased. The observation that berberine from Hydrastis has a longer intracellular retention time in hepatocytes than berberine alone suggests the existence of an unknown multidrug resistance pump inhibitor in the herb.[67]

The innate effects of Hydrastis and Astragalus on pro-inflammatory cytokines produced by cultured macrophages were examined using two different commercial preparations.[158] Both Hydrastis and Astragalus were found to exhibit little to no direct effect on stimulation of mouse macrophages, with only Astragalus able to affect production of TNF-alpha when used in high concentrations. However, both herbs were able to modify responses from LPS-stimulated macrophages, reducing production of TNF-alpha, IL-6, IL-10 and IL-12 in a dose-dependent manner.

The antigen-specific immunomodulatory potential of Hydrastis (6.6 g/L of drinking water) was assessed in rats over 6 weeks.[159] The rats were periodically injected with an antigen (keyhole limpet haemocyanin) over this time period. Hydrastis caused an increase in the primary IgM response in the first 2 weeks only, but had no major impact on IgG production.

Berberis vulgaris is widely used in Pakistan for the treatment of kidney stones. To evaluate its antiurolithic potential, the aqueous-methanol extract of Berberis root bark was tested in an animal model of urolithiasis in male Wistar rats.[160] The extract (50 mg/kg/day, ip) inhibited calcium crystal deposition in renal tubules and protected against associated changes including polyuria, weight loss, impaired renal function and the development of oxidative stress in the kidneys (see also a study by the same group in the berberine section of this monograph).

Pharmacokinetics

An early study found that oral administration of 500 mg/kg of berberine to rabbits resulted in a maximum level in the blood after 8h. Berberine was still found in the blood after 72h. Levels were highest in the heart, pancreas and liver and it was excreted through the stools and urine.[161] Another early study investigated the concentration of berberine in rat plasma after oral administration of aqueous extracts of *Coptis spp.* Co-administration with aqueous extract of Glycyrrhiza did not influence the bioavailability of berberine from the Coptis extract.[162]

Human studies have established that the oral bioavailability of berberine is relatively low, but the phytochemical has a long residence time in the body.[163,164] One study found that the average half-life of a single oral 400 mg dose of berberine in 20 healthy volunteers was 28.6 ± 9.5 h.[163] The same study recorded a Cmax of 0.44 ± 0.42 ng/mL with a corresponding Tmax of 9.8 ± 6.6 h.

The metabolism of berberine has also been studied. An investigation in rats found that intravenously administered berberine mainly underwent hepatobiliary excretion after metabolism in the liver with phase I demethylation and phase II glucuronidation.[165] A study in conventional and germ-free rats (treated with antibiotics) found that orally administered berberine was converted into four main metabolites that were present in the free state or as glucuronide conjugates.[166] These were the products of phase I demethylation (berberrubine and thalifendine) or ring cleavage (demethyleneberberine and jatrorrhizine). These metabolites achieved significantly higher concentrations than berberine and were more persistent in plasma (as a result of enterohepatic circulation), suggesting that they might be more important than berberine itself for any systemic pharmacological activity. Interestingly, the four metabolites and their conjugates were much lower in the germ-free rats, which the authors suggested indicated a significant role of intestinal flora in their enterohepatic circulation.

Despite the fact that berberine and its metabolites are largely excreted via the bile, some studies have determined the main urinary metabolites of the alkaloid. An earlier study found sulphates of jatrorrhizine, demethyleneberberine and thalifendine in the urine of healthy volunteers following the administration of 900 mg/day berberine chloride for 3 days.[167] This was confirmed in humans and rats in a later study, which additionally found free thalifendine and other metabolites (including glucuronides).[168]

One reason for the low bioavailability of berberine could be due to P-glycoprotein (P-gp) in the intestinal wall, which might pump absorbed berberine back into the lumen. This was supported by an in vitro study which found that P-gp inhibitors improved the intestinal uptake of berberine by a factor of 6.[169]

Clinical trials (mainly using berberine)

Diarrhoea and cholera

As noted previously, berberine possesses broad antimicrobial activity in vitro. Of interest to intestinal health, Chinese researchers found that berberine may have a selective antimicrobial effect. Using the more comprehensive microcalorimetric method (which measures the energy changes of bacterial growth), they measured IC_{50} values of berberine towards *Bacillus shigae* (a harmful bacterium), *Bifidobacterium adolescentis* (a commensal or probiotic) and *E. coli* (a bacterium of the intermediate flora). IC_{50} values were 75 μg/mL for *Bacillus shigae*, 101 μg/mL for *E. coli* and 806 μg/mL for *Bifidobacterium adolescentis*. This suggests that, at an intestinal concentration sufficient to inhibit the growth of harmful and intermediate flora, berberine would have little effect on probiotic flora.[170] Due to the low oral bioavailability of berberine, the intestine is exposed to most of the dose and hence relevant enteric antimicrobial concentrations could well be achieved.

Results from an early uncontrolled clinical study suggested that berberine hydrochloride therapy (50 mg orally every 8h for the first 2 days, and then tapering off) might be useful for cholera and severe diarrhoea.[171] Data collected for 620 patients suggested berberine was superior to chloramphenicol in some respects. A parallel, open clinical trial comparing berberine and a variety of antidiarrhoeal drug combinations was conducted in 100 children suffering from gastroenteritis of less than 5 days' duration. Fifty children up to 6 months old received 25 mg of berberine four times a day; older children received 50 mg initially and 25 mg every 6h; another 50 children received one of several antidiarrhoeal drugs. The state of hydration and number of stools passed were used to assess the treatment. Berberine demonstrated effective antidiarrhoeal action and compared well with the standard antidiarrhoeal drugs. Patients on berberine improved faster, although the lack of a placebo group weakens the value of this finding.[172]

In a randomised, placebo-controlled, double blind clinical trial, the effects of berberine, tetracycline and tetracycline plus berberine were studied in 400 patients presenting with acute watery diarrhoea. Of this number, 185 patients had cholera and 215 non-cholera diarrhoea. At the dosage used (100 mg four times daily) berberine did not show significant anti-secretory activity in either group. A reduction in stool volume and cAMP concentrations in stools was observed, although not significant.[173] In a later trial, a larger dose of berberine of 200 mg four times daily plus tetracycline (2 g/day) was compared with tetracycline alone using a randomised, double blind clinical design involving 74 patients infected with *V. cholerae*. No statistically significant differences were observed between the two groups.[174]

One hundred and sixty-five adult men with diarrhoea caused by enterotoxigenic *E. coli* or *Vibrio cholerae* were treated in a randomised, controlled clinical trial. In patients with *E. coli* diarrhoea, mean stool volume decreased significantly (p<0.05) in the first 8h after treatment with 400mg berberine sulphate, compared with controls. Over the first 24h period significantly more patients taking berberine stopped having diarrhoea compared with controls (42% versus 20%, p<0.05). Only limited effects against diarrhoea caused by *V. cholerae* were observed, with no significant difference found between patients treated with 1200mg berberine sulphate plus tetracycline and those treated with tetracycline alone.[175]

The conclusion to draw from these clinical studies is that berberine is probably valuable for some forms of acute infectious diarrhoea, particularly *E. coli* infection, but has no value in the treatment of *V. cholerae* infection (cholera).

Other gastrointestinal effects

Small intestinal transit time in 20 healthy human volunteers was significantly delayed after oral administration of 1.2g of berberine (p<0.01). Hence the antidiarrhoeal property of berberine might be further mediated by its ability to delay small intestinal transit.[176]

A clinical trial compared the effects of the antiulcer drug ranitidine and four antibacterial drugs, one of which was berberine (300mg twice daily), in patients with *H. pylori*-associated duodenal ulcer disease. Although the antibacterial drugs were more effective at *H. pylori* clearance and improving gastritis, ranitidine was more effective for ulcer healing.[177]

Trachoma

Fifty-one patients with clinically active trachoma lesions (stages I and II) were treated for 8 weeks with eyedrops containing either 0.2% berberine chloride or 20% of the antitrachoma drug sulfacetamide in an open label trial. Sulfacetamide eyedrops gave the better clinical results, but the infective agent (*Chlamydia trachomatis*) remained present in the conjunctiva and relapses of symptoms occurred. Berberine-treated patients showed only very mild ocular symptoms after treatment and were negative for the infective agent. No relapses occurred among these patients.[178]

A single blind, placebo-controlled clinical trial was conducted in 96 children with trachoma stage IIa or IIb over a period of 3 months. Berberine eyedrops (0.2%) were compared with berberine plus neomycin ointment, sulfacetamide or a placebo. In patients treated with berberine alone, 83% were clinically cured (p<0.001), but only 50% were microbiologically cured. The response rate was higher in those treated with berberine plus neomycin (88%) and lower in the sulfacetamide (73%) and placebo (0%) groups (no p values provided). The berberine treatment was better tolerated than sulfacetamide.[179]

Giardiasis

After berberine was administered at a dose of 5mg/kg/day for 6 days to 25 giardiasis patients between the ages of 1 and 10 years, 68% became negative for the presence of Giardia cysts.

In a similar group receiving placebo, only 25% experienced a parasitological cure. Metronidazole at a dose of 10mg/kg/day for 6 days was 100% effective in another nine patients.[180]

A clinical trial involving children (ages from 5 months to 14 years) with giardiasis compared the effect of berberine with established antigiardial drugs. Of the group of 42 patients who received 10mg/kg/day of berberine orally for 10 days, 90% had negative stool specimens upon completion of treatment, although a small number of cases relapsed 1 month later. This result compared favourably with the three other antigiardial drugs investigated, including metronidazole.[181]

Liver cirrhosis

Patients with cirrhosis of the liver have high plasma concentrations of tyramine, resulting in cardiovascular and neurologic complications. An uncontrolled clinical trial investigated the effect of oral berberine on hypertyraminaemia in cirrhotic patients over several months. Oral administration of berberine (600 to 800mg/day) corrected hypertyraminaemia and prevented the elevation of plasma tyramine levels following chemical tyramine stimulation. This effect was probably due to inhibition by berberine of bacterial tyrosine decarboxylase in the intestine.[182]

Diabetes mellitus

In an early uncontrolled clinical trial, the effect of berberine was investigated in 60 patients with varying levels of type 2 diabetes mellitus. Oral doses (300 to 500mg three times a day) were prescribed for 1 to 3 months, together with a therapeutic diet for 1 month. Major symptoms of diabetes disappeared, strength improved, blood pressure normalised and blood lipids decreased. Fasting glycaemic levels in 60% of patients were better controlled.[183]

More recent trials have delivered impressive results, although they did involve the use of relatively high doses of berberine. In a randomised, double blind, placebo-controlled trial in 116 type 2 diabetes patients with dyslipidaemia, berberine (1000mg/day) for 3 months significantly improved a range of metabolic parameters.[184] Relative to placebo, berberine significantly lowered body weight, systolic blood pressure, fasting blood glucose (FBG), postload blood glucose, HbA_{1c}, triglycerides, total and LDL-cholesterol, liver transaminases and IL-6 (p<0.0001 to p=0.038). Compared with baseline, berberine lowered fasting plasma glucose by 20%, HbA_{1c} by 12%, triglycerides by 36% and LDL-cholesterol by 21%. No serious adverse events occurred, but five patients in the berberine group complained of constipation, compared to just one in the placebo group (p=0.207 for frequency of constipation between the two groups).

Two different trials were described in the one publication.[185] In the first controlled (and presumably open label) trial, 36 adults with newly diagnosed type 2 diabetes were randomly assigned to berberine or metformin (1500mg/day of each) over 3 months, with 31 patients completing the study. Berberine demonstrated similar activity to metformin in terms of reductions in HbA_{1c}, FBG and PBG and had reduced these significantly by the end of the trial, compared with baseline (p<0.01). In the second open label trial,

48 adults with poorly controlled type 2 diabetes received berberine (1500 mg/day) in addition to their current treatments for 3 months. If gastrointestinal side effects occurred, the dose of berberine was reduced to 900 mg/day. Compared with baseline, by the end of the trial there were significant reductions (p<0.01 to p<0.001) in HbA_{1c} (10%), FBG (21%), PBG (34%), fasting insulin (28%), HOMA-IR (a measure of insulin resistance, 45%) and LDL-cholesterol (14%). The incidence of functional gastrointestinal adverse events in both trials for berberine was 34.5% (mainly in the first 4 weeks), with flatulence the most common complaint (19%). Berberine was decreased in 14 (24%) patients in the second trial as a consequence of gastrointestinal side effects, with a successful resolution.

In a randomised, double blind, three-arm controlled trial involving 97 patients with type 2 diabetes, berberine treatment (1000 mg/day) was compared with metformin (1500 mg/day) and rosiglitazone (4 mg/day) over a 2-month period.[186] All three treatments significantly lowered FBG and HbA_{1c} by a similar amount, but only berberine significantly lowered plasma triglycerides compared with baseline. Following berberine therapy, liver transaminases were significantly lowered (p<0.01), serum insulin had declined by 28.2% (p<0.01) and insulin receptor expression on peripheral blood lymphocytes was significantly elevated by 3.6-fold (p<0.01). A second trial in patients with liver disease was also included in this publication, motivated by the observation that current drugs for type 2 diabetes can cause adverse hepatic effects. This open label trial included 35 patients with either type 2 diabetes or insulin resistance (impaired fasting glucose) in conjunction with chronic hepatitis B or C. They were administered berberine (1000 mg/day) for 2 months. Berberine significantly lowered FBG, triglycerides and transaminases in all patient subgroups (p<0.01 or p 0.001).

A comprehensive metabonomic analysis was performed to understand the potential mechanisms of action of berberine in patients with both type 2 diabetes and dyslipidaemia.[187] Sixty patients were randomly selected for analysis from the trial described above.[184] Compared with placebo, patients before and after berberine treatment could be separated into distinct clusters in terms of changes in global serum metabolites. There was a highly significant decrease in the serum concentration of 13 FFAs following berberine, 10 of these also differed statistically from placebo. These results suggest that berberine downregulates the high level of FFAs seen in type 2 diabetes.

Cardiovascular disease

Twelve patients with refractory congestive heart failure (CHF) were studied before and during berberine intravenous infusion (at rates of 0.02 and 0.2 mg/kg/min for 30 min) in an acute single-dose study. The lower infusion dose produced no significant circulatory changes, apart from a reduction in heart rate. The higher dose produced marked and significant changes indicative of cardiotonic activity.[188] Some time later, a randomised, placebo-controlled clinical trial was instigated to evaluate the safety and efficacy of oral berberine in congestive heart failure.[189] One hundred and 56 patients were randomised into two groups and all received appropriate conventional medications such as ACE (angiotensin-converting enzyme) inhibitors, diuretics, digoxin and nitrates. The active group was also given 1.2 to 2.0 g/day of berberine. After 8 weeks, the berberine group displayed a significant improvement in left ventricular ejection fraction and exercise capacity, less dyspnoea and a decrease in the frequency and complexity of ventricular premature complexes (a marker of CHF). Additionally, the mortality rate of patients in the berberine group was almost half that of the control group during the 24-month follow-up period. A prior 2-week study in 56 patients with CHF found more significant decreases in the frequency and complexity of ventricular premature complexes and increases in left ventricular ejection fraction when plasma concentrations of berberine reached levels higher than 0.11 μg/mL (after oral doses of berberine of 1200 mg/day).[190]

Berberine also lowers elevated blood lipids, including those in patients with type 2 diabetes (see above). A single blind clinical trial compared the effects of daily oral administration of berberine (500 mg/day) with a combination including berberine, policosanol, red yeast extract, folic acid and astaxanthin for 4 weeks in 40 patients with moderate hypercholesterolaemia. Compared with baseline readings, the berberine and the berberine combination significantly reduced total cholesterol (16% and 20%), LDL-cholesterol (20% and 25%), apolipoprotein B (15% and 29%) and triglycerides (22% and 26%). Both treatments also increased HDL-cholesterol (by 6.6% and 5.1%, respectively, p<0.05 for both).[191]

Even more striking results were obtained in an earlier randomised, placebo-controlled trial that investigated the effects of oral berberine (1000 mg/day) in 43 hypercholesterolaemic patients. After 3 months of treatment, berberine reduced total cholesterol by 29%, LDL-cholesterol by 25% and triglycerides by 35% (p<0.0001 compared with baseline).[69]

One clinical trial assessed the value of combining berberine with simvastatin. In this randomised, controlled (presumably open) three-arm trial, 63 patients with hyperlipidaemia received either berberine (1000 mg/day), simvastatin (20 mg/day) or their combination for 2 months.[70] All patient groups exhibited significant reductions in total cholesterol, LDL-cholesterol and triglycerides compared with baseline readings (p<0.05 to p<0.001). The effect of the combination on these parameters was significantly better than either berberine (p<0.05) or simvastatin (p<0.01) alone. In terms of LDL-cholesterol, the reductions after berberine, simvastatin and their combination were 23.8%, 14.3% and 31.8%, respectively.

In an open label comparative trial, 86 hyperlipidaemic patients also suffering from chronic hepatitis B (n=51), chronic hepatitis C (n=18) or alcoholic liver cirrhosis (n=17) were given either berberine (1000 mg/day, n=70) or silymarin (210 mg/day, n=16 and only in hepatitis B patients) for 3 months.[192] Compared with baseline, berberine significantly reduced total cholesterol, LDL-cholesterol and triglycerides in all patient groups (p<0.001 or p<0.0001), whereas silymarin in the hepatitis B patients only lowered triglycerides (p<0.05). Both silymarin and berberine significantly lowered hepatic transaminases (p<0.001 or p<0.0001). The authors concluded that, unlike some current conventional treatments, berberine appeared well-suited as a treatment for lipid dysfunction in liver patients. It should be noted that the dose of silymarin used in the trial was relatively low.

The lipid-lowering effects of berberine (500 mg/day) and ezetimibe (10 mg/day) were compared in 195 patients with hypercholesterolaemia in a 3-month (presumably open label) clinical trial.[193] Berberine was more effective than ezetimibe in terms of lowering total cholesterol (24.1% versus 21.7%, p=0.002) and LDL-cholesterol (31.7% versus 29.3%, p=0.03) from baseline. Both treatments lowered triglycerides by about 17%. Only two patients reported gastrointestinal intolerance to berberine. No significant adverse effects, including AST, ALT and CPK levels, were observed during the two treatments.

Radioprotective activity

Given the traditional role of berberine-containing herbs in China for the treatment of diarrhoea, the impact of berberine on radiation-induced acute intestinal syndrome (RIAIS) was explored.[194] RIAIS includes side effects such as nausea, vomiting, abdominal pain, loss of appetite, diarrhoea, colitis and proctitis. Thirty-six patients with seminoma (a type of testicular cancer) or lymphoma, and another 42 with cervical cancer, were randomly administered either berberine (900 mg/day) or a placebo for 4 and 5 weeks, respectively. The berberine was given just prior to and during abdominal or pelvic radiotherapy. Berberine had significantly improved the incidence and severity of RIAIS in both patient groups by the end of the trial (p<0.05). Berberine (900 mg/day) also reduced existing RIAIS in a separate group of eight patients. The treatment was well tolerated.

In a prior randomised, double blind, placebo-controlled study, the effect of 6 weeks of berberine (20 mg/kg/day) on radiation-induced lung injury (RILI) was assessed in 90 patients undergoing treatment for non-small cell lung cancer.[195] The incidence of RILI was significantly lower in the berberine group compared with the placebo group at 6 weeks and at a 6-month follow-up (45.2% versus 72.1% and 35.7% versus 65.1%, respectively, both p<0.05). Two measures of radiation-induced lung tissue damage (soluble intercellular adhesion molecule-1 and transforming growth factor beta 1) were also significantly reduced at 6 weeks compared with the placebo (p<0.01 for both), and two measures of lung function were significantly improved at 6 months.

Other effects

Ten patients with cutaneous leishmaniasis received a 1% berberine salt solution intralesionally at weekly intervals for a period of 2 months. A blood sample was taken from the patients before and after treatment. The lesions showed evidence of healing after the second injection. Two patients dropped out of this uncontrolled trial, and of the remaining eight, healing was complete by 4 to 8 weeks.[196]

Berberine sulphate, given on its own and in a combined treatment at a dose of 15 mg/day for 15 days, increased platelet count in patients with primary and secondary thrombocytopenia.[197]

Two hundred and fifteen patients with chloroquine-resistant malaria were randomised into three groups: 82 patients received pyrimethamine and berberine chloride (1500 mg/day), 64 patients received pyrimethamine and tetracycline, and 69 patients received pyrimethamine and co-trimoxazole, all for 3 days. The clearance rate of asexual parasitaemia after treatment was 74% in the berberine group, 67% in the tetracycline group and 48% in the co-trimoxazole group. Berberine was more effective in clearing the parasite than the other antimicrobial agents when used in conjunction with pyrimethamine.[198]

Toxicology and other safety data

Toxicology

Early acute toxicological studies have established the following LD_{50} values: berberine 329 mg/kg (oral, mice) and 18 mg/kg (sc, mice),[146] berberine 23 mg/kg (ip, mice),[199] hydrastine 104 mg/kg (ip, rats)[200] and Hydrastis extract 1.62 g/kg (oral, mice).[146]

A recent study in mice suggests that berberine has extremely low oral toxicity as a result of its relatively low gastrointestinal absorption. LD_{50} values for berberine chloride after iv and ip injection were 9.0 and 57.6 mg/kg, respectively, but no LD_{50} could be determined for intragastric (oral) administration.[201] A 30% mortality rate was found among mice in the two highest oral dose groups (41.6 and 83.2 g/kg), which was related to the level achieved in their blood (with around 0.43 µg/mL being a potentially toxic concentration). An oral dose of 20.8 g/kg of berberine exhibited no acute toxic effects in mice, which corresponds to about 3 g/kg for a human. This is more than 100 times above the typical doses used in published clinical trials (up to around 30 mg/kg). A much earlier study found an oral LD_{50} for berberine sulphate in rats of >1 g/kg, confirming its low toxicity by this route.[202] A single oral dose of berberine given to mice (4 mg/kg) 1 h prior to the administration of a sub-lethal dose of strychnine enhanced the effect of strychnine, causing 100% mortality. The authors suggest that the berberine had an inhibitory effect upon cytochrome P450 enzymes.[203]

Berberine has been found to partially insert into DNA in vitro.[204] Berberine hydrochloride was weakly mutagenic in *Salmonella typhimurium* strain TA98 in the absence of S9 mix, but was inactive towards strain TA100 under these conditions. In the presence of S9 mix (metabolic activation) it was non-mutagenic towards both strains.[205] Berberine did not show genotoxic activity with or without metabolic activation in the SOS chromotest. It was inactive in treatments performed under non-growth conditions, but showed mild mutagenic activity in dividing cells.[206]

An in vitro study demonstrated that berberine exhibits phosphorescence in ethanol. UVA irradiation of keratinocytes in the presence of berberine resulted in a decrease in cell viability and an increase in DNA damage.[207] The effect of the topical application of berberine or berberine-containing preparations and subsequent skin exposure to UVA irradiation or to natural light has not been studied.

In vitro berberine has caused mitochondrial depolarisation and fragmentation, with a simultaneous increase on oxidative stress.[208] This has relevance to its antitumour activity as well as any potential toxicity.

Human lens epithelial cells were damaged when incubated with berberine and exposed to UVA. Under the same conditions palmatine was less phototoxic and hydrastine, canadine and hydrastinine were inactive.[209] At much higher concentrations berberine also damaged human retinal pigment epithelial cells following irradiation with visible light. The authors suggested that eyewashes and lotions derived from Hydrastis or containing berberine should be used with caution when the eyes are exposed to bright sunlight, but oral preparations are unlikely to cause ocular phototoxicity.

The US National Institute of Environmental Health Services (NIEHS) has published the results of its short- and long-term genetic toxicology and carcinogenesis studies of Hydrastis.[210] A significant incidence of liver tumours was observed in rats and male mice at doses of 50 000 and 25 000 ppm of diet, respectively, corresponding to doses at least 10 times higher than normal human doses over the lifespan of the animals. Moreover, the vast majority of the tumours were benign, and it is debated if such tumours do actually demonstrate carcinogenic potential. In support of this, the same study also found that Hydrastis lacked mutagenic and genotoxic activities using standard in vitro and in vivo tests. Nonetheless, the National Toxicology Program concluded that there was 'clear evidence' of liver carcinogenicity in the rats and 'some evidence' for the male mice. The short-term toxicity studies found evidence of Hydrastis inducing hepatocellular hypertrophy in rats and mice, but without apparent adverse health effects.

Contraindications

Use of berberine-containing plants is best avoided during pregnancy[211,212] or for jaundiced neonates.[211] The *British Herbal Pharmacopoeia* 1983 advises that Hydrastis is contraindicated in pregnancy and hypertensive conditions.[6] The contraindication for hypertension may be based on the cardiovascular activity of berberine. The *British Herbal Compendium* 1992 does not list hypertension as a contraindication.[22] An Eclectic text notes that 'the whole drug … arterial tension is augmented, and blood pressure in the capillaries increased, rendering it valuable, like belladonna and ergot, in overcoming blood stasis'.[7] This contraindication of Hydrastis in hypertension is unjustified on current information.

Although berberine-containing plants have been used in traditional Chinese medicine for the treatment of jaundiced neonates, berberine is thought to cause severe acute haemolysis and neonatal jaundice in babies with glucose-6-phosphate dehydrogenase (G6PD) deficiency.[213] However, a review published in 2001 questioned the causal relationship between the berberine-containing herb *Coptis chinensis* and haemolysis in G6PD-deficient infants (see also the Pregnancy and lactation section below).[214]

The *British Herbal Pharmacopoeia* 1983 also advises that Berberis is contraindicated in diarrhoea and early pregnancy.[6]

The contraindication for diarrhoea is probably not valid. Berberis bark was used by Eclectic practitioners for the treatment of chronic diarrhoea and dysentery,[5] and berberine has been administered in clinical trials for the treatment of diarrhoea (see previously).

Special warnings and precautions

None required.

Interactions

A Chinese study investigating the effect of berberine on the protein binding of bilirubin in vitro found that berberine exerted a 10-fold effect compared with phenylbutazone, a potent displacer of bilirubin. Chronic ip administration of berberine (10 to 20 mg/kg/day for 7 days) to rats resulted in a significant decrease in mean bilirubin serum protein binding.[211] Hence, berberine may reinforce the effects of other drugs that displace the protein binding of bilirubin. This might also explain the contraindication for pregnancy, rather than any reputed uterine-contracting effects (see also the discussion under Pregnancy and lactation).

Berberine appears to interact with cyclosporin. A randomised, placebo-controlled clinical trial investigated the effect of berberine (600 mg/day) in 52 renal transplant patients and found that levels of cyclosporin A were increased by 29.3% in the berberine group.[215] In a separate pharmacokinetic study, co-administration of berberine with cyclosporin (6 mg/kg/day) in six patients for 12 days resulted in a 34.5% increase in plasma cyclosporin.[215] Berberine (600 mg/day for 10 days) did not increase blood levels of cyclosporin A (6 mg/kg/day) in six healthy male volunteers, but in another six volunteers 300 mg/day berberine increased the bioavailability of 3 mg/kg/day of cyclosporin A.[216] Combined use of cyclosporin A and berberine increased the blood concentration of cyclosporin A in heart transplant recipients and reduced the dosage required of the drug.[217]

The notion that ingestion of Hydrastis could mask illicit drugs in urinalysis has appeared in the popular literature since the late 1970s. A number of scientific studies have verified that this is a fallacy.[218,219] For example, the performance of a particular assay (CEDIA) for screening amphetamines, barbiturates, benzodiazepines, cocaine, opiates, phencyclidine and tetrahydrocannabinol in urine was evaluated. Only minimal or selective interferences were observed with the presence of adulterants, which were added to urine to potentially invalidate the screening results. These included Hydrastis tea, lemon juice, Visine and low concentrations of bleach and Drano.[220] This notion is likely to have come from a novel written in 1900 by the well-known American herbalist John Uri Lloyd.[219] It has been suggested that the copious water consumed with Hydrastis tea might in fact lead to false negative drug tests.[221]

Chronic use of Hydrastis is said to decrease absorption of vitamin B.[222] There is no further information available to support this claim.

In vitro, Hydrastis decreased the activity of several cytochrome P450 enzymes, including CYP2C8, CYP2C9,

CYP2D6, CYP2E1 and CYP3A4.[223–227] When individual alkaloids were tested, hydrastine was substantially more potent than berberine, but both were active.

These findings have led to in vivo and human studies. Berberine (30 and 100 mg/kg/day, oral for 14 days) did not influence the pharmacokinetics of oral carbamazepine or iv-administered digoxin in rats.[228] However, berberine did substantially increase the bioavailabilities of oral digoxin and cyclosporin A, probably by inhibition of intestinal P-gp. No significant changes in CYP3A activity were observed.

In 12 healthy volunteers given Hydrastis (2700 mg/day of dried extract) for 28 days, probe drug cocktails determined that CYP2D6 and CYP3A4/5 were moderately but significantly inhibited.[229] Similarly, Hydrastis extract (3969 mg/day containing 132 mg hydrastine and 77 mg berberine) for 14 days moderately inhibited CYP3A4 in 16 healthy volunteers.[230] The extract (3210 mg/day, similar alkaloid doses) for 14 days also significantly inhibited CYP2D6 in 18 healthy volunteers.[231] However, Hydrastis root (2280 mg/day) for 14 days had no influence on the pharmacokinetics of indinavir.[232] Based on this finding the authors suggested that the interaction of Hydrastis with other drugs metabolised by CYP3A4 is unlikely. The apparent discrepancy between this and the above three studies can be explained by dose (use of extract, which is more concentrated than the root by at least a factor of 3, versus use of the root). Furthermore, the above positive studies (in terms of CYP inhibition) employed doses of Hydrastis much higher than those recommended in this monograph, notwithstanding the authors' adherence to label recommendations for dosage.

In 20 healthy volunteers given Hydrastis extract (3210 mg/day) for 14 days, no impact on the pharmacokinetics of 0.5 mg digoxin was observed, other than a 14% increase in Cmax.[233] Based on these findings the authors suggested that Hydrastis is not a potent modulator of P-gp in humans at the dosage tested.

Use in pregnancy and lactation

Category C – Berberine-containing plants have caused or are associated with a substantial risk of causing harmful effects on the fetus or neonate without causing malformations (on the basis of the presence of berberine and related alkaloids).

On this basis, Hydrastis is best avoided during pregnancy except for short-term use to assist labour (see above and below). Hydrastine (500 mg) induced labour when taken orally by pregnant women.[234]

At the high oral dosage of 1.86 g/kg (65 times normal human dose) administered from days 1 to 15 of gestation, Hydrastis did not have any adverse effect on reproductive outcome in rats. Fetal weights were slightly increased when the herb was administered from days 1 to 8 and days 8 to 15 of gestation.[235,236] There was no difference in placental weight, the number of resorptions or litter size and there were no externally visible malformations. The herb was administered as an ethanol extract and the dose administered was the highest possible at which the ethanol remained below the teratogenic threshold.[237] Hydrastis did induce toxicity when embryos were cultured for 26 h in rat serum to which

the extract was added.[236] Poor oral absorption of the alkaloids probably explains this discrepancy.

A reduction in average fetal body weight per litter was observed in the offspring of mated mice fed Hydrastis root powder (7.7 g/kg/day) from days 6 to 17. No significant developmental toxicity was observed below this dosage. Maternal liver weights were increased at greater than 2 g/kg/day, but histopathological lesions were absent.[238]

Berberine has caused uterine contraction in both non-pregnant and pregnant experimental models.[212] In another study that investigated 10 berberine-containing plant extracts, stimulation or relaxation of isolated uterus occurred depending upon the extract tested. Results did not correlate with berberine content. This suggests that a berberine-containing herb will not necessarily produce uterine contractions merely because of the presence of berberine.[146] An alcohol extract of the bark of branches and stem of Berberis enhanced the contractility of isolated uterus.[239] Also see p. 414.

The maternal LOAEL (lowest observed adverse effect level) for mated rats fed berberine chloride dihydrate from gestational day 6 to day 20 was measured at 531 mg/kg/day. Maternal NOAEL (no observed adverse effect level) was 282 mg/kg/day. The developmental LOAEL was 1313 mg/kg/day and the NOAEL was 531 mg/kg/day.[240] A follow-up study using the same protocol (except for administration by gavage) found similar results, but there was an absence of a significant effect for berberine on developmental toxicity. It was suggested the developmental toxicity NOAEL could be raised in rats to approximately 1100 mg/kg/day berberine.[241,242] This indicates that doses less than 1 g/kg of berberine chloride dihydrate had no observable effect on offspring in the model used.

In mice fed berberine chloride dihydrate (BCD) by gavage on gestation days 6 to 17, a maternal toxicity LOAEL of 841 mg/kg/day was determined, with a developmental toxicity LOAEL of 1000 mg/kg/day. Corresponding NOAEL values were 569 and 841 mg/kg/day, respectively.[242] Levels for berberine chloride would be about 20% lower (accounting for the waters of hydration in BCD).

The incidence of kernicterus in premature Chinese infants with neonatal jaundice has been reported to be associated in some cases with exposure to Coptis chinensis, either by direct administration, transplacental absorption or via breast milk.[211] (Coptis contains 7% to 9% berberine.) This suggests that berberine-containing plants are best avoided during pregnancy and lactation. However, this association with neonatal jaundice has been challenged by two Chinese authors, who provided data from their experiments in newly born rats and mice indicating that Coptis did not increase serum bilirubin.[243] More research is needed on this topic.

Effects on ability to drive and use machines

No negative influence is expected for either herb.

Side effects

No adverse reactions have been documented for Berberis. In popular literature Hydrastis is often described as toxic in large doses and/or that it should be restricted to short-term use. It is possible that this information comes from a misinterpretation of the writings of the homeopath Dr Edwin Hale, who noted side effects (such as exhaustion of the mucous membranes) after many homeopathic provings in the mid-nineteenth century.[218] The results of homeopathic provings do not necessarily translate to herbal practice.

Native Americans and Eclectic physicians have used golden seal topically, particularly for ophthalmias (eye inflammation). One objection to this use was its ability to stain the conjunctiva.[7]

A case has been reported of the hospitalisation of an 11-year-old girl with diabetic ketoacidosis and severe hypernatraemia in conjunction with newly diagnosed type 1 diabetes.[244] Despite the fact that diabetic ketoacidosis is commonly associated with hypernatraemia, its severe nature led the authors to link it to the concurrent use of Hydrastis (1000 to 1500 mg/day for at least 2 weeks prior to admission). The Hydrastis was used to treat her polyuria, which the family attributed to a bladder infection. The authors incorrectly attributed aquaretic properties to Hydrastis and also failed to confirm the identity of the herb being taken.

The use of berberine for diarrhoea in children has resulted in cases of poor tolerance due to emesis. However, the berberine was often given in combination with other compounds that might have contributed to this adverse reaction.[212]

At doses higher than 500 mg, berberine may cause dizziness, nose bleeds, dyspnoea, skin and eye irritation, gastrointestinal irritation, nausea, diarrhoea, nephritis and urinary tract disorders.[245] However, apart from moderate gastrointestinal side effects, it was generally well tolerated in clinical trials.

Overdosage

Hydrastis has been said to cause irritation of the mouth, throat and stomach as well as convulsions when taken in toxic (undefined) doses.[222]

The Commission E notes that no reports of poisoning with Berberis are known, but that death from berberine poisoning has (possibly) occurred.[245]

Safety in children

Berberine has been used to treat diarrhoea and giardiasis in children, which suggests that berberine-containing plants, such as Hydrastis and Berberis, may also be used in this way. Treatment of neonates and very young children should be avoided until further information becomes available.

Regulatory status in selected countries

Berberis bark is covered by a negative Commission E monograph. In the opinion of the Commission E there is no evidence for the efficacy of the herb and there are risks associated with plant parts containing berberine. Side effects are possible if more than 500 mg of berberine is ingested.

Berberis is on the UK General Sale List.

Berberis does not have GRAS status. However, it is freely available as a 'dietary supplement' in the USA under DSHEA legislation (1994 Dietary Supplement Health and Education Act).

Berberis is not included in Part 4 of Schedule 4 of the Therapeutic Goods Act Regulations of Australia and is freely available for sale.

Hydrastis canadensis is official in the *United States Pharmacopea – National Formulary* USP31 NF26 2008.

Hydrastis is not covered by a Commission E monograph but it is on the UK General Sale List.

Hydrastis does not have GRAS status. However, it is freely available as a 'dietary supplement' in the USA under DSHEA legislation (1994 Dietary Supplement Health and Education Act). Hydrastis has been present in the following over-the-counter (OTC) drug products: digestive aid products, weight control products, orally administered menstrual products, antiseptic products and counterirritant products. Hydrastis has also been present as an ingredient in products offered OTC for use as an aphrodisiac. However, the FDA advises: 'that based on evidence currently available, there is inadequate data to establish general recognition of the safety and effectiveness of these ingredients for the specified uses'.

Hydrastis is not included in Part 4 of Schedule 4 of the Therapeutic Goods Act Regulations of Australia and is freely available for sale.

References

1. Mabberley DJ. *The Plant Book*, 2nd ed. Cambridge: Cambridge University Press; 1997. p. 84.

2. Osol A, Farrar GE, et al. *The Dispensatory of the United States of America*, 24th ed. Philadelphia: JB Lippincott; 1947. pp. 543–545.

3. Mabberley DJ. *The Plant Book*, 2nd ed. Cambridge: Cambridge University Press; 1997. p. 352.

4. Concannon JA, DeMeo TE. *Endangered Species Bull*. 1997;22(6):10–12.

5. Felter HW, Lloyd JU. *King's American Dispensatory*. 18th ed., rev 3, vol. 1, 1905. Portland, reprinted by Eclectic Medical Publications; 1983. pp. 345–346.

6. British Herbal Medicine Association's Scientific Committee. *British Herbal Pharmacopoeia*. West York: BHMA; 1983. pp. 39–40.

7. Felter HW, Lloyd JU. *King's American Dispensatory*, 18th ed., vol. 2, Portland; Eclectic Medical Publications; 1983. pp. 1020–1030.

8. Spaich W. *Moderne Phytotherapie*. Heidelberg: Karl F. Haug Verlag; 1977. pp. 232–234.

9. Grieve M. *A Modern Herbal*, vol. 1. New York: Dover Publications; 1971. pp. 82–84.

10. Leung AY, Forster S. *Encyclopedia of Common Natural Ingredients Used in Food, Drugs and Cosmetics*, 2nd ed. New York: John Wiley; 1996. pp. 67, 282.

11. Chiej R. *The Macdonald Encyclopaedia of Medicinal Plants*. London: Macdonald; 1984. Entry no. 54.

12. Launert EL. *The Hamlyn Guide to Edible and Medicinal Plants of Britain and Northern Europe*. London: Hamlyn; 1981. p. 24.

13. Veringa L, Zaricor BR. *Goldenseal/etc. A Pharmacognosy of Wild Herbs*. Santa Cruz: Ruka Publications; 1978. pp. 20–22.

14. Govindan M, Govindan G. *Fitoterapia*. 2000;71(3):232–235.

15. Weber HA, Zart MK, Hodges AE, et al. *J Agric Food Chem*. 2003;51(25): 7352–7358.

16. Bannerman J. *HerbalGram*. 1997;41: 51–52.

17. Chopra RN, Chopra IC, Handa KL, et al. *Chopra's Indigenous Drugs of India*, 2nd ed. Calcutta; 1958. Reprinted Academic Publishers; 1982. p. 289.

18. Lange D. *Europe's Medicinal and Aromatic Plants: Their Use, Trade and Conservation*. TRAFFIC International; 1998. p. IV.

19. Wagner H, Bladt S. *Plant Drug Analysis: A Thin Layer Chromatography Atlas*, 2nd ed. Berlin: Springer-Verlag; 1996. p. 10.

20. Brown PN, Roman MC. *J AOAC Int*. 2008;91(4):694–701.

21. Simeon S, Rios JL, Villar A. *Plantes Méd Phytothér*. 1989;23(3):202–250.

22. British Herbal Medicine Association. *British Herbal Compendium*, vol. 1. Bournemouth: BHMA; 1992. pp. 119–120.

23. Sun D, Abraham SN, Beachey EH. *Antimicrob Agents Chemother*. 1988;32(8):1274–1277.

24. Domadia PN, Bhunia A, Sivaraman J, et al. *Biochemistry*. 47(10):3225–3234.

25. Yu HH, Kim KJ, Cha JD, et al. *J Med Food*. 2005;8(4):454–461.

26. Wang D, Yu L, Xiang H, et al. *FEMS Microbiol Lett*. 2008;279(2):217–225.

27. Wang X, Qiu S, Yao X, et al. *J Orthop Res*. 2009;27(11):1487–1492.

28. Wang X, Yao X, Zhu Z, et al. *Int J Antimicrob Agents*. 2009;34(1):60–66.

29. Mahajan VM, Sharma A, Rattan A. *Sabouraudia*. 1982;20(1):79–81.

30. Iwazaki RS, Endo EH, Ueda-Nakamura T, et al. *Antonie Van Leeuwenhoek*. 2010;97(2):201–205.

31. Vennerstrom JL, Klayman DL. *J Med Chem*. 1988;31(6):1084–1087.

32. Kaneda Y, Torii M, Tanaka T, et al. *Ann Trop Med Parasitol*. 1991;85(4):417–425.

33. Ghosh AK, Rakshit MM, Ghosh DK. *Indian J Med Res*. 1983;78:407–416.

34. Saha P, Sen R, Hariharan C, et al. *Free Radic Res*. 2010;43(11):1101–1110.

35. Vennerstrom JL, Lovelace JK, Waits VB, et al. *Antimicrob Agents Chemother*. 1990;34(5):918–921.

36. Ahuja A, Purohit SK, Yadav JS, et al. *Indian J Public Health*. 1993;37(1):29–31.

37. Dutta NK, Iyer SN. *J Indian Med Assoc*. 1968;50(8):349–352.

38. Sun D, Courtney HS, Beachey EH. *Antimicrob Agents Chemother*. 1988;32(9):1370–1374.

39. Scazzocchio F, Cometa MF, Tomassini L, et al. *Planta Med*. 2001;67(6):561–564.

40. Mahady GB, Pendland SL, Stoia A, et al. *Phytother Res*. 2003;17(3):217–221.

41. Chen QM, Ye YC, Chai FL, et al. *Chung Kuo Chi Sheng Chung Hsueh Yu Chi Sheng Chung Ping Tsa Chih*. 1991;9(2):137–139.

42. Chin LW, Cheng YW, Lin SS, et al. *Arch Virol*. 2010 [Epub ahead of print].

43. Hayashi K, Minoda K, Nagaoka Y, et al. *Bioorg Med Chem Lett*. 2007;17(6): 1562–1564.

44. Amin AH, Subbaiah TV, Abbasi KM. *Can J Microbiol*. 1969;15:1067–1076.

45. Palasuntheram C, Sangara Iyer K, De Silva LB, et al. *Indian J Med Res*. 1982;76(suppl):71–76.

46. Pizzorno JE, Murray MT. *A Textbook of Natural Medicine*, vol. 1. Seattle: John Bastyr College Publications; 1987. p. V. Hydras-2.

47. Takase H, Yamamoto K, Ito K, et al. *Nippon Yakurigaku Zasshi*. 1993;102(2):101–112.

48. Zhang MF, Shen YQ. *Chung Kuo Yao Li Hsueh Pao*. 1989;10(2):174–176.

49. Donowitz M, Wicks J, Sharp GW. *Rev Infect Dis*. 1986;8(suppl 2):S188–S201.

50. Swabb EA, Tai YH, Jordan L. *Am J Physiol*. 1981;241(3):G248–G252.

51. Tai YH, Feser JF, Marnane WG, et al. *Am J Physiol*. 1981;241(3):G253–G258.

52. Sack RB, Froehlich JL. *Infect Immun*. 1982;35(2):471–475.

53. Khin-Maung U, Nwe-Nwe-Wai J. *Diarrhoeal Dis Res*. 1992;10(4):201–204.

54. Palasuntheram C, Sangara IK, De Silva LB, et al. *Indian J Med Res*. 1982;76(suppl):71–76.

55. Taylor CT, Baird AW. *Br J Pharmacol*. 1995;116(6):2667–2672.

56. Cheng ZF, Zhang YQ, Liu FC. *Regul Pept*. 2009;155(1–3):145–149.

57. Lau CW, Yao XQ, Chen ZY, et al. *Cardiovasc Drug Rev*. 2001;19(3): 234–244.

58. Hua Z, Wang XL. *Yao Hsueh Hsueh Pao*. 1994;29(8):576–580.

59. Wang YX, Yao XJ, Tan YH. *J Cardiovasc Pharmacol*. 1994;23(5):716–722.

60. Hong Y, Hui SC, Chan TY, et al. *Am J Chin Med*. 2002;30(4):589–599.

61. Hong Y, Hui SC, Chan TY, et al. *Life Sci*. 2003;72(22):2499–2507.

62. Zhao HP, Hong Y, Xie JD, et al. *Yao Xue Xue Bao*. 2007;42(3):336–341.

63. Ziablitskii VM, Romanovskaia VN, Umurzakova RZ, et al. *Eksp Klin Farmakol*. 1996;59(1):37–39.

64. Wu JF, Liu TP. *Yao Hsueh Hsueh Pao*. 1995;30(2):98–102.

65. Chu ZL, Huang CG, Lai FS. *Chin Pharmacol Bull*. 1994;10(2):114–116.

66. Abidi P, Zhou Y, Jiang JD, et al. *Arterioscler Thromb Vasc Biol*. 2005;25(10):2170–2176.

67. Abidi P, Chen W, Kraemer FB, et al. *J Lipid Res*. 2006;47(10):2134–2147.

68. Brusq JM, Ancellin N, Grondin P, et al. *J Lipid Res*. 2006;47(6):1281–2188.

69. Kong W, Wei J, Abidi P, et al. *Nat Med*. 2004;10(12):1344–1351.

70. Kong WJ, Wei J, Zuo ZY, et al. *Metabolism*. 2008;57(8):1029–1037.

71. Jia X, Chen Y, Zidichouski J, et al. *Atherosclerosis*. 2008;201(1):101–107.

72. Suckling KE, Jackson B. *Prog Lipid Res*. 1993;32(1):1–24.

73. Wang Y, Jia X, Ghanam K, et al. *Atherosclerosis*. 2010;209(1):111–117.

74. Holy EW, Akhemdov A, Luscher TF, et al. *J Mol Cell Cardiol*. 2009;46(2):234–240.

75. Li K, Yao W, Zheng X, et al. *Cell Res*. 2009;19(8):1006–1017.

76. Cho BJ, Im EK, Kwon JH, et al. *Mol Cells*. 2005;20(3):429–434.

77. Liang KW, Yin SC, Ting CT, et al. *Eur J Pharmacol*. 2008;590(1–3):343–354.

78. Hsieh YS, Kuo WH, Lin TW, et al. *J Agric Food Chem*. 2007;55(25):10437–10445.

79. Huang Z, Wang L, Meng S, et al. *Int J Cardiol*. 2009 [Epub ahead of print].

80. Wang Y, Huang Y, Lam KS, et al. *Cardiovasc Res*. 2009;82(3):484–492.

81. Xu MG, Wang JM, Chen L, et al. *J Hum Hypertens*. 2008;22(6):389–393.

82. Xu MG, Wang JM, Chen L, et al. *Cardiology*. 2009;112(4):279–286.

83. Wang JM, Yang Z, Xu MG, et al. *Eur J Pharmacol*. 2009;614(1–3):77–83.

84. Sun Y, Xun K, Wang Y, et al. *Anticancer Drugs*. 2009;20(9):757–769.

85. Tang J, Feng Y, Tsao S, et al. *J Ethnopharmacol*. 2009;126(1):5–17.

86. Fukuda K, Hibiya Y, Mutoh M, et al. *J Ethnopharmacol*. 1999;66(2):227–233.

87. Kuo CL, Chi CW, Liu TY. *Cancer Lett*. 2004;203(2):127–137.

88. Fukuda K, Hibiya Y, Mutoh M, et al. *Planta Med*. 1999;65(4):381–383.

89. Ckless K, Schlottfeldt JL, Pasqual M, et al. *J Pharm Pharmacol*. 1995;47(12A): 1029–1031.

90. Jeong HW, Hsu KC, Lee JW, et al. *Am J Physiol Endocrinol Metab*. 2009;296(4):E955–E964.

91. Lee CH, Chen JC, Hsiang CY, et al. *Pharmacol Res*. 2007;56(3):193–201.

92. Luo CN, Lin X, Li WK, et al. *J Ethnopharmacol*. 1998;59(3):211–215.

93. Luo CN, Lin X, Li WK, et al. *Phytother Res*. 1997;11(8):585–587.

94. Ivanovska N, Philipov S. *Int J Immunopharmacol*. 1996;18(10): 553–561.

95. Zhou H, Mineshita S. *J Pharmacol Exp Ther*. 2000;294(3):822–829.

96. Kupeli E, Kosar M, Yesilada E, et al. *Life Sci*. 2002;72(6):645–657.

97. Shen YB, Piao XS, Kim SW, et al. *Poult Sci*. 2010;89(1):13–19.

98. Zhang HQ, Wang HD, Lu DX, et al. *Shock*. 29(5):617–622.

99. Kulkarni SK, Dhir A. *Phytother Res*. 2010;24(3):317–324.

100. Zhu F, Qian C. *BMC Neurosci*. 2006;7:78.

101. Kulkarni SK, Dhir A. *Eur J Pharmacol*. 2008;589(1–3):163–172.

102. Peng WH, Lo KL, Lee YH, et al. *Life Sci*. 2007;81(11):933–938.

103. Peng WH, Wu CR, Chen CS, et al. *Life Sci*. 2004;75(20):2451–2462.

104. Bhutada P, Mundhada Y, Bansod K, et al. *Epilepsy Behav*. 2010;18(3):207–210.

105. Peng WH, Hsieh MT, Wu CR. *Jpn J Pharmacol*. 1997;74(3):261–266.

106. Yin J, Hu R, Chen M, et al. *Metabolism*. 2002;51(11):1439–1443.

107. Zhou L, Yang Y, Wang X, et al. *Metabolism*. 2007;56(3):405–412.

108. Turner N, Li JY, Gosby A, et al. *Diabetes*. 2008;57(5):1414–1418.

109. Al-Masri IM, Mohammad MK, Tahaa MO. *J Enzyme Inhib Med Chem*. 2009;24(5):1061–1066.

110. Yi P, Lu FE, Xu LJ, et al. *World J Gastroenterol*. 2008;14(6):876–883.

111. Kong WJ, Zhang H, Song DQ, et al. *Metabolism*. 2009;58(1):109–119.

112. Chen Y, Li Y, Wang Y, et al. *Metabolism*. 2009;58(12):1694–1702.

113. Liu LZ, Cheung SC, Lan LL, et al. *Mol Cell Endocrinol*. 2010;317(1–2):148–153.

114. Liu W, Liu P, Tao S, et al. *Arch Biochem Biophys*. 2008;475(2):128–134.

115. Liu W, Tang F, Deng Y, et al. *Mol Cell Biochem*. 2009;325(1–2):99–105.

116. Leng SH, Lu FE, Xu LJ. *Acta Pharmacol Sin*. 2004;25(4):496–502.

117. Lee YS, Kim WS, Kim KH, et al. *Diabetes*. 2006;55(8):2256–2264.

118. Tang LQ, Wei W, Chen LM, et al. *J Ethnopharmacol*. 2006;108(1):109–115.

119. Zhou J, Zhou S, Tang J, et al. *Eur J Pharmacol*. 2009;606(1–3):262–268.

120. Zhou JY, Zhou SW, Zhang KB, et al. *Biol Pharm Bull*. 2008;31(6):1169–1176.

121. Zhang W, Xu YC, Guo FJ, et al. *Chin Med J (Engl)*. 2008;121(21):2124–2128.

122. Zhang M, Lv XY, Li J, et al. *Exp Diabetes Res*. 2008; 2008: 704045.

123. Wang Y, Campbell T, Perry B, et al. *Metabolism*. 2010 [Epub ahead of print].

124. Yin J, Gao Z, Liu D, et al. *Am J Physiol Endocrinol Metab*. 2008;294(1): E148–156.

125. Zhou L, Wang X, Shao L, et al. *Endocrinology*. 2008;149(9):4510–4518.

126. Gao Z, Leng S, Lu F, et al. *J Huazhong Univ Sci Technolog Med Sci*. 2008;28(3):261–265.

127. Liu L, Deng Y, Yu S, et al. *Pharmazie*. 2008;63(5):384–388.

128. Pan GY, Wang GJ, Sun JG, et al. *Yao Xue Xue Bao*. 2003;38(12):911–914.

129. Liu L, Yu YL, Yang JS, et al. *Naunyn Schmiedebergs Arch Pharmacol*. 2010;381(4):371–381.

130. Liu WH, Hei ZQ, Nie H, et al. *Chin Med J (Engl)*. 2008;121(8):706–712.

131. Zhou JY, Zhou SW. *Yao Xue Xue Bao*. 2007;42(12):1243–1249.

132. Lin WC, Change HL. *Res Commun Mol Pathol Pharmacol*. 1995;90(3):333–346.

133. Imaseki I, Kitabatake Y, Taguchi H. *Yakugaku Zasshi*. 1961;81:1281–1284.

134. Cao JW, Luo HS, Yu BP, et al. *Digestion*. 2001;64(3):179–183.

135. Chan MY. *Comp Med East West*. 1977;5(2):161–168.

136. Seki T, Morohashi M. *Skin Pharmacol*. 1993;6(1):56–60.

137. Hu JP, Nishishita K, Sakai E, et al. *Eur J Pharmacol*. 2008;580(1–2):70–79.

138. Lee HW, Suh JH, Kim HN, et al. *J Bone Miner Res*. 2008;23(8):1227–1237.

139. Wei P, Jiao L, Qin LP, et al. *Zhong Xi Yi Jie He Xue Bao*. 2009;7(4):342–348.

140. Hu Y, Davies GE. *Fitoterapia*. 2010;81(5):358–366.

141. Kim WS, Lee YS, Cha SH, et al. *Am J Physiol Endocrinol Metab*. 2009;296(4):E812–E819.

142. Bashir S, Gilani AH. *Eur J Pharmacol*. 2011;651(1–3):168–175.

143. Pepeljnjak S, Petricic J. *Pharmazie*. 1992;47(4):307–308.

144. Cwikla C, Schmidt K, Matthias A, et al. *Phytother Res*. 2010;24(5):649–656.

145. Gibbs OS. *Fed Proc*. 1947;6:322.

146. Haginiwa J, Harada M. *Yakugaku Zasshi*. 1962;82:726–731.

147. Palmery M, Leone MG, Pimpinella G, et al. *Pharmacol Res*. 1993;27(suppl 1):73–74.

148. Palmery M, Cometa MF, Leone MG. *Phytother Res*. 1996;10(suppl 1): S47–S49.

149. Cometa MF, Galeffi C, Palmery M. *Phytother Res*. 1996;10(suppl 1):S56–S58.

150. Cometa MF, Abdel-Haq H, Palmery M. *Phytother Res*. 1998;12(suppl 1):S83–S85.

151. Bolle P, Cometa MF, Palmery M, et al. *Phytother Res*. 1998;12(suppl 1):S86–S88.

152. Rentz E. *Arch Exp Pathol Pharmakol*. 1948;205:332–338.

153. Tripathi YB, Shukla SD. *Phytother Res*. 1996;10(7):628–630.

154. Nikoronow M. *Acta Polon Pharm*. 1939;3:23–56.

155. Khattak SG, Gilani SN, Ikram M. *J Ethnopharmacol*. 1985;14(1):45–51.

156. Wolf S, Mack M. *Drug Stand*. 1956;24(3):98–101.

157. Karmakar SR, Biswas SJ, Khuda-Bukhsh AR. *Asian Pac J Cancer Prev*. 2010;11(2):545–551.

158. Clement-Kruzel S, Hwang SA, Kruzel MC, et al. *J Med Food*. 2008;11(3): 493–498.

159. Rehman J, Dillow JM, Carter SM. *Immunol Lett*. 1999;68(2–3):391–395.

160. Bashir S, Gilani AH, Siddiqui AA, et al. *Phytother Res*. 2010;24(8):1250–1255.

161. Bhide MB, Chavan SR, Dutta NK. *Indian J Med Res*. 1969;57(11):2128–2131.

162. Ozaki Y, Suzuki H, Satake M. *Yakugaku Zasshi*. 1993;113(1):63–69.

163. Hua W, Ding L, Chen Y, et al. *J Pharm Biomed Anal*. 2007;44(4):931–937.

164. Yu C, Zhang H, Ren JY, et al. *Chinese J Clin Pharm*. <http://en.cnki.com.cn/Article_en/CJFDTotal–GLYZ200001010.htm>. Accessed 5.11.10.

165. Tsai PL, Tsai TH. *Drug Metab Dispos*. 2004;32(4):405–412.

166. Zuo F, Nakamura N, Akao T, et al. *Drug Metab Dispos*. 2006;34(12):2064–2072.

167. Pan JF, Yu C, Zhu DY, et al. *Acta Pharmacol Sin*. 2002;23(1):77–82.

168. Qiu F, Zhu Z, Kang N, et al. *Drug Metab Dispos*. 2008;36(11):2159–2165.

169. Pan GY, Wang GJ, Liu XD, et al. *Pharmacol Toxicol*. 2002;91(4):193–197.

170. Yan D, Wei L, Xiao XH, et al. *Chin Sci Bull*. 2009;54(3):369–373.

171. Lahiri SC, Dutta NK. *J Indian Med Assoc*. 1967;48(1):1–11.

172. Sharda DC. *J Indian Med Assoc*. 1970;54: 22–24.

173. Khin-Maung U, Myo-Khin Nyunt-Nyunt-Wai, et al. *Br Med J (Clin Res Ed)*. 1985;291(6509):1601–1605.

174. Khin-Maung-U Myo-Khin Nyunt-Nyunt-Wai. *J Diarrhoeal Dis Res*. 1987;5(3): 184–187.

175. Rabbani GH, Butler T, Knight J, et al. *J Infect Dis*. 1987;155(5):979–984.

176. Yuan J, Shen XZ, Zhu XS. *Chung Kuo Chung Hsi I Chieh Ho Tsa Chih*. 1994;14(12):718–720.

177. Hu FL. *Chung Hua I Hsueh Tsa Chih*. 1993;73(4):217–219, 253.

178. Babbar OP, Chhatwal VK, Ray IB, et al. *Indian J Med Res*. 1982;76(suppl):83–88.

179. Mohan M, Pant CR, Angra SK, et al. *Indian J Ophthalmol*. 1982;30(2):69–75.

180. Choudhry VP, Sabir M, Bhide VN. *Indian Pediatr*. 1972;9(3):143–146.

181. Gupte S. *Am J Dis Child*. 1975;129(7):866.

182. Watanabe A, Obata T, Nagashima H. *Acta Med Okayama*. 1982;36(4):277–281.

183. Ni YX, Liu AQ, Gao YF, et al. *Chin J Integr Med*. 1988;8(12):71–713.

184. Zhang Y, Li X, Zou D, et al. *J Clin Endocrinol Metab*. 2008;93(7):2559–2565.

185. Yin J, Xing H, Ye J. *Metabolism*. 2008;57(5):712–717.

186. Zhang H, Wei J, Xue R, et al. *Metabolism*. 2010;59(2):285–292.

187. Gu Y, Zhang Y, Shi X, et al. *Talanta*. 2010;81(3):766–772.

188. Marin-Neto JA, Maciel BC, Secches AL, et al. *Clin Cardiol.* 1988;11(4):253–260.

189. Zeng XH, Zeng XJ, Li YY. *Am J Cardiol.* 2003;92(2):173–176.

190. Zeng X, Zeng X. *Biomed Chromatogr.* 1999;13(7):442–444.

191. Cicero AF, Rovati LC, Setnikar I. *Arzneimittelforschung.* 2007;57(1):26–30.

192. Zhao W, Xue R, Zhou ZX, et al. *Biomed Pharmacother.* 2008;62(10):730–731.

193. Pisciotta L, Ivaldi C, Borrini C, et al. *Nutr Metab Cardiovasc Dis.* 2009;19(suppl 1):S22.

194. Li GH, Wang DL, Hu YD, et al. *Med Oncol.* 2010;27(3):919–925.

195. Liu Y, Yu H, Zhang C, et al. *Eur J Cancer.* 2008;44(16):2425–2432.

196. Purohit SK, Kochar DK, Lal BB, et al. *Indian J Public Health.* 1982;26(1):34–37.

197. Chekalina SI, Umurzakova RZ, Saliev KK, et al. *Gematol Transfuziol.* 1994;39(5): 33–35.

198. Sheng WD, Jiddawi MS, Hong XQ, et al. *East Afr Med J.* 1997;74(5):283–284.

199. Schmeller T, Latz-Bruning B, Wink M. *Phytochemistry.* 1997;44(2):257–266.

200. Poe CF, Johnson CC. *Acta Pharmacol Toxicol.* 1954;10:338–346.

201. Kheir MM, Wang Y, Hua L, et al. *Food Chem Toxicol.* 2010;48(4):1105–1110.

202. Kowalewski Z, Mrozikiewicz A, Bobkiewicz T, et al. *Acta Pol Pharm.* 1975;32(1):113–120.

203. Janbaz KH, Gilani AH. *Fitoterapia.* 2000;71(1):25–33.

204. Saran A, Srivastava S, Coutinho E, et al. *Indian J Biochem Biophys.* 1995;32(2): 74–77.

205. Nozaka T, Watanabe F, Tadaki S, et al. *Mutat Res.* 1990;240(4):267–279.

206. Pasqual MS, Lauer CP, Moyna P, et al. *Mutat Res.* 1993;286(2):243–252.

207. Inbaraj JJ, Kukielczak BM, Bilski P, et al. *Chem Res Toxicol.* 2001;14(11):1529–1534.

208. Pereira CV, Machado NG, Oliveira PJ. *Toxicol Sci.* 2008;105(2):408–417.

209. Chignell CF, Sik RH, Watson MA, et al. *Photochem Photobiol.* 2007;83(4):938–943.

210. National Toxicology Program *Natl. Toxicol Program Tech Rep Ser.* 2010;562:1–188.

211. Chan E. *Biol Neonate.* 1993;63(4): 201–208.

212. De Smet P.A.G.M.Keller K, Hansel R, editors. *Adverse Effects of Herbal Drugs,* vol. 1. Berlin: Springer-Verlag; 1992. pp. 97–104.

213. Ho NK. *Singapore Med J.* 1996;37(6): 645–651.

214. Fok TF. *J Perinatol.* 2001;21(suppl 1): S98–S100.

215. Wu X, Li Q, Xin H, et al. *Eur J Clin Pharmacol.* 2005;61(8):567–572.

216. Xin HW, Wu XC, Li Q, et al. *Methods Find Exp Clin Pharmacol.* 2006;28(1): 25–29.

217. Huang XS, Yang GF, Pan YC. *Zhongguo Zhong Xi Yi Jie He Za Zhi.* 2008;28(8):702–704.

218. Bergner P. *Med Herbalism.* 1996–1997;8(4):1, 4–6. Available via <www.mediherb.com.au>.

219. Foster S. *HerbalGram.* 1989;21:735.

220. Wu AHB, Forte E, Casella G, et al. *J Forensic Sci.* 1995;40(4):614–618.

221. Cone EJ, Lange R, Darwin WD. *J Anal Toxicol.* 1998;22(6):460–473.

222. Hamon NW. *Can Pharm J.* 1990;123(11):508–510.

223. Budzinski JW, Foster BC, Vandenhoek S, et al. *Phytomedicine.* 2000;7(4):273–282.

224. Budzinski JW, Trudeau VL, Drouin CE, et al. *Can J Physiol Pharmacol.* 2007;85(9):966–978.

225. Raner GM, Cornelious S, Moulick K, et al. *Food Chem Toxicol.* 2007;45(12): 2359–2365.

226. Etheridge AS, Black SR, Patel PR, et al. *Planta Med.* 2007;73(8):731–741.

227. Chatterjee P, Franklin MR. *Drug Metab Dispos.* 2003;31(11):1391–1397.

228. Qiu W, Jiang XH, Liu CX, et al. *Phytother Res.* 2009;23(11):1553–1558.

229. Gurley BJ, Gardner SF, Hubbard MA, et al. *Clin Pharmacol Ther.* 2005;77(5):415–426.

230. Gurley BJ, Swain A, Hubbard MA, et al. *Clin Pharmacol Ther.* 2008;83(1):61–69.

231. Gurley BJ, Swain A, Hubbard MA, et al. *Mol Nutr Food Res.* 2008;52(7): 755–763.

232. Sandhu RS, Prescilla RP, Simonelli TM, et al. *J Clin Pharmacol.* 2003;43(11):1283–1288.

233. Gurley BJ, Swain A, Barone GW, et al. *Drug Metab Dispos.* 2007;35(2):240–245.

234. Grismondi GL, Scivoli L, Cetera C. *Min Ginecol.* 1979;31(1/2):19–32.

235. Ernst E, Schmidt K. *BMC Cancer.* 2005;5:69.

236. Yao M, Ritchie HE, Brown-Woodman PD. *Birth Defects Res B Dev Reprod Toxicol.* 2005;74(5):399–404.

237. Yao M, Brown-Woodman PDC, Ritchie H. *Teratology.* 2001;64(6):323–324.

238. NTP Study TER99004. Final Study Report: Developmental Toxicity Evaluation for Goldenseal (Hydrastis canadensis) Root Powder Administered in the Feed to Swiss (CD1®) Mice on Gestational Days 6–17. Available from the National Toxicology Program website: <http://ntp-server.niehs.nih.gov>. Accessed November, 2010.

239. Aliev RK, Yuzbashinskaya NA. *Doklady Akad Nauk Azerbaidzhan SSR.* 1953;9(4):231–237.

240. Price CJ, George JD, Marr MC, et al. *Teratology.* 2001;63(6):279.

241. NTP Study TER20102. Final Study Report: Developmental Toxicity Evaluation for Berberine Chloride Dihydrate (Cas No. 5956–60–5) Administered by Gavage to Sprague-Dawley (CD®) Rats on Gestational Days 6 through 19. Available from the National Toxicology Program website: <http://ntp-server.niehs.nih.gov>. Accessed November, 2010.

242. Jahnke GD, Price CJ, Marr MC, et al. *Birth Defects Res B Dev Reprod Toxicol.* 2006;77(3):195–206.

243. Yang S, Wang X. *J Tradit Chin Med.* 2008;28(3):235–240.

244. Bhowmick SK, Hundley OT, Rettig KR. *Clin Pediatr (Phila).* 2007;46(9):831–834.

245. Blumenthal M, ed. *The Complete German Commission E Monographs: Therapeutic Guide to Herbal Medicines.* Austin: American Botanical Council; 1998. pp. 309–310.

Bilberry fruit

(*Vaccinium myrtillus* L.)

Synonyms

Whortleberry (Engl), Myrtilli fructus (Lat), Heidelbeeren, Blaubeeren (Ger), Petit myrte, Baies de myrtille (Fr), Baceri mirtillo (Ital), Blåbær (Dan).

What is it?

The *Vaccinium* genus contains hundreds of species, many with edible berry-like fruits (including the American cranberry, *V. macrocarpon*). Bilberry fruit is well known as a food, and in particular as a jam. The name is derived from a Danish word meaning dark berry, possibly because, unlike the blueberry, its pulp as well as skin is dark blue. Bilberry has been used in Europe to colour wine and to dye wool. During World War II, bilberry jam or wine was consumed by RAF pilots to improve their night vision. Both the leaves and the ripe blue-black fruits are used medicinally, but this monograph only covers the use of the fruit. It is available as fresh or dried fruit, fluid extract or in solid dose form as a tablet or capsule.

Effects

Assists vision, decreases vascular permeability, supports the microcirculation, protects against oxidative stress; astringent and anti-inflammatory to mucosa of the gastrointestinal tract.

Traditional view

Bilberry fruit was used to treat diarrhoea, dysentery, gastro-intestinal inflammation, haemorrhoids and vaginal discharges and to 'dry up' breast milk. It has also been used to treat scurvy and for urinary complaints.[1]

Summary of actions

Vasoprotective, anti-oedema, antioxidant, anti-inflammatory, astringent.

Can be used for

Indications supported by clinical trials

Peripheral vascular disorders of various origin, including Raynaud's syndrome; venous insufficiency, especially of the lower limbs; venous disorders during pregnancy, including haemorrhoids; symptoms caused by decreased capillary resistance; conditions involving increased capillary fragility, such as nosebleed; diabetic and hypertensive retinopathies; postoperative complications of minor surgery (such as ear, nose, throat); vision disorders due to impaired photosensitivity or altered microcirculation of the retina, including myopia, retinitis, hemeralopia and simple glaucoma. Many of the studies supporting these uses are open label trials.

Traditional therapeutic uses

Digestive disorders (diarrhoea, dyspepsia, dysentery, gastrointestinal infections and inflammations), haemorrhoids.

May also be used for

Extrapolations from pharmacological studies

For capillary repair and to protect damaged capillaries; to treat and protect against ischaemic injury; antioxidant including inhibition of lipid peroxidation; wound healing (internal and topical); stabilisation of connective tissue; gastric disorders requiring repair of gastric mucosal barrier (ulceration, gastritis, oesophagitis).

Other applications

Topical treatment for inflammation of the mucous membranes of the mouth and throat;[2] inclusion in cosmetics (toners and skin products).[3]

Preparations

Dried or fresh fruit as a decoction, fluid extract and tablets or capsules for internal use. Decoction or extract for topical use. Available as a concentrated extract standardised for anthocyanin content and prepared from the fresh fruit. Due to the instability of the anthocyanins on drying, preparations made from the fresh fruit are preferable.

Testing of solid and liquid forms of purified bilberry extract under drastic conditions (such as mild and strong acidic solutions at elevated temperatures) did not produce important changes in the relative anthocyanin composition. Mild conditions did not result in significant degradation of the anthocyanins.[4] However, a more recent study found heating at 100°C or more rapidly degraded bilberry anthocyanins.[5] One in vitro study found that exposure of bilberry anthocyanins to physiological conditions that mimic those in the body may stimulate the conversion of monomeric anthocyanins to their polymeric forms.[6]

Dosage

- 3 to 6 mL of 1:1 fluid extract per day.

Tablets or capsules containing dried extracts of the fresh berries delivering 60 to 160 mg or more of anthocyanins per day (equivalent to about 20 to 50 g of fresh fruit).

Duration of use

May be taken long term for most applications.

Summary assessment of safety

No significant adverse effects from ingestion of bilberry are expected, although ingestion of the whole fresh fruit (as opposed to extracts) may irritate the intestinal lining in sensitive individuals. High doses may have clinical antiplatelet activity.

Technical data

Botany

Vaccinium myrtillus, a member of the Ericaceae (heath) family, is a small shrub approximately 30 to 40 cm high with erect, branched flowering stems. The alternate, light green leaves are flat, oval and pointed with a toothed margin; flowers contain four to five white or pink petals. The fruit is a deep violet, fleshy berry enclosing crescent-shaped seeds.[7]

Adulteration

High-performance liquid chromatography (HPLC) mass spectroscopy and nuclear magnetic resonance have been used to detect adulteration of bilberry extracts with a synthetic dye amaranth. This adulteration is not detected by simple analytical techniques.[8]

Vaccinium uliginosum and *V. vitis-idaea* have been noted as adulterant species.

Key constituents

- Anthocyanins (0.5%), also known as anthocyanosides, including C-3 glucosides of the anthocyanidins delphinidin, malvidin, pelargonidin, cyanidin and petunidin;[9] some of these are blue pigments responsible for the colour of the ripe fruits.
- Catechin, epicatechin, condensed tannins,[10] oligomeric procyanidins (procyanidin B1–B4).[11]
- Resveratrol[12] (moderate levels in uncooked products).[13]
- Flavonoids,[14] phenolic acids, pectins.[10,11]

Analysis of bilberry fruits collected in different locations from cultivated and wild plants in Sweden revealed a significant variation in anthocyanin content.[15] Higher values were observed for fruit from northern latitudes or from a more northerly origin of parent plants.

	R¹	R²
Delphinidin 3-O-glycoside	OH	OH
Cyanidin 3-O-glycoside	OH	H
Petunidin 3-O-glycoside	OH	OCH₃
Peonidin 3-O-glycoside	OCH₃	H
Malvidin 3-O-glycoside	OCH₃	OCH₃

glyc = arabinoside, glucoside or galactoside

Anthocyanins

Pharmacodynamics

Vascular protective and anti-oedema activity

Anthocyanins improved functional disturbances of the fine blood vessels, especially capillaries,[16] were more effective in protecting damaged capillaries than flavonoids[17] and stimulated capillary repair.[18] Anthocyanin-rich bilberry extracts demonstrated endothelium-dependent relaxation in coronary arteries in vitro. Extract concentrations too low to directly alter coronary vascular tone still protected the arteries from reactive oxygen species.[19]

Oral administration of bilberry extract in vivo reduced microvascular impairments due to ischaemia-reperfusion injury, resulting in preservation of endothelium, attenuation of leucocyte adhesion and improvement of capillary perfusion.[20] A separate study indicated that increased arteriolar vasomotion might also contribute to these effects.[21]

Oral administration to rats of bilberry extract (equivalent to 180 mg/kg anthocyanins per day) for 12 days maintained normal permeability of the blood-brain barrier and limited the increase in vascular permeability in the skin and aorta wall after induced hypertension. Interaction with collagen within blood vessel walls is believed to be partly responsible for this vasoprotective activity.[22]

Oral administration of bilberry extract (equivalent to 72 to 144 mg/kg anthocyanins) demonstrated significant vasoprotective and anti-oedema effects in vivo. Activity was stronger and longer lasting than that of rutin, and was not due to a specific antagonism of inflammatory mediators such as histamine or bradykinin. The anti-oedema activity was also observed after topical application (but resulted in persistent colouration due to the anthocyanins).[23]

Effects on vision

Anthocyanins have demonstrated an affinity for the pigmented epithelium of the retina in vitro.[24] Bilberry hastened the regeneration of rhodopsin (visual purple) in vitro and in vivo after injection.[25]

Senescence-accelerated OXYS rats were given either control diets or those supplemented with 25% bilberry extract (equivalent to 20 mg/kg body weight). After 3 months, more than 70% of control rats had cataract and macular degeneration, while the bilberry completely prevented such damage in the lens and retina.[26]

Bilberry extract improved the viability of cultured human corneal epithelial cells.[27] Neuroprotective activity against retinal neuronal damage was demonstrated in vitro and in mice for bilberry and its main anthocyanin constituents. The bilberry extract was administered to the mice by intravitreous injection (10 or 100 μg per eye).

Antioxidant activity

Anthocyanins have demonstrated in vitro antioxidant activity in a number of models, including scavenging of superoxide anions, inhibition of lipid peroxidation,[28] and upregulation of haeme-oxygenase and glutathione-S-transferase-pi.[29] Fifteen bilberry anthocyanins, particularly as aglycones,[30] and bilberry catechins and procyanidins[31] have all shown appreciable activity.

Bilberry extract also demonstrated antioxidant activity in vitro by inhibiting the potassium ion loss induced by free radicals in human erythrocytes, and by inhibiting cellular reactions induced by oxidant compounds.[32,33] A concentration-dependent inhibition of oxysterol formation (cholesterol oxides) was observed in vitro for bilberry extract after photo-induced oxidation of human low-density lipoproteins (LDL).[34] Aqueous extract of bilberry also demonstrated potent protective activity on human LDL particles during in vitro copper-mediated oxidation.[35] Dietary bilberry powder supplementation (1.6 g/mouse) protected against intestinal oxidative damage following ischaemia-reperfusion injury.[36]

A US team investigating the effects of antioxidant foods on mental ageing found that, while some fruits such as strawberries gave promising results, blueberry supplementation was particularly effective at reversing the negative effects of ageing on balance and coordination.[37] The team found that anthocyanins in blueberries showed the most activity in penetrating cells and providing antioxidant protection,[38] and were even present in the brains of elderly rats after they were fed blueberries for 8 weeks. The more anthocyanins found in the brains of the rats, the better they were at negotiating a complex maze.[39] In fact, blueberries in the diet appeared to exert a rejuvenating effect on the brain cells of elderly rats, making them behave more like young rats.[40] Such effects are also likely for the anthocyanins in bilberry.

Wound healing activity

Anthocyanins have demonstrated collagen-stabilising activity in vitro.[41] Two anthocyanins from bilberry protected collagen against non-enzymatic proteolytic activity in vitro and therefore may protect collagen from degradation during inflammatory processes.[42] Anthocyanins stimulated mucopolysaccharide biosynthesis in experimentally induced granuloma in vivo.[43] Bilberry extract induced active phagocytosis and intense cell regeneration from human umbilical cord and demonstrated growth-promoting activity for fibroblasts and smooth muscle cells in vitro.[44,45]

Bilberry extract was reported to accelerate the process of spontaneous healing of experimental wounds after topical application.[46] Topical bilberry extract significantly improved the healing of experimental skin wounds after it had been delayed by a steroidal anti-inflammatory agent. The wound healing activity was more potent than that of the selected triterpenoids of *Centella asiatica* (gotu kola).[47]

Cardiovascular activity

Bilberry extract exhibited a significant, dose-dependent inhibition of angiotensin-converting enzyme in cultured endothelial cells from human umbilical veins.[48] The anthocyanin myrtillin chloride was also active, but not anthocyanin aglycones (anthocyanidins).

Addition of either bilberries or yeast-fermented bilberries at 0.02% to the diet of apoE-deficient mice led to a significant inhibition of atherosclerotic plaque development, whereas no effect on oxidative stress or lipid profiles was observed.[49] Later work by the same group using just a fermented bilberry extract at 0.02% of diet demonstrated a reduction in serum cholesterol together with altered expression of aortic genes related to atherosclerosis development.[50]

Bilberry anthocyanins (0.01 to 1.0 mg/L) significantly attenuated ischaemia-reperfusion injury in isolated rat hearts.[51]

Bilberry extract demonstrated strong antiplatelet activity in vitro and, at dosages equivalent to up to 144 mg/kg anthocyanins, prolonged bleeding time without affecting blood coagulation in vivo.[52] Inhibition of platelet aggregation was demonstrated from the blood of healthy volunteers after oral administration of an extract equivalent to 173 mg anthocyanins/day for 30 to 60 days. The mechanism of action may depend on an increase in the concentration of cAMP and/or a decrease in the concentration of platelet thromboxane.[53]

Gastrointestinal effects

Several biomarkers of colon cancer including colonic cell proliferation were reduced in Fischer 344 male rats by a diet supplemented with a bilberry extract.[54] These findings were supported by another study in mice that supplemented bilberry at the high level of 10% of diet. Similarly, dietary bilberry extract reduced colon tumour number in a mouse model, an effect that was not related to ellagic acid.[55]

Cyanidin chloride (an anthocyanin from bilberry) demonstrated promising antiulcer activity in vivo. Gastric mucus production was increased without affecting gastric secretion.[56,57] Bilberry extract (equivalent to 9 to 72 mg/kg anthocyanins) demonstrated significant dose-dependent antiulcer activity, in some cases exhibiting stronger activity than carbenoxolone or cimetidine.[47] More recently, oral administration of bilberry anthocyanins (30 and 100 mg/kg) significantly protected against ethanol-induced gastric ulceration in mice.

Bilberry extract (1, 5 and 10 mg/kg, ip) helped to induce the resolution of liver fibrosis in mice with chemical liver injury, partially by downregulating fibrogenic cytokines.[58] The extract (50 to 200 mg/kg, oral) also reduced restraint-induced liver injury in mice.[59] Attenuation of mitochondrial dysfunction was identified as a key mechanism. In addition, the bilberry extract increased glutathione and ascorbate levels and decreased oxidative parameters in the same model at the same doses.[60]

Other activity

Phenolic compounds present in bilberries and other berries (cranberry, cloudberry, raspberry and strawberry) selectively inhibit the growth of human gastrointestinal pathogens such as salmonella and staphylococcus.[61] An effect in reducing bacterial adherence to gut epithelium may be a factor.

Oral administration of 500 mg/kg bilberry extract for 10 days to mice treated with doxorubicin (10 mg/kg) partially restored the toxicity-induced changes by increasing red blood cell and bone marrow counts. Dietary supplementation with the extract at 1% also significantly suppressed doxorubicin-induced myocardial damage.[62]

Five-day oral administration of bilberry extract (50 to 200 mg/kg) attenuated potassium bromate-induced kidney damage in mice.[63] Oxidative parameters were also improved, indicating reduced oxidative stress. Bilberry extract (2.7% of diet) reduced blood glucose and enhanced insulin sensitivity in type 2 diabetic mice via activation of AMP-activated protein kinase.[64]

Pharmacokinetics

Animal pharmacokinetic studies following oral administration of bilberry extract suggest that, although the anthocyanins have low bioavailability, plasma peak levels are within the therapeutic range.[65,66] Absorption from the gastrointestinal tract was about 5% and there was no hepatic first-pass effect. Plasma concentrations of anthocyanins reached peak levels after 15 minutes and then rapidly declined within 2 h. Elimination occurred mainly through the bile.[67]

A more recent study in mice found that, after oral administration of bilberry extract (100 mg/kg) both unmodified and methylated anthocyanins appeared in plasma.[68] The concentration of total anthocyanins reached a maximum of 1.18 μM after 15 minutes and then sharply decreased. About 1.9% of the total dose of bilberry anthocyanins was excreted in the urine, all within 24 h. Malvidin-3-glucoside and malvidin-3-galactoside were the main anthocyanins observed. With prolonged dosing, anthocyanins were detected in body tissues, but only in the liver, kidney, testes and lung.

General human studies on anthocyanin bioavailability (not specifically related to bilberry) have shown that only a small percentage (<1%) is found in plasma or in urine, typically as phase II conjugates via glucuronidation or methylation pathways.[69,70] More recently, a bilberry-lingonberry puree was given to six healthy volunteers in order to investigate the absorption of phenolic acids resulting from the bowel flora fragmentation of anthocyanins.[71] Methylated phenolic acids

such as vanillic and homovanillic acids were the most abundant metabolites in urine, although other expected fragments were not found, suggesting a significant part of anthocyanin metabolism remains unknown.

In a later pilot study, anthocyanins and their metabolites were analysed in the urine of two patients with colorectal liver metastases, each given a single dose of 1.88 g of bilberry extract.[72] The dose was administered via either nasogastric or nasojejunal tube intraoperatively during liver resection. More anthocyanins and metabolites were observed in the urine of the patient who received the extract via the stomach (greater than 20 times), suggesting that the stomach is a primary site of absorption (consistent with rodent studies). Intact glycosides were identified in urine, suggesting that a percentage of each anthocyanin is absorbed and excreted unchanged. Absorption efficiency was influenced by the nature of the aglycone and the sugar moiety. In addition, the bilberry anthocyanins underwent metabolic conjugation via glucuronidation or methylation pathways (consistent with the above).

Clinical trials

Peripheral vascular disorders and venous disorders

In open trials, bilberry extract (equivalent to 86 to 173 mg anthocyanins per day) improved oedema and subjective symptoms of lower limb varicose syndrome,[73] reduced protein exudate of varicose ulcers[43] and decreased the total drainage time after reactive hyperaemia in chronic venous insufficiency.[74] Bilberry extract (57 to 115 mg anthocyanins per day for 2 to 3 months) provided relief for venous disorders including haemorrhoids during pregnancy.[75,76] A review of open trials from 1979 to 1985 involving a total of 568 patients with venous insufficiency of the lower limbs concluded that bilberry extract caused rapid disappearance of symptoms and improvements in venous microcirculation and lymph drainage.[77] Mobilisation of finger joints was improved in patients with Raynaud's syndrome.[78]

Bilberry extract (equivalent to 173 mg anthocyanins per day) or placebo was administered for 30 days in a single blind, placebo-controlled clinical trial in 60 patients with venous insufficiency. Significant reduction in the severity of symptoms (oedema, sensation of pain, paraesthesia, cramping pain) was observed for the treated group after 4 weeks' treatment (p<0.01).[79]

In a double blind, placebo-controlled trial, 47 patients with peripheral vascular disorders of various origins were treated with bilberry extract (equivalent to 173 mg anthocyanins per day) or placebo for 30 days. The treated group experienced a reduction in subjective symptoms including paraesthesia, pain, heaviness and oedema.[78]

Microcirculation disorders including retinopathy

In open trials, bilberry extract (equivalent to 57 to 288 mg anthocyanins per day) improved symptoms caused by decreased capillary resistance (petechiae, bruising and faecal occult blood),[44] reduced the microcirculatory changes induced by cortisone therapy in patients with asthma and chronic bronchitis,[80] and improved diabetic retinopathy with a marked reduction or even disappearance of retinic haemorrhages.[81] Post-operative complications from surgery of the nose were reduced in patients who received bilberry extract (equivalent to 115 mg anthocyanins per day) administered for 7 days before and 10 days after surgery.[82]

In a placebo-controlled trial, bilberry extract (equivalent to 115 mg anthocyanins per day for 12 months) improved early phase diabetic retinopathy, as indicated by a reduction of hard exudate at the posterior pole.[83]

In a double blind, placebo-controlled clinical trial, 14 patients with diabetic and/or hypertensive retinopathy received bilberry extract (equivalent to 115 mg anthocyanins per day) or placebo for 1 month. Significant improvements in the ophthalmoscopic and angiographic patterns were observed in 77% to 90% of treated patients.[84]

Visual disorders

In open trials conducted as early as 1964, bilberry extract (including isolated anthocyanins), alone or in combination with beta-carotene and retinol, improved vision in healthy subjects and in patients with visual disorders such as myopia.[85,86] Enlargement of visual range was observed for patients with pigmentary retinitis[87] and retinal sensitivity was improved in patients with hemeralopia (defective vision in bright light).[88]

Visual perception improved in 76% of myopic patients receiving 150 mg/day bilberry extract and retinol for 15 days.[89] Similar results were obtained for patients with simple glaucoma.[90]

Three placebo-controlled trials[91–93] and two open studies[85,94] have demonstrated improvement in night vision in a number of settings. However more recent research[95] and a systematic review[96] have cast doubt on the validity of such findings.

Other conditions

In open trials, bilberry extract was administered post-operatively in conjunction with anti-inflammatory and analgesic drugs to patients who had undergone haemorrhoidectomy. Bilberry reduced post-operative symptoms (itching and oedema).[97,98]

In a placebo-controlled trial, bilberry extract (equivalent to 115 mg anthocyanins per day for 180 days) was effective in reducing nosebleed caused by abnormal capillary fragility of the mucous membranes.[99]

In a double blind, placebo-controlled trial, 30 women with chronic primary dysmenorrhoea were treated with bilberry extract (equivalent to 115 mg anthocyanins per day) for 3 days before and during menstruation. Bilberry significantly reduced symptoms of dysmenorrhoea such as pelvic and lumbosacral pain, mammary tension, headache, nausea and heaviness of lower limbs ($p<0.01$).[100]

In a controlled trial, 62 volunteers at increased risk of cardiovascular disease were randomised to receive either 330 mL/day of bilberry juice or water for 4 weeks.[101]

Supplementation with bilberry juice resulted in significant decreases in plasma levels of several inflammatory factors or measures regulated by NF-kappaB. Unexpectedly, an increase of TNF-alpha was observed. Plasma quercetin and *p*-coumaric acid increased in the bilberry group.

Naturally occurring anthocyanins possess colorectal cancer chemopreventive properties in rodent models. Hence, a human investigation was undertaken to determine if an anthocyanin-rich standardised bilberry extract caused pharmacodynamic changes consistent with chemopreventive efficacy, and generated measurable levels of anthocyanins in blood, urine and target tissue.[102] Twenty-five colorectal cancer patients scheduled to undergo resection of the primary tumour or liver metastases received extract containing 0.5 to 2.0 g anthocyanins daily for 7 days before surgery. Anthocyanins and their methyl and glucuronide metabolites were identified in plasma, colorectal tissue and urine, but not in liver. Anthocyanin concentrations in plasma and urine were roughly dose-dependent, reaching approximately 179 ng/g in tumour tissue at the highest dose. Proliferation in tumour tissue was decreased by an average of 7% for all patients on bilberry compared with pre-intervention values. The authors concluded that repeated administration of bilberry anthocyanins exerts pharmacodynamics effects and generates concentrations of anthocyanins in humans resembling those active in a murine adenoma model sensitive to the chemopreventive properties of anthocyanins. Studies of doses containing less than 0.5 g bilberry anthocyanins are necessary to determine if they may be appropriate as colorectal cancer chemopreventive agents.

Toxicology and other safety data

Toxicology

LD$_{50}$ data recorded in rats and mice for bilberry extract and its anthocyanins indicate very low oral acute toxicity.[103] Oral administration of a single dose of bilberry extract (equivalent to 1.08 g/kg anthocyanins) to dogs did not result in adverse effects, apart from darkening of the urine and faeces which was attributed to absorption of the extract.[104] No toxic effects were observed in chronic oral toxicity studies where anthocyanins (600 mg/day) were administered to rats for 90 days and to guinea pigs for 15 days,[105] or where bilberry extract was administered to rats and dogs for 6 months at doses equivalent to 45 to 180 mg/kg/day and 29 to 115 mg/kg/day anthocyanins, respectively.[104]

Weak activity was observed for bilberry extract in the Ames mutagenicity test, probably due to the presence of quercetin.[106] However, bilberry extract (standardised to 36% anthocyanins) failed to demonstrate mutagenic activity in other in vitro studies with or without metabolic action, or in vivo after oral administration of up to 5 g/kg to rats.[104,107]

Contraindications

None known.

Special warnings and precautions

High doses (>100 mg/day anthocyanins) should be used cautiously in patients with haemorrhagic disorders and in those taking warfarin or antiplatelet drugs, because of the observed human antiplatelet activity.

Interactions

Possible interaction with warfarin and antiplatelet drugs, but only for high doses. (See Special warnings and precautions.)

Use in pregnancy and lactation

Category A – no proven increase in the frequency of malformation or other harmful effects on the fetus despite consumption by a large number of women.

A number of uncontrolled studies involving over 200 pregnant women have reported that bilberry extract is a safe and effective treatment for venous disorders, including haemorrhoids, with no adverse effects observed in mothers or infants. Doses of extract equivalent to 57 to 173 mg/day of anthocyanins were administered for 60 to 102 days.[75,76,108,109]

Bilberry extract (standardised to 36% anthocyanins) did not demonstrate teratogenic activity or adversely influence fertility in rats.[104] Oral administration of anthocyanins (360 mg/kg) failed to demonstrate teratogenic activity in three successive generations of rats and rabbits.[105]

Bilberry is listed in one traditional Western herbal as an anti-galactogogue.[1] This is not otherwise supported and it is considered compatible with breastfeeding.[110]

Effects on ability to drive and use machines

No adverse effects expected.

Side effects

A post-marketing surveillance study was conducted on 2295 patients with venous disorders and retinal microcirculation disorders who consumed bilberry extract (standardised to 36% anthocyanins). Dosages ranged from the equivalent of 29 to 288 mg/day of anthocyanins for 14 to 60 days, with most patients (69.5%) consuming 115 mg/day of anthocyanins for 30 to 60 days. Ninety-four patients (4.1%) reported mild side effects affecting the gastrointestinal system (gastric pain, pyrosis and nausea in 3.3% of cases), skin (0.2%) or nervous system (0.2%).[111]

Ingestion of the whole fruit (as opposed to extracts) may irritate the intestinal lining of sensitive individuals due to the presence of fruit fibre and acids.

Overdosage

No incidents found in published literature.

Safety in children

Concentrated bilberry powder in a study of infants with acute dyspepsia was well tolerated.

Regulatory status in selected countries

Bilberry is official in the *European Pharmacopoeia* (2006).

Bilberry fruit is covered by a positive Commission E monograph and has the following applications:

* Non-specific, acute diarrhoea
* Topical treatment of mild inflammation of the mucous membranes of the mouth and throat.

Bilberry does not have GRAS status. However, it is freely available as a 'dietary supplement' in the USA under DSHEA legislation (1994 Dietary Supplement Health and Education Act).

Bilberry is not included in Part 4 of Schedule 4 of the Therapeutic Goods Act Regulations of Australia and is freely available for sale.

References

1. Grieve M. *A Modern Herbal*. New York: Dover Publications; 1971. pp. 99–100.
2. German Federal Minister of Justice (ed). *German Commission E for Human Medicine Monograph*, Bundes-Anzeiger (German Federal Gazette) no. 76, dated 23.04.1987, no. 50, dated 13.03.1990.
3. Smeh NJ. *Creating Your Own Cosmetics – Naturally*. Garrisonville: Alliance; 1995. pp. 81, 142.
4. Martinelli EM, Scilingo A, Pifferi G. *Anal Chim Acta*. 1992;259(1):109–113.
5. Yue X, Xu Z. *J Food Sci*. 2008;73(6):C494–4499.
6. Nalliah RE, Phillips JS, Gaier AJ, et al. *Int J Food Sci Nutr*. 2009;60(suppl 1):209–219.
7. Chiej R. *The Macdonald Encyclopedia of Medicinal Plants*. London: Macdonald; 1984. Entry No. 321.
8. Penman KG, Halstead CW, Matthias A, et al. *J Agric Food Chem*. 2006;54(19):7378–7382.
9. Wagner H, Bladt S. *Plant Drug Analysis: A Thin Layer Chromatography Atlas*, 2nd ed. Berlin: Springer-Verlag; 1996. p. 282.
10. Bisset NG, Wichtl M, eds. *Herbal Drugs and Phytopharmaceuticals* (German edition). Stuttgart: Medpharm Scientific Publishers; 1994.
11. Brenneisen R, Steinegger E. *Pharm Acta Helv*. 1981;56(7):180–185.
12. Rimando AM, Kalt W, Magee JB, et al. *J Agric Food Chem*. 2004;52(15):4713–4719.
13. Lyons MM, Yu C, Toma RB, et al. *J Agric Food Chem*. 2003;51(20):5867–5870.
14. Erlund I, Marniemi J, Hakala P, et al. *Eur J Clin Nutr*. 2003;57(1):37–42.
15. Akerstrom A, Jaakola L, Bang U, et al. *J Agric Food Chem*. 2010;58(22):11939–11945.
16. Terrasse J, Moinade S. *Presse Med*. 1964;72:397–400.
17. Demure G. PhD Thesis in Medicine: *Etude expèrimentale et clinique d'un nouveau facteur vitaminique P: les Anthocyanosides*. France 1964, Clermont.
18. Bombardelli E. *Therapia Angiol*. 1976;5:177.
19. Bell DR, Gochenaur K. *J Appl Physiol*. 2006;100(4):1164–1170.

20. Bertuglia S, Malandrino S, Colantuoni A. *Pharmacol Res*. 1995;31(3–4): 183–187.

21. Colantuoni A, Bertuglia S, Magistretti MJ, et al. *Arzneimittelforschung*. 1991;41(9):905–909.

22. Detre Z, Jellinek H, Miskulin M, et al. *Clin Physiol Biochem*. 1986;4:143–149.

23. Lietti A, Cristoni A, Picci M. *Arzneimittelforschung*. 1976;26(1): 829–835.

24. Wegmann R, Maeda P, Tronche P, et al. *Ann Histochim*. 1969;14:237–256.

25. Cluzel C, Bastide P, Wegman R, et al. *Biochem Pharmacol*. 1970;19:2295–2302.

26. Fursova A, Gesarevich OG, Gonchar AM, et al. *Adv Gerontol*. 2005;16:76–79.

27. Song J, Li Y, Ge J, et al. *Phytother Res*. 2010;24(4):520–524.

28. Meunier MT, Duroux E, Bastide P. *Plantes Méd Phytothér*. 1989;23(4):267–274.

29. Milbury PE, Graf B, Curran-Celentano J, et al. *Invest Ophthalmol Vis Sci*. 2007;48(5):2343–2349.

30. Rahman MM, Ichiyanagi T, Komiyama T, et al. *Free Radic Res*. 2006;40(9): 993–1002.

31. Maatta-Riihinen KR, Kahkonen MP, Torronen AR, et al. *J Agric Food Chem*. 2005;53(22):8485–8491.

32. Maridonneau I, Braquet P, Garay RP. In: Farkas L, Gabor M, Kallay F, eds. *Flavonoids and Bioflavonoids, 1981*. Amsterdam: Elsevier; 1982. pp. 427–436.

33. Mavelli I, Rossi L, Autuori F, et al. In: Cohen G, Greenwald RA, eds. *Oxy Radicals Their Scavenger Systems. Proceedings International Conference Superoxide Dismutase*, 3rd ed. New York: Elsevier; 1982. pp. 326–329.

34. Francesca Rasetti M, Caruso D, Galli G, et al. *Phytomedicine*. 1996/1997;3(4): 335–338.

35. Laplaud PM, Lelubre A, Chapman MJ. *Fundam Clin Pharmacol*. 1997;11(1): 35–40.

36. Jakesevic M, Aaby K, Borge GI, et al. *BMC Complement Altern Med*. 2011;11:8.

37. Joseph JA, Shukitt-Hale B, Denisova NA, et al. *J Neurosci*. 1999;19(18):8114–8121.

38. Galli RL, Shukitt-Hale B, Youdim KA, et al. *Ann N Y Acad Sci*. 2002;959: 128–132.

39. Andres-Lacueva C, Shukitt-Hale B, Galli RL, et al. *Nutr Neurosci*. 2005;8(2): 111–120.

40. de Rivera C, Shukitt-Hale B, Joseph JA, et al. *Neurobiol Aging*. 2006;27(7): 1035–1044.

41. Ronziere MC, Herbage D, Garrone R, et al. *Biochem Pharmacol*. 1981;30: 1771–1776.

42. Monboisse JC, Braquet P, Randoux A, et al. *Biochem Pharmacol*. 1983;32:53–58.

43. Mian E, Curri SB, Leitti A, et al. *Minerva Med*. 1977;68(52):3565–3581.

44. Piovella C, Curri BS, Piovella M, et al. *Therapia Angiol*. 1979;35:119.

45. Piovella F, Ricetti MM, Almasio P, et al. *Minerva Angiol*. 1981;6:135.

46. Curri SB, Leitti A, Bombardelli E. *Giorn Minerva Derm*. 1976;111:509.

47. Cristoni A, Magistretti MJ. *Il Farmaco Ed Pr*. 1987;42(2):29–43.

48. Persson IA, Persson K, Andersson RG. *J Agric Food Chem*. 2009;57(11): 4624–4629.

49. Mauray A, Milenkovic D, Besson C, et al. *J Agric Food Chem*. 2009;57(23): 11106–11111.

50. Mauray A, Felgines C, Morand C, et al. *Nutr Metab Cardiovasc Dis*. 2010 [Epub ahead of print].

51. Ziberna L, Lunder M, Moze S, et al. *Cardiovasc Toxicol*. 2010;10(4):283–294.

52. Morazzoni P, Magistretti MJ. *Fitoterapia*. 1990;61(1):13–21.

53. Pulliero G, Montin S, Bettini V, et al. *Fitoterapia*. 1989;60(1):69–75.

54. Lala G, Malik M, Zhao C, et al. *Nutr Cancer*. 2006;54(1):84–93.

55. Mutanen M, Pajari AM, Paivarinta E, et al. *Asia Pac J Clin Nutr*. 2008;17 (suppl 1):123–125.

56. Magistretti MJ, Conti M, Cristoni A. *Arzneimittelforschung*. 1988;38(5):686–690.

57. Cristoni A, Malandrino S, Magistretti MJ. *Arzneimittelforschung*. 1989;39(5):590–592.

58. Domitrovic R, Jakovac H. *Food Chem Toxicol*. 2011;49(4):848–854.

59. Bao L, Abe K, Tsang P, et al. *Fitoterapia*. 2010;81(8):1094–1101.

60. Bao L, Yao XS, Yau CC, et al. *J Agric Food Chem*. 2008;56(17):7803–7807.

61. Puupponen-Pimia R, Nohynek L, Alakomi HL, et al. *Biofactors*. 2005;23(4):243–251.

62. Choi EH, Park JH, Kim MK, et al. *Biofactors*. 2010;36(4):319–327.

63. Bao L, Yao XS, Tsi D, et al. *J Agric Food Chem*. 2008;56(2):420–425.

64. Takikawa M, Inoue S, Horia F, et al. *J Nutr*. 2010;140(3):527–533.

65. Ichiyanagi T, Shida Y, Rahman MM, et al. *J Agric Food Chem*. 2006;54(18): 6578–6587.

66. He J, Magnuson BA, Lala G, et al. *Nutr Cancer*. 2006;54(1):3–12.

67. Morazzoni P, Livio S, Scilingo A, et al. *Arzneimittelforschung*. 1991;41(1):128–131.

68. Sakakibara H, Ogawa T, Koyanagi A, et al. *J Agric Food Chem*. 2009;57(17): 7681–7686.

69. Bitsch I, Janssen M, Netzel M, et al. *Int J Clin Pharmacol Ther*. 2004;42(5): 293–300.

70. Kay CD, Mazza G, Holub BJ. *J Nutr*. 2005;135(11):2582–2588.

71. Nurmi T, Mursu J, Neinonen M, et al. *J Agric Food Chem*. 2009;57(6):2274–2281.

72. Cai H, Thomasset SC, Berry DP, et al. *Biomed Chromatogr*. 2011;25(6):660–663.

73. Ghiringhelli C, Gregoratti F, Marastoni F. *Minerva Cardioang*. 1977;26:255–276.

74. Corsi C, Pollastri M, Tesi C, et al. *Fitoterapia*. 1985;56(suppl 1):23.

75. Grismondi GL. *Minerva Gin*. 1981; 33(2–3):221–230.

76. Teglio L, Tronconi R, Mazzanti C, et al. *Quad Clin Ostet Ginecol*. 1987;42(3):221–231.

77. Berta V, Zucchi C. *Fitoterapia*. 1988;59(suppl 1):27.

78. Allegra C, Pollari G, Criscuolo A. *Minerva Angiol*. 1982;7:39–44.

79. Gatta L. *Fitoterapia*. 1988;59(suppl 1):19.

80. Carmignani G. *Lotta Contro La Tuberce Malattie Polm Soc*. 1983;53:732.

81. Orsucci PL, Rossi M, Sabbatini G, et al. *Clin Ocul*. 1983;4:377.

82. Mattioli L, Dallari S, Galetti R. *Fitoterapia*. 1988;59(suppl 1):41.

83. Repossi P, Malagola P, de Cadihac C. *Ann Ottal Clin Ocul*. 1987;113(4):357–361.

84. Perossini M, Guidi G, Chiellini S, et al. *Ann Ottal Clin Ocul*. 1987;113(12): 1173–1190.

85. Morazzoni P, Bombardelli E. *Fitoterapia*. 1996;67(1):3–29.

86. Gandolfo E. *Boll Ocul*. 1990;69(1):57–72.

87. Fiorini G, Biancacci A, Graziano FM. *Ann Ottal Clin Ocul*. 1965;91(6):371–386.

88. Zavarise G. *Ann Ottalmol Clin Ocul*. 1968;94(2):209–214.

89. Virno M, Recori Giraldi J, Auriemma L. *Boll Ocul*. 1986;65(4):789–796.

90. Caselli L. *Arch Med Intern*. 1985;37: 29–35.

91. Jayle GE, Aubert L. *Therapie*. 1964;19:171–185.

92. Jayle GE, Aubury M, Gavini G, et al. *Ann Ocul*. 1965;198:556–562.

93. Vannini L, Samuelly R, Coffano M, et al. *Boll Ocul*. 1986;65(suppl 6):569.

94. Contestabile MT, Appolloni R, Suppressa F, et al. *Boll Ocul*. 1991;70(6): 1157–1169.

95. Muth ER, Laurent JM, Jasper P. *Altern Med Rev*. 2000;5(2):164–173.

96. Canter PH, Ernst E. *Surv Ophthalmol*. 2004;49(1):38–50.

97. Pezzangora V, Barina R, De Stefani R, et al. *Gaz Med Ital*. 1984;143(6):405–409.

98. Oliva E, Nicastro A, Sorcini A, et al. *Aggior Med Chir*. 1990;8:1.

99. Massenzo D, Gentile A, Mosciaro O. *Riv Ital Otl Aud Fon*. 1992;12(1):65–68.

100. Colombo D, Vescovini R. *Giorn Ital Ost Gin*. 1985;7(12):1033–1038.

101. Karlsen A, Paur I, Bohn SK, et al. *Eur J Nutr*. 2010;49(6):345–355.

102. Thomasset S, Berry DP, Cai H, et al. *Cancer Prev Res*. 2009;2(7):625–633.

103. Mills S, Bone K, eds. St Louis: Elsevier Churchill Livingstone; 2005.

104. Eandi M. Cited in Morazzoni P, Bombardelli E. *Fitoterapia* 1996;67(1):3–29.

105. Pourrat H, Bastide P, Dorier P, et al. *Chim Ther*. 1967;2:33–38.

106. Schimmer O, Kruger A, Paulini H, et al. *Pharmazie*. 1994;49(6):448–451.

107. American Herbal Pharmacopoeia. Bilberry Fruit – Vaccinium myrtillus L.: Standards of Analysis, Quality Control and Therapeutics. Santa Cruz: American Herbal Pharmacopoeia; 2001.

108. Baisi F. Report on clinical trial of bilberry anthocyanosides in the treatment of venous insufficiency in pregnancy and of post-partum hemorrhoids [in Italian]. Livorno Hospital, 1987, Obstetrics and Gynecology Operating Unit.

109. Baudon J, Bruhat M, Plane C, et al. *Lyon Mediterr Med*. 1969:46.

110. Blumenthal M, ed. *The Complete German Commission E Monographs: Therapeutic Guide to Herbal Medicines*. Austin: American Botanical Council; 1998.

111. Eandi M. Cited in Morazzoni P, Bombardelli E. *Fitoterapia* 1996;67(1): 3–29.

(*Actaea racemosa* var. *racemosa* L.)

Synonyms

Cimicifuga racemosa (L.) Nutt. (botanical synonym), bugbane, black snakeroot (Engl), Cimicifugae rhizoma (Lat), schwarzes Wanzenkraut, Cimicifugawurzelstock (Ger), cimicaire, actée à grappes (Fr), sølvlys (Dan).

What is it?

Black cohosh is still widely referred to by its former botanical name, *Cimicifuga racemosa*. However, a taxonomic revision published in 1998 reclassified the genus *Actaea* to include *Cimicifuga*.[1] The common names of black snakeroot and rattle snakeroot refer to its former use in North America, where it is native, to treat snakebite including that of rattlesnake. The old generic name *Cimicifuga* comes from the Latin 'to chase insects away' and reflects on a reputed use of the European species. Black cohosh rhizome is a popular treatment for menopausal symptoms, and proprietary medicines based on black cohosh are registered in Germany. The part used therapeutically consists of the fresh or dried rhizome with attached roots.[2,3]

Effects

Suppresses luteinising hormone (LH), allays inflammation, promotes fertility, improves bone density.

Traditional view

Black cohosh, a favourite of the Eclectic physicians, was used for myalgia, neuralgia (not of spinal origin), chorea, female reproductive tract disorders (amenorrhoea, dysmenorrhoea, ovarian pain and menorrhagia) and rheumatic conditions (arthralgia, muscular rheumatism). Other conditions treated included whooping cough, tinnitus and mastitis.[4,5] Black cohosh is also used to treat premenstrual syndrome and secondary amenorrhoea in Germany.[3,6]

Summary actions

Hormone modulating, antirheumatic, spasmolytic.

Can be used for

Indications supported by clinical trials

Treatment of menopausal symptoms; to promote fertility.

Traditional therapeutic uses

Used particularly for arthritis and rheumatism, neuralgia, sciatica, menstruation disorders (amenorrhoea, dysmenorrhoea, menorrhagia, ovarian pain), respiratory tract disorders, (whooping cough, asthma), tinnitus.

May also be used for

Extrapolations from pharmacological studies

Adjunct in the treatment of conditions requiring reduction in LH levels (e.g. infertility, miscarriage, cyst formation, ovarian tumorigenesis and polycystic ovary syndrome). Potentially as an aid in the treatment of osteoporosis.

Preparations

Dried or fresh rhizome for decoction, liquid extract or solid dose forms for internal use.

Dosage

Typical adult dosage ranges used by Western herbalists are:
* 0.9 to 6 g/day of dried root and rhizome or by decoction
* 0.9 to 6 mL/day of a 1:1 liquid extract
* 1.5 to 3 mL/day of a 1:2 liquid extract, 3.0 to 7.5 mL/day of the 1:5 tincture, or equivalent doses in tablet or capsule form.

However, herbalists typically now recommend doses at the lower end of these ranges. In addition doses at the higher end have been linked to adverse reactions such as headaches (see Overdosage section).

Typical adult dosage ranges used in most clinical trials of German products:[2]
* Standardised extract equivalent to 40 to 140 mg/day of dried root and rhizome and containing approximately 3% triterpene glycosides.

Duration of use

May be taken long term within the recommended dosage, although the Commission E recommends not for more than 6 months.

Summary assessment of safety

Generally no adverse effects are expected from ingestion of black cohosh when used at the lower end of the recommended dosage. Dosage at the higher end may cause headaches. Black cohosh has been associated with rare cases of liver damage, although this link is disputed. It is not recommended during pregnancy except for assisting childbirth, although there is no strong indication of harm.

Technical data

Botany

Black cohosh is a member of the Ranunculaceae (buttercup) family and grows to an average height of 150 cm.[7] It produces white blossoms in slender, feathery drooping racemes and a dry fruit containing numerous seeds. The leaves have three-pointed, trilobate leaflets. The fleshy, dark brown/black rhizome is a creeping underground stem, from which follow dark brown roots.[2,8]

Adulteration

Other *Actaea/Cimicifuga* species, particularly *C. americana*, have been unintentionally mixed with black cohosh due to the similarity in aboveground appearance. Occasionally black cohosh is adulterated with the underground portions of baneberry (*Actaea pachypoda* and *A. rubra*).[2] In August 1998, Australian manufacturers were alerted to the possibility of substitution of black cohosh by other *Cimicifuga spp*. In May 2001 the Therapeutic Goods Administration Laboratories advised that 35% of the Australian products they tested indicated the presence of species other than *Cimicifuga racemosa*. Manufacturers were advised to verify their raw materials to ensure the correct *Cimicifuga* species is used. Other medicinal *Cimicifuga* species were implicated such as *C. foetida*, *C. dahurica*, *C. heracleifolia* and *C. simplex*.[9] See also the findings of Health Canada regarding adulteration (cited under Side effects in the safety section later in this monograph).

Key constituents

Constituents of black cohosh include at least 20 triterpene glycosides (saponins) of the cycloartane type, including actein, 23-epi-26-deoxyactein, cimiracemoside A and cimicifugoside.

Other constituents include aromatic acids (including ferulic, isoferulic and acyl caffeic acids), resins (cimicifugin), tannins and fatty acids.[10,11] Despite earlier reports, the herb does not contain significant quantities of isoflavones (see below).

	R
Actein	β-D-xylosyl
Acetylacteol	H

Pharmacodynamics

The pharmacology of black cohosh is poorly understood. The question of whether the herb has oestrogenic activity in particular remains unresolved and conflicting results from many studies on this topic are available. While the majority of more recent studies indicate that black cohosh extracts do not contain compounds that are potent agonists at either of the two known oestrogen receptors, black cohosh appears to possess several pharmacological effects that are consistent with oestrogen-like activity, including lowering of LH levels (by injection) and protection against menopausal bone loss. Meanwhile, other potential mechanisms of action have emerged such as serotonergic, dopaminergic and opioid receptor activity, all of which could potentially play a part in the ameliorating effects of black cohosh on menopausal symptoms. In addition, anti-inflammatory activity has been demonstrated in vitro, supporting some traditional uses of the herb. Any oestrogenic effects from the herb are likely to be complex and mild.

Hormonal activity

In early research, prolonged injections of black cohosh extract in rats and mice increased the weight of the uterus and established menstrual cycles in juvenile and climacteric animals.[12] Black cohosh extract demonstrated a selective reduction of serum LH in ovariectomised rats. FSH (follicle-stimulating hormone) and prolactin levels were unchanged. Intraperitoneal administration of black cohosh extract (24 mg dried extract per day) resulted in significant inhibition of LH secretion after the third day. Fractionated extraction of black cohosh and subsequent testing with three fractions indicated that the LH-suppressive substances resided in the dichloromethane extract. The intact glycosidal components of this extract were more active with regard to LH suppression than the aglycone form. Oral administration of the non-hydrolysed extract demonstrated a significant inhibition of LH, although much lower than that achieved by injection.[13] (This does not necessarily mean the aglycone is inactive, as the glycoside may provide enhanced bioavailability with cleavage of the sugars yielding an active aglycone.)[14]

A subsequent study by the same group found serum levels of LH in ovariectomised rats were reduced after intraperitoneal administration of a trichloromethane fraction of a black cohosh methanolic extract, whereas the ethanolic fraction of the extract did not affect LH levels. The trichloromethane fraction also demonstrated an ability to bind to oestrogen receptors in vitro. This fraction was further separated into three subfractions, two of which suppressed LH secretion in vivo and displaced oestrogen in vitro. This indicates that at least two groups of compounds may be responsible for the endocrine activity of black cohosh.[15] One active compound identified was the isoflavone formononetin. However, five more recent studies have failed to detect formononetin in black cohosh,[2] a fact that casts some doubt on the extract used in the study.

In other early research, water and chloroform fractions prepared from a black cohosh methanol extract were tested in ovariectomised rats by intraperitoneal injection over several days (chronic administration). The chloroform fraction demonstrated a strong LH-suppressing effect after 3 days; the water fraction was inactive. Further fractionation of the chloroform extract led to the conclusion that the LH-suppressive effect of black cohosh extract was caused by at least three different synergistically acting compounds.[16]

Another later study in ovariectomised rats showed that a dichloromethane (lipophilic) extract (60 mg subcutaneously for 7 days) produced effects similar to those of oestradiol on LH levels and other biomarkers influenced by oestrogen receptors.[17]

Two commercial black cohosh extracts were tested for their ability to compete with oestradiol for antigen binding sites on an antibody (IgG) directed against oestradiol (radioimmunoassay). Both extracts ran parallel with the displacement curve obtained with oestradiol, which supports the presence of oestrogenic compounds in black cohosh.[18] However, no oestrogenic activity was found after oral or subcutaneous administration of black cohosh extract (6, 60, 600 mg/kg) to groups of immature mice and ovariectomised rats respectively.[19]

A 50% aqueous ethanolic extract of black cohosh did not bind to oestrogen or progesterone receptors of human breast cancer cell lines (MCF7 and T47D) in vitro (100 µg/mL) and did not affect cell proliferation.[20] Similarly, a methanolic extract (200 µg/mL) did not bind to human recombinant alpha and beta oestrogen receptors in vitro.[21] Gene expression studies in MCF7 cells found that a lipophilic black cohosh extract had no oestrogenic activity, but instead exerted anti-proliferative and pro-apoptotic effects at the transcriptional level.[22] (See also below under Effects on human breast cancer cells.)

Only the lipophilic subfraction of a dry, hydroethanolic extract of black cohosh was able to activate the human alpha oestrogen receptor, but neither the total extract nor the lipophilic sub-fraction showed any in vivo uterotrophic effects in 21-day-old rats.[23]

One hundred and ten women experiencing menopausal symptoms, who had received no hormone replacement therapy (HRT) for at least 6 months, received either a standardised black cohosh extract or placebo. After 8 weeks of treatment, LH levels were significantly reduced (p<0.05) in the black cohosh group, but FSH was unchanged.[16]

Effects on menopausal bone loss

Several studies have indicated that black cohosh might protect against menopausal bone loss (see also under Clinical trials).

An in vitro study investigated the effects of an ethanolic black cohosh extract on bone nodule formation in mouse pre-osteoblast cells.[24] The extract did not stimulate osteoblast proliferation, but significantly increased bone nodule formation (500 ng/mL), an effect that was shown to result from enhanced gene expression of osteocalcin and Runx2 (a transcription factor involved in osteoblast differentiation). Interestingly, co-treatment with a selective oestrogen receptor antagonist abolished the effects on gene expression, demonstrating the involvement of an oestrogen receptor-dependent mechanism.

An experimental model was designed to understand the mechanism of action of black cohosh on bone tissue and to compare its effects with oestrogen and testosterone.[25] RANK (receptor activator of nuclear factor-kappaB, NF-kappaB) and its ligand RANKL largely regulate osteoclast activity and hence bone breakdown. Crosslaps (or Ratlaps in rats), specifically the metabolic products of bone-specific collagen-1 alpha1, are markers of such bone degradation. When black cohosh, oestradiol and testosterone were given to castrated rats of both sexes, oestradiol and black cohosh reduced levels of RANKL and Ratlaps, the latter parameter only in female rats. The authors suggested that the bone sparing effect of black cohosh is therefore partly mediated by inhibition of RANKL. However, the receptors involved in mediating this effect are not thought to be oestrogen receptors.

In a 35-day study of metaphyseal fracture healing in ovariectomised rats with early stage osteoporosis, the effects of a black cohosh supplemented diet (dried aqueous ethanolic extract, average 24.9 mg/day) was compared with oestrogen treatment (average 0.03 mg/kg/day).[26] A high rate of metaphyseal callus formation was observed in the animals receiving black cohosh, but oestrogen improved fracture healing more, with the authors commenting that the 5-week treatment period was possibly too short for black cohosh to demonstrate its full potential.

The triterpenoid glycoside 25-acetylcimigenol xylopyranoside isolated from black cohosh was shown in vitro to potently block osteoclastogenesis induced by tumour necrosis factor-alpha (TNF-alpha) and a related cytokine. The compound was also found to reduce bone loss induced by TNF-alpha in vivo.[27]

Effects on human breast cancer cells

Because of the potential oestrogen-like action of black cohosh, the issue of its safety in oestrogen-dependent tumours is of significant clinical interest, and a number of studies have been undertaken in an attempt to clarify this issue.

Unlike oestradiol, black cohosh extract did not stimulate growth of mammary tumour cells in vitro. In fact, a dosage of 2.5 mg/mL led to a strong inhibition of proliferation.[28] The simultaneous incubation of tumour cells with tamoxifen (anti-carcinogenic agent, oestrogen antagonist) and black cohosh displayed a much stronger inhibition of growth than for either substance alone.[29] (Oestrogen is contraindicated in patients with oestrogen receptor-positive breast carcinoma, since it promotes the growth of the tumour cells.)

Several other studies have demonstrated that black cohosh does not promote the growth of human breast cancer cells in vitro. A 50% aqueous ethanolic extract (100 μg/mL) did not promote cell proliferation of T47D cells.[20] In another study, a methanol-water extract was fractionated. A fraction rich in triterpenoid glycosides inhibited the growth of two human breast cancer cell lines (IC$_{50}$ values of 10 to 20 μg/mL).[30] The same fraction also caused cell cycle arrest at G1 (30 μg/m and G2 (60 μg/mL), suggesting that different compounds are involved in causing cell cycle arrest. The triterpene glycosides actein, 23-epi-26-deoxyactein and cimiracemoside A were shown to be involved in these effects.

In a subsequent gene expression study conducted by the same group, actein was shown to activate transcription factors that enhance apoptosis.[31] It also repressed cell cycle genes and acted synergistically with two chemotherapy agents, doxorubicin and 5-fluorouracil, in causing growth inhibition of the breast cancer cell line MDA-mB 453.[32] The same study also showed that actein enhanced the induction of apoptosis by paclitaxel, 5-fluorouracil and doxorubicin.

A review of the safety and efficacy of black cohosh for cancer patients assessed data from clinical (n=5) and pre-clinical (n=21) studies as well as case reports.[33] The five clinical studies all involved women with breast cancer or a history of the disease. None of the adverse effects reported from these trials (including one case of breast cancer recurrence) was linked to the black cohosh treatment. The authors of the review concluded that black cohosh does not have phyto-oestrogenic activity, appears to be safe for breast cancer patients and may potentially be protective against breast cancer, as it appears to inhibit the growth of tumour cells in vitro (See also under Clinical trials and Toxicology.)

Effects on prostate cancer cells

In vitro studies have demonstrated that black cohosh can inhibit proliferation of prostate cancer cells. In one study, the cell growth inhibitory effects of an isopropanolic extract of black cohosh on androgen-sensitive LNCaP and androgen-insensitive PC-3 and DU 145 prostate cancer cells were investigated. Results showed the extract caused a significant dose- and time-dependent downregulation of all prostate cancer cell lines after 72 h (IC$_{50}$ values between 37.1 and 62.7 μg/mL). Further, the study demonstrated that the extract killed prostate cancer cells by induction of apoptosis and activation of caspases, regardless of the hormone responsive status of the cells.[34]

A phenolic compound isolated from black cohosh, peta-siphenone, was studied in vitro with regard to its effects on the proliferation of LNCaP cells (incubated with 10 nM oestradiol, 1 nM dihydrotestosterone, or without either) and their secretion of prostate-specific antigen (PSA). A dose-dependent inhibition of the LNCaP cells was observed regardless of hormone treatment, while PSA release was not altered.[35]

In an in vivo study, a black cohosh extract was tested in immunodeficient mice inoculated sc with LNCaP cells. Inoculation with the prostate cancer cells resulted in formation of solid tumours in 12 of 18 control animals, compared with only five of 18 animals treated with dietary black cohosh extract (2 to 2.8 mg extract/ day). After 10 weeks, the amount of tumour tissue in the black cohosh-treated animals was significantly less than in controls. Serum testosterone levels were not significantly affected by the treatment.[36]

Other activity possibly contributing to menopausal effects

While the nature and degree of any oestrogenic activity of black cohosh remains unresolved, other potential mechanisms of action have emerged. That several mechanisms might be at play in a chemically complex herbal medicine is of course unsurprising.

A commercial black cohosh extract demonstrated in vitro dopaminergic activity in the dopamine receptor D2 assay,[37] and there are suggestions that serotonergic effects might play a role in the therapeutic effects of black cohosh. Researchers at the University of Illinois at Chicago working on black cohosh extract did not find evidence of oestrogen receptor binding or oestrogenic effects in animals, but did observe strong binding to several serotonin receptor subtypes in vitro, with partial agonist activity at the 5-HT$_7$ receptor.[38] The same group has also shown that black cohosh acts as a mixed competitive ligand and partial agonist at the human mu opioid receptor.[39]

Central opioid activity has also been shown in a mechanistic study involving 11 postmenopausal women.[40] The study employed two methods to examine the effects on central opioid function: naloxone challenge (n=6) and positron emission tomography with a selective micro-opioid receptor radioligand (n=5), before and after 12 weeks of standard treatment with a black cohosh isopropanolic extract (40 mg/day). Treatment did not affect oestrogen levels or spontaneous LH pulsatility, but administration of naloxone (a competitive mu opioid receptor antagonist) caused suppression of mean LH pulse frequency. This was most marked during sleep, when the mean interpulse interval was prolonged by 90 minutes. Positron emission tomography showed significant increases in mu opioid receptor binding potential in parts of the brain involved with emotional and cognitive function.

Because of the close relationship between the central nervous and hormone systems, it is plausible that mechanisms involving serotonergic, dopaminergic and opioid receptors are at least partly responsible for the effects of black cohosh on menopausal symptoms.

Anti-inflammatory and antioxidant activities

Several recent in vitro studies have lent some support to the traditional use of black cohosh in the treatment of inflammatory conditions. An aqueous extract (up to 6 mg/mL) was found to inhibit the generation of nitric oxide in lipopolysaccharide (LPS)-stimulated macrophages in a concentration-dependent manner. The mechanism for this was shown to be the reduced expression of inducible nitric oxide synthase (iNOS) rather than inhibition of iNOS activity. The triterpenoid glycoside 23-epi-26-deoxyactein was identified as the active compound.[41]

Another black cohosh compound, cimiracemate A (140 μM), has been shown to suppress the in vitro production of the inflammatory cytokine TNF-alpha induced by LPS in macrophages.[42]

Aqueous black cohosh extracts (3 and 6 mg/mL) have also been shown to reduce the release of TNF-alpha and the interleukin IL-6 (another inflammatory cytokine) and almost completely block the release of interferon-gamma in LPS-stimulated whole human blood. In contrast, IL-8 (also an inflammatory chemokine) was stimulated. Among five prevalent compounds isolated from the extract, isoferulic acid was found to be responsible for the inhibition of TNF-alpha and IL-6, but not for the stimulation of IL-8.[43]

Black cohosh showed potent antioxidant activity in the oxygen radical absorption capacity (ORAC) assay in a study that applied a sequential three solvent (ethyl acetate, methanol and 50% aqueous methanol) extraction process and combined the antioxidant activity of the three extracts. Black cohosh was the second most potent of 53 medicinal plants tested, being second only to olive leaf.[44]

Another in vitro study found black cohosh to be an effective scavenger of 1,1-diphenyl-2-picrylhydrazyl free radicals. Nine compounds with activity in this assay were isolated and six of these (methyl caffeate>caffeic acid>ferulic acid>cimiracemate A>cimiracemate B>fukinolic acid) were found to also reduce menadione-induced DNA damage in cultured S30 breast cancer cells.[45]

Other activity

Pretreatment with cimicifugoside inhibited blastogenesis in mouse splenic lymphocytes and brought about a decrease in the number of plaque-forming colonies using sheep erythrocytes (SRBC). The anti-SRBC response in the plaque-forming assay was suppressed in mice after pretreatment by intraperitoneal administration, and delayed hypersensitivity was suppressed after intravenous administration. The immunosuppressive activity of cimicifugoside is directed toward B-cell function, with larger doses being required for suppression of T-cell function.[46]

Black cohosh extract, and several fractions obtained from it, demonstrated hypotensive activity after intravenous administration at 1 mg/kg to rabbits. The hypotensive activity was observed in particular with the resinous part and may be due to actein. A hypotensive effect was not observed in human volunteers (by intravenous administration), although a peripheral vasodilatory effect was evident, even in subjects with peripheral arterial disease.[47] Oral administration of black cohosh extract (2 g/kg) inhibited 5-hydroxytryptophan-induced diarrhoea in mice.[48]

Pharmacokinetics

The triterpene glycoside actein has been shown to be bioavailable in rats when administered by gastric intubation (37.5 mg/ kg). Serum levels of actein peaked after 6 h at 2.4 μg/mL, dropping to 0.1 μg/mL 24 h post administration. The urine level of actein at 24 h was 0.8 μg/mL.[49]

The pharmacokinetics of one of the most abundant triterpenoid glycosides in black cohosh, 23-epi-26-deoxyactein, was studied in 15 healthy, postmenopausal women. They received single oral doses of a 75% ethanolic extract containing 1.4, 2.8 or 5.6 mg of 23-epi-26-deoxyactein. Serial blood and 24 h urine samples were collected and analysed. Peak plasma levels (2.2 to 12.4 ng/mL) and area under the time-concentration curve (a measure of bioavailability) of 23-epi-26-deoxyactein increased proportionally with dosage, and the half-life was 2 to 3 h. Less than 0.01% of the compound was recovered in the urine 24 h after administration, but metabolites were not detected.[50]

Clinical trials

Menopause

In phytotherapy, black cohosh is predominantly used in the treatment and management of menopausal symptoms. Menopause is the permanent cessation of menstruation and fertility defined as the absence of ovarian follicular activity for at least 12 months. The symptom picture associated with the transition from peri- to postmenopause can range from mild to debilitating, and the duration of symptoms can range from a few months up to 10 years.

Experts on menopause refer to a wide variety of physical symptoms including hot flushes, cardiac complaints, fatigue, vertigo, sweating, muscle pain, muscle spasm, joint pain, urinary incontinence, vaginal dryness and vaginal epithelium atrophy, and psychological symptoms: depression, anxiety, nervousness, irritability, forgetfulness, sleep disturbances and decreased libido. Vasomotor symptoms of hot flashes and night sweats are the most common physical manifestation, occurring in up to 80% of menopausal women.[51] Women who experience vasomotor symptoms are also more likely to suffer sleep disturbances and depressive symptoms and experience a negative impact on their quality of life.

A broad array of treatments including hormone therapy, antidepressant medications, herbal and nutritional therapies, and diet and lifestyle modifications are utilised by women to ameliorate unwanted menopausal symptoms.

Black cohosh is the herbal medicine most commonly recommended for managing psychological and physical symptoms of menopause. Standardised black cohosh extract was used with success in the 1950s and 1960s for the treatment of menopausal symptoms, menstrual disturbances in young women (secondary but not primary amenorrhoea) and symptoms arising from ovarian dysfunction or insufficiency.

Research interest in black cohosh has gained momentum since the publication of the Women's Health Initiative study in 2002. This study found an association between the long-term use of HRT and increased breast cancer and cardiovascular risk.[52] As a result of these findings, prescribers and users of HRT began to explore non-hormonal alternatives, the most common being black cohosh. Black cohosh is prescribed alone in a number of proprietary formulas, but is also used in combination with other herbs and nutrients in formulations for menopausal symptoms.

Black cohosh for menopausal symptoms has been investigated extensively in clinical trials, but not all trials have been convincing. This may in part be due to poor trial design, including small sample size and variability in the dose used. Many trials (including several with positive outcomes) have used an extract dose equivalent to 40 mg/day of dried herb, a dose which is low in comparison to the more traditional one recommended in the *British Herbal Pharmacopoeia* 1983 (0.9 to 6 g/day dried root and rhizome).[4]

A number of recent comprehensive monographs,[53] systematic reviews[54,55] and a meta-analysis[56] have examined the efficacy and safety of black cohosh for menopausal symptoms; this body of literature represents the most rigorous and global assessment of black cohosh currently available.

A systematic review published in 2008 included six double blind, randomised, controlled trials (n=1112) of black cohosh for the relief of menopausal symptoms.[55] Trials that included women suffering medically induced menopause were excluded. Each of the included trials focused on menopausal symptoms, and used a placebo or a standard drug treatment as control. Three of the six trials used an isopropanolic extract in a daily dose equivalent to 40 mg herb, one trial used 160 mg of a 70% ethanolic extract (equivalent to 5 mg of triterpene glycosides), another used a 58% ethanolic extract equivalent to 40 mg of herb, and the sixth used 6.5 mg of a 60% ethanolic extract. Despite the authors' conclusion that the evidence for the efficacy of black cohosh was still inconclusive, five of the six trials produced some positive outcomes. Details of these six studies are provided below.

In an early trial, Stoll used a randomised, double blind design in 75 women with symptoms of menopause. The 3-month study compared treatment with black cohosh with conjugated oestrogens and placebo. The Kupperman Menopausal Index (KMI), Hamilton anxiety scale, and proliferation status of vaginal epithelium were the outcome measures, and results demonstrated that black cohosh improved all parameters compared with placebo.[57]

Another 3-month randomised, double blind, multicentre trial involving 62 postmenopausal women also compared black cohosh (equivalent to 40 mg/day), conjugated oestrogens and placebo. Outcome measures included the Menopause Rating Scale (MRS), markers of bone formation and degradation, and endometrial thickness. Results of this trial showed that both active treatments were effective in reducing menopausal symptoms and both had beneficial effects on bone metabolism. Unlike treatment with conjugated oestrogens, black cohosh did not affect endometrial thickness.[58]

Osmers and co-workers conducted a 12-week randomised, double blind, placebo-controlled multicentre trial involving 304 women with menopausal symptoms. Women in the black cohosh group received extract equivalent to 40 mg/day, and the MRS was again the primary outcome measure. The women receiving black cohosh experienced significantly greater improvement in menopausal symptoms, especially hot flushes, compared with the placebo group. Women in early menopause benefited the most.[59]

A multicentre, randomised, placebo-controlled, double blind study was conducted by Frei-Kleiner and co-workers in 122 menopausal women experiencing at least three hot flushes daily. They were treated over 12 weeks with a black cohosh extract (equivalent to 42 mg herb) or placebo. Outcome measures were a weekly score for hot flushes, the *Kupperman Index* and the MRS. Overall the results showed no significant difference between the two groups. However, significant benefits of black cohosh were evident in women with more severe symptoms (*Kupperman Index* score of at least 20), and the effects of black cohosh over placebo almost reached significance (p=0.052) for the subgroup comprising perimenopausal women.[60]

In the HALT study, a 12-month randomised, double blind, trial was undertaken with 351 peri or postmenopausal women. They received either black cohosh (160 mg of a 70% ethanolic extract equivalent to 5 mg triterpene glycosides daily), a multi-botanical preparation (alfalfa, chaste tree, dong quai, false unicorn, licorice, oats, pomegranate, Siberian ginseng, boron; 200 mg daily), the multi-botanical plus telephone counselling to increase dietary soy intake, conjugated oestrogens with or without medroxyprogesterone acetate, or placebo. The main outcome measures were frequency and intensity of vasomotor symptoms. The study found no difference between the herbal interventions and placebo at 3, 6 or 12 months, whereas the HRT resulted in a significant decrease in vasomotor symptoms compared with placebo (p<0.001).[61]

Bai and colleagues conducted a 3-month double blind, multicentre, non-inferiority trial in China in 244 women with menopausal symptoms. They were randomised to receive either black cohosh extract (equivalent to 40 mg/day) or the synthetic steroid drug tibolone (2.5 mg/day), which has been shown in numerous placebo-controlled trials to be effective in the treatment of menopausal symptoms. The main outcome measures were the KI and the frequency of adverse events. The effects of the two treatments were similar and clinically relevant: in the black cohosh group mean KI decreased from 24.7 at baseline to 11.2 and 7.7 after 4 and 12 weeks, respectively, while the corresponding scores for the tibolone group were 11.2 and 7.5. These results demonstrated that the black cohosh treatment was as effective as tibolone treatment (non-inferiority was statistically significant, p=0.002), with the benefit-risk balance for black cohosh being significantly superior to tibolone (p=0.01).[62]

A 2010 meta-analysis by researchers at McGill University in Montreal included nine randomised, placebo-controlled trials of black cohosh-containing preparations for menopausal symptoms. Four of the included trials have been reviewed above; the additional five trials used black cohosh in combination with other active ingredients such as St John's wort, isoflavones, lignans or other herbs. Overall, the authors of this meta-analysis found that six of the nine studies demonstrated a significant effect for the black cohosh-containing intervention over placebo. Combining the data from seven trials, they calculated an estimated improvement in menopausal vasomotor symptoms of 26% (95% CI 11–40%) with black cohosh treatment.[56] However, the value of comparing different treatments in a meta-analysis is questionable. The five trials of black cohosh in combination with other active ingredients are reviewed below.

The efficacy of black cohosh in combination with St John's wort was assessed in 89 symptomatic peri- and postmenopausal women in a 12-week double blind, randomised, placebo-controlled, multicentre study. The main outcome measure was the Kupperman Index (KI); biochemical parameters (hormone levels and lipid profiles) and pathology (vaginal atrophy) were also measured. The active treatment consisted of a 264 mg tablet containing 0.0364 mL of extract from black cohosh rhizome (equivalent to 1 mg terpene glycosides) and 84 mg of dried extract from *Hypericum perforatum*, equivalent to 0.25 mg hypericin. Treatment with the herbal preparation resulted in significantly greater reduction in KI scores after 4 (p=0.002) and 12 (p<0.001) weeks, compared with placebo. There were no other clinically significant differences between the two groups (although HDL levels decreased marginally in the placebo group). The results demonstrated this combination of black cohosh and St John's wort to be effective in alleviating menopausal symptoms.[63]

A second study also examined the efficacy of the fixed combination of black cohosh and St John's wort in women with menopausal symptoms. The double blind, randomised, placebo-controlled study included 301 women experiencing menopausal symptoms with a pronounced psychological component. They were treated with ethanolic St John's wort extract and isopropanolic black cohosh extract or placebo for 16 weeks. The MRS and the Hamilton Depression Rating Scale were used to measure outcomes. The mean MRS score decreased 50% (0.46 to 0.23) in the treatment group and 19.6% (0.46 to 0.37) in the placebo group, whereas the Hamilton Depression Rating Scale total score decreased 41.8% (18.9 to 11.0) in the treatment group compared with 12.7% (18.9 to 16.5) in the placebo group. The herbal treatment was significantly (p<0.001) better than placebo for both measures.[64]

Another randomised, double blind, placebo-controlled trial in 50 healthy peri- and postmenopausal women assessed a formula containing standardised extracts of black cohosh, dong quai, milk thistle, red clover, American ginseng and chaste tree berry for 3 months. Frequency and intensity of menopausal symptoms were monitored by way of a structured questionnaire, administered weekly. Biochemical tests, breast checks and transvaginal ultrasonography were also performed. Women receiving the herbal formula reported a significant and progressive reduction in menopausal symptoms over the placebo group. After 3 months there was a 73% decrease in hot flushes and a 69% reduction of night sweats, with a decrease in symptom intensity and improved sleep quality in the herbal group. Complete cessation of hot flushes was reported by 47% of women in the herbal group compared with 19% in the placebo group. Vaginal ultrasonography, hormone levels (oestradiol, FSH), liver enzymes or thyroid-stimulating hormone showed no change in either group.[65]

A study by an Italian group evaluated the short-term effects of a combination of black cohosh with isoflavones and lignans on acute menopause-related symptoms in postmenopausal women using a double blind, randomised, placebo-controlled design. Eighty healthy, postmenopausal women were randomly assigned to receive either the combination formula or a placebo (calcium supplement). The groups were similar at baseline, but after 3 months of treatment the KI was significantly lower (p<0.05) in the black cohosh-phyto-oestrogen group compared with the placebo group.[66]

A supplement containing black cohosh and soy isoflavones was studied in a randomised, placebo-controlled, double blind multicentre 12-week trial involving 124 women who experienced at least five vasomotor symptoms every 24 h. They were randomised to receive daily either the black cohosh-isoflavone supplement or placebo. The modified KI and the Greene Climacteric Scale were used to measure outcomes. After 6 and 12 weeks of treatment, all scores had improved in both groups compared with baseline, and there was no statistically significant difference between the supplement and placebo groups.[67]

A large scale, observational study comparing the effect of black cohosh alone and black cohosh in combination with St John's wort also deserves mention. The study was conducted in Germany between March 2002 and March 2004, and included 6141 women with any menopausal symptoms and who had not taken HRT in the 4 weeks preceding the study. The participants had mostly mild to moderate symptoms and were treated with recommended doses of black cohosh monotherapy (isopropanolic extract equivalent to 20 mg herb per tablet) or combination therapy (isopropanolic extract of black cohosh equivalent to 30 mg herb plus St John's wort extract equivalent to 245 to 350 mg herb per tablet). The treating physician determined the choice and dose of treatment. Patients were evaluated at baseline, 3 and 6 months, with some patients electing to continue for a further 6 months. The primary outcome measures were the MRS and the PSYCHE sub-score of the MRS. In women receiving black cohosh monotherapy, total MRS scores declined from baseline by 0.10 and 0.14 after 3 and 6 months, respectively, whereas the corresponding decreases were 0.12 and 0.18 for the combination therapy, suggesting that the addition of St John's wort provided an additional effect. Similarly, the changes on the PSYCHE sub-score were significantly greater with the combination therapy than with black cohosh alone (p<0.001). However, the data are potentially confounded by the fact that baseline scores for the two groups were not equal and doses were not fixed. Improvements were sustained by both treatments at 6 and 12 months.[68]

In a small double blind, placebo-controlled trial, black cohosh had no significant anxiolytic activity in women with anxiety disorder due to menopause.[69]

Breast cancer patients with menopausal symptoms

Black cohosh used in the management of hot flushes in patients with breast cancer has also been studied in clinical trials. Two such studies, with conflicting results, are summarised below. In an open label randomised trial, 136 breast cancer survivors (35 to 52 years) were treated over 12 months with a black cohosh extract for hot flushes caused by tamoxifen therapy. The patients had all been treated with segmental or total mastectomy, chemotherapy and radiation therapy and were receiving tamoxifen 20 mg/day (n=46) or tamoxifen 20 mg/day plus black cohosh (equivalent to 20 mg herb per day) (n=90). Results revealed those in the intervention (black cohosh) group had fewer and less severe hot flushes compared with controls. After 12 months' treatment nearly half of those receiving black cohosh were completely free of hot flushes, while 24.4% of the black cohosh group versus 73.9% of the tamoxifen group were still reporting severe hot flushes (p<0.01).[70]

An earlier randomised, placebo-controlled trial involving 85 breast cancer survivors stratified for tamoxifen use (59 on tamoxifen and 26 not on tamoxifen) did not find any effect of black cohosh over placebo in terms of number and severity of hot flushes. The dose of black cohosh used in this trial was not provided in the report. Subjects completed a 4-day hot flush diary at baseline and at 30 and 60 days, as well as a menopause symptom questionnaire at baseline and at the final visit. FSH and LH levels were measured in a subset of patients at the first and final visits, but no significant differences were detected between the two groups.[71]

Bone loss prevention

Bone mineral loss (osteoporosis) is a major consideration for postmenopausal women, as it is a major age-related source of morbidity and mortality. A 12-week double blind study in 62 postmenopausal women compared the effects of a black cohosh preparation (equivalent to 40 mg herb per day), conjugated oestrogens or placebo on bone metabolism and other parameters. Black cohosh and conjugated oestrogens were found to have beneficial effects of similar magnitude on bone metabolism. Black cohosh treatment significantly increased serum levels of bone-specific alkaline phosphatase, indicative of increased osteoblast activity. Treatment with conjugated oestrogens, however, did not produce this effect, but appeared to decrease the activity of osteoclasts. Hence, while the net effects on bone of the two treatments were comparable, it appeared that the mechanism of action differed.[58]

This effect of black cohosh on bone density parameters appears to be mild and, on current evidence, it could not be credibly proposed as a treatment for osteoporosis. However, it probably should play a role as part of an appropriate diet, supplementation and lifestyle regime for the prevention of osteoporosis in both men and women, especially those with borderline osteopenia.

A study in 128 women found that, while an exercise programme favourably affected bone health, adjuvant supplementation with black cohosh (40 mg/day) did not enhance this effect.[72] Perhaps a higher dose might have been necessary for this experimental design.

Arthritis

In a randomised, double blind, placebo-controlled trial, 82 male and female patients with osteoarthritis and rheumatoid arthritis received a licensed over-the-counter (OTC) herbal medicine (two tablets/day) or placebo for a period of 2 months. The formula contained black cohosh, willow bark, guaiacum resin, sarsaparilla and poplar bark. Although there was no significant difference between the two groups for most symptoms, a significant decrease (p<0.05) in pain scores occurred for those taking the herbal formula. Many patients reported a decline in health related to the cold, damp, windy weather experienced near the end of the trial, which may have altered the findings. A relative improvement in mood scores was also noted for those taking the herbal tablets.[73] The authors of this study advised that the results may not be relevant to the activity of black cohosh, as the formulation predominantly comprised herbs containing salicylate derivatives.

Infertility

Unexplained infertility is typically defined as the failure to conceive over 1 year for couples exhibiting no apparent abnormalities. It is believed to occur in 15% to 30% of couples trying to conceive. Medically it is often treated with the fertility drug clomiphene citrate, which can be used in conjunction with gonadotropins to help trigger ovulation. In a controlled clinical trial, patients with unexplained infertility who had not responded to clomiphene therapy alone were randomly divided into two groups. The first group was given black cohosh dry extract at 120 mg/day (500 mg of dried root) from days 1 to 12 of the cycle. Both groups received clomiphene from days 3 to 7 and human chorionic gonadotropin (HCG) injection close to ovulation. All were recommended to have timed intercourse every day for the corresponding week. Endometrial thickness was measured on the day of the HCG injection and was found to be significantly thicker for the group receiving black cohosh (8.9±1.4 mm versus 7.5±1.3 mm, p<0.001). Serum progesterone concentrations measured in the luteal phase (days 21 to 23) were significantly higher in the black cohosh group (13.3±3.1 ng/mL versus 9.3±2.0 ng/mL, p<0.01). The pregnancy rate was also significantly higher for the group given black cohosh (36.7% versus 13.6%, p<0.01), even after one treatment cycle. These results suggest a benefit to including black cohosh in the medical management of infertility.[74]

A follow-up trial by the same group using a similar design found that follicular-phase black cohosh exerted a better activity than ethinyloestradiol in terms of improving cycle characteristics in 134 infertile women treated with clomiphene citrate. No significant difference was found regarding clinical pregnancy rates.[75]

Toxicology and other safety data

Toxicology

No toxic effects were observed from oral administration of standardised black cohosh extract (up to 5 g/kg/day) for 26 weeks in rats.[76] A constituent isolated from the chloroform fraction of black cohosh extract, likely to be actein, did not provoke acute toxicity when administered by intragastric and hypodermic routes to rabbits. The minimum lethal dose of this constituent was greater than 500 mg/kg (ip) in mice, 1000 mg/kg (oral) in rats and 70 mg/kg (iv) in rabbits. In subchronic toxicity studies over 30 days, the minimum lethal dose was greater than 10 mg/kg (ip) in mice and 6 mg/kg (oral) in rabbits.[77]

Standardised black cohosh extract did not show mutagenic activity in the Ames test.[78] Scientists from Duquesne University observed that the incidence of metastasis increased in sexually mature female transgenic (MMTV-neu, genetically engineered) mice fed black cohosh (at amounts said to reflect the normal human dose, about 0.3 mg/mouse) for 12 months. The incidence of mammary tumours was not increased.[79] This experimental model, in which female mice spontaneously develop mammary tumours through the activation of an oncogene common in human breast cancer, is still highly controversial in terms of providing reproducible and relevant results. The experimental conditions were highly artificial (for example, feeding black cohosh to mice for 12 months is the equivalent of a woman taking it continuously for at least 30 years).

The relevance of using a mouse model to assess the safety of a treatment that is already widely used in the community can be queried; it could be that this in vivo study is nothing more than a scientific curiosity. The best way to assess any risks associated with black cohosh consumption is to study the health of women already taking it.

Such studies have now been published. The association between a range of 'hormone-related supplements' (including black cohosh) containing 'phyto-oestrogens' and breast cancer incidence was reassessed in a retrospective case-control epidemiological study.[80] The US study examined 949 cases of women with breast cancer and 1524 controls and specifically targeted use of black cohosh, American ginseng (*Panax quinquefolius*), red clover (*Trifolium pratense*), dong quai (*Angelica sinensis*) and yam products (*Dioscorea* species). After adjusting for variables such as age, education, age at full-term pregnancy, menopause status, family history of breast cancer and use of HRT, intake of the above herbal products (as a group) was associated with a reduced incidence of breast cancer (adjusted odds ratio (OR) 0.65, 95% confidence interval (CI): 0.49 to 0.87). However, it was only black cohosh that demonstrated a highly significant breast cancer protective effect (adjusted OR 0.39, 95% CI: 0.22 to 0.70). The authors concluded that additional confirmatory studies are required to determine whether black cohosh could be used as a treatment to prevent breast cancer.

Within a German case-control study, associations between patterns of herbal product use and incidence of breast cancer were investigated in 10121 postmenopausal women.[81] Use of herbal products was inversely associated with invasive breast cancer (OR 0.74) in a dose-dependent manner. The two black cohosh subgroups (isopropanolic and other types of extracts) demonstrated moderate protection, but it was most marked for chaste tree (*Vitex agnus-castus*, OR 0.4). As part of the VITAL epidemiological study, 35016 postmenopausal women were queried on their use of dietary supplements and followed for up to 7 years.[82] Black cohosh use was not found to be associated with an increased risk of invasive breast cancer.

However, questions remain as to whether black cohosh can be safely used by women with diagnosed breast cancer. While more information is required, findings from one clinical study strongly imply that black cohosh lacks any oestrogenic activity in breast or endometrial tissue. This was a prospective, open, uncontrolled safety study in which baseline status was compared by blinded observers with status after 6 months of treatment.[83] A total of 74 women were treated with black cohosh extract daily (40 mg/day), and 65 women completed the study. Mammograms were performed and breast cells were collected by percutaneous fine needle aspiration biopsies at baseline and after 6 months. Breast cell proliferation was assessed using the Ki-67/MIB-1 monoclonal antibody (cells positive for this marker are in a state of active proliferation). Safety was monitored by adverse event reporting, laboratory assessments and measurement of the endometrium by vaginal ultrasound.

None of the women showed any increase in mammographic breast density. Furthermore, there was no increase in breast cell proliferation. The mean change in the proportion of Ki-67-positive cells was 0.5%±2.4% for paired samples. The mean change in endometrial thickness was 0.0±0.9 mm. A modest number of adverse events were possibly related to treatment, but none of these was serious. Laboratory findings and vital signs were normal. The findings suggest that the isopropanolic extract of black cohosh tested did not cause adverse effects on breast tissue. Furthermore, the data did not indicate any endometrial or general safety concerns during 6 months of treatment.

This finding was supported by another study published at around the same time that found 12 weeks of black cohosh given to postmenopausal women had no impact on oestrogen markers in serum and no effect on pS2 (a potential marker of breast cancer activity) or cellular morphology in nipple aspirate fluid.[84]

An observational retrospective cohort study investigated breast cancer patients treated at German institutions.[85] Of 18861 patients, a total of 1102 had received therapy with an isopropanolic extract of black cohosh. The mean overall observation time was 3.6 years. Black cohosh was not linked with an increased risk of recurrence, but instead was associated with prolonged disease-free survival (hazard ratio 0.83).

Contraindications

A traditional contraindication is pregnancy and lactation (see below), except to assist with childbirth.

A systematic review of the safety and efficacy of black cohosh in patients with cancer concluded that black cohosh appears to be safe in breast cancer patients without risk for liver disease, although further research is needed.[33]

Black cohosh is contraindicated in patients with pre-existing liver disease.

Special warnings and precautions

As noted above, caution should be exercised in patients with oestrogen-sensitive malignant tumours, especially when using doses at the higher end of the range.

Patients on long-term black cohosh therapy should be monitored for signs and symptoms of liver damage.

Interactions

The antiproliferative effect of black cohosh extract in combination with tamoxifen was assessed in vitro on 17-beta-oestradiol-stimulated MCF-7 human breast cancer cells.[86] Dilutions of black cohosh extract in the range 10^{-3} to 10^{-5} augmented the antiproliferative action of 10^{-5} tamoxifen. Whether this interaction also applies in vivo has not been established.

Although a black cohosh extract and six triterpenoid glycosides isolated from it were shown to inhibit the key drug metabolising cytochrome P450 enzyme CYP3A4 in vitro,[87] two human drug interaction studies have indicated this does not occur in people. One study found that a black cohosh extract (40 mg twice daily, standardised to 2.5% triterpene glycosides) did not affect CYP3A, which is involved in the metabolism of about half of all pharmaceutical drugs.[88] The other study screened a black cohosh extract (1090 mg twice daily, each capsule standardised to 0.2% triterpene glycosides) for effects on the drug metabolising enzymes CYP3A4/5, CYP1A2, CYP2E1 and CYP2D6 in 12 healthy volunteers who took the extract for 28 days. There was a statistically significant inhibition of only CYP2D6, but the magnitude of the effect was small (around 7%) and deemed unlikely to be of clinical relevance.[89] A subsequent study conducted by the same group, in which 18 healthy volunteers took a standardised black cohosh extract for 14 days, found no evidence for an effect on CYP2D6.[90] A separate drug interaction study (using digoxin as a probe drug) found no evidence for effects on the drug transporter P-glycoprotein in 16 healthy volunteers who took a black cohosh extract (equivalent to 40 mg herb per day) for 2 weeks.[91]

The potential for black cohosh to alter the response to radiation therapy and four common anticancer drugs (docetaxel, doxorubicin, cisplatin and 4-hydroperoxycyclophosphamide – 4-HC, an analogue of cyclophosphamide that is active in cell culture) was studied in vitro in a mouse breast cancer cell line. Black cohosh extract increased the cytotoxicity of docetaxel and doxorubicin, decreased the cytotoxicity of cisplatin and did not alter the effects of 4-HC or radiation.[92] The relevance of these findings to the human use of black cohosh is uncertain.

Use in pregnancy and lactation

Category B2 – no increase in frequency of malformation or other harmful effects on the fetus from limited use in women. Animal studies are lacking.

The traditional position is generally that black cohosh should not be taken during pregnancy except to assist with birth. According to the British Herbal Compendium black cohosh is contraindicated in pregnancy;[93] however, this restriction is not listed in the Commission E.[94] Black cohosh was widely used by the Eclectics in traditional Western herbal medicine as a partus preparator, if taken in the last weeks of pregnancy.[5]

In a 1999 survey of certified nurse-midwives in the US, black cohosh was used by 45% of the 90 respondents who used herbal medicine to stimulate labour. Adverse effects attributed to use of blue cohosh and black cohosh were not separately assigned and included nausea, increased meconium-stained fluid and transient fetal tachycardia.[95]

After a normal labour, a female infant was not able to breathe spontaneously and sustained CNS hypoxic-ischaemic damage. A midwife had attempted induction of labour using a combination of blue cohosh and black cohosh given orally (dosage undefined) at around 42 weeks' gestation.[96] It was not possible to identify the herbal preparation as the causative agent; however, this reaction may have been due to the blue cohosh (Caulophyllum thalictroides) rather than to the black cohosh (see Chapter 5).

A prospective, epidemiological study investigated the influence of first trimester use of medications and vaccines in the 1950s on the occurrence of congenital malformations and fetal survival in approximately 3200 pregnancies. Black cohosh was used in 1 of 266 pregnancies where a malformation occurred and in 2 of 532 pregnancies from the comparison groups. The dose and duration of use of black cohosh and the nature of the malformation were not specified.[97] Black cohosh could not be identified as a causative agent.

Black cohosh use should be strongly discouraged during breastfeeding. This consideration is based on a possible oestrogenic effect. The British Herbal Compendium contraindicates black cohosh during lactation.[93] However, the Commission E does not list this restriction.[94]

Effects on ability to drive or operate machinery

No adverse effects expected.

Side effects

General side effects

High doses of black cohosh can cause a frontal headache, with a dull, full or bursting feeling. This headache is the most characteristic effect observed when giving even therapeutic doses.[98] A review published in 2000 found that mild gastrointestinal upset was the most frequent minor adverse event reported in clinical studies (average of 5.6% of patients across five studies). Other minor adverse events reported in clinical studies included headache, vertigo, weight gain, mastalgia, heavy feeling in the legs and a stimulant effect. Vaginal bleeding has also been reported.[2]

Two reviews published in 2003 confirm that adverse events with black cohosh are rare, mild and reversible. Gastrointestinal upsets and rashes are the most common adverse events. There is record of a few serious adverse events, including hepatic and circulatory conditions, but causality could not be determined.[99,100] Details of some of the case reports follow.

A case was reported in 2001 of a woman diagnosed with grade 1 endometrioid adenocarcinoma of the endometrium 'whose history was notable for extensive use of supplemental phytoestrogens'. Herbs included chaste tree, dong quai, black cohosh and licorice.[101] No causality was demonstrated.

A 45-year-old woman who had been taking separate bottled products of black cohosh, Vitex agnus-castus and evening primrose oil for 4 months had three nocturnal seizures within a 3-month period. The patient had also consumed one to two beers 24 to 48h prior to each incident.[102] It was not established whether the herbal preparations caused the seizures.

A 26-year-old woman presented at a hospital with chest pain. Her heart rate and blood pressure dropped temporarily during the course of monitoring. Her urine digoxin level was 'elevated' at 0.9 ng/mL (but within the normal therapeutic range – 0.5 to 2.0 ng/mL). However, she was not taking digoxin. In addition to the contraceptive pill, she was taking a herbal preparation containing black cohosh, skullcap (*Scutellaria lateriflora*), lousewort (*Pedicularis canadensis*), hops (*Humulus lupulus*), valerian (*Valeriana officinalis*) and cayenne pepper (*Capsicum annuum*). The product was not available for analysis. The chest pain had started during her shift as a topless dancer, during which she had consumed four alcoholic drinks, but no illicit drugs.[103] This study inappropriately speculated on 'digoxin-like factors' with cardiotonic activity claimed to be 'commonly' found in herbal teas. The source of the patient's symptoms remains a mystery, but factors that interfere with digoxin assays, yet are without cardiotonic activity, have been reported in some herbs. (Refer to the Ginseng (*Eleutherococcus senticosus*) monograph by way of example.)

A case report exists of a 54-year-old woman who developed severe asthenia and high blood levels of creatine phosphokinase (230 to 237 U/L), lactate dehydrogenase (504 to 548 U/L) and total cholesterol, while taking a supplement derived from black cohosh for the management of vasomotor symptoms related to menopause. Notably the woman had previously taken the product for 12 months with no alteration in biochemistry and had restarted the product after a 3-month break. The black cohosh tablets contained 20 mg of dried rhizome and root extract. No other cause could be identified for her symptoms and she was advised to discontinue the product, after which a progressive normalisation of biochemical parameters and improvement in clinical symptoms occurred.[104]

A case report described a 56-year-old woman diagnosed with cutaneous pseudolymphoma after taking a black cohosh product for 12 months. The localised erythematous plaques on her arms and legs appeared after 6 months and completely disappeared with withdrawal of the product for 3 months.[105]

Other adverse reactions attributed to black cohosh use include cutaneous vasculitis[106] and coagulation activation with fluid retention (secondary to a transient autoimmune hepatitis).[107]

Liver injury

On the 9 February 2006, the Australian TGA announced the following:

> The Therapeutic Goods Administration (TGA) reviewed the safety of Black cohosh (*Cimicifuga racemosa*) following reports of possible liver problems internationally and in Australia. At the time of the review, there were 47 cases of liver reactions worldwide, including 9 Australian cases. In Australia, 4 patients were hospitalised, including two who required liver transplantation. Although some reports are confounded by multiple ingredients, by more than

one medication or by other medical conditions, there is sufficient evidence of a causal association between Black cohosh and serious hepatitis. However, considering the widespread use of Black cohosh, the incidence of liver reaction appears to be very low. Following the safety review, the TGA has decided that medicines containing Black cohosh should include the following label statement: 'Warning: Black cohosh may harm the liver in some individuals. Use under the supervision of a healthcare professional'.

On July 18, 2006, the Medicines and Healthcare Products Regulatory Agency (MHRA) in the UK issued a press release stating that all black cohosh products sold there should carry the following label warning: 'Black cohosh may rarely cause liver problems. If you become unwell (yellowing eyes/skin, nausea, vomiting, dark urine, abdominal pain, unusual tiredness) stop taking immediately and seek medical advice. Not suitable for patients with a previous history of liver disease.'

Notwithstanding the Australian TGA's claim at the time concerning the number of cases of liver damage linked to black cohosh (which include the adverse reaction reports filed with the UK MHRA and other health authorities) only five papers or letters had been published purporting to demonstrate a link between black cohosh (*Actaea racemosa*) ingestion and subsequent liver injury. It is important to closely examine these published reports since, because of the process of peer review, these represent the best-documented evidence of any association with liver injury. The first publication, from doctors at the Princess Alexandra Hospital in Brisbane, Australia, described six patients with evidence of severe hepatitis that was linked to taking a range of herbal products.[108] Two of these patients were taking black cohosh, although one was also taking other herbs including skullcap, a herb which can be substituted by *Teucrium* species, a known hepatotoxic genus.[109]

The one case attributed to black cohosh alone (Case 1) was truly dramatic. Of the cases reported, the most serious illness occurred in this 47-year-old woman who was taking black cohosh for menopausal symptoms. She required liver transplantation even though, according to the publication, the patient had been taking the black cohosh for just 1 week. Histological examination of her liver confirmed severe hepatitis and early fibrosis. The patient did not exhibit eosinophilia and had no signs of any systemic disturbance. Serology for hepatitis A, B and C was negative, but rechallenge with the herb was not performed 'for ethical reasons'. The dose of black cohosh taken was not specified, neither was the product.

The second publication, also from Australia, describes a 52-year-old woman with acute liver failure (Case 2).[110] She had been taking an herbal formula containing 1:1 liquid extracts prescribed by a pharmacist. Black cohosh 1:1 was 10% of the mixture and the daily dose of the combination was 7.5 mL twice a day. The patient underwent successful liver transplantation. Although the authors stated that: 'Extensive investigation excluded other recognised causes of liver failure', they provided no details of what these investigations were. Analysis by the TGA was said to confirm the presence of golden seal, black cohosh and Ginkgo in the herbal mixture. Other stated ingredients were ground ivy and oats seed.

The phenomenon of idiosyncratic hepatic reactions to drugs is well documented. It also appears that this reaction does occur to certain herbs, for example chaparral (*Larrea tridentata*) and germander (*Teucrium* species). By definition, such reactions are rare and unpredictable and are not dose related. There are two types of idiosyncratic hepatic injury: hypersensitivity and aberrant metabolism. The former develops 1 to 5 weeks after exposure to the drug and, since it is immune-mediated and acute, also involves a systemic reaction including rash, fever and eosinophilia. The latter takes weeks to months to develop and symptoms are confined to the liver. Diagnosis of drug-induced idiosyncratic liver injury (DILI) is very difficult and relies largely on circumstantial evidence. Factors taken into account include a temporal association, exclusion of other possible causes, a consistent latency period to those described above, presence or absence of hypersensitivity (systemic) features, positive response to drug removal (dechallenge), positive response to rechallenge and a positive lymphocyte stimulation test (this last factor is quite controversial). Complicating this is the fact that DILI can mimic every known human liver disease.[111] There are many confounding factors that could lead to incorrect associations between ingested medications or herbs and idiosyncratic liver injury. Many viruses that cause liver disease are still to be identified[112] and there are no tests for them. Even known viruses are not always tested for. For example, a Dutch study published this year found that hepatitis E virus was a significant cause of unexplained hepatitis.[113] Occult coeliac disease has been suggested as a cause of unexplained raised ALT and AST.[114] Rare liver diseases may not be excluded.[115,116] Other environmental factors could be implicated.

The experience of a liver transplant unit highlights some key issues behind the history and incidence of severe acute hepatitis (fulminant hepatic failure, FHF). All adult cases of FHF presenting to the Victorian Liver Transplant Unit (Australia) from 1988 to 2002 were analysed. Eighty patients (mostly female) were referred, at a rate of approximately one case per million population per year. Mean age was about 38 years. Most cases were due to paracetamol poisoning (36%) or idiopathic hepatitis (34%).[110] Only five of the 80 cases were classified as drug induced, making this causality a rare factor. Other main causes included hepatitis A (three cases), hepatitis B (eight cases) and Wilson's disease (six cases). The 27 cases (34%) of hepatitis due to unknown causes (idiopathic) is a surprising rate. These cases are also described as non-A non-B hepatitis, since patients are not positive for hepatitis A or B. In the USA one study found that the most common cause of FHF was non-A non-B (idiopathic) hepatitis.[117] (Note that this US study was published in 1995, well before the dramatic rise in herbal use in that country.) Presumably unidentified infectious or environmental factors could cause these cases of idiopathic hepatitis. However, the authors of the Australian study state: 'The strong female predominance of cases argues against a viral cause and raises the possibility that hormonal factors are involved, or that the condition is linked to autoimmune liver diseases. There is clearly a need for large, detailed, multicentre epidemiological studies, to provide further clues to a possible aetiology/ies of this syndrome.'

The demographics of idiopathic hepatitis (female, late 30s to early 50s) and black cohosh use strongly overlap. Hence, there is a distinct possibility that some patients who develop idiopathic hepatitis might also be coincidentally taking black cohosh. The herb could then be mistakenly attributed as the cause.

Since these initial series of cases attributing idiosyncratic hepatotoxicity to black cohosh, more cases have been reported. There have also been several publications analysing these and the earlier case reports, especially from the team headed by Teschke.

In 2009 the group rigorously analysed all 69 reported cases (at the time) and found no likelihood of causality in 68.[118] Most cases were marred by confounding variables, misreported data and a lack of critical information.[119] In particular, there was a lack of identification of the herb involved in the initial cases.[120]

Of high relevance here are the findings of Health Canada. From January 2005 to March 2009, Health Canada received six domestic reports of liver adverse reactions suspected of being associated with black cohosh. Analysis of three products associated with these reports revealed that they did not contain authentic black cohosh. Their phytochemical profiles were consistent with the presence of other related herbal species. A review of the authenticity of all licensed products containing black cohosh resulted in the voluntary withdrawal of several products not containing authentic black cohosh, including the products reported in four of the adverse reaction cases.[121]

Studies in black cohosh users have also sought to understand its impact on the liver. A prospective, longitudinal study recruited 100 healthy postmenopausal women from a hospital in Egypt. The women received black cohosh extract (40 mg/day) for relief of menopausal symptoms and were followed up for 12 months. Eighty-seven women completed the study, which included evaluation of total hepatic blood flow and liver function. The study sought to investigate potential mechanisms of hepatotoxicity: compromise of blood flow to the liver or a direct toxic effect on liver cells. The following results were obtained after 12 months of treatment:

- No significant changes in hepatic artery blood flow, portal vein blood flow or total hepatic blood flow
- No significant changes in any liver function tests
- A significant reduction in the prevalence, daily frequency and severity of hot flushes, compared with baseline.[122]

A meta-analysis of five trials involving 1117 women found no evidence that the isopropanolic extract of black cohosh has an adverse effect on liver function.[123]

Overdosage

According to early data, ingestion of 5 g of the herb or 12 g of the fluid extract can cause nausea, vomiting, violent headache, vertigo, joint pain, red eyes and weak pulse. Visual and nervous disturbances have also been noted.[8,124,125] Some of these effects may have been due to the past adulteration of black cohosh with the poisonous plants red baneberry (*Actaea spicata*) and white cohosh or white baneberry (*A. panchypoda* (*A. alba*)).[126] However, in the absence of any further information such doses of black cohosh are not recommended.

Safety in children

No information available, although the Eclectics did describe use in children for fever.[5]

Regulatory status in selected countries

Black cohosh is covered by a positive Commission E monograph with the following applications: neurovegetative complaints of premenstrual, dysmenorrhoeic or climacteric origin.

Black cohosh is on the UK General Sale List, with a maximum single dose of 200 mg. However, it does require a warning statement as noted above. Black cohosh products have achieved Traditional Herbal Registration in the UK with the traditional indication of relief of symptoms of the menopause.

Black cohosh does not have GRAS status. However, it is freely available as a 'dietary supplement' in the USA under DSHEA legislation (1994 Dietary Supplement Health and Education Act). Black cohosh has been present in OTC menstrual drug products. The FDA advises: 'based on evidence currently available, there is inadequate data to establish general recognition of the safety and effectiveness of these ingredients for the specified uses'.

Black cohosh is not included in Part 4 of Schedule 4 of the Therapeutic Goods Act Regulations of Australia and is freely available for sale provided products carry a warning regarding possible liver damage.

References

1. Compton JA, Culham A, Jury SL. *Taxon.* 1998;47:593–634.
2. American Herbal Pharmacopoeia. Black cohosh rhizome: Actaea racemosa L. syn. Cimicifuga racemosa (L.) Nutt.: Analytical, Quality Control, and Therapeutic Monograph. Santa Cruz: American Herbal Pharmacopoeia; 2002.
3. German Federal Minister of Justice. *German Commission E for Human Medicine Monograph*, Bundes-Anzeiger (German Federal Gazette) no. 43, dated 02.03.1989.
4. British Herbal Medicine Association. *British Herbal Pharmacopoeia*. Cowling: BHMA; 1983. p. 66.
5. Felter HW, Lloyd JU. *King's American Dispensatory*, 18th ed., rev 3. Portland: 1905. Reprinted by: Eclectic Medical Publications, 1983;1:528–533.
6. Harnischfeger G, Stolze H. *Erfahrungsheilkunde.* 1981;30(6):439–444.
7. Chiej R. *The Macdonald Encyclopedia of Medicinal Plants*. London: Macdonald; 1984. Entry no. 87.
8. Grieve MA. *A Modern Herbal*, vol 1. New York: Dover Publications; 1971. p. 211.
9. Information on file. Warwick, Queensland 4072, Australia: MediHerb Pty Ltd; 2003.
10. Hostettmann K, Marston A. *Chemistry & Pharmacology of Natural Products: Saponins*. Cambridge: Cambridge University Press; 1995. p. 280.
11. Wagner H, Bladt S. *Plant Drug Analysis: A Thin Layer Chromatography Atlas*, 2nd ed. Berlin: Springer-Verlag; 1996. p. 336.
12. Gizycki H. *Z Exp Med.* 1944;113:635–644.
13. Jarry H, Harnischfeger G. *Planta Med.* 1985;51(1):46–49.
14. Jarry H, Ch Gorkow, Wuttke W. In: Loew D, Rietbrock N, eds. *Phytopharmaka in Forschung und klinischer Anwendung*. Darmstadt: Steinkopff (Verlag); 1995. p. 104.
15. Jarry H, Harnischfeger G, Düker EM. *Planta Med.* 1985;51(4):316–319.
16. Duker EM, Kopanski L, Jarry H, et al. *Planta Med.* 1991;57(5):420–424.
17. Jarry H, Leonhardt S, Duls C, et al. *23rd International LOF-Symposium on Phyto-Oestrogens.* Belgium: University of Gent; 1999.
18. Jarry H, Ch Gorkow, Wuttke W. In: Loew D, Rietbrock N, eds. *Phytopharmaka in Forschung und klinischer Anwendung*. Darmstadt: Steinkopff (Verlag); 1995. pp. 109–110.
19. Einer-Jensen N, Zhao J, Andersen KP, et al. *Maturitas.* 1996;25(2):149–153.
20. Zava DT, Dollbaum CM, Blen M. *Proc Soc Exp Biol Med.* 1998;217(3):369–378.
21. Liu J, Burdette JE, Xu H, et al. *J Agric Food Chem.* 2001;49(5):2472–2479.
22. Gaube F, Wolfl S, Pusch L, et al. *BMC Pharmacol.* 2007;7:11.
23. Bolle P, Mastrangelo S, Perrone F, et al. *J Steroid Biochem Mol Biol.* 2007;107(3–5):262–269.
24. Chan BY, Lau KS, Jiang B, et al. *Bone.* 2008;43(3):567–573.
25. Seidlová-Wuttke D, Jarry H, Wuttke W. *Planta Med.* 2007;73:995.
26. Kolios L, Schumann J, Sehmisch S, et al. *Planta Med.* 2010;76(9):850–857.
27. Qiu SX, Dan C, Ding LS, et al. *Chem Biol.* 2007;14(7):860–869.
28. Nesselhut T, Schellhase C, Dietrich R, et al. *Arch Gynecol Obstet.* 1993;254(1–4):817–818.
29. Nesselhut T. *Expert Forum on Remifemin®: Report and Results From Endocrinology Expert Forum in Luneburg.* Salzgitter (Ringelheim): Schaper & Brummer GmbH & Co.; 1993.
30. Einbond LS, Shimizu M, Xiao D. *Breast Cancer Res Treat.* 2004;83(3):221–231.
31. Einbond LS, Su T, Wu HA. *Int J Cancer.* 2007;121(9):2073–2083.
32. Einbond LS, Shimizu M, Nuntanakorn P, et al. *Planta Med.* 2006;72(13):1200–1206.
33. Walji R, Boon H, Guns E, et al. *Support Care Cancer.* 2007;15:913–921.
34. Hostanska K, Nisslein T, Freudenstein J, et al. *Anticancer Res.* 2005;25(1A):139–147.
35. Jarry H, Stromeier S, Wuttke W, et al. *Planta Med.* 2007;73(2):184–187.
36. Seidlová-Wuttke D, Thelen P, Wuttke W. *Planta Med.* 2006;72(6):521–526.
37. Jarry H, Metten M, Spengler B, et al. *Maturitas.* 2003;44(Suppl 1):S31–S38.
38. Burdette JE, Liu J, Chen SN, et al. *J Agric Food Chem.* 2003;51(19):5661–5670.
39. Rhyu MR, Lu J, Webster DE, et al. *J Agric Food Chem.* 2006;54(26):9852–9857.
40. Reame NE, Lukacs JL, Padmanabhan V, et al. *Menopause.* 2008;15(5):832–840.
41. Schmid D, Gruber M, Woehs F, et al. *J Pharm Pharmacol.* 2009;61(8):1089–1096.
42. Yang CL, Chik SC, Li JC, et al. *J Med Chem.* 2009;52(21):6707–6715.
43. Schmid D, Woehs F, Svoboda M, et al. *Can J Physiol Pharmacol.* 2009;87(11):963–972.
44. Wojcikowski K, Stevenson L, Leach D, et al. *J Altern Complement Med.* 2007;13(1):103–109.
45. Burdette JE, Chen SN, Lu ZZ, et al. *J Agric Food Chem.* 2002;50(24):7022–7028.
46. Hemmi H, Ishida N. *J Pharmacobiodyn.* 1980;3(12):643–648.
47. Genazzani E, Sorrentino L. *Nature.* 1962;194:544–545.
48. Yoo JS, Jung JS, Lee TH, et al. *Korean J Pharmacogn.* 1995;26(4) 355.
49. Einbond LS, Soffritti M, Esposti DD, et al. *Fundam Clin Pharmacol.* 2009;23(3):311–321.
50. van Breemen RB, Liang W, Banuvar S, et al. *Clin Pharmacol Ther.* 2010;87(2):219–225.
51. Bachmann GA. *J Reprod Med.* 2005;50(3):155–165.

52. Rossouw JE, Anderson GL, Prentice RL, et al. *JAMA*. 2002;288(3):321–333.
53. Knöss W. *Assessment Report on Cimicifuga racemosa (L.) Nutt., rhizoma*. London: European Medicines Agency; 2010.
54. Palacio C, Masri G, Mooradian AD. *Drugs Aging*. 2009;26(1):23–36.
55. Borrelli F, Ernst E. *Pharmacol Res*. 2008;58(1):8–14.
56. Shams T, Setia MS, Hemmings R, et al. *Altern Ther Health Med*. 2010;16(1):36–44.
57. Stoll W. *Therapeuticum*. 1987;1:23–31.
58. Wuttke W, Seidlová-Wuttke D, Gorkow C. *Maturitas*. 2003;44(suppl 1):S67–S77.
59. Osmers R, Friede M, Liske E, et al. *Obstet Gynecol*. 2005;105(5 Pt 1):1074–1083.
60. Frei-Kleiner S, Schaffner W, Rahlfs VW, et al. *Maturitas*. 2005;51(4):397–404.
61. Newton KM, Reed SD, LaCroix AZ, et al. *Ann Intern Med*. 2006;145(12):869–879.
62. Bai W, Henneicke-von Zepelin HH, Wang S, et al. *Maturitas*. 2007;58(1):31–41.
63. Chung DJ, Kim HY, Park KH, et al. *Yonsei Med J*. 2007;48(2):289–294.
64. Uebelhack R, Blohmer JU, Graubaum HJ, et al. *Obstet Gynecol*. 2006;107(2 Pt 1):247–255.
65. Rotem C, Kaplan B. *Gynecol Endocrinol*. 2007;23(2):117–122.
66. Sammartino A, Tommaselli GA, Gargano V, et al. *Gynecol Endocrinol*. 2006;22(11):646–650.
67. Verhoeven MO, van der Mooren MJ, van de Weijer PH, et al. *Menopause*. 2005;12(4):412–420.
68. Briese V, Stammwitz U, Friede M, et al. *Maturitas*. 2007;57(4):405–414.
69. Amsterdam JD, Yao Y, Mao JJ, et al. *J Clin Psychopharmacol*. 2009;29(5):478–483.
70. Hernández Muñoz G, Pluchino S. *Maturitas*. 2003;44(suppl 1):S59–S65.
71. Jacobson JS, Troxel AB, Evans J, et al. *J Clin Oncol*. 2001;19(10):2739–2745.
72. Bebenek M, Kemmler W, von Stengel S, et al. *Menopause*. 2010;17(4):791–800.
73. Mills SY, Jacoby RK, Chacksfield M, et al. *Br J Rheumatol*. 1996;35(9):874–878.
74. Shahin AY, Ismail AM, Zahran KM, Makhlouf AM. *Reprod Biomed Online*. 2008;16(4):580–588.
75. Shahin AY, Ismail AM, Shaaban OM. *Reprod Biomed Online*. 2009;19(4):501–507.
76. Korn WD. *Six-month Oral Toxicity Study with Remifemin Granulate in Rats Followed by an Eight-week Recovery Period*. Hannover, Germany: International Bioresearch; 1991.
77. Genazzani E, Sorrentino L. *Nature*. 1962;194(4828):544–545.
78. Beuscher N. *Z Phytother*. 1995;16:301–310.
79. Davis VL, Jayo MJ, Ho A, et al. *Cancer Res*. 2008;68(20):8377–8383.
80. Rebbeck TR, Troxel AB, Norman S, et al. *Int J Cancer*. 2007;120:1523–1528.
81. Obi N, Chang-Claude J, Berger J, et al. *Cancer Epidemiol Biomarkers Prev*. 2009;18(8):2207–2213.
82. Brasky TM, Lampe JW, Potter JD, et al. *Cancer Epidemiol Biomarkers Prev*. 2010;19(7):1696–1708.
83. Hirschberg AL, Edlund M, Svane G, et al. *Menopause*. 2007;14(1):89–96.
84. Ruhlen RL, Haubner J, Tracy JK, et al. *Nutr Cancer*. 2007;59(2):269–277.
85. Zepelin HH, Meden H, Kostev K, et al. *Int J Clin Pharmacol Ther*. 2007;45(3):143–154.
86. German Patent DE 196 52 183 CI. *Verwendung eines Extraktes aus Cimicifuga racemosa*: Schaper & Brümmer.
87. Tsukamoto S, Aburatani M, Ohta T. *Evid Based Complement Alternat Med*. 2005;2(2):223–226.
88. Gurley B, Hubbard MA, Williams DK, et al. *J Clin Pharmacol*. 2006;46(2):201–213.
89. Gurley BJ, Gardner SF, Hubbard MA, et al. *Clin Pharmacol Ther*. 2005;77(5):415–426.
90. Gurley BJ, Swain A, Hubbard MA, et al. *Mol Nutr Food Res*. 2008;52(7):755–763.
91. Gurley BJ, Barone GW, Williams DK, et al. *Drug Metab Dispos*. 2006;34(1):69–74.
92. Rockwell S, Liu Y, Higgins SA. *Breast Cancer Res Treat*. 2005;90(3):233–239.
93. British Herbal Medicine Association. *British Herbal Compendium*. Bournemouth, BHMA; 1992. pp. 34–36.
94. Blumenthal M, ed. *The Complete German Commission E Monographs: Therapeutic Guide to Herbal Medicines*. Austin: American Botanical Council; 1998.
95. McFarlin BL, Gibson MH, O'Rear J, et al. *J Nurse Midwifery*. 1999;44(3):205–216.
96. Gunn TR, Wright IM. *N Z Med J*. 1996;109(1032):410–411.
97. Mellin GW. *Am J Obst Gynec*. 1964;90(7, Pt 2):1169–1180.
98. Felter HW. *The Eclectic Materia Medica, Pharmacology and Therapeutics, 1922*. Portland: Eclectic Medical Publications; 1983. pp. 466–469.
99. Dog TL, Powell KL, Weisman SM. *Menopause*. 2003;10(4):299–313.
100. Huntley A, Ernst E. *Menopause*. 2003;10(1):58–64.
101. Johnson EB, Muto MC, Yanushpolsky EH, et al. *Obstet Gynecol*. 2001;98(5 Pt 2):947–950.
102. Shuster J. *Hosp Pharm*. 1996;31(12):1553–1554.
103. Scheinost ME. *J Am Osteopathic Assoc*. 2001;101(8):444–446.
104. Minciullo PL, Saija A, Patafi M, et al. *Phytomedicine*. 2006;13(1–2):115–118.
105. Meyer S, Vogt T, Obermann EC, et al. *Dermatology*. 2007;214(1):94–96.
106. Ingraffea A, Donohue K, Wilkel C, Falanga V. *J Am Acad Dermatol*. 2007;56(suppl 5):S124–S126.
107. Zimmermann R, Witte A, Voll RE, et al. *Climacteric*. 2010;13(2):187–191.
108. Whiting PW, Clouston A, Kerlin P. *MJA*. 2002;177(8):440–443.
109. Mills S, Bone K. *The Essential Guide to Herbal Safety*. USA: Churchill Livingstone; 2005. pp. 581–584.
110. Lontos S, Jones RM, Angus PW, et al. *MJA*. 2003;179(7):390–391.
111. Pishvaian AC, Trope BW, Lewis JH. *Curr Opin Gastroenterol*. 2004;20(3):208–219.
112. Bowden D, Moaven LD, Locarnini S. *MJA*. 1996;164:87–89.
113. Waar K, Herremans M, Vennema H. *J Clin Virol*. 2005;33(2):145–149.
114. Bardella M, Vecchi M, Conte D. *Hepatology*. 1999;29(3):654–657.
115. Tordjmann T, Grimbert S, Genestie C. *Gastroenterol Clin Biol*. 1998;22(3):305–310.
116. Gaya D, Thorburn D, Oien K. *J Clin Pathol*. 2003;56(11):850–853.
117. Hoofnagle J, Carithers R, Shapiro C. *Hepatology*. 1995;21:240–252.
118. Teschke R, Bahre R, Genthner A, et al. *Maturitas*. 2009;63(4):302–314.
119. Teschke R. *Menopause*. 2010;17(2):426–440.
120. Teschke R, Schwarzenboeck A, Schmidt-Taenzer W, et al. *Ann Hepatol*. 2011;10(3):249–259.
121. Black cohosh products and liver toxicity: update. *Canadian Adverse Reaction Newsletter*. 2010:1–2.
122. Nasr A, Nafeh H. *Fertil Steril*. 2009;92(5):1780–1782.
123. Naser B, Schnitker J, Minkin MJ, et al. *Menopause*. 2011;18(4):366–375.
124. Mills SY. *The A-Z of Modern Herbalism*. London: Thorsons; 1989. p. 39.
125. Blaschek W, Ebel S, Hackenthal E, et al. *HagerROM 2002: Hagers Handbuch der Drogen und Arzneistoffe*. Heidelberg: Springer; 2002.
126. Grieve M. *A Modern Herbal*, vol 1. New York: Dover Publications; 1971. pp. 81–82.

Boswellia

(*Boswellia serrata* Roxb. ex Colebr.)

Synonyms

Boswellia glabra Roxb. (botanical synonym), Boswellia, Indian frankincense, Indian olibanum (Engl), Salaibaum (Ger), Baswellie-dentelee (Fr), (Dan) Sallaki (Sanskrit) Salai guggal (Hindi).

What is it?

The Boswellia shrubs and small trees belong to the same family (Burseraceae) as the trees that produce myrrh and are native to the dry tropics of Africa (especially the northeast) and Asia. The fragrant resins exuded from many species of Boswellia are known as frankincense or oleo-gum olibanum and have been used since antiquity for incense and embalming liquids. (*Boswellia serrata* resin is closely related to the Biblical frankincense (*B. carterii*).) As well as a long tradition of therapeutic use, particularly in Ayurveda, *Boswellia serrata* has recently been tested in clinical studies for a wide range of inflammatory conditions. Research has centred on the triterpenoids, especially the boswellic acids, which are considered to be responsible for the observed anti-inflammatory and antiarthritic activities of the resin. Studies on *B. carterii* have generally not been included in this review.

Effects

Reduces inflammation in a variety of body tissues; possibly disease modifying in osteoarthritis.

Traditional view

In Ayurveda, Boswellia resin, known as Salai guggal, is mainly used as an astringent and anti-inflammatory agent (when applied topically) and as a stimulant and expectorant (internal use).[1] Therapeutic applications include pulmonary diseases, especially if chronic, rheumatic disorders, diarrhoea, dysentery, piles, dysmenorrhoea, gonorrhoea, syphilis and liver disorders. It is also used for general weakness and to improve appetite.[2,3]

Summary actions

Anti-inflammatory, antiarthritic.

Can be used for

Indications supported by clinical trials

As an anti-inflammatory agent in asthma, inflammatory bowel disease (Crohn's and ulcerative colitis), rheumatoid arthritis (mixed results) and osteoarthritis. There is some clinical evidence to suggest Boswellia may reduce oedema in patients with certain malignant brain tumours.

May also be used for

Extrapolation from pharmacological studies

Other conditions where leukotrienes and cytokines play an important role as inflammatory mediators. Disorders characterised by elevated levels of leukotrienes include cystic fibrosis, psoriasis, allergic rhinitis, lupus, gout, urticaria, liver cirrhosis, multiple sclerosis and chronic smoking. The value of Boswellia for these conditions has not been established and recently the clinical relevance of the in vitro inhibition of 5-lipoxygenase by boswellic acids has been questioned. Boswellia may have clinically significant anti-tumour activity.

Other applications

Its anti-inflammatory properties and ability to cross the blood-brain barrier (especially for beta-boswellic acid) suggest a possible role for Boswellia in the prevention of Alzheimer's disease.

Preparations

The dried oleo-gum resin or a dry extract standardised for boswellic acids in tablet or capsule form. Boswellia resin requires a high content of alcohol for extraction (usually 90%) similar to myrrh and ginger. For this reason, Boswellia is more conveniently dispensed as a tablet or capsule rather than as a tincture, given the relatively high doses required.

Dosage

The dosage for Boswellia is 200 to 400mg of extract three times a day, taken with meals. This extract is typically standardised to have a boswellic acid content of 60% to 70% and the dose corresponds to an equivalent resin intake of 2.4 to 4.8 g.

Duration of use

There are no known problems with long-term consumption. However, wherever possible the cause of the inflammation should be addressed, rather than relying only on palliation with Boswellia.

Summary assessment of safety

No major problems have been associated with the ingestion of normal doses and there are no documented interactions with conventional drugs. Typical adverse reactions occur with a low frequency and include diarrhoea and allergy.

Technical data

Botany

The Burseraceae family, to which both the Boswellia and Commiphora genera belong, contains trees or shrubs with prominent resin ducts in the bark. When the bark is cut, the secretion exudes and solidifies to a gum-like consistency after exposure to the air. *Boswellia serrata* is a deciduous, medium-sized tree native to the dry hills of India. The leaves are opposite, sessile and have serrated edges. Flowers occur in auxiliary racemes, shorter than the leaves, and are small, aromatic and white. The fruit is three-angled, splits into three valves and contains a single compressed seed.[1-4]

Adulteration

There are no documented adulterants, but presumably other species of Boswellia are possible candidates. The assessment of boswellic acid levels in standardised extracts is sometimes determined by simple acid-base titration. This leads to the possibility that a common food acid such as citric acid could be added as an adulterant to falsely elevate the level of boswellic acids measured by this means.

Key constituents

The oleo-gum-resin of *Boswellia serrata* contains pentacyclic triterpene acids (mainly beta-boswellic acid and the acetyl-boswellic acids: acetyl-beta-boswellic acid, acetyl-11-keto-beta-boswellic acid (AKBA) and 11-keto-beta-boswellic acid),[5] and tetracyclic triterpene acids.[6]

Other constituents include an essential oil, terpenols, monosaccharides, uronic acids, sterols and phlobaphenes.[7] The oils from *Boswellia species* consist of monoterpenes and sesquiterpenes: alpha-thujene can be a major component of the oil obtained from *Boswellia serrata*.[8] The tetracyclic triterpenoid 3-oxo-tirucallic acid (unrelated to the boswellic acids) has also been identified as a component of Boswellia.[9]

beta-Boswellic acid

Pharmacodynamics

The relevant pharmacodynamics of Boswellia (including *B. carterii*) and the boswellic acids have been the subject of two comprehensive reviews.[10,11]

Anti-inflammatory and related activity

Laboratory studies on Boswellia extract and boswellic acids have demonstrated their ability to both prevent and relieve inflammation. Anti-inflammatory and antiarthritic activity was demonstrated in several models:[12] carrageenan-, histamine- and dextran-induced oedema, carrageenan-induced pleurisy,[13] adjuvant arthritis, formaldehyde- and bovine serum albumin (BSA)-induced arthritis[14] and sodium urate gouty arthritis. Oral doses of Boswellia extract from 25 to 200 mg/kg were typically tested. The anti-inflammatory effect was not affected by removal of the adrenal glands, indicating the pituitary-adrenal axis was not involved. No significant activity occurred in cotton pellet-induced granuloma, which is more sensitive to steroidal than non-steroidal anti-inflammatory agents. In the developing adjuvant polyarthritis model, boswellic acids significantly reduced the development of secondary lesions. The reversal of syndromes of established arthritis indicated that it could control damage arising from immunological mechanisms.[12]

In adjuvant arthritis, administration of Boswellia extract or boswellic acids decreased the urinary excretion of connective tissue metabolites[15] and had a beneficial effect on glycohydrolases and lysosomal stability.[16,17] Treatment also reduced the degradation of glycosaminoglycans. From these results it is likely that Boswellia has beneficial effects in inflammatory conditions by suppressing proliferating tissue and preventing the degradation of connective tissue.[18] Anti-inflammatory activity was also observed for *B. carterii* extract (450 to 900 mg/kg/day for 7 days, oral) in inflammation induced by complete Freund's adjuvant.[19] Topical application of a boswellic acid ointment demonstrated a dose-dependent anti-inflammatory effect in both acute and chronic experimental models, including croton-oil-induced mouse ear oedema and adjuvant arthritis in rats.[20]

Oral administration of boswellic acids reduced the development of 24 h delayed-type hypersensitivity reaction and complement fixing antibody in mice.[21] Oral administration of boswellic acids, particularly AKBA, before treatment with galactosamine/

endotoxin significantly reduced serum enzyme activity and potential liver damage in mice.[22] (This is a model of increased leukotriene synthesis.) A pain-relieving activity was reported for Boswellia extract,[23,24] but this finding was not confirmed in later studies.[12] Weak antipyretic activity was, however, observed.[12] AKBA (50 to 200 mg/kg, oral doses) produced a dose-dependent and significant analgesic effect in several different experimental models of nociception and potentiated the analgesic effect of selective cyclo-oxygenase inhibitors such as nimesulide.[25]

Conflicting results were observed in experimental models of gastrointestinal inflammation. One study found that Boswellia extract did not ameliorate symptoms of colitis in mice,[26] whereas in another AKBA and high-dose Boswellia extract significantly reduced tissue injury in rats with experimental ileitis.[27] AKBA was also found to confer protection in experimental murine colitis induced by dextran sodium sulphate, possibly by interfering with P-selectin-mediated recruitment of inflammatory cells.[28]

Boswellic acids were described as belonging to the group of slow-acting antiarthritic medications and inhibited latex-induced rat paw inflammation at oral doses of 50 to 100 mg/kg.[29] Unlike conventional non-steroidal anti-inflammatory drugs (NSAIDs), ulcerogenic effects were not detected for Boswellia extract in animal models, and the extract even exhibited a protective effect on experimentally induced ulcers in rats.[30] Other side effects of NSAIDs, such as prolonged gestation and parturition and diarrhoea, were not observed for the boswellic acids.[12]

Mechanism of action

The clinically relevant anti-inflammatory mechanisms for Boswellia are not fully understood. It appears to possess activity across a wide range of inflammatory diseases. While earlier studies have suggested the basis for anti-inflammatory activity is 5-lipoxygenase inhibition, this understanding has been challenged in recent times.

In early research, boswellic acids significantly inhibited the stimulated release of leukotrienes from intact human neutrophils, with AKBA being the most potent.[31] Boswellia extract also reduced the formation of leukotrienes by inhibiting the enzyme 5-lipoxygenase in vitro.[32]

Boswellic acids appeared to exert a specific in vitro inhibitory activity on 5-lipoxygenase, with little effect on cyclo-oxygenase (which produces prostaglandins) or 12-lipoxygenase, although some inhibitory activity on both these enzymes has been recently found in human platelets.[33] The mechanism of action is therefore quite distinct from conventional NSAIDs, which inhibit prostaglandin production. Compounds that inhibit 5-lipoxygenase usually do so because they are antioxidants. However, the action of the boswellic acids does not rely on antioxidant properties and for these reasons it is described as novel and specific.[34,35] It was concluded that Boswellia could be a useful treatment in leukotriene-mediated inflammation and hypersensitivity-based disorders. Some degradation products of boswellic acids are also potent inhibitors of 5-lipoxygenase.[36]

There is a suggestion from in vitro research that the action of Boswellia on 5-lipoxygenase is biphasic.[37] Concentrations greater than 10 to 15 μg/mL inhibited the enzyme in stimulated neutrophils, as noted previously. In contrast, lower concentrations of extracts (1 to 10 μg/mL) potentiated 5-lipoxygenase product formation. It was proposed in one study that this stimulatory effect on 5-lipoxygenase activity may be due (at least in part) to 3-oxo-tirucallic acid and related compounds, rather than the boswellic acids.[38,39]

A 2009 study found that while the 11-keto-boswellic acids efficiently suppressed 5-lipoxygenase activity in isolated neutrophils, this effect was absent in whole human blood.[40] A single dose (800 mg) of Boswellia extract to 12 healthy male volunteers failed to suppress leukotriene B4 (a product of 5-lipoxygenase) in plasma. The authors suggested that, since leukotrienes do not play a major role in osteoarthritis and inflammatory bowel disease, a lack of clinical activity on 5-lipoxygenase is actually consistent with the observed value of Boswellia for these disorders. Their findings certainly question the relevance of 5-lipoxygenase inhibition to the pharmacological activity of Boswellia. However, unpublished results quoted in a recent review claimed inhibition of cysteine-leukotriene formation in stimulated granulocytes ex vivo from healthy humans given 1200 mg of a commercial Boswellia extract.[11] The inhibitory effect was more than 90% with a maximum 6 h after intake, which corresponds with the known pharmacokinetics of boswellic acids.

That the anti-inflammatory mechanism of Boswellia is not confined to the inhibition of leukotriene formation was highlighted in a 2006 review.[41] There is suggestion from in vitro studies that Boswellia can alter the production of pro-inflammatory cytokines. AKBA and acetyl-alpha-boswellic acid downregulated tumour necrosis factor alpha (TNF-alpha) in stimulated peripheral monocytes by inhibiting NF-kappaB signalling.[42] A related species (Boswellia carterii) inhibited Th1 cytokines and promoted Th2 cytokines in vitro.[43] One mechanism by which TNF-alpha causes inflammation is by potently inducing the expression of adhesion molecules such as VCAM-1 (vascular cell adhesion molecule 1). This was completely prevented by Boswellia extract in vitro for isolated human microvascular endothelial cells.[44]

Boswellic acids were also found to inhibit another pro-inflammatory enzyme in vitro: human leukocyte elastase (HLE). The dual inhibition of both 5-lipoxygenase and HLE is apparently unique to these compounds.[45] They also possess anticomplementary activity in the classical and alternative complement pathways. A key enzyme of the classical complement pathway (C3-convertase) was inhibited.[46,47] (Complement is a blood-based enzymatic cascade that serves to amplify, or complement, other inflammatory processes in the body. It is particularly implicated in the inflammation that occurs in rheumatoid arthritis.)

Like HLE, cathepsin G (catG) is another serine protease found in neutrophil granules that may participate in the breakdown of ingested pathogens and other inflammatory responses. CatG inhibitors have potential in the treatment of inflammatory conditions such as asthma, emphysema, psoriasis and rheumatoid arthritis.[10] Boswellic acids exhibited a high and specific binding affinity for catG in vitro and potently suppressed the proteolytic activity of catG in a competitive and reversible manner.[48] Related serine proteases were significantly less sensitive in vitro, including HLE, or not affected at all. Boswellic acids inhibited chemoinvasion but not chemotaxis of challenged neutrophils in vitro and suppressed catG induced calcium mobilisation in human platelets in vitro. Oral administration of a defined Boswellia extract to 12 healthy volunteers (800 mg single dose) and to five patients with Crohn's disease (2400 mg/day) significantly lowered the catG activity of various blood samples.[11] This research represents an intriguing development in the understanding of the anti-inflammatory activity of Boswellia.

Anti-allergic activity

An extract of Boswellia containing 60% AKBA was evaluated for anti-allergic and mast cell stabilising activity using passive rat paw anaphylaxis and induced degranulation of mast cells as the experimental in vivo models.[49] The extract inhibited the anaphylaxis reaction in a dose-dependent manner at oral doses of 20, 40 and 80 mg/kg, but was not as strong as dexamethasone (0.27 mg/kg). Similarly, a dose-dependent inhibition of mast cell degranulation was observed at the above doses.

Anticancer activity

Boswellia extract and boswellic acids have shown anticancer activities in cell cultures, including inhibition of cell growth and DNA synthesis.[50,51] The induction of differentiation and apoptosis (possibly due to topoisomerase I inhibition) suggests that boswellic acids may be useful in the treatment of leukaemia.[52–54]

The ability of boswellic acids (such as boswellic acid acetate and AKBA) to induce in vitro apoptosis has been demonstrated in the following tumour cell lines: myeloid leukaemia cells,[55] metastatic melanoma and fibrosarcoma cells,[56] various leukaemia, haematological and brain tumour cell lines,[57] colon cancer cells,[58] liver cancer Hep G2 cells[59] and malignant glioma.[60] In addition AKBA was found to be cytotoxic towards meningioma cells in vitro.[61,62] A useful and extensive review of the anticancer activity of the boswellic acids is available,[63] as is a discussion of their molecular targets in this context.[64]

Topical application of Boswellia extract with the tumour promoter 12-O-tetradecanoylphorbol-13-acetate (TPA) inhibited the expected formation of skin tumours in mice.[65,66] Boswellic acids have also been shown to inhibit tumour growth in vivo using a rat brain tumour model (glioma), albeit at quite high doses (720 mg/kg boswellic acids).[67] The effect was dose dependent. In mice carrying prostate cancer cell tumours, systemic doses of AKBA inhibited tumour growth and triggered apoptosis in the absence of systemic toxicity.[68]

Other activity

Boswellia resin demonstrated lipid lowering activity in vivo.[69–71] It is interesting that another Ayurvedic remedy, the resin from a plant in the same family, *Commiphora mukul*, has demonstrated hypocholesterolaemic activity both in vivo and in clinical trials, although a recent trial has cast doubt on its clinical efficacy.[72]

Oral doses of AKBA (100 mg/kg) and nimesulide (2.42 mg/kg) for 15 days significantly reversed the age-induced deterioration of memory, cognitive performance and meta-function in mice.[73]

The 11-methylene analogue of 11-keto-boswellic acid (KBA), namely beta-boswellic acid, potently induced calcium mobilisation in platelets in vitro.[74] Pivotal protein kinases were activated, resulting in functional platelet responses such as thrombin generation, liberation of arachidonic acid and aggregation.

Pharmacokinetics

Boswellic acids have also been shown to cross the blood-brain barrier in rats.[75] Permeation studies of Boswellia extract in the in vitro Caco-2 model of intestinal absorption found poor permeability for AKBA and moderate absorption of KBA.[76] Most of these compounds were retained in the Caco-2 monolayer. In rat liver microsomes and hepatocytes, as well as in human liver microsomes, KBA but not AKBA, underwent extensive phase I metabolism.[77] This was verified in vivo, where it was found that KBA undergoes extensive first-pass metabolism, whereas AKBA does not. Hence, metabolism (e.g. deacetylation) is not mainly responsible for the relatively low bioavailability of AKBA.

The human bioavailability of boswellic acids has been established in several pharmacokinetic studies. These indicate that beta-boswellic acid exhibits relatively better bioavailability than KBA and AKBA. Twelve healthy adult men were given capsules containing 333 mg of Boswellia extract after a 7-day washout period.[78] Venous blood samples, drawn at various times after administration of the herb, were analysed for KBA. A mean peak plasma level of 2.72±0.18 μM was reached at 4.50±0.55 h, with an elimination half-life of 5.97±0.95 h. These results suggested that Boswellia is best taken orally every 6 h and that this should achieve steady-state plasma levels after approximately 30 h.

In a randomised, open, single-dose, two-way crossover study, 12 healthy male volunteers received 786 mg of Boswellia extract either with or without a standard high-fat meal.[79] Plasma concentrations of boswellic acids were measured up to 60 h after oral dosing. Administration in conjunction with a high-fat meal led to a substantial improvement in the bioavailability of the boswellic acids. For example, the maximum concentration for AKBA and KBA respectively was 6.0 and 83.8 ng/mL for the fasted conditions versus 28.8 and 227 ng/mL with food. However, as might be expected, the time at which this and other maxima were reached was delayed by the meal. In contrast, a pilot study involving six healthy volunteers found an average concentration of KBA of 43 ng/mL 2 h after the administration of 500 mg of a Boswellia extract.[80] No relationship to meals was specified.

Steady-state concentrations of boswellic acids in the plasma of Crohn's disease patients receiving 2400 mg/day of a Boswellia extract were 6.35±1.0 μM for beta-boswellic acid, 0.33±0.1 μM for KBA and 0.04±0.01 μM for AKBA.[11]

As part of a method validation process, 10 different boswellic acids were found in the plasma of a brain tumour patient (glioblastoma multiforme) who took 3144 mg/day of Boswellia extract for 10 days.[81] The highest concentration was found for beta-boswellic acid at 10.1 μM.

Clinical trials

Arthritis

A significant improvement in symptoms was observed for 60 rheumatoid arthritis (RA) patients after receiving 6 to 8 weeks of treatment with boswellic acids in an open label study.[82] After reviewing the successful results of preclinical toxicology and efficacy studies, an uncontrolled clinical trial was undertaken at the orthopaedic department of Government Medical College, Jammu, India.[83,84] Results for 175 RA patients were 'excellent' for 14% and 'good' for 44%. Most patients taking Boswellia had some improvement in symptoms such as pain, stiffness and poor grip strength. Improvement occurred after 2 to 4 weeks of treatment.

In another uncontrolled study, Boswellia extract was given to 30 patients with RA.[85] The percentage of patients with detectable C-reactive protein was 63% initially, but this decreased to 47% after 6 months of treatment, a significant finding. This suggests that Boswellia may have a disease-modifying effect in RA.

The clinical efficacy of a herbomineral formulation containing *Withania somnifera*, *Boswellia serrata*, *Curcuma longa* (turmeric) and a zinc complex was evaluated in a randomised, double blind, placebo-controlled, crossover study in 42 patients with osteoarthritis.[86] The treatment period was 3 months, with a 15-day washout period before crossover and then another 3 months of treatment. Clinical efficacy was evaluated every fortnight on the basis of such findings as severity of pain, morning stiffness, joint score, disability score and grip strength. Treatment with the herbomineral formulation produced a significant drop in pain ($p<0.001$) and disability ($p<0.05$). However, X-ray assessment of joints did not show any significant changes.

The above herbomineral formulation was also evaluated in a randomised, double blind, placebo-controlled, cross-over trial of 20 RA patients for a period of 3 months. Significantly greater relief of pain, decreased morning stiffness, Ritchie Articular Index, joint score and erythrocyte sedimentation rate (ESR) were observed for those treated with the product. Seroconversion occurred for most of the treated patients, but radiological assessment did not show significant changes in either group.[87]

Etzel in 1996 reviewed 12 controlled clinical trials conducted in Germany or India (including those cited above) that assessed the effects of Boswellia in the treatment of RA.[88] Of these studies, only two were double blind, placebo-controlled trials, so results were difficult to interpret overall. However, summarising the results of different studies, Etzel suggested the following:

* There was a benefit from Boswellia treatment over placebo in patients suffering from RA for several years and in patients who responded poorly to conventional treatment.
* Boswellia was apparently as effective as gold therapy for RA.
* Some children suffering from chronic juvenile arthritis particularly benefited from Boswellia treatment.
* Tolerance was good and side effects were mild, such as diarrhoea and urticaria.

These positive outcomes contrast with a subsequent German study that found, under double blind, placebo-controlled conditions, that Boswellia was not more effective than placebo in patients with chronic polyarthritis (presumably mainly RA).[89] The authors of this study reserved their judgement, suggesting that a larger trial than the one they conducted was necessary to confirm or reject the use of Boswellia in RA sufferers, especially since the dropout rate in their trial was quite high.

An extract of Boswellia standardised to 40% boswellic acids by HPLC (high-performance liquid chromatography) yielded good results in the treatment of osteoarthritis.[90] A randomised, double blind, placebo-controlled, crossover study was conducted to assess the efficacy, safety and tolerability of the Boswellia extract (1000mg/day) in 30 patients with osteoarthritis of the knee, 15 each receiving active treatment or placebo for 8 weeks. After the first intervention, washout was given and then the groups were crossed over to receive the opposite intervention for 8 weeks. All patients receiving herbal treatment reported a significant decrease in knee pain, increased knee flexion and increased walking distance. The frequency of swelling in the knee joint was substantially decreased, but radiologically there was no change. Boswellia was well tolerated by the patients, except for minor gastrointestinal adverse reactions.

Since the boswellic acids were considered to be specific, non-redox inhibitors of 5-lipoxygenase and hence leukotriene biosynthesis, research attention as noted above had previously focused on the effects of Boswellia in inflammatory joint diseases such as RA. Despite this research focus on RA, herbal clinicians also favoured the use of Boswellia in osteoarthritis. The results of the above trial provided the first good evidence to support this application. What was striking about the trial was the substantial clinical benefit observed. Results were highly statistically significant ($p<0.001$) and changes in treatment parameters were quite large. For example, in the first 8-week treatment period before crossover, the pain index in the Boswellia group fell from 2.7 ± 0.45 to 0.26 ± 0.45, the loss of movement index was reduced from 2.8 ± 0.41 to 0.30 ± 0.48 and the swelling index went from 1.1 ± 0.91 to zero. The group receiving the placebo treatment after crossover showed substantial deterioration over the ensuing 8 weeks, suggesting that the 21-day washout period before crossover was insufficient. Although this is a flaw in the experimental design, it suggests a substantial residual therapeutic benefit after stopping Boswellia.

A prospective, randomised study conducted in India assessed the efficacy and tolerability of Boswellia extract in comparison to valdecoxib, a selective COX-2 inhibitor.[91] Sixty-six patients aged between 40 and 70 years with primary osteoarthritis of the knee, diagnosed according to the criteria of the American College of Rheumatology, were recruited. X-rays confirmed the diagnosis. Patients were assessed by the WOMAC scale at baseline and at monthly intervals until 1 month after discontinuation of 6 months' therapy. The WOMAC (Western Ontario and McMaster Universities Osteoarthritis Index) scale consists of questions based on the three symptoms (pain, stiffness and difficulty in performing daily activities), to which the patient assigns a number between 0 and 100. Patients received either 1000mg standardised Boswellia extract (containing 40% boswellic acids, which corresponded to a dose of 400mg/day of boswellic acids) or valdecoxib 10mg/day. There were 33 patients in each treatment group. During the trial patients were permitted to continue receiving physiotherapy and take a rescue medication (ibuprofen).

Results indicated that Boswellia extract was as effective as valdecoxib for knee osteoarthritis. In comparison with valdecoxib, Boswellia had a slower onset of action but the effect persisted after the discontinuation of therapy (unlike valdecoxib). The implications of this trial are that Boswellia is effective for knee osteoarthritis but needs to be taken for at least 2 months to establish the full clinical effect. Furthermore, the slow onset and slow washout of benefit suggests it could be disease modifying.

In a trial published in 2008, 75 patients with knee osteoarthritis received either Boswellia extract (containing 100 or 250 mg/day of an AKBA-enriched selective boswellic acid extract) or placebo for 90 days. Boswellia conferred a clinically and statistically significant dose-response improvement in pain and physical function scores. Symptom alleviation was faster in the higher dose Boswellia group (as early as 7 days) and a significant reduction in synovial fluid levels of matrix metalloproteinase-3 (a cartilage-degrading enzyme) was also observed for the Boswellia groups.[92]

A later study evaluated the activity of this AKBA-enriched selective boswellic acid extract at 100 mg/day against a similar extract with enhanced bioavailability (also at 100 mg/day) and a placebo in 60 patients with knee osteoarthritis.[93] A double blind, randomised, placebo-controlled design was used, with a trial period of 90 days. At the end of the study, both Boswellia extracts conferred clinically and statistically significant improvements in pain and physical function scores versus placebo (various p values). Significant improvements were recorded as early as 7 days for the enhanced bioavailability extract, which demonstrated better activity than the other extract. By 90 days, some clinical changes for the enhanced bioavailability extract were particularly marked. For example, the WOMAC pain subscale fell by 69% (p<0.0001 versus placebo) and the WOMAC stiffness subscale by 70.1% (p<0.0001 versus placebo) from baseline.

A formulation containing Withania, Boswellia, turmeric and ginger was shown to be effective in osteoarthritis in a double blind, randomised, placebo-controlled trial involving 99 patients.[94] Concurrent NSAIDs or analgesics were not permitted. Significant improvements were noted for pain (visual analogue scale) (p<0.05) and a modified WOMAC score (p<0.01) by the end of trial (32 weeks). There was no significant difference in type and number of adverse effects between active and placebo, although 28 patients did not complete the trial.

Ulcerative colitis

A group of Indian and German scientists conducted an open, non-randomised pilot study to test the hypothesis that Boswellia might be beneficial for the treatment of ulcerative colitis. For the study, 34 patients (18 with grade II and 16 with grade III colitis) were given 350 mg of Boswellia resin three times a day, and eight patients (five with grade II and three with grade III colitis) were given the drug sulfasalazine, 1 g three times a day. The authors commented that the cost of the drug was responsible for the small control group. Symptoms such as abdominal pain, loose stool, mucus and blood improved in both groups, with results for the control sulfasalazine group slightly better than the Boswellia group. Sigmoidoscopic examination for the grading of the disease and rectal biopsies both showed substantial improvements in the two treatment groups, and there was no statistically significant difference between them. About 80% of the patients receiving Boswellia went into remission. The authors concluded that, although they could not statistically confirm the superiority of Boswellia over sulfasalazine, the data suggest that it is at least not inferior.[95]

Twenty patients with chronic colitis received Boswellia gum resin (900 mg/day for 6 weeks) and another 10 patients were given sulfasalazine (3 g/day for 6 weeks) in an open label trial.[96] Out of 20 patients treated with Boswellia, 18 went into remission (90% compared with 60% for sulfasalazine).

Asthma

In a double blind, placebo-controlled clinical study, 80 patients with chronic asthma were treated with 900 mg/day of Boswellia, gum resin or placebo for 6 weeks.[97] Only 27% of patients in the control group showed improvement, whereas 70% of patients taking Boswellia improved. After taking Boswellia, positive changes were observed for shortness of breath, number of attacks and respiratory capacity as well as indicators of inflammation. Comparing the Boswellia group with the placebo group, there was a significant improvement in forced expiratory volume (in 1 second), a measure of bronchial obstruction (p=0.0001). Peak expiratory flow rate, a measure of lung capacity, was also significantly increased (p=0.0001). The number of asthma attacks was lower in the Boswellia group (p=0.0001). Additionally, Boswellia treatment showed substantial improvements (compared with placebo) in secondary outcome parameters such as rhonchi, eosinophil count, ESR and respiratory rate (p<0.05). Two patients who received Boswellia complained of epigastric pain and nausea.

It should not be assumed that inhibition of leukotrienes is the only mechanism by which Boswellia might provide beneficial effects for asthma, especially given the antiallergic activity from experimental models.

Crohn's disease

The safety and efficacy of a Boswellia extract was compared against mesalazine for the treatment of 102 patients with active Crohn's disease in an 8-week randomised, double blind European study.[98] The primary clinical outcome measured was the change in Crohn's Disease Activity Index (CDAI). After therapy with Boswellia extract (3.6 g/day) the average CDAI was reduced by 90, compared with a reduction of 53 for the mesalazine group (4.5 g/day). The authors concluded that the Boswellia extract was as effective as mesalazine, which is the current anti-inflammatory treatment for this disorder. Considering the observed fewer side effects and better safety profile of Boswellia, they suggested that this novel herbal treatment appears to be superior to mesalazine in terms of a risk-benefit evaluation.

In contrast, a 52-week double blind, placebo-controlled randomised trial in 108 patients with Crohn's disease found 2400 mg/day of a Boswellia extract was not superior to placebo in terms of maintaining remission.[99] However, only 66 patients completed the trial due to early termination and the extract did not seem to deliver high plasma levels of boswellic acids relative to other studies (see under Pharmacokinetics).[11] Boswellia treatment was well tolerated.

Brain tumours

Malignant brain tumours produce highly active forms of leukotrienes and this causes localised fluid build-up in the brain around the tumour, which damages healthy nerve cells. Twelve patients with malignant glioma, a type of brain tumour, were given 3600 mg/day of Boswellia extract (standardised to 60% boswellic acids) for 7 days prior to surgery.[100] Ten patients showed a decrease in fluid around the tumour, with an average reduction of 30% in eight of the 12 patients. Signs of brain damage decreased during the treatment; one patient became worse. Vomiting as a side effect was observed in one patient. This resulted in the European Commission declaring Boswellia as an orphan drug (a drug with no sponsors to fund the registration process) for the treatment of oedema resulting from brain tumours.[75]

Nineteen children and adolescents with intracranial tumours received palliative therapy with Boswellia extract at a maximum dose of 126 mg/kg/day for up to 26 months.[101] All patients were previously treated with conventional therapy. An anti-oedematous effect was demonstrated by MRI in one patient. Five of the 19 children reported an improvement of general health (perhaps a placebo effect). Some objective improvement, sometimes transient, was observed in seven patients.

Twelve patients with brain tumours and progressive oedema caused by either the tumour or treatment were given 3600 mg/day Boswellia extract for 4 weeks.[102] Oedema was reduced in five patients. Of five patients with treatment-related leukoencephalopathy, the clinical improvement following Boswellia was sustained for several months.

Forty-four patients with primary or secondary malignant cerebral tumours were randomly assigned to radiotherapy plus either 4200 mg/day Boswellia extract or placebo in a double blind trial.[103] Compared with baseline and measured immediately after the end of radiotherapy, a greater than 75% reduction in cerebral oedema was observed in 60% of the patients receiving Boswellia versus 26% receiving placebo (p=0.023). The dexamethasone dose during radiotherapy did not significantly differ between groups. The tumour/oedema volume ratio decreased only in the Boswellia group, suggesting an antitumour effect in addition to the anti-oedema activity. However, progression-free survival did not differ between the groups. Nonetheless, the better tumour response to radiotherapy was an unexpected finding. Common adverse events associated with radiotherapy were similar in both groups, although gastrointestinal discomfort was probably higher in the Boswellia group. While boswellic acids could be detected in patients' serum, the level of AKBA was quite low and could not be detected. Compliance with the high dose of extract used was an issue.

Other conditions

Collagenous colitis is a form of microscopic colitis of unknown aetiology and pathogenesis. The main symptom is chronic watery diarrhoea with few or no endoscopic abnormalities. Patients (n=31) with proven collagenous colitis were randomised to receive either 400 mg of Boswellia extract three times daily or placebo for 6 weeks in a double blind, randomised placebo-controlled trial.[104] Clinical remission at the end of the trial was higher in the Boswellia group (64% versus 26% for protocol, p=0.04; 44% versus 27% intention-to-treat, p=0.25). The authors concluded that results were promising and larger trials are necessary to confirm any benefit from Boswellia for this disorder.

A multicentre veterinary clinical trial was conducted by 10 practising veterinarians in Switzerland involving 29 dogs with degenerative chronic joint and spinal osteoarthritis.[105] An extract of Boswellia was administered in food at a dose of 400 mg/10 kg/day over 6 weeks. A statistically significant reduction in signs such as intermittent lameness and stiff gait were reported after 6 weeks. In five dogs reversible brief episodes of diarrhoea and flatulence occurred, but only in one case was a relationship to the Boswellia treatment suspected.

Toxicology and other safety data

Toxicology

Toxicity studies have generally shown that boswellic acids possess very low acute toxicity and cause no adverse effects after chronic administration. The oral and intraperitoneal LD_{50} was greater than 2 g/kg in mice and rats. No significant changes were observed in general behaviour, or in clinical, haematological, biochemical and pathological data after chronic oral administration.[106] A Boswellia extract enriched with 30% AKBA exhibited an oral LD_{50} >5 g/kg in rats and was classified as non-irritant to the skin.[107] A subacute toxicity study of the same extract over 90 days at up to 2.5% of feed indicated no adverse effects. However, one study involving experimentally induced colitis in mice found hepatotoxic effects for a methanolic extract at 1% of feed for 21 days, which was also supported by in vitro data.[26]

Contraindications

None known.

Special warnings and precautions

Caution in patients with a known allergic tendency. This is based on the fact that other resinous herbs such as myrrh are known to cause various allergic reactions and that allergic reactions have been reported for Boswellia (see below).

Interactions

No interactions have been reported in the literature.

Extracts of the oleo-gum, resin of Boswellia carterii, Boswellia frereana, Boswellia sacra and Boswellia serrata, were identified as equally potent, non-selective inhibitors of the major drug-metabolising CYP enzymes 1A2/2C8/2C9/2C19/2D6 and 3A4 in vitro.[108] Although the boswellic acids could be identified as moderate to potent inhibitors of the applied CYP enzymes, they were not the major CYP inhibitory principles. The clinical significance of these in vitro findings is uncertain.

Use in pregnancy and lactation

Category B1 – no increase in frequency of malformation or other harmful effects on the fetus from limited use in women. No evidence of increased fetal damage in animal studies.

Treatment of pregnant rats with a boswellic acid fraction (250 to 1000 mg/kg, oral route) revealed no significant effects on gestation period, litter size and weight of offspring at birth. No gross morphological or skeletal abnormalities were recorded. This generation of offspring in turn produced a normal number of normal offspring.[106]

Boswellia is likely to be compatible with breastfeeding.

Effects on ability to drive and use machines

No adverse effects are expected.

Side effects

Contact dermatitis has been caused by *Boswellia spp.*[109] Boswellia was well tolerated in clinical trials for the treatment of RA and Crohn's disease. Very mild side effects such as diarrhoea and urticaria were reported.[88]

Overdosage

No incidents found in the published literature.

Safety in children

No information available but adverse effects are not expected.

Regulatory status in selected countries

In the UK Boswellia is not included on the General Sale List and it was not included in the Commission E assessment in Germany.

Boswellia does not have GRAS status in the USA. However, it is freely available as a 'dietary supplement' in the USA under DSHEA legislation (Dietary Supplement Health and Education Act of 1994).

In Australia Boswellia is not included in Part 4 of Schedule 4 of the Therapeutic Goods Regulations and is freely available for sale.

References

1. Thakur RS, Puri HS, Husain A. *Major Medicinal Plants of India*. Lucknow: Central Institute of Medicinal and Aromatic Plants; 1989. p. 123.
2. Kapoor LD. CRC *Handbook of Ayurvedic Medicinal Plant*. Boca Raton: CRC Press; 1990. p. 83.
3. Bharatiya Vidya Bhavan's Swami Prakashananda Ayurveda Research Centre. *Selected Medicinal Plants of India*, Bombay, Chemexcil, 1992;67–68.
4. Mabberley DJ, ed. *The Plant Book*, 2nd ed. Cambridge: Cambridge University Press; 1997. pp. 99, 107.
5. Pardhy RS, Bhattacharyya SC. *Indian J Chem Sect B*. 1978;16(3):176–178.
6. Pardhy RS, Bhattacharyya SC. *Indian J Chem Sect B*. 1978;16(3):174–175.
7. Ammon HPT. *Eur J Med Res*. 1996;1(8):369–370.
8. Lawrence BM. Progress in essential oils. In: *Essential Oils 1992–1994*. Carol Stream: Allured Publishing Corporation; 1995. pp. 20–23.
9. Boden SE, Schweizer S, Bertsche T, et al. *Mol Pharmacol*. 2001;60(2):267–273.
10. Abdel-Tawab M, Werz O, Schubert-Zsilavecz M. *Clin Pharmacokinet*. 2011;50(6):349–369.
11. Ammon HP. *Phytomedicine*. 2010;17(11): 862–867.
12. Singh GB, Singh S, Bani S. *Phytomedicine*. 1996;3(1):81–85.
13. Sharma ML, Khajuria A, Kaul A, et al. *Agents Actions*. 1988;24(1–2):161–164.
14. Sharma ML, Bani S, Singh BG. *Int J Immunopharmacol*. 1989;11(6):647–652.
15. Kesava Reddy G, Dhar SC, Singh GB. *Agents Actions*. 1987;22(1–2):99–105.

16. Kesava Reddy G, Dhar SC, Singh GB. *Leather Sci*. 1986;33:192–199.
17. Kesava Reddy G, Dhar SC. *Ital J Biochem*. 1987;6(4):205–217.
18. Kesava Reddy G, Chandrakasan G, Dhar SC. *Biochem Pharmacol*. 1989;38(20):3527–3534.
19. Fan AY, Lao L, Zhang RX, et al. *J Altern Complement Med*. 2005;11(2):323–331.
20. Singh S, Khajuria A, Taneja SC, et al. *Phytomedicine*. 2008;15(6–7):400–407.
21. Sharma ML, Kaul A, Khajuria A, et al. *Phytother Res*. 1996;10(2):107–112.
22. Safayhi H, Mack T, Ammon HPT. *Biochem Pharmacol*. 1991;41(10):1536–1537.
23. Kar A, Menon MK. *Life Sci*. 1969;8(19):1023–1028.
24. Menon MK, Kar A. *Planta Med*. 1971;19(4):333–341.
25. Bishnoi M, Patil CS, Kumar A, et al. *Indian J Exp Biol*. 2006;44(2):128–132.
26. Kiela PR, Midura AJ, Kuscuoglu N, et al. *Am J Physiol Gastrointest Liver Physiol*. 2005;288(4):G798–G808.
27. Krieglstein CF, Anthoni C, Rijcken EJ, et al. *Int J Colorectal Dis*. 2001;16(2): 88–95.
28. Anthoni C, Laukoetter MG, Rijcken E, et al. *Am J Physiol Gastrointest Liver Physiol*. 2006;290(6):G1131–G1137.
29. Gupta OP, Sharma N, Chand D. *J Pharmacol Toxicol Methods*. 1994;31(2):95–98.
30. Singh S, Khajuria A, Taneja SC, et al. *Phytomedicine*. 2008;15(6–7):408–415.
31. Wildfeuer A, Neu IS, Safayhi H, et al. *Arzneimittelforschung*. 1998;48(6):668–674.
32. Ammon HP, Mack T, Singh GB, et al. *Planta Med*. 1991;57(3):203–207.

33. Siemoneit U, Hofmann B, Kather N, et al. *Biochem Pharmacol*. 2008;75(2):503–513.
34. Safayhi H, Mack T, Sabieraj J, et al. *J Pharmacol Exp Ther*. 1992;261(3): 1143–1146.
35. Safayhi H, Sailer ER, Ammon HP. *Mol Pharmacol*. 1995;47(6):1212–1216.
36. Schweizer S, von Brocke AF, Boden SE, et al. *J Nat Prod*. 2000;63(8):1058–1061.
37. Safayhi H, Boden SE, Schweizer S, et al. *Planta Med*. 2000;66(2):110–113.
38. Altmann A, Poeckel D, Fischer L, et al. *Br J Pharmacol*. 2004;141(2):223–232.
39. Altmann A, Fischer L, Schubert-Zsilavecz M, et al. *Biochem Biophys Res Commun*. 2002;290(1):185–190.
40. Siemoneit U, Pergola C, Jazzar B, et al. *Eur J Pharmacol*. 2009;606(1–3):246–254.
41. Ammon HP. *Planta Med*. 2006;72(12):1100–1116.
42. Syrovets T, Buchele B, Krauss C, et al. *J Immunol*. 2005;274(1):498–506.
43. Chevrier MR, Ryan AE, Lee DY, et al. *Clin Diagn Lab Immunol*. 2005;12(5):575–580.
44. Roy S, Khanna S, Shah H, et al. *DNA Cell Biol*. 2005;24(4):244–255.
45. Safayhi H, Rall B, Sailer ER, et al. *J Pharmacol Exp Ther*. 1997;281(1): 460–463.
46. Kapil A, Moza N. *Int J Immunopharmacol*. 1992;14(7):1139–1143.
47. Knaus U, Wagner H. *Phytomedicine*. 1996;3(1):77–81.
48. Tausch L, Henkel A, Siemoneit U, et al. *J Immunol*. 2009;183(5):3433–3442.
49. Pungle P, Banavalikar M, Suthar A, et al. *Indian J Exp Biol*. 2003;41(12): 1460–1462.
50. Han R. *Stem Cells*. 1994;12(1):53–63.

51. Huang M-T, Shao Y, Ma W, et al. *Proc Ann Meet Am Assoc Cancer Res.* 1997;38:A2465.

52. Jing Y, Nakajo S, Xia L, et al. *Leuk Res.* 1999;23(1):43–50.

53. Hoernlein RF, Orlikowsky T, Zehrer C, et al. *J Pharmacol Exp Ther.* 1999;288(2):613–619.

54. Syrovets T, Buchele B, Gedig E, et al. *Mol Pharmacol.* 2000;58(1):71–81.

55. Xia L, Chen D, Han R, et al. *Mol Cancer Ther.* 2005;4(3):381–388.

56. Zhao W, Entschladen F, Liu H, et al. *Cancer Detect Prev.* 2003;27(1):67–75.

57. Hostanska K, Daum G, Saller R. *Anticancer Res.* 2002;22(5):2853–2862.

58. Liu JJ, Nilsson A, Oredsson S, et al. *Carcinogenesis.* 2002;23(12):2087–2093.

59. Liu JJ, Nilsson A, Oredsson S, et al. *Int J Mol Med.* 2002;10(4):501–505.

60. Glaser T, Winter S, Groscurth P, et al. *Br J Cancer.* 1999;80(5–6):756–765.

61. Park YS, Lee JH, Harwalkar JA, et al. *Adv Exp Med Biol.* 2002;507:387–393.

62. Park YS, Lee JH, Bondar J, et al. *Planta Med.* 2002;68(5):397–401.

63. Shah BA, Qazi GN, Taneja SC. *Nat Prod Rep.* 2009;26(1):72–89.

64. Poeckel D, Werz O. *Curr Med Chem.* 2006;13(28):3359–3369.

65. Huang M-T, Badmaev V, Xie J-G, et al. *Proc Ann Meet Am Assoc Cancer Res.* 1997;8:A2464.

66. Huang MT, Badmaev V, Ding Y, et al. *Biofactors.* 2000;13(1–4):225–230.

67. Winking M, Sarikaya S, Rahmanian A, et al. *J Neurooncol.* 2000;46(2):97–103.

68. Syrovets T, Gschwend JE, Buchele B, et al. *J Biol Chem.* 2005;280(7):6170–6180.

69. Zutshi U, Rao PG, Kaur S, et al. *Indian J Pharmacol.* 1986;18(3):182–183.

70. Singh GB, Singh S. *J Molec Cell Cardiol.* 1994;25(suppl 3):188.

71. Pandey RS, Singh BK, Tripathi YB. *Indian J Exp Biol.* 2005;43(6):509–516.

72. Szapary PO, Wolfe ML, Bloedon LT, et al. *JAMA.* 2003;290(6):765–772.

73. Bishnoi M, Patil CS, Kumar A, et al. *Methods Find Exp Clin Pharmacol.* 2005;27(7):465–470.

74. Poeckel D, Tausch L, Altmann A, et al. *Br J Pharmacol.* 2005;146(4):514–524.

75. Reising K, Meins J, Bastian B, et al. *Anal Chem.* 2005;77(20):6640–6645.

76. Krüger P, Kanzer J, Hummel J, et al. *Eur J Pharm Sci.* 2009;36(2–3):275–284.

77. Krüger P, Daneshfar R, Eckert GP, et al. *Drug Metab Dispos.* 2008;36(6):1135–1142.

78. Sharma S, Thawani V, Hingorani L, et al. *Phytomedicine.* 2004;11(2–3):255–260.

79. Sterk V, Buchele B, Simmet T. *Planta Med.* 2004;70(12):1155–1160.

80. Shah SA, Rathod IS, Suhagia BN, et al. *J Chromatogr B.* 2007;848(2):232–238.

81. Büchele B, Simmet T. *J Chromatogr B.* 2003;795(2):pp. 355–362.

82. Singh, Hardayal, Singh GP, et al. Abstract presented at International Conference on Clinical Pharmacology and Therapeutics, Bombay: 1987; pp. 20–22.

83. Proceedings of the Symposium of Recent Advances in Mediators of Inflammation and Anti-Inflammatory Agents. Jammu: Council of Scientific and Industrial Research, Regional Research Laboratory; 1984.

84. Gupta VN, Yadav DS, Jain MP, et al. *Indian Drugs.* 1987;24(5):221–231.

85. Eleventh European Congress of Rheumatology. 1987; 5 (supplement issue):175.

86. Kulkarni RR, Patki PS, Jog VP, et al. *J Ethnopharmacol.* 1991;33(1–2):91–95.

87. Kulkarni RR, Patki PS, Jog VP, et al. *Indian J Pharmacol.* 1992;24(2):98–101.

88. Etzel R. *Phytomed.* 1996;3(1):91–94.

89. Sander O, Herborn G, Rau R. *Z Rheumatol.* 1998;57(1):11–16.

90. Kimmatkar N, Thawani V, Hingorani L, et al. *Phytomedicine.* 2003;10(1):3–7.

91. Sontakke S, Thawani V, Pimpalkhute S, et al. *Indian J Pharmacology.* 2007;39(1):27–29.

92. Sengupta K, Alluri KV, Satish AR, et al. *Arthritis Res Ther.* 2008;10:R85.

93. Sengupta K, Krishnaraju AV, Vishal AA, et al. *Int J Med Sci.* 2010;7(6):366–377.

94. Chopra A, Lavin P, Patwardhan B, et al. *J Clin Rheumatol.* 2004;10(5):236–245.

95. Gupta I, Parihar A, Malhotra P, et al. *Eur J Med Res.* 1997;2(1):37–43.

96. Gupta I, Parihar A, Malhotra P, et al. *Planta Med.* 2001;67(5):391–395.

97. Gupta I, Gupta V, Parihar A, et al. *Eur J Med Res.* 1998;3(11):511–514.

98. Gerhardt H, Seifert F, Buvari P, et al. *Z Phytother.* 2001;22:69–75.

99. Holtmeier W, Zeuzem S, Preiss J, et al. *Inflamm Bowel Dis.* 2011;17(2):573–582.

100. Winking M, Boeker DK, Simmet TH. *J Neurooncol.* 1996;30(2):P39.

101. Janssen G, Bode U, Breu H, et al. *Klin Padiatr.* 2000;212(4):189–195.

102. Streffer JR, Bitzer M, Schabet M, et al. *Neurology.* 2001;56(9):1219–1221.

103. Kirste S, Treier M, Wehrle SJ, et al. *Cancer.* 2011;117(16):3788–3795.

104. Madisch A, Miehlke S, Eichele O, et al. *Int J Colorectal Dis.* 2007;22(12):1445–1451.

105. Reichling J, Schmokel H, Fitzi J, et al. *Schweiz Arch Tierheilkd.* 2004;146(2):71–79.

106. Singh GB, Bani S, Singh S. *Phytomedicine.* 1996;3(1):87–90.

107. Lalithakumari K, Krishnaraju A, Sengupta K, et al. *Toxicol Mech Methods.* 2006;16(4):199–226.

108. Frank A, Unger M. *J Chromatogr A.* 2005;1112(1–2):255–262.

109. Mitchell J, Rook A. *Botanical Dermatology: Plants and Plant Products Injurious to the Skin.* Vancouver: Greengrass; 1979. pp. 144–145.

Buchu

(*Agathosma betulina* (Bergius) Pill.)

Synonyms

Barosma betulina (Bergius) Bartl. et Wendl. (botanical synonym), bucco (Engl), Barosmae folium (Lat), Bukkostrauch, Buccoblätter (Ger), buchu (Fr), diosma (Ital), bukko (Dan).

What is it?

Buchu is a South African herb extensively employed as a urinary antiseptic and may also be used in laxative and carminative formulas. The Hottentots use buchu leaves to perfume their bodies. (The Agathosma genus is native to South Africa, especially the southwest Cape region.) The essential oil is a component of artificial fruit flavours, especially blackcurrant, and it may be found in trace amounts in a wide variety of food products and beverages.

The leaves are the part most commonly used for therapeutic purposes and should be harvested whilst the plant is flowering and fruiting. They possess a strongly aromatic taste and a curious blackcurrant-peppermint-like odour.

Effects

Disinfects the urinary tract and acts as a mild diuretic.

Traditional view

Buchu was used to treat gravel, inflammation and catarrh of the bladder.[1] According to the Eclectics, buchu is an aromatic stimulant and tonic that promotes the appetite, relieves nausea and flatulence, and acts as a diuretic and diaphoretic. Its principal use was in the treatment of chronic diseases of the genitourinary tract including chronic inflammation of the mucous membranes of the bladder, irritable conditions of the urethra, for urinary discharges (particularly mucopurulent discharges), abnormally acidic urine with a constant desire to urinate and little relief from micturition, and incontinence associated with a diseased prostate.[2]

Summary actions

Urinary antiseptic, mild diuretic.

Can be used for

Traditional therapeutic uses

Urinary tract infection, dysuria, cystitis, urethritis and prostatitis.

May also be used for

Other applications

Buchu may be included as an aroma or taste enhancer in herbal tea mixtures.[3]

Preparations

Dried leaf as a decoction, liquid extract, tincture, tablets or capsules for internal use. As with all essential oil-containing herbs, use of the fresh plant or carefully dried herb is advised. Keep covered if infusing the herb to retain the essential oil.

Dosage

* 3 to 6 g/day of the dried leaf or as an infusion
* 2 to 4 mL/day of 1:2 liquid extract, 5 to 10 mL/day of 1:5 tincture.

Duration of use

May be taken long term for most applications.

Summary assessment of safety

May occasionally cause gastrointestinal irritation if taken on an empty stomach. Other species of Agathosma contain high levels of pulegone and are contraindicated in pregnancy.

Technical data

Botany

Agathosma betulina, a member of the Rutaceae (citrus) family, is a low shrub that can grow to a height of 2 m. The leaves are rhomboid-obovate in shape, 12 to 20 mm long and 4 to 25 mm broad, with a blunt and recurved apex. Numerous small oil glands are scattered throughout the lamina and large oil glands are situated at the base of each marginal indentation and at the apex. The flowers have five whitish petals and the brown fruits contain five carpels.[4] The leaves become brittle and coriaceous when dried and when moistened become mucilaginous.[4] They have a spicy odour and a pungent and spicy taste.[5]

Adulteration

The Khoi-San (a native South African tribe) name 'buchu' is applied to any aromatic herb or shrub that they find suitable for use as a dusting powder. Hence many species, including those not in the Agathosma genus, are recorded as buchu. The genus Diosma is often referred to as wild buchu, but was only used in cases where true buchu (Agathosma) was unprocurable.[6]

Adulterants include: *Agathosma crenulata*, *A. serratifolia*, *A. ericifolia*, *Adenandra fragrans*,[7] *Empleurum serrulatum*, *Psoralea olbiqua* and *Myrtus communis*.[8] Other species also traded as medicinal buchu have included *Diosma oppositifolia* (*Diosma succulentum*), *Agathosma pulchella*, *Empleurum unicapsulare* (*Empleurum ensatum*) and the so-called anise buchu (possibly *A. variabilis*).[9]

Although *A. crenulata* has been used traditionally as true buchu, it is not suitable for therapeutic use due to the lower diosphenol and higher pulegone and isopulegone contents of the essential oil.[10,11]

The preferred medicinal buchu (*Agathosma betulina*) may be distinguished from *A. crenulata* and *A. serratifolia* by the ratio of leaf length to leaf width.[7] This distinction does not hold for buchu hybrids (considerable hybridisation has taken place between *A. betulina* and *A. crenulata*), where chemical analysis of the essential oil is required.[12] Use of buchu hybrids is not generally acceptable, since the level of pulegone in the essential oil varies enormously.[13]

From chemotaxonomic studies, two chemotypes of *A. betulina* have been identified[11]:

* Diosphenol chemotype: high concentration of diosphenol (total diosphenol isomers ≥22%), low isomenthone content (<29%)
* Isomenthone chemotype: high concentration of isomenthone (>31%), low diosphenol content (total diosphenol isomers ≤0.3 %).

No chemotypes of *A. crenulata* have been found. The diosphenol chemotype is probably preferable for therapeutic use.

Key constituents

* Essential oil (2%), consisting mainly of the monoterpene diosphenol. Other components include: limonene, (−)-isomenthone, (+)-menthone, (−)-pulegone, terpinen-4-ol and the sulphur-containing p-menthan-3-on-8-thiol, which is responsible for the blackcurrant flavour[5]
* Flavonoids, especially diosmin and rutin.[14]

As noted under Adulteration, other species such as *Agathosma crenulata* are not suitable for medicinal use due to the lower diosphenol and higher pulegone contents in their essential oils.[10]

Diosmin

(−)-Pulegone   Diosphenol

Pharmacodynamics

Antimicrobial activity

An early in vitro study demonstrated some activity for the alcoholic extract of buchu against microflora typical of urinary tract infections.[15] However, only the essential oil showed considerable activity against all the test organisms.

More recently poor or absent antimicrobial activity was observed for buchu essential oil against five different microorganisms using the zone of inhibition technique.[16] This finding was somewhat supported by a later study that found only moderate activity, with minimum inhibitory concentrations (MIC) for the oil varying from 4 to 32 mg/mL (depending on the microorganism tested for *Bacillus cereus*, *Staphylococcus aureus*, *Klebsiella pneumoniae* and *Candida albicans*), as determined by a microtitre plate dilution method.[17] In fact, the methanol:dichloromethane (1:1) extract of buchu leaf was more active than its hydrodistilled essential oil in this test model (MIC range against the same organisms 2 to 4 mg/mL).[18]

In an attempt to better reflect in vivo activity, extracts of buchu were treated with simulated gastric and intestinal fluids. The water extract showed a doubling of antimicrobial activity after it was subjected to simulated intestinal conditions. Intestinal transport simulation using the Caco-2 cell monolayer revealed good bioavailability for the compounds present in this extract.[19,20]

Other activity

At a high concentration buchu essential oil had an initial spasmogenic action on isolated guinea pig ileum, followed by spasmolysis. Cyclic AMP generation and the blocking of calcium channels were suggested as possible mechanisms for the spasmolytic activity, based on the experimental probes used.[16]

A relatively strong inhibition of 5-lipoxygenase was observed in vitro for the essential oil (IC$_{50}$=50.4 μg/mL), but not the methanol:dichloromethane (1:1) extract.[17,20]

Pharmacokinetics

No human or animal data available. See above under Antimicrobial activity for limited in vitro information.

Clinical trials

No clinical studies on the urinary antiseptic and diuretic effects traditionally attributed to buchu are available.

Unpublished results from a double blind, placebo-controlled clinical trial involving 30 healthy male volunteers found that a buchu oil gel applied three times daily reduced swelling following exercise-induced muscle damage.[20]

Toxicology and other safety data

Toxicology

There are no reports of cases of poisoning and only in vitro toxicology data are available. Here the toxicities of buchu essential oil and extract were evaluated using the MTT (3-(4,5-dimethylthiazol-2-yl)-2,5-diphenyltetrazolium bromide) cellular viability assay in Graham cells (transformed human kidney epithelial cells).[17,18,20] While the extract demonstrated no toxicity at the concentrations tested ($IC_{50}>100\,\mu g/mL$), the oil was highly active in disrupting the viability of test cells.

Contraindications

None required on current evidence.

Special warnings and precautions

Best not used during lactation without professional advice.

Interactions

No precautions required on current evidence.

Use in pregnancy and lactation

Category B2 – no increase in frequency of malformation or other harmful effects on the fetus from limited use in women. Animal studies are lacking.

The British Herbal Compendium 1992 suggests that buchu is contraindicated in pregnancy.[14] However, this would only be the case for buchu substitutions (such as A. crenulata) that contain much higher levels of pulegone in their essential oil (see above).

Buchu is compatible with breastfeeding but caution should be exercised as it contains an essential oil that may pass into breast milk. As the therapeutic effects provided by buchu are rarely required in infants, its effects in this patient group are unknown, but probably benign.

Effects on ability to drive and use machines

None known.

Side effects

Occasional gastrointestinal intolerance and irritation if taken on an empty stomach.[14]

Overdosage

No reports of poisoning occur in published literature.[9]

Safety in children

No information available, but adverse effects are not expected.

Regulatory status in selected countries

Buchu is covered by a null Commission E monograph. It is on the UK General Sale List.

Buchu does not have GRAS status. However, it is freely available as a 'dietary supplement' in the USA under DSHEA legislation (1994 Dietary Supplement Health and Education Act). Buchu has been present as an ingredient in OTC weight control drug products and orally administered menstrual drug products. The FDA, however, advises that: 'based on evidence currently available, there is inadequate data to establish general recognition of the safety and effectiveness of these ingredients for the specified uses'.

Buchu is not included in Part 4 of Schedule 4 of the Therapeutic Goods Act Regulations of Australia and is freely available for sale.

References

1. Grieve M. A Modern Herbal, Vol 1. New York: Dover Publications; 1971. pp. 133–134.
2. Felter HW, Lloyd JU. King's American Dispensatory, 18th ed. 3rd rev, Vol 1. 1905, Portland: Reprinted by Eclectic Medical Publications; 1983. pp. 891–892.
3. German Federal Minister of Justice. German Commission E for Human Medicine Monograph, Bundes-Anzeiger (German Federal Gazette), No. 22a, dated 01.02.1990.
4. Evans WC. Trease and Evans' Pharmacognosy, 14th ed. London: WB Saunders; 1996. p. 272.
5. Bisset NG, ed. Herbal Drugs and Phytopharmaceuticals. Stuttgart: Medpharm Scientific Publishers; 1994. pp. 102–103.
6. Watt JM, Breyer-Brandwijk MG. The Medicinal and Poisonous Plants of Southern and Eastern Africa: Being an Account of Their Medicinal and Other Uses, Chemical Composition, Pharmacological Effects and Toxicology in Man and Animal, 2nd ed. Edinburgh: Livingstone; 1962. pp. 909–910.
7. Spreeth AD. J S Afr Bot. 1976;42(2):109–119.
8. Anonymous. Flavour Ind. 1970;1(6): 379–382.
9. Blaschek W, Ebel S, Hackenthal E, et al. HagerROM 2002: Hagers Handbuch der Drogen und Arzneistoffe. Heidelberg: Springer; 2002.
10. Kaiser R, Lamparsky D, Schudel P. J Agric Food Chem. 1975;23(5):943–950.

11. Collins NF, Graven EH, van Beek TA, et al. *J Essent Oil Res*. 1996;8(3):229–235.

12. Blommaert KLJ, Bartel E. *J South Afr Bot*. 1976;42(2):121–126.

13. Mills S, Bone K, eds. *The Essential Guide to Herbal Safety*. St Louis: Elsevier Churchill Livingstone; 2005. p. 296.

14. British Herbal Medicine Association. *British Herbal Compendium*, Vol 1. Bournemouth: BHMA; 1992. pp. 43–45.

15. Didry N, Pinkas M. *Plantes Med Phytother*. 1982;16(4):249–252.

16. Lis-Balchin M, Hart S, Simpson E. *J Pharm Pharmacol*. 2001;53:579–582.

17. Viljoen AM, Moolla A, van Vuuren SF, et al. *J Essent Oil Res*. 2006;18(suppl):2–16.

18. Moolla A, van Vuuren SF, van Zyl RL, et al. *South Afr J Bot*. 2007;73:588–592.

19. Viljoen AM, Vermaak I, Hamman J, et al. *South Afr J Bot*. 2007;73:319–320.

20. Moolla A, Viljoen AM. *J Ethnopharmacol*. 2008;119(3):413–419.

Bugleweed and European bugleweed

(*Lycopus virginicus* L., *Lycopus europaeus* L.)

Synonyms

Lycopus europaeus: gipsywort, bitter bugle, gypsy herb, marsh horehound. *Lycopus virginicus*: Virginia bugleweed, sweet bugleweed, Virginia horehound.

What is it?

Two main species of Lycopus are used therapeutically. Bugleweed (*L. virginicus*) is a native of the eastern United States and European bugleweed (*L. europaeus*) is one of the two European species.[1] The traditional uses of hyperthyroidism and heart palpitations were given some scientific support by experiments in the 1940s and 1950s that found influences on dampening thyroid function. Since then there have been several studies investigating the mode of action and active constituents. While these investigations have been informative, the relevance of their findings is hampered by the dominance of in vitro studies and animal models where the herb was administered by injection. Also lacking at present are properly designed and conducted clinical trials. Hence, despite the scientific interest and theoretically plausible mechanisms, the rationale for the use of this herb still largely rests on traditional treatises, both from the United States and Europe, with a positive Commission E monograph.

Effects

May interfere with the effects of thyroid stimulating hormone (TSH) leading to reduced thyroxine production by the thyroid; alleviates palpitations and tachycardia caused by an overactive thyroid; possible inhibition of female fertility.

Traditional view

Traditional uses, especially for *L. virginicus*, included nervous tachycardia, Graves' disease with cardiac involvement, thyrotoxicosis with difficult breathing, tachycardia and tremor[2] and exophthalmic goitre.[3] It was also recommended for organic and functional cardiac disease, abnormally active circulation and rapid pulse with high temperature.[3] Other clinical uses included chronic cough, irritating and wet cough, pneumonia, bronchitis,[2,3] restlessness, insomnia and anxiety.[3]

Bugleweed, particularly *L. europaeus*, is considered in European herbal medicine to have antithyroid activity.[4] Being less powerful than conventional drugs, it is recommended for mild thyroid hyperfunction and can be used as a long-term treatment.[5]

Summary actions

TSH antagonist, antithyroid, mild sedative, possible antigonadotropic agent.

Can be used for

Indications supported by clinical trials

Hyperthyroidism, especially Graves' disease and associated symptoms such as tachycardia and rapid pulse (open label trials, weak evidence). 'Vegetative dystonia' which is essentially anxiety characterised by cardiac and digestive symptoms (open label trials, weak evidence).

Traditional therapeutic uses

Hyperthyroidism as above, but especially with cardiac involvement; also for restlessness, insomnia and anxiety.

Preparations

Dried herb for an infusion, tincture or liquid extract for internal use.

Dosage

- 3 to 9 g/day of dried aerial parts or by infusion
- 2 to 6 mL/day of a 1:2 liquid extract or equivalent in tablet or capsule form
- 6 to 18 mL/day of a 1:5 tincture.

Duration of use

May be taken long-term, but only if appropriate.

Summary assessment of safety

Contraindicated in pregnancy and lactation and in patients with an underactive thyroid. Do not administer with thyroid hormone preparations or during the application of thyroid diagnostic procedures using radioactive isotopes.

Technical data

Botany

L. europaeus is a perennial herb spreading by branching stolons. The quadrangular, pubescent stems are erect, simple or branched, 30 to 100 cm tall. Leaves are opposite, short-petioled and ovate-lanceolate to elliptic, up to 12 cm long; the lower leaves are pinnate, the upper leaves crenate. Flowers are about 4 mm long, white with purple dots and grow in dense whorls at the base of the uppermost leaves.[1,6]

L. virginicus is a perennial, 15 to 60 cm tall. Stems are quadrangular, erect and pubescent, producing stolons at the base. The leaves are opposite, ovate or oblong-lanceolate, coarsely serrate but entire near the base, 2 to 5 cm long. Flowers are small, purplish, growing in axillary whorls, with a mint-like odour.

Adulteration

Leonurus marrubiastrum L. may be mistaken for *L. europaeus*, especially when wildcrafted.[7]

Key constituents

L. virginicus and *L. europaeus* aerial parts contain flavonoids and phenolic acids, such as derivatives of cinnamic acid (including caffeic acid), although the pattern varies in each plant.[8–10]

Pharmacodynamics

Antithyroid and antigonadotropic activities

It is probably most useful to review the pharmacological research into the antihormonal activity of Lycopus in an approximate chronological order, as there is certainly an aspect of unfolding discovery to the story.

Madaus, Cook and Albus in 1941 were able to show in experimental investigations that the effects of *L. europaeus* and *L. virginicus* L. were similar.[11] Lycopus countered the typical weight decrease and tachycardia from thyroxine in the rabbit in an acute model. Results from another model also suggested a direct thyroxine antagonism: thyroxine antagonises the temperature fall induced by novocaine injection in the guinea pig and this effect was cancelled by Lycopus administration. Thyroxine causes an increased oxygen requirement as a result of increased metabolism and Lycopus countered this effect in rats. Next to this direct antithyroxine effect, the authors also showed effects on TSH activity. After repeated injection of TSH, oxygen consumption in the guinea pig increased by around 25%. Simultaneous administration of Lycopus extract reduced this to about 10%, but only at the highest dosage.[12]

Pharmacodynamic research on Lycopus began in earnest in the early 1960s when Kemper and co-workers found that an aqueous extract of *L. virginicus* inhibited the actions of gonadotropic hormones and TSH in vivo (based on organ

weights) after administration by injection to guinea pigs and rats.[13,14] However, a preparation of *L. europaeus* had no influence on thyroid metabolism in rats after oral doses, as assessed using radioactive iodine.[15]

A paper published in 1970 claimed, on the basis of in vivo experiments using doses administered by injection, that an oxidised form of lithospermic acid was the antigonadotropic principle in *L. virginicus*.[16] However, it was the work of the late Dr Hilke Winterhoff and team that found a different basis for this and the antithyroid activity in a series of studies published from 1976 to recently. Lithospermic acid was shown to have little antihormonal activity compared to the freeze-dried extract of Lycopus.[17,18] This freeze-dried aqueous extract of Lycopus (species not specified) given alone by injection or with TSH to infant female rats led to a marked fall in circulating thyroid hormones.[19] When TRH and *L. virginicus* extract were co-administered (at different sites) by injection to rats, TSH levels were significantly lower after 10 minutes when compared to the TRH and saline controls.[20] As a result, thyroid hormone levels were suppressed and significantly lower 3 h later. Pretreatment of rats with dried extract for 4 days resulted in a drop in peripheral thyroid hormone levels.[20]

In the euthyroid rat, injections (50 mg/kg) of freeze-dried extracts of both *L. europaeus* and *L. virginicus* greatly reduced serum and pituitary TSH levels.[21] Effects were less clear in hypothyroid rats. Serum prolactin was also reduced by *L. virginicus* injection, but only at 400 mg/kg. *L. europaeus* injection (50 mg/kg) did significantly lower pituitary (but not serum) prolactin levels.

The active components suggested by Winterhoff and team as responsible for these effects were the oxidation products of phenolic compounds such as rosmarinic acid, which are abundant in *Lycopus* species.[22] These showed marked antigonadotropic activity in a rat model after injection. This line of research was further progressed by this group in collaboration with others, including several in vitro investigations conducted in the 1980s. The antigonadotropic activity of ether-extracted fractions of *L. virginicus* aqueous extracts was tested in a suitable model (details not specified).[23] Within the ether extracts, significant activity was only found after the addition of an oxidising agent (up to a 10-fold increase). This oxidised and active form was identified to contain oxidation products of rosmarinic acid. Freeze-dried aqueous extracts of *L. virginicus* and *L. europaeus* inhibited the binding of bovine TSH to human thyroid plasma membranes and inhibited the stimulation of adenylate cyclase.[24] Auto-oxidation products of the 3,4-dihydroxycinnamic acid derivatives (such as caffeic, rosmarinic, chlorogenic and ellagic acids) were also active in the same model.[25] It was suggested that these compounds form adducts with TSH, resulting in a greatly reduced or absent ability to bind to the TSH receptor.[26] In later research, rosmarinic acid and a freeze-dried aqueous extract of *L. virginicus* also inhibited forskolin-induced activation of adenylate cyclase in cultured rat thyroid cells.[27]

The impact of Lycopus on the peripheral conversion of T4 to T3 was investigated in vitro using iodothyronine deiodinases from rat liver microsomes.[28] Preparations of *L. virginicus*, especially the ether fraction of hot aqueous extracts, markedly inhibited the enzyme in a dose-dependent manner. Subsequent investigation found that the active principles exhibited chemical characteristics of phenolcarboxylic acids (e.g. rosmarinic acid). Curiously, oxidation of extracts with potassium permanganate decreased this activity.[29]

In all samples of Graves' immunoglobulin G (IgG) tested, incubation with *L. virginicus* or *L. europaeus* or their auto-oxidised constituents decreased the TSH-binding inhibitor activity in vitro. This was in a dose-dependent manner and with some degree of specificity.[30] The plant extracts and their auto-oxidised constituents also inhibited the biological responses to Graves' IgG in vitro.

The efficacy of injections of *L. virginicus* extracts for up to 3 days at inhibiting thyroid hormone levels and thyroid weight varied with the method of preparation.[31] Extraction with boiling water or ethanol yielded inactive extracts, whereas oxidation with potassium permanganate re-established activity. The reduction in prolactin levels observed in an earlier study was also confirmed (as assessed by assay 6 h after a single intravenous injection). It was shown in a subsequent study that several phenolic plant ingredients mentioned already, but additionally luteolin-7-beta-glucuronide,[32] confer antigonadotropic activity. However, their oxidation products are likely to be more active.[33] The suggestion that *L. europaeus* contains lithospermic acid was also refuted. Oligomeric (short polymers) oxidation products of caffeic acid (cyclolignan derivatives) with antigonadotropic activity were subsequently identified as likely active components.[34,35]

As well as the previously noted antagonism of TSH, results from a series of experiments suggested that injections of *L. europaeus* are capable of suppressing thyroid hormone secretion by a direct intrathyroidal attack.[36] Additional phenolic acids (including isoferulic acid and ferulic acid) as well as caffeic acid were active in this TSH-antagonism model.

One reservation that can be expressed about the above research is that most of the results have been generated using in vitro models or in vivo models following injection of the herbal extracts or relevant compounds. This was addressed by Winterhoff's team in a 1994 publication where a 70% ethanolic extract *L. europaeus* was administered by oral means to rats, albeit at quite high doses of 200 and/or 1000 mg/kg.[37] Diverse endocrine parameters were measured between 3 and 24 h after oral doses and compared with intraperitoneal doses (of *L. virginicus*). Oral application of the extract caused a long-lasting decrease in T3 levels, presumably due to reduced peripheral T4 deiodination. A pronounced reduction of T4 and TSH was observed, as well as LH (luteinising hormone), indicating a central action for the extract.

The impact of oral *L. europaeus* (2×5 mg or 2×200 mg/kg per day for up to 8 weeks of a dried aqueous-ethanolic extract) on cardiac symptoms in hyperthyroid rats was compared with the beta-blocking drug atenolol.[38] Even the lower dose of the herb countered the raised body temperature, whereas the reduced body weight and increased food intake was not influenced by any treatment. No significant changes in thyroid hormone levels or TSH were observed. Lycopus (in general both doses) and atenolol reduced the increased heart rate, blood pressure and heart size, but the drug was considerably more active with respect to heart rate. Interestingly,

Lycopus given to normal rats at 2×200 mg/kg per day had no impact on any of the above parameters. Collectively the above findings suggest that the herb only antagonises the **effects** of increased thyroid hormone levels, and does this without altering depressed TSH and elevated thyroxine levels, at least in the model used.

This work was subsequently extended in two publications using three rat models of differing severity of hyperthyroidism induced by differing applications of T4. Findings were similar to the above study in both publications, with Lycopus extract, extract fractions and powdered herb having almost the same potency as beta-blockers (atenolol and propranolol) in reducing body temperature.[39,40] The effects on beta-adrenoreceptor density, blood pressure and heart rate were less distinct, but still significant. In the later publication there was some suggestion that Lycopus powder had inhibited T4 to T3 conversion.[40] (Note that this result may have been more determined by the model used than the form of Lycopus, since the powder was only tested in one model of hyperthyroidism.)

Summarising the research to date, results from in vitro experiments or in vivo models with dosage by injection suggest that Lycopus extracts or its components at relatively high doses antagonised or reduced pituitary hormones (TSH, gonadotropins, prolactin), reduced thyroxine production, reduced peripheral conversion of T4 to T3 and antagonised the binding and effects of Graves' IgG. In terms of phytochemical components responsible for these effects, oligomeric oxidation products of phenolic acids such as caffeic acid were found to be most active. As a consequence, freshly prepared aqueous-ethanolic extracts were not found to be active, as they are devoid of such products. However, some of the above results (TSH, T4 and T3 reductions) were confirmed in an oral-dose model using high doses of a commercial aqueous-ethanolic extract. Perhaps this extract was active because phenolic acid oxidation products had formed in the time since its manufacture. More recently, animal models using realistic oral doses of a commercial aqueous-ethanolic extract have provided quite a different perspective. Here it was found that Lycopus could antagonise the cardiac effects of induced hyperthyroidism without any corresponding change in thyroid hormones or TSH. Lycopus given orally to normal rats at such doses had no impact on thyroid function. The phytochemical components responsible for the activities observed in these later experiments have not been explored to date.

Other activity

A methanolic extract of *L. europaeus* was one of the three most active of 122 traditional Chinese herbs screened for in vitro activity against xanthine oxidase (the enzyme that catalyses purine metabolites to uric acid) with an IC_{50} of 26 µg/mL.[41] Two new isopimarane diterpenes were isolated from *L. europaeus* that were capable of potentiating the in vitro activities of tetracycline and erythromycin against resistant strains of *Staphylococcus aureus* possessing multidrug efflux mechanisms.[42] Aqueous and methanolic extracts of *L. europaeus* showed high radical scavenger capacity compared to 17 other medicinal Labiatae species tested.[43]

Pharmacokinetics

No relevant data found.

Clinical trials

Early clinical studies were largely observational in nature and, while they could be construed to provide weak evidence by modern standards, some interesting and sometimes striking results were documented. The following brief review is not comprehensive, as many such studies were published in the 1950s and early 1960s. Throughout these and the later trials, the doses of Lycopus administered were quite low.

Mattausch reported in 1943 on the treatment of about 200 patients with mild hyperthyroidism. A decline in pulse frequency was observed and, following a longer treatment duration, also a normalisation of other symptoms.[44] A group of 50 patients with symptoms of hyperthyroidism, or 'vegetative dystonia' that with more exacting clinical investigation turned out to be latent hyperthyroidism, were treated with Lycopus.[45] The thyroid uptake of radioactive iodine was evaluated in 32 of these patients. This demonstrated an objective improvement in thyroid function in 15 cases; eight of the other 17 exhibited symptom improvement with no corresponding objective change. Overall for the 50 cases, pulse rates were normalised and insomnia was alleviated. Another study found reduced symptoms and pulse rate, and increased body weight in 53 hyperthyroid patients treated with Lycopus.[46]

One hundred patients with severe hyperthyroidism were treated with Lycopus prior to surgery, rather than with Lugol's solution.[47] The appearance of the gland in the operation field showed relatively less vascularisation, and postoperative reactions were notably mild.

As alluded to above, Lycopus has been used to treat 'vegetative dystonia', a disturbance of autonomic nervous system function. In a series of 123 cases this disturbance was attributed to elevated thyroid function.[48] Patients were treated with a commercial Lycopus tincture (12 drops twice a day). After 14 days, the pulse rate had dropped by an average of 11%. Based on subjective symptoms there was a clear improvement in 83 patients after 14 days, which by 28 days had increased to 102 patients. Symptoms such as dermographism, tremor, hair loss and sweating were improved. A significant weight gain was also observed.

In a more recent observational study of 43 patients (21 with latent hyperthyroidism and 22 with 'vegetative dystonia'), Lycopus dried extract (10 mg/day equivalent to 40 mg of herb) was given for 21 days.[49] Of the 34 patients with cardiac symptoms, 27 reported improvement in palpitations and/or benign arrhythmias. However, thyroid parameters were unchanged, including in another 20 healthy volunteers who received the herbal treatment.

A controlled, open study examined the effect of 40 mg/day L. europaeus extract on thyroid function and associated symptoms in 62 patients with hyperthyroidism of unspecified causes.[50] The study population consisted of patients with a TSH <1.0 mU/L and hyperthyroidism-associated symptoms. The main clinical outcome measured was 24-h urinary T3 and T4 excretion after around 12 days of therapy. The study found that T4 excretion was significantly increased by Lycopus (p=0.032). There was also a trend to increased T3 excretion that did not achieve clinical significance. This occurred in conjunction with a reduction of some symptoms, specifically increased heart rate in the morning. However, TSH and serum T3 and T4 levels were not changed. The authors proposed that a renal mechanism was responsible for the increased T4 clearance. Apart from the lack of a placebo group, a key weakness of this study was the entry point of TSH <1.0 mU/L, which meant that patients with both clinical and sub-clinical hyperthyroidism were included. Also the causes of hyperthyroidism were not differentiated.

Toxicology and other safety data

Toxicology

Pressed juice of L. europaeus was lethal to male mice (0.75 mL corresponding to 7.5 g fresh plant, route unknown but probably injection). Intravenous injection of 1 mL of L. virginicus pressed juice was lethal, but 3 mL given orally caused no toxic symptoms.[51]

Caffeic acid has been listed as a possible carcinogen on the basis of in vivo studies in mice and rats using two oral dosage regimes: 2.1 g/kg (males), 3.1 g/kg (females) for 96 weeks; 0.7 g/kg and 0.8 g/kg over 104 weeks.[52] Given the small amount present in the herb, this research is unlikely to be relevant to the therapeutic application of bugleweed.[7] Moreover, caffeic acid is a common constituent of many plant foods, including fruit, vegetables and coffee, principally in conjugated forms such as chlorogenic acid.

Contraindications

Thyroid hypofunction, enlargement of the thyroid without functional disorder,[53] pregnancy and lactation.[51]

Special warnings and precautions

Caution is advised in women wishing to conceive.

Interactions

Interference with uptake of radioactive isotopes has been observed in humans.[51] Bugleweed should not be administered concurrently with preparations containing thyroid hormone and iodine supplements, although those concerns are largely theoretical and, given the therapeutic uses of Lycopus, their co-administration is clinically unlikely.[53]

Use in pregnancy and lactation

Category C – has caused or is associated with a substantial risk of causing harmful effects on the fetus or neonate without causing malformations.

Reduction in serum thyroid hormones in vivo suggests that Lycopus should not be taken during pregnancy. Treatment with Lycopus in mice and rats has reduced the number of offspring.[51]

Lycopus is contraindicated in breastfeeding. Decreased milk supply has been observed after administration of *L. virginicus* in suckling rats.[51] Although the human relevance of the effects of Lycopus on serum prolactin in experimental models is not clear, these herbs should not be taken while breastfeeding due to the possibility of both prolactin reduction in the mother and antithyroid constituents passing into breast milk.

Effects on ability to drive and use machines

No negative influence is expected.

Side effects

In rare cases, extended therapy and high (undefined) dosages of bugleweed preparations have resulted in an enlargement of the thyroid. Sudden discontinuation of bugleweed preparations can cause increased symptoms of the disease (hyperthyroid function).[53] The following side effects have been reported in the literature between 1941 to 1968 from clinical usage of bugleweed alone or combined with motherwort (*Leonurus cardiaca*): headache, increase in size of thyroid, and occasionally an increase in hyperthyroid symptoms including nervousness, tachycardia and loss of weight. Increase in thyroid size was observed in patients with goitre not due to thyroid malfunction. The incidence of headache could probably be avoided by reducing the dosage.[51] Not all trials resulted in such side effects.

Overdosage

No incidents found in published literature.

Regulatory status in selected countries

In the UK bugleweed is included on the General Sale List and is covered by a positive Commission E Monograph.

In the USA bugleweed does not have GRAS status. However, it is freely available as a 'dietary supplement' under DSHEA legislation (Dietary Supplement Health and Education Act of 1994).

Bugleweed is not included in Part 4 of Schedule 4 of the Therapeutic Goods Regulations in Australia and is freely available for sale.

References

1. Applequist W. *The Identification of Medicinal Plants: A Handbook of the Morphology of Botanicals in Commerce.* USA: American Botanical Council; 2006.
2. British Herbal Medicine Association's Scientific Committee. *British Herbal Pharmacopoeia.* Bournemouth: BHMA; 1983.
3. Felter HW, Lloyd JU. *King's American Dispensatory*, 18th ed. rev 3, 1905, Portland. Reprinted Eclectic Medical Publications; 1983.
4. Madaus G. *Lehrbuch der biologischen Heilmittel*, Vol 2, Leipzig, 1938. Reprinted New York Verlag; 1976. pp. 1807–1809.
5. Weiss RF. *Herbal Medicine*, translated by Meuss AR from the 6th German Edition of Lehrbuch der Phytotherapie. Beaconsfield: Beaconsfield Publishers; 1988.
6. Harvey R. *Br J Phytother.* 1995/96;4(2): 55–65.
7. Blaschek W, Ebel S, Hackenthal E, et al. *HagerROM 2002: Hagers Handbuch der Drogen und Arzneistoffe.* Heidelberg: Springer; 2002.
8. Kartnig T, Bucar F. *Planta Med.* 1995;61(4):392.
9. Bucar F, Kartnig T, Paschek G, et al. *Planta Med.* 1995;61(5):489.
10. Kartnig T, Bucar F, Neuhold S. *Planta Med.* 1993;59(6):563–564.
11. Madaus G, Koch E, Albus G. *Z Gesamte Exp Med.* 1941;109:411–424. In: Vonhoff C, Winterhoff H. *Z Phytother.* 2006;27(3):110–119.

12. Koch FE. *Madaus Jahresbericht VI* 107–112. In: Vonhoff C, Winterhoff H. *Z Phytother* 2006;27(3):110–119.
13. Kemper F, Loeser A. *Acta Endocrinol.* 1961;38(2):200–206.
14. Kemper F, Loeser A, Richter A. *Arzneimittelforschung.* 1961;11:92–94.
15. Hartenstein H, Müller WA. *Hippokrates.* 1961;32:284–288.
16. Wagner H, Hörhammer L, Frank U. *Arzneimittelforschung.* 1970;20(5):705–713.
17. Kemper FH, Winterhoff H, Sourgens H, et al. *Planta Med.* 1978;33(3):311.
18. Niehaus KD, Winterhoff H, Kemper FH. *Naunyn Schmiedebergs Arch Pharmacol.* 1976;293(suppl):R39.
19. Winterhoff H, Sourgens H, Gumbinger HG, et al. *Acta Endocrinol.* 1979;91(suppl 225):43.
20. Sourgens H, Winterhoff H, Gumbinger HG, et al. *Acta Endocrinol.* 1980;94(suppl 234):49.
21. Sourgens H, Winterhoff Gumbinger HF, et al. *Planta Med.* 1982;45(2):78–86.
22. Gumbinger HG, Winterhoff H, Sourgens H, et al. *Contraception.* 1981;23(6): 661–666.
23. Gumbinger HG, Winterhoff H. *Naunyn Schmiedebergs Arch Pharmacol.* 1980;311(suppl1):R52. Abstract 208.
24. Auf'mkolk M, Ingbar JC, Amir SM. *Endocrinology.* 1984;115(2):527–534.
25. Auf'mkolk M, Amir SM, Kubota K, et al. *Endocrinology.* 1985;116(5):1687–1693.

26. Auf'mkolk M, Amir SM, Kubota K, et al. *Endocrinology.* 1985;116(5):1677–1686.
27. Kleemann S, Winterhoff H. *Planta Med.* 1990;56(6):683.
28. Köhrle J, Auf'mkolk M, Winterhoff H, et al. *Acta Endocrin.* 1981;96(suppl 240):15–16.
29. Auf'mkolk M, Köhrle J, Gumbinger H, et al. *Horm Metab Res.* 1984;16(4): 188–192.
30. Auf'mkolk M, Ingbar JC, Kubota K, et al. *Endocrinology.* 1985;116(5):1687–1693.
31. Sourgens H, Winterhoff H, Gumbinger HG, et al. *Planta Med.* 1982;45(6):78–86.
32. Gumbinger HG, Winterhoff H, Wylde R, et al. *Planta Med.* 1992;58(1):49–50.
33. Winterhoff H, Gumbinger HG, Sourgens H. *Planta Med.* 1988;54(2):101–106.
34. Nahrstedt A, Albrecht M, Wray V, et al. *Planta Med.* 1990;56(4):395–398.
35. John M, Gumbinger HG, Winterhoff H. *Planta Med.* 1990;56(1):14–18.
36. Frömbling-Borges A. *Z Phytother.* 1990;11(1):1–6.
37. Winterhoff H, Gumbinger HG, Vahlensieck U, et al. *Arzneimittelforschung.* 1994;44(1):41–45.
38. Vonhoff C, Baumgartner A, Hegger M, et al. *Life Sci.* 2006;78(10):1063–1070.
39. Vonhoff C, Biller A, Nahrstedt A. et al., 51st Annual Congress of the Society for Medicinal Plant Research, Germany, 217: August 31–September 4, 2003. Abstract P267.
40. Vonhoff C, Winterhoff H. *Z Phytother.* 2006;27(3):110–119.

41. Kong LD, Cai Y, Huang WW, et al. *J Ethnopharmacol*. 2000;73(1–2):199–207.

42. Gibbons S, Oluwatuyi M, Veitch NC, et al. *Phytochemistry*. 2003;62(1):83–87.

43. López V, Akerreta S, Casanova E, et al. *Plant Foods Hum Nutr*. 2007;62(4):151–155.

44. Mattausch F. *Kippokrates*. 1943;10:168–170. In: Vonhoff C, Winterhoff H. *Z Phytother* 2006;27(3):110–119.

45. Lobenhofer G. *Münch Med Wochenschr*. 1953;95(51):1375–1376.

46. Gottlieb J. *Folia Clin Int*. 1952;2(9):420–423.

47. Sittig H. *Münch Med Wochenschr*. 1995;97(25):826, 829–832.

48. Ackermann VJ. *Dtsch Med J*. 1959;10(12):409–411.

49. Scheck R, Biller A. *Natura Med*. 2000;15(5):31–36.

50. Beer A-M, Wiebelitz KR, Schmidt-Gayk H. *Phytomed*. 2008;15(1–2):16–22.

51. De Smet P.A.G.M.Keller K, Hansel R, eds. *Adverse Effects of Herbal Drugs*, Vol 2. Berlin: Springer-Verlag; 1993. pp. 245–251.

52. WHO, International Agency for Research on Cancer. *IARC Working Group on the Evaluation of Carcinogenic Risks to Humans*, Vol 56. Lyon: IARC; 1993. p. 115.

53. Blumenthal M, ed. *The Complete German Commission E Monographs: Therapeutic Guide to Herbal Medicines*. Austin: American Botanical Council; 1998. pp. 98–99.

Bupleurum

(*Bupleurum falcatum* L.)

Synonyms

Hare's ear root (Engl), Bupleuri radix (Lat), chai hu (Chin), saiko (Jap), siho (Kor), segl-hareøre (Dan).

What is it?

Several species of Bupleurum have been officially used in traditional Chinese medicine (TCM), mainly *B. falcatum* L., *B. chinense* DC and *B. scorzonerifolium* Willd. Although other species may be used, the toxic plant *B. longiradiatum* should not be used medicinally. Pharmacological research on Bupleurum root highlights an anti-inflammatory activity that appears to be mediated through the enhanced release and potentiation of hormones from the adrenal cortex. There are still many gaps in the research evidence, but it is possible that Bupleurum acts to mobilise the body's own equivalent of steroidal anti-inflammatory mechanisms.

Effects

Supports the body's anti-inflammatory responses; modulates immune function; protects the liver, stomach and kidneys from toxic damage.

Traditional view

In TCM Bupleurum is classified as a herb that resolves *Lesser Yang Heat* patterns, relaxes constrained *Liver Qi*, disharmony between the *Liver* and the *Spleen* and raises the *Yang Qi* in *Spleen* or *Stomach Deficiency*. Hence Bupleurum is used to treat alternating chills and fever, liver enlargement, prolapse of the uterus and rectum and irregular menstruation.[1] Traditional texts list its properties as bitter and cool and it acts as a diaphoretic (in fever management) and to regulate and restore gastrointestinal and liver function.

Summary actions

Anti-inflammatory, hepatoprotective, antitussive, diaphoretic.

Can be used for

Indications supported by clinical trials

Influenza, common cold, feverish conditions (uncontrolled studies).

Traditional therapeutic uses

Alternating chills and fever; liver enlargement; prolapse of the uterus and rectum; epigastric pain, nausea, indigestion; irregular menstruation. Often combined with Astragalus for debility and prolapse.

May also be used for

Extrapolations from pharmacological studies

Chronic inflammatory disorders, especially autoimmune disease involving the liver or kidneys; acute or chronic liver diseases, chemical liver damage, poor liver function.

Preparations

Dried root for decoction, liquid extract, tablets and capsules; powdered root.

Dosage

- 3 to 12 g/day of the dried root by decoction
- 4 to 8 mL/day of the 1:2 liquid extract or its equivalent.

Duration of use

May be used in the long term if taken within the recommended dosage.

Summary assessment of safety

Minor side effects may occur in sensitive individuals.

Technical data

Botany

The Bupleurum genus is a member of the Umbelliferae (Apiaceae, carrot) family and consists of shrubs and herbs with entire leaves, often parallel veined, hence the name hare's ear.[2] *Bupleurum chinensis* grows 45 to 85 cm high and may or may not be branched. Leaves are alternate, broad-linear to broad-lanceolate (3 to 9 cm long, 0.6 to 1.3 cm wide) with a marginal vein. Umbels are compound, axillary and terminal and contain yellow flowers. Fruit is ovoid, the brown root is conical, 6 to 15 cm long and 0.3 to 0.8 cm in diameter.[3]

Key constituents

Bupleurum falcatum:

- Triterpenoid saponins (saikosaponins a, b_1, b_2, b_3, b_4, c, d, e and f) and their sapogenins[4]
- Phytosterols,[4] pectin-like polysaccharides (bupleurans).[5]

Since the highest levels of saikosaponins are found in *Bupleurum falcatum* (2.8%) and *B. chinensis* (1.7%), these species are preferred.[6,7] Saikosaponins a and d are considered to be the most biologically active.

Adulteration

Although other species of Bupleurum may be used, the toxic plant *B. longiradiatum* should not be used medicinally.[6,8]

	R
Saikosaponin a	β-OH
Saikosaponin d	α-OH

Pharmacodynamics

Many pharmacological studies have been conducted on the isolated saikosaponins. Although these studies have relevance to the medicinal use of Bupleurum, some important qualifications should be considered. In much of the research, saikosaponins were tested in vitro or administered by injection. Since a major active form of saikosaponins in the bloodstream is probably the sapogenins (i.e. saponin aglycones), the relevance of the in vitro research to the oral use of Bupleurum is uncertain. Similarly, the relevance of injected saikosaponins to the oral use of Bupleurum is not entirely clear, although it appears that oral doses do have some similar but milder activity.[9–11]

Anti-inflammatory activity

The anti-inflammatory activity of the saikosaponins appears to be related, at least in part, to their ability to both induce secretion of endogenous corticosterone and potentiate its anti-inflammatory activity. Saikosaponins and some of their gastric and intestinal metabolites have demonstrated this activity following oral doses in mice.[10] Saikosaponin d caused an increase

in serum corticosterone in rats when administered orally.[9] Combined oral administration of Bupleurum extract and corticosterone acetate increased anti-inflammatory activity compared with corticosterone alone, as indicated by the increase in activity of liver tyrosine aminotransferase (LTA).[4] This effect was also demonstrated clinically[4] and confirmed in a later study on rats that found individual injection of saikosaponins a, d or f (ssa, ssd, ssf) or cortisone acetate did not induce LTA activity in adrenalectomised rats.[12] However, co-administration of the same dose of cortisone acetate with either ssa, ssd or ssf significantly induced LTA activity, suggesting that these saikosaponins potentiate the action of cortisone.[11]

Saikosaponins a, b_1, b_2, b_3, b_4, d and saikogenins F and G were all found to increase plasma corticosterone levels in rats 30 minutes after ip injection.[9] Ssa and ssd had the strongest effect and the activity of the saikosaponins was considerably greater than the saikogenins. Saikosaponin c (ssc) was inactive.[9]

Injection of ssa and ssd, but not ssc, raised plasma corticosterone and ACTH levels in rats pretreated with dexamethasone.[13] Dexamethasone is a potent and long-lasting inhibitor of ACTH secretion via negative feedback to the hypothalamus and pituitary. This suggests that the site of action of saikosaponins is the hypothalamic-pituitary system. The use of an antihistamine showed that the saponin-induced corticosterone secretion was not due to histamine release.[12] Another study found that injection of saikogenin A (sgA) increased plasma ACTH levels, possibly through its effect of increasing cyclic AMP levels in the pituitary, but not the hypothalamus.[14] Injections of ssd significantly increased adrenal weight and decreased thymus weight in both dexamethasone-treated and normal rats.[15] However, this effect was abolished in rats with no pituitary, suggesting a mechanism of action involving the pituitary or hypothalamus.[14] The authors suggested that saikosaponins may be used to reduce the dose of glucocorticoid drugs and to prevent glucocorticoid-induced adrenal suppression.

The anti-inflammatory action of oral saikosaponins has been demonstrated in several experimental models. Oral doses of a mixture of saikosaponins were shown to have significant anti-inflammatory activity using the granuloma pouch,[4,16] dextran-induced oedema[15] and cotton pellet methods.[8] (In one study plasma corticosteroid levels decreased and adrenal weight remained unchanged, contrary to previous findings.)[8] However, some negative in vivo results have also been recorded for oral doses of saikosaponins in tests for anti-inflammatory activity.[4]

In contrast, saikosaponins administered by injection demonstrated potent anti-inflammatory activities in several models.[6,8] Saikosaponins a and d antagonised the inflammatory effects of implanted cotton pellets and were as active as prednisolone.[6] Combined injection of doses of ssd and dexamethasone produced an anti-inflammatory effect on cotton-induced granuloma in rats.[17] However, individual administration of the same doses of ssd and dexamethasone were inactive.[16] An in vitro study found that some saikosaponins inhibit the production of prostaglandins[18,19] while another found that they increased prostaglandin E_2 (PGE_2).[20] Saikogenin D inhibited PGE_2 production in vitro.[21]

The ability of saikosaponins to raise blood glucose levels was demonstrated in several pharmacological studies following both oral and injected doses.[6,9,12] This is probably a direct consequence of their ability to increase levels of endogenous glucocorticoids. Since saikosaponins also increase liver glycogen stores,[6] Bupleurum might prove to be useful in the treatment of reactive hypoglycaemia (dysglycaemia).

Immune-modulating activity

Saikosaponins and saikogenins given by injection in vivo stimulate immune function. However, some in vitro studies on saikosaponins suggest immune suppression.

Injections of ssa, ssd and saikogenin D caused a marked increase in the number and activation of macrophages in the peritoneum of mice.[22] Since saikogenin D is a metabolite of ssd, it is probable that ssd also possesses oral activity in this regard. The same compounds were found to enhance the non-specific resistance of mice infected with *Pseudomonas aeruginosa*, but not *Listeria monocytogenes*.[23] Peritoneal macrophages from mice treated with ssd showed intense spreading and significantly increased phagocytic activity.[24] In contrast ssd suppressed murine T cell activation in vitro via multiple mechanisms.[25,26] Also ssa inhibited the proliferation and activation of stimulated T cells in vitro and induced apoptosis of activated T cells, suggesting immunosuppressive activity.[27]

Pretreatment of mice with ssd injections increased the antibody response after immunisation with sheep red blood cells (SRBC).[28] Ssd also enhanced spleen cell proliferative responses to Tcell mitogens both before and after immunisation with SRBC, but decreased the response to B-cell mitogens.[21] Macrophages from ssd-treated mice showed increased spreading activity and lysosomal enzyme activity. Interleukin-1 production was also increased in a dose-dependent manner.[21] Similar results were also found in another study by the same research group, who also observed increased intracellular killing of yeasts by macrophages obtained from ssd-treated mice.[29]

Hot water extracts of Bupleurum demonstrated mitogenic activity on lymphocytes in vitro. The mitogenic substances were likely to be large molecular weight polyphenolic compounds and polysaccharides.[30] Further testing determined that the mitogenic substance was indeed a polyphenolic compound and the structure had been modified by the extraction to increase the stable free radical components.[31] Bupleurum polysaccharides (bupleurans) have also demonstrated T cell-independent B cell mitogenic activity and antibody stimulation in vitro.[32,33] Bupleuran 2IIc appears to be most active.[34,35] In contrast crude Bupleurum polysaccharides (15 or 30 mg/kg/day for 35 days, oral) prevented glomerular injury and lowered serum autoantibodies in a murine model of autoimmune disease.[36]

Hepatoprotective activity

Although Bupleurum is traditionally used as a liver treatment, the hepatoprotective activity of saikosaponins after oral doses has only been recently demonstrated.[4] Oral administration of ssa (at 0.004% of diet) improved hepatic antioxidant capacity and protected against carbon tetrachloride-induced liver injury in rats.[37] A similar model and dose found that ssa significantly reduced hepatic collagen and inhibited NF-kappaB expression. Hepatic pro-inflammatory cytokines were also inhibited.[38] Injected doses of ssa and ssd have demonstrated marked hepatoprotective activity in several animal models.[39–42] Decoctions of Bupleurum administered subcutaneously were also hepatoprotective.[43] Saponins isolated from *B. scorzonerifolium* demonstrated hepatoprotective activity on D-galactosamine-induced cytotoxicity in cultured rat hepatocytes.[44] Saikosaponin d attenuated liver fibrosis in vitro[45] and in vivo following subcutaneous injection at 1 to 2 mg/kg.[46]

The hepatoprotective mechanism of the saikosaponins is not known. However, they have been shown to increase hepatic protein synthesis in vivo and in vitro.[47,48] Increased protein synthesis may enhance the ability of the hepatocyte to withstand a toxic insult. The anti-inflammatory and antioxidant effects noted above may also play a role.

Nephroprotective activity

Injection of ssd significantly decreased urinary protein excretion in rats with chemically induced proteinuria (and symptoms similar to nephrotic syndrome).[49] Urinary protein was reduced by up to 48% after ssd treatment and the degree of abnormality in glomerular epithelial cells was lowered. It was suggested that ssd protects the basement membrane of the glomerulus.[32]

Injection of various saikosaponins demonstrated antinephritic activity following administration of an antiglomerular basement membrane serum to rats.[50] In the same model (but using oral doses) ssd at 10 mg/kg/day suppressed the increased urinary protein excretion and histopathological changes in adrenalectomised rats, possibly by an agonistic action on the glucocorticoid receptor.[51] Other experimentation suggested that the antinephritic mechanisms of saikosaponins were partly due to antiplatelet and corticosterone-releasing activities and an inhibition of the decrease in free radical scavengers such as glutathione peroxidase.[33] Ssd (1.8 mg/kg/day, ip) inhibited the progression of experimental mesangioproliferative glomerulonephritis in rats via a reduction in both transforming growth factor beta-1 and the infiltration of macrophages and CD8+ T lymphocytes.[52]

Ssd has also demonstrated antiproliferative activity on rat glomerular mesangial cells and inhibited synthesis of extracellular matrix proteins in vitro.[53,54] Bupleurum inhibited cytokine production in human mesangial cells in vitro, but there was no additional effect from concurrent angiotensin II receptor blockade.[55]

Antineoplastic activity

Research into the antineoplastic activity of Bupleurum components is at an early stage and largely based on in vitro models. Ssa and ssd induced differentiation of rat C6 glioma cells in vitro.[56] In vitro ssd upregulated the expression of the glucocorticoid receptor, inhibited cell growth and induced apoptosis in HL-60 cells.[57] The potent cytotoxicity of ssd against HepG2 human hepatocellular carcinoma cells was due to induction of apoptosis.[58,59] Similar activity was observed for ssa on human breast cancer cell lines.[60] Ssd inhibited the proliferation of human non-small cell lung cancer A549 cells in vitro by inducing apoptosis and blocking cell cycle progression in the G1 phase.[61] Bupleurum extract increased the cytotoxicity of 5-fluorouracil in HepG2 cells in vitro, but protected normal blood lymphocytes against this agent.[62] Ssb$_2$ induced differentiation without growth inhibition in cultured B16 melanoma cells.[63] However, in an earlier study ssb$_2$ inhibited the proliferation of B16 melanoma cells in vitro. Apoptosis induced by this compound may be due to downregulation of protein kinase C activity.[64,65]

Ssc lacks growth-inhibiting activity in vitro and promoted angiogenesis in human umbilical vein endothelial cells.[66] In contrast, ssd inhibited angiogenesis in chicken embryos in vitro.[67] Bupleurum was among the six most active of 232 Chinese herbs tested for inhibition of adhesion of solid tumour cell lines in vitro.[68] Ssa, ssd and sse also exhibited potent anti-cell adhesive activity and a strong haemolytic action in this study.

The formulation Sho-saiko-to contains Bupleurum and has shown cancer preventative properties in vivo, but did not reduce the risk of spontaneous hepatocarcinogenesis in rats after oral dosing via the diet.[69]

Other activity

Both bupleurans and saikosaponins exhibit decreased gastric ulcer development in a number of models.[5,6,70] The saikosaponins may act by inhibiting gastric secretion.[71] Saikosaponins have also been found to decrease the corrosive and protein-denaturing effects of tannic acid and to improve the integrity of the gastric mucosa of rats.[72] However, as might be expected of saponins, high doses of saikosaponins cause gastric irritation.[6] The antiulcer polysaccharide BR-2 from Bupleurum healed chronic ulcers in rats (50 to 200 mg/kg, oral).[73]

Many saponins are known to lower cholesterol and this activity has also been demonstrated for the saikosaponins.[6,30] It has been suggested that saikosaponins and saikogenins lower cholesterol by increasing cholesterol excretion in bile.[6]

Oral administration of Bupleurum decoction and saikosaponins demonstrated antipyretic activity.[6] Injection of saikosaponins demonstrated a potent antitussive effect on guinea pigs.[74] Intranasal administration of a Bupleurum essential oil gel decreased body temperature in rabbits, suggesting possible antipyretic activity.[75]

Ssd inactivated enveloped viruses such as measles and herpes viruses but had no effect on a naked virus (polio).[76] Despite this, a toxic effect on host cells was noted, leading to the conclusion that ssd is not a useful antiviral agent.[38] In contrast ssc was effective against hepatitis B virus (HBV) in vitro[58] and ssb$_2$ exhibited potent anticoronaviral activity by possibly interfering with the early stage of viral replication.[77] The crude saponin fraction of Bupleurum also inhibited HBV replication in vitro.[78]

Oral doses of saikosaponins from Bupleurum inhibited slow kindling and seizures (an epilepsy model) induced in rats by pentetrazole.[79] Proposed mechanisms included correction of neurotransmitter anomalies[80] and inhibition of glial fibrillary acidic protein overexpression.[81] Bupleurum (150 to 600 mg/kg, oral) countered the stress-induced impairment of spatial working memory in rats and demonstrated anxiolytic activity.[82] After oral administration a Bupleurum extract (150 and 300 mg/kg) exhibited antidepressant activity in a rat model via a mechanism that possibly involves the serotonergic and noradrenergic systems.[83]

Ssa at doses more than 1 mg/kg (iv) significantly inhibited passive cutaneous anaphylaxis in rats in a dose-dependent manner.[84] At 3 and 10 mg/kg it also suppressed asthmatic bronchoconstriction in sensitised guinea pigs. Ssa administered during the induction phase inhibited contact sensitivity in a murine model.[85]

Ssd has a similar structure to oestradiol and stimulated the proliferation of MCF-7 cells in vitro by acting as a weak phyto-oestrogen, possibly mainly via oestrogen receptor alpha.[86] Ssd also demonstrated weak oestrogenic activity in ovariectomised mice (5 and 50 mg/kg, ip).[87]

Pharmacokinetics

The pharmacokinetics of oral doses of saponins are complex and not completely understood. While low levels of triterpenoid saponins may be absorbed into the bloodstream unchanged, it is also likely on current evidence that significant quantities of triterpenoid saponin metabolites are absorbed in most cases. These metabolites are usually formed by the action of gastric and intestinal secretions and/or bowel flora. The pharmacological implications of these observations are not fully understood.

Oral administration of saikosaponins at a dosage which was 10 times that of intramuscular injection demonstrated a similar anti-inflammatory activity in the granuloma pouch method.[8] This indicates that the saponins and/or their metabolites probably exhibit poor absorption profiles (about 10% absorption). Ssa, ssc and ssd are transformed into 27 metabolites in the gastrointestinal tract of mice.[10,88] Therefore 30 compounds are potentially available for absorption into the bloodstream. However, only ssa and its monoglycoside (prosaikogenin F) and aglycone (saikogenin F) were detected in the plasma of rats when ssa was administered orally.[31] The plasma concentration of ssa peaked after 30 minutes at 74 µg/L and ssa was undetectable after 1.5 h.[31] In contrast, the ssa metabolites were both found to peak after 8 h at about 2 µg/L and were undetectable after 12 h.[31] This implies that after oral doses of ssa there is a short but intense plasma concentration (and therefore activity) of ssa itself, followed by more prolonged and less intense activities of its metabolites. These findings need to be confirmed in human studies. Total faecal excretion of injected doses of saikosaponins after 2 and 7 days accounted for about 50% and 85% respectively of the administered dose.[6] This suggests that saikosaponin metabolites undergo enterohepatic recycling.

An in vitro study found that ssc is transformed into four saikogenins by human intestinal bacteria.[89] Bacterial enzymes responsible for saikosaponin metabolism could include a beta-D-glucosidase and a beta-D-fucosidase isolated from *Eubacterium spp.*[90] Supporting this concept, the oral administration of ssb$_1$ to germ-free and *Eubacterium spp.* A-44-infected rats was investigated.[91] After a dose of

50 mg/kg, no metabolite was detected in the plasma, caecal contents or faeces of the germ-free rats. In contrast, considerable quantities of the metabolites prosaikogenin A and saikogenin A were found in the plasma of the rats containing the *Eucobacterium spp.*

Clinical trials

Despite the considerable number of pharmacological studies on the saikosaponins, controlled clinical studies on both Bupleurum and saikosaponins are lacking. However, formulations containing Bupleurum have been tested in controlled clinical trials such as the prevention of hepatocellular carcinoma in hepatitis C patients.[92,93]

In an uncontrolled clinical study of 143 patients treated with *B. chinensis*, fever subsided within 24 h in 98.1% of influenza cases and 87.9% of common cold cases. In another study of 40 patients with pathological fever, Bupleurum produced an antipyretic effect in 97.5% and achieved a reduction of 1 to 2°C in body temperature in 77.5%.[6] Intravenous injection of *B. chinensis* (10 to 20 mL, one to two times a day for adults, 5 to 10 mL per day for children) was found to give satisfactory therapeutic effects in 100 cases of infectious hepatitis in an uncontrolled study.[6] In chronic hepatitis with hepatomegaly, an injection of Bupleurum and *Salvia miltiorrhiza* was used, with vitamins B and C taken orally. Each course lasted 10 days, with a 4- to 5-day interval between courses. After treatment, patients usually showed marked improvement in mental state, appetite and subjective symptoms. Amelioration or disappearance of pain over the liver area was achieved in 4 to 5 days in most patients.[6]

Toxicology and other safety data

Toxicology

Like most saponins, crude saikosaponins show moderate toxicity after ip administration (LD_{50} 112 mg/kg in mice, 58.3 mg/kg in guinea pigs) but low toxicity by the oral route (LD_{50} 4.7 g/kg in mice).[16,72] Aqueous extract of Bupleurum root did not show any toxic effect in rats and mice at oral doses of 6 g/kg.[65] Repeated oral administration at 1.5 and 3.0 g/kg/day over 21 days caused slight decreases in red blood cell count and liver weight.[94]

Bupleurum methanolic extract did not demonstrate mutagenic activity in vitro in the Ames test.[95] Bupleurum extract decreased the mutagenicity of the mutagens benzo(a)-pyrene and aflatoxin B in the Ames test in one study,[65] but hot water extracts enhanced the mutagenic activity of benzo(a)pyrene in other studies.[96,97] Hot water extracts of Bupleurum also demonstrated antimutagenic activity in vivo.[98]

Chronic oral administration of Sho-saiko-to (2 g/kg/day) containing Bupleurum to male and female rats did not affect their general condition, body weight, food consumption, reproductive ability or gross anatomy. Neither did it cause any abnormalities in the F1 generation or F2 fetuses.[99]

Contraindications

Bupleurum is contraindicated in *Deficient Yin* cough (i.e. cough in debility) or *Liver Fire* ascending to the head (i.e. some cases of headache and hypertension). Bupleurum can occasionally cause nausea or vomiting; if this happens, use the smallest dose possible.[1]

Special warnings and precautions

Saponin-containing herbs are best kept to a minimum in patients with pre-existing cholestasis. Bupleurum has a sedative effect in some patients and is used in a popular insomnia formulation in Taiwan.[100]

Interactions

None known.

Use in pregnancy and lactation

Category B1 – no increase in frequency of malformation or other harmful effects on the fetus from limited use in women. No evidence of increased fetal damage in animal studies.

Subcutaneous administration of Bupleurum aqueous extract (0.1 to 0.4 mL/day) for 5 days did not affect fertility or exhibit teratogenic effects in mice.[101] Oral administration to female rats, from 2 weeks before mating until day 21 after delivery, of a TCM herbal formula (2 g/kg/day) containing Bupleurum did not exert teratogenic effects in the F1 generation or F2 fetuses.[99] This formula, also known as Sho-saiko-to, contains Bupleurum as the main ingredient (26 to 29% by weight) as well as six other herbs. Another Japanese herbal formula containing Bupleurum abolished the teratogenicity of sodium valproate in rats. Oral administration of this formula (up to 3 g/kg/day) to rat fetuses during organogenesis also resulted in no abnormalities.[102]

Bupleurum is compatible with breastfeeding. Oral administration of Sho-saiko-to to female rats from 2 weeks prior to mating until day 21 after delivery (which includes the lactation period) did not result in any abnormalities in growth, development, behaviour or reproductive ability in the F1 generation or F2 fetuses.[99]

Effects on ability to drive and use machines

Bupleurum has a sedative effect in some patients, especially in larger doses,[6] therefore sensitive patients should exhibit caution when driving or operating machinery.

Side effects

Large doses of Bupleurum may have a sedative effect, increase bowel movements and flatulence or decrease appetite in some patients.[6] As with all herbs rich in saponins, oral use may cause irritation of the gastric mucous membranes and reflux.

Three cases of allergic reaction have been reported in patients given intramuscular injections of Bupleurum.[6]

The formula Sho-saiko-to has been associated with eosino-philic pneumonia,[103] pulmonary oedema,[104] liver damage[105] and multiple cases of pneumonitis.[106–108] In Japan, Sho-saiko-to is mainly used to treat liver disease and is the most frequently used herbal remedy for this condition, which may explain the high number of reported reactions. Pneumonitis induced by herbs is suspected to be caused by an allergic mechanism rather than a toxic mechanism.[106] A review of the literature found that, in addition to reports of hepatotoxic-ity, Sho-saiko-to is hepatoprotective in humans and animals and has beneficial effects on the liver.[109] Cases of liver tox-icity[110] and adult respiratory distress syndrome[111] have also been reported after the use of other TCM herbal prepara-tions containing Bupleurum. However, Sho-saiko-to and these preparations contain seven or more different herbs, and the particular herb or herbs responsible for these adverse reac-tions are currently unknown. A provocation test with Baical skullcap (*Scutellaria baicalensis*) suggested that this herb was responsible for a case of drug-induced pneumonitis caused by a TCM formula that also contained Bupleurum.[112] Baical skullcap is also present in Sho-saiko-to. A case was reported of a man who developed acute hepatitis with jaun-dice after he was given a Japanese herbal medicine, Sairei-to (Bupleurum and Hoelen combination).[113] Unusually, the component thought to be responsible for the observed drug-induced liver injury was able to be identified. Lymphocyte migration inhibition testing indicated that *Pinellia ternata* was the causative agent.

A study was undertaken to determine the association between the use of TCM formulas containing Bupleurum and the risk of hospitalisation related to liver injury among HBV-infected patients in Taiwan.[114] From data for a total of 639 779 patients between 1997 and 2004, case-control and case-crossover designs were used to assess the risk of

hospitalisation. Cumulative doses of TCM formulas and Bupleurum were assessed for any dose-response relation-ship. An odds ratio of 1.9 was found, indicating an increased risk of liver damage from TCM Bupleurum formulas. The risk from prescribing Sho-saiko-to was significantly high and a dose-response relationship was observed.

Overdosage

No incidents found in the published literature.

Safety in children

No adverse effects anticipated, although specific information is lacking.

Regulatory status in selected countries

Bupleurum is official in the *Pharmacopoeia of the People's Republic of China* (English edition, 2000) and the *Japanese Pharmacopoeia* (English 14th edition, 2001).

Bupleurum is not covered by a Commission E Monograph and is not on the UK General Sale List.

Bupleurum does not have GRAS status. However, it is freely available as a 'dietary supplement' in the USA under DSHEA legislation (1994 Dietary Supplement Health and Education Act).

Bupleurum is not included in Part 4 of Schedule 4 of the Therapeutic Goods Act Regulations of Australia and is freely available for sale.

References

1. Bensky D, Gamble A. *Chinese Herbal Medicine Materia Medica*. Seattle: Eastland Press; 1986. pp. 68–69.
2. Mabberley DJ. *The Plant Book*, 2nd ed. Cambridge: Cambridge University Press; 1997. p. 107.
3. World Health Organization. *Medicinal Plants in China*. Manilla: Regional Office for the Western Pacific, World Health Organization; 1989. p. 61.
4. Tang W, Eisenbrand G. *Chinese Drugs of Plant Origin*. Berlin: Springer Verlag; 1992. pp. 223–232.
5. Yamada H, Sun XB, Matsumoto T, et al. *Planta Med*. 1991;57(6):555–559.
6. Chang H, But P. *Pharmacology and Applications of Chinese Materia Medica*, Vol 2. Singapore: World Scientific; 1987. pp. 967–974.
7. Dong YY, Luo SQ. *Chung Kuo Chung Yao Tsa Chih*. 1989;14(11):678–681, 703–704.
8. *Pharmacopoeia Commission of the People's Republic of China*, English edn , Vol 1.

Beijing: Chemical Industry Press; 1997. pp. 143–144.
9. Yamamoto M, Kumagai A, Yamamura Y. *Arzneimittelforschung*. 1975;25(7):1021–1023.
10. Yokoyama H, Hiai S, Oura H. *Chem Pharm Bull (Tokyo)*. 1981;29(2):500–504.
11. Nose M, Amagaya S, Ogihara Y. *Chem Pharm Bull (Tokyo)*. 1989;37(10):2736–2740.
12. Hashimoto M, Inada K, Ohminami H, et al. *Planta Med*. 1985;51(5):401–403.
13. Hiai S, Yokoyama H, Nagasawa T, et al. *Chem Pharm Bull (Tokyo)*. 1981;29(2):495–499.
14. Cheng JT, Tsai CL. *Biochem Pharmacol*. 1986;35(15):2483–2487.
15. Hiai S, Yokoyama H. *Chem Pharm Bull (Tokyo)*. 1986;34(3):1195–1202.
16. Shibata M. *Yakugaku Zasshi*. 1970;90(3):398–404.
17. Abe H, Sakaguchi M, Arichi S. *Nippon Yakurigaku Zasshi*. 1982;80(2):155–161.

18. Ohuchi K, Watanabe M, Ozeki T, et al. *Planta Med*. 1985;51(3):208–212.
19. Kumazawa Y, Takimoto H, Nishimura C, et al. *Int J Immunopharmacol*. 1989;11(1):21–28.
20. Kyo R, Nakahata N, Kodama Y, et al. *Biol Pharm Bull*. 1999;22(12):1385–1387.
21. Kodama Y, Xiaochuan L, Tsuchiya C, et al. *Planta Med*. 2003;69(8):765–767.
22. Kumazawa Y, Kawakita T, Takimoto H, et al. *Int J Immunopharmacol*. 1990;12(5):531–537.
23. Ushio Y, Abe H. *Int J Immunopharmacol*. 1991;13(5):493–499.
24. Ushio Y, Oda Y, Abe H. *Int J Immunopharmacol*. 1991;13(5):501–508.
25. Wong VK, Zhou H, Cheung SS, et al. *J Cell Biochem*. 2009;107(2):303–315.
26. Leung CY, Liu L, Wong RN, et al. *Biochem Biophys Res Commun*. 2005;338(4):1920–1927.
27. Sun Y, Cai TT, Zhou XB, et al. *Int Immunopharmacol*. 2009;9(7–8):978–983.

28. Ushio Y, Abe H. *Jpn J Pharmacol.* 1991;56(2):167–175.

29. Oka H, Ohno N, Iwanaga S, et al. *Biol Pharm Bull.* 1995;18(5):757–765.

30. Ohtsu S, Izumi S, Iwanaga S, et al. *Biol Pharm Bull.* 1997;20(1):97–100.

31. Abe H, Sakaguchi M, Yamada M, et al. *Planta Med.* 1980;40(4):366–372.

32. Sakurai MH, Matsumoto T, Kiyohara H, et al. *Immunology.* 1999;97(3):540–547.

33. Guo Y, Matsumoto T, Kiluchi Y, et al. *Immunopharmacology.* 2000;49(3):307–316.

34. Matsumoto T, Hosono-Nishiyama K, Yamada H. *Biol Pharm Bull.* 2008;31(5):931–934.

35. Matsumoto T, Moriya M, Sakurai MH, et al. *Int Immunopharmacol.* 2008;8(4):581–588.

36. Wang Z, Li H, Xu H, et al. *J Ethnopharmacol.* 2009;124(3):481–487.

37. Wu SJ, Lin YH, Chu CC, et al. *J Med Food.* 2008;11(2):224–229.

38. Wu SJ, Tam KW, Tsai YH, et al. *Am J Chin Med.* 2010;28(1):99–111.

39. Abe H, Sagaguchi M, Odashima S, et al. *Naunyn Schmiedebergs Arch Pharmacol.* 1982;320(3):266–271.

40. Abe H, Orita M, Konishi H, et al. *J Pharm Pharmacol.* 1985;37(8):555–559.

41. Lin CC, Chiu HF, Yen MH, et al. *Am J Chin Med.* 1990;18(3–4):105–112.

42. He Y, Hu ZF, Li P, et al. *Zhongguo Zhong Yao Za Zhi.* 2008;33(8):915–919.

43. Matsuda H, Murakami T, Ninomiya K, et al. *Bioorg Med Chem Lett.* 1997;7(17):2193–2198.

44. Yamamoto M, Kumagai A, Yamamura Y. *Arzneimittelforschung.* 1975;25(8):1240–1243.

45. Fan J, Li X, Li P, et al. *Biochem Cell Biol.* 2007;85(2):189–195.

46. Dang SS, Wang BF, Cheng YA, et al. *World J Gastroenterol.* 2007;13(4):557–563.

47. Fujiwara K, Ogihara Y. *Life Sci.* 1986;39(4):297–301.

48. Abe H, Orita M, Konishi H, et al. *Eur J Pharmacol.* 1986;120(2):171–178.

49. Hattori T, Ito M, Suzuki Y. *Nippon Yakurigaku Zasshi.* 1991;97(1):13–21.

50. Sun XB, Matsumoto T, Yamada H. *J Pharm Pharmacol.* 1991;43(10):699–704.

51. Hattori T, Hishimura H, Kase Y, et al. *Nephron Physiol.* 2008;109(2):19–27.

52. Li P, Gong Y, Zu N, et al. *Nephron Exp Nephrol.* 2005;101(4):3111–3118.

53. Zu N, Li P, Li N, et al. *Biochem Cell Biol.* 2007;85(2):169–174.

54. Zu N, Dong X, Fu GX. *Zhongguo Zhong Xi Yi Jie He Za Zhi.* 2007;27(4):321–325.

55. Cho BS, Kim SD, Park JK, et al. *Phytother Res.* 2010;24(3):339–343.

56. Tsai YJ, Chen IL, Horng LY, et al. *Phytother Res.* 2002;16(2):117–121.

57. Bu S, Xu J, Sun J. *Zhonghua Xue Ye SXue Za Zhi.* 1999;20(7):354–356.

58. Chiang LC, Ng LT, Liu LT, et al. *Planta Med.* 2003;69(8):705–709.

59. Hsu YL, Kuo PL, Chiang LC, et al. *Cancer Lett.* 2004;213(2):213–221.

60. Chen JC, Chang NW, Chung JG, et al. *Am J Chin Med.* 2003;31(3):363–377.

61. Hsu YL, Kuo PL, Lin CC. *Life Sci.* 2004;75(10):1231–1242.

62. Kang SJ, Lee YJ, Kim BM, et al. *Basic Clin Pharmacol Toxicol.* 2008;103(4):305–313.

63. Zong Z, Fujikawa-Yamamoto K, Ota T, et al. *Cell Struct Funct.* 1998;23(5):265–272.

64. Shimizu K, Amagaya S, Ogihara Y. *J Pharmacobiodyn.* 1985;8(9):718–725.

65. Tanaka S, Takahashi A, Onoda K, et al. *Yakugaku Zasshi.* 1986;106(8):671–686.

66. Shyu KG, Tsai SC, Wang BW, et al. *Life Sci.* 2004;76(7):813–826.

67. Wang BF, Cheng YA, Dang SS. *Zhongguo Zhong Xi Yi Jie He Za Zhi.* 2009;29(5):425–429.

68. Ahn BZ, Yoon YD, Lee YH, et al. *Planta Med.* 1998;64(3):220–224.

69. Watanabe S, Kitade Y, Masaki T, et al. *Nutr Cancer.* 2001;39(1):96–101.

70. Shibata M, Yoshida R, Motoashi S, et al. *Yakugaku Zasshi.* 1973;93(12):1660–1667.

71. Hung CR, Wu TS, Chang TY. *Chin J Physiol.* 1993;36(4):211–217.

72. Takagi K, Shibata M. *Yakugaku Zasshi.* 1969;89(5):712–720.

73. Matsumoto T, Sun XB, Hanawa T, et al. *Phytother Res.* 2002;16(1):91–93.

74. Ushio Y, Abe H. *Planta Med.* 1992;58(2):171–173.

75. Cao SL, Chen E, Zhang QZ, et al. *Arch Pharm Res.* 2007;30(8):1014–1019.

76. Motoo Y, Sawabu N. *Cancer Lett.* 1994;86(1):91–95.

77. Cheng PW, Ng LT, Chiang LC, et al. *Clin Exp Pharmacol Physiol.* 2006;33(7):612–616.

78. Chang JS, Wang KC, Liu HW, et al. *Am J Chin Med.* 2007;35(2):341–351.

79. Xie W, Bao Y, Yu LJ, et al. *Nan Fang Yi Ke Da Xue Xue Bao.* 2006;26(2):177–180.

80. Xie W, Li CZ, Bao Y, et al. *Nan Fang Yi Ke Da Xue Xue Bao.* 2006;26(8):1132–1135.

81. Xie W, Bao Y, Yu LJ, et al. *Nan Fang Yi Ke Da Xue Xue Bao.* 2006;26(4):452–455.

82. Lee B, Shim I, Lee H, et al. *Biol Pharm Bull.* 2009;32(8):1392–1398.

83. Kwon S, Lee B, Kim M, et al. *Prog Neuropsychopharmacol Biol Psychiatry.* 2010;34(2):265–270.

84. Park KH, Park J, Koh D, et al. *Phytother Res.* 2002;16(4):359–363.

85. Zhang L, Dong Y, Sun Y, et al. *Pharm Pharmacol.* 2006;58(9):1257–1264.

86. Wang P, Ren J, Tang J, et al. *Eur J Pharmacol.* 2010;626(2–3):159–165.

87. Li Y, Wang P, Ren JL, et al. *Zhong Xi Yi Jie He Xue Bao.* 2009;7(7):657–660.

88. Kim JM, Ji HW, Jung YM. *Korean J Vet Public Health.* 1994;18(3):261–268.

89. Yu KU, Jang IS, Kang KH, et al. *Arch Pharm Res.* 1997;20(5):420–424.

90. Kida H, Akao T, Meselhy MR, et al. *Biol Pharm Bull.* 1997;20(12):1274–1278.

91. Kida H, Akao T, Meselhy MR, et al. *Biol Pharm Bull.* 1998;21(6):588–593.

92. Shimizu I. *J Gastroenterol Hepatol.* 2000;15(suppl):D84–D90.

93. Ikegami F, Sumino M, Fujii Y, et al. *Hum Exp Toxicol.* 2006;25(8):481–494.

94. Tsukiyama K, Tasaka Y, Nakajima M, et al. *Nippon Kyobu Shikkan Gakkai Zasshi.* 1989;27(12):1556–1561.

95. Yamamoto H, Mizutani T, Nomura H. *J Pharm Soc Jap.* 1982;102(6):596–601.

96. Sakai Y, Nagase H, Ose Y, et al. *Mutat Res.* 1988;206(3):327–334.

97. Niikawa M, Sakai Y, Ose Y, et al. *Chem Pharm Bull (Tokyo).* 1990;38(7):2035–2039.

98. Liu DX. *Chung Kuo Tung Yao Tsa Chih.* 1990;15:640–642.

99. Shimazu H, Katsumata Y, Takamatsu T, et al. *Yakuri To Chiryo.* 1997;25(6):29–42.

100. Chen LC, Chen IC, Wang BR, et al. *J Clin Pharm Ther.* 2009;34(5):555–560.

101. Matsui AS, Rogers J, Woo YK, et al. *Med Pharmacol Exp.* 1967;16:414–424.

102. Minematsu S, Taki M, Watanabe M, et al. *Nippon Yakurigaku Zasshi.* 1990;96(5):265–273.

103. Kobashi Y, Nakajima M, Niki Y, et al. *Nihon Kyobu Shikkan Gakkai Zasshi.* 1997;35(12):1372–1377.

104. Miyazaki E, Ando M, Ih K, et al. *Nihon Kokyuki Gakkai Zasshi.* 1998;36(9):776–780.

105. Itoh S, Marutani K, Nishimina T, et al. *Dig Dis Sci.* 1995;40(8):1845–1848.

106. Mizushima Y, Oosake R, Kobayashi M. *Phytother Res.* 1997;11(4):295–298.

107. Sato A, Toyoshima M, Kondo A, et al. *Nihon Kyobu Shikkan Gakkai Zasshi.* 1997;35(4):391–395.

108. Hatakeyama S, Tachibana A, Morita M, et al. *Nihon Kyobu Shikkan Gakkai Zasshi.* 1997;35(5):505–510.

109. Stickel F, Egerer G, Seitz HK. *Public Health Nutr.* 2000;3(2):113–124.

110. Kane JA, Kane SP, Jain S. *Gut.* 1995;36(1):146–147.

111. Shiota T, Wilson JG, Matsumoto H, et al. *Intern Med.* 1996;35(6):494–496.

112. Takeshita K, Saisho Y, Kitamura K, et al. *Intern Med.* 2001;40(8):764–768.

113. Aiba T, Takahashi T, Suzuki K, et al. *J Gastroenterol Hepatol.* 2007;22(5):762–763.

114. Lee CH, Wang JD, Chen PC. *PLoS One.* 2011;6(1):e16064.

Butcher's broom

(*Ruscus aculeatus* L.)

Synonyms

Knee holly, box holly, pettigree, *R. ponticus* Woron., *R. hyrcanus* Stankov & Taliev, Mäusedorn (Ger), petit houx (Fr).

What is it?

The butcher's broom (*Ruscus aculeatus*) is a small evergreen shrub native to western Europe.[1,2] The tough leaf-like branches (known as phylloclades) have been used to assemble makeshift brooms, hence the common name. However, the part used therapeutically is the rootstock and rhizome.

In recent times, butcher's broom has been the subject of several scientific investigations, including clinical trials. The research has focused on its anti-oedema and venotonic properties, which make it an effective therapy for symptoms associated with varicose veins and haemorrhoids (similar to the horsechestnut with which it combines well). In Europe, proprietary preparations of butcher's broom are commonly used for varicose veins and haemorrhoids. The extract is often combined with other ingredients, especially hesperidin methylchalcone and ascorbic acid. (Hesperidin is a flavonoid that has beneficial activity on capillaries.)

Effects

Improves venous tone, decreases oedema associated with venous stagnation and inflammation.

Traditional view

Butcher's broom root was traditionally regarded in Western herbal medicine as a diuretic, diaphoretic, laxative and expectorant, and was used to treat dropsy, urinary obstruction or gravel, dysuria, oedema, ascites, jaundice, difficult breathing and for the removal of phlegm. For the treatment of haemorrhoids it was used both orally and locally.[3,4] The oedema-reducing effect of this plant is clearly highlighted in the traditional literature, with reference to butcher's broom as 'much recommended by Dioscorides and other ancient physicians as an aperient and diuretic'.[3]

Summary actions

Venotonic, antio-edematous, anti-inflammatory.

Can be used for

Indications supported by clinical trials

Chronic venous insufficiency, varicose veins, varicose ulcers, lymphoedema, haemorrhoids, congestive symptoms of premenstrual syndrome (most of these trials in combination with other agents). Possibly useful in cases of retinopathy.

Traditional therapeutic uses

Oedema and haemorrhoids.

May also be used for

Extrapolation from pharmacological studies

May be useful in orthostatic hypotension.

Preparations

Decoction of the dried root, liquid extract and tablets or capsules for internal use. Extracts of the herb can also be applied topically as a cream, ointment or gel.

Dosage

- 1.5 to 3 g/day of dried root
- Butcher's broom tablets or capsules (200 mg of a 4:1 concentrate standardised to contain 20 mg of saponins expressed as ruscogenin), two to three per day
- 3 to 6 mL/day of 1:2 liquid extract; 7.5 to 15 mL/day of 1:5 tincture

In most of the clinical trials, butcher's broom extract was used in combination. The typical daily doses of the components used in many trials were 300 mg of butcher's broom extract, 300 mg of hesperidin methylchalcone and 200 mg of ascorbic acid (corresponding usually to two capsules per day).

Duration of use

There is no suggestion that the long-term use of butcher's broom should be limited.

Summary assessment of safety

In rare cases the herb has been implicated in the development of lymphocytic colitis after long-term use. However, these cases were all recorded for the combination product and the identification of butcher's broom root and rhizome as the causative agent has not been confirmed.

Technical data

Botany

A sub-shrub which, in some instances, may grow to 1 m. It has a fibrous, oblique, whitish rhizome from which emerge green, striate stems. The branches take on a leaf-like form and are known as cladodes or phylloclades; they are green, leathery and ovate-lanceolate with a spine at the top. The true leaves are represented by scales. The greenish-white, six-petalled flowers are borne on a lanceolate bract on the first half of the cladode. The fruit is an almost spherical, red berry with one to two seeds and a viscous pulp. This unusual type of shrub can often be seen wild throughout Britain and Europe on the outskirts of woods and in moist, uncultivated ground. It is collected in September, but as it is a protected plant special permission is needed.[2]

Adulteration

No adulterants known.

Key constituents

The rhizome contains steroidal compounds (0.5% to 1.5%) comprising the aglycones ruscogenin and neoruscogenin and their glycosides (which are of the spirostanol and furostanol saponin types).[5] One study has also identified the presence of triterpene and sterol compounds.[6]

Pharmacodynamics

A preparation containing butcher's broom extract, hesperidin methylchalcone and ascorbic acid has been extensively studied in recent decades. Throughout this monograph this formulation will be referred to as 'butcher's broom extract combination'.

A 1994 review of published pharmacological studies indicated that butcher's broom extract exerted activity on the three circulatory compartments involved in chronic venous insufficiency. The venoconstrictor effect is explained by its peripheral post-synaptic alpha-noradrenergic action. This action also possibly explains the lymphatic activity observed in experimental models assessing lymphatic flow. A microcirculatory activity is also involved: this combines an inhibitory effect on capillary permeability, a protective action on the endothelium against hypoxia via stimulation of mitochondrial enzymes, and an inhibition of the endothelial leukocyte adhesion observed in models of ischaemia/reperfusion. The other

components in the proprietary butcher's broom extract combination, namely hesperidin methylchalcone and ascorbic acid, exert their effects mainly by reducing capillary permeability and increasing capillary resistance.[7]

Anti-inflammatory activity

In research conducted in the 1950s and 1960s, butcher's broom extract demonstrated activity against experimental paw inflammation and peritonitis in vivo.[8]

Saponin constituents isolated from butcher's broom displayed anti-inflammatory activity on rat paw oedema, but did not influence capillary fragility. A strong vasoconstrictor activity was observed on isolated blood vessels and the ruscogenins also decreased capillary permeability in a rabbit model.[9] However, the ruscogenins failed to inhibit hyaluronidase activity in vitro, but did exhibit a remarkable anti-elastase activity.[10] An in vivo study in mice found that ruscogenin significantly suppressed zymosin A-evoked leukocyte migration, possibly through an anti-adhesive activity via inhibition of the NF-kappaB pathway.[11]

Venotonic activity

In an experimental microcirculation model, butcher's broom extract caused constriction in venules, but not arterioles, after intravenous administration.[12] The inhibitory effect of butcher's broom extract on histamine-induced microvascular permeability was attributed to the blocking of calcium and a selective activation of alpha1-adrenoceptors (and to a lesser extent alpha2-receptors).[12–14] Butcher's broom extract potentiated the activity of norepinephrine (noradrenaline) released at nerve endings.[15] The vasoconstriction is independent of the endothelium and, as indicated above, is mediated by the activation of smooth muscle adrenergic receptors, but not by endothelin receptors.[16] This adrenergic action of butcher's broom extract enhances venous return.[17]

The venoconstriction induced by butcher's broom in isolated vessels was increased by heat.[12,18] This effect of temperature on the response to butcher's broom resembled that noted during partial alpha1-adrenergic activation.[19] A venotonic effect was also observed in diabetic animals, and treatment with butcher's broom extract combination reversed an experimentally impaired venoarteriolar reflex (which is a hallmark of diabetic microangiopathy).[20]

Studies utilising isolated human veins indicated that butcher's broom extract caused dose-dependent contractions in leg veins from patients with primary varicosity. Varicose tributaries were more sensitive to the contractile effects of butcher's broom extract than segments of the greater saphenous vein removed from the same patient. Contractions following butcher's broom exposure were independent of the endothelium and mediated by the activation of adrenergic receptors on the smooth muscle, but not endothelin-A.[21]

Butcher's broom extract increased the cyclic AMP concentration in isolated human varicose veins, but did not affect cyclic GMP levels. In the presence of the extract, the ratios of 6-ketoprostaglandin-F_{1a} to thromboxane B_2 in varicose veins were rendered identical to normal vein tissue. (Segments of vein were obtained from patients who had undergone surgery.)[22] Contractions initiated by butcher's broom extract were enhanced following chronic exposure to progesterone, an effect that could be reversed by oestrogen. These contractions were mediated by an adrenergic and a non-adrenergic component. The adrenergic component was enhanced by progesterone and decreased by oestrogen.[23]

A venoconstrictive activity of a butcher's broom cream under orthostatic conditions was demonstrated by ultrasonography in a randomised, double blind study involving 18 healthy volunteers. Within 2.5 h of applying a quantity of butcher's broom cream containing 64 to 96 mg of extract, the diameter of the femoral vein decreased by an average of 1.25 mm, compared with a diameter increase of 0.5 mm for the placebo cream ($p < 0.05$).[24]

As noted earlier, the mechanism of action of the combination of butcher's broom extract and hesperidin methylchalcone in the treatment of venous diseases is thought to involve an increase in venous tone (by butcher's broom extract) and protection of capillary integrity (by hesperidin methylchalcone). In a double blind study involving 20 healthy volunteers, the efficacy of the individual agents, their combination and a placebo were assessed. Butcher's broom decreased venous capacity ($p < 0.01$), reduced the blood pool in the lower leg under orthostatic conditions and decreased tissue volume in the foot and ankle ($p < 0.01$). Hesperidin methylchalcone lowered the capillary filtration rate ($p < 0.01$) and increased the blood pool (due to dehydration of the lower leg tissue). Blood volume after use of the combination was between the values for butcher's broom and hesperidin methylchalcone alone, and effects on other parameters corresponded to those obtained for the individual substances.[25] Some of the 20 volunteers administered the butcher's broom extract combination showed a significantly reduced venous capacity, whereas others developed an increase in venous storage ability.

Haemorheological and haemostasis parameters

The influence of combined treatment with butcher's broom extract (450 mg/day containing 11.16 mg ruscogenin) and hesperidin methylchalcone (450 mg/day) on fibrinolytic activity of the vein wall was investigated ex vivo in patients with venous insufficiency.[26] Patients received treatment for 14 days in a double blind, placebo-controlled design: 10 were given active treatment and 10 were given placebo. The fibrinolytic activity of the intima of the greater saphenous vein was significantly increased in the active group ($p < 0.01$). Activity in the adventitia layer also showed a significant increase after an incubation time of 60 minutes ($p < 0.05$). These results suggest that the combination might reduce the risk of venous thrombosis in patients with varicose veins.

The effect of an extract of butcher's broom on haemorheological parameters was also investigated under double blind, placebo-controlled conditions.[27] Forty-five participants took part in the clinical trial. There were 20 volunteers who acted as a normal, untreated control group, 13 patients with venous insufficiency who received oral doses of butcher's broom extract (amount not specified) and another 12 patients who were given a placebo. Venous blood samples were collected before and after 30 days of treatment, each time before and after 10 minutes of venous stasis induced by a hyperpressure of 10 mmHg. Results demonstrated that butcher's broom treatment was accompanied by a significant improvement in several rheological parameters under these conditions of venous stasis, including a decrease in plasma viscosity ($p < 0.01$), a reduction in red cell deformability ($p < 0.001$), a reduction in red cell aggregation ($p < 0.01$), an increase in red cell aggregation time ($p < 0.01$) and a reduction in the red cell disaggregation shear rate ($p < 0.05$).

Anti-oedema activity

Oral administration of the butcher's broom extract combination inhibited histamine-induced plasma exudation in hamsters with mild diabetes, without affecting blood glucose.[28] In addition to reducing experimentally induced capillary permeability, a combination of butcher's broom extract, hesperidin methylchalcone, methylesculetin and ascorbic acid decreased experimentally induced hyperaemia, UV erythema and dextran or carrageenin local oedemas after either oral dosing or intraperitoneal injection.[29]

The anti-oedematous effect of a combination containing butcher's broom extract and hesperidin methylchalcone was tested in a randomised, double blind study using water plethysmography.[30] Forty patients with permanent oedema caused by chronic venous insufficiency were treated for 15 days orally with 450 mg butcher's broom extract and 450 mg hesperidin methylchalcone (n=20) or placebo (n=20). After placebo, the oedema volume caused by orthostatic stress increased slightly (16.3 mL). However, in patients receiving active treatment the extent of the provoked venous oedema was significantly reduced (53.4 mL, $p < 0.01$).

Other activity

Butcher's broom extract inhibited the activation of endothelial cells induced by hypoxia (which mimics venous blood stasis), as evidenced by its effect on several parameters. Hesperidin methylchalcone was also able to inhibit the hypoxia-induced decrease in ATP content.[31] Butcher's broom extract combination and each of its components demonstrated a dose-dependent protection against hypoxia in endothelial cells in vitro. A synergistic effect between the components was observed.[32]

Pharmacokinetics

The oral bioavailability of butcher's broom extract was found to be 'good' after administration of a radiolabelled extract in an experimental model. The sapogenins were excreted mainly in the urine.[33] The relative bioavailability of butcher's broom extract following oral, intravenous or topical administration was assessed in rats. Absorption was estimated at 65% by the oral route and 25% after topical application. Biliary excretion was also observed, with enterohepatic cycling.[34,35]

The major spirostanol glycosides of butcher's broom (degluconeoruscin and deglucoruscin) were detected in human plasma after oral administration of 1 g of butcher's broom extract. Three healthy volunteers took part in the study.[36]

Clinical trials

Chronic venous insufficiency/varicose veins

More than 30 clinical trials over the past 30 years have demonstrated the benefit of the butcher's broom extract combination in the management of chronic venous insufficiency. A recent meta-analysis included 20 placebo-controlled, randomised, double blind studies, five studies randomised against a comparison treatment and six single-arm surveillance studies.[37] (Several of the individual studies included in this meta-analysis are also reviewed below.) In total there was information from 10 246 patients. On a 4-point symptom severity scale, the butcher's broom extract combination significantly reduced pain severity (0.44 ± 0.12), cramps (0.26 ± 0.08), heaviness (0.53 ± 0.11) and paraesthesia (0.29 ± 0.10) compared with placebo. There was also a significant reduction in venous capacity of $0.7 \pm 0.19 \, \text{mL/100mL}$. Reductions in the severity of oedema and decreases in calf and ankle circumference did not achieve statistical significance. The authors concluded that their analysis was a strong and objective demonstration of the clinical efficacy of the butcher's broom extract combination in chronic venous insufficiency.

A study published after this meta-analysis examined the activity of butcher's broom extract alone. In a well-designed multicentre, double blind, randomised, placebo-controlled trial, 166 women suffering from chronic venous insufficiency received either butcher's broom extract (72 to 75 mg/day of a 15 to 20:1 extract) or a placebo for 12 weeks.[38] Analysis of the 148 women who completed the trial revealed the herbal treatment significantly reduced leg volume, ankle and leg circumferences (all $p < 0.001$) and subjective symptoms such as heavy tired legs ($p = 0.0022$). Tolerability of both treatments was assessed as good to very good. The authors concluded that butcher's broom was a safe and effective treatment for patients suffering chronic venous insufficiency.

Significant decreases in the venous diameter of deep veins (for example $p = 0.02$ for the common femoral vein), a significant increase in flow parameters in these veins ($p = 0.05$) and a non-significant decrease in the flow parameters in superficial veins was observed when 12 patients with primary varicose vein disease were treated with butcher's broom extract combination and assessed in the standing position.[39] Measurements were taken using ultrasonography at baseline, 2 h after the intake of the combination on the first day of the study and at the end of the 7-day study period. (Most of the above venotonic outcomes occurred at the 2-h measurement.) In terms of the primary endpoint (venous diameter of the greater saphenous vein in the supine position after 7 treatment days), the study failed to demonstrate a significant effect. (Two hours was assumed to be the time of the peak concentration of the herbal treatment.)

During a 2-month treatment with butcher's broom extract combination, a significant decrease or regression of clinical symptoms and a reduction in ankle circumference was observed.[40] This randomised, double blind, placebo-controlled trial involved 60 patients with uncomplicated chronic venous insufficiency. Clinical symptoms that were significantly reduced included heavy legs ($p < 0.01$ at 30 and 60 days), tired legs ($p < 0.01$ at 30 and 60 days), sensation of evening oedema ($p < 0.01$ at 30 and 60 days, $p < 0.05$ at 15 days), pain ($p < 0.01$ at 30 and 60 days), pruritus ($p < 0.01$ at 60 days) and cramp ($p < 0.05$ at 30 and 60 days). The reduction in average ankle circumference for the treatment group compared with placebo was significant at the end of the trial ($p < 0.05$). Global assessment of efficacy in the 30 patients in the butcher's broom group showed an excellent result in 15 patients, good in 13 and satisfactory in two. Of the 30 patients receiving placebo, results were rated as excellent in four, good in 17, satisfactory in eight and insufficient in one. The tolerability of butcher's broom extract combination was found to be similar to the placebo.

In a double blind, placebo-controlled, crossover trial, 40 patients with chronic venous disorders of the lower limbs evaluated butcher's broom extract combination.[41] The trial involved two treatment periods of 2 months, with an interim washout phase of 15 days. During active treatment, patients received capsules each day containing butcher's broom extract (99 mg), hesperidin (450 mg) and ascorbic acid (300 mg). An overall tendency for improvement occurred that was more distinct during active treatment than during placebo treatment. Pruritus and plethysmographic parameters changed significantly with active treatment compared to placebo ($p < 0.01$ or $p < 0.05$, depending on the parameter). Tolerability was deemed to be excellent.

A significant improvement in venous tone ($p < 0.05$) was measured after 2 weeks in a randomised, double blind, placebo-controlled trial involving 50 patients with varicose veins.[42] Active treatment consisted of the butcher's broom extract combination. To assess venous function, venous capacity, venous distensibility and expelled blood volume were measured by plethysmography. The authors suggested that, despite the improvements observed, the treatment period was probably too short to obtain a full therapeutic effect since not all parameters achieved statistical significance.

In patients with post-thrombotic syndrome, the median blood velocity in the femoral vein increased by 24% on the diseased side 2 h after the oral administration of butcher's broom extract combination.[43] The ratio of the middle arterial inflow to venous outflow velocities showed a favourable decrease of 40% after medication ($p < 0.05$). Measurements were conducted using ultrasound and the study was an open design, with results compared against baseline.

In a double blind, placebo-controlled trial involving 100 patients, butcher's broom extract combination for a period of 1 to 3 months improved the following symptoms: heavy and painful legs, nocturnal cramps, oedema of the lower limbs.[44] The overall improvement was significant, as measured by global assessment ($p < 0.05$).

A clinical trial comparing the therapeutic efficacy of butcher's broom extract combination with micronised diosmin found the two treatments produced similar effects by the conclusion of the trial (2 months).[45] The onset of action for the butcher's broom extract combination appeared to be earlier, since benefits were observed at 15 days.

In a randomised, multicentre study, butcher's broom extract combination was more effective than hydroxyethyl rutoside after 90 days of treatment for chronic venous insufficiency.[46,47] More rapid and complete regression of symptoms occurred for the butcher's broom group (p<0.01). A significant reduction in the affected limb size was observed in both groups, but only persisted for 90 days with the butcher's broom extract combination (p<0.01).

Several other double blind, placebo-controlled or comparative trials published in the 1980s or early 1990s demonstrated significant clinical benefit for the butcher's broom extract combination in the management of chronic venous insufficiency.[48–51] Similarly, a group of more recent open label trials from Mexico and South America have shown positive clinical outcomes in patients with chronic venous disorders.[52–55]

The safety and efficacy of the butcher's broom extract combination was evaluated in a multicentre surveillance study involving 886 cases.[56] After 30 and 60 days of treatment, the number of patients reporting mild and absent symptoms (pain, cramping, paraesthesia, heaviness) was substantially increased. Tolerance was rated as excellent for 85.4% of patients and side effects were reported in 5.6%. These were essentially minor digestive troubles or transient problems that did not necessitate the cessation of treatment except in three cases.

Topical and oral use during pregnancy

A significant reduction in the dilatation of the femoral vein (p<0.05) in pregnancy was observed in an uncontrolled study in 18 women that assessed the use of a butcher's broom cream.[57] Similar beneficial results were also observed in an earlier study.[58]

A therapeutic trial involving 20 pregnant women (21 to 24 weeks) found that the oral use of butcher's broom extract combination improved symptoms of venous insufficiency and was innocuous to the fetus, as assessed by the usual clinical and ultrasonographic criteria of pregnancy surveillance, including umbilical artery flow and the state of the infant and placenta following birth.[59] In a much larger earlier study, the efficacy and tolerability of the butcher's broom extract combination were assessed in an uncontrolled multicentre clinical trial.[60] The product was administered for 2 months to 214 women who presented with chronic venous insufficiency as a result of their pregnancy. Symptoms (including pain, cramps and paraesthesia) and signs (such as varices and oedema) were significantly improved compared to baseline at 30 and 60 days of treatment (no p values were provided). Tolerability was rated as excellent, with only nine patients reporting mild gastrointestinal or skin reactions. No information regarding pregnancy outcomes was provided.

Varicose ulcers

In a randomised, double blind trial, 23 patients with venous leg ulcers were treated over a period of 6 weeks with six capsules daily of the butcher's broom extract combination (n=12) or a placebo (n=11).[61] The treatment was in addition to basic ulcer therapy. In the placebo group five patients did not show any improvement or healing of the ulcer during the observation period, whereas in 11 of 12 patients treated with the active combination the ulcer area was markedly reduced (p<0.001). Parallel to the change in the ulcer size,

venous haemodynamics were improved and venous drainage increased significantly (p<0.05). The results showed that this additional therapy favourably affects the healing rate of venous ulcers.

Lymphoedema

Fifty-seven patients with secondary lymphoedema of the upper limb after previous treatment for breast cancer participated in a double blind, placebo-controlled trial of butcher's broom extract combination for a period of 3 months. All patients also underwent manual lymphatic drainage twice a week for at least 1 month. A significant reduction in the volume of arm oedema (12.9%, p<0.01) was observed in the treatment group compared with placebo. Decreased oedema was more marked in the forearm compared to the upper arm, where there was increased fat deposition.[62]

Haemorrhoids

The efficacy of butcher's broom extract combination for the treatment of acute attacks of haemorrhoids was investigated in an open label multicentre study.[63] One hundred and twenty-four patients were treated for 1 week. The treatment protocol was six capsules of the combination daily for the first 3 days, then four capsules daily. Each capsule contained 150 mg of butcher's broom extract, 150 mg of hesperidin methylchalcone and 100 mg of ascorbic acid. Parameters studied were painful symptoms (discomfort, sensation of heaviness, burning, pruritus, tenesmus), accompanying symptoms (rectal bleeding, altered intestinal motility, abdominal pains), local signs (prolapse, congestive state, inflammation), overall severity score of symptoms and clinical efficacy and safety. Analysis of results demonstrated a statistically significant decrease in all scores between day 0 and day 7. The main results were: an average decrease of 4.9 points in painful symptoms (p=0.0001 compared against baseline), a decrease of 1.3 points in the assessment of accompanying symptoms (p=0.0001), a decrease of 3.6 points in local signs (p=0.0001) and a decrease of 9.8 points in the overall severity score of the symptoms (p=0.0001). Sixty-nine per cent of the patients rated the efficacy of the treatment as good or excellent (>75% for the physicians' rating).

Premenstrual syndrome

In a randomised, double blind trial, 40 women suffering premenstrual syndrome received either butcher's broom extract combination (n=20) or an identical placebo (n=20) for 90 days.[64] Mastalgia (p<0.02), menstrual pain (p<0.05) and mood (p<0.05) were significantly improved in the treatment group compared with placebo.

Orthostatic hypotension

It has been postulated that butcher's broom may counter the blood pooling in the lower limbs associated with orthostatic hypotension by virtue of its vasoconstrictive and venotonic properties.[65]

Diabetic retinopathy

The effects of a combination of buckwheat leaf (1.5 g/day) and troxerutin (90 mg/day) or butcher's broom extract (75 mg/day) on ophthalmological and biochemical parameters in patients with non-proliferative diabetic retinopathy were compared with that of the synthetic rutin derivative troxerutin (1 g/day).[66] During the study period of 3 months, 60 diabetic patients were divided into three equal groups: group I received troxerutin, group II received butcher's broom and group III received buckwheat plus troxerutin. The amplitude of oscillating potentials decreased in patients receiving only the troxerutin, and increased in group II and III patients. Regression of changes in the fundus of the eye was demonstrated in 23.1% to 27.8% of all treated patients; however, deterioration in 5.6% of patients in group I, 3.3% of those in group III and none in group II was also observed. Troxerutin seemed to be less effective than the herbs, especially when oscillating potentials were considered.

Toxicology and other safety data

Toxicology

The following LD_{50} data have been recorded for butcher's broom extract and its constituents:

Substance	Route, model	LD_{50}	Reference
Butcher's broom rhizome, fluid extract	Oral, mice	4.6 g/kg*	67
Butcher's broom rhizome, fluid extract	Oral, rat	>4.6 g/kg*	67
Ruscogenins (ruscogenin, neoruscogenin)	Oral, mice	>3.0 g/kg	9
Ruscogenins (ruscogenin, neoruscogenin)	Oral, rats	>3.0 g/kg	9

*Value expressed as dried herb equivalent.

Intravenous administration of dried butcher's broom extract to dogs resulted in a slowing of the heart rate, a marked drop in arterial pressure, and at high doses increased respiration and blood glucose levels. Intraperitoneal doses of 1.5 to 2.0 g/kg of dried ethanolic extract of butcher's broom were lethal in guinea pigs. The authors estimated that the upper level of a safe dose for a human would be about 10 g of extract by injection.[68]

Prolonged oral administration of high doses (300 mg/kg) of saponosides, prosapogenins and ruscogenins isolated from butcher's broom were well tolerated by rats.[9]

Contraindications

Because of the irritant effect of the saponins, butcher's broom should not be applied to broken or ulcerated skin.

Special warnings and precautions

The use of herbs rich in saponins is possibly inappropriate in coeliac disease, fat malabsorption and vitamin A, D, E and K deficiency, and some upper digestive irritations. Saponin-containing herbs are best kept to a minimum in patients with pre-existing cholestasis.

Interactions

None identified in the literature.

Use in pregnancy and lactation

Category B1 – no increase in frequency of malformation or other harmful effects on the fetus from limited use in women. No evidence of increased fetal damage in animal studies.

Animal studies have not produced any evidence of embryotoxic activity for butcher's broom extract. Butcher's broom combined with sweet clover (*Melilotus officinalis*) or hesperidin methylchalcone has been used topically to treat varicose veins in pregnant women.[57,67] An uncontrolled trial (noted earlier) observed that oral administration of butcher's broom combined with hesperidin methylchalcone and ascorbic acid to pregnant women (21 to 24 weeks' gestation) had no adverse effect on their infants. The 20 women involved in the study received the herbal treatment for at least 6 weeks and not more than 13 weeks. Postprandial digestive heaviness was noted by eight patients and was ascribed to the herbal treatment.[59]

The herb is rated as compatible with breastfeeding.

Effects on ability to drive and use machines

No adverse effects expected.

Side effects

As with all herbs rich in saponins, oral use may cause irritation of the gastric mucous membranes and reflux. The use of an enteric-coated preparation is preferred in sensitive patients.

Contact allergy to ruscogenins occurs rarely, but may be underestimated. In the 10 years to 1998 eight cases were reported to the French medical authorities.[69] Contact allergy to butcher's broom extract has also been reported.[70,71] In one of these cases the cream contained butcher's broom extract and the excipient thimerosal, and positive patch test results were obtained for both ingredients.[70]

Adverse reactions associated with the oral intake of butcher's broom extract combined with hesperidin methylchalcone and ascorbic acid have been reported. In particular, lymphocytic colitis (one case associated with ileal villous atrophy and most with chronic diarrhoea) were observed, many after long-term use of the product.[72–75] Faecal fluid measurements were not consistent with an osmotic mechanism.[75] Other cases of chronic diarrhoea[76–79] including diarrhoea without mucus or blood,[80] and watery diarrhoea mimicking coeliac disease, have been reported.[81] These earlier reports are probably also cases of lymphocytic colitis that were recorded before this association was more widely recognised. The lymphocytic colitis may be secondary to a chronic activation of the mucosal immune system by one or several components of the combination.[82] It has not been determined if the butcher's broom extract is implicated in this adverse reaction.

A case of cytolytic hepatitis associated with the ingestion of a preparation containing ruscogenins, hesperidin, ascorbic acid and aesculetol has been reported.[83]

All the clinical trials noted previously indicate that the risk of side effects for butcher's broom is relatively low and that such side effects are likely to be minor.

Overdosage

No incidents found in the literature.

Safety in children

No information available.

Regulatory status in selected countries

In the UK butcher's broom is not included on the General Sale List. In Germany it is covered by a positive Commission E Monograph. Butcher's broom is official in the *European Pharmacopoeia* 2006.

In the USA butcher's broom does not have GRAS status. However, it is freely available as a 'dietary supplement' in the USA under DSHEA legislation (Dietary Supplement Health and Education Act of 1994).

In Australia butcher's broom is not included in Part 4 of Schedule 4 of the Therapeutic Goods Regulations and is freely available for sale.

References

1. Mabberley DJ. *The Plant Book*, 2nd ed. Cambridge: Cambridge University Press; 1997. p. 628.
2. Chiej R. *The Macdonald Encyclopedia of Medicinal Plants*. London: Macdonald; 1984. Entry No. 269.
3. Grieve M. *A Modern Herbal*, Vol 1. New York: Dover Publications; 1971. pp. 128–129.
4. Leclerc H. *Précis de Phytothérapie*, 5th ed. Paris: Masson; 1983. pp. 46–47.
5. Wagner H, Bladt S. *Plant Drug Analysis: A Thin Layer Chromatography Atlas*, 2nd ed. Berlin: Springer-Verlag; 1996. p. 309.
6. Dunouau C, Bellé R, Oulad-Ali A, et al. *Planta Med*. 1996;62:189–190.
7. Domange JR, Bougaret S, Yubero L. *Clin Hemorheol*. 1994;14(suppl 1):S7–S13.
8. Chevillard L, Ranson M, Senault B. *Med Pharmacol Exp*. 1965;12(2):109–114.
9. Capra C. *Fitoterapia*. 1972;43(4):99–113.
10. Facino RM, Carini M, Stefani R, et al. *Arch Pharm (Weinheim)*. 1995;328(10):720–724.
11. Huang YL, Kou JP, Ma L, et al. *J Pharmacol Sci*. 2008;108(2):198–205.
12. Bouskela E, Cyrino FZ, Marcolon G. *J Cardiovasc Pharmacol*. 1993;22(2):221–224.
13. Bouskela E, Cyrino FZ, Marcolon G. *J Cardiovasc Pharmacol*. 1994;24(2):281–285.
14. Bouskela E, Cyrino FZ, Marcolon G. *J Cardiovasc Pharmacol*. 1994;24(1):165–170.
15. Marcelon G, Vanhoutte PM. *Phlebology*. 1988;3(suppl 1):51–54.
16. Miller VM, Rud K, Gloviezki P. *Clin Hemorheol*. 1994;14(suppl 1):S34–S37.
17. Anon. *Dtsch Apoth Ztg*. 1985;125(6):295.
18. Rubanyi G, Marcelon G, Vanhoutte PM. *Gen Pharmacol*. 1984;15(5):431–434.
19. Barton D, Ollis WD, eds. *Advances in Medicinal Phytochemistry*. London: John Libbey Eurotext; 1986. pp. 187–194.
20. Bouskela E, Cyrino FZ, Bougaret S. *Clin Hemorheol Microcirc*. 1997;17(5):351–356.
21. Miller VM, Rud K, Gloviczki P. *Clin Hemorheol*. 1994;14(suppl 1):S37–S45.
22. Nemcova S, Gloviczki P, Rud KS, et al. *J Vasc Surg*. 1999;30(5):876–883.
23. Miller VM, Marcelon G, Vanhoutte PM. *Phlebology*. 1991;6(4):261–268.
24. Berg D. *Fortschr Med*. 1990;108(24):473–476.
25. Rudofsky C. *Fortschr Med*. 1989;107(19):52. 55–58
26. Haas S, Lill G, Stiller A, et al. In: Vanhoutte PM, ed. *Return Circulation and Norepinephrine: An Update*. Paris-London: John Libbey Eurotext; 1991. pp. 157–162.
27. Le Devehat C, Khodabandehlou T, Vimeux M, Bondoux G.. In: Vanhoutte PM, ed. *Return Circulation and Norepinephrine: An Update*. Paris-London: John Libbey Eurotext; 1991. pp. 225–236.
28. Svensjo E, Bouskela E, Cyrino FZ, et al. *Clin Hemorheol Microcirc*. 1997;17(5):385–388.
29. Tarayre JP, Lauressergues H. *Ann Pharm Franc*. 1976;34:375–382.
30. Strauss AL, Rieger H. *Phlebologie*. 1992;21:247–251.
31. Bouaziz N, Michiels C, Janssens D, et al. *Int Angiol*. 1999;18(4):306–312.
32. Baurain R, Dom G, Trouet A. *Clin Hemorheol*. 1994;14(suppl 1):S15–S21.
33. Benard P, Cousse H, Rico AG, et al. *Ann Pharm Fr*. 1986;43(6):573–584.
34. Chanal JL, Mbatchi B, Sicart MT, et al. *Trav Soc Pharm Montpellier*. 1981;41(4):263–272.
35. Chanal JL, Cousse H, Sicart MT, et al. *Trav Soc Pharm Montpellier*. 1978;38(1):43–48.
36. Rauwald HW, Grunwidl J. *Planta Med*. 1991;57(suppl 2):A75–A76.
37. Boyle P, Diehm C, Robertson C. *Int Angiol*. 2003;22(3):250–262.
38. Vanscheidt W, Jost V, Wolna P, et al. *Arzneimittelforschung*. 2002;52(4):243–250.
39. Jager K, Eichlisberger R, Jeanneret Ch, et al. *Clin Drug Invest*. 1999;17(4):265–273.
40. Parrado F, Buzzi A. *Clin Drug Invest*. 1999;18(4):255–261.
41. Cappelli R, Nicora M, Di Perri T. *Drugs Exp Clin Res*. 1988;14(4):277–283.
42. Weindorf N, Schultz-Ehrenburg U. *Z Hautkr*. 1987;62(1):28–38.
43. Marshall M. *Fortschr Med*. 1984;102(29–30):772–774.
44. Elbaz C, Nebot F, Reinharez D. *Phlebology*. 1976;29(1):77–84.
45. Monteil-Seurin J. *C R Ther Pharmacol Clin*. 1993;109:3–7.
46. Beltramino R, Penenory A, Buceta AM. *Int Angiol*. 1999;18(4):337–342.
47. Beltramino R, Penenory A, Buceta AM. *Angiology*. 2000;51(7):535–544.
48. Rudofsky G, Diehm C, Gruss JD, et al. *MMW*. 1990;132:205–210.
49. Le Devehat C, Lemoine A, Roux E, et al. *Angiologie*. 1984;34(3):119–122.
50. Lozes A, Boccalon H. *Int Angiol*. 1984;3:99–102.
51. Braun R, Hirche H, Van Laak H-H. *Z Allgemeinm*. 1985;61:309–313.
52. Guex JJ, Avril L, Enrici E, et al. *Int Angiol*. 2010;29(6):525–531.
53. Guex JJ, Enriquez Vega DM, Avril L, et al. *Phlebology*. 2009;24(4):157–165.
54. Porto CL, Milhomens AL, Pires CE, et al. *Int Angiol*. 2009;28(3):222–231.
55. Guex JJ, Enrici E, Boussetta S, et al. *Dermatol Surg*. 2008;34(12):1666–1675.
56. Leutenegger E, Martinaggi P. *Gazette Med*. 1988;95(13):66–69.
57. Berg D. *Fortschr Med*. 1992;110(3):67–68. 71–72.
58. Berg D. In: Vanhoutte PM, ed. *Return Circulation and Norepinephrine: An Update*.

Paris: John Libbey Eurotext; 1991. pp. 55–61.

59. Baudet JH, Collet D, Aubard Y, et al. In: Vanhoutte PM, ed. *Return Circulation and Norepinephrine: An Update*. Paris: John Libbey Eurotext; 1991. pp. 63–71.

60. Leutenegger E, Martinaggi P. *Gazette Med*. 1988;95(33):83–85.

61. Leyh F. *Therapiewoche*. 1988;36: 2325–2331.

62. Cluzan RV, Alliot F, Ghabboun S, et al. *Lymphology*. 1996;29(1):29–35.

63. Bennani A, Biadillah MC, Cherkaoui A, et al. *Phlebologie*. 1999;52(1):89–95.

64. Monteil-Seurin J, Ladure Ph. Efficacy of Ruscus extract in the treatment of the premenstrual syndrome. In: Vanhoutte PM, ed. *Return Circulation and Norepinephrine: An Update*. Paris: John Libbey Eurotext; 1991. pp. 43–53.

65. Redman DA. *J Altern Complement Med*. 2000;6(6):539–549.

66. Archimowicz-Cyrylowska B, Adamek B, Drozdzik M, et al. *Phytother Res*. 1996;10(8):659–662.

67. Seidenberger AV, Muller I, Heindl HJH. *Therapiewoche*. 1974;24(8):866–881.

68. Caujolle F, Meriel P, Stanislas E. *Ann Pharm Fr*. 1953;11:109–120.

69. Elbadir S, El-Sayed R, Renaud F, et al. *Rev Fr Allergol*. 1998;38(1):37–40.

70. Breuil K, Patte F, Meurice JC, et al. *Rev Fr Allergol Immunol Clin*. 1989;29(4):215.

71. Landa N, Aguirre A, Goday J, et al. *Contact Dermatitis*. 1990;22(5):290–291.

72. Dharancy S, Dapvril V, Dupont-Evrard F, et al. *Gastroenterol Clin Biol*. 2000;24(1):134–135.

73. Pierrugues R, Saingra B. *Gastroenterol Clin Biol*. 1996;20(10):916–917.

74. Bouaniche M, Chassagne P, Landrin I, et al. *Rev Med Interne*. 1996;17(9):776–778.

75. Ouyahya F, Codjovi P, Machet MC, et al. *Gastroenterol Clin Biol*. 1993;17(1):65–66.

76. Mornet M, Boiserie P, Jonville AP, et al. *Therapie*. 1991;46(3):254.

77. Anon. *Presc Int*. 1993;2(7):123.

78. Gendreau-Tranquart C, Barbieux JP, Furet Y, et al. *Presse Med*. 1989;18(29):1439.

79. Oliver JM, Bacq Y, Dorval ED, et al. *Gastroenterol Clin Biol*. 1991;15(2): 160–162.

80. Thomas-Anterion C, Guy C, Vial F, et al. *Rev Med Interne*. 1993;14(4): 215–217.

81. Widgren S, De Peyer R, Geissbuhler P, et al. *Schweiz Med Wochenschr*. 1994;124(8):313–318.

82. Beaugerie L, Luboinski J, Brousse N, et al. *Gut*. 1994;35(3):426–428.

83. Sgro C, Taque R, Zoll A, et al. *J Hepatol*. 1995;22(2):251.

Chamomile, German

(*Matricaria recutita* (L.) Rauschert)

Synonyms

Matricaria chamomilla L., *Chamomilla recutita* (L.) Rauschert (botanical synonyms), German chamomile, wild chamomile, matricaria (Engl), Matricariae flos (Lat), Kamillenblüten, Feldkamille (Ger), fleur de camomile, matricaire (Fr), camomilla (Ital), kamille (Dan).

What is it?

A number of plants have 'chamomile' as part of their common name, such as the corn chamomile (*Anthemis arvensis*). Although sweet or Roman chamomile (*Chamaemelum nobile = Anthemis nobilis*) is also used medicinally, the German chamomile (*Matricaria recutita*) is the medicinal chamomile covered by this monograph. German chamomile has been known and utilised since ancient times: the flower heads were widely included in pharmaceutical and medicinal preparations, beverages and cosmetics, and the essential oil in perfumery. In the Mediterranean it is common to order chamomile tea in restaurants or bars, even in a concentrated 'espresso' form. The Eclectic physicians preferred the use of German over Roman chamomile; the latter is also known to cause allergic reactions such as contact dermatitis and anaphylaxis. The use of German chamomile chemotypes rich in bisabolol (levomenol) is preferred, as this will confer maximum anti-inflammatory and spasmolytic activities.

Effects

Anti-inflammatory; inhibits spasm in the digestive tract; inhibits the occurrence of ulceration; promotes wound healing; stimulates skin metabolism.

Traditional view

Chamomile was considered to have two specific fields of action: the nervous system (as a calming treatment) and the gastrointestinal tract (decreasing irritation and as a carminative and spasmolytic). It is believed to affect both sensory and motor nerves and was used to treat nervous manifestations of dentition, and conditions with a morbid susceptibility to pain. Other important applications were amenorrhoea and nervous conditions involving the gastrointestinal tract. Large doses of chamomile infusion produce free diaphoresis, which was even said to relieve dysmenorrhoea and prevent clotting.[1] Chamomile was also considered to be anticatarrhal and used to treat catarrhal conditions of the ears, nose and eyes.[1,2] It was commonly employed in external applications for haemorrhoids, mastitis, mammary abscess, leucorrhoea and leg ulcers. The traditional use in children indicates chamomile

was considered a very gentle and safe herb.[2,3] Eclectic physicians also prescribed chamomile for therapeutic use during pregnancy.[1]

Summary of actions

Anti-inflammatory, spasmolytic, mild sedative, antiulcer, carminative, vulnerary, diaphoretic.

Can be used for

Indications supported by clinical trials

- Topical application: eczema, including neurodermatitis; wound healing.
- Internal use: anxiety, non-specific gastrointestinal complaints; in combination with pectin for the treatment of acute, non-complicated diarrhoea; in combination with dong quai for treatment of menopause; in combination with other herbs for the treatment of infantile colic.

Traditional therapeutic uses

Flatulent and nervous dyspepsia, travel sickness, nervous diarrhoea; nasal catarrh; dysmenorrhoea, amenorrhoea; restlessness and anxiety; during dentition.

May also be used for

Extrapolations from pharmacological studies

Spasm or ulceration of the gastrointestinal tract; restlessness, anxiety, mild sleep disorders.

Other applications

Cosmetics (for sensitive skin, anti-inflammatory and anti-acne products), bath preparations and hair care products.[4]

Preparations

Infusion of dried herb or liquid extract for internal use; infusion of dried herb, liquid extract or essential oil for external use or as an ingredient in ointments, creams, bath additives, mouthwashes and sprays. As with all essential oil-containing herbs, use of the fresh plant or carefully dried herb is advised. Keep covered when infusing the herb to retain the essential oil.

Topical use studies have generally used chamomile extracts from high-bisabolol chemotypes. Given the pharmacological properties of (–)-alpha-bisabolol and matricine (chamazulene), it is important to prefer these varieties.

Dosage

- 2 to 4g three times per day of dried flower heads or in an infusion
- 3 to 6mL/day of 1:2 liquid extract, 7 to 14mL/day of 1:5 tincture; 50% ethanol is the preferred extraction solvent
- Infusions or semisolid preparations containing 3% to 10% (w/w) of the flowers or equivalent for external use as a compress, wash or gargle.

Duration of use

No restriction on long-term use.

Summary assessment of safety

Except in extremely rare cases of allergy and contact dermatitis in susceptible patients, chamomile is a safe herb.

Technical data

Botany

Matricaria recutita, a member of the Compositae (Asteraceae, daisy) family, is an annual that can grow as tall as 1m in the right soil (usually up to 60cm). The alternate leaves are bipinnatisect, delicately lobed and thread-like, ending in a point. The flower consists of 12 to 16 white ligules (ray florets, 10 to 15mm long) surrounding the central mound of tiny yellow flowers (disc florets, five-lobed), which are embedded in a hollow, conical receptacle. The flower head is 1.2 to 2.4cm in diameter. The light-coloured fruits are very small achenes, without outside oil glands.[5,6]

Adulteration

There has been much contention over the appropriate botanical classification of chamomile. There are various genotypes and it is also easily confused with related species of similar appearance or odour, especially from the genera Anthemis, Matricaria, Chamomilla, Chrysanthemum and Tanacetum. One authoritative review of the literature suggested that most cases of allergic contact dermatitis involving chamomile may actually be from related species, particularly *Anthemis cotula* (stinking dog fennel), which contains much higher levels of a particularly potent potential allergen, anthecotulide.[7,8]

Key constituents

- Essential oil (0.5% to 1.5%), containing (–)-alpha-bisabolol (also known as levomenol), chamazulene, bisabolol oxides A, B, C and cis- and trans-en-yn-dicycloethers.[9] The

intensely blue phytochemical chamazulene is an artefact formed from matricine during steam distillation[10]
- Flavonoids (0.5% to 3%), particularly apigenin-7-glucoside, flavonoid aglycones,[9] coumarins (herniarin and umbelliferone), phenolic acids, mucilage,[11] GABA (gamma-aminobutyric acid).[12]

The content of these constituents varies considerably between different chemical races or varieties of chamomile.[13] Weather and where the plant is grown also affect the content and composition of the essential oil.[14,15] The *British Pharmacopoeia* recommends that chamomile contain not less than 4mL/kg of blue essential oil.[16]

(–)-α-Bisabolol

cis-En-yn-dicycloether

Matricine

Chamazulene

Apigenin-7-glucoside

	R
Herniarin	CH$_3$
Umbelliferone	H

Pharmacodynamics

Anti-inflammatory activity

Chamazulene inhibited the formation of leukotriene B4 in intact neutrophils in a dose-dependent manner and blocked the chemical peroxidation of arachidonic acid. Matricine did not show these effects, even at higher concentrations. Matricine had no effect on cyclo-oxygenase (COX) and 12-lipoxygenase activities in human platelets.[17] However, other in vitro studies have determined that at least part of the anti-inflammatory activity of chamomile extracts is due to constituents that inhibit the formation of 5-lipoxygenase and COX, and have antioxidant activity. Bisabolol and apigenin appear to be responsible for this.[18]

An aqueous chamomile extract inhibited the release of prostaglandin E$_2$ from lipopolysaccharide (LPS)-activated macrophages in vitro. The activity was due to a dose-dependent inhibition of COX-2 activity. Chamomile reduced COX-2 mRNA and protein expression, without affecting COX-1 expression or activity. The species was not defined, but is likely to be *Matricaria recutita*.[19] Apigenin also inhibited COX-2 and nitric oxide synthase (NOS) activity in LPS-activated macrophages.[20]

In terms of a possible influence on cytokine activity, apigenin inhibited LPS-induced interleukin-6 production in macrophages. Oral pretreatment (50 mg/kg) inhibited LPS-induced interleukin-6 and tumour necrosis factor-alpha production in mice.[21]

Oral intake of matricine demonstrated anti-inflammatory activity in the carrageenan test on rat paw.[22] Matricine was nearly as effective as (–)-alpha-bisabolol up to 3 h after oral administration. Chamazulene was significantly less active than both these compounds.[23] Matricine, together with most of the components in chamomile oil but especially bisabolol, demonstrated anti-inflammatory activity when tested topically on skin.[24]

(–)-alpha-Bisabolol demonstrated anti-inflammatory activity in a number of experimental inflammatory models: rat paw oedema, adjuvant arthritis of the rat, ultraviolet erythema of the guinea pig and yeast fever in rats.[25] *cis*-En-yn-dicycloether inhibited the development of dextran-induced oedema in rats.[26] Several polysaccharides in chamomile have demonstrated anti-inflammatory activity when applied topically.[27]

The anti-inflammatory activity of an aqueous-alcoholic extract of fresh chamomile, an aqueous-alcoholic extract of dried chamomile, the essential oil and isolated components of the essential oil were investigated by topical administration using croton oil-induced dermatitis in mouse ear. The extract prepared from dried flowers showed a mild but significant anti-inflammatory activity (24%), but the extract based on fresh chamomile was more active (32%) and equalled the activity of the reference drug, benzydamine. The essential oil solution did not show any significant inhibition of oedema. The anti-inflammatory activity of apigenin was 10 times higher than matricine, which was 10 times higher than chamazulene. The differences in anti-inflammatory activity of the various preparations might be attributable to the varying concentrations of matricine.[28]

An aqueous-alcoholic extract of dried chamomile demonstrated a significant reduction of oedema (23.4%) compared with controls after topical administration to mice in the croton oil ear test. The non-steroidal anti-inflammatory agent benzydamine produced a similar reduction at a dose corresponding to twice its usual clinical dose. Hydrocortisone was the most active agent (56.4%).[29] Anti-inflammatory effects were demonstrated for topical administration of standardised chamomile extract, the flavone fraction and isolated flavones (apigenin, luteolin and quercetin) in the same model. The lipophilic flavone fraction demonstrated stronger activity than the total chamomile extract, and the action of apigenin was superior to the reference drugs indomethacin and phenylbutazone.[30]

The anti-inflammatory efficacies of topical compounds were measured directly and objectively on the skin of healthy volunteers using the Tesafilm stripping technique. Three pharmaceutical formulations were investigated: a chamomile cream, its cream base and a hydrocortisone ointment. Chamomile cream exhibited 70% of the activity of the hydrocortisone ointment.[31] Experimentally induced toxic contact dermatitis was topically treated with a chamomile ointment and compared with ointment base and 1% hydrocortisone acetate. The chamomile ointment demonstrated a superior soothing effect in comparison to the cortisone cream on human skin.[32]

Spasmolytic activity

Chamomile extract and some of its constituents demonstrated a dose-dependent spasmolytic effect on isolated guinea pig ileum. (–)-alpha-Bisabolol, bisabolol oxides A and B and chamomile oil showed a papaverine-like antispasmodic activity, with the essential oil showing the lowest effect. The *cis*-en-yn-dicycloether component also showed activity, although it was not dose dependent. The flavones apigenin, luteolin, patuletin and quercetin demonstrated marked antispasmodic effects, with apigenin significantly more potent than the other flavones, but less active than papaverine. The coumarins only demonstrated a weak effect.[33] Freeze-dried, ethanol-free extract of chamomile completely blocked slow wave activity in isolated mouse small intestine.[34] Inhibition of cAMP phosphodiesterase was a likely mechanism for the spasmolytic activity.[35]

Spasmolytic activity has also been observed following oral administration of apigenin.[36] *cis*-En-yn-dicycloether demonstrated a more pronounced antispasmodic effect than papaverine on isolated guinea pig and rabbit intestine.[26] Chamomile extract (25 mL/L)[37] and chamomile oil (0.2 mL diluted in 400 mL methanol)[38] inhibited acetylcholine- and histamine-induced contractions in guinea pig ileum in vitro.

Chamomile extract showed moderate inhibitory activity in experimentally induced hyperperistalsis. The inhibition (56%) was greater than that of the control drug loperamide (34% at doses of 10 mg/kg). Rats were treated orally with the methanol extract of the aerial parts (5:1, 300 mg/kg).[39]

Sedative and CNS activity

Several fractions from the aqueous extract of chamomile, including apigenin, have demonstrated significant affinity for the central benzodiazepine receptor in vitro. Apigenin also demonstrated clear antianxiety activity (10 mg/kg) and slight sedative activity without muscle relaxant effects after intraperitoneal administration in mice.[40] However, a later study in rats found that apigenin (doses from 0.5 to 10 mg/kg, ip) did not demonstrate antianxiety activity. In vitro investigations suggest that any sedative effect demonstrated in vivo for apigenin (by injection), is not mediated by benzodiazepine receptors.[41] Fractions isolated from the methanol extract of chamomile were able to selectively bind to both central and peripheral benzodiazepine receptors in vitro. The displacing activity on radiolabelled muscimol binding observed for several of the fractions was found to be due to the presence of GABA in micromolar concentrations. The identity of other active compounds was not established. However, some of the fractions not containing GABA produced a statistically significant reduction of locomotor activity in rats after intracerebroventricular injection.[12] Chamomile extract significantly inhibited GAD (glutamic acid decarboxylase) activity in vitro (brain homogenate). GAD is a rate-limiting enzyme that determines GABA levels in normal nervous tissues, such as the brain.[42]

Oral administration of chamomile extract (300 mg/kg) caused a significant shortening in sleep latency in rats. Flumazenil (a benzodiazepine receptor antagonist) at a dose that caused no obvious effect when used alone showed a significant antagonistic effect on the shortening of sleep latency induced by the chamomile extract.[43]

A dried preparation of a chamomile infusion demonstrated a depressive effect on the CNS after intraperitoneal administration in mice. A dose-dependent decrease of basal locomotor activity was observed (90 to 360 mg/kg) without involving motor coordination and muscle relaxation. A significant sleeping-time potentiating effect was only observed at the two highest doses (160 and 320 mg/kg).[44] Inhalation of chamomile oil vapour decreased stress-induced increases in plasma ACTH (adrenocorticotropic hormone) in ovariectomised rats, compared with placebo. The plasma ACTH level decreased further when diazepam was administered with chamomile oil vapour, and the decrease was blocked by flumazenil. This suggests that chamomile oil may have an effect on GABA ergic systems in rat brain and perhaps an activity similar to benzodiazepine agonists.[45]

A series of clinical tests in Japan found that an increase in mental activity was observed just after eating warmed chamomile jelly. There was also a decrease in heart rate and an increase in 'pleasantness' and good mood. Compared with control nights, eating the warmed jelly improved aspects of sleep in men and women. Skin temperature increased more when drinking chamomile tea than when drinking hot water.[46–48] No exact details of dosage were provided in these studies.

The effect of olfactory stimulation on fluency, vividness of imagery and associated mood was studied with 22 volunteers after exposure to either chamomile oil or placebo. Participants were asked to visualise positive and negative images after exposure to one oil then the other. Chamomile oil did not affect the vividness of imagery ratings, but significantly prolonged the time taken for participants to visualise both positive and negative phrases, suggesting a sedative effect. Negative mood ratings following negative phrase presentation were less extreme after chamomile (p=0.042). Overall mood rating was significantly higher (mean=+1) after chamomile compared with placebo (mean=0) (p=0.001).[49]

Co-administration of extract of *Matricaria chamomilla* (25 mg/kg) with morphine (both by ip injection) greatly reduced the development of morphine dependence in rats. Administration of chamomile extract before induction of withdrawal syndrome by naloxone injection inhibited the expression of abstinence syndrome in morphine-dependent animals.[50] Pretreatment with an aqueous-methanolic extract of chamomile (200 mg/kg, ip) increased the latency of seizure onset in experimentally induced seizure in mice.[51]

Antiulcer activity

Chamomile extract demonstrated antipeptic activity in vitro.[52] (–)-alpha-Bisabolol inhibited the occurrence of ulceration induced by indomethacin, stress or ethanol in rats. A decrease in healing time of ulcers was also observed. A standardised chamomile extract also demonstrated ulcer-protective activity.[53] Oral administration of (–)-alpha-bisabolol demonstrated a significant protective effect (p<0.05) against gastric toxicity produced by acetylsalicylic acid in rats.[54] Several more recent studies have confirmed that an aqueous-ethanolic extract of chamomile and alpha-bisabolol can reduce experimentally induced gastric lesions.[55–57] The mechanism of gastroprotection may involve a reduction in oxidation (chamomile extract, alpha-bisabolol),[55,57] and activation of ATP-sensitive potassium channels (alpha-bisabolol).[56]

In an interesting series of experiments, the antiulcerogenic activity of chamomile in rats was compared with a number of other herbs.[58] A liquid aqueous-ethanolic extract of chamomile demonstrated a dose-dependent protection (2.5, 5 and 10 mL/kg, oral) against indomethacin-induced ulcers, but was not as active as many of the other herbs, including licorice and caraway. However, chamomile extract (10 mL/kg, oral) was the most potent herb at decreasing gastric acidity and acid output. It also significantly increased gastric mucin content, activity shared with licorice, St Mary's thistle and caraway.

Antimicrobial activity

Antimicrobial activity has been demonstrated for (–)-alpha-bisabolol in vitro[59] and chamomile oil (<0.05%, v/v) against *Staphylococcus aureus*, *Bacillus subtilis* and *Candida albicans*[60] and for herniarin in the presence of near UV light. Chamomile extracts demonstrated similar activity against *Escherichia*.[61] The growth of *Staphylococcus aureus*, *Streptococcus mutans*, group B Streptococcus and *Streptococcus salivarius* was completely inhibited by chamomile extract at 10 mg/mL. The extract showed strong antibacterial activity against *Bacillus megatherium* and *Leptospira icterohaemorrhagiae*. The effective concentration of each component (alpha-bisabolol, bisabolol oxides, dicycloethers and chamazulene) was much lower when the component was in combination with the others, as in the natural extract, indicating a possible synergistic effect.[62]

The antibacterial activity of chamomile against *Helicobacter pylori* was tested in vitro. Activity ranged from no activity (infusion,[63] aqueous-ethanolic extract standardised for alpha-bisabolol,[64] methanol extract[65]) to some activity (olive oil extract,[66] essential oil,[67] concentrated aqueous-methanolic extract[68]). Test methods varied, making comparison difficult. The methanol extract was described as having no activity (MIC greater than 100 μg/mL). In comparison, the MIC of amoxicillin was 0.002 to 0.06 μg/mL.[65] The MIC_{90} of chamomile olive oil extract (1:10) was 125 mg/mL (no standard comparison),[66] while the MIC for the essential oil was 36 to 70 μg/mL (in comparison, the MIC of amoxicillin was 0.02 μg/mL).[67] (The minimum inhibitory concentration (MIC) is the lowest concentration at which there is no visible bacterial growth. MIC_{90} is the minimum concentration at which 90% of the bacterial growth is inhibited.)

An aqueous-ethanolic extract of chamomile, standardised for alpha-bisabolol, inhibited the growth of *Campylobacter jejuni* by approximately 100% at both 1:25 and 1:100 dilutions. The IC_{50} (for dry weight of herb) against the bacteria was 2 mg/mL. In comparison, the IC_{50} for gentamicin was 0.08 μg/mL. (IC_{50} is the concentration of a compound needed to reduce the growth of an organism by 50%.[64])

Quorum sensing is a process of intercellular communication among bacterial cells, which occurs with the use of signalling molecules. Inhibition of quorum sensing may reduce infections. Chamomile essential oil was ineffective in inhibiting quorum sensing of two sensor strains in vitro.[69]

Chamomile essential oil demonstrated significant virucidal activity towards herpes simplex virus type 2 (HSV-2) in vitro with an IC_{50} of 1.5 μg/mL.[70] The oil was also active against an acyclovir-sensitive HSV-1 strain and against acyclovir-resistant clinical HSV-1 isolates.[71] Chamomile essential oil affected the viruses by interrupting the adsorption of virus onto the host cell.[70,71]

Bisabolol (500 and 1000 μg/mL) achieved 100% inhibition of *Leishmania infantum* promastigote in vitro.[72]

Wound healing, itching

Aqueous extract of chamomile (120 mg/kg/day) in the drinking water of rats resulted in an increased rate of wound contraction, increased wound-breaking strength and hydroxyproline content, and improved histology of experimentally induced wounds.[73] Topical application of chamomile extract accelerated the healing of burns and incisions in rats.[74,75] A chamomile ointment was effective in the treatment of oral mucositis in a hamster model. The ointment contained a fluid extract of chamomile (10%) and tincture of myrrh.[76] The same preparation promoted faster wound healing of tongue lesions compared with topical corticosteroids in rats.[77]

The wound-healing activity of chamomile is closely linked to its anti-inflammatory activity. (–)-alpha-Bisabolol promotes granulation and tissue regeneration.[59] Application of chamomile extract altered the metabolism of guinea pig skin cells, indicating possible stimulation of cellular regeneration and inhibition of inflammation.[78] Extracts of chamomile showed moderate activity in stimulating proliferation and migration of fibroblasts in vitro.[79]

The impact of oral administration of chamomile in reducing experimentally induced itch was investigated in mice. A diet containing 30% (w/w) of dried, powdered chamomile for 11 days reduced itch by about 30%, which was not significant. Of the other extracts tested, significant inhibition of itch occurred for an ethyl acetate extract (dosage adjusted to 30% (w/w) of dried chamomile). Removal of water-soluble substances from the ethanol extract appeared to significantly enhance its antipruritic activity.[80] In the same model, oral administration of ethyl acetate extract of chamomile extract (25:1, 300 mg/kg) combined with antihistamines was more effective for the suppression of scratching behaviour in mice than administration of antihistamines alone. At least part of the antipruritic activity was due to the essential oil, present at approximately 30% in the extract.[81] Topical application of chamomile essential oil (3% oil, 70 μL, daily for six times per week) alleviated some altered immune parameters in mice with experimentally induced atopic dermatitis. The elevation in serum immunoglobulin E (IgE), IgG1 and histamine were significantly reduced compared with control groups. Scratching frequency was significantly lower than in either control group (saline, jojoba oil).[82]

Other activity

Chamazulene and (–)-alpha-bisabolol, within the concentration range 10^{-9} to 10^{-5} M, demonstrated very little influence on histamine release in isolated rat mast cells. At concentrations higher than 10^{-5} M they stimulated histamine release. En-yn-dicycloether exhibited a moderate stimulating effect at concentrations lower than 10^{-4} M and a strong inhibiting effect on histamine release at higher concentrations.[83]

Extracts and infusion (species undefined) of chamomile have shown antioxidant activity in vitro. The activity was moderate compared with other herbs.[84,85] Chamazulene inhibited membrane lipid peroxidation in vitro in a concentration- and time-dependent manner. It also demonstrated hydroxyl radical scavenging activity.[86] Chamomile may protect against global cerebral ischaemia/reperfusion-induced brain injury in rats. Oral administration of methanol extract decreased lipid peroxidation and increased superoxide dismutase, catalase, glutathione and total thiol levels compared with the untreated group. Cerebral infarction area was also significantly reduced in chamomile-treated groups. The activity was dose-dependent (100 to 300 mg/kg body weight, 9.3:1 extract).[87]

Chamomile extract strongly stimulated the proliferation of lymphocytes, as determined by the mixed lymphocyte reaction, an in vitro stimulatory system involving T cell activation.[88]

Diets containing chamomile flower (1.5% and 7%), several chamomile oils (0.2% to 0.35%) or guaiazulene (0.2%) stimulated liver regeneration in rats.[89] Intragastric administration of a mixture of flavonoids of chamomile normalised sphingolipid metabolism in the liver of old rats. (An increase in sphingolipid turnover in the liver is associated with elevation of free radical production and state of chronic inflammation in old age.) Animals were fed 160 mg/kg of a mixture consisting of apigenin, luteolin, apigenin-7-glucoside, luteolin-7-glucoside, isorhamnetin and quercetin.[90] The same mixture and dosage normalised the elevated ceramide content in carbon tetrachloride-damaged livers of rats via neutral sphingomyelinase inhibition and ceramidase activation. Alterations in sphingolipid turnover induced by administration of the flavonoids coincided with the stabilisation of the damaged hepatocyte membranes.[91] This mixture (40 to 80 mg/kg) induced a dose-dependent increase in bile flow and bile acid secretion in adult and old rats. Cholesterol bile secretion was increased and hepatic lipid content reduced in old rats, but not in adult rats.[92]

In a long-term feeding test, the hot water extract of chamomile (500 mg/kg/day) significantly suppressed blood glucose levels in streptozotocin-induced diabetic rats. The hypoglycaemic effect of chamomile was independent of the inhibition of intestinal alpha-glycosidases, but depended on the inhibition of hepatic glycogen phosphorylase. Chamomile extract also showed strong inhibition against aldose reductase in vitro.[93] In the same model, oral administration of an aqueous-ethanolic extract of the aerial parts of chamomile reduced hyperglycaemia and oxidative stress in a dose-dependent manner. Significant results were obtained for daily dosages of 280 and 560 mg/kg (dried herb equivalent). Histological investigation indicated that treatment with chamomile protected the majority of the pancreatic islet cells, in comparison with the control group.[94]

An ethanol extract of chamomile showed weak activity against a cancer cell line in vitro.[95] In another test, a significant decrease in cell viability was observed in several cancer cell lines for chamomile extracts. Chamomile exposure resulted in differential apoptosis in cancer cells.[96] Bisabolol oxide A at a concentration of $10\,\mu M$ inhibited the growth of leukaemia cells in vitro. Combination with 5-fluorouracil further inhibited the growth of leukaemia.[97] Bisabolol oxide A at 5 to $10\,\mu M$ did not exert a cytotoxic action on normal non-proliferative cells (rat thymocytes) in a previous study.[98] Luteolin (5 mg/kg, ip) suppressed prostate tumour growth in mice by inhibiting insulin-like growth factor 1 receptor signalling.[99] Luteolin inhibited platelet-derived growth factor (PDGF)-induced proliferation by inhibiting PDGF receptor phosphorylation in vascular smooth muscle cells.[100] Bisabolol efficiently and selectively induced apoptosis in malignant tumour cells in vitro by targeting lipid rafts on cell membranes.[101]

Chamomile extract stimulated osteoblastic cell differentiation and exhibited an anti-oestrogenic effect on breast cancer cells in vitro, without proliferative effects on cervical adenocarcinoma cells.[102] Using an in vitro tissue culture indicator system, chamomile (species undefined) was found to have weak oestrogen agonist activity and weak progestogenic activity.[103]

An aqueous-ethanolic extract of chamomile was superior to 2.5% sodium hypochlorite solution as a cleaning agent to remove the smear layer of teeth. A smear layer is produced by cutting the enamel or dentin in cavity preparation. Extracted, single-rooted teeth were used for this in vitro investigation. Chamomile extract was not better than sodium hypochlorite solution combined with EDTA (ethylenediaminetetraacetic acid), but was more effective than tea tree oil.[104]

Pharmacokinetics

Chamazulene is formed from matricine in the gut of rats by the action of gastric acid following oral administration.[23] When volunteers were given matricine orally (500 mg, in suspension), peak plasma levels of chamazulene carboxylic acid were determined at 0.9 to $2.2\,\mu g/mL$.[105]

Topical application of radioisotope-labelled (–)-alpha-bisabolol to the skin of nude mice resulted in half the radioactivity being found on the skin, with the remainder present in tissue and organs. Of the level measured in the tissues and organs, 90% was intact (–)-alpha-bisabolol. Further measurements indicated that (–)-alpha-bisabolol penetrated quickly into the skin. Five hours after the topical application, it was displaced from outermost to innermost areas. Hence a fast cutaneous absorption and a long therapeutic effect might be expected from (–)-alpha-bisabolol.[106] In contrast, a similar earlier study found that most of the bisabolol had been metabolised to a polar metabolite. Bisabolol was mainly excreted in the urine in the form of polar metabolites and to a slight extent as carbon dioxide in exhaled air.[107]

Skin penetration studies of the chamomile flavones apigenin, luteolin and apigenin 7-O-beta-glucoside were carried out with nine healthy female volunteers. Apigenin showed the greatest flux (the greatest amount of flavonoid per time and area), followed by luteolin. Penetration of apigenin 7-O-beta-glucoside was negligible. A steady state was attained after 3 h, indicating that the flavonoids penetrated through further skin layers. It was concluded that these flavonoids are not only adsorbed at the skin surface, but penetrate into deeper skin layers.[108,109]

Clinical trials

Eczema, dermatitis and ulceration

Topical application of chamomile preparations helped relieve eczema[110] and varicose eczema.[111] In a survey conducted in the early 1980s, 95% of 2477 general practitioners described good tolerance and therapeutic efficacy for a chamomile cream (containing 2% standardised chamomile extract) in the treatment of eczema.[110] The herbal treatment decreased inflammation[111] and facilitated a reduction in the level of topical corticosteroids used.[110]

Chamomile cream was compared to steroidal and non-steroidal dermal preparations in the maintenance therapy of hand, forearm and lower leg eczema in an open bilateral comparative trial involving 161 patients. During maintenance therapy over 3 to 4 weeks, the chamomile cream showed similar efficacy to 0.25% hydrocortisone and superior activity to the non-steroidal anti-inflammatory agent (5% bufexamac) and a glucocorticoid preparation (0.75% fluocortin butyl ester).[112] After 2 weeks of treatment, a standardised chamomile cream showed mild superiority over 0.5% hydrocortisone cream and marginal improvement compared with placebo in medium-degree atopic eczema. This was a partially blinded, randomised trial carried out as a half-side comparison (one side of the body compared with the other).[113] Eight patients with neuro-dermatitis in the stage of subacute eczema were treated with ointments containing 1% of a carbon dioxide extract of chamomile or 1% hydrocortisone, in a randomised, double blind trial. Global clinical impression was used to assess the results. Hydrocortisone was significantly more effective than chamomile ($p < 0.001$). Nearly all the patients had been pretreated topically with steroids. In cases of pretreatment with weak or moderately potent steroids, hydrocortisone was much more effective than chamomile, but not in patients pretreated with potent or very potent steroids. The carbon dioxide extract contained constituents similar to the essential oil, with the exception of chamazulene, which was absent.[114]

In an open, uncontrolled clinical trial, patients with varicose ulcers were treated with a chamomile ointment alone or the ointment and a chamomile wash. The therapeutic response was good at 83% and 78%, respectively.[115]

Wound healing

Standardised chamomile ointment had similar efficacy to 5% dexpanthenol cream in healing episiotomy wounds in an open, controlled, randomised trial.[116] An open, randomised trial compared several procedures for second degree haemorrhoid treatment and found best results in the group receiving application of a standardised chamomile ointment in conjunction with surgical procedures (ligature and anal dilation).[117]

Chamomile extract demonstrated a statistically significant improvement in wound healing in a double blind, placebo-controlled clinical trial involving 14 patients. The significant decrease in weeping of the wound area and the drying tendency after dermabrasion of tattoos (p<0.05) indicated the therapeutic efficacy of chamomile.[118] In a randomised, single blind, controlled trial involving 48 women, chamomile cream was not statistically more effective than almond cream at reducing erythema and moist desquamation acquired after receiving radiotherapy for breast cancer. However, there was a trend to fewer and later appearances of grade 2 reactions for the chamomile treatment.[119]

A physiotherapist and a medical doctor carried out a small study involving five patients with chronic wounds. The patients were treated with a mixture of chamomile and *Lavandula angustifolia* essential oils in a grape seed oil carrier base and compared with three controls. One of the controls, who had wounds on his left and right legs, started the study as both a control and a member of the experimental group. Fifty-six days into treatment he discontinued conventional treatment and used essential oils only. The recipients of the essential oils did better than those who only received conventional treatments.[120]

Colostomy patients seeking treatment for a peristomal skin lesions were assigned to one of two treatments: hydrocortisone (1%) ointment applied once a day or chamomile compress in an open label trial involving 72 patients.[121] A chamomile solution was prepared by infusing dried and powdered flowers (6g) in 150mL of boiling water for 10 minutes in a closed glass container. The filtered solution was applied to gauze and the compress placed on the wound for 1 hour twice a day. The lesions were evaluated every 3 days for a maximum of 28 days. Lesions healed significantly faster in the chamomile than in the hydrocortisone group (mean time to healing: 8.9 and 14.5 days respectively; p=0.001). Complete healing was achieved in 100% of the chamomile group by day 15, while 76% of the hydrocortisone group achieved complete healing by day 21. Pain intensity and itching were lower in the chamomile group.

Oral inflammation

In an uncontrolled trial involving 36 patients, a chamomile mouthwash provided a cooling and astringent effect in the treatment of chronic oral inflammation, except in the case of glossodynia.[122] A chamomile preparation was used therapeutically and prophylactically as an oral rinse in the treatment of oral mucositis caused by head and neck irradiation and systemic chemotherapy in an uncontrolled trial. Resolution of mucositis was accelerated by the chamomile rinse and prophylactic use was also favourable.[123]

In a double blind, placebo-controlled clinical trial involving 164 patients, a chamomile mouthwash did not decrease the incidence of stomatitis resulting from 5-fluoruracil-based chemotherapy. The mouthwash was administered three times per day for 2 weeks.[124] This may have been too short a period to detect improvement.[125] A later, randomised trial conducted in Iran found that allopurinol

and chamomile mouthwashes were superior to placebo (saline) for the treatment of chemotherapy-induced stomatitis. Both active mouthwashes were equally effective. The chamomile mouthwash was prepared from an infusion (8g powdered flower per 50mL water) and filtered.[126] A case of methotrexate-induced oral mucositis in a patient with rheumatoid arthritis was successfully treated with a chamomile mouthwash. The patient refused standard mouthwash treatment and was instead administered an infusion of *Matricaria recutita* (8g dried flower in 1 litre of boiling water). The suggested dosage was 20mL kept in the mouth or gargled for 1 to 2 minutes and repeated four times daily. By the 13th day the oral mucositis had reduced from grade 3 (oral ulcers, liquid diet only) to grade 2 (oral erythema, ulcers, able to eat solids) and was completely healed within 4 weeks.[127]

Fluid extract of chamomile provided an analgesic effect in patients with aphthous stomatitis and other painful ulcers of the mouth in an open label trial. The analgesic effect was considered excellent by 82% and good by 18% of patients. The efficacy of chamomile was considered excellent in 67% of patients and good in 33%. Pain was assessed using a visual analogue scale and 34 patients were evaluated.[128]

Anxiety

Fifty-seven outpatients with mild to moderate generalised anxiety disorder were randomised via a double blind design to receive chamomile (*Matricaria recutita*) extract or placebo for 8 weeks. Treatment was initiated at one capsule per day for the first week and increased to two per day during the second week. Patients with a 50% reduction or less in total Hamilton Anxiety Rating (HAM-A) score (compared with baseline) were increased to three capsules per day during week 3, and then to four per day during week 4. Patients who continued to only have a 50% reduction or less in baseline HAM-A score were increased to five capsules/day during weeks 5 to 8. The chamomile extract (220mg/capsule, undefined strength) was standardised to contain 1.2% apigenin. There was a significantly greater reduction over time in the mean total HAM-A score for chamomile versus placebo (p=0.047). Secondary outcomes included changes in the Beck Anxiety Inventory, Psychological Well Being and Clinical Global Impression Severity scores and the proportion of patients with 50% reduction or more in baseline HAM-A score. There were no statistically significant differences observed between the groups for any secondary outcome measure. One patient in each treatment group discontinued therapy because of adverse events. The proportion of patients experiencing adverse events was not significantly different between groups (p=0.417).[129]

Gastrointestinal conditions

In an uncontrolled study, 104 patients with non-specific gastrointestinal complaints (probably functional dyspepsia) were treated with an aqueous-ethanolic preparation of chamomile (standardised for alpha-bisabolol and apigenin-7-glucoside) at 25 drops four times a day (in a cup of hot water) for a period of 6 weeks. The following symptoms were assessed: stomach and abdominal pain, burping, fullness, heartburn, loss of appetite, nausea and vomiting. Symptoms completely disappeared in 44.2% of patients. The success rate for single symptoms ranged from 61% for loss of appetite to 84.5% for stomach and abdominal pain and 88.7% for nausea.[130]

In a prospective, double blind, randomised, multicentre, parallel group study, 79 children with acute, non-complicated diarrhoea received either a preparation containing apple pectin and chamomile extract or placebo for 3 days in addition to the usual rehydration and realimentation diet. At the end of treatment, the diarrhoea had stopped significantly more frequently (p<0.05) in the pectin/chamomile group (85%) compared with the placebo group (58%). The pectin/chamomile combination also significantly reduced the duration of diarrhoea by at least 5.2 h (p<0.05). In contrast to placebo, a trend of continuous improvement was observed by parents for the pectin/chamomile group. The parents expressed their satisfaction more frequently (82%) with pectin/chamomile than with placebo (60%).[131] A follow-up trial (also of double blind design) with a larger number of patients found that the combination significantly reduced stool frequency compared with placebo. This multicentre, randomised trial enrolled 255 children aged between 6 months and 6 years with acute diarrhoea. Two hundred and forty-one children were available for final analysis: 121 received the active medication and 120 received placebo. Stool frequency on the third day was significantly lower in the treatment group compared with placebo (decreases of 49% and 36%, respectively; p=0.0012). Each child also received a glucose-electrolyte solution on the first day of treatment.[132]

The effect of a herbal instant tea preparation containing chamomile, vervain, licorice, fennel and lemon balm on infantile colic was assessed in a prospective, double blind study on babies about 3 weeks old. Tea or placebo up to 150 mL per dose was given to each infant with every episode of colic, but not more than three times a day. After the 7 days of the trial, the colic improvement scores were significantly better in the herbal tea group: 1.7 versus 0.7 for the placebo group (p<0.05). In addition, more babies in the treatment group had their colic eliminated: 57% compared with 26% for placebo (p<0.01).[133] A randomised, double blind, placebo-controlled trial showed that colic in infants improved within 1 week of treatment with a combination of chamomile, fennel (*Foeniculum vulgare*) and lemon balm (*Melissa officinalis*). The preparation also contained vitamin B1, calcium pantothenate and vitamin B6.[134] An experimental study found that the activity of the combination in reducing upper gastrointestinal motility was due to the chamomile and lemon balm.[135]

Other activity

Oral administration of chamomile tea during cardiac catheterisation induced a deep sleep in 10 of 12 patients tested, despite the pain and anxiety experienced from the procedure. The chamomile tea had essentially no cardiac effects.[136]

Fifty-five postmenopausal women were randomly assigned to receive tablets containing *Matricaria recutita* (150 mg/day of an undefined extract) and dong quai (*Angelica sinensis*, 375 mg/day of an undefined extract) or placebo for a period of 12 weeks. There were significant and dramatic differences observed between the study and control groups in terms of the number and intensity of hot flushes (both p<0.001). In the herbal treatment group, a response was already in evidence by the first month (68% reduction of hot flushes during the day and 74% during the night). There was also a marked alleviation of sleep disturbance and fatigue.[137]

Mean scores improved for Conners' hyperactivity, inattention and immaturity factors in three young men (14 to 16 years old) diagnosed with attention-deficit hyperactivity disorder who received treatment with chamomile. Two participants received chamomile for 4 weeks and then placebo for 4 weeks; the others received placebo first followed by chamomile. The observed improvement was lower than reported in stimulant trials, but was similar to that found in non-stimulant trials, such as for desipramine.[138] Treatment with chamomile also led to a slight improvement in irritability and stereotypic behaviour in three male patients with autism. The standardised extract used provided 200 mg/day of alpha-bisabolol.[139]

A randomised, double blind trial found no significant impact on post-operative sore throat and hoarseness for a herbal spray containing standardised chamomile extract administered before intubation, compared with a normal saline spray (placebo). One hundred and sixty-one elective surgery patients were recruited for this study.[140]

Sixty outpatients with uncomplicated common cold were randomly assigned to test whether a chamomile inhalation would provide symptomatic relief in an open label, controlled trial. The control group used a solution containing 35% alcohol, while three different treatment groups used increasing doses of an alcoholic extract of chamomile. The steam inhalation was prepared with boiled water cooled to 50°C, with the chamomile extract then added. Patients inhaled slowly and deeply, breathing through the nose and mouth for 10 minutes, with their heads above the container and below a towel. Chamomile reduced symptoms of the common cold in a dose-dependent manner, especially those of the upper and middle respiratory tract. Onset of action was within 15 minutes, the maximum effect was reached between 20 to 30 minutes. The benefit then declined over 2 to 3 h.[141]

A preliminary study found that use of chamomile baths and a chamomile bladder wash as an adjunct to antibiotic treatment provided a faster alleviation of the symptoms of haemorrhagic cystitis than use of antibiotics alone.[142]

A study in the UK investigated the use of aromatherapy within a healthcare setting for 8058 women in childbirth. A total of 10 essential oils were used, plus carrier oil, and were administered via skin absorption and inhalation. Two essential oils, namely chamomile and clary sage, were effective in alleviating pain.[143] It is not clear whether the oils were administered individually or in combination. They were described only by common name.

A metabonomic strategy was applied to the study of human biological responses to chamomile tea ingestion. Daily urine samples were collected from 14 volunteers during a 6-week period incorporating a 2-week baseline period, 2 weeks of daily chamomile tea ingestion, and a 2-week post-treatment phase. Although strong intersubject variation in metabolite profiles was observed, a clear differentiation between the samples obtained before and after chamomile ingestion was achieved.[144] It was found that depletion of creatinine and elevation of hippurate, glycine and other molecules in urine were strongly associated with chamomile intake. In addition, the metabolic consequences of chamomile ingestion were prolonged in the 2-week post-dosing period, implying a persistent change of resident gut microflora activities. The clinical significance of these findings is not known.

Twenty-five cancer patients with phlebitis from intravenous infusion of antineoplastic chemotherapy were divided into five treatment groups using an open label design.[145] The patients received compresses of chamomile infusion (1.25%, 2.5%, 5.0% or 10.0%) or water (control group) three times a day for 20 minutes each time. Phlebitis (erythema) regression times were significantly shorter for the 1.25%, 2.5% and 5% concentration groups compared with the control group ($p<0.001$). The average regression time for the 2.5% concentration group was 29.2 h versus 110.4 h for the control group.

Toxicology and other safety data

Toxicology

No toxic effects were observed in mice administered up to 1440 mg/kg of a dried preparation of chamomile infusion by intraperitoneal injection. (Reversible depressive effects on the CNS occurred after long-term use at doses beyond 90 mg/kg.) There were no gastrointestinal effects observed in rats for doses up to 5 g/kg.[44] See Table 1 below for LD_{50} values recorded for chamomile essential oil and alpha-bisabolol.

Long-term oral administration of chamomile extract produced no observable toxicity and no teratogenicity in rats. Daily cutaneous application of chamomile to rabbits, or inhalation of chamomile extract by guinea pigs, produced no observable toxicity over 3 weeks.[111]

Chamomile infusion did not show significant genotoxicity in the Somatic Mutation and Recombination Test in *Drosophila melanogaster*, and may have exerted an antimutagenic action against hydrogen peroxide (used as the oxidative genotoxicant in the test).[146] Daunorubicin and methyl methane sulphonate may potentially cause genotoxic damage. Oral administration of chamomile essential oil (5, 50 and 500 mg/kg) to mice demonstrated a dose-dependent inhibitory effect on sister chromatid exchanges produced by daunorubicin and methyl methane sulphonate in bone marrow cells.[147] The methodology of this experiment has been questioned.[148]

The mutagenicity and antimutagenicity of alpha-bisabolol were evaluated in the Salmonella/microsome assay. The phytochemical was not found to be mutagenic and inhibited the effects of aflatoxin B1 and some indirect-acting mutagens. The

antimutagenic effect demonstrated by alpha-bisabolol might be explained, at least in part, by inhibition of the activity of some cytochrome P450 enzymes (CYP1A and CYP2B subfamilies) involved in the metabolic activation of promutagens.[149]

Chamomile essential oil did not cause irritation when applied undiluted to the highly sensitive hen's egg chorioallantoic membrane.[71]

Contraindications

Despite reports of skin reactions and dermatitis from topical use of chamomile, the likelihood of chamomile preparations causing contact allergy is low. However, persons with known sensitivity to other members of the Compositae family (such as ragweed, daisies and chrysanthemums) should avoid topical application of chamomile or chamomile products.

Since ingestion of chamomile has been linked to anaphylaxis, its intake should clearly be avoided in cases of known allergy.

Special warnings and precautions

Best avoided in patients with known hypersensitivity to plants in the Compositae family.

Interactions

The activity of CYP1A2 in the liver microsomes of rats receiving chamomile tea (2%, w/v) was significantly decreased by 39%. No alterations were observed in the activities of CYP2D and CYP3A.[153] The effect of chamomile essential oil and its major constituents on cytochrome P450 enzymes was investigated using microsomes (in vitro). The essential oil inhibited each of the enzymes, with CYP1A2 being more sensitive than the other isoforms. Three constituents of the oil, namely chamazulene, cis-spiroether and trans-spiroether, strongly inhibited CYP1A2, and were active towards CYP3A4. CYP2C9 and CYP2D6 were less affected and only chamazulene and alpha-bisabolol significantly inhibited the latter.[154] The clinical relevance of such in vitro findings is uncertain.

Three cases of an interaction between herbal teas and cyclosporin in renal transplant patients have been reported. The dosages were 2 L/day of herbal tea (containing peppermint (*Mentha piperita*), rose hip (*Rubus fruticosus*), chamomile (*Matricaria recutita*), lemon balm (*Melissa officinalis*), coriander (*Coriandrum sativum*), sandalwood (*Santalum album*), orange peel (*Citrus aurantium*), ratanhia root (*Krameria triandra*) and anise (*Pimpinella anisum*)); 1 to 1.5 L/day of chamomile tea (species undefined), and 'large quantities' of fruit tea containing hibiscus (2%) and rose hip extract (0.1%), and another drink containing black tea extract (1.3%)). The interaction was confirmed by rechallenge in one case, but there were no signs of rejection.[155]

Speculative interactions with NSAIDs and analgesics,[156] antiepileptics[157] and warfarin[158] are based on a misunderstanding of the implications of the coumarin content of the herb. Hence, the following case report needs to be viewed with caution. A patient on warfarin was admitted to hospital with internal haemorrhage. She had been using chamomile tea (five cups/day; one teaspoon dried chamomile leaves) and a

Table 1 LD_{50} data recorded for chamomile essential oil and alpha-bisabolol

Substance	Route, model	LD_{50}	Reference
Chamomile essential oil	Oral, rats	>5 g/kg	150
Chamomile essential oil	Dermal, rabbits	>5 g/kg	150
alpha-Bisabolol	Oral, mice	15.1 mL/kg	151
alpha-Bisabolol	Oral, rats	>5 g/kg	152

chamomile-based body lotion. The patient was taking several drug medications, which were ruled out as the cause of the adverse event by the authors.[159]

A clinical study indicated a potential interaction between *Matricaria recutita* ingestion and reduced iron absorption. An infusion of chamomile reduced the absorption of iron by 47% from a bread meal (compared to a water control) in adult volunteers. The inhibition was dose dependent and related to polyphenol content (phenolic acids, monomeric flavonoids, polymerised polyphenols). Inhibition by black tea was 79% to 94%.[160] A randomised clinical trial conducted in Latin America measured the iron bioavailability of meals based on wheat flour and fortified with ferrous sulphate in 13 women of child-bearing age. In contrast to the above trial, iron absorption from bread given alone or with chamomile infusion was not significantly different. The infusion was sweetened with pan-ela, a traditional unrefined whole sugar cane preparation, and the authors noted that it cannot be discounted that panela may have a promoting effect on iron absorption that could have counteracted any inhibitory effect from the chamomile.[161]

Until further information becomes available, chamomile should not be taken simultaneously with meals or iron supplements in anaemia and cases where iron supplementation is required.

Use in pregnancy and lactation

Category A – no credible proven increase in the frequency of malformation or other harmful effects on the fetus despite consumption by a large number of women.

Chamomile is widely consumed as a tea in many countries and adverse effects on pregnancy have not been credibly documented. Three hundred and 92 Italian women from the maternity wards of two hospitals were interviewed during January to October 2009. One hundred and nine women (27.8%) reported taking one or more herbal products during pregnancy. The most frequently used herbs were chamomile (oral and topical), licorice, fennel, aloe (oral and topical), valerian, Echinacea, almond oil (topical), propolis (oral and inhalatory) and cranberry. Forty women were defined as 'regular users', as they consumed herbs (chamomile, licorice, fennel) every day throughout their pregnancies. A statistically significant difference in morbidities was found between users of herbs and nonusers (52.3% versus 37.8%, p=0.013). Neonates of users were more frequently small for their gestational age (11.9% versus 5.3%, p=0.039). By examining separate herb usage, a higher frequency of threatening miscarriages (21.6%) and preterm labours (21.6%) was observed among the 37 regular users of chamomile.[162] The statistical significance of this finding in such a small group was not provided, and the species of the herbs involved were not verified.

In contrast, after adjusting for potential confounders no association was found in another study between chamomile use in the last two trimesters of pregnancy and prematurity. This was a more rigorous case-control study conducted in Canada involving 3191 women.[163] The species of the herbs were also not verified.

Two cases of premature constriction of the fetal ductus arteriosus have been incorrectly reported as associated with maternal consumption of 'camomile tea'. However, the tea was apparently made from the leaves of *Camellia sinensis*, which is green tea.[164] The authors further confused the issue by discussing the properties of green tea root extract.

Long-term oral administration of chamomile extracts to rats produced no teratogenicity or signs of changes in prenatal development.[165] A herbal formula containing chamomile, sage and yeast plasmolysate did not produce teratogenic effects in rats. The administered dose of chamomile extract was 0.4mL/day.[166,167]

Prenatal development was not affected in rats and rabbits orally administered up to 1mL/kg of alpha-bisabolol. Teratogenic effects were also not observed at this dosage. A dose of 3mL/kg did increase the number of resorptions.[151] alpha-Bisabolol administered orally (250 to 500mg/kg) to pregnant rats had no effect on the fetus.

There is a reference to chamomile infusion having a stimulating effect on the uterus,[168] but the relevance of this to normal human use is uncertain.

Chamomile use is compatible with breastfeeding.

Effects on ability to drive and use machines

No negative influence is expected.

Side effects

An observational study recruited German physicians to evaluate prescribing patterns and adverse reactions (ARs) for remedies containing plants from the Asteraceae (Compositae, daisy) family.[169] From September 2004 to September 2006 all prescriptions and suspected ARs for both conventional and complementary therapies were documented. Thirty-eight physicians participated by reporting any suspected serious ARs, and a subgroup of seven reported minor and serious ARs. Overall assessment of the results concluded that treatment with Compositae-containing remedies is not associated with a high risk of ARs, including allergic reactions. A total of 50 115 patients were evaluated and 344 ARs for conventional and complementary remedies were reported. Altogether, 18 830 patients (58.0% female, 60.3% children) received 42 378 Compositae-containing remedies. The most frequently prescribed were German chamomile (*Matricaria recutita*, 23%), followed by *Calendula officinalis* (20%) and *Arnica montana* (20%, homeopathic). No serious ARs for Compositae-containing remedies were reported and the few minor ARs were not indicative of any increased risk.

Contact allergy and hypersensitivity reactions

Hypersensitivity reactions have been confirmed as the basis for contact dermatitis to chamomile,[170,171] but are relatively rare. Chamomile tea allergy,[172] and contact dermatitis,[173–176] as well as urticaria,[177] including from cosmetics, have been reported.[178] Occasional hypersensitivity reactions, including asthma, to chamomile dust have been reported among tea packers.[179,180] A 20-year-old woman with a proven allergy to chamomile suffered from short-lasting rhinitis when using a chamomile-scented toilet paper. The plant species was not disclosed.[181] Contact dermatitis with asthma and rhinitis was reported in a beautician using chamomile in face masks.[182] Recurrent facial dermatitis from drinking German chamomile tea has been reported.[183]

Chamomile was described as a trigger for eczema as early as 1921. However, varying reports of chamomile causing iatrogenic contact dermatitis have been published since. In a 1936 study on 539 patients, 3.1% displayed sensitivity to chamomile on epidermal testing. No occurrences were reported in 260 patients over a period from 1957 to 1963. From 1964 to 1967, 1.3% of 237 patients demonstrated an adverse reaction to external applications containing chamomile. Other authors concluded that chamomile was not a causative factor in their studies of 265 and 240 cases of iatrogenic contact dermatitis. However, a 1967 report indicated that 7.1% of 338 patients demonstrated contact dermatitis from chamomile preparations. It is unknown whether the chamomile preparation was the single identifiable harmful substance.[184]

Later studies suggest that genuine contact dermatitis from chamomile has a lower incidence. One clinical investigation was undertaken to clarify possible adverse reactions to chamomile preparations. Among 200 patients, 21 (10.5%) reacted positively on epicutaneous tests to chamomile preparations, though only three patients reacted to chamomile extract. Only one patient had exhibited a clinical contact reaction to a chamomile ointment used previously. Of the other 18 patients, 13 had a provable hypersensitivity to the preservatives and five patients probably to ointment bases and/or other constituents of the preparations. The authors felt that genuine chamomile allergy was not as prevalent as first thought.[185]

This conclusion was also supported in a study of 830 patients with contact dermatitis. Only one patient with very high exposure to chamomile tested positive when patch tested with chamomile extract. One hundred and fifty-two patients were tested with chamomile cream and chamomile ointment. Results were negative, even in one patient with oral allergy syndrome and immediate hypersensitivity to many plants, including chamomile.[186]

A high (–)-alpha-bisabolol-containing chamomile extract demonstrated negative results in a contact allergy study in 540 patients with eczema. These results suggest that the extract does not contain allergenic components, such as might be found in other chamomile products.[185] However, allergic contact dermatitis to bisabolol has been reported twice in European adults (1995 and 2008). Bisabolol was also regarded as the likely allergen in three children who presented with recalcitrant atopic dermatitis.[187] The coumarin herniarin, which is present in German chamomile, may also be a sensitiser. Among 36 patients with known or suspected Compositae contact allergy who were patch tested, there was one positive and three doubtful positive reactions to herniarin.[188]

To investigate Compositae dermatitis, sesquiterpene lactones and ether extracts of five European Compositae plants (Arnica, feverfew, German chamomile, yarrow and tansy) were added to routine patch testing of patients over 1 year; 4.5% of the 686 patients demonstrated Compositae sensitivity. Testing with the individual ingredients of the extract in

these 31 Compositae-allergic patients resulted in 75% positive reaction to chamomile.[189] In a later study, patch testing in 190 Danish Compositae-allergic patients found that feverfew caused positive reactions most frequently (81%), followed by tansy (77%), German chamomile (64%), yarrow (41%) and Arnica (23%). A large proportion of the positive reactions to feverfew, tansy and chamomile are likely to be due to chrysanthemum (Dendranthema cultivar) sensitivity, that is they are cross-reactions.[190]

Chamomile allergies are also likely to follow previous sensitisation to mugwort (*Artemisia vulgaris*). Cross-reactivity with mugwort has been confirmed by skin patch tests using chamomile in 21 out of 24 affected individuals. Positive inhalation reactions to chamomile pollen occurred in 16 of these individuals, and positive reactions to oral consumption of chamomile in 13 out of the 24.[191]

A study of 30 patients with atopic dermatitis found that nine were positive in patch tests to a mix of Compositae or Compositae mix and sesquiterpene lactone mix. Five were positive to chamomile. Among Compositae-sensitive patients, 78.8% had other contact allergies, most often to nickel.[192] When chamomile-sensitive patients were patch tested with a range of preparations, although positive reactions occurred most frequently to the plant, fragrances, emulsifiers and preservatives also tested positive. Avocado oil and witch hazel tincture were unexpectedly detected as sensitisers as well.[193]

Allergic conjunctivitis was observed in seven hay fever sufferers who had used chamomile tea as an eyewash; all cases had positive skin tests to chamomile, but there were no reactions after oral consumption. The pollens were judged to be the sensitising components.[194]

The above data suggest that the likelihood of chamomile preparations causing a contact allergy is low, but persons with known sensitivity to other members of the Compositae family should generally avoid contact with chamomile or chamomile products. However, it may be that chamomile is in part a victim of misidentification, as suggested in the Adulteration section above.

Anaphylactic reaction

Severe anaphylaxis occurred in a man 1h after consuming chamomile tea. Laboratory examination demonstrated a total serum IgE of 123kU/L, with specific IgE against chamomile (4.94kU/L, class 3). Skin prick test and labial provocation test with chamomile both showed a strong positive reaction.[195]

Two cases of anaphylactic shock associated with the use of chamomile as an enema have been reported (1998 and 2001). The enemas were prepared using an oily extract of chamomile (*Matricaria recutita*) and tea (species unknown).[196,197] One case of severe anaphylactic reaction was observed in an atopic child after taking chamomile tea for the first time. Mugwort was identified as one of the predisposing allergens.[198]

Over a 2-year period, 14 patients with sensitivity to chamomile (as proven by RAST (radioallergoabsorbent test) and/or the skin prick test) were identified in an allergy unit serving approximately 4000 patients/year. Ten of these patients had a positive history of anaphylaxis to chamomile. The most severe symptoms were observed in two women who had received chamomile-containing enemas, in one case an oily extract of chamomile (case mentioned above). Eleven of the 14 patients exhibited positive RAST and skin prick test reactions to mugwort; six patients had a history of a mugwort-celery-spice syndrome and eight were sensitised to birch pollen. Bet v 1 (homologue of birch pollen allergen) and non-carbohydrate high molecular weight proteins were found to be allergens and responsible for cross-reactivity with other foods and pollen.[199]

Given the widespread consumption of chamomile tea and the few reported cases of anaphylaxis, this type of reaction is quite rare. Moreover, the use of ethanolic extracts denatures the proteins in chamomile and renders this type of reaction unlikely.

Other reactions

One thousand, four hundred and twenty people completed questionnaires regarding their use of herbal medicines from pharmacies in a north-eastern town in Italy. Two consumers noted an adverse reaction (hypotension, tachycardia) to a product containing chamomile, valerian and Melissa.[200] The species of the herbs were not verified.

Overdosage

No incidents found in published literature.

Safety in children

Chamomile is judged as generally benign when taken by children.[201] As discussed above, a chamomile and pectin combination was beneficial for the treatment of diarrhoea in children aged between 6 months and 5.5 years in a placebo-controlled clinical trial.[131]

Regulatory status in selected countries

Chamomile is official in the *European Pharmacopoeia* 7.0 (2011). Chamomile is also listed in the *United States Pharmacopeia-National Formulary* (USP31–NF26, 2008).

Chamomile is covered by a positive Commission E Monograph and has the following applications:

* Externally: inflammation of the skin and mucous membranes and bacterial skin conditions, including those of the mouth and gums
* Inhalations: inflammation and irritation of the respiratory tract
* Baths and washes: complaints in the anal and genital regions
* Internally: gastrointestinal spasms and inflammatory conditions of the gastrointestinal tract.

Chamomile is on the UK General Sale List.

Chamomile and chamomile oil have GRAS status. Chamomile is also freely available as a 'dietary supplement' in the USA under DSHEA legislation (1994 Dietary Supplement Health and Education Act). Chamomile has been present in over-the-counter (OTC) digestive aid drug products. The FDA, however, advises: 'based on evidence currently available, there is inadequate data to establish general recognition of the safety and effectiveness of these ingredients for the specified uses'.

Chamomile is not included in Part 4 of Schedule 4 of the Therapeutic Goods Act Regulations of Australia and is freely available for sale.

References

1. Felter HW, Lloyd JU. *King's American Dispensatory*, ed 18, rev 3, vol 2, 1905. Portland, Reprinted by Eclectic Medical Publications; 1983: pp. 1246–1247.
2. British Herbal Medicine Association's Scientific Committee. *British Herbal Pharmacopoeia*. West York: BHMA; 1983. pp. 139–140.
3. Grieve M. *A Modern Herbal*, Vol 1. New York: Dover Publications; 1971. pp. 187–188.
4. Smeh NJ. *Creating Your Own Cosmetics – Naturally*. Garrisonville: Alliance Publishing; 1995. pp. 81, 82, 137.
5. Chiej R. *The Macdonald Encyclopedia of Medicinal Plants*. London: Macdonald; 1984. Entry no. 191.
6. Launert EL. *The Hamlyn Guide to Edible and Medicinal Plants of Britain and Northern Europe*. London: Hamlyn; 1981. pp. 192–194.
7. De Smet PAGM, Keller K, Hansel R, eds. *Adverse Effects of Herbal Drugs*, Vol 1. Berlin: Springer-Verlag; 1993. pp. 243–248.
8. Hausen BM, Busker E, Carle R. *Planta Med.* 1984;50:229–234.
9. Wagner H, Bladt S. *Plant Drug Analysis: A Thin Layer Chromatography Atlas*, 2nd ed. Berlin: Springer-Verlag; 1996. pp. 159, 199.
10. Schmidt PC, Weibler K, Soyke B. *Dtsch Apoth Ztg.* 1991;131:175–181.
11. British Herbal Medicine Association. *British Herbal Compendium*, Vol 1. BHMA, Bournemouth; 1992. pp. 154–157.
12. Avallone R, Zanoli P, Corsi L, et al. *Phytother Res.* 1996;10(suppl 1):S177–S179.
13. Carle R, Isaac O. *Dtsch Apoth Ztg.* 1985;125(43 suppl 1):2–8.
14. Gosztola B, Sárosi S, Németh E. *Nat Prod Commun.* 2010;5(3):465–470.
15. Orav A, Raal A, Arak E. *Nat Prod Res.* 2010;24(1):48–55.
16. *British Pharmacopoeia vol IV Herbal Drugs, Herbal Drug Preparations and Herbal Medicinal Products – Matricaria Flowers*, 2011 [online].
17. Safayhi H, Sabieraj J, Sailer E–R, et al. *Planta Med.* 1994;60(5):410–413.
18. Ammon HPT, Sabieraj J, Kaul R. *Dtsch Apoth Ztg.* 1996;136(22):17–30.
19. Srivastava JK, Pandey M, Gupta S. *Life Sci.* 2009;85(19–20):663–669.
20. Liang YC, Huang YT, Tsai SH, et al. *Carcinogenesis.* 1999;20(10):1945–1952.
21. Smolinski AT, Pestka JJ. *Food Chem Toxicol.* 2003;41(10):1381–1390.
22. Shipochliev T, Dimitrov A, Aleksandrova E. *Vet Med Nauki.* 1981;18:87–94.
23. Jakovlev V, Isaac O, Flaskamp E. *Planta Med.* 1983;49(10):67–73.
24. Della Loggia R. *24th International Symposium on Essential Oils*. Berlin. July 1993.
25. Jakovlev V, Isaac K, Thiemer K, et al. *Planta Med.* 1979;35(2):125–140.
26. Breinlich J, Scharnagel K. *Arzneimittelforschung.* 1968;18:429–431.
27. Fuller E, Sosa S, Tubaro A, et al. *Planta Med.* 1993;59(suppl 1):A666–A667.
28. Della Loggia R, Carle R, Sosa S, et al. *Planta Med.* 1990;56(6):657–658.
29. Tubaro A, Zilli C, Redaelli C, et al. *Planta Med.* 1984;50(4):359.
30. Della Loggia R. *Dtsch Apoth Ztg.* 1985;125(suppl 1):9–11.
31. Albring M, Albrecht H, Alcorn G, et al. *Meth Find Exp Clin Pharmacol.* 1983;5(8):575–577.

32. Nissen HP, Biltz H, Kreysel HW. *Z Hautkr.* 1988;63(3):184–190.
33. Achterrath-Tuckermann U, Kunde R, Flaskamp E, et al. *Planta Med.* 1980;39(1):38–50.
34. Sibaev A, Yuece B, Kelber O, et al. *Phytomedicine.* 2006;13(suppl 5):80–89.
35. Maschi O, Cero ED, Galli GV, et al. *J Agric Food Chem.* 2008;56(13):5015–5020.
36. Redaelli C. Formentini L., Santaniello E. Cited in Carle R, Isaac O. *Z Phytother* 1987;8:67–77.
37. Forster HB, Niklas H, Lutz S. *Planta Med.* 1980;40(4):309–319.
38. Lis-Balchin M, Hart S, Deans SG, et al. *J Herbs Spices Med Plants.* 1996;4(2):69–86.
39. Calzada F, Arista R, Pérez H. *J Ethnopharmacol.* 2010;128(1):49–51.
40. Viola H, Wasowski C, Levi de Stein M, et al. *Planta Med.* 1995;61:213–215.
41. Avallone R, Zanoli P, Puia G, et al. *Biochem Pharmacol.* 2000;59(11):1387–1394.
42. Awad R, Levac D, Cybulska P, et al. *Can J Physiol Pharmacol.* 2007;85(9):933–942.
43. Shinomiya K, Inoue T, Utsu Y, et al. *Biol Pharm Bull.* 2005;28(5):808–810.
44. Della Loggia R, Traversa U, Scarcia V, et al. *Pharmacol Res Commun.* 1982;14(2):153–162.
45. Yamada K, Miura T, Mimaki Y, et al. *Biol Pharm Bull.* 1996;19(9):1244–1246.
46. Kakuta H, Yano E, Maeda T, et al. *Aroma Res.* 2002;3(2):131–136.
47. Yano E, Hashimoto K, Haeno H, et al. *J Physiol Anthropol Appl Human Sci.* 2004;23(5):183–184.
48. Nakamura H, Moriya K, Oda S, et al. *Aroma Res.* 2002;3(3):251–255.
49. Roberts A, Williams JM. *Br J Med Psychol.* 1992;65(2):197–199.
50. Gomaa A, Hashem T, Mohamed M, et al. *J Pharmacol Sci.* 2003;92(1):50–55.
51. Heidari MR, Dadollahi Z, Mehrabani M, et al. *Ann N Y Acad Sci.* 2009;1171:300–304.
52. Thiemer K, Stadler R, Isaac O. *Arzneimittelforschung.* 1972;22(6):1086–1087.
53. Szelenyi I, Isaac O, Thiemer K. *Planta Med.* 1979;35(3):218–227.
54. Torrado S, Torrado S, Agis A, et al. *Pharmazie.* 1995;50(2):141–143.
55. Cemek M, Yilmaz E, Büyükokurolu ME. *Pharm Biol.* 2010;48(7):757–763.
56. Bezerra SB, Leal LK, Nogueira NA, et al. *J Med Food.* 2009;12(6):1403–1406.
57. Moura Rocha NF, Venâncio ET, Moura BA, et al. *Fundam Clin Pharmacol.* 2010;24(1):63–71.
58. Khayyal MT, el-Ghazaly MA, Kenawy SA. *Arzneimittelforschung.* 2001;51(7):545–553.
59. Carle R, Isaac O. *Z Phytother.* 1987;8:67–77.

60. Aggag ME, Yousef RT. *Planta Med.* 1972;22:140–144.
61. Ceska O, Chaudhary SK, Warrington PJ, et al. *Fitoterapia.* 1992;58(5):387–394.
62. Cinco M, Banfi E, Tubaro A, et al. *Int J Crude Drug Res.* 1983;21(4):145–151.
63. Annuk H, Hirmo S, Türi E, et al. *FEMS Microbiol Lett.* 1999;172(1):41–45.
64. Cwikla C, Schmidt K, Matthias A, et al. *Phytother Res.* 2010;24(5):649–656.
65. Mahady GB, Pendland SL, Stoia A, et al. *Phytother Res.* 2005;19(11):988–991.
66. Shikov AN, Pozharitskaya ON, Makarov VG, et al. *Phytother Res.* 2008;22(2):252–253.
67. Weseler A, Geiss HK, Saller R, et al. *Pharmazie.* 2005;60(7):498–502.
68. Stamatis G, Kyriazopoulos P, Golegou S, et al. *J Ethnopharmacol.* 2003;88(2–3):175–179.
69. Szabó MA, Varga GZ, Hohmann J, et al. *Phytother Res.* 2010;24(5):782–786.
70. Koch C, Reichling J, Schneele J, et al. *Phytomedicine.* 2008;15(1–2):71–78.
71. Koch C, Reichling J, Kehm R, et al. *J Pharm Pharmacol.* 2008;60(11):1545–1550.
72. Morales-Yuste M, Morillas-Márquez F, Martín-Sánchez J, et al. *Phytomedicine.* 2010;17(3–4):279–281.
73. Nayak BS, Raju SS, Rao AV. *J Wound Care.* 2007;16(7):298–302.
74. Jarrahi M. *Nat Prod Res.* 2008;22(5):422–427.
75. Jarrahi M. *Nat Prod Res.* 2010;24(8):697–702.
76. Pavesi VC, Lopez TC, Martins MA, et al. *Support Care Cancer.* 2011;19(5):639–646.
77. Martins MD, Marques MM, Bussadori SK, et al. *Phytother Res.* 2009;23(2):274–278.
78. Thiemer K, Stadler R, Isaac O. *Arzneimittelforschung.* 1973;23(6):756–759.
79. Fronza M, Heinzmann B, Hamburger M, et al. *J Ethnopharmacol.* 2009;126(3):463–467.
80. Kobayashi Y, Nakano Y, Inayama K, et al. *Phytomedicine.* 2003;10(8):657–664.
81. Kobayashi Y, Takahashi R, Ogino F. *J Ethnopharmacol.* 2005;101(1–3):308–312.
82. Lee SH, Heo Y, Kim YC. *J Vet Sci.* 2010;11(1):35–41.
83. Miller T, Wittstock U, Lindequist U, et al. *Planta Med.* 1996;62(1):60–61.
84. Pereira RP, Fachinetto R, de Souza Prestes A, et al. *Neurochem Res.* 2009;34(5):973–983.
85. Campanella L, Bonanni A, Tomassetti M. *J Pharm Biomed Anal.* 2003;32(4–5):725–736.
86. Rekka EA, Kouroundakis AP, Kourounakis PN. *Res Commun Mol Pathol Pharmacol.* 1996;92(3):361–364.
87. Chandrashekhar VM, Ranpariya VL, Ganapaty S, et al. *J Ethnopharmacol.* 2010;127(3):645–651.

88. Amirghofran Z, Azadbakht M, Karimi MH. *J Ethnopharmacol.* 2000;72(1–2):167–172.
89. Gershbein LL. *Food Cosmet Toxicol.* 1977;15:173–181.
90. Babenko NA, Shakhova EG. *Exp Gerontol.* 2006;41(1):32–39.
91. Babenko NA, Shakhova EG. *Lipids Health Dis.* 2008;28(7):1.
92. Babenko NO, Shakhova OH. *Fiziol Zh.* 2005;51(4):65–69.
93. Kato A, Minoshima Y, Yamamoto J, et al. *J Agric Food Chem.* 2008;56(17):8206–8211.
94. Cemek M, Ka a S, Sim ek N, et al. *J Nat Med.* 2008;62(3):284–293.
95. Mazzio EA, Soliman KF. *Phytother Res.* 2009;23(3):385–398.
96. Srivastava JK, Gupta S. *J Agric Food Chem.* 2007;55(23):9470–9478.
97. Ogata–Ikeda I, Seo H, Kawanai T, et al. *Phytomedicine.* 2010 [Epub ahead of print].
98. Ogata I, Kawanai T, Hashimoto E, et al. *Arch Toxicol.* 2010;84(1):45–52.
99. Fang J, Zhou Q, Shi XL, et al. *Carcinogenesis.* 2007;28(3):713–723.
100. Kim JH, Jin YR, Park BS, et al. *Biochem Pharmacol.* 2005;69(12):1715–1721.
101. Darra E, Abdel-Azeim S, Manara A, et al. *Arch Biochem Biophys.* 2008;476(2):113–123.
102. Kassi E, Papoutsi Z, Fokialakis N, et al. *J Agric Food Chem.* 2004;52(23):6956–6961.
103. Rosenberg Zand RS, Jenkins DJ, Diamandis EP. *Clin Chim Acta.* 2001;312(1–2):213–219.
104. Sadr Lahijani MS, Raoof Kateb HR, Heady R, et al. *Int Endod J.* 2006;39(3):190–195.
105. Ramadan M, Goeters S, Watzer B, et al. *J Nat Prod.* 2006;69(7):1041–1045.
106. Hahn B, Hölzl J. *Arzneimittelforschung.* 1987;37(6):716–720.
107. Hölzl J, Hahn B. *Dtsch Apoth Ztg.* 1985;125(suppl 1):32–38.
108. Merfort I, Heilmann J, Hagedorn-Leweke U, et al. *Pharmazie.* 1994;49(7):509–511.
109. Heilmann J, Merfort I, Hagedorn U, et al. *Planta Med.* 1993;59(suppl 1):A638.
110. Patzelt-Wenczler R. *Dtsch Apoth Ztg.* 1985;125(suppl 1):12–13.
111. Homberg Pharma Germany, Division of Degussa: Kamillosan Scientific Information, Frankfurt, Main.
112. Aertgeerts P, Albring M, Klaschka F, et al. *Z Hautkr.* 1985;60(3):270–277.
113. Patzelt-Wenczler R, Ponce-Poschl E. *Eur J Med Res.* 2000;5(4):171–175.
114. Hempel B. *Acta Hort.* 1999;503:15–17.
115. Aertgeerts J. *Arztl Kosmetol.* 1984;14(6):502–504.
116. Kaltenbach FJ.. In: Nasemann Th, Patzelt-Wenczler R, eds. *Kamillosan im Spiegel der Literatur.* Frankfurt: Pmi Verlag; 1991.
117. Forster CF, Sussmann HE, Patzelt-Wenczler R. *Schweiz Rundsch Med Prax.* 1996;85(46):1476–1481.

118. Glowania HJ, Raulin Chr, Swoboda M. *Z Hautkr.* 1987;62(17):1262–1271.
119. Maiche AG, Grohn P, Maki-Hokkonen H. *Acta Oncol.* 1991;30:395–396.
120. Hartman D, Coetzee JC. *J Wound Care.* 2002;11(8):317–320.
121. Charousaei F, Dabirian A, Mojab F. *Ostomy Wound Manage.* 2011;57(5):28–36.
122. Nasemann T. *Z Allgemeinmed.* 1975;51(25):1105–1106.
123. Carl W, Emrich LS. *J Prosthet Dent.* 1991;66:361–369.
124. Fidler P, Loprinzi CL, O'Fallon JR, et al. *Cancer.* 1996;77(3):522–525.
125. O'Hara M, Kiefer D, Farrell K, et al. *Arch Fam Med.* 1998;7(6):523–536.
126. Shabanloei R, Ahmadi F, Vaez J, et al. *J Clin Diagn Res.* 2009;3(3):1537–1542.
127. Mazokopakis EE, Vrentzos GE, Papadakis JA, et al. *Phytomedicine.* 2005;12(1–2):25–27.
128. Ramos-e-Silva M, Ferreira AF, Bibas R, et al. *J Drugs Dermatol.* 2006;5(7):612–617.
129. Amsterdam JD, Li Y, Soeller I, et al. *J Clin Psychopharmacol.* 2009;29(4):378–382.
130. Stiegelmeier H. *Kassenarzt.* 1978;18:3605–3606.
131. De La Motte S, Bose-O'Reilly S, Heinisch M, et al. *Arzneimittelforschung.* 1997;47(11):1247–1249.
132. Becker B, Kuhn U, Hardewig–Budny B. *Arzneimittelforschung.* 2006;56(6):387–393.
133. Weizman Z, Alkrinawi S, Goldfarb D, et al. *J Pediatr.* 1993;122(4):650–652.
134. Savino F, Cresi F, Castagno E, et al. *Phytother Res.* 2005;19(4):335–340.
135. Capasso R, Savino F, Capasso F. *Phytother Res.* 2007;21(10):999–1101.
136. Gould L, Reddy RCV, Gomprecht RF. *J Clin Pharmacol.* 1973;13:475–479.
137. Kupfersztain C, Rotem C, Fagot R, et al. *Clin Exp Obstet Gynecol.* 2003;30(4):203–206.
138. Niederhofer H. *Phytomedicine.* 2009;16(4):284–286.
139. Niederhofer H. *Z Phytother.* 2008;29(6):275–276.
140. Kyokong O, Charuluxananan S, Muangmingsuk V, et al. *J Med Assoc Thai.* 2002;85(suppl 1):S180–S185.
141. Saller R, Beschorner M, Hellenbrecht D, et al. *Eur J Pharmacol.* 1990;183(3):728–729.
142. Barsom VS, Moosmayr A, Sakka M. *Erfahungsheilkunde.* 1993;3:159–164.
143. Burns E, Blamey C, Ersser SJ, et al. *Complement Ther Nurs Midwifery.* 2000;6(1):33–34.
144. Wang Y, Tang H, Nicholson JK, et al. *J Agric Food Chem.* 2005;53(2):191–196.

145. Reis PE, Carvalho EC, Bueno PC, et al. *Rev Lat Am Enfermagem.* 2011;19(1):3–10.
146. Romero-Jiménez M, Campos-Sánchez J, Analla M, et al. *Mutat Res.* 2005;585(1–2):147–155.
147. Hernandez-Ceruelos A, Madrigal-Bujaidar E, de la Cruz C. *Toxicol Lett.* 2002;135(1–2):103–110.
148. Nersesyan AK. *Toxicol Lett.* 2004;150(2):229–230.
149. Gomes-Carneiro MR, Dias DM, De-Oliveira AC, et al. *Mutat Res.* 2005;585(1–2):105–112.
150. Opdyke DLJ. *Food Cosmet Toxicol.* 1974;12:851–852.
151. Habersang S, Leuschner F, Isaac C, et al. *Planta Med.* 1979;37(10):115–123.
152. Bhatia SP, McGinty D, Letizia CS, et al. *Food Chem Toxicol.* 2008;46(suppl 11):S72–S76.
153. Maliakal PP, Wanwimolruk S. *J Pharm Pharmacol.* 2001;53(10):1323–1329.
154. Ganzera M, Schneider P, Stuppner H. *Life Sci.* 2006;78(8):856–861.
155. Nowack R, Nowak B. *Nephrol Dial Transplant.* 2005;20(11):2554–2556.
156. Abebe W. *J Clin Pharm Ther.* 2002;27:391–401.
157. Spinella M. *Epilepsy Behav.* 2001;2:524–532.
158. Heck AM, DeWitt BA, Lukes AL. *Am J Health Syst Pharm.* 2000;57:1221–1227.
159. Segal R, Pilote L. *CMAJ.* 2006;174(9):1281–1282.
160. Hurrell RF, Reddy M, Cook JD. *Br J Nutr.* 1999;81:289–295.
161. Olivares M, Pizarro F, Hertrampf E, et al. *Nutrition.* 2007;23(4):296–300.
162. Cuzzolin L, Francini-Pesenti F, Verlato G, et al. *Pharmacoepidemiol Drug Saf.* 2010 [Epub ahead of print].
163. Moussally K, Bérard A. *Eur J Obstet Gynecol Reprod Biol.* 2010;150(1):107–108.
164. Sridharan S, Archer N, Manning N. *Ultrasound Obstet Gynecol.* 2009;34(3):358–359.
165. Mann C, Staba EJ. The *Chemistry, Pharmacology, and Commercial Formulations of Chamomile Herbs, Spices, and Medicinal Plants,* Vol 1. Phoenix: Oryx Press; 1986.p. 265.
166. Leslie GB, Salmon G. *Swiss Med.* 1979;1:43–45.
167. Bio-Strath AG. Personal communication; September 2003.
168. Shipochliev T. *Vet Med Nauki.* 1981;18:94–98.
169. Jeschke E, Ostermann T, Luke C, et al. *Drug Saf.* 2009;32(8):691–706.
170. Anliker MD, Borelli S, Wuthrich B. *Contact Dermatitis.* 2002;46(2):72–74.

171. Bossuyt L, Dooms-Goossens A. *Contact Dermatitis.* 1994;31(2):131–132.
172. Casterline CL. *JAMA.* 1980;244:330–331.
173. Giordano-Labadie F, Schwarze HP, Bazex J. *Contact Dermatitis.* 2000;42(4):247.
174. Pereira F, Santos R, Pereira A. *Contact Dermatitis.* 1997;36(6):307.
175. Rodriguez-Serna M, Sanchez-Motilla JM, Ramon R, et al. *Contact Dermatitis.* 1998;39(4):192–193.
176. Rudzki E, Rebandel P. *Contact Dermatitis.* 1998;38(3):164–184.
177. Foti C, Nettis E, Cassano N, et al. *Contact Dermatitis.* 2000;42(6):360–361.
178. Schempp CM, Schopf E, Simon JC. *Hautarzt.* 2002;53:93–97.
179. Abramson MJ, Sim MR, Fritschi L, et al. *Occup Med (Lond).* 2001;51:259–265.
180. Vandenplas O, Pirson F, D'Alpaos V, et al. *Allergy.* 2008;63(8):1090–1092.
181. Scala G. *Int Arch Allergy Immunol.* 2006;139(4):330–331.
182. Rudzki E, Rapiejko P, Rebandel P. *Contact Dermatitis.* 2003;49(3):162.
183. Rycroft RJ. *Contact Dermatitis.* 2003;48(4):229.
184. Von Beetz D, Cramer H, Melhorn HC. *Derm Mschr.* 1971;157:505–510.
185. Jablonska S, Rudzki E. *Z Hautkr.* 1996;71(7):542–546.
186. Rudzki E, Jablonska S. *J Dermatol Treat.* 2000;11(3):161–163.
187. Jacob SE, Hsu JW. *Pediatr Dermatol.* 2010;27(1):103–104.
188. Paulsen E, Otkjaer A, Andersen KE. *Contact Dermatitis.* 2010;62(6):338–342.
189. Paulsen E, Andersen KE, Hausen BM. *Contact Dermatitis.* 1993;29(1):6–10.
190. Paulsen E, Andersen KE, Hausen BM. *Contact Dermatitis.* 2001;45(4):197–204.
191. de la Torre Morin F, Sanchez Machin I, Garcia Robaina JC, et al. *J Investig Allergol Clin Immunol.* 2001;11:118–122.
192. Jovanovi M, Poljacki M, Duran V, et al. *Med Pregl.* 2004;57(5–6):209–218.
193. Paulsen E, Chistensen LP, Andersen KE. *Contact Dermatitis.* 2008;58(1):15–23.
194. Subiza J, Subiza JL, Alonso M, et al. *Ann Allergy.* 1990;65:127–132.
195. Andres C, Chen WC, Ollert M, et al. *Allergol Int.* 2009;58(1):135–136.
196. Jensen-Jarolim E, Reider N, Fritsch R, et al. *J Allergy Clin Immunol.* 1998;102:1041–1042.
197. Thien FC. *Med J Aust.* 2001;175:54.
198. Subiza J, Subiza JL, Hinojosa M, et al. *J Allergy Clin Immunol.* 1989;84:353–358.
199. Reider N, Sepp N, Fritsch P, et al. *Clin Exp Allergy.* 2000;30(10):1436–1443.
200. Cuzzolin L, Benoni G. *Phytother Res.* 2009;23(7):1018–1023.
201. Fugh-Berman A. *Nutr Today.* 2002;37:122–124.

Chaste tree

(*Vitex agnus-castus* L.)

Synonyms

Monk's pepper (Engl), Agni casti fructus (Lat), Keuschlammfrüchte (Ger), agneau chaste, gatillier (Fr), kyskhedstræ (Dan).

What is it?

The ripe berries of chaste tree have long been regarded as a symbol of chastity, and were used in the Middle Ages and earlier to suppress sexual excitability. The name 'agnus' derives from the Greek 'agnes' meaning pure or chaste.[1] The dried fruits have a peppery taste and were apparently used in monasteries instead of pepper, supposedly to suppress libido. Hence the common name 'monk's pepper'. Another account suggests that monks carried the seeds with them.[1] Hippocrates, Theophrastus and Dioscorides all mentioned the plant.[1] As a remedy it was considered primarily a herb for women's complaints, especially from the mid-1900s throughout Europe. Modern scientific interest developed in Germany in the 1930s.

Effects

Enhances corpus luteal development (thereby correcting a relative progesterone deficiency) via a dopaminergic activity on the anterior pituitary (which inhibits prolactin); normalises the menstrual cycle, encourages ovulation. Indicated for any kind of premenstrual aggravation. The inhibition of prolactin contrasts with the traditional use to promote breast milk.

Traditional view

A tincture of the fresh berries was traditionally used by the Eclectics as a galactagogue and emmenagogue and was also said to 'repress the sexual passions'. Other suggested uses from the Eclectics included impotence (paradoxical, but there are indirect references to such properties in ancient Spartan culture[1] and chaste tree could indeed be relevant here if hyperprolactinaemia is the cause), sexual melancholia, sexual irritability with nervousness, melancholia or mild dementia.[2] The main traditional use of chaste tree occurred in Europe, where it was widely used by women for a variety of gynaecological problems. Details of such use by women are scant (as is often the case with such remedies). However, the herb appears to have enjoyed a wide variety of applications and was an archetypal 'women's herb' in some Mediterranean traditions. Ironically, the most persistent traditional indication is insufficient lactation.[3,4]

In addition to dysmenorrhoea, chaste tree is used traditionally in France to relieve minor sleep disorders in adults and children.[5] In Jordan and Israel, it is used for headaches, stomach-ache and joint pains.[6,7]

A survey of current practice among 155 herbalists conducted in the UK and Ireland and published in 1997 found the following therapeutic uses (in order of decreasing prevalence): premenstrual syndrome (PMS), perimenopausal complaints, female acne, uterine fibroids, breast cysts, fibrocystic breast disease, female infertility, menstrual irregularities, endometriosis, male acne and PCOS (polycystic ovary syndrome).[8] Interestingly, only around 3% of those who responded to the survey noted milk flow disturbance as a potential use. The average dose used was 2.2 mL/day of a 1:5 tincture, which corresponds to 440 mg of the dried berry.

Summary actions

Prolactin inhibitor, dopamine agonist, indirectly progesterogenic, possible galactagogue.

Can be used for

Indications supported by clinical trials

Menstruation disorders including secondary amenorrhoea, metrorrhagia (from functional causes), oligomenorrhoea (lengthened cycle), polymenorrhoea (shortened cycle), especially when marked by progesterone deficiency (cystic hyperplasia of the endometrium) and latent hyperprolactinaemia; PMS (except perhaps type C, which is characterised by symptoms such as headache, craving for sweets, palpitations and dizziness), especially premenstrual mastalgia and fluid retention; other premenstrual aggravations (such as mouth ulcers, orofacial herpes, epilepsy); insufficient lactation (very low doses only, certainly less than 150 mg/day); infertility due to decreased progesterone levels or hyperprolactinaemia; acne (in both sexes); perimenopausal PMS-like syndromes; poor sleep maintenance, insomnia (indirect evidence via melatonin stimulation); restless legs syndrome.

Most of these indications come from low-level, uncontrolled trials, with the most robust data being for PMS.

Traditional therapeutic uses

Promotion of lactation; menstrual irregularities; to decrease male libido; perimenopausal symptoms; to enhance female fertility.

May also be used for

Extrapolations from pharmacological studies

Possible roles in relative progesterone deficiency or conditions where unopposed oestrogen plays a role: uterine fibroids, endometriosis, follicular ovarian cysts; additional conditions caused by hyperprolactinaemia (such as some cases of erectile dysfunction or infertility in men, hypogonadism, galactorrhoea or irregular menstruation) and conditions in which raised prolactin secretion is implicated: breast cysts, fibrocystic breast disease, benign prostatic hyperplasia. Any activity for chaste tree in Parkinson's disease could depend on whether its dopaminergic compounds cross the blood-brain barrier in sufficient quantity.

Several autoimmune diseases have been linked to higher levels of prolactin in the blood, including systemic lupus erythematosus (SLE),[9] rheumatoid arthritis (RA),[10] Sjögren's syndrome[11] and juvenile arthritis.[12] For SLE, serum prolactin concentrations have been correlated with both clinical activity and remission.[9,13] Studies on dopaminergic drugs such as bromocriptine suggest that lowering elevated prolactin levels of pituitary origin can lead to clinical improvement in SLE,[14] RA,[15,16] psoriatic arthritis and Reiter's syndrome.[16] (Prolactin is also produced peripherally in inflammatory diseases.) One study involving 79 patients with SLE, 23 with RA and 28 healthy controls, found significant elevations in around 40% of patients in a pattern resembling latent hyperprolactinaemia.[17] In other words, the stress of taking the first blood sample significantly raised prolactin, which was lower in subsequent samples. This pattern was not observed in healthy controls. Hence chaste tree at lower doses (see below) may be of value for the above autoimmune diseases.

Preparations

Dried or fresh ripe berries for decoction, or tinctures, tablets or capsules for internal use.

Dosage

Low doses are typically used in Germany, equivalent to 30 to 40 mg/day of herb as an aqueous-ethanolic extract. However, clinicians in English-speaking countries tend to use the following doses: daily dose of 1 to 5 mL of a 1:5 tincture or 1 to 4 mL of a 1:2 extract, or equivalent doses in tablet or capsule form. In severe cases or certain disorders, higher doses may be used in the short term. Prolonged use of high doses can also be appropriate for some health problems (see below). Table 1 lists suggested dosages for a number of different conditions.

In Table 1 the term 'clinical observation' refers to traditional use, the experience of the authors and their colleagues and surveys of usage in the UK[8] and Australia.[18] The authors do not recommend and have no clinical experience of the low doses used in some clinical trials and referred to above and below.

Table 1 Recommended doses of chaste tree for various health conditions

Condition	Dosage (dry herb equivalent)	Rationale
Mastalgia, premenstrual symptoms, menstrual cycle irregularities and perimenopausal complaints	200 to 500 mg/day	Based on clinical trials and clinical observation
Corpus luteal insufficiency	200 to 500 mg/day	Based on clinical trials and clinical observation
Latent hyperprolactinaemia (LHP) and infertility associated with LHP or other issues	200 to 500 mg/day	Based on clinical trials and clinical observation
Uterine fibroids, endometriosis, acne, excessive male sex drive	Up to 2500 mg/day in divided doses given two to three times per day	This higher dosage may be required to exert a significant oestrogen/testosterone antagonist effect. Based on clinical observation
Hyperprolactinaemia, breast cysts	Up to 2500 mg/day in divided doses given two to three times per day (the dosage will be influenced by the prolactin level)	To exert a significant dopaminergic effect, thereby reducing prolactin secretion. Based on clinical observation
Polycystic ovary syndrome	200 to 1000 mg/day	In cases of moderate prolactin/androgen excess, from clinical observation
	1000 to 2500 mg/day in divided doses given two to three times per day	In cases of higher prolactin or androgen levels. Based on clinical observation
Sleep disorders including poor sleep maintenance and problems associated with shift work and jet lag	1000 to 2400 mg/day in divided doses given two to three times per day	Based on a clinical trial assessing melatonin secretion

It is common practice, and also recommended by some German manufacturers, that chaste tree is taken as a single dose each morning before breakfast throughout the cycle. It is considered that hormonal regulation via the pituitary is more receptive to this regime, although there is no pharmacological or clinical evidence to support this proposition.

Duration of use

May be used long term if prescribed within the recommended therapeutic range. Chaste tree should be discontinued or the dose reduced if the length of the menstrual cycle is excessively changed.

Summary assessment of safety

Only mild adverse effects from ingestion of chaste tree are expected when taken within the recommended dosage range.

Technical data

Botany

Vitex agnus-castus, a member of the Verbenaceae (verbena) family, was indigenous to southern Europe but is now widely cultivated.[19] The shrub grows to 3 to 5 m and produces large dark green leaves radiating from a long, hairy stalk. The shoots terminate in a slender spike and are composed of whorls of violet flowers. The black spherical berries are about 5 mm in size and contain four seeds.[20]

Adulteration

Common adulterants of *V. agnus-castus* are *V. negundo*, *V. rotundifolia* and *V. trifolia*, which are Asiatic species used in Chinese or Ayurvedic medicine.[21]

Key constituents

- Essential oil, about 0.7%, containing monoterpenes and sesquiterpenes such as sabinene, cineole, beta-caryophyllene and trans-beta-farnesene[22,23]
- Flavonoids including methoxylated flavones such as casticin, eupatorin and penduletin; together with other flavonoids including vitexin and orientin[24]
- Iridoid glycosides, including aucubin (0.3%) and agnuside (0.6%).[25]
- Diterpenes of the labdane and halimane types including rotundifuran (0.04% to 0.3%), vitexilactone (0.016% to 0.167%),[26] vitetrifolin B and C[24] and viteagnusins A to I[27-29]
- Other constituents include vitexlactam A, triterpenic acids, phenolic acids[29] and cleroda-7,14-dien-13-ol.[30]

Casticin

Pharmacodynamics

Hormonal activity

From the 1960s up to the 1990s the conventional wisdom was that chaste tree corrected a clinical situation of oestrogen excess or relative progesterone deficiency by acting on the pituitary to increase luteinising hormone (LH) and decrease follicle-stimulating hormone (FSH). This was promoted in the literature and in the product information from German suppliers of chaste tree products. The apparent basis for this thinking was some early pharmacological research.[31] The study in question found that low doses of chaste tree tincture (0.75 and 1.5 drops/kg, oral) given to female guinea pigs for 90 days decreased oestrogenic and promoted progesterogenic effects. Corpus luteal development and glandular proliferation in breast tissue were enhanced and follicular development and uterine weight were slightly decreased. These findings were interpreted by the authors to be the result of increased LH and decreased FSH, but these pituitary hormones were never measured. The same publication also examined the effect of 10 to 20 times the above doses (15 drops/kg, oral) and found results that were interpreted as an inhibition of all gonadotrophic hormones and growth hormone. In other words, anterior pituitary function was suppressed by the high dose, with decreases in pituitary, adrenal and uterine weights and signs of atrophy in breast tissue. One small, uncontrolled trial published many years later in 1990 did observe an increase in LH and an inconsistent decrease in FSH in 15 patients with secondary amenorrhoea, with subsequent onset of menstruation after 6 months of chaste tree.[32]

Later research has challenged this perspective. It is now known that chaste tree has dopaminergic activity. This can also explain its activity in treating gynaecological conditions (including PMS) because many of these can be related to high prolactin levels. Dopamine inhibits prolactin secretion from the anterior pituitary. Increased prolactin levels inhibit corpus luteal development, thereby indirectly reducing the secretion of progesterone in the luteal phase of the menstrual cycle. Therefore, chaste tree may increase progesterone by reducing prolactin secretion, rather than by increasing LH. Increased prolactin levels are associated with premenstrual mastalgia, corpus luteal insufficiency, benign breast tumours and infertility. In many cases the hyperprolactinaemia may not be constant and is referred to latent hyperprolactinaemia. Here prolactin is typically elevated by stress and/or premenstrually. The active dopaminergic compounds in chaste tree appear to be mainly diterpenes. Although there are other factors involved in PMS and other menstrual disturbances (and, indeed, the hormonal action of chaste tree is probably more than just dopaminergic), this finding provides a coherent rationale for the role of this herb in a range of female hormonal problems.

Prolactin secretion from the anterior pituitary is under the dual control of a hypothalamic factor (thyroxin-releasing hormone, TRH) which stimulates prolactin release, and the catecholamine dopamine, which acts as a prolactin inhibiting factor. Several intrinsic (such as sleep) and extrinsic (such as stress) stimuli enhance prolactin release. The prolactin-producing cells of the pituitary, the lactotropes, express the D2 subtype of the dopamine receptor, which is coupled to adenylate cyclase. Activation of the D2 receptor by either dopamine, or compounds with aspects of their molecular structure similar to dopamine, reduces the synthesis of cAMP resulting in an inhibition of prolactin secretion.

In some of the earliest research on this topic, chaste tree extract and a synthetic dopamine agonist (lisuride) were found to significantly inhibit basal and TRH-stimulated prolactin secretion in isolated rat pituitary cells. This inhibition could be blocked by the addition of a dopamine receptor blocker, confirming the dopaminergic effect of the herb.[33] In addition, a dopamine agonist (haloperidol) was able to counteract the prolactin-lowering effect of chaste tree, providing further proof a dopaminergic mode of action.[34] Using the corpus striatum membrane dopamine receptor binding assay, it was determined that chaste tree extract contained several active principles that bind to the dopamine D2 receptor. The action of chaste tree on pituitary hormone secretion in vitro was selective, since both basal and LH releasing hormone (LHRH)-stimulated gonadotropin (FSH, LH) release remained unaffected.[35]

A chaste tree extract (containing 3.3 mg/mL water-soluble substances) markedly reduced stress-induced prolactin release in rats after intravenous injection.[36] Other early research found that administration of chaste tree extract (0.3 to 2.3 g/kg, sc) to suckling rats resulted in a clear increase in offspring without milk. This effect was comparable to rats given bromocriptine, a drug that suppresses prolactin secretion. The authors believed the reduction in prolactin levels by chaste tree led to a significant reduction in milk production. There were no indications of toxicity, including no change in the body weight of the adults.[37]

An aqueous-ethanolic extract of chaste tree displaced sulpiride (a dopamine receptor antagonist) from dopamine D2 receptors. Only the hexane subfraction (containing diterpenes and fatty acids) demonstrated dopamine D2 receptor affinity. Further investigation indicated that the diterpenes rotundifuran and 6-beta,7-beta-diacetoxy-13-hydroxy-labda-8,14-diene, and the unsaturated fatty acid linoleic acid were active. Agnuside, aucubin and casticin and other flavonoids did not show any effect.[38]

Another research group published a series of papers concerning the identity of dopaminergic compounds in chaste tree.[39–41] Bio-guided fractionation of an ethanolic chaste tree extract resulted in the isolation of a mixture of bicyclic diterpenes of the clerodane type. Based on their dopaminergic

potency and concentration in the chaste tree extract, these appeared to be the most significant compounds, although other labdane dopaminergic diterpenes such as rotundifuran also contributed to the overall in vitro activity. Both dopamine and the clerodane diterpenes reduced cAMP formation in, and prolactin secretion from, lactotropic cells.[41] The in vitro dopaminergic activity of commercial chaste tree preparations showed considerable variation.[41]

Injection of either a hydroethanolic chaste tree extract (65 to 465 mg/kg) or dopamine decreased LH and testosterone in male mice.[42] This suggests that dopamine regulates the gonadotroph-Leydig cell axis and provides an interesting rationale for the traditional use of chaste tree to decrease male libido. Relatively high doses of a dried 70% ethanol extract of chaste tree (0.6 and 1.2 g/kg, oral) reduced plasma prolactin levels in ovariectomised rats, but had no such effect in normal female rats.[43]

Other compounds in chaste tree might also influence prolactin levels. The flavone-enriched fraction of *Vitex rotundifolia* (which was high in casticin) decreased prolactin levels in mice with induced hyperprolactinaemia at oral doses of 25 and 50 mg/kg.[44] Casticin was also active at the same doses, as were other fractions of the herbal extract. A subsequent publication from the same group found that casticin (10 to 40 mg/kg, ip) also inhibited prolactin release in rats with induced hyperprolactinaemia, and countered the in vitro prolactin release from pituitary cells stimulated with oestradiol.[45] However, casticin had no effect on prolactin release from unstimulated primary pituitary cells in vitro, consistent with the findings quoted above.[38]

Human data also support effects on prolactin levels. In a placebo-controlled trial, 20 male volunteers received a special extract of chaste tree (120, 240 or 480 mg/day) or placebo for 14 days. Men were chosen because they do not have a fluctuating hormonal cycle. There was a significant increase in a 24 h prolactin secretion at the lowest dosage, in contrast to the higher dosages, which caused a small drop. On the last day of the trial, prolactin release over a 1 h period after TRH stimulation was measured compared with placebo. A significant increase of prolactin at the lowest dosage and a significant drop at the highest dosage were recorded. This suggests the activity of chaste tree is dependent on dose and the initial level of the prolactin concentration. Chaste tree did not alter the serum concentrations of the gonadotropins (LH, FSH) or testosterone.[46,47]

A case was described of a prolactinoma (a benign pituitary tumour that secretes prolactin) in an 18-year-old girl who had a history of oligomenorrhoea and galactorrhoea.[48] On review by an endocrinologist 6 months later, the patient reported a regular 28-day menstrual cycle and was negative for galactorrhoea, with a concurrent decrease in her serum prolactin (although it was still elevated). She had been taking 15 drops each morning of a chaste tree tincture for 3 months. The concern was expressed that chaste tree could mask a prolactinoma.[48] However, another group suggested that the herb might instead prove to be a useful treatment for this condition.[49] They described another case of prolactinoma treated with a chaste tree tincture (20 drops twice a day) by a 31-year-old woman. While this time the chaste tree did not alter the typical symptoms noted above, it did reduce prolactin levels.

In terms of other hormonal activity, early research found pretreatment before mating with powdered chaste tree (1 to 2 g/kg) had no antifertility effect (as measured by a reduction in the number of fetuses) in male and female rats and guinea pigs.[50] The flavonoid-rich fraction from the seeds of *Vitex negundo*, which mainly contain methoxylated flavones similar to *Vitex agnus-castus*, showed antiandrogenic effects in vivo by the intraperitoneal route.[51] This effect may be related to the casticin research cited above.

Chaste tree and its phytochemical components could also possibly modulate oestrogen effects, although some experimental findings need to be interpreted with caution. For example, one study using in vitro techniques identified linoleic acid as an oestrogenic compound from chaste tree.[52] While this is a perfectly valid finding, it adds little to our understanding of the hormonal activity of chaste tree, since the linoleic acid is only present at low levels in the herb and is far more abundant in other plants. A similar argument can be applied to the in vitro finding that apigenin is the most active component in chaste tree in terms of binding to oestrogen receptor-beta.[41,53] Apigenin is a widely distributed flavonoid. Perhaps of more relevance were the concurrent findings that chaste tree extract did not bind to oestrogen receptor-alpha, and that other flavonoids such as vitexin and pendulitin exhibited an affinity for the beta receptor. However, even for these results there is the confounding issue that flavonoids typically exhibit poor intact bioavailability.

Relatively high doses of a dried 70% ethanolic extract of chaste tree (0.6 and 1.2 g/kg, oral) substantially increased uterine weight and vaginal cornification in ovariectomised rats, but had no effect on uterine and ovarian weights in normal rats.[43] Chaste tree extract also increased plasma oestrogen and progesterone in both normal and ovariectomised rats, while FSH and LH levels were unchanged (except LH decreased slightly in the ovariectomised animals).

A dried 70% ethanol extract of chaste tree (133.3 mg/kg, oral) demonstrated an osteoprotective effect in castrated male rats.[54] The effects on bone matrix were similar to the oestrogen control group and superior to the testosterone control group, with both cortical and trabecular bone preserved. Earlier research found that oral chaste tree extract had a minor nonsignificant positive effect on osteoporosis and decreased serum leptin after 3 months in ovariectomised rats.[40]

Interestingly, wild female baboons that consume the African black plum (*Vitex doniana*) exhibit substantially higher faecal progesterone excretion.[55] The plant appears to act on cycling females as both a physiological contraceptive (like the oral contraceptive pill) and a social contraceptive (preventing sexual swelling, thus reducing association with males). Similarly, hyperprogesteronaemia was observed in female wild chimpanzees in association with consumption of *Vitex fischeri*.[56] Female oestrogen levels were not significantly impacted, nor were male testosterone levels.

Seasonally elevated faecal progesterone excretion was found in wild female Phayre's leaf monkeys, with higher levels when *Vitex* species leaves and fruits were abundant.[57] Females had longer cycle lengths and follicular phases, while receptive periods did not change. They were more likely to conceive at these times, but that also correlated with improving physical condition due to seasonal factors. The authors suggested that the active constituents in Vitex might not be phytosteroids at all, but rather phytochemicals that influence steroid levels downstream.

Antimicrobial activity

Ethanolic and etheric extracts of chaste tree demonstrated weak in vitro antimicrobial activity against the following species using the dilution method: *Staphylococcus aureus, Streptococcus faecalis* (6.5% to 20% extracts), *Salmonella spp., Escherichia coli* (10% to 20%), *Candida albicans, C. tropicalis, C. pseudotropicalis* and *C. krusei* (10% to 40%). High toxicity against the mycelial growth of *Trichophyton mentagrophytes, Epidermophyton floccosum, Microsporum canis, M. gypseum* (1.5% to 12%) and *Penicillium viridicatum* (9% to 23%) was also found.[58] Essential oil from chaste tree ripe fruit showed greater antimicrobial activity against *E. coli* and *Candida albicans* than against *Staph. aureus* or *Bacillus anthracoides*.[59] Chaste tree essential oil has also exhibited antifungal activity against dermatophyte strains, although the leaf essential oil had the highest activity.[60]

Antitumour activity

Chaste tree extracts or some isolated components have demonstrated antitumour activity against a range of cancer cells in vitro. For the extract, cytotoxicity and induction of apoptosis has been observed for ovarian, cervical, breast, gastric, colon, small cell lung and prostate cancer cell lines.[61–63] However, the antitumour activity of the herb compared with other plants such as *Dioscorea villosa* and *Sanguinaria canadensis* was relatively low.[64] Rotundifuran induced apoptosis in human myeloid leukaemia cells,[65] and flavonoids found in the herb, including luteolin, have demonstrated in vitro activity against cell lines such as human colon cancer and mouse lymphocytic leukaemia.[66]

Other activity

Chaste tree extract exhibited pronounced binding to mu- and kappa-opioid receptor subtypes in vitro, especially the lipophilic fractions of the extract.[38] The aqueous extract was more active at binding to delta receptors. A later investigation established that this activity was not just due to the free fatty acids in chaste tree extract, and determined that the extract was in fact agonistic at the mu-opiate receptor, which is a primary target of beta-endorphin.[67] Follow-up research found that a methanolic extract of chaste tree bound and activated mu- and delta-, but not kappa-opioid receptor subtypes in vitro.[68] Biological evaluation identified four flavonoids, including apigenin and casticin, as weak ligands of mu- and delta-opioid receptors, exhibiting dose-dependent receptor binding.[29,68] Only casticin acted as a delta-opioid receptor agonist. Since beta-endorphin assists in regulating the menstrual cycle, this might provide an additional mechanism behind the clinical effects of chaste tree. However, it is difficult to see how such mild in vitro activities of compounds with relatively low oral bioavailability could translate into significant clinical effects.

Chaste tree extract (60 to 180 mg/kg, ip) exhibited dose-dependent antiepileptic activity on amygdala-kindled seizures in male rats.[69]

Pharmacokinetics

No data available.

Clinical trials

Hyperprolactinaemia is one of the most frequent causes for cyclical disorders, from corpus luteal insufficiency (shortened luteal phase, extended PMS and/or reduced progesterone secretion) to secondary amenorrhoea and premenstrual mastalgia. While latent hyperprolactinaemia (LHP) can be present throughout the cycle, the removal of the inhibitory effect of progesterone at the end of the luteal phase can result in the release of high quantities of prolactin under minor stress conditions, as well as during deep sleep phases at night. Hyperprolactinaemia and corpus luteum insufficiency may both be implicated in PMS, but there is insufficient evidence to link them invariably with the condition.

Menstruation disorders

Early uncontrolled clinical studies on chaste tree date back to 1954. Improvement was noted in patients suffering from a variety of menstruation disorders, including secondary amenorrhoea. Results were particularly marked for patients suffering from cystic hyperplasia of the endometrium (a disorder due to a relative progesterone deficiency) over treatment periods of 5 to 24 months after a dose of 45 drops of tincture per day. Ovulatory cycles were re-established in a number of these patients. Chaste tree was considered to be particularly indicated for patients with deficient corpus luteum function.[70] This work was supported by another uncontrolled study that demonstrated improvement in 63% of patients.[71] Beneficial effects were also observed in 66% patients with heavy or frequent bleeding.[72] For 33 cases of polymenorrhoea (shortened cycle), treatment with chaste tree (45 drops/day of tincture) lengthened the average cycle from 20 to 26 days. For 35 cases of oligomenorrhoea (infrequent menstruation) the average cycle was shortened from 39 to 31 days, and for 58 cases of menorrhagia the average duration of bleeding decreased from 8 to 5 days. Treatment with chaste tree was over at least 2 to 3 months.[73] Such results were confirmed in a later uncontrolled, 6-month trial involving 120 women with irregular cycles. Chaste tree (20 mg extract/day) normalised the cycle of 63% of women in one trial, and 29% fell pregnant.[74]

In a large, uncontrolled trial, 1592 women with various conditions collectively defined as corpus luteum insufficiency were treated with chaste tree. After an average treatment period of 6 months of chaste tree tincture (45 drops/day), 33% were observed to be free of complaints and 51% were in satisfactory condition, according to the physician's assessment. In the patient's assessment, 61% rated the treatment as good and 29% as satisfactory. Of 145 patients attempting to conceive, 56 became pregnant.[75] Thirteen patients with hyperprolactinaemia and cyclic disorders were treated for

3 months with a chaste tree tincture (60 drops/day). The menstrual cycle returned to normal in all patients and prolactin levels were significantly reduced or normalised.[76] Of 20 patients with secondary amenorrhoea, treatment with chaste tree (40 drops/day of tincture, equivalent to around 33 mg/dried herb) restored menstruation in 10 after 6 months.[77]

Observation of 551 patients by 153 gynaecologists over several menstrual cycles found the efficacy of chaste tree treatment (40 drops/day of tincture, equivalent to around 33 mg dried herb) to be good in 68.8% of cases. Three hundred and sixty-nine patients had symptoms of corpus luteal insufficiency or cyclic disorders; 210 had PMS. A majority of patients (81.1%) were relieved of their complaints or stated that their condition had improved.[78]

Thirty-seven women (from an original 52) with luteal phase defects due to LHP completed a 3-month double blind, placebo-controlled trial testing the efficacy of a chaste tree preparation (20 mg/day dried herb equivalent). With this disorder, basal blood levels of prolactin may only be slightly raised, but there is an excessive prolactin response following iv injection of TRH. The menstrual cycle is also abnormal: the luteal phase is much shorter, although the total length of the cycle can be normal. Blood for hormonal analysis was taken at days 5 to 8 and day 20 of the menstrual cycle, before and after 3 months of therapy. Following the chaste tree treatment, prolactin release following TRH was significantly reduced compared with placebo ($p<0.001$). Shortened luteal phases were normalised ($p<0.005$ compared with placebo) and luteal phase progesterone deficiencies were only corrected in the chaste tree group. There were no changes in any other hormones except that luteal phase 17-beta-oestradiol levels were higher in the chaste tree group ($p<0.05$ compared with placebo). Two women receiving chaste tree became pregnant and PMS symptoms were also significantly reduced in the chaste tree group ($p<0.05$).[79] In another study, frequent blood samples were drawn from patients with premenstrual mastalgia.[40] As a result of the stress of blood withdrawal, prolactin levels in the pathological range were observed, indicative of LHP. There were also pathological surges of prolactin associated with LH pulses. These responses were no longer evident after 3 months of a chaste tree formulation.

Premenstrual syndrome

The pharmacological and clinical studies cited above suggest that chaste tree can correct a relative progesterone deficiency created by LHP. Many patients with premenstrual symptoms demonstrate LHP in conjunction with corpus luteum insufficiency and this might be the only aetiological factor in PMS that responds to chaste tree treatment. Therefore the reputation of chaste tree in the treatment of PMS may be based solely on its dopaminergic activity. This could explain the negative finding in one PMS clinical trial cited below (due to the selected patient cohort possibly having a low prevalence of LHP), but the high placebo effect in PMS makes such trials difficult to design and conduct in any case.

Uncontrolled trials in PMS provide only weak evidence of efficacy due to the high placebo effect in this condition. However, such trials in the early 1960s at least tended to indicate that chaste tree exerts a favourable effect on a variety of unusual premenstrual aggravations, including post-traumatic epilepsy,[80] mouth ulcers[81] and orofacial herpes simplex.[82] Since then, there have been several other uncontrolled, observational studies, some involving large numbers of patients. Because of their weak evidentiary nature, only a brief review of these trials follows. In a study involving 36 women with PMS, 40 drops/day of chaste tree tincture relieved physical and psychological symptoms and normalised the luteal phase from an average of 5.4 to 11.4 days.[83] Another study using the same preparation and similar dosage (corresponding to 33 mg of dried herb) found improvement in 80% of 1542 women after an average treatment period of 166 days.[84] A similar trial (design, preparation and dosage) in 1571 patients yielded similar results.[85] Striking results were found in a study involving 1634 women with PMS where chaste tree (20 mg dried herb equivalent per day) improved symptoms in 93% over three menstrual cycles.[86] In a study involving 132 women, of whom about half were taking the contraceptive pill, chaste tree extract (20 mg/day, equivalent to around 180 mg dried herb) for 3 months improved symptoms in more than half, with no real difference between those taking the pill or not.[87] The same preparation, dose and design saw 38 of 43 patients judge the treatment of their PMS as moderate to excellent.[88] Swiss physicians judged the same preparation at an average dose of 40 mg/day of extract to be successful, or partially successful, over a 3-month period in 86% of 428 women with PMS.[89] PMS symptoms significantly improved in 409 patients after receiving chaste tree extract (20 mg/day, equivalent to around 180 mg herb) for three cycles.[90] A different chaste tree extract (4 mg/day, equivalent to 40 mg dried herb) induced a positive response by the third treatment cycle in 68% of 118 women with PMS.[91] Finally, a chaste tree extract (40 mg/day) approximately halved the incidence of headaches in 36 women suffering from migraines in conjunction with PMS.[92]

In a pilot controlled clinical trial, significant benefit was observed for all types of PMS, except type PMS-C (characterised by symptoms such as headache, craving for sweets, palpitations and dizziness).[93] This pilot was followed up by a double blind, placebo-controlled trial, where 217 patients with PMS received chaste tree (1.8 g/day) or a soya-based placebo for 3 months. There was little difference found between chaste tree and placebo for the majority of symptoms associated with PMS. However, there was a tendency to improvement in the fluid retention group of symptoms, especially for mastalgia, although it did not quite reach statistical significance (p=0.09).[94] The soya-based placebo may have exerted significant pharmacological activity and the trial exhibited a high dropout rate (600 women began the study). See also the comments above regarding LHP in PMS.

In a multicentre, randomised, double blind, comparative trial, 127 women with PMS received either chaste tree or vitamin B6 (pyridoxine) over three menstrual cycles. Patients either received a chaste tree extract capsule (4 mg/day, equivalent to around 40 mg dried herb) and a placebo capsule throughout the cycle, or one capsule of placebo twice daily on days 1 to 15 followed by one capsule of pyridoxine (100 mg) twice daily on days 16 to 35 of the menstrual cycle.

Some patients did not complete the trial or were excluded from analysis. Premenstrual Tension Scale (PMTS) scores decreased for both treatments, but chaste tree was superior to pyridoxine overall. Characteristic symptoms (breast tenderness, oedema, abdominal tension, headache, constipation, depressed mood) were more significantly reduced by chaste tree than by pyridoxine. The efficacy of treatment was rated as excellent by about 25% of physicians for chaste tree, but only by 12% for pyridoxine. Thirty-six per cent of women treated with chaste tree felt they were free of complaints, compared with 21% of the pyridoxine-treated patients. Nine patients recorded adverse events, four from the pyridoxine group and five receiving chaste tree. Of these adverse events, gastrointestinal disturbances were approximately equally distributed between the two study groups. Two chaste tree-treated patients experienced skin reactions and one reported transient headache.[95] The significance of this study is difficult to assess because a placebo control group was not included, and pyridoxine is not widely regarded as an effective treatment for PMS.

The best designed and conducted trial of chaste tree in PMS was the prospective, randomised, double blind, placebo-controlled study published in the *BMJ* in 2001.[96] In all, 178 women (of whom 170 were evaluated) with PMS according to the DSM-IIIR received either chaste tree extract (20 mg/day, equivalent to around 180 mg dried herb) or placebo for three menstrual cycles. Self-assessment of typical PMS symptoms using a visual analogue scale resulted in a significantly lower average score for the chaste tree group by the end of the trial (p<0.001 versus placebo). Attending physicians also rated the chaste tree as superior (p<0.001). Responder rates (at least a 50% reduction in symptoms) were 52% for chaste tree compared with 24% for placebo. Mild adverse events were noted for seven women, four in the chaste tree group.

Premenstrual dysphoric disorder (PMDD) as defined by the DSM-IV is characterised by markedly depressed mood, marked anxiety, affective lability and decreased interest in daily activities during the last week of luteal phase in most menstrual cycles during the past year.[97] (PMDD is hence a severe form of PMS.) At the completion of an 8-week, randomised, single-blind trial (n=41) a similar percentage of PMDD patients (around 60%) responded to chaste tree (20 to 40 mg/day, undefined extract) as did to fluoxetine (serotonin reuptake inhibitor, 20 to 40 mg/day). However, there were differences in the specific treatment outcomes. Fluoxetine was more effective for the psychological symptoms, and chaste tree better reduced the physical symptoms of PMDD. Both treatments were well tolerated, although two patients experienced sexual dysfunction in the fluoxetine group, whereas no patients receiving chaste tree experienced any sexual side effect.

A clinical trial conducted in China assessed the value of chaste tree extract (4 mg/day, equivalent to 40 mg dried herb) in women suffering from moderate to severe PMS.[98] A prospective, double blind, placebo-controlled, parallel-group, clinical trial design was employed. After a screening and preparation phase lasting three cycles, 217 eligible patients were randomly assigned to receive the herb or placebo for up to three menstrual cycles. Efficacy was assessed using the Chinese version PMSdiary (PMSD) and the PMTS. The difference in the mean PMSD score from baseline to the third cycle in the treatment group (22.71±10.33) was significantly higher than the difference in the placebo group (15.50±12.94, p<0.0001). Results for PMTS were similar, with the total scores for PMTS being significantly different between the two groups (p<0.01). A placebo effect of 50% was found in the study, consistent with other studies. No serious adverse event occurred in either group.

A second study conducted in China utilised the same product, dosage and basic design to assess the value of chaste tree in 67 women with moderate to severe PMS.[99,100] Based on a Chinese version of a 17-item diarised symptom score (PMSD) and also the PMTS sum score, chaste tree treatment was significantly superior to placebo by the third treatment cycle (p=0.015 and p=0.040, respectively). A significant difference was also evident for the PMSD score by the second cycle (p=0.030). The efficacy rate was 84.9% in the treatment group versus 55.9% in the placebo group (p=0.010). Most individual symptoms showed a significantly greater improvement with chaste tree than placebo (p<0.05). There was no significant change in basal serum prolactin after treatment. However, the presence of LHP was not assessed. No information concerning side effects was provided.

A systematic review of herbal treatments for PMS found that chaste tree was the most investigated treatment and, after excluding trials because of poor quality or unsuitable diagnostic criteria, identified four eligible trials involving 500 women.[101] (These trials are reviewed above.[96–99]) The review concluded that chaste tree seemed useful for PMS, but more trials are required in order to fully account for the heterogeneity of the condition.

Menopausal conditions

A review of chaste tree in the treatment of menopause-related complaints concluded that such use is relatively recent.[102] Several studies were described where chaste tree was included in complex herbal formulations, with varying outcomes. One of these was the HALT trial, which is reviewed in this book in the dong quai and black cohosh monographs. The trial failed to find any difference between various herbal interventions and placebo. The review authors suggested that chaste tree might have a role in alleviating the PMS-like symptoms associated with perimenopause.

A randomised, double blind trial conducted in Australia included 100 late-perimenopausal or postmenopausal women experiencing hot flushes and other menopausal symptoms.[103] Ninety-three women completed the study. They received chaste tree (1 g/day) and St John's wort (Hypericum perforatum) or placebo for 16 weeks. The St John's wort tablets contained 900 mg/day of extract corresponding to 5.4 g of dried herb flowering top (containing 2.97 mg of hypericins, 27 mg of hyperforin and 54 mg of flavonoid glycosides). The trial measured hot flushes (number and severity of hot flushes and sweating episodes experienced each day and night), menopausal symptoms (using the Greene Climacteric Scale), depression (using the Hamilton Depression Inventory) and quality of life (using the Utian Quality of Life Scale). There was no

difference observed between the herbal intervention and placebo for any of these measures.

Data on premenstrual syndrome-like symptoms were collected from a small subgroup (14) of late-perimenopausal women who took part in the above clinical trial.[104] Participants recorded the severity of their PMS-like symptoms at entry by recall and during the premenstrual phase whenever the impending onset of menstruation was evident throughout the 16 weeks of treatment. Eight women received herbal treatment and six were in the placebo group. At the end of treatment, the herbal combination was found to be superior to placebo for total PMS-like scores (p=0.02).

Chaste tree essential oil demonstrated some efficacy in two observational trials for the alleviation of menopausal symptoms.[105,106] However, the lack of a placebo group, the variable use of oils (from leaf and fruit) and the different routes of administration (at least in the first study) render these findings of uncertain relevance to the oral use of chaste tree fruit.

Female infertility

Some uncontrolled trials already included above under *Menstruation disorders* also observed improved fertility in some patients. The influence of chaste tree on corpus luteal function was investigated in two early uncontrolled trials. When the data from these two trials are combined, the effect of chaste tree was studied on 45 infertile women aged between 23 and 39. These women were considered to be capable of reproduction and had normal basal prolactinaemia (less than 20 ng/mL), but showed pathologically low serum progesterone levels of between 7.0 and 12.0 ng/mL at day 20 of the menstrual cycle. After 3 months, chaste tree treatment (equivalent to about 33 mg/day dried herb) was considered to be successful in 39 of 45 cases. Seven women became pregnant, 25 women exhibited normal serum progesterone levels at day 20 and another seven tended towards normal levels. These results generally coincided with a lengthening of the luteal (hyperthermic) phase and a positive change in the LHRH test dynamic.[107,108] The findings indicate an enhancement of corpus luteal function, which may have been inhibited as part of LHP.

The effect of a homeopathic formula containing chaste tree mother tincture (60 drops/day) was investigated in 96 women with fertility disorders in a 3-month randomised, placebo-controlled, double blind study.[109] A positive outcome (pregnancy, improved concentrations of luteal phase hormones or spontaneous menstruation if amenorrhoea was present) was achieved in 58% of treated women versus 36% in the control group (p=0.069). In women with amenorrhoea or luteal insufficiency, pregnancy occurred more than twice as often in the treated group. Only minor side effects occurred.

A complex dietary supplement containing chaste tree resulted in a significantly higher conception rate than placebo (p=0.01) in a 3-month randomised, double blind trial involving 93 women with fertility problems.[110]

Mastalgia

Mastalgia or mastodynia can be a typical symptom of PMS, especially if it is cyclical. However, a number of chaste tree studies have examined this condition alone. In the period 1968 to 1976, 1480 women with mastodynia were treated with a homeopathic formula containing chaste tree mother tincture (hereafter referred to as HCTMT) for 3 to 6 months. An analysis of 444 women found 58% achieved a symptom-free state and 25% experienced a clear improvement.[111] In another early uncontrolled trial, 52 patients with mastalgia received chaste tree extract (60 drops/day, equivalent to 33.4 mg of herb) over a period of at least three menstrual cycles. No pain was experienced by 46% of patients, and in 29% the pain was decreased to a minimum.[112] These results from such uncontrolled trials should be interpreted with caution, because a high placebo effect is likely.

In a double blind clinical trial, 160 patients with cyclic mastalgia received HCTMT (60 drops/day), gestagen therapy (lynestrenol) or placebo. Significant differences were observed between the groups, with the phytotherapy conferring good relief of symptoms in 74.5% of patients, compared with 82.1% for lynestrenol and 36.8% for placebo. Treatment with HCTMT was considered superior because of the lower incidence of side effects.[113] In an earlier trial with 20 patients using the same design but including crossover, a statistically significant reduction of symptoms was observed with HCTMT treatment. Short-lived nausea was also reported.[114]

The effect of two preparations of HCTMT (a tablet and a liquid) over three menstrual cycles was compared against a placebo in a randomised, double blind trial involving 104 patients with cyclical mastalgia.[115] Both treatment arms contained equivalent doses (equal to around 32 mg/day of chaste tree dried herb) and significantly reduced breast pain compared with placebo (p<0.01). Relative to the placebo group, basal prolactin levels fell significantly by an average of 4.35 ng/mL for the liquid and 3.70 ng/mL for the tablet (p=0.05).

In a placebo-controlled, randomised, double blind study, HCTMT (60 drops/day, containing around 32 mg of dried chaste tree) for one and two menstrual cycles significantly reduced pain intensity compared with a placebo in 97 women with cyclic mastalgia (p=0.018 and p=0.006, respectively).[116,117] After three cycles the difference against placebo was of borderline significance (p=0.064). The frequency of adverse events was the same in both groups.

In what was essentially two small 3-month, open label trials, chaste tree (40 mg/day) was compared with the dopaminergic drug bromocriptine (5 mg/day) in 40 patients with mild hyperprolactinaemia (Group 2) and 40 with mastalgia (Group 1).[118] For Group 1, both treatments significantly reduced mastalgia from baseline (p<0.0001), with no difference between them. Similarly, prolactin levels for Group 2 dropped significantly after both treatments (p<0.0001). There were no side effects with chaste tree, but 12.5% of the patients given bromocriptine suffered nausea and vomiting.

It should also be noted that mastalgia was also among the clinical endpoints in many of the PMS trials involving chaste tree. This point was noted in a 2007 review that concluded, based on five clinical trials (all reviewed above under PMS (mainly) or mastalgia), chaste tree is an efficient agent in the management of mastalgia.[119]

Other conditions

In a 2-year, controlled, open label trial involving 161 patients (both male and female) with various forms of acne, a minimum of 3 months' treatment with chaste tree (40 drops/day tincture for 4 to 6 weeks followed by 30 drops/day) in conjunction with a mild topical disinfectant resulted in an improvement for 70% of patients, a result which was significantly better than standard therapy.[120] The mechanism for the beneficial effect of chaste tree on acne is not known, but may be due to a mild antiandrogenic effect.

A favourable effect was observed on milk production in 80% of 125 nursing women treated with chaste tree in a case observation study.[121] In an open, controlled trial involving 817 postnatal patients, a significant effect was observed from chaste tree treatment (45 drops/day of tincture, equivalent to around 38 mg dried herb), with average milk production about three times that of controls after 20 days of treatment.[122] These early trials involved the use of quite low doses of chaste tree and higher doses might in all probability be counterproductive, given the potential dopaminergic activity.

The role of melatonin in human health and disease is being extensively investigated. In particular, melatonin functions in the regulation of circadian rhythms, mood and tumour growth.[123] Since the effects of melatonin can be biphasic, for example some concentrations can inhibit tumour growth while other concentrations have a stimulating effect, it makes sense to investigate natural means of manipulating the melatonin output by the pineal gland. The circadian rhythm of melatonin secretion was measured in 20 healthy males aged 20 to 32 years after the intake of placebo or various doses of an extract of chaste tree for 14 days. In an open, placebo-controlled study, the doses investigated were 120 to 480 mg/day of this extract (corresponding to at least 0.6 to 2.4 g of dried herb).[123] The concentration of melatonin in serum showed the typical nocturnal increase, beginning approximately 1 h after the light was turned off. Administration of chaste tree caused a dose-dependent increase of melatonin secretion, especially during the night (compared with placebo treatment). Total melatonin output was approximately 60% higher in the group receiving chaste tree. The authors observed that the feeling of fatigue or the promotion of sleepiness observed by some patients taking chaste tree during the trial might be a result of the stimulation of endogenous melatonin secretion and speculated that chaste tree may have value in the treatment of sleep-maintenance insomnia and jet lag.

Given the above, and the fact that dopaminergic drugs are used in the management of restless legs syndrome, the effect of chaste tree extract (40 mg/day, equivalent to 360 mg dried herb) in this disorder was investigated in an uncontrolled, practitioner-based pilot study involving 12 patients.[124] Of seven patients receiving chaste tree alone, five responded positively. Another five with more severe symptoms received chaste tree with conventional dopaminergic agents, with four responding favourably by being able to reduce their dosage of the drugs. One patient was able to cease pramipexol altogether. No side effects were observed from the chaste tree.

Toxicology and other safety data

Toxicology

The oral and intraperitoneal LD_{50} of chaste tree extract exceeded 2g/kg in rats and mice, indicating low toxicity. No animals died at this dose. The no-observed-effect level of chaste tree extract was 50mg/kg in a subacute oral toxicity study lasting 28 days, and 40mg/kg in a chronic oral toxicity study lasting 26 weeks.[21]

Genotoxic-mutagenic activity was not observed for a homeopathic mother tincture preparation of chaste tree in the Ames test in vitro or in the micronucleus test in vivo after oral administration of a dose corresponding to 370mg/kg chaste tree.[125]

Contraindications

None known.

Special warnings and precautions

In general, chaste tree is best not taken in conjunction with progesterone drugs and hormone replacement therapy. The herb is quite safe in low doses in conjunction with the contraceptive pill and several of the PMS trials included patients on this treatment without apparent harm. Chaste tree may aggravate pure spasmodic dysmenorrhoea not associated with PMS (clinical observation of the authors). This may be due to the priming effect of progesterone on endometrial prostaglandin release during the initial stages of menstruation. However chaste tree is usually beneficial for spasmodic dysmenorrhoea associated with PMS and also for congestive dysmenorrhoea.

Interactions

Chaste tree may interact antagonistically with dopamine receptor antagonists.[126] However, this has not been observed clinically.

A survey of UK herbalists found that 93.8% of 145 respondents reported that they had not found any conventional medications to interact with chaste tree, whilst 70.5% of 149 respondents answered that they did not prescribe chaste tree in conjunction with conventional oestrogenic/progesterogenic medications.[8] Chaste tree did not demonstrate any interactions with the low-dose contraceptive pill in clinical trials, as noted above.

Use in pregnancy and lactation

Category B1 – no increase in frequency of malformation or other harmful effects on the fetus from limited use in women. No evidence of increased fetal damage in animal studies. Use cautiously in pregnancy and only in the early stages for insufficient corpus luteum function.

There were no significant differences in maternal toxicity, reproductive outcome or fetal developmental parameters compared with placebo in rats and rabbits orally administered a homeopathic preparation containing chaste tree tincture during the organogenesis period of gestation. The dosages administered corresponded to 6.3 to 51.1mg/kg of chaste tree in rats and 3.7 to 37mg/kg in rabbits. A non-significant increase in fetal body weight, placental weight and number of resorptions was observed in the high dose group for rabbits. For rabbits, three external deformities occurred in the low dose group and one skull deformity (hydrocephalus) in each of the medium dose and high dose groups. It was not determined whether these results were due to chaste tree, the homeopathic preparation, the alcohol content or spontaneous occurrences.[125]

Oral administration of the same preparation to female rats from 2 weeks before mating until up to 28 days postpartum at doses corresponding to 4 to 40mg/kg of chaste tree had no effects on body weight or development, mating behaviour, fertility, reproductive outcome or lactation. No teratogenic effects were observed in F1 or F2 fetuses and F1 and F2 offspring did not differ from controls.[125] Oral administration of chaste tree seeds (1 or 2g/kg/day) to pregnant rats from day 1 to day 10 of pregnancy did not reduce the number of fetuses compared with controls.[50] Chaste tree (part unspecified) tested negative for antizygotic, anti-implantation and early abortifacient activity.[127] One review expressed concerns over the lack of conclusive data for the safety of chaste tree in pregnancy and advised caution.[128]

Although the dopaminergic activity of chaste tree might suggest that it is best avoided during lactation,[33,34] clinical trials have demonstrated its positive activity on milk production, albeit at low doses of the berry and in poorly designed trials.[121,129] Hence, higher doses (greater than 250mg/day) should certainly be avoided during lactation.

As described above, a homeopathic preparation containing chaste tree tincture orally administered to female rats (4 to 40mg/kg chaste tree) during their lactation period did not exert toxic adverse effects on either the dams or their F1 and F2 offspring.[125] However, injection of chaste tree in suckling rats did deprive offspring of milk.[37]

Effects on ability to drive and use machines

No adverse effects expected.

Side effects

A 2001 review of the literature found that chaste tree was well tolerated in the majority of clinical studies. Side effects were reported in only 1% to 2% of participants in most studies and severe side effects were only rarely reported. Gastrointestinal disturbances (particularly nausea) and skin conditions (acne, pruritus and rashes) were the most common adverse effects reported. Side effects occasionally reported included headache, fatigue and hormone-related symptoms, such as menstrual cycle changes, mastalgia and weight gain.[21] Chaste tree extract (120 to 480mg/day) was administered to healthy males for 14 days in a placebo-controlled trial. There were no undesired effects on blood pressure, heart rate, blood count, clinical laboratory parameters or testosterone, FSH and LH values.[46]

A 2005 systematic review of adverse events from the published literature, herbal manufacturers and drug authority databases found that adverse reactions from chaste tree are mild and reversible.[130] The most frequent side effects include nausea, headache, gastrointestinal disturbances, menstrual disorders, acne, pruritus and rash. No drug interactions were reported.

A 32-year-old woman with tubal infertility undergoing unstimulated IVF treatment had signs and symptoms suggestive of a mild ovarian hyperstimulation syndrome after commencing a herbal preparation containing chaste tree, *Mitchella repens* and *Viburnum opulus* for 13 days (dose not specified). The preparation was discontinued and her next two menstrual cycles were endocrinologically normal. The authors stated that there was no conclusive evidence that the patient's unusual response was due to the herbal preparation.[131,132]

A 45-year-old woman who had been taking separate bottled products of chaste tree, black cohosh and evening primrose oil for 4 months had three nocturnal seizures within a 3-month period. The patient had also consumed one to two beers 24 to 48h prior to each incident.[133] It was not established if any of the herbal preparations contributed to the seizures.

A case was reported in 2001 of a woman diagnosed with grade 1 endometrioid adenocarcinoma of the endometrium 'whose history was notable for extensive use of supplemental phytoestrogens'. Herbs consumed included chaste tree, dong quai, black cohosh and licorice.[134] No causality was demonstrated.

As noted previously in this monograph, concerns have been expressed that chaste tree use might mask a prolactinoma.[48]

Overdosage

No incidents found in the published literature.

Safety in children

No information available.

Regulatory status in selected countries

Chaste tree is covered by a positive Commission E Monograph and can be used for the treatment of menstrual problems, premenstrual syndrome and mastodynia.

Chaste tree is now on the UK General Sale List. Chaste tree products have achieved Traditional Herbal Registration in the UK with the traditional indication of relief of symptoms associated with premenstrual syndrome.

Chaste tree does not have GRAS status. However, it is freely available as a 'dietary supplement' in the USA under DSHEA legislation (1994 Dietary Supplement Health and Education Act).

Chaste tree is not included in Part 4 of Schedule 4 of the Therapeutic Goods Act Regulations of Australia and is freely available for sale.

References

1. Tsoulogiannis IN, Spandidos DA. *Hormones (Athens)*. 2007;6(1):80–82.
2. Felter HW, Lloyd JU. *King's American Dispensatory*. Vol 2. 18th ed., rev 3, Portland: 1905. Reprinted by: Eclectic Medical Publications; 1983:p. 2056.
3. Mills SY. *Out of the Earth: The Essential Book of Herbal Medicine*. London: Viking Arkana (Penguin); 1991. pp. 522–524.
4. Mills SY. *Woman Medicine: Vitex Agnus-Castus, the Herb*. Christchurch, UK: Amberwood; 1992. pp. 10–15.
5. British Herbal Medicine Association. *A Guide to Traditional Herbal Medicines: A Sourcebook of Accepted Traditional Uses of Medicinal Plants Within Europe*. Bournemouth: BHMA;2003.
6. Lev E, Amar Z. *J Ethnopharmacol*. 2002;82(2–3):131–145.
7. Lev E, Amar Z. *J Ethnopharmacol*. 2000;72(1–2):191–205.
8. Christie S, Walker AF. *Eur J Herbal Med*. 1997;3(3):29–45.
9. Vera-Lastra O, Mendez C, Jara LJ, et al. *J Rheumatol*. 2003;30(10):2140–2146.
10. Ram S, Blumberg D, Newton P, et al. *Rheumatology (Oxford)*. 2004;43(10): 1272–1274.
11. El Meidany YM, Ahmed I, Mooustafa H, et al. *Joint Bone Spine*. 2004;71(3):203–208.
12. Picco P, Gattorno M, Buoncompagni A, et al. *Ann N Y Acad Sci*. 1999;876:262–265.
13. Pacilio M, Migliaresi S, Meli R, et al. *J Rheumatol*. 2001;28(10):2216–2221.
14. Walker SE. *Lupus*. 2001;10(10):762–768.
15. Figueroa F, Carrion F, Martinez ME, et al. *Rev Med Chil*. 1998;126(1):33–41.
16. Mader R. *Harefuah*. 1997;133(11):527–529.
17. Dostál C, Moszkorzová L, Musilová L, et al. *Ann Rheum Di*. 2003;62:487–488.
18. Burgoyne B. *MediHerb eNewsletter*. 2011.
19. Mabberley DJ, ed. *The Plant Book*. Cambridge: Cambridge University Press; 1997. p. 749.
20. Thomson WAR, ed. *Healing Plants*. London: Macmillan; 1980. p. 111.
21. Upton R, Petrone C, Graff A, eds. *Chaste Tree Fruit: Vitex agnus-castus, American Herbal Pharmacopoeia and Therapeutic Compendium*. Santa Cruz, CA: American Herbal Pharmacopoeia; 2001.
22. Zwaving JH, Bos R. *Planta Med*. 1996;62(1):83–84.
23. Sorensen JM, Katsiotis ST. *Planta Med*. 2000;66(3):245–250.
24. Hajdu Z, Hohmann J, Forgo P, et al. *Phytother Res*. 2007;21(4):391–394.
25. Gorler K, Oehlke D, Soicke H. *Planta Med*. 1985;50(6):530–531.
26. Hoberg E, Meier B, Sticher O. *Planta Med*. 2000;66(4):352–355.
27. Ono M, Yamasaki T, Konoshita M, et al. *Chem Pharm Bull (Tokyo)*. 2008;56(11):1621–1624.
28. Ono M, Nagasawa Y, Ikeda T, et al. *Chem Pharm Bull (Tokyo)*. 2009;57(10):1132–1135.
29. Chen SN, Friesen JB, Webster D, et al. *Fitoterapia*. 2011;82(4):528–533.
30. van Rensen I. *Z Phytother*. 2010;31:322–326.
31. Haller J. *Z Geburtsh Gynakol*. 1961;156(3):274–302.
32. Loch E, Kaiser E. *Gynakol Praxis*. 1990;14:489–495.
33. Sliutz G, Speiser P, Schultz AM, et al. *Horm Metab Res*. 1993;25(5):253–255.
34. Winterhoff H. *Abstracts of papers of the American Chemical Society*.1996;212 (1–2):AGFD 105.
35. Jarry H, Leonhardt S, Gorkow C, et al. *Exp Clin Endocrinol*. 1994;102(6):448–454.
36. Wuttke W, Ch Gorkow, Jarry H. In: Loew D, Rietbrock N, eds. *Phytopharmaka in Forschung und klinischer Anwendung*. Darmstadt: Steinkopff (Verlag); 1995. pp. 83–90.
37. Winterhoff H, Gorkow C, Behr B. *Z Phytother*. 1991;12(6):175–179.
38. Meier B, Berger D, Hoberg E, et al. *Phytomedicine*. 2000;7(5):373–381.
39. Christoffel V, Spengler B, Abel G, et al. *FACT*. 2000;5(1):87–88.
40. Wuttke W, Jarry H, Christoffel V, et al. *Phytomedicine*. 2003;10(4):348–357.
41. Jarry H, Spengler B, Wuttke W, et al. *Maturitas*. 2006;55(suppl 1):S26–S36.
42. Nasri S, Oryan S, Rohani AH, et al. *Pak J Biol Sci*. 2007;10(14):2300–2307.
43. Ibrahim NA, Shalaby AS, Farag RS, et al. *Nat Prod Res*. 2008;22(6):537–546.
44. Hu Y, Xin HL, Zhang QY, et al. *Phytomedicine*. 2007;14(10):668–674.
45. Ye Q, Zhang QY, Zheng CJ, et al. *Acta Pharmacol Sin*. 2010;31(12): 1564–1568.

46. Loew D, Gorkow C, Schrodter A, et al. *Z Phytother*. 1996;17(4):237–240, 243.

47. Merz PG, Schrodter A, Rietbrock S, et al. In: Loew D, Rietbrock N, eds. *Phytopharmaka in Forschung und klinischer Anwendung*. Darmstadt: Steinkopff (Verlag); 1995. pp. 93–97.

48. Gallagher J, Lynch FW, Barragry J. *Eur J Obstet Gynecol Reprod Biol*. 2008;137(2):257–258.

49. Tamagno G, Burlacu MC, Daly AF, et al. *Eur J Obstet Gynecol Reprod Biol*. 2007;135(1):139–140.

50. Lal R, Sankaranarayanan A, Mathur VS, et al. *Bull Postgrad Inst Med Educ Res Chandigarh*. 1985;19(2):44–47.

51. Bhargava SK. *J Ethnopharmacol*. 1989;27(3):327–339.

52. Liu J, Burdette JE, Sun Y, et al. *Phytomedicine*. 2004;11(1):18–23.

53. Jarry H, Spengler B, Porzel A, et al. *Planta Med*. 2003;69(10):945–947.

54. Sehmisch S, Boeckhoff J, Wille J, et al. *Phytother Res*. 2009;23(6):851–858.

55. Higham JP, Ross C, Warren Y, et al. *Horm Behav*. 2007;52(3):384–390.

56. Emery Thompson M, Wilson ML, Gobbo G, et al. *Am J Primatol*. 2008;70(11): 1064–1071.

57. Lu A, Beehner JC, Czekala NM, et al. *Horm Behav*. 2011;59(1):28–36.

58. Pepeljnjak S, Antolic A, Kustrak D. *Acta Pharm*. 1996;46(3):201–206.

59. Mishurova SS, Malinovskaya TA, Akhmedov IB, et al. *Rastitel'Nye Resursy*. 1986;22(4):526–530.

60. Marongiu B, Piras A, Porcedda S, et al. *Nat Prod Res*. 2010;24(6):569–579.

61. Ohyama K, Akaike T, Hirobe C, et al. *Biol Pharm Bull*. 2003;26(1):10–18.

62. Weisskopf M, Schaffner W, Jundt G, et al. *Planta Med*. 2005;71(10):910–916.

63. Ohyama K, Akaike T, Imai M, et al. *Int J Biochem Cell Biol*. 2005;37(7):1496–1510.

64. Mazzio EA, Soliman KF. *Phytother Res*. 2009;23(3):385–398.

65. Ko WG, Kang TH, Lee SJ, et al. *Phytother Res*. 2001;15(6):535–537.

66. Imai M, Kikuchi H, Denda T, et al. *Cancer Lett*. 2009;276(1):74–80.

67. Webster DE, Lu J, Chen SN, et al. *J Ethnopharmacol*. 2006;106(2):216–221.

68. Webster DE, He Y, Chen SN, et al. *Biochem Pharmacol*. 2011;81(1):170–177.

69. Saberi M, Rezvanizadeh A, Bakhtiarian A. *Neurosci Lett*. 2008;441(2):193–196.

70. Probst V, Roth OA. *Dtsch Med Wochen schr*. 1954;79(35):1271–1274.

71. Roth OA. *Med Klin*. 1956;51:1263–1265.

72. Kayser HW, Istanbulluoglu S. *Hippokrates*. 1954;25:717–719.

73. Bleier W. *Zbl Gynakol*. 1959;81(18):701–709.

74. Bubenzer R. *Therapiewoche*. 1993;43 (32–33):1705–1706 [Article in German].

75. Propping D, Bohnert KJ, Peeters M, et al. *Therapeutikon*. 1991;5:581–585.

76. Roeder D. *Z Phytother*. 1994;15(3):157–163.

77. Loch EG, Kaiser E. *Gynakol Prax*. 1990;14:489–495.

78. Peters-Welte C, Albrecht M. *TW Gynakol*. 1994;7(1):49–52.

79. Milewicz A, Gejdel E, Sworen H, et al. *Arzneimittelforschung*. 1993;43(7):752–756.

80. Ecker G. *Landarzt*. 1964;40:872–874.

81. Hillebrand H. *Landarzt*. 1964;40(36):1577–1578.

82. Albus GA. *Z Hautkr Geschlkrkh*. 1964;36(7):220–223.

83. Coeugnier E, Elek E, Kühnast R. *Arztezeitchr Naturheilverf*. 1986;27:619–622.

84. Dittmar F, Böhnert K. *TW Gynakol*. 1992;5:60–68.

85. Feldmann HU, Albrecht M, Lamertz M, et al. *Gyne*. 1990;12:421–425.

86. Loch EG, Selle H, Boblitz N. *J Womens Health Gend Based Med*. 2000;9(3):315–320.

87. Berger D, Aebi S, Samochowiec E, et al. *Z Phytother*. 1999;20:155–157. [Article in German].

88. Berger D, Schaffner W, Schrader E, et al. *Arch Gynecol Obstet*. 2000;264(3):150–153.

89. Falch BS, Bitzer J, Polasek W. *Therapiewoche*. 2003;19:287–288.

90. Widmer R, Baez Y, Kreuter *GanzheitsMedizin*. 2005;17:351–354.

91. Priplepskaya VN, Ledina AV, Tagiyeva AV, et al. *Maturitas*. 2006;55(suppl 1):S55–S63.

92. Di Lorenzo C, Goppola G, Pierelli F, et al. *Cephalalgia*. 2007;27(6):747. Poster F088.

93. Promotional Brochure. UK: Gerard House; 1988.

94. Turner S, Mills S. *Complement Ther Med*. 1993;1:73–77.

95. Lauritzen CH, Reuter HD, Repges R, et al. *Phytomedicine*. 1997;4(3):183–189.

96. Schellenberg R. *BMJ*. 2001;322(7279):134–137.

97. Atmaca M, Kumru S, Tezcan E. *Hum Psychopharmacol*. 2003;18(3):191–195.

98. He Z, Chen R, Zhou Y, et al. *Maturitas*. 2009;63(1):99–103.

99. Ma L, Lin S, Chen R, et al. *Aust NZ J Obstet Gynaecol*. 2010;50(2):189–193.

100. Ma L, Lin S, Chen R, et al. *Gynecol Endocrinol*. 2010;26(8):612–616.

101. Dante G, Facchinetti F. *J Psychosom Obstet Gynaecol*. 2011;32(1):42–51.

102. Van Die MD, Burger HG, Teede HJ, Bone KM. *J Altern Complement Med*. 2009;15(8):853–862.

103. Van Die MD, Burger HG, Bone KM, et al. *Menopause*. 2009;16(1):156–163.

104. Van Die MD, Bone KM, Burger HG, et al. *J Altern Complement Med*. 2009;15(9):1045–1048.

105. Chopin Lucks B. *Complement Ther Nurs Midwifery*. 2003;9(3):157–160.

106. Lucks BC, Sørensen J, Veal L. *Complement Ther Nurs Midwifery*. 2002;8(3):148–154.

107. Propping D, Katzorke T. *Z Allge Med*. 1987;63(31):932–933.

108. Propping D, Katzorke T, Belkien L. *Therapiewoche*. 1988;38(41):2992–3001.

109. Gerhard II, Patek A, Monga B, et al. *Forsch Komplementarmed*. 1998;5(6): 272–278.

110. Westphal LM, Polan ML, Trant AS. *Clin Exp Obstet Gynecol*. 2006;33(4): 205–208.

111. Gregl A. *Med Welt*. 1979;30:264–268.

112. Kress D, Thanner E. *Med Klin*. 1981;76(20):566–567.

113. Kubista E, Muller G, Spona J. *Rev Fr Gynecol Obstet*. 1987;82(4):221–227.

114. Kubista E, Muller G, Spona J. *Zentralbl Gynakol*. 1983;105(18):1153–1162.

115. Wuttke W, Splitt G, Gorkow C, et al. *Geburtsh Frauenheilk*. 1997;57(10): 569–574.

116. Halaska M, Beles P, Gorkow C, et al. *Breast*. 1999;8(4):175–181.

117. Halaska M, Raus K, B les P, et al. *Ceska Gynekol*. 1998;63(5):388–392.

118. Kilicdag EB, Tarim E, Bagis T, et al. *Int J Gynecol Obstet*. 2004;85(3):292–293.

119. Carmichael AR. *Evid Based Complement Altern Med*. 2008;5(3):247–250.

120. Giss G, Rothenburg W. *Z Haut Geschlechtskr*. 1968;43(15):645–647.

121. Noack M. *Dtsch Med Wochen schr*. 1943; 9:204–206.

122. Mohr W. *Hippokrates*. 1957;28:586–591.

123. Dericks-Tan JS, Schwinn P, Hildt C. *Exp Clin Endocrinol Diabetes*. 2003;111(1):44–46.

124. Brattström A, Kaiser WF. *Z Phytother*. 2010;31(5):247–250.

125. Blaschek W, Ebel S, Hackenthal E, et al. *HagerROM 2002: Hagers Handbuch der Drogen und Arzneistoffe*. Heidelberg: Springer; 2002.

126. Blumenthal M, ed. *The Complete German Commission E Monographs: Therapeutic Guide to Herbal Medicines*. Austin: American Botanical Council; 1998.

127. Chaudhury RR. *Plants with Possible Antifertility Activity, Special Report Series No. 55*. New Delhi: Indian Council of Medical Research; 1966. pp. 3–19.

128. Dugoua JJ, Seely D, Perri D, et al. *Can J Clin Pharmacol*. 2008;15(1): e74–e79.

129. Mohr W. *Dtsch Med Wochen schr*. 1954;79(41):1513–1516.

130. Daniele C, Thompson-Coon J, Pittler MH, et al. *Drug Saf*. 2005;28(4):319–332.

131. Cahill DJ, Fox R, Wardle PG, et al. *Hum Reprod*. 1994;9(8):1469–1470.

132. Cahill DJ. *Hum Reprod*. 1995; 10(8):2175–2176.

133. Shuster J. *Hosp Pharm*. 1996;31(12):1553–1554.

134. Johnson EB, Muto MC, Yanushpolsky EH, et al. *Obstet Gynecol*. 2001;98 (5 Pt 2):947–950.

(*Chelidonium majus* L.)

Synonyms

Greater celandine (Engl), Chelidonii herba (Lat), Schöllkraut, Goldwurz (Ger), chélidoine (Fr), cinerognolle (Ital), svaleurt (Dan), baiqucai (Chin).

What is it?

Chelidonium has a long history of use as a therapeutic plant. It was mentioned by Pliny, to whom we owe the tradition of calling the plant Chelidonium, derived from the Greek *chelidon* (a swallow). This is apparently because it comes into flower when the swallows arrive and fades when the swallows depart. Pliny reported that its acrid juice was used to remove films from the cornea of the eye and alchemists believed it was beneficial for jaundice because of its intense yellow colour. Although the root also contains the characteristic alkaloids and is utilised to a limited extent medicinally, the aerial parts are more widely used and are the main focus of this monograph.

Effects

Assists liver and gallbladder function, protects against hepatic injury; spasmolytic to the gastrointestinal tract; stimulates bile flow; active topically against fungal infections and warts; decreases benign and malignant tumours (topically and internally).

Traditional view

Chelidonium was employed to treat conditions of the liver such as jaundice, hepatic congestion and biliary dyspepsia. It was also used for bilious and migraine headaches and haemorrhoids.[1] The herb was often used in the form of a poultice or ointment for the treatment of cutaneous problems and traumatic inflammation,[1] and the fresh milky juice was used topically in the treatment of warts, ringworm and corns.[1,2]

Summary actions

Choleretic, cholagogue, spasmolytic, mild laxative, anti-inflammatory, antineoplastic, antiviral and vulnerary (topically).

Can be used for

Indications supported by clinical trials

Disorders of the liver and gallbladder; cramp-like pain of the gastrointestinal tract and gall ducts, including irritable bowel syndrome; as an enema for colonic polyposis; as a topical application for warts (mostly uncontrolled studies); functional dyspepsia (alone and in combination).

Traditional therapeutic uses

Gallbladder disease, gallstones; liver disease, jaundice; to aid detoxification via the liver and bowel; hepatic and splenic congestion; migraine, bilious headaches and supraorbital neuralgia; skin conditions including warts, fungal growths and ringworm (especially the fresh juice).[1]

In China Chelidonium is also used for gastritis, gastric ulcer, enteritis, jaundice and abdominal pain as well as bronchitis and whooping cough.[3,4]

May also be used for

Extrapolations from pharmacological studies

Inhibition of keratinocyte proliferation in psoriasis (topical use).

Preparations

Dried herb as a decoction, liquid extract and tablets or capsules for internal use. Decoction, extract or fresh juice for external use.

Dosage

1 to 2 mL/day of 1:2 liquid extract, 2 to 4 mL/day of 1:5 tincture. Short-term use of higher doses up to the equivalent of 3 to 4 g per day may be necessary (as per the Berlin clinical trial).

The dose used in China is 3 to 9 g per day or even higher. However, these doses are generally administered by decoction and this method may not extract the Chelidonium alkaloids as efficiently as alcohol and water.

Duration of use

High doses should be restricted to short-term use; long-term use of normal doses is not recommended.

Summary assessment of safety

No significant adverse effects have been noted for short-term use, but excessive intake of the decoction may cause nausea and other gastrointestinal symptoms. Long-term use is associated with a low risk of a moderate idiosyncratic hepatotoxic reaction. The herb should not be given to patients with pre-existing liver damage.

Technical data

Botany

Chelidonium majus is a member of the Papaveraceae (poppy) family and is a perennial herb approximately 50 to 90 cm in height with a branched woody taproot. The fragile stems are branched, with scattered hairs and contain an orange latex. The leaves are pinnatisect, with up to seven oblong or ovate leaflets with a bluish green underside. The flowers contain four bright yellow petals and are grouped in small clusters. The fruit capsule is one-celled, up to 5 cm long and contains black seeds with a white appendage.[5]

Adulteration

No adulterants known.

Key constituents

- Isoquinoline alkaloids (0.35 to 1.3%),[6] including the major alkaloids chelidonine (>0.07%), chelerythrine, sanguinarine, berberine, coptisine and dl-stylopine
- Other alkaloids: sparteine (which is usually found in the Leguminosae (pea) family)[6,7]
- Flavonoids, phenolic acids.[7]

The isoquinoline group of alkaloids contains many structural types including the benzophenanthridines (chelidonine, chelerythrine, sanguinarine) and protoberberines (berberine, coptisine). An analysis of 20 Chelidonium samples from different parts of China found the total alkaloids varied from 0.89% to 1.70%, with coptisine the highest alkaloid present (average content of 0.5%) and berberine the lowest at 0.013%.[8]

The milky orange sap of Chelidonium contains defensive proteins, including an extracellular peroxidase with nuclease activity.[9,10]

Chelidonine

Chelerythrine

Sanguinarine

Pharmacodynamics

Hepatoprotective and choleretic activity

Oral administration of an alcohol extract of dried Chelidonium reduced carbon tetrachloride-induced liver injury in rats.[11] Significant reductions in elevated plasma levels of liver enzymes and bilirubin occurred in the treated group. A follow-up study was undertaken to clarify the underlying aspects of tissue recovery. There was an absence of fibrotic changes in the Chelidonium-treated rats (125 mg/kg/day for 3 weeks, oral), which was thought to be related to a reduced degree of cellular necrosis and a reduction in fibroblast-stimulating factors.[12]

Extracts of dried Chelidonium were tested for choleretic activity using the isolated perfused rat liver. The 70% ethanolic extract of the herb significantly induced choleresis (bile flow). However, it did this without increasing the total output of bile acids (that is, there was an increased flow of more dilute bile). In contrast, the phenolic and alkaloidal fractions of the total extract, tested individually and in combination, did not significantly increase bile flow, although small increases were observed. The authors concluded that the increased bile flow is due to an additive effect from all compounds in the total extract of Chelidonium, not one or two specific active constituents or fractions.[13]

Antimicrobial activity

Isolated chelerythrine and an alkaloid fraction from the dried roots of Chelidonium containing chelerythrine and sanguinarine were found to be ineffective against Gram-negative bacteria in vitro. However, a significant antimicrobial effect was observed against Gram-positive bacteria such as *Staphylococcus aureus* and two strains of *Streptococcus*, and also against the fungus *Candida albicans*.[14] Chelerythrine inhibited the adherence of *Streptococcus mutans* and was thereby considered to possess significant anticariogenic activity.[15] This alkaloid also inhibited the growth of this organism in vitro with an MIC (minimum inhibitory concentration) of 0.78 mg/mL, but chelidonine was inactive.[16] Sanguinarine is also well described as an alkaloid with activity against dental plaque.[17–19]

In an in vitro screening of the ethanolic extracts from 12 Siberian herbs for antimicrobial activity against five common pathogenic organisms, the extract of Chelidonium aerial parts was not active. In contrast, the root extract demonstrated marked activity against *Bacillus cereus*, *Candida albicans* and *Salmonella enteritidis*.[20]

Extracts of Chelidonium were found to exert antiviral effects in vitro against adenovirus types 12 and 5 and herpes simplex virus type 1 (HSV-1). The most promising antiviral alkaloid was found in greater concentrations in the fresh and aerial plant samples. This alkaloid, which belonged to the benzophenanthridine group, was not identified.[21] A crude extract of Chelidonium was found to inhibit HIV-1 from infecting cells in vitro.[22] A low sulphated polyglycosaminoglycan appeared to be responsible for this action and protected mice from the negative effects of murine retrovirus infection after iv administration. Such a large molecule is unlikely to have oral activity.

Alkaloids from Chelidonium and sanguinarine inhibited the growth of *Trichomonas vaginalis* in vitro. Sanguinarine also caused the protozoa to undergo deformation followed by disintegration within 2 h.[23]

An in vitro study demonstrated that the alkaloids extracted from Chelidonium, chelerythrine, and a mixture of chelerythrine and sanguinarine, exerted an antifungal effect on some Trichophyton strains, *Microsporum canis*, *Epidermophyton floccosum* and *Aspergillus fumigatus*.[24] Another in vitro study investigated the effect of Chelidonium extracts on several *Candida* species and other dermatophytes. Liquid extracts of Chelidonium prepared from dried plant material collected in late July and early September (Europe) were compared. Both extracts showed greater than average antifungal activity against some organisms involved in skin infections. The July extract was active against *Candida albicans*, but the September extract showed no activity.[25]

When six species of clinically resistant yeast fungi were exposed to isolated Chelidonium alkaloids, 8-hydroxydihydrosanguinarine and 8-hydroxydihydrochelerythrine demonstrated potent activity, with MIC ranges of 2 to 80 and 4 to 100 μg/mL, respectively.[26] Other alkaloids also had some degree of antifungal activity. The two above compounds were also quite active against methicillin-resistant *Staph. aureus*.[27]

Fusarium species have the capacity to cause opportunistic human infections. Extracts of Chelidonium showed some activity against certain strains of this organism in vitro, with Chelidonium root extracts being more active than shoot extracts.[28]

Antitumour activity

An ethanolic extract of rhizomes and roots of Chelidonium exhibited cytotoxicity against a carcinoma of the nasopharynx in vitro. One of the cytotoxic principles was found to be the alkaloid coptisine.[29] Chelidonium exerted an antimutagenic effect in vitro against several mutagens in the Ames test.[30] The extract caused changes in the mitotic index of transplanted ascitic cells, showing marked antimitotic activity.[3]

Chelidonine and sanguinarine induce apoptosis in leukaemia cells in vitro, but only the former induced cell cycle arrest.[31] Sanguinarine and chelerythrine induce DNA damage and cytotoxic effects in normal and cancer cells, whereas chelidonine does not.[32] Chelidonine may inhibit tumour cell growth by reducing telomerase activity.[33] A methanolic extract of Chelidonium also induced apoptosis in two leukaemia cell lines.[34]

The milky sap from fresh Chelidonium contains two nuclease enzymes with apoptotic activity against the HeLa tumour cell line, but not CHO cells.[35] A lectin isolated from Chelidonium inhibited growth of two tumour cell lines, but not normal mouse fibroblasts.[36]

The activities of aqueous and alcoholic extracts of Chelidonium, the partially purified methanol extract and chelidonine and protopine were screened using transplanted tumours in mice. The water-soluble, purified methanol extract of dried Chelidonium demonstrated high tumour inhibition with relatively mild cytotoxic side effects. Intraperitoneal administration of 700 mg/kg for 7 days resulted in 55% inhibition of sarcoma 180 and Ehrlich carcinoma. The aqueous extract showed insignificant activity, and chelidonine and protopine (both of which are insoluble in water) showed negligible tumour inhibition and were associated with cytotoxic side effects. The crude methanol extract also showed more pronounced toxic side effects.[37]

The numbers of stomach tumours in rats treated with oral doses of a Chelidonium extract after initial exposure to a carcinogen were significantly lower, compared with untreated but exposed animals.[38] An ethanolic whole plant extract of Chelidonium (0.1 mL/mouse of a 1:20 diluted extract) reduced the incidence of chemically induced liver cancer in mice after 60 and 120 days.[39]

Ukrain is described as a semi-synthetic eastern European anticancer drug derived from Chelidonium. It purportedly contains one molecule of thiophosphoric acid conjugated (bonded) to three molecules of chelidonine and is administered by intravenous injection.[40] However, chemical analysis revealed that some commercial samples of Ukrain were just a mixture of Chelidonium alkaloids, with no trimeric structure evident.[41] This was also the case 6 years later in 2006, when another research team found that the Ukrain sample they tested lacked the purported trimeric 'Ukrain molecule' and instead resembled an alkaloidal extract of Chelidonium, with chelidonine, sanguinarine and chelerythrine present as major components.[42] Their in vitro studies suggested chelidonine was a particularly active inducer of tumour cell apoptosis.

A 2005 review of the anticancer research on Ukrain identified 36 in vitro studies and 46 in vivo experiments. These publications suggest that it has the capacity to exert selective cytotoxic and cytostatic effects on tumour cells, while favourably modifying the immune response.[43] Specifically, diminished DNA, RNA and protein synthesis, inhibition of cellular oxygen consumption, inhibition of tubulin polymerisation[44] and induction of apoptosis have all been described.[45] Ukrain also modifies the host immune response via an increase in T cells and normalisation of the T-helper/T-suppressor lymphocyte ratio. Tumour mass reductions have also been demonstrated in vivo.[45] More recent examples of in vivo studies include growth inhibitory effects against B16 melanoma cells[46] and Ehrlich's carcinoma,[47] both in mice. It is uncertain how much, if any, of this research would have relevance to the oral use of Chelidonium extracts.

Anti-inflammatory activity

The alkaloids sanguinarine and chelerythrine are potent in vitro inhibitors of 5-lipoxygenase in polymorphonuclear leucocytes and 12-lipoxygenase in mouse epidermis. An extract of Chelidonium also inhibited 5-lipoxygenase. The inhibitory effects against lipoxygenase enzymes appear to be due to a specific enzyme interaction, rather than a non-specific redox mechanism.[48]

The Chelidonium alkaloids chelerythrine and sanguinarine (5 and 10 mg/kg, oral and sc) demonstrated anti-inflammatory activity in the carrageenan rat paw oedema test.[14] A Chelidonium extract (40 and 400 mg/kg/day for 28 days, oral) suppressed the progression of collagen-induced arthritis in mice. Decreased levels of cytokines and activated immune cells were observed, together with increased numbers of regulatory T cells.[49]

Other effects

Chelidonium extract and isolated components (coptisine and caffeoylmalic acid) weakly antagonised experimentally induced contraction of isolated rat ileal smooth muscle.[50] Two ethanolic dry extracts of Chelidonium and their three main alkaloids were studied in different antispasmodic test models on isolated guinea-pig ileum.[51] Both extracts induced relaxation in barium chloride, carbachol and electric field stimulated ileum, as did the alkaloids.

Radioreceptor assays suggest that the alkaloids sanguinarine, chelerythrine, stylopine, allcryptopine and particularly protopine interact with the chloride channel of the GABA-A receptor.[52] Chelidonium extract inhibited GABA-activated current via G proteins in vitro, suggesting an analgesic mechanism (see below).[53] Studies in mice found that allocryptopine and protopine increased the brain concentration of the neurotransmitter GABA and the activity of its synthesising enzyme GAD.[54]

Chelidonium alkaloids acted as irreversible inhibitors of liver mitochondrial monoamine oxidase in vitro. Chelidonine was the strongest inhibitor.[55] The same alkaloids also reversibly inhibited acetylcholinesterase in vitro, with sanguinarine and berberine exhibiting the strongest activity.[56] Of the minor alkaloids, 8-hydroxydihydrochelerythrine and 8-hydroxydihydrosanguinarine had potent acetylcholinesterase inhibitory activity.[57]

Chelerythrine chloride exerted an in vitro antiplatelet effect that was believed to be due to inhibition of thromboxane formation and phosphoinositide breakdown.[58]

An extract of Chelidonium inhibited human keratinocyte proliferation, with sanguinarine being the most potent constituent. The mechanism of action appears to be inhibition of the inflammatory mediators leukotriene B4 and 12(S)-HETE, both of which have a known role in stimulating epidermal keratinocyte proliferation. Although the alkaloids have demonstrated cytotoxic activity in low concentrations, sanguinarine and chelerythrine did not cause more damage to cell membranes than the antipsoriatic drug anthralin, as observed by the release of lactate dehydrogenase activity (an indicator of plasma membrane damage).[59]

The antinociceptive action of aminophenazone in mice was potentiated by the Chelidonium alkaloids allocryptopine, chelidonine and sanguinarine.[60] Chelidonium extract suppressed glycine-induced responses and elevated those induced by glutamate in isolated rat periaqueductal grey neurons.[61] This might activate the descending pain control system leading to an analgesic effect.

A liquid extract of Chelidonium (2.5, 5 and 10 mL/kg, oral) dose-dependently protected against indomethacin-induced gastric ulceration in rats.[62] However, it was not as active as other digestive herbs such as licorice and peppermint.

High doses of Ukrain caused slight osteopenic effects in rats, possibly due to inhibition of locomotor activity.[63] However, it was anabolic on bone in ovariectomised female rats (doses 7, 14 and 28 mg/kg, ip).

Pharmacokinetics

No data available.

Clinical trials

Spasmolytic and cholagogue effects

In an early uncontrolled trial, a Chelidonium extract exerted good to very good results in two-thirds of patients treated for cholangitis, cholelithiasis and cholecystitis without stones. Forty patients received 3 mL/day (for 43 to 50 days) of a fresh plant tincture standardised to 20 mg alkaloids/100 mL.[64] An early clinical trial investigated the effect of a suspension of Silybum marianum, Chelidonium and Curcuma on 28 patients. Compared to a control liquid, the herbal mixture demonstrated a greater increase in bile flow and pancreatic secretion.[65]

In 60 Berlin practices, 608 patients were treated in an uncontrolled study over a 3-month period with a standardised preparation of dried Chelidonium, which acted as a plant-based spasmolytic. The main presenting symptoms were cramp-like pains in the gastrointestinal tract (43%) or gall ducts (48.2%), but also included dyspeptic symptoms. Each Chelidonium tablet contained 125 mg of a 5:1 to 7:1 hydroethanolic extract with 2.85 mg of total alkaloids, including 0.79 mg of chelidonine. The dose was initially 5 tablets/day and this was reduced to 3 tablets/day in patients who responded to treatment. The average duration of treatment was 22 days and the longest treatment time was 2.5 months. A good or very good therapeutic effect on symptoms with a quick response was observed in 87.4% of cases. In most cases symptom relief occurred within 30 minutes of taking the herbal medication (62.3%). In 46.1% of patients, the average duration of efficacy of each tablet dose was more than 3 h.

This study suggests value for Chelidonium in the treatment of cramp-like abdominal pains associated with irritable bowel syndrome and other causes.[66]

In a retrospective, open label study conducted over a 6-month period, 206 patients with epigastric complaints related to gallstones or gallbladder removal were evaluated.[67] Patients received either a Chelidonium capsule (125 mg/day of a hydromethanolic extract containing 0.68 mg of chelidonine) or a liquid (three times 20 drops daily containing 0.15 mg chelidonine). There was a noted improvement in symptoms such as flatulence, diarrhoea, constipation and upper abdominal pain. Pain-free intervals were increased and inflammatory markers decreased.

The efficacy and tolerability of a standardised Chelidonium extract was investigated in a randomised, placebo-controlled, double blind trial involving 60 patients with functional epigastric symptoms.[68] These included cramp-like pains, sensation of pressure or fullness, flatulence and nausea. Patients receiving active treatment took 6 tablets/day, each containing 66 to 167 mg of a Chelidonium dry extract (5.3:1 to 7.5:1) delivering 4 mg of total alkaloids calculated as chelidonine. Following 6 weeks of treatment, there was a clear difference in physician-rated response rates: 60% in the Chelidonium group versus 27% in placebo (p=0.0038). The treatment was without significant side effects compared with the placebo.

A double blind, placebo-controlled trial investigated the impact of a Chelidonium and turmeric root combination in 76 patients with upper abdominal pain attributed to functional disorders of the biliary system.[69] Patients received either 3 capsules/day (each containing Chelidonium (104 to 131 mg of a 5:1 to 10:1 extract containing 4 mg of alkaloids calculated as chelidonine) and turmeric (45 mg of a 12.5:1 to 25:1 extract)) or a matching placebo for 3 weeks. In the first week there was a significant reduction in pain for the patients receiving the herbal treatment, compared with placebo. No other symptoms changed significantly relative to placebo.

A proprietary formula known as STW 5 contains liquid extracts of Chelidonium, *Matricaria recutita* (chamomile) flower, *Iberis amarus* (bitter candywort) herb, *Carum carvi* (caraway) fruit, *Angelica archangelica* (garden angelica) root, *Glycyrrhiza glabra* (licorice) root, *Silybum marianum* (milk thistle) fruit, *Melissa officinalis* (lemon balm) leaf and *Mentha × piperita* (peppermint) leaf and has been extensively researched for indigestion and functional dyspepsia. Two meta-analyses of the clinical studies on this formula have been published.[70,71] They found that STW 5, at a dose of 1 mL 3 times per day, significantly reduced symptoms compared with placebo. It also demonstrated similar efficacy to cisapride and metoclopramide.

Warts, polyps

In a small, uncontrolled trial, an infusion of dried Chelidonium was administered as an enema for colonic polyposis. Administration of 10 or more enemas resulted in the complete disappearance of colonic polyps in several cases.[72] In a later study, the fresh plant was made into a paste and administered 2 or 3 h after an evacuant enema. In most cases, two or three courses (consisting of 10 to 20 enemas each) were deemed to be necessary. This regime was ineffective for treating malignant regenerated or degenerated polyps. Over a 2-year period treating 149 patients with various forms of polyposis, 59% showed improvement with 27% making a complete recovery.[73]

An ethanolic extract of Chelidonium was used as a topical application to treat nursing mothers for warts, papillomas, condylomas and nodules in an uncontrolled trial. The extract was applied to the affected area approximately 200 times per day for 2 to 3 weeks or until improvement was observed. Complete resolution of the warts occurred after 15 to 20 days in 135 women.[74]

Respiratory conditions

Chelidonium was given as a syrup or extract (equivalent to 15 g of herb per day) to patients with chronic bronchitis in an uncontrolled study. The effective response rate was around 80%. It was more effective in the simple type than the asthmatic type.[3] Chelidonium syrup or a decoction of the fresh herb was used to treat whooping cough in an uncontrolled study. Dosages were: infants under 6 months, 5 to 8 mL; 6 to 12 months, 8 to 10 mL; 1 to 3 years, 10 to 15 mL; 3 to 6 years, 5 to 20 mL; and above 6 years, 20 to 30 mL. Treatment was for a course of 8 to 10 days. Of 500 cases so treated, 355 were 'cured' and 116 improved.[3]

Chelidonium tincture improved tonsillar function and immunity and reduced recurrence of infection in an open comparative study in children with tonsillitis (article in Russian).[75]

Anticancer activity

Chelidonium was one of three herbs used to examine the efficacy of traditional Chinese herbs on squamous cell carcinoma of the oesophagus. A 30 mL dose of a decoction of Chelidonium (equivalent to 30 g of crude herb) was given orally to 30 patients twice daily for 2 weeks prior to surgery. Histological examination of the excised tissue demonstrated a greater degree of stromal lymphoid cell infiltration and cancer tissue degeneration in the patients given Chelidonium than in those given the herb plus endoxan or in the control group. The antitumour action of Chelidonium was thought to be due to the activation of an immunological rejection mechanism.[76]

A systematic review of seven clinical trials on Ukrain given intravenously to patients with colorectal, pancreatic, bladder and breast cancer found benefit in improving survival compared with various control groups.[40] Trials were generally of low quality and clear interpretation of results was difficult due to various methodological and reporting flaws. As noted previously, the relevance of Ukrain to the clinical use of Chelidonium is uncertain.

HIV infection

An uncontrolled trial reported on the efficacy of a combination of freeze-dried Chelidonium, *Ulmus rubra* (slippery elm) bark and *Sanguinaria canadensis* (bloodroot) in 13 HIV positive patients.[77] Each capsule contained 175 mg Chelidonium, 20 mg slippery elm and 5 mg bloodroot. The dose used was 9 capsules per day. The most dramatic response was a general improvement in lymphadenopathy in the patients affected by this. Minor improvements in CD4+ T cell counts and energy levels were also noted.

Toxicology and other safety data

Toxicology

No harmful or toxic effects from therapeutic doses have been established. The LD_{50} of the decoction in mice by intraperitoneal injection is $9.5\,g/kg^3$ and the LD_{50} of the alkaloids in mice is $300\,mg/kg$ (subcutaneous).[4]

In an antitumour experiment, intraperitoneal administration of a methanol extract of Chelidonium ($350\,mg/kg/day$ for 7 days) to mice resulted in a 20% mortality rate.[37] After 4 weeks of feeding Chelidonium (1.5 and $3\,g/kg/day$) to rats, no toxic or hepatotoxic effects were observed.[78] This suggests the herb is not inherently hepatotoxic and that the observed adverse hepatic reactions are rare, idiosyncratic responses.

Contraindications

Pre-existing serious liver disease or damage.

Special warnings and precautions

Given the nature of the alkaloid content of this herb and the rare hepatotoxic reactions, long-term use (except topical) is not preferred. Caution should be observed during pregnancy and lactation and in patients with gallstones. Use of Chelidonium should not be combined with heavy alcohol consumption.

Interactions

None documented.

Use in pregnancy and lactation

Category C-has caused or is associated with a substantial risk of causing harmful effects on the fetus or neonate without causing malformations.

Intramuscular injection of Ukrain on days 6 to 11 of gestation to hamsters and on days 6 to 15 of gestation to rats (0.1 to $28\,mg/kg/day$) did not produce teratogenic effects in either species compared with controls. Slight embryotoxic effects (increased post-implantation losses), and in consequence decreased number of average litter size, were noted in hamsters exposed to Ukrain at doses that were otherwise not embryotoxic to rats.[79]

Chelidonium use is strongly discouraged during breastfeeding.

Effects on ability to drive and use machines

No adverse effects expected.

Side effects

The potential association of Chelidonium with idiosyncratic hepatotoxicity was first reported in 1996. A 69-year-old woman developed symptoms of acute hepatitis after taking tablets containing several herbs including Chelidonium over a period of 6 weeks. Symptoms returned with rechallenge.[80] Three additional cases were then reported (1997, 1998).[81–83] In one series of observations over 2 years (1997–1999) in an area of approximately 1 million inhabitants in Germany, preparations of Chelidonium apparently induced 10 cases of acute hepatitis. Investigations and tests excluded viral causes, alcohol intake and hereditary causes. Although immunological factors could not be safely excluded, the evidence, including liver biopsy, suggested a treatment-related pathology. Cholestasis was observed in half the cases, but there were no cases of liver failure and the condition improved quickly in all cases when the Chelidonium was stopped. In one case a rechallenge led to a second attack of hepatitis.[84] Three cases of acute hepatitis associated with Chelidonium were then reported in the literature in 2002 and May 2003,[85,86] and another in 2006.[87] Again, patients returned to normal when the herbal treatment was ceased. Another case report of cholestatic hepatitis (with complete recovery) including a review of 16 cases documented in the literature, was published in 2009.[88] Assessment of causality for this case suggested a probable relationship with Chelidonium consumption. Generally these hepatotoxic reactions have been observed after using higher-dose German products.

A case of contact dermatitis has been linked to exposure to the plant.[89]

A case of haemolytic anaemia was reported after the oral ingestion of Chelidonium extract. The patient was treated with corticosteroids, blood transfusions and haemodialysis and recovered after about 12 days.[90]

When Chelidonium was used in traditional Chinese medicine studies, various degrees of dry mouth, dizziness, gastric discomfort, diarrhoea, abdominal distension, nausea and mild leucopenia were reported in a minority of patients. Symptoms generally disappeared within 3 to 5 days without the discontinuation of treatment.[3]

Overdosage

Critical consideration of the often-cited fatal case of poisoning in a 4-year-old boy recorded in 1936 suggests that it is by no means certain that Chelidonium was involved. More than $500\,g$ of Chelidonium is said to be required to cause toxic effects in horses and cattle.[91]

Safety in children

No information available, but prolonged use is probably unsuitable in children, although it has been used to treat chronic tonsillitis.

Regulatory status in selected countries

Chelidonium is covered by a positive Commission E Monograph and can be used for cramp-like disorders of the biliary and gastrointestinal tracts.

Chelidonium is not on the UK General Sale List. Under the terms of the British Medicines Act 1968 and the Statutory Instrument SI 2130 (Retail Sale or Supply of Herbal Remedies) Order 1977 (Schedule Part III), the sale of Chelidonium is restricted to herbal practitioners. It may be prescribed at a maximum dosage of 2 g three times per day.

Chelidonium does not have GRAS status. However, it is freely available as a 'dietary supplement' in the USA under DSHEA legislation (1994 Dietary Supplement Health and Education Act).

Chelidonium is not included in Part 4 of Schedule 4 of the Therapeutic Goods Act Regulations of Australia and is freely available for sale. However, Chelidonium-containing products must contain the following warning: 'Greater Celandine may harm the liver in some people. Use only under the supervision of a healthcare practitioner.'

References

1. Felter HW, Lloyd JU. *King's American Dispensatory*, Vol 1. 18th ed., rev 3. Portland: 1905. Reprinted by Eclectic Medical Publications; 1983. pp. 491–493.

2. Grieve M. *A Modern Herbal*, Vol 1. New York: Dover Publications; 1971. pp. 178–179.

3. Chang HM, But PP. *Pharmacology and Applications of Chinese Materia Medica*, vol 1. Singapore: World Scientific; 1987. pp. 390–394

4. Huang KC. *The Pharmacology of Chinese Herbs*. Boca Raton: CRC Press; 1993. pp. 144–145.

5. Launert EL. *The Hamlyn Guide to Edible and Medicinal Plants of Britain and Northern Europe*. London: Hamlyn; 1981. p. 26.

6. Wagner H, Bladt S. *Plant Drug Analysis: A Thin Layer Chromatography Atlas*, 2nd ed. Berlin: Springer-Verlag; 1996. p. 10.

7. Colombo ML, Bosisio E. *Pharmacol Res*. 1996;33(2):127–134.

8. Gu Y, Qian D, Duan JA, et al. *J Sep Sci*. 2010;33(8):1004–1009.

9. Nawrot R, Kalinowski A, Gozdzicka-Jozefiak A. *Phytochemistry*. 2007;68(12):1612–1622.

10. Nawrot R, Lesniewicz K, Pienkowska J, et al. *Fitoterapia*. 2007;78(7-8):496, 501.

11. Mitra S, Gole M, Samajdar K, et al. *Int J Pharmacog*. 1992;30(2):125–128.

12. Mitra S, Sur RK, Roy A, et al. *Phytother Res*. 1996;10(4):354–356.

13. Vahlensieck U, Hahn R, Winterhoff H, et al. *Planta Med*. 1995;61(3):267–271.

14. Lenfeld J, Kroutil M, Marsalek E, et al. *Planta Med*. 1981;43(10):161–165.

15. Cheng RB, Chen X, Liu SJ, et al. *Shanghai Kou Qiang Yi Xue*. 2007;16(1):68–72.

16. Cheng RB, Chen X, Liu SJ, et al. *Shanghai Kou Qiang Yi Xue*. 2006;15(3):318–320.

17. Kuftinec MM, Mueller-Joseph LJ, Kopczyk RA. *J Can Dent Assoc*. 1990;15(suppl 7):31–33.

18. Laster LL, Lobene RR. *J Can Dent Assoc*. 1990;56(suppl 7):19–30.

19. Hannah JJ, Johnson JD, Kuftinec MM. *Am J Orthod Dentofacial Orthop*. 1989;96(3):199–207.

20. Kokoska L, Polesny Z, Rada V, et al. *J Ethnopharmacol*. 2002;82(1):51–53.

21. Kery A, Horvath J, Nasz I, et al. *Acta Pharm Hung*. 1987;57(1–2):19–25.

22. Gerencer M, Turecek PL, Kistner O, et al. *Antiviral Res*. 2006;72(2):153–156.

23. Bodalski T, Pelozarska H, Ujec M. *Arch Immunol Terapii Doswiadcjalny*. 1958;6(4):705–711.

24. Hejtmánková N, Walterova D, Preininger V. *Fitoterapia*. 1984;55(5):291–294.

25. Vukusic I, Pepeljnjak S, Kustrak D, et al. *Planta Med*. 1991;57(suppl 2):A46.

26. Meng F, Zuo G, Hao X, et al. *J Ethnopharmacol*. 2009;125(3):494–496.

27. Zuo GY, Meng FY, Hao XY, et al. *J Pharm Pharm Sci*. 2008;11(4):90–94.

28. Matos OC, Baeta J, Silva MJ, et al. *J Ethnopharmacol*. 1999;66(2):151–158.

29. Kim HK, Farnsworth NR, Blomster RN, et al. *J Pharm Sci*. 1969;58(3):372–374.

30. Shi GZ. *Chung-Hua Yu Fang I Hsueh Tsa Chih*. 1992;26(3):165–167.

31. Pilchenkov A, Kaminskyy V, Zavelevich M, et al. *Toxicol In Vitro*. 2008;22(2):287–295.

32. Kaminskyy V, Lin KW, Filyak Y, et al. *Cell Biol Int*. 2008;32(2):271–277.

33. Noureini SK, Wink M. *World J Gastroenterol*. 2009;15(29):3603–3610.

34. Nadova S, Miadokova E, Alfoldiova L, et al. *Neuro Endocrinol Lett*. 2008;29(5):649–652.

35. Nawrot R, Wolun-Cholewa M, Gozdzicka-Jozefiak A. *Folia Histochem Cytobiol*. 2008;46(1):79–83.

36. Fik E, Wolun-Cholewa M, Kistowska M, et al. *Folia Histochem Cytobiol*. 2001;39(2):215–216.

37. Sokoloff B, Saelhof CC, Yoshichi MD, et al. *Growth*. 1964;28:225–231.

38. Kim DJ, Ahn B, Han BS, et al. *Cancer Lett*. 1997;112(2):203–208.

39. Biswas SJ, Bhattacharjee N, Khuda-Bukhsh AR. *Food Chem Toxicol*. 2008;46(5):1474–1487.

40. Ernst E, Schmidt K. *BMC Cancer*. 2005;5:69.

41. Panzer A, Joubert AM, Eloff JN, et al. *Cancer Lett*. 2000;160(2):237–241.

42. Habermehl D, Kammerer B, Handrick R, et al. *BMC Cancer*. 2006;6:14.

43. Uglyanitsa KN, Nefyodov LI, Doroshenko YM, et al. *Drugs Exp Clin Res*. 2000;26(5–6):341–356.

44. Panzer A, Hamel E, Joubert AM, et al. *Cancer Lett*. 2000;160(2):149–157.

45. Jagiello-Wojtowicz E, Kleinrok Z, Urbanska EM. *Drugs Exp Clin Res*. 1998;24(5–6):213–219.

46. Skivka L, Susak Y, Trompak O, et al. *J Oncol Pharm Pract*. 2010 [Epub ahead of print].

47. Susak YM, Skivka LM, Rudik MP, et al. *Exp Oncol*. 2010;32(2):107–110.

48. Vavreckova C, Gawlik I, Müller K. *Planta Med*. 1996;62(5):397–401.

49. Lee YC, Kim SH, Roh SS, et al. *J Ethnopharmacol*. 2007;112(1):40–48.

50. Boegge SC, Kesper S, Verspohl EJ, et al. *Planta Med*. 1996;62(2):173–174.

51. Hiller KO, Ghorbani M, Schilcher H. *Planta Med*. 1998;64(8):758–760.

52. Häberlein H, Tschiersch KP, Boonen G, et al. *Planta Med*. 1996;62(3):227–231.

53. Kim Y, Shin M, Chung J, et al. *Am J Chin Med*. 2001;29(2):265–279.

54. Jagiello-Wójtowicz EWA, Feldo M, Kleinrok Z. *Polish J Pharmacol Pharm*. 1992;44(suppl):144.

55. Iagodina OV, Mikol'skaia EB, Faddeeva MD. *Tsitologiia*. 2003;45(10):1032–1037.

56. Kuznetsova LP, Sochilina EE, Faddeeva MD, et al. *Ukr Biokhim Zh*. 2005;77(2):147–153.

57. Cho KM, Yoo ID, Kim WG. *Biol Pharm Bull*. 2006;29(11):2317–2320.

58. Ko FN, Chen IS, Wu SJ, et al. *Biochim Biophys Acta*. 1990;1052:360–365.

59. Vavreckova C, Gawlik I, Müller K. *Planta Med*. 1996;62(6):491–494.

60. Jagiello-Wójtowicz EWA, Feldo M, Chodkowska A, et al. *Polish J Pharmacol Pharm*. 1992;44(Suppl):143.

61. Shin MC, Jang MH, Chang HK, et al. *Clin Chim Acta*. 2003;337(1–2):93–101.

62. Khayyal MT, el-Ghazaly MA, Kenawy SA, et al. *Arzneimittelforschung*. 2001;51(7):545–553.

63. Jablonski M. *Drugs Exp Clin Res*. 2000;26(5–6):317–320.

64. Neumann-Mangoldt P. *Med Welt*. 1977;28(4):181–185.

65. Baumann JC, Heintze K, Muth HW. *Arzneimittelforschung*. 1971;21(1):98–101.

66. Kniebel R, Urlacher W. *Zeit Allg Med*. 1993;69(25):680–684.

67. Ardjah H. *Fortschr Med Suppl*. 1991;115:2–8.

68. Ritter R, Schatton WFH, Gessner B, et al. *Comp Ther Med*. 1993;1:189–193.

69. Niederau C, Gopfert E. *Med Klin (Munich)*. 1999;94(8):425–430.

70. Melzer J, Rösch W, Reichling J, et al. *Aliment Pharmacol Ther*. 2004; 20(11–12):1279–1287.

71. Rösch W, Liebregts T, Gundermann KJ, et al. *Phytomedicine*. 2006;13(suppl 1): 114–121.

72. Aminev AM, Stoliarenko AI. *Vop Onkol*. 1960;6(8):81–82.

73. Aminev AM. *Am J Proctol*. 1963;14(1):25–27.

74. Demchenko PF. *Vrachebn Delo*. 1957;12:1335–1338.

75. Khmel'nitsakaia NM, Vorob'ev KV, Kliachko LL, et al. *Vestn Otorinolaringol*. 1998(4):39–42.

76. Xian MS, Hayashi K, Lu JP, et al. *Acta Med Okayama*. 1989;43(6):345–351.

77. D'Adamo P. *J Naturopathic Med*. 1992;3(1):31–34.

78. Mazzanti G, Di Sotto A, Franchitto A, et al. *J Ethnopharmacol*. 2009;126(3): 518–524.

79. Juszkiewicz T, Minta M, Wlodarczyk B, et al. *Drugs Exp Clin Res*. 1992;18(suppl):23–29.

80. De Smet PA, Van den Eertwegh AJ, Lesterhuis W, et al. *BMJ*. 1996;313(7049):92.

81. Greving I, Niedereichholz U, Meister V, et al. Poster No. PO19, Europäischer Pharmakovigilanz Kongress, Berlin: 1997.

82. Greving I, Meister V, Monnerjahn C, et al. *Pharmacoepidemiol Drug Saf*. 1998;7: S66–S69.

83. Strahl S, Ehret V, Dahm HH, et al. *Dtsch Med Wochenschr*. 1998;123(47):1410–1414.

84. Benninger J, Schneider HT, Schuppan D, et al. *Gastroenterology*. 1999;117(5): 1234–1237.

85. Crijns AP, de Smet PA, van den Heuvel M, et al. *Ned Tijdschr Geneeskd*. 2002;146(3):124–128.

86. Stickel F, Poschl G, Seitz HK, et al. *Scand J Gastroenterol*. 2003;38(5):565–568.

87. Rifai K, Flemming P, Manns MP, et al. *Internist (Berl)*. 2006;47(7):749–751.

88. Moro PA, Cassetti F, Giugliano G, et al. *J Ethnopharmacol*. 2009;124(2):328–332.

89. Etxenagusia MA, Anda M, Gonzales-Mahave I, et al. *Contact Dermatitis*. 2000;43(1):47.

90. Pinto Garcia V, Vicente PR, Barez A, et al. *Sangre (Barc)*. 1990;35(5):401–403.

91. Frohne D, Pfander HJ. *A Colour Atlas of Poisonous Plants: A Handbook for Pharmacists, Doctors, Toxicologists, and Biologists*. London: Wolfe Publishing; 1984. translated from the 2nd German edition by NG Bisset. pp. 160–162.

Devil's claw

(*Harpagophytum procumbens* DC ex Meissner)

Synonyms

Grapple plant (Engl), Harpagophyti radix (Lat), Teufelskralle, Trampelklette, Sudafrikanische (Ger), tubercule de griffe du diable (Fr), venustorn (Dan), duiwelsklou (Afrik).

What is it?

Harpagophytum procumbens, a native to the savannah of the Kalahari of South Africa, Namibia and Botswana, has been wildcrafted and imported into Europe and subsequently elsewhere since 1953. The fruit is a capsule protected by numerous curved spines which, after the splitting of the fruit, take on a claw-like appearance. The names Harpagophytum (from the Greek *harpagos*, a grappling hook) and devil's claw are derived from this. However, the secondary root tuber is the part used medicinally. Devil's claw is also known as wood spider, grapple plant, burdock and Windhoeks' root. Recognition of the medicinal value of the plant by Europeans is apparently traced to German soldiers, and later to GA Menhert during the Hottentot rebellion in 1904. Menhert observed the recovery of a Hottentot (who had been given up as lost by doctors) when treated by a local witch doctor. He then followed the witch doctor and discovered what plant was used, subsequently promoting the use of the root under the name 'harpagophytum tea'.

Effects

Reduces inflammation and pain; acts as a bitter tonic.

Traditional view

Not much is known about the use of the herb in early traditional African medicine. Devil's claw has been used in recent times in South Africa by Europeans, Euro-Africans, Bushmen, Hottentots and the Bantu for its purgative action, as a bitter tonic for digestive disturbances, and for febrile illnesses, allergic reactions and migraine. Externally it has been used in the form of an ointment for ulcers, wounds, cutaneous lesions and boils. Amongst the Bushmen, Hottentots and Bantu, women ingest the pulverised root and apply an ointment to the abdomen during labour to alleviate pain.[1,2]

Summary actions

Anti-inflammatory, analgesic, antirheumatic, bitter.

Can be used for

Indications supported by clinical trials

Rheumatic and arthritic conditions, including muscle pain. Possible value for pain in endometriosis.

Traditional therapeutic uses

Digestive disturbances, febrile illnesses, allergic reactions and to relieve pain. Externally for wounds, ulcers, boils and the relief of pain.

May also be used for

Extrapolations from pharmacological studies

Cardiac arrhythmias.

Preparations

Decoction of dried root, tablets, capsules or liquid extract for internal use; dried root or liquid extract for external use as an ingredient in ointments and creams.

Dosage

In tablet form, devil's claw has been used in doses up to 6g/day without side effects.[3] In view of this and other recent clinical trials, the doses given in the *British Herbal Pharmacopoeia* 1983 are inadequate for antirheumatic and analgesic activity.[4] For these applications the equivalent of 3 to 6g/day of the dried herb should be prescribed.[5,6] This corresponds to 6 to 12mL/day of a 1:2 extract or 15 to 30mL/day of 1:5 tincture. Even higher doses have been used in some clinical trials. Tablets containing a 3:1 powdered extract should be taken at the rate of 1000 to 2000mg/day of extract. For gastrointestinal complaints, much lower doses can be used.

Some studies have indicated that the analgesic and anti-inflammatory effects of devil's claw are decreased by the acidity of the stomach. While these findings do not necessarily discount the use of galenical preparations (such as teas and liquid extracts), they do suggest that enteric-coated extracts of devil's claw may be more beneficial clinically. At the very least, devil's claw preparations should be administered between meals when gastric activity is at its lowest.

Duration of use

No restriction on long-term use.

Summary assessment of safety

No adverse effects are expected if used as recommended, but, given its bitter properties, devil's claw should be prescribed with caution in patients with peptic ulcers.

Technical data

Botany

Harpagophytum procumbens, a member of the Pedaliaceae family, is a weedy, perennial plant with creeping stems spreading from a tuberous rootstock. The greyish-green leaves are placed either alternately or directly opposite each other. Red-violet, yellow-violet or violet flowers are found at the juncture between leaf and stem. The characteristic fruits have long branching arms with anchor-like hooks (which assist their dissemination by animals). The primary root descends up to 2 m with secondary roots spreading out for up to 1.5 m on all sides, which allows it to conserve water.[2,7] Two subspecies are defined: *Harpagophytum procumbens* subsp. *procumbens* and *Harpagophytum procumbens* subsp. *transvaalensis*.[8]

Adulteration

Occasionally the harpagoside-poor primary roots of devil's claw are found as an adulterant, as are the roots of other intensely bitter tasting African plants, such as *Elephantorrhiza spp.* and *Acanthosicyos naudinianus* and *Harpagophytum zeyheri*.[9] Even though *Harpagophytum procumbens* and *H. zeyheri* can easily be distinguished in the field, it is impossible to tell them apart visually when in the form of dried and sliced tubers. Both species are harvested and traded as devil's claw in Namibia. Between 1985 and 1986 it was estimated that about 50% of the harvested wild material was mixed *H. procumbens* and *H. zeyheri*.[10] Devil's claw was proposed for inclusion in Appendix II of the Convention on International Trade in Endangered Species (CITES) in April 2000, but the proposal was not accepted,[11] and it remains off the list as of August 2011.

Key constituents

- Iridoid glycosides (0.5% to 3.0%), primarily harpagoside (which has a bitter taste), isoharpagoside, harpagide (which has a slightly sweet taste), procumbide[12]
- Sugars (over 50%), triterpenes, phytosterols, phenolic acids and glycosides, flavonoids.[6,13,14] The sugars lead to an unusually high water-soluble fraction of 50% to 70%.[6,14]

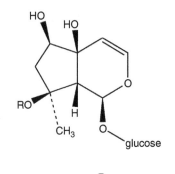

	R
Harpagoside	*trans*-cinnamoyl
Harpagide	H

The *European Pharmacopoeia* recommends that devil's claw contain not less than 1.2% harpagoside, calculated with reference to the dried herb.[15] *H. zeyheri* is physically similar to *H. procumbens* and is considered an inferior substitution species. Chemical testing indicates that harpagoside can be completely absent from *H. zeyheri*[8] and the ratio of harpagoside to 8-p-coumaroylharpagide can be used to readily distinguish between *H. procumbens* and *H. zeyheri*.[16]

Pharmacodynamics

Anti-inflammatory and antirheumatic activity

Many of the studies undertaken to examine the anti-inflammatory effects of devil's claw have demonstrated limited activity in standard inflammatory models. The anti-inflammatory effect varies with the route of administration and nature of the condition (acute or subacute).

Most non-steroidal anti-inflammatory drugs (NSAIDs) act by inhibiting prostaglandin biosynthesis by cyclo-oxygenase (COX). Despite earlier studies suggesting no activity in such models,[17] more recent in vitro assays indicate that harpagoside and/or devil's claw extracts inhibit the expression of COX-2 and inducible nitric oxide,[18–22] the production of inflammatory cytokines (for example, interleukin-1beta, interleukin-6, tumour necrosis factor-alpha),[23,24] and leukotriene,[25] the activity of COX-1,[21,22] and the production of matrix metalloproteinases (cartilage-degrading enzymes)[26] and elastase.[27] However, a study that examined the effect of devil's claw (2 g/day of powder for 21 days) on prostaglandin production during blood clotting in healthy humans found no significant differences in prostaglandin levels between the before and after measurements.[28] Three known triterpenoids from devil's claw root showed significant inhibitory activity against experimentally stimulated neutrophil respiratory burst.[29] Several iridoids from devil's claw also showed inhibitory activity against macrophage respiratory burst in vitro.[30]

Anti-inflammatory effects have been more convincingly demonstrated in subacute animal models rather than acute, but overall results have been mixed.[5] In subacute animal models utilising formaldehyde-, Freund's adjuvant- and granuloma-induced experimental arthritis, aqueous and methanolic extracts of devil's claw appear to be efficient in reducing inflammation. In one study using the croton oil-induced granuloma pouch test in rats, the reduction in inflammation produced by the 12-day oral administration of aqueous and methanolic extracts of devil's claw (200 mg/kg/day) was similar to phenylbutazone.[31] In the formaldehyde-induced arthritis test, an effect comparable to 40 mg/kg/day of phenylbutazone was demonstrated for an aqueous extract of devil's claw (20 mg/kg/day for 10 days, ip).[32] Another study using different but similar models found that oral administration of devil's claw did not produce significant effects on primary or secondary inflammatory reactions in rats.[33] More recently, devil's claw extract reduced the acute inflammation of fresh egg albumin-induced paw oedema (50 to 800 mg/kg, ip),[34] and reduced oedema in Freund's adjuvant-induced arthritis (assessing acute and chronic inflammation; extract administered orally).[35]

Devil's claw extract administered by intraperitoneal injection reduced the intensity of carrageenan-induced inflammatory response in hindpaws of normal and adrenalectomised rats. The extract was ineffective when administered orally. Two and four hours after ip injection of the extract there was a significant reduction in the number of circulating leukocytes in normal rats, indicative of a hyperactive response by the adrenal cortex. No change was observed after oral administration. Overall, these results suggest that the anti-inflammatory response observed for devil's claw after injection does not depend on the release of adrenal corticosteroids. For both routes the devil's claw extract was administered at doses of 100 to 800 mg/kg (extract strength undefined).[36]

Oral administration of standardised devil's claw extract exerted a potential chondroprotective effect in an experimental model (joint destabilisation). There was a trend toward chondroid regeneration and increased elastic and collagen fibres in the hip cartilage of the surgically altered limb of devil's claw treated rabbits. Investigation of RNA activity suggests the effect may be due to the inhibition of matrix metalloproteinase-2.[37]

Little or no activity of oral doses of aqueous extracts of devil's claw or harpagoside was demonstrated in studies using acute models, such as carrageenan-induced oedema.[5,17,31,32] However, intraperitoneal pretreatment with an aqueous extract of devil's claw produced significant, dose-dependent anti-inflammatory effects in this model.[38] The highest dose tested (equivalent to 400 mg/kg of root) was more effective than pretreatment with 10 mg/kg of indomethacin.[38] Harpagoside does not appear to be involved in this anti-inflammatory effect, since it did not protect against carrageenan inflammatory effects at levels corresponding to 400 mg of dried root. When devil's claw root was treated with acid at similar levels to the stomach, it lost all activity via intraperitoneal injection.[38] A later study confirmed the loss of anti-inflammatory activity following passage through the stomach.[39]

Topical anti-inflammatory activity has been demonstrated using an ex vivo porcine skin model. An ethanolic extract of devil's claw and some constituents (including harpagoside) decreased COX-2 expression. Another constituent, harpagide, caused an increase in the levels of COX-2 expression after 6 hours. The overall anti-inflammatory activity of a topically applied extract may depend upon the ratio of these compounds.[40–42] Topical application of methanol extract of devil's claw inhibited 12-O-tetradecanoylphorbol-13-acetate-induced COX-2 expression in mouse skin. (12-O-Tetradecanoylphorbol-13-acetate has tumour-promoting activity.)[43]

Analgesic activity

Injection of devil's claw extract and harpagoside exhibited dose-dependent peripheral analgesic effects comparable to aspirin.[38] This activity was abolished by acid pretreatment of the herbal extract. In earlier work, intraperitoneal administration of harpagoside (20 mg/kg) produced an analgesic effect comparable to phenylbutazone (50 mg/kg).[32] However, harpagoside hydrolysed by emulsion (which would produce harpagogenin) was inactive.[32] No consistent analgesic effects were found in mice after oral doses of devil's claw extracts.[31] In a later study, oral pretreatment with devil's claw extract (30 to 300 mg/kg, standardised to contain 1.9% harpagoside) did produce significant analgesic effects in the formalin test of mice. Naloxone (5 mg/kg, sc) significantly attenuated the analgesic effect of devil's claw, suggesting that the opioidergic system may be involved.[44] Devil's claw extract has also demonstrated analgesic activity against heat- and chemical-induced pain in mice (50 to 800 mg/kg, 64:1 extract, ip injection)[34] and against heat-induced pain in rats (extract administered orally).[35]

Cardiovascular activity

In conscious normotensive rats, the dried methanolic extract of devil's claw caused a significant dose-dependent reduction of arterial blood pressure, and a concomitant decrease of heart rate. The reduction of blood pressure was only significant at the higher oral dosage of 400 mg/kg. Under the same experimental conditions, an equivalent quantity of harpagoside was not as effective as the full plant extract. The methanolic extract of devil's claw caused a mild decrease in heart rate with a concomitant mild positive inotropic effect at lower concentrations in vitro, and marked negative inotropic effect at higher concentrations.[45] Devil's claw extract also demonstrated a dose-dependent protective effect against arrhythmias induced by aconitine and particularly those provoked by calcium and epinephrine-chloroform, both in vivo (100 to 400 mg/kg, oral) and in vitro.[45]

In another study on isolated rat hearts, methanolic extracts of devil's claw showed a significant, dose-dependent protection against hyperkinetic ventricular arrhythmias induced by reperfusion following ischaemia. Additionally, it was demonstrated that both the methanolic extract and harpagoside inhibited hyperkinetic arrhythmias triggered by digitoxin. The mechanism of action of devil's claw was thought to be analogous to that of verapamil. Thus devil's claw may modify the cellular metabolism that causes transmembrane ionic fluxes, thereby producing a calcium antagonistic effect.[46]

Another in vivo study demonstrated that the iridoids, triterpenes and the flavonoids (luteolin and kaempferol) were all responsible for the electrophysiological and haemodynamic effects of devil's claw. The oral doses used in this study were 20 and 40 mg/kg of a methanolic extract.[47]

Other activity

Devil's claw extract and tincture inhibited free radical generation in vitro.[48] Water-soluble constituents of devil's claw extract were antioxidant, but harpagoside did not contribute significantly to the antioxidant activity.[49]

The effect of an aqueous extract of devil's claw root on longitudinal, tubular uterine horn muscle strips taken from both non-pregnant and pregnant young adult, female rats was investigated. Devil's claw extract (10 to 800 µg/mL, 28:1 extract) increased the tone and induced contraction of oestrogen-dominated rat longitudinal uterine horn muscle strips taken from stilboestrol-pretreated, non-pregnant female rats. The same effect was observed for longitudinal, tubular uterine horn muscle strips taken from female rats in the early, middle and late stages of pregnancy. Moderate to high concentrations (200 to 1000 µg/mL, 28:1 extract) provoked powerful contractions of isolated longitudinal, tubular uterine horn muscle preparations of both non-pregnant and pregnant rats.[50]

The potential anticonvulsant activity of a devil's claw aqueous extract (28:1) administered by intraperitoneal injection was investigated against pentylenetetrazole-, picrotoxin- and bicuculline-induced seizures in mice. At the dosage of 100 to 800 mg/kg, the average onset of convulsions was delayed and the average duration of convulsions reduced. The activity was greater in the pentylenetetrazole and picrotoxin models. Two reference drugs were also tested. By comparison, animals were 90% protected after administration of the reference drug diazepam (0.5 mg/kg, ip) against convulsions caused by picrotoxin, while the highest dose of devil's claw (800 mg/kg) resulted in 70% protection.[51]

Intraperitoneal injection of devil's claw aqueous extract (50 to 800 mg/kg, 64:1 extract) produced dose-dependent, significant reductions in blood glucose concentrations of both fasted normal and fasted diabetic rats.[34]

The antimicrobial activity of plant extracts against 29 species of aerobic and anaerobic bacteria and yeasts was tested in vitro. An aqueous standardised extract of devil's claw was effective against all microbes tested, but generally only at higher concentrations (100 µg/mL of a stock solution comprising 200 mg/mL of the 1.5:1 to 2.5:1 extract). Harpagoside was not active.[52]

Pharmacokinetics

There has been controversy over the effects of stomach and acid hydrolysis on devil's claw extract and its active ingredients, as suggested by some of the above studies. Some authors have proposed that the compounds obtained after acid hydrolysis, especially harpagogenin, are the true active compounds producing the anti-inflammatory and antiarthritic properties. In contrast, other studies suggest that the extract, and harpagoside in particular, may be partially inactivated by the acid milieu of the stomach.[7,39] In other words, the basic issue is whether harpagoside and other iridoid glycosides (and perhaps other compounds in the root) are more active after

oral doses than their respective hydrolysis products, such as harpagogenin.[38,39]

An in vitro experiment investigating the simulated gastric disintegration of devil's claw extract tablets was published in 2000. The tablets (which were not enterically coated) disintegrated after around 18 minutes in artificial gastric fluid. The harpagoside content was decreased by about 10% in this medium after periods of 1 and 3 h. Harpagoside remained stable in artificial intestinal fluid for a period of 6 h.[53]

Another consideration complicates this picture. The main iridoids of devil's claw, namely harpagide, harpagoside and 8-O-p-coumaroylharpagide, were transformed into the pyridine monoterpene alkaloid aucubinine B by human faecal flora and by specific bacterial species isolated from the flora. Aucubinine B was also generated from harpagide, harpagoside and 8-O-p-coumaroylharpagide by beta-glucosidase in the presence of the ammonium ion.[54] Hence this alkaloid could be an active agent after oral doses of devil's claw.

The hepatobiliary excretion of harpagoside was investigated in rats. The bile-to-blood distribution ratio (AUC_{bile}/AUC_{blood}) was 986 for an intravenous dose of 3 mg/kg. The ratio dropped significantly to 6.41 or 221.2 after co-administration of cyclosporin A (10 mg/kg) or verapamil (1.2 mg/kg), respectively. In other words, both drugs increased the concentration of harpagoside in the blood. Elimination of harpagoside via the bile is probably regulated by P-glycoprotein (P-gp), since cyclosporin A and verapamil are P-gp inhibitors.[55]

The pharmacokinetics of devil's claw was investigated in three pilot, single-dose studies with small numbers of healthy volunteers. Three different standardised extracts were orally administered at varying doses. Maximum concentrations of harpagoside in plasma (Cmax) were reached after 1.3 to 2.5 h and ranged from around 8 to 50 ng/mL. The half-life was short, ranging between 3.7 and 6.4 h, and clearance was about 15 L/min. A linear relationship between the dose of harpagoside and the first Cmax and area under the concentration (AUC) curve was observed.[25]

Clinical trials

Antirheumatic activity

There are several reports of uncontrolled and controlled trials in the late 1970s to 1990 investigating the oral administration of devil's claw for the treatment of rheumatic conditions.[7] Examples of two early uncontrolled trials follow. In one large, open study involving 630 patients with various rheumatic illnesses, 42% to 85% of the patients showed a significant improvement after 6 months of devil's claw (3 to 9 g/day). Efficacy varied with the site of the arthritis; 80% of patients with arthritis in the large joints or spinal column experienced a significant improvement in symptoms, whilst the remaining 20% experienced no therapeutic effect even at maximum dosage.[56] However, one small open study involving 13 patients with rheumatoid arthritis and psoriatic arthropathy found no benefit from devil's claw treatment.[57]

Several reviews have assessed the quality of the clinical trial data. The most comprehensive systematic review was published in 2003 and examined 20 trials of devil's claw in the treatment of chronic musculoskeletal pain, including low back pain and arthritis.[58] Of the 20 trials included in the review, eight were uncontrolled or observational studies, two were open comparisons with conventional treatments (phenylbutazone or various conventional treatments) and 10 were randomised, double-blinded comparisons: eight against placebo and two against non-steroidal anti-inflammatory drugs (NSAIDs: diacerhein and rofecoxib).

In the opinion of the reviewers, the uncontrolled studies provided mainly preliminary information. The two open label trials were subject to performance, detection and/or selection bias. Of the eight randomised, double blind comparisons against placebo, six were affected by lack of transparency; one trial[3] could not provide definitive evidence in terms of its pre-selected principal outcome measure (consumption of the rescue analgesic drug tramadol), and the remaining trial[59] provided good-quality evidence of a dose-dependent superiority over placebo. One of the randomised controlled comparison trials (devil's claw versus rofecoxib) was intended only as a pilot study.[60] The other comparative trial[61] provided evidence that devil's claw powder is as effective as the weak NSAID diacerhein.[58]

More details are provided below for the latter four trials:

* For the secondary outcome measure – the number of patients with low back pain who were pain free – treatment with devil's claw extract (containing 60 mg/day of harpagoside for 4 weeks) was significantly better than placebo (p=0.008) in a randomised trial involving 118 patients.[3]

* More patients with an exacerbation of chronic low back pain receiving devil's claw extract (equivalent to 4.5 g/day or 9 g/day of root and containing 50 mg/day or 100 mg/day of harpagoside, respectively) for 4 weeks were pain-free compared with placebo. Treatment with extract containing 100 mg/day of harpagoside was more effective than 50 mg/day in terms of the number of pain-free patients, but not in terms of improvement in the pain component of the Arhus low back pain index. This was a randomised, double blind study involving 197 patients.[59]

* Devil's claw extract (containing 60 mg/day of harpagoside) over a 6-week period reduced pain in patients with low back pain to about the same extent as rofecoxib (12.5 mg/day).[60] This was a randomised, double-dummy, double blind trial involving 88 patients.

* Devil's claw powder (2.6 g/day, containing 57 mg/day of harpagoside) taken over a period of 4 months significantly reduced both spontaneous pain and functional disability, and exhibited similar efficacy to diacerhein (100 mg/day) in a trial involving 122 patients with osteoarthritis of the knee or hip. The number of patients using other NSAIDs and analgesic drugs (diclofenac or paracetamol-caffeine) at the completion of the study was significantly lower in the devil's claw group.[61]

A 2006 Cochrane review of herbal medicine for low back pain[62] included three of these devil's claw trials,[3,59,60] considering them to be of high quality.

Three postmarketing surveillance studies[63–65] and a retrospective analysis of existing trial data[66] have been undertaken subsequent to the 2003 systematic review. Some of these studies were a continuation of prior work, or involved subgroups of patients from previous surveillance studies. Patients had low back pain or osteoarthritis of the knee or hip. Results were obtained in some cases for up to 54 weeks of treatment. In general, treatment with devil's claw extract (50 to 60 mg/day harpagoside) was clinically beneficial. For example, in one trial maximum pain relief occurred after 3 to 4 months[66] and in another trial 34% of patients had responded to treatment by month 1, with 51% responding by month 2.[64]

An uncontrolled trial involving 259 patients was conducted in the UK, with results published in 2007. Patients with mild to moderate rheumatic disorders were treated for 8 weeks with devil's claw extract (about 2.2 g/day dried herb equivalent). There were statistically significant (p<0.0001) improvements in patients' assessment of global pain, stiffness and function, with significant reductions in mean pain scores for the hand, wrist, elbow, shoulder, hip, knee and back.[67]

In one interesting study, patients with slight to moderate muscular tension or pain in the back, shoulder and neck were enrolled in a randomised, double blind, placebo-controlled trial: 63 patients received either a placebo or devil's claw (960 mg/day of a 5:1 60% ethanolic extract) for 4 weeks.[68] By the end of the trial, devil's claw treatment was significantly better than placebo in terms of muscle pain (visual analogue scale), muscle tenderness (pressure algometer test) and muscle stiffness (all p<0.001).

Other activity

A preliminary observational study found that devil's claw extract (400 mg capsules, four per day for 12 weeks) was beneficial in 12 patients with histologically proven endometriosis. A reduction of symptoms such as dysmenorrhoea and dyspareunia was observed after 4 weeks of treatment in six patients. All patients reported improvement in symptoms after 8 weeks and quality of life was also enhanced.[69] A patent lodged for this application[70] indicates the capsule contained a 30% aqueous ethanolic concentrate (2.6:1 to 3.1:1), suggesting a daily dose of about 4.5 g dried herb equivalent.

Regression of follicular lymphoma occurred in two patients who self-treated with devil's claw (dosage undefined). One patient was also taking the herbal formulation known as Essiac. CT scan images at baseline and follow-up (10 and 11 months later) provided objective evidence of regression of the tumours. Spontaneous regression of low-grade lymphoma has been previously reported in seven of 44 patients taking neither herbal medicines nor COX-2 inhibitors. However, the timing of the response in these two patients suggests a possible therapeutic effect. The chance of observing spontaneous regression in two consecutive lymphoma patients is approximately 2%.[71]

Devil's claw has also generated interest for its veterinary applications. The effect of devil's claw on degeneration of the proximal intertarsal, distal interdistal and tarsometatarsal joints and of muscular disorders was investigated in ten race horses by comparison with a control group of ten horses treated with phenylbutazone.[72] The horses were given 0.5 mg/kg of an approximately 3:1 extract of devil's claw for 60 days. Six horses receiving the devil's claw showed a marked improvement of symptoms, even compared with the control group receiving the drug. The dose used in this study appears to be relatively low.

Toxicology and other safety data

Toxicology

Devil's claw demonstrated low toxicity in acute and subacute toxicity studies.[17,31] No significant haematological or gross pathological findings were evident in rats after oral administration of 7.5 g/kg of devil's claw for 21 days. Hepatotoxic effects could not be demonstrated in terms of liver weight, levels of microsomal protein and liver enzymes after 7 days of oral treatment with 2 g/kg.[31] Table 1 lists the LD$_{50}$ data recorded for devil's claw extract and its constituents.

Contraindications

None advised, but see below.

Special warnings and precautions

The Commission E advises that the use of devil's claw is contraindicated in patients with gastric or duodenal ulcers and should only be used with professional supervision in patients with gallstones.[74] However, any health risks are theoretical in nature and are projected from the bitter tonic activity of the herb. Bitters should be used with caution in oesophageal reflux and in states of hyperacidity.

Interactions

The in vitro inhibitory activity of a devil's claw extract (undefined) towards the cytochrome P450 enzymes 1A2 and 2D6 was relatively low (IC$_{50}$>900 μg/mL). CYP 2C8, CYP 2C9, CYP 2C19 and CYP 3A4 were moderately inhibited, with IC$_{50}$ values in the range of 100 to 350 μg/mL. (IC$_{50}$ is the concentration that is required to produce 50% inhibition.)[75] Three standardised extracts of devil's claw inhibited P-gp activity in vitro (using two tests: calcein-AM and esterase). Harpagoside was almost inactive. Expression of P-gp was also tested. In cells cultured for 3 days in the presence of devil's claw extracts or pure harpagoside, a dose-dependent increase in P-gp expression was observed.[76]

Devil's claw may potentiate the effect of warfarin. A case of purpura was reported in a patient taking warfarin and devil's claw.[77] The patient's medical condition, other medications, and the doses and duration of the warfarin and devil's claw ingestion were not reported.

Devil's claw has demonstrated a protective effect against arrhythmia in vitro and in vivo[45,46] and it has been proposed that it may interact with antiarrhythmic drugs.[5] However, this is a theoretical concern of unknown clinical relevance.

Use in pregnancy and lactation

Category B2 – no increase in frequency of malformation or other harmful effects on the foetus from limited use in women. Animal studies are lacking.

In South African traditional medicine, low doses of the dried tuber (such as 0.25 g three times daily) are administered to pregnant women to relieve pain, and this is continued postpartum at a reduced dose. The fresh tuber is also made into an ointment and applied to the abdomen of women who anticipate a difficult birth.[78] While devil's claw has increased the contraction of isolated uterine strips,[50] the clinical relevance of this is uncertain.

Devil's claw is probably compatible with breastfeeding, since it has been used in low doses in the postpartum period in traditional South African medicine.[78]

Effects on ability to drive and use machines

No adverse effects expected.

Side effects

A systematic review published in 2008 investigated the safety of devil's claw preparations. Twenty-eight clinical studies (uncontrolled, observational and controlled) were identified from 1985 up to early 2007 involving a total of 6892 patients. Twenty-one of the studies were of short duration (up to 8 weeks) and two postmarketing surveillance studies were carried out over 54 weeks. Double blind trials assessed 615 patients, uncontrolled and observational studies included 6277 patients. For the double blind trials, the incidence of adverse events during treatment with devil's claw was not higher than during placebo treatment. Minor adverse events were described in 20 studies (n=4274) in a total of 138 patients, which corresponds to an overall adverse event rate of around 3%. Some of the adverse events, such as gastrointestinal complaints and allergies, were probably related to intake of devil's claw.[79]

One case of conjunctivitis, rhinitis and asthma has been reported after occupational exposure to devil's claw. Allergy was confirmed by a provocation test.[80]

Overdosage

No incidents found in published literature.

Safety in children

No information available, but adverse effects are not expected.

Table 1 LD$_{50}$ data recorded for devil's claw extract and its constituents

Substance	Route, model	LD$_{50}$ (g/kg)	Reference
Devil's claw	oral, mice	>13.5	17
Devil's claw purified extract (85% harpagoside)	iv, mice	0.511	31
Harpagoside	ip, mice	1.0	73

Regulatory status in selected countries

Devil's claw is official in the *European Pharmacopoeia* 2001 and the *British Pharmacopoeia* 2011.

Devil's claw is covered by a positive Commission E Monograph and has the following applications:

- Lack of appetite, dyspeptic complaints
- In supportive therapy for degenerative disorders of the musculoskeletal system.

Devil's claw is on the UK General Sale List. Products have achieved Traditional Herbal Registration in the UK with the traditional indication of relief of symptoms (aches and pains) associated with the muscles and joints.

Devil's claw does not have GRAS status. However, it is freely available as a 'dietary supplement' in the USA under DSHEA legislation (1994 Dietary Supplement Health and Education Act).

Devil's claw is not included in Part 4 of Schedule 4 of the Therapeutic Goods Act Regulations of Áustralia and is freely available for sale.

References

1. Ragusa S, Circosta C, Galati EM, et al. *J Ethnopharmacol.* 1984;11(3):245–257.
2. Van Wyk B-E, Van Oudtshoorn B, Gericke N. *Medicinal Plants of South Africa.* Arcadia: Briza Publications; 1997: pp. 144–145.
3. Chrubasik S, Zimpfer CH, Schutt U, et al. *Phytomedicine.* 1996;3(1):1–10.
4. British Herbal Medicine Association's Scientific Committee. *British Herbal Pharmacopoeia.* Cowling: BHMA; 1983. p. 111.
5. Scientific Committee of ESCOP (European Scientific Cooperative on Phytotherapy). *ESCOP Monographs: Harpagophytum radix.* UK: European Scientific Cooperative on Phytotherapy Secretariat; 1996.
6. British Herbal Medicine Association. *British Herbal Compendium,* Vol 1. Bournemouth: BHMA; 1992. pp. 78–80.
7. Wenzel P, Wegener T. *Dtsch Apoth Ztg.* 1995;135(13):1131–1144.
8. van Wyk BE. *J Ethnopharmacol.* 2008;119(3):342–355.
9. Bisset NG, ed. *Herbal Drugs and Phytopharmaceuticals: A Handbook for Practice on a Scientific Basis.* Stuttgart: Medpharm Scientific Publishers; 1994. p. 250.
10. Hachfeld B, Schippmann U. *Medicinal Plant Conservation,* vol 6. Bonn: Bundesamt fur Naturschutz; 2000. pp. 3–9.
11. Convention of International Trade in Endangered Species of Wild Fauna and Flora, Eleventh meeting of the Conference of the Parties, Gigiri (Kenya): 2000. pp. 10–20.
12. Wagner H, Bladt S. *Plant Drug Analysis: A Thin Layer Chromatography Atlas,* 2nd ed. Berlin: Springer-Verlag; 1996: p. 76.
13. Burger JFW, Brandt EV, Ferreira D. *Phytochemistry.* 1987;26(5):1453–1457.
14. Ziller KH, Franz G. *Planta Med.* 1979;37(12):340–348.
15. *European Pharmacopoeia,* 3rd ed. Strasbourg: European Department for the Quality of Medicines within the Council of Europe; 1996. pp. 716–717.
16. Baghdikian B, Lanhers MC, Fleurentin J, et al. *Planta Med.* 1997;63(2):171–176.
17. Whitehouse LW, Znamirowska M, Paul CJ. *Can Med Assoc J.* 1983;129(3):249–251.
18. Huang TH, Tran VH, Duke RK, et al. *J Ethnopharmacol.* 2006;104(1–2):149–155.
19. Kaszkin M, Beck KF, Koch E, et al. *Phytomedicine.* 2004;11(7–8):585–595.
20. Jang MH, Lim S, Han SM, et al. *J Pharmacol Sci.* 2003;93(3):367–371.
21. Anauate MC, Torres LM, de Mello SB. *Phytother Res.* 2010;24(9):1365–1369.
22. Bermejo Benito P, Díaz Lanza AM, Silván Sen AM, et al. *Planta Med.* 2000;66(4):324–328.
23. Inaba K, Murata K, Naruto S, et al. *J Nat Med.* 2010;64(2):219–222.
24. Fiebich BL, Heinrich M, Hiller KO, et al. *Phytomedicine.* 2001;8(1):28–30.
25. Loew D, Möllerfeld J, Schrödter A, et al. *Clin Pharmacol Ther.* 2001;69(5):356–364.
26. Schulze-Tanzil G, Hansen C, Shakibaei M. *Arzneimittelforschung.* 2004;54(4):213–220.
27. Boje K, Lechtenberg M, Nahrstedt A. *Planta Med.* 2003;69(9):820–825.
28. Moussard C, Alber D, Toubin MM, et al. *Prostagland Leuk Essent Fatty Acids.* 1992;46(4):283–286.
29. Qi J, Li N, Zhou JH, et al. *Planta Med.* 2010;76(16):1892–1896.
30. Qi J, Chen JJ, Cheng ZH, et al. *Phytochemistry.* 2006;67(13):1372–1377.
31. Erdos A, Fontaine R, Friehe H, et al. *Planta Med.* 1978;34(1):97–108.
32. Eichler O, Koch C. *Arzneimittelforschung.* 1970;20:107–109.
33. McLeod DW, Revell P, Robinson BV. *Br J Pharmacol.* 1979;66(1):140P–141P.
34. Mahomed IM, Ojewole JA. *Phytother Res.* 2004;18(12):982–989.
35. Andersen ML, Santos EH, Seabra Mde L, et al. *J Ethnopharmacol.* 2004;91(2–3):325–330.
36. Catelan SC, Belentani RM, Marques LC, et al. *Phytomedicine.* 2006;13(6):446–451.
37. Chrubasik JE, Lindhorst E, Neumann E, et al. *Phytomedicine.* 2006;13(8):598–600.
38. Lanhers MC, Fleurentin J, Mortier F, et al. *Planta Med.* 1992;58(2):117–123.
39. Soulimani R, Younos C, Mortier F, et al. *Can J Physiol Pharmacol.* 1994;72(12):1532–1536.
40. Abdelouahab N, Heard C. *J Nat Prod.* 2008;71(5):746–749.
41. Ouitas NA, Heard CM. *Int J Pharm.* 2009;376(1–2):63–68.
42. Ouitas NA, Heard C. *Phytother Res.* 2010;24(3):333–338.
43. Kundu JK, Mossanda KS, Na HK, et al. *Cancer Lett.* 2005;218(1):21–31.
44. Uchida S, Hirai K, Hatanaka J, et al. *Biol Pharm Bull.* 2008;31(2):240–245.
45. Circosta C, Occhiuto F, Ragusa A, et al. *J Ethnopharmacol.* 1984;11(3):259–274.
46. Costa de Pasquale R, Busa G, Circosta C, et al. *J Ethnopharmacol.* 1985;13(2):193–199.
47. Occhiuto F, de Pasquale A. *Pharmacol Res.* 1990;22(suppl 3):72–73.
48. Grant L, McBean DE, Fyfe L, et al. *Phytother Res.* 2009;23(1):104–110.
49. Betancor-Fernández A, Pérez-Gálvez A, Sies H, et al. *J Pharm Pharmacol.* 2003;55(7):981–986.
50. Mahomed IM, Ojewole JA. *J Smooth Muscle Res.* 2009;45(5):231–239.
51. Mahomed IM, Ojewole JA. *Brain Res Bull.* 2006;69(1):57–62.
52. Weckesser S, Engel K, Simon-Haarhaus B, et al. *Phytomedicine.* 2007;14(7–8):508–516.
53. Chrubasik S, Sporer F, Dillmann-Marschner R, et al. *Phytomedicine.* 2000;6(6):469–473.
54. Baghdikian B, Guiraud-Dauriac H, Ollivier E, et al. *Planta Med.* 1999;65(2):164–166.
55. Wu Q, Wen XD, Qi LW, et al. *J Chromatogr B Analyt Technol Biomed Life Sci.* 2009;877(8–9):751–756.
56. Belaiche P. *Phytotherapy.* 1982;1:22–28.
57. Grahame R, Robinson BV. *Ann Rheum Dis.* 1981;40(6):632.
58. Chrubasik S, Conradt C, Black A. *Phytomedicine.* 2003;10(6–7):613–623.

59. Chrubasik S, Junck H, Breitschwerdt H, et al. *Eur J Anaesthesiol.* 1999;16(2): 118–129.

60. Chrubasik S, Model A, Black A, et al. *Rheumatology.* 2003;42(1):141–148.

61. Chantre P, Cappelaere A, Leblan D, et al. *Phytomedicine.* 2000;7(3):177–183.

62. Gagnier JJ, van Tulder M, Berman B, et al. *Cochrane Database Syst Rev.* 2006;2: CD004504.

63. Chrubasik S, Künzel O, Thanner J, et al. *Phytomedicine.* 2005;12(1–2):1–9.

64. Chrubasik S, Chrubasik C, Künzel O, et al. *Phytomedicine.* 2007;14(6):371–376.

65. Wegener T, Lüpke NP. *Phytother Res.* 2003;17(10):1165–1172.

66. Thanner J, Kohlmann T, Künzel O, et al. *Phytother Res.* 2009;23(5):742–744.

67. Warnock M, McBean D, Suter A, et al. *Phytother Res.* 2007;21(12):1228–1233.

68. Göbel H, Heinze A, Ingwersen M, et al. *Schmerz.* 2001;15(1):10–18.

69. Arndt D, Bobermien K, Heyer H, et al. *Geburtsh Frauenheilk.* 2006;67(S1): PO-E-03-10.

70. WO/2006/114422. *Use of Devil's Claw (Harpagophytum procumbens) Root Extracts for Endometriosis Treatment.* 2006.

71. Wilson KS. *Curr Oncol.* 2009;16(4): 67–70.

72. Montesano D, Ferrara L. *Rev Fitoterapia.* 2002;2(S1):105. Abstract A045.

73. Van Haelen M, Van Haelen-Fastre R, Samaey-Fontaine J, et al. *Phytotherapy.* 1983;5:7–13.

74. Blumenthal M et al., eds. *The Complete German Commission E Monographs: Therapeutic Guide to Herbal Medicines.* Austin: American Botanical Council; 1998. p. 120.

75. Unger M, Frank A. *Rapid Commun Mass Spectrom.* 2004;18(19):2273–2281.

76. Romiti N, Tramonti G, Corti A, et al. *Phytomedicine.* 2009;16(12):1095–1100.

77. Shaw D, Leon C, Kolev S, et al. *Drug Saf.* 1997;17(5):342–356.

78. Watt JM, Breyer-Brandwijk MG. *The Medicinal And Poisonous Plants of Southern and Eastern Africa: Being an Account of Their Medicinal and Other Uses, Chemical Composition, Pharmacological Effects and Toxicology in Man and Animal.* Edinburgh: Churchill Livingstone; 1962. p. 830.

79. Vlachojannis J, Roufogalis BD, Chrubasik S. *Phytother Res.* 2008;22(2):149–152.

80. Altmeyer N, Garnier R, Rosenberg N, et al. *Arch Mal Prof.* 1992;53:289–291.

Dong quai

(*Angelica sinensis* (Oliv.) Diels)

Synonyms

Angelica polymorpha var. *sinensis* (botanical synonym), dong quai (Engl), Radix Angelica sinensis (Lat), dang gui (Chin), toki (Jap), tanggwi (Kor), kinesisk kvan (Dan).

What is it?

The root of dong quai is an extremely popular herb that has been used by the Chinese for thousands of years as a tonic and a spice. Its reputation in the West as a Chinese herb is second only to ginseng. Women have especially used dong quai to maintain their health and it is sometimes regarded as a 'women's ginseng'. *Angelica acutiloba*, which is indigenous to Japan, became a substitute in that country for genuine dong quai, but probably has some different phytochemistry (see Adulteration below). The popular use of dong quai in the West as a herb to treat menopausal symptoms such as hot flushes appears to be ill advised (although there are some positive trials for its use in combination). Nonetheless, it may have value in menopause as a tonic.

Effects

Regulates menstruation, alleviates dysmenorrhoea; treats blood deficiency; relieves constipation by lubricating the bowel; treats and prevents cardiovascular disorders; protects the liver; has blood-building and tonic effects (in combination with Astragalus).

Traditional view

Dong quai is sweet, acrid, bitter and warm. It strengthens the heart, lung and liver meridians and lubricates the bowel. Dong quai tonifies the *Blood*, regulates menstruation, invigorates and harmonises the *Blood* and is used to treat congealed blood conditions, blood deficiency and *Deficient Blood* patterns. It is an important herb in the treatment of gynaecological problems.[1]

Summary actions

Antianaemic, antiplatelet, female tonic, mild laxative, antiarrhythmic, anti-inflammatory.

Can be used for

Indications supported by clinical trials

To relieve dysmenorrhoea and treat infertility (uncontrolled trials); chronic hepatitis and cirrhosis (uncontrolled trial), chronic obstructive pulmonary disease and cor pulmonale (uncontrolled trials). No benefits were found in the treatment of menopausal symptoms with the use of dong quai alone; trials where it was used in combination have yielded mixed results.

Traditional therapeutic uses

Irregular menstruation, amenorrhoea, dysmenorrhoea; constipation; congealed blood (abdominal pain, traumatic injuries, swellings, contusions, bruising); blood deficiency (tinnitus, blurred vision, palpitations); as a tonic, especially for women.

May also be used for

Extrapolations from pharmacological studies

For the prevention of atherosclerosis; as an antiplatelet agent.

Preparations

Dried root as a decoction; liquid extract, tablets or capsules for internal use.

Dosage

* 3 to 15 g/day of the dried root by decoction
* 4 to 8 mL/day of a 1:2 liquid extract; 10 to 20 mL/day of 1:5 tincture; or equivalent doses as tablets or capsules.

Duration of use

May be taken long term.

Summary assessment of safety

No adverse effects from ingestion of dong quai are expected, providing the suggested contraindications are observed.

Technical data

Botany

Dong quai, a member of the Umbelliferae (Apiaceae, carrot) family, is a fragrant, perennial herb native to China, Korea and Japan that grows to a height of 0.5 to 1 m. The inferior leaves are tripinnate, superior leaves are pinnate, on long, sheathed petioles. The umbels number 10 to 14, with irregular rays, each umbel containing 12 to 36 white flowers. The root's exterior is grey-dark brown in colour and its surface is covered in wrinkles. The root consists of a head, body and tail.[2] Different properties are ascribed to these parts: the head is most tonic and the tail moves the blood most strongly. Such preparations are very expensive and the entire root is usually prescribed.

Adulteration

Ligusticum glaucescens and *Levisticum officinale* are regarded as substitutes of lower quality for dong quai.[2] *Angelica acutiloba* is a therapeutically interchangeable species for *A. sinensis* in Japan (but in China would be regarded as a substitute of lower quality).[2,3] *A. dahurica*, *A. pubescens* and *Ligusticum chuanxiong* are also used in traditional Chinese medicine, *Ligusticum porteri* is traditionally used in Mexico and is sold in the USA. These plants are morphologically similar to *Angelica sinensis* and may occur as substitutes.[3]

A. acutiloba contains phthalides as main constituents and can be difficult to distinguish from *A. sinensis* by thin layer chromatography,[4] although ferulic acid was detected in *A. sinensis* and not in *A. acutiloba*.[5] Senkyunolide A, analysed using a high performance liquid chromatography method, is a useful standard compound for quality evaluation and chemical differentiation between *Ligusticum chuanxiong* rhizome and *Angelica sinensis* root.[6]

Key constituents

- Essential oil (0.4% to 0.7%), mainly consisting of the phthalides ligustilide and n-butylidenephthalide[2] (n-butylidenephthalide has a penetrating characteristic fragrance,[7] like all plant phthalides)
- Phytosterols, ferulic acid, coumarins (angelol, angelicone).[2]

Ligustilide

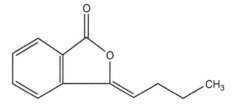

n-Butylidenephthalide

Pharmacodynamics

Effects on sexual function

The essential oil relaxed the isolated uterus, but other components increased uterine contraction.[8] Butylidenephthalide demonstrated spasmolytic activity by inhibiting rat uterine contractions. Its effect was non-specific, similar to papaverine, but with a different mechanism of action.[9] In vitro tests with isolated rat uterus suggest that ligustilide has a non-specific antispasmodic activity.[10] Some experiments on the whole root of dong quai have shown a stimulant activity in vivo, while others have shown that it can relax or coordinate (make more rhythmic) uterine contractions, depending on uterine tone. Different parts of the root exhibited a similar spasmolytic action on isolated rabbit uterus.[11]

A review suggested that the in vitro experiments provide conflicting evidence concerning the oestrogenicity of dong quai.[11] In contrast, oral administration of a standardised ethanolic dong quai extract at 'doses based on typical clinical human doses' produced oestrogenic activity in ovariectomised rats. The uterine cellular structure was stimulated, vaginal cornification provoked and serum luteinising hormone decreased.[12] However, dong quai had no effect on uterine weight when administered orally to mice for a period of 4 days.[13]

One study showed increased sexual activity in female animals and a reduction in signs of vitamin E deficiency in male mice.[2] Intraperitoneal injection of dong quai protected mice ovaries from the damaging effects of gamma radiation.[14]

An aqueous extract of dong quai stimulated the growth of breast cancer cells in vitro.[15] In an earlier study this activity was also demonstrated for the ethanolic extract.[13] Clinical implications (such as adverse effects from the use of dong quai during breast cancer) cannot yet be drawn from this research.

Cardiovascular activity

Dong quai has a quinidine-like action on the isolated heart. It can prolong the refractory period and correct experimental atrial fibrillation induced by atropine, pituitrin, strophanthin, acetylcholine or electrical stimulation.[8] Extracts of dong quai relaxed isolated aorta[16] and promoted the growth of vascular endothelial cells in vitro and in vivo.[17,18] Dong quai increased the production of vascular endothelial growth factor (VEGF) in a rat model of myocardial infarction.[19] It had an antioxidant activity in vitro and reversed the morphological changes induced in vascular endothelial cells by hyperlipidaemic serum.[20,21] Ferulic acid and ligustilide exhibit antiplatelet activity in vitro or in vivo, as does the aqueous extract.[8] Both the aqueous extract of dong quai and ferulic acid inhibited platelet aggregation and serotonin release.[22]

Dong quai lowered blood pressure, dilated coronary vessels, increased coronary flow, reduced serum cholesterol and reduced respiratory rate. Mixed in feed at 5%, it reduced atherosclerosis formation in animals.[23] The herb exerted a stimulating action on haematopoiesis in vitro in bone marrow,[23] and a recent in vitro and in vivo (oral doses) publication observed that polysaccharide components might be responsible for this effect.[24] A decoction of dong quai (15 g/kg orally to mice) for 4 weeks reduced the mortality rate and cardiotoxicity following subsequent administration of the chemotherapeutic drug doxorubicin.[25]

Renal effects

Danggui Buxue Tang (DBT) is a combination of dong quai and Astragalus in the ratio of 1:5, usually prepared by decoction. This decoction given orally alleviated hyperlipidaemia in nephrotic rats. The combination also retarded the progression of renal fibrosis and deterioration of renal function.[26,27] Renoprotective effects were demonstrated in both an in vitro[28] and an in vivo model,[29] including positive microvasculature changes with an increase of VEGF production in vivo.[30] DBT is a traditional antifibrotic agent in China. Combined treatment with the ACE (angiotensin-converting enzyme) inhibitor enalapril was significantly more effective than the drug alone in decreasing tubulointerstitial fibrosis in a rat model of obstructive uropathy.[31] The antifibrotic activity might be associated with the enhanced production of nitric oxide that was observed in a similar model following oral doses of DBT (14 g/kg/day).[32]

DBT induced the mRNA expression of erythropoietin (EPO) in vitro (albeit in cultured human hepatocellular carcinoma cells rather than renal cells) in a dose-dependent manner.[33] Use of a myelosuppression mouse model found that DBT (10 mg/kg/day) significantly increased the recovery of megakaryocytes.[34] DBT also enhanced EPO gene expression in cyclophosphamide-induced anaemia in rats and somewhat countered the reduced levels of red and white blood cells, platelets and vitamin B12.[35]

Cytotoxic effects

An antitumour action for n-butylidenephthalide was demonstrated in vitro and in vivo for the brain tumour cell glioblastoma multiforme. The survival rate of inoculated rats was significantly prolonged.[36] Dong quai extracts (20 or 60 mg/kg of different extracts, ip) also showed activity in vivo against the same cancer.[37] Phthalides from dong quai exhibited in vitro cytotoxic activity against human colon cancer HT-29 cells, but their effect was greater when combined with other ingredients in the herb extract.[38] Cytotoxic bioassay-guided fractionation of a methanolic extract of dong quai demonstrated that the phthalides in particular, and also

two polyacetylenes, possessed significant in vitro activity.[39] A recent study found only weak in vitro activity for an aqueous extract of dong quai against a range of tumour cell lines, perhaps as might be expected from the above focus on relatively non-polar components of the herb.[40]

An in vitro and in vivo study found that dong quai reduced the metastasis of BL16-BL6 mouse melanoma cells, possibly by inhibiting their adherence and migration characteristics.[41] In contrast, dong quai promoted proliferation of normal melanocytes, melanin synthesis and tryosinase activity in vitro.[42]

Immune function

Some studies have shown a pronounced inhibition of antibody production, while others have shown a sometimes weak stimulation of phagocytosis and lymphocyte proliferation.[8] Dong quai can somewhat counter the immunosuppressive effects of hydrocortisone in vivo, but is not as effective as Astragalus.[43] Combined with Astragalus as DBT, it improved thrombocytopenic purpura in rabbits[43] and markedly induced cell proliferation, secretion of interleukin-2 and macrophage phagocytosis in vitro.[44] The immunomodulating impact of DBT was revealed to be strongest at the traditionally used 1:5 ratio.[44]

Other activity

Ligustilide demonstrated an antiproliferative effect on smooth muscle cells in vitro[45] and a muscle relaxing activity in rats, which was believed to be of central origin.[46] The compound given to guinea pigs (0.14 mL/kg, ip) inhibited the asthmatic reaction induced by acetylcholine and histamine.[47]

Feeding rats 5% dong quai for 4 weeks increased metabolism and oxygen utilisation in the liver. Glutamic acid and cysteine oxidation were also enhanced.[8]

Sodium ferulate pretreatment (via intragastric administration) demonstrated hepatoprotective activity in mice.[48] A water extraction of dong quai protected the liver from carbon tetrachloride toxic hepatitis and prevented loss of liver glycogen.[2] Dong quai protected against experimentally induced injury in rat lungs by decreasing alveolitis and the release of inflammatory factors.[49]

Injection of dong quai extract inhibited the progress of radiation-induced pulmonary fibrosis in mice, possibly by downregulating the expression of the pro-inflammatory cytokine transforming growth factor beta-1.[50,51]

Aqueous extract of dong quai stimulated the proliferation, alkaline phosphatase activity, protein secretion and type I collagen synthesis of bone cells in vitro.[52] An unidentified multicomponent factor from an aqueous extract of dong quai enhanced the deposition of hyaluronic acid and proliferation of osteoblasts in vitro, as well as bone regeneration in the rat calvarial defect model.[53] Together these results suggest a beneficial effect in periodontal regeneration.

Dong quai essential oil (30 mg/kg, oral) had a modest anxiolytic activity in mice.[54] Butylidenephthalide (100 mg/kg by injection) reduced the impairment of inhibitory avoidance performance induced by drugs in rats. This finding reflected on activation of the central cholinergic neuronal system via muscarinic and nicotinic receptors.[55] Phthalide dimers from the herb were found to be active in an in vitro GABA-A receptor-binding assay.[56] Ligustilide (5 and 20 mg/kg by injection) protected against neuronal damage induced by transient cerebral ischaemia in mice.[57] An ethanolic extract of dong quai also protected against beta-amyloid peptide-induced neurotoxicity in vitro.[58]

Pharmacokinetics

When an ethanol extract of dong quai was orally administered to a rabbit, 32 compounds (including ligustilide and butylidenephthalide) present in the extract were also found in the blood. At least 10 other components not in the original extract were found in plasma, indicating that these compounds were metabolites.[59] The bioavailability of ferulic acid from dong quai in mice was substantially increased by combination with cinnamon bark.[60]

Clinical trials

Female reproductive tract conditions

Ligustilide at 450 mg/day was used to treat 112 cases of dysmenorrhoea in an uncontrolled trial. The effective rate was 77% compared to 38% for aqueous extract of dong quai.[61] In combination with Corydalis, Paeonia lactiflora and Ligusticum, dong quai showed a 93% improvement rate for the treatment of dysmenorrhoea in an uncontrolled trial. The decoction was given daily, starting 5 days before and until cessation of menstruation. (After treatment for about four cycles, 72% were 'cured'.[62])

Infertility due to tubal occlusion was treated for up to 9 months with uterine irrigation of dong quai extract in an uncontrolled trial; 79% of patients regained tubal patency and 53% became pregnant.[63]

In November 2007 a case of a woman with atypical polypoid adenomyoma (APA) and infertility was reported. Oral use of dong quai (dose not specified) for 4 months corrected her endometrium to that of a normal secretory endometrium. (APA is an unusual form of precancerous endometrial proliferation.) Pregnancy soon followed. Her doctors suggested that dong quai may have acted as an ovulation inducer.[64]

In a randomised, double blind, placebo-controlled clinical trial, 71 postmenopausal women (FSH levels of >30 mIU/mL with hot flushes) received either dong quai (4.5 g dried root per day) or placebo for 24 weeks. Dong quai did not produce oestrogen-like responses in endometrial thickness or in vaginal maturation. The incidence of symptoms dropped in both groups but there was no significant difference between dong quai and placebo.[65]

In a controlled clinical trial, 55 postmenopausal women were randomly assigned to receive either a herbal tablet containing dong quai and chamomile (Matricaria recutita) or a placebo over 12 weeks. The average number per week of daytime and night hot flushes declined significantly in the herbal group compared with the placebo patients (p<0.001). There was also a significant decline in the intensity of hot flushes for the herbal group versus placebo (p<0.001), and they were almost completely eliminated by the third month of the herbal treatment. There were no differences in serum levels of oestrogen, FSH or LH recorded, nor was there any morphological change noted on vaginal ultrasound scans. The authors concluded that the herbal combination appeared to be an effective and safe treatment for the vasomotor symptoms of menopause.[66] The details provided on the dong quai and chamomile product used in this successful trial are vague. Daily doses were 375 mg for dong quai and 150 mg for chamomile in tablet form, but it is not clear if these were doses of dried extract or dried herb. If it is the latter then the doses used in the trial were quite low.

Treatment with a preparation containing extracts of dong quai, soy and black cohosh reduced the frequency and severity of menstrual migraine in a randomised, double blind trial. The average number of migraines (weeks 9 to 24) compared to baseline for the treatment group was 4.7%, and for the placebo group was 10.3%. The difference in the results between the two groups was significant (p<0.01). The differences in the results (favouring herbal treatment) were also significant for headache severity score and doses of triptan and analgesics (weeks 20 to 24). Although the extract strengths were not defined, the daily dose of actives corresponded to 1 mg ligustilide (dong quai), 60 mg soy isoflavones and 4 mg triterpenes (black cohosh).[67]

A complex formulation containing extracts of black cohosh, dong quai, milk (St Mary's) thistle, red clover, American ginseng and chaste tree was tested in a randomised, placebo-controlled, double blind pilot study in 50 healthy but symptomatic peri- and postmenopausal women.[68] There was a high dropout rate and only 35 women completed the 3-month study. Statistical analysis (not using intention-to-treat) revealed a significant 73% reduction in hot flushes for the herbal group versus 38% for placebo (p=0.026), with similar results for night sweats. There were no changes in vaginal ultrasonography, or levels of oestradiol and FSH.

In contrast, DBT failed to demonstrate any superiority over placebo in a 6-month randomised, double blind study involving 103 women suffering hot flushes.[69] However, the formulation was statistically superior to placebo in the treatment of mild flushes.

The HALT study (Herbal Alternatives for Menopause Trial) used a 1-year randomised, double blind, placebo-controlled design to assess the impact of various herbal treatments in 351 peri- and postmenopausal women.[70,71] The trial consisted of five treatment arms: black cohosh 160 mg/day, a complex herbal formulation that included black cohosh (200 mg/day) and dong quai (400 mg/day), the formulation plus dietary soya intake, conjugated equine oestrogen (with or without medroxyprogesterone acetate) and placebo. At 3, 6 and 12 months patients receiving the herbal interventions had the same change in vasomotor symptoms (hot flushes, night sweats) as those receiving placebo (except for more severe symptoms in the soya plus herbal formulation group). In contrast oestrogen substantially decreased vasomotor symptoms.[71] None of the herbal treatments exhibited any effects on vaginal epithelium, endometrium or reproductive hormones.[72]

A randomised, double blind, placebo-controlled trial was conducted in 22 men receiving luteinising hormone-releasing hormone agonist therapy for prostate cancer and experiencing hot flushes.[73] After 3 months there was no significant influence on the severity, frequency or duration of hot flushes from dong quai treatment compared with placebo.

Other conditions

Dong quai has been successfully used to treat Buerger's disease and constrictive aortitis[8] and is often combined with dan shen in the treatment of angina, peripheral vascular disorders and stroke. This information is based on case studies and uncontrolled trials.

Dong quai improved abnormal protein metabolism, improved abnormal thymol turbidity test and increased plasma protein level in 60% of patients with chronic hepatitis or hepatic cirrhosis after 1 to 3 weeks of treatment in an uncontrolled trial.[74]

Dong quai extract, given orally to patients with chronic obstructive pulmonary disease for 50 to 60 days in an uncontrolled trial, significantly increased the forced expiratory volume. In cases of chronic cor pulmonale (pulmonary heart disease) dong quai lowered the mortality rate, improved blood gas measurements and improved ECG (electrocardiogram).[75]

A case report described a 56-year-old man with end-stage renal disease and chronic anaemia due to resistance to EPO.[76] He experienced marked improvement in his anaemia and well-being after self-initiating once-weekly consumption of a herbal decoction prepared from about 12 g dong quai and 52 g *Paeonia lactiflora* root.

Toxicology and other safety data

Toxicology

The following LD_{50} data have been recorded for dong quai and its constituents:

Substance	Route, model	LD_{50}	Reference
Concentrated dong quai extract*	Oral, rats	100 g/kg	4
3-n-Butylidene-phthalide	Oral, rats	2.45 g/kg	77

*According to information supplied by the author, this concentrated extract was 8:1 to 16:1.[4]

The minimum lethal dose of dong quai root was 30 to 90 g/kg in mice (route unknown). Respiration was inhibited and blood pressure fell in anaesthetised rabbits, cats and dogs intravenously administered the essential oil (1 mg/kg).[8]

Ferulic acid, which also occurs naturally in many fruits and vegetables, demonstrated chromosome-damaging activity in vitro at a concentration of 25 mg/mL.[78,79] However, it has also demonstrated antigenotoxic and anticarcinogenic activity in vivo after oral and intraperitoneal administration and topical application.[79] In any case, it occurs at quite low levels in dong quai.

Safrole, a carcinogenic compound, has been detected in dong quai root,[2] although not confirmed. If present it is likely to occur at very low levels.

Subcutaneous administration of dong quai aqueous extract (0.1 to 0.4 mL/day) for 5 days did not affect fertility or exhibit teratogenic effects in mice.[80]

At concentrations higher than 2500 µg/mL, aqueous extracts of dong quai root exerted a general cytotoxicity to melanocytes in culture. Prior treatment of the dong quai extract to reduce its coumarin content resulted in reduced cytotoxicity.[81]

Contraindications

Contraindications according to traditional Chinese medicine are as follows: diarrhoea caused by weak digestion, haemorrhagic disease, bleeding tendency or very heavy periods, first trimester of pregnancy, tendency to spontaneous abortion and acute viral infections such as colds and influenza.[2] At the doses used in the West, the main concern would be in the first trimester of pregnancy.

Special warnings and precautions

Caution is advised for patients receiving chronic treatment with warfarin.

Interactions

The effects of dong quai on the pharmacodynamics and pharmacokinetics of warfarin were studied in rabbits. Single subcutaneous doses of warfarin (2 mg/kg) were administered with or without 3 days' treatment with oral dong quai extract (2 g dried herb/kg, twice daily). The dong quai treatment did not affect prothrombin time on its own, but significantly lowered the value 3 days after co-administration with warfarin. No significant variation in the pharmacokinetic parameters of warfarin was observed after dong quai treatment for both single-dose administration or steady-state concentrations of warfarin.[82] Caution is therefore advised for patients receiving chronic treatment with warfarin.

One female patient stabilised on warfarin presented with widespread bruising and an increased international normalised ratio (INR),[83] and another developed an increased INR and prothrombin time after taking dong quai concurrently for 4 weeks.[84]

A survey completed by 28 professional members of the American Herbalists Guild in 2004 found that of the 25 who regularly used dong quai, only one respondent reported having seen potentiation of an anticoagulant drug when combined with the herb. Nineteen reported no evidence of potentiation and five had not combined the two agents.[85]

Use in pregnancy and lactation

Category C – has caused or is associated with a substantial risk of causing harmful effects on the fetus or neonate without causing malformations. (Apparently, based on traditional considerations, dong quai is contraindicated in the first trimester of pregnancy and in women with a tendency to spontaneous abortion.[2])

The essential oil relaxed the isolated uterus, but other components of dong quai increased uterine contraction. Some experiments on the whole root have shown a stimulant action in vivo, while others have shown that it can relax or coordinate uterine contractions, depending on uterine tone.[8,75] Subcutaneous administration of dong quai aqueous extract (0.1 to 0.4 mL/day) for 5 days did not affect fertility or exhibit teratogenic effects in mice.[80]

Dong quai is considered compatible with breastfeeding.

Effects on ability to drive and use machines

No adverse effects expected.

Side effects

A 35-year-old man developed gynaecomastia (mammary glandular hyperplasia) after ingestion of dong quai capsules for 1 month. The label indicated '100% dong quai (*Angelica sinensis*) root powder. No fillers or additives'. The patient discontinued the pills and the gynaecomastia had regressed completely when he was reviewed 3 months later.[86]

'Angelica-Paeonia Powder' has been reported to cause mild lassitude, drowsiness and urticaria after oral administration.[8] The species of Angelica and the formula was not defined.

A case of liver toxicity in a female patient was reported after the ingestion of a Chinese herbal preparation for 6 months. Dong quai was one of nine herbs in the formula. The patient's liver function normalised within several months of ceasing the herbal mixture.[87] It is not known if the dong quai was implicated.

A case was reported in 2001 of a woman diagnosed with grade 1 endometrioid adenocarcinoma of the endometrium 'whose history was notable for extensive use of supplemental phytoestrogens'. Herbs used included chaste tree, dong quai, black cohosh and licorice.[88] No causality was demonstrated.

A survey completed by 28 professional members of the American Herbalists Guild in 2004 found that of the 25 who regularly used dong quai, 11 respondents reported observing side effects with the use of dong quai. The most notable side effects included bleeding gums, increased menstrual flow, headaches, digestive disturbance and increased hot flushes rash.[85]

Overdosage

No effects known.

Safety in children

No information available, but adverse effects are not expected.

Regulatory status in selected countries

Dong quai is official in the *Pharmacopoeia of the People's Republic of China* (English edition, 1997). It is not covered by a Commission E Monograph and is not on the UK General Sale List.

Dong quai does not have GRAS status. However, it is freely available as a 'dietary supplement' in the USA under DSHEA legislation (1994 Dietary Supplement Health and Education Act). Dong quai has been used as an ingredient in products offered over the counter for use as an aphrodisiac. The FDA, however, advises that: 'based on evidence currently available, any OTC drug product containing ingredients for use as an aphrodisiac cannot be generally recognised as safe and effective'.

Dong quai is not included in Part 4 of Schedule 4 of the Therapeutic Goods Act Regulations of Australia and is freely available for sale.

References

1. Bensky D, Gamble A. *Chinese Herbal Medicine Materia Medica*. Seattle: Eastland Press; 1986: pp. 474–476.
2. Zhu DP. *Am J Chin Med*. 1987;15(3–4):117–125.
3. Zschocke S, Liu JH, Stuppner H, et al. *Phytochem Anal*. 1998;9:283–290.
4. Wagner H. Bauer R, Peigen X, eds. *Chinese Drug Monographs and Analysis: Radix Angelicae sinensis – Danggui*, vol. 3, no.14. Kotzting/Bayer: Verlag fur Ganzheitliche Medizin; 2001.
5. Sheu SJ, Ho YS, Chen YP, et al. *Planta Med*. 1986;53:377–378.
6. Yi T, Leung KS, Lu GH, et al. *Chem Pharm Bull*. 2005;53(11):1480–1483.
7. Lin M, Zhu GD, Sun QM, et al. *Yao Hsueh Hsueh Pao*. 1979;14(9):529–534.
8. Chang HM, But PP. *Pharmacology and Applications of Chinese Materia Medica*, vol 1. Singapore: World Scientific; 1987. pp. 489–505.
9. Ko WC. *Jpn J Pharmacol*. 1980;30(1):85–91.
10. Du J, Bai B, Kuang X, et al. *J Ethnopharmacol*. 2006;108(1):54–58.
11. Piersen CE. *Integr Cancer Ther*. 2003;2(2):120–138.
12. Circosta C, Pasquale RD, Palumbo DR, et al. *Phytother Res*. 2006;20(8):665–669.
13. Amato P, Christophe S, Mellon PL. *Menopause*. 2002;9(2):145–150.
14. Zhang D, Shan S, Zhang L. *Acta Acad Med Hubei*. 1996;17(3):216–218.
15. Lau CB, Ho TC, Chan TW, et al. *Menopause*. 2005;12(6):734–740.
16. Rhyu MR, Kim JH, Kim EY. *J Cardiovasc Pharmacol*. 2005;46(1):99–104.
17. Lei Y, Gao Q, Li YS. *Zhongguo Zhong Xi Yi Jie He Za Zhi*. 2003;23(10):753–756.
18. Lam HW, Lin HC, Lao SC, et al. *J Cell Biochem*. 2008;103(1):195–211.
19. Meng H, Guo J, Sun JY, et al. *Am J Chin Med*. 2008;36(3):541–554.
20. Wang BH, Ouyang JP, Liu YM, et al. *Sheng Li Xue Bao*. 2001;53(3):240–243.
21. Xiaohong Y, Jing-Ping OY, Shuzheng T. *Clin Hemorheol Microcirc*. 2000;22(4):317–323.
22. Yin ZZ, Zhang LY, Xu LN. *Yao Hsueh Hsueh Pao*. 1980;15(6):321–326.
23. Huang KC. *The Pharmacology of Chinese Herbs*. Boca Raton: CRC Press; 1993. pp. 247–248.
24. Liu PJ, Hsieh WT, Huang SH, et al. *Exp Hematol*. 2010;38(6):437–445.
25. Xin YF, Zhou GL, Shen M, et al. *Basic Clin Pharmacol Toxicol*. 2007;101(6):421–426.
26. Li J, Yu L, Li N, et al. *Chin Med J*. 2000;113(4):310–314.

27. Wang H, Li J, Yu L, et al. *Life Sci.* 2004;74(13):1645–1658.

28. Li B, Tang JW, Cai SQ, et al. *Beijing Da Xue Xue Bao.* 2006;38(4):381–384.

29. Song JY, Li S, Meng LQ, et al. *Beijing Da Xue Xue Bao.* 2009;41(2):196–202.

30. Song J, Meng L, Li S, et al. *Vascul Pharmacol.* 2009;50(5–6):185–193.

31. Wojcikowski K, Wohlmuth H, Johnson DW, et al. *Phytother Res.* 2010;24(6):875–884.

32. Meng L, Qu L, Tang J, et al. *Vascul Pharmacol.* 2007;47(2–3):174–183.

33. Gao QT, Cheung JK, Choi RC, et al. *Planta Med.* 2008;74(4):392–395.

34. Yang M, Chan GC, Deng R, et al. *J Ethnopharmacol.* 2009;124(1):87–97.

35. Chang MS, Kim do R, Ko EB, et al. *J Med Food.* 2009;12(3):637–642.

36. Tsai NM, Chen YL, Lee CC, et al. *J Neurochem.* 2006;99(4):1251–1262.

37. Lee WH, Jin JS, Tsai WC, et al. *Pathobiology.* 2006;73(3):141–148.

38. Kan WL, Cho CH, Rudd JA, et al. *J Ethnopharmacol.* 2008;120(1):36–43.

39. Chen QC, Lee J, Jin W, et al. *Arch Pharm Res.* 2007;30(5):565–569.

40. Chu Q, Satoh K, Kanamoto T, et al. *Anticancer Res.* 2009;29(8):3211–3219.

41. Gu Q, Xu JY, Cheng LG, et al. *Zhong Yao Cai.* 2007;30(3):302–305.

42. Deng Y, Yang L. *Di Yi Jun Yi Da Xue Xue Bao.* 2003;23(3):239–241.

43. Luo B, Li SC, Cui WY, et al. *J Beijing Med Univ.* 1987;19(6):419–422.

44. Gao QT, Cheung JK, Li J, et al. *Planta Med.* 2006;72(13):1227–1231.

45. Kobayashi S, Mimura Y, Notoya K, et al. *Jpn J Pharmacol.* 1992;60(4):397–401.

46. Ozaki Y, Sekita S, Harada M. *Yakugaku Zasshi.* 1989;109(6):402–406.

47. Tao JY, Ruan YP, Mei QB, et al. *Yao Xue Xue Bao.* 1984;19(8):561–565.

48. Wang H, Peng RX. *Chung Kuo Yao Li Hsueh Pao.* 1994;15(1):81–83.

49. Xu Q, Liu W, Lin Y. *Acta Acad Med Hubei.* 1997;18(1):20–23.

50. Han G, Zhou YF, Zhang MS, et al. *Radiat Res.* 2006;165(5):546–552.

51. Zhong YH, Han G, Zhou YF, et al. *Zhonghua Yu Fang Yi Xue Za Zhi.* 2007;41(2):105–109.

52. Yang Q, Populo SM, Zhang J, et al. *Clin Chim Acta.* 2002;324(1–2):89–97.

53. Zhao H, Alexeev A, Sharma V, et al. *Phytother Res.* 2008;22(7):923–928.

54. Chen SW, Min L, Li WJ, et al. *Pharmacol Biochem Behav.* 2004;79(2):377–382.

55. Hsieh MT, Wu CR, Lin LW, et al. *Planta Med.* 2001;67(1):38–42.

56. Deng S, Chen SN, Lu J, et al. *Phytochem Anal.* 2006;17(6):398–405.

57. Kuang X, Yao Y, Du JR, et al. *Brain Res.* 2006;1102(1):145–153.

58. Huang SH, Lin CM, Chiang BH. *Phytomedicine.* 2008;15(9):710–721.

59. Wang YL, Liang YZ, Chen BM, et al. *Anal Bioanal Chem.* 2005;383(2):247–254.

60. Yang ZY, Pei J, Liu RM, et al. *Zhongguo Zhong Yao Za Zhi.* 2006;31(12):1012–1015.

61. Gao YM, Zhang H, Duan ZX. *J Lanzhou Med Coll.* 1988;1:36–38.

62. Liu MA, Qi CH, Yang JC. *Beijing J Trad Chin Med.* 1988;5:30–31.

63. Fu YF, Xia Y, Shi YP, et al. *Jiangsu J Trad Chin Med.* 1988;9(1):15–16.

64. Wong AY, Chan KS, Lau WL, et al. *Fertil Steril.* 2007;88(5):1438. e7–1438,e9.

65. Hirata JD, Swiersz LM, Zell B, et al. *Fertil Steril.* 1997;68(6):981–986.

66. Kupfersztain C, Rotem C, Fagot R, et al. *Clin Exp Obstet Gyn.* 2003;30(4):203–206.

67. Burke BE, Olson RD, Cusack BJ. *Biomed Pharmacother.* 2002;56(6):283–288.

68. Rotem C, Kaplan B. *Gynecol Endocrinol.* 2007;23(2):117–122.

69. Haines CJ, Lam PM, Chung TK, et al. *Climacteric.* 2008;11(3):244–251.

70. Newton KM, Reed SD, Grothaus L, et al. *Maturitas.* 2005;52(2):134–146.

71. Newton KM, Reed SD, LaCroix AZ, et al. *Ann Intern Med.* 2006;145(12): 869–879.

72. Reed SD, Newton KM, LaCroix AZ, et al. *Menopause.* 2008;15(1):51–58.

73. Al-Bareeq RJ, Ray AA, Nott L, et al. *Can Urol Assoc J.* 2010;4(1):49–53.

74. Zhou QJ. In: Chang HM, ed. *Advances in Chinese Medicinal Materials Research.* Singapore: World Scientific; 1985. p. 217.

75. Mei QB, Tao JY, Cui B. *Chin Med J.* 1991;104(9):776–781.

76. Bradley RR, Cunniff PJ, Pereira BJ, et al. *Am J Kidney Dis.* 1999;34(2):349–354.

77. Opdyke DL. *Food Cosmet Toxicol.* 1979;17(3):251.

78. Stich HF, Rosin MP, Wu CH, et al. *Cancer Lett.* 1981;14(3):251–260.

79. Stich HF. *Mutat Res.* 1991;259(3–4): 307–324.

80. Matsui AS, Rogers J, Woo YK, et al. *Med Pharmacol Exp.* 1967;16:414–424.

81. Raman A, Lin ZX, Sviderskaya E, et al. *J Ethnopharmacol.* 1996;54(2–3): 165–170.

82. Lo AC, Chan K, Yeung JH, et al. *Eur J Drug Metab Pharmacokinet.* 1995;20(1):55–60.

83. Ellis GR, Stephens MR. *BMJ.* 1999;319:650.

84. Page RL, Lawrence JD. *Pharmacotherapy.* 1999;19(7):870–876.

85. Romm A, Upton R. *J Am Herbalists Guild.* 2004;5(2):40–45.

86. Goh SY, Loh KC. *Singapore Med J.* 2001;42(3):115–116.

87. Kane JA, Kane SP, Jain S. *Gut.* 1995;36(1):146–147.

88. Johnson EB, Muto MC, Yanushpolsky EH, et al. *Obstet Gynecol.* 2001;98(5 Pt 2): 947–950.

Echinacea root

(*Echinacea angustifolia* (DC.) Hell. and/or *purpurea* (L.) Moench)

Synonyms

Echinacea radix (Lat), Sonnenhut, Igelkopf (Ger), racine d'échinaeace (Fr), Echinacea (Ital), solhat (Dan).

What is it?

Three main species of Echinacea, commonly known as purple coneflower, are used medicinally: *Echinacea angustifolia* (narrow-leaved purple coneflower), *E. purpurea* (common or broad-leaved purple coneflower) and *E. pallida* (Nutt.) Nutt. (pale purple coneflower). *E. purpurea* has become the most cultivated and widely used of the various species because the whole plant (root, leaf, flower, seed) can be used and also because it is more easily cultivated. The root and rhizome of *E. angustifolia* and *E. pallida* are typically used medicinally, although *E. pallida* is sometimes considered to be less active, because it is low in alkylamides. In the past *E. pallida* preparations have been incorrectly labelled as *E. angustifolia*, particularly in Europe. *Parthenium integrifolium*, the Missouri snakeroot, is a documented adulterant of commercial Echinacea.

Echinacea has been the subject of a considerable amount of misinformation and misunderstanding concerning its active principles, mode of action, clinical efficacy and cautions and contraindications. One important reason behind such confusion is the many types of Echinacea products on the market. This has an historical background. The Native Americans, and the Eclectics physicians who adopted their use of Echinacea, preferred the root (see below). In fact, the Eclectics only used an aqueous-ethanolic (lipophilic) extract of dried *E. angustifolia* root high in alkylamides. After oral intake, these phytochemicals impart a persistent tingling sensation in the mouth and stimulate the flow of saliva, a sign of good quality according to *King's American Dispensatory*.[1] In Europe during the 1930s, the German herbalist Madaus promoted *E. purpurea* as it was easier to grow. Being somewhat influenced by the homeopathic approach of using fresh plant tinctures, his firm eventually developed a hydrophilic product prepared from the stabilised juice of fresh *E. purpurea* tops (aerial parts). This is still the most popular form of Echinacea in Germany. Another popular European product is a fresh plant tincture of the whole plant of *E. purpurea*.

As might be expected, these different products exhibit substantial variations in their phytochemical content (and hence by definition their pharmacological and clinical properties). Yet they are typically discussed in the literature under the generic term 'Echinacea' as if they shared identical properties. Hence a rudimentary concept of phytotherapy, the overriding importance of the part of the plant being used, appears to have been overlooked or ignored. The mode of preparation also creates phytochemical differences. Specifically the hydrophilic type of product will be low in alkylamides and higher in water-soluble compounds such as polysaccharides, whereas a lipophilic product will be much higher in alkylamides (especially if prepared from the root).

As a counter to this poor academic rigour in the discussion of Echinacea, the decision has been made to limit this monograph to the roots of *E. angustifolia* and *E. purpurea*. These are, after all, the species and plant part still preferred by herbal clinicians in the English-speaking world. Accordingly, scientific investigations of other plant parts or other Echinacea species have not been included, except by way of contrast. Furthermore, studies where the plant part used is not clear from the publication (as can sometimes be the case) and studies where mixed plant parts were used (for example root combined with aerial parts) have also been omitted from review (in most cases).

Effects

Immune enhancing, mainly acting on innate immunity, hence may modulate immune function in allergy and autoimmunity; enhances resistance to infections, particularly of the upper respiratory tract; assists in recovery from chemotherapy; anti-inflammatory, particularly after topical application.

Traditional view

As noted above, information about the use of Echinacea root first came from Native American tribes. Their use was adopted by the Eclectics, a group of practitioners who were prominent around the late 19th and early 20th centuries in the USA. By 1921 Echinacea (specifically the root of *E. angustifolia*) was by far the most popular treatment prescribed by Eclectic physicians. The Eclectics used Echinacea root for about 50 years. Given that their use was based on tribal knowledge and that they accumulated extensive clinical experience, their traditional use data is of a high quality. The best sources of these data are *King's American Dispensatory*[1] and Ellingwood.[2] The extensive range of conditions in these texts for which Echinacea root was prescribed included snakebite, syphilis, typhus, septic wounds, diphtheria, scarlet fever, dysentery and even cancer. It is clear from these writers that the limitations on Echinacea use suggested by some modern authors are not supported. The conditions treated were mainly infections and envenomations of various kinds, which probably attest to Echinacea's influence on the immune system. However, the inclusion of tuberculosis and disorders related to autoimmunity such as diabetes, exophthalmic goitre, psoriasis and renal haemorrhage contrasts with contraindications proposed by some modern writers.

The Eclectics were also not averse to using Echinacea root long term. For example, according to Ellingwood, it was recommended for the following chronic conditions: cancer, chronic mastitis, chronic ulceration, tubercular abscesses, chronic glandular indurations and syphilis. With regard to syphilis, Ellingwood wrote: 'The longest time of all cases yet reported, needed to perfect the cure, was nine months.' He cites a dramatic case history of a vaccination reaction where Echinacea root was taken every 2 h for up to 6 weeks.

Summary actions

Immunomodulatory, anti-inflammatory, vulnerary, lymphatic adaptogenic. Any significant clinical antibacterial and antiviral activity probably follows indirectly from immune enhancement.

Can be used for

Indications supported by clinical trials

Treatment of upper respiratory tract infections (clinical evidence is controversial); beneficial for the prophylaxis of upper respiratory tract infections and infections in general; to promote immune function.

Traditional therapeutic uses

Bacterial, viral and protozoal infections, including infections of the digestive, respiratory and urinary tracts; mild septicaemia; states of weakened, suppressed or imbalanced immunity, including allergies and autoimmune disease; inflammatory and purulent conditions, including acne, abscess, furunculosis; envenomation. Topically for poorly healing wounds, inflamed skin conditions and bacterial infections.

May also be used for

Extrapolations from pharmacological

To increase phagocytosis; antiviral activity, probably indirect; for benign prostatic hyperplasia; to control anxiety. Topically: to improve wound healing, increase resistance to infection and to increase connective tissue regeneration.

Preparations

Echinacea purpurea or *E. angustifolia* root preparations include liquid extracts of fresh or dried root and rhizome and tablets and capsules based on these.

Dosage

Preventative doses or doses for chronic conditions are recommended as follows:

- 1 to 3 g/day of *E. angustifolia* dried root
- 1.5 to 4.5 g/day of *E. purpurea* dried root

- 2 to 6 mL/day of 1:2 liquid extract of *E. angustifolia* root
- 3 to 9 mL/day of 1:2 liquid extract of *E. purpurea* dried root
- 5 to 15 mL/day of 1:5 tincture of *E. angustifolia* root
- 7.5 to 22.5 mL/day of 1:5 tincture of *E. purpurea* dried root.

Equivalent doses to these can also be used in tablet or capsule form as long as these have been carefully dried to preserve the alkylamide content.

These dosages may be substantially increased in the short term for acute conditions; for example, *E. angustifolia* root can be taken up to 10 to 15 g/day (or its equivalent in a liquid, capsule or tablet preparation).

Duration of use

Despite suggestions to the contrary, there is no evidence to suggest that long-term usage of Echinacea root will have an adverse effect on immune function. Echinacea root is most likely a benign agent acting mainly on innate immunity (although there is still much to be understood about its mode of action).

Summary assessment of safety

Echinacea root preparations may be safely prescribed for oral and topical use if the recommended dosage is not exceeded. Despite many reputed contraindications in the literature, the herb is unlikely to cause adverse effects in a wide range of applications including asthma, allergies and autoimmunity. However, care should be exercised when prescribing any preparation of Echinacea (including the root) to patients with known allergy to members of the Compositae (Asteraceae, daisy) family.

Technical data

Botany

Echinacea is a member of the Compositae (Asteraceae, daisy) family and grows to a maximum height of 50 to 180 cm, depending on the species. The distinctive flower head consists of white, rose or purple drooping ray florets and a conical disc made up of numerous tubular florets. *E. angustifolia* is most easily identified by its low habit and the coarse hair and relatively straight ray florets; *E. purpurea* by the large, egg-shaped, serrated leaves and the bright purple ray florets; *E. pallida* by the white pollen and the longer length of the paler ray florets.[3,4]

In 1968 the botanist McGregor reported on a 15-year journey studying wild Echinacea plants from populations throughout its entire geographical range in North America.[5] As a result of this work McGregor recognised nine species and four varieties of the genus Echinacea and the classification and names suggested are still currently used by both herbal clinicians and regulatory authorities (e.g. *E. angustifolia*, *E. purpurea*, *E. pallida* and so on).

In 2001 and 2002, a group of US botanists undertook an extensive review of the Echinacea genus using morphometric analysis and the taxonomic results have recently been republished.[5] Their analysis found that the genus contained two subgenera, namely *Echinacea* subgenus *Echinacea* (containing a single species *E. purpurea*) and *Echinacea* subgenus *Pallida* (containing three species: *E. pallida*, *E. atrorubens* and *E. laevigata*). The botanists' classification also agreed with the earlier work of Cronquist.[5] Perhaps the most important outcome of this work from a herbal perspective is that under the new classification *E. angustifolia* does not exist as a separate species, but becomes a subspecies of *E. pallida*, namely *E. pallida* var. *angustifolia*.[5] However, there is still controversy over this attribution.

Adulteration

Echinacea has been readily adulterated, particularly in the USA, by species of Parthenium such as *P. integrifolium*.[6] The roots of *E. angustifolia* and *E. pallida* are very similar both macroscopically and microscopically[7] and are often confused. They can, however, be chemically differentiated.[8]

In the USA native species of Echinacea are dwindling in the wild due to loss of habitat and over-harvesting. *E. purpurea* is not as threatened as *E. angustifolia*, since the former is the most widely used species for cultivation.[9] Hence the use of *E. purpurea* root should be encouraged, either alone or preferably in combination with *E. angustifolia* root.

Key constituents

Roots

- Alkylamides (alkamides), mostly isobutylamides (which cause the characteristic tingling in the mouth).[10–13] Largely absent from *E. pallida*[11]
- Caffeic acid esters: echinacoside (not present in *E. purpurea*), chicoric acid (significant quantities in *E. purpurea* only),[14] cynarin (in *E. angustifolia* only)[15]
- Essential oil;[16] polyacetylenes (including a distinctive series in *E. pallida*);[10,17] polysaccharides,[18] non-toxic pyrrolizidine alkaloids.[19]

Aerial parts

- Alkylamides as above[20]
- Caffeic acid esters: including echinacoside (not present in *E. purpurea*), chicoric acid (abundant in *E. purpurea*), verbascoside (*E. angustifolia*, *E. pallida*), caftaric acid (*E. purpurea*, *E. pallida*), chlorogenic and isochlorogenic acids (*E. angustifolia*, *E. pallida*)[20]
- Flavonoids,[20] essential oil;[16] polysaccharides (notably in *E. purpurea*).[21]

The phytochemistry of Echinacea has been extensively reviewed, demonstrating considerable variation between species and plant part (as noted above).[22] One key difference is for the alkylamides, which are highest in *E. angustifolia* and

absent from *E. pallida*. The roots of *E. angustifolia* and *E. purpurea* contain a much higher concentration of alkylamides than their respective aerial parts.[23] Cynarin is found mainly in *E. angustifolia* roots.[23] Qualitative differences also exist for the alkylamides; those in *E. angustifolia* mainly exhibit 2-monoene and dodecatetraene structures, whereas the 2,4-diene and dodecatetraene types predominate in *E. purpurea*.[24]

Studies have shown considerable phytochemical variation in Echinacea commercial products, with the concentrations of alkylamides especially exhibiting a particularly wide range.[25] One study found that alkylamides levels in stored *E. purpurea* roots dropped significantly over 64 weeks.[26] However, another found the major alkylamide in *E. purpurea* root hydro-alcoholic extract was quite stable, whereas the alkylamide content reduced over time in the dried powdered root.[27] Degradation of the major alkylamides in *E. purpurea* extracts was monitored under different conditions.[28] Alkylamides degraded faster in dry films than in solution and the Echinacea phenolic compounds acted as protective antioxidants. Predicted half-lives for alkylamides in extracts suggested very good stability.

Polysaccharides in *Echinacea spp.* have received considerable research attention as possible immunologically active components. However, much of the research has been conducted on polysaccharides isolated from cell cultures rather than from the naturally growing plant. The term 'polysaccharide' is generic in nature, and encompasses starches and other potentially inert plant compounds. Indeed, some of the non-specific techniques used to analyse the polysaccharide content of plants also detect simple sugars. Hence, commercial Echinacea products claiming quantified levels of immunologically active polysaccharides should be viewed with caution, depending on the quantification methodology used.

While the polysaccharide research is more relevant to the aerial parts of Echinacea, the roots also contain these compounds. One study isolated arabinogalactan-proteins from the high-molecular-weight fraction of an aqueous extract of the root of *E. purpurea*.[29]

However, the true polysaccharides (as opposed to starches and sugars misidentified as polysaccharides) appear to be difficult to extract from Echinacea plant parts. An extensive research project isolated two polysaccharides (respectively named I and II) from *E. purpurea* aerial parts that were structurally characterised as a heteroxylan (molecular weight 35 000) and an acidic arabinorhamnogalactan (molecular weight 450 000. Polysaccharide (PS) I resembled other xylans found in plants and contained arabinose, xylose and 4-O-methylglucuronic acid in a molar ratio of 1:4.9:0.9. PS II was composed of arabinose, galactose, glucuronic acid and galacturonic acid in a molar ratio of 0.8:0.6:1:0.6.[30] These polysaccharides were determined at around 15 mg/g in both the root and leaf of the freshly harvested senescent plant, with less than half this level in root and leaf from the freshly harvested mature plant. However, storage for just a few days resulted in substantial losses of PS II. Any solvent mixture containing more than 40% of ethanol was unable to extract the polysaccharides, while less than 4% of PS I and 17% of PS II was extracted by water at pH 5.5 from any dried plant part. Water extraction of the fresh plant was substantially more efficient for PS II, but PS I was absent from fresh plant root preparations. These results imply that polysaccharides are probably not present in sufficient quantities to influence the pharmacology of aqueous (hydrophilic) extracts of Echinacea dried root (even if the polysaccharides were bioavailable). They will certainly be absent from aqueous-ethanolic (lipophilic) extracts of Echinacea root prepared using more than 40% ethanol, unlike the alkylamides.

Dodeca-2,4,8,10-tetraenoic acid
isobutylamides (mixture)

Pharmacodynamics

Immunomodulating activity

There is still much to understand about the way Echinacea root impacts the human immune system. Each in vitro study by its nature can provide just a narrow insight into a few specific aspects of immune function, with any clinical relevance potentially confounded by bioavailability, dosage issues and local tissue factors. The in vitro studies probably of most relevance are the ones investigating alkylamides, since these compounds have proven bioavailability (see later).

Indeed, one discussion paper has challenged the relevance of in vitro studies to the study of plant immunostimulants, suggesting that the whole concept may be a myth originating from such studies.[31] (This is of course notwithstanding the traditional uses of Echinacea, which certainly seem to point to enhanced immune function, as noted earlier.) The authors state: 'From a historical prospective, these first reports on plant immunostimulants may have "seduced" a whole generation of researchers to adopt uncritically the view that certain plants strengthen the immune system by activating it'.[31]

As this discussion paper points out, several in vitro studies of herbs on immune function (and possibly in vivo studies if the extract was administered by injection) have been confounded by endotoxin contamination from bacteria.[31] This is certainly the case for Echinacea, especially if aqueous extracts are used.[32] Based on their findings, one research group asserted that the majority of in vitro macrophage activation exhibited by extracts of some immune-enhancing plants is due to bacterial lipoproteins and lipopolysaccharides.[33] The majority of such activities for a range of samples of E. angustifolia root and aerial parts were abolished by treatment with agents that break down endotoxins.[34]

With these limitations in mind, the in vitro and in vivo data for Echinacea are reviewed below.

In early research, ethanolic extracts of the roots of all three main Echinacea species demonstrated an increase in phagocytic activity in vitro and after oral administration in vivo using the carbon clearance test. Of the three tested extracts, E. purpurea was the most active, both in vitro and in vivo.[35,36] Lipophilic (fat-soluble) and hydrophilic (water-soluble) fractions of these ethanol extracts also demonstrated activity, although this was weaker than the complete ethanolic extracts. The lipophilic fractions from E. angustifolia and E. pallida were considerably more active than their hydrophilic fractions, both in vitro and in vivo. In contrast, the hydrophilic fraction of the ethanol extract of E. purpurea significantly stimulated phagocytosis in vitro and showed activity in vivo after oral doses, although not as great as the whole extract. Components of the lipophilic fraction included polyacetylenes, essential oil and alkylamides; the hydrophilic fraction contained caffeic acid derivatives. Polysaccharides were not present.[37] Immunostimulatory principles of Echinacea were therefore said to be present in both the lipophilic and the hydrophilic fractions of a pure ethanolic extract.

Some in vitro studies have compared lipophilic and hydrophilic extracts of Echinacea root. One study used a highly complex experimental design to conclude, on the basis of immunological responses in human whole blood samples, that the main immunostimulating activity of Echinacea plant parts (including root) resided in the water-soluble materials.[38] The authors assumed these water-soluble extracts contained polysaccharides, but did not confirm their presence. Also, no assessment was made of the confounding impact of bacterial endotoxins on their results. Ironically, the authors of this study suggest that their findings are consistent with the traditional use of Echinacea, but have at the same time completely discounted such traditional use by declaring the inactivity of the traditionally preferred lipophilic extracts.

Cytokine antibody arrays were used to investigate changes in pro-inflammatory cytokines released from human bronchial epithelial cells exposed to a rhinovirus.[39] Virus infection stimulated the release of at least 31 cytokine-related molecules and most of these were reversed by simultaneous exposure to the Echinacea extracts. The lipophilic extract of E. purpurea root was less active than the expressed juice of the aerial parts in this regard. However, in uninfected cells these cytokines were stimulated by Echinacea, with the lipophilic extract being more active. A follow-up study by the same investigators using gene array analysis suggested that production of various transcription factors involved in proliferative and differentiation signalling pathways were stimulated by the Echinacea extracts.[40]

A comparison of five Echinacea species using various in vitro models of immunological activity, such as monocyte cytokine secretion and mononuclear cell proliferation, suggested that the 50% ethanolic tincture of E. angustifolia was most active.[32] In another study, the alkylamide-rich Echinacea species were more active at stimulating cytokine production by peripheral blood mononuclear cells (PBMCs) taken from older volunteers 6 months after influenza vaccination.[41] This was confirmed in a second study for blood samples from unvaccinated volunteers.[42] However, cytokines from stimulated PBMCs taken from recently vaccinated individuals were not impacted by E. purpurea and E. angustifolia root extracts.[42]

Dendritic cells (DCs) are antigen-presenting cells that play a key role in mediating activities of various immune responses. Lipophilic extracts of the alkylamide rich plant parts of

E. purpurea (root or flower) upregulated expression of CD83 on DCs in vitro, whereas the leaf extract had the opposite effect.[43] CD83 is a key marker for DC maturation. Downregulation of mRNA expression of specific chemokines and their receptors was observed in the leaf-treated DCs, whereas other chemokines and regulatory molecules involved in the c-Jun pathway were upregulated in root-treated DCs.

Several in vitro studies have investigated the effects of alkylamide fractions or isolated alkylamides in immune models. Alkylamides inhibited lipopolysaccharide (LPS)-mediated activation of a murine macrophage line (anti-inflammatory activity).[44–46] They also countered the decrease in NF-kappaB production by LPS-stimulated T cells in vitro, as did chicoric acid,[47] and reduced interlevkin (IL-2) production in stimulated T cells.[48] Liver enzyme-mediated oxidation of *E. purpurea* alkylamides produced metabolites that were less active in terms of suppressing IL-2 secretion by stimulated T cells.[49]

Cynarin binds to CD28 in vitro, a receptor on T cells, and downregulated CD-28 IL-2 expression in a T cell culture line.[50] Cynarin also effectively blocked the binding between CD80 on B cells and CD28 on T cells, thereby potentially exerting an immunomodulatory effect.[51]

In early in vivo research, chicoric acid or an enriched alkylamide fraction from *E. angustifolia* and *E. purpurea* roots increased phagocytic activity after oral doses. Extracts of the aerial parts of the three species demonstrated lower activity than that of the roots.[36] In contrast, echinacoside from *E. angustifolia* and *E. pallida* roots (which is often used as a quality marker for these species) did not demonstrate immune-enhancing activity.[35]

A significant proportion of the in vivo investigations of Echinacea root (specifically *E. purpurea*) have been conducted by the research team of Sandra Miller in Canada. In an unusually entitled paper, 'Echinacea: a miracle herb against aging and cancer', Dr Miller reviewed her team's research on Echinacea, specifically *E. purpurea* root.[52] Their interest in Echinacea was triggered by research on the drug indomethacin, which is a cyclo-oxygenase inhibitor that reduces the endogenous suppressors of natural killer (NK) cells, namely the prostaglandins.[53,54] The drug resulted in statistically significant increases in NK cell numbers and function in leukaemic mice. This led to the search for a safe agent without dangerous side effects that might function in the same way.

The observation that alkylamides in Echinacea can inhibit prostaglandin production in vitro, and the general reputation of Echinacea as an immune herb, led to the investigation of the potential of Echinacea in NK cell enhancement using in vivo laboratory models. In healthy young adult mice, oral doses of *E. purpurea* root (0.45 mg/25 g body weight, similar to human dose rates) stimulated NK cell production by bone marrow in the first 7 days, which resulted in significantly higher levels (around 25% more) of NK cells in the spleen by 2 weeks.[55] In addition, the accessory cells for NK cells, the monocytes, were also about 25% more numerous in both the bone marrow and spleen of mice consuming Echinacea. The Echinacea treatment influenced no other white blood cell counts. Polysaccharides, even by injection, were not found to be responsible for this effect.[56]

NK cells decline in number and function with age and this is thought to be one factor behind the increase of various cancers with age. Experiments conducted in healthy, elderly mice found that 2 weeks of oral doses of Echinacea root returned NK cell numbers in bone marrow and spleen to the levels of young adults and also resurrected their functional capacity (target cell binding, lysis).[57] On this result Dr Miller writes:

> These observations appear to apply uniquely to this herb since we could never rejuvenate the NK cell-mediated component of the immune system in elderly mice by any of the other typical NK cell enhancers ...

One of the persistent controversies about Echinacea is whether it is safe to be taken consistently for long periods of time. The answer, at least in mice, appears to be in the affirmative. Mice were fed *E. purpurea* root from 7 weeks of age to 13 months at the dose previously described.[58] Long-term use of Echinacea was in fact beneficial. By 13 months of age 46% of the control mice fed the standard chow were still alive, compared with 74% of those consuming Echinacea. As in previous experiments, the NK cell levels in the Echinacea-fed mice were considerably elevated compared with controls. On this Miller writes:

> Given that the key immune cells acting as the first line of defence against developing neoplasms in mice and humans are NK cells, it is not difficult to conclude that sustained enhancement of NK cells alone, throughout life, could readily account for the reduced frequency in deaths with advancing age. Spontaneous neoplasms, clinically undetectable, are well known to increase with advancing age in humans and mice. Thus, the logical corollary from this study indicates that chronic daily intake of Echinacea, is clearly not detrimental to the immune system, but rather prophylactic.

Finally, the team investigated the question of whether Echinacea is effective once a cancer is in progress. Leukaemias and lymphomas are well known as targets for NK cell attack, and these cells are established as the first line of defence against these types of malignancies. Leukaemia-induced mice typically died after 3.5 weeks, whereas one-third of mice additionally fed Echinacea survived until 3 months after leukaemia onset and went on to live a normal lifespan.[59]

While these findings need to be regarded as work in progress, the implications are intriguing. In addition to helping to dispel some of the common myths about what is active in Echinacea and how it is best used (including the contraindication in leukaemia from the German Commission E), the research provides a possible insight into perhaps one of the key aspects of Echinacea's mode of action on the immune system. This is the boost in NK and monocyte number and function. NK cells and monocytes represent the innate immunity. Any agent acting largely on innate immunity will be beneficial in a range of areas including infection prevention and therapy, cancer prevention and therapy and even autoimmune disease (if stealth pathogens are involved as triggers via processes such as molecular mimicry). Above all, the consistent use of an agent that promotes innate immunity could well extend lifespan, since immunosenescence is a key aspect of poor health with ageing.

The NK cell connection for Echinacea root needs to be confirmed in humans.

The impact of *E. purpurea* root extract (2 mg/mouse/day) consumption was investigated in non-obese diabetic (NOD) mice, which are a model of human type 1 diabetes. NKT (natural killer T) cells are believed to be implicated in type 1 diabetes and their functional and/or numerical deficiency is thought to be largely responsible for the development of this disease in NOD mice.[60] When NOD mice were fed Echinacea for varying times, there was a substantial and significant increase in NK cell numbers. This was the only type of immune cell influenced by the Echinacea in these mice. The authors concluded:

> The observations of the present study have, at least in the animal model of human type 1 diabetes, led to 2 conclusions. First, daily consumption of Echinacea by animals afflicted with this particular autoimmune disease, leads to no negative repercussions, and indeed, may provide all the advantages, in vivo, that consuming this herb does for normal, unafflicted mice (humans). Second, the study may provide evidence for a possible new approach to the treatment of type 1 diabetes. That is, immuno-stimulation only of those cells (NK/NKT) involved in modulating the disease. Echinacea is one such uniquely tailored, immunostimulant, whose effect is on NK cells.

Other in vivo studies support the activity of Echinacea root on the macrophage/monocyte system. E. purpurea demonstrated a dose-dependent increase in the phagocytic activity of alveolar macrophages after oral administration to rats.[61] Alkylamides (12 μg/kg/day, oral) significantly increased phagocytic activity and the phagocytic index of alveolar macrophages in rats.[62] These alveolar macrophages also produced significantly more tumour necrosis factor (TNF)-alpha and nitric oxide (NO) after LPS stimulation in vitro. Chicoric acid and polysaccharides (oral doses) were not as active.

Rats given E. angustifolia root extract (equivalent to 3.3 g/L root in drinking water) for 6 weeks demonstrated a significantly higher primary and secondary IgG response to a novel antigen.[63] In contrast, 6 weeks of various Echinacea root extracts (tinctures and in glycerol) showed no activity in male rats in terms of NK cell activity, T cell-mediated delayed-type hypersensitivity, or specific antibody formation.[64] E. purpurea root at 2% and 4% of diet did not exhibit antiviral effects or show any evidence of immune-enhancing properties in respiratory syndrome virus infected nursery pigs.[65]

Alcohol extracts from roots of the three widely used Echinacea species, E. angustifolia, E. pallida, and E. purpurea, were investigated for immunomodulating properties.[66] Mice were gavaged once a day (for 7 days) with one of the Echinacea extracts (130 mg/kg) or vehicle and immunised with sheep red blood cells (SRBC) 4 days prior to collection of immune cells for multiple immunological assays. The three herb extracts induced similar, but different, changes in the percentage of immune cell populations and their biological functions, including increased percentage of CD49+ and CD19+ lymphocytes in spleen and NK cell cytotoxicity. The antibody response to SRBC was significantly increased equally by extracts of all three Echinacea species. Concanavalin A-stimulated splenocytes from E. angustifolia- and E. pallida-treated mice demonstrated significantly higher T cell proliferation. In addition, the Echinacea treatment significantly altered the cytokine production by mitogen-stimulated splenic cells. The three herbal extracts significantly increased interferon-gamma production, but inhibited the release of TNF-alpha and interleukin (IL)-1beta.

Only E. angustifolia- and E. pallida-treated mice demonstrated significantly higher production of IL-4 and increased IL-10 production. The authors suggested Echinacea is a wide-spectrum immunomodulatory agent that modulates both innate and adaptive immune responses. In particular, E. angustifolia or E. pallida may have more anti-inflammatory potential.

Following the observation that E. angustifolia and E. purpurea root extracts reduced cytokine production and intracellular killing activity by macrophages in vitro (although E. angustifolia enhanced bacterial phagocytosis), these effects were investigated in mice.[67] The Echinacea root extracts (130 mg/kg/day for 7 days, oral) did not substantially influence NO production and phagocytosis by LPS-stimulated peritoneal exudate cells (PECs) extracted from the mice. In addition, the antibacterial function of PECs was not affected, although NO production was somewhat decreased.

Twenty-four healthy men received 4.5 mL/day of standardised alcoholic extract of E. purpurea root (equivalent to 1 mg each of chicoric acid and alkylamides per day) or placebo for 5 days. A maximum stimulation of granulocyte phagocytosis was observed on the fifth day at 120% of the starting value. The rate of immune stimulation was much higher than that observed for administration by intramuscular injection.[68]

This study has been widely misinterpreted as demonstrating that Echinacea causes immune system tachyphylaxis if taken for more than a few days. A cursory examination of the figures published in this paper might lead to the conclusion that the use of Echinacea for more than a few days depletes the phagocytic response. However, this would be a misinterpretation of the results. The arrows at the bottom of the figures indicated the application of the test dose, which was administered for only the first 5 days. While the Echinacea was given, phagocytic activity remained high. Only when the Echinacea was stopped did the phagocytic activity decline to normal levels, a typical washout effect.

So the study in fact demonstrated the following:

- Phagocytic activity remained higher than normal while Echinacea was given.
- Oral doses of Echinacea stimulated phagocytic activity more than injected doses.
- When Echinacea was stopped, phagocytic activity remained well above normal for a few days, indicating that, far from causing depletion, there was a residual stimulating effect when Echinacea was stopped.
- Phagocytic activity only returned to normal, that is there was no depleting effect, when activity dropped to less than normal.

In terms of other probable misconceptions from the Echinacea research, immune-enhancing activity has been demonstrated for Echinacea polysaccharides in vitro.[69–72] However, these results may not be translatable to effects in a living organism after oral administration because of the gastrointestinal breakdown, poor absorption and poor tissue mobility of the large polysaccharides. As noted previously, polysaccharides are probably not present in pharmacologically significant quantities in Echinacea preparations and are not absorbed in levels sufficient to achieve the concentrations used for in vitro studies.

In the only clinical trial to date on Echinacea polysaccharides, they were administered by injection because of the uncertainties over their oral bioavailability. If the trial scientists had believed that the polysaccharides were orally active, then they would certainly have administered them by this simpler way. In this open, prospective study with matched historical controls, a polysaccharide fraction isolated from *E. purpurea* cell cultures was tested to see if it could counter the undesired side effects of cancer chemotherapy.[73] Fifteen patients with advanced gastric cancer undergoing palliative chemotherapy with a range of cytotoxic drugs also received daily intravenous injections of 2 mg of a polysaccharide fraction from Echinacea. While the polysaccharide treatment did appear to increase white cell counts, there were no clinically relevant effects on phagocytic activity or lymphocyte subpopulations. The authors suggested that this form of treatment should be investigated in further studies.

Interestingly, there is a new voice in the Echinacea polysaccharide debate. An LPS-free preparation of a commercial aqueous extract of *E. angustifolia* has demonstrated immune activity in vitro and in vivo.[74–76] For example, it reduced *Candida albicans*-induced mortality in both normal and in cyclosporine-A-treated mice.[76] This polysaccharide-targeted extract is being marketed as having superior immune activity to the traditional lipophilic extracts of *E. angustifolia* because it contains only low levels of alkylamides, which are being represented as inhibiting T cell function. Such assertions would be best supported by human data.

Excessive extrapolations of the early pharmacological research, especially the in vitro studies on Echinacea polysaccharides, have led to unsupported statements concerning the immunological activity of Echinacea. These include that Echinacea is mitogenic to T lymphocytes, that ethanolic extracts of Echinacea are ineffective, that Echinacea will accelerate pathology in HIV/AIDS and that Echinacea will aggravate asthma.[77]

Cannabinoid receptor activity

A significant discovery, first presented at the International Congress on Natural Products 2004, was the observation by two separate research teams that the immune effects of Echinacea may be mediated by the interaction of Echinacea alkylamides with cannabinoid receptors. Two papers were presented on this topic. A Swiss research team found that an in vitro immunomodulating effect of a lipophilic *E. purpurea* extract (and individual alkylamides) on monocytes/macrophages could be neutralised by the presence of agents that block CB2 cannabinoid receptors.[78] Bauer, in collaboration with US scientists, found that alkylamides from *E. angustifolia* bound to both CB1 and CB2 cannabinoid receptors.[79] In particular, certain alkylamides exhibited selectivity for CB2 receptors. The most potent binding to CB2 receptors (binding as strongly as THC from Cannabis) was exhibited by a monoene alkylamide found only in *E. angustifolia* (tetradeca-2E-ene-10,12-diynoic acid isobutylamide).[80]

CB1 receptors are highly localised in the central nervous system (CNS) and are believed to primarily modulate behaviour,

while CB2 receptors predominate in immune tissues outside the CNS, especially in the spleen, and are believed to modulate immune function.[81] Cannabinoid receptors are remarkably preserved across the animal kingdom, which suggests they play an important developmental and physiological role.[82,83] Much of the immune activity of the cannabinoid system appears to be mediated by the cytokine network. Cytokines include the interleukins (IL-3, IL-6, etc.), TNF-alpha and the interferons. Both receptors mediate analgesic effects and CB2 effects can be mainly classed as anti-inflammatory.

The Swiss team mentioned above followed on from this ground-breaking research and confirmed that certain Echinacea alkylamides bind strongly to CB2 receptors.[84] In addition they have found that alkylamides exert additional effects on immune cells that are independent of CB2.[84] Their research has been particularly insightful into one aspect of the mode of action of Echinacea alkylamides.[85] A lipophilic extract of *E. purpurea* strongly stimulated TNF-alpha mRNA synthesis in peripheral monocytes, but not TNF-alpha protein production. In other words, the Echinacea-induced new TNF-alpha transcripts (mRNA) were not translated into TNF-alpha itself. When monocytes were treated with LPS (lipopolysaccharide or endotoxin, a powerful stimulator of the immune system), TNF-alpha protein production was substantially increased. However, co-incubation of monocytes with LPS and Echinacea extract resulted in a strong inhibition of this effect of LPS. Investigation over a longer time-span revealed that the lipophilic Echinacea extract, via interaction with CB2 receptors, modulated and prolonged TNF-alpha production following immune stimulation. The results of this study suggest that Echinacea acted more as a modulator or facilitator of the immune response than as an immune stimulant. In resting monocytes it prepared them for a quicker immune response by inducing TNF-alpha mRNA. However, in overstimulated monocytes (as in the case of LPS) it first reduced and then extended their response in terms of TNF-alpha production. In particular, these key findings challenge the concept that traditional Echinacea extracts will 'overstimulate and wear out' the immune system if taken continuously.

One point worth emphasising is that the strong binding (and partial agonist effects) of certain Echinacea alkylamides at CB2 receptors is not shared by alkylamides from other plant species. As well as the monoene mentioned above, the tetraene alkylamides from both *E. purpurea* and *E. angustifolia*, especially the ZZ isomer, also bind strongly to the CB2 receptor.[86] The binding of both synthetic and natural alkylamides to type 1 and 2 CB receptors was investigated in vitro.[87] Naturally occurring alkylamides from herbs such as maca (*Lepidium meyenii*) and *Spilanthes spp*. showed a poor affinity for both CB1 and CB2 receptors. In contrast, the above alkylamides from *E. angustifolia* and *E. purpurea* bound more strongly to CB2 receptors than the endogenous cannabinoid anandamide.[84] Anandamide binds strongly to CB1 (as strongly as THC from Cannabis), whereas the Echinacea alkylamides only have a weak affinity for CB1 receptors (but perhaps sufficient to promote the sense of well-being that many patients report after taking Echinacea consistently).

An ethanolic root and herb extract of *E. purpurea* produced synergistic pharmacological effects at the CB2 receptor.[88] In particular, superadditive effects of alkylamide combinations were seen at the level of intracellular calcium release as a consequence of CB2 receptor activation.

A review of fatty acid amides and the human endocannabinoid system noted that alkylamides also partially inhibit the action of fatty acid amide hydrolase (FAAH), which controls the breakdown of endocannabinoids.[89] Hence they could exert also indirect agonistic effects at CB2 receptors. The CB2 receptor binding of alkylamides and their FAAH inhibition do not correlate.

An alkylamide from *E. angustifolia* that lacked affinity for the CB2 receptor inhibited IL-2 secretion in T cells through activation of PPARgamma, suggesting that cytokine modulation by alkylamides is not due just to CB2 effects.[90]

Antiviral activity

Given the immune system attacks viruses, there is a degree of overlap between the antiviral and immune system activities of Echinacea root. In fact, it is most likely that any direct effects of Echinacea root on disabling viruses are relatively modest.

In early research, chicoric acid demonstrated antiviral activity against vesicular stomatitis viruses in vitro.[91] Later chicoric acid was found to inhibit HIV-1 integration into a host chromosome and was a non-competitive, but reversible, inhibitor of HIV-1 integrase in vitro.[92] Purified root extracts from the three *Echinacea* species demonstrated antiviral activity towards herpes simplex virus (HSV) and influenza virus in vitro. An indirect antiviral effect was also observed via stimulation of alpha- and beta-interferon production.[93]

Extracts of eight species of Echinacea were found to have antiviral activity against HSV-1 in vitro when exposed to visible and UV light.[94] n-Hexane extracts of roots containing alkylamides and alkenes were more active than ethyl acetate extracts containing caffeic acids. Potent inhibitors included chicoric acid (MIC 45 μg/mL) and *E. purpurea* root n-hexane extract (MIC 120 μg/mL).

Interferons are cytokines that limit viral replication. The influence of Echinacea root extracts on virus-induced cell death and interferon secretion was investigated using HSV infection in murine macrophages.[95] Cells incubated with extracts prior to infection showed very modest enhancement of viability, and no increase in the secretion of interferons alpha or beta compared with control cells. Virus-infected macrophages treated with extracts from *E. purpurea* showed a small (<2-fold) induction of guanylate binding protein production, but no effect of extracts from other species was observed. In virus-infected cells, all the extracts increased the amount of inducible nitric oxide synthase (iNOS) protein, and this effect varied by type of extraction preparation. Together, these results suggested that any potential antiviral activities of Echinacea root extracts are likely not mediated through large inductions of interferon, but may involve iNOS.

Anti-inflammatory and wound-healing activity

In early research an anti-inflammatory effect was observed after the topical application of a crude polysaccharide fraction from *E. angustifolia* roots in the croton oil mouse ear test.[96] Topical application of an extract of *E. angustifolia* root inhibited oedema in the croton oil mouse ear test both at the maximum (6h) and in the decreasing phase (18h). Echinacea was more potent than the topical NSAID benzydamine.[97] Alkylamides from Echinacea demonstrated inhibitory activity against cyclo-oxygenase (COX) and 5-lipoxygenase (LOX) in vitro. The structure of the alkylamide determined the degree of activity, and most alkylamides were more active on COX-1 than COX-2.[98,99]

Alkylamides isolated from *E. angustifolia* root also inhibited COX-2-dependent prostaglandin E_2 (PGE_2) formation in vitro in human neuroglioma cells, but did not inhibit COX-2 expression at the transcriptional or translational level.[100] Extracts of the roots from four of six *Echinacea* species at 15 μg/mL inhibited PGE_2 production by macrophages.[101] Synergy between alkylamides was suggested to be largely responsible. Ketones from Echinacea were also found to contribute to this activity.[102]

See also under Immunomodulating activity above for additional studies demonstrating anti-inflammatory effects for Echinacea root and its components.

Antimicrobial activity

In early research echinacoside demonstrated weak antimicrobial activity against *Staphylococcus aureus* in vitro.[103] Polyacetylenes from *E. angustifolia* and *E. purpurea* root also demonstrated bacteriostatic and fungistatic activity against *Escherichia coli* and *Pseudomonas aeruginosa*.[17] *E. angustifolia* extract showed weak inhibitory activity in vitro against *Trichomonas vaginalis*[104] and *E. purpurea* extract inhibited the growth of *Epidermophyton interdigitale* in vitro.[105]

Results from an in vitro study suggest that any antifungal activity of *E. purpurea* root extract could be the result of disruption of the fungal cell wall.[106] Both lipophilic and hydrophilic extracts of Echinacea (including a lipophilic extract of *E. angustifolia* root) exhibited dose-dependent antileishmanial and trypanocidal activities in vitro.[107] Differences in anti-adhesion activity against *Campylobacter jejuni* in vitro were found for the two main *Echinacea* species, with *E. purpurea* root displaying higher activity than *E. angustifolia* root.[108]

Other effects

Caffeic acid esters obtained from *E. angustifolia* root demonstrated antihyaluronidase activity in vitro.[109] The possible antihyaluronidase activity may help increase the resistance of tissue to the spread of certain infections and, in conjunction with the increased presence of fibroblasts, facilitate connective tissue regeneration. This effect would most likely be observed for topical application of Echinacea preparations.

Caffeic acid esters protected collagen from free radical damage in vitro. The protection occurred via a scavenging effect on reactive oxygen species. The authors concluded that topical Echinacea preparations may be useful in the prevention or treatment of photodamage of the skin by UV radiation.[110]

A synergistic antioxidant effect on human low-density lipoprotein was demonstrated in vitro for alkylamides, caffeic acid derivatives and polysaccharide fractions from *E. purpurea* root.[111]

Young rats were fed *E. purpurea* root extract (50 mg/kg) for 30 and 60 days.[112] Assessment of prostate glands indicated a decrease in prostate weight and an increase in tissue lymphocytes. Results were more marked after 60 days of treatment. The same research group followed up these findings using an experiment rat model of benign prostatic hyperplasia (BPH).[113] Using the same dose and treatment times as above, *E. purpurea* root extract progressively reduced prostate size and degenerative changes.

The anxiolytic activities of five different Echinacea preparations were investigated in mice.[114] Most consistently effective was a lipophilic extract of *E. purpurea* root, active at oral doses of 4 mg/kg. The authors described its anxiolytic potential as 'considerable'.

Splenic lymphocytes from mice treated with *E. purpurea* root extract and *Hypericum perforatum* herb extract (both at 30 and 100 mg/kg/day for 14 days, oral) were shown to be significantly more resistant to apoptosis.[115]

Hexane extracts of Echinacea root demonstrated cytotoxic activity against human pancreatic and colon cancer cells in vitro.[116] *E. pallida* was the most active, with the polyacetylenes exhibiting a significant portion of such activity.[117]

Pharmacokinetics

Using the Caco-2 monolayer as an in vitro model of intestinal permeability, the tetraene alkylamides demonstrated rapid passive diffusion across this artificial membrane.[118] A later study using the Caco-2 monolayer confirmed the ready permeability of both diene and monoene Echinacea alkylamides and also found that caffeic acid derivatives (caffeoylquinics) such as chicoric acid and echinacoside exhibited poor permeability.[119]

Alkylamides have also exhibited significant bioavailability in vivo. The tetraene alkylamides exhibited rapid absorption after a single oral dose in rats (2.5 mg/kg) and appeared in the brain within 8 minutes.[120] The Cmax in plasma was 26.4 ng/mL, while the Cmax in different brain regions varied between 33.8 and 46.0 ng/mL. This provides clear evidence that Echinacea alkylamides cross the blood-brain barrier. A study in rats found that the absolute bioavailability of a tetraene alkylamide was 29.2%, which was increased to 47.1% by administration as part of a 60% ethanol *E. purpurea* root extract.[121] However, the administration of the Echinacea extract had no impact on the Cmax of the alkylamide, instead increasing blood exposure by prolonging half-life.

The majority of the pharmacokinetic studies on Echinacea, however, have been human trials. The first trial dates from Germany in 2001, where a tetraene alkylamide was detected in the blood of a single healthy volunteer after a 65 mL dose of a concentrated *E. purpurea* mother tincture.[122] Two more comprehensive studies were published close together in 2005. The first, a follow-up from the German study, used a single 2.5 mL dose of a 60% ethanol *E. angustifolia* root extract in 11 healthy volunteers.[123] The maximum concentration reached by the tetraene alkylamides was 10.9 ng/mL and occurred after 30 minutes. The second study was Australian and examined the pharmacokinetics in nine healthy volunteers of a single dose of a tablet preparation containing lipophilic extracts of *E. purpurea* and *E. angustifolia*.[124] Caffeic acid conjugates could not be identified in any plasma sample at any time after tablet ingestion. Alkylamides were rapidly absorbed and remained detectable for up to 12 h. Tmax occurred at 2 to 3 h and Cmax was 336 ng/mL for the sum of alkylamides. There was no difference observed in alkylamide absorption between fasted volunteers and those who consumed a high fat breakfast prior to intake. Another study by the German team using a different preparation administered as a single dose to eight healthy volunteers found considerably lower Cmax values for alkylamides, probably as a reflection of the lower doses given.[125]

Another pharmacokinetic study from the Australian team compared the relative bioavailabilities of single doses of a tablet and a liquid preparation of *E. purpurea* and *E. angustifolia* extracts delivering the same dose of alkylamides.[126] Alkylamides were rapidly absorbed from both preparations, with no quantitative difference between the two. Tmax increased from 20 minutes for the liquid to 30 minutes for the tablet. The same team also investigated pharmacokinetic parameters following repeated doses of the Echinacea tablets (two tablets twice a day for 14 days) in six healthy volunteers.[127] There was no evidence for either the induction or inhibition of alkylamide metabolism, as evidenced by a consistent elimination half-life of around 1.5 h and similar Cmax values (of around 100 ng/mL) at the beginning and the end of the trial.

The relative bioavailability of the major alkylamides, the dodeca-2E,4E,8Z,10E/Z-tetraenoic acid isobutylamides, from *E. purpurea* root lozenges at three different dosage levels (0.07, 0.21 and 0.9 mg) was evaluated in a human pharmacokinetic study.[128] Alkylamides were found to be rapidly absorbed and measurable in plasma 10 minutes after administration of 0.21 and 0.9 mg via the lozenges and remained detectable for more than 3 h for the latter. Results of pharmacokinetic analysis revealed that a Cmax of 8.88 ng/mL was reached at 19 minutes with the 0.9 mg lozenges. Other results suggested that a fraction of the alkylamides was directly absorbed through the oral mucosa.

Following their initial pharmacokinetic study indicating a substantial first-pass metabolism of alkylamides, the Australian group investigated the in vitro hepatic metabolism of these compounds using human liver microsomes.[129] No significant degradation of alkylamides was evident in cytosolic fractions. Time- and NADPH-dependent degradation of alkylamides was observed in microsomal fractions, suggesting they are metabolised by cytochrome P450 enzymes in human liver. There was a difference in the susceptibility of monoene and diene pure synthetic alkylamides to microsomal degradation, with (2E)-N-isobutylundeca-2-ene-8,10-diynamide (compound 1, a monoene) metabolised to only one-tenth the extent of the diene (2E,4E,8Z,10Z)-N-isobutyldodeca-2,4,8,10-tetraenamide (compound 2) under identical incubation conditions. Markedly less degradation of the diene was evident in the mixture of alkylamides present in an ethanolic Echinacea extract, suggesting that metabolism by liver P450s was dependent both on their chemistry and the combination present in the incubation. Co-incubation of compound 1 with 2 at equimolar concentrations resulted in a significant decrease in the metabolism of compound 2 by liver microsomes. This inhibition of metabolism by the monoene, which has a terminal alkyne moiety, was found to be time- and concentration-dependent, and due to a mechanism-based inactivation of the P450s involved. Alkylamide metabolites were detected and found to be the predicted epoxidation, hydroxylation and dealkylation products. The monoene alkylamides are predominant in *E. angustifolia* root.

Hence, put in simple language, the bioavailability of alkylamides in *E. angustifolia* root can be expected to be better than for *E. purpurea* root because of reduced first-pass hepatic metabolism. Moreover, a combination of *E. angustifolia* with *E. purpurea* could be expected to improve the bioavailability of the *E. purpurea* alkylamides.

Further metabolic studies evaluated the human cytochrome P450 enzymes involved in the metabolism of an alkylamide mixture using recombinant P450s, human liver microsomes and a pure synthetic compound.[130] Epoxidation, N-dealkylation and hydroxylation products were detected, with different relative amounts produced by recombinant P450s and microsomes. The major isoforms showing activity toward the metabolism of N-isobutyldodeca-2E,4E,8Z,10Z-tetraenamide were CYP1A1, CYP1A2 (both producing the same epoxide and N-dealkylation product), CYP2A13 (producing two epoxides) and CYP2D6 (producing two epoxides and a hydroxylated metabolite). Several other forms showed less activity. In incubations with human liver microsomes and selective inhibitors, CYP2E1 was found to be principally responsible for producing the dominant, hydroxylation product, whereas CYP2C9 was the principal source of the epoxides and CYP1A2 was responsible for the dealkylation product.

Clinical trials

Treatment of upper respiratory tract infections

There are relatively few clinical trials of Echinacea root in the treatment of acute respiratory infections and the results of such trials are mixed. Acute viral respiratory infections were certainly not the mainstay of the traditional use of Echinacea root by the Eclectic physicians. This common conception (or perhaps misconception) of the role of Echinacea has developed in modern times, probably as an extrapolation of its immune system reputation and driven by companies wishing to exploit a ready over-the-counter sale. Such a popular use of Echinacea also fitted in well with the ill-advised notion that the herb could only be taken for a few days at a time. In fact, the clinical trial evidence is considerably more supportive of the value of Andrographis in the treatment of colds and mild influenza (see the Andrographis monograph).

However, it should be noted that several trials (both positive and negative) have been excluded from this monograph because they used the aerial parts, sometimes in combination with the root. One exception is a Canadian product from *E. purpurea* that may include aerial parts (see below). This was included because its phytochemical profile resembles one that could be achieved from the root alone.

The issue of the use of differing plant parts, with their substantially different phytochemical profiles, calls into question the value of most published systematic reviews and meta-analyses of Echinacea trials for the treatment of respiratory infections, including the Cochrane review.[131] In other words, the heterogeneity of the different treatments works against any meaningful analysis.

In an early randomised, double blind, placebo-controlled trial, 180 patients with upper respiratory tract infections received the equivalent of 1800 mg/day or 900 mg/day of *E. purpurea* root as a tincture, or a placebo. Patients receiving the high dose experienced significant relief of symptoms. Patients receiving the lower dose were not significantly different from the control.[132] (Based on this trial result, the therapeutic dose for a 1:5 tincture of *E. purpurea* root would therefore begin at 9 mL/day during an infection.)

The Canadian product mentioned above has been assessed in two clinical trials. This is a liquid formulation prepared from 'various parts' of freshly harvested *E. purpurea* and contains 0.25, 2.5 and 25 mg/mL respectively of alkylamides, chicoric acid and polysaccharides. (No information was provided on how the 'polysaccharides' were measured. However, since the liquid was formulated in 40% ethanol the presence of true polysaccharides is questionable.) In the first trial, 282 people were randomly assigned to Echinacea or placebo using a double blind design.[133] At the onset of the first symptom related to a cold they took 10 doses on the first day (4 mL each) and four doses per day thereafter for 6 days. A total of 128 participants contracted a common cold (59 Echinacea, 69 placebo) and the total daily symptom scores were 23.1% lower in the Echinacea group (p<0.01). However, Echinacea did not impact the duration of symptoms. The herbal treatment was well tolerated.

In the second double blind, placebo-controlled trial, 150 volunteers were recruited and randomised. Of these, 62 participants (26 Echinacea, 36 placebo) contracted a common cold and completed the study.[134] The timing and doses were similar to above, with eight doses on the first day (5 mL each) and three doses per day thereafter for 6 days. A modest decrease in daily symptoms was more evident in the Echinacea group (p<0.05) and Echinacea use was associated with a significant and sustained increase in circulating white blood cells, monocytes, neutrophils and NK cells.

In a well-designed trial involving 719 patients, a combination of *E. purpurea* and *E. angustifolia* roots standardised to 4.2 mg alkylamides per tablet did not substantially alter the course of the common cold.[135] Patients were assigned to one of four parallel groups: no tablets, placebo tablets (blinded), Echinacea tablets (blinded), or Echinacea tablets (unblinded, open label). Echinacea groups received the equivalent of 10.2 g of dried Echinacea root during the first 24 hours and 5.1 g during each of the next 4 days. The primary outcome was the area under the curve for global severity, with severity assessed twice daily by self-report using the Wisconsin Upper Respiratory Symptom Survey (WURSS), short version. Secondary outcomes included IL-8 levels and neutrophil counts from nasal wash, assessed at intake and 2 days later.

Of the 719 patients enrolled, 713 completed the protocol. Mean global severity was 236 and 258 for the blinded and unblinded Echinacea groups, respectively; 264 for the blinded placebo group; and 286 for the no-pill group. A comparison of the two blinded groups showed a 28-point trend (95% CI, −69 to 13 points) toward benefit for Echinacea (p=0.089). Mean illness duration in the blinded and unblinded Echinacea groups was 6.34 and 6.76 days, respectively, compared with 6.87 days in the blinded placebo group and 7.03 days in the no-pill group. A comparison of the blinded groups showed a nonsignificant 0.53-day (C1, −1.25 to 0.19 days) benefit for the herbal treatment (p=0.075). Median change in IL-8 levels and neutrophil counts were also not statistically significant.

In a randomised, double blind, controlled trial, a total of 154 patients (133 analysed in the per protocol collective) with acute sore throat present for not more than 72 hours were included in the study. They used either an Echinacea/sage spray or a chlorhexidine/lidocaine spray with two puffs every 2 hours, in a double-dummy blinded manner, up to 10 times daily until they were symptom-free, for a maximum of 5 days. The main outcome measure was the comparison of response rates during the first 3 days. A response was defined as a decrease of at least 50% of the total symptoms compared to baseline. The Echinacea/sage treatment exhibited similar efficacy to the chlorhexidine/lidocaine treatment in reducing sore throat symptoms during the first 3 days. Response rates after 3 days were 63.8% in the Echinacea/sage group and 57.8% in the chlorhexidine/lidocaine group. For all secondary parameters, such as time to becoming symptom free, throat pain, and global assessments of efficacy by the physician and patient, no difference between the two treatments was seen. They were both very well tolerated.[136]

Infection prevention

Given the difficulties involved in undertaking infection prevention studies, the data on Echinacea root in this regard are reasonably good (especially if the experimental rhinovirus study is excluded). This is certainly consistent with the clinical experience of the authors (see also Chapter 8). In fact, the main value of Echinacea root probably lies in its capacity to prevent acute infections and resolve subacute or chronic infections, rather than to alter the course of short acute infections such as the common cold (where the immune system is probably functioning at its maximum anyway).

The safety and efficacy of two root extracts of Echinacea (*E. purpurea* or *E. angustifolia*) for preventing upper respiratory tract infections were assessed in a three-armed, randomised, double blind, placebo-controlled trial involving 302 healthy volunteers over 12 weeks.[137] Although there was a numerical tendency towards a lower infection rate in both Echinacea groups, statistical significance was not achieved. Participants in the treatment groups believed they had more benefit from Echinacea than those in the placebo group (p=0.04). Adverse effects reports were 18 for *E. angustifolia*, 10 for *E. purpurea* and 11 for placebo. One problem with this trial was the relatively low doses of Echinacea used (about 200 mg of dried root per day).

Three preparations with distinct phytochemical profiles were produced by extraction of *E. angustifolia* roots with supercritical carbon dioxide, 60% ethanol or 20% ethanol.[138] A total of 437 volunteers were randomly assigned to receive either prophylaxis (beginning 7 days before the virus challenge) or treatment (beginning at the time of the challenge) either with one of these preparations or with placebo. The results for 399 volunteers who were challenged with rhinovirus type 39 and observed in a sequestered setting for 5 days were included in the data analysis.

There were no statistically significant effects of any of the three Echinacea extracts on rates of infection or severity of symptoms. Similarly, there were no significant effects of treatment on the volume of nasal secretions, on polymorphonuclear leukocyte or IL-8 concentrations in nasal-lavage specimens or on quantitative virus titre. The dose of *E. angustifolia* root used was 900 mg/day and the dose was not adjusted for the acute infection phase of the study. This is a relatively low dose for either prevention or treatment.

In an unpublished study presented by the late Dr Anna Macintosh at the 1999 Convention of the American Association of Naturopathic Physicians, an Echinacea root formulation was compared against a herbal adaptogenic formulation and a placebo in the prevention of winter colds over a 90-day period.[139] The trial recruited 260 medical students who were under stress from their studies. The placebo group averaged an infection rate of 10%, whereas this dropped to as low as 2% by day 70 (p=0.013) in the Echinacea group. The daily dose of Echinacea root was 1.7 or 3.5 g (two doses were consecutively trialled in the study).

A randomised, double blind placebo-controlled clinical trial was undertaken with 175 participants travelling return from Australia to America, Europe or Africa for a period of 1 to 5 weeks on commercial flights via economy class.[140] Participants were administered *E. purpurea* and *E. angustifolia* extract tablets (containing the equivalent of 1.275 g of root and standardised to 4.4 mg/tablet alkylamides) or placebo tablets, and trial dosing consisted of three protocols (priming, travel and sick), depending on the phase of travel of the participants and their health status. The priming dose was two tablets/day, travel dose four tablets/day and the dose when ill was six tablets/day.

Outcomes were assessed using questions about upper respiratory symptoms related to quality of life (based on WURSS-44). Each participant completed the survey before travel (baseline), less than 1 week after travel (return) and at 4 weeks after return from travel (follow-up). Compared with baseline, the average WURSS-44 scores for both groups increased immediately after travel (return) (p<0.0005). However, the placebo group had a significantly higher average WURSS-44 score (around double) compared with the Echinacea group (p=0.05). WURSS-44 scores tended to return to baseline levels for both groups at the 4-week follow-up. Hence, supplementation with Echinacea, if taken before and during travel, appears to have a protective effect against the development of respiratory symptoms during travel periods associated with long haul flights.

Other immunological effects

Two open label pilot studies using four healthy volunteers found that *E. purpurea* root (0.93 g/day for 7 days) significantly increased CD25 and CD69 expression on T cells.[141,142] These results suggest a possible activation and regulation of T cell function.

In an open label pilot trial, 11 healthy volunteers were evaluated at baseline (day 1) and on day 15 after consuming two Echinacea root tablets per day (containing 1.275g of *E. purpurea* and *E. angustifolia* root, standardised to 4.4mg alkylamides per tablet) for 14 days.[143] Echinacea root enhanced the increase in leucocyte heat shock protein (hsp70) expression after mild heat shock (p=0.029). White cell counts were mildly increased (p=0.043) and there was a preventative effect against free radical induced erythrocyte haemolysis (p=0.006), indicative of a clinical antioxidant effect.

A follow-up open label trial in 24 healthy volunteers conducted by the same research team used the same design, except the Echinacea root dose was twice the above.[144] While Echinacea did not significantly change basal hsp70 expression in lymphocytes, it increased CD4, CD8 and NK cell stress-induced hsp70 expression. The effect was most marked in NK cells (p<0.05). The authors suggested, since the differences were most evident when cells were exposed to a stressor (mild heat shock), that this implies that Echinacea root may play a role in activating the immune system when the body encounters a challenge such as a virus.

Idiopathic autoimmune uveitis is usually treated by oral corticosteroids. It is an inflammation of part or all of the uvea, the middle (vascular) tunic of the eye, although it also commonly involves the sclera, cornea and the retina. On the basis of the known interaction of Echinacea alkylamides with cannabinoid CB2 receptors, which implies immunomodulating and anti-inflammatory activities, a group of Italian clinicians investigated the safety and efficacy of *E. purpurea* (plant part not specified) in this autoimmune disease.[145] Fifty-one patients with low-grade autoimmune uveitis were treated with conventional therapy, including oral prednisone. In addition, 32 of these patients were given Echinacea as an add-on therapy. At the last follow-up, which was 9 months later, 87.5% of patients receiving Echinacea were in clinical remission compared with 82.3% of the control group. However, steroid-off time was significantly higher in the Echinacea group (indicating that patients receiving Echinacea needed less prednisone to induce remission). The authors concluded that the oral intake of Echinacea appeared safe and effective in the control of low-grade autoimmune uveitis. No patient showed any side effects or aggravation from the use of Echinacea for their autoimmune disease.

In the study of Echinacea lozenges in six healthy volunteers cited in the Pharmacokinetics section, inflammatory cytokine levels in collected plasma samples were downregulated 24h after lozenge administration.[128]

Toxicology and other safety data

Toxicology

The acute toxicity of an *E. purpurea* root extract has been determined at a level of more than 3000mg/kg in mice.[146] Male rats given *E. purpurea* root extract (50mg/kg) for 4 or 8 weeks exhibited a reduction in testicular mass after 8 weeks as well as changes in histological structure.[147]

Contraindications

Long-term use of Echinacea root is contraindicated in patients taking immunosuppressant medication (for example transplant patients). Short-term therapy only is suggested in this instance.

The German Commission E Monograph states that, in principle Echinacea should not be used in 'progressive conditions' such as tuberculosis, leukaemia, collagen disorders, multiple sclerosis, AIDS, HIV infection and other autoimmune disease.[148] However, the key words here are 'in principle'. There are no clinical studies or case reports that credibly document any adverse effect resulting from Echinacea use in any of these conditions. Other authoritative sources do not support these restrictions.[149,150] In fact, their suggestion of use of Echinacea in infection prophylaxis implies long-term use.

A 1999 publication suggested that Echinacea is not beneficial for the immune systems of people living with HIV.[151] The basis for this recommendation appears to be extrapolated from the results of an in vitro study in which incubation with fresh expressed juice of *E. purpurea* stimulated the production of cytokines from human peripheral blood macrophages.[152] Seven other in vitro and two in vivo studies also reported stimulation of cytokines after application of Echinacea. However, six of the seven in vitro studies used either purified polysaccharides or extracts containing glycoproteins and polysaccharides; these same extracts were administered by intravenous injection to mice in the in vivo studies.[152–154] How the results of such studies relate to oral use of Echinacea is not known, particularly since the polysaccharides and glycoproteins may not be bioavailable. Echinacea root and alkylamides tend to reduce cytokine production in stimulated immune cells in vitro (see under Pharmacodynamics).

The above in vitro research may have triggered the concern expressed in a 1997 article published in the *Australian Medical Observer* which cautioned that Echinacea is a danger to asthmatic patients.[155] There is currently no sound evidence to suggest that Echinacea root cannot be used for the treatment of HIV, or that it should be used with caution in asthma.

The suggestion that Echinacea root is contraindicated in autoimmune disease assumes that any enhancement of any aspect of immune function is detrimental for these disorders. There is growing evidence that an inappropriate response to infectious microorganisms, through phenomena such as molecular mimicry, may be a factor in the pathogenesis of autoimmune disorders. If so, Echinacea root may be beneficial in these disorders because it may decrease the chronic presence of microorganisms. There are many herbal clinicians who routinely prescribe Echinacea root in autoimmune disease without apparent adverse effects in their patients.

Special warnings and precautions

Allergic reactions, mainly contact dermatitis, may occur rarely in susceptible patients sensitised to Echinacea aerial parts and to plants from the Compositae family. The likelihood of Echinacea root preparations causing allergy is low.

There is no sound evidence that it is detrimental to use Echinacea root for long periods. Indications listed in traditional sources (such as prophylaxis and treatment of chronic infections) suggest long-term usage is warranted.[149,150] A randomised, double blind, placebo-controlled trial investigating the efficacy of two herbal formulas in preventing the common cold in highly stressed medical students over a period of 15 weeks also found *E. angustifolia* root and *E. purpurea* root blend to be effective and well-tolerated (see under Clinical trials).

There is no evidence to suggest that Echinacea causes immune system tachyphylaxis. In a clinical study the oral administration of *E. purpurea* root tincture over a 5-day period increased phagocytic activity compared with controls.[156] Only when the Echinacea was stopped did phagocytic activity decline to normal (pre-test) values, demonstrating a typical washout effect (see above).

Interactions

Echinacea should not be prescribed long term with immunosuppressant medication as it may decrease the effectiveness of the drug. This is a theoretical concern based on the immune-enhancing activity of Echinacea. No case reports of this interaction have been published.

A 2008 review located eight papers containing primary data relating to potential drug interactions for Echinacea (mainly *E. purpurea*).[157] Four of these papers included studies on Echinacea root. The authors of the review suggested that herbal products made from *E. purpurea* appear to have a low potential to generate cytochrome P450 (CYP 450)-mediated herb-drug interactions, including effects on CYP1A2 and CYP3A4. Studies published subsequent to this review noted no significant effects in human volunteers of an *E. purpurea* product high in alkylamides on CYP2D6[158] and P-glycoprotein.[159]

A 2009 in vitro study confirmed that Echinacea and selected alkylamides did not induce CPY3A4 mRNA expression in vitro.[160] However, an earlier study suggested that alkylamides can exert inhibitory effects on CYP3A4, 2D6 and 2C19 in vitro,[161] although the human studies cited above[157,158] suggest that these effects do not have clinical relevance.

Other human studies have found no impact of Echinacea root on warfarin pharmacodynamics[162] (although it did reduce plasma concentrations of S-warfarin) and the overall pharmacodynamics of the anti-HIV drugs darunavir and ritonavir in combination.[163]

Use in pregnancy and lactation

Category A – no proven increase in the frequency of malformation or other harmful effects on the fetus despite consumption by a large number of women.

Echinacea is commonly consumed by pregnant women, as has been demonstrated in several surveys.[164,165]

Pregnant mice were fed daily *E. purpurea* (0.45 mg/mouse, plant part not specified, probably root) from pregnancy onset until gestational days 10, 11, 12, 13 and 14.[166] The pregnancy-induced elevations in splenic lymphocytes and nucleated erythroid cells were all but eliminated by Echinacea and

the number of viable fetuses was reduced. The authors suggested caution with Echinacea during the early/mid stages of pregnancy.

However, a prospective, controlled study published in 2000 concluded that gestational use of Echinacea (typically for 5 to 7 days) during organogenesis was not associated with an increased risk of major malformations. There were no significant differences in pregnancy outcomes between the study group consisting of 206 women who had used Echinacea during pregnancy (112 during the first trimester, 17 for all three trimesters) and their matched controls (206).[167] It should be noted that no differentiation between Echinacea plant parts was undertaken in this study.

On available information Echinacea is compatible with breastfeeding. In contrast, a 2006 review recommended caution with Echinacea during breastfeeding.[168] However, a study in a breastfeeding woman found that only small quantities of alkylamides (about 0.5% of the maternal dose) are passed to the infant during feeding[169] and these may in fact confer health benefits.

Effects on ability to drive and use machines

No adverse effects anticipated.

Side effects

In many published case reports the plant part(s) of the Echinacea product involved was not specified. Hence they need to be viewed in the context of this limitation.

Side effects are generally not expected for oral or topical administration of Echinacea root. As indicated below, contact dermatitis may occur rarely in susceptible patients. Unsubstantiated reports of three deaths attributed to Echinacea products over a 6-year period occurred in the German media in 1996. However, no action was taken by the authorities as no causal link between the deaths and the taking of Echinacea could be established.[170]

A total of 1032 patients randomly chosen from six patch test clinics were patch tested with a series of five ointments and the components of the ointment bases. Two patients demonstrated a positive reaction to Echinacea. However, it is not certain that the reaction was to the plant material itself.[171] Anaphylaxis was attributed by an Australian immunologist to a woman with allergy after taking, among other dietary supplements, a commercial extract of *E. purpurea* and *E. angustifolia*.[172] However, it was suggested that the pharyngeal irritation experienced by the patient may have been due to the alkylamide content of the preparation (the patient took twice the recommended amount).[173]

A subsequent 2002 publication by the Australian immunologist evaluated five cases of adverse reactions to Echinacea.[174] Two patients experienced anaphylaxis, another two aggravation of asthma, and the fifth developed a rash. Three of the patients had a positive skin prick test (SPT) to Echinacea. Twenty per cent of 100 atopic subjects who had never taken Echinacea also exhibited a positive SPT to this herb when tested. However, it is unclear if any of the products involved contained Echinacea root. Allergic reaction is far more likely to the aerial parts of Echinacea because of the likely presence of pollen proteins. Moreover, such a high risk of allergy has not been borne out by subsequent case reports.

Other published case reports attributed to Echinacea (species and plant part usually not specified) include erythema nodosum,[175] leukopenia,[176] aggravation of autoimmunity,[177,178] acute hepatitis[179] and hypereosinophilia.[180]

Misinformation exists that Echinacea is potentially hepatotoxic due to the presence of pyrrolizidine alkaloids (PAs). However, the PAs found in Echinacea do not contain the 1,2-unsaturated necrine ring system which is essential for such reactions.

Overdosage

No incidents found in the published literature.

Safety in children

No specific information is available for Echinacea root, but adverse effects are not expected.

Regulatory status in selected countries

Monographs of *E. angustifolia* and *E. purpurea* roots appear in the *United States Pharmacopeia-National Formulary* USP31 NF26 2008 and the *British Pharmacopoeia* 2012 edition.

Echinacea angustifolia/pallida herb, *E. angustifolia* root and *E. purpurea* root are covered by null and negative Commission E monographs. *E. pallida* root and *E. purpurea* herb are covered by positive monographs. These herbs are listed with the following uses:

- To support the immune system with infections of the respiratory and lower urinary systems (*E. purpurea* herb)
- In supportive treatment of influenza-like infections (*E. pallida* root)
- Externally for poorly healing wounds and chronic ulcerations (*E. purpurea* herb).

E. purpurea root is listed in the unapproved component characteristics section. The negative status of *Echinacea angustifolia/pallida* herb, *E. angustifolia* root and *E. purpurea* root is due to poor benefit-risk ratio and concerns about the risk from parenteral application (injection). The null status is due to a lack of substantiation of its activity for the listed conditions, leading to its therapeutic use not being recommended.

Echinacea is on the UK General Sale List. Echinacea root products have achieved Traditional Herbal Registration in the UK with the traditional indication of relief of symptoms of the common cold and influenza.

Echinacea does not have GRAS status. However, it is freely available as a 'dietary supplement' in the USA under DSHEA legislation (1994 Dietary Supplement Health and Education Act).

Echinacea root is not included in Part 4 of Schedule 4 of the Therapeutic Goods Act Regulations of Australia and is freely available for sale.

References

1. Felter HW, Lloyd JU. 18th ed. *King's American Dispensatory*, vol. 1. Portland: Eclectic Medical; 1983. pp. 671–677.
2. Ellingwood F. *American Materia Medica, Therapeutics and Pharmacognosy*, vol. 2. Portland: Eclectic Medical Publications; 1993. pp.358–376.
3. Bauer R, Wagner H. *Echinacea Handbuch für Ärzte, Apotheker und andere Naturwissenschaftler*. Stuttgart: Wissenschaftliche Verlagsgesellschaft; 1990. pp. 30–32.
4. Lust J. *The Herb Book*. New York: Bantam Books; 1974. p. 177.
5. Baum BR, Binns SE, Arnason JT. *HerbalGram*. 2006;72:32–46.
6. Hobbs C. *Echinacea: The Immune Herb*. Santa Cruz: Botanica Press; 1990. p. 70.
7. Bisset NG, ed. *Herbal Drugs and Phytopharmaceuticals: A Handbook for Practice on a Scientific Basis*. Stuttgart: Medpharm Scientific Publishers; 1994. pp. 182–184.
8. Blaschek W, Ebel S, Hackenthal E, et al. *HagerROM 2002: Hagers Handbuch der Drogen und Arzneistoffe*. Heidelberg: Springer; 2002.
9. Natural Resources Conservation Service. *Plant Guide: Eastern Purple Coneflower Echinacea purpurea (L.) Moench*. United States Dept of Agriculture. Available via http://plants.usda.gov/. Accessed May 2003.
10. Bauer R, Khan IA, Wagner H. *Planta Med.* 1988;54:426–430.
11. Bauer R, Remiger P. *Planta Med.* 1989;55:367–371.
12. Bauer R, Remiger P, Wagner H, et al. *Phytochemistry.* 1989;28:505–508.
13. Bohlmann F, Grenz M. *Chem Ber.* 1966;3:197–3200.
14. Bauer R, Wagner H. *Echinacea. Handbuch für Ärzte, Apotheker und andere Naturwissenschaftler*. Stuttgart: Wissenschaftliche Verlagsgesellschaft; 1990. pp. 94–95.
15. Bauer R, Alstat E. *Planta. Med.* 1990;56:533–534.
16. Bauer R, Wagner H. In: Farnsworth NR, ed. *Economic and Medicinal Plant Research*, vol. 5. London: Academic Press; 1991. pp. 266–267.
17. Schulte KE, Ruecker G, Perlick J. *Arzneimittelforschung.* 1967;17:825–829.
18. Giger E, Keller F, Baumann TW. Poster, 37th Annual Congress of the Society of Medicinal Plant Research, Braunschweig, September 5–10, 1989.
19. Röder E, Wiedenfeld H, Hille T, et al. *Dtsch Apoth Ztg. 1984;124:2316–2318.
20. Bauer R, Remiger P, Wagner H. *Dtsch Apoth Ztg.* 1988;128:174–180.
21. Bauer R, Wagner H. Farnsworth NR, ed. *Economic and Medicinal Plant Research*, vol. 5. London: Academic Press; 1991. pp. 280–282.
22. Harborne JB, Williams CA. In: Miller SC, ed. *Echinacea: The Genus Echinacea*. Boca Raton, USA: CRC Press; 2004. pp. 55–71.
23. Perry NB, Wills RBH, Stuart DL. Factors effecting Echinacea quality: agronomy and processing. In: Miller SC, ed. *Echinacea The Genus Echinacea*. Boca Raton, USA: CRC Press; 2004: 116.
24. Pietta P, Mauri P, Fuzzati N. In: Miller SC, ed: *Echinacea: The Genus Echinacea*. Boca Raton, USA: CRC Press; 2004. pp. 95–99.
25. Perry NB, Wills RBH, Stuart DL. In: Miller SC, ed. *Echinacea: The Genus Echinacea*. Boca Raton, USA: CRC Press; 2004. pp. 123.

26. Perry NB, van Klink JW, Burgess EJ, et al. *Planta Med.* 2000;66(1):54–56.

27. Livesey J, Awang DV, Arnason JT, et al. *Phytomedicine.* 1999;6(5):347–349.

28. Lui Y, Murphy PA. *J. Agric Food Chem.* 2007;55(1):120–126.

29. Bossy A, Blaschek W, Classen B. *Planta Med.* 2009;75(14):1526–1533.

30. Stuart DL, Wills RBH, Dickeson TM. *Optimisation of Polysaccharides in Processed Echinacea purpurea.* RIRDC Publication No. 04/118, 2004.

31. Gertsch J, Viveros–Paredes JM, Taylor P. *J Ethnopharmacol.* 2011;136:385–391.

32. Senchina DS, McCann DA, Asp JM, et al. *Clin Chim Acta.* 2005;355 (1–2):67–82.

33. Pugh ND, Tamta H, Balachandran P, et al. *Int Immunopharmacol.* 2008;8(7): 1023–1032.

34. Tamta H, Pugh ND, Balachandran P, et al. *J Agric Food Chem.* 2008;56(22): 10552–10556.

35. Bauer R, Jurcic K, Puhlmann J, et al. *Arzneimittelforschung.* 1988;38(2): 276–281.

36. Bauer R, Remiger P, Jurcic K, et al. *Z Phytother.* 1989;10:43–48.

37. Bauer R, Wagner H. In: Farnsworts NR, ed. *Economic and Medicinal Plant Research,* vol. 5. London: Academic Press; 1991. pp. 292–296, 304–306.

38. Pillai S, Pillai C, Mitscher LA, et al. *J Altern Complement Med.* 2007;13(6):625–634.

39. Sharma M, Arnason JT, Burt A, et al. *Phytother Res.* 2006;20(2):147–152.

40. Altamirano-Dimas M, Hudson JB, Cochrane D, et al. *Can J Physiol Pharmacol.* 2007;85(11):1091–1098.

41. Senchina DS, Wu L, Flindd GN, et al. *Planta Med.* 2006;72(13):1207–1215.

42. McCann DA, Solco A, Lui Y, et al. *J Interferon Cytokine Res.* 2007;27(5): 425–436.

43. Wang CY, Chiao MT, Yen PH, et al. *Genomics.* 2006;88(6):801–808.

44. Chen Y, Fu T, Tao T, et al. *J Nat Prod.* 2005;68(5):773–776.

45. Matthias A, Banbury L, Stevenson LM, et al. *Immunol Invest.* 2007;36(2): 117–130.

46. Stevenson LM, Matthias A, Banbury L, et al. *Molecules.* 2005;10(10):1279–1285.

47. Matthias A, Banbury L, Bone KM, et al. *Fitoterapia.* 2008;79(1):53–58.

48. Asagawa M, Cech NB, Gray DE, et al. *Int Immunopharmacol.* 2006;6(7): 1214–1221.

49. Cech NB, Tutor K, Doty BA, et al. *Planta Med.* 2006;72(15):1372–1377.

50. Dong GC, Chuang PH, Forrest MD, et al. *J Med Chem.* 2006;49(6): 1845–1854.

51. Dong GC, Chuang PH, Chang KC, et al. *Pharm Res.* 2009;26: (2)375–381.

52. Miller SC. *eCAM.* 2005;2(3):309–314.

53. Christopher FL, Dussault I, Miller SC. *Immunobiology.* 1991;184:37–52.

54. Dussault I, Miller SC. *Nat Immun.* 1993;12:66–78.

55. Sun LZ–Y, Currier NL, Miller SC. *J Altern Complement Med.* 1999;5:437–446.

56. Currier NL, Lejtenyi D, Miller SC. *Phytomedicine.* 2003;10:145–153.

57. Currier NL, Miller SC. *Exp Gerontol.* 2000;35:627–639.

58. Brousseau M, Miller SC. *Biogerontology.* 2005;6:157–163.

59. Currier NL, Miller SC. *J Altern Complement Med.* 2001;7:241–251.

60. Delorme D, Miller SC. *Autoimmunity.* 2005;38(6):453–461.

61. Goel V, Chang C, Slama J, et al. *J Nutr Biochem.* 2002;13(8):487.

62. Goel V, Chang C, Slama JV, et al. *Int Immunopharmacol.* 2(2–3):381–387.

63. Rehman J, Dillow JM, Carter SM. *Immunol Lett.* 1999;68(2–3):391–395.

64. South EH, Exon JH. *Immunopharmacol Immunotoxicol.* 2001;23(3):411–421.

65. Hermann JR, Honeyman MS, Zimmerman JJ, et al. *J Anim Sci.* 2003;81(9):2139–2144.

66. Zhai Z, Lui Y, Wu L, et al. *J Med Food.* 2007;10(3):423–434.

67. Zhai Z, Haney D, Wu L, et al. *Food Agric Immunol.* 2007;18(3–4):221–236.

68. Jurcic K, Melchart D, Holzmann M, et al. *Z Phytother.* 1989;10:67–70.

69. Wagner H, Proksch A, Riess-Maurer I, et al. *Arzneimittelforschung.* 1985;35:1069–1075.

70. Stimpel M, Proksch A, Wagner H, et al. *Infect Immunol.* 1984;46:845–849.

71. Luettig B, Steinmüller G, Gifford GE, et al. *J Nat Cancer Inst.* 1989;81:669–675.

72. Bauer R, Wagner H. In: Farnsworth NR, ed. *Economic and Medicinal Plant Research,* vol. 5. London: Academic Press; 1991. pp. 286–288, 301.

73. Melchart D, Clemm C, Weber B, et al. *Phytother Res.* 2002;16:138–142.

74. Wu H, Narfone A, Lacetera N. *Res Vet Sci.* 2009;87(3):396–398.

75. Farinacci M, Colitti M, Stefanon B. *Vet Immunol Immunopathol.* 2009;128(4):366–373.

76. Morazzoni P, Cristoni A, Di Pierro F, et al. *Fitoterapia.* 2005;76(5):401–411.

77. Bone K. *Alternat Med Rev.* 1997;2(2):87–93.

78. Gertsch J, Schoop R, Kuenzle U, et al. International Congress on Natural Products Research, Phoenix, Arizona USA, July 31–August 4, 2004. Lecture O:9.

79. Woelkart K, Xu W, Makriyannis A, et al. International Congress on Natural Products Research, Phoenix, Arizona

USA, July 31–August 4, 2004. Poster P:342.

80. Woelkart K, Xu W, Pei Y, et al. *Planta Med.* 2005;71(8):701–705.

81. Ralevic V. *Eur J Pharmacol.* 2003;472(1–2):1–21.

82. Salzet M, Breton C, Bisogno T, et al. *Eur J Biochem.* 2000;267(16):4917–4927.

83. Fride E. *Neuro Endocrinol Lett.* 2004;25(1–2):24–30.

84. Raduner S, Majewska A, Chen J-Z, et al. *J Biol Chem.* 2006;281(2):14192–14206.

85. Gertsch J, Schoop R, Kuenzle U, et al. *FEBS Lett.* 2004;577(3):563–569.

86. Matovic N, et al. *Org Biomol Chem.* 2007;5(1):169–174.

87. Gertsch J, Raduner S, Chicca A, et al. *Planta Med.* 2007;73:843.

88. Chicca A, Raduner S, Pellati F, et al. *Int Immunopharmacol.* 2009;9(7–8): 850–858.

89. Gertsch J. *Planta Med.* 2008;74(6): 638–650.

90. Spelman K, Iiams-Hauser K, Cech NB, et al. *Int Immunopharmacol.* 2009;9(11):1260–1264.

91. Cheminat A, Zawatsky R, Becker H, et al. *Phytochem.* 1988;27:2787–2794.

92. Reinke RA, Lee DJ, McDougall BR, et al. *Virology.* 2004;326(2):203–219.

93. Beuscher N, Bodinet C, Willigmann I, et al. *Z Phytother.* 1995;16(3):157: 165–166.

94. Binns SE, Hudson J, Merali S, et al. *Planta Med.* 2001;68(9):780–783.

95. Senchina DS, Martin AE, Buss JE, et al. *Phytother Res.* 2010;24(6):810–816.

96. Tubaro A, Tragni E, Del Negro P, et al. *J Pharm Pharmacol.* 1987;39(7):567–569.

97. Tragni E, Tubaro A, Melis C, et al. *Food Chem Toxicol.* 1985;23(2):317–319.

98. Wagner H, Breu W, Willer F, et al. *Planta Med.* 1989;55:566–567.

99. Wagner H, Jurcic K. *Arzneimittelforschung.* 1991;41: 1072–1076.

100. Hinz B, Woelkart K, Bauer R. *Biochem Biophys Res Commun.* 2007;360(2):441–446.

101. LaLone CA, Hammer KD, Wu L, et al. *J Agric Food Chem.* 2007;55(18):7314–7322.

102. LaLone CA, Rizshsky L, Hammer KD, et al. *J Agric Food Chem.* 2009;57(19):8820–8830.

103. Stoll A, Renz J, Brack A. *Helv Chim Acta.* 1950;33:1877–1893.

104. Samochowiec E, Urbanska L, Manka W, et al. *Wiad Parazytol.* 1979;25:77–81.

105. Jung H-D, Schröder H. *Arch Dermatol Syphilis.* 1954;197:1144–1300.

106. Mir-Rashed N, Cruz I, Jessulat M, et al. *Med Mycol.* 2010;48(7):949–958.

107. Canlas J, Hudson JB, Sharma M, et al. *Pharm Biol.* 2010;48(9): 1047–1052.

108. Bensch K, Tiralongo J, Schmidt K, et al. *Phytother Res*. 2011;25(8):1125–1132.

109. Facino RM, Carini M, Aldini G, et al. *Farmaco*. 1993;48(10):1447–1461.

110. Facino RM, Carini M, Aldini G, et al. *Planta Med*. 1995;61(6):510–514.

111. Dalby-Brown L, Barsett H, Landbo AK, et al. *J Agric Food Chem*. 2005;53(24):9413–9423.

112. Skaudickas D, Kondrotas AJ, Baltrusaitis K, et al. *Medicina*. 2003;39(8):761–766.

113. Skaudickas D, Kondrotas AJ, Kevelaitis E, et al. *Phytother Res*. 2009;23(10):1474–1478.

114. Haller J, Hohmann J, Freund TF. *Phytother Res*. 2010;24(11):1605–1613.

115. Di Carlo G, Nuzzo I, Capasso R, et al. *Pharmacol Res*. 2003;48(3):273–277.

116. Chicca A, Adinolfi B, Martinotti E, et al. *J Ethnopharmacol*. 2007;110(1):148–153.

117. Chicca A, Pellati F, Adinolfi B, et al. *Br J Pharmacol*. 2008;153(5):879–885.

118. Jager H, Meiner L, Dietz B, et al. *Planta Med*. 2002;68(5):649–671.

119. Matthias A, Blanchfield JT, Penman KG, et al. *J Clin Pharm Ther*. 2004;29(1):7–13.

120. Woelkart K, Frye RF, Derendorf H, et al. *Planta Med*. 2009;75(12):1306–1313.

121. Ardjomand-Woelkart K, Kollroser M, Magnes C, et al. *Planta Med*. May 20, 2011 [ePub ahead of print].

122. Dietz B, Heilmann J, Abuer R. *Planta Med*. 2001;67(9):863–864.

123. Woelkart K, Koidl C, Grisold A, et al. *J Clin Pharmacol*. 2005;45(6):683–689.

124. Matthias A, Addison RS, Penman KG, et al. *Life Sci*. 2005;77(16):2018–2029.

125. Woelkart K, Marth E, Suter A, et al. *Int J Clin Pharmacol Ther*. 2006;44(9):401–408.

126. Matthias A, Addison RS, Agnew LL, et al. *Phytomedicine*. 2007;14(9):587–590.

127. Agnew L, Addison R, Matthias A, et al. *Planta Med*. 2010;76(12):P617, 1351.

128. Guiotto P, Woelkart K, Grabnar I, et al. *Phytomedicine*. 2008;15:544–547.

129. Matthias A, Gillam EM, Penman KG, et al. *Chem Biol Interact*. 2005;155(1–2):62–70.

130. Toselli F, Matthias A, Bone KM, et al. *Phytother Res*. 2010;24(8):1195–1201.

131. Linde K, Barrett B, Wolkart K, et al. *Cochrane Database Syst Rev*. 2006;1:CD000530.

132. Bräunig B, Dorn M, Knick E. *Z Phytother*. 1992;13:7–13.

133. Goel V, Lovlin R, Barton R, et al. *J Clin Pharm Ther*. 2004;(1):75–83.

134. Goel V, Lovlin R, Chang C, et al. *Phytother Res*. 2005;19(8):689–694.

135. Berrett B, Brown R, Rakel D, et al. *Ann Intern Med*. 2010;153(12):769–777.

136. Schapowal A, Berger D, Klein P, et al. *Eur J Med Res*. 2009;14(9):406–412.

137. Melchart D, Walther E, Linde K, et al. *Arch Fam Med*. 1998;7:541–545.

138. Ronald B, Turner MD, Bauer R, et al. *N Engl J Med*. 2005;33(4):341.

139. McIntosh A, D'Huyretter K, Goldberg B, et al. Infections prevention by herbal formulas in a high stress population. AANP Convention, Coeur d' Arlene, 1999.

140. Tiralongo E, Lea R, Wee S, et al. *Planta Med*. 2010;76(12):1190. SL–49

141. Zwickey H, Brush J, Tacullo CM, et al. *Phytother Res*. 2007;21(11):1109–1112.

142. Brush J, Medenhall E, Guggenheim A, et al. *Phtother Res*. 2006;20(8):687–695.

143. Agnew LL, Guffogg SP, Matthias A, et al. *J Clin Pharm Ther*. 2005;30(4):363–369.

144. Agnew L, Matthias A, Shipp C, et al. *Planta Med*. 2010;76(12):P629, 1354.

145. Neri PG, Stagni E, Filippello M, et al. *J Ocul Pharmacol Ther*. 2006;22(6):431–436.

146. German Federal Minister of Justice: German Commission E for human medicine monograph. Bundes–Anzeiger (German Federal Gazette), no. 162, dated 29.08.1992.

147. Skaudickas D, Kondrotas A, Baltrusaitis K. *Medicina*. 2004;40(12):1211–1218.

148. Blumenthal M, etal., eds. *The Complete German Commission E Monographs: Therapeutic Guide to Herbal Medicines*. Austin: American Botanical Council; 1998. pp. 327–328, 391–393.

149. British Herbal Medicine Association Scientific Committee. *British Herbal Pharmacopoeia*. Bournemouth: BHMA; 1983. pp. 80–81.

150. British Herbal Medicine Association. *British Herbal Compendium*, vol. 1. Bournemouth: BHMA; 1992. pp. 81–83.

151. No authors listed. *Treatmentupdate*. 1999;11(1):3.

152. Burger RA, Torres AR, Warren RP, et al. *Int J Immunopharmacol*. 1997;19(7):371–379.

153. Bauer R. In: Wagner H, ed. *Immunomodulatory Agents from Plants*. Basel: Birkauser Verlag; 1999. pp. 49–53, 56–57, 62–65, 73–77.

154. Rininger JA, Kickner S, Chigurupati P, et al. *J Leukoc Biol*. 2000;68(4):503–510.

155. Sharp R. Echinacea a danger to asthmatics. *Medical Observer*, 8 August 1997. p. 1.

156. Jurcic K, Melchart D, Holzmann M, et al. *Z Phytother*. 1989;10:67–70.

157. Freeman C, Spelman K. *Mol Nutr Food Res*. 2008;52(7):789–798.

158. Gurley BJ, Swain A, Hubbard MA, et al. *Mol Nutr Food Res*. 2008;52(7):755 p. 763.

159. Gurley BJ, Swain A, Williams DK, et al. *Mol Nutr Food Res*. 2008;52(7):772–779.

160. Modari M, Silva E, Suter A, et al. *Evid Based Complement Alternat Med*. 2009 [Epub ahead of print].

161. Modari M, Gertsch Suter A, et al. *J Pharm Pharmacol*. 2007;59(4):567–573.

162. Abdul MI, Jiang X, Williams KM, et al. *Br J Clin Pharmacol*. 2010;69(5):508–515.

163. Molto J, Valle M, Miranda C, et al. *Antimicrob Agents Chemother*. 2011;55(1):326–330.

164. Cuzzolin L, Francini-Presenti F, Verlato G, et al. *Pharmac Drug Saf*. 2010;19(11):1151–1158.

165. Tsui B, Dennehy CE, Tsourounis C. *Am J Obstet Gynecol*. 2001;185(2):433–437.

166. Chow G, Johns T, Miller SC. *Biol Neonate*. 2006;89(2):133–138.

167. Gallo M, Sarkar M, Au W, et al. *Arch Intern Med*. 2000;160(20):3141–3143.

168. Perri D, Dugoua JJ, Mills E, et al. *Can J Clin Pharmacol*. 2006;13(3):e262–e267.

169. Matthias A, Bone K, Lehmann R. Safety and interactions with Echinacea: risks and benefits. UNE International Conference: Evidence-Based Complementary Medicine, Armidale, Australia, 2009.

170. Bauer R, Wagner H. *Z Phytother*. 1996;17:251–252.

171. Bruynzeel DP, Van Ketel WG, Young E, et al. *Contact Derm*. 1992;27:278–279.

172. Mullins RJ. *MA*. 1998;168:170–171.

173. Myers SP, Wohlmuth H. *MJA*. 1998;168:583.

174. Mullins RJ, Heddle R. *Ann Allergy Asthma Immunol*. 2002;88(1):42–51.

175. Soon S, Crawford RI. *J Am Acad Dermatol*. 2001;44(2):298–299.

176. Kemp DE, Franco KN. *J Am Board Fam Pract*. 2002;15(5):417–419.

177. Lee AN, Werth VP. *Arch Dermatol*. 2004;140(6):723–727.

178. Logan JL, Ahmed J. *Clin Rheumatol*. 2003;22(2):158–159.

179. Kocaman O, Hulagu S, Senturk O. *Eur J Intern Med*. 2008;19(2):148.

180. Maskatia ZK, Baker K. *South Med J*. 2010;103(11):1173–1174.

Evening primrose oil

(Oenothera biennis **L.)**

Synonyms

Echte Nachtkerze (Ger), herbe aux ânes, onagre bisannuelle (Fr), stella di sera (Ital), kaempe natlys (Dan).

What is it?

Evening primrose oil (EPO) is the fixed (fatty) oil obtained from the seed of the common evening primrose, *Oenothera biennis*. Flowers of this genus often open and release their scent in the evenings and are pollinated by moths.[1] The seeds were recommended as a coffee substitute in wartime and have an aromatic flavour reminiscent of poppy seed oil.[2] Other parts of the plant have been used medicinally: the leaves for dyspepsia, liver and female complaints; the root can be eaten as a vegetable.[3] Evening primrose oil was developed as a source of gamma-linolenic acid (GLA) in response to an increased understanding of the role of eicosanoids in human disease processes.

Effects

Anti-inflammatory; corrects omega-6 EFA deficiency; improves vasodilator eicosanoid synthesis; helps to correct nerve blood flow and conduction velocity deficits in diabetes.

Traditional view

Evening primrose oil was not used traditionally.

Summary actions

Anti-inflammatory, antiallergic, corrects omega-6 EFA deficiency, hypotensive.

Can be used for

Indications supported by clinical trials

Indications supported by trials using evening primrose oil: diabetic neuropathy; atopic dermatitis. However, both these uses of EPO are controversial. EPO may also be beneficial in the treatment of premenstrual syndrome, mastalgia, rheumatoid arthritis, schizophrenia, Raynaud's phenomenon and ulcerative colitis, although the overall results of clinical trials are inconsistent. Single clinical trials support the use of EPO for dry eye in contact lens wearers, alcohol withdrawal (some benefits), cardiovascular risk reduction and some instances of cancer palliation.

Indications suggested by trials using evening primrose oil with fish oil include hypertension, dyslexia, postviral fatigue syndrome and osteoporosis, although more studies are necessary to fully confirm efficacy.

May also be used for

Extrapolations from pharmacological studies

Impaired omega-6 essential fatty acid (EFA) metabolism (especially in diabetes); inflammatory disorders (including rheumatoid arthritis, ulcerative colitis, systemic lupus erythematosus); alcoholism.

Other applications

Use in cosmetic products such as hand lotions, soaps and shampoos.[4] Veterinary applications include skin disorders such as papulocrustous dermatitis, crusting dermatoses and non-seasonal atopic dermatitis.

Preparations

Oils such as EPO (containing the polyunsaturated cis fatty acid, GLA) are difficult to preserve, as they can easily be oxidised and become rancid. Hence, EPO is best administered with a preservative such as vitamin E and protected from oxygen in soft gelatin capsules.

Dosage

Low to medium dosage should be used for conditions such as atopic dermatitis and mastalgia: 250 to 500 mg GLA per day (approximately 2.6 to 5.2 g/day of EPO).

Medium to high doses should be used for conditions such as diabetes, alcoholism, inflammatory disorders (including arthritis, ulcerative colitis) or cardiovascular disorders (hyperlipidaemia, hypertension): 0.4 to 2 g GLA per day (approximately 4.2 to 21 g/day of EPO). A suitable dose to begin treatment for rheumatoid arthritis is 500 to 600 mg GLA per day (approximately 5.2 to 6.3/day of EPO).

Duration of use

Evening primrose oil should be used cautiously in the long term for patients with rheumatoid arthritis. Otherwise long-term use appears to be safe.

Summary assessment of safety

Evening primrose oil is well tolerated, with very few side effects reported in clinical trials when administered at therapeutic doses over the short and medium term. Long-term use may potentiate the risk of arachidonate build-up in the treatment of rheumatoid arthritis. There is concern expressed in some quarters regarding the administration of EPO where there is a history of epilepsy, but this is not well supported by fact.

Technical data

Botany

Evening primrose is a member of the Onagraceae (willow herb) family, which grows to a height of about 1 m. It is an annual or biennial plant with lanceolate leaves and large, showy yellow flowers arranged in a terminal leafy spike. The flowers consist of four petals; the fruit is cylindrical and opens lengthwise by four valves.[5,6]

Adulteration

No adulteration known.

Key constituents

- Fixed oil (15% to 20%), containing EFAs: linoleic acid (65%), GLA (8% to 10%)[7,8]
- Triacylglycerols in the oil, mainly comprising trilinolein (linoleic acid in all three esterified positions on the glycerol molecule) and dilinoleoyl-mono-gamma-linolenin (two linoleic acids, one GLA). The latter triglyceride, known as DLMG, accounts for over half the total amount of GLA.[9]

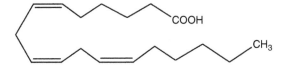

gamma-Linolenic acid

Pharmacodynamics

Essential fatty acids (EFAs) are nutrients that play a role in the structure of cell membranes, helping to ensure their fluidity and flexibility, and consequently modulate the behaviour of membrane-bound proteins. They are also precursors of the eicosanoids (prostaglandins, leukotrienes and thromboxanes) that function in regulating platelet aggregation and inflammatory processes. Since they contain two or more double bonds, EFAs are classified as polyunsaturated fatty acids (PUFAs). There are two types of EFA: the omega-6 series derived from linoleic acid and the omega-3 series derived from alpha-linolenic acid (ALA). These are so named for the position of the double bond nearest to the methyl (CH_3) group at the end of the molecule. Omega-3 fatty acids are found in fish oils and certain seeds (e.g. linseed).

Within the body, linoleic and ALA are metabolised by a series of alternating desaturations and elongations, as shown below.

omega-6 series	omega-3 series
linoleic acid	alpha-linolenic acid (*ALA*)
↓	↓
gamma-linolenic acid (*GLA*)	
↓	↓
dihomogamma-linolenic acid (*DGLA*)	
↓	↓
arachidonic acid (*AA*)	eicosapentaenoic acid (*EPA*)
↓	↓
↓	↓
↓	docosahexaenoic acid (*DHA*)

AA forms prostaglandin products of the 2-series (e.g. PGE_2) and leukotrienes with subscript 4 (LTB_4). DGLA and EPA can be converted to metabolites closely related to these eicosanoids: DGLA producing prostaglandins of the 1-series and leukotrienes of the 3-series, EPA producing prostaglandins of the 3-series and leukotrienes of the 5-series. The presence of these EFAs can result in decreased production of some arachidonate metabolites and increased levels of the other less inflammatory eicosanoids.

Although GLA has been found in higher concentrations from other sources, including borage oil, blackcurrant oil and fungal lipids, there is less clinical evidence to support their efficacy compared to EPO.

Diabetes

Reduced nerve perfusion, indicated by a nerve conduction velocity deficit and reduced nerve blood flow, is an important factor in the aetiology of diabetic neuropathy, a common complication of diabetes. Metabolic changes include a high polyol pathway flux (mediated by aldose reductase), increased advanced glycation endproducts, elevated oxidative stress and impaired omega-6 EFA metabolism. GLA improves vasodilator eicosanoid synthesis, correcting nerve blood flow and nerve conduction velocity deficits. Combined treatment of EPO with aldose reductase inhibitors or antioxidants (such as ascorbate) markedly enhanced neuroactivity.[10] Depletion of PUFAs derived from the omega-6 pathway may also lead to abnormalities of myelin turnover and membrane-bound proteins (e.g. enzymes, receptors) and other axonal structural abnormalities.[11]

Treatment with EPO can prevent or reverse motor nerve conduction velocity deficit (an indicator of peripheral neuropathy) in diabetic animals. This was achieved without changing the sorbitol, fructose or myoinositol levels in peripheral nerves and without having any effect on the control of blood sugar.[12,13] Evening primrose oil outperformed blackcurrant oil, borage oil and fungal oils in ameliorating nerve conduction velocity deficits in diabetic rats.[14] Treatment with EPO improved nerve blood flow measurements in rats with experimentally induced diabetes. Reduced production of nitric oxide may be responsible for the development of endoneurial ischaemia in diabetes, and EPO may correct this deficiency in vivo.[15] Aspirin enhanced the neuroactivity of EPO in experimental diabetes, indicating that prostanoids are unlikely to mediate this effect.[16] Daily treatment with EPO caused oscillation of nerve conduction velocity in diabetic rats needing 10 days to stabilise. The latency suggests that neuroactivity of EPO may be mediated by its metabolic products synthesised in the body and not by ready-made constituents of the oil.[17]

The positive effect of EPO on nerve conduction velocity was further demonstrated in a 2001 study in rats with streptozotocin-induced diabetes. The study, which assessed 2 weeks' treatment, also demonstrated that EPO improved endoneurial blood flow.[18] A 2004 study examined the effect of a combined alpha-lipoic acid (LA)/EPO treatment on diabetic-induced changes in the enteric nerves of rats with streptozotocin-induced diabetes. Nerves supplying the ileum containing vasoactive intestinal polypeptide (VIP), calcitonin gene-related peptide (CGRP) and noradrenaline (norepinephrine) (NA) were examined. Diabetes caused a significant increase in VIP-containing cell bodies, a decrease in NA content and loss of CGRp immunoreactivity. LA/EPO treatment totally prevented diabetes-induced changes in VIP and CGRP, and partially reversed these changes after they had been allowed to develop. In contrast, NA-containing nerves did not respond to treatment. This study demonstrated that LA/EPO treatment was only effective for treating diabetes-induced changes in some enteric nerves.[19]

Short-term biochemical changes have been noted from GLA treatment in type 2 diabetic patients. At the 2 g/day dosage of GLA over 6 weeks, a decrease in serum triglycerides, cholesterol and plasma beta-thromboglobulin was observed. No changes were observed on platelet aggregation or thromboxane B_2 and PGE_1 released from platelets.[20]

Anti-inflammatory activity

GLA and DGLA inhibited inflammation and excessive immune reactivity in a variety of models: adjuvant arthritis, experimental allergic encephalomyelitis, autoimmune disease (systemic lupus erythematosus), salmonella-associated arthritis and subacute, acute and chronic inflammation induced by Freund's adjuvant or urate crystal.[21–23] The GLA-enriched diet significantly suppressed the cellular phase of inflammation, but had little effect on the fluid phase.[22] EPO raised gastric mucosal prostaglandin synthesis in humans but not in

rats.[24,25] EPO, however, protected rats but not humans against aspirin-induced damage.[24,26] Four different doses of GLA, in the form of either borage oil or EPO, were fed to rats over 6 weeks and compared with corn oil. DGLA and GLA levels were dose-dependently increased in liver, red blood cell and aorta phospholipids. The AA:DGLA ratio in tissues decreased with increasing intake of GLA. There was no significant difference in GLA or DGLA levels within groups given borage oil or EPO. The dose of GLA did not influence PGE_2 production in stimulated aortic rings or thromboxane levels in serum, although an increase in PGE_1 occurred in the stimulated aorta.[27] In rats supplemented with EPO, fish oil or virgin olive oil, all three oils resulted in significantly reduced production of PGE_2 by neutrophils ex vivo.[28]

Bone metabolism

GLA and EPA were administered orally to different groups of rats in several ratios. Intestinal calcium absorption, calcium balance and bone calcium all increased significantly in the 3:1 (GLA:EPA) ratio group, compared with controls.[29] Several different ratios of GLA and EPA were administered to young rats, as a mixture of EPO and fish oil. Bone calcium content increased significantly in the group receiving the high GLA:EPA diet compared with controls receiving LA and ALA.[30]

Reproductive function

In a placebo-controlled trial during the reproductive period, male and female blue foxes were fed either a standard diet or one supplemented with EPO, zinc sulphate and vitamin E. A tendency for an increased litter size in the treatment group was found, mainly as an effect of male treatment.[31] Control male minks were mated with control and test female minks and test males were mated with control and test females. For those males supplemented with EPO, there was a tendency for a reduced rate of stillborns and loss of life during the first 21 days of life. EPO did not affect reproductive performance in females, but there was a tendency for lower weight losses during lactation.[32]

Cytotoxic effects

The cytotoxicity of GLA and other fatty acids containing two, four, five and six double bonds was examined on human breast cancer cells in vitro. GLA and arachidonate, with three and four double bonds respectively, were the most cytotoxic fatty acids, compared to acids with six double bonds, which were the least effective. The efficacy of a given fatty acid in killing cancer cells correlated with the extent of lipid peroxidation of the added fatty acid in the cells.[33] GLA, AA and EPA were highly effective in killing human breast, lung and prostate tumour cells in vitro, while leaving normal cells viable.[34] GLA, AA and EPA enhanced free radical generation in tumour cells, but not in normal cells in vitro.[35]

The growth of human breast carcinoma xenografts was studied in mice treated with dietary supplements of EPO and fish oil and compared with controls. Animals in the treatment group developed tumours that were significantly smaller than controls.[36]

Hypotensive effects

Vegetable oils including sunflower oil, linseed oil and EPO enhanced the hypotensive effect of antihypertensive drugs (dihydralazine, clonidine and captopril) in rats under experimental conditions.[37] Hypertension induced in rats was reversed by the addition of DGLA (5.0%) to the diet.[38] LA bioconversion to AA was decreased in the liver microsomes of spontaneously hypertensive rats compared with controls, due to a decrease in the desaturase enzymes.[39] The effect of salt loading on blood pressure development and its modification by dietary omega-3 and omega-6 fatty acids was studied in the borderline hypertensive rat. EPO abolished the pressor response, reducing blood pressure below control levels.[40] GLA supplementation reduced cardiovascular responses to chronic stress in normal and borderline hypertensive rats.[41,42]

Other effects

Early stage cyclosporine A (CsA)-induced nephrotoxicity was prevented by EPO (9% GLA) or fish oil (5.6% EPA) supplementation of the diet of rats. The animals were fed a diet of standard chow consisting of either 1% EPO or 10% fish oil for 70 days prior to the administration of CsA.[43] CsA is widely used as an immunosuppressant to prevent allograft rejection in transplant patients and in the treatment of some autoimmune diseases. It provokes intense vasoconstriction in the kidneys by enhancing the production of many vasoconstrictor substances including thromboxane A_2. In addition CsA also reduces the synthesis of the vasodilator prostaglandins PGE_2 and PGI_2. Supplementation with EPO resulted in an increase of PGE_1 and redirected PGH_2 conversion to PGE_2 and PGI_2 metabolites, instead of thromboxane A_2.[44]

EPO given to mice as 10% of their diet reduced the development of diet-induced atherosclerosis in an experimental model. Aortic vessel wall medial layer thickness was significantly reduced and there was suppression of the number of proliferating aortic smooth muscle cells.[45]

In comparison to a corn oil placebo, EPO produced significant inhibition of gastric mucosal damage induced by pylorus ligation, NSAIDs or hypothermic restraint and had a marked cytoprotective effect against all necrotising agents used.[46]

Treatment of pregnant rats with ethanol and EPO led to a significant reduction in the embryopathic activity of ethanol.[47] EPO slowed the progression of renal failure in rats[48] and reduced the severity of experimental autoimmune glomerulonephritis.[49]

Pharmacokinetics and metabolism

EFAs are hydrolysed by lipases in the gastric and intestinal lumen. Long-chain PUFAs are taken up by tissues less rapidly than short-chain PUFAs. The liver is one of the most active organs in producing long-chain PUFAs (by a series of desaturation and elongation reactions). In this way less active organs such as the brain are provided with long-chain PUFAs secreted in very low density lipoprotein. Insulin and thyroxine are necessary for the desaturation process, but glucagon, adrenaline (epinephrine), ACTH (adrenocorticotropin) and glucocorticoids inhibit desaturation.[50]

The pharmacokinetics of GLA in six healthy volunteers after the administration of EPO was recorded. EPO capsules were administered to each subject in the morning and the evening over several days. The values for accumulated concentration (24h) and Cmax (maximum concentration) for GLA were significantly increased over baseline values. Other fatty acids such as DGLA and AA did not show a significant increase in their concentration. After the evening administration, Tmax (time to reach maximum concentration) was shorter than after the morning dose. An influence of the administration of GLA on serum concentrations of DGLA and AA (and hence on the biosynthesis of prostaglandin PGE_1 and PGE_2) could not be clearly established in these healthy volunteers.[51]

Analysis of the fatty acid composition of the plasma of children with atopic bronchial asthma showed significantly higher levels of LA and lower levels of AA in comparison to healthy controls. No differences were observed for GLA and DGLA. It was suggested that there is therefore no justification for GLA supplementation on the basis of a 6-desaturation step defect (and subsequently low levels of eicosanoid precursors from DGLA).[52] However, other clinical studies have shown DGLA increases (see below and the Clinical trials section). The concept of a defect in 6-desaturation is widely proposed as a key rationale for EPO therapy.

In a study investigating the metabolism of GLA, 29 volunteers either adhered to a fat-controlled diet and received GLA supplementation, or maintained a typical Western diet. Supplementation with GLA at 3 to 6g/day resulted in increased GLA and DGLA in serum lipids. AA increased in all subjects. Neutrophil phospholipids were higher in DGLA but not GLA or AA. Neutrophils obtained from those supplemented with GLA synthesized less LTB_4 and platelet activating factor. The increase in DGLA relative to AA within inflammatory cells such as neutrophils may decrease the production of inflammatory AA metabolites and thereby explain how GLA exerts its anti-inflammatory activity.[53]

Veterinary studies

Eleven cats with papulocrustous dermatitis randomly received either EPO or sunflower oil for 12 weeks. Cats in both groups improved during the treatment period and the concentration of LA in erythrocyte phospholipid increased in the cats fed EPO. Six weeks after the treatment was withdrawn, the cats fed EPO had deteriorated less than those fed sunflower oil.[54] Fourteen cats with crusting dermatoses were treated with various combinations of EPO and fish oil. The cutaneous symptoms improved in those treated with either EPO alone or the combination. The subsequent administration of the two oils resulted in a resolution of the dermatosis.[55]

A significant effect was observed on erythema in dogs with non-seasonal atopic dermatitis. They were treated with EPO in a double blind, placebo-controlled crossover study. Plasma LA and AA levels were significantly higher for the EPO group, both in the first and second phases of the study. There was also a significant treatment effect for EPO given in the second phase.[56]

Clinical trials

Clinical trials have shown benefits in diabetic neuropathy, hypertension, PMS (premenstrual syndrome), osteoporosis and dementia. Mixed results have been obtained in trials for mastalgia, atopic eczema and dermatitis, rheumatoid arthritis, ulcerative colitis, diabetic lipid metabolism and alcoholism. The benefits of EPO therapy are disputed in schizophrenia and cancer. No benefit was observed in the treatment of menopausal hot flushes.

Atopic dermatitis and related skin disorders

Preliminary results from uncontrolled or open label trials were promising. For example, in an open label trial, 20 patients with dry skin and an atopic disposition (but not actual atopic dermatitis) received a 12.5% EPO cream applied to their lower right leg for 3 weeks. The other leg served as a control. The treated leg showed a significant increase in sebum content (p<0.01) and no change in transepidermal water loss. Transepidermal water loss was significant on the untreated side (p<0.05). Improvement in skin smoothness was observed on the treated side.[57] In an uncontrolled trial, infants with atopic dermatitis were treated with GLA (3g/day) for 28 days. A gradual improvement in erythema, excoriations and lichenification was observed. Significant differences from baseline were shown for itching (p<0.01) and for the reduced use of antihistamines (p<0.01). A significant rise in the percentage of circulating CD8 cells was found.[58] In other studies GLA reduced the requirement for topical steroids (by about 70%) and other medications such as oral steroids, antihistamines and antibiotics.[59,60] Two independent studies using different methodologies demonstrated that skin roughness was also significantly reduced.[61,62]

More significantly, a number of controlled clinical trials have been conducted for EPO in the treatment of atopic dermatitis. Proof of efficacy is controversial. These trials are listed below, grouped according to the positive or negative results obtained, and with the most recent work listed first.

A highly significant difference was observed for EPO (doses varying from 500mg to 6g/day, depending on the age of the child) versus a corn oil placebo in 50 patients with atopic dermatitis treated for 5 months in a randomised trial.[63] Using a scoring system based on extent, intensity, itch and dryness of the rash, improvement was noted in 96% of patients in the EPO group compared with 32% of control patients (p<0.0001). No significant adverse effects were reported.

A 2002 clinical trial involving 14 atopic dermatitis patients concluded that EPO (160mg/day of GLA) could be effective in the treatment of a non-inflammatory type of atopic dermatitis. EPO treatment resulted in an increase in serum interferon (IFN)-gamma levels and a reduction of serum IgE levels. The authors suggested that the restoration of IFN-gamma levels indicated that EPO might exert its effect through a modulation of the immunological mechanism involving this cytokine.[64]

A double blind, placebo-controlled study conducted in children with atopic dermatitis found a significant improvement in the overall severity of the condition after GLA treatment, independent of the occurrence of IgE-mediated allergy.

GLA increased the amount of omega-6 fatty acids in red blood cell membranes, particularly in those treated with the highest dose. A significant increase in DGLA occurred in the high-dose group.[65] In a double blind, placebo-controlled trial, 52 adults with atopic eczema completed 4 months' treatment with EPO. Patients were divided into three groups: women with premenstrual exacerbation of their eczema, women without the exacerbation and men. Results for the three groups combined indicated a significant effect of EPO on erythema and surface damage compared with placebo. No significant effect was observed for lichenification. Women with premenstrual flare of their eczema showed the greatest improvement with EPO treatment compared with placebo.[66]

Four weeks' treatment with EPO in children with atopic eczema resulted in significant improvement compared with those treated with an olive oil placebo. There were significant changes in plasma fatty acid composition before and after treatment and also between the placebo and EPO-treated groups.[67] Patients receiving EPO showed a greater reduction in inflammation than those receiving placebo in a double blind trial conducted over 12 weeks, although patients in the placebo group also showed a significant reduction. A statistically significant improvement was observed in the overall severity, grade of inflammation, dryness and itch and in the percentage of the body surface with eczema.[60]

A meta-analysis published in 1989 investigated nine placebo-controlled trials for the efficacy of a specific proprietary EPO product in the treatment of atopic eczema. Four of the trials were parallel and five were crossover design. Clinicians and patients assessed the severity of eczema by scoring measures of inflammation, dryness, scaliness, pruritus and overall skin involvement. Individual symptom scores were combined to give a single global score at each assessment point. In the parallel studies, both patient and clinician scores showed a highly significant improvement over baseline for EPO, which was also significantly better than placebo. Similar results were obtained in the crossover trials, except that the clinicians' global score, although favouring EPO, did not reach significance. The effect on itch was striking, with a highly significant response to EPO occurring (p<0.0001), and no placebo response. A positive correlation between an improvement in clinical score and a rise in the plasma fatty acid level was observed.[68] The validity of this meta-analysis has been subsequently questioned.[69]

A review of clinical trials for the treatment of atopic eczema with EPO published in 1992 noted that placebo-controlled trials of parallel design demonstrated marked improvement for EPO. Patients treated with EPO demonstrated less inflammation, dryness, scaling and overall severity compared with controls. Although these findings were supported by meta-analysis (see above), there was still conflicting evidence in trials based on a crossover design alone.[70] Since the publication of both the meta-analysis and the review, a number of trials yielding negative results have been conducted. Several of these are reviewed below.

In a double blind, placebo-controlled trial, 60 children with atopic dermatitis received either EPO or placebo for 16 weeks. Improvement was observed in the eczema symptoms, although no significant difference was found between the two groups. No therapeutic effect was observed on asthma symptoms in the 22 patients who also had asthma.[71] In a double blind, placebo-controlled, crossover trial, 24 children with atopic dermatitis received GLA (360 mg/day). After 10 to 14 weeks of treatment there was no improvement in the treatment compared with placebo (corn oil). Both groups improved while taking placebo.[72]

A double blind, placebo-controlled trial for the treatment of chronic hand dermatitis in 39 patients over 24 weeks found that EPO (600 mg/day GLA equivalent) was not superior to placebo (sunflower oil 500 mg/day).[73] The choice of placebo may have masked the results, due to the linoleic acid content of the sunflower oil. In a double blind, placebo-controlled, parallel trial, patients with atopic dermatitis were randomised to receive EPO, EPO plus fish oil or placebo for 16 weeks. One hundred and two patients completed the trial and no improvement was demonstrated by either EFA treatment.[74]

These negative outcome trials and apparent flaws in the 1989 meta-analysis[69] have led to some authors expressing doubts about the efficacy of EPO in atopic eczema, as assessed by systematic review.[75] In contrast, a 2006 update of the 1989 meta-analysis reaffirmed the efficacy of a proprietary EPO product.[76] In an analysis of 26 clinical studies including 1207 patients, it was suggested that EPO has a beneficial effect on pruritus, crusting, oedema and erythema that becomes apparent between 4 and 8 weeks after treatment is initiated. However, the magnitude of this effect was reduced with increasing frequency of potent steroid use, which might have been a confounding factor in some of the studies that did not show any benefit for EPO.

Psoriasis

A double blind, parallel trial of a combination of EPO and fish oil in the treatment of 37 patients with chronic stable plaque psoriasis was undertaken. There was no significant improvement in the clinical severity of psoriasis or change in transepidermal water loss.[77]

Female reproductive system disorders

Clinical trials conducted in the 1980s suggested that EPO demonstrated better activity than placebo in the treatment of premenstrual syndrome (PMS). Physical and psychological symptoms of PMS were significantly improved with EPO treatment, albeit only slightly compared with placebo.[78] More information on several of these trials is outlined below.[79,80] However, a review of seven placebo-controlled trials of EPO in the treatment of PMS published in 1996 found inconsistent scoring and response criteria, making a rigorous meta-analysis inappropriate. The two best controlled trials failed to show any beneficial effects for EPO. These two trials were relatively small, however, and the authors noted that modest effects could not be ruled out.[81]

EPO treatment alleviated premenstrual symptoms and depression better than placebo in 30 women with severe PMS. The capacity of platelets to release thromboxane B_2 during spontaneous clotting was also decreased in patients receiving EPO compared with those receiving placebo.[79] Results from three double blind, placebo-controlled studies,

one large uncontrolled study on women who had failed other therapies for PMS, and one large uncontrolled study on new patients, all suggested EPO was an effective treatment for depression, breast pain and tenderness and fluid retention associated with PMS.[80]

Over 17 years up to 1992 at the Cardiff Mastalgia Clinic, 324 patients with cyclical and 90 with non-cyclical mastalgia received a variety of drug treatments in clinical trials. In patients who responded to therapy, danazol was found to be the most effective drug (approximately 70%), with bromocriptine and EPO having equivalent efficacy (approximately 45%). Patients taking EPO reported fewer adverse events.[82,83]

Two reviews published in 2002 and 2003 suggested that EPO provides modest benefit in women with moderate symptoms of breast tenderness[84] and benign cyclical breast pain.[85] However, a 2006 review of mastalgia treatments conducted by the Breast Disease Committee and approved by the Executive and Council of the Society of Obstetricians and Gynaecologists of Canada found there is presently insufficient evidence to recommend the use of oral EPO for the treatment of mastalgia. Of the five trials reviewed, serious methodological flaws were found in two randomised controlled trials, with neither having been published in a peer review journal. Three randomised, double blind, placebo-controlled trials failed to demonstrate efficacy. This review did not include the findings from the Cardiff Mastalgia Clinic (see previous paragraph) and the latest publication date of the papers reviewed was only 1993.[86] Further to this, a randomised, double blind clinical trial (2002) found that EPO at a dose of 3 g/day (9.6% GLA) had no effect on mastalgia compared with a placebo (corn oil).[87]

A 2005 open, non-randomised, comparative study of a topical non-steroidal anti-inflammatory (NSAI) gel verses oral dosing of EPO (500 mg twice daily) demonstrated some benefit for EPO.[88] Fifty female patients between the ages of 15 and 50 years with a history of moderate to severe breast pain took part in the trial. Treatment with EPO resulted in a clinically significant improvement in 64% of patients after 3 months' use. There was a 92% improvement rate in the group using the NSAI gel. Results of this trial are difficult to interpret because of the lack of a placebo group.

In a complex randomised, double blind, placebo-controlled clinical trial also published in 2005, 426 women were assigned to one of four groups and received either EPO plus a multivitamin and mineral antioxidant supplement, EPO plus a placebo supplement, a placebo fatty acid (hydrogenated coconut oil) plus antioxidant supplement or a placebo fatty acid plus placebo supplement. The blinded phase of the trial lasted for four menstrual cycles and was followed by an open phase over eight menstrual cycles. Each EPO capsule contained 500 mg EPO (40 mg GLA) and they were given at a dosage of four capsules twice daily. Patients in all four groups experienced a statistically significant improvement compared against baseline for breast pain, overall mastalgia symptoms, sleep disturbance, restriction of daily activities, effect on physical relationships and overall response. However, there was no statistically significant difference between the four groups. The authors, surprised at the high placebo response, suggested that the hydrogenated coconut oil used as the placebo may have exhibited some beneficial effects.[89]

A randomised, double blind, placebo-controlled study investigated the efficacy of GLA in the treatment of menopausal hot flushes and sweating. Thirty-five women suffering hot flushes at least three times a day received either four capsules of 500 mg EPO plus 10 mg vitamin E or a placebo twice a day for 6 months. The only significant improvement for the women taking GLA was a reduction in the maximum number of night-time flushes ($p<0.05$). Overall there was no benefit over placebo in treating menopausal flushing.[90]

Diabetes

In a randomised, double blind, placebo-controlled, parallel trial conducted over seven centres in the UK and Finland, 111 patients with mild diabetic neuropathy received GLA (480 mg/day) or placebo over 1 year and were assessed by standard tests. A significant favourable change was noted in the treatment group for 13 of the 16 parameters investigated, demonstrating a clear beneficial effect on the course of mild diabetic neuropathy. Sex, age, diabetes type, age of onset or duration of diabetes did not significantly affect the result. The treatment was, however, more effective in relatively well-controlled diabetic patients.[91] Patients could continue in the trial for a further 12 months and all those who participated in this received GLA (unknowingly). Improvement continued over this period.[92]

Twenty-two patients with distal diabetic polyneuropathy who participated in a double blind, placebo-controlled study received either 360 mg GLA per day or placebo capsules for 6 months. Patients in the treatment group showed significant improvement in symptoms of distal diabetic polyneuropathy.[93] However, in a randomised, double blind, placebo-controlled study, 51 patients with type 1 or 2 diabetes and autonomic peripheral neuropathy were given EPO containing 480 mg/day of GLA or placebo for 1 year. At the end of the study patients receiving EPO showed no improvements in vibratory perception threshold compared with the placebo group.[94]

Inflammatory arthritis

A review of the clinical trials marked with asterisks (**) below has noted a limited applicability for their results in rheumatoid arthritis. Overall, these studies were not well controlled (olive oil may itself produce beneficial results and may not be the best choice of placebo; the effect of vitamin E has not been completely ascertained). The trials did not run for long enough (at least 6 months is required to assess symptomatic improvement, longer than 1 year for disease-modifying potential). The concomitant use of medications was not standardised (some of the drugs may have influenced the patients' subjective assessment) and abrupt discontinuation of NSAIDs may have aggravated patients' symptoms early on, thus masking the effect of GLA. The most appropriate statistical tests were not conducted and drop-out rates were high.[95] In contrast, a meta-analysis that included seven studies with seed oils from blackcurrant, borage and evening primrose at GLA doses greater than or equal to 1400 mg/day showed symptomatic benefit, whereas lower doses (about 500 mg/day) were ineffective.[96]

In a randomised, double blind, placebo-controlled 24-week trial, 37 patients with rheumatoid arthritis and active synovitis received 1400 mg/day GLA or placebo. Treatment with GLA resulted in significant reduction in the signs and symptoms of disease activity ($p<0.05$) compared with the placebo group, which showed no change or worsened.[97]

**In a placebo-controlled clinical trial, 18 patients with rheumatoid arthritis received 20 mL/day of EPO (1500 mg GLA perday) or olive oil for 12 weeks. Plasma levels of PGE_2 decreased and thromboxane B_2 increased in both treatment groups, but no significant improvement in laboratory findings or clinical signs occurred in either group.[98] **In a double blind, placebo-controlled clinical trial, 49 rheumatoid arthritis patients were treated with EPO (540 mg GLA perday), EPO plus fish oil (240 mg GLA plus 450 mg EPA perday) or placebo, over a period of 12 months. Significant improvement was demonstrated in subjective symptoms. There was a significant reduction in NSAID therapy for those receiving EPO and EPO plus fish oil, compared with placebo. After this treatment period, placebo was given to all patients for 3 months. After 3 months of placebo, the condition of those originally receiving the EPO/fish oil treatment had relapsed. Despite changes in the subjective assessment of symptoms and NSAID use throughout the treatment, EPO did not alter any of the biochemical indicators of the disease.[99] **Forty patients with rheumatoid arthritis and upper gastrointestinal lesions caused by NSAIDs took part in a double blind, placebo-controlled study over a 6-month period. Patients received either 6 g/day EPO or 6 g/day of olive oil. Three patients in each group also reduced their dose of NSAIDs. A significant reduction in morning stiffness occurred in the EPO group at 3 months. A significant reduction in pain and the articular index occurred at 6 months for those taking olive oil.[100]

In a double blind, placebo-controlled clinical trial, 56 patients with active rheumatoid arthritis received either GLA (2.8 g/day) or placebo (sunflower oil) over a period of 6 months. Following this, all patients received GLA for 6 months in single blind fashion. Treatment with GLA resulted in significant reductions in the signs and symptoms of disease activity. At least 25% improvement in four measured parameters occurred for more patients in the treatment group (14 of 22) than in the placebo group (4 of 19). During the second 6-month period, both groups exhibited improvement in disease activity.[101] In a double blind, placebo-controlled trial, 38 patients with psoriatic arthritis received a combination of EPO and fish oil daily for 9 months. All patients then received placebo capsules for a further 3 months. At the third month of the study, patients reduced their intake of NSAIDs and maintained the decrease, symptoms permitting. All measures of skin and joint symptoms were unchanged by the treatment. The requirement for NSAIDs was unchanged for both the treatment and placebo groups.[102]

Schizophrenia

Studies in groups of schizophrenics from England, Ireland, Scotland, Japan and the USA have indicated an association with lower levels of linoleic acid in patients' plasma phospholipids, with a variable pattern for the other EFAs.[103–105] In one study, omega-6 EFA levels were significantly reduced, whereas omega-3 EFA levels were elevated compared with controls.[103]

In a randomised, single blind, placebo-controlled trial, 21 inpatients with a schizophrenic illness resistant to neuroleptic drug treatments received either neuroleptic medication and DGLA, placebo and DGLA, or two placebo medications. No marked treatment effects were noticed on ratings of the patients' behaviour or symptomatology, although some positive clinical effects were noted in dyskinetic patients.[106]

In a double blind, placebo-controlled, crossover trial, 37 psychiatric patients, predominantly schizophrenics with tardive dyskinesia (abnormal involuntary movements), received capsules containing EPO over 16 weeks. A further 37 people in two groups, a psychiatric control group and a normal control group, were given a placebo. Although EFA supplementation did not produce improvement in abnormal movement measurements, there was significant improvement in mental state, schizophrenic symptoms and memory. In the open phase at the end of the trial, addition of co-factors (zinc, niacin and vitamins C and B6) to EPO treatment produced an increase in omega-3 and omega-6 EFA incorporation into red cell membranes. During this phase, marked and significant clinical improvements in memory, schizophrenic symptoms and abnormal movement were observed in comparison to placebo or EPO-only treatment.[107–109]

Despite this benefit, the overall data are not strong. A systematic review published by the Cochrane Collaboration found there was no clear benefit for the use of GLA in the treatment of schizophrenia and, while there is currently no reason for clinicians to either encourage or discourage the use of PUFAs, the review goes on to state: 'If a person with schizophrenia wishes to use one (PUFA) then, perhaps, an omega-3 preparation should be the preferred option'.[110]

Cardiovascular effects

In an open pilot study of 3 months' duration, a dose of 4000 mg/day of EPO (320 mg/day GLA) was given to 10 elderly subjects with an age range of 69 to 90 years (mean age 83 years). All participants were without specific metabolic or degenerative diseases and were in a satisfactory mental state. Supplementation with EPO was associated with a beneficial reduction of cardiovascular risk factors including a moderate decrease in arterial blood pressure and total cholesterol, and an increase in HDL-cholesterol and apolipoprotein A-I. However, these changes were not statistically significant, possibly due to the low patient number. There was also an increased biosynthesis of PGE_2, which has a vasodilatory action in the kidneys. This might contribute to a decrease in arterial blood pressure and maintenance of renal function.[111]

Another pilot open study assessed the effects of combined aspirin and dietary fatty acids on platelet angiotensin II (AII) binding. In pregnancy-induced hypertension and pre-eclampsia there is an imbalance in arachidonic metabolites resulting in increased AII binding. Sixty non-pregnant women were given one of the following treatments: aspirin 75 mg/day, EPO 4 g/day (7% to 11% GLA), fish oil 4 g/day (18% EPA, 12.8% DHA), aspirin plus EPO, aspirin plus fish oil. The control group received no treatment. After 1 month there was no change in platelet AII binding in the control group or in those taking EPO or fish oil alone. Aspirin with or without EPO caused a non-significant increase in AII binding. In the fish oil plus aspirin group there was a statistically significant decrease in AII binding.[112]

In a partially double-blinded, three-arm, placebo-controlled clinical trial, a combination of EPO and fish oil, magnesium oxide or a placebo was administered to pregnant women for 6 months; 21% of the women had personal or family histories of hypertension. Those taking the EPO and fish oil exhibited a significantly lower incidence of oedema (13%) compared with the control group (29%) (p=0.004). Significantly fewer women developed hypertension in the group receiving magnesium oxide. Three cases of eclampsia occurred, all in the control group.[113]

In an uncontrolled clinical trial, 12 hyperlipidaemic patients received 3 g/day GLA for 4 months. After treatment, plasma triglyceride levels were decreased by 48% (p<0.001), HDL-cholesterol levels increased by 22% (p<0.01) and total cholesterol and LDL-cholesterol levels were significantly decreased. Experimentally induced platelet aggregation and serum thromboxane B_2 levels decreased, with a significant increase in bleeding time.[114] These results were similar to those found in an earlier placebo-controlled, crossover clinical trial. Supplementation with EPO at a dose of 3.6 g/day resulted in an increase of DGLA in plasma lipids and red blood cells, and a significant decrease in LDL-cholesterol by 9.3% (p<0.01).[115]

In a double blind, placebo-controlled crossover study, 25 non-obese patients with uncomplicated essential hypertension received placebo for 4 weeks followed by EPO plus fish oil or sunflower seed and linseed oil for 12 weeks. The mean systolic blood pressure of patients receiving EPO plus fish oil was significantly lower after 8 and 12 weeks, while those receiving sunflower/linseed oil exhibited no significant reduction in blood pressure.[116]

In a double blind, placebo-controlled study, 21 patients with Raynaud's phenomenon received a 2-week course of placebo, after which 11 received EPO for 8 weeks and 10 received placebo. Patients receiving EPO experienced a significant improvement in symptoms, but there was no change in blood flow, despite changes in platelet behaviour and thromboxane B_2 levels.[117]

Cancer therapy

In a case-control study, 96 patients with advanced cancer of the gastrointestinal tract (oesophageal, gastric, hepatocellular, pancreas, colorectal, etc.) were given either EPO (up to 3000 mg/day GLA) or placebo in conjunction with palliative radiotherapy or chemotherapy. There was an obvious benefit for the EPO group, with a highly statistically significant survival difference between the two groups (p=0.0009).[118]

In an uncontrolled clinical trial, GLA was administered by intracerebral injection (1 mg/day for 10 days) to 15 patients with malignant gliomas. The cerebral gliomas regressed, as evidenced by computed tomography, and patients' survival was increased by 1.5 to 2 years.[119]

In a double blind, placebo-controlled trial, 62 patients with very advanced primary liver cancer were given either EPO capsules (supplying 1440 mg/day GLA) or olive oil capsules as a placebo. There was no statistically significant difference between the two groups for liver size or survival time, which was an average of 42 days in both groups. However, in the EPO group there was a significant decrease in serum gamma-glutamyltransferase which, according to the authors, can be interpreted as showing an effect on the tumour. The authors also comment that the large tumour size (up to 3 kg in some patients) may account for the lack of significant effect on survival time.[120]

EPO and vitamin C given to six patients with primary liver cell cancer demonstrated some clinical improvement and reduction in tumour size (three patients). One patient demonstrated a marked reduction of liver and tumour size and liver damage.[121]

Bone metabolism

In a clinical trial conducted in care homes for the aged, 40 women with confirmed osteoporosis were divided into four groups and received either fish oil, EPO, fish oil plus EPO, or olive oil (control) over 16 weeks. Serum alkaline phosphatase levels dropped in both the fish oil and the combined oil groups, indicating a favourable effect on bone metabolism. Osteocalcin levels, an indicator of bone growth, rose in the fish oil group and more significantly in the combined oil group. Although the EPO had no effect on its own, it appeared to increase the effect of the fish oil on these bone formation markers, possibly due to a more balanced plasma fatty acid profile.[122]

Similar beneficial effects were demonstrated in a 1998 controlled study. Sixty-five women (mean age 79.5 years), were given capsules containing either a combination of GLA + EPA or coconut oil (placebo). The active treatment was 6 g/day of a mixture of EPO and fish oil (8% GLA, 4% EPA, 3% DHA). All the women had confirmed osteoporosis or osteopenia. During the trial they were also supplemented with 600 mg/day of calcium carbonate. After 18 months there was an increase of 1.3% in femoral bone density in the treatment group, while in the placebo group there was a decrease of 2.1%. Lumbar spine density remained the same in the treatment group, but decreased by 3.2% in the placebo group. Twenty-one participants continued for a further 18 months, during which time all took the active treatment. At the end of this period lumbar spine density had increased by a further 3.1% in the patients who remained on the active treatment and by 2.3% in the group who switched from placebo to active treatment. Deoxypyridinoline levels fell significantly in both groups, indicating decreased bone degradation.[123]

However, such findings were not observed in a 12-month double blind, placebo-controlled trial published in 2000. In this trial, 43 premenopausal women (aged 25 to 40 years) and 42 postmenopausal women (aged 50 to 65 years) were given an active treatment consisting of 4000 mg EPO, 440 mg fish oil and 1000 mg calcium or a 'placebo' of 1000 mg/day calcium. There were no significant differences in total body bone mineral density between the active and placebo groups.[124] Perhaps the ratio of EPO to fish oil was not optimal.

Other effects

In a randomised, double blind, placebo-controlled trial lasting 6 months, patients with Sjögren's syndrome were given either 800 or 1600 mg/day of GLA as the free fatty acid or a placebo (corn oil with no GLA). There was no statistically significant change in fatigue (the primary outcome parameter) at evaluation after 3 or 6 months. There were also no statistically significant changes in other symptoms such as eye and mouth dryness or depression and no change in analgesic use.[125]

In a randomised, placebo-controlled study, 43 patients with stable ulcerative colitis received either EPO, fish oil or olive oil (placebo) for 6 months in addition to their usual medication. Alteration of cell membrane fatty acids was observed in those taking EPO and fish oil compared with the control group. Although there was no difference in stool frequency, rectal bleeding, disease relapse, sigmoidoscopic appearance or rectal histology in the three groups, EPO significantly improved stool consistency compared with fish oil and placebo at 6 months, and this difference was maintained 3 months after treatment was discontinued ($p<0.05$).[126]

In a double blind, placebo-controlled study, 63 patients with postviral fatigue syndrome received a preparation containing EPO (80%) and fish oil (20%) or placebo (8×500 mg capsules per day) over a 3-month period. At the end of the trial, 85% of patients in the treatment group compared to 17% in the control group assessed themselves as improved ($p<0.0001$). A normalisation of EFA levels in red blood cell membranes was observed in the treatment group.[127]

In a double blind, placebo-controlled clinical trial, the effect of giving EPO to alcoholics was investigated. In the early weeks of withdrawal from alcohol, EPO significantly reduced the severity of withdrawal syndrome and improved liver function. Relapse rates over 6 and 12 months did not improve. However, in those who did not relapse, several parameters of cerebral function (such as memory and visual motor coordination) improved significantly with EPO treatment.[78] A review of the role of EFAs in alcohol dependence notes that if alcohol-induced tissue damage is associated with impaired fatty acid and phospholipid metabolism, EFAs may be beneficial in the treatment of alcoholics.[128]

In a double blind, placebo-controlled study, 89 renal transplantation patients received either EPO or placebo, together with standard immunosuppressive medication. Graft survival was significantly better in the EPO group compared with controls during the first 3 to 4 months post-transplant, but not significantly different at 6 months.[129]

In the treatment of attention deficit hyperactivity disorder, EPO was of benefit in patients with borderline zinc levels in a small double blind, placebo-controlled, crossover trial.[130] An open pilot study investigated the effects of a high DHA fish oil plus EPO (providing 480 mg DHA, 108 mg EPA and 96 mg GLA per day) in 20 dyslexic children aged between 9 and 17 years.[131] Subjective parent and child assessments demonstrated increasing numbers of positive responders over the 5 months of the trial, in terms of reading speed, general schoolwork and overall benefit. Average reading speed increased by 60% from baseline ($p<0.01$), 13 of 17 children had a significant improvement on the word-chain test ($p<0.04$) and letter decoding (motoric-perceptual speed) was up by 23% ($p<0.05$).

Using a randomised, double blind, placebo-controlled design, 76 women wearing soft contact lenses suffering from dry eye symptoms were treated for 6 months with either EPO (containing 300 mg GLA per day) or a placebo (olive oil).[132] Compared with placebo treatment the EPO group showed a significant improvement in dryness at 3 and 6 months (p<0.01) and a slight but significant gain in overall lens comfort at 6 months (p<0.01). Tear meniscus height was increased in the EPO group at 6 months relative to baseline. Only 52 women completed the trial (p<0.01) and this relatively high dropout rate was attributed to non-compliance.

Toxicology and other safety data

Toxicology

Being an intermediate of normal human metabolism, GLA is unlikely to be harmful or toxic if it is consumed in quantities comparable to those formed within the human body; 20 mg/kg/day of GLA is likely to be formed from linolenic acid in a normal adult woman and 23 to 65 mg/kg/day of GLA may be consumed by a breastfed baby.[12]

In two sets of toxicity studies, effects of oral administration of EPO (containing 8.5 to 9% GLA, and 70% to 73% LA) were compared with corn oil (60% LA) and controls receiving no oil.[133,134] In rats (fed up to 2.5 mL/kg/day over 53 weeks) and dogs (fed up to 5 mL/kg/day over 52 weeks) there were no significant differences between tested groups in terms of clinical signs, food consumption or body weight changes. No consistent differences were seen in haematology or urinalysis results for rats or dogs, or in clinical chemistry for male rats. Serum potassium was marginally increased in female rats on the highest EPO dose. Male EPO-treated rats showed modestly reduced liver weights and a greater proportion showed testicular shrinkage or softening than in the control group. The authors concluded that no important adverse effects were produced by EPO administration and it is as safe as corn oil as a nutritional supplement.[1] No significant effect on tumour incidence was observed in the rats fed EPO compared with the other groups.[2]

Contraindications

None required.

Special warnings and precautions

EPO may have potential to instigate undiagnosed temporal lobe epilepsy, especially in those patients receiving phenothiazines.[135] This is unlikely on current evidence, but caution should apply (see Side effects).

Interactions

There is insufficient evidence to suggest avoiding concomitant use of EPO with phenothiazines (see Side effects).

There are no reports of an interaction between EPO and anticoagulants or antiplatelet drugs.

Use in pregnancy and lactation

Category B1 – no increase in frequency of malformation or other harmful effects on the fetus from limited use in women. No evidence of increased fetal damage in animal studies.

A retrospective study involving 108 nulliparous women found that oral administration of EPO from the 37th gestational week until birth did not shorten gestation or decrease the overall length of labour. There was a trend for the EPO group to have a more protracted active phase, prolonged rupture of membranes, oxytocin augmentation and arrest of descent. The prescribed dosage of EPO was 1500 mg/day for the first week, then 500 mg/day until labour began. The babies were slightly larger in the EPO group, but this is unlikely to account for the differences observed.[136] EPO has been trialled in pre-eclampsia with mixed results.[137,138] Diastolic pressor response to A II was significantly reduced in mid-trimester pregnant women who received EPO (320 mg/day of GLA) and vitamins compared to controls.[139]

In a 1999 survey of certified nurse-midwives in the US, EPO was reported to be used by 60% of the 90 respondents who used herbal medicine to stimulate labour. It was often applied topically for this purpose. There were no reported complications from the use of EPO.[140]

The diet of male and female blue foxes was supplemented with EPO (4.5 g/day), zinc sulphate (2.5 mg/day) and vitamin E (90 mg/day) to observe effects on reproduction. Compared with the control group, there was an increased rate of abortion in the EPO group, but simultaneously a non-significant decrease in the frequency of barren females. A tendency for increased litter size in the EPO group was found mainly as an effect of male treatment (suggesting an effect on semen quality).[141] EPO supplementation had a beneficial effect in pregnant zinc-deficient rats and subsequently in their newborn pups.[142] EPO had no effect on parturition or postnatal growth when fed to rats prior to mating.[143]

EPO is compatible with breastfeeding and GLA and LA are normally found in human milk.[144–146] A comparative study noted that the breast milk of allergic mothers contained less GLA than that of healthy mothers. The serum lipid fatty acid levels in atopic infants did not correlate with those in maternal breast milk.[147]

A placebo-controlled trial observed that maternal supplementation with EPO during breastfeeding raised the EFA and total fat content of breast milk.[148]

Effects on ability to drive and use machines

No adverse effects expected.

Side effects

General

The most common adverse effects reported in trials using GLA for the treatment of various conditions are headache, mild nausea and abdominal discomfort.[95]

Arachidonate build-up

The potential risk of arachidonate build-up associated with long-term use of GLA in the treatment of rheumatoid arthritis has been raised. Several tests have shown GLA administration increased arachidonate levels: 2 g/day of GLA given to previously obese women increased the arachidonate content of their serum phospholipids. With prolonged administration of GLA over more than a year, arachidonate could accumulate in tissue, thus possibly counteracting early therapeutic effects of GLA. Tissue build-up of arachidonate might promote subsequent inflammation, thrombosis and immunosuppression. Symptoms may rebound in patients after discontinuation of GLA.[149]

Epilepsy

Often repeated in the literature are concerns about the use of EPO in patients with a history of epilepsy. Originally this arose from three case reports and a trial in patients with schizophrenia who were being treated concomitantly with antischizophrenic drugs (phenothiazines and related compounds). Episodes of epilepsy were reported, but no definite link to EPO treatment was established. Rather, the nature of the illness and side effects of the conventional medication were the more likely cause. Similar events have been reported in patients not taking EPO.[78,150] Moreover, it can be extremely difficult to distinguish between schizophrenia and temporal lobe epilepsy. Three hospitalised schizophrenics who failed to respond to conventional drug therapy became substantially worse when treated with EPO. A later diagnosis of temporal lobe epilepsy resulted in successful treatment (with conventional drugs).[151] In two clinical trials conducted since this time, psychiatric patients (predominantly schizophrenics) who received EPO (540 to 600 mg/day GLA) did not experience such adverse effects.[152,153]

Perhaps in response to the trials in patients with schizophrenia, the British Epilepsy Association warned those with epilepsy to avoid EPO because of a possible lowering of the threshold for seizures.[135,154-156] This position is probably excessively cautious.

A 45-year-old woman who had been taking herbal preparations containing black cohosh, chaste tree and EPO for 4 months had three seizures within a 3-month period. The herbal preparations were stopped and the patient was treated with anticonvulsants.[157] No causal link between the seizures and the herbal treatment was established, much less the EPO.

Antiplatelet effect

Blood tests of patients with Raynaud's phenomenon who received EPO (6 g/day EPO, containing 8% GLA) indicated an antiplatelet effect. This was significant during the first 2 to 6 weeks of treatment, and there was a 'fall off' in effect by week 8.[158] In multiple sclerosis patients treated with EPO for 6 weeks (20 g/day EPO, containing 8% GLA), only platelet aggregation to thrombin was significantly reduced compared with controls. Overall, EPO did not show a significant effect on platelets of multiple sclerosis patients.[159] In hypertriglyceridaemic patients, GLA supplementation did not affect platelet function.[160]

Safety in children

Adverse effects are not expected. EPO and GLA have been administered to children in clinical trials.

Of the randomised clinical trials for the treatment of atopic eczema examined to the year 2000, seven trials involved children, with ages ranging from 0.8 to 16 years and treatment from 4 to 16 weeks. In most cases 0.5 to 4 g/day of EPO was administered. In one of these trials, 48 atopic children aged 2.2 to 8.5 years received placebo, low dose EPO or high dose EPO for 8 weeks. The high dose amounted to 500 mg/kg/day of EPO. No adverse effects were observed.[161]

In other early trials EPO was administered to children with atopic eczema,[162] hyperactivity,[163-166] type 1 diabetes (90 mg/day GLA for 4 months increasing to 180 mg/day for 4 months)[167] and cystic fibrosis (20 g/day EPO for 12 months).[168]

Overdosage

No incidents found in published literature. It is known that an excess of omega-6 EFAs can reduce the metabolism of ALA, possibly leading to a deficit of eicosapentaenoic acid and other metabolites.[169]

Regulatory status in selected countries

Evening primrose oil is not covered by a Commission E Monograph and is not on the UK General Sale List.

Evening primrose oil does not have GRAS status. However, it is freely available as a 'dietary supplement' in the USA under DSHEA legislation (1994 Dietary Supplement Health and Education Act).

Evening primrose oil is not included in Part 4 of Schedule 4 of the Therapeutic Goods Act Regulations of Australia and is freely available for sale.

References

1. Mabberley DJ. *The Plant Book*, 2nd ed. Cambridge: Cambridge University Press; 1997. p. 499.
2. Weiss RF. *Herbal Medicine*. Beaconsfield: Beaconsfield Publishers; 1988. p. 333.
3. Grieve M. *A Modern Herbal*, vol. 2. New York: Dover Publications; 1971. p. 657.
4. Leung AY, Foster S. *Encyclopedia of Common Natural Ingredients Used in Food, Drugs and Cosmetics*, 2nd ed. New York: John Wiley; 1996. p. 236.
5. Launert EL. *The Hamlyn Guide to Edible and Medicinal Plants of Britain and Northern Europe*. London: Hamlyn; 1981. p. 86.
6. Chiej R. *The Macdonald Encyclopedia of Medicinal Plants*. London: Macdonald; 1984. Entry no. 208.
7. Therapeutic Goods Administration. *Approved Terminology for Drugs*. Canberra: Australian Government Publishing Service; 1995.

8. Tyler VE, Brady LR, Robbers JE. *Pharmacognosy*, 9th ed. Philadelphia: Lea & Febiger; 1988. p. 471.
9. Redden PR, Lin X, Horrobin DF. *Chem Phys Lipids*. 1996;79(1):9–19.
10. Cameron NE, Cotter MA. *Diabetes*. 1997;46(suppl 2):S31–37.
11. Jamal GA. *Diabet Med*. 1994;11(2):145–149.
12. Julu POJ. *Diabetic Complicat*. 1988;2(4):185–188.
13. Tomlinson DR, Robinson JP, Compton AM, et al. *Diabetologia*. 1989;32(9):655–659.
14. Dines KC, Cotter MA, Cameron NE. *Prostagland Leukot Essent Fatty Acids*. 1996;55(3):159–165.
15. Omawari N, Dewhurst M, Vo P, et al. *Br J Pharmacol*. 1996;118(1):186–190.
16. Julu PO, Gow JW, Jamal GA. *J Lipid Mediat Cell Signal*. 1996;13(2):115–125.
17. Julu PO. *J Lipid Mediat Cell Signal*. 1996;13(2):99–113.
18. Ford I, Cotter MA, Cameron NE, et al. *Metabolism*. 2001;50(8):868–875.
19. Shotton HR, Broadbent S, Lincoln J. *Auton Neurosci*. 2004;111(1):57–65.
20. Chaintreuil J, Monnier L, Colette C, et al. *Hum Nutr Clin Nutr*. 1984;38(2):121–130.
21. Karmali RA. *Prostagland Leukot Med*. 1987;29(2–3):199–204.
22. Tate GA, Mandell BF, Karmali RA, et al. *Arthritis Rheum*. 1988;31(12):1543–1551.
23. Tate GA, Mandell BF, Laposata M, et al. *J Rheumatol*. 1989;16(6):729–734.
24. Prichard P, Brown G, Bhaskar N, et al. *Aliment Pharmacol Ther*. 1988;2(2):179–184.
25. De La Hunt MN, Hillier K, Jewell R. *Prostaglandins*. 1988;35(4):597–608.
26. Huang YS, Drummond R, Horrobin DF. *Digestion*. 1987;36(1):36–41.
27. Raederstorff D, Moser U. *Lipids*. 1992;27(12):1018–1023.
28. de La Puerta Vazquez R, Martinez-Dominguez E, et al. *Metabolism*. 2004;53(1):59–65.
29. Claassen N, Coetzer H, Steinmann CM, et al. *Prostagland Leukot Essent Fatty Acids*. 1995;53(1):13–19.
30. Claassen N, Potgieter HC, Seppa M, et al. *Bone*. 1995;16(4 suppl):385S–392S.
31. Tauson AH, Forsberg M. *Acta Vet Scand*. 1991;32(3):345–351.
32. Tauson AH, Neil M, Forsberg M. *Acta Vet Scand*. 1991;32(3):337–344.
33. Begin ME, Ells G, Horrobin DF. *J Natl Cancer Inst*. 1988;80(3):188–194.
34. Begin ME, Ells G, Das UN. *Anticancer Res*. 1986;6(2):291–295.
35. Das UN, Begin ME, Ells G, et al. *Biochem Biophys Res Commun*. 1987;145(1):15–24.
36. Pritchard GA, Jones DL, Mansel RE. *Br J Surg*. 1989;76(10):1069–1073.
37. Hoffmann P, Taube C, Bartels T, et al. *Biomed Biochim Acta*. 1984;43(8–9):S195–S198.
38. Hassall CH, Kirtland SJ. *Lipids*. 1984;19(9):699–703.
39. Narce M, Poisson JP. *Arch Mal Coeur Vaiss*. 1996;89(8):1025–1028.
40. Mills DE, Ward RP, Mah M, et al. *Lipids*. 1989;24(1):17–24.
41. Mills DE, Summers MR, Ward RP, et al. *Lipids*. 1985;20(9):573–577.
42. Mills DE, Ward RP. *Lipids*. 1986;21(2):139–142.
43. Morphake P, Bariety J, Darlametsos I, et al. *Prostaglandins Leukot Essent Fatty Acids*. 1994;50(1):29–35.
44. Darlametsos IE, Varonos DD. *Prostaglandins Leukot Essent Fatty Acids*. 2001;64(4&5):231–239.
45. Fan YY, Ramos KS, Chapkin RS. *J Nutr*. 2001;131(6):1675–1681.
46. Al-Shabanah OA. *Food Chem Toxicol*. 1997;35(8):769–775.
47. Varma PK, Persaud TV. *Prostaglandins Leukot Med*. 1982;8(6):641–645.
48. Barcelli UO, Miyata J, Ito Y, et al. *Prostaglandins*. 1986;32(2):211–219.
49. Papanikolaou N. *Prostaglandins Leukot Med*. 1987;27(2–3):129–149.
50. Bezard J, Blond JP, Bernard A, et al. *Reprod Nutr Dev*. 1994;34(6):539–568.
51. Martens-Lobenhoffer J, Meyer FP. *Int J Clin Pharmacol Ther*. 1998;36(7):363–366.
52. Leichsenring M, Kochsiek U, Paul K. *Pediatr Allergy Immunol*. 1995;6(4):209–212.
53. Johnson MM, Swan DD, Surette ME, et al. *J Nutr*. 1997;127(8):1435–1444.
54. Harvey RG. *Vet Rec*. 1993;133(23):571–573.
55. Harvey RG. *Vet Rec*. 1993;133(9):208–211.
56. Scarff DH, Lloyd DH. *Vet Rec*. 1992;131(5):97–99.
57. Janossy IM, Raguz JM, Rippke F, et al. *H & GJ*. 1995;70:498–502.
58. Fiocchi A, Sala M, Signoroni P, et al. *J Int Med Res*. 1994;22(1):24–32.
59. Stewart JCM, Morse PF, Moss M, et al. Cited in Horrobin DF. *Rev Contemp Pharmacother*. 1990;1:1–45.
60. Schalin-Karrila M, Mattila L, Jansen CT, et al. *Br J Dermatol*. 1987;117(1):11–19.
61. Marshall RJ, Evans RW. Cited in Horrobin DF, ed. *Omega-6 Essential Fatty Acids: Pathophysiology and Roles in Clinical Medicine*, New York: Wiley Liss; 1990: pp. 81–98.
62. Nissen HP, Wehrmann W, Kvoll U, et al. *Fat Sci Technol*. 1988;7:247.
63. Senapati S, Sanerjee S, Gangopadhyay DN. *Indian J Dermatol Venereol Leprol*. 2008;74(5):447–452.
64. Yoon S, Lee J, Lee S. *Skin Pharmacol Appl Skin Physiol*. 2002;15(1):20–25.
65. Biagi PL, Bordoni A, Hrelia S, et al. *Drugs Exp Clin Res*. 1994;20(2):77–84.
66. Humphreys F, Symons JA, Brown HK, et al. *Eur J Dermatol*. 1994;4(8):598–603.
67. Bordoni A, Biagi PL, Masi M, et al. *Drugs Exp Clin Res*. 1988;14(4):291–297.
68. Morse PF, Horrobin DF, Manku MS, et al. *Br J Dermatol*. 1989;121(1):75–90.
69. Williams HC. *BMJ*. 2003;327(7428):1358–1359.
70. Kerscher MJ, Korting HC. *Clin Invest*. 1992;70(2):167–171.
71. Hederos CA, Berg A. *Arch Dis Child*. 1996;75(6):494–497.
72. Borrek S, Hildebrande A, Forster J. *Klin Paediatr*. 1997;209(3):100–104.
73. Whitaker DK, Cilliers J, De Beer C. *Dermatology*. 1996;193(2):115–120.
74. Berth-Jones J, Graham-Brown RA. *Lancet*. 1993;341(8860):1557–1560.
75. Williams HC, Grindlay DJ. *Clin Exp Dermatol*. 2008;33(6):685–688.
76. Morse NL, Clough PM. *Curr Pharm Biotechnol*. 2006;7(6):503–524.
77. Oliwiecki S, Burton JL. *Clin Exp Dermatol*. 1994;19(2):127–129.
78. Horrobin DF. *Rev Contemp Pharmacother*. 1990;1:1–45.
79. Puolakka J, Makarainen L, Viinikka L, et al. *J Reprod Med*. 1985;30(3):149–153.
80. Horrobin DF. *J Reprod Med*. 1983;28(7):465–468.
81. Budeiri D, Li Wan Po A, Dornan JC. *Control Clin Trials*. 1996;17(1):60–68.
82. Gateley CA, Miers M, Mansel RE, et al. *J Roy Soc Med*. 1992;85(1):12–15.
83. Pye JK, Mansel RE, Hughes LE. *Lancet*. 1985;2(8451):373–377.
84. Dickerson LM, Mazyck PJ, Hunter MH. *Am Fam Physician*. 2003;67(8):1743–1752.
85. Norlock FE. *J Am Med Womens Assoc*. 2002;57(2):85–90.
86. Rosolowich V, Saettler E, et al. *J Obstet Gynaecol Can*. 2006;28(1):49–57.
87. Blommers J, Elisabeth SM, et al. *Am J Ostet Gynecol*. 2002;187(5):1389–1394.
88. Qureshi S, Sultan N. *Surgeon*. 2005;3(1):7–10.
89. Goyal A, Mansel RE. *Breast J*. 2005;11(1):41–47.
90. Chenoy R, Hussain S, Tayob Y, et al. *Br Med J*. 1994;308(6927):501–503.
91. Keen H, Payan J, Allawi J, et al. *Diabetes Care*. 1993;16(1):8–15.
92. Scotia Pharmaceuticals Ltd. *Pioneering Research in Diabetic Neuropathy. The EF4 Project: The Role of Gamma-Linolenic Acid*. England: Scotia Pharmaceuticals; 1991. pp. 11–16.
93. Jamal GA, Carmichael H. *Diabet Med*. 1990;7(4):319–323.
94. Purewal TS, Evans PMS, et al. *Diabetologia*. 1997;40(suppl 1): Abstract 2187, A556. Cited in Halat KM, Denneby CE. *J Am Board Fam Pract*. 2003;16(1):47–57.
95. Joe LA, Hart LL. *Ann Pharmacother*. 1993;27(12):1475–1477.
96. Cameron M, Gagnier JJ, Little CV, et al. *Phytother Res*. 2009;23(12):1647–1662.

97. Leventhal LJ, Boyce EG, Zurier RB. *Ann Intern Med.* 1993;119(9):867–873.

98. Jantti J, Seppala E, Vapaatalo H, et al. *Clin Rheumatol.* 1989;8(2):238–244.

99. Belch JJ, Ansell D, Madhok R, et al. *Ann Rheum Dis.* 1988;47(2):96–104.

100. Brzeski M, Madhok R, Capell HA. *Br J Rheumatol.* 1991;30(5):370–372.

101. Zurier RB, Rossetti RG, Jacobson EW, et al. *Arthritis Rheum.* 1996;39(11): 1808–1817.

102. Veale DJ, Torley HI, Richards IM, et al. *Br J Rheumatol.* 1994;33(10):954–958.

103. Horrobin DF, Manku MS, Morse-Fisher N, et al. *Biol Psychiatry.* 1989;25(5): 562–568.

104. Bates C, Horrobin DF, Ells K. *Schizophr Res.* 1991;6(1):1–7.

105. Kaiya H, Horrobin DF, Manku MS, et al. *Biol Psychiatry.* 1991;30(4):357–362.

106. Vaddadi KS, Gilleard CJ, Mindham RH, et al. *Psychopharmacology (Berl).* 1986;88(3):362–367.

107. Vaddadi KS. *Prostaglandins Leukot Essent Fatty Acids.* 1992;46(1):67–70.

108. Vaddadi KS, Courtney P, Gilleard CJ, et al. *Psychiatry Res.* 1989;27(3):313–323.

109. Vaddadi K. *Prostaglandins Leukot Essent Fatty Acids.* 1996;55(1–2):89–94.

110. Joy CB, Mumby-Croft R, Joy LA. *Cochrane Database Syst Rev.* 2006;3 CD001257

111. Hornych A, Oravec S, et al. *Bratisl Lek Listy.* 2002;103(3):101–107.

112. Walker T, Singh PK, et al. *J Obstet Gynaecol.* 1999;19(1):56–58.

113. D'Almeida A, Carter JP, Anatol A, et al. *Women Health.* 1992;19(2–3): 117–131.

114. Guivernau M, Meza N, Barja P, et al. *Prostaglandins Leukot Essent Fatty Acids.* 1994;51(5):311–316.

115. Ishikawa T, Fujiyama Y, et al. *Atherosclerosis.* 1989;75(2–3):95–104.

116. Venter CP, Joubert PH, Booyens J. *Prostaglandins Leukot Essent Fatty Acids.* 1988;33(1):49–51.

117. Belch JJ, Shaw B, O'Dowd A, et al. *Thromb Haemost.* 1985;54(2):490–494.

118. Manolakis G, van der Merwe C, Hager E. *Dtsch Z Onkol.* 1995;27(5):124–129. Cited in Boon H, Wong J. *Expert Opin Pharmacother.* 2004;5(12):2485–2501

119. Das UN, Prasad VV, Reddy DR. *Cancer Lett.* 1995;94(2):147–155.

120. van der Merwe CF, Booyens J, et al. *Prostaglandins Leukot Essent Fatty Acids.* 1990;40(3):199–202.

121. Booyens J, Louwrens C, Engelbrecht P. *S Afr J Sci.* 1984;80:144.

122. Van Papendorp DH, Coetzer H, Kruger MC. *Nutr Res.* 1995;15(3):325–334.

123. Kruger MC, Coetzer H, et al. *Aging (Milano).* 1998;10(5):385–394.

124. Bassey EJ, Littlewood JJ, et al. *Br J Nutr.* 2000;83(6):629–635.

125. Theander E, Horrobin DF, et al. *Scand J Rheumatol.* 2002;31:72–79.

126. Greenfield SM, Green AT, Teare JP, et al. *Aliment Pharmacol Ther.* 1993;7(2): 159–166.

127. Behan PO, Behan WM, Horrobin D. *Acta Neurol Scand.* 1990;82(3):209–216.

128. Glen I, Skinner F, Glen E, et al. *Alcohol Clin Exp Res.* 1987;11(1):37–41.

129. McHugh MI, Wilkinson R, Elliott RW, et al. *Transplantation.* 1977;24(4): 263–267.

130. Arnold LE, Pinkham SM, Votolato N. *J Child Adolesc Psychopharmacol.* 2000;10(2):111–117.

131. Lindmark L, Clough P. *J Med Food.* 2007;10(4):662–666.

132. Kokke KH, Morris JA, Lawrenson JG. *Cont Lens Anterior Eye.* 2008;31(3):141–146.

133. Everett DJ, Greenough RJ, Perry CJ, et al. *Med Sci Res.* 1988;16:863–864.

134. Everett DJ, Perry CJ, Bayliss P. *Med Sci Res.* 1988;16:865–866.

135. Lin Wan Po A. *Pharmaceut J.* 1991: 676–678.

136. Dove D, Johnson P. *J Nurse Midwifery.* 1999;44(3):320–324.

137. Laivuori H, Hovatta O, Viinikka L, et al. *Prostaglandins Leukot Essent Fatty Acids.* 1993;49(3):691–694.

138. D'Almeida A, Carter JP, Anatol A, et al. *Women Health.* 1992;19(2–3):117–131.

139. O'Brien PMS, Morrison R, Pipkin FB. *Br J Clin Pharmacol.* 1985;19:335–342.

140. McFarlin BL, Gibson MH, O'Rear J, et al. *J Nurse Midwifery.* 1999;44(3):205–216.

141. Tauson AH, Forsberg M. *Acta Vet Scand.* 1991;32(3):345–351.

142. Dib A, Carreau JP. *Ann Nutr Metab.* 1987;31(5):312–319.

143. Leaver HA, Lytton FD, Dyson H, et al. *Prog Lipid Res.* 1986;25:143–146.

144. Gibson RA, Kneebone GM. *Am J Clin Nutr.* 1981;34(2):252–257.

145. Harzer G, Haug M, Dieterich I, et al. *Am J Clin Nutr.* 1983;37(4):612–621.

146. Carter JP. *Food Technol.* 1988;42(6):72–82.

147. Kankaanpaa P, Nurmela K, Erkkila A, et al. *Allergy.* 2001;56(7):633–638.

148. Cant A, Shay J, Horrobin DF. *J Nutr Sci Vitaminol.* 1991;37(6):573–579.

149. Phinney S. *Ann Intern Med.* 1994;120(8):692.

150. Holman CP, Bell AFJ. *J Orthomol Psychiatry.* 1983;12:302–304.

151. Vaddadi KS. *Prostagland Med.* 1981;6(4):375–379.

152. Vaddadi KS, Courtney P, Gilleard CJ, et al. *Psychiatry Res.* 1989;27(3):313–323.

153. Wolkin A, Jordan B, Peselow E, et al. *Am J Psychiatry.* 1986;143(7):912–914.

154. Dobbin SN. *Vet Rec.* 1992;131(25–26):591.

155. Arundel BL. *Vet Rec.* 1992;131(23):543.

156. Editorial *Curr Therapeut.* 1992;67

157. Shuster J. *Hosp Pharm.* 1996;31: 1553–1554.

158. Belch JJ, Shaw B, O'Dowd A, et al. *Thromb Haemost.* 1985;54(2):490–494.

159. McGregor L, Smith AD, Sidey M, et al. *Acta Neurol Scand.* 1989;80(1):23–27.

160. Boberg M, Vessby B, Selinus I. *Acta Med Scand.* 1986;220(2):153–160.

161. Biagi PL, Bordoni A, Hrelia S, et al. *Drugs Exp Clin Res.* 1994;20(2):77–84.

162. Biagi PL, Bordoni A, Masi M, et al. *Drugs Exp Clin Res.* 1988;14(4):285–290.

163. Aman MG, Mitchell EA, Turbott SH. *J Abnorm Child Psychol.* 1987;15(1): 75–90.

164. Arnold LE, Kleykamp D, Votolato NA, et al. *Biol Psychiatry.* 1989;25:222–228.

165. Colquhoun I, Bunday S. *Med Hypotheses.* 1981;7(5):673–679.

166. Gibson RA. *Proc Nutr Soc Aust.* 1985;10:196.

167. Arisaka M, Arisaka O, Yamashiro Y. *Prostaglandins Leukot Essent Fatty Acids.* 1991;43(3):197–201.

168. Horrobin DF. *Prog Lipid Res.* 1992;31(2):163–194.

169. Belch JJF, Hill A. *Am J Clin Nutr.* 2000;71(suppl 1):352S–356S.

Eyebright

(*Euphrasia officinalis* L.)

Synonyms

Euphrasia rostkoviana Hayne (botanical synonym), Euphrasiae herba (Lat), Augentrostkraut (Ger), herbe d'euphraise officinale, casse-lunettes (Fr), eufrasia (Ital), lægeøjentrøst (Dan).

What is it?

The name Euphrasia is derived from the Greek word *euphrosyne*, meaning gladness, due to its use in folk medicine for the treatment of eye complaints. It is this use that also gave rise to the vernacular name eyebright. The aerial parts of eyebright can be used topically as a poultice or eyewash for external eye problems and as a nasal douche for inflamed or catarrhal mucous membranes. It can also be taken orally for these conditions.

Effects

Relieves conjunctivitis, itchy, irritated eyes; reduces excessive upper respiratory secretions and catarrh.

Traditional view

Eyebright was used in the 14th century as an eye medicine and was said to 'cure all evils of the eye'.[1] It was considered slightly tonic and astringent and was employed for all mucous diseases attended with increased discharges, specifically for the nasal membranes and lacrimal apparatus (acute catarrhal diseases of the eyes, nose and ears). Catarrhal diseases of the digestive tract were also treated with eyebright.[2]

Summary of actions

Astringent, anticatarrhal, anti-inflammatory.

Can be used for

Indications supported by clinical trials

Indication supported by a trial using a topical homeopathic form of eyebright (D2, a 1:10 dilution of mother tincture) and rose oil: conjunctivitis.

Traditional therapeutic uses

Eye conditions such as irritation and redness, infection, inflammation, particularly conjunctivitis and blepharitis;[2] nasal catarrh, particularly where there is profuse watery flow;[2] sinusitis, chronic sneezing, hayfever and middle ear problems; sore throat; the catarrhal phase that occurs during and after measles.[3]

May also be used for

Extrapolations from pharmacological studies

Because of its aucubin content, eyebright may be useful in the treatment of bacterial infections and liver toxicity. It may also possess antiviral and nerve-regenerating activity for the same reason.

Preparations

Dried or fresh herb as an infusion, poultice or liquid extract for topical use. Infusion, extract, capsules or tablets for internal use. For use in eyebaths, decoctions of greater than 10 minutes at boiling point, with transfer to a sterile container, are recommended.

Dosage

- 6 to 12 g/day or as an infusion
- 3 to 6 mL/day of 1:2 liquid extract; 7.5 to 15 mL/day of 1:5 tincture or equivalent doses in tablets or capsules.

For topical use a solution of approximately five to six drops of a 1:2 extract can be added to an eyebath containing recently boiled water or saline. The mixture should be allowed to cool before applying to the eye as a 30 to 60 second bath. (Allowing much of the alcohol to evaporate before applying to the eye is important).

Duration of use

May be taken long term.

Summary assessment of safety

No significant adverse effects from topical use or ingestion of eyebright are expected; however, the requirement for sterility of topical preparations for the eye should be observed.

Technical data

Botany

Euphrasia officinalis, in the narrow sense equivalent to *E. rostkoviana*,[4] is a small plant that grows to approximately 15 cm in height and is a member of the Orobanchaceae (broomrape) family. The leaves are opposite, ovate or cordate, downy, strongly ribbed and furrowed. The inodorous flowers are axillary, solitary and very abundant. They are most commonly white, with deep purple streaks and a yellowish palate. The oblong, flattened seed pods contain numerous seeds that are oblong and grooved lengthwise.[2]

Adulteration

The nomenclature for this species is under debate. Medicinal eyebright includes various *Euphrasia* species, but especially the taxa grouped around *E. rostkoviana* Hayne (including *E. officinalis* L. – an ambiguous name) and *E. stricta* D. Wolff ex J.F. Lehm, as well as their hybrids. The classification of the genus *Euphrasia* differs greatly in the literature.[5] The US Department of Agriculture lists *E. rostkoviana* Hayne as preferred to the previous *E. officinalis* L., nom. ambig.[6] The *Flora Europaea* continues to list *Euphrasia officinalis* L., nom. ambig., albeit with a provisional name status.

A nomenclature study published in 1991 suggested *Euphrasia officinalis* L. may be divided into several subspecies including *E. officinalis* spp. *rostkoviana* (Hayne) Townsend (synonym *Euphrasia rostkoviana* Hayne).[7] In addition to the species listed here, many other species of *Euphrasia* are regarded as medicinal. Due to the different systematic organisations of the genus *Euphrasia* and/or the ambiguity of some species or varieties within the species, adulteration is probable. The significance of substitution with other *Euphrasia* species is not known.[8]

Key constituents

- Iridoid glycosides, including aucubin, catalpol, euphroside and ixoroside[9]
- Flavonoids, including quercetin and apigenin glycosides; lignans.[9]

Aucubin   **Euphroside**

Pharmacodynamics

Most of the published pharmacodynamic studies have examined the constituent aucubin or its aglycone. Aucubin is common to many other plants, including *Plantago lanceolata*. The fact that plants containing aucubin have been used in many different traditions for the treatment of respiratory catarrh suggests that aucubin may possess clinically relevant antimicrobial and anticatarrhal activities.

Antimicrobial activity

Aucubigenin, the aglycone of aucubin, was shown to be antibacterial against organisms such as *Micrococcus aureus*, *Escherichia coli*, *Bacillus subtilis* and *Mycobacterium phlei*, and to a lesser extent showed modest antifungal activity against a small number of fungi, with *Penicillium italicum* being the most sensitive.[10] Petroleum ether, ethanolic and aqueous extracts of eyebright had no activity against strains of *Candida albicans* in vitro.[11]

Aucubin alone had no antiviral activity in vitro. However, when aucubin (100 to 1000 μM/mL) was mixed with beta-glucosidase (an enzyme that releases the aglycone from the glycoside), it had significant antiviral activity against hepatitis B.[12]

Hepatoprotective activity

In vivo studies demonstrated that aucubin exerted hepatoprotective activity against such liver toxins as carbon tetrachloride,[13] alpha-amanitin[14] and an aqueous extract of amanita mushroom. Even post-administration of aucubin after amanita mushroom ingestion led to complete survival.[15]

An in vitro study demonstrated that aucubigenin inhibited cytochrome P450 in isolated rat hepatocytes. Aucubin had no effect. The authors commented that the reported hepatoprotection of aucubin against carbon tetrachloride would appear to be due to inactivation of P450 by the aglycone aucubigenin, which is probably formed in vivo through hydrolysis in the gut.[16]

Antitumour activity

When administered intraperitoneally at a dose of 100 mg/kg, the aglycone of aucubin was found to have antitumour activity in mice bearing the experimental tumour leukaemia P388. Aucubin, also administered intraperitoneally (100 mg/kg), showed no antitumour activity. It therefore appears that the hemiacetal aglycone structure is important for the antitumour activity.[17]

Spasmolytic activity

Peracetylated aucubin in vitro exerted a non-specific spasmolytic effect on contractions of rat uterus induced by acetylcholine and calcium chloride. In vitro spasmolytic activity was also found for rat vas deferens depolarised by potassium. The degree of activity was similar to papaverine.[18]

Anti-inflammatory activity

The aglycone of aucubin, but not aucubin itself, suppressed tumour necrosis factor-alpha (TNF-alpha) production in vitro.[19] This contrasts with an earlier study that found aucubin did inhibit TNF-alpha,[20] but such a finding is unlikely as the intact glycoside (aucubin) does not readily penetrate cell membranes.[19] Aucubin ($100\,\mu$M) inhibited leukotriene C_4 release from stimulated mouse peritoneal macrophages and inhibited thromboxane B_2 release from stimulated platelets, but had no effect on prostaglandin E_2 release.[21] Aucubin, administered orally at a dose of $100\,mg/kg$, had an anti-inflammatory effect in carrageenan-induced mouse paw oedema.[22] An anti-inflammatory effect was also shown on TPA-induced mouse ear oedema with topical application of $1\,mg/ear$ of aucubin.[22]

Other activity

The most important feature in neuronal cell differentiation is outgrowth of neurites. Regulation of this outgrowth is considered to be one of the most basic mechanisms in the development and regeneration of nerve tissue. Discovery of agents that increase the outgrowth of neurites could lead to the development of antidementia drugs, since dementia is characterised by progressive neuronal degeneration.[23] The aglycone of aucubin (at a dose of 1 and $10\,\mu g/mL$), but not aucubin itself, was effective in inducing a cultured cell line of paraneuron PC12h to differentiate, causing a morphological change characterised by extended neurites and promotion of neurite outgrowth.[23,24]

Pharmacokinetics

Anaerobic incubation of aucubin with defined strains of human intestinal bacteria and with human faeces resulted in its transformation into aucubigenin and the pyridine monoterpene alkaloids aucubinine A and aucubinine B. Among the 25 species isolated from human faeces that were examined, 21 species produced aucubinine A and a trace of aucubinine B. Aucubin may be initially hydrolysed to aucubigenin and glucose by bacterial beta-glucosidase, followed by a series of reactions, the first involving ammonia, to yield the aucubinines. The nitrogen atom could originate from the ammonia produced by bacteria (some species such as *Klebsiella pneumoniae* contain high levels of intracellular ammonia).[25] This finding suggests that, in order to convert aucubin into the active aglycone aucubigenin, there must be high levels of favourable gut bacteria. There is also the distinct possibility that other bacterial metabolites of aucubin, such as the aucubinines, might contribute to its oral activity.

In another pharmacokinetic study, aucubin was given intravenously, orally, intraperitoneally and hepatoportally to rats. The bioavailability of aucubin after administration at a dose of $100\,mg/kg$ through hepatoportal, intraperitoneal and oral routes was 83.5%, 76.8% and 19.3% respectively. The moderate oral bioavailability of aucubin is probably due to its metabolism by gut flora as outlined above.[26]

Clinical trials

A prospective, open label multicentre trial conducted in Germany and Switzerland evaluated the efficacy of eyebright eyedrops in patients with inflammatory or catarrhal conjunctivitis. One drop was prescribed one to five times per day. Of the 65 patients that completed the study, 53 patients had a complete recovery, and 11 patients experienced a clear improvement. Efficacy parameters were redness, swelling, secretion, burning of the conjunctiva, foreign body sensation and veiled vision. The degree of severity was assessed relative to baseline after approximately 7 and 14 days. Efficacy and tolerability were evaluated by patients and clinicians as good to very good in more than 85%. The eye drops contained a homeopathic form of eyebright (D2, a 1:10 dilution of mother tincture) and rose oil.[27] However, this dilution is still likely to be pharmacologically active after direct topical application.

Toxicology and other safety data

Toxicology

No symptoms indicative of toxicity were observed over a 72-hour period in rats orally administered an aqueous extract of *E. officinalis* leaf (0.1 to $6\,g/kg$).[28] Respiratory depression and hypothermia were observed after the intraperitoneal administration of aucubin ($100\,mg/kg$) to rats.[29]

Eyebright tincture demonstrated in vitro mutagenic activity in the Ames test.[30]

Contraindications

None known.

Special warnings and precautions

Topical eye preparations need to be sterile. Normal herbal tinctures or extracts should never be applied directly to the eyes because of their ethanol content.

Interactions

No adverse interactions known.

Use in pregnancy and lactation

Category B – no increase in frequency of malformation or other harmful effects on the fetus from limited use in women. Animal studies are lacking.

Eyebright is compatible with breastfeeding on available information.

Effects on ability to drive and use machines

No adverse effects expected.

Side effects

None known.

Overdosage

No effects known.

Safety in children

No information available, but adverse effects are not expected.

Regulatory status in selected countries

Eyebright is covered by a null Commission E Monograph. The Commission E recommends that, as the efficacy has not been documented, the topical application of eyebright cannot be recommended because of hygienic reasons.

Eyebright is on the UK General Sale List.

Eyebright does not have GRAS status. However, it is freely available as a 'dietary supplement' in the USA under DSHEA legislation (1994 Dietary Supplement Health and Education Act).

Eyebright is not included in Part 4 of Schedule 4 of the Therapeutic Goods Act Regulations of Australia and is freely available for sale.

References

1. Grieve M. *A Modern Herbal*, vol 1. New York: Dover; 1971. pp. 290–293.
2. Felter HW, Lloyd JU. *King's American Dispensatory*, ed 18, vol 2, rev 3, 1905, Portland. Reprinted by Eclectic Medical Publications; 1983. pp. 751–752.
3. Bartram T. *Encyclopedia of Herbal Medicine*. Dorset: Grace Publishers; 1995. p. 177.
4. Mabberley DJ, ed. *The Plant Book*. 2nd ed. Cambridge: Cambridge University Press; 1997.
5. Bisset NG, ed. *Herbal Drugs and Phytopharmaceuticals: A Handbook for Practice on a Scientific Basis*. Stuttgart: Medpharm Scientific; 1994.
6. Wiersema JH, Leon B. *World Economic Plants: A Standard Reference*. Florida: CRC Press; 1999. p. 221.
7. Silverside AJ. *Watsonia*. 1991;18:343–350.
8. Blaschek W, Ebel S, Hackenthal E, et al. *Hagers Handbuch der Drogen und Arzneistoffe*. Heidelberg: Springer; 2002.
9. Wagner H, Bladt S. *Plant Drug Analysis: A Thin Layer Chromatography Atlas*, 2nd ed. Berlin: Springer-Verlag; 1996. p. 75.
10. Rombouts JE, Links J. *Experientia*. 1956;12(2):78–80.
11. Trovato A, Monforte MT, Forestieri AM, et al. *Boll Chim Farm*. 2000;139(5):225–227.
12. Chang I. *Phytother Res*. 1997;11:189–192.
13. Chang IM, Ryu JC, Park YC, et al. *Drug Chem Toxicol*. 1983;6(5):443–453.
14. Chang IM, Yun HS, Kim YS, et al. *J Toxicol Clin Toxicol*. 1984;22(1):77–85.
15. Chang IM, Yamaura Y. *Phytother Res*. 1993;7:53–56.
16. Bartholomaeus A, Ahokas J. *Toxicol Lett*. 1995;80:75–83.
17. Isiguro K, Yamaki M, Takagi S, et al. *Chem Pharm Bull*. 1986;34(6):2375–2379.
18. Ortiz de Urbina AV, Martin ML, Fernandez B, et al. *Planta Med*. 1994;60:512–515.
19. Park KS, Chang IM. *Planta Med*. 2004;70(8):778–779.
20. Jeong HJ, Koo HN, Na HJ, et al. *Cytokine*. 2002;18(5):252–259.
21. Bermejo Benito P, Diaz Lanza AM, Silvan Sen AM, et al. *Planta Med*. 2000;66(4):324–328.
22. Recio M, Giner RM, Manez S, et al. *Planta Med*. 1994;60:232–234.
23. Yamazaki M, Hirota K, Chiba K, et al. *Biol Pharm Bull*. 1994;17(12):1604–1608.
24. Yamazaki M, Chiba K, Mohri T. *Biol Pharm Bull*. 1996;19(6):791–795.
25. Hattori M, Kawata Y, Inoue K, et al. *Phytother Res*. 1990;4(2):66–70.
26. Suh N, Shim C, Lee MH, et al. *Pharm Res*. 1991;8(8):1059–1063.
27. Stoss M, Michels C, Peter E, et al. *J Altern Complement Med*. 2000;6(6):499–508.
28. Porchezhian E, Ansari SH, Shreedharan NKK. *Fitoterapia*. 2000;71:522–526.
29. Ortiz de Urbina AV, Martin ML, Fernandez B, et al. *Planta Med*. 1994;60:512–515.
30. Schimmer O, Kruger A, Paulini H, et al. *Pharmazie*. 1994;49:448–451.

(*Foeniculum vulgare* Mill.)

Synonyms

Foeniculum officinale Mill. (botanical synonym), Foeniculi fructus (Lat), Fenchel, Bitterfenchel (Ger), aneth fenouil, fenouil (Fr), finocchio (Ital), fennikel frø (Dan), xian hui xiang (Chin).

What is it?

Fennel is a well-known culinary herb and vegetable. It was cultivated by the ancient Romans for its aromatic fruit and succulent edible shoots and was frequently listed in Anglo-Saxon cookery and medical recipes prior to the Norman Conquest. Fennel shoots, fennel seed and fennel water were all mentioned in ancient Spanish agricultural records. In medieval times fennel, in conjunction with St John's wort and other herbs, was hung over doors on Midsummer's Eve to ward off evil spirits. Similarly, it was used as a condiment for the salt fish consumed during Lent. Fennel seeds were discovered amongst the personal chattels salvaged from the tombs of Egyptian pharaohs.

The fruit (often called the seed) and root are the parts most commonly used for medical purposes (although the root is no longer used as it is considered inferior to the fruit). The exact species definition varies between different authorities, but it is agreed that *Foeniculum vulgare* Miller is represented by two varieties in cultivation (with common names designated as bitter fennel and sweet fennel).[1,2] These different varieties of fennel are difficult to separate, mainly due to their tendency to hybridise.[3]

Effects

Relaxes sphincters and decreases spasm of the gastrointestinal tract; acts as an expectorant in the respiratory tract, increases the mucociliary activity of the ciliary epithelium; exerts oestrogenic activity, increases milk flow.

Traditional view

Fennel was used as a carminative to treat flatulent colic, windy colic in infants, irritable bowel syndrome and to increase appetite.[4] It had an ancient reputation for strengthening eyesight and was used topically to treat conjunctivitis and blepharitis.[5,6] The fruits are said to benefit nausea, hiccups, shortness of breath and wheezing. Syrup made from the fresh juice was used for chronic coughs. The leaves were once used by poor people to satisfy the cravings of hunger on fasting days.[5] It has also been used for the treatment of amenorrhoea and to increase milk production in nursing mothers.[7] A gargle is used to treat mouth and throat inflammation.[6] Paradoxically, fennel has been used in both anorexia[4,6] and obesity.[5,8]

In traditional Chinese medicine, fennel is used to treat *Cold* hernia-like disorders and any kind of lower abdominal pain from *Cold* and *Cold Stomach* patterns with symptoms such as abdominal pain, indigestion, decreased appetite and vomiting.[9]

Summary actions

Carminative, spasmolytic, galactagogue, oestrogenic, antimicrobial, expectorant.

Can be used for

Indications supported by clinical trials

Fennel fruit: irritable bowel syndrome (weak data) and topically to inhibit facial hair growth and hair size in women with idiopathic hirsutism. Fennel fruit essential oil: dysmenorrhoea, infantile colic. Fennel fruit in combination with other herbs: dyspeptic conditions of the upper gastrointestinal tract, including pain, nausea, belching and heartburn; chronic non-specific colitis with diarrhoea or constipation; infantile colic; chronic constipation; cough.

Traditional therapeutic uses

Digestive disorders (windy colic in infants, flatulent colic, griping pain, irritable bowel); suppressed lactation; obesity; topically for conjunctivitis, pharyngitis. Internal use and as an eyebath to strengthen eyesight and for inflammatory conditions of the external eye (such as conjunctivitis). Fennel has been added to herbal powders to allay their tendency to gripe[10] and is a constituent of 'Gripe Water',[5] a popular proprietary liquid for infants.

May also be used for

Extrapolations from pharmacological studies

To reduce vaginal fragility and other symptoms in postmenopausal women.

Other applications

Fennel is also used as a flavouring agent in tea mixtures,[11] alcoholic and non-alcoholic beverages and food products.[12] Fennel oil can be used as an antiseptic ingredient in toothpastes and mouthwashes, an ingredient in antiwrinkle and antiageing skin products and cellulite products,[13] and in soaps, detergents, creams, lotions and perfumes.[12]

Preparations

Fruit as a decoction, syrup (including honey), liquid extract, essential oil and tablets or capsules for internal use. Decoction, extract or essential oil for topical use.

As with all essential oil-containing herbs, use of the fresh plant or carefully dried herb is advised. Keep covered if infusing the herb to retain the essential oil.

Dosage

* 900 to 1800 mg/day of the dried fruit or as an infusion
* 3 to 6 mL/day of 1:2 liquid extract, 7 to14 mL/day of 1:5 tincture or equivalent in tablet or capsule form
* 5 to 20 drops/day of the essential oil.

Duration of use

The Commission E advised that fennel preparations should not be taken for more than several weeks without medical advice.[14] Despite this unexplained caution, fennel is safe for use in the long term, although prolonged intake should be avoided in children due to potential oestrogenic side effects.

Summary assessment of safety

Except in rare cases of contact allergy in susceptible patients, fennel is an extremely safe herb.

Technical data

Botany

Foeniculum vulgare, a member of the Umbelliferae (Apiaceae, carrot) family, is a bluish green biennial or perennial herb that can grow to a height of 2 m. The leaves have a thick, fleshy edible sheath at the base, are three to four times pinnate, triangular and consist of threadlike segments up to 5 cm long. The flowers are 1 to 2 mm in diameter, have five yellow petals and are grouped in small umbels, which in turn are grouped into larger umbels. The fruit consists of two prominently ribbed ovoid achenes 4 to 6 mm long.[15,16]

Adulteration

Adulteration with other plant species has not been documented.

Key constituents

The chemical composition differs between the two varieties and different authors report varying levels. The *European Pharmacopoeia* limits are defined below:

* *Foeniculum vulgare* subsp. *vulgare* var. *vulgare* (bitter fennel): essential oil (>4%), containing >60% *trans*-anethole, >15% fenchone, <5% estragole.[17]
* *Foeniculum vulgare* subsp. *vulgare* var. *dulce* (sweet fennel): essential oil (>2%), containing >80% *trans*-anethole, <7.5% fenchone, <10% estragole.[17]

Additional constituents found in fennel include a fixed oil, flavonoids, organic acids,[1] stilbene trimers[18] and plant sterols, including beta-sitosterol.[19] There are only low levels of furanocoumarins such as 5-methoxypsoralen in fennel fruit.[20]

The sweetness of fennel is due to the presence of *trans*-anethole and estragole, either alone or in combination. Sweet varieties of fennel taste sweeter than bitter varieties because they contain more *trans*-anethole and less fenchone.[21]

The chemical profile of dosage forms varies according to the method of preparation. Fennel tea prepared by 2-minute decoction in a covered cup containing water and heated in a microwave contained a higher content of *p*-anisaldehyde than the tea prepared by infusion. This may be due to the different extraction conditions, and/or to degradation of *trans*-anethole to *p*-anisaldehyde.[22]

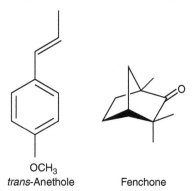

OCH$_3$
trans-Anethole   Fenchone

Pharmacodynamics

Anethole bears a certain chemical resemblance to the catecholamines adrenaline (epinephrine), noradrenaline (norepinephrine) and dopamine. This structural similarity appears to be responsible for the various sympathomimetic effects exerted by fennel and anise. Like adrenaline, fennel and anise have exhibited bronchodilating properties and, like amphetamine, fennel is said to facilitate weight loss, although these effects have not been clinically tested. Psychoactive and psychedelic effects of fennel, anise and anethole have been noted in the past.[8]

Effects on smooth muscle

Fennel oil and alcoholic extracts of fennel demonstrated significant spasmolytic activity in several in vitro models using isolated smooth muscle, such as the histamine and carbachol-induced contractility of isolated guinea pig ileum.[23–27] This action appears to be due to an effect on calcium metabolism in the smooth muscle cells[24] and was confirmed in an in vivo model by injection.[23] One in vitro study found that fennel oil and anethole increased smooth muscle tone under certain conditions.[25] Fennel oil reduced the intensity of oxytocin- and prostaglandin E_2-induced contractions in isolated rat uterus.[28]

Oral administration of a combined stomachic formulation (containing many ingredients including herbs and antacids) reduced the inhibition of stomach movement caused by sodium pentobarbitone in rabbits. The effective (stimulating) ingredients were found to be fennel (active at 24 mg/kg, oral doses), gentian and l-menthol. The stimulating effect of the combined stomachic was abolished by atropine sulphate or hexamethonium bromide, suggesting that the action is due to an increase in the cholinergic nerve activity, not the direct stimulation of the smooth muscle itself.[29] Hence, it appears that fennel relaxes smooth muscle by direct local activity, but also stimulates such activity via the sympathetic nervous system. (See also the section on Respiratory activity below.)

Antimicrobial activity

Fennel oil demonstrated bacteriostatic activity against the following bacteria using the agar diffusion and serial dilution methods: *Aerobacter aerogenes*, *Bacillus subtilis*, *Escherichia coli*, *Proteus vulgaris*, *Pseudomonas aeruginosa*, *Staphylococcus albus* and *Staph. aureus*.[30] Fennel oil (0.02 mL/7 mm filter) also demonstrated antibacterial activity in vitro against the following organisms isolated from patients with urinary tract infections: *E. coli*, *Streptococcus pyogenes*, *Staph. aureus*. The antibacterial activity of fennel oil was equal to or greater than the standard antibiotics tested (streptopenicillin, penicillin and tetracycline).[31] Since these early studies, antibacterial activity has continued to be demonstrated in vitro for fennel oil, with varying results[32,33] perhaps due to the test method or specific essential oil tested. Rising fennel oil steam exerted antibacterial activity in vitro against *Mycobacterium avium*.[34] Fennel oil (0.1%) inhibited mould growth in agar for 6 days. Anethole was also effective at 0.1%.[35] The growth of *Staph. aureus* and *Bacillus subtilis* was prevented by 1 mg/mL of the ethanol extract of fennel, but other tested organisms were not affected at any of the concentrations used.[36] However, the chloroform extract exhibited antibacterial activity against *Bacillus subtilis* and *Proteus vulgaris*, with other bacteria unaffected.[37] Strong inhibition of fungal growth in vitro was demonstrated for fennel oil (against *Aspergillus spp.*), with only mild inhibition found for fennel seed aqueous extract (*Candida albicans*, *Saccharomyces cerevisiae*).[38,39]

Plant extracts were tested in vitro for antibacterial activity against fifteen *Helicobacter pylori* strains. Methanol extract of fennel seed demonstrated a minimum inhibitory concentration (MIC) of 50 μg/mL, which was better than the MIC of the antibiotic metronidazole.[40] Fennel extract was one of the most active of 21 herbs tested in vitro against *Campylobacter jejuni*.[41]

Oestrogenic and related activity

Fennel oil demonstrated a favourable influence on the fat content and total quantity of milk in goats.[42] Lactating mice fed fennel produced pups that consumed a significantly higher quantity of fennel-containing food than controls (mothers not fed fennel during lactation).[43] This indicates that the flavour (and hence at least some chemical constituents) of fennel are passed in breast milk.

The structural resemblance of anethole to catecholamines may have a bearing on the galactagogue activity of fennel. Anethole may influence milk secretion by competing with dopamine at appropriate receptor sites, thereby reducing the inhibition of prolactin secretion by dopamine. Dianethole and photoanethole (polymers of anethole), which resemble the oestrogenic compounds stilbene and diethylstilbestrol, have also demonstrated oestrogenic activity.[8]

Injection of fennel oil triggered a mating response in sexually immature female rats and in ovariectomised mice.[44] Extracts of fennel can induce oestrus, cause growth of mammary glands and oviducts in adult ovariectomised rats and exert an antiandrogenic effect in adult male rats.[45] Fennel extract increased the organ weight of the cervix and vagina of ovariectomised rats, as well as increasing RNA, DNA and protein concentrations. Fennel caused the growth of the cervix and vagina by inducing both hyperplasia and hypertrophy. The most potent dose was 250 μg/100 g bodyweight, which produced changes similar to oestrus-intact females.[45] Moderate oral doses of an acetone extract of fennel (0.5 mg/kg) increased the weight of mammary glands, whilst higher doses (2.5 mg/kg) increased the weight of the oviduct, endometrium, myometrium, cervix and vagina.[46] A follow-up study demonstrated that the acetone extract induced cellular growth and proliferation in the endometrium and stimulated metabolism in the myometrium in rats. Changes induced by fennel provided a more favourable environment for the survival of spermatocytes and the implantation of the zygote in the uterus.[47]

Oral administration of the acetone extract of fennel fruit to male rats for 15 days produced a significant reduction in the total protein concentration of testes and vas deferens and an increase in the seminal vesicles and prostate gland.[46]

Intragastric administration of aqueous extract of fennel seed (50 mg/day or about 2 g/kg for 25 days) significantly reduced female fertility in mice compared with controls (p<0.025). No effect was observed on male mice fertility.[48] (See also the Safety section of this monograph.)

Respiratory activity

Fennel oil administered by inhalation exerted a mild antitussive or cough suppressant effect on cough generated by mechanical stimulation in guinea pigs.[49] In an earlier study, the volume and thickness of expelled respiratory tract fluid (RTF) was measured after administration of anethole and fenchone in various doses to rabbits. A dose-dependent increase in RTF volume was observed for fenchone, with the maximum response at 9 mg/kg. The increase in volume for anethole was not dose-dependent, and the maximum response occurred at 3 mg/kg. A comparison of seasonal results indicated a strong increase in RTF volume in autumn. Thickness of RTF was reduced in a dose-dependent manner, with minima occurring at 9 to 27 mg/kg.[50] Application of bitter fennel tea (equivalent to 9.1 mg of fruit) increased mucociliary transport velocity by 12% in isolated oesophageal mucosal membranes from frogs. The reference drug bromhexine (20 mg) produced an increase of 34%.[51] Fennel ethanolic extract and essential oil showed a relatively potent bronchodilatory effect on isolated tracheal chains of the guinea pig.[52,53]

Effects on digestion

An aqueous extract of fennel increased gastric acid secretion in rats.[54] A single oral dose of fennel seed (250 mg/kg) enhanced the activity of amylase in pancreatic tissue and lipase in the small intestine. Dietary intake (0.5% for 8 weeks) resulted in an increase in pancreatic trypsin and intestinal amylase.[55]

Fennel fruit extract caused a significant increase (33%) of collected bile after oral administration (500 mg/kg) to rats. The bilirubin content of the bile was similar in both treated and control groups.[36]

Fennel at 0.5% of diet over 6 weeks shortened food transit time in rats by 12%.[56] Pretreatment with aqueous extract of fennel (75 to 300 mg/kg by oral gavage) significantly reduced ethanol-induced gastric damage in rats.[57]

Other effects

Administration of a methanol extract of fennel fruit (200 mg/kg of 5:1 extract) reduced the amnesic effect of scopolamine and age-induced memory deficit in mice.[58]

Fennel oil (0.4 mL/kg) by oral administration demonstrated hepatoprotective activity in the carbon tetrachloride-induced liver injury model in rats.[59] The subcutaneous injection of fennel oil (100 mg/day or approximately 300 mg/kg) to partially hepatectomised rats for 7 days produced a significant increase (p<0.05) in the regeneration of liver tissue, as expressed by an increase in wet and dry liver weights in relation to total body weight.[60] Fennel reduced the toxicity of strychnine in mice, indicating that it might increase the activity of liver microsomal drug metabolising enzymes.[61] In contrast, a methanol extract of fennel fruit inhibited cytochrome P450 3A4 in human liver microsomes[62] and 5-methoxypsoralen was later identified as a key active constituent.[63] It is not known whether this will cause any clinically relevant herb-drug interaction.

Fennel extracts exhibited antioxidant activity in vitro.[64,65] Fennel oil demonstrated antioxidant activity in soybean oil,[66] and in sunflower oil the effect was stronger than vitamin E.[67] Fennel inhibited lipid peroxidation (rancidity) in slated cooked ground fish. Dried fennel was a more effective antioxidant than fresh fennel in this context.[68]

The acetone extract of fennel exhibited strong in vitro cytotoxic activity against murine leukaemia cells and human colon cancer cells.[69] Water extract of fennel inhibited the growth of mouse leukaemia cells in vitro. The ethanol extract was inactive.[48]

Oral doses of an aqueous extract of fennel fruit lowered systolic blood pressure in spontaneously hypertensive rats. Fennel also increased water, sodium and potassium excretion (i.e. had a diuretic effect), which was the probable basis of its hypotensive action.[70] The ethanol extract of fennel fruit (500 mg/kg) demonstrated significant diuretic activity 5 and 24 h after oral administration to rats (when compared with controls). The diuresis in this case was not associated with changes in sodium and/or potassium excretion.[36] Hydroalcoholic extracts of fennel root demonstrated diuretic activity in rats, producing an increase in urinary flow and urinary sodium excretion.[71]

In previous screening, fennel oil was identified as having significant antiplatelet activity among 24 essential oils tested. Anethole was subsequently shown to be as potent as fennel oil in vitro.[72] It also prevented thrombin-induced clot retraction at concentrations similar to fennel oil. Both fennel oil and anethole (30 mg/kg/day orally for 5 days) showed significant antithrombotic activity in mice without haemorrhagic side effects, unlike the reference drug aspirin.[72]

The ethanol extract of fennel fruit demonstrated significant but moderate analgesic activity 90 and 150 minutes after oral administration (500 mg/kg) to mice. Antipyretic activity was also evident at 30 and 90 minutes, but not at 150 minutes.[36] A methanol extract of fennel fruit by oral administration (200 mg/kg of 15:1 extract) demonstrated anti-inflammatory activity in acute and subacute inflammation and type IV allergic reactions in mice and rats.[73] Previously, 100 mg/kg (oral) of an 80% ethanolic extract inhibited carrageenan-induced paw oedema in rats.[74]

Feeding rats 1 g/day of dry fennel leaf inhibited bone resorption, but this may not be relevant to the use of the fruit.[75]

Pharmacokinetics

Anethole was absorbed very slowly in mice after oral administration (200 mg/kg). After 30 and 120 minutes, 60% and 23% of the administered dose, respectively, were still present in the stomach.[76] After 72 h, 2% of an orally administered dose was found in the faeces of rats.[77]

The metabolic fate of 1 mg of *trans*-anethole has been investigated in human volunteers using the radioactively labelled compound.[78] The main routes of elimination were the urine and expired air. The major urinary metabolite was 4-methoxyhippuric acid (56% of dose). Another study found that doses up to 250 mg had no systematic effect on the rate and route of excretion and on the pattern of urinary metabolites.[79]

Clinical trials

Effects on the gastrointestinal tract

Five patients with irritable bowel syndrome (IBS) defined as meeting the Rome criteria, who were also poor responders to available therapies, were selected for treatment with fennel fruit in a small, open label pilot trial. Patients were given four sugar coated fennel fruits to chew and swallow after meals for 1 week. The dose was increased gradually to 8 to 12 fruits three times a day. After 2 weeks of therapy there were marked clinical improvements, with fewer abdominal cramps, less dependence on medication (laxative, antidiarrhoeal drug, analgesics) and fewer visits to physicians.[80]

A liquid herbal formula (25 drops three times daily) containing, in increasing proportions, wormwood, caraway, fennel and peppermint was found to be superior to the spasmolytic drug metoclopramide (p=0.02) in terms of relief of symptoms such as pain, nausea, belching and heartburn in a randomised, double blind clinical trial of the treatment of dyspepsia. Sixty patients took part in the trial, which consisted of 2 weeks' treatment.[81] In another placebo-controlled, randomised, double blind clinical trial, 70 patients with strongly marked chronic digestive problems such as flatulence or bloating were treated with either a herbal formula containing caraway, fennel, peppermint and gentian in tablet form or a placebo over a 14-day period. Analysis of the trial results established a significant improvement in gastrointestinal complaint scores in the group receiving the herbal tablets, compared with the placebo group (p<0.05). Ultrasound results evaluating the amount of gas present also demonstrated a significant benefit from the herbal formula (p<0.05).[82]

In two randomised, double blind trials, a tablet containing 100 mg each of fennel fruit, peppermint and caraway and 30 mg gentian was evaluated against placebo in patients with idiopathic dyspepsia. In the acute trial involving 12 patients, a single dose of three tablets relieved acute symptoms (p=0.014, compared with placebo). The longer-term trial involved 70 patients over 2 weeks at six tablets per day. There was a statistically significant reduction in symptoms for the herbal combination compared with placebo (p value not stated).[83]

Twenty-four patients with chronic non-specific colitis were treated with a herb combination containing *Taraxacum officinale*, *Hypericum perforatum*, *Melissa officinalis*, *Calendula officinalis* and fennel in an open label trial. By the 15th day of treatment, spontaneous and palpable pains along the large intestine had disappeared in 96% of the patients. Defaecation was normalised in patients with diarrhoea syndrome.[84]

The effect of a herbal instant tea preparation containing chamomile, vervain, licorice, fennel and lemon balm on infantile colic was assessed in a prospective double blind study on babies about 3 weeks old. Tea or placebo up to 150 mL per dose was given to each infant with every episode of colic, but not more than three times a day. After the 7 days of the trial, the colic improvement scores were significantly better in the herbal tea group: 1.7 versus 0.7 for the placebo group (p<0.05). In addition, more babies in the treatment group had their colic eliminated: 57% compared with 26% for placebo (p<0.01).[85] A herbal preparation containing dry extracts of fennel, chamomile and lemon balm, together with small quantities of vitamins B1 and B6 and calcium pantothenate, was administered twice a day to breastfed colicky infants. This randomised, double blind, placebo-controlled trial found that crying time reduced from 201.2 minutes to 76.9 minutes in the active group, compared to a fall from 198.7 minutes to just 169.9 minutes in the placebo group (p<0.005). A higher incidence of vomiting was reported for the herb group compared with placebo, which might be expected, given that these herbs are also carminatives.[86]

Emulsion of fennel essential oil was superior to placebo in decreasing the intensity of infantile colic. In this placebo-controlled, randomised trial, parents were instructed to administer a minimum of 5 mL and a maximum of 20 mL of either a water emulsion of 0.1% fennel fruit essential oil or placebo up to four times a day. Colic according to the Wessel criteria was eliminated in 65% of those in the treatment group, compared with 23.7% in the placebo group (p<0.01).[87]

A proprietary herbal tea (containing fennel, licorice, sweet orange peel, cinnamon, coriander fruit, ginger and sweet orange oil dried on acacia gum) was tested in nursing home residents with chronic constipation using a double blind, placebo-controlled design.[88] Residents were randomly assigned to receive the herbal tea (n=42) or placebo (n=44) once daily for 28 days in addition to standard constipation treatment. In the intention to treat analysis there was a statistically significant increase in bowel movements in the herbal group (about one extra per week, p=0.017) compared with placebo.

Dysmenorrhoea

Thirty women (15 to 24 years old) with moderate to severe dysmenorrhoea participated in an open clinical study in Iran. They were evaluated for three menstrual cycles: no medication in the first (which served as a control), mefenamic acid (a non-steroidal anti-inflammatory drug, 250 mg every 6h) in the second cycle and fennel essential oil (25 drops every 4h) in the third. Both treatments effectively relieved menstrual pain compared with the control cycle. The mean duration of initiation of action (time period between ingestion and pain relief) was 67.5 minutes for mefenamic acid and 75 minutes for fennel oil. Mefenamic acid was more potent than fennel oil on the second and third menstrual days, with the difference on the other days not being significant. (See also the Side effects section below.[89])

In another open trial also conducted in Iran, adolescent girls were randomised to receive either fennel oil (30 drops) or mefenamic acid (250 mg) for 2 months. Each treatment was taken at the onset of menses and then continuously every 6h for the first 3 days. Both the treatments were equally effective in reducing pain intensity, limitation in activity and the need for rest.[90]

Other conditions

One case has been reported where chewing fennel fruit relieved the cough induced by the angiotensin-converting enzyme inhibitor enalapril. The severe irritating cough stopped within 2 to 3 days following an accidental chewing of fennel fruit (1 to 1.5 g). The fennel was retained between the teeth and cheek for half an hour. This regime was continued three times daily for 3 days. After improvement of the cough, fennel fruit was used twice daily for a week and then once a day. The patient remained free of cough despite regular use of 20 mg/day enalapril.[91]

Significant improvements for sleep discomfort, cough frequency and cough intensity were observed in allergic asthma patients who used a herbal tea. One cup of tea (200 mL) was taken twice daily. The tea was prepared as a decoction from 2.5 g each of powdered fennel, anise, cardamom and caraway fruits, 7.5 g chamomile flowers, 0.3 g saffron and licorice root and 1.3 g black seeds (*Nigella sativa*). The ratio of FEV1/FVC (a measure of lung function) was also increased in the treatment group compared with placebo (p=0.022).[92] (FEV1 is forced expiratory volume in 1 second and FVC is forced vital capacity.) The 'placebo' tea used was *Camellia sinensis* (normal tea) and the study was not blinded.

In a randomised, double blind clinical study, 38 patients with mild to moderate facial idiopathic hirsutism were treated with creams containing 1% or 2% of fennel extract (12.5:1) or placebo. The cream was prepared from fennel fruit extracted with ethanol and reduced in solvent. None of the patients had polycystic ovaries and all had normal serum androgen levels. The duration of treatment was 12 weeks and the cream was applied twice a day. Throughout the course of the treatment, density and hair growth were noted and hair diameter was measured. Reduction in hair diameter was greatest for the 2% cream (18.3%) compared against the 1% cream (7.8%) and placebo (−0.5%, a slight increase). These results demonstrated statistically significant differences (p<0.001) between each group. The rate of hair growth was also reduced in patients using the fennel cream, but not in the placebo group. No adverse effects were observed.[93]

Toxicology and other safety data

Toxicology

The oral LD_{50} of fennel oil in rats varied from 1.33g/kg to 4.5mL/kg.[3,94] Acute or chronic poisoning with fennel oil has not been reported in humans.[3] The acute oral LD_{50} of anethole in rats was found to be 2.09g/kg.[8] No phototoxic effects were reported for the application of undiluted bitter fennel oil on hairless mice and pigs. Bitter fennel oil (4% in petrolatum) produced no irritation in a 48h closed-patch test and no sensitisation reactions on human subjects.[95]

It is desirable to have low estragole-containing fennel. High-dosage estragole studies in rats indicate potential hepatocarcinogenicity. However, since estragole is metabolised differently in humans and has only limited absorption,[96,97] any posited carcinogenic risk in humans was suggested to be tenuous.

However, later data imply that humans do produce potentially carcinogenic metabolites from estragole, albeit in quite low amounts. The proximate carcinogenic metabolite of estragole is 1′-hydroxyestragole. There is considerable variation in the production of this metabolite by humans.[98] The sulphate conjugate of this metabolite is hepatotoxic and is the ultimate carcinogen.[99] The metabolism of estragole was investigated in humans after consumption of fennel tea.[100] Less than 0.41% of the administered dose was briefly converted to 1′-hydroxyestragole and the presence of the sulphate conjugate could not be confirmed. As noted above, fennel can contain varying amounts of estragole, and this was also reflected in a study on fennel tea that found a range of between 9 and 2058μg/L for teas prepared in different ways.[101] Based on these findings, a maximum exposure to estragole for adults drinking fennel teas was estimated at just 10μg/kg/day. In contrast, the very high doses of estragole used in carcinogenic studies in rodents may favour the production of carcinogenic metabolites by overloading the protective metabolic pathways.[102]

No toxic effects were observed in mice administered single oral doses of 0.5, 1 and 3g/kg of fennel ethanolic extract (equivalent to 5, 10 and 30g of fennel seed respectively). In a chronic toxicity study, 100mg/kg/day of fennel extract orally administered over 90 days caused no significant differences in mortality, external morphology, haematology or spermatogenesis compared with controls. After 40 days, alopecia in the snout area developed in some male animals. The average body weight of the male animals increased, while that of the female mice decreased or remained the same.[103] In another study using the same dosages, only the 3g/kg dose group showed signs of reduced locomotor activity and piloerection in mice. All other parameters were negative.[36]

Methanolic and water extracts of bitter and sweet fennel were not mutagenic in the Ames test and had no DNA-damaging activity in the *Bacillus subtilis* rec-assay.[103] In contrast fennel fruit extract prepared by percolation with 95% ethanol and concentrated by vacuum demonstrated intermediate mutagenic results in the Ames test and significant toxic activity in the brine shrimp bioassay.[104]

The mutagenic potential of fennel oil is not conclusive, as indicated by conflicting results obtained from in vitro tests. Fennel oil, sweet fennel oil and estragole were negative, but anethole was positive in Ames tests.[105,106] In another study, fennel oil and anethole showed weakly positive results.[107] Sweet fennel oil and anethole were negative in the *E. coli* reversion test. Sweet fennel oil but not anethole demonstrated DNA-damaging activity in the *Bacillus subtilis* rec-assay; however, the authors indicate problems with this test with respect to the testing of oils.[106] Fennel oil demonstrated negative results in the chromosomal aberration test on hamster fibroblasts.[105] The available mutagenicity and genotoxicity data indicate that *trans*-anethole is not genotoxic[108] and is even antigenotoxic in vivo.[109]

Contraindications

Fennel has been categorised as a spice allergen, with some publications reporting a cross-reaction with fennel in the so-called 'celery-carrot-mugwort-spice' syndrome. It is therefore contraindicated in these patients. However, even in this context allergic reactions to fennel are rare and seem to be limited to occupational exposure.[3]

Special warnings and precautions

Very high doses of fennel essential oil should be avoided in hepatic disorders.

Interactions

Concomitant oral dosing of the aqueous fennel extract (2g dried herb per kg) reduced the bioavailability of the antibiotic ciprofloxacin in rats. None of the phytochemical components of fennel seemed to cause this interaction, which may have been due to the presence of relatively large amounts of metal cations in the extract.[110] As noted earlier, fennel contains 5-methoxypsoralen, a furanocoumarin that can inhibit CYP 450 drug metabolising enzymes.

The bioavailability of paeoniflorin (present in Paeonia root) was enhanced by oral administration of fennel fruit to mice.[111]

Interaction between fennel essential oil and other drugs in humans is not expected.[3] Dermal application of the infusion of fennel in humans results in an aggravation of the inflammation caused by mustard oil, UV irradiation and the subcutaneous injection of tuberculin.[3]

Use in pregnancy and lactation

Category B3 – no increase in frequency of malformation or other harmful effects on the fetus from limited use in women. Evidence of negative effects in animal studies exists, although the relevance to humans is unknown.

Intragastric administration of water extract of fennel (0.05 g/day of dried herb) reduced the fertility of female mice. Of the six treated females only three became pregnant.[48] Anethole given orally to female rats at 50, 70 and 80 mg/kg in early pregnancy reduced successful implantation.[112]

Fennel essential oil reduced limb bud differentiation in vitro. (The limb bud micromass culture system used in this study provided the opportunity to evaluate chondrocyte differentiation, because changes in extracellular matrix composition parallel those seen in the intact limb.) There was no evidence of teratogenicity.[113]

Fennel is compatible with breastfeeding and traditionally used to enhance lactation.

Effects on ability to drive and use machines

No adverse effects expected.

Side effects

Cross-sensitivity to fennel and other members of the Umbelliferae (Apiaceae) has been found in a high proportion of patients with positive skin tests to birch, mugwort and celery.[114] (The 'celery-carrot-mugwort-spice' syndrome is well known in Europe. People sensitised to carrot, for example, may also have allergic reactions to other vegetables or spices of the Umbelliferae family.[115,116]) A 2002 analysis of 589 cases of food allergies found frequent sensitisation to Umbelliferae spices. In those who were tested, a positive prick test towards fennel seed was found in 9.9% of children and 7.4% of adults. Only adults were allergic to spices and allergy to spices accounted for 6.4% of food allergies. Investigation of case reports suggests that the reaction to fennel seed is greater than for fennel leaf, due to the higher protein content of the former.[117] In one study, fennel sensitivity was found in just one case among 202 food challenges performed in 142 children with food allergies.[118] However, some diagnosed 'spice allergies' to Umbelliferae such as fennel, anise, coriander and cumin may not have an immunological component and may be best characterised as food intolerances.[119]

Immediate hypersensitivity reactions to the ingestion of fresh fennel have been reported. Skin prick tests indicated the patient typically had strong reactivity to several pollens as well as to most vegetable foods tested (cucumber, tomato, potato, orange, pea, beans, celery, carrot, onion, garlic).[120] Skin prick tests also showed a positive immediate response to a range of other spices in one subject allergic to aniseed. These comprised asparagus, caraway, coriander, cumin, dill and fennel extracts.[121] A positive skin test to fresh fennel seed was found in one case of occupational asthma,[122] and in one case of childhood atopic dermatitis (as a partial allergen).[123]

No substantial adverse effects were reported in one cohort study of 30 young women with primary dysmenorrhoea treated with fennel essential oil. Five patients (16.6%) withdrew due to the odour; one patient (3.1%) reported a mild increase in the amount of menstrual flow.[89]

Premature thelarche is defined as isolated breast development with no other clinical signs of sexual maturation in girls before the age of 8 years. The mechanism is unknown, although increased oestrogen levels can be detected in the serum. A Turkish study describes four cases of premature thelarche apparently linked to the long-term consumption of fennel tea.[124] The four cases were observed between January 2001 and December 2007 in a paediatric department in Ankara. The first case was a 5-month-old infant girl exhibiting premature thelarche and elevated oestradiol. Around the same time a 65-year-old postmenopausal woman was under investigation because her menstrual cycle had recommenced. Her history revealed the long-term consumption of fennel tea. This prompted the authors to search for a link between fennel and the thelarche case and also in three other subsequent cases (aged 3 to 5 years). All four girls had been given fennel tea two to three times a day for several months to eliminate colic. Physical and genital examination of the girls was unremarkable. However, serum oestradiol levels were 15 to 20 times higher than normal for their ages. After the fennel tea was stopped the premature thelarche resolved within 3 to 6 months and oestradiol levels returned to normal. Prolonged intake of fennel should be avoided by boys and girls. Clinicians should also be watchful for potential oestrogenic side effects from the use of this herb in either sex.

Overdosage

No effects known.

Safety in children

Apart from the rare case of allergic reaction, no adverse effects are expected in children from short-term use of fennel.[125] However, as noted above, prolonged intake should be avoided in children due to potential oestrogenic effects.

Regulatory status in selected countries

Bitter and sweet fennel are official in the *European Pharmacopoeia* (2006) and the *British Pharmacopoeia* (2007). Fennel is also official in the *Pharmacopoeia of the People's*

Republic of China (English edition, 2000) and fennel and its oil are official in the *Japanese Pharmacopoeia* (English edition, 2001). Fennel and fennel oil were official in the second edition of the *Indian Pharmacopoeia* (1966), but were not included in the third edition (1985).

Fennel and fennel oil are covered by positive Commission E monographs and both have the following applications:

- dyspeptic complaints, such as mild cramp-like gastrointestinal disorders, a feeling of distension, flatulence
- catarrh of the upper respiratory tract
- fennel syrup and fennel honey for catarrh of the upper respiratory tract in children.

Fennel is on the UK General Sale List.

Fennel and fennel oil have GRAS status. They are also freely available as a 'dietary supplement' in the USA under DSHEA legislation (1994 Dietary Supplement Health and Education Act). Fennel has been present as an ingredient in products offered over the counter (OTC) for use as an aphrodisiac. The FDA, however, advises that: 'based on evidence currently available, any OTC drug product containing ingredients for use as an aphrodisiac cannot be generally recognised as safe and effective'.

Fennel is not included in Part 4 of Schedule 4 of the Therapeutic Goods Act Regulations of Australia and is freely available for sale.

References

1. Bisset NG, ed. *Herbal Drugs and Phytopharmaceuticals*. Stuttgart: Medpharm Scientific Publishers; 1994. pp. 200–202.
2. Mabberley DJ. *The Plant Book*, 2nd ed. Cambridge: Cambridge University Press; 1997. p. 286.
3. De Smet PAGM, ed. *Adverse Effects of Herbal Drugs*, vol. 1. Berlin: Springer-Verlag; 1992. pp. 135–142.
4. Bartram T. *Encyclopedia of Herbal Medicine*. Dorset: Grace Publishers; 1995. p. 181.
5. Grieve M. *A Modern Herbal*, vol. 1. New York: Dover Publications; 1971. pp. 293–297.
6. British Herbal Medicine Association Scientific Committee. *British Herbal Pharmacopoeia*. Cowling: BHMA; 1983. pp. 92–93.
7. Felter HW, Lloyd JU. *King's American Dispensatory*, ed 18, rev 3, vol 1, 1905, Portland, Reprinted by Eclectic Medical Publications; 1983. pp. 891–892.
8. Albert-Puleo M. *J Ethnopharmacol*. 1980;2:337–344.
9. Bensky D, Gamble A. *Chinese Herbal Medicine Materia Medica*. Seattle: Eastland Press; 1986. pp. 440–441.
10. Pharmaceutical Society of Great Britain. *British Pharmaceutical Codex 1934*. London: Pharmaceutical Press; 1934. p. 471.
11. Weiss RF. *Herbal Medicine*. Beaconsfield: Beaconsfield Publishers; 1988. p. 68.
12. Leung AY, Foster S. *Encyclopedia of Common Natural Ingredients Used in Food, Drugs and Cosmetics*, 2nd ed. New York: John Wiley; 1996. pp. 240–243.
13. Smeh NJ. *Creating Your Own Cosmetics – Naturally*. Garrisonville: Alliance Publishing; 1995. p. 88.
14. German Federal Minister of Justice. *German Commission E for Human Medicine Monograph*. Bundes-Anzeiger (German Federal Gazette), no. 74, dated 18.04.1991.
15. Chiej R. *The Macdonald Encyclopedia of Medicinal Plants*. London: Macdonald; 1984. Entry no. 133.
16. Launert EL. *The Hamlyn Guide to Edible and Medicinal Plants of Britain and Northern Europe*. London: Hamlyn; 1981. p. 98.
17. European Department for the Quality of Medicines Within the Council of Europe. *European Pharmacopoeia*, 3 ed. Strasbourg: 1996. pp. 848–850.
18. Ono M, Ito Y, Kinjo J, et al. *Chem Pharm Bull*. 1995;43(5):868–871.
19. Mendez J, Castro Poceiro J. *Rev Latinoam Quim*. 1981;12(2):91–92.
20. Hänsel R, Keller K, Rimpler H, Schneider, eds. Foeniculum. In: *Hagers Handbuch der Pharmazeutischen Praxis*, 5th ed., vol. 5. Berlin: Springer-Verlag; 1992. pp. 156–181.
21. Hussain RA, Poveda LJ, Pezzuto JM, et al. *Econ. Bot.* 1990;44(2):174–182.
22. Bilia AR, Fumarola M, Gallori S, et al. *J Agric Food Chem*. 2000;48(10): 4734–4738.
23. Gunn JWC. *J Pharmacol Exp Ther*. 1921;16:39–47.
24. Saleh MM, Hashem FA, Grace MH. *Pharm Pharmacol Lett*. 1996;6(1):5–7.
25. Reiter M, Brandt W. *Arzneimittelforschung*. 1985;35(1A):408–414.
26. Forster HB, Niklas H, Lutz S. *Planta Med*. 1980;40(4):309–319.
27. Forster HB. *Z Allgemeinmed*. 1983;59:1327–1333.
28. Ostad SN, Soodi M, Shariffzadeh M, et al. *J Ethnopharmacol*. 2001;76(3): 299–304.
29. Niiho Y, Takayanagi I, Takagi K. *Jpn J Pharmacol*. 1977;27(1):177–179.
30. Kivanc M, Akgul A. *Flavour Fragrance J*. 1986;1:175–179.
31. Afzal H, Akhtar MS. *J Pak Med Assoc*. 1981;31(10):230–232.
32. Singh G, Kapoor IP, Pandey SK, et al. *Phytother Res*. 2002;16(7):680–682.
33. Schelz Z, Molnar J, Hohmann J. *Fitoterapia*. 2006;77(4):279–285.
34. Maruzzella JC, Sicurella A. *J Am Pharm Assoc*. 1960;49:692–694.
35. Lord CF, Husa WJ. *J Am Pharm Assoc*. 1954;43:438–440.
36. Tanira MOM, Shah AH, Mohsin A, et al. *Phytother Res*. 1996;10:33–36.
37. Jawad ALM, Dharhir ABJ, Hussain AM, et al. *J Biol Sci Res*. 1985;16(2):17–21.
38. Lis-Balchin M, Hart S, Deans SG, et al. *J Herb Spice Med Plants*. 1996;4(2):69–86.
39. Metwali MR. *Egypt J Microbiol*. 2003;38(1):105–114.
40. Mahady GB, Pendland SL, Stoia A, et al. *Phytother Res*. 2005;19(11):988–991.
41. Cwikla C, Schmidt K, Matthias A, et al. *Phytother Res*. 2010;24(5):649–656.
42. Fingerling F. *Landw Vers Sta*. 67:253–289 (CAS 2:6758).
43. Shukla HS, Upadhyay PD, Tripathi SC. *Pesticides*. 1989;23(1):33–35.
44. Zondek B, Bergmann E. *Biochem J*. 1938;32:641–645.
45. Annusuya S, Vanithakumari G, Megala N, et al. *Indian J Med Res*. 1988;87:364–367.
46. Malini T, Vanithakumari G, Megala N, et al. *Indian J Physiol Pharmacol*. 1985;29(1):21–26.
47. Mekala N, Annusuya K, Devi G, et al. *Indian Drugs*. 1989;27(2):93–100.
48. Alkofahi A, Al-Hamood MH, Elbetieha AM. *Arch STD/HIV Res*. 1996;10(3): 189–196.
49. Misawa M, Kizawa M. *Pharmacometrics*. 1990;39(1):81–93.
50. Boyd EM, Sheppard EP. *Pharmacology*. 1971;6:65–80.
51. Muller-Limmroth W, Frohlich HH. *Fortschr Med*. 1980;98(3):95–101.
52. Boskabady MH, Khatami A. *Pharm Biol*. 2003;41(3):211–215.
53. Boskabady MH, Khatami A, Nazari A. *Pharmazie*. 2004;59(7):561–564.
54. Vasudevan K, Vembar S, Veeraraghavan K, et al. *Indian J Gastroenterol*. 2000;19(2):53–56.
55. Platel K, Srinivasan K. *J Food Sci Technol*. 2001;38(4):358–361.
56. Platel K, Srinivasan K. *Nutr Res*. 2001;21:1309–1314.
57. Birdane FM, Cemek M, Birdane YO, et al. *World J Gastroenterol*. 2007;13(4): 607–611.

58. Joshi H, Parle M. *J Med Food.* 2006;9(3):413–417.

59. Ozbek H, Ugras S, Dulger H, et al. *Fitoterapia.* 2003;74(3):317–319.

60. Gershbein LL. *Food Cosmet Toxicol.* 1977;15:173–181.

61. Han YB, Shin KH, Woo WS. *Annual Report of Natural Products Research Institute.* Seoul National University; 1984;23:46–49.

62. Subehan Usia T, Iwata H, et al. *J Ethnopharmacol.* 2006;105(3):449–455.

63. Subehan Zaidi SF, Kadota S, et al. *J Agric Food Chem.* 2007;55(25):10162–10167.

64. Mimica-Dukic N, Kujundzic S, Kouladis M. *51st Annual Congress of the Society for Medicinal Plant Research,* August 31st-September 4th, 2003, Kiel, Germany. p. 66. Abstract No. SL22.

65. Satyanarayana S, Sushruta K, Sarma GS, et al. *J Herb Pharmacother.* 2004;4(2):1–10.

66. Zygadlo JA, Lamarque AL, Maestri DM, et al. *Grasay Aceites.* 1995;46(4–5):285–288.

67. Stashenko EE, Puertas MA, Martinez JR. *Anal Bioanal Chem.* 2002;373(1–2):70–74.

68. Ramanathan L, Das NP. *J Food Sci.* 1993;58(2):318–320.

69. Kim KS, Paik JM, Hwang WI. *Korean Univ Med J.* 1988;25(3):759–770.

70. El Bardai S, Lyoussi B, Wibo M, et al. *Clin Exp Hypertens.* 2001;23(4):329–343.

71. Beaux D, Fleurentin J, Mortier F. *Phytother Res.* 1997;11(4):320–322.

72. Tognolini M, Ballabeni V, Bertoni S, et al. *Pharmacol Res.* 2007;56(3):254–260.

73. Choi EM, Hwang JK. *Fitoterapia.* 2004;75(6):557–565.

74. Mascolo N, Autore G, Capasso F, et al. *Phytother Res.* 1987;1:28–31.

75. Muhlbauer RC, Lozano A, Reinli A, et al. *J Nutr.* 2003;133(11):3592–3597.

76. Le Bourhis B. *Ann Biol Clin.* 1968;26:711–715.

77. Sangster SA, Cladwell J, Smith RL. *Food Chem Toxicol.* 1984;22:695–706.

78. Sangster SA, Caldwell J, Hutt AJ, et al. *Xenobiotica.* 1987;17(10):1223–1232.

79. Caldwell J, Sutton JD. *Fd Chem Toxic.* 1988;26(2):87–91.

80. Amjad H, Jafary HA, Beckly WV. *Am J Gastroenterol.* 2000;95(9) 2491. Abstract No. 273.

81. Westphal J, Hörning M, Leonhardt K. *Phytomedicine.* 1996;2(4):285–291.

82. Silberhorn H, Landgrebe N, Wohling D, et al. *6th Phytotherapy Conference,* Berlin, October 5–7, 1995.

83. Uehleke B, Silberhorn H, Wohling H. *Fortschr Med.* 2002;144(27/28):695.

84. Chakurski I, Matev M, Koichev A, et al. *Vutr Boles.* 1981;20(6):51–54.

85. Weizman Z, Alkrinawi S, Goldfarb D, et al. *J Pediatr.* 1993;122(4):650–652.

86. Savino F, Cresi F, Castagno E, et al. *Phytother Res.* 2005;19:335–340.

87. Alexandrovich I, Rakovitskaya O, Kolmo E, et al. *Altern Ther Health Med.* 2003;9(4):58–61.

88. Bub S, Brinckmann J, Cicconetti G, et al. *J Am Med Dir Assoc.* 2006;7(9):556–561.

89. Namavar Jahromi B, Tartifizadeh A, Khabnadideh S. *Int J Gynaecol Obstet.* 2003;80(2):153–157.

90. Modaress Nejad V, Asadipour M. *East Mediterr Health J.* 2006;12(3–4):423–427.

91. Arya SC. *Indian J Pharmacol.* 1999;31(2):159.

92. Haggag EG, Abou-Moustafa MA, Boucher W, et al. *J Herb Pharmacother.* 2003;3(4):41–54.

93. Javidnia K, Dastgheib L, Mohammadi Samani S, et al. *Phytomedicine.* 2003;10(6–7):455–458.

94. Opdyke DL. *Food Cosmet Toxicol.* 1974;12:309.

95. Opdyke DLJ. *Food Cosmet Toxicol.* 1979;17:529.

96. Sangster SA, Caldwell J, Smith RL. *Food Chem Toxicol.* 1984;22:707–713.

97. Caldwell J, Sutton JD. *Food Chem Toxicol.* 1988;26:87–91.

98. Punt A, Jeurissen SM, Boersma MG, et al. *Toxicol Sci.* 2010;113(2):337–348.

99. Smith RL, Adams TB, Doull J, et al. *Food Chem Toxicol.* 2002;40(7):851–870.

100. Zeller A, Horst K, Rychlik M. *Chem Res Toxicol.* 2009;22(12):1929–1937.

101. Raffo A, Nicoli S, Leclercq C. *Food Chem Toxicol.* 2011;49(2):370–375.

102. Punt A, Freidic AP, Delatour T, et al. *Toxicol Appl Pharmacol.* 2008;231(2):248–259.

103. Shah AH, Qureshi S, Ageel AM. *J Ethnopharmacol.* 1991;34(2–3):167–172.

104. Mahmoud I, Alkofahi A, Abdelaziz A. *Int J Pharmacog.* 1992;30(2):81–85.

105. Ishidate Jr M, Sofuni T, Yoshikawa K, et al. *Food Chem Toxicol.* 1984;22(8):623–636.

106. Sekizawa J, Shibamoto T. *Mutat Res.* 1982;101(2):127–140.

107. Marcus C, Lichtenstein EP. *J Agric Food Chem.* 1982;30(3):563–568.

108. Newberne P, Smith RL, Doull J, et al. *Food Chem Toxicol.* 1999;37(7):789–811.

109. Abraham SK. *Food Chem Toxicol.* 2001;39:493–498.

110. Zhu M, Wong PY, Li RC. *J Pharm Pharmacol.* 1999;51(12):1391–1396.

111. Yang ZY, Pei J, Liu RM, et al. *Zhongguo Zhong Xi Yi Jie He Za Zhi.* 2005;25(9):822–824.

112. Dhar SK. *Indian J Physiol Pharmacol.* 1995;39:63–67.

113. Ostad SN, Khakinegad B, Sabzevari O. *Toxicol In Vitro.* 2004;18(5):623–627.

114. Stager J, Wuthrich B, Johansson SG. *Allergy.* 1991;46(6):475–478.

115. Helbling A, Lopez M, Schwartz HJ, et al. *Ann Allergy.* 1993;70(6):495–499.

116. Muhlemann RJ, Wuthrich B. *Schweiz Med Wochenschr.* 1991;121(46):1696–1700.

117. Moneret-Vautrin DA, Morisset M, Lemerdy P, et al. *Allerg Immunol.* 2002;34(4):135–140.

118. Rance F, Dutau G. *Pediatr Allergy Immunol.* 1997;8(1):41–44.

119. Jensen-Jarolim E, Leitner A, Hirshwerh R, et al. *Clin Exp Allergy.* 1997;27(11):1299–1306.

120. Asero R. *Ann Allergy Asthma Immunol.* 2000;84(4):460–462.

121. Garcia-Gonzalez JJ, Bartolome-Zavala B, Fernandez-Melendez S, et al. *Ann Allergy Asthma Immunol.* 2002;88(5):518–522.

122. Schwartz HJ, Jones RT, Rojas AR, et al. *Ann Allergy Asthma Immunol.* 1997;78(1):37–40.

123. Ottolenghi A, De Chiara A, Arrigoni S, et al. *Pediatr Med Chir.* 1995;17(6):525–530.

124. Turkyilmaz Z, Karabulut R, Sonmez K, et al. *J Pediatr. Surg.* 2008;43(11):2109–2111.

125. Fugh-Berman A. *Nutr Today.* 2002;37(3):122–124.

Feverfew

(*Tanacetum parthenium* (L.) Schulz-Bip.)

Synonyms

Chrysanthemum parthenium (L.) Bernh., (botanical synonym), Tanaceti parthenii herba/folium (Lat), Mutterkraut (Ger), camomille grande (Fr), matrem (Dan).

What is it?

Feverfew, a herb with long traditional use, received much attention in the UK during the 1980s when it became popular as a migraine remedy. It has been given many botanical names including *Chrysanthemum parthenium*, *Pyrethrum parthenium* and *Matricaria pyrethrum*. The plant looks somewhat similar to chamomile at first glance and has a strong smell particularly disliked by bees. The common name is believed to be derived from the Latin *febris* (a fever) and *fugare* (to drive away), as it was used to cure fevers in the past. The part used medicinally is the leaf, with or without stem, collected when or after the plant flowered.

Effects

Antisecretory (inhibition of platelet aggregation, granule secretion from polymorphonuclear leucocytes); anti-inflammatory (inhibits NF-kappaB activation and prostaglandin biosynthesis).

Traditional view

Warm infusions were traditionally prescribed to purge choler, to treat colds and febrile diseases, to cleanse the kidneys and to bring on menstruation and expel worms.[1] The decoction, sweetened with honey or sugar, was given for coughs, wheezing and difficult breathing.[2] Cold infusions were considered an excellent tonic, including for 'those who have taken Opium too liberally'.[1] This preparation was also used to relieve facial and ear pain in dyspeptic or rheumatic patients.[2] The leaves were applied as a poultice to ease pain and swelling of the bowel and for wind or colic.[1] Eclectic physicians regarded feverfew as a tonic that influenced the entire intestinal tract, increased appetite, improved digestion, promoted secretion and acted upon the renal and cutaneous functions.[3] Although not widespread, there is reference to the traditional use of feverfew for headache in Welsh herbal literature.[4]

Summary actions

Anti-inflammatory, bitter, emmenagogue (only in high doses), anthelmintic.

Can be used for

Indications supported by clinical trials

Prophylaxis and treatment of migraine, tension headache and associated symptoms.

Traditional therapeutic uses

Coughs, colds; febrile diseases; atonic dyspepsia; nervous debility.

May also be used for

Extrapolations from pharmacological studies

Conditions requiring antiallergic or anti-inflammatory activity; inflammatory arthritis.[5]

Other applications

Anecdotal evidence suggests feverfew is beneficial for psoriasis.[6]

Preparations

Fresh or dried plant tincture; tablets or capsules from the dried leaf or leaf extracts.

Although one clinical trial was conducted using freeze-dried feverfew leaf and many users take the fresh leaves, some promoters of feverfew are of the opinion that the air-dried herb is less likely to cause side effects.[7] The results of one clinical trial clearly demonstrated efficacy for conventionally dried feverfew leaves grown in Israel and given as a capsule.[8]

Dosage

- 0.7 to 2 mL of 1:1 fresh plant tincture per day (but see below)
- 1 to 2 mL of 1:5 dried plant tincture per day (but see below)
- One tablet (say 150 mg dried herb, standardised to contain at least 0.6 mg parthenolide), one to two times per day (but see below).

The adequate dose varies with the quality of the herb and the severity and frequency of migraines. In addition, it is more likely that a higher starting dose establishes the prophylactic effect more rapidly. Probably because of the initial use and promotion of a low dose of the fresh leaves, there is a tendency to recommend quite low doses of feverfew for migraine prophylaxis. However, the use of such doses often means that it can take 6 to 9 months before any effective prophylaxis occurs. With this length of time, the patient might give up treatment before any benefit is established. Hence, the early use of higher doses of feverfew in migraine prevention is recommended for a faster clinical effect. Also, it can be combined with other relevant herbs to maximise the magnitude and speed of the onset of such prophylaxis. Typically, doses of at least 3 to 5 mL per day of the 1:5 tincture in 60% ethanol (to extract the lactones) or its equal in tablets or capsules (600 to 1000 mg/day of dried herb equivalent) are recommended initially. Once sufficient prophylaxis takes place the dose can be reduced to a suitable level (see above) to maintain the clinical effect.

Duration of use

There is no restriction on long-term use. Information from clinical surveys suggests treatment in excess of 4 to 6 months may be required to assess any beneficial effect.

Summary assessment of safety

Except in cases of allergy in susceptible patients, feverfew is a safe herb. Some uncomfortable side effects, such as mouth ulcers, may occur in a percentage of patients, especially those who chew the fresh leaves.

Technical data

Botany

Feverfew is a perennial plant that may grow up to 70 cm. Its light green leaves (2 to 9 cm long) are ovate in outline, pinnate with pinnatifid lobed or toothed leaflets. The flower heads (1 to 2.4 cm in diameter) consist of ray florets of white, short ligules and inner, yellow disc florets. The fruit is a ribbed achene approximately 1.5 mm long.[9,10] (Tanacetum and Chrysanthemum are two separate genera of the Anthemideae tribe of the Compositae (daisy) family,[11] so *Chrysanthemum parthenium* is not technically a synonym of *Tanacetum parthenium* but rather a former name.)

Adulteration

No adulterants known. However, parthenolide levels in feverfew can vary considerably. A US study found that none of four feverfew products tested contained the level of parthenolide claimed on the label.[12] Parthenolide instability might have contributed to this finding.[13]

Key constituents

- Sesquiterpene lactones containing an alpha-methylene-gamma-lactone group: in particular those of the germacranolide type,[14] including parthenolide (0.06% to 0.6%)[15] and 3-beta-hydroxyparthenolide; the guaianolide type[14] and others containing chlorine[16]
- Sesquiterpenes, monoterpenes, polyacetylene compounds,[17] essential oil,[18] flavonoids,[19–21] dicaffeoylquinic acids[22]
- Melatonin has also been detected in trace amounts (1.37 to 2.45 μg/g) in feverfew leaf samples and in a commercial preparation.[23]

As noted above, the parthenolide content of feverfew can vary considerably.[24,25] Tests conducted on Mexican- and Yugoslavian-grown plants yielded no parthenolide,[26] although a later study did find parthenolide in Mexican samples.[27] The post-flowering leaves can contain up to four times the levels of pre-flowering leaves.[26] Harvesting during the afternoon and subjecting plants to a single water stress event can increase parthenolide levels.[28] Varieties with light green/yellow leaf colour yield higher levels of this compound.[29]

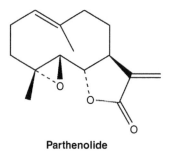

Parthenolide

Pharmacodynamics

Most of the pharmacological research has been conducted on parthenolide. The alpha-methylene-gamma-lactone (MGL) group probably provides much of the biological activity of this compound. Since the nucleophile in biological systems is very often a thiol (sulphydryl) group, this MGL group can act as an alkylating agent of such thiol residues,[30] thereby disrupting cell function. (Thiol groups, such as cysteine residues in proteins or enzymes, are important constituents of the plasma membrane and cytoskeleton.[31] The assembly of microtubules in the cytoskeleton is known to be involved in phagocytosis and the degranulation of neutrophils.[32])

The pathophysiology of migraine is not fully understood; hence feverfew's mechanism of action in migraine prophylaxis remains to be adequately defined. It had been proposed that a significant increase in serotonin release from platelets triggers the complex chain of events leading to a migraine attack,[33] and that migraine is caused by abnormal platelet activity and serotonin metabolism.[34] However, this theory no longer holds widespread currency. In accordance with this earlier theory, the observation that feverfew interacts with the protein kinase C pathway causing an inhibition of granule secretion from platelets was suggested as an antimigraine effect (with inhibition of degranulation from polymorphs as an antiarthritic effect).[35] Another theory is that feverfew exerts an anti-inflammatory activity in migraines, due in part to its parthenolide content. Parthenolide certainly has a unique anti-inflammatory profile that is now known to be largely mediated by inhibition of NF-kappaB activation. The mechanism involved is so specific that parthenolide is currently used as a pharmacological probe for in vitro experiments exploring the role of NF-kappaB in a variety of biochemical pathways. (The numerous studies where parthenolide has been employed in this way have not been included in this monograph.)

Antisecretory activity

Chloroform/methanol and aqueous extracts of feverfew inhibited the secretory activity of blood platelets and polymorphonuclear leucocytes in vitro. Release of serotonin from platelets induced by aggregating agents was inhibited. The pattern of effects of feverfew on platelets is different to that obtained with other inhibitors of platelet aggregation and the impact on polymorphs is more pronounced than that observed for very high concentrations of NSAIDs.[35] Aqueous extract of feverfew inhibited platelet aggregation induced by ADP, collagen and thrombin, but aggregation induced by arachidonic acid was not affected. Synthesis of thromboxane B_2 from platelets incubated with arachidonic acid was also not inhibited. However, feverfew extract did inhibit platelet phospholipase A_2, suggesting its antiplatelet activities are due to a phospholipase inhibitor that prevents the release of arachidonic acid.[36]

Eleven fractions obtained from a chloroform extract of feverfew demonstrated antisecretory activity in vitro; two fractions were devoid of activity. All the active fractions contained compounds with an MGL group. Five such compounds were isolated.[14] Feverfew and parthenolide dramatically reduced the number of acid-soluble sulphydryl groups in platelets at concentrations similar to those that inhibited platelet secretory activity. Feverfew itself did not induce the formation of disulphide-linked protein polymers in platelets, but polymer formation occurred when aggregating agents were added to feverfew-treated platelets.[37] In vitro studies also show that there are marked similarities between the inhibitory effects of feverfew extract and parthenolide on both serotonin secretion and platelet aggregation induced by several activating agents in human platelets. Results suggest an interaction with the protein kinase C pathway.[38] However, parthenolide neither activated nor inhibited protein kinase C type 1 from a bovine brain preparation in concentrations up to 200 µg/mL in vitro, nor did it affect the activity of membrane-associated protein kinase C in isolated lymphoma cell membranes.[39]

Several feverfew extracts were tested for antisecretory activity in a bioassay of platelets and compared with parthenolide. There was a close correlation between the parthenolide content of the extracts and their antisecretory activity.[40] Other sesquiterpene lactones from feverfew were also active. The content of parthenolide and bioactivity of feverfew plants varied enormously when grown under identical conditions using seeds from 10 different regions of Europe.[41] A selection of feverfew commercial preparations (leaves, tablets, drops) in the UK inhibited secretory activity in platelets, albeit at lower levels than expected (compared to freshly prepared feverfew).[42] Feverfew extracts modified the interaction of platelets with collagen substrates and inhibited both platelet spreading and formation of thrombus-like platelet aggregates on the collagen surface.[43] A chloroform extract of feverfew was a powerful inhibitor of platelet-collagen interaction in an in vitro model used for testing antithrombotic drugs. Feverfew also prevented the endothelial cell monolayer of perfused rabbit aorta from spontaneous injury.[44] While the platelets of patients taking feverfew aggregated normally to ADP and thrombin, aggregation in response to serotonin was greatly reduced.[45]

Feverfew extract inhibited the activity of polymorphonuclear leucocytes (PMNL) in vitro, probably via blockade of cellular sulphydryl groups (since cell lysis was ruled out).[46] Whole and fractionated acetone extracts of feverfew (and other *Tanacetum spp*) demonstrated inhibitory effects in vitro using a human PMNL-based bioassay. Although parthenolide was clearly an important determinant of activity, it was found not to be the sole factor.[47,48] Feverfew extracts markedly inhibited phagocytosis of *Candida guilliermondii* in vitro, but intracellular killing was not affected.[49] The fact that feverfew can inhibit phagocytosis as well as degranulation gives it increased potential as an anti-inflammatory agent.

A chloroform extract of feverfew dose-dependently inhibited histamine release induced by stimulating rat peritoneal mast cells via an IgE-anti-IgE reaction. The data suggest that this effect of feverfew is different to the inhibitory action on mast cells of both cromoglycate and quercetin. In addition, feverfew extract did not inhibit histamine release by interfering with oxidative phosphorylation.[50] Parthenolide inhibited IgE-mediated mast cell degranulation in vitro and inhibited passive cutaneous anaphylaxis in mice (10 mg/kg, ip).[51] Inhibition of microtubule formation was suggested as the mechanism,[51] although prevention of the increase in intracellular calcium levels has also been observed.[52]

Anti-inflammatory activity

Earlier research found parthenolide inhibited cyclo-oxygenase (COX, which converts arachidonic acid to prostaglandins) in vitro.[53] Parthenolide also inhibited the expression of inducible cyclo-oxygenase (COX-2) and proinflammatory cytokines in lipopolysaccharide (LPS)-stimulated macrophages in vitro, which correlated with the inhibition of mitogen-activated protein kinases. The MGL group was suggested to be behind the inhibitory activity.[54] However, aqueous extracts of whole plant and leaf inhibited prostaglandin biosynthesis, but not COX.[55] Parthenolide also did not inhibit COX activity in vitro using enzyme derived from sheep seminal vesicles.[39] Other evidence suggested that sesquiterpene lactones, including parthenolide, inhibited the release of arachidonic acid from membrane phospholipid stores rather than its conversion into thromboxane B_2 via the COX pathway.[39]

A chloroform extract of feverfew evoked changes in the metabolism of arachidonic acid similar to those observed in glutathione-depleted platelets.[37] It also inhibited the uptake and liberation of arachidonic acid from platelet membrane phospholipids,[56] which may be the result of an altered cytoskeletal-membrane interaction.[32] SH groups (sulphydryls) are essential for phospholipase A_2 activity (and the liberation of arachidonic acid),[57] and may have been influenced by feverfew in this context.[56] Chloroform extracts of feverfew produced dose-dependent inhibition of the generation of thromboxane B_2 and leukotriene B_4 by stimulated leucocytes. The activity was due to other lactones as well as sesquiterpene lactones.[58]

However, the most significant finding for feverfew in the context of inflammation is the specific inhibition of NF-kappaB activation by parthenolide. NF-kappaB is an inducible transcription factor that is an important mediator of immune and inflammatory responses. Its activation can lead to induction of COX-2 and production of proinflammatory prostaglandins. This pronounced in vitro activity of parthenolide was first discovered in the context of screening Mexican Indian traditional plants.[59] Isohelenin, which like feverfew is a sesquiterpene lactone (STL) with an MGL group, also inhibited NF-kappaB activation. Other STLs without this specific chemical group were not active.[60] Prevention of the degradation of the inhibitory proteins IkappaB-alpha and -beta was suggested as the possible underlying mechanism.[60] Shortly afterwards, it was also discovered that parthenolide inhibits NF-kappaB activation by targeting the IkappaB kinase (IKK) complex.[61] Parthenolide in fact binds directly to and inhibits IKK in vitro.[62]

This property of parthenolide might be relevant to the antimigraine activity of feverfew, since targeting NF-kappaB as a therapy for migraine has been suggested as a possible strategy (in the context of discussing parthenolide).[63] Nitric oxide (NO) generated from inducible NO synthase (iNOS) might be a relevant inflammatory mediator in this context. The NO donor glyceryl trinitrate (GTN) produces delayed migraine attacks in migraine sufferers. Expression of iNOS is preceded by significant NF-kappaB activity, as reflected by a reduction in the inhibitory protein IkappaB-alpha. Parthenolide (3 mg/kg, ip, to rats) inhibited IkappaB-alpha degradation, NF-kappaB activation and iNOS expression after GTN infusion.[63]

Further to this line of argument, a feverfew extract with 26% parthenolide (100 mg/kg/day for 6 days, ip) and parthenolide (15 mg/kg/day for 6 days, ip) reduced GTN-induced c-Fos activation in the brains of rats.[64] A parthenolide-depleted feverfew extract (0.8%) was inactive. Expression of c-Fos is an indirect measure of neuronal activity. The activity occurred in a key area of the brain involved in migraine pathogenesis, the nucleus trigeminalis caudalis. Purified parthenolide was better tolerated than the enriched herbal extract.

Parthenolide has demonstrated anti-inflammatory activity via inhibition of NF-kappaB activation in many in vitro and in vivo models. For example, it inhibited LPS-stimulated inflammatory responses via inhibition of NF-kappaB in vitro[65–67] and was especially effective in this regard compared with other natural products.[66] However, parthenolide also inhibited LPS-induced maturation of human dendritic cells independently of NF-kappaB.[68] Activity of iNOS was also inhibited in vitro,[69] as was IL-4 gene expression in stimulated human peripheral blood T cells (a mechanism involved in allergies).[70]

Parthenolide inhibited NF-kappaB activation and inflammatory responses in cystic fibrosis cells[71] and inhibited Nod2 signalling and target gene expression in human colonic epithelial cells, leading to reduced NF-kappaB activation (with possible implications for Crohn's disease).[72] NF-kappaB inhibitors such as parthenolide also have potential in the treatment of atherosclerotic plaque instability and rupture.[73]

Cyclophosphamide is associated with inducing haemorrhagic cystitis and voiding symptoms, probably mediated by NF-kappaB activation. Pretreatment with parthenolide (4 mg/kg/day for 3 days, sc) inhibited bladder inflammation and overactivity in rats given cyclophosphamide.[74] Parthenolide also dose-dependently suppressed tumour necrosis factor (TNF)-alpha induced COX-2 expression and prevented NF-kappaB phosphorylation and nuclear translocation, and IkappaB-alpha phosphorylation/degradation.[74] Protective effects were also observed in rats after myocardial reperfusion injury (0.25 or 0.5 mg/kg, ip, 10 minutes before reperfusion).[75] In a mouse model of cystic fibrosis, parthenolide (3 μcg/g, ip) inhibited lung NF-kappaB activation and resultant inflammatory responses following LPS challenge.[71] In (apoE) apolipoprotein E mice prone to arterial disease, long-term treatment with parthenolide (2, 4 and 10 mg/kg every second day for 10 to 20 weeks depending on dose, ip) reduced the size of the aortic lesion and plaque inflammatory responses.[76]

Parthenolide pretreatment exerted protective effects during endotoxic shock in rats (0.25, 0.5 and 1.0 mg/kg, ip) and mice (0.25 and 0.5 mg/kg, ip) through inhibition of NF-kappaB.[77] Such work led to an interest in NF-kappaB inhibition, and specifically the use of parthenolide, for limiting the inflammatory injury during sepsis. However, studies examining survival in LPS-challenged mice using such a strategy have exhibited only modest benefits, according to a recent review.[78]

Oral administration of a feverfew extract led to significant antinociceptive and anti-inflammatory effects against acetic acid-induced writhing in mice and carrageenan-induced paw oedema in rats, respectively.[79] These responses were dose-dependent (10, 20, 40 mg/kg). Parthenolide (1 and 2 mg/kg, ip) also produced antinociceptive and anti-inflammatory effects. Naloxone (1 mg/kg, ip), an opiate antagonist, failed to reverse feverfew- and parthenolide-induced antinociception. Feverfew extract in higher doses (40 and 60 mg/kg, oral) neither altered locomotor activity nor potentiated pentobarbitone-induced sleep time in mice. It also did not change the rectal temperature in rats. The authors concluded that feverfew extract exerted antinociceptive and anti-inflammatory effects without altering normal behaviour.

Topical application of a 1% solution of a parthenolide-depleted (PD) feverfew extract reduced UV-induced epidermal hyperplasia, DNA damage and apoptosis in hairless mice and pigs.[80] This extract was developed to eliminate the risk of skin sensitisation, a well-known property of sesquiterpene lactones. PD-feverfew directly inhibited activity of the pro-inflammatory enzymes 5-lipoxygenase, phosphodiesterase-3 and phosphodiesterase-4.[81] PD-feverfew also inhibited the release of the pro-inflammatory mediators nitric oxide, PGE_2 and TNF-alpha from macrophages, and TNF-alpha, IL-2, IFN-gamma and IL-4 from human peripheral blood mononuclear cells (PBMC). Additionally, PD-feverfew inhibited TPA-induced release of PGE_2 from human skin equivalents. In mice, topical application at 0.1 and 1.0% of PD-feverfew inhibited oxazolone-induced dermatitis, and was more potent than whole feverfew in reducing (TPA-induced dermatitis.[81] TPA is phorbol myristate acetate, a skin irritant.)

Interaction with contractile agonists

Parthenolide exhibited little activity at serotonin receptors.[82,83] However, it inhibited the contractile (serotonin release-mediated) responses of rat stomach fundus to two indirect-acting serotonin agonists, but not to serotonin itself.[84]

Extracts of fresh feverfew caused a dose- and time-dependent inhibition of the contractile responses of isolated smooth tissue to receptor-acting agonists such as serotonin and phenylephrine. Chloroform extracts of dried feverfew (which in this case did not contain parthenolide or other MGLs) were not inhibitory, but instead elicited contraction.[85] Chloroform extracts of feverfew and parthenolide inhibited smooth muscle contractility in isolated tissue in a time-dependent, non-specific and irreversible manner. The inhibition required the presence of the MGL group.[86,87] The inhibitory effects are non-specific and may result from interference with postreceptor contractile mechanisms. The irreversible nature of the inhibition implies a long-lasting toxic effect on the tissue.[88]

Isometric responses to serotonin and the indirect serotonergic agent D-fenfluramine were obtained on rat fundus and ileum. Parthenolide antagonised the effects of fenfluramine, but exhibited only slow activity on serotonin receptors in these tissues, whereas feverfew extract exerted potent activity.[89] Thermal degradation of the extract saw a loss of activity. Similar results were observed in rats fed orally with undegraded and degraded feverfew power (20 mg/kg/day for 30 days, equivalent to a human dose of 500 µg/day of parthenolide for the undegraded powder) and injected ip with parthenolide (23.4 µg/rat/day for 7 days). Feverfew powder was a more effective antiserotonergic agent than either its extracts or pure parthenolide. All these results suggest the presence of other compounds acting on serotonin receptors.

Anticancer activity

A 2010 review noted that sesquiterpene lactones such as parthenolide have been investigated as anticancer agents since the 1960s.[90] Numerous studies have demonstrated the activity of parthenolide against a range of tumour cell lines. Again, inhibition of NF-kappaB activity (via either interaction with IKK or more directly with its p65 subunit), which is constitutive in many types of cancers, is considered one of the main mechanisms of action.[91] In addition, inhibition of STAT (signal transducer and activator of transcription) and MAP (mitogen-activated protein) kinase activities, and the induction of sustained JNK (c-Jun N-terminal kinase) activity, can lead to increased susceptibility of cancer cells to chemotherapy and radiotherapy after treatment with feverfew.[91]

At the epigenetic level, parthenolide reduces HDAC1 (histone deacetylase 1) levels and, by inhibiting DNMT2 activity (a DNA methyltransferase), induces global hypomethylation of DNA, thereby restoring the expression of some suppressor genes.[91] In addition, parthenolide reduces the cellular level of glutathione in cancer cells, followed by accumulation of reactive oxygen species and apoptosis. A unique property is its ability to selectively induce cell death in cancer cells, sparing healthy cells. It also seems to have the potential to target certain cancer stem cells, such as breast and prostate.[91]

Examples of more recent in vitro studies of parthenolide include activity against liver cancer cells,[92] cholangiocarcinoma cells,[93] leukaemia stem cells,[94] melanoma cells[95] and gastric cancer cells.[96] Feverfew extracts have also shown anticancer activity in vitro. Activity was demonstrated against two human breast cancer cell lines and one human cervical cancer cell line.[97] Flavonoids in the herb might exhibit a weak synergistic activity with parthenolide.

A 2008 review of the molecular basis of parthenolide-dependent pro-apoptotic activity in cancer cells suggested several likely mechanisms.[98] Parthenolide inhibits NF-kappaB and STAT-mediated anti-apoptotic gene transcription. The pro-apoptotic activity includes intrinsic and extrinsic mechanisms. Stimulation of the intrinsic pro-apoptotic pathway involves higher levels of reactive oxygen species and modification of Bcl-2 family proteins. Parthenolide also amplifies the apoptotic signal through the sensitisation of cancer cells to extrinsic apoptosis induced by TNF-alpha. These effects are specific to tumour cells.

The in vivo anticancer activity of parthenolide has also been investigated, although there have been fewer studies. Most of the in vivo outcomes have been linked to parthenolide's role in inhibiting NF-kappaB activation. Parthenolide (40 mg/kg/day, oral) in combination with docetaxol reduced metastasis and improved survival in a murine xenograft model of breast cancer[99] and at the same dose restored chemotherapy and hormone therapy sensitivity in a murine xenograft model of hormone-refractory prostate cancer.[100] Inhibition of lung colonisation by murine osteosarcoma cells was inhibited by concurrent administration of parthenolide (mice, 0.01 µg to 1 mg/kg, ip), but it had no effect when given after the inoculation of tumour cells.[101] Tumour growth in a xenograft model of renal cell carcinoma was inhibited by parthenolide (mice, 3 µg/mouse, sc).[102] Renal damage induced by the anticancer drug cisplatin was also reduced by parthenolide (rats, 3 mg/kg/day, ip).[103] Treatment with parthenolide (20 mg/kg/day, ip) increased the efficacy of taxol in a murine xenograft model of non-small cell lung cancer.[104] Parthenolide (1 mg/kg/day, ip) reduced osteolytic metastatic bone lesions following the injection of W256 tumour cells in rats.[105]

Chemopreventative activity was observed for parthenolide (1 mg/mouse/day) in a model of UVB-induced skin cancer.[106]

Antimicrobial activity

Eudesmanolides (10 mg/mL) isolated from feverfew demonstrated antibacterial activity towards *Staph. aureus*, *E. coli* and *Salmonella spp.*[107] Parthenolide inhibited the growth of Gram-positive bacteria, yeasts and filamentous fungi in vitro. Species of *Bacillus* without endospores were particularly sensitive.[108]

The essential oil obtained from feverfew flowers showed bactericidal and fungicidal activity against most of the

27 microorganisms tested using the agar diffusion and broth dilution methods.[109] Two extracts of feverfew were tested in a similar way using many of the same test species, including *Staph. aureus*, *Strep. haemolyticus*, *Sarcina flava* and *E. coli*. Gram-negative species were much less sensitive than the Gram-positive species, fungi and dermatophytes.[110]

Parthenolide showed significant in vitro activity against the promastigote form of *Leishmania amazonensis*, with 50% inhibition at 0.37 μg/mL.[111] For the intracellular amastigote form, parthenolide at 0.81 μg/mL reduced the survival index of the parasite in macrophages by 50%. A guaianolide from feverfew was also active against this parasite species in vitro.[112]

In vitro activity against the epimastigote form of *Trypanosoma cruzi* was observed for crude extracts of feverfew and parthenolide (IC_{50} 0.5 μg/mL).[113] Parthenolide also exhibited synergistic activity with benznidazole against this parasite in vitro.[114]

Other activity

Addition of feverfew extract protected the endothelial cell monolayer from perfusion-induced injury and led to a reversible increase in the cyclic AMP content of aorta segments. This indicates that feverfew may exert a vasoprotective effect.[43] Parthenolide given ip reduced ischaemia-reperfusion injury in rat hearts, an effect thought to be mediated by inhibition of NF-kappaB activation.[115]

Feverfew extract inhibited mitogen-induced human PBMC proliferation and cytokine-mediated responses in vitro. Both the extract and parthenolide proved cytotoxic to mitogen-induced PBMC (after incubation for 48 to 72 h). If feverfew is cytotoxic in vivo to lymphocytes or macrophages that are overactive, this could possibly explain a beneficial effect in rheumatoid arthritis sufferers.[116]

Intraperitoneal administration of feverfew extract inhibited collagen-induced bronchoconstriction in guinea pigs. The authors concluded that this was a consequence of phospholipase A_2 inhibition.[117] Parthenolide protected against experimentally induced nephrocalcinosis in rats.[118]

Parthenolide injection (0.5 and 1 mg/kg) blocked LPS-induced osteolysis in the mouse calvarium model through suppression of NF-kappaB activity.[119] This suggests a possible role in bacteria-induced bone destruction, a theme expanded in a review that suggested NF-kappaB inhibitors might also be valuable in periprosthetic osteolysis, arthritis, Paget's disease and periodontitis.[120]

NF-kappaB inhibitors might improve healing and exert anti-ageing effects. Parthenolide (0.5 mg/kg, oral) improved the healing and mechanical stability of colonic anastomoses in rats during the early postoperative period[121] and inhibited UVB-mediated skin photoageing in vitro,[122] probably via inhibition of NF-kappaB.[123]

The antiserotonergic effects of parthenolide in platelets prompted an investigation into its role in depression. In mice, parthenolide (0.5 to 2.0 mg/kg, ip) exhibited dose-dependent depressant-like effects, possibly mediated by platelet/neuronal hyposerotonergic effects.[124]

Pharmacokinetics

It has been postulated that the actively alkylating MGL group (such as in parthenolide) would be rapidly inactivated via glutathione upon entering the bloodstream, perhaps raising doubts over the in vivo relevance of the in vitro studies using parthenolide. However, it has been observed that sequential treatment of old samples of dried powdered feverfew leaf (which contained no 'free' parthenolide) with an oxidant and a weak base caused the regeneration of substantial amounts of parthenolide. This process may also occur in vivo with cytochrome P450 enzymes as oxidants, with conversion back into 'free' parthenolide at the cellular level.[30] In vivo activity has certainly been demonstrated for parthenolide, even after oral doses.

Investigations using the Caco-2 in vitro model of the human intestinal wall found that parthenolide is effectively absorbed via a passive diffusion mechanism.[125] In vitro experiments found that parthenolide binds strongly to proteins in human plasma.[126]

A phase I dose escalation trial of feverfew containing standardised doses of parthenolide in 12 cancer patients also included an assessment of plasma pharmacokinetics.[127] Parthenolide could not be detected in plasma after a feverfew dose containing 4 mg/day of this compound. The feverfew was well tolerated. Preliminary murine metabolism studies found plasma concentrations of parthenolide of 28 ng/mL and 42 ng/mL 1 hour after oral doses of 4 mg/kg and 40 mg/kg, respectively. The 0.4 mg/kg dose in mice did not provide any detectable plasma parthenolide (and approximately corresponds to a 4 mg human dose).[127]

Clinical trials

Migraine

In 1973, at the suggestion of a friend and apparently based on the advice of a traditional Welsh healer, a Welsh woman Mrs Anne Jenkins tried taking three fresh leaves of feverfew each day in an attempt to rid herself of severe and recurrent migraines. After 10 months Mrs Jenkins' headaches had vanished and did not return as long as she kept taking feverfew. Her enthusiasm rapidly led to the widespread use of feverfew in the UK. Dr Stewart Johnson a London migraine specialist became interested and initiated a survey that was followed up by a clinical trial. The survey revealed some interesting findings:[128]

- About 72% of those surveyed (253 suffering from true migraine) found that feverfew was helpful for the prevention of their headaches; 78% of the 23 people suffering from tension headaches also found that feverfew reduced headache frequency and severity. Of 242 patients who recorded the frequency, 33% no longer had attacks and 76% had fewer migraines each month, compared with before taking feverfew.

- Associated nausea and vomiting decreased or disappeared. A proportion of patients experienced the migraine aura without the attack.

- When attacks did occur, they responded better to conventional painkillers (e.g. aspirin). Feverfew users experienced no adverse interactions with their orthodox medication.
- Many patients also suffering from arthritis found their symptoms somewhat relieved by feverfew.
- The onset of the effect was slow and gradual, often taking several months, and the average dose used was very low – about two and a half fresh leaves (4 cm long by 3 cm wide) per day. The average duration of treatment was 2.3 and 2.6 years for men and women respectively. When respondents stopped taking feverfew their migraines tended to return soon after.
- The survey also revealed some side effects in a small percentage of users. Adverse effects included mouth ulcers or inflammation. In contrast, a percentage of users experienced improved digestion, a sense of well-being and improved sleep.

This work was followed up by a double blind, placebo-controlled pilot clinical trial involving 17 patients who had been self-medicating with raw feverfew every day for 3 months. Eight of these patients received two capsules per day containing freeze-dried feverfew leaf powder (25 mg each) and nine received placebo for 24 weeks. Prior to the trial, the reduction in the frequency and migraines during self-treatment with feverfew was significant for both groups. Compared with the migraine frequency while self-medicating, there was no change in the frequency or severity of symptoms in the feverfew group during the trial. The placebo group, however, experienced a significant increase ($p<0.05$) in the frequency and severity of headaches when the results of the previous 3 months were considered. The placebo group also experienced a higher incidence and severity of nausea and vomiting than the feverfew group ($p<0.05$). The authors claimed a prophylactic benefit for feverfew in preventing migraine attacks. Curiously, fewer adverse events were reported by those taking feverfew (four patients reported none) compared with placebo (all patients taking reported at least one event).[129,130] Apparently, the trial had this unusual design because of ethical reasons (feverfew was considered to have unknown safety by the scientists). The patients were already using feverfew, so the trial therefore observed the results of patients unknowingly stopping their herbal treatment. As noted above, such an abrupt discontinuance led to the recurrence of severe migraines in some patients. Perhaps more importantly, the study showed that long-term feverfew users were normal in terms of a large number of biochemical and haematological parameters.

A few years later, 59 patients with classical or common migraine completed a randomised, double blind, placebo-controlled, crossover study. Only 17 of these patients had previously tried feverfew. After a 1-month single blind placebo run-in, patients were randomly allocated to receive either one capsule of freeze-dried powdered feverfew (averaging 82 mg and containing 2.2 mmol parthenolide, approximately two medium-sized leaves) or placebo for 4 months, then crossed over to the other treatment for a further 4 months. Feverfew was associated with a 24% reduction in the mean number of

attacks and a significant reduction in the degree of vomiting ($p<0.02$) for each 2-month assessment period. There was also a trend towards a reduction in severity of attacks, although the duration of individual attacks was unaltered. Significant improvement in the feverfew group was also observed for visual analogue scores ($p<0.0001$). Treatment with feverfew did not produce any adverse effects. Although there was no washout period between feverfew and placebo treatments, patients receiving placebo after feverfew did not experience a decreased deterioration compared with the placebo levels from the first phase of the trial.[131] No ex vivo reduction in serotonin secretion from platelets after ingestion of feverfew for 4 months could be demonstrated.[132]

A team of Dutch scientists active in the field of feverfew research tested the efficacy of a standardised extract for the prevention of migraine headaches. In a randomised, placebo-controlled, double blind, crossover design, 50 patients who had never taken feverfew before and who experienced at least one migraine attack per month were followed for 4 months of active treatment and 4 months of placebo. Active treatment consisted of 143 mg/day of a granulated ethanolic extract of feverfew containing 0.5 mg of parthenolide, corresponding to about 170 mg of original dried herb. The feverfew preparation used in this study did not exert any significant preventative effect on the frequency of migraine attacks, although patients appeared to have a tendency to use fewer analgesic drugs while they were using feverfew.[133]

The authors suggested the negative finding might be because previous studies were conducted in patients who had already found feverfew to be beneficial (which is not actually the case – see above). Other reasons speculated by the authors were the dried plant preparation used, or the fact that an extract was prescribed, rather than the crude leaf. (The original popularity of feverfew was based on consumption of the fresh leaves, although the two earlier clinical trials used freeze-dried leaves.) Initial users of raw feverfew found that it took 6 months use or longer to establish a reduction in migraine frequency, so perhaps the duration of the trial was insufficient. It is also possible that only a subset of migraine sufferers are feverfew responders and a benefit in this subset might be missed in a randomised clinical trial.

In a subsequent double blind, placebo-controlled trial, 57 chronic migraine sufferers (43% suffered more than 10 attacks per month) were selected at random and divided into two groups. Both groups received powdered feverfew capsules (total of 100 mg/day of dried leaves containing 0.2 mg parthenolide) in the preliminary phase, which lasted 2 months. In the second and third phases, which continued for an additional 2 months, a double blind, placebo-controlled, crossover study was conducted. The difference in pain intensity of migraines before and after treatment with feverfew (measured in phase I) was highly significant ($p<0.001$). In phase II, patients receiving feverfew continued to experience a decrease in pain intensity, while it increased in those on placebo. The difference between the two groups was significant ($p<0.01$). Moreover, a profound reduction was observed in typical migraine symptoms such as vomiting, nausea and sensitivity to noise and light ($p<0.001$). Transferring the feverfew-treated group to placebo in phase III resulted in an increase in pain intensity and other symptoms. In contrast, shifting the placebo group to feverfew therapy resulted in an improvement in pain and other symptoms. However, no information was provided about the frequency of migraine attacks.[8] In this trial, rather than acting to reduce the frequency of migraines, it appeared that feverfew reduced their severity. A longer treatment time or higher doses may have also seen an impact on migraine frequency.

A German research team next studied the efficacy of a supercritical CO_2 extract of feverfew in two randomised, double blind, placebo-controlled trials. In the first trial, the efficacy and tolerability of three different doses per day of the extract (6.24 mg, 18.75 mg and 56.25 mg corresponding to 0.5 mg, 1.5 mg and 4.5 mg of parthenolide) were compared with a placebo.[134] The patients (n=147) suffered from migraine with and without aura according to International Headache Society (IHS) criteria and were treated with one of the study medications for 12 weeks after a 4-week baseline period. The primary efficacy parameter was the number of migraine attacks during each 28 days of treatment, compared with the baseline period. Secondary endpoints were the total and average duration and intensity of migraine attacks, mean duration of a single attack, number of days with accompanying migraine symptoms, number of days with inability to work due to migraine, as well as type and amount of additional medication for the treatment of migraine attacks. With respect to the primary and secondary efficacy parameters, a statistically significant difference was not found. The frequency of migraine attacks for a predefined confirmatory subgroup of patients (n=49) with at least four migraine attacks during the baseline period decreased in a dose-dependent manner (p=0.001). The highest absolute change of migraine attacks was observed for treatment with 18.75 mg/day (-1.8 ± 1.5 per 28 days) compared with placebo (-0.3 ± 1.9; p=0.02). Overall, 52 of 147 (35%) patients reported at least one adverse event. The incidence of these in the active treatment groups was similar to that in the placebo group, and no dose-related effect was observed for any safety parameter.

This study was followed up by the second trial that assessed the efficacy of only the 18.75 mg/day dose against placebo.[135] Patients (n=170) suffering from migraine according to the IHS criteria were treated for 16 weeks after a 4-week baseline period. The primary endpoint was the average number of migraine attacks per 28 days during treatment months 2 and 3 compared with baseline. Safety parameters included adverse events, laboratory parameters, vital signs and physical examination. Migraine frequency decreased by 1.9 attacks per month in the feverfew group and by 1.3 attacks in the placebo group (p=0.0456). Logistic regression of responder rates showed an odds ratio of 3.4 in favour of feverfew (p=0.0049). Adverse events possibly related to study medication were 9/107 (8.4%) with feverfew versus 11/108 (10.2%) with placebo (p=0.654). The authors concluded that the feverfew extract was effective and shows a favourable risk-benefit ratio.

The authors claimed that 6.25 mg of extract containing 0.5 mg parthenolide corresponded to 1.05 g of feverfew leaf (presumably dried),[134] so doses used in both the above studies appear to be high. However, since feverfew can contain up to 1.6% lactones as parthenolide, the dried herb equivalence of

the CO_2 extract doses might be somewhat overstated in relation to good quality leaf.[136]

Findings of a later study have suggested that a higher dose of feverfew (600 mg/day) than those used in the earliest studies, together with a relatively small dose of willow bark (Salix alba, 600 mg/day) might bring on a quicker result in migraine prophylaxis. The herbal combination was standardised for parthenolide (0.2%) and salicin (1.5%).[137] A prospective, open label study was undertaken over 12 weeks in 12 patients diagnosed with migraine without aura. Two patients were excluded for reasons unrelated to treatment. With the herbal treatment, attack frequency was reduced by 57.2% at 6 weeks (p<0.029) and by 61.7% at 12 weeks (p<0.025) in nine out of 10 patients, with 70% having a reduction of at least 50%. Attack intensity was reduced by 38.7% at 6 weeks (p<0.005) and by 62.6% at 12 weeks (p<0.004) in all of the 10 patients, with 70% of patients having a reduction of at least 50%. Attack duration decreased by 67.2% at 6 weeks (p<0.001) and by 76.2% at 12 weeks (p<0.001) in all of 10 patients. Self-assessed general health, physical performance, memory and anxiety also improved by the end of the study. The herbal treatment was well tolerated and no adverse events occurred.

Although this was an open label trial and hence lacking a placebo group, results are quite striking. They suggest that combining feverfew in higher doses with willow bark might result in significant clinical improvement in migraine frequency within 6 weeks. The obvious next step is to conduct a placebo-controlled trial for this combination.

Feverfew (100 mg/day containing 0.7 mg parthenolide) in combination with 300 mg/day magnesium (as the citrate and oxide) and 400 mg/day riboflavin was compared against a 'placebo' containing 25 mg of riboflavin in a 30-month randomised, double blind, placebo-controlled trial involving 49 patients with migraine.[138] The placebo contained riboflavin because of the yellow colour it gives to urine, which might have alerted patients that they were receiving active treatment. Both interventions showed comparable clinical effects in reducing migraine frequency. Since the placebo response exceeded that reported for other migraine prophylaxis studies, the authors suggested that 25 mg riboflavin may have been an active comparator. Nonetheless, there seemed to be little additional benefit from the feverfew.

The reported clinical trials for a proprietary sublingual combination of feverfew and ginger[139,140] have not been reviewed in this monograph as this is a homeopathic preparation containing feverfew 3X and ginger 2X.

A 2004 Cochrane review[141] of feverfew in the prevention of migraine included five studies published up to 2002[8,129,131,133,134] involving a total of 343 patients. It concluded that results up to that time point were mixed and did not convincingly establish that feverfew was effective in migraine prevention. Dosage variation may have been a reason for the mixed results. Positive studies have been published after this review was conducted (see above).

Other activity

In a randomised, double blind, placebo-controlled trial, 40 patients with symptomatic rheumatoid arthritis received either dried, chopped feverfew (70 to 86 mg/day) or placebo capsules for 6 weeks. Patients continued with their NSAID and analgesic drug treatment throughout the trial. No important differences between clinical or laboratory variables were observed for the two groups during the treatment period.[142]

In a placebo-controlled, randomised, double blind study involving 12 volunteers, a parthenolide-depleted 1% feverfew emulsion significantly reduced UVB-induced erythema (p<0.05).[80] Methyl nicotinate induces a rapid vasodilatory response when applied topically. A randomised, controlled trial in eight volunteers found that prior application of a parthenolide-depleted feverfew emulsion (0.5% to 1.0% strength) dose-dependently reduced the erythema induced by application of methyl nicotinate to the forearm.[81]

Toxicology and other safety data

Toxicology

No toxic effects were observed in rats and guinea pigs fed 100 to 150 times the human daily dose of feverfew each day for 5 to 7 weeks.[143] The highest non-toxic oral dose of feverfew in rats was 0.86 g/kg/day as an alcohol extract in a subacute study.[144]

Detailed haematological analysis found no significant differences between 60 migraine patients who were feverfew users, non-user migraine patients and non-user healthy volunteers. Some feverfew users had taken feverfew daily for more than 1 year.[143]

No significant differences in the frequency of chromosomal aberrations or sister chromatid exchanges were found in the circulating peripheral lymphocytes of chronic feverfew users (over 11 consecutive months) and non-user migraine patients. The mutagenicity of urine from feverfew users was not different to urine from non-users.[145,146] Parthenolide at concentrations up to 800 μM was found to be non-mutagenic in a forward mutation assay using *Salmonella typhimurium*.[39]

Contraindications

Patients with a known hypersensitivity to either feverfew, parthenolide or other members of the Compositae family, should not take feverfew internally.[147]

Special warnings and precautions

Doses during pregnancy should be kept to a minimum, especially in the first trimester.

Interactions

None known.

Use in pregnancy and lactation

Category B3 – no increase in frequency of malformation or other harmful effects on the fetus from limited use in women. Evidence of increased fetal damage in animal studies

exists (at very high doses), but the relevance to humans is unknown.

Doses during pregnancy should be kept to a minimum (no more than 500 mg/day or equivalent). A decoction of the flowers in wine was combined with nutmeg or mace in traditional Western herbal medicine to bring on menstruation and to expel the afterbirth and stillborn children.[148]

High oral doses of feverfew (0.839 g/kg/day) reduced fetal weights when administered to rats from days 8 to 15 of gestation and caused enlarged placentas when administered from days 1 to 8 or days 8 to 15 of gestation. The percentages of implantation loss and litter size were not significantly different from controls and major malformations were relatively rare. The herb was administered as an ethanol extract and the dose administered was the highest possible for which the ethanol remained below the teratogenic threshold.[149,150]

According to one source, feverfew is reputed to cause abortion in grazing cows (presumably after intake of large amounts), but no specific information was provided.[151]

There are no data available concerning the suitability of feverfew during lactation.

Effects on ability to drive and use machines

No adverse effects expected.

Side effects

A review in 2000 of six randomised, double blind, placebo-controlled trials found that feverfew use was associated with only mild and transient adverse effects.[152] Adverse reactions were reported in four of the trials and included mild gastrointestinal symptoms, mouth ulceration, heavier periods, palpitations, dizziness, weight gain and skin rash. Feverfew was administered in capsule form or as an extract in these trials.[129,131,133,134] Reactions were reported more frequently in the placebo group than in the feverfew group in two of the trials,[129,131] including the incidence of mouth ulceration.[131]

A survey conducted in the early 1980s of 270 migraine patients who had eaten fresh feverfew leaves every day for prolonged periods found that side effects occurred in 17.9%. They included mouth ulcers/sore tongue (6.4%), abdominal pain/indigestion (3.9%), unpleasant taste (3.0%), tingling sensation (0.9%), urinary problems (0.9%), headache (0.9%), swollen lips/mouth (0.4%) and diarrhoea (0.4%). Symptoms were reported in the first week of treatment in some users, whereas in others they appeared gradually over the first 2 months. Of an additional 164 users who had stopped taking fresh feverfew, 21% did so because of side effects, which mainly involved the gastrointestinal tract.[143,153]

Migraine patients who had used feverfew long-term to control their symptoms found that the frequency and severity of headache, nausea and vomiting increased when they ceased using feverfew. Other symptoms reported by these patients after ceasing feverfew included increased nervousness, tension headache, insomnia/disturbed sleep and joint stiffness. These symptoms have been described as 'post-feverfew syndrome'.[129]

A 27-year-old woman who had been taking feverfew for 6 months had an abnormally high prothrombin time reading and was refused surgery.[154]

Cases of allergic contact dermatitis from feverfew, particularly with occupational exposure and creams, have been reported.[155] The sesquiterpene lactones are responsible. Cross-reactivity with other members of the Compositae family is very common.[156–159] Clinical tolerance testing of formulations containing PD feverfew in over 1200 people demonstrated that they did not elicit allergic responses.[160] However, another study did find that such creams could elicit positive patch test reactions in feverfew-sensitive patients.[161] The reactivity was lost over time, probably because of the degradation of the small amount of parthenolide left in these PD products. Some feverfew-allergic patients are sensitive to airborne particles released from the plant, with parthenolide most likely the responsible allergen.[162]

Safety in children

No information available.

Overdosage

No incidents found in the published literature.

Regulatory status in selected countries

Feverfew is listed in the *United States Pharmacopeia-National Formulary* (USP31–NF26, 2008). Feverfew is not covered by a Commission E monograph. It is on the UK General Sale List. Feverfew products have achieved Traditional Herbal Registration in the UK with the traditional indication of prevention of migraine.

Feverfew does not have GRAS status. However, it is freely available as a 'dietary supplement' in the USA under DSHEA legislation (1994 Dietary Supplement Health and Education Act).

Feverfew is not included in Part 4 of Schedule 4 of the Therapeutic Goods Act Regulations of Australia and is freely available for sale.

References

1. Le Strange R. *A History of Herbal Plants*. London: Angus & Robertson; 1977. p. 74.
2. Grieve M. *A Modern Herbal*, vol. 1. New York: Dover Publications; 1971. pp. 309–310.
3. Felter HW, Lloyd JU. *King's American Dispensatory*, ed 18, rev 3, vol 2, 1905. Portland, Reprinted by Eclectic Medical Publications; 1983. pp. 1438–1439.
4. Johnson ES. *Feverfew (Overcoming Common Problems)*. London: Sheldon Press; 1984. pp. 26–27.
5. Johnson ES. *Feverfew (Overcoming Common Problems)*. London: Sheldon Press; 1984. pp. 51, 52, 56–70.
6. Hancock K. *Feverfew. Your Headache May Be Over*. New Canaan: Keats Publishing; 1986. pp. 36, 47–51.
7. Hancock K. *Feverfew, Your Headache May Be Over*. Connecticut: Keats Publishing; 1986. p. 23.
8. Palevitch E, Earon G, Carasso R. *Phytother Res*. 1997;11(7):508–511.
9. Chiej R. *The Macdonald Encyclopedia of Medicinal Plants*. London: Macdonald; 1984. Entry no. 85.
10. Launert EL. *The Hamlyn Guide to Edible and Medicinal Plants of Britain and Northern Europe*. London: Hamlyn; 1981. p. 194.
11. Mabberley DJ. *The Plant Book*, 2nd ed. Cambridge: Cambridge University Press; 1997. pp. 176, 699.
12. Jin P, Madieh S, Augsburger LL. *AAPS PharmSciTech*. 2008;9(1):22–30.
13. Jin P, Madieh S, Augsburger LL. *AAPS PharmSciTech*. 2007;8(4):E105.
14. Groenewegen WA, Knight DW, Heptinstall S. *J Pharm Pharmacol*. 1986;38(9):709–712.
15. Fontanel D, Bizot S, Beaufils P. *Plantes Méd Phytother*. 1990;24(4):231–237.
16. Wagner H, Fessler B, Lotter H, et al. *Planta Med*. 1988;54(2):171–172.
17. Bohlmann F, Zdero C. *Phytochemistry*. 1982;21(10):2543–2549.
18. Hendriks H, Bos R, Woerdenbag HJ. *Flavour Fragrance J*. 1996;11(6):367–371.
19. Williams CA, Hoult JR, Harborne JB, et al. *Phytochemistry*. 1995;38(1):267–270.
20. Williams CA, Harborne JB, Geiger H, et al. *Phytochemistry*. 1999;51(3):417–423.
21. Long C, Sauleau P, David B, et al. *Phytochemistry*. 2003;64(2):567–569.
22. Wu C, Chen F, Wang X, et al. *Phytochem Anal*. 2007;18(5):401–410.
23. Murch SJ, Simmons CB, Saxena PK. *Lancet*. 1997;350(9091):1598–1599.
24. El-Shamy AM, El-Hawary SS, Rateb ME. *J AOAC Int*. 2007;90(1):21–27.
25. Nelson MH, Cobb SE, Shelton J. *Am J Health Syst Pharm*. 2002;59(16):1527–1531.
26. Awang DVC, Dawson BA, Kindack DG. *J Nat Prod*. 1991;54(6):1516–1521.
27. Avula B, Navarrete A, Joshi VC, et al. *Pharmazie*. 2006;61(7):590–594.
28. Fonseca JM, Rushing JW, Rajapakse NC, et al. *J Plant Physiol*. 2005;162(5):485–494.
29. Cutlan AR, Bonilla LE, Simon JE, et al. *Planta Med*. 2000;66(7):612–617.
30. Knight DW. *Nat Prod Rep*. 1995;12(3):271–276.
31. Abad MJ, Bermejo P, Villar A. *Phytother Res*. 1995;9(2):79–92.
32. Groenewegen WA, Knight DW, Heptinstall S. *Prog Med Chem*. 1992;29:217–238.
33. Hanington E, Jones RJ, Amess JA, et al. *Lancet*. 1981;2(8249):720–723.
34. Damasio H, Beck D. *Lancet*. 1978;1(8058):240–242.
35. Heptinstall S, White A, Williamson L, et al. *Lancet*. 1985;1(8437):1071–1074.
36. Makheja AN, Bailey JM. *Prostagland Leukot Med*. 1982;8(6):653–660.
37. Heptinstall S, Groenewegen WA, Spangenberg P, et al. *J Pharm Pharmacol*. 1987;39(6):459–465.
38. Groenewegen WA, Heptinstall S. *J Pharm Pharmacol*. 1990;42(8):553–557.
39. Marles RJ, Pazos-Sanou L, Compadre CM, et al.. In: Arnason JT, ed. *Recent Advances in Phytochemistry*, vol 29, *Phytochemistry of Medicinal Plants*. New York: Plenum Press; 1995. pp. 333–356.
40. Heptinstall S, Awang DV, Dawson BA, et al. *J Pharm Pharmacol*. 1992;44(5):391–395.
41. Marles RJ, Kaminski J, Arnason JT, et al. *J Nat Prod*. 1992;55(8):1044–1056.
42. Groenewegen WA, Heptinstall S. *Lancet*. 1986;1(8474):44–45.
43. Voyno-Yasenetskaya TA, Loesche W, Groenewegen WA, et al. *J Pharm Pharmacol*. 1988;40(7):501–502.
44. Loesche W, Mazurov AV, Voyno-Yasenetskaya TA, et al. *Folia Haematol Int Mag Klin Morphol Blutforsch*. 1988;115(1–2):181–184.
45. Biggs MJ, Johnson ES, Persaud NP, et al. *Lancet*. 1982;2(8301):776.

46. Losche W, Michel E, Heptinstall S, et al. *Planta Med*. 1988;54(5):381–384.

47. Brown AM, Edwards CM, Davey MR, et al. *J Pharm Pharmacol*. 1997;49(5):558–561.

48. Brown AMG, Edwards CM, Davey MR, et al. *Phytother Res*. 1997;11(7):479–484.

49. Williamson LM, Harvey DM, Sheppard KJ, et al. *Inflammation*. 1988;12(1):11–16.

50. Hayes NA, Foreman JC. *J Pharm Pharmacol*. 1987;39(6):466–470.

51. Miyata N, Gon Y, Nunomura S, et al. *Int Immunopharmacol*. 2008;8(6):874–880.

52. Hong J, Aoyama S, Hirasawa N, et al. *Planta Med*. 2010 [Epub ahead of print].

53. Pugh WJ, Sambo K. *J Pharm Pharmacol*. 1988;40(10):743–745.

54. Hwang D, Fischer NH, Jang BC, et al. *Biochem Biophys Res Commun*. 1996;226(3):810–818.

55. Collier HO, Butt NM, McDonald-Gibson WJ, et al. *Lancet*. 1980;2(8200):922–923.

56. Loesche W, Groenewegen WA, Krause S, et al. *Biomed Biochim Acta*. 1988;47(10–11):S241–S243.

57. Silk ST, DeMarco ME. *Biochem Biophys Res Commun*. 1987;146(2):582–588.

58. Summer H, Salan U, Knight DW, et al. *Biochem Pharmacol*. 1992;43(11):2313–2320.

59. Bork PM, Schmitz ML, Kuhnt M, et al. *FEBS Lett*. 1997;402(1):85–90.

60. Hehner SP, Heinrich M, Bork PM, et al. *J Biol Chem*. 1998;273(3):1288–1297.

61. Hehner SP, Hofmann TG, Dröge W, et al. *J Immunol*. 1999;163(10):5617–5623.

62. Kwok BH, Koh B, Ndubuisi MI, et al. *Chem Biol*. 2011;8(8):759–766.

63. Reuter U, Chiarugi A, Bolay *Ann Neurol*. 2002;51(4):507–516.

64. Tassorelli C, Greco R, Morazzoni P, et al. *Cephalalgia*. 2005;25(8):612–621.

65. Kang BY, Chung SW, Kim TS. *Immunol Lett*. 2001;77(3):159–163.

66. Shah VO, Ferguson JE, Hunsaker LA, et al. *Nat Prod Res*. 2010;24(12):1177–1188.

67. Smolinski AT, Pestka JJ. *Food Chem Toxicol*. 2003;41(10):1381–1390.

68. Uchi H, Arrighi JF, Aubry JP, et al. *J Allergy Clin Immunol*. 2002;110(2):269–276.

69. Fukuda K, Hibiya Y, Mutoh M, et al. *Biochem Pharmacol*. 2000;60(4):595–600.

70. Li-Weber M, Giaisi M, Treiber MK, et al. *Eur J Immunol*. 2002;32(12):3587–3597.

71. Saadane A, Masters S, DiDonato J, et al. *Am J Respir Cell Mol Biol*. 2007;36(6):728–736.

72. Huang S, Zhao L, Kim K, et al. *Mol Pharmacol*. 2008;74(1):274–281.

73. Gómez-Hernández A, Martín-Ventura JL, Sánchez-Galán E, et al. *Atherosclerosis*. 2006;187(1):139–149.

74. Kiuchi H, Takao T, Yamamoto K, et al. *J Urol*. 2009;181(5):2339–2348.

75. Zingarelli B, Hake PW, Denenberg A, et al. *Shock*. 2002;17(2):127–134.

76. López-Franco O, Hernández-Vargas P, Ortiz-Muñoz G, et al. *Arterioscler Thromb Vasc Biol*. 2006;26(8):1864–1870.

77. Sheehan M, Wong HR, Hake PW, et al. *Mol Pharmacol*. 2002;61(5):953–963.

78. Li X, Su J, Cui X, et al. *Expert Opin Investig Drugs*. 2009;18(8):1047–1060.

79. Jain NK, Kulkarni SK. *J Ethnopharmacol*. 1999;68(1–3):251–259.

80. Martin K, Sur R, Liebel F, et al. *Arch Dermatol Res*. 2008;300(2):69–80.

81. Sur R, Martin K, Liebel F, et al. *Inflammopharmacology*. 2009;17(1):42–49.

82. Weber JT, Hayataka K, O'Connor MF, et al. *Comp Biochem Physiol C Pharmacol Toxicol Endocrinol*. 1997;117(1):19–24.

83. Weber JT, O'Connor MF, Hayataka K, et al. *J Nat Prod*. 1997;60(6):651–653.

84. Bejar E. *J Ethnopharmacol*. 1996;50(1):1–12.

85. Barsby RW, Salan U, Knight DW, et al. *Planta Med*. 1993;59(1):20–25.

86. Hay AJ, Hamburger M, Hostettmann K, et al. *Br J Pharmacol*. 1994;112(1):9–12.

87. Barsby RW, Salan U, Knight DW, et al. *J Pharm Pharmacol*. 1992;44(9):737–740.

88. Barsby R, Salan U, Knight DW, et al. *Lancet*. 1991;338(8773):1015.

89. Mittra S, Datta A, Singh SK, et al. *Acta Pharmacol Sin*. 2000;21(12):1106–1114.

90. Ghantous A, Gali-Muhtasib H, Vuorela H, et al. *Drug Discov Today*. 2010;15(15–16):668–678.

91. Koprowska K, Czyz M. *Postepy Hig Med Dosw (Online)*. 2010;64:100–114.

92. Carlisi D, D'Anneo A, Angileri L, et al. *J Cell Physiol*. 2010 [Epub ahead of print].

93. Yun BR, Lee MJ, Kim JH, et al. *Exp Mol Med*. 2010;42(11):787–797.

94. Hassane DC, Sen S, Minhajuddin M, et al. *Blood*. 2010 [Epub ahead of print].

95. Czyz M, Lesiak-Mieczkowska K, Koprowska K, et al. *Br J Pharmacol*. 2010;160(5):1144–1157.

96. Zhao LJ, Xu YH, Li Y. *J Dig Dis*. 2009;10(3):172–180.

97. Wu C, Chen F, Rushing JW, et al. *J Med Food*. 2006;9(1):55–61.

98. Pajak B, Gajkowska B, Orzechowski A. *Folia Histochem Cytobiol*. 2008;46(2):129–135.

99. Sweeney CJ, Mehrotra S, Sadaria MR, et al. *Mol Cancer Ther*. 2005;4(6):1004–1012.

100. Shanmugam R, Jayaprakasan V, Gokmen-Polar Y, et al. *Prostate*. 2006;66(14):1498–1511.

101. Kishida Y, Yoshikawa H, Myoui A. *Clin Cancer Res*. 2007;13(1):59–67.

102. Oka D, Nishimura K, Shiba M, et al. *Int J Cancer*. 2007;120(12):2576–2581.

103. Francescato HD, Costa RS, Scavone C, et al. *Toxicology*. 2007;230(1):64–75.

104. Zhang D, Qiu L, Jin X, et al. *Mol Cancer Res*. 2009;7(7):1139–1149.

105. Idris AI, Libouban H, Nyangoga H, et al. *Mol Cancer Ther*. 2009;8(8):2339–2347.

106. Won YK, Ong CN, Shi X, et al. *Carcinogenesis*. 2004;25(8):1449–1458.

107. Stephanovic M, Ristic N, Vukmiorovic M. *Sci Nat*. 1988;23:23–40.

108. Blakeman JP, Atkinson P. *Physiol Plant Pathol*. 1979;15(2):183–192.

109. Kalodera Z, Pepeljnjak S, Blazevic N, et al. *Pharmazie*. 1997;52(11):885–886.

110. Kalodera Z, Pepeljnjak S, Petrak T. *Pharmazie*. 1996;51(12):995–996.

111. Tiuman TS, Ueda-Nakamura T, Garcia Cortez DA, et al. *Antimicrob Agents Chemother*. 2005;49(1):176–182.

112. da Silva BP, Cortez DA, Violin TY, et al. *Parasitol Int*. 2010;59(4):643–646.

113. Izumi E, Morello LG, Ueda-Nakamura T, et al. *Exp Parasitol*. 2008;118(3):324–330.

114. Pelizzaro-Rocha KJ, Tiuman TS, Izumi E, et al. *Phytomedicine*. 2010;18(1):36–39.

115. Konia MR, Schaefer S, Liu H. *Eur J Anaesthesiol*. 2009;26(6):496–503.

116. O'Neill LA, Barrett ML, Lewis GP. *Br J Clin Pharmacol*. 1987;23(1):81–83.

117. Keery RJ, Lumley P. *Br J Pharmacol*. 1986;89:834P.

118. Buck AC, Pugh J, Davies R, et al. Cited in Groenewegen WA, Knight DW, Heptinstall S. *Prog Med Chem*. 1992;29:217–238.

119. Yip KH, Zheng MH, Feng HT, et al. *J Bone Miner Res*. 2004;19(11):1905–1916.

120. Xu J, Wu HF, Ang ES, et al. *Cytokine Growth Factor Rev*. 2009;20(1):7–17.

121. Bedirli A, Salman B, Pasaoglu H, et al. *J Surg Res*. 2010 [Epub ahead of print].

122. Tanaka K, Hasegawa J, Asamitsu K, et al. *J Pharmacol Exp Ther*. 2005;315(2):624–630.

123. Tanaka K, Asamitsu K, Uranishi H, et al. *Curr Drug Metab*. 2010;11(5):431–435.

124. Pandey DK, Rajkumar R, Mahesh R, et al. *J Pharm Pharmacol*. 2008;60(12):1643–1650.

125. Khan SI, Abourashed EA, Khan IA, et al. *Planta Med*. 2003;69(11):1009–1012.

126. Wagner S, Kratz F, Merfort I. *Planta Med*. 2004;70(3):227–233.

127. Curry III EA, Murry DJ, Yoder C, et al. *Invest New Drugs*. 2004;22(3):299–305.

128. Johnson ES. *Feverfew (Overcoming Common Problems)*. London: Sheldon Press; 1984. pp. 42–55.

129. Johnson ES, Kadam NP, Hylands DM, et al. *Br Med J (Clin Res Ed)*. 1985;291(6495):569–573.

130. Hylands DM, Hylands PJ, Johnson ES, et al. *Br Med J (Clin Res Ed)*. 1985;291(6502):1128.

131. Murphy JJ, Heptinstall S, Mitchell JR. *Lancet*. 1988;2(8604):189–192.

132. Groenewegen WA. Cited in Groenewegen WA, Knight DW, Heptinstall S. *Prog Med Chem*. 1992;29:217–238.

133. De Weerdt CJ, Bootsma HPR, Hendriks H. *Phytomedicine*. 1996;3(3):225–230.

134. Pfaffenrath V, Diener HC, Fischer M, et al. *Cephalalgia*. 2002;22:523–532.

135. Diener HC, Pfaffenrath V, Schnitker J, et al. *Cephalalgia*. 2005;25:1031–1041.

136. Cutlan AR, Bonilla LE, Simon JE, et al. *Planta Med*. 2000;66(7):612–617.

137. Shrivastava R, Pechadre JC, John GW. *Clin Drug Invest*. 2006;26(5):287–296.

138. Maizels M, Blumenfeld A, Burchette R. *Headache*. 2004;44(9):885–890.

139. Cady RK, Schreiber CP, Beach ME, et al. *Med Sci Monit*. 2005;11(9):PI65–PI69.

140. Aurora SK, Vermaas AR, Barrodale PM. American Academy of Neurology, 58th Annual Meeting, San Diego, April 6, 2006.

141. Pittler MH, Ernst E. *Cochrane Database Syst Rev*. 2004;1 CD002286.

142. Pattrick M, Heptinstall S, Doherty M. *Ann Rheum Dis*. 1989;48(7):547–549.

143. Johnson ES. *MIMS Mag*. 1983;15:32–35.

144. Yao M, Brown-Woodman PD, Ritchie H. *Teratology*. 2001;64(6):323–324.

145. Anderson D, Jenkinson PC, Dewdney RS, et al. *Hum Toxicol*. 1988;7(2):145–152.

146. Johnson ES, Kadam NP, Anderson D, et al. *Hum Toxicol*. 1987;6(6):533–534.

147. De Smet PAGM, ed. *Adverse Effects of Herbal Drugs*, vol. 1. Berlin: Springer-Verlag; 1992. p. 257.

148. Culpeper N. *Culpeper's Complete Herbal and English Physician*. First published 1826, Bath. Reprinted by Harvey Sales; 1981. p. 58.

149. Yao M, Brown-Woodman PDC, Ritchie H. *Birth Defects Res (Part A)*. 2003;67:141–147. Abstract No. 9.

150. Yao M, Ritchie HE, Brown-Woodman PD. *Reprod Toxicol*. 2006;22(4):688–693.

151. Johnson S. *Feverfew: A Traditional Herbal Remedy for Migraine and Arthritis*. London: Sheldon Press; 1984. p. 89.

152. Ernst E, Pittler MH. *Public Health Nutr*. 2000;3(4A):509–514.

153. Johnson S. *Feverfew: A Traditional Herbal Remedy for Migraine and Arthritis*. London: Sheldon Press; 1984. pp. 78–83.

154. Murphy LM. *Assoc Operat Room Nurses J*. 1999;69(1):173–183.

155. Killoran CE, Crawford GH, Pedvis-Leftick A. *Dermatitis*. 2007;18(4):225–229.

156. Hausen BM. In:De Smet PAGM, Keller K, Hansel R, ed. *Adverse Effects of Herbal Drugs*, vol. 1. Berlin: Springer-Verlag; 1992. p. 257.

157. Baldwin CA, Anderson LA, Phillipson JD. *Pharm J*. 1987;239:237–238.

158. Paulsen E, Andersen KE, Hausen BM. *Contact Dermatitis*. 2001;45(4):197–204.

159. Lundh K, Hindsén M, Gruvberger B, et al. *Contact Dermatitis*. 2006;54(4):196–201.

160. Kurtz E, Walczak VR. *J Am Acad Dermatol*. 2005;52(suppl 3):P87. Abstract No. 1016.

161. Paulsen E, Christensen LP, Fretté XC, et al. *Contact Dermatitis*. 2010;63(3):146–150.

162. Paulsen E, Christensen LP, Andersen KE. *Br J Dermatol*. 2007;156(3):510–515.

Ginger

(*Zingiber officinale* Roscoe)

Synonyms

Zingiberis rhizoma (Lat), Ingwer (Ger), Gingembre (Fr), Zerzero (Ital), Ingefær (Dan), Ardhrakam (Sanskrit). Dried ginger: Gan jiang (Chin), Kankyo (Jap). Fresh ginger: Sheng jiang (Chin), Shokyo (Jap).

What is it?

Ginger root (actually the rhizome) is a familiar pungent and aromatic kitchen spice widely available either as the dried root or powder or as the whole fresh root ('green ginger'). Ginger has been valued as a spice and medicine for thousands of years. Its use is recorded in early Sanskrit and Chinese texts and is documented in ancient Greek, Roman and Arabic medical literature. Ginger was actually exploited to extinction in the wild in ancient times, and is probably among the first vegetatively cultivated plants.[1] The plant is currently grown commercially in India, China, Southeast Asia, West Indies, Mexico, Africa, Fiji and Australia. The biomedical research on ginger is unique in that the volume of human studies almost exceeds the volume of pharmacological research (for at least the research on the whole herb, as opposed to its constituents).

Effects

Reduces nausea and vomiting; stimulates circulatory activity; inhibits arachidonic acid metabolism, reduces platelet aggregation, reduces arthritic pain and has other inflammatory effects.

Traditional view

In traditional medicine around the world, ginger has been one of the most valued of remedies, primarily for its heating properties and as an antidote to diseases associated with cold, such as chest congestion, cough, dropsy and diarrhoea.[2] In Western traditions it has been utilised particularly for congestive chest problems, dyspepsia, flatulent colic, gastritis and diarrhoea associated with depletion. As a circulatory stimulant, a hot infusion of ginger was considered beneficial for amenorrhoea due to cold. It was also applied topically as a rubefacient.[3,4] The Eclectics used ginger particularly as a stimulating tonic, stomachic, carminative and antispasmodic. It was employed to treat nausea, gastrointestinal cramping, loss of appetite and cold extremities. The hot infusion was said to 'break up' colds and relieve painful menstruation.[5]

As alluded to above, in Eclectic and other 19th century North American traditions, ginger was described as a diffusive stimulant.[6] Here the term 'stimulant' refers to metabolic (heating) and circulatory enhancing properties that can also reinforce the therapeutic activity of other remedies. This diffusive property was associated with a reputation for opening up circulation to the peripheral tissues and a diaphoretic activity.

In traditional Chinese medicine, ginger is divided into three preparation types: *sheng jiang*, fresh raw rhizome; *gan jiang*, dried raw rhizome; and *pao jiang*, dried, quick-fried rhizome. All three are considered warming remedies with particular affinity for the bowel and lungs. The fresh rhizome is considered the most 'dispersing' of the three, meaning it has a broad spectrum of influence, but short-lived effects. It is used to disperse *Exterior Cold* brought on by 'external' agents, for vomiting, cough, debilitating sweating and to reduce the poisonous effect of other herbs.[7] Other applications include the common cold due to pathogenic *Wind Cold*, characterised by severe intolerance to cold, slight fever, headache, general ache, nasal congestion and a runny nose.[8] In comparison, the dried rhizome is more hot and with longer lasting benefits, used for cold conditions characterised by pallor, poor appetite and digestion, cold limbs, vomiting, diarrhoea, pale tongue, or thin, watery or white sputum. It is better matched with patterns of atony (lack of muscle tone), congestion or debility, which might manifest as cold limbs, pale complexion or diarrhoea and undigested food in the stool. The fried rhizome is employed in much the same way, although it is considered a stronger remedy and is also applied locally to stop bleeding.

In India, ginger is referred to as *vishwabhesaj*, 'the universal medicine'. As in Chinese medicine, Ayurvedic tradition also utilises the rhizome in a variety of forms (fresh, dried, peeled and unpeeled). Again, it is consistently used for digestive complaints, including nausea, diarrhoea, flatulence, dyspepsia and gastrointestinal spasm. It is also valued for chronic rheumatic complaints, venomous bites, for colds and influenza and applied topically for headache, toothache and to improve circulation to the limbs.[9,10]

In Thai traditional texts the main uses described for ginger rhizome include sweetening the voice, enhancing the appetite and for dyspepsia, flatulence, fever, mouth ulcers and intestinal infections.[11]

Summary actions

Carminative, antiemetic, peripheral circulatory stimulant, spasmolytic, anti-inflammatory, antiplatelet, diaphoretic, digestive stimulant.

Can be used for

Indications supported by clinical trials

Treatment and prophylaxis of nausea and emesis in cases of motion sickness, nausea of pregnancy and postoperative and drug-induced nausea (good evidence, but not entirely consistent); osteoarthritis; dysmenorrhoea; gastroparesis.

Traditional therapeutic uses

To enhance digestion, expectoration and diaphoresis; digestive problems, especially colic, flatulent dyspepsia, cramping, peptic ulcer, loss of appetite, gastrointestinal infections; fever, colds (especially the fresh rhizome); menstrual problems such as amenorrhoea and dysmenorrhoea.

May be used for

Extrapolations from pharmacological studies

Treatment of peptic ulceration; inflammatory conditions; thrombocytosis; migraine headaches; to enhance the bioavailability of other treatments; as an antiplatelet agent.

Preparations

Fresh or dried rhizome as an infusion, decoction, fluid extract, oleoresin or tablets and capsules for internal use. As with all essential oil-containing herbs, use of the fresh or carefully dried rhizome is advised.

Dosage

Fresh rhizome 500 to 1000 mg three times a day; dried rhizome 500 mg two to four times a day.

From 0.7 to 3 mL/day of a 1:2 liquid extract or 1.7 to 7.5 mL/day of a 1:5 tincture, or the equivalent in tablet or capsule form.

Higher doses than these may be needed for some clinical applications (see the Clinical trials section).

Duration of use

There are no known problems with long-term consumption and ginger is widely consumed around the world as a spice. However, for many of its therapeutic purposes only short-term use is needed.

Summary assessment of safety

No problems known from ingestion in moderate doses. Ginger may enhance the bioavailability of other medications and high doses may cause heartburn and have a blood-thinning effect.

Technical data

Botany

Ginger, a member of the Zingiberaceae family, is thought to be a cultigen of Indian origin.[12] It grows with erect leafy stems 0.6 to 1.2 m high. The leaves are narrow, linear-lanceolate (2 to 3 cm long, 1 to 2 cm wide). The inflorescence is a terminal spike with irregular flowers, coloured yellowish-green and streaked with purple. The fruit is a capsule. It has a stout, tuberous rhizome which is branched and laterally compressed. The surface of the rhizome is greyish-white with light-brownish rings.[13] It is commonly, but erroneously, referred to as ginger root (instead of rhizome).

Adulteration

There is a history of adulteration in the commercial spice trade, with substitutions such as turmeric and cayenne to bolster flavour and ferric oxide to add colour. There is also a tradition of washing with lime. Hence, sourcing whole roots is advisable. Substitution by other species of Zingiber and Alpinia is occasionally reported.

'Jamaican ginger paralysis' has entered the literature as an apparent toxic event associated with ginger. However, it has little to do with the spice. In 1930, thousands were poisoned by an illicit extract of Jamaica ginger ('jake' used to circumvent the Prohibition laws in America. A neurotoxic organophosphate compound, triorthocresyl phosphate, had been used as an adulterant.[14]

Key constituents

- Essential oil (1% to 3%), including zingiberene, sesquiphellandrene and beta-bisabolene.[15]
- Pungent (hot) principles: 1% to 2.5% gingerols and shogaols, the most abundant of which is 6-gingerol.[16]

The components beta-sesquiphellandrene and (−)-zingiberene are highest in fresh ginger, and decompose on drying and storage. This understanding may provide a basis for the preference in traditional Chinese medicine for the fresh rhizome in the treatment of the common cold. The gingerols gradually decompose into the shogaols on storage. The oleoresin of ginger contains mainly the essential oil and pungent principles.

Zingiberene

Gingerols

	n
6-Gingerol	4
8-Gingerol	6
10-Gingerol	8

Variations of up to 140% were found in the levels of 6-gingerol, 6-shogaol, 8-gingerol and 10-gingerol in nine different ginger products.[16] In another study, 10 different ginger dietary supplements were purchased randomly at local pharmacies and health food stores in the USA. The 6-gingerol concentrations ranged from 0.0 to 9.43 mg/g, 6-shogaol from 0.16 to 2.18 mg/g, 8-gingerol from 0.00 to 1.1 mg/g and 10-gingerol from 0.00 to 1.40 mg/g. Suggested ginger dosages varied from 250 mg to 4.77 g/day.[17]

Pharmacodynamics

Antiemetic and antinausea activity

Conventional antiemetics have potential teratogenic effects during the critical embryogenic period of pregnancy, so there has been considerable interest in the potential of a remedy that is also widely consumed as a food.

Acetone and ethanol extracts of ginger exhibited significant protection against cisplatin-induced emesis in dogs at oral doses of 25 to 200 mg/kg, but an aqueous extract at these doses was ineffective.[18] Presumably, the aqueous extract was not active because it contained only low levels of the pungent principles. In vitro and in vivo studies do suggest that the pungent principles are in fact responsible for the antinausea activity of ginger, including via weak 5-HT3 and cholinergic M3 receptor inhibition.[19–23] In contrast, Chinese pharmacological investigations have concluded that gingerols or ginger produce an antiemetic action via central and peripheral anticholinergic and antihistaminic effects and the inhibition of the expression of substance P and NK1.[24] (Substance P–neurokinin-1 (NK1) receptor pathways have been implicated in the pathophysiology of emesis and depression.)

From studies on radiation-induced conditioned taste aversion in Sprague-Dawley rats, researchers concluded that ginger extract (200 mg/kg, ip) was effective and had potential for clinical application in the mitigation of radiation-induced emesis in humans.[25]

This is one area fortunately where pharmacodynamic studies on human volunteers have been widespread, although with mixed conclusions. Mowrey and Clayson compared the effects of 1.88 g of dried powdered ginger, 100 mg dimenhydrinate and placebo on the symptoms of motion sickness in 36 healthy volunteers who reported a very high susceptibility to motion sickness. Motion sickness was induced by placing the blindfolded person in a tilted rotating chair. Ginger was found to be superior to dimenhydrinate and placebo in preventing the gastrointestinal symptoms of motion sickness and the authors postulated a local effect in the gastrointestinal tract for ginger. This was particularly likely since it was given as a powder only 25 minutes before the test.[26] The gingerols and shogaols were subsequently identified as the main antiemetic compounds.[27]

Several subsequent clinical studies investigated the mechanism of action. In a double blind, randomised, placebo-controlled, crossover study involving 13 healthy volunteers with a history of motion sickness, pretreatment with 1 and 2 g powdered ginger root reduced the increased nausea, tachygastria and plasma vasopressin caused by circular vection. Ginger also

prolonged the latency before nausea onset and shortened the recovery time.[28]

Earlier, a double blind, crossover, placebo trial on healthy volunteers by Grøntved and Hentzer found that ginger significantly reduced vertigo induced by heat stimulation of the vestibular system (that is, the irrigation of the left ear with water at 44°C). It had no effect on the duration or maximum slow phase velocity of nystagmus (involuntary, rhythmic movement of the eyeball). In three out of 24 tests, nausea was present after placebo, but it did not occur after ginger at all. At that time, two classes of drugs were used to treat motion sickness: antihistamines reduced nystagmus, but the second class comprising parasympatholytics and sympathomimetics (which basically reinforce the activity of the sympathetic nervous system) did not. Grøntved and Hentzer concluded that ginger root, like sympathomimetics and parasympatholytics, also dampens the induced vestibular impulses to the autonomic centres of the central nervous system (CNS).[29]

Although a second research group verified the finding that ginger had no effect on nystagmus, they disputed the interpretation of Grøntved and Hentzer and concluded that a CNS mechanism can be excluded for ginger.[30] A more accurate interpretation of their findings would be that ginger lacks central anticholinergic effects. It was suggested any reduction of motion sickness was derived from the influence of ginger on the digestive tract.

There have also been disputes about any effect on motion sickness at all. In one study, 28 human volunteers were placed in a rotating chair until they reached an endpoint of motion sickness short of vomiting (malaise III or M-III). Each person was tested with either ginger or scopolamine and a placebo. A substance was judged to possess antimotion sickness activity if it allowed a greater number of rotations compared to placebo control. Gastric electrical activity was monitored by cutaneous electrodes positioned over the abdominal area. The authors concluded that powdered ginger (whole root, 500 or 1000 mg) and fresh ginger root (1000 mg) did not possess antimotion sickness activity, nor did they significantly alter gastric function during motion sickness.[31]

The effect of dried ginger on the gastric emptying rate was discounted in a study using the oral paracetamol absorption model. In a randomised, double blind, crossover trial, 16 healthy volunteers received 1 g of ginger or placebo. It was concluded that any antiemetic effect of ginger in healthy people was not associated with increased gastric emptying (but also see below).[32]

Effects on digestive function

The traditional uses of ginger as a digestive remedy was supported in early Chinese and Japanese animal research, which *inter alia* found oral and intragastric application of fresh ginger decoction produced a stimulant action on gastric secretion, including free acid and lipase activity while, however, the activity of pepsin was decreased.[8] Fresh ginger was also found to contain a proteolytic enzyme.[33] Subsequent investigations have shown that dietary ginger (50 mg/100 g food) enhanced intestinal lipase activity and the disaccharidases sucrase and maltase in rats.[34] Intraduodenal doses of ginger extract also increased bile secretion in rats. Total secretion of bile solids was also increased, but not to the same extent as bile flow; 6-gingerol and 10-gingerol were identified as the active components.[35] German scientists found that chewing 9 g of crystallised ginger had a profound effect on saliva production in healthy volunteers.[36] Amylase activity was also increased and the saliva was not more watery, although it contained slightly less mucoprotein.

Ginger also appears to influence gastrointestinal motility, with positive results from both animal and human investigations. Oral doses of 6-shogaol (35 mg/kg) accelerated intestinal transit, and both 6-shogaol and 6-gingerol suppressed gastric contraction in rats.[37] An extract of ginger, and isolated 6-shogaol and gingerols, enhanced gastrointestinal motility in mice after oral doses. The effects of the ginger components were comparable to the antinausea drugs metoclopramide and domperidone.[38] Acetone and ethanol extracts of ginger (oral doses: 100, 200, 500 mg/kg) and ginger juice (2, 4 mL/kg) significantly reversed the delay in gastric emptying in rats induced by the emetic drug cisplatin. Ginger juice and acetone extract were more effective than the ethanol extract, and both were similar or superior to the reversal caused by the 5HT3 receptor antagonist ondansetron.[39]

Ginger rhizome extract (200 mg) increased both digestive and fasting gastroduodenal motility in 12 healthy volunteers.[40] Acute hyperglycaemia evokes gastric slow wave dysrhythmias via endogenous prostaglandin generation. In 22 healthy people it was shown that that this effect was prevented by 1 g of ginger root. Conversely, ginger had no effect on dysrhythmias elicited by the prostaglandin E_1 analogue misoprostol, indicating that ginger may reduce the production of prostaglandins in hyperglycaemia, rather than inhibit their action.[41]

Twenty-four healthy volunteers were studied on two afternoons, separated by at least 7 days, in a randomised, double blind design.[42] Following a fast of 8 h the volunteers took capsules containing a total of 1.2 g of ginger root powder or placebo. One hour later, they consumed 500 mL of chicken and corn soup. Ultrasonographic scanning performed prior to commencement of the study provided fasting motility patterns. Antral area (bottom of stomach, near the duodenum), fundus area (top, near the oesophagus) and diameter, and the frequency of antral contractions were then measured at intervals over 90 minutes. The gastric half-emptying time was calculated from the change in antral area. Gastric half-emptying time was less after ginger than placebo (13.1 minutes versus 26.7 minutes), and the frequency of antral contractions was greater. This accelerated gastric emptying could reduce gastroparesis and the risk of gastro-oesophageal reflux. (See also under Clinical trials.)

The carminative activity of ginger is supported by a human study. In a randomised, open label, controlled trial, 14 healthy male volunteers consumed either 1 g of ginger suspended in 100 mL of water or just the 100 mL water.[43] After ginger, the lower oesophageal resting pressures were unchanged, but the degree of relaxation at swallowing was significantly increased. The amplitude and duration of oesophageal contractions were not changed, but the velocity of contraction waves decreased. The authors suggested that these effects favoured the expulsion of gastric gas (without any increased risk of gastro-oesophageal reflux).

In contrast to enhanced gastric emptying, anticathartic activity is also known to be one of the effects of ginger. In a Japanese study, an acetone ginger extract (75 mg/kg, oral) significantly inhibited serotonin-induced diarrhoea in mice.[44] The pungent principles were found to be the active components.

Research suggests that ginger is one of a number of hot spices that in combination can increase the bioavailability of other drugs, either by enhancing their absorption from the gastrointestinal tract or by protecting the drug from being metabolised/oxidised in its first passage through the liver after being absorbed.[45] However, piperine from long or black pepper is probably the most active component in this regard.

Antiulcer activity

Ginger and 6-gingerol inhibited experimental gastric ulcers in rats.[46,47] From in vivo studies, several antiulcer compounds have been isolated from ginger including 6-gingesulfonic acid,[48] 6-shogaol and ar-curcumene.[49] Most notable is 6-gingesulfonic acid, which showed weaker pungency and more potent antiulcer activity than 6-gingerol and 6-shogaol.[50] Oral administration of spray-dried ginger extract (500 mg/kg), licorice extract (500 mg/kg) or the combination of the two extracts (Rikkunshi-to, 1000 mg/kg) significantly prevented gastric mucosal damage induced by ethanol in rats. Pretreatment with ginger extract or Rikkunshi-to inhibited the reduction in the deep corpus mucin content caused by the ethanol.[51]

However, high doses of ginger probably act as a gastric irritant. Fresh ginger in quantities of 6 g or more caused a significant increase in exfoliation of gastric surface epithelial cells in human volunteers.[52]

Anti-inflammatory activity

Ginger and its pungent components are dual inhibitors of arachidonic acid metabolism in vitro. That is, they inhibit both cyclo-oxygenase (COX) and lipoxygenase (LOX) enzymes of the prostaglandin and leukotriene biosynthetic pathways.[53-58] Dual inhibitors of COX and 5-LOX may have a better therapeutic profile and fewer side effects than non-steroidal anti-inflammatory drugs. Gingerols are more potent inhibitors of prostaglandin biosynthesis in vitro than indomethacin,[55] and are also potent inhibitors of 5-LOX.[56] However, one component of ginger actually promotes prostaglandin production. Zingerone was found to share a prostaglandin synthetase promoting activity with a number of other emetic, purgative and irritant drugs in the digestive system.[59] In later work, a ginger extract (in combination with *Alpinia galanga*) was shown to inhibit the induction of several genes encoding cytokines, chemokines and COX-2.[60]

Reviewers of the relevant literature have also concluded that ginger constituents interact with the vanilloid nociceptor.[61] A 2008 review also noted in vitro inhibition of stimulated macrophages and specifically iNOS (inducible nitric oxide synthase) for ginger components.[62] In contrast to feverfew (*Tanacetum parthenium*), ginger did not inhibit serotonin release from bovine platelets.[63]

A hydroalcoholic extract of ginger at the dose of 200 mg/kg/day (ip) was superior to indomethacin (2 mg/kg/day) at reducing inflammation in rat collagen-induced arthritis, for most of the measured parameters.[64] Ginger extract (50 and 100 mg/kg, oral) inhibited carrageenan-induced paw swelling and was as active as aspirin. However, ginger was devoid of analgesic activity at the doses used.[53] Essential oil of ginger (33 mg/kg, oral) inhibited chronic adjuvant arthritis in rats.[65,66] Oral administration of the essential oil of ginger at doses of 0.125, 0.25 and 0.5 g/kg dose-dependently weakened the delayed type hypersensitivity response to 2,4-dinitro-1-fluorobenzene in sensitised mice (p<0.05).[67] Other in vivo models have also demonstrated anti-inflammatory activity for ginger and its components.[61]

Antiplatelet and cardiovascular activity

Srivastava and co-workers found that aqueous extract of ginger inhibited platelet aggregation induced by ADP, adrenaline (epinephrine), collagen and arachidonic acid in vitro; it also inhibited prostacyclin synthesis in rat aorta[68] and thromboxane synthesis.[69,70] The in vitro antiplatelet action of 6-gingerol was found to be mainly due to the inhibition of thromboxane formation.[71]

Srivastava followed up this laboratory work with a clinical trial in healthy volunteers.[72] Danish women consumed either 70 g fresh onion or 5 g fresh ginger daily for a period of 7 days. Thromboxane was determined in serum obtained after blood clotting. Onion intake slightly increased production of thromboxane, whereas ginger caused a 37% inhibition. However, with only seven participants, this finding did not achieve statistical significance (p<0.1).

Dietary supplementation with 100 g/day of butter for 7 days in 20 healthy males was found to enhance platelet aggregation. Addition of 5 g of dried ginger in two divided doses to the fatty meal significantly inhibited platelet aggregation (p<0.001) compared to placebo.[73] In another similar study, supplementation of 5 g of ginger powder significantly reversed the decrease in fibrinolytic activity induced by 50 g of fat in 30 healthy adult volunteers (p<0.001).[74]

However, in a randomised double blind study involving eight healthy male volunteers, bleeding time, platelet count and platelet aggregation were found to be unaffected by a single dose of 2 g of dried ginger.[75] Another study published in 1996 also questioned the clinical antiplatelet activity of ginger. Eighteen patients consumed either 15 g of raw ginger root, 40 g of cooked stem ginger or placebo for 2 weeks in a randomised, crossover design.[76] Ginger consumption did not decrease thromboxane production by platelets ex vivo. Unfortunately, the study was a crossover design, with each participant consuming the test substances and placebo in a random order over three consecutive 2-week periods, but without a washout period. An effect of ginger might be sufficiently sustained to carry over into a following placebo phase. There was also little attempt at blinding subjects to the tastes. Another consideration was that the doses used in these two negative studies were relatively lower than for the positive studies. (Also, see the Clinical trials section.)

One conclusion might also be that the impact of ginger on platelet aggregation is most apparent when accompanying fatty foods. There are other potential benefits in such circumstances. Ginger decreased serum and hepatic cholesterol in cholesterol-fed rats,[77] and stimulated the conversion of cholesterol to bile acids.[78] However, ginger at '5 times normal human intake' had no effect on serum and liver cholesterol levels in one study in hypercholesterolaemic rats.[79] Oral administration of ginger extract reduced total cholesterol and serum LDL-cholesterol in hyperlipidaemic rabbits. Tissue lipid profiles of liver, heart and aorta showed similar changes. Ginger feeding increased the faecal excretion of cholesterol, which suggests a modulation of absorption.[80]

A 2009 review noted that ginger significantly lowered blood lipids, reduced atherosclerotic lesions and associated foam cell formation, and raised HDL-cholesterol as effectively as conventional drugs.[81] Models used included animals that were diabetic, deficient in the apolipoprotein E gene or fed a high lipid diet. Possible mechanisms included reduced hepatic cholesterol biosynthesis and increased faecal excretion.

Ginger exerted a powerful positive inotropic effect on isolated guinea pig left atria: gingerols were identified as the active components,[82,83] and later 6- and 8-shogaol were found to show a positive inotropic activity of about the same potency as 8-gingerol.[84] 8-Gingerol stimulated the Ca^{2+}-pumping ATPase in skeletal and cardiac sarcoplasmic reticulum in vitro.[85] Further investigation indicated that this activity was increased in a concentration-dependent manner by 6-gingerol, 8-gingerol and 10-gingerol.[86] Zingeronolol, a substance derived from zingerone, demonstrated beta-adrenergic blocking activity in rats (0.1 to 1.0 mg/kg, iv).[87] This contradicts the cardiotonic effect demonstrated by the whole extract in vitro.

The average systolic and diastolic blood pressures of normal volunteers given 1.0 g of fresh ginger to chew without swallowing were increased by 11.2 and 14 mmHg, respectively.[88] This pressor effect may be a short-term reflex response to the pungent effect of ginger. The component 6-shogaol also demonstrated a pressor response in pharmacological studies after intravenous administration to rats (0.5 mg/kg).[89] However, a 2005 study found that ginger extract (0.3 to 3.0 mg/kg, iv) induced a dose-dependent fall in the arterial blood pressure of rats via blockage of voltage-dependent calcium channels.[90]

Thermogenic activity

In traditional herbal therapy ginger is regarded as a warming and stimulating medicine. This also provides the probable basis for its diaphoretic activity in febrile states. Several studies have sought to understand a potential thermogenic role for ginger. European studies proposed that the pungent principles of ginger act to stimulate thermoregulatory receptors.[35,91] In addition ginger and its pungent components were thermogenic in the perfused rat hindlimb.[92]

Zingerone (like capsaicin from chillies and piperine from pepper, but unlike sulphur-containing pungent principles from garlic and mustard) increased the secretion of catecholamines, especially adrenaline, from the adrenal medulla after intravenous injection in rats, this possibly accounting in part for the warming effect.[93] These effects may be mediated by an interaction of the pungent principles in ginger with vanilloid receptors.[62] However, more sustained effects may arise from different mechanisms. Ginger extract stimulated cytokine secretion by human peripheral blood mononuclear cells.[94] A pyrogenic effect from these cytokines might play a role in any thermogenic effect of ginger. Ginger and its pungent principles also significantly inhibited serotonin-induced hypothermia.[44]

Not all experimental evidence is clear on the stimulant effect. In one study, in contrast to earlier studies on chilli and mustard sauce, a ginger sauce (prepared from fresh ginger) did not increase metabolic rate in human participants.[95]

Antimicrobial and antiparasitic activity

Some of the minor pungent components of ginger have been shown to have antifungal activity in vitro,[96] as have the gingerols.[62] Ginger extract demonstrated mild growth inhibition of Gram-positive and Gram-negative bacteria in vitro,[53] including *Escherichia coli*, *Proteus vulgaris*, *Salmonella typhimurium*, *Staphylococcus aureus* and *Streptococcus viridans*.[97] In vitro studies demonstrate that combinations of ginger extract and clarithromycin synergistically augmented inhibition of *Helicobacter pylori* cultures.[98]

Sesquiterpenes in ginger essential oil were found to have significant antirhinoviral activity in vitro.[99] The most active components were beta-sesquiphellandrene and zingiberene, and since these are highest in fresh ginger this might provide a basis for the preference in traditional Chinese medicine for the fresh rhizome in the treatment of the common cold. Acyclovir-resistant clinical isolates of herpes simplex virus type 1 (HSV-1) were analysed in vitro for their susceptibilities to the essential oils of ginger, thyme, hyssop and sandalwood. All essential oils exhibited high levels of virucidal activity against the acyclovir-sensitive strain KOS and acyclovir-resistant HSV-1 clinical isolates and significantly reduced plaque formation.[100]

There are also observations of a direct antiparasitic activity.[101] Gingerol completely abolished the infectivity of the parasite *Schistosoma mansoni* in snails and mice.[102] Further work with mice demonstrated antischistosomal activity for a crude aqueous extract of ginger. As well as reduced worm burden and egg density in liver and faeces of mice treated with an aqueous extract of ginger (500 mg/kg, oral), histopathological data indicated a reduction in the number and size of granulomatous inflammatory infiltrations in the liver and intestine.[103] A moderate anthelmintic activity in sheep was demonstrated for ginger powder and aqueous extract (1 to 3 g/kg, oral).[104]

An extract from ginger effectively destroyed lavae of the fish parasite Anisakis in vitro. The most active antinematodal constituent was 6-gingerol, although a synergistic action with 6-shogaol (also a potent constituent) was observed.[105]

Antitumour activity

Ginger extract and its components have demonstrated antitumour activity in a limited number of studies, as noted in two reviews on this topic.[106,107] Given that it is commonly consumed as a food, the observation that ginger might prevent cancer probably has more practical relevance. A 2007 review noted that topical application of ginger extract, 6-gingerol and 6-paradol suppressed initiation and promotion of mouse skin carcinogenesis in several models.[107] One study noted in the review found that gingerol (0.02% in diet) significantly reduced the multiplicity of azoxymethane-induced intestinal carcinogenesis. In other studies, spontaneous mammary tumorigenesis was also significantly inhibited in mice (0.125% ginger in drinking water), as was 1,2-dimethylhydrazine-induced colon carcinogenesis in rats (various doses). Antimetastatic activity has also been observed in mice for 6-gingerol.[107]

Other activity

Both 6-gingerol and 8-gingerol potentiated the contraction induced by prostaglandins (except PGD_2) and inhibited that produced by PGD_2, thromboxane A_2 and leukotrienes in vitro.[108] There is a structural requirement for this activity, as other gingerol-related derivatives do not necessarily produce the same effect.[109]

Antihepatotoxic activities for the gingerols and shogaols were observed in vitro for carbon tetrachloride- and galactosamine-induced cytotoxicity in cultured rat hepatocytes.[110] 6-Shogaol, 8-shogaol and 8-gingerol showed dose-dependent inhibitory activities on experimentally induced histamine release from rat peritoneal mast cells. Other tested compounds from fresh ginger showed no inhibitory activity. In addition, 6-shogaol and 6-gingerol exhibited antiallergic activity in vivo.[84]

Ginger, ginger extract and pungent principles (gingerol and zingerone) have demonstrated significant antioxidant activity in vitro.[111–116] Such antioxidant activity might be expected, since many inhibitors of lipoxygenase are also strong antioxidants.

The radioprotective activity of ginger extract has been demonstrated in vivo in several studies.[62] However, it was administered by intraperitoneal injection.

Pharmacokinetics

After intravenous injection in rats, 90% of 6-gingerol was bound to serum protein and eliminated mainly via the bile.[117] Oral administration of 6-gingerol to rats confirmed that biliary excretion of the glucuronide was the major metabolic pathway.[118] Oral or intraperitoneal dosage of zingerone resulted in the urinary excretion of metabolites within 24 h, mainly as glucuronide and/or sulphate conjugates. Appreciable biliary excretion (40% in 12 h) also occurred.[119] Evidence from a rat study also suggests that 6-shogaol is mostly metabolised and excreted via the bile as metabolites.[120]

Human volunteers were given ginger as a single oral dose ranging from 100 mg to 2.0 g and blood samples were obtained to 72 h. No participant had detectable free 6-gingerol, 8-gingerol, 10-gingerol or 6-shogaol in plasma, but their glucuronides were detected. The 6-gingerol sulphate conjugate was also detected, but only above the 1.0 g dose.[121] Cmax values for the 2.0 g dose were 0.85, 0.23, 0.53 and 0.15 µg/mL for 6-gingerol, 8-gingerol, 10-gingerol and 6-shogaol, respectively.

Clinical trials

Nausea and emesis

The antiemetic and antinausea effects of ginger have been assessed in many clinical trials. These are summarised in Table 1.

Table 1

First author and year	Total participants	Preparation and daily dose	Study design	Study duration	Symptom/condition	Tolerability/safety	Efficacy versus control
Grontved 1988[177]	80	1 g powdered ginger	Double blind, randomised, placebo-controlled trial	Single dose study	Sea sickness		Ginger significantly reduced the tendency to vomiting and cold sweating versus placebo (p<0.05)
Fischer-Rasmussen 1990[178]	30	250 mg capsules ginger powder four times daily	Double blind, randomised, crossover trial	Four days	Hyperemesis gravidarum	One subsequent spontaneous abortion not considered to be linked	A significantly greater relief of symptoms such as nausea and vomiting was found after ginger treatment (p = 0.035)
Bone 1990[179]	60	1 g powdered ginger	Double blind, randomised study against metoclopramide and placebo	Postoperative	Postoperative nausea and vomiting (after gynaecological surgery)		There were statistically significantly fewer incidences of nausea in the ginger group compared with placebo (p<0.05). The incidences of nausea in the ginger and metoclopramide groups were similar. The need for an antiemetic after surgery was significantly greater in the placebo group compared with the other two groups (p-<0.05)
Phillips 1993[180]	120	1 g powdered ginger	Prospective double blind, randomised study against 10 mg metoclopramide and placebo	Postoperative day basis	Postoperative nausea and vomiting (after gynaecological laparoscopy)	There was no difference in the incidence of possible side effects such as sedation, abnormal movement, itch and visual disturbance between the three groups	The incidences of nausea in the ginger and metoclopramide groups were similar (27% and 21%) and less than for placebo (41%). The requirement for postoperative antiemetics was lower in the patients receiving ginger.
Schmid 1994[181]	1489	250 mg of ginger	Randomised, double blind study of seven treatments	One dose 2 h prior to departure	Travel sickness		80% of subjects receiving ginger reported no seasickness. Ginger was found to be as effective as the antiemetic drugs tested
Arfeen 1995[182]	108	0.5 and 1 g ginger	Double blind, randomised, controlled trial against placebo (all with oral diazepam premedication)	One hour pre-operatively; assessment at 3 h postoperatively	Postoperative nausea and vomiting (after gynaecological laparoscopy)		Ginger in doses of 0.5 or 1.0 g was not effective in reducing the incidence of postoperative nausea and vomiting. (However there was only one reading at 3 h after intervention)

Study	n	Intervention	Design	Duration	Condition	Adverse effects	Results
Meyer 1995[183]	11	1590 mg ginger powder 30 minutes prior to drug ingestion	Open label with patients acting as their own controls	Single dose study	Nausea following 8-methoxypsoralen		The average nausea score (out of 4) was 2.05 without ginger and 0.73 with ginger
Careddu 1996[184]	24	1.25 powdered ginger	Double blind trial against metoclopramide	Acute dose study, 500 mg every 4 h	Children with hyperketonaemia		Ginger was significantly more effective in the opinion of the physicians ($p < 0.0005$) and significantly better at preventing vomiting ($p < 0.05$)
Visalyaputra 1998[185]	120	2 g of ginger	Randomised, controlled trial comparing ginger, placebo, droperidol and ginger plus droperidol	Single dose study	Postoperative nausea and vomiting (after gynaecological laparoscopy)		There were no significant differences in the incidences of postoperative nausea or vomiting across the four groups
Vutyavanich 2001[186]	70	1 g ginger	Double blind, randomised, placebo-controlled	Four days plus follow-up at day 7	Nausea and vomiting in pregnancy	No adverse effects	Visual analogue symptom scale of nausea decreased significantly in the ginger group (2.1 ± 1.9) compared with placebo (0.9 ± 2.2, $p = 0.014$)
Keating 2002[187]	26	Ginger syrup (or placebo), 1 tablespoon in 4 to 8 ounces of hot or cold water four times daily (equivalent to 1 g/day ginger)	Double blind, placebo-controlled, randomised clinical trial	Two weeks	Nausea and vomiting in first trimester of pregnancy		77% patients receiving ginger (20% placebo) had at least a 4-point improvement on a 10-point nausea scale; 67% of ginger takers stopped vomiting (20% placebo)
Eberhart 2003[188]	180	0.3 to 0.6 g ginger root extract (10 to 20:1) extracted using acetone	Randomised, double blind, placebo-controlled trial	100 or 200 mg preoperatively as well as 3 and 6 h postoperatively	Postoperative nausea and vomiting (after gynaecological laparoscopy)		No effect from the ginger extract
Pongrojpaw 2003[189]	80	1.0 g ginger powder 1 h before procedure	Double blind, randomised, placebo-controlled trial	Single dose study	Postoperative nausea and vomiting (after gynaecological laparoscopy)		There was a significant difference in visual analogue nausea scores and vomiting times between groups taking ginger and placebo at 2 and 4 h after surgery ($p < 0.05$). No difference at 24 h was found. Incidence and frequency of vomiting were similar in both groups
Sripramote 2003[190]	128	1500 mg of ginger compared with 30 mg of vitamin B6	Double blind, randomised, controlled trial against vitamin B6	Three days	Nausea and vomiting in first 16 weeks of pregnancy	Minor side effects in both groups such as sedation and heartburn	No significant difference in reduced nausea scores and vomiting incidents between the two treatments. Both treatments reduced nausea score from baseline ($p < 0.001$) and vomiting episodes ($p < 0.01$)

Table 1 (Continued)

First author and year	Total participants	Preparation and daily dose	Study design	Study duration	Symptom/condition	Tolerability/safety	Efficacy versus control
Willetts 2003[191]	120	125 mg ginger extract (equivalent to 1.5 g of dried ginger) or placebo given four times per day	Double blind, randomised, placebo-controlled trial	Four days	Nausea and vomiting in first 20 weeks of pregnancy, in patients who had experienced morning sickness daily for at least a week and had no relief of symptoms through dietary changes	Follow-up of the pregnancies revealed normal ranges of birth weight, gestational age, Apgar scores and frequencies of congenital abnormalities in treatment group	Nausea as measured by the Rhodes Index of Nausea, Vomiting and Retching was significantly less for ginger (p>0.05) on each treatment day; there was less effect on retching and none on vomiting
Sontakke 2003[192]	50	1 g powdered ginger	Double blind, randomised, crossover trial against metoclopramide or ondansetron	One dose prior to chemotherapy and a second dose 6 h after	Nausea and vomiting in cancer patients receiving chemotherapy with cyclophosphamide in conjunction with other agents	No adverse effects attributable to ginger were recorded	Complete control of nausea was achieved in 62% of patients on ginger, 58% with metoclopramide and 86% with ondansetron. Similar results for control of vomiting
Manusirivithaya 2004[193]	48	1 g of ginger powder	Randomised, double blinded, crossover study against placebo and oral metoclopramide	Five days	Emesis in gynaecological cancer patients receiving cisplatin-based chemotherapy	Restlessness occurred more often in metoclopramide arm compared to ginger (p = 0.109)	Addition of the ginger to a standard antiemetic regimen had no advantage in reducing nausea or vomiting in the acute phase of cisplatin-induced emesis; in the delayed phase, ginger and metoclopramide had comparable efficacy
Smith 2004[194]	291	1.05 g of ginger daily	A randomised, controlled equivalence trial against 75 mg of vitamin B6	Three weeks	Nausea and vomiting in first 16 weeks of pregnancy		Ginger was equivalent to vitamin B6 in reducing nausea, retching and vomiting across the duration of the trial
Nanthakomon 2006[195]	120	1 g ginger powder 1 h before the procedure	Double blind, randomised, placebo controlled	Single dose study	Nausea and vomiting after major gynaecological surgery	Side effects not observed	A visual analogue nausea score and frequency of vomiting at 0, 2, 6, 12 and 24 h after surgery showed a statistically significant improvement for the ginger group, especially at 2 and 6 h
Tavlan 2006[196]	120	500 mg of ginger 1 h prior to surgery	Randomised, double blind, placebo-controlled comparing dexamethasone plus ginger with dexamethasone alone	Single dose study	Postoperative nausea and vomiting (after thyroidectomy)		There was no additional advantage from adding ginger to dexamethasone treatment. The dose used was lower than many other trials

Study	N	Intervention	Study design	Duration	Condition	Results
Apariman 2006[197]	60	1500 mg of ginger powder 1 h prior to surgery	Randomised, double blind, placebo-controlled	Single dose study	Postoperative nausea vomiting (after gynaecological laparoscopy)	Visual analogue symptom scale of nausea was significantly lower at 6 h postoperatively for ginger versus placebo ($p = 0.015$). Reduction in vomiting incidence was borderline significant for ginger versus placebo at 6 h ($p = 0.058$)
Chittumma 2007[198]	126	1950 mg ginger	Double blind, randomised, controlled trial against vitamin B6 (75 mg/day)	Four days	Nausea and vomiting in the first 16 weeks of pregnancy	Ginger was superior to vitamin B6 for nausea and vomiting as assessed by the Rhodes Index ($p<0.05$) and both treatments effected significant improvements from baseline ($p<0.05$). There were minor side effects, with no difference between the two groups. These included sedation, heartburn and arrhythmia
Pongrojpaw 2007[199]	170	1 g of ginger powder	Randomised, controlled trial against dimenhydrinate (100 mg/day)	Seven days	Nausea and vomiting in pregnancy	There was no significant difference in the visual analogue nausea scores and vomiting episodes between the two treatment groups. Drowsiness was significantly higher for dimenhydrinate ($p<0.01$)
Levine 2008[200]	28	Protein supplemented meals (high or normal) with added ginger 1 g	Controlled clinical trial against normal diet	Three days immediately after chemotherapy	Delayed nausea after chemotherapy	Diary reports of nausea and recourse to antiemetic medication were significantly less common for higher doses of protein with ginger than for lower doses and the control group
Zick 2009[201]	162	1 or 2 g ginger daily	Randomised, double blind, placebo-controlled trial of two doses of ginger given with 5-HT3 receptor antagonists and/or aprepitant	Three days	Chemotherapy-induced nausea and vomiting	Blinding failed and there were no differences between groups in the prevalence and severity of acute or delayed nausea or vomiting. Well tolerated, with no difference in all adverse events and significantly less fatigue in the ginger group
Ensiyeh 2009[202]	70	1 g of ginger	Double blind, randomised, controlled trial against vitamin B6 (40 mg/day)	Four days	Nausea and vomiting in pregnancy	The decrease in the visual analogue score of nausea in the ginger group was significantly greater than for the B6 group ($p = 0.024$). The number of vomiting episodes decreased for both groups, but with no difference between them

Table 1 (Continued)

First author and year	Total participants	Preparation and daily dose	Study design	Study duration	Symptom/condition	Tolerability/safety	Efficacy versus control
Ozgoli 2009[203]	67	1 g of ginger powder	Double blind, randomised, placebo-controlled	Four days	Nausea and vomiting in pregnancy		The decrease in vomiting episodes among ginger users was significantly greater than for placebo ($p<0.05$) and ginger effected a higher rate of improvement versus placebo ($p<0.01$)
Pillai 2011[204]	60	Ginger root powder (1 or 2 g depending on the weight of the child)	Double blind, randomised, placebo-controlled trial, comparing ginger as an additional antiemetic to ondansetron and dexamethasone	Days 1 to 3 of chemotherapy cycle	Chemotherapy-induced nausea and vomiting in children with bone sarcoma		Ginger was superior to placebo for all key measures. Acute moderate to severe nausea was observed in 93.3% of treatment cycles in the control group as compared to 55.6% cycles in the ginger group ($p = 0.003$). The respective rates for acute moderate to severe vomiting were 76.7% versus 33.3% ($p = 0.002$), for delayed moderate to severe nausea 73.3% versus 25.9% ($p<0.001$), and for delayed moderate to severe vomiting 46.67% versus 14.81% ($p = 0.022$)
Ryan 2011[205]	744	0.5, 1.0 or 1.5 g powdered ginger	Double blind, randomised, four-arm, placebo-controlled trial	Six days, starting three days before chemotherapy	Nausea in cancer patients receiving chemotherapy		A total of 576 patients were included in the final analysis. All doses of ginger significantly reduced nausea compared to placebo on day 1 of chemotherapy ($p = 0.003$). The largest reduction in nausea occurred with 0.5 and 1.0 g of ginger

This table of 29 clinical studies represents an impressive body of evidence.

Two recent meta-analyses of this clinical research have come to different verdicts. In one conducted in Thailand, five randomised trials including 363 patients were pooled for analysis. A benefit in preventing postoperative nausea and vomiting was demonstrated. Only one side effect, abdominal discomfort, was reported.[122] This positive conclusion followed the elimination of studies that used low doses of ginger or short-term observations, and this may have accounted for the difference between the findings of an earlier (2005) systematic review and meta-analysis from Germany, which was more reluctant to confirm the efficacy of ginger.[123] Published systematic reviews have tended to favour a benefit of ginger over placebo in pregnancy-related nausea,[124,125] with some caution as to the extent that the approach can be universally recommended. Of course, more positive trials have been published since all of the above reviews.[125]

In order to assess the efficacy and safety of treatments for nausea, vomiting and retching in early pregnancy (up to 20 weeks' gestation), a Cochrane review team (updating their earlier report of 2003) reviewed relevant published randomised, controlled trials. Trials of interventions for hyperemesis gravidarum were excluded, as were quasi-randomised trials and trials using a crossover design. Twenty-seven trials involving 4041 women met their inclusion criteria. These trials covered several interventions, including acupressure, acustimulation, acupuncture, ginger, vitamin B6 and several antiemetic drugs. In all, nine studies on ginger were included, and none were excluded. Evidence for the efficacy of ginger was considered limited and not consistent.[126] However, no meta-analysis was conducted.

One key omission from the published clinical research might be contributing to the above controversy. Only occasionally in published papers is the provenance and analysis of the ginger treatment provided. Given the noted variability in constituent levels in ginger (see Key constituents above), it is incumbent on future researchers to appropriately quantify their treatments so that sound assessments of benefit can be made.

Digestive conditions

Ginger accelerated gastric emptying and stimulated antral contractions in patients with functional dyspepsia in a preliminary investigation. Nine patients with functional dyspepsia were studied on two separate days in a randomised, double blind design.[127] Following a fast of 8h the patients took capsules containing a total of 1.2g of ginger root powder or placebo. One hour later they consumed 500mL of a low-nutrient soup. Antral area (bottom of stomach, near the duodenum), fundus area (top, near the oesophagus) and diameter, and the frequency of antral contractions were then measured using ultrasound at intervals over 90 minutes. Gastric half-emptying time was significantly less after ginger than placebo (11.9 minutes versus 21.1 minutes), and the frequency of antral contractions was significantly greater. Antral area decreased more rapidly with ginger. However, there was no difference observed in fundus dimensions, serum peptides or gastrointestinal symptoms.

An extension of this study that included data for 11 patients yielded similar results.[128] Gastric emptying was more rapid after ginger than placebo (12.3 minutes versus 16.1 minutes, $p<0.05$), but fundus dimensions, serum peptides and gastrointestinal symptoms did not differ.

Respiratory conditions

Delayed gastric emptying is a major problem in intensive care unit patients receiving enteral nutrition. It can lead to aspiration and subsequent development of ventilator associated pneumonia (VAP). A group of Iranian scientists investigated the impact of ginger on nosocomial (hospital-associated) pneumonia in 32 patients with adult respiratory distress syndrome who were dependent on mechanical ventilation and fed via a nasogastric tube.[129] Patients were randomised into two groups: the control group received 1g/day of coconut oil as a placebo and the study group received 120mg/day of a ginger extract (undefined). The supplements were added during tube feeding three times a day. The nurse was unblinded to treatment assignment, whereas the patients and investigators remained blinded to the randomisation. Treatment was continued for 21 days unless death or discharge from the intensive care unit (ICU) occurred. The diagnosis of VAP was made based on the International Sepsis Consensus Conference 2005.

While the small patient numbers limited the statistical power of the trial, some significant results were still observed. The average number of ICU-free days was significantly lower in the ginger group (7.0 ± 0.8 versus 4.4 ± 0.8, $p = 0.02$), as was the average number of ventilator-free days (11.3 ± 1.1 versus 7.1 ± 1.1, $p = 0.04$). The incidence of VAP saw a distinct trend in favour of ginger that just failed to reach statistical significance (6.3% versus 31.3%, $p = 0.07$). There was also a significant improvement in the ginger group compared with the control group in terms of the amount of feeding tolerated at the first 48h ($p<0.005$). The authors discussed current drug treatments such as metoclopramide and erythromycin for prevention of VAP in ICU patients and concluded that the evidence for their efficacy was scant. Given the positive impact of ginger, they suggested that a larger study was warranted.

A reduction in delayed gastric emptying was suggested by the authors as the mechanism of action of ginger. If the contents of nasogastric feeding spend less time in the stomach, there would be less risk of regurgitation and aspiration. There certainly is additional clinical evidence to support this hypothesis (see elsewhere in this monograph). Ginger should be considered for any patient experiencing symptoms associated with delayed gastric emptying (gastroparesis).

A randomised, placebo-controlled clinical trial conducted in Iran investigated the use of ginger for the treatment of asthma.[130] In all, 92 patients received either ginger (tincture containing 150mg of rhizome every 8h) or placebo for 2 months. The results indicated that ginger was effective in reducing asthmatic symptoms, but had no effect on the severity of the disease, as assessed by spirometry. Those receiving ginger had fewer nocturnal coughing attacks, fewer dyspnoeic attacks and reduced usage of inhaled medication. These reductions were significantly different from that experienced in the placebo group ($p<0.05$ for each parameter). The authors noted that the prescribed dosage (about 0.5g/day) was below the standard therapeutic dose of 1 to 4g/day. Blinding was probably an issue, given that a liquid dose of ginger was used.

Inflammatory conditions

Ginger has long been used as a popular treatment for arthritic and other inflammatory pains. Modern evidence of such prospects has been relatively recent and, although still mixed, is promising.

In a controlled, double blind, crossover study, 3 weeks of a combination of ginger and *Alpinia galanga* extracts (510mg/day) was compared to placebo and ibuprofen in a randomised sequence in patients with osteoarthritis of the hip or knee. A statistically significant effect of the herbal combination over placebo could only be demonstrated in the first period of treatment before crossover, and a significant difference was not observed in the study as a whole.[131]

Two hundred and forty-seven patients with osteoarthritis of the knee and moderate-to-severe pain received a highly purified and standardised combination of ginger and *Alpinia galanga* extracts (510mg/day) or placebo twice daily for 6 weeks in a randomised, double blind, placebo-controlled trial. The primary efficacy variable was the proportion of responders experiencing a reduction in 'knee pain on standing', using an intent-to-treat analysis. In all, 63% of those taking the ginger combination experienced a clinically significant reduction on a visual analogue scale for knee pain on standing, compared with 50% in the control group (p = 0.048). Analysis of the secondary efficacy variables revealed a consistently greater response in the herbal group compared with the control group. Patients receiving the herbal extract combination experienced more gastrointestinal adverse events than the placebo group (59 versus 21 patients), although these adverse events were mostly mild.[132]

Twenty-nine patients (6 men and 23 women) with symptomatic gonarthritis were randomised into a double blind, placebo-controlled, crossover study over 24 weeks. The treatment group was given a ginger extract (1000mg/day).There were no significant differences in visual analogue scales for handicap and pain on movement at crossover at 12 weeks, but by the end of 24 weeks there was a statistically significant difference in favour of the ginger group (p<0.001).[133] The study was limited by the lack of a washout (no treatment) period before crossover.

Cardiovascular activity

In an open study involving both normal human volunteers and hypertensive patients, ginger (1g/day for 7 days) demonstrated a synergistic effect with nifedipine (10mg/day) in terms of reducing platelet aggregation (using collagen, ADP and adrenaline (epinephrine) as agonists) in hypertensive patients, and potentiated the antiplatelet effect of nifedipine in normal volunteers.[134] (See also the Interactions section in this monograph).

Powdered ginger given at a dose of 4g/day to 30 patients with coronary artery disease (CAD) did not affect platelet aggregation measured after 1.5 and 3 months of administration. In addition, no changes in fibrinolytic activity and fibrinogen were observed. No information was provided for controls. However, a single dose of 10g of ginger given to each of 10 CAD patients produced a significant reduction in platelet aggregation after 4h (p<0.05). There was a small non-significant rise in platelet aggregation for the placebo group. Ginger did not affect blood lipids and blood sugar when administered at 4g/day for 3 months. The doses used in these studies were relatively high and lower doses are probably unlikely to offer any significant risk protection. In this context, it is interesting to note that 4g of dried ginger powder (of unspecified quality) did not have a significant effect on platelet aggregation, even after regular intake for 3 months, but a dose of 10g significantly reduced platelet aggregation.[135]

In a 45-day double blind, placebo-controlled clinical trial, 85 patients with hyperlipidaemia and without other complications were randomised to receive ginger (3g/day in three divided doses) or placebo. There was a significantly higher reduction in triglyceride and total cholesterol levels demonstrated for the ginger group versus placebo (p<0.05).[136] However, overall reductions from baseline with ginger treatment were modest, in the order of 10%.

Analgesic activity

Inhibition of thromboxane and prostaglandin activity provides a plausible mechanism for traditional reputation of ginger in pain relief, particularly in the case of migraine[137] and dysmenorrhoea.[138]

In a double blind, comparative trial conducted in Iran, 150 female students (mean age of about 21 years) with primary dysmenorrhoea were assigned to one of three groups: ginger, mefenamic acid or ibuprofen.[139] Students in the ginger group took 250mg capsules of ginger rhizome powder four times a day for 3 days from the start of their menstrual period. The other groups received 250mg mefenamic acid or 400mg ibuprofen capsules under the same protocol. Severity of dysmenorrhoea was assessed before and after treatment by a scoring system (0 to 3).

At the end of treatment (one menstrual period), severity of dysmenorrhoea decreased in all groups; for example, the incidence of severe dysmenorrhoea decreased from 28% to 8% in the ginger group, 32% to 6% in the mefenamic acid group and 38% to 18% in the ibuprofen group. No significant differences were found between the groups in terms of the severity of dysmenorrhoea. The change in pain severity was similar in all three groups; for example, 36% were considerably relieved in the ginger group, with 30% and 36% considerably relieved in the mefenamic acid and ibuprofen groups, respectively. No severe side effects occurred. In this trial of short duration, ginger was as effective as mefenamic acid and ibuprofen in relieving pain in women with primary dysmenorrhoea.

A single dose of ginger (2g of fresh ginger 30 minutes prior to exercise) had no effect on quadriceps muscle pain, rating of perceived exertion, work rate, heart rate and oxygen uptake (VO$_2$) during and after 30min of cycling at 60% of VO$_2$ peak exercise in 25 college-age participants. This was a placebo-controlled, double blind, crossover study.[140]

Twenty-seven participants performed 24 eccentric actions of the non-dominant elbow flexors. Then, in a double blind, crossover design, participants ingested a 2g dose of fresh ginger or placebo 24h and 48h after this exercise.[141] Overall, ginger consumption demonstrated no effect on muscle pain, dysfunction or metabolic rate compared with placebo. In the sub-set of participants who consumed ginger 24h after exercise, arm pain was reduced the following day, 48h after exercise. Participants who ingested placebo 24h post-exercise exhibited no change in pain the following day. The authors concluded that a single 2g dose of ginger does not attenuate eccentric exercise-induced muscle pain, inflammation or dysfunction 45min after its ingestion, but ginger may attenuate the day-to-day progression of muscle pain.

The same research group examined the effect of 11 days of 2g/day fresh (study 1) or 2g/day heat-treated (study 2) ginger on muscle pain.[142] Studies 1 and 2 were identical double blind, placebo-controlled, randomised experiments with 34 and 40 volunteers, respectively. On day 8, participants performed 18 eccentric actions of the elbow flexors to induce pain and inflammation. Pain intensity, perceived effort, plasma prostaglandin E_2, arm volume, range-of-motion and isometric strength were assessed prior to and for 3 days after exercise. Fresh and heat-treated ginger resulted in similar pain reductions 24h after eccentric exercise compared to placebo (25%, p = 0.041 and 23%, p = 0.049, respectively). Smaller effects were noted between both types of ginger and placebo on other measures. In conclusion, daily supplementation with ginger reduced muscle pain caused by eccentric exercise, and this effect was not changed by heat-treating the ginger.

Toxicology and other safety data

Toxicology

The acute oral LD_{50} for ginger oil in rats and the acute dermal LD_{50} in rabbits both exceeded 5 g/kg.[143]

Ginger extract caused no mortality at doses of up to 2.5g/kg in mice (equivalent to about 75g/kg of fresh rhizome).[19] This low acute toxicity was confirmed in a separate study that also found ginger extract caused no signs of chronic toxicity at 100mg/kg per day for 3 months.[144]

Components in ginger have both mutagenic[145] and antimutagenic activity.[146–149] Depending on the test model, ginger extract has also shown mutagenic[150] and antimutagenic[151] and anticarcinogenic effects.[152,153]

Contraindications

According to the Commission E, use of ginger is contraindicated in patients with gallstones, except under close supervision and should not be administered for morning sickness during pregnancy.[154]

However, the dictate from traditional Chinese medicine that dried ginger preparations can be used cautiously during pregnancy is probably a more rational approach.[7] A daily dose of 2g of dried ginger should not be exceeded in pregnancy (see below and the Clinical trials section).

Special warnings and precautions

Daily doses of ginger in excess of 4g should be prescribed with caution in patients who are already taking blood-thinning

drugs such as warfarin or aspirin or who have an increased risk of haemorrhage (see the Interactions section below).[135]

Proceed with caution in cases of peptic ulceration or other gastric diseases. However, any exacerbation in such cases should be immediately apparent and transient. It is best not to proceed if symptoms such as heartburn occur.

Interactions

There is a suggestion that ginger is one of a number of hot spices that increase bioavailability of other drugs, either by increasing their absorption rate from the gastrointestinal tract or by protecting the drug from being metabolised/oxidised in its first passage through the liver after being absorbed.[45] This means that concurrent administration of ginger, and other hot spices, might increase the activity of other medication.

There is a theoretical possibility that ginger may increase the chance of bleeding especially when combined with anticoagulants.[155–158] In one report a 76-year-old European woman on long-term phenprocoumon therapy with an international normalised ratio of prothrombin time (INR) within the therapeutic range began using ginger products. Several weeks later she developed an elevated INR (up to 10) and epistaxis. Her INR returned to normal after ginger was stopped and vitamin K1 was given. An objective assessment revealed that causality due to an interaction of phenprocoumon and ginger was 'probable'.[159]

However, powdered ginger given at 4g daily to 30 patients with CAD did not affect platelet aggregation, fibrinolytic activity and fibrinogen level after 1.5 and 3 months of administration.[135] In another study, ginger had no effect on S-warfarin concentration and response (prothrombin complex activity) in healthy volunteers who were given a single warfarin dose (25mg).[160]

In a related open label, three-way crossover randomised study, 12 healthy male volunteers received a single 25mg dose of warfarin alone, or after 7 days of pretreatment with recommended doses of Ginkgo or ginger (from reliable sources). Dosing with Ginkgo or ginger was continued for 7 days after the administration of the warfarin dose. There was no significant effect of either herb on observed platelet aggregation, INR, warfarin enantiomer protein binding, warfarin enantiomer concentration in plasma and S-7-hydroxywarfarin concentration in urine.[161]

On the other hand, there is always the possibility of interactions occurring less frequently (as perhaps is relevant to the case report above). In a prospective, longitudinal Canadian study, 171 adults prescribed warfarin anticoagulation therapy for at least 4 months completed a 16-week diary, recording bleeding events and exposure to factors known to increase the risk of bleeding or a supratherapeutic INR. In all, 87 (51%) reported at least one bleeding event and 36 (21%) had a supratherapeutic INR. Ginger was one of two natural remedies (with coenzyme Q10) independently associated with an increased risk of self-reported bleeding.[162]

There is one case report of a reduction in platelet count from 1.8 million to 240000 in a patient with Kawasaki disease the day after consuming a ginger beverage (comprising a half-teaspoon of ground ginger plus sugar steeped in boiling water, which had soda water added to it after cooling). The effect was believed to be due to ginger and carbon dioxide, both regarded as thromboxane synthetase inhibitors.[163]

The best practice is to keep ginger levels relatively low when there is a risk of increased bleeding, probably below 2 g/day (certainly no greater than 4 g/day). In the case of anti-coagulant medication, there should be close monitoring for danger signs and changes in coagulation parameters.

Use in pregnancy and lactation

Category A – no proven increase in the frequency of malformation or other harmful effects on the fetus despite consumption by a large number of women.

Ginger is in fact one of the most popular remedies for self-medication among pregnant women.[164–166]

After a systematic search of the literature for the use of ginger as an antiemetic, 15 studies were considered eligible for a review of potential side effects. These included data for 777 patients, and of these a total of 136 patients were treated with ginger within the first trimester of pregnancy. Ginger was not associated with complications, with the exception of an abortion that occurred in the 12th week of gestation, but was not considered to be linked.[167] Pregnant women who called the Canadian Motherisk Program and were taking ginger during the first trimester of their pregnancy were enrolled in a safety study.[168] From 187 pregnancies, there were 181 live births with three major malformations, two stillbirths, three spontaneous abortions and one therapeutic abortion. There were no statistical differences in pregnancy outcomes between this ginger group and a comparison group, with the exception of more infants weighing less than 2.5 kg in the comparison group (12 versus 3, p<0.001).

However, expert views on the safety of ginger in pregnancy are not consistent; in accordance with good practice, the herb should not be used during pregnancy and lactation without expert advice, particularly at doses above 2 g/day.

Ginger included in the drinking water of pregnant rats (at levels of 20 and 50 g/L) led to increased embryo loss compared with controls, but increased the weight and development of fetuses, with no other adverse effects observed on developed fetuses or mothers.[169] However, a study of a ginger-Alpinia standardised extract showed no effect on organogenesis or any other adverse effects on pregnancy in rats.[170]

Ginger is considered compatible with breastfeeding.

Effects on ability to drive and use machines

No adverse effects expected.

Side effects

In the review of the antiemetic literature cited above, 3.3% of the 777 total patients suffered from slight side effects, mainly mild gastrointestinal symptoms and sleepiness, neither requiring specific treatments.[167]

At higher doses a blood-thinning effect and an increase in gastric secretory activity leading to heartburn is possible.

Occupational allergic contact dermatitis from spices is relatively rare, but needs to be taken into consideration in patients who have hand dermatitis and work with spices and foods. Acute spice reactions may also be linked to respiratory symptoms (although the possibility is that these are due to direct irritation of the lungs).[171] Ginger is known to be a significant contributor to such allergies.[172,173] Patients at risk of spice allergy are young adults sensitised to mugwort and birch allergens, sharing cross-sensitisation with various food plant allergens: this group makes up 6.4% of all food allergies in adults.[174] There are, however, doubts about the consistency of a link with celery-birch allergy patterns.[175]

Overdosage

No incidents found in the published literature.

Safety in children

Ginger is generally considered a safe remedy for children.[176]

Regulatory status in selected countries

Ginger is official in the *European Pharmacopoeia* (2001), the *British Pharmacopoeia* (2011), the *United States Pharmacopeia – National Formulary* (USP 34–NF 29, 2011), the *Chinese Pharmacopoeia* (English edition, 1997) and the *Japanese Pharmacopoeia* 15th edition (English edition, 2006). It was official in the second edition of the *Indian Pharmacopoeia* (1966), but was not included in the third edition (1985).

Ginger is covered by a positive Commission E Monograph and can be used for dyspepsia and the prevention of motion sickness.

Ginger is on the UK General Sale List.

Ginger and ginger oil have GRAS status. Ginger is also freely available as a 'dietary supplement' in the USA under DSHEA legislation (1994 Dietary Supplement Health and Education Act). It has been present in the following over-the-counter (OTC) drug products: digestive aid drug products and as an ingredient in products offered for use as a smoking deterrent. The FDA however advises that 'based on evidence currently available, there is inadequate data to establish general recognition of the safety and effectiveness of these ingredients for the specified uses'.

Ginger is not included in Part 4 of Schedule 4 of the Therapeutic Goods Act Regulations of Australia and hence is freely available for sale. However, products containing ginger with an equivalent dry weight per dosage unit of 2 g and above are required to carry warnings regarding concomitant use with anticoagulants and advising that those with bleeding problems seek medical advice.

References

1. Dalby A. *Dangerous Tastes: The Story of Spices*. UK: British Museum Press; 2000. pp. 21–26.

2. Perry LM. *Medicinal Plants of East and Southeast Asia: Attributed Properties and Uses*. USA: MIT Press; 1980. p. 443.

3. Grieve M. *A Modern Herbal*, vol. 1. New York: Dover Publications; 1971. pp. 353–354.

4. British Herbal Medicine Association Scientific Committee *British Herbal Pharmacopoeia*. Cowling: BHMA; 1983. pp. 239–240.

5. Felter HW, Lloyd JU. *King's American Dispensatory*, vol. 2, 18th ed., rev. 3. Portland: Eclectic Medical Publications; 1905. pp. 2109–2112.

6. Lyle TJ. *Physio-Medical Therapeutics, Materia Medica and Pharmacy*, London. Reprinted by the National Association of Medical Herbalists of Great Britain, 1932.

7. Bensky D, Clavey S, Stoger E. *Chinese Herbal Medicine Materia Medica*, 3rd ed. Seattle: Eastland Press; 2004.

8. Chen JK, Chen TT. *Chinese Medical Herbology and Pharmacology*. California: Art of Medicine Press: City of Industry; 2004.

9. Nadkarni KM., 1st ed. *Indian Materia Medica*, vols. 1 & 2. Bombay: Bombay Popular Prakashan; 1908. Reprinted 1991.

10. Bhattacharjee SK. *Handbook of Medicinal Plants*. Jaipur: Pointer; 2000.

11. Farnsworth NR, Bunyapraphatsara N, eds. *Thai Medicinal Plants*. Bangkok: Medicinal Plant Information Center; 1992. pp. 253–260.

12. Mabberley DJ. *The Plant Book*, 2nd ed. UK: Cambridge University Press; 1997. p. 767.

13. World Health Organization. *Medicinal Plants in China*. Regional Office for the Western Pacific, Manila, World Health Organization; 1989. p. 297.

14. Morgan JP, Penovich *Arch Neurol*. 1978;35(8):530–532.

15. Wagner H, Bladt S. *Plant Drug Analysis: A Thin Layer Chromatography Atlas*, 2nd ed. Berlin: Springer-Verlag; 1996. p. 293.

16. Schwertner HA, Rios DC. *J Chromatogr B Analyt Technol Biomed Life Sci*. 2007;856(1–2):41–47.

17. Schwertner HA, Rios DC, Pascoe JE. *Obstet Gynecol*. 2006;107(6):1337–1343.

18. Sharma SS, Kochupillai V, Gupta SK, et al. *J Ethnopharmacol*. 1997;57(2):93–96.

19. Lumb AB. *Anaesthesia*. 1993;48(12):1118.

20. Yang Y, Kinoshita K, Koyama K, et al. *Phytomedicine*. 2002;9(2):146–152.

21. Abdel-Aziz H, Nahrstedt A, Petereit F, et al. *Planta Med*. 2005;71(7):609–616.

22. Abdel-Aziz H, Windeck T, Ploch M, et al. *Eur J Pharmacol*. 2006;530(1–2):136–143.

23. Pertz HH, Lehmann J, Roth-Ehrang R, et al. *Planta Med*. 2011 [Epub ahead of print].

24. Qian QH, Yue W, Chen WH. *Chin Med J*. 2010;123(4):478–484.

25. Sharma A, Haksar A, Chawla R, et al. *Pharmacol Biochem Behav*. 2005;81(4):864–870.

26. Mowrey DB, Clayson DE. *Lancet*. 1982;1(8273):655–657.

27. Kawai T, Kinoshita K, Koyama K, et al. *Planta Med*. 1994;60(1):17–20.

28. Lien HC, Sun WM, Chen YH, et al. *Am J Physiol Gastrointest Liver Physiol*. 2003;284(3):481–489.

29. Grontved A, Hentzer E. *ORL J Otorhinolaryngol Relat Spec*. 1986;48(5):282–286.

30. Holtmann S, Clarke AH, Scherer H, et al. *Acta Oto Laryngologica*. 1989;108(3/4):168–174.

31. Stewart JJ, Wood MJ, Wood CD, Mims ME. *Pharmacology*. 1991;42(2):111–120.

32. Phillips S, Hutchinson S, Ruggier R. *Anaesthesia*. 1993;48(5):393–395.

33. Thompson EH, Wolf ID, Allen CE. *J Food Sci*. 1973;38(4):652–655.

34. Platel K, Srinivasan K. *Int J Food Sci Nutr*. 1996;47(1):55–59.

35. Yamahara J, Miki K, Chisaka T, et al. *J Ethnopharmacol*. 1985;13(2):217–225.

36. Blumberger W, Glatzel H. *Nutr Dieta*. 1964;6:181–192.

37. Suekawa M, Ishige A, Yuasa K, et al. *J Pharmacobiodyn*. 1984;7(11):836–848.

38. Yamahara J, Huang QR, Li YH, et al. *Chem Pharm Bull (Tokyo)*. 1990;38(2):430–431.

39. Sharma SS, Gupta YK. *J Ethnopharmacol*. 1998;62(1):49–55.

40. Micklefield GH, Redeker Y, Meister V, et al. *Int J Clin Pharmacol Ther*. 1999;37(7):341–346.

41. Gonlachanvit S, Chen YH, Hasler WL, et al. *J Pharmacol Exp Ther*. 2003;307(3):1098–1103.

42. Wu KL, Rayner CK, Chuah SK, et al. *Eur J Gastroenterol Hepatol*. 2008;20(5):436–440.

43. Lohsiriwat S, Rukkiat M, Chaikomin R, et al. *J Med Assoc Thai*. 2010;93(3):366–372.

44. Huang Q, Matsuda H, Sakai K, et al. *Yakugaku Zasshi*. 1990;110(12):936–942.

45. Atal CK, Zutshi U, Rao PG, et al. *J Ethnopharmacol*. 1981;4(2):229–232.

46. Yamahara J, Mochizuki M, Rong HQ, et al. *J Ethnopharmacol*. 1988;23(2–3):299–304.

47. al-Yahya MA, Rafatullah S, Mossa JS, et al. *Am J Chin Med*. 1989;17(1–2):51–56.

48. Yoshikawa M, Hatakeyama S, Taniguchi K, et al. *Chem Pharm Bull*. 1992;40(8):2239–2241.

49. Yamahara J, Hatakeyama S, Taniguchi K, et al. *Yakugaku Zasshi*. 1992;11(9):645–655.[Article in Japanese].

50. Yoshikawa M, Yamaguchi S, Kunimi K, et al. *Chem Pharm Bull*. 1994;42(6):1226–1230.

51. Goso Y, Ogata Y, Ishihara K, et al. *Comp Biochem Physiol C Pharmacol Toxicol Endocrinol*. 1996;113(1):17–21.

52. Yamahara J, Huang QR, Li YH, et al. *Chem Pharm Bull (Tokyo)*. 1990;38(2):430–431.

53. Mascolo N, Jain R, Jain SC, et al. *J Ethnopharmacol*. 1989;27(1–2):129–140.

54. Flynn DL, Rafferty MF, Boctor AM, et al. *Prostagland Leuko Med*. 1986;24(2–3):195–198.

55. Kiuchi F, Shibuya M, Sankawa U. *Chem Pharm Bull*. 1982;30(2):754–757.

56. Iwakami S, Shibuya M, Tseng CF, et al. *Chem Pharm Bull*. 1986;34(9):3960–3963.

57. Kiuchi F, Iwakami S, Shibuya M, et al. *Chem Pharm Bull*. 1992;40(2):387–391.

58. Suekawa M, Yuasa K, Isono M, et al. *Nippon Yakurigaku Zasshi*. 1986;88(4):263–269.

59. Collier HO, McDonald-Gibson WJ, Saeed SA. *Br J Pharmacol*. 1976;58(2):193–199.

60. Grzanna R, Lindmark L, Frondoza CG. *J Med Food*. 2005;8(2):125–132.

61. Chrubasik S, Pittler MH, Roufogalis BD. *Phytomedicine*. 2005;12(9):684–701.

62. Ali BH, Blunden G, Tanira MO, et al. *Food Chem Toxicol*. 2008;46(2):409–420.

63. Marles RJ, Kaminski J, Arnason JT, et al. *J Nat Prod*. 1992;55(8):1044–1056.

64. Fouda AM, Berika MY. *Basic Clin Pharmacol Toxicol*. 2009;104(3):262–271.

65. Sharma JN, Srivastava KC, Gan EK. *Pharmacology*. 1994;49(5):314–318.

66. Sharma JN, Ishak FI, Yusof APM, et al. *Asia Pac J Pharmacol*. 1997;12(1–2):9–14.

67. Zhou HL, Deng YM, Xie QM. *J Ethnopharmacol*. 2006;105(1–2):301–305.

68. Srivastava KC. *Prostagland Leuko Med*. 1984;13:227.

69. Srivastava KC. *Biomed Biochim Acta*. 1984;43(8–9):S335–S346.

70. Srivastava KC. *Prostagland Leuko Med*. 1986;25:187.

71. Guh JH, Ko FN, Jong TT, et al. *J Pharm Pharmacol*. 1995;47(4):329–332.

72. Srivastava KC. *Prostaglandins Leukot Essent Fatty Acids*. 1989;35:183.

73. Verma SK, Singh J, Khamesra R, Bordia A. *Indian J Med Res*. 1993;98:240–242.

74. Verma SK, Bordia A. *Indian J Med Sci*. 2001;55(2):83–86.

75. Lumb AB. *Thromb Haemost*. 1994;71(1):110–111.

76. Janssen PL, Meyboom S, van Staveren WA, et al. *Eur J Clin Nutr*. 1996;50(11):722–724.

77. Giri J, Sakthidevi TK, Meerarani S. *Indian J Nutr Diet*. 1984;21(12):433–436.

78. Srinivasan K, Sambaiah K. *Int J Vit Nutr Res*. 1991;61:364.

79. Sambaiah K, Srinivasan K. *Nahrung*. 1991;35(1):47–51.

80. Sharma I, Gusain D, Dixit VP. *Phytother Res*. 1996;10(6):517–518.

81. Nicoll R, Henein MY. *Int J Cardiol*. 2009;131(3):408–409.

82. Shoji N, Iwasa A, Takemoto T, et al. *J Pharm Sci*. 1982;71(10):1174–1175.

83. Kobayashi M, Ishida Y, Shoji N, et al. *J Pharmacol Exp Ther*. 1988;246(2):667–673.

84. Yamahara J, Matsuda H, Yamaguchi S, et al. *Nat Med*. 1995;49(1):76–83.

85. Kobayashi M, Shoji N, Ohizumi Y. *Biochim Biophys Acta*. 1987;903(1):96–102.

86. Ohizumi Y, Sasaki S, Shibusawa K, et al. *Biol Pharm Bull*. 1996;19(10):1377–1379.

87. Wu BN, Ho WC, Chiang LC, et al. *Asia Pac J Pharmacol*. 1996;11(1):5–12.

88. Chang HM, But PP. *Pharmacology and Applications of Chinese Materia Medica*. Singapore: World Scientific; 1987.

89. Suekawa M, Aburada M, Hosoya E. *J Pharmacobiodyn*. 1986;9(10):842–852.

90. Ghayur MN, Gilani AH. *J Cardiovasc Pharmacol*. 2005;45(1):74–80.

91. Westerterp-Plantenga M, Diepvens K, Joosen AM, et al. *Physiol Behav*. 2006;89(1):85–91.

92. Eldershaw TP, Colquhoun EQ, Dora KA, et al. *Int J Obes Relat Metabol Dis*. 1992;16(10):755–763.

93. Kawada T, Sakabe SI, Watanabe T, et al. *Proc Soc Exp Biol Med*. 1988;188(2):229–233.

94. Chang CP, Chang JY, Wang FY, et al. *J Ethnopharmacol*. 1995;48(1):13–19.

95. Henry CJ, Piggott SM. *Hum Nutr Clin Nutr*. 1987;41(1):89–92.

96. Endo K, Kanno E, Oshima Y. *Phytochemistry*. 1990;29(3):797–799.

97. Gugnani HC, Ezenwanze EC. *J Commun Dis*. 1985;17(3):233–236.

98. Nostro A, Cellini L, Di Bartolomeo S, et al. *Phytother Res*. 2006;20(3):187–190.

99. Denyer CL, Jackson P, Loakes DM, et al. *J Nat Prod*. 1994;57(5):658–662.

100. Schnitzler P, Koch C, Reichling J. *Antimicrob Agents Chemother*. 2007;51(5):1859–1862.

101. Guerin JC, Reveillere HP. *Ann Pharm Fr*. 1984;42(6):553–559.

102. Adewunmi CO, Oguntimein BO, Furu P. *Planta Med*. 1990;56(4):374–376.

103. Mostafa OM, Eid RA, Adly MA. *Parasitol Res*. 2011 [Epub ahead of print].

104. Iqbal Z, Lateef M, Akhtar MS, et al. *J Ethnopharmacol*. 2006;106(2):285–287.

105. Goto C, Kasuya S, Koga K, et al. *Parasitol Res*. 1990;76(8):653–656.

106. Oyagbemi AA, Saba AB, Azeez OI. *Biofactors*. 2010;36(3):169–178.

107. Shukla Y, Singh M. *Food Chem Toxicol*. 2007;45(5):683–690.

108. Kimura I, Kimura M, Pancho LR. *Jpn J Pharmacol*. 1989;50(3):253–261.

109. Kimura I, Pancho LR, Koizumi T, et al. *J Pharmacobiodyn*. 1989;12(4):220–227.

110. Hikino H, Kiso Y, Kato N, et al. *J Ethnopharmacol*. 1985;14(1):31–39.

111. Govindarajan VS. *Crit Rev Food Sci Nutr*. 1982;17(3):189–258.

112. Aeschbach R, Loliger J, Scott BC, et al. *Food Chem Toxicol*. 1994;32(1):31–36.

113. Krishnakantha TP, Lokesh BR. *Indian J Biochem Biophys*. 1993;30:133.

114. Reddy AC, Lokesh BR. *Mol Cell Biochem*. 1992;111:117.

115. Cao ZF, Chen ZG, Guo P, et al. *Chung-Kuo Chung Yao Tsa Chih*. 1993;18(12):750–751, 764. [Article in Chinese].

116. Zhou Y, Xu R. *Chung-Kuo Chung Yao Tsa Chih*. 1992;17:368–373.

117. Naora K, et al. *Chem Pharm Bull*. 1992;40:1295.

118. Nakazawa T, Ohsawa K. *Life Sci*. 2002;70(18):2165–2175.

119. Monge P, Scheline R, Solheim E, *Xenobiotica*. 1976;6(7):411–423.

120. Asami A, Shimada T, Mizuhara Y, et al. *J Nat Med*. 2010;64(3):281–287.

121. Zick SM, Djuric Z, Ruffin MT, et al. *Cancer Epidemiol Biomarkers Prev*. 2008;17(8):1930–1936.

122. Chaiyakunapruk N, Kitikannakorn N, Nathisuwan S, et al. *Am J Obstet Gynecol*. 2006;194(1):95–99.

123. Betz O, Kranke P, Geldner G, et al. *Forsch Komplementarmed Klass Naturheilkd*. 2005;12(1):14–23.

124. Borrelli F, Capasso R, Aviello G, et al. *Obstet Gynecol*. 2005;105(4):849–856.

125. Boone SA, Shields KM. *Ann Pharmacother*. 2005;39(10):1710–1713.

126. Matthews A, Dowswell T, Haas DM, et al. *Cochrane Database Syst Rev*. 2010;8(9): CD007575.

127. Hu ML, Wu KL, Chuah SK, et al. *J Gastroenterol Hepatol*. 2009;24(suppl 1):A31.

128. Hu ML, Rayner CK, Wu KL, et al. *World J Gastroenterol*. 2011;17(1):105–110.

129. Shariatpanahi ZV, Taleban FA, Mokhtari M, et al. *J Crit Care*. 2010;25(4):647–650.

130. Rouhi H, Ganji F, Nasri H. *Pakistan J Nutr*. 2006;5(4):373–376.

131. Bliddal H, Rosetzsky A, Schlichting P, et al. *Osteoarthritis Cartilage*. 2000;8(1):9–12.

132. Altman RD, Marcussen KC. *Arthritis Rheum*. 2001;44(11):2531–2538.

133. Wigler I, Grotto I, Caspi D, et al. *Osteoarthritis Cartilage*. 2003;11(11):783–789.

134. Young HY, Liao JC, Chang YS, et al. *Am J Chin Med*. 2006;34(4):545–551.

135. Bordia A, Verma SK, Srivastava KC. *Prostaglandins Leukot Essent Fatty Acids*. 1997;56(5):379–384.

136. Alizadeh-Navaei R, Roozbeh F, Saravi M. *Saudi Med J*. 2008;29(9):1280–1284.

137. Mustafa T, Srivastava KC. *J Ethnopharmacol*. 1990;29:267.

138. Backon J. *Med Hypotheses*. 1991;36:223.

139. Ozgoli G, Goli M, Moattar F. *J Altern Complement Med*. 2009;15(2):129–132.

140. Black CD, O'Connor PJ. *Int J Sport Nutr Exerc Metab*. 2008;18(6):653–664.

141. Black CD, O'Connor PJ. *Phytother Res*. 2010;24(11):1620–1626.

142. Black CD, Herring MP, Hurley DJ, et al. *J Pain*. 2010;11(9):894–903.

143. Opdyke DLJ. *Food Cosmet Toxicol*. 1974;12:901–902.

144. Qureshi A, Shah AH, Tariq M, et al. *Am J Chin Med*. 1989;17(1–2):57–63.

145. Nakamura H, Yamamoto T. *Mutat Res*. 1983;122(2):87–94.

146. Nagabhushan M, Amonkar AJ, Bhide SV. *Cancer Lett*. 1987;36(2):221–233.

147. Nakamura H, Yamamoto T. *Mutat Res*. 1982;103(2):119–126.

148. Soudamini KK, Unnikrishnan MC, Sukumaran K, et al. *Indian J Physiol Pharmacol*. 1995;39(4):347–353.

149. Surh YJ, Lee E, Lee JM. *Mutat Res*. 1998;402(1–2):259–267.

150. Srivastava KC, Mustafa T. *Med Hypotheses*. 1992;39(4):342–348.

151. Soudamini KK, Unnikrishnan MC, Sukumaran K, et al. *Indian J Physiol Pharmacol*. 1995;39(4):347–353.

152. Tarjan V, Csukas I. *Mutat Res*. 1989;216:297.

153. Sivaswamy SN, Balachandran B, Balanehru S, et al. *Indian J Exp Biol*. 1991;29(8):730–737.

154. German Federal Minister of Justice. *German Commission E for Human Medicine Monographs*. Bundes-Anzeiger (German Federal Gazette) no. 85, dated 05.05.1988, no. 50, dated 13.03.1990, no.164, dated 01.09.1990.

155. USP Drug Information. *US Pharmacopeia Patient Leaflet Ginger (Oral)*. Rockville: The United States Pharmacopeial Convention, Inc. 1998.

156. Abebe W. *J Clin Pharm Ther*. 2002;27(6):391–401.

157. Heck AM, DeWitt BA, Lukes AL. *Am J Health Syst Pharm*. 2000;57(13):1221–1227.

158. Pribitkin ED, Boger G. *Arch Facial Plast Surg*. 2001;3(2):127–132.

159. Krüth P, Brosi E, Fux R, et al. *Ann Pharmacother*. 2004;38(2):257–260.

160. Jiang X, Blair EY, McLachlan AJ. *J Clin Pharmacol*. 2006;46(11):1370–1378.

161. Jiang X, Williams KM, Liauw WS, et al. *Br J Clin Pharmacol*. 2005;59(4):425–432.

162. Shalansky S, Lynd L, Richardson K, et al. *Pharmacotherapy*. 2007;27(9):1237–1247.

163. Backon J. *Med Hypotheses*. 1991;34(3):230–231.

164. Hollyer T, Boon H, Georgousis A, et al. *Complement Altern Med*. 2002;2(1):5.

165. Tiran D. *Complement Ther Nurs Midwifery*. 2002;8(4):191–196.

166. Tsui B, Dennehy CE, Tsourounis C. *Am J Obstet Gynecol*. 2001;185(2):433–437.

167. Betz O, Kranke P, Geldner G, et al. *Forsch Komplementarmed Klass Naturheilkd*. 2005;12(1):14–23.

168. Portnoi G, Chng LA, Karimi-Tabesh L, et al. *Am J Obstet Gynecol*. 2003;189(5):1374–1377.

169. Wilkinson JM. *Reprod Toxicol.* 2000;14(6):507–512.

170. Weidner MS, Sigwart K. *Reprod Toxicol.* 2001;15(1):75–80.

171. Zuskin E, Kanceljak B, Skuric Z, et al. *Environ Res.* 1988;47(1):95–108.

172. Futrell JM, Rietschel RL. *Cutis.* 1993;52(5):288–290.

173. Kanerva L, Estlander T, Jolanki R. *Contact Dermatitis.* 1996;35(3):157–162.

174. Moneret-Vautrin DA, Morisset M, Lemerdy P, et al. *Allerg Immunol (Paris).* 2002;34(4):135–140.

175. Stager J, Wuthrich B, Johansson SG. *Allergy.* 1991;46(6):475–478.

176. Fugh-Berman A. *Nutr Today.* 2002;37(3):122–124.

177. Grontved A, Brask T, Kambskard J, et al. *Acta Otolaryngol.* 1988;105(1–2):45–49.

178. Fischer-Rasmussen W, Kjaer SK, Dahl C, et al. *Eur J Obstet Gynecol Reprod Biol.* 1990;38(1):19–24.

179. Bone ME, Wilkinson DJ, Young JR, et al. *Anaesthesia.* 1990;45(8):669–671.

180. Phillips S, Ruggier R, Hutchinson SE. *Anaesthesia.* 1993;48(8):715–717.

181. Schmid R, Schick T, Steffen R, et al. *J Travel Med.* 1994;1(4):203–206.

182. Arfeen Z, Owen H, Plummer JL. *Anaesth Intensive Care.* 1995;23(4):449–452.

183. Meyer K, Schwartz J, Crater D, et al. *Dermatol Nurs.* 1995;7(4):242–244.

184. Careddu P. Unpublished Pharmaton report 1986, cited in Scientific Committee of ESCOP: ESCOP Monographs: Zingiberis rhizoma. Exeter: European Scientific Cooperative on Phytotherapy; March 1996.

185. Visalyaputra S, Petchpaisit N, Somcharoen K, et al. *Anaesthesia.* 1998;53(5):506–510.

186. Vutyavanich T, Kraisarin T, Ruangsri R. *Obstet Gynecol.* 2001;97(4):577–582.

187. Keating A, Chez RA. *Altern Ther Health Med.* 2002;8(5):89–91.

188. Eberhart LH, Mayer R, Betz O, et al. *Anesth Analg.* 2003;96(4):995–998.

189. Pongrojpaw D, Chiamchanya C. *J Med Assoc Thai.* 2003;86(3):244–250.

190. Sripramote M, Lekhyananda N. *J Med Assoc Thai.* 2003;86(9):846–853.

191. Willetts KE, Ekangaki A, Eden JA. *Aust N Z J Obstet Gynaecol.* 2003;43(2):139–144.

192. Sontakke S, Thawani V, Naik MS. *Indian J Pharmacol.* 2003;35:32–36.

193. Manusirivithaya S, Sripramote M, Tangjitgamol S, et al. *Int J Gynecol Cancer.* 2004;14(6):1063–1069.

194. Smith C, Crowther C, Willson K, et al. *Obstet Gynecol.* 2004;103(4):639–645.

195. Nanthakomon T, Pongrojpaw D. *J Med Assoc Thai.* 2006;89(suppl 4):130–136.

196. Tavlan A, Tuncer S, Erol A, et al. *Clin Drug Invest.* 2006;26(4):209–214.

197. Apariman S, Ratchanon S, Wiriyasirivej B. *J Med Assoc Thai.* 2006;89(12):2003–2009.

198. Chittumma P, Kaewkiattikun K, Wiriyasiriwach B. *J Med Assoc Thai.* 2007;990(1):15–20.

199. Pongrojpaw D, Somprasit C, Chanthasenanont A. *J Med Assoc Thai.* 2007;90(9):1703–1709.

200. Levine ME, Gillis MG, Koch SY, et al. *J Altern Complement Med.* 2008;14(5):545–551.

201. Zick SM, Ruffin MT, Lee J, et al. *Support Care Cancer.* 2009;17(5):563–572.

202. Ensiyeh J, Sakineh MA. *Midwifery.* 2009;25(6):649–653.

203. Ozgoli G, Goli M, Simbar M. *J Altern Complement Med.* 2009;15(3):243–246.

204. Pillai AK, Sharma KK, Gupta YK, et al. *Pediatr Blood Cancer.* 2011;56(2):234–238.

205. Ryan JL, Heckler CE, Roscoe JA, et al. *Support Care Cancer.* 2011 [Epub ahead of print].

Ginkgo

(*Ginkgo biloba* L.)

Synonyms

Maidenhair tree (Engl), Ginkgoblätter (Ger), arbre aux quarante écus (forty coin tree) (Fr), Ginkgo (Ital), tempeltrae (Dan).

What is it?

Ginkgo biloba is a deciduous tree that has survived unchanged for about 150 million years from when dinosaurs walked the earth. Described by Charles Darwin as a living fossil, it may have been saved from extinction by the Chinese who revered the tree and planted it around their temples. While Ginkgo nuts are used in traditional Chinese medicine (TCM, see below), the modern use of the green leaf (not the yellow autumn leaf) is entirely due to scientific discovery. In the 1960s a group of German scientists were investigating the effects of exotic herbs on circulation in vivo and found that the leaves of Ginkgo were particularly active. A special, highly concentrated extract standardised for flavonoid content was developed and patented soon after. In the years that followed, standardised extracts of Ginkgo leaf became widely used in Europe and elsewhere.

When the standardised extract of Ginkgo leaf was first developed by German scientists, the original therapeutic focus was improving peripheral circulation to the legs and brain. Later the neuroprotective effects were recognised and Ginkgo became an important herbal treatment for Alzheimer's disease. In addition, a wide variety of other clinical effects have been discovered, making Ginkgo one of the most clinically versatile plants in the modern herbal materia medica, with all such uses underpinned by human evidence.

Effects

Increases blood flow, tissue oxygenation and tissue nutrition; platelet-activating factor (PAF) antagonism; prevention of cellular damage caused by free radicals; protects mitochondrial function during cellular stress; enhances memory and cognitive function, especially in the elderly; protects nervous tissue against damage; helps adaptation to stressors; modulates cardiovascular risk; allays anxiety.

Traditional view

Only Ginkgo nuts were widely used in TCM as an antiasthmatic and against polyuria.[1] The main information on the therapeutic use of Ginkgo leaf comes from clinical trials on the standardised extract conducted over the past 5 decades, backed up by data from experimental models. However, the Chinese have now incorporated the use of Ginkgo leaf into their materia medica.

Summary actions

Anti-PAF activity, antioxidant, tissue perfusion enhancer, circulatory stimulant, nootropic, neuroprotective, anxiolytic, adaptogen.

Can be used for

Indications supported by clinical trials

Disorders and symptoms due to restricted cerebral blood flow (memory and/or cognitive impairment, dizziness, tinnitus, headaches, anxiety/depression, fatigue, stroke); vertigo, acute cochlear deafness, tinnitus of vascular origin (mixed results); peripheral arterial disease (particularly intermittent claudication, mixed results); favourable modification of cardiovascular risk; early stages of primary degenerative dementia (Alzheimer-type); multi-infarct dementia; disorders due to reduced retinal blood flow and normal tension glaucoma, age-related macular degeneration (preliminary data); congestive dysmenorrhoea and premenstrual syndrome; effects of high altitude or hypoxia; anxiety, adjunct therapy in chronic schizophrenia; to improve cognitive function (mixed results); diabetic retinopathy and neuropathy; symptoms associated with multiple sclerosis; allergic conjunctivitis (topically), asthma; protection from radiation damage; idiopathic oedema; vitiligo; improving adaptation to stress.

Traditional therapeutic uses

Ginkgo leaf does not have well-documented traditional use.

May also be used for

Extrapolations from pharmacological studies

Disorders due to restricted peripheral blood flow (including diabetic vascular disease, atherosclerosis); anti-PAF activity (useful in the treatment of asthma, allergic reactions, immunological reactions, shock, ischaemia, thrombosis); antioxidant activity, protection against ischaemia and reperfusion injury. New uses may follow from the anti-PAF activity, such as prevention of migraine headaches.

Preparations

Standardised extract for internal and topical application.

Dosage

The dose of liquid extracts is uncertain if they have not been standardised for major active constituents. Because of potential adverse reaction to the ginkgolic acids, the use of normal galenical extracts (tinctures or fluid extracts) is not recommended.

The daily dose is typically 120 to 240 mg of a 50:1 Ginkgo standardised extract (containing 24% ginkgo flavone glycosides and about 6% terpenoids). This corresponds to 4 to 16 g of leaf, depending on the quality of original leaf. Ginkgolic acids are usually specified to be less than 5 parts per million. The extract can be incorporated into liquids or tablets, usually at 40 mg/mL or 40 to 60 mg/tablet, making the daily dose 3 to 6 mL or two to six tablets, depending on their strength.

Duration of use

There is no restriction on the long-term use of Ginkgo. Moreover, for most applications it should be given to patients for at least 6 weeks before any clinical benefit is assessed.

Summary assessment of safety

There is very low risk associated with the administration of Ginkgo. The risk of a bleeding event or interaction with blood thinning drugs is overstated in most articles and texts and not supported by controlled clinical trials.

Technical data

Botany

Ginkgo biloba is a member of the Ginkgoaceae family, a gymnosperm that has survived unchanged from the Triassic period. It can grow to a height of over 100 m, living for 1000 years. Ginkgo is dioecious (possessing male and female flowers on separate trees) and its leaves have open dichotomous venation and a characteristic fan-like appearance with two lobes (hence the species name, *biloba*). The leaf shape has been likened to the cerebral hemispheres The naked seed (or nut) is oily and edible, but the seed coat and embryo are bitter.[2,3]

Adulteration

Considerable variability has been found in total terpene content and in individual terpene levels in commercial Ginkgo leaf extracts.[4] A 2002 study by the Hong Kong Consumer Council found that 13 of 14 commercial products contained levels of ginkgolic acids exceeding WHO (World Health Organization) recommendations by 16 to 733 times.[5] (Ginkgolic acid is potentially allergenic.) See also under Key constituents below.

Key constituents

- 0.5% to 1% mono-, di- and triglycosides of the flavonols quercetin, kaempferol and isorhamnetin, quercetin-3-beta-D-glucoside, quercitrin and rutin,[6,7] including coumaric acid esters of these flavonoids

- Terpene lactones (terpenoids), including bilobalide and ginkgolides A, B, C and J.[8]

- Biflavonoids, ginkgolic acids, sterols, procyanidins, polysaccharides.[7,9]

The majority of the pharmacological studies and clinical trials have been conducted using a chemically complex, concentrated extract containing at least 26 identified components and standardised to 24% flavonol glycosides (ginkgo flavone glycosides) and 6% terpenoids (ginkgolides and bilobalide). The standardised extract allows the concentration of potentially active constituents and the elimination of undesirable substances. For this reason, many of the known constituents of Ginkgo leaves are present only in minute amounts or absent from these extracts, including the ginkgolic acids, biflavonoids and sterols. The German Commission E and WHO stipulate that extracts should contain less than 5 ppm ginkgolic acids.[10,11]

The standardised extract also contains approximately 7% proanthocyanidins, 13% carboxylic acids, 2% catechins, 20% non-flavonol glycosides and 4% high molecular weight compounds.[12] Around 5% of its content is inorganic in nature and about 13% contains other phytochemical constituents.

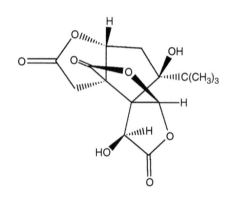

Flavonol diglycosides

	R
kaempferol-3-O-rutinoside	H
quercetin-3-O-rutinoside	OH
isorhamnetin-3-O-rutinoside	OCH₃

Ginkgolides

	R¹	R²
Ginkgolide A	H	H
Ginkgolide B	OH	H
Ginkgolide C	OH	OH
Ginkgolide J	H	OH

Coumaric esters of flavonoids

	R
kaempferol-3-O-α-(6'''-*trans*-p-coumaroylglucosyl)-β-1,2-rhamnoside	H
quercetin-3-O-α-(6'''-*trans*-p-coumaroylglucosyl)-β-1,2-rhamnoside	OH

Bilobalide

A 2003 quality control assessment of commercial standardised Ginkgo extracts using analysis of intact flavonol glycosides found one product had been adulterated with rutin in order to elevate the total flavonol levels.[13]

A total of 16 Ginkgo products were assessed in a 2005 Belgian study, including four that were registered medicines, the others being food supplements.[14] All the examined medicines complied with the pharmacopoeial standards and eight of the 12 food supplements contained the claimed level of flavonoids. The remaining four did not, and two of these contained unexpectedly low amounts. Seven food supplement products had an unexpectedly high proportion of rutin present, indicating that adulteration with this flavonoid had likely occurred.

Following this knowledge of the potential adulteration of Ginkgo extracts with rutin (and possibly other flavonoids), a test method was developed for its reliable detection. The application of this method in the quality control of standardised Ginkgo extracts is now a requirement of the *United States Pharmacopoeia–National Formulary* (USP32-NF27) and for product registration (listing) with the Australian Therapeutic Goods Administration.

Pharmacodynamics

The considerable number of pharmacological studies on *Ginkgo biloba* extract have not been comprehensively reviewed in this monograph. Rather, the results from important, unique or representative studies and reviews have been included.

PAF antagonism

Platelet-activating factor (PAF) is an ether-linked phospholipid formed by platelets, basophils, neutrophils, monocytes and macrophages. It is a potent platelet-aggregating agent (more so in animals than humans), inflammatory factor and inducer of systemic anaphylactic symptoms. The ginkgolides (particularly ginkgolide B) are potent and specific PAF receptor antagonists.[15,16] Their effects are long-lived and are rapidly established after oral doses.[17] No side effects have been recorded, even when given in high doses (120 mg of a ginkgolide mixture) to healthy human volunteers.[15]

High doses of ginkgolides control mast cell degranulation,[18] and have been used to treat systemic mastocytosis (high blood levels of mast cells).[19] Ginkgolides partially countered PAF-induced and antigen-induced bronchoconstriction[20,21] and inhibited the induction of airway hyperreactivity by PAF in vivo.[22] Ginkgolides inhibit the response of eosinophils to PAF[23] and decrease the IgE-mediated cytotoxicity of eosinophils.[16] Ginkgolides and the standardised extract of Ginkgo have demonstrated a potent thrombolytic effect on the PAF-induced thrombus.[24,25] Standardised Ginkgo extract has improved peak flow rates in asthmatic children and caused significant clinical improvement in adults.[25] More recent research has focused on analogues (chemical derivatives) of the ginkgolides as potential new drugs with PAF-inhibiting activity.[26]

Effects on ischaemia and blood flow

Ginkgolides prevent the metabolic damage caused by experimental cerebral ischaemia and have a normalising effect when given 1 h after the event. They can reduce the infarct size in experimental myocardial occlusion. Arrhythmias induced by experimental myocardial ischaemia are significantly countered by the prior administration of ginkgolides.[27] Bilobalide has demonstrated a potent neuroprotective effect against ischaemic damage, which was stronger than ginkgolide B.[28]

There is experimental evidence to support the view that Ginkgo extracts have neuroprotective properties under conditions such as hypoxia/ischaemia, seizure activity and peripheral nerve damage (see also below).[29] Standardised Ginkgo extract, as well as its non-flavonol fraction (probably the ginkgolides), but not the flavonol glycosides, conferred protection in mice against brain damage caused by hypoxia and retarded the breakdown of brain energy metabolism.[30] Oral administration of Ginkgo extract produced slight to moderate changes in glucose utilisation in the brain structures of rats. Glucose utilisation was significantly decreased in the frontoparietal somatosensory cortex, nucleus accumbens, cerebellar cortex and pons when a 50 mg/kg dose of

extract was administered. This may help explain the clinical efficacy of Ginkgo extract in treating problems associated with deficient somatosensory processing (such as impairment of vigilance) and vestibular mechanisms (such as vertiginous syndromes).[31] One study investigated the effect of Ginkgo extract (up to 15 mg/kg) on the dynamic equilibrium of free radicals and amino acids in rats with cerebral ischemia/reperfusion injury. Ginkgo reduced levels of gamma-aminobutyric acid (GABA), glycine, glutamine, aspartate and malondialdehyde (a measure of oxidation) and increased antioxidant enzymes. These results indicate that Ginkgo can protect damaged neurons via balancing inhibitory/excitatory amino acids and enhancing the removal of free radicals.[32]

Ginkgo has favourably influenced a number of the metabolic events that accompany cerebral ischaemia, including a preventative effect on ischaemic damage by inhibiting vasospasm and thrombus formation and improving cerebral blood flow to underperfused areas without robbing adjacent areas. It has increased cerebral perfusion after oral administration[33] and improved hypoxia tolerance[34] in humans. Also, Ginkgo has inhibited thrombus formation,[35] promoted prostacyclin synthesis,[36] reduced cerebral oedema,[37–39] normalised brain ATP and glucose following ischaemia,[38,40] improved neuronal function following infarction[37] and inhibited arteriolar spasm[41] in animals. A recent review concluded that the main mechanisms behind the protective effects of Ginkgo extract in brain ischaemia/reperfusion injury were antioxidation, enhanced free radical clearance, inhibition of excitatory amino acids, reduced inflammation and inhibition of neuronal apoptosis.[42]

However, a recent study suggests that heme oxygenase 1 (HO-1) could represent a key aspect of the neuroprotective role of Ginkgo in transient ischaemia/reperfusion. HO-1 is an inducible enzyme (by the Nrf2/ARE pathway) that plays a vital role in cellular homeostasis in response to oxidative stress. Mice pretreated with Gingko extract (25 to 100 mg/kg, oral) had 50.9% less neurological dysfunction and 48.2% smaller infarct volumes, but this benefit was abolished in HO-1 knockout mice (lacking the enzyme).[43] Acute post-treatment with Ginkgo also reduced infarct size. The same group had previously shown that Ginkgo extract induced HO-1 levels in neuronal cell cultures.[44]

Standardised Ginkgo extract and bilobalide inhibited the hypoxia-induced decrease in ATP content in endothelial cells in vitro. After oral administration in an in vivo model of hypoxia, both compounds increased the respiratory control ratio of mitochondria isolated from rat hepatocytes. The authors concluded that these agents helped to retain the ability to form ATP, thereby reducing the cell's need to induce glycolysis, probably via preserving ATP regeneration by mitochondria as long as oxygen was available.[45] A protective effect of standardised Ginkgo extract on the hypoxic myocardium was demonstrated by the changes in enzyme activities in rat myocardium after pretreatment with Ginkgo for 3 months.[46]

In a comparative study on stroke victims, intravenous standardised Ginkgo extract was more active at improving cerebral blood flow compared with 28 conventional drugs (see also under Clinical trials).[47]

Gingko biloba extract (240 mg/day) was evaluated in a 3-week randomised, double blind, placebo-controlled study of skin blood flow in 27 healthy middle-aged volunteers.[48] Skin blood flow was measured on the forefoot using laser Doppler flowmetry. Ginkgo exerted a modulating effect on haemodynamics, enhancing the skin blood flow of participants with impaired circulation, normalising excess skin blood flow in cases of hypercirculation, while not affecting normal flow. A randomised controlled study on the effect of Ginkgo extract on forearm haemodynamics in 16 healthy volunteers was conducted over 6 weeks.[49] Forearm blood flow and venous capacity were measured by strain-gauge plethysmography. Forearm blood flow was significantly higher during active treatment after 3 and 6 weeks, as compared with placebo treatment ($p<0.05$), while mean arterial blood pressure was unchanged. In an earlier randomised placebo-controlled crossover study in 10 healthy volunteers, Ginkgo markedly decreased erythrocyte aggregation and increased blood flow in nail-fold capillaries.[50]

Other neuroprotective effects

A 2007 review noted that ginkgolide B has demonstrated neuroprotective activity in several in vitro models including nitric-oxide-induced neurotoxicity and against beta-amyloid.[51] An earlier review observed that bilobalide in vivo can reduce cerebral oedema produced by triethyltin and decrease cortical infarct volume in stroke models.[52] Possible protective mechanisms included preservation of mitochondrial function, inhibition of apoptotic damage and suppression of hypoxia-induced cell membrane deterioration in the brain. Neurochemical modulation may also be responsible for neuroprotection, with an ex vivo study demonstrating that bilobalide antagonised the GABA-A receptor binding of TBPS (t-butylbicyclophosphorothionate), a molecule with a high affinity for GABA-A, to rat cortical membranes. TBPS binding was competitively inhibited by bilobalide in the low micromolar range (IC_{50} 3.7 μM).[53]

Research in one laboratory has focused on understanding the mechanism of action of Ginkgo in protecting against Alzheimer's disease (AD) and this was reviewed in 2006.[54] Ginkgo extract protects against beta-amyloid aggregation in vitro, attenuates beta-amyloid-induced reactive oxygen species in the roundworm and reduces its neuronal toxicity. Several other in vitro studies have observed that Ginkgo extract protects against beta-amyloid neurotoxicity.[55–57]

Ginkgo has also demonstrated protective activity in murine models of AD.[58,59] One study used a transgenic mouse model and found that Ginkgo extract (300 mg/kg diet) given for 16 months significantly lowered amyloid precursor protein levels in the cerebral cortex.[58]

Ginkgo biloba may possess a preventative role in Parkinson's disease. A standardised extract of Ginkgo was tested on a Parkinson's disease animal model (6-hydroxydopamine (6-OHDA)-induced neurotoxicity in the nigrostriatal dopaminergic system of the rat brain). At 8 weeks after the induced lesion, the number of contralateral forepaw adjusting steps was significantly higher in rats treated with the high dose of Ginkgo (100 mg/kg/day, ip) than in those treated with a low dose (50 mg/kg, ip) or with the control, denoting a neuroprotective and anti-Parkinson effect.[60]

Antioxidant activity

As noted above, much of the neuroprotective activity of Ginkgo extract is probably predicated on its antioxidant activity. Flavonoids from Ginkgo extract scavenged free radicals and antagonised lipid peroxidation and cell necrosis of rat hepatocytes more potently than the terpene lactones (ginkgolides, bilobalide) in vitro.[61] Ginkgo extract scavenged various reactive oxygen species, such as hydroxyl and superoxide radicals, and also peroxyl radicals, which are involved in the propagation step of lipid peroxidation.[62] Standardised Ginkgo extract inhibited or reduced functional and morphological retinal impairments observed after lipoperoxide release.[63] The extract has demonstrated powerful antioxidant effects on copper-mediated human low-density lipoprotein oxidation in vitro.[64]

Such passive in vitro antioxidant effects probably do not underlie the in vivo antioxidant activity of Ginkgo, which is more likely based on its activation of specific protector pathways, such as Nrf2/ARE. For example, an increase in catalase and superoxide dismutase (SOD) activities in the hippocampus, striatum and substantia nigra and a decrease of lipid peroxidation in the hippocampus was displayed in rats treated with Ginkgo.[65] Ginkgo extract (100 mg/kg, oral) prevented mobile phone-induced oxidative stress in the brains of rats exposed to 900 MHz radiation for 7 days (1 h/day).[66] Cellular brain injury was also reduced.

Volunteers given standardised Ginkgo extract (200 mg/day) for 1 week also exhibited red blood cells that were more resistant to oxidative damage.[67] Ginkgo extract decreased the clastogenic activity (a marker of oxidative stress) of blood taken from salvage personnel working on the Chernobyl reactor accident.[68] In a further study, 30 recovery workers were treated with standardised Ginkgo extract (120 mg/day) for 2 months. The clastogenic activity of their plasma was reduced to control levels at the end of the treatment period and persisted for at least 7 months thereafter.[69] This study also implies a radioprotective activity (see also under Clinical trials).

Mitochondrial effects

It has been suggested that effects on mitochondria exerted by Ginkgo extract could underpin several of its observed pharmacological activities, including AD prevention, neuroprotection, cardioprotection, attenuation of ischaemia/reperfusion injury and antioxidant activity.[70,71]

Cardioprotective activity observed in vitro using cardiomyocytes and isolated heat have been attributed to favourable effects on mitochondrial function.[72–75] This cardioprotective aspect of Ginkgo extract has also been confirmed in vivo for the hearts of older rats.[76]

Treatment of two different age groups of mice with Ginkgo extract (100 mg/kg/day for 14 days, oral) showed beneficial effects on complexes I, IV and V of the mitochondrial respiratory chain in brain cells against nitric oxide stress.[77] Interestingly, these effects were only observed in the aged mice. In another study, favourable effects on mitochondrial dysfunction in the hippocampi of a senescence-accelerated strain of mice were observed after Ginkgo extract

(100 mg/kg, oral), but again only in old mice.[78] The authors attributed this enhanced effect to an age-associated increase in the permeability of the blood-brain barrier.

Neurotransmitter and other CNS effects

A review of the chemistry and biology of the terpene trilactones from Ginkgo observed that ginkgolide B is a potent and selective antagonist of the glycine receptor chloride channel in vitro.[26] Glycine receptors are found primarily in the spinal cord and brain stem, but also in higher brain regions such as the hippocampus. The implications of this novel finding for ginkgolide B are not clear. Other ginkgolides also possess this activity, as well as being antagonists of the ion channels for GABA.[79] Studies have also shown that the ginkgolides and bilobalide particularly modulate the peripheral benzodiazepine receptor (now called translocator protein).[26] This may increase the risk of seizures. Several in vitro studies indicate that bilobalide also affects the major neurotransmitters in the brain, namely glutamate and GABA.[26]

Another review noted that Ginkgo extract has exhibited mixed results on noradrenaline (norepinephrine) levels and receptor density in rats, inhibited the degeneration of dopaminergic neurons in the striatum of mice (an antiparkinsonism effect) and ameliorated the natural decline in acetylcholine receptors with age in rats.[80] Favourable activity on serotonergic mechanisms in the brains of rats was also observed, especially with respect to 5-HT$_{1A}$ receptor density and function.[80]

A single oral dose of Ginkgo extract (100 mg/kg) had no effect on monoamine levels in the prefrontal cortex and striatum of conscious rats.[81] However, following chronic treatment for 14 days, the same daily dose significantly increased extracellular dopamine and noradrenaline (norepinephrine) levels, while serotonin levels were unaffected. Chronic treatment with Ginkgo showed dose-dependent increases in frontocortical dopamine levels and, to a lesser extent, in the striatum. Treatment with the main constituents of the herb revealed that the increase in dopamine levels was mostly caused by the flavonol glycosides and ginkgolide fractions, whereas bilobalide treatment was without effect. These observations may have implications for the effect of Ginkgo on cognitive function.

Ginkgo has demonstrated anxiolytic activity in several animal models, especially under conditions of stress (see also Antistress activity below). In an early study, intragastric administration of a preparation containing standardised extracts of Ginkgo and ginger demonstrated anxiolytic effects comparable to diazepam (by injection) in vivo. However, the herbal preparation demonstrated an anxiety-promoting effect at a higher dosage (100 mg/kg).[82] A similar effect to diazepam was observed in a social interaction model in mildly stressed rats for Ginkgo extract (48 or 96 mg/kg/day for 8 days, oral) and there was an additive effect from its combination with the drug.[83]

The anxiolytic-like effects of Ginkgo extract and its four key terpenoid components were assessed using the elevated plus-maze test in mice.[84] Administration of Ginkgo extract as an acute oral dose (0.5 or 1 g/kg) caused a state of suppressed motor activity and shortened the time spent in the open-sided arms. However, when Ginkgo extract (0.063 to 1 g/kg, oral) was administered daily for 7 days and the plus-maze test carried out, the time spent in the open-sided arms was prolonged, with the peak anxiolytic-like effect at the 0.125 g/kg dose. A combination of 7-day administration of Ginkgo extract (0.125 g/kg) and a single dose of diazepam (1 mg/kg, oral, 10 min before testing) enhanced the anxiolytic-like effect. Flumazenil blocked the effect of diazepam, but not of Ginkgo. Daily administration of ginkgolide A (1 or 2 mg/kg, oral) resulted in an anxiolytic-like effect, but neither ginkgolide B, C, nor bilobalide produced any such activity. These results suggest that Ginkgo produces a significant anxiolytic-like effect following repeated administration, and that ginkgolide A is most likely responsible for this effect. Ginkgo exerts a sedative effect at comparatively higher doses.

There is also a suggestion from animal models that Ginkgo might possess antidepressant activity. This does not appear to be due to monoamine oxidase inhibition, despite some in vitro activity in that regard.[85,86] Ginkgo demonstrated clear antidepressant effects in two behavioural models in rats at oral doses ranging between 10 and 100 mg/kg.[87]

Antistress effects

Several animal studies have observed an antistress activity for Ginkgo extract. In fact, one group of researchers suggested that the improved cognitive functioning following sustained treatment with Ginkgo extract (see below) may be secondary to neuroprotective properties that buffer the animal from the harmful effects of stress.[88]

A review of the research up to 2000 indicated that Ginkgo possesses an antistress action that differs from conventional drugs (antidepressants, anxiolytics).[89] This action of Ginkgo appears to be linked to a modulation of adrenal activity, as it reduced circulating concentrations of adrenaline (epinephrine), noradrenaline (norepinephrine) and corticosterone in stressed old and young rats after chronic administration at oral extract doses ranging from 50 to 100 mg/kg/day. Such effects were demonstrated in various experimental models of stress, including studies that observed a suppression of the downregulation of hippocampal glucocorticoid receptors induced by prednisolone or amphetamine, with a normalisation of learning and behavioural parameters. These studies demonstrate that Ginkgo in fact meets the definition of an adaptogen. These effects were due in part to the ginkgolides, and it appears that peripheral glucocorticoid biosynthesis serves as their molecular target.[89]

Studies published since 2000 have confirmed these findings and added new insights. For example, catecholamines (norepinephrine, dopamine), serotonin and plasma corticosterone levels were studied in rat brains following 1, 2 and 4 h restraint stress.[90] Ginkgo extract (14 mg/kg, oral) restored the restraint stress-induced elevations of catecholamines, serotonin and plasma corticosterone to near normal levels in the brain.

Like most adaptogens, Ginkgo has demonstrated effects on the immune response. Stress-induced suppression of the cellular immune response in rats was countered by Ginkgo extract (100 mg/kg/day for 7 days, oral).[91] Another similar study using the same dose confirmed this result and also found that Ginkgo improved innate immune responses in stressed rats.[92]

A comparison of Ginkgo (30 mg/kg, oral) and *Panax ginseng* (100 mg/kg, oral) extracts in stressed rats found that Ginkgo was more effective in reversing the biochemical changes induced by acute stress, whereas ginseng was superior in chronic stress.[93]

Exposure to chronic stress in humans alters cognitive function, possibly as a result of elevated glucocorticoids. One group has found that Ginkgo extract (100 mg/kg, oral) normalised stress- and corticosterone-induced impairment of recall and spatial memory in rats.[94–96]

The adaptogenic activity of Ginkgo has been demonstrated in healthy volunteers. One study evaluated the effects of Ginkgo on salivary cortisol and blood pressure responses during stress in 70 healthy young volunteers in a double blind, placebo-controlled design.[97] A stress model involving a combination of static exercise (handgrip) and mental stimuli was used. Single treatment with Ginkgo extract (120 mg) reduced the stress-induced rise in blood pressure without affecting heart rate. Salivary cortisol responses showed differences with respect to gender and time of day of the stress exposure, with the activation only in men in the afternoon. This activation was absent if they were first treated with Ginkgo.

Ginkgo extract at 120 mg/day for 3 months significantly dropped plasma cortisol levels during the stress caused by the glucose tolerance test in healthy volunteers.[98] According to the scientists involved in the trial, Ginkgo might also reduce blood levels of cortisol in other types of stress.

Effect on memory and/or learning

Many in vivo models have demonstrated a positive effect of Ginkgo on cognitive function. In a controlled animal study, Ginkgo treatment (100 mg/kg/day, for 4 to 8 weeks prior to training and 10 weeks prior to testing, oral) enhanced performance on the tested task, indicating improved retrieval of the learned response.[99] However, it did not affect performance in a passive avoidance test.[100] Oral administration of Ginkgo extract to young and old rats facilitated behavioural adaptation, despite adverse environmental influences. Stress-induced detrimental changes in both discrimination learning and plasma hormones became significant after the third day of learning. Ginkgo was more effective in decreasing the number of inefficient lever presses and reaction times in the older animals.[101]

A review of other studies up to 2000 indicated that Ginkgo had been found to enhance cognitive performance and learned responses in an eight-arm radial maze, to improve short-term memory in a passive avoidance paradigm and increase brain neuronal membrane fluidity.[89] Results were most marked with chronic administration and in older animals, as noted in a slightly later review.[102]

In later studies Ginkgo (50 to 200 mg/kg, oral) acutely reversed yohimbine-induced spatial working memory deficit in rats[103] and with chronic administration (60 mg/kg/day for 30 days, oral) enhanced spatial learning and memory and hippocampal synaptic plasticity in aged rats.[104] The countering effect on yohimbine was attributed to the action of Ginkgo on alpha-2-adrenoceptors.

A 2003 review provided an overview of much of this research and its relationship to key aspects of the other pharmacological research above. It observed that, while individual effects of cognition and behavioural assessment in all areas have been reported for adult animals and acute dosing, more pronounced effects are usually seen in aged animals and after subchronic treatment.[105] Specifically for the cognition improving properties, pronounced beneficial effects are mainly present in those situations where cognition was impaired by ageing or other noxious stimuli. Since all these conditions are associated with mitochondrial dysfunction, the stabilising or even protective effect of Ginkgo on mitochondrial function seems to be a major mechanism associated with many of its behavioural effects. Bilobalide is most important in this respect. Moreover, bilobalide and the ginkgolides have been shown to affect chloride conductance by interfering with the function of membrane proteins related to receptor-gated chloride channels. These mechanisms are probably associated with behavioural effects requiring acute changes of neuronal activity, but might indirectly also improve mitochondrial function.

Most of the recent investigations on the cognitive activity of Ginkgo extract have been human studies. These are reviewed in the Clinical trials section under the relevant heading.

Other activity

The inflammatory response induced by intracolonic administration of acetic acid in rats was inhibited by 2 days of oral pretreatment with Ginkgo (30, 60, 120 mg/kg), significantly decreasing colonic myeloperoxidase activity, tumour necrosis factor (TNF)-alpha and interleukin (IL)-1beta levels and increasing the glutathione concentration. Ginkgo treatment also attenuated macroscopic colonic damage, as assessed by histopathological examination. An antioxidant action was regarded as being responsible for this antiulcerogenic activity.[106] Another study involving an ethanol-induced gastric lesion rat model demonstrated that intravenous Ginkgo extract (8.75, 17.5 and 26.25 mg/kg) inhibited gastric ulcer formation.[107]

The effects of various fractions of Ginkgo extract on human (obtained from impotent men) and rabbit penis corpus cavernosal tissue were investigated in vitro.[108] One fraction was particularly active at relaxing corpus cavernosal tissues, suggesting a possible benefit in erectile dysfunction.

Oral administration of Ginkgo extract (10 mg/kg/day, for 12 weeks) in conjunction with a high-fat diet reduced disturbances of lipid metabolism and the severity of plaque formation in rabbits. In addition to hypolipidaemic and antioxidant (antiatherosclerotic) activities, Ginkgo also affected metabolic processes in the liver and may modify lipid deposition in major arteries.[109]

Ginkgo extract showed a promoting effect on hair regrowth after cutaneous administration to shaved mice in a 1993 study.[110] There appear to be no further studies on this theme. Ginkgo extract demonstrated an anti-inflammatory activity with potency comparable to that of indomethacin after topical application in the croton oil test in mice.[111]

Unilateral vestibular deafferentation (UVD) causes ocular motor and postural disorders, some of which disappear over time in a process of behavioural recovery known as vestibular compensation. Vestibular compensation may be enhanced either by reducing the initial symptoms of UVD or by accelerating the compensation process. The positive impact of injected Ginkgo extract in UVD in vivo was suggested to be due to acceleration of compensation.[112]

Pharmacokinetics

The first attempt to understand the pharmacokinetics of Ginkgo was undertaken using a radioactively labelled extract (with the carbon-14 isotope).[113] After oral administration to rats, absorption of at least 60% was determined. The half-life of the radioactivity was about 4.5h and after 72h 22% was found in urine and 29% in faeces. Glandular and neuronal tissues and the eyes demonstrated a high affinity for the labelled substances (possibly ginkgolides and bilobalide). A site of absorption in the upper gastrointestinal tract was suspected, since specific activity in blood peaked after 1.5h.

However, no flavonoid glycosides or aglycones were detected in urine, faeces or blood within 24h of intragastric administration of Ginkgo extract to rats in another early study. Seven metabolites of flavonoid degradation were found.[114] These were phenylalkyl acids formed by C-ring fission of the flavonoids by gut microorganisms (see Chapter 2).

Consistent with the above, Ginkgo flavonoids have exhibited a low bioavailability in mice. Oral administration of Ginkgo extract (about 36mg/kg via the diet) resulted in plasma concentrations of quercitin, kaempferol and isorhamnetin (after hydrolysis with glucuronidase/sulphatase) of 12, 7 and 50ng/mL, respectively, compared with levels of 5, 3 and 0ng/mL in control mice.[115] This low bioavailability of the intact flavonoids was confirmed in a later study in a beagle dog, after plasma concentrations following injection were compared against concentrations resulting from an oral dose.[116,117]

A recent German study investigated the ability of Ginkgo flavonoid constituents to cross the blood-brain barrier in rats, after single (600mg/kg) or repeated (8 days, 100 or 600mg/kg) oral administration of Ginkgo extract.[118] A highly sensitive method for the determination of the Ginkgo flavonoid metabolites (quercetin, kaempferol and isorhamnetin derivatives) in the brain and plasma was developed. The single dose of 600mg/kg resulted in maximum plasma concentrations of 176, 341, and 183ng/mL for quercetin, kaempferol, and isorhamnetin/tamarixetin, respectively, and in maximum brain concentrations of 291ng/g protein for kaempferol and 161ng/g protein for isorhamnetin/tamarixetin. In comparison, the repeated administration of the same dose for 8 days led to an approximate 4.5-fold increase in the plasma concentration of quercetin, an 11.5-fold increase for kaempferol and a 10-fold increase for isorhamnetin/tamarixetin. In the brain, an approximate 2-fold increase was observed for kaempferol and isorhamnetin/tamarixetin. About 90% of the determined flavonoids were distributed in the hippocampus, frontal cortex,

striatum and cerebellum, which together represent only 38% of the whole brain.

The bioavailabilities of ginkgolides A and B and bilobalide were determined in rats after a single oral administration of 30, 55 and 100mg/kg of Ginkgo extract.[119] Their pharmacokinetics were found to be dose-linear, with maximum plasma concentrations for the lowest dose of 68, 40 and 159ng/mL and half-lives of 1.7, 2.0 and 2.2h, respectively. A study in rats found that ginkgolide B was metabolised to its hydroxyl metabolite, mainly via CYP2D6.[120] Another rat study observed that ginkgolide B can pass through the blood-brain barrier, especially after ischaemia-reperfusion injury.[121]

Results from human studies of the pharmacokinetics of Ginkgo extract tend to reflect the animal findings. After Ginkgo extract (4g) was given to healthy volunteers observing a flavonoid-free diet, urine samples were collected for 3 days, and blood samples were withdrawn every 30min for 5h.[122] Only urine samples contained detectable amounts of substituted benzoic acids, including a 4-hydroxybenzoic acid conjugate, 4-hydroxyhippuric acid, 3-methoxy-4-hydroxyhippuric acid, 3,4-dihydroxybenzoic acid, 4-hydroxybenzoic acid, hippuric acid and 3-methoxy-4-hydroxybenzoic acid (vanillic acid). In contrast to rats, no phenylacetic acid or phenylpropionic acid derivatives were found in urine, thus indicating that a more extensive metabolism takes place in humans. As for rats, the metabolites found in human urine accounted for less than 30% of the flavonoids given. When the same test procedure was applied to blood samples, no metabolites could be detected. A review of early pharmacokinetic studies of the Ginkgo flavonoids described evidence that intact flavonols could in fact be identified in human urine following oral doses of Ginkgo extract, apparently as glucuronide metabolites.[123] A later study did confirm the presence of quercetin and kaempferol, mainly as glucuronides, in human urine after a single dose of Ginkgo.[124]

The pharmacokinetic properties of the terpenoids in humans have been more extensively studied than the flavonoids, probably because they exhibit better bioavailability and possibly also because they are more likely to explain much of the pharmacological activity of Ginkgo. Data obtained from an early human investigation suggested that ginkgolides A and B and bilobalide are excreted unchanged in the urine (70%, 40% and 30%, respectively of the administered dose) and exhibited relatively high bioavailability after oral ingestion (>80%, >80% and 70%, respectively).[125] Ginkgolide C was not bioavailable.

This high bioavailability was also observed after the oral administration of 120mg of Ginkgo extract to 12 healthy human volunteers. Elimination half-lives (after oral dosing while fasting) of 4.5, 10.6 and 3.2h were measured for the three compounds, respectively.[126] There was no relevant influence of food on the pharmacokinetics of the terpenoids. A 2003 review paper also included data from unpublished work.[123] A study in 12 healthy male volunteers found that maximum plasma concentrations were reached within 1h following a single dose of 80, 120 or 240mg of Ginkgo extract. These concentrations were 15.2, 25.3 and 42.9ng/mL, respectively, for ginkgolide A, 6.5, 9.1 and 18.1ng/mL for ginkgolide B and 30.2, 35.2 and 58.6ng/mL for bilobalide, indicating an approximately dose-linear response. Another unpublished study included in the review investigated pharmacokinetics in 12 elderly volunteers after single (60 mg) and multiple (60 mg twice a day for 8 days) Ginkgo extract administration.[123] There was no change in pharmacokinetics (for example, no accumulation) after multiple-dose administration. The steady-state concentrations of ginkgolide A and B and bilobalide were 9.4, 6.2 and 8.7 ng/mL, respectively, and clearance rates in the elderly were lower than young volunteers, as might be expected.

A 2002 pharmacokinetic study of two different doses of Ginkgo extract involving 12 healthy volunteers discovered that twice daily administration of 40 mg of the extract produced a higher serum half-life ($t\frac{1}{2}$) and mean residence time of bilobalide B than a single 80 mg daily dose. A higher concentration peak (Cmax) was reached however with the 80 mg dosage, while both dosages yielded a maximum concentration 2.3 h (Tmax) after administration.[127]

Several studies have shown that the bioavailability of Ginkgo extracts (both in terms of flavonoids and terpenoids) can vary according to the pharmaceutical preparation. Complexing with soy phospholipids appears to enhance bioavailability based on animal[128,129] and human[130] studies. Higher dissolution rates of Ginkgo solid dose products also improved bioavailability in humans.[131]

Clinical trials

Cerebral insufficiency and stroke

Cerebral (not cerebrovascular) insufficiency is not strictly a medical condition and it is not accepted as being associated with any pathological change. Rather, it is a collection of symptoms associated with mental deterioration from ageing, and affects many elderly people who do not necessarily have dementia or a history of strokes. Typical symptoms of cerebral insufficiency include difficulties in concentration and memory, absentmindedness, confusion, lack of energy, tiredness, decreased physical performance, depressive mood, anxiety, dizziness, tinnitus and headaches. These symptoms can also be associated with the early stages of dementia, of either the Alzheimer (degenerative) or multi-infarct (circulatory) types.

The focus of the early Ginkgo clinical trials on cerebral insufficiency was a barrier to its wider acceptance as a treatment for the elderly. Subsequent trials have demonstrated the benefit of Ginkgo in dementia (see later); hence the review immediately below should be viewed in its historical context. One development in the field of pathology that could be relevant to the concept of cerebral insufficiency is the concept of 'white matter ischaemia'. After computed tomography was introduced in clinical practice, it was realised that rarefaction or low attenuation of the white matter of the brain (the axons) was more common than previously thought. Although this can occur for several reasons (for example after head injury), age and ischaemia to the white matter are regarded as the commonest causes.[132]

The vulnerability of the white matter to ischaemia is due to the fact that it is supplied by long penetrating end arterioles from the surface and base of the brain that travel for a long distance with very few interconnections. Computed tomography of the brain shows that 30% of people aged 85 years have evidence of low attenuation of white matter. Magnetic resonance imaging (MRI) shows an incidence approaching 100% at age 85. Studies demonstrate that normal people with white matter ischaemia could have subtle neuropsychological deficits, such as a slower rate of mental processing and impaired attention and concentration. Hence a tentative link between white matter ischaemia and cerebral insufficiency has been established. Since Ginkgo has anti-ischaemic activity, it may prevent or ameliorate symptoms associated with white matter ischaemia. White matter ischaemia is also closely associated with vascular or so-called multi-infarct dementia. The key difference is that a patient need not show a history of strokes to have a cognitive impairment brought about by such ischaemia. A recent review has concluded that abnormalities in the small vessels caused by ageing and hypertension, together with systemic circulatory disturbances such as heart disease or abrupt variations in blood pressure, may lead to selective white matter injury. The damage is structurally characterised by incomplete infarction or selective cellular injury.[133]

A critical review of 40 clinical trials conducted from 1975 to 1991 on Ginkgo and cerebral insufficiency and other conditions found eight to be well conducted.[134] Trials under this general heading also included the following conditions: primary degenerative dementia, dizziness associated with labyrinth and/or vestibular disorders, acute cochlear deafness, senile cognitive decline, vertigo, hearing loss and tinnitus.

The trials included Ginkgo versus placebo or registered drugs, mostly by oral route, and in one case combined with physical training. Shortcomings of the 40 trials included limited numbers of patients and incomplete description of randomisation procedures, patient characteristics, effect measurement and data presentation. All except one of the 40 trials showed positive results, 26 trials demonstrated significant results. The inconclusive result was obtained for a trial on senile dementia of vascular origin.[135] In most trials the dosage was 120 to 160 mg/day of Ginkgo extract, given for at least 4 to 6 weeks. No serious side effects were reported in any trial, and those that were reported were not significantly different from side effects observed in placebo-treated patients.

Eleven double blind, placebo-controlled trials using, in most cases, 150 mg/day of standardised Ginkgo extract over 12 weeks for cerebral insufficiency were evaluated by meta-analysis. Global efficacy was confirmed in five studies, compared to one study that was inconclusive.[135] Three studies were excluded on the basis of methodological or objective reasons and two were excluded because assessment by physician or patients was missing. Analysis of the total score of clinical symptoms from eight of the 11 studies indicated similar results (seven studies demonstrated Ginkgo was significantly better than placebo, one study was inconclusive).[133] It was concluded that treatment with Ginkgo extract provided a better therapeutic effect compared with placebo in the treatment of cerebral insufficiency.[136]

In other early trials (uncontrolled, double blind, placebo and comparative), standardised Ginkgo extract was found to be of benefit in the treatment of recent stroke victims. Improvement was observed in cerebral blood flow, motor recovery, intellectual performance, memory, mood and behaviour.[137–140]

A 2005 Cochrane review was conducted primarily to determine whether Ginkgo improved cognitive deficit and the functional outcome of patients with acute ischaemic stroke without causing deleterious side effects. The secondary outcome of effects on neurological impairment and quality of life in stroke sufferers was also reviewed. Ten trials involving a total of 792 patients met methodological standards and were included in the review (nine were conducted in China, where Ginkgo is used as a treatment for stroke). Analysing the trials together, Ginkgo was observed to significantly improve functional outcome in acute ischaemic stroke (OR 2.66; 95% CI −8.9 to 10.52). The authors concluded that, although Ginkgo shows promise in improving the functional outcome of stroke victims, most of the studies had some methodological failings, such as inadequate blinding and/or randomisation and an insufficient follow-up time (14 to 35 days).[141] It should be noted that Ginkgo was administered by injection in four of the 10 trials and for several trials treatment was instituted within 48 h.

In an early double blind, placebo-controlled trial not considered in the meta-analysis, 47 patients with acute ischaemic stroke received either Ginkgo extract (40 mg) or placebo at 6-hourly intervals along with routine management over 4 weeks. Both groups showed significant improvement, with negligible difference in degree of change in either group. The study group did, however, consist of patients who were treated more than 48 h after stroke and the treatment time was relatively short (4 weeks).[142]

The prevention of deleterious change in cerebral architecture and cognitive deficit in ageing humans was examined in a double blinded, controlled study involving 48 men (aged 60 to 70 years). Single photon emission computed tomography (SPECT) and measurement of blood viscosity were employed after 8 months of Ginkgo extract (80 mg/day). After the 8-month treatment period, the Ginkgo group showed a reduction in blood viscosity, improved cerebral perfusion in specific areas and improved global cognitive functioning. In contrast, the control group demonstrated the opposite (higher blood viscosity, a reduction in cerebral perfusion in specific areas and cognitive deterioration in different functions).[143] A follow-up study compared a macerated garlic oil against Ginkgo extract (80 mg/day) and placebo over 180 days in men and women and found Ginkgo was more effective in reducing blood viscosity from baseline.

Nine healthy men, of mean age 61±10 years, underwent a series of MRI scans at baseline and again after 4 weeks of treatment with Ginkgo extract (120 mg/day).[144] Cerebral blood flow was analysed at three different levels of spatial resolution in 10 brain regions. A small but statistically significant increase in cerebral blood flow was found in the left parietal-occipital white matter after Ginkgo administration (p≤0.001). The left parietal-occipital region has been implicated in visual memory and cognition. In other regions there was a (non-significant) trend of higher blood flow. There was also a small and statistically significant increase in global

cerebral blood flow (all regions combined): 15% in white matter and 13% in grey matter (p≤0.0001).

Alzheimer's disease and vascular dementia

Treatment

Ginkgo has been used successfully in the treatment of senile dementia of both the Alzheimer and vascular types. As a vast amount of literature exists regarding Ginkgo and dementia, only clinical trials and reviews of note are subsequently discussed.

A review published in 2008 assessed the efficacy of standardised Ginkgo extract in the treatment of dementia of vascular origin (VaD) and Alzheimer's disease (AD) by considering the external validity (such as everyday life activities, patient evaluation, quality of life of patients and carers) in addition to the usual criteria of randomisation and trial blinding. The authors assessed 34 placebo-controlled clinical trials to 2002. Despite some methodological limitations, there was sufficient evidence indicating the efficacy of Ginkgo for these conditions. The most frequent dosage was 120 mg/day, up to a maximum of 240 mg/day.[145] Three randomised, placebo-controlled trials published since this review have reported mixed results,[146–148] although subgroup analysis of one trial,[147] and the results of a trial with rigorous patient selection,[146] indicate standardised Ginkgo extract may be most beneficial to patients with neuropsychiatric symptoms. (The most frequent neuropsychiatric symptoms in dementia (Alzheimer and vascular) are apathy, depression and agitation/aggression. Up to 80% of patients with dementia, irrespective of cause, exhibit such symptoms.) A further subgroup analysis of this trial found that Ginkgo was equally effective for VaD and AD.[149]

In late 2008, the German Institute for Quality and Efficiency in Health Care (IQWiG) assessed trials for meta-analysis and noted there is evidence of a benefit for high-dose standardised Ginkgo extract (240 mg/day, for at least 16 weeks) in patients with AD, particularly for the goal of coping with daily activities. The results of the high-dose trials are of greater relevance as they are more homogeneous (not much deviation in results).[150] Four trials were included in the IQWiG meta-analysis of Ginkgo versus placebo.[151]

An alternative interpretation of the published data is provided by the Cochrane Collaboration (2009). A meta-analysis of randomised, placebo-controlled trials concluded the evidence for Ginkgo having a predictable and clinically significant benefit for people with dementia or cognitive impairment was inconsistent and unreliable.[152] The analysis incorporated trials mentioned above, including those covered in the 2008 review and the IQWiG meta-analysis. Criticism of some aspects of the methodology and conclusions of this Cochrane meta-analysis has been noted below and in the feedback section of the review article.

In terms of specific results, 36 trials were included, but most were small and of less than 3 months' duration. Results of the more recent trials showed inconsistent results. Of the four most recent trials, three found no difference between Ginkgo and placebo and one reported very large treatment effects in favour of Ginkgo. A subgroup analysis of only AD patients (925 from nine trials) also showed no consistent pattern of benefit.

Unlike the Cochrane meta-analysis, a meta-analysis published in 2010 only included trials evaluating specifically defined dementia and AD; trials of just cognitive impairment were excluded. Results indicated Ginkgo extract to be more effective than placebo in improving cognition in these patients. The trials were at least 12 weeks in duration and nine trials were included (2372 patients).[153] Effect sizes were moderate. Another 2010 meta-analysis that considered the influence of baseline risk on the treatment effect found Ginkgo extract for 6 months was effective in dementia. As mentioned, this meta-analysis took into account the variation of changes in the placebo groups across the included trials.[154] (Baseline risk is the risk of the event (in this case, cognitive decline) occurring without the active treatment (i.e. in the placebo group).) Six trials were included in the analysis.

A retrospective analysis of one of the trials included in these 2010 meta-analyses investigated whether the effect of treatment correlated with the extent of neuropsychiatric symptoms at baseline. Standardised Ginkgo extract (240 mg/day) was found to be effective in the treatment of dementia irrespective of the severity of neuropsychiatric symptoms. However, due to a faster decline in the placebo group, the net effect of Ginkgo was larger in patients with more pronounced neuropsychiatric symptoms, similar to observations noted above.[155]

A 2009 review identified 10 randomised, controlled, double blind clinical trials of Ginkgo in the treatment of AD and VaD.[156] In three of the four large trials, conducted in accordance with recent guidelines, Ginkgo extract was significantly superior to placebo with respect to cognitive performance and one or more further (global, functional or behavioural) outcomes. Only one trial was inconclusive, but was deemed to be of questionable external validity due to excessively rigorous patient selection.

Some of the key clinical trials included in the above reviews are discussed below.

The efficacy and safety of Ginkgo extract in the treatment of patients with mild-to-severe AD or VaD were assessed in a 52-week, randomised, double blind, placebo-controlled clinical trial.[157] Patients received either 120 mg/day of the extract or placebo. Primary outcome measures were the Alzheimer's Disease Assessment Scale (ADAS), Geriatric Evaluation by Relative's Rating Instrument (GERRI) and Clinical Global Impression of Change (CGIC). Of the 309 patients who began the trial, 202 provided useful data for the endpoint analysis, with 27% of patients treated with Ginkgo achieving at least a 4-point improvement on the ADAS compared with 14% taking placebo (p=0.005). On the GERRI, 37% of patients were considered improved with Ginkgo, compared with 23% taking placebo (p=0.003). No difference was seen in the CGIC and no significant difference compared with placebo was observed in the number of patients reporting adverse events or in the incidence and severity of these events. The authors concluded that Ginkgo extract was safe and appears capable of stabilising and, in a substantial number of cases, improving the cognitive performance and social function of patients with dementia.

A later retrospective statistical analysis of this study used intent-to-treat (ITT) evaluation of all 309 patients that began the trial. It concluded that the placebo group showed a statistically significant worsening in all domains of assessment, while the group receiving Ginkgo was considered to be slightly improved on cognitive assessment, daily living and social behaviour. Mean treatment differences favoured Ginkgo, with 1.3 and 0.12 points, respectively, on the ADAS-Cog (p=0.04) and the GERRI (p=0.007). In the group receiving Ginkgo, 26% of the patients achieved at least a 4-point improvement on the ADAS-Cog, compared to 17% with placebo (p=0.04). On the GERRI, 30% of the Ginkgo group improved and 17% worsened, while the placebo group displayed an opposite trend with 37% of patients worsening and 25% improved (p=0.006).[158]

A later stratification of the ITT data set collected during this 52-week trial (using cut-off points of 23 and 14 for the Mini-Mental State Examination (MMSE) score) yielded interesting results.[159] In the severity stratum 1 (MMSE >23), the placebo group did not demonstrate significant changes, while the Ginkgo group improved significantly by 1.7 points on the ADAS-Cog and by 0.09 points on the GERRI. In the severity stratum 2 (MMSE <24), the placebo group worsened by 4.1 points on the ADAS-Cog and 0.18 points on the GERRI, whereas the Ginkgo group showed 60% less decline on the ADAS-Cog (a treatment difference of 2.5 points) and no change on the GERRI (a treatment difference of 0.25 points). The most severely impaired subgroup (MMSE <15) displayed a slightly more pronounced worsening in both treatment groups. However, compared with placebo, Ginkgo induced virtually the same magnitude of effect as was observed in the entire stratum 2.

The results of this retrospective analysis further indicated that a treatment effect favourable to Ginkgo could be observed with respect to cognitive performance (p=0.02) and social functioning (p=0.001) regardless of the stage of dementia, whether mild or moderately severe. The authors believed their results reflected that Ginkgo ameliorated cognitive decline in cases of mild impairment, while in more severe cases it exerted a stabilisation or slowing-down of degeneration.

A 24-week randomised, controlled trial compared the efficacy of a standardised Ginkgo extract (160 mg/day) against a positive control group (donepezil, a cholinesterase inhibitor, 5 mg/day) and placebo in patients aged 50 to 80 years with mild to moderate dementia.[160] Results demonstrated a comparable efficacy between donepezil and Ginkgo in attenuating the progression of dementia, as assessed by the Syndrom Kurztest (SKT), the MMSE and CGI score.

In a prospective, randomised, double blind, placebo-controlled multicentre study, 216 outpatients with presenile and senile dementia of Alzheimer type and VaD received either Ginkgo extract (240 mg/day) or placebo for 24 weeks. The data from the 156 patients who completed psychopathological, attention, memory and behavioural assessment indicated that the groups differed significantly in favour of Ginkgo.[161] A later retrospective analysis of the ITT data estimated

ADAS-Cog and CGI-2 scores based on measured SKT scores.[162] After 24 weeks of treatment, the ITT analysis of the SKT and estimated ADAS-Cog scores revealed a mean decrease in the total score by −2.1 (95% CI −2.7 to −1.5) points and −2.7 (95% CI −3.5 to −1.9) points, respectively, for the Ginkgo group, indicating an improvement in cognitive function. In contrast, the placebo group exhibited only a minimal change of −1.0 (95% CI −1.6 to −0.3) and −1.3 (95% CI −2.0 to −0.4) points, respectively. The changes from baseline differed significantly between treatment groups by 1.1 (SKT) and 1.4 (estimated ADAS-Cog) points, respectively (p=0.01). The CGI-2 score favoured the Ginkgo group compared with placebo, with a mean difference of 0.4 points (p=0.007). The results of this ITT analysis reflected the results of the 1996 trial, although such results should be interpreted cautiously, as the estimated ADAS-Cog and CGI-2 scores were reached via a subjective ITT analysis.[161]

In contrast to the majority of trials displaying efficacy for Ginkgo in attenuating the progression of cognitive decline, a 24-week, randomised, double blind, placebo-controlled, parallel-group, trial involving 214 elderly participants with dementia (AD or VaD) or age-associated memory impairment, demonstrated equivocal results.[163] Patients were randomly allocated Ginkgo (either 240 mg/day or 160 mg/day) or placebo after a 3-week placebo run-in. After 12 weeks, the patients in the two Ginkgo groups were randomised to continue Ginkgo treatment or placebo. No statistically significant differences in mean change of scores between Ginkgo and placebo were observed, as assessed via the primary outcomes measures involving the SKT, CGI-2 and the Nuremberg Gerontopsychological Rating Scale for Activities of Daily Living. Although the authors noted there was a positive difference in favour of Ginkgo treatment, neither the dementia subgroup (n=36), nor the age-associated memory impairment subgroup (n=87), achieved a significant effect from Ginkgo treatment. The lack of a positive finding for the results of this methodologically rigorous study could be due to an 'outlier by chance', the fact that the study did not use the ADAS-Cog subtest (commonly used in dementia trials), or that this particular sub-population were non-responders to Ginkgo (as detailed in a neurological profile study of Ginkgo by Le Bars in 2003).[164]

One interesting trial (not included in any of the reviews) examined the impact of a combination of Ginkgo and donepezil. A randomised, double blind, exploratory clinical trial was undertaken to compare Ginkgo against donepezil in patients with confirmed AD also exhibiting neuropsychiatric symptoms.[165] Patients received either Ginkgo extract (240 mg/day for 22 weeks, n=31), donepezil (5 mg/day for 4 weeks and then 10 mg/day for 18 weeks, n=33) or both treatments (n=32). The presence of neuropsychiatric symptoms was required, as indicated by a minimum score of 3 in at least one item (other than delusions or hallucinations) of the Neuropsychiatric Inventory (NPI) and a total composite score of at least 5. To exclude patients with severe depression, the total score of the 17-item Hamilton Rating Scale for Depression (HAM-D) had to be below 20.

Seven patients dropped out from the trial before week 12 and one after, but only one of these was from the Ginkgo group. At the end of the trial patients were assessed according to the HAM-D, NPI and a battery of cognitive tests assessing memory, attention/concentration, visuospatial abilities, executive functioning and verbal fluency. Activities of daily living and severity of tinnitus and dizziness were also evaluated.

During the 22 weeks of double blind treatment, patients in all three treatment groups showed, on average, improvements over baseline values in all tests and rating scales. No statistically significant or clinically relevant differences could be detected between treatments. However, on the short cognitive performance test (SKT) there was a trend (p=0.08) to greater improvement for the combined herbal and drug treatments. During the trial, 26 adverse events (AEs) were documented for 10 patients (32%) treated with Ginkgo, 51 AEs for 24 patients (73%) taking donepezil and 29 AEs for 18 patients (56%) receiving combined treatment. For three AEs in three patients in the Ginkgo group and 38 AEs in 21 patients in the donepezil group, a causal relationship to the treatment could not be ruled out. Of the AEs reported for the combined treatment group, four events in four patients were considered as possibly related to Ginkgo and 21 events in 14 patients as possibly related to donepezil. For treatment with Ginkgo alone significantly fewer patients suffered from adverse events potentially related to the study medication than under the other treatments (p<0.01). No serious treatment-related AEs were recorded.

The authors concluded that their exploratory findings have helped to develop three hypotheses that will need to be tested in further studies: (1) there is no significant difference in efficacy between Ginkgo and donepezil, (2) a combination therapy will be superior in efficacy to therapy with either one of both substances and (3) there will be fewer side effects for a combination therapy than under therapy with donepezil alone.

The authors noted in their discussion:

> Relying on the proven efficacy of donepezil we did not include a placebo group. Estimating the natural deterioration of each patient of our sample using the relationship between deterioration and baseline severity as reported by Stern and co-workers a mean deterioration by 3.61 SKT points would result. The equation found by Stern and colleagues may tend to overestimate the natural progression of disease, but it highlights the fact that the real effect of drug treatment is not just the improvement over baseline, but improvement *versus* natural deterioration.

In other words, the observed average improvements in SKT scores of 1.8 points for the Ginkgo group and 3.5 points for the Ginkgo plus donepezil group must be added to a natural deterioration of up to 3.6 points over the treatment period. (SKT scores range between 0 and 27, with 27 being the weakest score).

Prevention

Despite its promising pharmacological properties, trials investigating the preventative role of Ginkgo in dementia and cognitive decline have yielded mixed results. A 2005 review concluded that standardised Ginkgo extract is likely to be of similar efficacy to cholinesterase inhibitors in delaying progression of cognitive impairment in AD. The review compared a trial of standardised Ginkgo extract with eight trials evaluating drugs (rivastigmine, donepezil, galantamine) published to 2000.[166] A 2006 trial tended to confirm this conclusion.[160]

Two trials have investigated standardised Ginkgo extract (240 mg/day) for prevention of dementia in elderly individuals with normal cognition and those with mild cognitive impairment. Ginkgo was not effective, although in one trial a protective effect was found when medication compliance was taken into account (see below).[167,168]

An earlier nested prospective case-controlled trial in the EPIDOS (EPIDemiology of OSteoporosis) study involving 1462 community-dwelling elderly women aged over 75 years was conducted to determine Ginkgo extract's efficacy in attenuating cognitive decline over a 7-year period.[169] Pfeiffer's test was conducted at the start of the study to determine cognitive function, with volunteers being included with a reading of ≥8 (indicating normal cognitive function). A cohort of 714 women with assessed cognitive function was analysed after follow-up. Multivariate analysis including potential confounding factors showed that fewer women developed Alzheimer's dementia if they had been prescribed pharmacological dementia treatment, including Ginkgo, for at least 2 years (OR 0.31, 95% CI 0.12 to 0.82, p=0.018).

Results for the longest and largest European study for prevention of AD ever conducted are emerging (the GuidAge study). Treatment with standardised Ginkgo extract (240 mg/day) did not significantly delay conversion to clinical disease in the randomised, double blind trial. However, in this ITT analysis, all patients, including those who did not complete the trial, were considered. A further analysis considering patients treated for at least 4 years found a clinically and statistically significant difference for treatment with Ginkgo (1.6% developed AD versus 3.0% in the placebo group).[170] Interestingly the protective effect in this subset was most marked in men: AD incidence was 2.9% for the Ginkgo group versus 7.0% for placebo (p=0.007). The compliance rate for those who continued in the study was 93%.

However, the preventative study that received the most media attention was the GEM (Ginkgo Evaluation of Memory) trial. This study was designed as a dementia prevention trial and the final results were published in the *Journal of the American Medical Association* (*JAMA*) in 2008.[167] The study failed to find any preventative effect for Ginkgo, but has been criticised because of the advanced age of participants (72 to 96 years), the relatively short treatment time (about 6 years) and the poor patient compliance with the treatment (only about 60%), which was 240 mg/day of Ginkgo extract.

In late 2009 a secondary analysis of the original GEM data was again published in *JAMA*.[171] In this analysis, the impact of Ginkgo on cognitive decline among the participants in the GEM study was assessed. No benefit was found for Ginkgo.

A considered examination of the study design and results readily shows that they were not suitable to support any conclusions about the impact of regular Ginkgo intake on cognitive decline. There were five major weaknesses in the second published study:[172,173]

- It was not originally designed to assess cognitive decline, hence for about the first 4 of the 6 years of treatment most participants were only assessed by very basic dementia scales, such as the MMSE, which are neither sensitive nor accurate measures of cognitive function.
- There was a very high dropout rate over the course of the study (approximately one-third) and yet the ITT analysis used would have included these dropouts as non-responders.
- There was poor compliance with the Ginkgo (as noted earlier), with only about 60% of participants actually taking the tablets regularly.
- The participants were of an advanced age (average 79 years at the beginning of the trial) and hence might not represent the effects of Ginkgo on cognition in younger people.
- Despite their high age, trial participants showed only a very low rate of cognitive decline in both the Ginkgo and placebo groups: the rate was in fact seven times slower than the reference rate used by the authors to plan their study. It would be very difficult for any active treatment to realistically impact a rate of cognitive decline that was already seven times lower than the typical norm for that age group.

A prospective, cohort study conducted in Vienna from 2000 to 2002 examined 526 individuals without dementia aged 75 years to investigate the influence of medication on plasma levels of amyloid beta protein 42 (Abeta42). Plasma Abeta42 levels are elevated in both late onset AD patients and their cognitively normal first-degree relatives. Users of Ginkgo for at least 2 years had significantly decreased Abeta42 plasma levels compared with non-users. This reduction was also independent of medial temporal lobe (brain) atrophy, as assessed by MRI scanning.[174] At follow-up 2.5 years later, longer use of Ginkgo seemed to decrease plasma Abeta42 levels to a greater extent than shorter use. There was a weak association of Ginkgo use with the ability to remain cognitively healthy for the observation period.[175]

Peripheral arterial disease

A 2004 systematic review of randomised, double blind, placebo-controlled clinical trials in patients with peripheral arterial occlusive disease (intermittent claudication) in stage II (according to Fontaine) treated with Ginkgo extract suggested positive benefit.[176] Nine studies were found to be eligible for review. Although the methodological quality and design of the trials were heterogeneous, the majority of the studies reflected an advantage of Ginkgo in the increase of pain-free walking distance compared with placebo. For seven studies, the advantage was found to be statistically significant.

An earlier 2000 meta-analysis of eight randomised, placebo-controlled, double blind trials observed a statistically significant difference in the increase in pain-free walking distance in favour of Ginkgo extract compared with placebo (weighted mean difference 34 m, 95% CI 26 to 43 m).[177] In studies with similar methodological features (ergometer speed 3 km/h, inclination 12%) this difference was 33 m in favour of Ginkgo (95% CI 22 to 43 m). Although the effect size was considered by the authors as modest, the results of the meta-analysis supported the use of Ginkgo in the treatment of intermittent claudication.

In placebo-controlled trials published since the 2004 review, standardised Ginkgo extract:

- produced a modest, but not statistically significant, increase in maximal walking time (300 mg/day)[178]
- did not provide additional benefit when combined with supervised exercise training (240 mg/day).[179]

A 2009 meta-analysis of randomised trials (those mentioned above, including from the 2004 review) conducted by the Cochrane Collaboration concluded that there was no evidence that Ginkgo has a clinically significant benefit for patients with peripheral arterial disease. People using standardised Ginkgo extract could walk 64.5 m further, which was not considered to be significant in comparison with the placebo group.[180]

A standardised Ginkgo extract (360 mg/day) was assessed in the treatment of Raynaud's disease. In a 2-week assessment period, 22 patients recorded the frequency, severity and duration of attacks in diaries. Patients were then randomised to active or placebo treatments for 10 weeks, during which time ischaemic attacks were recorded in their diaries. The number of ischaemic attacks per day was significantly reduced after Ginkgo treatment versus placebo (56% versus 27%, respectively, $p<0.00001$). The mean duration of attacks reduced from 28 min pre-treatment to 17 min in the placebo intervention and to 10.3 min after Ginkgo administration.[181]

Many doctors in South Korea prescribe Ginkgo extract for primary Raynaud's disease. A clinical trial found patients treated for 8 weeks with slow release nifedipine showed a 50% improvement in the rate of attacks, and those treated with Ginkgo extract (120 to 240 mg/day), showed a 30% improvement.[182] Hence the drug was more effective.

Addition of Ginkgo extract to existing and/or local treatment healed an ischaemic ulcer in a man with peripheral arterial disease (120 mg/day, case report),[183] and significantly decreased the ulcer area in patients with chronic leg ulcers (160 mg/day, randomised controlled trial).[184]

Other vascular disorders

When the standardised extract of Ginkgo was developed by German scientists in the 1960s, the original therapeutic focus was on improving peripheral circulation to the legs and the brain. Later the neuroprotective effects of Ginkgo were recognised and it became an important herbal treatment to boost brain function and provide a benefit in AD. Always missing from the scenario was any potential impact of Ginkgo on heart function, especially in the prevention of heart disease. Given its known circulatory effects and its capacity to help body tissues survive a poor oxygen environment, it is likely that Ginkgo would exert some benefit here. Now some preliminary studies are suggesting that such a benefit might be unexpectedly profound.

A German and Swedish research team conducted an open label pilot trial in eight patients who had undergone coronary bypass surgery.[185] They examined the impact of Ginkgo extract (240 mg/day) for 2 months on the capacity of blood samples to form nanoplaques. Nanoplaques are considered to be the very first stage of degeneration of the arterial wall that leads to atherosclerosis and eventually heart disease. In the case of bypass patients, the tendency to nanoplaque formation can determine how quickly the replacement blood vessels will become diseased.

The reduction in nanoplaque formation from the Ginkgo amounted to 11.9±2.5% ($p<0.008$) and nanoplaque size was reduced by 24.4±8.1% ($p<0.023$). Given these marked findings, the authors suggested that Ginkgo could be regularly consumed by heart patients as a complement to statin drugs to help prevent the redevelopment of atherosclerotic plaque following bypass surgery. They stressed that its mechanism of action and effects were unlike statin drugs.

But perhaps a more significant finding was the Ginkgo treatment lowered lipoprotein(a) by 23.4±7.9% ($p<0.023$). In a subsequent letter to the editor, another research group highlighted that this might represent a clinically remarkable outcome. This is because no conventional therapeutic approach has been identified so far capable of efficiently and safely lowering the plasma concentration of this intriguing lipoprotein.[186]

Lipoprotein(a) is considered to be a significant independent cardiovascular risk factor.[187,188] Despite this, it has not received much research attention until recently, presumably because there are no available drugs that can influence its levels. Attention has been on LDL-cholesterol (low-density lipoprotein cholesterol) and the statin drugs that lower this.

In the pilot study the Ginkgo treatment also upregulated superoxide dismutase (SOD) activity by 15.7±7.0% ($p<0.039$) and lowered the percentage of oxidised LDL by 17.0±5.5% ($p<0.023$). The authors concluded that the atherosclerosis-inhibiting effect of Ginkgo is possibly due to an upregulation of the body's own radical scavenging enzymes (perhaps via the Nrf2/ARE pathway) and a reduction in the risk factors of oxidised LDL and lipoprotein(a).

A letter to the editor on the study mentioned above suggested that the reduction in lipoprotein(a) might represent an anti-inflammatory effect, especially a reduction in IL-6 (interleukin-6).[186] In response, the authors agreed with this possibility, but also stressed that a reduction in levels of reactive oxygen species might also play a role.[189]

Continuing with the theme of Ginkgo coming into prominence as a herb for the heart, Chinese research is moving in this direction. In a clinical study in patients with coronary artery disease, Ginkgo extract (via injection) significantly improved distal left anterior descending (LAD) coronary blood flow.[190] A similar trial in healthy elderly adults also observed an improvement in LAD blood flow.[191] In both cases the increased response was proposed to result from an improved endothelium-dependent vasodilatory capacity, which is regulated by the enhanced release of nitric oxide.

The beneficial effects of Ginkgo on nanoplaque formation were investigated in a second observational trial involving 11 patients with metabolic syndrome.[192] After 2 months of treatment with Ginkgo extract (240 mg/day), nanoplaque formation and nanoplaque size were reduced by 14.7% and 21.5% respectively. These results were highly statistically significant.

Ginkgo lowered the percentage of oxidised LDL (by 21.0%), lowered lipoprotein(a) concentration (by 26.3%) and upregulated the activities of SOD and glutathione peroxidase (19.6% and 11.6%, respectively).

An extensive range of other biomarkers were measured, which led the authors to conclude that the atherosclerosis-inhibiting effect of Ginkgo can be attributed to:

- a stimulation of radical scavenging enzymes in the body
- a restriction of certain risk factors (lipoprotein(a), percentage of oxidised LDL)
- an increase in nitric oxide/cyclic GMP release (having a vasodilatory effect).

Interestingly, treatment with Ginkgo resulted in a significant increase in both mean corpuscular haemoglobin levels and concentration. In conjunction with the observed vasodilation, this will result in improved oxygen supply and enhanced organ perfusion.

In an earlier double blind, placebo-controlled trial, 15 patients undergoing aortic valve replacement (in cardiopulmonary bypass) received either Ginkgo extract (320 mg/day) or placebo for 5 days before surgical intervention. Plasma samples taken at crucial stages of the operation indicated that Ginkgo limited free radical-induced oxidative stress generated throughout the surgery. Recovery of the Ginkgo patients was improved (but not significantly) compared with placebo, and Ginkgo was considered useful in limiting oxidative stress. The protective activity was attributed to a membrane-protective mechanism rather than a direct scavenging effect.[193] (Earlier in vitro and in vivo studies suggest the cardioprotective effects of the Ginkgo terpenoids involve an inhibition of free radical formation rather than direct free radical scavenging.)[194]

In an early uncontrolled trial, 20 outpatients with a long history of elevated plasma viscosity and fibrinogen levels and a variety of underlying diseases received 240 mg/day Ginkgo extract for 12 weeks. Steady and significant reductions in fibrinogen levels and blood viscosity were observed over the treatment period.[195]

A short-term 7-day, crossover, placebo-controlled, double blind study found that Ginkgo extract (240 mg/day) had no impact on blood pressure, heart rate or electrocardiographic variables in young, healthy volunteers.[196]

Ear, nose, throat problems

Ginkgo extract is the most clinically tested herbal therapy for disorders involving the ear. However, results from clinical trials have not always been consistent.

Hearing loss

Deafness of sudden onset (acute cochlear deafness) is often due to ischaemia of the cochlea and the metabolic derangement that accompanies this. The first study on the use of Ginkgo in acute cochlear deafness was published in 1986.[197] The author suggested that prognosis in acute cochlear deafness is entirely dependent on the rapid initiation of an effective treatment. Hence a relatively high dose of Ginkgo extract of 320 mg/day was employed in the study. The efficacy of Ginkgo was compared to nicergoline, an alpha-adrenoreceptor blocker, and the study involved 18 patients in a double blind design over 30 days. Audiometric analyses and labyrinth tests demonstrated that all of the patients in the Ginkgo group had normal values at the end of the trial, whereas one-third of the patients in the nicergoline group still had inconclusive tests. The significance of this trial was hampered by the small patient numbers.

In another trial, Ginkgo extract (intravenous 200 mg/day for 9 days, followed by oral 160 mg/day for 6 weeks) was found to be superior to the drug piracetam for the treatment of sudden deafness (one-sided hearing loss).[198] Median values for hearing thresholds in the range 250 to 3000 Hz were significantly lower with Ginkgo treatment.

In a randomised comparative study, 80 patients with idiopathic sudden hearing loss of no longer than 10 days were treated with either Ginkgo extract or naftidrofuryl (a vasodilator). After 1 week, 40% of patients in each group experienced a complete remission. After 3 weeks there was a significant borderline benefit for Ginkgo over naftidrofuryl. Ginkgo treatment was preferred due to a lack of side effects, unlike the naftidrofuryl.[199]

A study conducted in India examined the value of Ginkgo extract against a combined drug treatment for acquired sensorineural hearing loss in 52 patients.[200] Probable aetiologies included presbycusis (36.5%), followed by unknown causes (28.8%). Outcomes for Ginkgo were better than the conventional treatment in responding patients. Response rates were similar between the two treatments.

In a relatively large trial involving 106 patients, the efficacies of two different dosages of Ginkgo for unilateral idiopathic sudden hearing loss were compared in a randomised, double blind design.[201] The higher dose of Ginkgo (240 mg/day) appeared to accelerate and secure the recovery of patients, with a good chance for complete recovery (p=0.006). Positive results were observed after 1 week of treatment.

In a randomised, prospective, double blind study involving 72 patients, the therapeutic efficacy of Ginkgo extract (n=37) was compared with pentoxifylline (n=35) for the treatment of sudden deafness.[202] The dose of Ginkgo extract was 200 mg/day via intravenous infusion. The two treatments were equally well tolerated and showed a statistically significant equivalence in terms of either improvement or a return to normal of the auditory thresholds. Subjective assessment of the treatment (with regard to improvement in hearing and reduction in tinnitus) suggested that Ginkgo extract was more beneficial than pentoxifylline.

Vestibular disorders

Most of the trials assessing the value of Ginkgo in vertigo date to the 1980s, although there is one trial of more recent origin. In one early trial, which had an open phase with Ginkgo extract followed by a double blind, placebo-controlled phase, results were compiled for 50 patients complaining of dizziness. These results showed a clear benefit for Ginkgo in the open phase as well as over the placebo, except for patients with Ménière's disease.[203]

A randomised, placebo-controlled, double blind trial in 35 patients assessed the value of Ginkgo extract at 160 mg/day for vestibular vertigo.[204] The primary outcome measured was performance using posturography (assessment of body sway with eyes open or closed) and there was a statistically significant benefit from baseline observed for therapy with Ginkgo, which was also superior to placebo.

A study conducted in three centres included 70 patients with vertigo of recent and idiopathic onset in a double blind, placebo-controlled trial.[205] The efficacy of Ginkgo extract (160 mg/day) on both the frequency and duration of vertigo achieved statistical significance, with 47% of patients in the Ginkgo group free of symptoms at the end of the trial compared with 18% for the placebo group (p<0.05).

A trial conducted in Poland compared Ginkgo extract plus physical therapy against physical therapy alone for the treatment of vestibular organ peripheral lesion syndrome in an open label design.[206] Patients in both groups improved, but improvement was more marked and faster, as assessed by dynamic posturography, for the group receiving Ginkgo.

A 2007 systematic review of randomised, double blind clinical trials identified five studies (including those reviewed above) and concluded that Ginkgo extract (120 to 240 mg/day) was a beneficial treatment for vestibular and non-vestibular vertigo (see also below).[207]

Tinnitus or combined syndromes

After vertigo, nausea and hearing loss, tinnitus is one of the most important symptoms in the field of disorders of the ear. In most cases the origin of the tinnitus is not identifiable, although it is recognised that it can arise in any part of the hearing pathway. It is frequently associated with vertigo, nausea and hearing loss. An age predominance exists and identifiable causes include presbycusis, atherosclerosis, chronic otitis media, otosclerosis, acoustic trauma, Ménière's disease and ototoxicity. Given such a wide range of causes, known and unknown, it is likely that clinical trials in this field will be fraught with difficulties and prone to conflicting results. This is certainly the case for trials involving Ginkgo treatment.

Since the pathophysiology and treatment of tinnitus is still under debate and is relatively obscure, it is likely that Ginkgo may assist in the treatment of specific sub-populations of tinnitus sufferers. The difficulty is determining potential responders to Ginkgo treatment.

An early trial conducted in 1979 included 60 patients with hearing loss and/or vertigo and tinnitus.[208] Ginkgo extract (120 mg/day) was compared with nicergoline and found to be superior. Another early open design trial found good efficacy for Ginkgo extract in patients with hearing impairment and tinnitus due to a variety of causes, mainly involving ischaemia.[209]

In 1986 Meyer conducted a defining study on 103 patients that clearly established a reputation for Ginkgo in the treatment of tinnitus (deserved or otherwise).[210] A randomised, double blind, placebo-controlled trial with Ginkgo extract included only patients with tinnitus of recent onset (less than one year). Improvement or cure was observed after an average of 70 days in patients treated with Ginkgo compared with 119 days in patients receiving placebo. Tinnitus of recent onset, unilateral and intermittent seemed to be particularly responsive to Ginkgo.

Soft laser therapy in combination with Ginkgo for the treatment of tinnitus was found to be effective in one open trial[211] and ineffective in another.[212] In a double blind, placebo-controlled trial involving 100 elderly patients (with at least four symptoms out of poor memory, anxiety, vertigo, tinnitus and headaches), therapy with Ginkgo extract (112 mg/day) or placebo was assessed after 12 weeks.[213] Improvement in tinnitus from baseline was 37% for the Ginkgo group versus 12% for the placebo group.

The 20 patients reporting a positive effect on persistent severe tinnitus in an open study involving 80 patients were included in a double blind placebo-controlled crossover study.[214] They received either Ginkgo extract (29.2 mg/day, 2 weeks) or placebo. The success of the treatment was based on patient preference (as there is no objective measurement) and on this basis Ginkgo did not demonstrate a significant effect. However, the dose of Ginkgo extract used was subtherapeutic.

A study published in the *BMJ* found no advantage for Ginkgo extract (150 mg/day) in treating tinnitus in a double blind, placebo-controlled trial using postal questionnaires in 1121 healthy people with a comparatively stable condition.[215]

In contrast, a trial involving 60 patients with chronic tinnitus observed a positive result for Ginkgo extract (200 mg/day by intravenous infusion for 10 days followed by oral therapy of 160 mg/day) compared with placebo after 12 weeks of therapy.[216] While results achieved statistical significance, the absolute difference between the two treatment groups was only moderate.

A systematic search of the literature identified 19 clinical trials (many early) investigating the effect of Ginkgo extract on tinnitus.[217] The results of eight controlled studies were found for the most part to show a statistically significant superiority of Ginkgo extract over placebo or reference drugs. Tinnitus of recent onset had a better prognosis.

A 12-week randomised, double blind trial of Ginkgo extract (120 mg/day, slow release tablet) involving 66 patients with tinnitus was conducted with Tinnitus Handicap Inventory (THI), Glasgow Health Status Inventory (GHSI) and average of hearing threshold at 0.5, 1, 2, 4 kHz being used as the outcome measures.[218] Results showed that the mean differences in changes of the THI, GHSI and hearing between Ginkgo (n=31) and placebo (n=29) were 2.51 (CI −10.1 to 5.1, p=0.51), 0.58 (CI −4.8 to 3.6, p=0.38) and 0.68 db (CI −4.13 to 2.8, p=0.69), respectively, indicating no statistical difference between Ginkgo and placebo. The researchers conducted and published a meta-analysis in the same paper of five previously conducted studies. Meta-analysis revealed 21.6% of Ginkgo-treated patients (107 of 552) gained benefit versus 18.4% (87 of 504) of placebo-treated patients with an odds ratio of 1.24 (CI 0.89 to 1.71) indicating only a small benefit.[218]

A 2004 Cochrane systematic review of Ginkgo in the treatment of tinnitus was conducted to determine evidence of efficacy.[219] Although 12 trials were initially located, 10 were excluded from the review on methodological grounds. The interventions assessed were Ginkgo versus placebo, with no 'gold standard' treatment available for an active control. Most studies involved a dosage of 120 to 200 mg/day of standardised Ginkgo extract, using outcome measures such as changes in loudness of tinnitus, severity and impact on quality of life. The exclusion of 10 of the studies was due to a variety of methodological failings, including a high drop-out rate, cohort number reporting and concealment, and unsatisfactory rating scales. After a later update, another acceptable study was located and three randomised placebo-controlled studies were included. One was a 12-week trial involving 99 patients given 120 mg/day Ginkgo extract that demonstrated improvement in the sound volume (5 to 10 dB) of the ear with the worst tinnitus in the Ginkgo group, while the placebo group remained unchanged.[220] The other two studies have been reviewed above. The Cochrane review concluded that limited evidence does not demonstrate Ginkgo was effective for tinnitus.

Part of a double blind, placebo-controlled trial of Ginkgo extract in dementia investigated effects on dizziness and tinnitus. The trial involved outpatients aged 50 years or older with mild-to-moderate dementia with neuropsychiatric symptoms.[221] After receiving Ginkgo extract (240 mg/day) for 22 weeks, the mean severity score for dizziness improved from 4.35 to 2.09 and the severity score for tinnitus decreased from 4.02 to 1.91. There were only slight improvements in the placebo group, from 4.22 to 3.88 for dizziness and from 3.90 to 3.75 for tinnitus. Dizziness was improved in 86% of Ginkgo recipients and in 28% of the placebo group. Improvement rates for tinnitus were 84% of the Ginkgo-treated patients versus 20% of the placebo group. The differences were significant between Ginkgo and placebo on all measures ($p<0.001$).

Since hypercholesterolaemia might promote the development of tinnitus, a retrospective study was performed to assess whether simvastatin might impact this disorder. Remission rates in 58 patients were investigated after 4 months of simvastatin (40 mg/day) and compared to results for Ginkgo (120 mg/day) in 36 patients as a control group.[222] Only small reductions in tinnitus scores were observed in both groups, casting doubt on the efficacy of either treatment.

In an address to Australian clinicians in September 2007, a spokesperson of the European Federation of Tinnitus Associations advised that European doctors had a high degree of success treating tinnitus with standardised Ginkgo extract. It is most successful if administered within the first 3 months of onset,[223] and a dose of 240 mg/day was recommended.[224]

Olfactory disorders

Seventy-one patients who were diagnosed with postviral olfactory loss participated in a randomised trial conducted in South Korea.[225] Patients did not have sinus inflammation, nasal discharge, allergic rhinitis or chronic rhinosinusitis. They were treated with oral prednisolone (2 weeks) or oral prednisolone (2 weeks) plus Ginkgo extract (240 mg/day, 4 weeks).

All patients could take two puffs of mometasone furoate (a corticosteroid) nasal spray per nostril twice daily for 4 weeks. Olfactory function tests, including the butanol threshold test (tests odour threshold) and the cross-cultural smell identification test (CCSIT, tests odour identification) were performed at baseline and after treatment.

Although not statistically different between the two groups, the addition of Ginkgo showed a tendency toward greater efficacy (for example, for CCSIT response rate p=0.08). The results of CCSIT are considered more relevant, as odour identification is a more complex and higher-level olfactory function than odour threshold.

Eye disorders

As Ginkgo exerts vascular protective, antioxidant and circulatory enhancing activity, it is posited that it can have a therapeutic role in treating age-related macular degeneration. A 2000 Cochrane review was conducted evaluating its efficacy in treating macular degeneration.[226] Two studies were identified by the review. A trial involving 20 people found that visual acuity improved in Ginkgo treated patients more than the control over a 6-month period.[227] The other study reviewed tested the visual acuity of 99 participants with macular degeneration, finding no statistical difference between the low-dose (60 mg/day) and high-dose (240 mg/day) Ginkgo groups.[228] Further work is needed in this area, given that these trials did indicate some benefits.

A US research team evaluated a possible therapeutic effect of Ginkgo extract that might benefit glaucoma patients through improvement in ocular blood flow.[229] A phase I crossover trial of Ginkgo with placebo control in 11 healthy volunteers was performed. Patients were treated with either Ginkgo extract (120 mg/day) or placebo for 2 days. Colour Doppler imaging was used to measure ocular blood flow before and after treatment. There was a 2-week washout period between Ginkgo and placebo treatments. Ginkgo extract significantly increased end diastolic velocity in the ophthalmic artery (baseline versus Ginkgo treatment; 6.5±0.5 versus 7.7±0.5 cm/sec, 23% change, p=0.023), with no change seen in placebo (baseline versus placebo; 7.2±0.6 versus 7.1±0.5 cm/sec, 3% change, p=0.892). No side effects related to Ginkgo were found. Ginkgo extract did not alter arterial blood pressure, heart rate or intraocular pressure. The authors concluded that the extract deserves further investigation for possible application in the treatment of optic neuropathy linked to glaucoma as well as other ischaemic ocular diseases.

Significant improvements in visual field indices, but not intraocular, pressures were recorded in a randomised, double blind, placebo-controlled trial involving patients with normal tension glaucoma (a form of primary open-angle glaucoma). Patients received standardised Ginkgo extract (120 mg/day) for 4 weeks.[230] Beneficial results with Ginkgo were demonstrated in another controlled trial of the same disorder, with tests conducted over a period of at least 4 years.[231]

Ginkgo extract (80 mg/day) for at least 6 months did not improve visual field indices in patients with primary open-angle glaucoma. In this trial, treated patients were retrospectively matched with control patients.[232]

In earlier research in 24 patients suffering from blockage of veins in the retina, Ginkgo extract produced improvements in blood vessels, visual acuity and field of vision in a double blind, placebo-controlled trial. Where the blood supply to the retina was deficient, Ginkgo improved many aspects of vision such as near and far vision, colour recognition and field of vision.[233] In an uncontrolled trial, 35 patients with poor blood supply to the retina, or to those parts of the brain that interpret the signals from the eyes, were treated with Ginkgo extract (120 mg/day) over a 3-month period; 86% of patients with reduced vision improved markedly.[234]

Two open label studies demonstrated that standardised extract of Ginkgo (120 to 240 mg/day for 3 months) reduced the abnormal blood parameters seen in diabetic retinopathy including a decrease in lipid peroxidation,[235,236] a decrease in clotting factors and red blood cell deformity, and improved blood viscosity and elasticity, resulting in improved retinal capillary blood flow rate.[236]

A total of 60 patients with symptomatic allergic conjunctivitis were enrolled and randomly assigned to 15 days of treatment with Ginkgo and hyaluronic acid (GB-HA) eye drops or hyaluronic acid ophthalmic solution (HA) alone for 1 month.[237] Clinical symptoms such as conjunctival hyperaemia (redness), conjunctival discharge and chemosis (swelling or oedema of the conjunctiva), and subjective signs as itching, photophobia, stinging and lacrimation were evaluated before and after the treatment. Patients treated with GB-HA, compared with patients treated with HA alone, showed a significant decrease in the appearance of conjunctival hyperaemia, conjunctival discharge and chemosis. Hyperaemia was particularly responsive to the GB-HA eye drops, dropping by 85%. In addition, all patients treated with GB-HA showed a significant improvement in subjective symptoms. Itching was substantially reduced.

Psychiatric and learning disorders

Although Ginkgo is commonly used to treat dementia, cognitive decline, peripheral arterial disease and tinnitus, studies have noted that mood modulation can also occur in cognitively impaired patients. A 2006 randomised, double blind trial (n=107) was conducted using Ginkgo extract (480 mg or 240 mg/day) or placebo for 4 weeks in adults with general anxiety disorder or adjustment disorder with anxious mood as assessed via DSM-III-R.[238] ITT analyses were performed on the primary outcome measure the Hamilton anxiety scale (HAMA-A), and the secondary outcome measures, the CGI, the Erlangen anxiety tension and aggression scale and the patient's global rating of change. The patients' HAM-A total scores decreased by −14.3 (±−8.1), −12.1 (±−9.0) and −7.8 (±−9.2) in the 480 mg/day Ginkgo group, the 240 mg/day Ginkgo group and the placebo group, respectively. Results indicated dose-dependent anxiolysis compared with placebo (p=0.0003 in the higher-dose group, p=0.01 in the lower-dose group).

A methodologically rigorous 10-week pilot study involving 27 adults assessed whether a Ginkgo extract may prevent the symptoms of winter depression in patients with seasonal affective disorder.[239] Results demonstrated that Ginkgo did not prevent the seasonally provoked depressive symptoms as assessed via an extended Montgomery-Asberg Depression Rating Scale and various self-assessed key symptoms on a visual analogue scale.

A systematic review and meta-analysis of the role of Ginkgo as an adjunct therapy in chronic schizophrenia found six clinical trials published between 1996 and 2008 comprising a total of 828 patients.[240] Five of the trials were placebo-controlled and the dose of Ginkgo extract ranged from 120 to 360 mg/day. The trials lasted from 8 to 16 weeks, with four being conducted in East Asia and the remainder in Eastern Europe. Ginkgo treatment was combined with the following drugs: chlorpromazine, haloperidol, olanzapine and clozapine.

All trials used the Scale for the Assessment of Negative Symptoms to measure negative symptoms, and the Scale for the Assessment of Positive Symptoms or the Brief Psychiatric Rating Scale to measure total symptoms. The difference between Ginkgo and control groups from their pre- and post-trial scores and the pooled standard deviation were used to compute the standardised mean difference (SMD). Ginkgo as an add-on therapy to antipsychotic medication produced a statistically significant moderate improvement (SMD=−0.50) in total and negative symptoms associated with chronic schizophrenia. The authors concluded that Ginkgo has a statistically significant moderate therapeutic benefit with acceptable safety limits as an add-on therapy for chronic schizophrenia, but that more research is needed, especially in terms of its potential interactions with psychotropic drugs.

Ginkgo extract improved word recognition and reading in children with dyslexia (80 mg/day, pilot trial),[241] and improved cognitive function and social behaviour in children with Down syndrome (80 to 120 mg/day, two cases).[242] Ginkgo extract (200 mg/day) improved behaviour, hyperactivity, inattention and immaturity in six young adults with attention deficit hyperactivity disorder (ADHD).[243] In an open trial, 56% of ADHD children improved with Ginkgo treatment.[244] However, Ginkgo was not as effective as methylphenidate in a randomised, double blind trial conducted in Iran.[245]

Asthma and PAF-related disorders

Platelet activating factor (PAF) is a phospholipid formed by platelets, basophils, neutrophils, monocytes and macrophages. Anti-PAF activity is regarded as useful in the treatment of asthma, allergic reactions, immunological reactions, shock, ischaemia and thrombosis.

Ginkgo extract protected asthmatic patients exposed to challenge with an inhaled allergen (600 mg single dose pretreatment; uncontrolled trial).[25] It also improved asthma in adults, some of whom were able to stop corticosteroid therapy, and normalised pulmonary function in children with atopic asthma, which was correlated with a significant improvement in flow parameters (uncontrolled trial).[34] Compared with those treated only with inhaled corticosteroid, addition of Ginkgo extract (oral, 240 mg/day) for 4 weeks decreased airway inflammation in asthmatic patients in a trial conducted in China.[246] In a placebo-controlled trial, also from China, concentrated Ginkgo leaf liquor reduced airway hyper-reactivity, improved clinical symptoms and pulmonary function in asthmatic patients.[247,248]

Treatment with Ginkgo leaf tablets for 3 months significantly lowered elevated serum PAF levels in chronic hepatitis B patients. Indices of liver fibrosis were also significantly lowered. The daily dose of Ginkgo provided 86.4 mg/day of ginkgo flavonol glycosides and 21.6 mg/day of ginkgolides. A control group received a tablet containing mostly silybin, at a daily dose of 315 mg/day. Gingko treatment was deemed superior to the control.[249]

Acute mountain sickness

Two randomised, double blind, placebo-controlled clinical trials were undertaken to assess the efficacy of 240 mg/day of two different Ginkgo standardised extracts in reducing the incidence and severity of acute mountain sickness (AMS) following rapid ascent to a high altitude.[250] The trial was conducted at Pike's Peak in Colorado, which has over 300 000 visitors a year who rapidly ascend from 2000 to 4300 m in 2 h via train or car. As might be expected, many of these visitors experience AMS, which includes symptoms such as extreme shortness of breath (due to pulmonary oedema) and confusion (due to cerebral oedema) in its more severe manifestations. Symptoms associated with mild-to-moderate AMS include difficulty sleeping, dizziness, fatigue, headache, loss of appetite, nausea, rapid pulse and shortness of breath with exertion. The cause is unknown, although theories implicating oxidative stress have been suggested.[251] The drug acetazolamide is used as a preventative treatment, but is not tolerated by some people and is associated with side effects such as nausea and paraesthesia.

An oral dose of 120 mg of Ginkgo or placebo was self-administered by participants twice per day, morning and evening, for 4 days (study 1) or 3 days (study 2) prior to ascent and during 24 h at altitude, for a total treatment time of 5 days in study 1 and 4 days in study 2. Results were conflicting: Ginkgo significantly reduced the incidence and severity of AMS in study 1 but not in study 2 (p=0.027 versus p=0.247 for incidence, p=0.029 versus p=0.272 for severity, respectively). The authors suggested that despite the weaknesses in their study design, which included low patient numbers (40 in study 1 and 37 in study 2), differing pretreatment times (4 versus 3 days) and a greater placebo effect in study 2, the main reason for the observed difference between the two studies was the source of Ginkgo. The extract used in study 1 contained a much higher level of ginkgolides A, B and C than the one used in study 2, even though the total level of terpene lactones was similar at around 6.5%. They concluded that the source and composition of the Ginkgo extract may determine the efficacy of Ginkgo for the prevention of AMS.[250]

This study adds to the controversy around using Ginkgo for the prevention of AMS, a controversy that was highlighted by the same authors when they published a review of all the other Ginkgo trials in this context.[251] From this review it was concluded that, given the mixed results, more studies are required in AMS, especially focusing on what is active in Ginkgo extracts.

Cognitive function

A review published in 2009 sought to find differential effects for the cognition-enhancing activity of standardised Ginkgo extract.[252] Included in the analysis were 29 randomised, double blind, placebo-controlled studies of chronic (greater than 4 weeks) administration providing data on function-specific cognitive tests in healthy and cognitively impaired volunteers of any age. (Some of the trials in this review are also covered individually or by review below.) Objective psychometric test results were examined for four cognitive domains (memory, attention, executive functions, intelligence) comprising 14 subfunctions (for example, for the domain of memory, the subfunctions were short- and long-term, visual and verbal memory). There was consistent evidence found from studies investigating mild cognitive impairment, depression, multiple sclerosis and healthy young and elderly volunteers that Ginkgo improves selective attention, some executive processes (working memory, cognitive flexibility) and long-term memory for verbal and non-verbal (visual) material. Little specific information could be obtained from trials for treatment of dementia. Except for one trial, standardised extract providing 24% to 25% ginkgo flavone glycosides and 6% terpenoids was administered. Daily doses ranged from 80 to 240 mg/day, with 120 mg/day the most common dosage (14 trials). The reviewers suggested that future trials should be more comprehensive and use psychometric standards to evaluate cognitive function. A lack of investigation of some functions (such as divided attention, an early feature of AD) tends to penalise Ginkgo and make it difficult to identify its strengths and weakness in terms of functions sensitive to its influence.

However, a systematic review that assessed clinical research to January 2007 concluded that standardised Ginkgo extract did not have a beneficial effect on cognitive function in healthy people under the age of 60 years. The review assessed randomised clinical trials in which Ginkgo was ingested as a single dose (seven trials) or over longer periods of time (eight trials, ranging from 2 days to 12 weeks).[253]

One placebo-controlled trial not included in this review measured the effect of Ginkgo (240 mg/day for 4 weeks) on vision-related neural function using electroencephalography in healthy adults aged from 41 to 83 years. No effect was found on the lower level physiological function of the visual system, but significant improvement was found when assessing higher order neural changes. The higher order visual system relies on additional cognitive processing, and may include cognitive aspects such as attention, recognition and memory.[254] Other key trials are reviewed below.

To elucidate the mechanism of clinical benefit of Ginkgo in the treatment of symptoms of impaired brain function in advanced age, its effect on cognitive information processing was investigated by means of long-latency auditory event-related potentials (P300). In a double blind, placebo-controlled study, 48 elderly patients with age-associated memory impairment received 120 mg/day of Ginkgo extract or placebo for 57 days. P300 latency was shortened in the Ginkgo group and this may reflect shorter stimulus-evaluation times.[255]

A 12-week, double blind, placebo-controlled study assessed the effects of Ginkgo extract (120 mg/day) on a wide range of cognitive abilities, executive function, attention and mood in 93 healthy older adults (55 to 79 years) and in 104 young adults (18 to 43 years). An enhancement of long-term memory in older adults (p=0.04) was demonstrated, while no other changes occurred in other cognitive measures.[256] A placebo-controlled, double blind trial involving 52 healthy students was conducted to assess the impact of Ginkgo on attention, memory and executive function.[257] Participants were randomly allocated to receive a single 120 mg dose of Ginkgo extract (n=26) or placebo (n=26), and were tested 4h later during the acute phase of the trial. Results demonstrated that an acute dose of Ginkgo significantly improved performance on the sustained-attention task and pattern-recognition memory task; however, there were no effects on working memory, planning, mental flexibility or mood. In the second part of the study, 40 of the students were randomly allocated to receive Ginkgo (120 mg/day; n=20) or placebo (n=20) for a 6-week period. After 6 weeks of treatment, there were no significant effects of Ginkgo on mood or any of the cognitive tests, with the authors commenting that tolerance may develop in young healthy people with normal cognition. A 4-week, randomised, double blind, placebo-controlled, parallel-group, monocentric study involving 66 healthy volunteers (aged 50 to 65 years) testing Ginkgo extract (240 mg/day) revealed that self-estimated quality of life significantly favoured Ginkgo treatment.[258]

A 6-week randomised, double blind, placebo-controlled, parallel-group trial was conducted involving 98 men and 132 women (>60 years of age) in general good health with MMSE scores greater than 26.[259] Participants were randomly assigned to receive a standardised Ginkgo extract (120 mg/day, n=115), or matching placebo (n=115) and were evaluated by a variety of cognitive outcome measures. Analysis of the modified ITT population of 219 participants indicated that there were no significant differences between treatment groups on any cognitive outcome measures as assessed via standard neuropsychological tests of learning, memory, attention, concentration and verbal fluency. A double blind, placebo-controlled study testing the acute effects of Ginkgo extract (120 mg) on the memory function in healthy older volunteers using the cognitive drug research battery of memory tests and the Rey auditory verbal learning task, discovered no acute effects of Ginkgo in any of the memory tests conducted.[260]

A short-term double blind, placebo-controlled design involving 60 healthy male volunteers was conducted to determine the nootropic effect of Ginkgo extract (120 mg/day for 5 days).[261] On the fifth day, after a 2h waiting period, all volunteers were given the Sternberg Memory Scanning Test, a reaction time control test, the vocabulary and digit span subtests of the WAIS-R and a prose recall test. No significant changes occurred with Ginkgo intervention on all the tests except the Sternberg Memory Scanning Test. A 30-day randomised, double blind, placebo-controlled clinical trial involving 61 participants was conducted using Ginkgo extract to assess nootropic activity.[262] Volunteers were administered a battery of validated neuropsychological tests before and after treatment, with results indicating significant improvements in speed of information processing working memory and executive processing.

A placebo-controlled, multi-dose, double blind, crossover study using 20 participants receiving Ginkgo extract (120 mg, 240 mg and 360 mg) or a matching placebo was conducted to assess cognitive performance via the Cognitive Drug Research computerised test battery immediately prior to dosing, and at 1, 2.5, 4 and 6h after.[263] Compared with the placebo, the acute administration of Ginkgo produced a number of significant changes in performance measures, most noticeably in speed of attention which was evident at 2.5h and was still present at 6h. Another study investigated the effects of acute doses of Ginkgo extract on memory and psychomotor performance in a randomised, double blind and placebo-controlled five-way crossover design.[264] Thirty-one volunteers with normal cognition (aged 30 to 59 years) received varying dosages of Ginkgo extract (120, 150, 240 or 300 mg/day) for 2 days. Psychometric tests concluded a more pronounced effect occurred on memory (particularly working memory) in the Ginkgo group compared with placebo. The study noted that the cognitive-enhancing effects of Ginkgo were more apparent in the 50 to 59 year-old sub-population.

Although the overall evidence of Ginkgo's nootropic effect on healthy volunteers is equivocal, it is likely that acute or short-term Ginkgo administration (which was assessed in the majority of studies) may not be long enough to influence cognitive enhancement in people with pre-existing optimum cognition. Ginkgo also appears to demonstrate the most profound enhancement in cases of cognitive deficit, which presents more commonly in older patients.

A number of clinical trials have found a beneficial effect on cognitive function for a combination of Ginkgo and ginseng (*Panax ginseng*). (These studies are reviewed in the ginseng monograph.)

Diabetes

Ginkgo extract improved peripheral nerve function and blood supply in patients with diabetic neuropathy (120 mg/day; controlled trial)[265] and enhanced nerve conduction and thermal perception in patients with diabetic neuropathy (dosage undefined; controlled trial).[266] It also improved colour vision in children and adolescents with type 1 diabetes not yet exhibiting retinopathy (120 mg/day; uncontrolled trial).[267]

Ginkgo extract (120 mg/day, taken for 12 weeks) improved motor nerve conduction velocities in diabetic patients with peripheral neuropathy in a small, placebo-controlled trial conducted in Korea.[268]

In a randomised, controlled trial from China, Ginkgo extract taken for 3 months had a protective effect on early diabetic nephropathy.[269] In a later trial, also from China, treatment with standardised Ginkgo extract (providing 57.6 mg/day of Ginkgo flavone glycosides and 14.4 mg/day of terpenoids) for 8 weeks improved vascular endothelial function in 64 patients with early stage diabetic nephropathy.[270]

Multiple sclerosis

After limited success in an open trial using intravenous ginkgolide B with multiple sclerosis (MS) patients in acute relapse, a double blind, placebo-controlled study was undertaken with 104 patients. There was no significant difference between placebo and the low or high-dose ginkgolide B groups.[271,272]

A blinded, controlled pilot trial using a Ginkgo extract (240 mg/day) in ameliorating the presentation of MS was conducted with 22 patients diagnosed via Poser criteria.[273] Results demonstrated that the Ginkgo group contained significantly more improved patients compared with placebo, as assessed via the outcome measures of fatigue (p>0.024), symptom severity (p>0.06) and functionality. Although the results should be interpreted with caution due to the small sample size, they indicate a therapeutic role of Ginkgo in treating MS. Another small trial (n=38) found that Ginkgo (240 mg/day for 12 weeks) significantly improved cognitive function in the Stroop test compared with placebo (p=0.008) in MS patients.[274]

Cancer

Regular use of Ginkgo extract was associated with a reduced risk of ovarian cancer, especially of the non-mucinous type, in an epidemiological study.[275] Ginkgo improved cognitive function, mood and quality of life in long-term survivors (6 months or more) of brain tumour who had received radiation therapy and were radiographically stable. The beneficial effect on mood was mostly due to reductions in fatigue and confusion (120 mg/day; uncontrolled trial).[276,277] Ginkgo also neutralised genotoxic damage (induced by radioiodine treatment) in Graves' disease patients (120 mg/day; randomised controlled trial)[278] and in Chernobyl accident recovery workers (120 mg/day; uncontrolled trial).[69]

The former trial assessed the effect of standardised Ginkgo extract on the appearance of micronuclei (MN) in lymphocytes from patients with Graves' disease after radioactive iodine therapy.[278] Twenty-five patients were randomly assigned to receive Ginkgo extract (120 mg/day) or placebo from 3 days before and up to 30 days after iodine therapy. During this time period all patients took the same dose of methimazole (an antithyroid drug).

The peak increase of MN and the mean increase of MN were significantly higher in the placebo group than in Ginkgo-treated patients. An early and sustained MN increase was observed in the placebo group, but in the Ginkgo-treated patients the increase never reached statistical significance. The protective effect of Ginkgo extract was still present after correcting the data for age, gender, thyroid hormone profile and bone marrow dose. Administration of Ginkgo did not have any adverse effect on the efficacy of the radiotherapy.

The summary results of a phase II, uncontrolled trial investigating Ginkgo in irradiated brain tumour survivors were published in 2010. Ginkgo extract (120 mg/day) was prescribed to 34 patients for 24 weeks. There was a high drop-out rate (56% completed the trial) due to perceived lack of efficacy and development of either intercurrent medical illness or brain tumour progression. Of the 19 remaining patients, there were significant improvements in some measures of cognitive function and quality of life.[279]

Premenstrual syndrome

In a controlled, multicentre, double blind study involving 165 women with congestive symptoms of premenstrual syndrome (PMS), patients received either 160 mg/day of Ginkgo extract or placebo. The medication was taken from day 16 of the menstrual cycle to day 5 of the following cycle. Ginkgo significantly improved breast tenderness. There were marked improvements in other symptoms for the Ginkgo group including oedema, anxiety, depression and headaches.[280]

The efficacy of 120 mg/day of Ginkgo standardised extract for the amelioration of the symptoms of PMS was also assessed in a later randomised, single blind, placebo-controlled clinical trial.[281] Trial participants were 90 students (average age around 22 years) with PMS living in dormitories of a medical university (Tehran). Participants took the Ginkgo or placebo from the day 16 of the menstrual cycle to the fifth day of the next cycle for two consecutive cycles.

Eighty-five (94.4%) participants completed the study. The two groups were similar in terms of demographic characteristics and overall severity of symptoms at baseline. After the intervention, there was a significant decrease in the overall severity of symptoms and physical and psychological symptoms in both the Ginkgo (23.68%) and placebo (8.74%) groups (p<0.001). However, the mean decrease in the severity of symptoms was significantly more in the Ginkgo group compared with the placebo group (p<0.001). The authors concluded that Ginkgo can reduce the severity of PMS symptoms.

Antidepressant-induced sexual dysfunction

A triple blind (investigator, patient, statistician), randomised, placebo-controlled, trial of Ginkgo extract (240 mg/day) was conducted in 24 patients (male and female) with sexual impairment due to antidepressant drugs.[282] A validated, sex (gender)-orientated questionnaire was recorded throughout the 12-week trial. The researchers commented that, although spectacular individual responses occurred in both groups, no statistically significant differences between Ginkgo and placebo were apparent. Another 8-week controlled study involving 37 men examined Ginkgo in the treatment of SSRI-evoked sexual dysfunction. (SSRI is selective serotonin reuptake inhibitor.) It revealed a high response in both placebo and Ginkgo groups, with no difference between the two.[283] In an uncontrolled trial, Ginkgo extract (average dose 207 mg/day) was found to be 84% effective in alleviating sexual dysfunction secondary to antidepressant drug use in 33 female and 30 male patients.[284] No adverse effects were reported. The inconsistency of results involving sexual dysfunction is conceivably due to small sample sizes, differing classes of antidepressants, the psychological component of the condition yielding a high placebo effect and individual psycho-physiological sexual responses. Essentially, the promising results of an earlier uncontrolled trial have not been supported by controlled studies.

Other conditions

An epidemiological study conducted in France assessed 3534 elderly people from 1988 to 2001. Participants aged 65 years or over and without dementia were included in the study. Those who took Ginkgo had a significantly lower risk of mortality in the long term, compared with non-users, even after adjustment for confounding factors.[285]

Ginkgo extract had a beneficial effect on sleep patterns in patients with major depression being treated with trimipramine (240 mg/day, pilot trial).[286]

In two separate trials, Ginkgo extract decreased capillary hyperpermeability in women with idiopathic oedema (160 to 240 mg/day, uncontrolled study)[287,288] and helped prevent retinal oedema following cataract surgery (160 mg/day, uncontrolled study).[289]

In a double blind, placebo-controlled trial involving 52 patients with vitiligo (with 47 evaluated), Ginkgo extract (120 mg/day) for 6 months induced a significant cessation of active progression and depigmentation (p=0.006).[290] Repigmentation was observed in 10 patients in the Ginkgo group versus two patients receiving placebo. The extract was well tolerated.

Toxicology and other safety data

Toxicology

The following LD_{50} data have been recorded for Ginkgo extract and its constituents:

Substance	Route, model	LD_{50}	Reference
Standardised Ginkgo extract	Oral, mice	7.7 g/kg	291,292
Standardised Ginkgo extract	ip mice	1.9 g/kg	292
Standardised Ginkgo extract	iv mice	1.1 g/kg	292
Standardised Ginkgo extract	ip rats	2.1 g/kg	292
Standardised Ginkgo extract	iv rats	1.1 g/kg	292
Ginkgo leaf extract fraction (ginkgolic acids 16%; biflavones 6.7%)	Injection, hen's eggs	1.8 mg/egg (33 ppm)	293
Ginkgo leaf extract fraction (ginkgolic acids 58%; biflavones 0.02%)	Injection, hen's eggs	3.5 mg/egg (64 ppm)	293
Ginkgo leaf extract fraction (ginkgolic acids 1%; biflavones 16%)	Injection, hen's eggs	250 mg/egg (4540 ppm)	293

The toxicity data indicate standardised Ginkgo extract has very low toxicity. No deaths occurred in rats orally administered up to 10 g/kg of standardised extract. Chronic oral toxicity studies indicated no evidence of biochemical, haematological or histological damage or impairment of hepatic or renal function in rats and dogs orally administered standardised Ginkgo extract for 6 months. Doses began at 20 and 100 mg/kg/day and gradually increased to 500 mg/kg/day in rats and 400 mg/kg/day in dogs. Light and transient vasodilatory effects were observed in dogs at the 100 mg/kg dose and became more pronounced with increasing dose.[291,292,294]

No carcinogenic effects were observed in rats orally administered standardised leaf extract for 104 weeks at doses of 4, 20 and 100 mg/kg,[292] or in rats fed Ginkgo seed for almost a year.[295] Standardised leaf extract did not demonstrate mutagenic activity using in vitro tests with and without metabolic activation, or in vivo tests in mice after oral administration of doses up to 20 g/kg.[291,292]

No adverse effects were observed in human volunteers administered pure ginkgolides at doses of 720 mg (acute) or 360 mg/day for 1 week.[296]

Fractions of Ginkgo leaf extract containing high concentrations of ginkgolic acids have been shown to be cytotoxic against human and animal cell lines in vitro[297] and immunotoxic in vivo after subplantar injection.[298,299] They were also embryotoxic in the hen's egg test (see left). The authors of the last study did not exclude the possibility that other constituents such as the biflavones may amplify the adverse effects of ginkgolic acids.[292] Ginkgolic acids demonstrated neurotoxic,[300] genotoxic and tumour promoting[301] activities in vitro.

Contraindications

Ginkgo preparations are contraindicated in those with a known sensitivity.

Special warnings and precautions

Caution should be observed when prescribing Ginkgo to patients with coagulation disorders or concomitantly with anticoagulant or antiplatelet medication. (See Side effects and Interactions.) This is based on poorly described case reports and adverse effects are not typically expected.

Patients about to undergo surgery are advised to stop taking Ginkgo 5 to 7 days beforehand due to possible (but very minor) risk of increased bleeding tendency.[302,303]

Ginkgo preparations that contain appreciable quantities of ginkgolic acids may pose a risk of allergic reaction.

Interactions

See Appendix C for the data and recommendations regarding potential herb-drug interactions for Ginkgo that are deemed to be clinically relevant.

A 2002 publication listed 185 reports of adverse effects in connection with Ginkgo, with 20 reports related to bleeding disorders. It was concluded that patients using Ginkgo extracts are at risk of suffering complications during surgery or spontaneous bleeding, and there is an increased danger of bleeding with concomitant use of anticoagulant or antiplatelet agents.[304] However, there is still no strong evidence for this. Treatment with standardised Ginkgo extract (100 mg/day) for 4 weeks in patients who were stabilised on long-term warfarin had no significant influence on their response to warfarin in a randomised, double blind, placebo-controlled, crossover trial (average age of patients was 64.5 years). The stability of international normalised ratio (INR) values was confirmed and major bleedings or thromboembolic events were not observed.[305]

Another clinical study investigated the effect of Ginkgo on the pharmacokinetics and pharmacodynamics of warfarin and clotting status.[306] The open label, three-way crossover, randomised study involved 12 healthy male volunteers who received a single 25 mg dose of warfarin alone or after 7 days of pretreatment with Ginkgo. The trial determined that INR values and platelet aggregation were not affected by administration of Ginkgo. The mean ratio of apparent clearance for S-warfarin was 1.05 and for R-warfarin was 1.00 when co-administered with Ginkgo. Other pharmacokinetic parameters for warfarin were not affected by Ginkgo. These results were replicated later in a similar trial by the same research team, demonstrating that the S-warfarin concentration and response (prothrombin complex activity) data from 24 healthy volunteers who received a single warfarin dose (25 mg) were not altered by Ginkgo administration.[307]

A randomised, controlled study involving 24 outpatients on stable, long-term warfarin treatment was undertaken, assessing the impact of Ginkgo extract (100 mg/day) on INR over a 4-week period. Results indicated that INR was stable during all treatment periods, with no bleeding episodes occurring.[308]

A substudy within the National Institutes of Health-funded Dementia Prevention (GEM) Study investigated whether Ginkgo standardised extract would affect platelet function. Fifty-one patients had platelet function analysis performed at baseline and at 6-month follow-up. Patients were randomised to receive Ginkgo (240 mg/day) or placebo. There was no significant difference between the placebo and Ginkgo groups. Fifteen patients were taking aspirin but there was no difference in closure time at either time point, and aspirin did not show any interaction with Ginkgo.[309] A double blind, double-dummy procedure involving 50 healthy male volunteers (20 to 44 years) using 120 or 240 mg/day of Ginkgo extract in combination with acetylsalicylic acid (aspirin) demonstrated no additional effect on bleeding time, coagulation parameters or platelet activity in response to various anticoagulant-provoking agonists.[310] Aspirin given alone clearly prolonged bleeding time, whereas the combination of aspirin and Ginkgo exerted similar effects to aspirin alone on all coagulation parameters measured, including bleeding time (aspirin alone: 4.1 min before therapy, 6.2 min after therapy; aspirin plus Ginkgo: 4.2 min before therapy, 6.3 min after therapy; ratio of means: 1.01, 90% CI 0.86 to 1.19) and agonist-induced platelet aggregation (collagen-induced platelet aggregation: 84.5% before therapy, 81.0% after aspirin therapy; aspirin plus Ginkgo: 86.6% before therapy, 81.0% after therapy; ratio of means: 1.00, 90% CI 0.95 to 1.05; adenosine diphosphate-induced platelet aggregation with aspirin: 72.6% before therapy, 47.2% after therapy; with aspirin plus Ginkgo: 71.7% before therapy, 44.8% after therapy; ratio of means: 0.95, 90% CI 0.85 to 1.06).

A study in Taiwan in 2002 found no clinically significant change in coagulation parameters (including INR, bleeding time and clotting time) in healthy volunteers taking standardised Ginkgo extract (120 mg/day) and warfarin. In 21 clinical cases, no significant change in INR was found after adding Ginkgo to existing warfarin therapy.[311]

A 2008 review of studies published up to March 2007 found four trials (included above) and seven case reports pertaining to the potential interaction of drugs that can elevate the risk of bleeding with Ginkgo.[312] As noted above, the trials did not provide any evidence for an interaction of aspirin or warfarin with Ginkgo. Establishing causality from the case reports was difficult due to the generally low quality of the reports and the presence of confounding factors, with scant evidence to suggest any adverse interaction. An excerpt from the Mediplus database in Germany failed to show any increased bleeding risk from the combination of Ginkgo with antiplatelet or anticoagulant drugs.

Studies published since the March 2007 cut-off date of this review are consistent with its overall conclusions. For example, it was confirmed that standardised Ginkgo extract (300 mg/day) combined with aspirin did not have an impact on bleeding parameters among older adults at risk of cardiovascular disease.[313]

An interaction was observed in one clinical study for a single dose of Ginkgo extract (120 mg) combined with the antiplatelet drug cilostazol. The bleeding time prolongation of cilostazol was extended by Ginkgo. There was no change in platelet aggregation ex vivo or clotting time. Also there was no significant correlation between prolongation of bleeding time and inhibition of platelet aggregation. No interaction was found between Ginkgo and the antiplatelet drug clopidogrel.[314] Dosing of Ginkgo (extract undefined, 160 mg/day) to healthy volunteers over 7 days found no effect on the pharmacokinetics of cilostazol or on platelet aggregation or bleeding time.[315]

In Korea, Ginkgo extract is administered with ticlopidine (an antiplatelet drug, chemically similar to clopidogrel) for the prevention of ischaemic stroke and acute coronary syndrome.[316] In a single-dose study, standardised Ginkgo extract (80 mg) combined with ticlopidine exerted no significant additional effect on bleeding time or platelet aggregation.[317] No effect on the pharmacokinetics of the drug was found when Ginkgo extract (120 mg/day) was taken for 3 days.[318] Both trials involved healthy volunteers.

Concerns have also been expressed about the potential interaction of Ginkgo with antiepileptic drugs. In an innocuously entitled paper, 'Ginkgo biloba and Ginkgotoxin', two German scientists drew the rather radical conclusion that the low levels of ginkgotoxin found in products containing Ginkgo leaf extracts '… can have a detrimental effect on a person's health condition'. Ginkgotoxin should not be confused with the ginkgolic acids. The latter are irritant and allergenic compounds controlled to quite low levels in appropriately made standardised extracts of Ginkgo leaves (as noted previously). Ginkgotoxin is 4'-O-methylpyridoxine, a vitamin B6 antagonist. It occurs in relatively high levels in Ginkgo nuts and is believed to be responsible for the poisoning that occurs after the ingestion of unprocessed nuts. It is also found at much lower levels in Ginkgo leaves.

On the basis of their in vitro research, the authors proposed that ginkgotoxin primarily acts as a toxicant by inhibiting vitamin B6 phosphorylation.[319] This could deplete the brain of phosphorylated B6 vitamers, resulting in a reduction of glutamate metabolism which in turn would increase neuronal excitability due to lower levels of GABA. Poisoning with Ginkgo nuts certainly causes epileptiform seizures, unconsciousness and leg paralysis.[319] Children are especially vulnerable to the toxin and vitamin B6 administration typically leads to full recovery with no serious complications.

The major thesis of the authors was that even the very low levels of ginkgotoxin found in typical daily doses of standardised Ginkgo leaf extract, estimated by them to be 11.4 to 58.6 μg, might increase the risk of seizures in epileptic patients. In support of this, they cited adverse event reports linking Ginkgo leaf to seizures. In the closing paragraphs, a rather tangential argument was proposed that Ginkgo leaf might also present a risk to epileptic patients by interacting with their medications.

One commentary expressed doubts over the relevance of conclusions from test tube research involving high doses of ginkgotoxin, when a pharmacokinetic study found that the compound was below detection limits (1 nM/mL) in human plasma after normal oral doses of Ginkgo extract. Supporting this contention, documentation from extensive clinical trial experience and records for 150 million daily doses per year for more than two decades have not recorded one case of epileptic seizure attributed to Ginkgo extract.[320]

Reports of seizures linked to Ginkgo essentially come from three sources: the US FDA Nutritionals database, which has been shut down due to its poor accuracy and reliability, and the articles by Granger in 2001[321] and Kupiec and Raj in 2005.[322] However, the latter two publications could be describing a herb-drug interaction. Kupiec and Raj certainly provide some evidence that Ginkgo might reduce the levels of some anticonvulsant drugs via increased hepatic metabolism.[322] Ginkgo has been found in a clinical trial to induce CYP2C19 activity, an enzyme involved in the metabolism of some anticonvulsants.[323] For this reason the herb should be used with caution in epileptic patients controlled by medication, despite the relatively low number of reported cases.

A brief review of the potential interaction of Ginkgo with other drugs follows. An elderly patient with AD developed a coma a few days after starting the SSRI antidepressant trazodone (40 mg/day), which has hypnotic and sedative effects, in conjunction with Ginkgo extract (160 mg/day). Previously she had been taking bromazepam (3.5 mg/day), donepezil (5 mg/day) and vitamin E (1200 mg/day). It was postulated that sedation was caused by increased GABAergic activity via ginkgo flavonols acting directly at the benzodiazepine receptor and indirectly by inducing CYP34A to increase the metabolism of trazodone to an active compound that also has GABAergic activity.[324] However, this case certainly does not provide conclusive evidence of a drug interaction with Ginkgo.

An elderly patient started treatment with a thiazide diuretic for elevated blood pressure. She then started taking Ginkgo and after a week her blood pressure was found to have increased further. Her blood pressure decreased gradually when both medications were ceased.[325] It was unclear how soon the Ginkgo was started after the thiazide diuretic and the interpretation of this case as a herb-drug interaction is highly questionable, although it has been widely recorded as such.

Concerns have been raised that Ginkgo extract may increase the hepatic metabolic clearance rate of insulin and hypoglycaemic agents in type 2 diabetes mellitus patients, resulting in reduced insulin-mediated glucose metabolism and elevated blood glucose.[326] However, no adverse effects of any significance have been reported for blood glucose levels and for laboratory results of glucose control in 10 trials conducted from 1980 to 1998 where Ginkgo extract was administered to diabetic and non-diabetic patients.[4,327]

There are many published in vitro, in vivo and human studies investigating the potential impact of Ginkgo extract on the metabolism of drugs (some are mentioned above and several are included in Appendix C). A 2010 review concluded that the findings in humans (which must be given priority) were conflicting and further studies are needed to elucidate the role of Ginkgo in altered drug absorption due to cytochrome P450 (CYP) and P-glycoprotein (P-gp) inhibition.[328] Three clinical studies excluded any effect of Ginkgo on CYP3A4, but two other studies with the probe drugs alprazolam and midazolam suggest an inhibition of this enzyme. Ginkgo did not interact with drug substrates of CYP1A2, CYP2E1 or CYP2D6 (as reported in three studies). One study found that Ginkgo altered the metabolism of the CYP2C19 substrate omeprazole in a genotype-dependent manner, but a different study did not find this for a different CYP2C19 probe drug (voriconazole).

The review did note that drugs that are P-gp substrates should be monitored in conjunction with Ginkgo. Some studies have reported a high between-subject variability of the bioavailability of digoxin (a P-gp substrate) and the pharmacokinetics of talinol (another P-gp substrate) was modified by long-term intake of Ginkgo in two different studies by the same research group.[328]

Use in pregnancy and lactation

Category B1 – no increase in frequency of malformation or other harmful effects on the fetus from limited use in women. No evidence of increased fetal damage in animal studies.

One review hypothesised that Ginkgo may be a risk factor for excessive blood loss during delivery, but there are no reports of this in the literature.[4]

Oral administration of standardised Ginkgo extract to rats (up to 1600 mg/kg/day) and rabbits (up to 900 mg/kg/day) did not cause teratogenicity or embryotoxicity or affect reproduction.[291,292] In contrast, a study from Pakistan attributed malformations in the offspring of mice to Ginkgo extract at 100 mg/kg/day, but found no teratogenic effects at 78 mg/kg/day.[329]

A commercial Ginkgo extract and fractions of Ginkgo extract containing high concentrations of ginkgolic acids demonstrated embryotoxic effects in the hen's egg test when injected into freshly fertilised chick eggs (see Toxicology).[293,330] The dose of the commercial Ginkgo extract was not specified.[330]

A study claimed to have identified the highly toxic alkaloid colchicine in a commercial Ginkgo preparation and linked this to their discovery of the presence of colchicine in the placental blood of women who had used herbal supplements. The herbal supplements taken by the women were not identified and it was not clear whether Ginkgo was one of them.[331] Colchicine has never been detected in Ginkgo previously and studies conducted since the findings were released have failed to detect colchicine in commercial preparations.[332–334] The validity of the colchicine findings and the conclusions drawn from them have been vigorously criticised.[332,335] (See Chapter 5 for a further discussion of this issue.)

Pretreatment of hamster oocytes in vitro with Ginkgo (1 mg/mL) significantly reduced penetration by human sperm compared to a control. However, significant reduction of sperm penetration was not observed at a concentration of 0.1 mg/mL, which represents typical human exposure for in vitro research.[336] (See Chapter 5 for further discussion of this issue.)

No data are available regarding the use of Ginkgo in breastfeeding mothers. However, only small amounts of flavonol glycosides and terpene lactones accumulate in the serum and the serum half-life of terpene lactones is relatively short. This would reduce the amount available to enter the breast milk and the possibility of accumulation in the infant.[4]

A 2006 systematic review examined the literature for evidence on the use, safety and pharmacology of Ginkgo in the context of pregnancy and lactation.[337] The review found some weak scientific evidence that Ginkgo has antiplatelet activity that might be of concern during labour because of prolonged bleeding times. It concluded that the safety of Ginkgo in lactation is unknown and recommended that it be avoided during breastfeeding until more safety information is generated.

Effects on ability to drive or operate machinery

Possible improvement of these functions, especially in older subjects.

Side effects

Reviews and meta-analyses of clinical trials have shown that standardised Ginkgo extract has a remarkably low incidence of side effects[177,291,338,339] and there were no differences between Ginkgo and placebo in adverse event profiles.[291,340,341] Two adverse events were reported in 314000 patient years of use in 1988. Only 0.5% of 9772 patients reported adverse events over 44 clinical trials. Adverse events reported have included mild gastrointestinal complaints, headache, dizziness, allergic skin reactions and palpitations.[291] Palpitations and ventricular arrhythmia have been associated with Ginkgo use in a case report.[342]

More than 5 million units of Ginkgo preparations were sold in Germany in 1998 alone.[343] German authorities recorded 117 reports of adverse effects in connection with preparations containing Ginkgo from 1990 to 2000, including non-standardised extracts, homeopathics and multi-ingredient preparations. Ginkgo was indicated as the only medication in 65 cases.[344] By 2002 the number of adverse reactions was 185. In fact, given the widespread use of Ginkgo, the number of published adverse reactions is remarkably low.

The primary concern of an adverse reaction occurring with Ginkgo commonly expressed in the literature is an increase of bleeding or an initiation of spontaneous bleeding, as documented in several case studies (discussed below). A 2005 review of spontaneous bleeding associated with Ginkgo use reported 15 published cases of purported Ginkgo-induced bleeding events, including one new case report described in the publication. The review, however, commented there was very limited evidence to support Ginkgo being a risk factor for bleeding due the documented cases involving concomitant drug use, inadequate reporting or a lack of re-challenge to establish causation.[345] The review did document a new case, where re-challenge with Ginkgo evoked spontaneous bleeding in a 73-year-old Caucasian male who reported haemorrhoidal bleeding and increased bleeding from minor skin trauma. He was taking a standardised Ginkgo preparation (75 mg/day). After stopping Ginkgo (6-week washout period) his bleeding time was assessed via a 'blinded' laboratory test at 5.5 min (normal range 2.5 to 9.5 min). When Ginkgo use was reinitiated, his bleeding time increased to >15 min and he started noticing occasional ecchymoses, although coagulation studies were still normal. After discontinuing Ginkgo, the patient experienced no further haematological abnormalities (although over the next few years he developed Alzheimer's dementia).

Other cases of spontaneous cerebral or extracerebral bleeding[346–351] attributed to the intake of Ginkgo preparations have also been reported. It was not possible to establish Ginkgo as the cause in any of these cases. Prolonged bleeding times were noted in two of the bleeding cases,[346,348] although the bleeding time quoted in one is widely considered to be within the normal range.[348] In another case involving spontaneous hyphema, the authors state that, after extensive ophthalmological and haematological investigations, no putative causes were recorded other than Ginkgo intake.[352] Use of Ginkgo has also been attributed to one case of postoperative bleeding following laparoscopic cholecystectomy.[303] Other isolated cases of spontaneous bleeding have been attributed to drug interactions with Ginkgo (see Interactions above).

Contrary to these isolated case histories, a 7-day haematological study involving 40 elderly subjects (65 to 79 years of age) who were administered a Ginkgo extract (240 mg/day) demonstrated no change on primary haemostasis.[353] The complete set of PFA-100 in vitro bleeding time and coagulation parameters including prothrombin time, activated partial thromboplastin time and INR confirmed no statistically significant prolongation in bleeding time or coagulation parameters in patients. A prospective, double blind, randomised, placebo-controlled trial tested a Ginkgo extract (120, 240 or 480 mg over 14 days) in 32 healthy men to evaluate any haematological changes.[354] Results revealed no alterations of platelet function or coagulation and no adverse bleeding events.

Another 2005 systematic review of case reports concluded that the causality between Ginkgo intake and bleeding is unlikely.[355] A systematic review of eight randomised controlled trials, also published in 2005, concluded that the available evidence does not demonstrate that Ginkgo extract causes significant changes in blood coagulation parameters.[356]

The 2008 review cited under Interactions also sought to understand the evidence for the impact of Ginkgo on haemostasis and the case reports of increased bleeding.[312] None of the trials reviewed (including some summarised above) demonstrated any convincing evidence for the impact of Ginkgo on haemostasis. The 21 case reports identified were of low quality. Not only was there variability in Ginkgo products, but also the documentation of key factors such as product name, standardisation and other potentially active ingredients were generally absent. The low quality of these case reports casts doubts on causality. The large Mediplus database study found the frequency of reported bleeding events in patients taking Ginkgo was the same as in patients not taking Ginkgo. The review concluded that, similar to most medicinal herbs, the possibility of a rare idiosyncratic bleeding event due to Ginkgo use is very unlikely, but cannot be excluded.[312]

From 2000 to 2008 the GEM study assessed 3069 healthy volunteers treated with standardised Ginkgo extract (240 mg/day) or placebo for incident dementia. There were no statistically significant differences in the rate of major bleeding, and no difference between the groups for the incidence of bleeding in the patients taking aspirin. However, compliance during the trial was low.[167]

To date, the balance of the evidence indicates that Ginkgo has an extremely low chance of provoking spontaneous bleeding, if at all. Rare cases of idiosyncratic increases in bleeding may occur in certain individuals, hence monitoring is advised in cases of known haematological abnormalities, close to surgery or in high-dosage with concomitant use of anticoagulants and antiplatelet drugs.

A substantial part of the misunderstanding that Ginkgo alters haemostasis probably arises from knowledge of its capacity to enhance tissue perfusion and inhibit PAF. But these are both quite separate phenomena.

PAF is a weak activator of platelets not of primary importance to the process of haemostasis, and its inhibition is unlikely to cause haemorrhage.[312] PAF-mediated aggregation of human platelets in vitro was half-maximally inhibited by ginkgolide B at a concentration of 2.5 μg/mL. (Ginkgolide B is present at about 0.5% in standardised Ginkgo extract.) Higher concentrations were required for the other ginkgolides. These concentrations are more than 100 times higher than peak plasma levels measured after oral intake of Ginkgo extract at doses of 120 to 240 mg.

Some clinical studies show that standardised Ginkgo extract increases blood flow to and within an organ, and to tissues, or it may have a regulatory effect (dilating or constricting blood vessels depending upon the condition). Increases in blood flow mean Ginkgo improves oxygen and nutrient supply to the organs and tissues, but this does not mean it increases the risk of haemorrhage.

Ginkgo has also decreased blood viscosity in healthy volunteers[143,357] and patients (often with initially elevated levels),[195,267,358,359] but blood viscosity is related to friction among red blood cells and is a measure of blood flow and tissue perfusion. In a trial involving healthy elderly volunteers, in addition to reducing blood viscosity, Ginkgo improved cerebral perfusion and cognitive function.[360]

Ginkgo has been shown to modify circulating platelet aggregates in pathological conditions. In a small, randomised, placebo-controlled trial, Ginkgo extract (120 mg/day) over a period of 12 weeks reduced the elevated platelet reactivity index (a measure of platelet aggregates) in elderly patients with cerebral insufficiency and 'cerebral vascular risk' (risk of stroke).[360] Ginkgo appears to have shifted elevated platelet aggregates towards normal. Note that the test system used did not assess the capacity of platelets to aggregate under normal physiological conditions.

Cases of Stevens-Johnson syndrome associated with the use of preparations containing Ginkgo have been reported.[344,361] Stevens-Johnson syndrome is an acute inflammatory skin disease that affects the skin and mucous membranes of the face and mouth.

Severe circulatory disturbances, local phlebitis, allergic skin reactions and anaphylactic shock may occur with parenteral use of standardised Ginkgo extracts.[338] Injectable preparations have been disallowed in some European countries.[362]

Hypersensitivity reactions to standardised extracts of Ginkgo leaf are extremely rare, indicating that it has a very low potential for sensitisation.[291,363] However, cases of allergic contact dermatitis to Ginkgo fruit pulp have been repeatedly reported.[364] Gastrointestinal disturbances (tenesmus, stomatitis and proctitis) have also been reported after consumption of the fruit.[338,365] Provocation tests in patients and animal experiments have identified alkylphenols such as ginkgolic acids as the causative constituents.[298] Tests in guinea pigs have shown that, although sensitisation developed with purified ginkgolic acids, it failed to occur to leaf extract containing approximately 1000 ppm ginkgolic acids,[364] which is 200 times higher than the level deemed acceptable for standardised extracts. Nonetheless, consumption of Ginkgo extracts containing ginkgolic acids above acceptable levels may constitute a risk to those who are allergic to plants from the Anacardiaceae family, such as poison ivy and cashew, because of cross-reactivity between the alkylphenols of the two families.[299]

A diffuse morbilliform eruption occurred in a 66-year-old woman about 1 week after the ingestion of a Ginkgo preparation that was suspected to be due to alkylphenols.[366] The alkylphenol level of the preparation was not measured.

Manic psychosis has been questionably associated with the use of Ginkgo in two sisters who had been consuming the herb for approximately 2 years at a dosage twice that recommended. A few months before onset of symptoms the dose had been further increased. Family psychiatric history was significant for paranoid schizophrenia on the paternal side. They were stabilised on medication and 6 months later were free of all medications and were not manifesting psychiatric symptoms. Almost 1 year after the first episode one sister had a relapse while not taking Ginkgo.[367] One case of hypomania has been reported; however, the patient (with a history of mild traumatic brain injury) combined an unknown Ginkgo preparation with St John's wort, fluoxetine and buspirone. Hence the exact cause of the adverse reaction cannot be determined.[294]

Overdosage

Intoxication generally occurs after ingestion of large numbers of Ginkgo seeds and young children are more vulnerable to poisoning. Those under the age of 6 comprise about 74% of cases.[368] Symptoms include vomiting, diarrhoea, irritability, seizure and in some cases death.[369-372] The number of seeds consumed in reported fatalities ranged from 15 to 574 pieces.[369] The neurotoxin 4'-O-methylpyroxidine, which can cause vitamin B6 deficiency symptoms as noted previously, is thought to be responsible.[371,372] Intravenous vitamin B6 (2 mg/kg) has been used to treat Ginkgo seed poisoning.[369]

As mentioned previously, the stems and leaves of Ginkgo also contain 4'-O-methylpyroxidine (ginkgotoxin).[373,374] This toxin has been measured at levels of 42 µg/g fresh weight of stem[209] and up to 80 µg/g in raw seed.[208] The highest concentration of 4'-O-methylpyroxidine in medicinal preparations tested conferred a daily dose of 60 µg.[374] In contrast, the acute oral toxic dose was measured at 11 mg/kg in guinea-pigs.[371,372] The ingestion of normal quantities of Ginkgo extracts and of boiled Ginkgo seeds (eaten in Japan) is not expected to cause detrimental effects,[373,374] although ingestion of seeds should be limited, particularly in children. In extreme cases of overdosage of Ginkgo extract the phytochemicals noted above may cause toxic effects, but even this is unlikely given the low toxicity observed for the extract.

Safety in children

No side effects were observed in infants (2 to 7 months old) with hypoxic-ischaemic encephalopathy treated with standardised Ginkgo extract (0.5 mL/day, oral) for 2 months.[375]

Standardised Ginkgo extract has also been used to treat asthma in children (see previous).

Cases of poisoning have been reported in young children after ingestion of a large number of Ginkgo seeds, 50 or more in some cases (see Overdosage).[369-372] Japanese authorities advise that children should not eat more than five seeds (nuts) per day and that they should not eat seeds every day.[368] However, the risk of toxic or adverse effects in children for Ginkgo leaf extract is very low.

Regulatory status in selected countries

Ginkgo is included on the General Sale List in the UK.

Standardised Ginkgo leaf extract is covered by a positive German Commission E monograph, but Ginkgo leaf is covered by a negative Commission E monograph.

Ginkgo is official in the *British Pharmacopoeia* 2012 and the *European Pharmacopoeia* 2012.

In the USA Ginkgo is official in the *United States Pharmacopeia-National Formulary* (USP 34-NF 29, 2011).

Ginkgo does not have GRAS status. However, it is freely available as a 'dietary supplement' in the USA under DSHEA legislation (Dietary Supplement Health and Education Act of 1994).

Ginkgo is not included in Part 4 of Schedule 4 of the Therapeutic Goods Act Regulations of Australia and is freely available for sale.

References

1. Bensky D, Gamble A. *Chinese Herbal Medicine Materia Medica*. Seattle: Eastland Press; 1986. pp. 560–561.
2. Allaby M, ed. *The Concise Oxford Dictionary of Botany*. Oxford: Oxford University Press; 1992. p. 177.
3. Willard T. *The Wild Rose Scientific Herbal*. Calgary: Wild Rose College Natural Healing; 1991. p. 142.
4. McKenna DJ, Jones K, Hughes K, et al. *Botanical Medicines: The Desk Reference for Major Herbal Supplements*, 2nd ed. New York: The Haworth Herbal Press; 2002. pp. 480–448.
5. Hong Kong Consumer Council. *Test Casts Doubt on Clinical Benefits of Ginkgo Leaf Products with Non-Standardized Extract*. Choice No. 289, 15 November 2002.
6. Ding S, Dudley E, Plummer S, et al. *Rapid Commun Mass Spectrom*. 2006;20(18):2753–2760.
7. Wagner H, Bladt S. *Plant Drug Analysis: A Thin Layer Chromatography Atlas*, 2nd ed. Berlin: Springer-Verlag; 1996. p. 237.
8. DeFeudis FV. *Ginkgo Biloba Extract (Egb 761): Pharmacological Activities and Clinical Applications*. Amsterdam: Elsevier; 1991. pp. 10–13.
9. Singh B, Kaur P, Gopichand *Fitoterapia*. 2008;79(6):401–418.
10. Blumenthal M, ed. *The Complete German Commission E Monographs: Therapeutic Guide to Herbal Medicines*. Austin: American Botanical Council; 1998. p. 137.
11. World Health Organization. *WHO Monographs on Selected Medicinal Plants*, vol. 1. Geneva: WHO; 1999. p. 158.
12. van Beek TA, Montoro P. *J Chromatogr A*. 2009;1216(11):2002–2032.
13. Duff Sloley B, Tawfik SR, Scherban KA, Tam YK. *J Food Drug Anal*. 2003;11(2):102–107.
14. Saevels J, Corthout J. *J Pharm Belg*. 2005;60(4):129–134.
15. Chung KF, Dent G, McCusker M, et al. *Lancet*. 1987;1(8527):248–251.
16. Braquet P, Touqui L, Shen TY, et al. *Pharmacol Rev*. 1987;39:97–145.
17. Lane HC, Fauci AS. *Ann Intern Med*. 1985;103(5):714–718.
18. Stanworth DR, Griffiths HR, Braquet P. *New Trends Lipid Mediat Res*. 1988;2:18–25.
19. Guinot P, Summerhayes C, Berdah L, et al. *Lancet*. 1988;2(8602):114.
20. Roberts NM, McCusker M, Chung KF, et al. *Br J Clin Pharmacol*. 1988;26:65–72.
21. Braquet P, Etienne A, Touvay C, et al. *Lancet*. 1985;1:1501.
22. Vilain B, Lagente V, Touvay C, et al. *Pharmacol Res Commun*. 1986;18(suppl):119–126.
23. Barnes PJ, Chung KF, Page CP. *Pharmacol Rev*. 1988;40(1):49–84.
24. Bourgain RH, Maes L, Andries R, et al. *Prostaglandins*. 1986;32(1):142–144.
25. Braquet P. *Adv Prostagland Thromboxane Leukot Res*. 1986;16:179–198.
26. Strømgaard K, Nakanishi K. *Angew Chem Int Ed Engl*. 2004;43(13):1640–1658.
27. Braquet P, Paubert-Braquet M, Koltai M, et al. *Trends Pharmacol Sci*. 1989;10(1):23–30.
28. Krieglstein J, Ausmeier F. *International Congress on Phytotherapy*, Munich, September 10–13, 1992.

29. Smith PF, Maclennan K, Darlington CL. *J Ethnopharmacol*. 1996;50:131–139.

30. Oberpichler H, Beck T, Abdel-Rahman MM, et al. *Pharmacol Res Commun*. 1988;20(5):349–368.

31. Duverger D, DeFeudis FV, Drieu K. *Gen Pharmacol*. 1995;26(6):1375–1383.

32. Hu B, Sun SG, Mei YW. *Zhongguo Zhong Xi Yi Jie He Za Zhi*. 2003;23(6):436–440.

33. Safi N, Galley P. *Bordeaux Med*. 1977;10:171–176.

34. Schaffler K, Reeh PW. *Arzneimittelforschung*. 1985;35:1283–1286.

35. Borzeix MG, Labos M, Hartl C, et al. *Sem Hop (Paris)*. 1980;56:393–398.

36. Hansel R, Haas H. *Therapie Mit Phytopharmaka*. Berlin: Springer-Verlag; 1984. p. 76.

37. Spinnewyn B, Blavet N, Clostre F. *Presse Med*. 1986;15:1511–1515.

38. Le Poncin-Laffitte M, Rapin J, Rapin JR. *Arch Int Pharmacodyn*. 1980;243: 236–244.

39. Gabard B, Chatterjee SS. *Naunyn Schmiedebergs Arch Pharmacol*. 1980;311(suppl):R68, Abstract 271.

40. Hansel R, Haas H. *Therapie Mit Phytopharmaka*. Berlin: Springer-Verlag; 1984. pp. 68–69.

41. Reuse-Blom S, Drieu K. *Presse Med*. 1986;15:1520–1523.

42. Zhou QP, Lu JF, Wang HP, Xia Q. *Zhejiang Da Xue Xue Bao Yi Xue Ban*. 2010;39(4):442–447.

43. Saleem S, Zhuang H, Biswal S, et al. *Stroke*. 2008;39(12):3389–3396.

44. Zhuang H, Pin S, Christen Y, Doré S. *Cell Mol Biol (Noisy-le-grand)*. 2002;48(6):647–653.

45. Janssens D, Michiels C, Delaive E, et al. *Biochem Pharmacol*. 1995;50(7):991–999.

46. Punkt K, Welt K, Schaffranietz L. *Acta Histochem*. 1995;97(1):67–79.

47. Heiss WD, Zeiler K. *Pharmakother*. 1978;1:137–144.

48. Boelsma E, Lamers RJ, Hendriks HF, et al. *Planta Med*. 2004;70(11):1052–1057.

49. Mehlsen J, Drabaek H, Wiinberg N, Winther K. *Clin Physiol Funct Imaging*. 2002;22(6):375–378.

50. Jung F, Mrowietz C, Kiesewetter H, et al. *Arzneimittelforschung*. 1990;40(5):589–598.

51. Xia SH, Fang DC. *Chin Med J (Engl)*. 2007;120(10):922–928.

52. Defeudis FV. *Pharmacol Res*. 2002;46(6):565–568.

53. Kiewert C, Kumar V, Hildmann O, et al. *Brain Res*. 2007;1128(1):70–78.

54. Luo Y. *Life Sci*. 2006;78(18):2066–2072.

55. Bastianetto S, Ramassamy C, Doré S, et al. *Eur J Neurosci*. 2000;12(6):1882–1890.

56. Rhein V, Giese M, Baysang G, et al. *PLoS One*. 2010;5(8) e12359.

57. Longpré F, Garneau P, Christen Y, Ramassamy C. *Free Radic Biol Med*. 2006;41(12):1781–1794.

58. Augustin S, Rimbach G, Augustin K, et al. *Arch Biochem Biophys*. 2009;481(2): 177–182.

59. Tchantchou F, Xu Y, Wu Y, et al. *FASEB J*. 2007;21(10):2400–2408.

60. Kim MS, Lee JI, Lee WY, Kim SE. *Phytother Res*. 2004;18(8):663–666.

61. Joyeux M, Lobstein A, Anton R, et al. *Planta Med*. 1995;61(2):126–129.

62. Maitra I, Marcocci L, Droy-Lefaix MT, et al. *Biochem Pharmacol*. 1995;49(11):1649–1655.

63. Hasenohrl RU, Nichau CH, Frisch CH, et al. *Pharmacol Biochem Behav*. 1996;53(2):271–275.

64. Yan LJ, Droy-Lefaix MT, Packer L. *Biochem Biophys Res Commun*. 1995;212(2):360–366.

65. Bridi R, Crossetti FP, Steffen VM, Henriques AT. *Phytother Res*. 2001;15(5):449–451.

66. Ilhan A, Gurel A, Armutcu F, et al. *Clin Chim Acta*. 2004;340(1–2):153–162.

67. Artmann GM, Schikarski C. *Clin Haem*. 1993;13(4):529–539.

68. Emerit I, Arutyunyan R, Oganesian N, et al. *Free Radic Biol Med*. 1995;18(6):985–991.

69. Emerit I, Oganesian N, Sarkisian T, et al. *Radiat Res*. 1995;144(2):198–205.

70. Eckert A, Keil U, Kressmann S, et al. *Pharmacopsychiatry*. 2003;36(suppl 1):S15–S23.

71. Leuner K, Hauptmann S, Abdel-Kader R, et al. *Antioxid Redox Signal*. 2007;9(10):1659–1675.

72. Shen J, Lee W, Gu Y, et al. *Chin Med*. 2011;6:8.

73. Bernatoniene J, Majiene D, Peciura R, et al. *Phytother Res*. 2011 [Epub ahead of print].

74. Liu TJ, Yeh YC, Ting CT, et al. *Cardiovasc Res*. 2008;80(2):227–235.

75. Baliutyte G, Baniene R, Trumbeckaite S, et al. *J Bioenerg Biomembr*. 2010;42(2):165–172.

76. Mozet C, Martin R, Welt K, Fitzl G. *Aging Clin Exp Res*. 2009;21(1):14–21.

77. Abdel-Kader R, Hauptmann S, Keil U, et al. *Pharmacol Res*. 2007;56(6):493–502.

78. Shi C, Xiao S, Liu J, et al. *Platelets*. 2010;21(5):373–379.

79. Jensen AA, Begum N, Vogensen SB, et al. *J Med Chem*. 2007;50(7):1610–1617.

80. Ahlemeyer B, Krieglstein J. *Cell Mol Life Sci*. 2003;60(9):1779–1792.

81. Yoshitake T, Yoshitake S, Kehr J. *Br J Pharmacol*. 2010;159(3):659–668.

82. Droy-Lefaix MT, Cluzel J, Menerath JM, et al. *Int J Tissue React*. 1995;17(3): 93–100.

83. Chermat R, Brochet D, DeFeudis FV, Drieu K. *Pharmacol Biochem Behav*. 1997;56(2):333–339.

84. Kuribara H, Weintraub ST, Yoshihama T, Maruyama Y. *J Nat Prod*. 2003;66(10):1333–1337.

85. Porsolt RD, Roux S, Drieu K. *Arzneimittelforschung*. 2000;50(3): 232–235.

86. Fowler JS, Wang GJ, Volkow ND, et al. *Life Sci*. 2000;66(9):PL141–PL146.

87. Sakakibara H, Ishida K, Grundmann O, et al. *Biol Pharm Bull*. 2006;29(8): 1767–1770.

88. Ward CP, Redd K, Williams BM, et al. *Pharmacol Biochem Behav*. 2002;72(4):913–922.

89. DeFeudis FV, Drieu K. *Curr Drug Targets*. 2000;1(1):25–58.

90. Shah ZA, Sharma P, Vohora SB. *Eur Neuropsychopharmacol*. 2003;13(5): 321–325.

91. Puebla-Pérez AM, Lozoya X, Villaseñor-García MM. *Int Immunopharmacol*. 2003;3(1):75–80.

92. Villaseñor-García MM, Lozoya X, Osuna-Torres L, et al. *Int Immunopharmacol*. 2004;4(9):1217–1222.

93. Rai D, Bhatia G, Sen T, Palit G. *J Pharmacol Sci*. 2003;93(4):458–464.

94. Walesiuk A, Trofimiuk E, Braszko JJ. *Pharmacol Res*. 2006;53(2):123–128.

95. Walesiuk A, Braszko JJ. *Phytomedicine*. 2009;16(1):40–46.

96. Walesiuk A, Braszko JJ. *Fitoterapia*. 2010;81(1):25–29.

97. Jezova D, Duncko R, Lassanova M, et al. *J Physiol Pharmacol*. 2002;53(3):337–348.

98. Kudolo GB. *Clin Chem*. 2007;53 (6 suppl S):A186.

99. Winter E. *Pharmacol Biochem Behav*. 1991;38(1):109–114.

100. Porsolt RD, Martin P, Lenegre A, et al. *Pharmacol Biochem Behav*. 1990;36(4):963–971.

101. Rapin JR, Lamproglou I, Drieu K, et al. *Gen Pharmacol*. 1994;25(5):1009–1016.

102. Maclennan KM, Darlington CL, Smith PF. *Prog Neurobiol*. 2002;67(3):235–257.

103. Zhang M, Cai J. *Behav Pharmacol*. 2005;16(8):651–656.

104. Wang Y, Wang L, Wu J, Cai J. *Br J Pharmacol*. 2006;148(2):147–153.

105. Müller WE, Chatterjee SS. *Pharmacopsychiatry*. 2003;36 (suppl 1):S24–S31.

106. Mustafa A, El-Medany A, Hagar HH, El-Medany G. *Pharmacol Res*. 2006;53(4):324–330.

107. Chen SH, Liang YC, Chao JC, et al. *World J Gastroenterol*. 2005;11(24):3746–3750.

108. JaeSeung P, JinHaeng L. *J Urol*. 1996;156(5):1876–1880.

109. Wojcicki J, Samochowiec L, Juzwiak S, et al. *Phytomedicine*. 1994;1:33–38.

110. Kobayashi N, Suzuki R, Koide C, et al. *Yakugaku Zasshi*. 1993;113(10): 718–724.

111. Della Loggia R, Sosa S, Tubaro A, et al. *Fitoterapia*. 1996;67(3):257–264.

112. Smith PF, Darlington CL. *J Vestib Res*. 1994;4(3):169–179.

113. Moreau JP, Eck CR, McCabe J, Skinner S. *Presse Med.* 1986;15(31):1458–1461. [Article in French].

114. Pietta PG, Gardana C, Mauri PL, et al. *J Chromatogr B Biomed Appl.* 1995;673(1):75–80.

115. Watanabe CM, Wolffram S, Ader P, et al. *Proc Natl Acad Sci USA.* 2001;98(12):6577–6580.

116. Zhao Y, Sun Y, Li C. *J Am Soc Mass Spectrom.* 2008;19(3):445–449.

117. Zhao Y, Wang L, Bao Y, Li C. *Rapid Commun Mass Spectrom.* 2007;21(6):971–981.

118. Rangel-Ordóñez L, Nöldner M, Schubert-Zsilavecz M, Wurglics M. *Planta Med.* 2010;76(15):1683–1690.

119. Biber A, Koch E. *Planta Med.* 1999;65(2):192–193.

120. Wang DL, Liang Y, Chen WD, et al. *Acta Pharmacol Sin.* 2008;29(3):376–384.

121. Fang W, Deng Y, Li Y, et al. *Eur J Pharm Sci.* 2010;39(1–3):8–14.

122. Pietta PG, Gardana C, Mauri PL. *J Chromatogr B Biomed Sci Appl.* 1997;693(1):249–255.

123. Biber A. *Pharmacopsychiatry.* 2003;36(suppl 1):S32–S37.

124. Wang FM, Yao TW, Zeng S. *J Pharm Biomed Anal.* 2003;33(2):317–321.

125. Kleijnen J, Knipschild P. *Lancet.* 1992;340(8828):1136–1139.

126. Fourtillan JB, Brisson AM, Girault J, et al. *Therapie.* 1995;50(2):137–144.

127. Drago F, Floriddia ML, Cro M, Giuffrida S. *J Ocul Pharmacol Ther.* 2002;18(2):197–202.

128. Mauri P, Minoggio M, Iemoli L, et al. *J Pharm Biomed Anal.* 2003;32(4–5):633–639.

129. Mauri P, De Palma A, Pozzi F, et al. *J Pharm Biomed Anal.* 2006;40(3):763–768.

130. Mauri P, Simonetti P, Gardana C, et al. *Rapid Commun Mass Spectrom.* 2001;15(12):929–934.

131. Kressmann S, Biber A, Wonnemann M, et al. *J Pharm Pharmacol.* 2002;54(11):1507–1514.

132. Amar K, Wilcock G. *Br Med J.* 1996;312(7025):227–231.

133. Pantoni L, Garcia JH. *Ann NY Acad Sci.* 1997;826:92–102.

134. Kleijnen J, Knipschild P. *Br J Clin Pharmacol.* 1992;34(4):352–358.

135. Hartmann A, Frick M. *MMW.* 1991;133(suppl):S23–S25.

136. Hopfenmuller W. *Arzneim-Forsch.* 1994;44(9):1005–1013.

137. Eckmann F, Schlag H. *Fortschr Med.* 1982;100(31–32):1474–1478.

138. Leroy H, Salaun P, Chovelon R, et al. *Vie Medicale.* 1978;28:2513–2519.

139. Boudouresques C, Vigouroux R, Boudouresques J. *Med Pract.* 1975;598:75–78.

140. Tea S, Celsis P, Clanet M, et al. *Gaz Med Fr.* 1979;86(35):4149–4152.

141. Zeng X, Liu M, Yang Y, et al. *Cochrane Database Syst Rev.* 2005;4:CD003691 [republished 2009].

142. Garg RK, Nag D, Agrawal A. *J Assoc Physicians India.* 1995;43(11):760–763.

143. Santos RF, Galduróz JC, Barbieri A, et al. *Pharmacopsychiatry.* 2003;36(4):127–133.

144. Mashayekh A, Pham DL, Yousem DM, et al. *Neuroradiology.* 2011;53(3):185–191.

145. Bornhöft G, Maxion-Bergemann S, Matthiessen PF. *Z Gerontol Geriatr.* 2008;41(4):298–312. [Article in German].

146. Napryeyenko O, Borzenko I. GINDEM-NP Study Group. *Arzneimittelforschung.* 2007;57(1):4–11.

147. Schneider LS, DeKosky ST, Farlow MR, et al. *Curr Alzheimer Res.* 2005;2(5):541–551.

148. McCarney R, Fisher P, Iliffe S, et al. *Int J Geriatr Psychiatry.* 2008;23(12):1222–1230.

149. Napryeyenko O, Sonnik G, Tartakovsky I. *J Neurol Sci.* 2009;283(1–2):224–229.

150. Institut für Qualität und Wirtschaftlichkeit im Gesundheitswesen (IQWiG). IQWiG Reports – Commission No. A05–19B, Executive Summary, version 1.0, September 2008. <http://www.iqwig.de/download/A05–19B_Executive_Summary_Ginkgo_in_Alzheimers_disease.pdf>. Accessed 29.09.11.

151. Winckler T. *Pharm Unserer Zeit.* 2009;38(5):454–461. [Article in German].

152. Birks J, Grimley Evans J. *Cochrane Database Syst Rev.* 2009;1:CD003120.

153. Weinmann S, Roll S, Schwarzbach C, et al. *BMC Geriatr.* 2010;10:14.

154. Wang BS, Wang H, Song YY, et al. *Pharmacopsychiatry.* 2010;43(3):86–91.

155. Ihl R, Tribanek M, Bachinskaya N. *J Neurol Sci.* 2010;299(1–2):184–187.

156. Kasper S, Schubert H. *Fortschr Neurol Psychiatr.* 2009;77(9):494–506. [Article in German].

157. Le Bars PL, Katz MM, Berman N, et al. *JAMA.* 1997;278(16):1327–1332.

158. Le Bars PL, Kieser M, Itil KZ. *Dement Geriatr Cogn Disord.* 2000;11(4):230–237.

159. Le Bars PL, Velasco FM, Ferguson JM, et al. *Neuropsychobiology.* 2002;45(1):19–26.

160. Mazza M, Capuano A, Bria P, Mazza S. *Eur J Neurol.* 2006;13(9):981–985.

161. Kanowski S, Herrmann WM, Stephan K, et al. *Pharmacopsychiatry.* 1996;29(2):47–56.

162. Kanowski S, Hoerr R. *Pharmacopsychiatry.* 2003;36(6):297–303.

163. van Dongen M, van Rossum E, Kessels A, et al. *J Clin Epidemiol.* 2003;56(4):367–376.

164. Le Bars PL. *Pharmacopsychiatry.* 2003;36(suppl 1):S50–S55.

165. Yancheva S, Ihl R, Nikolova G, et al. *Aging Ment Health.* 2009;13(2):183–190.

166. Hoerr R. *Phytomedicine.* 2005;12(8):598–600.

167. DeKosky ST, Williamson JD, Fitzpatrick AL, et al. *JAMA.* 2008;300(19):2253–2262.

168. Dodge HH, Zitzelberger T, Oken BS, et al. *Neurology.* 2008;70(19 Pt 2):1809–1817.

169. Andrieu S, Gillette S, Amouyal K, et al. *J Gerontol A Biol Sci Med Sci.* 2003;58(4):372–377.

170. Ipsen. Encouraging results of GuidAge®, large scale European trial conducted in the prevention of Alzheimer's Dementia. Available online: <http://www.ipsen.com/sites/default/files/communiques-presse/PR%20GuidAge%20Results%20FINAL%20EN.pdf>. Accessed 30.09.11.

171. Snitz BE, O'Meara ES, Carlson MC, et al. *JAMA.* 2009;302(24):2663–2670.

172. American Botanical Council, News Release December 29, 2009. <http://abc.herbalgram.org/site/MessageViewer?em_id=9801.0>. Accessed 11.02.10.

173. Yahoo! Finance, Schwabe Statement on Article by Snitz et al, *JAMA* 2009. <http://finance.yahoo.com/news/Schwabe-Statement-on-Article-bw-793688901.html?x=0&.v=1>. Accessed 11.02.10.

174. Blasko I, Kemmler G, Krampla W, et al. *Neurobiol Aging.* 2005;26(8):1135–1143.

175. Blasko I, Jungwirth S, Jellinger K, et al. *J Psychiatr Res.* 2008;42(11):946–955.

176. Horsch S, Walther C. *Int J Clin Pharmacol Ther.* 2004;42(2):63–72.

177. Pittler MH, Ernst E. *Am J Med.* 2000;108(4):276–281.

178. Gardner CD, Taylor-Piliae RE, Kiazand A, et al. *J Cardiopulm Rehabil Prev.* 2008;28(4):258–265.

179. Wang J, Zhou S, Bronks R, et al. *Clin Rehabil.* 2007;21(7):579–586.

180. Nicolai SP, Kruidenier LM, Bendermacher BL, et al. *Cochrane Database Syst Rev.* 2009;2:CD006888.

181. Muir AH, Robb R, McLaren M, et al. *Vasc Med.* 2002;7(4):265–267.

182. Choi WS, Choi CJ, Kim KS, et al. *Clin Rheumatol.* 2009;28(5):553–559.

183. Steins A, Zuder D, Hahn M, et al. *Eur J Dermatol.* 1997;7(2):109–111.

184. Maillet P, Bazex J, d'Arbingy P, et al. In: Clostre F, DeFeudis FV, eds. *Cardiovascular Effects of Ginkgo Biloba Extract (EGb 761) (Advances in Ginkgo Biloba Extract Research 3).* Paris: Elsevier; 1994. pp. 151–160.

185. Rodríguez M, Ringstad L, Schäfer P, et al. *Atherosclerosis.* 2007;192:438–444.

186. Lippi G, Targher G, Guidi GC. *Atherosclerosis.* 2007;195:417–418.

187. Pati U, Pati N. *Mol Genet Metab.* 2000;71(1–2):87–92.

188. Boffa MB, Marcovina SM, Koschinsky ML. *Clin Biochem.* 2004;37(5):333–343.

189. Schäfer P, Rodríguez M, Siegel G. *Atherosclerosis.* 2007;195:419–422.

190. Wu Y, Li S, Cui W, et al. *Planta Med.* 2007;73:624–628.

191. Wu Y, Li S, Cui W, et al. *Phytomedicine.* 2008;15:164–169.

192. Siegel G, Schafer P, Sauer F, et al. *Z Phytother.* 2008;29(S1):S16.

193. Pietri S, Seguin JR, D'Arbigny P, et al. *Cardiovasc Drugs Ther.* 1997;11(2): 121–131.

194. Israel L, Della' Accio E, Martin G, et al. *Psychol Med.* 1987;19:1431–1439.

195. Witte S, Anadere I, Walitza E. *Fortschr Med.* 1992;110(13):247–250.

196. Kalus JS, Piotrowski AA, Fortier CR, et al. *Ann Pharmacother.* 2003;37(3):345–349.

197. Dubreuil C. *Presse Med.* 1986;15(31):1559–1561.

198. Baschek V, Steinert W. In: Claussen CF, Kirtane MV, Schlitter K, eds. *Vertigo, Nausea, Tinnitus and Hypoacusia, in Metabolic Disorders.* Amsterdam: Elsevier; 1988. pp. 575–582.

199. Hoffmann F, Beck C, Schutz A, et al. *Laryngorhinootologie.* 1994;73(3): 149–152.

200. Kumar A, Raizada RM, Chaturvedi VN. *Indian J Otolaryngol Head Neck Surg.* 2000;52(3):212–219.

201. Burschka MA, Hassan HA, Reineke T, et al. *Eur Arch Otorhinolaryngol.* 2001;258(5):213–219.

202. Reisser CH, Weidauer H. *Acta Otolaryngol.* 2001;121(5):579–584.

203. Schwerdtfeger F. Elektronystagmographisch und klinisch dokumentierte Therapie-erfahrungen mit rokan bei Schwindelsymptomatick. *Therapiewoche.* 1981;31:8658–8667. In: DeFeudis FV. *Ginkgo Biloba Extract (EGb 761): Pharmacological Activities and Clinical Applications.* Paris: Elsevier; 1991.

204. Hamann KF. Physikalische Therapie des vestibularen Schwindels in Verbindung mit GBE. *Therapiewoche.* 1985;35:4586–4590. In: DeFeudis FV. *Ginkgo Biloba Extract (EGb 761): Pharmacological Activities and Clinical Applications.* Paris: Elsevier; 1991.

205. Haguenauer JP, Cantenot F, Koskas H, et al. *Presse Med.* 1986;15(31): 1569–1572.

206. Orendorz-Fraczkowska K, Pospiech L, Gawron W. *Otolaryngol Pol.* 2002;56(1):83–88.

207. Hamann KF. *HNO.* 2007;55(4):258–263. [Article in German].

208. Chesseboeuf L, Herard J, Trevin J. Etude comparative de deux vasoregulaterus dans les hypoacousies et les syndromes vertigineux. *Med Nord Est.* 1979;3: 534–539. In: DeFeudis FV. *Ginkgo Biloba Extract (EGb 761): Pharmacological Activities and Clinical Applications.* Paris: Elsevier; 1991.

209. Artieres J. Effets therapeutiques du Tanakan sur les hypoacousies et les acouphenes. *Lyon Mediterr Med.* 1978;14:2503–2515. In: DeFeudis FV. *Ginkgo Biloba Extract (EGb 761): Pharmacological Activities and Clinical Applications.* Paris: Elsevier; 1991.

210. Meyer B. *Presse Med.* 1986;15(31): 1562–1564.

211. Plath P, Olivier J. *Adv Otorhinolaryngol.* 1995;49:101–104.

212. Partheniadis-Stumpf M, Maurer J, Mann W. *Laryngorhinootologie.* 1993;72(1): 28–31.

213. Vorberg G, Schenk N, Schmidt U. *Herz Gefasse.* 1989;9:936–941.

214. Holgers KM, Azelsson A, Pringle I. *Audiology.* 1994;33(2):85–92.

215. Drew S, Davies E. *BMJ.* 2001;322(7278):73.

216. Morgenstern C, Biermann E. *Int J Clin Pharmacol Ther.* 2002;40(5):188–197.

217. Holstein N. *Fortschr Med Orig.* 2001;118(4):157–164.

218. Rejali D, Sivakumar A, Balaji N. *Clin Otolaryngol Allied Sci.* 2004;29(3): 226–231.

219. Hilton M, Stuart E. *Cochrane Database Syst Rev.* 2004;2:CD003852.

220. Morgenstern C, Biermann E. *Fortschr Med.* 1997;115(29):57–58.

221. Hoerr R, Napryeyenko O, Borzenko I. *Focus Altern Complement Ther.* 2007;12:26–27.

222. Canis M, Olzowy B, Welz C, et al. *Am J Otolaryngol.* 2011;32(1):19–23.

223. Schapowal S, Spokesperson of the European Federation of Tinnitus Associations. National Health News, Australian Healthcare & Hospitals Association, September 4, 2007. Available online: <http://www.aushealthcare.com.au/news/news_details.asp?nid=9688>. Accessed 22.07.09.

224. [No authors listed]. *Forsch Komplementarmed.* 2008;15(2):115–117.

225. Seo BS, Lee HJ, Mo JH, et al. *Arch Otolaryngol Head Neck Surg.* 2009;135(10):1000–1004.

226. Evans JR. *Cochrane Database Syst Rev.* 2000;2:CD001775.

227. Lebuisson DA, Leroy L, Rigal G. *Presse Med.* 1986;15(31):1556–1558.

228. Fies P, Dienel A. *Wien Med Wochenschr.* 2002;152(15–16):423–426.

229. Chung HS, Harris A, Kristinsson JK, et al. *J Ocul Pharmacol Ther.* 1999;15(3): 233–240.

230. Quaranta L, Bettelli S, Uva MG, et al. *Ophthalmology.* 2003;110(2):359–362.

231. Ha SJ, Rho SH. *J Korean Ophthalmol Soc.* 2003;44(9):2047–2057.

232. Vessaini RM, Medeiros F, Susanna FL, et al. *3rd International Glaucoma Symposium.* Prague, Czech Republic: March 21–25, 2001.

233. DeFeudis FV. *Ginkgo Biloba Extract (EGb 761): Pharmacological Activities and Clinical Applications.* Amsterdam: Elsevier; 1991. pp. 133–134.

234. Lagatz WH, Fies AM, Bartsch G. *Z Allg Med.* 1990;66:573–578.

235. Kudolo GB, Delaney D, Blodgett J. *Diabetes Res Clin Pract.* 2005;68(1): 29–38.

236. Huang SY, Jeng C, Kao SC, et al. *Clin Nutr.* 2004;23(4):615–621.

237. Russo V, Stella A, Appezzati L, et al. *Eur J Ophthalmol.* 2009;19(3):331–336.

238. Woelk H, Arnoldt KH, Kieser M, Hoerr R. *J Psychiatr Res.* 2007;41(6):472–480.

239. Lingaerde O, Føreland AR, Magnusson A. *Acta Psychiatr Scand.* 1999;100(1):62–66.

240. Singh V, Singh SP, Chan K. *Int J Neuropsychopharmacol.* 2010;13(2): 257–271.

241. Donfrancesco R, Ferrante L. *Phytomedicine.* 2007;14(6):367–370.

242. Donfrancesco R, Dell'umomo A. *Phytomedicine.* 2004;11(6):469.

243. Niederhofer H. *Phytother Res.* 2010;24(1):26–27.

244. Frei H. *Schweiz Z Ganzheitsmed.* 2002;14(1):10–13.

245. Salehi B, Imani R, Mohammadi MR, et al. *Prog Neuropsychopharmacol Biol Psychiatry.* 2010;34(1):76–80.

246. Tang Y, Xu Y, Xiong S, et al. *J Huazhong Univ Sci Technolog Med Sci.* 2007;27(4):375–380.

247. Li MH, Zhang HL, Yang BY. *Zhongguo Zhong Xi Yi Jie He Za Zhi.* 1997;17(4):216–218.

248. Huntley A, Ernst E. *Thorax.* 2000;55(11):925–929.

249. He Y, Yuan FY, Wang JB, et al. *Chin J Integr Med.* 2002;8(2):90–94.

250. Leadbetter G, Keyes LE, Maakestad KM, et al. *Wilderness Environ Med.* 2009;20(1):66–71.

251. Tissot van Patot MC, Keyes LE, Leadbetter G, et al. *High Alt Med Biol.* 2009;10(1):33–43.

252. Kaschel R. *Hum Psychopharmacol.* 2009;24(5):345–370.

253. Canter PH, Ernst E. *Hum Psychopharmacol.* 2007;22(5):265–278.

254. Page JW, Findley J, Crognale MA. *J Gerontol A Biol Sci Med Sci.* 2005;60(10):1246–1251.

255. Semlitsch HV, Anderer P, Saletu B, et al. *Pharmacopsychiatry.* 1995;28(4):134–142.

256. Burns NR, Bryan J, Nettelbeck T. *Hum Psychopharmacol.* 2006;21(1):27–37.

257. Elsabagh S, Hartley DE, Ali O, et al. *Psychopharmacology (Berl).* 2005;179(2):437–446.

258. Cieza A, Maier P, Pöppel E. *Arch Med Res.* 2003;34(5):373–381.

259. Solomon PR, Adams F, Silver A, et al. *JAMA.* 2002;288(7):835–840.

260. Nathan PJ, Ricketts E, Wesnes K, et al. *Hum Psychopharmacol.* 2002;17(1):45–49.

261. Moulton PL, Boyko LN, Fitzpatrick JL, Petros TV. *Physiol Behav.* 2001;73(4): 659–665.

262. Stough C, Clarke J, Lloyd J, Nathan PJ. *Int J Neuropsychopharmacol*. 2001;4(2): 131–134.

263. Kennedy DO, Scholey AB, Wesnes KA. *Psychopharmacology (Berl)*. 2000;151(4):416–423.

264. Rigney U, Kimber S, Hindmarch I. *Phytotherapy Res*. 1999;13(5):408–415.

265. Smirnova V, Strokov I, Ivanova L, Ichunina A. *Diabetologia*. 1999;42(suppl 1):A293. Abstract No. 1109

266. Thajeb P, Lin MS, Chen PH. *Neurol*. 1996;46(2, suppl):A132. Abstract No. PO1 060.

267. Bernardczyk-Meller J, Siwiec-Pro ci ska J, Stankiewicz W, et al. *Klin Oczna*. 2004;106(4–5):569–571.

268. Choi KM, Kim DR, Kim NH, et al. *J Korean Diabetes Assoc*. 2000;24(3): 375–384.

269. Zhu HW, Shi ZF, Chen YY. *Zhongguo Zhong Xi Yi Jie He Za Zhi*. 2005;25(10):889–891.

270. Li XS, Zheng WY, Lou SX, et al. *Chin J Integr Med*. 2009;15(1):26–29.

271. Brochet B, Orgogozo JM, Guinot P, et al. *Rev Neurol (Paris)*. 1992;148(4):299–301.

272. Brochet B, Guinot P, Orgogozo JM, et al. *J Neurol Neurosurg Psychiatry*. 1995;58(3):360–362.

273. Johnson SK, Diamond BJ, Rausch S, et al. *Explore (NY)*. 2006;2(1):19–24.

274. Lovera J, Bagert B, Smoot K, et al. *Mult Scler*. 2007;13(3):376–385.

275. Ye B, Aponte M, Dai Y, et al. *Cancer Lett*. 2007;251(1):43–52.

276. Gehring K, Sitskoorn MM, Aaronson NK, Taphoorn MJ. *Lancet Neurol*. 2008;7(6):548–560.

277. Shaw EG. *A Phase II Study of Ginkgo Biloba in Irradiated Brain Tumor Patients: Effects on Quality of Life and Cognitive Function*. Soc Integrative Oncology 2nd Intl. Conference, California, November, 2005. Abstract #61. Available online: <http://www.integrativeonc.org/index.php/final-program>. Accessed 05.10.11.

278. Dardano A, Ballardin M, Ferdeghini M, et al. *J Clin Endocrinol Metab*. 2007;92(11):4286–4289.

279. Attia A, Case LD, D'Agostino R, et al. *J Clin Oncol*. 2010;28(suppl):e12523.

280. Tamborini A, Taurelle R. *Rev Fr Gynecol Obstet*. 1993;88(7–9):447–457.

281. Ozgoli G, Selselei EA, Mojab F, et al. *J Alt Comp Med*. 2009;15(8):845–851.

282. Wheatley D. *Hum Psychopharmacol*. 2004;19(8):545–548.

283. Kang BJ, Lee SJ, Kim MD, Cho MJ. *Hum Psychopharmacol*. 2002;17(6):279–284.

284. Cohen AJ, Bartlik B. *J Sex Marital Therapy*. 1998;24:139–145.

285. Dartigues JF, Carcaillon L, Helmer C, et al. *J Am Geriatr Soc*. 2007;55(3): 395–399.

286. Hemmeter U, Annen B, Bischof R, et al. *Pharmacopsychiatry*. 2001;34(2):50–59.

287. DeFeudis FV. *Ginkgo Biloba Extract (EGb 761): Pharmacological Activities and Clinical Applications*. Amsterdam: Elsevier; 1991.

288. American Herbal Pharmacopoeia *Ginkgo Leaf, Ginkgo Leaf Dry Extract – Ginkgo biloba L.: Standards of Analysis, Quality Control, and Therapeutics*. Santa Cruz: American Herbal Pharmacopoeia; 2003.

289. Keita CT. *Med Afr Noire*. 1997;44(suppl 8–9):490–494. [Article in French].

290. Parsad D, Pandhi R, Juneja A. *Clin Exp Dermatol*. 2003;28(3):285–287.

291. DeFeudis FV. *Ginkgo Biloba Extract (EGb 761): Pharmacological Activities and Clinical Applications*. Amsterdam: Elsevier; 1991. pp. 143–146.

292. Blaschek W, Ebel S, Hackenthal E, et al. *HagerROM 2002: Hagers Handbuch der Drogen und Arzneistoffe*. Heidelberg: Springer; 2002.

293. Baron-Ruppert G, Luepke NP. *Phytomedicine*. 2001;8(2):133–138.

294. Spinella M, Eaton LA. *Brain Inj*. 2002;16(4):359–367.

295. Hirono I, Shibuya C, Shinizu M, et al. *Gann*. 1972;63(3):383–386.

296. Bonvoison B, Guinot P. In: Braquet P, ed. *Ginkgolides – Chemistry, Biology, Pharmacology and Clinical Perspectives*, vol. 2. Barcelona, JR: Prous Science Publishers; 1989. pp. 845–854.

297. Siegers CP. *Phytomedicine*. 1999;6(4): 281–283.

298. Koch E, Jaggy H, Chatterjee SS. *Int J Immunopharmacol*. 2000;22(3):229–236.

299. Jaggy H, Koch E. *Pharmazie*. 1997;52(10):735–738.

300. Ahlemeyer B, Selke D, Schaper C, et al. *Eur J Pharmacol*. 2001;430(1):1–7.

301. Westendorf J, Regan J. *Phytomedicine*. 2000;7(suppl 2):104.

302. Ang-Lee MK, Moss J, Yuan CS. *JAMA*. 2001;286(2):208–216.

303. Fessenden JM, Wittenborn W, Clarke L. *Am Surg*. 2001;67(1):33–35.

304. Arzneimittelkommission der deutschen Ärzteschaft. *Dtsch Ärztebl*. 2002;99(33):A2214.

305. Engelsen J, Nielsen JD, Winther K. *Thromb Haemost*. 2002;87(6): 1075–1076.

306. Jiang X, Williams KM, Liauw WS, et al. *Br J Clin Pharmacol*. 2005;59(4):425–432.

307. Jiang X, Blair EY, McLachlan AJ. *J Clin Pharmacol*. 2006;46(11):1370–1378.

308. Engelsen J, Nielsen JD, Hansen KF. *Ugeskr Laeger*. 2003;165(18):1868–1871.

309. DeLoughery TG, Kaye JA, Morris CD, et al. *Blood*. 2002;11 Abstract 3809.

310. Wolf HR. *Drugs R D*. 2006;7(3): 163–172.

311. Lai CF, Chang CC, Fu CH, et al. *Pharmacotherapy*. 2002;22(10):1326. Abstract No. 12.

312. Bone KM. *Mol Nutr Food Res*. 2008;52(7):764–771.

313. Gardner CD, Zehnder JL, Rigby AJ, et al. *Blood Coagul Fibrinolysis*. 2007;18(8):787–793.

314. Aruna D, Naidu MU. *Br J Clin Pharmacol*. 2007;63(3):333–338.

315. Yeo C, Cho H, Park S, et al. *Clin Pharm Ther*. 2010;87:S43.

316. Kim TE, Kim BH, Kim J, et al. *Clin Ther*. 2009;31(10):2249–2257.

317. Kim BH, Kim KP, Lim KS, et al. *Clin Ther*. 2010;32(2):380–390.

318. Lu WJ, Huang JD, Lai ML. *J Clin Pharmacol*. 2006;46(6):628–634.

319. Leistner E, Drewke C. *J Nat Prod*. 2010;73(1):86–92.

320. Kuenick C. *Dtsch Apoth Ztg*. 2010;150(5):60–61.

321. Granger AS. *Age Ageing*. 2001;30(6): 523–525.

322. Kupiec T, Raj V. *J Anal Toxicol*. 2005;29(7):755–758.

323. Yin OQ, Tomlinson B, Waye MM, et al. *Pharmacogenetics*. 2004;14(12):841–850.

324. Galluzzi S, Zanetti O, Binetti G, et al. *J Neurol Neurosurg Psychiatry*. 2000;68(5):679–680.

325. Shaw D, Leon C, Kolev S, et al. *Drug Saf*. 1997;17(5):342–356.

326. Kudolo GB. *J Clin Pharmacol*. 2001;41(6):600–611.

327. Appleton G. *Health Notes Rev Complement Integr Med*. 2000;7:298–300.

328. Colalto C. *Pharmacol Res*. 2010;62(3):207–227.

329. Zehra U, Tahir M, Lone KP. *J Coll Physicians Surg Pak*. 2010;20(2):117–121.

330. Flossiac M, Chopin S. *FASEB J*. 1999;13(5):A1031.

331. Petty HR, Fernando M, Kindzelskii AL, et al. *Chem Res Toxicol*. 2001;14(9): 1254–1258.

332. American Botanical Council. Herbal science group debunks research suggesting presence of toxin colchicine in Ginkgo. News release to national media, August 30, 2001.

333. Li W, Fitzloff JF, Farnsworth NR, et al. *Phytomedicine*. 2002;9(5):442–446.

334. Li W, Sun Y, Fitzloff JF, et al. *Chem Res Toxicol*. 2002;15(9):1174–1178.

335. Bone K. *Townsend Letter for Doctors & Patients*. 2002;225:143–144.

336. Ondriek RR, Chan PJ, Patton WC, et al. *Fertil Steril*. 1999;71(3):517–522.

337. Dugoua JJ, Mills E, Perri D, Koren G. *Can J Clin Pharmacol*. 2006;13(3):e277–e284.

338. Woerdenbag HJ, Van Beek TA. In: De Smet PAGM, Keller K, Hansel R et al, eds. *Adverse Effects of Herbal Drugs*, vol. 3. Berlin: Springer-Verlag; 1997. pp. 57–60.

339. Ernst E, Pittler MH. *Clin Drug Invest*. 1999;4:301–308.

340. Le Bars PL, Kastelan J. *Public Health Nutr*. 2000;3(4A):495–499.

341. Birks J, Grimley EV, Van Dongen M. *Cochrane Database Syst Rev*. 2002;4:CD003120.

342. Cianfrocca C, Pelliccia F, Auriti A, et al. *Ital Heart J.* 2002;3(11):689–691.

343. Schwabe U, Paffrath D. *Arzneiverordnungs-Report 1999.* Berlin: Springer Verlag; 2000.

344. Arzneimittelkommission der deutschen Ärzteschaft *Dtsch Ärztebl.* 2000;97(8):A474.

345. Bent S, Goldberg H, Padula A, Avins AL. *J Gen Intern Med.* 2005;20(7):657–661.

346. Rowin J, Lewis SL. *Neurology.* 1996;46:1775–1776.

347. Gilbert GJ. *Neurology.* 1997;48(4):1137.

348. Vale S. *Lancet.* 1998;352(9121):36.

349. Benjamin J, Muir T, Briggs K, et al. *Postgrad Med J.* 2001;77(904):112–113.

350. Purroy Garcia F, Molina C, Alvarez Sabin J. *Med Clin (Barc).* 2002;119(15):596–597.

351. Miller LG, Freeman B. *J Herbal Pharmacother.* 2002;2(2):57–63.

352. Schneider C, Bord C, Misse P, et al. *J Fr Ophtalmol.* 2002;25(7):731–732.

353. Halil M, Cankurtaran M, Yavuz BB, et al. *Blood Coagul Fibrinolysis.* 2005;16(5):349–353.

354. Bal Dit Sollier C, Caplain H, Drouet L. *Clin Lab Haematol.* 2003;25(4):251–253.

355. Ernst E, Canter PH, Coon JT. *Perfusion.* 2005;18(2):52–56.

356. Savovic J, Wider B, Ernst E. *Evid Based Integrative Med.* 2005;2(3):167–176.

357. Galduroz JC, Antunes HK, Santos RF. *Phytomedicine.* 2007;14(7–8):447–451.

358. Guo KF, Guo S, Yan KL. *Chin J Clin Rehab.* 2006;10(2):43–45.

359. Witte S. *Clin Hemorheol.* 1989;9:323–326.

360. Hofferberth B. In: Christen Y.Courtois Y, Droy-Lefaix MT, eds. *Advances in Ginkgo Biloba Research,* vol. 4. Paris: Elsevier; 1995. pp. 141–148.

361. Davydov L, Stirling AL. *J Herbal Pharmacother.* 2001;1(3):65–69.

362. Sticher O, Hasler A, Meier B. *Dtsch Apoth Ztg.* 1991;131:1827–1835.

363. Mossabeb R, Kraft D, Valenta R. *Wien Klin Wochenschr.* 2001;113(15–16):580–587.

364. Hausen BM. *Am J Contact Dermat.* 1998;9(3):146–148.

365. Becker LE, Skipworth GB. *JAMA.* 1975;231(11):1162–1163.

366. Chiu AE, Lane AT, Kimball AB. *J Am Acad Dermatol.* 2002;46(1):145–146.

367. La Monaca G, Klesmer J, Kata JL. *Prim Psychiat.* 2001;8(6):63–64.

368. Wada K.. In: van Beek TA, ed. *Ginkgo Biloba.* Amsterdam: Harwood Academic; 2000. pp. 453–465.

369. Kajiyama Y, Fujii K, Takeuchi H, et al. *Pediatrics.* 2002;109(2):325–327.

370. Yagi M, Wada K, Sakata M, et al. *Yakugaku Zasshi.* 1993;113(8):596–599.

371. Wada K, Ishigaki S, Ueda K, et al. *Chem Pharm Bull (Tokyo).* 1985;33(8):3555–3557.

372. Wada K, Ishiaki S, Ueda K, et al. *Chem Pharm Bull.* 1988;36(5):1779–1782.

373. Arenz A, Klein M, Fiehe K, et al. *Planta Med.* 1996;62:548–551.

374. Leistner E, Arenz A. *Z Phytother.* 1997;18:230–231.

375. Shprakh VV, Saiutina SB, Revezova TV, et al. *Zh Nevrol Psikhiatr Im S S Korsakova.* 2000;100(3):33–35.

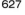

Ginseng

(*Panax ginseng* C. Meyer)

Synonyms

Korean ginseng, Panax, Man root (Engl), Ginseng radix (Lat), Ginsengwurzel, Kraftwurzel (Ger), Racine de ginseng (Fr), Ginseng (Dan), Ren shen (Chin), Ninjin (Jap), Insam (Kor).

What is it?

Ginseng (*Panax ginseng*), also commonly known as Korean or Asian ginseng, is one of the most valued (and expensive) medicinal plants. Originally part of traditional Chinese medicine, the root is now widely consumed in the West. The name Panax is apparently derived from the Greek word for panacea or cure-all. According to the Chinese sages, ginseng replenished the vital energy, increased the production of body fluids and promoted health and longevity. Since the 1960s, ginseng has been the subject of numerous scientific investigations. The great diversity of pharmacological properties now attributed to ginseng suggests that it might act in a unique and fundamental way on the body. In fact, sometimes its activity appears to be based on whole body effects, rather than particular organs or systems. This is notwithstanding the fact that ginseng can also profoundly influence the metabolism of the individual cell. These outcomes lend weight to the traditional view that ginseng is above all a tonic herb which can revitalise the functioning of the organism as a whole. There is no equivalent concept or treatment in contemporary conventional medicine.

Medicinal ginseng consists of the main and lateral roots. The smaller root hairs, which are used in the West, should be regarded as an inferior substitution. Most of the available root is from cultivated sources; roots sourced from the wild are superior in quality and attract a premium price. Two forms of the root are available in commerce: red ginseng, where the root is steamed before drying, and white ginseng, which is dried by normal processes.

Effects

Increases vitality and the ability to withstand stress by acting on the hypothalamus-pituitary-adrenal cortex axis; restores and strengthens the body's immune response; promotes longevity, metabolism and growth of normal cells; enhances insulin sensitivity; prevents cancer in regular users.

Traditional view

In traditional Chinese medicine ginseng is classified as a herb that tonifies the *Qi* (energy) and is used for severe collapsed *Qi* conditions marked by shallow respiration and shortness of breath. It benefits *Yin* and generates *Fluids* (used in high fevers, profuse sweating in very depleted individuals), tonifies the *Lungs*, the *Stomach* and strengthens the *Spleen* (used for laboured breathing, lethargy, chest and abdominal distension and prolapse). Ginseng also benefits and calms the *Spirit* (a manifestation of *heart* Qi-used for palpitations with anxiety, insomnia and restlessness). Traditionally ginseng would be taken as the powdered, dried root or as a decoction.[1,2]

Western herbalists have used ginseng traditionally as a mild stomachic, tonic and stimulant for anorexia and digestive complaints arising from mental and nervous exhaustion.[3] The *British Herbal Pharmacopoeia* 1983 recommends its use in the treatment of neurasthenia, neuralgia and for depressive states associated with sexual inadequacy.[4] In addition to the above conditions, the Eclectics used ginseng for cerebral anaemia, asthma, convulsions, paralysis and urinary gravel.[5]

Summary actions

Adaptogenic, tonic, immunomodulator, cardiotonic, cancer preventative, adjunct in the management of type 2 diabetes.

Can be used for

Indications supported by clinical trials

As a tonic for the elderly, to improve performance and well-being; to improve general performance under stress, improves cerebrovascular deficit and cognitive performance; congestive heart failure, elevates HDL-cholesterol; selected extracts decrease the risk of developing certain types of cancer when consumed for extended periods; protective effect on depressed bone marrow in cervical cancer patients undergoing radiation therapy; erectile dysfunction, male fertility problems; type 2 diabetes.

Traditional therapeutic uses

Prostration, heart failure, dyspnoea, asthma, organ prolapse, spontaneous sweating, cold limbs, digestive complaints, palpitations, neuralgia, convulsions, neurosis, anxiety, long-term debility, sexual inadequacy.

May also be used for

Extrapolations from pharmacological studies

Improves resistance to a wide variety of stressors; counters some effects of ageing; improves learning and memory and intellectual capacity; radioprotective;[6] improves ethanol clearance which may be beneficial in alcoholism; may be useful in drug-dependent states.

Preparations

Dried root for decoction, fluid extract, tablets and capsules; powdered root.

Dosage

The traditional dried dosage is 1 to 10 g/day of the dried root by decoction. Larger doses up to 30 g have been used in cases of haemorrhagic shock.[2]

The adult dose used in the West is from 0.5 to 3 g/day of the dried main or lateral roots (depending on the quality of the root and the application) or 1 to 6 mL/day of the 1:2 fluid extract or its equivalent in other dosage forms. Preparations from the root hairs are therapeutically inferior and should be avoided. Many clinical trials have been conducted using a daily dose of 200 mg of a 5:1 standardised extract in tablet or capsule form.

Duration of use

Generally up to 3 months, with a repeated course.[7] Continuous use in the unwell and elderly is appropriate.

Summary assessment of safety

No adverse effects are expected if used as recommended. Overstimulation may occur in susceptible individuals, especially at higher doses.

Technical data

Botany

Panax ginseng, a member of the Araliaceae (ginseng) family, is a perennial slow-growing herb native to the mountainous regions of China, Japan, Korea and the Soviet Union. The stem is erect, simple not branching, the leaves are verticillate and compound with five leaflets, the three terminal leaflets are larger than the lateral ones. The inflorescence is a small terminal, hemispherical umbel consisting of pink, polygamous flowers containing five petals. The fruit is a small berry which is red in colour when ripe. The root produces a branch root from its middle.[8]

Adulteration

The main and lateral roots of ginseng can be adulterated with the inferior root hairs and aerial parts (see below). Despite the rarity of wild ginseng, only the population of *Panax ginseng* from the Russian Federation is listed on Appendix II of the Convention on International Trade in Endangered Species (CITES) as of October 2011.

Key constituents

The main and lateral roots of ginseng contain:

* a complex mixture of triterpene dammarane and oleanane saponins (2 to 3%), called ginsenosides.[9,10] The ginsenosides can be divided into three classes-the predominant protopanaxatriol (PPT) class consisting mainly of Rg_1, Rg_2, Rf and Re, the protopanaxadiol (PPD) class consisting mainly of Rc, Rd, Rb_1 and Rb_2[11] and the minor ocotillol class.[10] Malonyl derivates of Rb_1, Rb_2, Rc and Rd are also found and are termed acidic ginsenosides[10]
* polysaccharides and essential oil[12]
* diacetylenes, peptides, trilinolein and other lipids,[13,14] arginine.[15]

The vast phytochemistry of ginseng has been extensively studied, with more than 200 ginsenosides and non-saponin constituents isolated and identified.[16] As can be seen from Table 1, the total level of ginsenosides cannot be the sole determinant of quality; otherwise the leaves and root hairs would be preferred. These ginsenoside profiles in root and leaf have been confirmed in later studies.[17] Clearly, the activity of ginseng must be attributable to the particular combination of ginsenosides found in the main and lateral roots. In particular, the ratio of Rg_1 to Rb_1 being greater than 0.5 is a marker of main and lateral root quality. However, it is also likely that other components found in the main root contribute significantly to the therapeutic activity of ginseng. On the other hand, there is significant product variability in the marketplace and it is likely that some samples of ginseng will have disappointing effects.[18]

Red ginseng is made by steaming and drying the fresh roots and contains some distinctive constituents, such as ginsenosides Rg_3, Rg_5, Rh_1, Rh_2 and Rk_1.[10,19] The malonyl group is released and there is a loss of the sugar at C20 to yield, for example, Rh_1, Rh_2 and Rg_3.[10] Some of the arginine in ginseng root is converted to Amadori products such as arginylfructose during the steaming process.[15]

The preference for wild ginseng is at least partly explained by the observed accumulation of ginsenosides as the plant matures (wild ginseng plants are usually harvested at a greater age than cultivated plants). The total content of ginsenosides in ginseng root increases significantly with age, with 4-year-old plants containing about three times the level of 1-year-old plants.[20] In contrast, total ginsenosides in the leaf decrease with age, although levels remain higher at any age than corresponding root samples (albeit Rg_1 and Rb_1 are significantly higher (four to five times) in the root of a mature plant compared with the leaf).

Table 1 Distribution of ginsenosides in *Panax ginseng* plant parts[21]

	Rg$_1$	Re	Rf	Rg$_2$	Rb$_1$	Rc	Rb$_2$	Rd	Total
Leaves	1.078	1.524	–	–	0.184	0.736	0.553	1.113	5.188
Leaf stalks	0.327	0.141	–	–	–	0.190	–	0.107	0.765
Stem	0.292	0.070	–	–	–	–	0.397	–	0.759
Main root	0.379	0.153	0.092	0.023	0.342	0.190	0.131	0.038	1.348
Lateral roots	0.406	0.668	0.203	0.090	0.850	0.738	0.434	0.143	3.532
Root hairs	0.376	1.512	0.150	0.249	1.351	1.349	0.780	0.381	6.148

glc = β-D-glucose
rha = α-L-rhamnose
ara = α-L-arabinose
p = pyranose
f = furanose

	R^1	R^2
20(S)-Protopanaxatriol	H	H
Ginsenoside Re	glc(2–1)rha	glc
Ginsenoside Rf	glc(2–1)glc	H
Ginsenoside Rg$_1$	glc	glc
Ginsenoside Rg$_2$	glc(2–1)rha	H

Protopanaxatriol class

	R^1	R^2
20(S)-Protopanaxadiol	H	H
Ginsenoside Rb$_1$	glc(2–1)glc	glc(6–1)glc
Ginsenoside Rb$_2$	glc(2–1)glc	glc(6–1)ara p
Ginsenoside Rc	glc(2–1)glc	glc(6–1)ara f
Ginsenoside Rd	glc(2–1)glc	glc

Protopanaxadiol class

Pharmacodynamics

Hundreds of studies have been published on the pharmacological activity of ginseng. The following information provides a broad review of the literature, with an emphasis on review papers and the more interesting studies.

One interpretative caution that should be observed for in vivo pharmacological studies is that in many cases the ginseng or ginsenosides were administered by injection. Since the original ginsenosides in the plant are most likely not the active forms reaching the bloodstream after oral doses of ginseng (see Pharmacokinetics), more weight should be given to the oral pharmacological studies, especially as it has been suggested that certain ginsenosides exert some biological activities only after being deglycosylated by intestinal bacteria.[22] The same caution also applies to the interpretation of the numerous in vitro investigations.

Adaptogenic and related activities

In many animal experiments, ginseng has increased resistance to a wide variety of physical, chemical and biological stressors.[23] Some of these studies are reviewed below:

- Oral administration of ginseng root saponins or ginsenoside Rb$_1$ antagonised the immunosuppression induced by cold water swim stress in mice and rats. Conflicting results were obtained for serum corticosterone levels. The increase in serum corticosterone was inhibited in stressed rats, but accentuated in stressed mice.[24,25]

- Ginseng or its components countered stress-induced changes from heat stress[26,27] and forced exercise,[28] sometimes posited as animal models of depression.[29]
- Other models where ginseng or its components demonstrated improved adaptation to stress included food deprivation,[30] and the cold-hypoxia-restraint model.[31]
- The effects of ginseng extract administered by injection prior to exercise in rats suggested that it could exert an antifatigue effect by increasing the biochemical capability of working skeletal muscle to better utilise free fatty acids, thus sparing body carbohydrate stores.[32] Oral administration to rats at 100 mg/kg reduced oxidative stress damage in muscles after acute exercise.[33]
- Ginseng extract (oral doses, 33 mg/kg) produced an increase in adrenal zona fasciculata cell size compared to controls. In mice treated with ginsenoside Rb_1 or Rg_1 (oral doses), the mean cell areas were unchanged, but the distribution of cell sizes differed from controls.[34]

Ginseng administration has also countered some effects of ageing in animal models. For example, ginseng extract at an oral dose of 600 mg/kg significantly stimulated granuloma collagen synthesis in an aged rat model and restored this parameter to near levels seen in young rats.[35] Repeated intraperitoneal injections of ginsenoside Rg_1 improved the performance of aged rats in the radial-arm maze, possibly through an increase of choline acetyltransferase activity in the brain.[36] Daily oral administration of ginseng extract (8 g/kg/day for 12 to 33 days) ameliorated the impaired learning performance of aged rats in a radial maze.[37] Oral intake of a water extract of ginseng for 4 weeks produced an increase in spontaneous motor activity during the dark period in old rats, while it caused a decrease in the activity of young rats (rats are nocturnal animals).[38]

Digestive metabolites of ginseng saponins have been shown to reduce acetylcholine receptor-induced production of catecholamines.[39] There is further evidence, albeit from intraperitoneal injections, of a complex effect on corticosteroid responses in stress.[40] IL-6, a marker of stress, was also reduced. Ginseng also raised plasma ACTH (adrenocorticotropic hormone) and cortisone in the relaxed (non-stressed) state when given by injection (thereby possibly generating a sense of alertness and well-being).[41] Ginseng saponins (100 mg/kg, oral) and ginsenosides Rg_3 and Rb_1 (10 mg/kg, oral) reduced the brain levels of the polyamine putrescine during immobilisation stress in mice. Polyamines are acknowledged as stress stimuli markers.[42]

This modern evidence supports an earlier hypothesis that ginseng acts on the hypothalamus, mediated through the anterior pituitary and ACTH release so as to improve the response of the adrenal cortex to stress. Based on human experience of ginseng, it was proposed that glucocorticoid production responses were sharper in acute stress and spared in chronic stress conditions.[43]

Memory, learning, neuroprotection and other neurological effects

The total effect of the root is stimulatory, but the diols such as Rb_1 are sedative and the triols such as Rg_1 are stimulatory.[44]

Evidence suggests that different doses have different effects on performance: standardised ginseng extract was administered orally at doses of 3 to 300 mg/kg for 10 days to 10 rats each dose. With the 'shuttle-box' method for active avoidance, the most pronounced effect on learning and memory was obtained by the dose of 10 mg/kg. With the 'step-down' method for passive avoidance, the 30 mg/kg dose significantly improved retention. In the staircase maze training with positive (alimentary) reinforcement, only the dose of 10 mg/kg significantly improved learning and memory. The dose of 100 mg/kg greatly increased the locomotor activity of mice.[45] Oral doses of ginsenosides Rb_1 and Rg_1 (each at about 50 mg/kg) accelerated brain and body development in young mice and facilitated memory acquisition in two models.[46] Oral administration of a ginseng ethanol extract 90 minutes before testing dose-dependently improved the maze performance of rats after disruption by scopolamine.[47]

The effects of oral doses of standardised extracts of ginseng (17, 50 and 150 mg/kg), Ginkgo and their combination were investigated on young and old rats in a series of behavioural tests. As before, effects varied with the dose and the test used, but both ginseng and Ginkgo extracts demonstrated properties similar to nootropic drugs (drugs that affect neurons favourably). The two extracts and their combination improved the retention of learned behaviour.[48]

The non-saponin fraction of red ginseng (50 mg/kg/day, oral) was investigated on learning deficits in aged rats.[49] It significantly ameliorated deficits in place-navigation learning in the aged rats, an effect partly attributed to an augmentation of long-term potentiation in the hippocampal CA3 subfield of the brain.

A 2009 review noted the in vitro evidence for a neuroprotective role of ginsenosides. They increased survival of cultured neuronal cells, enhanced neurite outgrowth and regenerated neuronal networks. Furthermore, it has been shown that Rb_1 and Rg_1 protect neurons from exitotoxicity induced by, for example, glutamate and from oxidative stress.[10] Another review discussed the in vitro evidence for ginsenoside Rg_3 protecting hippocampal neurons from NMDA (N-methyl-D-aspartate) and homocysteine neurotoxicity.[50]

The same review noted neuroprotective effects in vivo for ginseng and ginsenosides, both after oral doses and via injection.[50] These included protection against insults such as ischaemia, hyperbaric oxygen, kainic acid, homocysteine, 3-nitropropionic acid and rotenone.

Another review included the studies investigating the impact of ginseng or ginsenosides in Parkinson's disease models.[51] In vivo protection after oral administration of a ginseng extract was demonstrated against the neurotoxic effects of MPTP (1-methyl-4-phenyl-1,2,3,6-tetrahydropyridine) or its active metabolite. MPTP is a known inducer of parkinsonism in humans. The review also noted several relevant in vitro studies. It has been suggested that the lower incidence of Parkinson's disease in China might be a related observation.

The relatively recent discovery of the in vitro effects of ginsenosides on neuronal membrane proteins, such as voltage-dependent ion channels, has been reviewed.[50] Ginsenosides inhibit voltage-dependent Ca^{2+}, K^+ and Na^+ channel activities in a stereospecific manner. Certain ginsenosides (Rb_1 and Rg_3 in particular) also inhibit ligand-gated ion channels such as NMDA, some subtypes of nicotinic acetylcholine and serotonin type 3 receptors.[50]

Immune system effects

Immune system effects attributed to ginseng have been reviewed.[10,52] However, the majority of the included studies and subsequent investigations have employed in vitro tests, or in vivo models where ginseng or ginsenosides were given by injection.

Emphasising studies involving the oral administration of ginseng extract it was found to:

- enhance B and T lymphocyte and natural killer (NK) cell activities in mice and increase production of interferon following an interferon-inducer (the dose was 10 mg/mouse/day of ginseng for 4 consecutive days)[53]
- increase NK cell activity and dose-dependently enhance antibody formation in mice (in vitro it inhibited lymphocyte proliferation)[54]
- protect one particular mouse strain against *Candida albicans* infection[55]
- inhibit *Helicobacter pylori* adhesion to host cells.[56]

One early study observed a particular immunosuppressive effect. Saponins from ginseng, when injected into mice at approximately 10 mg/kg, had no significant effect on lymphocyte responses to a subsequent influenza virus infection. However, the saponins selectively suppressed delayed-type hypersensitivity to the virus when administered before, but not after, virus sensitisation. The authors suggested that this effect may be related to the steroid-like structure of the saponins (ginsenosides).[57]

A 2009 publication reviewed the in vitro immunomodulatory effects of the ginsenosides.[10] Depending on the ginsenoside and the model used, both immunostimulatory and immunosuppressive effects were observed. For example, ginsenosides Rb_1 and Re significantly enhanced mitogen-induced lymphocyte proliferation, Rg_1 had no effect and Rb_2 strongly blocked proliferation. In contrast, ginsenosides Rb_1 and Rb_2 did not suppress the proliferation of IL-2-stimulated T cells, whereas Re and Rg_1 were strongly suppressant. Perhaps more credibly, maturation of dendritic cells is promoted by intestinal metabolites of ginsenosides, such as compound K.

Ginseng may help to prevent cancer through effects on the immune system. The effects of long-term oral administration of ginseng extract (30 and 150 mg/kg/day) on levels of immunoglobulin types were studied in mice. Serum levels of gamma-globulin fell dose-dependently (p<0.05) after ginseng. Among the immunoglobulin isotypes, only serum IgG_1 was decreased (p<0.05). The authors suggested that since IgG_1 is rarely involved in killing cancer cells, and can act as a blocking antibody, this effect of ginseng may be beneficial for the prevention and inhibition of cancer.[58] Experiments have also shown that the anticarcinogenic activity of ginseng may be related to the augmentation of NK cell activity.[59]

Effects on cellular function

The effects of ginseng and its components on cultures of normal cells have been the subject of several studies, although more recent attention has focused on ginseng's influence on abnormal cells. The positive effects of ginseng in promoting the longevity, metabolism and growth of normal cells are seen by many investigating scientists as confirmation of its tonic activity. As early as 1969, aqueous extract of ginseng was found to delay degeneration of human amnion cells in vitro, an activity also exhibited by hydrocortisone and some of its analogues.[60] Fulder confirmed this observation using cell cultures of human fibroblasts. Ginseng promoted growth and delayed cellular necrosis, as did hydrocortisone.[61]

Subsequent in vitro studies have demonstrated the effects of ginseng or its components on the metabolism of a variety of cell types. These included the stimulation of DNA and protein synthesis in testes,[62] an increase in lactate levels[63] and a decrease in intracellular protein degradation in human fibroblasts.[64] Ginseng total saponins stimulated haematopoietic progenitor cell growth of cells taken from normal subjects and from 14 of 29 patients with aplastic anaemia.[65] Ginsenoside Rg_1 stimulated activity of tyrosine aminotransferase in hepatocytes.[66]

A tetrapeptide isolated from ginseng root stimulated the growth of several cell lines.[67] Based on immunoreactivity, a basic fibroblast growth factor-like molecule was identified in ginseng root.[68]

Ginseng or its components administered orally or by injection have also been found to stimulate cellular metabolism. Of a number of herbs tested, only injection of ginseng stimulated nuclear RNA synthesis in the liver cells of rats.[69] Injection of various components of ginseng root stimulated activities of nuclear RNA polymerase[70] and cytoplasmic RNA in rat liver cells,[71] increased RNA, protein and lipid synthesis in rat bone marrow cells,[72] and stimulated rat renal nuclear RNA synthesis.[73]

Oral doses of various ginseng components substantially increased rough endoplasmic reticulum and RNA synthesis in rat hepatocytes,[74] stimulated DNA, protein and lipid synthesis in rat bone marrow cells[75] and increased hepatic lactate dehydrogenase activity in mice.[76] This last finding, according to the authors of the study, could provide one explanation for the putative antifatigue properties of ginseng.[76]

A 2007 review emphasised the steroid-like effects of ginsenosides at a cellular level.[77]

Anticancer activity

Considerable interest has been shown among researchers in the ways that ginseng might prevent or assist in the treatment of cancer. It has been implied that the tonic, adaptogenic and immune-enhancing effects of ginseng could lead to improved natural resistance against malignant tumours.[78] However, the research summarised below suggests that more specific mechanisms could also apply.

In early research ginseng extract, ginsenosides and other components in the root, such as the diacetylenic alcohols, have inhibited the growth of various tumour cell lines in several test tube experiments.[79–82] Moreover, diol-type prosapogenins and sapogenins (which are likely to be among the active forms of ginsenosides after oral ingestion) were also active against several cancer cell lines.[83,84]

Since then, the cytotoxic and antiproliferative effects of ginsenosides towards human and animal cancer cell lines have been demonstrated in numerous investigations.[10] The potential ginsenoside metabolites (aglycones) 20(S)-PPD and 25(R)-25-OH-PPD demonstrated most marked activity in one series of experiments, via both increased apoptosis and cell-cycle arrest. Ginsenosides with fewer or no sugars seem to be more active than those with more, suggesting that greater lipid solubility enhances their activity.[10]

Ginsenosides of the 20(S)-PPD family are the best studied group, with a focus on Rh_2. The compound has been shown to suppress proliferation in vitro for a range of human cancer cell lines including breast, colorectal, prostate, hepatic, intestinal and melanoma. Again induction of apoptosis and arrest of cell cycle progression appear to be the operative mechanisms.[10] Compound K, the potential metabolite of some of the major PPD ginsenosides such as Rb_1, Rb_2, Rc and Rd, was cytotoxic and antiproliferative in a number of in vitro models.[10]

Much less is known regarding the antiproliferative and cytotoxic effects of members of the 20(S)-PPT family of ginsenosides, although it appears they are active as well (at least as their aglycone form).[10]

One interesting property of the ginsenosides is their ability to induce differentiation in cancer cell cultures. (Differentiation means that a tumour cell divides into daughter cells that show normal behaviour.) For example, this has been demonstrated for cultures of mouse melanoma cells[85] and teratocarcinoma cells: the activity may involve interaction of the ginsenoside with a glucocorticoid receptor in the cell.[86]

Ginseng extract[87] and ginsenosides Rb_1[88] and Rh_2[89] have exhibited antimutagenic activity against genotoxic agents in various in vitro models. In the first two cases the mechanism of action could involve enhanced DNA repair.

Early animal investigations of the antitumour activity of ginseng yielded mainly inconclusive or negative results.[90] Subsequently, one group of scientists focused on the activity of ginsenoside Rh_2, finding that oral doses prolonged survival of mice bearing human ovarian cancer cells[91] and acted synergistically with the anticancer drug cisplatin.[92] Another component of ginseng root, panaxytriol (a polyacetylenic alcohol), produced significant tumour growth delays (p<0.01) at an injected dose of 40 mg/kg in mice transplanted with B16 melanoma cells.[93] Oral administration of ginseng extract, radiation treatment and the combination of both increased the survival of intrahepatic sarcoma-180 tumour-bearing mice to 20.4%, 16.9% and 82.1% respectively. Radiation treatment destroyed both cancer and liver cells, but the ginseng extract seemed to help recovery of healthy liver cells from radiation treatment and inhibited the infiltration of cancer cells.[94]

Using athymic mice transplanted with ovarian cancer cells, ip injection of Rg_3 at 3 mg/kg/day for 10 days improved survival and decreased tumour weights and angiogenesis. It also added to the antitumour activity of cyclophosphamide.[95]

Oral doses of a lipid-soluble extract of red ginseng (0.1, 0.3 and 1.0 g/kg/day) dose-dependently inhibited the growth of human lung tumour xenografts in mice.[96]

Positive results have been demonstrated in cancer prevention experiments where ginseng was co-administered with a known cancer-causing agent. For example prolonged administration of red ginseng extract (1 mg/mL in drinking water) to mice significantly inhibited the incidence and proliferation of tumours produced by benzo-alpha-pyrene, 9,10-dimethyl-1,2-benz-alpha-anthracene, urethane and aflatoxin B1, but not N-2-fluorenylacetamide and tobacco smoke condensate. The same authors found that red ginseng had more activity than white ginseng (although both exhibited good cancer-preventing activity) and that activity increased with the age of the root.[97] Ginseng may exert its protective effect on benzo(a) pyrene by altering its metabolism.[98]

Rats fed ginseng powder (0.5 g or 2 g/kg) for 5 weeks were exposed to azoxymethane (an inducer of colon cancer) during weeks 2 to 3.[99] There were fewer progressed aberrant crypt foci at week 8 in the animals given ginseng, compared with the control group, indicating a cytostatic effect. Ginseng extract (10 mg/kg, oral) resulted in a significant reduction of lung tumours induced in mice by benzo(a)pyrene.[100] A 2000 review identified several additional studies demonstrating the chemopreventative action of ginseng extract (mainly) or ginsenosides. These included models of induction of lung, liver, stomach, ovarian, breast, renal, cervical and skin cancers in rodents.[101]

Some ginsenosides appear to inhibit metastasis. Injection of ginsenoside Rg_3 in rats significantly decreased the incidence of cancer metastases induced by the chemicals azoxymethane and bombesin,[102] and in other in vivo models. Ginsenoside Rg_3 was also found to be a potent inhibitor of invasion by various tumour cell lines when tested using an in vitro cell monolayer invasion model. However, other ginsenosides were inactive in this model.[103] Ginsenoside Rb_2 inhibited tumour angiogenesis and metastasis produced by melanoma cells in mice. Intravenous administration of ginsenoside Rb_2 after tumour inoculation achieved a remarkable reduction in the number of blood vessels oriented towards the tumour mass, but did not cause a significant inhibition of tumour growth. In contrast, intra tumoral or oral administration caused an inhibition of both neovascularisation and tumour growth.[104]

Subsequently, various ginsenosides including Rg_3 and compound K have demonstrated anti-angiogenic activity in different tumour models.[77] Rg_3 is the most extensively investigated compound, exerting activity in several in vivo models (xenografts of breast, ovarian and colon and melanoma cells) when administered alone or in combination with conventional agents. A significant reduction of intra tumoural microvessel density and (VEGF) vascular endothelial growth factor expression was observed. Similar results were also demonstrated when Rg_3 was combined with a low dose of cyclophosphamide in mice bearing Lewis lung carcinoma, all indicative of the key role of suppression of tumour-induced angiogenesis in the anti-metastatic activity of ginsenosides. Another key mechanism is inhibition of the basement membrane degrading enzymes MMP-2 and MMP-9.[77]

As alluded to above, ginseng extract or its components can potentiate the activity of cytotoxic drugs. This has additionally been demonstrated for the drug mitomycin C in both in vitro[105] and in vivo experiments.[106] The in vivo results suggest that this effect happens without an increase in toxicity to the host.[107]

In an acute myelogenous leukaemia in vitro model, PPT ginsenosides were found to exert a chemosensitising effect on P-glycoprotein-mediated multi-drug resistant cells by increasing intracellular accumulation of daunorubicin and doxorubicin.[77] Similar results have been observed for 20(S)-PPT, Rh_2, Rc, Rd and compound K. Ginsenosides (Rh_2, PPD and PPT) interacted directly with breast cancer resistance protein in MCF-7 cells, increasing the cytotoxicity of mitoxantrone.[77]

One review, noting that chronic inflammation is associated with a high cancer risk, linked the putative chemopreventative action of ginseng with its anti-inflammatory activities.[108] Mechanisms discussed included inhibition of cyclo-oxygenase (COX-2) and NF-kappaB induction, stimulation of (iNOS) inducible nitric oxide synthase and antioxidant effects.

Cardiovascular activity

According to a recent review, a major effect of ginsenosides on the cardiovascular system is a reduction of sympathetic nerve activity, leading to vascular relaxation and lowered blood pressure.[10] This is partially mediated by the release of endothelial nitric oxide (NO). Vasorelaxation may also involve Ca^{2+} activated K^+ channels in vascular smooth muscle cells.[10,109] Researchers have reported that the chronic feeding of ginsenosides to rabbits may have enhanced vasodilatation by preventing NO degradation.[110]

Ginsenosides enhanced cerebral blood flow in rats and reduced cholesterol levels and atheroma formation in rabbits fed a high cholesterol diet.[10] HDL was increased and lipid peroxidation reduced in the hyperlipidaemic rat.[109] Oral ginseng given to rats with surgically reduced livers reduced the resultant atherosclerosis by decreasing platelet adhesiveness. An antiatherosclerotic impact in rabbits fed ginseng was attributed to increased prostacyclin in the carotid artery and decreased thromboxane A_2 in platelets.[109] Ginsenosides are also relatively potent PAF antagonists in vitro.[10]

Blood sugar regulation

There is considerable research interest in the antidiabetic activity of ginseng, and potential hypoglycaemic constituents identified in ginseng have been reviewed.[111] These components include glycans, which are called panaxans (more have subsequently been identified[112]), adenosine and unidentified large molecules with insulin-like activity. However, hypoglycaemic activity has only been established after injection, and it is unlikely that any of these compounds would confer significant hypoglycaemic activity to oral doses of ginseng. These reservations would also apply to a polypeptide isolated from ginseng root and found to have hypoglycaemic activity.[113] Perhaps of greater interest are results for injection of ginsenoside Rb_2, which countered some of the unfavourable metabolic changes observed in diabetic rats. In particular it boosted intracellular ATP and decreased cyclic AMP,[114] and improved protein biosynthesis[115] and nitrogen balance.[116] Body weight was improved and diabetic symptoms such as polyuria were decreased.[117]

Recent research has indeed focused on the ginsenosides, with several in vivo studies demonstrating hypoglycaemic activity.[10] However, antidiabetic effects have only been generated for a few specific ginsenosides, including Rb_1, Re, Rh_2 and the aglycone 20(S)-PPT. For example, antidiabetic activity was demonstrated for ginsenoside Re in ob/ob diabetic mice and ginsenoside Rh_2 increased insulin secretion in rats. In vitro mechanistic studies suggest the antidiabetic activity of ginsenoside Rb_1 is probably related to activation of peroxisome PPAR-gamma. This transcription factor is involved in lipid and glucose metabolism and fat cell differentiation. Certain modern antidiabetic drugs are PPAR-gamma activators.[10] Some investigators suggest that the hypoglycaemic activity of ginseng depends not just on the total ginsenoside content, but also on the profile.[10]

Other activity

Ginseng extract or total saponins administered by injection countered the deleterious effects of repeated administration of narcotic drugs such as morphine,[118] cocaine,[119] methamphetamine and apomorphine[120] in animal models. Ginseng total saponins may inhibit the dopaminergic activation induced by morphine[121] and ginseng extract inhibited the development of tolerance to the analgesic and hyperthermic effects of morphine, depending on the administered doses of ginseng and morphine.[122] It is encouraging that oral doses of ginseng extract (ranging from 50 to 400 mg/kg) also significantly inhibited the development of morphine-induced tolerance and physical dependence, as well as inhibiting the decrease in hepatic glutathione induced by morphine multiple injections.[123]

A number of studies have been reviewed that suggest the antioxidant and organ-protective actions of ginseng are linked to enhanced NO synthesis in the endothelium of the lung, heart and kidney and in the corpus cavernosum.[124] It was suggested that enhanced NO synthesis could contribute to ginseng-associated vasodilation and perhaps also to an aphrodisiac action. However, these findings are largely based on in vitro tests. One in vivo study observed that feeding of red ginseng (50 mg/kg) to rabbits and rats for 3 months induced significant effects in corpus cavernosal muscle strips. Ginseng has also increased testosterone and decreased prolactin in rodents.[110]

A single oral dose of 200 mg/kg red ginseng increased ethanol clearance in rats,[125] a finding that might be relevant to humans. Fourteen healthy male volunteers were studied to assess the effects of ginseng on blood alcohol clearance, using each person as his own control. Participants received 72 g of 25% ethanol, and at another time 3 g of ginseng extract (about 6 g of root) with the ethanol, all doses per 65 kg of body weight. At 40 minutes after the last drink, the average blood alcohol level after ginseng and ethanol consumption was 35% lower than after ethanol alone.[126]

Pharmacokinetics

Pharmacokinetics of ginsenosides Rg_1, Rb_1 and Rb_2 in rats were reviewed in an early publication. Rg_1 was easily decomposed to its prosapogenin in both rat stomach and dilute hydrochloric acid, whereas Rb_1 and Rb_2 were little decomposed in rat stomach, but were easily converted to their prosapogenins by dilute hydrochloric acid. The ginsenosides were also metabolised to several prosapogenins by gut bacteria and enteric enzymes. The amount of Rg_1, Rb_1 and Rb_2 absorbed from the gastrointestinal tract of the rat was 1.9%, 0.1% and 3.7% respectively of the administered dose. Rb_1 and Rb_2 were mainly excreted in the urine, whereas Rg_1 was excreted in the urine and bile in a 2:5 ratio. Unabsorbed saponins were metabolised by gut flora.[127]

Early studies on humans tended to support the above picture that the ginsenosides have low bioavailability as such, but their decomposition products after the action of digestion and bowel flora are absorbed and may be the true active forms of the ginsenosides. Analysis of urine samples from 60 Swedish athletes who had consumed various ginseng preparations within 10 days before urine collection revealed that samples contained significant quantities of the sapogenin 20(S)-PPT.[128] The results after intake of single oral doses of ginseng preparations demonstrated a linear relationship between the amounts of ginsenosides consumed and the 20(S)-PPT glycosides excreted in the urine. Only about 1.2% of the dose was recovered in the glycosidic (ginsenoside) form over 5 days.[129] The main metabolites of ginsenosides after incubation with human faecal flora were identified as prosapogenins and sapogenins and these were also detected in the blood and urine of humans after oral administration of high doses of ginseng extract.[130] One organism implicated in hydrolysing ginsenosides was *Prevotella oris*.[131]

The metabolism and absorption of ginsenosides have been intensively studied in recent years, although relatively few investigations have been in humans.[10,132] A study in rats found that after oral administration of ginseng powder the absorption of ginsenosides was fast, but maximum concentrations of individual key ginsenosides were relatively low, ranging from 1.5 to 6.4 µg/mL.[132] Only 3.29% of Rg_1 and 0.64% of Rb_1 were detected in rat serum after oral administration of ginsenosides.[133] However, such findings seem to vary; for example another study found much higher numbers, although the higher bioavailability of Rg_1 (by a factor greater than 4) was confirmed.[134] In vitro investigations suggest that sodium-dependent glucose co-transporter 1 is involved in the intestinal transport of Rg_1.[135]

From the various in vitro and in vivo studies, a reasonably clear picture of the metabolism of ginsenosides has emerged.[10] Ginsenosides of the PPT type, such as Rg_1 and Re, are metabolised to ginsenosides Rh_1 and F_1, and then finally to 20(S)-PPT. For ginsenosides of the PPD type, such as Rb_1, Rb_2 and Re, the process is similar. The main metabolites are compound K (20-O-beta-glucopyranosyl-20(S)-PPD, sometimes named M1 or IH-901) and then finally 20(S)-PPD. The production of compound K requires the presence of bacterial beta-glucosidase enzymes, such as provided by *Eubacterium spp.*, *Prevotella oris* and *Bifidobacterium spp.*

Studies suggest that the production of compound K is likely to vary considerably between people, depending on their resident intestinal flora.[10]

It is a noteworthy observation that the concentrations of these deglycosylated ginsenosides in plasma after oral administration of ginseng are in a range where a significant physiological effect might be expected. Compound K is mostly excreted in the bile and is esterified with fatty acids in the liver, leading possibly to more active metabolites.[10]

In a small pilot study, two healthy volunteers received 700 mg of an extract standardised to 4% ginsenosides.[136] Ginsenosides Rh_1 and F_1 and compound K were the main compounds detected in plasma, confirming the above discussion. Ginsenoside Rb_1 was also clearly detected in one volunteer. Compound K was also detected in urine. A more recent study in 32 healthy men showed a strong effect of bowel flora on the metabolism of ginsenoside Rb_1 (via compound K) but not on its absorption after an oral dose of 12 g of ginseng powder.[137]

(See Chapter 2 for a further discussion of the pharmacokinetics of saponins in general and ginseng in particular.)

Clinical trials

Several clinical studies on ginseng have involved two preparations. The first is a 5:1 extract (G115) standardised for ginsenoside levels, so that 200 mg of extract (the typical dose used) corresponds to about 1 g of root. The second preparation involves the combination of this standardised extract with vitamins and minerals. While most of the clinical studies on ginseng have been included in this review, because of the potentially confounding effect of adding vitamins and minerals to ginseng only some of the studies on this second product have been reviewed.

Physical performance

If ginseng has tonic and adaptogenic properties, it might be expected to improve human performance and well-being in a variety of circumstances. Some clinical studies have supported this hypothesis. One German team has been prominent in these reports. For example, in a double blind, placebo-controlled trial, 30 elite male athletes (19 to 31 years of age) were subjected to a graded ergometric test. Ten athletes in each of three groups received either 200 mg of ginseng extract, 200 mg ginseng extract and 400 mg vitamin E, or placebo for 9 weeks. While there was no statistically significant difference between the groups receiving ginseng or ginseng plus vitamin E, there was a clear benefit of these two treatments over placebo for heart rate ($p<0.001$), blood lactate ($p<0.01$) and maximal oxygen uptake ($p<0.01$).[138] Ginseng in conjunction with vitamins and minerals improved parameters such as total workload, maximal oxygen uptake, heart rate and blood lactate levels in a randomised, double blind, placebo-controlled trial involving 50 male sports teachers. The authors suggested that their results indicate the ginseng preparation increased work capacity by improving muscular oxygen utilisation.[139] In a double blind, placebo-controlled crossover trial, 43 male triathletes received either 200 mg of ginseng extract (approx 1 g of root) or placebo for two consecutive training periods of 10 weeks. Although there were no significant changes in physical fitness during the first period, ginseng retarded the loss of fitness during the second 10-week period.[140]

A more recent study was also positive. Seven healthy male volunteers performed two exhaustive incremental exercises on the treadmill before and after 8 weeks of 6 g daily of ginseng extract. The extract increased time until exhaustion by 1.5 min ($p < 0.05$). Malondialdehyde rises were attenuated after ginseng administration, and catalase and superoxide dismutase activities following exercise were significantly elevated, suggesting an effect to facilitate recovery from exhausting exercise.[141]

One study was undertaken to determine whether administration of a standardised ginseng extract (standardisation not defined) at 300 mg/day for 8 weeks could enhance maximum aerobic and anaerobic exercise capabilities and whether any changes in such effects occurred when exercise training was added.[142] Forty-one male university students were randomly divided into four groups as ginseng-untrained (GU, n=10), ginseng-trained (GT, n=10), placebo-untrained (PU, n=10), and placebo-trained (PT, n=11). The trained groups underwent 8 weeks of aerobic exercise. Initially, all groups did not differ in average maximum oxygen consumption. After 8 weeks, this parameter increased significantly from the initial level by 12.6% in group GU, 14.5% in group PT and 24.5% in group GT, which was significantly higher than group GU but not group PT. Changes in all measured parameters related to maximum oxygen consumption were similar among the groups, except group PU. Leg strength was also significantly enhanced over group PU in groups PT, GU and GT. As a result of these findings it was concluded that, under the conditions of the study, ginseng administration at the prescribed dose exhibited training-like effects on maximum oxygen consumption as well as anaerobic power and leg muscle strength. However, no clear synergistic action on these physical fitness variables occurred when both ginseng administration and exercise training were combined. Body fat was significantly decreased in both ginseng groups compared with baseline ($p < 0.05$).

However, the weight of more recent reviews on the effect of ginseng on physical performance have cast doubt on these properties, citing methodological flaws in earlier research.[143–145] New original research is also negative. In one study 20 young men and eight young women were randomly assigned to either a ginseng or placebo group for a period of 3 weeks in a double blind design. Prior to and following treatment, the participants performed a symptom-limited graded exercise test. No significant treatment effect was observed.[146] Sixty men from the Royal Thai Navy were randomised into either 3 g ginseng or placebo for 8 weeks. There were no differences in lactic acid levels, heart rate, fat and carbohydrate oxidation rates detected after cycle ergometry.[147] A study on 36 healthy men given 200 to 400 mg/day of ginseng extract or placebo over 8 weeks failed to

show any favourable influence of ginseng intake on the same parameters during graded maximal aerobic exercise.[148] The same team randomly assigned 24 healthy, active women to a 400 mg/day G115 ginseng or placebo for 8 weeks. Before and after the trial period, each woman performed an all-out-effort, 30-second leg cycle ergometry test followed by a controlled recovery under constant laboratory conditions. No significant difference was found between the ginseng and placebo study groups for the following variables measured: peak anaerobic power output, mean anaerobic power output, rate of fatigue and immediate post-exercise recovery heart rates ($p > 0.05$).[149] Some of the negative studies, however, are handicapped by the small numbers of volunteers or short duration of the treatments.[150,151]

In an acute high-dose study, eight male college students were randomly given water or 20 g of ginseng root extract immediately after acute resistance exercise.[152] Responses of plasma hormones such as growth hormone, testosterone and cortisol were not influenced by the ginseng, compared with controls. Perhaps dosing of ginseng prior to exercise might have yielded a different result. The effects of a ginseng extract (equivalent to 2 g/day) or a placebo for 6 weeks were assessed in endurance athletes.[153] No impact on immune parameters, plasma testosterone and plasma cortisol was observed.

All the above studies were conducted on normal individuals, some of them very fit or undergoing intensive training. An interesting placebo-controlled study enlisting 92 patients found that standardised ginseng (G115, 300 mg/day for 3 months) significantly improved pulmonary functions and exercise capacity in patients with moderately severe chronic obstructive pulmonary disease.[154] The degree of the improvements was quite striking. For example, maximum oxygen consumption increased by 37.5% compared to the placebo group. This study implies that the benefits of ginseng on physical performance might be more marked in unwell or unfit people.

Psychomotor performance and cognitive function

A few studies have examined the influence of ginseng on psychomotor performance, and overall results to date indicate ginseng appears to be of limited value. The effect of ginseng (200 mg/day, approx 1 g of root) or placebo on reaction time to auditory and visual stimuli was investigated in a double blind study. Significant decreases in reaction times ($p < 0.01$) were seen only in older participants (40 to 60 years). In addition, significant improvements in subjective feelings related to well-being ($p < 0.01$) were observed in both older males and all females.[155] Various tests of psychomotor performance were carried out in a group of 16 healthy male volunteers given a ginseng extract (200 mg/day, approx. 1 g of root) for 12 weeks and in a similar group given an identical placebo under double blind conditions. Ginseng was only statistically superior to placebo in for the mental arithmetic test and did not enhance pure motor function, recognition and visual reaction time. No adverse effects were reported.[156]

Fifteen young soccer players were randomised to receive either 350 mg/day ginseng extract or a placebo for 8 weeks in a double blinded trial.[157] Before and after the treatment they performed an incremental bicycle ergometer test until exhaustion. The ginseng significantly improved psychomotor performance, as assessed by reaction time at rest and during exercise, but did not impact exercise capacity.

Several trials have examined the impact of ginseng on cognitive function. The effect of a ginseng extract (400 mg/day, approx. 2 g of root) on a variety of cognitive functions was compared with a placebo in a double blind, randomised, test-retest design. Trial participants (112) were healthy volunteers older than 40 years of age and the treatment duration was 8 to 9 weeks. The ginseng group showed a tendency to faster simple reaction times (not significant) and significantly better abstract thinking than controls (p=0.02, Wisconsin Card Sorting Test). However, baseline values were not established for this test, and it is conceivable that the significant difference was inherent between the two groups, rather than resulting from the ginseng treatment. There was no significant difference between ginseng and placebo for concentration or memory.[158]

A 2010 Cochrane review searched for blinded, randomised, placebo-controlled trials assessing the effects of ginseng on cognitive function.[159] Compound formulations were also evaluated if ginseng was the major component. Nine trials were identified and, of these, five were included in the analysis, as they provided extractable information. Two of these included trials are reviewed above.[156,158] One of the included trials was on a multi-herb formulation and all five involved healthy volunteers. Pooling of the data was not possible because of heterogeneity in outcome measures, trial duration and ginseng dose. Analysis suggested that some aspects of cognitive function, behaviour and quality of life were improved by ginseng, without serious adverse events. However, the authors considered that convincing evidence was lacking and more rigorously designed trials were needed.

An earlier 2003 review of the evidence for an effect of ginseng on cognitive performance concluded that single doses of ginseng most notably engender cognitive benefits in terms of improved memory, but can also be associated with 'costs' in terms of attention task deficits following less mnemonically beneficial doses.[160] As noted by the review, most of the studies of ginseng on cognition and mood have been single dose acute studies. Hence a study was designed to assess the impact of subacute dosing (over 8 days).[161] A three-arm placebo-controlled, double blind, crossover design was used in a trial involving 30 healthy young volunteers (200 mg and 400 mg ginseng extract and placebo). Results confirmed previous findings that an acute dose of ginseng can modulate cognitive function (and mood), but there was no additional effect conferred by the next 7 days of dosing. Both doses of ginseng significantly slowed the deterioration in subjective ratings of calmness in the last two testing sessions on day 1 (p<0.05). While the acute 400 mg dose significantly improved key aspects of working memory (as assessed by a mental arithmetic task), the 200 mg dose led to a significant slowing of performance. Again there was no additional cumulative effect from repeated dosing.

However, there appears to be a significant benefit on cognitive function by combining *Ginkgo biloba* with ginseng.

A placebo-controlled, double blind, crossover trial examined the acute effects of ginseng and Ginkgo on mental performance in 20 healthy volunteers.[162] College students were tested four times between 1 and 6 h after taking the herbs. Those receiving Ginkgo only demonstrated significantly improved concentration within 2.5 h. The highest dose tested (360 mg of 50:1 standardised extract) was the most effective. A dose of 400 mg of 5:1 ginseng extract (equivalent to 2 g of root) sharpened memory after just 1 h, with improvements in ability to store, hold and retrieve information. When both the Ginkgo extract (360 mg, equivalent to 18 g of leaf) and the ginseng extract (600 mg, equivalent to 3 g of root) were combined as a single treatment, results were striking. Not only was the effect on cognitive function more pronounced than treatment with either herb on its own, it was immediately evident when the volunteers were first tested. The lead researcher, Dr Andrew Scholey was quoted as saying: 'The results were incredible in terms of improvements in speed and accuracy-usually there is a trade-off and you improve one at the expense of the other'. Follow-up publications have elaborated on these experimental findings.[163,164]

Long-term dosing of these two herbs was also found to be beneficial in terms of cognitive function. A 14-week, double blind, placebo-controlled, randomised trial studied the cognitive effects of two different doses of the combination in 256 healthy volunteers between the ages of 38 and 66 years (60 mg/day of Ginkgo extract and 100 mg/day of ginseng extract, or double this dose).[165] Trial participants performed a battery of tests using the Computerised Cognitive Assessment system. Volunteers receiving the ginseng and Ginkgo combination demonstrated statistically significant improvements in memory compared with the placebo group, even after a 2-week washout. However, no beneficial effects from this combination on cognitive measures were seen in a 12-week double blind, placebo-controlled trial involving 57 postmenopausal women.[166]

Some preliminary investigations have explored the potential role of ginseng in Alzheimer's disease (AD). In an open label trial, 61 patients diagnosed with probable AD were randomised to one of three groups for a period of 12 weeks: low-dose red ginseng (4.5 g/day), high-dose red ginseng (9 g/day), or control.[167] Antidementia drugs (donepezil, galantamine, memantine or rivastigmine) that had been taken for at least 6 months prior to randomisation were continued during the 12-week trial. At the end of treatment, patients in the high-dose ginseng group showed significant improvement on the cognitive subscale of ADAS (Alzheimer's Disease Assessment Scale) and CDR (Clinical Dementia Rating) when compared with those in the control group (p=0.032 and 0.006, respectively). The same research group also published results of a larger 12-week open label trial in AD involving 97 patients and using a red ginseng dose of 4.5 g/day.[168] A significant outcome was observed for the cognitive subscale of ADAS (p=0.029 versus baseline). Scores declined to the levels of the control group after discontinuing ginseng.

A 2009 systematic review of ginseng in AD identified only these two studies.[169] The review concluded that both of these trials were burdened with methodological limitations.

However, given the stated preliminary nature of the above open label trials in AD, a systematic review is probably premature at this stage of the research.

Stress, well-being and quality of life

Ginseng has shown some benefit in a variety of trials assessing quality of life (QoL) or general performance under stress. In a randomised, double blind trial, 501 participants received either ginseng extract with vitamins and minerals or a preparation containing only the vitamins and minerals. After 4 months, the group receiving ginseng showed highly significant improvements (p<0.0001) in all of the 11 QoL questionnaire items, whereas the group receiving only vitamins and minerals showed no significant improvement in any of these items. Adverse effects were minimal in both groups.[170] The effect on QoL of ginseng extract in conjunction with vitamins and minerals was compared with placebo in a randomised, 12-week double blind study. Healthy employed volunteers (n=390) older than 25 years were included. Significant improvements above placebo were noted for alertness (p<0.05), relaxation (p=0.02), appetite (p=0.04) and overall score on 18 QoL factors (p=0.03). Among the subgroup with the 20% lowest score at baseline, the active treatment improved both vitality (p=0.03) and depressed mood (p=0.05).[171]

A 2003 review of all published studies of ginseng and QoL identified nine clinical trials, including the two above.[172] Doses evaluated were 80 to 400 mg/day extract over 2 to 9 months. The review found that eight studies demonstrated some degree of QoL improvement, but mainly on subscores. Improvement in overall composite scores of QoL was rarely seen, indicating the need for additional research to clarify this issue.

In a randomised, double blind trial on the treatment of fatigue, 232 patients between the ages of 25 and 60 years received either ginseng extract (80 mg/day, approximately 0.4 g of root) with vitamins and minerals or placebo over a period of 6 weeks. Patients were allowed to choose the five items that best described their condition from a pre-established list of 20 items. Analysis of these scores of fatigue levels at the end of the study indicated a statistically greater improvement for the active treatment. Side effects were minimal with only two patients withdrawing from active treatment.[173]

In a randomised, double blind study in 83 participants (average age 38 years) the effect of ginseng extract (200 mg/day, approximately 1 g of root) or placebo on several parameters related to well-being were assessed. After 4 months of treatment the following significant changes were observed for the ginseng group when compared to the placebo group: fall in systolic blood pressure (p<0.01), improvements in colds (p<0.005) and bronchitis (p<0.05) (whether this was frequency, severity or both was not specified), improvement in appetite (p<0.01) and improvements in sleep (p<0.025), well-being (p<0.005) and performance (p<0.005).[174]

The effects of ginseng (1.2 g/day) on 12 fatigued night nurses was assessed by self-rating scales in a double blind, placebo-controlled, crossover design. Shifts consisted of 3 or 4 consecutive nights followed by 3 days of rest, and participants received treatment for the first 3 consecutive nights of work. According to the crossover design, each nurse was tested after ginseng, placebo or a good night's sleep. Although ginseng improved 11 of the 16 mood variables and eight of the 14 somatic symptoms compared with placebo, none of the differences were statistically significant. This may reflect on the short duration of ginseng use or low patient numbers. Participants slept less and rated sleep quality as worse during ginseng use.[175]

Ginseng is particularly valued as a tonic for the elderly in China, and a number of studies have examined the benefits of ginseng use in elderly people. Ginseng extract with vitamins and minerals (dose not specified) caused a significant increase (p<0.05) in REM sleep compared with placebo in a 10-week double blind trial in 20 elderly subjects. Other treatment effects were noted which suggest a positive effect on sleep quality.[176] In a double blind, crossover trial to test whether ginseng improved depression and impaired performance associated with old age, 49 participants were given 1500 mg red ginseng root or an identical placebo each for 10 days, with a washout period between dosages. The major result was a highly significant improvement in reaction time and decision making, as assessed by the tapping test and the reaction timer. Participants felt slightly more alert and energetic when taking ginseng, but were also less happy. No major side effects were recorded and the treatment did not influence blood pressure.[177] Another study produced neutral results. Ginseng extract (80 mg/day, about 0.4 g of root) with vitamin and minerals for 8 weeks did not improve rehabilitation of geriatric patients in a randomised placebo-controlled, double blind design involving 49 patients.[178]

Infection and immunity

Korean scientists have examined the effects of red ginseng in patients with HIV infection in a series of open trials. These trials suffer from poor experimental design, but they do suggest that the value of ginseng in this disorder should be examined further. In one trial the influence of 5.4 g/day of red ginseng powder on prognostic markers was assessed in 23 patients after 3 and 6 months. The following significant changes were noted at 6 months: decreased lymphocyte percentage (p<0.05), mean CD4 T cell percentage increased from 16.3±5.2% at baseline to 20.1±9.0% (p<0.05), CD8 T cell percentage increased (p<0.01), and two patients with measurable serum p24 antigen levels seemed to have these suppressed during treatment.[179] These beneficial results were reflected in a second trial where ginseng therapy was compared with zidovudine[180] and in a third that conducted long-term follow-up over several years.[181]

Further to these findings, the researchers investigated whether 5.4 g/day of Korean ginseng root powder taken long term had any impact on the development of resistant HIV-1 strains in patients treated with the drug zidovudine.[182] Nine patients were treated with both ginseng and the drug; another nine acted as controls and received only the drug. In samples after 24 months of therapy, the incidence of six resistance mutations to zidovudine was 21.7% for the ginseng group, versus 56.3% for the controls (p<0.01). The authors concluded that the observed maintenance of CD4 T cell counts by the zidovudine and ginseng combination might be indirectly due to the delayed development of resistance to zidovudine.

Clinical parameters in 68 HIV-1 infected patients who lived for more than 5 years without antiretroviral therapy were analysed to assess any confounding effect of their HLA class on disease progression.[183] The average Korean red ginseng intake over 112 months was 4.1 g. Ginseng intake was shown to significantly slow the decrease in CD4 T cells even when the influence of HLA class I was statistically eliminated (p<0.05). There was also a significant correlation between ginseng intake and a decrease in serum-soluble CD8 antigen levels (p<0.001).

The effects of ginseng on cell-mediated immune function were studied in 60 healthy volunteers. Three groups received either placebo, 200 mg/day standardised ginseng extract (about 1 g of root) or 200 mg/day of ginseng aqueous extract. Significant improvements after 8 weeks were noted in both ginseng groups for chemotaxis, phagocytic activity and intracellular killing, whereas only the last parameter increased in the placebo group. Results tended to be better for the standardised ginseng extract.[184]

The same research team examined the effect of ginseng extract (200 mg/day, about 1 g of root) on the function of alveolar macrophages in 40 patients with chronic bronchitis in a placebo-controlled, single blind trial. The ginseng extract was able to improve the immune response of alveolar macrophages collected by bronchoalveolar lavage.[185] In a subsequent randomised, double blind study, 227 volunteers (average age 48 years) received either ginseng extract (200 mg/day, about 1 g of root) or placebo for a period of 12 weeks during which they also received an anti-influenza polyvalent vaccination at week 4. As a result, while the incidence of influenza or common cold between weeks 4 and 12 was 42 cases in the placebo group, it was only 15 cases in the ginseng group (p<0.0001). Also antibody titres (p<0.0001) and natural killer cell activity (p<0.0001) were significantly higher in the ginseng group. There were nine adverse events: two cases of nausea, one of epigastralgia, one of anxiety and four of insomnia in the ginseng group, compared to one case of insomnia in the placebo group.[186]

However, 300 mg/day of ginseng extract for 2 months failed to influence total and differential white blood cell count and lymphocyte subpopulations in a double blind, placebo-controlled trial involving 20 healthy men.[187] Likewise, salivary secretory IgA was not changed by 400 mg/day of ginseng extract for 8 weeks in another trial.[188]

Cardiovascular effects

Forty-five patients with advanced congestive heart failure were divided into three groups and received either digoxin, red ginseng or both treatments in an open label design. The group receiving ginseng and digoxin showed the best results in terms of biochemical and haemodynamic parameters, followed by the group receiving ginseng. There were no adverse effects.[189]

Shengmai is a traditional Chinese formula for congestive heart failure containing ginseng, *Ophiopogon japonicus* and *Schisandra chinensis*. It is mainly administered as an injection or as an oral infusion. A 2011 Cochrane review identified six eligible trials, five where it was administered by injection and one as an oral liquid.[190] Compared to conventional treatment alone, Shengmai plus conventional treatment resulted in an improvement in the New York Heart Association assessment of severity. The quality of trials was low, hence any evidence of benefit was deemed to be weak.

A randomised, double blind, placebo-controlled study of 30 healthy university students found that 200 mg/day of ginseng extract for 28 days had no clinically significant impact on electrocardiographic and haemodynamic parameters.[191] There was a small decrease in diastolic blood pressure and increase in the QT_c interval following the very first dose.

An open study in 15 postmenopausal women found that 500 mg/day of ginseng root for 12 weeks had no impact on serum lipid profiles.[192] Given the positive effect on HDL levels with higher doses in a study in men with erectile dysfunction (see Reproductive function below), there may be a dose-related effect. A small, high-dose open label trial (n=8) did find that ginseng extract (6 g/day) for 8 weeks significantly lowered total cholesterol, triglycerides and LDL-cholesterol and raised HDL-cholesterol (all p<0.05).[193] HDL-cholesterol was increased by around 40%. The study also found that malondialdehyde (a measure of oxidation) was lowered and erythrocyte superoxide dismutase and catalase levels were significantly increased (all p<0.01).

A 2005 systematic review of the effects of ginseng on cardiovascular risk factors identified around 30 studies yielding results for blood pressure, lipids and/or blood glucose.[194] Nine studies evaluated cholesterol outcomes over periods ranging from 7 days to 3 months, with ginseng alone trialed in six. Overall results were inconsistent, but five of nine studies demonstrated improvements in one or more lipid parameters that were statistically significant. Since the quality of several of these trials was poor, or they were just simply preliminary studies, the authors suggested that while ginseng may improve lipid profiles, better designed trials were needed.

One of the concerns about using ginseng is that many patients who would benefit from its use often have high blood pressure. The oft-quoted thinking is that ginseng is contraindicated in hypertension. However, clinical studies do not support such a broad contraindication for this valuable herb.

One Korean study evaluated changes in blood pressure after 8 weeks of treatment with red ginseng root (4.5 g/day) using 24h blood pressure monitoring.[195] Placebo was administered for 4 weeks followed by red ginseng, which implies that the study was unblinded from the perspective of the clinician (in other words it was a single blind study). In 26 patients with essential hypertension, average systolic blood pressure was significantly decreased (p=0.03), while diastolic pressure only showed a tendency to decline (p=0.17). In eight patients with 'white coat' hypertension, no significant blood pressure change was observed, which might be expected given the low number of patients. The authors suggested that red ginseng might be considered a relatively safe treatment in conjunction with antihypertensive drugs. Side effects from ginseng were considered to be trivial and temporary.

In contrast to the poorly documented case reports (in terms of doses and products taken), the above clinical trial does not support the contraindication of ginseng in hypertension. This implies that any hypertensive response to ginseng is probably idiosyncratic and the risk needs to be assessed on a case by case basis. This was well illustrated by an earlier clinical trial in which red ginseng intake (3 to 6 g/day) for an average of 10 months gave the following results:

- In hypertensive patients, 51% showed lowered blood pressure, 43% remained unchanged and 5% showed elevation.
- In normotensive patients, 95% were unchanged, 2% showed a decrease in blood pressure and 3% an increase.
- In hypotensive patients 63% were unchanged, 31% showed an increase in blood pressure and in 6% blood pressure fell further.[196]

Hence, while there is a strong tendency for red ginseng to either not influence or normalise blood pressure, it can apparently exert a contrary effect in only a very small percentage of patients.

The 2005 systematic review mentioned above identified 11 ginseng trials that included blood pressure outcomes, with five assessing ginseng as a monopreparation.[194] The authors concluded that, while there is no consistent evidence that ginseng lowers blood pressure, there is little evidence to suggest it elevates this parameter.

The effect of ginseng extract (200 mg/day) on mainly moderate cerebrovascular deficit in 45 patients (average age 58 years) was compared with the drug hydergine (3 mg/day) or placebo under double blind conditions over 3 months. Significantly improved cerebrovascular circulation was noted in both active treatment groups.[197] A combined Ginkgo and ginseng formula improved circulation and lowered blood pressure in a controlled single dose study involving 10 healthy young volunteers.[198]

A study assessed a formulation containing *Panax ginseng* and *Panax notoginseng* in patients with mild or moderate vascular dementia (due to a number of small strokes).[199] Twenty-five patients took the ginseng combination, while another 15 took a drug for dementia containing almitrine plus raubasine, which is thought to improve oxygen delivery to the brain. The scientists based at the University of Beijing conducted a battery of tests that measured patients' ability at recall and verbal and visual recognition. Patients taking the ginseng compound showed more improvement in overall memory than those taking the drug combination. However, such results are preliminary and placebo-controlled studies are needed.

In an acute randomised, controlled, double blind, crossover trial, 17 healthy fasted individuals received on separate occasions four treatments consisting of: 3 g of placebo, ginseng root, bioequivalent dose of ginsenosides (105 mg) or the equivalent polysaccharide fraction (172 mg). Blood pressure and the augmentation index (AI-an emerging method for measuring arterial elasticity to assess cardiovascular risk beyond conventional blood pressure measurements) were recorded with applanation tonometry at baseline and 1, 2 and 3 h post-treatment. Compared with placebo, ginseng significantly lowered radial AI by 4.6% (p=0.045), and the ginsenoside fraction comparably decreased AI by 4.8% (p=0.057). However, no effect was observed with the polysaccharides and there was no overall effect on blood pressure.[200] In contrast, a Korean double blind, placebo-controlled trial involving 80 medicated patients with hypertension found that Korean red ginseng (3 g/day) for 3 months did not improve arterial stiffness.[201] There was no additional impact of ginseng on blood pressure.

Cancer prevention and therapy

South Korea is in a unique position for epidemiological studies involving ginseng use. As the socioeconomic status of Korea began to improve in about the second half of the 20th century, and Koreans began to prefer their traditional herbal teas, many started to drink ginseng tea. Nowadays in Korea, ginseng tea is served as often as coffee and the use of other forms of this herb are equally widespread. A group of Korean clinicians and epidemiologists have taken advantage of this opportunity. In their first study, they found an inverse association between ginseng intake and cancer incidence.[202] The scientists extended this initial study to a case-control investigation involving 1987 pairs.[203] The cancer sites studied were all primary tumours classified according to WHO guidelines. Corrections for confounding factors such as age, sex, education, marital status, smoking and alcohol consumption were performed during the statistical analysis of results.

Overall, the relative risk of cancer for ginseng users was 50% lower than for ginseng non-users. Concerning the type of ginseng, the relative risk of cancer was 37% for fresh ginseng extract users, 57% for white ginseng extract users, 30% for white ginseng powder users and a remarkable 20% for red ginseng users. However, users of fresh ginseng slice, fresh ginseng juice and white ginseng tea showed no reduction in cancer risk.

There was also a decrease in risk with rising frequency and duration of ginseng intake, showing a clear dose–response relationship. Not all cancers were affected by ginseng. For cancers of the female breast, cervix, bladder and thyroid gland there was no association (positive or negative) with ginseng intake. Apparently smokers particularly benefited from ginseng intake, with incidences of cancers of the lung, lip, oral cavity and pharynx substantially lower in smokers who were ginseng users compared with smokers who were not. There was no significant difference in cancer risk between those who began to use ginseng between the ages of 30 to 39 and after age 60. In both groups, the preventative effect appeared 1 year after the first ginseng intake and increased with duration of consumption. The authors conceded that the greatest weakness of their study was the inability to adjust for diet for cancers of the digestive organs, and sexual behaviour for reproductive cancers.

The same authors conducted a cohort study in a ginseng-growing area of Korea on 4634 adults over 40 years of age.[204] There were 79 deaths from cancer over 5 years. Ginseng users had only a 48% chance of contracting cancer when compared with non-users.

A similar opportunity to observe the potential protective effects of ginseng has been taken in China. A cohort of 1455 breast cancer patients recruited to the Shanghai Breast Cancer Study between August 1996 and March 1998 were followed through until the end of 2002 by a US research team. Information on ginseng use before cancer diagnosis was collected at baseline recruitment. Survivors' ginseng use after cancer diagnosis was obtained at the follow-up survey and was correlated to QoL at the same time. The Kaplan-Meier method and Cox regression models were applied to evaluate the association of ginseng use with overall and disease-free survival. The relation between ginseng use and QoL was evaluated using multiple linear regression models. Approximately 27% of study participants were regular ginseng users before cancer diagnosis. Compared with patients who never used ginseng, regular users had a significantly reduced risk of death. Ginseng use after cancer diagnosis, particularly current use, was positively associated with QoL scores, with the strongest effect in the psychological and social well-being domains. Additionally, QoL improved as cumulative ginseng use increased.[205]

In the Kangwha Cohort Study, researchers in South Korea followed 6282 volunteers who were 55 years of age or older in March 1985 until December 31, 2003 to evaluate the effects of ginseng intake on mortality.[206] Intake of ginseng was found to significantly decrease all-cause mortality in older males. After adjusting for age, education, occupation, alcohol intake, smoking, chronic disease, body mass index and elevated blood pressure, men who used ginseng had a 10% reduction in risk of death from all causes, compared with nonusers. The risk decreased significantly with increasing frequency of ginseng intake. The association was not shown in women. However, intake of ginseng lowered the risk of mortality from cancer in women, with the relationship between greater ginseng intake and lower risk approaching statistical significance. Mortality caused by cardiovascular disease was not related to ginseng intake in men or women. Ginseng users were grouped into frequent users (taking ginseng often or very often), infrequent users (occasionally) and non-users (never). The dosage of ginseng as well as the exact frequency and duration of intake was not collected. The study also did not collect information on species and types, although it is highly likely that Korean ginseng was mainly consumed.

A randomised, double blind, placebo-controlled trial was conducted in China over 11 years to assess the impact of a period of regular Korean red ginseng intake on the development of primary cancers.[207] The trial was a collaboration between several research centres in Korea and China. In all, 643 patients with chronic atrophic gastritis were enrolled in the trial, because this condition is associated with an elevated risk of stomach cancer. About 60% of the participants were men, more than half were smokers and their average age at the beginning of the trial was around 47 years. The dose of Korean ginseng extract was 1g/week (taken as four discrete doses containing ginsenosides at 38mg/week) and its ginsenoside profile suggests that this would correspond to around 5g of root. This dose, or the matching placebo, was consumed for 3 years and the trial participants were followed-up 8 years later.

During the 11 years of the study, 16 cancer cases confirmed by pathological examination occurred in the placebo group versus eight in the ginseng group. The relative risk (RR) for development of cancer in the ginseng group was 0.54, but this failed to reach statistical significance (p=0.13), presumably because of the relatively low numbers in the trial. Of the 24 cancer patients, 21 were male and the RR for all cancers in men was found to be statistically significant (p=0.03) at 0.35. There were no differences in side effects between the two groups and the incidence of increasing blood pressure was actually higher in the placebo group. The authors concluded that Korean red ginseng exerted a non-organ-specific cancer preventative effect, consistent with previous epidemiological studies.

It should not be concluded from this study that Korean ginseng benefits only men in terms of cancer prevention. The likely reasons for the statistically significant protective effect in the men are their higher number in the trial and the greater incidence of cancers.

The effect of ginseng (5g/day) was assessed in 50 cervical cancer patients undergoing radiation therapy in a double blind, placebo-controlled study. After 5 weeks, a number of haematological parameters were tested. Results suggested that ginseng had a protective effect on depressed bone marrow only in terms of platelet count, which was significantly elevated in the ginseng group (p<0.05). A longer and more detailed study was recommended by the authors.[208]

In a long-term Korean study, the impact of red ginseng therapy on postoperative immunity and survival was investigated in patients with gastric cancer.[209] Forty-nine patients who had undergone gastric resection with lymph node removal by the same surgeon for histologically proven AJCC (American Joint Committee on Cancer) stage III gastric adenocarcinoma were enrolled in the trial. After the application of predefined exclusion criteria, 22 patients were given ginseng (4.5g/day) for the first 6 months after surgery and another 20 acted as placebo controls. All patients were also treated with chemotherapy each month for 6 months after surgery. Flow cytometry for peripheral T lymphocyte subsets showed that the ginseng powder restored CD4 T cell levels to the initial preoperative values during chemotherapy. Depression of CD3 lymphocytes was also inhibited. The study demonstrated 5-year disease-free survival and overall survival rates that were significantly higher in patients taking ginseng compared with controls (68.2% versus 33.3%; 76.4% versus 38.5%, respectively, p<0.05). In other words, the ginseng treatment significantly prolonged survival and reduced the incidence of metastases.

A form of ginseng known as sun ginseng was found to be beneficial at 3g/day on some aspects of mental and physical functioning after 12 weeks of therapy in a randomised, double blind, placebo-controlled trial involving 53 cancer patients.[175]

Reproductive function

Several clinical trials have reinforced traditional views that ginseng has particular relevance for sexual and fertility problems in men. Ginseng extract was assessed in an open study involving 66 male patients, of whom 20 were controls, 30 had an idiopathic low sperm count and 16 had a low sperm count associated with varicocele.[210] All received 4g/day of ginseng extract for 3 months. Sperm count, total testosterone, sperm motility, free testosterone and dihydrotestosterone rose in all groups after 3 months of ginseng treatment. The normal control participants only showed small increases, whereas increases in the low sperm count groups were substantial for these parameters (although only in the case of free testosterone did levels approach those of the control group). In contrast, prolactin levels, which were elevated in the low sperm count groups, fell in all treated groups. Gonadotrophins showed a progressive increase in the low sperm count groups, but in the control group a moderate decrease was observed, probably due to the corresponding increase in androgens. It was suggested that the ginseng, and specifically ginsenosides, may have an effect at different levels of hypothalamus-pituitary-testes axis to improve male fertility.

In a second clinical trial conducted in Korea, the effect of red ginseng on erectile dysfunction (ED) was compared with placebo and the drug trazodone.[211] A total of 90 patients were closely followed, with 30 patients in each group. The overall therapeutic efficacy on ED as evaluated by the patient was 60 % for the ginseng group and 30% for the placebo- and trazodone-treated groups (p<0.05). In particular, ginseng significantly improved libido. The ginseng dose used was 1.8g/day of extract.

There were design faults in both the above studies. In particular, there was no placebo control group in the first study and neither study was conducted under double blind conditions. In a more robust study, however, prospects for benefits in the management of male sexual disorders are reinforced. In a controlled study involving 35 elderly men with psychogenic impotence, 2.7 or 1.8g of ginseng root or placebo was given for 2 months. The overall therapeutic effect on erectile function was 67% for ginseng versus 28% for placebo (p<0.05) and results tended to be better in the higher dose ginseng group. HDL-cholesterol was significantly elevated by ginseng (p<0.05), but there was no other effect on serum lipids.[212]

In a study published in 2002, a total of 45 patients with clinically diagnosed ED were enrolled in a double blind, placebo-controlled, crossover trial (8 weeks on treatment, 2 weeks of washout and 8 weeks on treatment). The effects of Korean red ginseng root (2.7g/day) and a placebo were compared. The five-item version of the International Index of Erectile Function (IIEF-5) was used to assess patients at the beginning and end of the trial. Mean IIEF scores were significantly higher for patients taking red ginseng than for those who received the placebo (p<0.01). Scores on questions 3 (penetration) and 4 (maintenance) were also significantly higher in the ginseng group (p<0.01). In response to the overall efficacy question, 60% of the patients answered that red ginseng improved erection (p<0.01). Among other variables, penile tip rigidity using the RigiScan device showed significant improvement for ginseng against placebo.[213] No changes in serum testosterone were observed.

In a more recent study, a total of 60 patients with mild to moderate ED were recruited for a double blind, randomised, placebo-controlled trial conducted in Brazil.[214] Patients received either 3g/day of Korean red ginseng root or a matched placebo for 12 weeks. Other health problems included hypertension in nine patients (30.0%) in the ginseng group and 13 patients (43.3%) in the placebo group, and diabetes in four patients (13.3%) in the ginseng group and six patients (20%) receiving placebo. By the end of the trial the IIEF-5 was significantly higher in the group receiving the herbal treatment compared with baseline (p<0.0001). In contrast there was no change for placebo. In addition, 20 patients (67%) receiving Korean ginseng reported improved erection compared with none in the placebo group. Levels of serum testosterone, prolactin and cholesterol were not significantly altered by the herbal treatment.

A systematic review and meta-analysis identified seven randomised, controlled trials of red ginseng in the treatment of ED.[215] Some of the included trials are reviewed above.[212–214] Six of the trials compared the effect of ginseng against placebo, enabling a meta-analysis. This demonstrated a highly significant and clinically relevant effect of ginseng on ED (p<0.00001). The authors cautioned that the low methodological quality and small sample size precluded definitive conclusions.

In spite of its possibly erroneous reputation as a male only remedy, ginseng consumption during pregnancy is popular in Hong Kong. Eighty-eight patients taking ginseng during their pregnancy were matched with control patients with similar characteristics who delivered within the same period, but were not taking ginseng. Eight patients in the control group developed pre-eclampsia, but only one patient in the ginseng group suffered this condition (p<0.02). The control group also had higher mean blood pressures in the second and third trimesters, but the differences were not statistically significant. The authors suggested that further studies are necessary to clarify this possible benefit of ginseng during pregnancy.[216]

The effect of a Korean ginseng aqueous extract (3g/day, about 15g of root) on sexual arousal in menopausal women was evaluated in a clinical trial in Korea.[217] The randomised, double blind, crossover trial lasted 20 weeks: 2 weeks for collecting baseline data, two 8-week treatment periods (placebo, ginseng) with a 2-week washout period between the treatment periods. Thirty-two women were recruited, and four dropped out during the study due to a lack of subjective improvement.

The main outcome measures were the Female Sexual Function Index (FSFI) and Global Assessment Questionnaire (GAQ). The FSFI consisted of six domains (desire, arousal, lubrication, orgasm, global satisfaction, pain) assigned with 19 items. GAQ consisted of a single question, asking whether sexual function had improved at the end of each treatment. Ginseng improved scores on the FSFI in the sexual arousal domain from 3.1 to 3.5 (p=0.006). Significant improvements were shown for each of the three individual items of this domain: frequency, level and satisfaction of arousal. Korean ginseng did not have a significant effect on the other five domains. Also ginseng produced a significantly better effect than placebo for GAQ results (p=0.046). There were no severe adverse events in the ginseng group, although two cases of vaginal bleeding occurred during ginseng treatment (which was described as normal menstrual bleeding). It should be noted that the clinical effect appears to be small.

Earlier trials in menopausal women had undertaken to assess the effect of ginseng on psychological parameters and QoL. A small open label, placebo-controlled trial in 49 women found that 3 months of ginseng extract (200 mg/day) improved symptoms such as headache, depression and sleep disturbances.[218] There were no side effects and no changes in vaginal and cervical cytology. A small, open label trial conducted in Japan observed that 6 g/day of Korean red ginseng for 30 days improved fatigue, insomnia, depression and psychological tests in 12 postmenopausal women.[219] The cortisol/DHEA-S ratio decreased significantly.

In a large randomised, multicentre, double blind, placebo-controlled trial involving 384 symptomatic postmenopausal women, the impact of a ginseng extract (200 mg/day) for 16 weeks on the Psychological General Well-Being (PGWB) index, Women's Health questionnaire (WHQ) and Visual Analogue (VA) scale were assessed.[220] There was only a tendency for a slightly better overall symptomatic relief from ginseng ($p<0.1$). However, analysis of PGWB subsets demonstrated significant outcomes for depression, well-being and health ($p<0.05$). No impact was observed on the WHQ and VA scales, hormone levels, endometrial thickness and hot flushes.

Diabetes

Several studies, mostly involving a single acute dose, have investigated the impact of ginseng on blood glucose parameters under different experimental conditions in healthy volunteers. Results are inconsistent, which might reflect in part the different ginsenoside profiles of the various forms of ginseng tested. These are briefly summarised below. Pooled effects from a variety of single doses of ginseng (1 to 9 g) on blood glucose following the oral glucose tolerance test (OGTT) in 11 healthy volunteers found a significant increase in values at 2 h ($p=0.05$).[221] A trial of similar design in 12 healthy volunteers also found that 3 g of ginseng increased blood glucose during the OGTT, but red ginseng had no effect.[222] In contrast, single doses of 200 and 400 mg of a 5:1 ginseng extract lowered blood glucose in a study involving 30 healthy young adults.[223] This was confirmed in another study by the same group for a 200 mg extract dose.[224] Yet another similar study by the same research group confirmed this finding, but in this case co-administration of ginseng with 25 g glucose resulted in a blood sugar increase above glucose alone.[225] In contrast, these researchers found no impact of the same ginseng extract on blood glucose levels in healthy volunteers for both an acute and a longer team study.[226] An investigation in seven healthy volunteers found that 2 to 6 g of ginseng rootlets decreased blood glucose during the OGTT, but an aqueous extract and the main root were inactive.[227] Stepwise multiple regression models identified Rg_1 as the sole predictor of activity.

Results for long-term studies in diabetic patients are more consistent, although the main therapeutic impact appears to be on plasma insulin. In a double blind, placebo-controlled study, 30 patients with type 2 diabetes were treated for

8 weeks with ginseng extract (100 or 200 mg/day) or placebo. Ginseng improved patients' mood, vigour, well-being and psychomotor performance. Results were more significant for the higher dose. Both doses of ginseng caused a small but significant fall in fasting blood glucose ($p<0.05$).[228]

In another long-term study, 12 weeks' supplementation with Korean red ginseng (2 g before each meal) maintained glycaemic control and substantially improved fasting plasma insulin levels ($p=0.046$) in a randomised, double blind, placebo-controlled, crossover study involving 19 participants with well-controlled type 2 diabetes (average HbA_{1c} 6.5%).[229] The OGTT results reflected a similar pattern. There was a trend to lower plasma glucose levels of borderline statistical significance ($p=0.052$), but the reduction in plasma insulin was much more striking. Compared with baseline, mean plasma insulin fell by 31% in the ginseng group ($p=0.012$ compared with placebo) and peak plasma insulin fell by 32% ($p=0.011$). Insulin sensitivity index values (which are the inverse of insulin resistance) rose by 36% in the treated group ($p=0.025$). In other words, although the effects of ginseng on the plasma glucose parameters failed to reach significance, there was a significant and substantial reduction in insulin resistance. Treatment with ginseng had no impact on hepatic and renal function, haemostasis parameters and systolic and diastolic blood pressures.

A randomised, placebo-controlled, double blind, crossover study in 20 type 2 diabetic patients assessed the impact of 1.1 g/day of ginseng for 4 weeks.[230] By the end of the trial there was a significant decrease in insulin resistance (HOMA-IR) ($p<0.05$) and fasting plasma glucose ($p<0.05$) for the ginseng group compared with placebo.

Other conditions

A case history was described where a patient with severe postpartum hypopituitarism (Sheehan's syndrome) was successfully treated with high doses of ginseng and licorice over 50 days.[231]

A causal link has been suggested with *Helicobacter pylori* infection and halitosis. In an open label trial, 88 functional dyspepsia patients with subjective or objective (halimeter) halitosis received Korean red ginseng (2.7 g/day) for 10 weeks or acted as controls.[232] Thirty-eight of 68 *H. pylori*-positive patients became free of halitosis, accompanied with halimeter confirmation. Among the remaining 30 patients, 15 receiving triple therapy plus red ginseng responded better than the 15 receiving triple therapy alone. Of the 20 *H. pylori*-negative patients, 13 became free of halitosis with red ginseng. Red ginseng was also active against volatile sulphur compound generation by *H. pylori* in vitro.

Toxicology and other safety data

Toxicology

The toxicity of ginseng root is very low. A 5:1 extract was found to be safe up to 6 g/kg in mice when administered intraperitoneally and up to 30 g/kg given by the oral route as a single dose.[233] Subacute toxicity studies at 1.5 to 15 mg/kg/day for 90 days of the same extract revealed no treatment-related effects on body weight, food consumption, haematology, biochemical parameters and histopathological findings.[234]

A 5:1 extract of ginseng root administered to male rabbits and rats as part of their feed at 100 mg/kg/day for 30 to 60 days caused a reduction in testicular germ cell counts, size and number of Leydig cells and other features of reduced fertility.[235]

Contraindications

Ginseng is traditionally contraindicated in acute asthma, signs of heat, excessive menstruation or nose bleeds.

Special warnings and precautions

Concurrent use with stimulants such as caffeine and amphetamines is best avoided, as is use during acute infections.

Interactions

Two independent reports of a possible interaction of the monoamine oxidase inhibitor phenelzine with ginseng have been reported.[236,237] However, the identity of ginseng was not confirmed.

A case of a possible interaction between warfarin and ginseng has been described. Ginseng intake appeared to reduce the anticoagulant activity of the warfarin, but the mode of action was unclear and the patient was taking other medications.[238] However, no interaction with warfarin was observed for ginseng in two clinical trials, even at high doses.[239,240]

Interactions with sildenafil, hypoglycaemic drugs and CNS stimulants are also theoretically possible, but no cases have been reported.

Inhibition of one or more cytochrome P450 enzymes may lead to a drug interaction.[241] A cocktail of specific cytochrome P450 probes was administered to investigate potential interactions with ginseng and *Ginkgo biloba*. The probe drugs administered were specific for the following enzymes: CYP1A2, CYP2CP, CYP2D6, CYP3A4 and also for the cellular drug pump P-glycoprotein. Seventy-two healthy volunteers were randomised to the following groups: ginseng, Ginkgo, both herbs or placebo. There were no significant differences found between the treatment groups for any of the measured probe drug parameters. These results suggest that daily use of ginseng or Ginkgo, or the combination of both herbs, will not alter the pharmacokinetics of the majority of prescription or over-the-counter drugs. A similar study in 20 healthy, elderly volunteers confirmed no effect of ginseng on CYP1A2, CYP2D6, CYP2E1 and CYP3A4.[242]

(See also the recommendations regarding potential herb–drug interactions for 'Korean ginseng' in Appendix C.)

Use in pregnancy and lactation

Category A–no proven increase in the frequency of malformation or other harmful effects on the fetus despite consumption by a large number of women.

Ginseng has been given to pregnant women without apparent harm in clinical trials in Asia. A 2008 review of the literature concluded that, based on strong evidence from a cohort study, ginseng was not associated with adverse effects during pregnancy.[243]

The effect of a 5:1 extract of ginseng root on reproductive performance was studied in male and female rats at oral doses of 1.5, 5 and 15 mg/kg/day. No adverse effects were seen in two generations of offspring.[244]

The isolated ginsenoside Rb$_1$ caused significant morphological changes in vitro using a whole rat embryo culture model at a concentration of 30 µg/mL.[245] Despite the considerable publicity given to this finding at the time of its release, this study has little relevance to the oral use of normal doses of ginseng. It stands in stark contrast to the human and in vivo studies that have shown no adverse effects on pregnancy. This is because of the high levels of exposure and the uncertain bioavailability of the ginsenosides as such.

Ginseng is compatible with breastfeeding and has been traditionally prescribed as a tonic to lactating mothers.

Effects on ability to drive and use machines

No negative influence is expected.

Side effects

Results from controlled clinical trials using a daily dose of 1 g indicate that ginseng is generally safe and well-tolerated. However, higher doses may cause side effects, and ginseng abuse syndrome (GAS) has been described in the early literature.[231] GAS was defined as hypertension, together with nervousness, euphoria, insomnia, skin eruptions and morning diarrhoea, and was postulated to be related to ginseng's interaction with glucocorticoid production in the body. However, since this particular study did not differentiate the species of ginseng used, its reliability must be questioned. Moreover, a follow-up study found that many people with reported GAS were actually taking *Eleutherococcus senticosus* (Siberian ginseng).[246] Symptoms of GAS were reported in independent studies in the wake of this publication,[247,248] and there has been an unexplained report of a 64-year-old patient experiencing a hypertensive crisis leading to a transient ischaemic attack linked to ingestion of ginseng root for 2 weeks.[249] In the absence of more recent reports of GAS, and the clinical trials demonstrating no adverse impact of ginseng on blood pressure, its importance has diminished.

Ginseng may cause side effects related to an oestrogen-like activity in women.[250] Cases of mastalgia[251] and vaginal bleeding in a 72-year-old woman[252] have been reported. A case of postmenopausal bleeding attributed to the use of a ginseng face cream has also been published.[253] The potential adulteration of these products with hormonal agents needs to be considered.

Ginseng is widely used and several other severe adverse reactions have been reported that are at best possibly related to ginseng, or may otherwise reflect on contamination, adulteration or coincidence. These include Stevens-Johnson syndrome,[254,255] diuretic resistance, cerebral arteritis,[256] mania,[257,258] mydriasis[259] and bradyarrhythmia.[260]

A systematic review of adverse effects involving ginseng observed that the most commonly experienced events were mild and similar to those for placebo.[261]

Overdosage

Two women who had consumed around 25 g of ginseng root both apparently developed transient cerebral arteritis with severe headaches, nausea and vomiting.[262]

Safety in children

No information available but adverse effects are not expected

Regulatory status in selected countries

Ginseng is official in the *Chinese Pharmacopoeia* (2005) and the *Japanese Pharmacopoeia* (English edition, 2006), the *European Pharmacopoeia* 7.2 2011, the *United States Pharmacopeia-National Formulary* (USP 34-NF 29, 2011), and the *British Pharmacopoeia* 2012.

Ginseng is covered by a positive Commission E monograph and can be used as a tonic to combat feelings of lassitude and debility, lack of energy and ability to concentrate and during convalescence. It is on the UK General Sale list.

Ginseng does not have GRAS status. However, it is freely available as a 'dietary supplement' in the USA under DSHEA legislation (1994 Dietary Supplement Health and Education Act). Korean ginseng has been present as an ingredient in products offered over-the-counter (OTC) for use as an aphrodisiac. The FDA however advises that 'based on evidence currently available, any OTC drug product containing ingredients for use as an aphrodisiac cannot be generally recognised as safe and effective'.

Ginseng is not included in Part 4 of Schedule 4 of the Therapeutic Goods Act Regulations of Australia and is freely available for sale.

References

1. Chang HM, But PP. *Pharmacology and Applications of Chinese Materia Medica*, vol. 1. Singapore: World Scientific; 1986. pp. 17–31.
2. Bensky D, Gamble A. *Chinese Herbal Medicine Materia Medica*. Seattle: Eastland Press; 1986. pp. 450–454.
3. Grieve M. *A Modern Herbal*, vol. 1. New York: Dover Publications; 1971. pp. 354–357.
4. British Herbal Medicine Association's Scientific Committee *British Herbal Pharmacopoeia*. Cowling: BHMA; 1983. p. 152.
5. Felter HW. *The Eclectic Materia Medica, Pharmacology and Therapeutics*. 1922. Reprinted Portland: Eclectic Medical Publications; 1983. pp. 1429–1430.
6. Jagetia GC. *J Clinical Biochem Nutr*. 2007;40(2):74–81.
7. German Federal Minister of Justice. *German Commission E for Human Medicine Monograph. Bundes-Anzeiger* (German Federal Gazette), no. 11, dated 17.01.1991.
8. World Health Organization. *Medicinal Plants in China*. Manila: World Health Organization, Regional Office for the Western Pacific; 1989. pp. 194–195.
9. Wagner H, Bladt S. *Plant Drug Analysis: A Thin Layer Chromatography Atlas*, ed 2 Berlin: Springer-Verlag; 1996. p. 307.
10. Christensen LP. *Adv Food Nutr Res*. 2009;55:1–99.
11. Tang W, Eisenbrand G. *Chinese Drugs of Plant Origin*. Berlin: Springer Verlag; 1992. pp. 711–737.
12. Ng TB. *J Pharm Pharmacol*. 2006;58(8):1007–1019.
13. Kwon BM, Nam JY, Lee SH, et al. *Chem Pharm Bull*. 1996;44(2):444–445.
14. Choi KT. *Acta Pharmacol Sin*. 2008;29(9):1109–1118.
15. Joo KM, Park CW, Jeong HJ, et al. *J Chromatogr B Analyt Technol Biomed Life Sci*. 2008;865(1–2):159–166.
16. Attele AS, Wu JA, Yuan CS. *Biochem Pharmacol*. 1999;58(11):1685–1693.
17. Wang CZ, Ni M, Sun S, et al. *J Agric Food Chem*. 2009;57(6):2363–2367.
18. Harkey MR, Henderson GL, Gershwin ME, et al. *Am J Clin Nutr*. 2001;73(6):1101–1106.
19. Kim SN, Ha YW, Shin H, et al. *J Pharm Biomed Anal*. 2007;45(1):164–170.
20. Shi W, Wang Y, Li J, et al. *Food Chem*. 2007;102(3):664–668.
21. Soldati F, Sticher O. *Plant Med*. 1980;39(4):348–357.
22. Chu SF, Zhang JT. *Chin J Integr Med*. 2009;15(6):403–408.
23. Kaneko H, Nakanishi K. *J Pharmacol Sci*. 2004;95(2):158–162.
24. Luo YM, Cheng XJ, Yuan WX. *Chung Kuo Yao Li Hsueh Pao*. 1993;14(5):401–404.
25. Singh A, Saxena E, Bhutani KK. *Phytother Res*. 2000;14(2):122–125.
26. Yoshimatsu H, Sakata T, Machidori H, et al. *Physiol Behav*. 1993;53(1):1–4.
27. Yuan Wx Wu XJ, Yang FX, et al. *Chung Kuo Yao Li Hsueh Pao*. 1989;10(6):492–496.
28. Filaretov AA, Bogdanova TS, Podivigina TT, et al. *Exp Clin Endocrinol*. 1988;92(2):129–136.
29. Dang H, Chen Y, Liu X, et al. *Prog Neuropsychopharmacol Biol Psychiatry*. 2009;33(8):1417–1424.
30. Lee SP, Honda K, Rhee YH, et al. *Neurosci Lett*. 1990;111(1–2):217–221.
31. Ramachandran U, Divekar HM, Grover SK, et al. *J Ethnopharmacol*. 1990;29(3):275–281.
32. Avakian EV, Sugimoto RB, Taguchi S, et al. *Planta Med*. 1984;50(2):151–154.
33. Voces J, Cabral de Oliveira AC, Prieto JG, et al. *Braz J Med Biol Res*. 2004;37(12):1863–1871.
34. Buffi O, Ciaroni S, Guidi L, et al. *Boll Soc Ital Biol Sper*. 1993;69(12):791–797.
35. Metori K, Furutsu M, Takahashi S. *Biol Pharm Bull*. 1997;20(3):237–242.
36. Yamaguchi Y, Higashi M, Kobayashi H. *Eur J Pharmacol*. 1997;329(1):37–41.
37. Nitta H, Matsumoto K, Shimizu M, et al. *Biol Pharm Bull*. 1995;18(9):1286–1288.
38. Watanabe H, Ohta H, Imamura L, et al. *Jpn J Pharmacol*. 1991;55(1):51–56.
39. Tachikawa E, Kudo K. *J Pharmacol Sci*. 2004;95(2):140–144.

40. Kim DH, Moon YS, Jung JS, et al. *Neurosci Lett*. 2003;343(1):62–66.

41. Hiai S, Yokoyama H, Oura H, et al. *Endocrinol Jpn*. 1979;26(6):661–665.

42. Lee SH, Jung BH, Kim SY, et al. *Pharmacol Res*. 2006;54(1):46–49.

43. Fulder S. *The Root of Being*. London: Hutchinson & Co; 1980.

44. Shibata S, et al. In: Farnsworth NR, ed. *Economic and Medicinal Plant Research*, vol. 1. London: Academic Press; 1985.

45. Petkov VD, Mosharrof AH. *Am J Chin Med*. 1987;15(1–2):19–29.

46. Ying Y, Zhang JT, Shi CZ, et al. *Yao Hsueh Pao*. 1994;29(4):241–245.

47. Nitta H, Matsumoto K, Shimizu M, et al. *Biol Pharm Bull*. 1995;18(10):1439–1442.

48. Petkov VD, Kehayov R, Belcheva S, et al. *Planta Med*. 1993;59(2):106–114.

49. Kurimoto H, Nishijo H, Uwano T, et al. *Physiol Behav*. 2004;82(2–3):345–355.

50. Nah SY, Kim DH, Rhim H. *CNS Drug Rev*. 2007;13(4):381–404.

51. Radad K, Gille G, Liu L, Rausch WD. *J Pharmacol Sci*. 2006;100(3):175–186.

52. Zee-Cheng RK. *Methods Find Exp Clin Pharmacol*. 1992;14(9):725–736.

53. Singh VK, Agarwal SS, Gupta BM. *Planta Med*. 1984;50(6):462–465.

54. Jie YH, Cammisuli S, Baggiolini M. *Agents Actions*. 1984;15(3–4):386–391.

55. Akagawa G, Abe S, Tansho S, et al. *Immunopharmacol Immunotoxicol*. 1996;18(1):73–89.

56. Lee JH, Park EK, Uhm CS, et al. *Planta Med*. 2004;70(7):615–619.

57. Yeung HW, Cheung K, Leung KN. *Am J Chin Med*. 1982;10(1–4):44–54.

58. Kim YW, Song DK, Kim WH, et al. *J Ethnopharmacol*. 1997;58(1):55–58.

59. Yun YS, Moon HS, Oh YR, et al. *Cancer Detect Prev Suppl*. 1987;1:301–309.

60. Yuan GC, Chang RS. *J Gerontol*. 1969;24(1):82–85.

61. Fulder SJ. *Exp Gerontol*. 1977;12(3–4):125–131.

62. Yamamoto M, Kumagai A, Yamamura Y. *Arzneimittelforschung*. 1977;27(7):1404–1405.

63. Shia GT, Ali S, Bittles AH. *Gerontology*. 1982;28(2):121–124.

64. Lu ZQ, Dice JF. *Biochem Biophys Res Commun*. 1985;126(1):636–640.

65. Gao RL, Xu CL, Jin JM. *Chung Kuo Chung Hsi I Chieh Ho Tsa Chih*. 1992;12(5):285–287.

66. Kang SY, Lee KY, Lee SK. *Biochem Biophys Res Commun*. 1994;205(3):1696–1701.

67. Yagi A, Ishizu T, Okamura N, et al. *Planta Med*. 1996;62(2):115–118.

68. Takei Y, Yamamoto T, Higashira H, et al. *Biosci Biotechnol Biochem*. 1996;60(4):584–588.

69. Oura H, Hiai S, Nakashima S, et al. *Chem Pharm Bull*. 1971;19(3):453–459.

70. Hiai S, Oura H, Tsukada K, et al. *Chem Pharm Bull*. 1971;19(8):1656–1663.

71. Oura H, Tsukada K, Nakagawa H. *Chem Pharm Bull*. 1972;20(2):219–225.

72. Yamamoto M, Masaka M, Yamada Y, et al. *Arzneimittelforschung*. 1978;28(12):2238–2241.

73. Nagasawa T, Oura H, Hiai S, et al. *Chem Pharm Bull*. 1977;25(7):1665–1670.

74. Oura H, Hiai S, Nabetani S, et al. *Planta Med*. 1975;28(1):76–88.

75. Yamamoto M, Takeuchi N, Kumagai A, et al. *Arzneimittelforschung*. 1977;27(6):1169–1173.

76. Harper N, Osborne AJ, Makov VE, et al. *Biochem Pharmacol*. 1984;33(9):1571–1573.

77. Yue PYK, Mak NK, Cheng YK, et al. *Chin Med*. 2007;2:6.

78. Chang S, Seo E-K, Gyllenhaal C, et al. *Integr Cancer Ther*. 2003;2(1):13–33.

79. Kikuchi Y, Sasa H, Kita T, et al. *Anticancer Drugs*. 1991;2(1):63–67.

80. Motoo Y, Sawabu N. *Cancer Lett*. 1994;86(1):91–95.

81. Saita T, Katano M, Matsunaga H, et al. *Biol Pharm Bull*. 1995;18(7):933–937.

82. Matsunaga H, Saita T, Nagumo F, et al. *Cancer Chemother Pharmacol*. 1995;35(4):291–296.

83. Baek N-I, Kim DS, Lee YH, et al. *Arch Pharmacal Res*. 1995;18(3):164–168.

84. Abdrasilov BS, YuA K, Nurieva RI, et al. *Biochem Mol Biol Int*. 1996;38(3):519–526.

85. Ota T, Fujikawa-Yamamoto K, Zong ZP, et al. *Cancer Res*. 1987;47(14):3863–3867.

86. Lee YN, Lee HY, Chung HY, et al. *Eur J Cancer*. 1996;32A(8):1420–1428.

87. Rhee YH, Ahn JH, Choe J, et al. *Planta Med*. 1991;57(2):125–128.

88. Park HJ, Rhee MH, Park KM, et al. *J Ethnopharmacol*. 1995;49(3):157–162.

89. Zhu JH, Takeshita T, Kitagawa I, et al. *Cancer Res*. 1995;55(6):1221–1223.

90. Lee KD, Huemer RP. *Jpn J Pharmacol*. 1971;21(3):299–320.

91. Tode T, Kikuchi Y, Hirata J, et al. *Nippon Sanka Fujinka Gakkai Zasshi*. 1993;45(11):1275–1282.

92. Tode T, Kikuchi Y, Sasa H, et al. *Nippon Sanka Fujinka Gakkai Zasshi*. 1992;44(5):589–594.

93. Katano M, Yamamoto H, Matsunaga H, et al. *Gan To Kagaku Ryoho*. 1990;17(5):1045–1049.

94. You J-S, Hau D-M, Chen K-T, et al. *Phytother Res*. 1995;9(5):331–335.

95. Xu TM, Xin Y, Cui MH, et al. *Chin Med J (Engl)*. 2007;120(7):584–588.

96. Lee SD, Park SK, Lee ES, et al. *J Med Food*. 2010;13(1):1–5.

97. Yun TK. *Nut Rev*. 1996;54(11 pt 2):S71–S81.

98. Lee FC, Park JK, Ko JH, et al. *Drug Chem Toxicol*. 1987;10(3–4):227–236.

99. Wargovich MJ. *J Korean Med Sci*. 2001;16(suppl):S81–S86.

100. Panwar M, Samarth R, Kumar M, et al. *Biol Pharm Bull*. 2005;28(11):2063–2067.

101. Shin HR, Kim JY, Yun TK, et al. *Cancer Causes Control*. 2000;11(6):565–576.

102. Ishi H, Tatsuta M, Baba M, et al. *Clin Exp Metastasis*. 1997;15(6):603–611.

103. Shinkai K, Akedo H, Mukai M, et al. *Jpn J Cancer Res*. 1996;87(4):357–362.

104. Sato K, Mochizuki M, Saiki I, et al. *Biol Pharm Bull*. 1994;17(5):635–639.

105. Tong CN, Matsuda H, Kubo M. *Yakugaku*. 1992;112(11):856–865.

106. Matsuda H, Tong CN, Kubo M. *Yakugaku*. 1992;112(11):846–855.

107. Kubo M, Chun-Ning T, Matsuda H. *Planta Med*. 1992;58(5):424–428.

108. Hofseth LJ, Wargovich MJ. *J Nutr*. 2007;137(1 suppl):183S–185S.

109. Zhou W, Chai H, Lin PH, et al. *Med Sci Monit*. 2004;10(8):RA187–RA192.

110. Jia L, Zhao Y, Liang XJ. *Curr Med Chem*. 2009;16(22):2924–2942.

111. Ng TB, Yeung HW. *Gen Pharmacol*. 1985;16(6):549–552.

112. Oshima Y, Konno C, Hikino H. *J Ethnopharmacol*. 1985;14(2–3):255–259.

113. Wang BX, Yang M, Jin YL, et al. *Yao Hsueh Pao*. 1990;25(6):401–405.

114. Yokozawa T, Fujitsuka N, Yasui T, et al. *J Pharm Pharmacol*. 1991;43(4):290–291.

115. Yokozawa T, Oura H. *J Nat Prod*. 1990;53(6):1514–1518.

116. Yokozawa T, Oura H, Kawashima Y. *J Nat Prod*. 1989;52(6):1350–1352.

117. Yokozawa T, Kobayashi T, Oura H, et al. *Chem Pharm Bull*. 1987;35(10):4208–4214.

118. Kim HS, Kang JG, Oh KW. *Gen Pharmacol*. 1995;26(5):1071–1076.

119. Kim HS, Kang JG, Seong YH, et al. *Pharmacol Biochem Behav*. 1995;50(1):23–27.

120. Kim HS, Kang JG, Rheu HM, et al. *Planta Med*. 1995;61(1):22–25.

121. Kim HS, Jang CC, Oh KW, et al. *J Ethnopharmacol*. 1998;60:33–42.

122. Bhargava HN, Ramarao P. *Gen Pharmacol*. 1991;22(3):521–525.

123. Kim HS, Jang CG, Lee MK. *Planta Med*. 1990;56(2):158–163.

124. Gillis CN. *Biochem Pharmacol*. 1997;54(1):1–8.

125. Lee YJ, Pantuck CB, Pantuck EJ. *Planta Med*. 1993;59(1):17–19.

126. Lee FC, Ko JH, Park JK, et al. *Clin Exp Pharmacol Physiol*. 1987;14(6):543–546.

127. Takino Y. *Yakugaku Zasshi*. 1994;114(8):550–564.

128. Cui JF, Garle M, Bjorkhem I, et al. *Scand J Clin Lab Invest*. 1996;56(2):151–161.

129. Cui JF, Bjorkem I, Eneroth P. *J Chromatogr B Biomed Appl*. 1997;689(2):349–355.

130. Hasegawa H, Sung JH, Matsumiya S, et al. *Planta Med*. 1996;62(5):453–457.

131. Hasegawa H, Sung JH, Benno Y. *Planta Med*. 1997;63(5):436–440.

132. Lü JM, Yao Q, Chen C. *Curr Vasc Pharmacol*. 2009;7(3):293–302.

133. Leung KW, Wong AS. *Chin Med*. 2010;5:20.

134. Xu QF, Fang XL, Chen DF. *J Ethnopharmacol*. 2003;84(2–3):187–192.

135. Xiong J, Sun M, Guo J, et al. *J Pharm Pharmacol*. 2009;61(3):381–386.

136. Tawab MA, Bahr U, Karas M, et al. *Drug Metab Dispos*. 2003;31(8):1065–1071.

137. Lee J, Lee E, Kim D, et al. *J Ethnopharmacol*. 2009;122(1):143–148.

138. Forgo I. *MMW Munch Med Wochenschr*. 1983;125(38):822–824.

139. Pieralisi G, Ripari P, Vecchiet L. *Clin Ther*. 1991;13(3):373–382.

140. Van Schepdael P. *Acta Ther*. 1993;19(4):338–347.

141. Kim SH, Park KS, Chang MJ, Sung JH. *J Sports Med Phys Fitness*. 2005;45(2):178–182.

142. Cherdrungsi P, Rungroeng K. *Korean J Ginseng Sci*. 1995;19(2):93–100.

143. Palisin TE, Stacy JJ. *Curr Sports Med Rep*. 2006;5(4):210–214.

144. Bahrke MS, Morgan WP, Stegner A. *Int J Sport Nutr Exerc Metab*. 2009;19(3):298–322.

145. Bucci LR. *Am J Clin Nutr*. 2000;72(2 suppl):624–636.

146. Allen JD, McLung J, Nelson AG, Welsch M. *J Am College Nutr*. 1998;17(5):462–466.

147. Kulaputana O, Thanakomsirichot S, Anomasiri W. *J Med Assoc Thai*. 2007;90(6):1172–1179.

148. Engels HJ, Wirth JC. *J Am Diet Assoc*. 1997;97(10):1110–1115.

149. Engels HJ, Kolokouri I, Cieslak TJn, Wirth JC. *J Strength Cond Res*. 2001;15(3):290–295.

150. Morris AC, Jacobs I, McLellan TM, et al. *Int J Sport Nutr*. 1996;6(3):263–271.

151. Knapik JJ, Wright JE, Welch MJ, et al. *Fed Proc*. 1983;42(3):336.

152. Youl KH, Hwan KS, Jun LW, Byrne HK. *J Strength Cond Res*. 2002;16(2):179–183.

153. Gaffney BT, Hügel HM, Rich PA. *Life Sci*. 2001;70(4):431–442.

154. Gross D, Shenkman Z, Bleiberg B, et al. *Monaldi Arch Chest Dis*. 2002;56(5–6):242–246.

155. Forgo I, Kayasseh L, Staub JJ. *Med Welt*. 1981;32(19):751–756.

156. D'Angelo L, Grimaldi R, Caravaggi M, et al. *J Ethnopharmacol*. 1986;16(1):15–22.

157. Ziemba AW, Chmura J, Kaciuba-Uscilko H, et al. *Int J Sports Nutr*. 1999;9(4):371–377.

158. Sorensen H, Sonne J. *Curr Ther Res*. 1996;57(12):959–968.

159. Geng J, Dong J, Ni H, et al. *Cochrane Database Syst Rev*. 2010(12):CD007769.

160. Kennedy DO, Scholey AB. *Pharmacol Biochem Behav*. 2003;75(3):687–700.

161. Reay JL, Scholey AB, Kennedy DO. *Hum Psychopharmacol*. 2010;25(6):462–471.

162. Kennedy D, Scholey A, Wesnes K. *Nutr Neurosci*. 2001;4(5):399–412.

163. Scholey AB, Kennedy DO. *Hum Psychopharmacol*. 2002;17(1):35–44.

164. Kennedy DO, Scholey AB, Wesnes KA. *Physiol Behav*. 2002;75(5):739–751.

165. Wesnes K, Ward T, McGinty A, et al. *Psychopharmacology (Berl)*. 2000;152(4):353–361.

166. Hartley DE, Elsabagh S, File SE. *Nutr Neurosci*. 2004;7(5–6):325–333.

167. Heo JH, Lee ST, Chu K, et al. *Eur J Neurol*. 2008;15(8):865–868.

168. Lee ST, Chu K, Sim JY, et al. *Alzheimer Dis Assoc Disord*. 2008;22(3):222–226.

169. Lee MS, Yang EJ, Kim JI, Ernst E. *J Alzheimers Dis*. 2009;18(2):339–344.

170. Caso MA, Vargas RR, Salas VA, Begoña IC. *Drugs Exp Clin Res*. 1996;22(6):323–329.

171. Wiklund I, Karlberg J, Lund B. *Curr Ther Res*. 1994;55(1):32–42.

172. Coleman CI, Hebert JH, Reddy P. *J Clin Pharm Ther*. 2003;28(1):5–15.

173. Le Gal M, Cathebras P, Struby K. *Phytother Res*. 1996;10(1):49–53.

174. Gianoli AC, Riebenfeld D. *Cytobiol Rev*. 1984;8(3):177–186.

175. Kim JH, Park CY, Lee SJ. *J Clin Pharm Ther*. 2006;31(4):331–334.

176. Kerkhof GA, Middlekoop HAM, Van Der Hoeve R, et al. *J Interdisciplinary Cycle Res*. 1989;20(1):57–64.

177. Fulder S, Mohan K, Gethyn-Smith B. *Proceedings of the 4th International Ginseng Symposium*. Korea: Seoul: Korean Ginseng & Tobacco Research Institute; 1984. pp. 215–223.

178. Thommessen B, Laake K. *Aging (Milano)*. 1996;8(6):417–420.

179. Cho YK, Kim YB, Choi BS, et al. *J Korean Soc Microbiol*. 1994;29(4):371–379.

180. Cho YK, Kim YB, Lee I, et al. *J Korean Soc Microbiol*. 1996;31(3):353–360.

181. Cho Y, Lee H, Oh W, Kim Y. *Abstr Gen Meet Am Soc Microbiol*. 1997;97:247. Abstract No. E44.

182. Cho YK, Sung H, Lee HJ, et al. *Int Immunopharmacol*. 2001;1:1295–1305.

183. Sung H, Kang SM, Lee MS, et al. *Clin Diagn Lab Immunol*. 2005;12(4):497–501.

184. Scaglione F, Ferrara F, Dugnani S, et al. *Drugs Exp Clin Res*. 1990;16(10):537–542.

185. Scaglione F, Cogo R, Cocuzza C, et al. *Int J Immunother*. 1994;10(1):21–24.

186. Scaglione F, Cattaneo G, Alessandria M, et al. *Drugs Exp Clin Res*. 1996;22(2):65–72.

187. Srisurapanon S, Apibal S, Siripol R, et al. *J Med Assoc Thai*. 1997;80:S81–S85.

188. Engels HJ, Fahlman MM, Wirth JC. *Med Sci Sports Exerc*. 2003;35(4):690–696.

189. Ding DZ, Shen TK, Cui YZ. *Chung Kuo Chung His I Chieh Ho Tsa Chih*. 1995;15(6):325–327.

190. Zheng H, Chen Y, Chen J, et al. *Cochrane Database Sys Rev*. 2011(2):CD005052.

191. Caron MF, Hotsko AL, Robertson S, et al. *Ann Pharmacother*. 2002;36(5):758–763.

192. Punnonen R, Lukola A. *Asia Oceania J Obstet Gynaecol*. 1984;10(3):399–401.

193. Kim SH, Park KS. *Pharmacol Res*. 2003;48(5):511–513.

194. Buettner C, Yeh GY, Phillips RS, et al. *Ann Pharmacother*. 2006;40(1):83–95.

195. Han KH, Choe SC, Kim HS, et al. *Am J Chin Med*. 1998;26(2):199–209.

196. Yamamoto M, Tamura Y, Kuashima K, et al. *Ginseng Rev*. 1990;9:15–27.

197. Quiroga H. *Orientacion Med*. 1982;31(1281):201–202.

198. Kiesewetter H, Jung F, Mrowietz C, et al. *Int J Clin Pharmacol Ther Toxicol*. 1992;30(3):97–102.

199. Tian J, Yin J, Yang C, et al. *28th International Stroke Conference*. Phoenix, Arizona: 2003 [Abstract P327].

200. Jovanovski E, Jenkins A, Dias AG, et al. *Am J Hypertens*. 2010;23(5):469–472.

201. Rhee MY, Kim YS, Bae JH, et al. *J Altern Complement Med*. 2011;17(1):45–59.

202. Yun TK, Choi SY. *Int J Epidemiology*. 1990;19(4):871–876.

203. Yun TK, Choi SY. *Cancer Epidemiol Biomarkers Prev*. 1995;4(4):401–408.

204. Yun TK, Choi SY. *Korean J Ginseng Sci*. 1995;19(2):87–92.

205. Cui Y, Shu XO, Gao YT, et al. *Am J Epidemiol*. 2006;163(7):645–653.

206. Yi SW, Sull JW, Hong JS, et al. *J Altern Complement Med*. 2009;15(8):921–928.

207. Yun TK, Zheng S, Choi SY, et al. *J Med Food*. 2010;13(3):489–494.

208. Chang YS, Park CI. *Seoul J Med*. 1980;21(2):187–193.

209. Suh SO, Kroh M, Kim NR, et al. *Am J Chin Med*. 2002;30(4):483–494.

210. Salvati G, Genovesi G, Marcellini L, et al. *Panminerva Med*. 1996;38(4):249–254.

211. Choi HK, Seong DH, Rha KH. *Int J Impotence Res*. 1995;7(3):181–186.

212. Kim YC, Hong YK, Shin JS, et al. *Korean J Ginseng Sci*. 1996;20(2):125–132.

213. Hong B, Ji YH, Hong JH, et al. *J Urol*. 2002;168(5):2070–2073.

214. de Andrade E, de Mesquita AA, de Almeida Claro J, et al. *Asian J Androl*. 2007;9(2):241–244.

215. Jang DJ, Lee MS, Shin BC, et al. *Br J Clin Pharmacol*. 2008;66(4):444–450.

216. Chin RK. *Asia Oceania J Obstet Gynaecol*. 1991;17(4):379–380.

217. Oh KJ, Chae MJ, Lee HS, et al. *J Sex Med*. 2010;7(4 Pt 1):1469–1477.

218. Reinold E. *Natur-und Ganzheits Med*. 1990;4:131–134. [Article in German].

219. Tode T, Kikuchi Y, Hirata J, et al. *Int J Gynaecol Obstet*. 1999;67(3):169–174.

220. Wiklund IK, Mattsson LA, Lindgren R, Limoni C. *Int J Clin Pharmacol Res*. 1999;19(3):89–99.

221. Sievenpiper JL, Arnason JT, Leiter LA, Vuksan V. *J Am Coll Nutr*. 2003;22(6):524–532.

222. Sievenpiper JL, Arnason JT, Leiter LA, Vuksan V. *J Am Coll Nutr*. 2004;23(3):248–258.

223. Reay JL, Kennedy DO, Scholey AB. *J Psychopharmacol*. 2005;19(4):357–365.

224. Reay JL, Kennedy DO, Scholey AB. *J Psychopharmacol*. 2006;20(6):771–781.

225. Reay JL, Kennedy DO, Scholey AB. *Br J Nutr*. 2006;96(4):639–642.

226. Reay JL, Scholey AB, Milne A, et al. *Br J Nutr*. 2009;101(11):1673–1678.

227. Sievenpiper JL, Sung MK, Di Buono M, et al. *J Am Coll Nutr*. 2006;25(2):100–107.

228. Sotaniemi EA, Haapakoski E, Rautio A. *Diabetes Care*. 1995;18(10):1373–1375.

229. Vuksan V, Sung MK, Sievenpiper JL, et al. *Nutr Metab Cardiovasc Dis*. 2008;18(1):46–56.

230. Ma SW, Benzie IF, Chu TT, et al. *Diabetes Obes Metab*. 2008;10(11):1125–1127.

231. Siegel RK. *JAMA*. 1979;241(15):1614–1615.

232. Lee JS, Kwon KA, Jung HS, et al. *Digestion*. 2009;80(3):192–199.

233. Farnsworth NR, Kinghorn AD, Soefarto DD, et al. In: Farnsworth NR, ed. *Economic and Medicinal Plant Research*, vol. 1. London: Academic Press; 1985. pp. 167, 171, 172.

234. Hess Jr. FG, Parent RA, Stevens KR, et al. *Food Chem Toxicol*. 1983;21(1):95–97.

235. Sharma KK, Sharma A, Chaturvedi M, et al. *International Ginseng Conference '99*. July 8–11, 1999. Hong Kong: BDG Communications Management Ltd.

236. Jones BD, Runikis AM. *J Clin Psychopharmacol*. 1987;7(3):201–202.

237. Shader RI, Greenblatt DJ. *J Clin Psychopharmacol*. 1988;8(4):235.

238. Janetzky K, Morreale AP. *Am J Health-Syst Pharm*. 1997;54:692–693.

239. Lee SH, Ahn YM, Ahn SY, et al. *J Altern Complement Med*. 2008;14(6):715–721.

240. Jiang X, Williams KM, Liauw WS, et al. *Br J Clin Pharmacol*. 2004;57(5):592–599.

241. Reed GA, Sunega JM, Peterson KS, et al. *FASEB J*. 2007;21(891):6. [meeting abstract].

242. Gurley BJ, Gardner SF, Hubbard MA, et al. *Drugs Aging*. 2005;22(6):525–539.

243. Seeley D, Dugoua JJ, Perri D, et al. *Can J Clin Pharmacol*. 2008;15(1):e87–e94.

244. Hess Jr FG, Parent RA, Cox GE, et al. *Food Chem Toxicol*. 1982;20(2):189–192.

245. Chan LY, Chiu PY, Lau TK. *Hum Reprod*. 2003;18(10):2166–2168.

246. Siegel RK. *JAMA*. 1980;243(1):32.

247. Chen KJ. *J Trad Chin Med*. 1981;1(1):69–72.

248. Hammond TG, Whitworth JA. *Med J Aust*. 1981;1(9):492.

249. Martínez-Mir I, Rubio E, Morales-Olivas FJ, et al. *Ann Pharmacother*. 2004;38(11):1970.

250. Punnonen R, Lukola A. *Br Med J*. 1980;281(6248):1110.

251. Palmer BV, Montgomery ACV, Monteiro JCMP. *Br Med J*. 1978;1(6122):1284.

252. Greenspan EM. *JAMA*. 1983;249(15):2018.

253. Hopkins MP, Androff L, Benninghoff AS. *Am J Obstet Gynecol*. 1988;159(5):1121–1122.

254. Faleni R, Soldati F. *Lancet*. 1996;348(9022):267.

255. Dega H, Laporte JL, Frances C, et al. *Lancet*. 1996;347(9011):1344.

256. Becker BN, Greene J, Evanson J, et al. *JAMA*. 1996;276(8):606–607.

257. Gonzalez-Seijo JC, Ramos YM, Lastra I. *J Clin Psychopharmacol*. 1995;15(6):447–448.

258. Engelberg D, McCutcheon A, Wiseman S. *J Clin Psychopharmacol*. 2001;21(5):535–537.

259. Chan TY. *Vet Hum Toxicol*. 1995;37(2):156–157.

260. Lin GM, Han CL. *Am J Emerg Med*. 2010;28(8):978.

261. Coon JT, Ernst E. *Drug Saf*. 2002;25(5):323–344.

262. Ryu SJ, Chien YY. *Neurology*. 1995;45(4):829–830.

Globe artichoke

(*Cynara cardunculus* var. *scolymus* L.)

Synonyms

Cynara scolymus L., French artichoke, Cynara (Engl), Cynarae folium (Lat), Artischocke (Ger), artichaut (Fr), artichiocco, carciofo (Ital), artiskok (Dan).

What is it?

The use of the immature flower of the globe artichoke as a vegetable is widely appreciated. (It should not, however, be confused with another edible plant: the tuber of Jerusalem artichoke, *Helianthus tuberosus*, a species of sunflower.) In contrast, herbalists value other parts of the plant for their medicinal properties. In particular, the leaves of Cynara have a well-established reputation for stimulating bile and urine flow, restoring the liver and lowering cholesterol. Much attention has been centred on the active component cynarin found mainly in the leaves. However, it is likely that many other compounds, some related to cynarin, contribute to the observed therapeutic effects. In recent studies, clinical attention has centred on the globe artichoke extract and its value in non-ulcer dyspepsia. It has been suggested that the combination of antioxidant and unique cholesterol-lowering properties also make this herb a prime candidate for the natural prevention of atherosclerosis.[1]

The medicinal properties of Cynara have been known since antiquity. It was particularly prized in the 16th to 19th centuries, but was out of favour between 1870 to about 1925. Cynara is actually a variety of thistle and some writers believe that it was never found in the wild state, being a product of cultivation and selection from *Cynara cardunculus* L. (wild thistle, cardoon). The flower of *C. cardunculus* is used in South America to curdle milk; Cynara has also been used for this purpose.

Effects

Stimulates hepatorenal function; stimulates bile flow from the liver; reduces blood lipids, inhibits cholesterol biosynthesis; protects liver cells against toxins via antioxidant processes, promotes regeneration of liver cells; prevents cholestasis; reduces nausea of various origins.

Traditional view

The leaves of Cynara were traditionally used by the Eclectic physicians as a diuretic and depurative for the treatment of rheumatism, gout, jaundice and especially for dropsies.[2] In Europe, Cynara is considered to have choleretic, cholagogue, laxative and diuretic activities. It has been used to clear the complexion, stimulate appetite, alleviate the symptoms of arthritis and for uraemia and hypercholesterolaemia. According to Leclerc, the activity of Cynara depends on tonifying the liver, in particular the 'wringing out of the hepatic sponge',[3] thereby suggesting an antitoxic (hepatoprotective) action. Cynara was also traditionally used to treat nephrosclerosis, urinary stones and oliguria of toxic or infectious origin, hepatic insufficiency and as a depurative for simple itch in children. Taken internally it was said to produce a deodorant activity.[4]

Summary actions

Hepatoprotective, hepatic trophorestorative, choleretic, cholagogue, bitter, hypocholesterolaemic, anticholestatic, antiemetic, diuretic; the combination of choleretic and diuretic activities makes it an ideal depurative.

Can be used for

Indications supported by clinical trials

Hyperlipidaemia; non-ulcer dyspepsia and irritable bowel syndrome; conditions requiring an increase in choleresis and antiemetic activity (functional bowel disorders, constipation, dyspepsia, functional gallbladder conditions, nausea, vomiting, flatulence).

Traditional therapeutic uses

Rheumatism, arthritis, gout, uraemia, jaundice, oedema, nephrosclerosis, urinary stones, gallstones, oliguria, hepatic insufficiency and conditions requiring a depurative action (such as skin itch).

May also be used for

Extrapolations from pharmacological studies

Prevention and treatment of toxic conditions, particularly those involving the liver; long-term prevention and treatment of cardiovascular disease; to improve and regenerate hepatic function.

Preparations

Dried herb, tincture, liquid extract, pressed juice, tablets or capsules for internal use.

Dosage

3 to 8 mL/day of 1:2 liquid extract or its equivalent in other dosage forms.

Clinical studies indicate that doses need to be relatively high, especially to achieve a clinically relevant reduction in cholesterol levels (in the range of the equivalent of 4 to 9 g/day of dried leaves). However, doses for the other therapeutic applications can be about 1.5 to 4 g/day. It is unlikely that drop doses of tinctures will achieve the effects described below.

Duration of use

No restriction on long-term use.

Summary assessment of safety

No adverse effects from ingestion of Cynara are expected on current evidence.

Technical data

Botany

Cynara is a member of the Compositae (daisy, Asteraceae) family and in the same tribe as *Silybum marianum*. It is a cultigen, probably a form of *Cynara cardunculus* L. and this is recognised in its new botanical name[5] (although the older *C. scolymus* is still retained in the *European Pharmacopoeia* and other official texts). Cynara is a herbaceous plant that produces stems of 1 m or more in length. The basal, lobate-bipinnatisect leaves are very large; the stem leaves may be pinnatisect or entire. (These leaves are eaten as a vegetable.) The inflorescence is formed of purplish-blue flowers grouped in heads which have an involucre of several long bracts which may be spiny. The fruit is an oval achene with a plumed pappus (tuft of bristles).[6]

Adulteration

Occasionally Cynara is confused with Jerusalem artichoke (*Helianthus tuberosus*).[2]

Key constituents

- Sesquiterpene lactones (0.5% to 6%), including cynaropicrin (40% to 80% of the total),[7] and sesquiterpene glycosides cynarascolosides A, B and C[8]
- Caffeic acid derivatives (polyphenols): chlorogenic acid (3-caffeoylquinic acid), cynarin (1,3-dicaffeoylquinic acid),[7] and many other dicaffeoylquinic acid derivatives[9,10]
- Flavonoids (mainly glycosides of luteolin).[10]

Phenolic acids (such as the caffeic acid derivatives) are potentially unstable, but careful drying of the leaves ensures that losses are minimal.[11,12]

Pharmacodynamics

The most important active components in Cynara appear to be the dicaffeoylquinic acid derivatives including cynarin, with a 2003 study of four commercial Cynara extracts demonstrating that the extract with the highest content exhibited the greatest in vivo choleretic and hepatoprotective activity.[13]

In the 1930s to 1950s several scientific investigations were conducted by French and Italian scientists.[4] Although there was much debate about active components, these studies confirmed the choleretic (increased bile flow from the liver) and diuretic activity of Cynara leaves. Clinical and pharmacological research in the 1930s confirmed that Cynara was choleretic, lowered cholesterol and caused diuresis in conjunction with an increase in urea and other nitrogen-containing substances in the urine.[14] This last activity is of particular novel interest and was confirmed by other researchers.[4] Cynara also stimulated the antitoxic (hepatoprotective) activity of the liver in chronic arsenic poisoning and eliminated the signs of arsenobenzol poisoning in patients treated for syphilis.[4]

Cynarin

Cynaropicrin

Choleretic activity

Experiments in the 1950s found that cynarin given by intraperitoneal injection produced a marked choleretic activity of longer duration than sodium dehydrocholate (a bile salt), with an increase in the excretion of cholesterol and solids in the bile.[15] In contrast to other conventional choleretics such as bile salts, cynarin administered by intravenous injection to rats stimulated bile production without later impairing the excretory function of the liver.[16] Cynara extract increased the secretion of bile in liver cell cultures and from isolated perfused rat liver,[17] and re-established biliary secretion when this was inhibited by the addition of taurolithocholate to cultured rat hepatocytes.[18]

Cynarin caused an increase of faecal bile acid excretion in seven healthy individuals and four patients with fatty liver.[19] Total extract of Cynara (containing 19% caffeoylquinic acids; 25 mg/kg) and purified extract (containing 46% caffeoylquinic acids; 200 mg/kg) demonstrated marked choleretic effects in rats when administered by intraperitoneal injection. The choleretic activity mostly influenced bile salt secretion.[20] In an early study on 24 healthy subjects, Cynara extract caused stimulation of choleresis (see also under Clinical trials).[21]

A 2004 study in rats using Cynara leaf extract at oral doses up to 400 mg/kg demonstrated a marked dose-dependent increase in bile flow and total bile acid concentration comparable to the reference compound dehydrocholic acid, although no significant changes in cholesterol and phospholipid contents were found.[22]

Hepatoprotective and hepatorestorative activity

Several studies have investigated the protective effect of cynarin against damage to isolated liver cells in vitro. One study found that cynarin afforded significant protection against the toxin galactosamine and was more active than silybin from *Silybum marianum*.[23] However, it was less active than silybin against carbon tetrachloride (CCl$_4$) damage.[24] Caffeic acid was found to be much less active than cynarin against CCl$_4$ toxicity in vitro,[25] but cynarin and caffeic acid both showed significant hepatoprotective activity against CCl$_4$ in vivo.[26] This protective activity has also been demonstrated for Cynara extract and is apparently related to its antioxidant properties.[27]

Water-soluble extracts of Cynara demonstrated marked antioxidant and protective activities against hydroperoxide-induced oxidative stress in cultured rat hepatocytes. Chlorogenic acid and cynarin accounted for only part of the antioxidant effect of the extracts, which was resistant to tryptic digestion, boiling, acidification and other treatments, but was slightly sensitive to alkalinisation.[28] In an earlier study using the same model, standardised Cynara extract offered similar protective activity and strong antioxidant activity.[29]

Oral doses of an aqueous extract of Cynara leaves stimulated liver repair and regeneration in rats.[30] This was confirmed in a follow-up study that found that Cynara leaves were more active than roots.[31]

Hypolipidaemic activity

Cynarin (400 mg/kg, ip) was found to inhibit the hepatic synthesis of cholesterol and was of low toxicity.[15] Injection of cynarin in rats prevented the ethanol-induced increase in total esterified fatty acids (p<0.001). Administration of cynarin was followed by levels that were approximately 28% lower than those observed in the control group; total serum lipids were also lower.[32] Oral cynarin (6 g/kg/day for 3 days) administered simultaneously with ethanol produced a distinct reduction in serum and hepatic cholesterol levels.[33] In rats receiving ethanol and cynarin simultaneously, a marked reduction of serum and hepatic triglyceride levels occurred.[34]

Injection of Cynara extracts reduced plasma cholesterol in hyperlipidaemic rats. Oral administration of a purified extract of Cynara (containing 46% caffeoylquinic acids; 100 mg/kg) decreased plasma cholesterol levels in ethanol-fed rats.[19] Cynara extract inhibited the increase in serum lipids and the manifestation of atherosclerotic plaques induced by an atherogenic diet in rats.[35,36]

In an experimental study using a methanolic extract, Cynara was found to suppress serum triglyceride elevation in olive oil-loaded mice.[8] The inhibition of gastric emptying was posited as being partly involved in the antihyperlipidaemic activity, with no effect on pancreatic lipase observed.

Results of in vitro tests suggest that standardised Cynara extract produces its antiatherosclerotic activity via a dual mechanism: inhibiting cholesterol synthesis and acting as a free radical scavenger, inhibiting LDL oxidation.[1,37] However, in vitro mechanisms must be viewed with caution due to the uncertain bioavailability of many of the phytochemicals found in the herb.

Standardised Cynara extract significantly inhibited cholesterol biosynthesis in primary cultures of rat hepatocytes (p<0.001). This inhibition of the de novo synthesis was not due to cytotoxic effects.[38] The flavonoid luteolin has been identified as a possible key component in this process.[17] Globe artichoke contains glycosidic derivatives of luteolin, which are probably converted to free luteolin by the action of bowel flora. However, whether clinically significant quantities of luteolin are absorbed is unlikely (see under Pharmacokinetics). Cynara extract inhibited cholesterol synthesis in vitro at several levels in the biosynthetic sequence and therefore, unlike modern cholesterol drugs (the HMG-CoA reductase inhibitors), might not result in the accumulation of potentially undesirable intermediate metabolites.[17] A modulation of HMG-CoA reductase activity was later observed in a study using high-dose aqueous Cynara extract in primary cultured rat hepatocytes. The results indicated no direct inhibition of HMG-CoA enzymatic steps, instead an indirect modulation of HMG-CoA reductase activity was suggested as the most likely mechanism.[39]

Other activity

Two dicaffeoylquinic acid derivatives (3,5-dicaffeoylquinic acid, 4,5-dicaffeoylquinic acid) demonstrated anti-inflammatory activity in vitro.[40] Dicaffeoylquinic acids also exhibited activity against human immunodeficiency virus (HIV) integrase in vitro and prevented HIV replication in tissue culture.[41]

An ethanolic extract of Cynara displayed antifungal activity against a variety of organisms, as determined via an agar-well diffusion assay technique.[42] Another in vitro antimicrobial disk assay also confirmed activity against seven bacteria species, four yeasts and four moulds, with the phenolic compounds expressing the greatest activity.[43] However, the in vivo relevance of such studies conducted using high concentrations of test material is uncertain.

Antioxidant activity of Cynara extract was confirmed via DPPH scavenging, ferric-reducing antioxidant power (FRAP) and copper-catalysed in vitro human low-lipoprotein oxidation.[44] One gram of Cynara displayed DPPH and FRAP antioxidant activity equivalent to 29.2 mg and 62.9 mg of vitamin C and 77.9 mg and 159 mg of vitamin E, respectively.

Cynarin (50 to 125 mg/kg, ip) stimulated spontaneous diuresis and enhanced the excretion of a water or saline load. It antagonised the antidiuretic action of posterior pituitary extract (which contains antidiuretic hormone).[15]

An in vitro study showed that while Cynara caused only modest inhibition of xanthine oxidase, luteolin exhibited good activity that was somewhat attenuated in its derivates (such as luteolin 7-O-glucuronide). However, oral administration of Cynara, luteolin or its glycoside did not produce any observable lowering of uric acid in a rat model.[45]

No stimulatory effect on acid secretion was exerted by Cynara extract in cultured cells from rat gastric mucosa.[46] Aqueous extract of Cynara (35.7 and 150 mg/kg) administered to sexually mature male rats five times per week for 75 days did not lead to any significant change in the structure of semen.[47]

Oral administration of the total extract of Cynara (containing 19% caffeoylquinic acids; 400 mg/kg) or purified extract (containing 46% caffeoylquinic acids; 200 mg/kg) increased the small intestinal transit of rats by 11% and 14% respectively.[20]

Pharmacokinetics

A 2005 crossover study (n=14) administering two quantitatively different Cynara extracts discovered no free target compounds in the participants' urine and plasma (dicaffeoylquinic acids, luteolin, caffeic acid or other phenolics) as determined by HPLC analysis.[48] However, caffeic acid, ferulic acid, luteolin, isoferulic acid, dihydrocaffeic acid and dihydroferulic acid were detected in urine and plasma as post-hepatic phase II conjugates, mainly as sulphates or glucuronides. Peak plasma conjugate concentrations of caffeic acid, ferulic acid and isoferulic acid were reached within 1 h and declined over 24 h, showing almost biphasic profiles. In contrast, maximum conjugate concentrations for total dihydrocaffeic and dihydroferulic acids were observed only after 6 to 7 h, indicating two different metabolic pathways for the caffeoylquinic acids. Around 2% of the luteolin glycosides were absorbed and excreted as luteolin conjugates via the urine.

These findings suggest that while the caffeoylquinic acids and luteolin glycosides are appropriate marker compounds for the evaluation of the quality of Cynara raw materials, the extrapolation of in vitro pharmacological data for these components to efficacy in vivo needs to be questioned. In vitro studies should not focus on the non-absorbed parent compounds, but should instead investigate the bioavailable

metabolites of these compounds at the concentrations found after normal human doses.

Clinical trials

Hypolipidaemic activity

Many early clinical studies investigated cynarin, rather than extracts of Cynara. However, it is worth reviewing these briefly, since they probably also reflect the activity of the leaf extract. Uncontrolled studies found that cynarin at oral doses of 750 mg to 1500 mg/day substantially reduced levels of total serum cholesterol.[49,50] A significant decrease (15%) was observed in 17 patients who received cynarin at the dose of 1000 mg/day over 4 weeks (p<0.005).[51]

Double blind, placebo-controlled clinical trials also demonstrated significant reductions in serum cholesterol.[52-54] For example, 60 patients with elevated serum lipids were treated for 50 days with cynarin (500 mg) or placebo. Total cholesterol was significantly lowered by about 20% (p<0.001). Surprisingly, there was also a significant reduction in average body weight of about 5 kg in the treated group.[54] The reason for the weight loss is unknown, but may be related to the influence of Cynara on liver metabolism.

In a double blind, placebo-controlled study, cynarin at 500 mg/day also significantly lowered triglyceride levels in elderly patients with hypertriglyceridaemia.[55] Not all clinical studies on cynarin have been positive. An uncontrolled study involving 17 patients with type II familial hyperlipoproteinaemia found that cynarin had no effect over 3 to 6 months.[56]

Clinical studies of Cynara in the 1930s established its promise in lowering serum levels of cholesterol, urea and other nitrogen metabolites.[4] Cynara extract brought about a decrease of serum cholesterol and of triglycerides in an uncontrolled trial in 132 patients. The decreases were 59% and 82%, respectively, for 25 of these patients with type II hyperlipoproteinaemia.[57] A review of the clinical data from 1936 to 1994 indicated that Cynara extract lowered lipid levels (cholesterol and/or triglyceride) from between just below 5% to approximately 45%. However, this does not take into consideration the differences in experimental conditions between the various studies.[17] Several of these trials are outlined below.

A decrease in serum cholesterol of 12% to 25% followed administration of Cynara extract (900 mg/day, about 5 g of leaf) for 6 weeks.[58,59] A reduction of about 15% was observed in a large group of hyperlipidaemic patients from general practice treated with a herbal formula containing Cynara and rhubarb root.[60] A decrease in serum lipid levels in 84 patients with secondary hyperlipidaemia was observed in three connected uncontrolled clinical trials. Patients were treated for 6 to 12 weeks with the pressed juice of fresh leaves and flower buds (10 mL, three times a day). Reductions in triglycerides of 4.7%, 12.9% and 4.4% were observed in the three trials and a reduction of 15.5% in LDL-cholesterol was found in the second trial.[61]

In a randomised, controlled clinical trial, 640 mg Cynara leaf extract or placebo was administered three times a day to 44 healthy volunteers over 12 weeks. Total cholesterol when high was significantly decreased. When only moderate or normal, there were no changes, although in these cases triglyceride levels were reduced. There were no significant differences between the two treatment groups with respect to side effects.[62]

A randomised, double blind, placebo-controlled trial evaluated a Cynara dry extract (equivalent to 45 to 63g/day of fresh leaf for 6 weeks) in 143 hypercholesterolaemic patients.[63] Total cholesterol and LDL-cholesterol decreased from baseline by 18.5% and 22.9%, respectively. In comparison to the decrease demonstrated by the placebo group (8.6% and 6.3% respectively), treatment with Cynara was significantly different (p=0.0001). A 2002 systematic review by the Cochrane Collaboration found only two randomised trials met all inclusion criteria.[62,63] It was concluded that, while beneficial effects are recorded, there were few data from rigorous clinical trials assessing Cynara for hypercholesterolaemia and more studies were needed.[64] Additional studies have indeed been published since this review.

An antiatherosclerotic action was demonstrated in a study of 18 moderately hyperlipidaemic patients given 20mL/day of frozen artichoke leaf juice for 6 weeks.[65] Endothelial dysfunction was evaluated by ultrasound measurement of brachial flow-mediated vasodilation (FMV) and by the determination of several humoral markers such as vascular cell adhesion molecule-1 (VCAM-1), intercellular adhesion molecule-1 (ICAM-1) and E-selectin. After Cynara treatment there was an increase in triglycerides versus baseline (p<0.05), a reduction in total cholesterol (p<0.05) and LDL–cholesterol (p<0.05), and decreases in VCAM-1 (1633 ± 1293 versus 1139 ± 883 ng/mL, p<0.05) and ICAM-1 (477 ± 123 versus 397 ± 102 ng/mL, p<0.05). Brachial FMV increased (3.3 ± 2.7 versus $4.5 \pm 2.4\%$, p<0.01), while controls did not exhibit significant changes in any of the above parameters. It was concluded that Cynara positively modulated endothelial function in hypercholesterolaemia.

Adults with mild-to-moderate hypercholesterolaemia randomly received Cynara extract (equivalent to about 6.4g/day of dried leaf, containing 32mg/day of caffeoylquinic acids including cynarin and chlorogenic acid) or placebo for 12 weeks.[66] Only those patients with plasma total cholesterol of 6 to 8mmol/L were included. The mean body mass index for both groups was above the ideal range of 20 to 25kg/m^2 and the majority participated in light or moderate exercise and had a moderately stressful lifestyle. Treatment with Cynara resulted in a modest but significant decrease in plasma total cholesterol (4.2%, from 7.16mmol/L at baseline to 6.86mmol/L), compared with an increase observed in the placebo group (6.90mmol/L at baseline to 7.03mmol/L). The difference between the groups was also statistically significant (p=0.025). No effect was observed for other lipid levels. There were no significant differences between the groups in terms of diet, with both groups averaging approximately four servings of fruit and vegetables per day. General well-being improved in both groups.

Choleretic activity

In an early, open clinical study involving 198 patients with biliary fistula, Cynara extract demonstrated choleretic and cholagogue effects and clinical improvement.[67] The increase

in choleresis after intraduodenal administration of standardised Cynara extract was investigated in a randomised, placebo-controlled, double blind pilot study using a crossover design. Twenty healthy male volunteers were given a single dose of six capsules, each of which contained 320mg of 4.5:1 to 5:1 Cynara extract (equivalent to 1.5g of leaf and providing 0.2mg of cynarin). The amount of bile released into the duodenum was defined as the primary variable. A maximum effect from the Cynara extract was achieved after 1h (p<0.01). Significant and clinically relevant differences were still apparent 3h after the Cynara was administered (p<0.05), whereas secretion fell after 3h in the placebo group. The effective period of approximately 120 to 150minutes was regarded as satisfactory to favourably influence enzymatic digestion and intestinal motor function when Cynara was given postprandially. No side effects were observed.[68]

In another randomised, placebo-controlled, double blind study, 60 patients with non-ulcer dyspepsia were treated with placebo or a herbal formula containing Cynara extract. Bile secretion measured with a duodenal probe increased significantly and there was also a significant improvement in symptoms such as bloating, nausea and heartburn. The herbal formula contained extracts of Cynara (50%), *Peumus boldus* (30%) and *Chelidonium majus* (20%).[69]

Dyspepsia

The above studies support a commonly held opinion in Europe that the choleretic and possibly antiemetic properties of Cynara mean that it is a valuable treatment for a range of functional digestive disorders. The 2009 ESCOP Cynara monograph cites several open studies demonstrating effects in reducing functional dyspeptic complaints.[70] These are supported by two postmarketing surveillance studies as follows. In a multicentre trial, patients with symptoms such as nausea, constipation, dyspepsia and functional gallbladder conditions were treated with a Cynara extract (standardised for caffeoylquinic acids). The average dose corresponded to about 7g/day of leaf. After 6 weeks of treatment, results for 170 patients were analysed. Improvements in symptoms were most marked for nausea and vomiting (improvement in 95% of cases), nausea (85%), abdominal pain (75%) and cramping right-sided pain (25%). In addition, symptoms such as flatulence and fat intolerance were favourably influenced. There was also a significant reduction in mean total cholesterol from 267mg/dL to 228mg/dL (6.9 to 5.9mmol/L). Patient assessment of the treatment differed only slightly from that of the physicians (22% excellent, 67% good) and mild side effects were noted in only 1.2% of cases.[1]

An open study on 553 dyspeptic patients (related to the above study) also found that symptoms improved in a clinically relevant and statistically significant (p<0.001) manner after 6 weeks of treatment with an average dose of about 7g/day of leaf. The therapeutic efficacy of the standardised Cynara extract was rated by physicians as excellent or good in 87% of patients. Substantial improvement was recorded for the following symptoms: vomiting, nausea, abdominal pain, constipation, flatulence, belching and fat intolerance.

Mean cholesterol values were lowered from 264 to 215 mg/dL (p<0.001; 6.83 to 5.56 mmol/L) and triglycerides fell from 234 to 188 mg/dL (p<0.001; 2.64 to 2.12 mmol/L). Tolerability of the Cynara extract was good, with only 1.3% of patients experiencing mild adverse reactions including flatulence, feeling of weakness and hunger.[71,72]

Treatment with a standardised Cynara extract (equivalent to 8.6 g/day dried leaf) reduced the severity of symptoms of patients with irritable bowel syndrome (IBS) in a postmarketing surveillance study. The overall effectiveness of Cynara rated favourably with both physicians and patients. Ninety-six percent of patients rated the herb as better than or at least equal to previous therapies.[73]

Healthy patients with self-reported dyspepsia (n=516), as assessed via the Nepean Dyspepsia Index and the State-Trait Anxiety Inventory, were randomly allocated 320 or 640 mg/day of Cynara extract for months in an open study.[74] In both dosage groups there was a significant reduction of all dyspeptic symptoms, with an average reduction of 40% in the Global Dyspepsia Score as compared with baseline values. Health-related quality of life was also significantly enhanced in both groups compared with baseline. A follow-up post hoc analysis of the data was later conducted to assess the subset of patients with IBS symptoms, namely alternating constipation and diarrhoea and mucus in stools.[75] Two hundred and eight adults were identified as meeting the criteria for IBS. Analysis revealed that there was a significant fall in IBS incidence of 26.4% (p<0.001) after treatment, with a significant shift away from alternating constipation and diarrhoea (p<0.001).

A 6-week double blind, placebo-controlled, randomised trial involving 247 adults with functional dyspepsia was conducted to assess the efficacy of Cynara (extract equivalent to 7.3 to 10.6 g dried leaf per day) in ameliorating dyspeptic symptoms.[76] The primary outcome measure used was the sum score of the patient's weekly rating of the overall change in dyspeptic symptoms and quality of life as assessed by the Nepean Dyspepsia Index. Results demonstrated a significantly greater amelioration of dyspepsia with Cynara than with placebo (8.3±4.6 versus 6.7±4.8, p<0.01) and a significantly greater improvement in the global quality-of-life scores (-41.1±47.6 versus -24.8±35.6, p<0.01). The main improvements observed were for alleviation of the sensation of fullness, early satiety and flatulence. No statistical change occurred for nausea, vomiting and epigastric pain. Patients with predominant IBS symptoms were not eligible for the trial. However, subgroup analysis of the overall change in symptoms found that patients without additional IBS symptoms gained much more benefit from Cynara treatment than the patients with some IBS.

Other conditions

A novel randomised, controlled trial (n=15) conducted to determine whether Cynara was effective in preventing hangovers concluded equivocal results, with no difference observed against placebo in hangover outcomes.[77]

In an early trial, clinical application of Cynara extract in patients with ascites caused by portal stasis resulted in stimulation of diuresis.[78]

Sixty-two workers chronically exposed to carbon disulphide experienced a favourable outcome from prophylactic treatment with a Cynara preparation over 2 years. The treatment significantly reduced their platelet aggregation.[79] (One of the many symptoms of exposure to carbon disulphide is increased platelet adhesiveness, possibly resulting from lipid metabolism disturbances.)

A double blind, placebo-controlled trial in 22 members of the Polish rowing team found that 1200 mg/day of Cynara extract (about 6 g/day of leaf) for 5 weeks provided antioxidant effects after heavy exercise.[80] While plasma total antioxidant capacity was significantly increased compared with placebo (p<0.05), this did not limit oxidative damage to erythrocytes. At the end of the trial, serum total cholesterol was significantly lower in the Cynara group versus placebo (p<0.05), although this observation was mainly due to an increase for the placebo group.

An extract of Cynara flowering buds (as opposed to the leaves) improved glycaemic control and insulin resistance in overweight participants in a clinical trial.[81] A similar extract in conjunction with Phaseolus vulgaris extract reduced appetite and improved insulin resistance and glycaemic control, also in overweight patients.[82]

Toxicology and other safety data

Toxicology

The following LD_{50} data have been recorded for Cynara extract:

Substance	Route, model	LD_{50}	Reference
Purified Cynara extract	Oral, rats	>2 g/kg	20
Purified Cynara extract (containing 46% caffeoylquinic acids)	ip, rats	265 mg/kg	20
Total extract of Cynara (containing 19% caffeoylquinic acids)	ip, rats	1 g/kg	20

Cynara also has low chronic toxicity. No toxic effects were observed in rats after oral administration of Cynara extract (10 to 200 mg/kg) for 4 months[83] or dermal application (1 g/kg and 3 g/kg) for 21 days.[84] The dermal LD_0 was 6 g/kg in rats. (LD_0 is the highest dose at which none of the test organisms die.) Cynara extract did not demonstrate skin-irritant or eye-irritant activity in rabbits nor skin-sensitising potential in guinea pigs.[84]

Aqueous extract of Cynara (35.7 and 150 mg/kg) administered to sexually mature male rats five times a week for 75 days did not lead to any significant change in the structure of the semen.[48]

Cynara leaf extract was cytotoxic to rat hepatocytes in culture at concentrations greater than 1 mg/mL.[28]

Contraindications

Use only with professional supervision in cholelithiasis (gallstones) or closure of the gallbladder.[85]

Special warnings and precautions

The Commission E advises caution for patients with known allergy to Cynara and to other plants of the Compositae family.[86] The likelihood of Cynara preparations causing an allergic reaction is very low.

Interactions

None known.

Use in pregnancy and lactation

Category B2-no increase in frequency of malformation or other harmful effects on the fetus from limited use in women. Animal studies are lacking.

Cynara is compatible with breastfeeding.

Effect on ability to drive or operate machinery

No adverse effects expected.

Side effects

The safety and tolerability of Cynara recorded in clinical studies are good to very good. A 1997 review stated that Cynara leaf extract had good tolerability with a very low rate of side effects.[76] Mild side effects such as flatulence and a feeling of weakness and hunger have been reported in 1.3% of 553 dyspeptic patients in post-marketing surveillance studies.[71,72] However, as with other members of the Compositae family, contact with the fresh plant can cause contact dermatitis.[87,88] This is presumably due to the content of potentially allergenic sesquiterpene lactones.[89] One case of urticaria-angioedema

from ingestion of both raw and boiled Cynara has been described. Allergy was confirmed by skin prick testing.[90] Case studies have also documented rhinitis and bronchial asthma occurring in warehouse workers exposed to artichokes, with an IgE-based allergy confirmed via skin prick test.[91]

A case of hepatitis attributed to Cynara intake was published in 2007.[92] A 24-year-old French woman was hospitalised in late 2005 with weakness and urticaria. She had been taking a daily dose of two ampoules of a liquid preparation of Cynara (20 mL/day, herb dosage not defined). Her serum hepatic enzymes were highly elevated, but bilirubin was normal. Tests for a variety of viruses were normal. The patient improved markedly with cessation of the Cynara and made a full recovery. Her hepatic enzyme levels returned to normal in 2 to 3 weeks.

Overdosage

Not known.

Safety in children

No information available but adverse effects are not expected.

Regulatory status in selected countries

In the UK artichoke is included on the General Sale List. Globe artichoke products have achieved Traditional Herbal Registration in the UK with the indication of the relief of digestive complaints such as indigestion, upset stomach, nausea, feelings of fullness and flatulence (wind). Globe artichoke is covered by a positive German Commission E monograph.

Globe artichoke does not have GRAS status. However, it is freely available as a 'dietary supplement' in the USA under DSHEA legislation (Dietary Supplement Health and Education Act of 1994).

Globe artichoke is not included in Part 4 of Schedule 4 of the Therapeutic Goods Regulations in Australia and is freely available for sale.

References

1. Wegener T. *Z Phytother*. 1995;16:81.
2. Felter HW, Lloyd JU. *King's American Dispensatory*, ed 18, rev 3, vol 1, 1905. Portland: Reprinted by Eclectic Medical Publications; 1983. p. 641.
3. Leclerc H. *Précis de Phytothérapie*, 5th ed. Paris: Masson; 1983. pp. 143–144.
4. Rocchietta S. *Minerva Med*. 1959;50:612–618.
5. Mabberley DJ. *The Plant Book*, 2nd ed. Cambridge: Cambridge University Press; 1997. p. 175.
6. Chiej R. *The Macdonald Encyclopedia of Medicinal Plants*. London: Macdonald; 1984. Entry no. 107.
7. Wagner H, Bladt S. *Plant Drug Analysis: A Thin Layer Chromatography Atlas*, 2nd ed. Berlin: Springer-Verlag; 1996. p. 77.
8. Shimoda H, Ninomiya K, Nishida N, et al. *Bioorg Med Chem Lett*. 2003;13(2):223–228.
9. Puigmacia M, Adzet T, Ruviralta M, et al. *Planta Med*. 1986;52:529–530.
10. Hammouda FM, Seif El-Nasr MM, Ismail SI, et al. *Int J Pharmacog*. 1993;31(4):299–304.
11. Nichiforesco E. *Ann Pharm Fr*. 1967;25(4):285–290.
12. Nichiforesco E, Coucou V. *Ann Pharm Fr*. 1966;24(2):127–132.
13. Speroni E, Cervellati R, Govoni P, et al. *J Ethnopharmacol*. 2003;86(2–3):203–211.
14. Tixier L. *Presse Med*. 1939;4:880–883.
15. Preziosi P, Loscalzo B. *Arch Int Pharmacodyn*. 1958;117:63–80.
16. Preziosi P, Loscalzo B, Marmo E. *Experientia*. 1989;15:135–138.
17. Kraft K. *Phytomedicine*. 1997;4(4):369–378.
18. Gebhardt R. *Med Sci Monit*. 2001;7(suppl 1):316–320.
19. Schreiber J, Erb W, Wildgrube J, et al. *Z Gastroenterol*. 1970;8:230–239.
20. Lietti A. *Fitoterapia*. 1977;48:153–158.
21. Struppler A, Rossler H. *Med Monatsschr*. 1957;11:221–223.

22. Saenz Rodriguez T, Garcia Gimenez D, de la Puerta Vazquez R. *Phytomedicine.* 2002;9(8):687–693.

23. Kiso Y, Tohkin M, Hikino H. *J Nat Prod.* 1983;46(6):841–847.

24. Kiso Y, Tohkin M, Hikino H. *Planta Med.* 1983;49(4):222–225.

25. Adzet T, Camarasa J, Laguna JC. *J Nat Prod.* 1987;50(4):612–617.

26. Camarasa J, Laguna JC, Gaspar A, et al. *Med Sci Res.* 1987;15:91–92.

27. Gebhardt R. *Pharm Ztg.* 1995;140(43):3858–3861.

28. Gebhardt R. *Toxicol Appl Pharmacol.* 1997;144(2):279–286.

29. Gebhardt R. *Med Welt.* 1995;46(7): 393–395.

30. Maros T, Racz G, Katonai B, et al. *Arzneimittelforschung.* 1966;16(2):127–129.

31. Maros T, Seres-Sturm L, Racz G, et al. *Arzneimittelforschung.* 1968;18(7):884–886.

32. Samochowiec L, Wojcicki J, Kadykow M. *Pan Med.* 1971;13:87–88.

33. Wojcicki J. *Drug Alcohol Depend.* 1978;3(2):143–145.

34. Wojcicki J. *Arzneimittelforschung.* 1976;26(11):2047–2048.

35. Samochowiec L. *Diss Pharm.* 1959;11: 99–112.

36. Samochowiec L. *Fol Biol.* 1962;10:75–83.

37. Zapolska-Downar D, Zapolski-Downar A, Naruszewicz M, et al. *Life Sci.* 2002;71(24):2897–2908.

38. Gebhardt R. *Med Welt.* 1995;46(6): 348–350.

39. Gebhardt R. *J Pharmacol Exp Ther.* 1998;286(3):1122–1128.

40. De Feo V, De Simone R, Bresciano E, et al. *J Nat Prod.* 1995;58(5):639–646.

41. McDougall B, King PJ, Wu BW, et al. *Antimicrob Agents Chemother.* 1998;42(1):140–146.

42. Zhu XF, Zhang HX, Lo R. *Fitoterapia.* 2005;76(1):108–111.

43. Zhu X, Zhang H, Lo R. *J Agric Food Chem.* 2004;52(24):7272–7278.

44. Jimenez-Escrig A, Dragsted LO, Daneshvar B, et al. *J Agric Food Chem.* 2003;51(18):5540–5545.

45. Sarawek S, Feistel B, Pischel I, et al. *Planta Med.* 2008;74(3):221–227.

46. Gebhardt R. *Pharm Pharmacol Lett.* 1997;7(2–3):106–108.

47. Ilieva P, Khalkova Zh Zaikov Kh *Probl Khig.* 1994;19:105–111.

48. Wittemer SM, Ploch M, Windeck T, et al. *Phytomedicine.* 2005;12(1–2):28–38.

49. Cima G, Bonora R. *Minerva Med.* 1959;50:2288–2291.

50. Mancini M, Oriente P, D'Andrea L. *Minerva Med.* 1960;51:2460–2463.

51. Adam G, Kluthe R. *Therapiewoche.* 1979;29:5637–5640.

52. Cairella M, Volpari B. *Clin Ter.* 1971;57(6):541–552.

53. Montini M, Levoni P, Ongaro A, et al. *Arzneimittelforschung.* 1975;25:1311–1314.

54. Eberhardt G. *Z Gastroenterol.* 1973;11(3):183–186.

55. Mars G, Brambilla G. *Med Welt.* 1974;25(39):1572–1574.

56. Heckers H, Dittmar K, Schmahl FW, et al. *Atherosclerosis.* 1977;26(2):249–253.

57. Hammerl H, Kindler K, Kranzl C, et al. *Wien Med Wochenschr.* 1973;123:601–605.

58. Wojcicki J, Samochowiec K, Kosmider K. *Herba Pol.* 1981;27(3):265–268.

59. Wojcicki J, Winter S. *Med Pracy.* 1975;26:213–217.

60. Vorberg G. *Z Allg Med.* 1980;56(25): 1598–1602.

61. Dorn M. *Br J Phytother.* 1995/1996;4(1):21–26.

62. Petrowicz O, Gebhardt R, Donner M, et al. *Atherosclerosis.* 1997;129:147.

63. Englisch W, Beckers C, Unkauf M, et al. *Arzneimittelforschung.* 2000;50(3):260–265.

64. Pittler MH, Ernst E. *Cochrane Database Syst Rev.* 2002(Issue 3):CD003335.

65. Lupattelli G, Marchesi S, Lombardini R, et al. *Life Sci.* 2004;76(7):775–782.

66. Bundy R, Walker AF, Middleton RW, et al. *Phytomedicine.* 2008;15(9):668–675.

67. Hammerl H, Pichler O. *Wien Med Wochenschr.* 1957;107(25/26):545–546.

68. Kirchhoff R, Beckers Ch, Kirchhoff GM, et al. *Phytomedicine.* 1994;1(2):107–115.

69. Kupke D, Sanden HV, Trinzcej-Gartner H, et al. *Z Allg Med.* 1991;67(16):1046–1058.

70. European Scientific Cooperative on Phytotherapy *The ESCOP Monographs 2009 Supplement to 2nd Edition.* ESCOP, Exeter and Thieme Verlag Stuttgart; 2009.

71. Fintelmann V. *Z Allg Med.* 1996;72 (suppl 2):3–19.

72. Fintelmann V, Menben HG. *Dtsch Apoth Ztg.* 1996;136(17):63–74.

73. Walker AF, Middleton RW, Petrowicz O. *Phytother Res.* 2001;15(1):58–61.

74. Marakis G, Walker AF, Middleton RW, et al. *Phytomedicine.* 2002;9(8):694–699.

75. Bundy R, Walker AF, Middleton RW, et al. *J Altern Complement Med.* 2004;10(4): 667–669.

76. Holtmann G, Adam B, Haag S, et al. *Aliment Pharmacol Ther.* 2003;18(11–12): 1099–1105.

77. Pittler MH, White AR, Stevinson C, et al. *CMAJ.* 2003;169(12):1269–1273.

78. Beggi D, Dettori L. *Policlin Sez Prat.* 1931;41:489–490.

79. Woyke M, Cwajda H, Wojcicki J, et al. *Med Pr.* 1981;32(4):261–264.

80. Skarpanska-Stejnborn A, Pilaczynska-Szczesniak L, Basta P, et al. *Int J Sport Nutr Exerc Metab.* 2008;18(3):313–327.

81. Rondanelli M, Opizzi A, Riva A, et al. *Abstracts of the 4th International Congress on Prediabetes and Metabolic Syndrome,* 2011, p. 108.

82. Rondanello M, Giacosa A, Orsini F, et al. *Phytother Res.* 2011 [Epub ahead of print].

83. Halkova Z, Zaikov C, Shumkov N, et al. *Khig Zdraveopaz.* 1997;40(1):9–12.

84. Halkova Z. *Probl Khig.* 1996;21:74–80.

85. German Federal Minister of Justice. *German Commission E for Human Medicine Monograph.* Bundes-Anzeiger (German Federal Gazette), No. 122, dated 06.07.1988; No. 164, dated 01.09.1990.

86. Blumenthal M, ed. *The Complete German Commission E Monographs: Therapeutic Guide to Herbal Medicines.* Austin: American Botanical Council; 1998.

87. Meding B. *Contact Derm.* 1983;9(4):314.

88. Quirce S, Tabar AI, Olaguibel JM, et al. *J Allergy Clin Immunol.* 1996;97(2):710–711.

89. Mitchell JC, Dupuis G. *Br J Dermatol.* 1971;84(2):139–150.

90. Romano C, Ferrara A, Falagiani P. *J Investig Allergol Clin Immunol.* 2000;10(2): 102–104.

91. Miralles JC, García-Sells J, Bartolomé B, et al. *Ann Allergy Asthma Immunol.* 2003;91(1):92–95.

92. Sinayoko L, Mennecier D, El Jahir Y, et al. *Gastroenterol Clin Biol.* 2007;31(11): 1039–1040.

Gotu kola

(*Centella asiatica* (L.) Urban)

Synonyms

Gotu kola, marsh pennywort (Engl), Herba centellae (Lat), Asiatischer Wassernabel (Ger), centelle asiatique, hydrocotyle (Fr), erba delle tigri, idrocotile (Ital), ji xue cao (Chin), bemgsag, brahmi (Hindi), tsubo kusa (Jap), gotu kola (Rus), brahmi (Bengali), brahmi (Sanskrit), *Hydrocotyle asiatica L.*

What is it?

This plant, most likely native to southern Asia, is now widespread throughout the tropics. Gotu kola has been valued in Ayurvedic medicine since time immemorial and has been adopted by Western herbal medicine. Researchers in Europe and elsewhere have investigated traditional uses and been able to document a scientific foundation for many of these, especially for wound healing (administered both topically and internally) and enhancing cognitive function. The aerial parts are typically used, but the entire plant (including the below ground parts) can also be employed as a medicine. Gotu kola is from the Singhalese language of Sri Lanka and means 'cup-shaped leaf'.

Gotu kola is an important herb in the modern materia medica that appears to possess a unique activity, namely oral doses (as well as topical doses) are able to promote tissue healing, especially via epithelial connective tissue regeneration. This stimulatory action of gotu kola on connective tissue elements might also extend to deeper tissues, suggesting potential value in conditions such as osteopenia and osteoarthritis (both currently unexplored except for preliminary chondroprotective activity). There is also evidence from pharmacological and clinical studies that the herb has a regenerative effect on the vein wall and benefits the microcirculation. Some pharmacological studies appear to support neuroprotective and neuroregenerative activities which, if verified clinically, could open up a new chapter in the unfolding story of this humble weed.

Effects

Assists cognitive function; supports venous and microcirculatory function; modulates inflammation; moderates stress responses; calms the nervous system; regulates connective tissue function and promotes healing.

Traditional view

Gotu kola is one of the esteemed *rasayana* herbs in Ayurvedic medicine, meaning a tonic believed to rejuvenate and restore the mind, body and spirit.[1] Its Sanskrit name means 'from Brahma', a central diety in the Hindu pantheon. Gotu kola is widely used in the traditional medicine systems of South Asia, particularly for a variety of chronic skin conditions and infections[2] and is often included in antiageing formulas.[3] Generally viewed as a cooling, drying herb, it was seen to drive out heat or inflammation.

In China, gotu kola is used to clear *Damp Heat*, cool *Blood*, stop bleeding, clear the *Liver* and brighten the eyes. This means it is considered useful for enteritis and dysentery (especially with vomiting), uterine bleeding, conjunctivitis, glaucoma and cataract.[4] In the Western herbal tradition, gotu kola has been used primarily as a nervine, depurative, connective tissue promoter and healing agent. Traditional Western herbal uses include skin and rheumatic conditions, such as chronic eczema, chronic rheumatism, leprosy, ulcers[5,6] and topically for poor healing wounds, leprous ulcers and scar formation after surgery.[5]

Gotu kola has been used traditionally in many other countries. In Thailand the whole plant is used as a depurative, particularly to treat skin diseases and as a diuretic and antidiarrhoeal remedy.[7] In Indonesia it has been utilised for mouth ulcers and oral thrush.[8] In Fijian traditional medicine, gotu kola was employed as a tonic for wasting diseases such as tuberculosis, stomach problems and rheumatic swelling and pain. It was used both internally and topically to relieve pain.[9] In South Africa gotu kola has been employed to treat wounds, cancer, leprosy, fever and syphilis.[10] In Australia the fresh leaves of gotu kola (and closely related species) are consumed as a folk medicine for arthritis.

Summary actions

Vulnerary; anti-inflammatory; antifibrotic; nervine tonic; adaptogenic; venotonic; depurative.

Can be used for

Indications supported by clinical trials

Chronic venous insufficiency (CVI), diabetic microangiopathy; keloids and hypertrophic scars (oral and topical), to promote healing (oral and topical); to enhance cognitive function; for liver fibrosis, atherosclerotic plaque stabilisation, scleroderma (oral and topical), leg ulcers, leprosy (oral and topical), haemorrhoids, anxiety, psoriasis (topical) and periodontal disease (topical in combination). The quality of trials varies (see the Clinical trials section for more information).

Traditional therapeutic uses

Internal use as a general tonic and for leg ulcers, leprosy, chronic skin and rheumatic conditions and for improving cognition. Topical use for psorasis, ulcers, wounds and eczema.

May also be used for

Extrapolations from pharmacological studies

May possess neuroprotective and neuroregenerative properties; could be of value in osteoarthritis and peptic ulceration.

Other applications

Gotu kola is a common ingredient in skin rejuvenating cosmetics and topical treatments for cellulite.

Preparations

Fresh or dried herb as infusion, liquid extract, standardised extract and tablets or capsules for internal use. Decoction, extract and fresh juice for external use; these can be incorporated into creams and ointments.

Dosage

- 3 to 30g dried or fresh herb per day, as infusion or powder
- 3 to 9mL/day of a 1:1 liquid extract, preferably containing at least 15mg/mL total triterpenes.
- Gotu kola extract tablets or capsules delivering 60 to 180mg/day total triterpenes.

Various but similar extracted isolates of gotu kola have been used in clinical trials. Being isolates they are not recommended in the context of phytotherapy. However, their use in positive trials does give guidance for the doses of triterpenes that will be clinically effective in the matrix of the whole herb (galenical) extract (see the doses recommended above for the 1:1 liquid extract and tablets or capsules).

The total triterpenic fraction (TTF), with 40% asiaticoside, 30% asiatic acid and 30% madecassic acid was dosed at 60 to 180mg/day. The basically identical titrated extract of *Centella asiatica* (TECA), with 40% asiaticoside, 30% asiatic acid, 30% madecassic acid, and around 1% madasiatic acid was given up to 90mg/day. The extract of triterpenoids of *Centella asiatica* (ETCA) referred to sometimes in the literature is the same as TECA. Earlier clinical trials often used 'asiaticoside' or 'Madecassol', which is most likely TECA.

Duration of use

No restriction on long term use.

Summary assessment of safety

Gotu kola is a safe herb. Other than infrequent gastrointestinal upset or contact dermatitis, almost no adverse effects are seen with this herb.

Technical data

Botany

Centella asiatica, a member of the Apiaceae (Umbelliferae, celery) family, is a tropical, evergreen, perennial creeping herb with reddish stems. The 2 to 3cm long and 3 to 4cm wide fleshy leaves are reniform with crenated margins and long, thin petioles with sheating bases. Leaves cluster at each stem node. The plant produces tiny pale pink flowers in small white umbels from June to September (northern hemisphere). Its non-branching rhizomes have many root hairs. Gotu kola produces an intricate network of stolons. Fruit is a disk-shaped, reticulate, diachene. The whole plant is aromatic and tastes spicy and sweet.[11]

Adulteration

There is no common adulterant, although theoretically *Hydrocotyle spp.* adulteration could occur. Usually these plants have single leaves at nodes and separate stipules, not sheathing leaf bases. Unintentional adulteration may occur due to confusion over the identity of 'brahmi', a common name used for both gotu kola and *Bacopa monnieri* in India. Trade samples of gotu kola herb often contain unacceptably low levels of triterpenes.

Key constituents

- Triterpene saponins (centellosides), mainly madecassoside and asiaticoside, together with their respective aglycones madecassic and asiatic acids[12]
- Monoterpenoids and sesquiterpenoids, including myrcene, farnesene, germacrene, caryophyllene and pinene;[12] a range of polyacetylenes[12]
- Flavonoids, including quercetin and kaempferol glucosides.[12]

Asiatic acid	$R_1 = H$,	$R_2 = OH$
Madecassic acid	$R_1 = OH$,	$R_2 = OH$
Asiaticoside	$R_1 = H$,	$R_2 = $ rha-glc-glc
Madecassoside	$R_1 = OH$,	$R_2 = $ rha-glc-glc

Most work has focused on the three major triterpenoids in gotu kola, which comprise 1% to 8% of the plant.[13] One study found that leaves had the highest concentration of triterpenoids compared to roots and petioles.[14]

Pharmacodynamics

Wound-healing activity

Several in vitro studies have examined the impact of gotu kola or its components on cells involved in wound healing. Early research found that 'asiaticoside' (probably TECA) activated the dermal layer and stimulated keratinisation in the epidermis of cultured pig skin.[15] Fifty-four genes with known functions for cell proliferation and synthesis of extracellular matrix (ECM) were significantly upregulated when skin fibroblasts were exposed to pure asiaticoside in much later work.[16,17] Exposure of human foreskin fibroblasts to TECA and human skin fibroblasts to TTF led to increased collagen synthesis in both cases.[18,19] Both type I and type III collagen production was stimulated in human skin fibroblasts by gotu kola saponins.[20] The aglycones were also able to stimulate type I collagen synthesis in vitro.[21] Ageing of the skin is primarily related to reductions in the level of type I collagen.[22] Asiaticoside was found to induce human type I collagen synthesis via activation of the transforming growth factor beta (TGF-beta) receptor I kinase-independent Smad pathway. The Smad signalling cascade is known to perform an important function in human collagen production and this might explain how asiaticoside inhibits hypertrophic scar formation.[23]

Systemic doses of gotu kola extract or its phytochemical constituents have been shown to improve healing or strengthen connective tissue in various animal models. In an early study TECA (100 mg/kg, oral) shortened the healing time of iterative wounds in rats.[24] A crude ethanol extract of gotu kola (1 mL/day) was applied topically or given orally to rats for 24 days after wounding.[25] Increased cellular proliferation and collagen synthesis at the wound site was observed, as evidenced by increases in the DNA, protein and collagen content of granulation tissue. Quicker and better maturation and cross-linking of collagen were found and the wounds healed faster. Compared with topical application, the oral use of gotu kola was generally more active for the above parameters.

Topical and oral asiaticoside were significantly more effective at promoting wound healing in guinea pigs than vehicle controls.[26] Applications of 0.2% asiaticoside solution increased the proline and collagen content of the healing tissue, increased its tensile strength and enhanced epithelialisation. Diabetic animals also showed improved wound healing after the application of a 0.4% asiaticoside solution. In the chick chorioallantoic membrane assay, 40 μg/disk of asiaticoside increased angiogenesis.

Gotu kola extract (800 mg/kg/day, oral) significantly improved wound strength, connective tissue content and healing rates in rats.[27] It also overcame the suppressive action of dexamethasone on wound healing, something that was not observed for asiaticoside alone at oral doses of 2 mg/kg.[28] However, oral doses of asiaticoside alone did dose-dependently increase the tensile strength of wounds after 4 and 6 days.[28]

Osteoarthritis is a degenerative joint disease in which focal cartilage destruction is a primary feature. A triterpene isolate of gotu kola containing 42% asiaticoside and 55% aglycones (0.3 mg/mouse/day, oral for 11 days) inhibited zymosan-induced cartilage degeneration without affecting inflammatory cell filtration and joint swelling.[29] This suggests a chondroprotective activity, which was supported by additional in vitro experiments on bovine cartilage explants and chondrocytes.

The impact of oral asiaticoside (10 to 20 mg/day for 10 to 15 days) on parameters of dermal wound healing was studied in 15 patients in an early human pharmacological study.[30] The higher dose for longer periods tended to increase leucine aminopeptidase activity and decrease thiol groups in the skin, which were considered to be favourable for accelerated healing.

As already touched on above, gotu kola or its components have also enhanced wound healing when applied topically. Three formulations (ointment, cream and gel) of an aqueous extract of gotu kola increased wound cellular proliferation, collagen synthesis and rates of healing in rats.[31] The gel formulation appeared to confer greatest activity. Local application of TECA improved rates of connective tissue regeneration and remodelling in a rat model.[32] Glycosaminoglycan synthesis was also increased. Asiaticoside exerted a preferential stimulation of collagen synthesis and was active at low doses only.[32] A study in rats found that asiaticoside application (0.2%, topical) twice daily for 7 days led to increased enzymatic (such as catalase and superoxide dismutase) and non-enzymatic (ascorbic acid and vitamin E) antioxidants in the wounds of rats.[33] However, these differences were not apparent after 14 days of continuous application, leading the authors to suggest that enhancement of antioxidant levels by asiaticoside early in healing may be an important factor in its wound-healing ability.

Topical application of asiaticoside at 0.5 or 1.0% three times daily for 1 to 3 months remarkably alleviated scar formation in the rabbit ear model.[34] TGF-beta1 expression was decreased and inhibitory Smad7 expression was remarkably enhanced (see earlier).

One early study of burns failed to find any benefit of intraperitoneal injection of TECA on wound healing or mortality in mice compared with the control group.[35] However, the topical application of a 70% ethanolic extract of gotu kola or isolated asiaticoside (at quite low concentrations) significantly accelerated burn wound repair in mice, possibly via enhanced angiogenesis.[36] Oral doses of madecassoside (6, 12 and 24 mg/kg) facilitated burn wound closure in a dose-dependent manner in mice.[37] Investigations suggested that several mechanisms may be involved, including antioxidant activity, regulation of collagen synthesis and promotion of angiogenesis.

Oral doses of gotu kola may also improve healing of gastric ulcers. An aqueous extract of gotu kola (0.1 to 0.25 g/kg, oral) and asiaticoside (5 to 10 mg/kg, oral) accelerated healing in rats with acetic-acid-induced gastric ulcers.[38] This was associated with increased expression of basic fibroblast growth factor, faster epithelialisation and increased angiogenesis in the healing ulcer crater. The same research group found that the same doses of gotu kola given to rats before ethanol administration significantly inhibited gastric lesion formation and decreased mucosal myeloperoxidase activity (an indicator of neutrophil infiltration).[39] These results suggested that the herb strengthened the gastric mucosal barrier and indirectly reduced free radical damage. Later in vivo research by this group suggested that an anti-inflammatory activity might also be involved.[27] Increased mucosal defence was supported by another study that used fresh gotu kola juice.[40]

Antifibrotic effects

Interestingly, given the data cited above clearly showing that gotu kola and its constituents can increase collagen synthesis in wounds, other research suggests it can decrease collagen in situations of fibrosis. Using an in vitro model of overactive hepatic stellate cells, asiatic acid and asiaticoside both inhibited excessive collagen formation.[41] Antifibrotic effects were also seen after applying gotu kola extract in vitro to mammalian renal cells.[42] One in vitro study found that gotu kola and its saponins inhibited the growth of keratinocytes, suggesting antipsoriatic activity.[43] There is also the suggestion from one model that asiaticoside might decrease post-burn hypertrophic scars.[44] Rats given TTF by gastric lavage also exhibited significantly less liver fibrosis following administration of dimethylnitrosamine.[45] Given these amphoteric effects, gotu kola could perhaps act as a collagen modulator (see also the Clinical trials section regarding scleroderma and keloid formation).

Anti-inflammatory and analgesic activities

Asiatic acid has been shown in vitro to moderately inhibit multiple inflammatory pathways, including inhibiting NF-kappaB and the expressions of cyclo-oxygenase-2 and inducible nitric oxide synthase, and by blocking production of pro-inflammatory cytokines in stimulated macrophages.[46] Asiaticoside was less active than asiatic acid in this test system. Madecassic acid exerted similar activity in vitro using stimulated macrophages.[47]

Centellosides given orally (50 to 200 mg/kg) or subcutaneously (50 to 100 mg/kg) to rats after implantation of glass rods dose-dependently reduced granuloma after 3 weeks.[48] All four individual compounds tested in this model were more or less equally effective.

Aqueous extract of gotu kola (4 and 10 mg/kg, ip) was effective at inhibiting PGE_2-induced inflammation in rats (including more effectively than mefenamic acid in the case of the higher dose).[49] Pain was inhibited in mice by an aqueous extract of gotu kola (assessed by the acetic acid and hot plate tests) in this same study.

Madecassoside (3, 10 and 30 mg/kg/day, oral from days 21 to 42) attenuated the inflammatory response in collagen-induced arthritis in mice.[50] A similar study by a different research group confirmed this finding.[51] The latter authors suggested that gotu kola might have clinical value in rheumatoid arthritis.

Asiatic acid blocks the binding of angiotensin II to its receptor in vitro.[52] This may also have implications in terms of gotu kola reducing or preventing hypertension.

Central and peripheral nervous system activity

Various extracts of gotu kola and pure asiaticoside have demonstrated anxiolytic activity in rats and mice.[53,54] In mice, asiaticoside 10 mg/kg (oral) was as effective as diazepam 0.3 mg/kg.[54] Anxiolytic activity was not linked to sedation in rats.[53] Anxiolytic effects were seen in two older studies in rodents, as well as anticonvulsant activity (in one case as potent as that of diazepam).[55,56] In both of these studies, gotu kola extracts also potentiated the sedative effects of barbiturates. Mice given 10 to 20 mg/kg asiaticoside (oral) exhibited similar antidepressant effects to clomipramine at 50 mg/kg.[57] Some of these results suggested gotu kola acts as a GABAergic agent, although in other research aqueous gotu kola extracts appeared to acts by decreasing the turnover of catecholamines.[58]

In vitro, an aqueous extract of gotu kola increased phosphorylation of cAMP-response element binding protein (CREB) in neuroblastoma cells expressing beta-amyloid.[59] CREB is a crucial regulator of genes involved in memory formation. Various synthetic derivates of asiaticoside directly protected neurons against the toxic effects of beta-amyloid in vitro.[60] This potential activity in Alzheimer-type dementia has been further explored in animal models. An aqueous extract of gotu kola (100, 200 and 300 mg/kg/day, oral for 21 days) prevented streptozotocin-induced cognitive deficit and oxidative stress in rats.[61] In mice spontaneously expressing beta-amyloid plaque formation, an undefined extract of gotu kola (2.5 and 5.0 g/kg, oral) decreased beta-amyloid formation after 8 months, partially by modulating oxidative stress and protecting against DNA damage.[62]

The potential neuroprotective activity of gotu kola has also been explored in experimental models. Asiatic acid exerted a significant neuroprotective effect in cultured cortical cells challenged with glutamate-induced exitotoxicity.[63] In vivo, a chloroform-methanolic extract of gotu kola (100 and 200 mg/kg, oral) protected against the free radical generation and excitotoxicity induced by feeding monosodium glutamate to rats.[64] Asiatic acid (37, 75 and 165 mg/kg, oral) demonstrated neuroprotective activity in a mouse model of cerebral ischaemia[65] and a 50% ethanolic gotu kola extract (300 mg/kg, oral) protected against MPTP-induced neurotoxicity in aged rats (a model of parkinsonism).[66]

As alluded to above, much of the neuroprotective activity of gotu kola might result from its ability to enhance endogenous antioxidant protective mechanisms. This hypothesis was further examined in several experimental models. An aqueous extract of gotu kola (200 mg and 300 mg/kg, oral) increased brain levels of glutathione and catalase and decreased measures of oxidative damage in rats.[67] This was coupled with improved cognition in a series of tests, which the authors suggested was linked to the observed antioxidant effects. Age-related decline in cerebral antioxidant defences and commensurable increases in measures of brain oxidation were considerably countered in aged rats by a gotu kola extract (300 mg/kg/day, oral for 60 days).[68] Similar antioxidant findings were observed in the brains of young mice fed a gotu kola extract (0.5% and 1.0% of diet) for 4 weeks.[69] Short-term oral intake of an aqueous extract of gotu kola (5 mg/kg/day for 10 days) conferred marked resistance against 3-nitropropionic acid-induced oxidative stress and mitochondrial dysfunction in the brains of young mice.[70,71]

There is even a suggestion from experimental models that gotu kola might possess neuroregenerative and neurodevelopmental activities. A gotu kola ethanolic extract (300 to 330 mg/kg/day, oral for 18 days) accelerated peripheral nerve regeneration following damage in rats.[72] More rapid functional recovery and increased axonal regeneration (larger calibre axons and greater numbers of myelinated axons) were observed compared with controls, indicating that axons grew at a faster rate. The same investigation found that an ethanolic extract and asiatic acid increased neurite outgrowth in vitro, but an aqueous extract was inactive.

Fresh leaf extract of gotu kola (4 and 6 mL/kg/day) fed to rat pups for 4 to 6 weeks increased dendritic length and branching in hippocampal neurons, a region of the brain involved in learning and memory.[73,74] Similar findings were also observed by the same research group in adult rats.[75] This might explain observations of enhanced learning and memory in young rodents fed gotu kola juice or aqueous extract[76,77] and suggests neuroplastic effects from the herb.

Anticonvulsant activity for gotu kola has also been observed in a few studies. An aqueous extract of gotu kola (300 mg/kg, oral) decreased pentylenetetrazole-induced seizures in rats and showed improvement in the associated learning deficit.[78] A different research group found this activity was associated with a recovery of brain levels of acetylcholine and acetylcholinesterase. A study in mice found the ethyl acetate extract of gotu kola exerted an anticonvulsant effect that was additive to some antiepileptic drugs.[79]

Circulatory activity

A review of pharmacological investigations, including human pharmacological studies, discussed the desirable properties of gotu kola (specifically TTF) in the context of the management of CVI, a more severe clinical manifestation of varicose veins.[80] These included an action on fibroblasts in the vein wall (improving collagen synthesis and remodelling), enhanced microcirculation with decreased oedema, improved lymphatic drainage, and a possible decrease in endothelial cell damage.

More details of some of these studies in human volunteers follow. An early open study found that 60 mg/day of an unspecified gotu kola extract (probably an isolate) for 30 days increased venous return in patients with CVI.[81] In 20 patients with varicose veins, TTF (60 mg/day for 90 days) significantly lowered the elevated serum levels of uronic acids and lysosomal enzymes.[82] These results were interpreted as an indirect confirmation of improved connective tissue metabolism in the vein wall.

The vacuum suction chamber produces a wheal on the skin, with the disappearance time (DT) determined by capillary filtration and permeability. After 2 weeks of 180 mg/day of TTF there was a significant decrease in DT in the limbs of patients with either superficial (n=22) or deep (n=12) venous incompetence. This was confirmed by laser Doppler flowmetry and clinical signs and symptoms.[83] TTF (90 mg/day for 3 weeks)

also reduced the number of circulating endothelial cells in the veins of 15 patients with a history of deep vein thrombosis in an open, controlled study.[84] This finding was interpreted as indicating a reduction of endothelial cell injury and an improvement in vascular integrity in these patients with diseased veins.

Some cardioprotective activity has been observed for gotu kola and madecassoside. Pretreatment with a hydroethanolic extract of gotu kola whole plant (100, 500 and 1000 mg/kg/day, oral for 7 days) dose-dependently reduced left ventricular necrosis and measures of oxidative stress in a rat model of myocardial ischaemia-reperfusion injury.[85] Madecassoside demonstrated similar protective activity in analogous models in rats[86] and rabbits.[87] Pretreatment with an aqueous extract of gotu kola (200 mg/kg, oral) protected against the cardiotoxicity of doxorubicin in rats by improving mitochondrial function[88] and improving antioxidant responses.[89]

Antimicrobial and antiparasitic activities

Aqueous but not ethanolic extracts (and pure asiaticoside) of gotu kola were active against herpes simplex virus I and II in vitro.[90,91] Two in vitro studies failed to find any activity for gotu kola extracts against *Mycobacterium leprae* or *M. tuberculosis*.[92,93] One study found that liposomal asiaticoside was significantly more active against *M. leprae* in vitro.[94] A tincture of gotu kola administered orally to dogs (30 mg/kg/day) dramatically reduced blood levels of infection with the microfilarial parasite *Dirofilaria immitis* without causing any adverse effects.[95]

Antitumour activity

Gotu kola extracts and triterpenoids have demonstrated activity against a range of cancer cells in vitro, including melanoma, uterine cancer and gastric cancer.[96,97] Asiaticoside in vitro induced apoptosis in a human colon cancer cell line.[98] A methanolic extract of gotu kola exerted the same effect on MCF-7 human breast cancer cells.[99] Asiaticoside has also been shown to enhance the lethality of vincristine against a range of multidrug resistant cancer cell lines.[100] Lifespan was increased in mice with solid and ascites tumours when they were fed gotu kola crude (1 g/kg) and purified (40 mg/kg) extracts.[101] Only simultaneous or prophylactic dosing was protective. Aqueous gotu kola extract (10 and 100 mg/kg, oral) decreased the incidence of colon cancers formed in rats exposed to the carcinogen azoxymethane.[102]

Other activity

The aqueous extract[103] (10, 100 and 300 mg/kg/day, orally for 7 days in mice) or suspension (100 mg/kg/day, orally for 7 days in rats)[104] of gotu kola enhanced both cellular and humoral immune responses. In mice, injections of a methanolic extract of gotu kola enhanced phagocytic activity without affecting B lymphocytes or antibody responses.[105]

Traditionally, gotu kola has been regarded as somewhat of an adaptogen and there is experimental support for this. Cold and restraint stress effects were countered in rats[106] and an ethanolic extract (100 mg/kg, oral) exhibited significant antistress activity in rats in a range of experimental models.[107,108]

Gotu kola may exert antitoxic activity against arsenic. Its aqueous extract (100, 200 or 300 mg/kg, oral) protected against arsenic toxicity in rats, especially in terms of measures of oxidative stress.[109] Arsenic concentrations in tissues were not changed.[110]

Protection against radiation-induced taste aversion was noted in a study in rats (100 mg/kg gotu kola extract, ip).[111] Gotu kola extract (100 mg/kg, oral) improved survival against radiation in mice[112] and protected against radiation-induced liver damage.[113]

Pretreatment with asiaticoside (5 to 20 mg/kg/day, oral for 3 days) demonstrated 'remarkable' hepatoprotective activity following lipopolysaccharide and galactosamine administration to mice, possibly related to inhibition of TNF (tumour necrosis factor)-alpha and cell kinases.[114]

Pharmacokinetics

An early study in rats using radioactively labelled compounds found that asiatic and madecassic acids were well absorbed, up to 50% of a single oral dose.[115] Once absorbed, the acids were subject to phase II conjugation to form glucuronides and sulphates and largely excreted via the bile. Oral asiaticoside is first converted to asiatic acid by the bowel microflora, leading to the slow and prolonged appearance of asiatic acid in rat plasma.

Oral administration of a gotu kola extract to beagles (containing 540 mg saponins of which asiaticoside was about 72%) revealed the following pharmacokinetic parameters for asiatic acid: half-life 4.29 h, Tmax 2.7 h and Cmax 0.74 μg/mL.[116]

In a double blind, randomised, crossover, multiple-dose study, six healthy male and six healthy female volunteers each received asiatic acid (6 mg) or asiaticoside (12 mg) twice daily for 9 days, with a single dose on the tenth day.[117] Pharmacokinetic parameters (for asiatic acid in plasma) were assessed only after the single dose on the tenth day and were as follows: Cmax 0.98 μg/mL and 0.65 mg/mL, Tmax 4.0 and 5.4 h and pre-dose level 0.39 and 0.50 μg/mL for administration of asiatic acid and asiaticoside, respectively. Despite these differences, the steady state area-under-the-curve values (reflecting total absorption) were similar for the two compounds. (Note that although the mg doses of the two compounds differed, their molar quantities were similar, owing to the higher molecular weight of asiaticoside compared to its aglycone asiatic acid.)

After oral administration of TTF at 30 or 60 mg twice daily for 7 days to 12 healthy men, the time to maximum plasma concentrations of asiatic acid was stable at just over 4 h, while the half-life and area-under-the-curve increased significantly from baseline to the end of study, reaching 6.3 or 10.3 h and 10.5 or 20.8 μg/mL/h for the 30 or 60 mg doses, respectively.[118] There were significant intra-individual differences in all parameters studied. Steady state Cmax values for asiatic acid were 1.03 and 1.69 μg/mL, respectively. Asiaticoside was determined to be converted to asiatic acid.

Clinical trials

Vascular diseases

In more than any other patient group, gotu kola has demonstrated a clinical ability to help people with chronic problems with varicose veins in the lower limbs accompanied by oedema, itch, skin atrophy and ulceration, and discomfort or pain (known as chronic venous insufficiency or CVI). The larger clinical trials have been summarised in Table 1. Unfortunately, all key studies to date have been conducted by the same research group and have not been well designed. As noted in the table, apparently one of those studies has been published twice and another essentially three times, with considerable time having elapsed between the first and last publications. Several less rigorous trials have also been reported using TTF for CVI patients, but only those including 40 or more patients were included in this review and Table 1.

The reasonably methodologically sound randomised clinical trials compared TTF to placebo in 99 and 40 patients (both used 60 mg twice per day, and one study also included a group receiving only 60 mg/day).[119,120] However, both were only single blind trials. A more rigorous double blind, randomised trial assessed TECA, 60 or 120 mg/day against placebo.[121] This trial found a modest benefit for both doses of the extract over placebo at improving symptomatology. However, this benefit was not as clinically significant as reported in the less rigorous trials.

It is useful to reflect here on why a herb with a well-established reputation for promoting healing has developed into a treatment for CVI. Varicose veins and CVI have long been regarded as disorders of valvular incompetence. However, recent evidence suggests that changes in the vein wall could well precede such incompetence. For example, varicosities are often observed below competent valves and often can occur before valvular incompetence.[128] Defects in ECM and collagen composition in the vein wall are thought to be part of this process.[129] Endothelial damage from abnormally sustained venous pressure could contribute as well. Given the above, the noted pharmacological properties of gotu kola in terms of effects on fibroblasts, collagen and ECM in the vein wall, together with its potential for reducing endothelial damage and improving microcirculation, would suggest that it is indeed a plausible (and perhaps disease-modifying) treatment for CVI.

Two controlled trials have investigated the activity of oral TTF in patients with microvascular damage due to diabetes. The largest trial involved 100 patients with or without neuropathy and compared TTF (120 mg/day) with placebo over 12 months and also in 40 healthy controls.[130] TTF was significantly more effective at improving microcirculatory parameters and oedema (p<0.05). A smaller trial with 50 patients compared 60 mg TTF twice daily with placebo or no treatment for 6 months.[131] TTF resulted in significant improvement in parameters linked to microscopic vascular damage, including capillary permeability (p<0.01 to p<0.05).

In a randomised trial, the impact of TTF (180 mg/day) for 2 days before, the day of, and 1 day after, a long airline flight (up to 14 h) against no treatment was compared in patients

Table 1 Summary of trials of gotu kola extracts in patients with chronic venous insufficiency

Trial design and reference	Number of patients	Preparation and daily dose (mg)	Control	Study duration (days)	Efficacy versus control
SBRCT[119,122,123]	99	TTF 60 or 120	Placebo	60	A dose-response effect was observed for most parameters. Substantial reduction in subjective symptom score (p<0.05), improvements in limb perfusion parameters (p<0.05)
DBRCT[121]	94	TECA 60 or 120	Placebo	60	Reductions in limb heaviness (p=0.033), oedema (p=0.026). Improvement in patient-rated overall efficacy (p=0.032, high dose only significant). Trend to improvement in venous distensibility (p=0.055 to 0.08)
SBRCT[124,125]	62	TTF 90 or 180	Placebo	28	A dose-response effect was observed. Reductions in subjective symptom score (p<0.05) and lower limb capillary filtration rate (p<0.05)
SBRCT[120]	40	TTF 120	Placebo	42	Significant improvements in limb perfusion parameters versus placebo (p<0.05), significant reduction in leg volume (p<0.05)
DBRCT[126]	40	ETCA (TECA) 60	HER 1000 mg/day	30	Similar efficacy to the reference treatment for most objective parameters, except ETCA superior for reduction in calf circumference (p<0.01) and improvements in venous distensibility (p<0.05) and flow (p<0.05). Apparent superiority over reference treatment for subjective symptoms (no p values provided)
SBRCT[127]	40	TTF 120	Placebo	56	Improvement in microcirculatory parameters in patients with venous hypertensive microangiopathy: resting flux (p<0.05), rate of ankle swelling (p<0.05)

DB = double blind; HER = hydroxyethylrutosides; RCT = randomised controlled trial; SB = single blind.

with mild-to-moderate chronic venous insufficiency.[132] Ankle oedema was significantly less in the TTF group (p<0.05), as were microcirculatory parameters such as rate of ankle swelling and venoarteriolar reflex (p<0.05). All parameters deteriorated with the length of flight, a phenomenon that was only partially compensated by the herbal treatment.

An open trial of TTF (60 mg/day) combined with bulk-forming laxatives (as appropriate) was rated as effective in relieving symptoms in over 90% of 210 patients with first or second degree haemorrhoids.[133]

Two interesting trials suggest that gotu kola may be able to stabilise vulnerable arterial plaque, indicating a possible role for the herb in modifying cardiovascular outcomes. Most atherosclerotic plaques do not trigger life-threatening events. A vulnerable plaque is one that is at high short-term risk of rupture. Plaque rupture is by far the most frequent cause of arterial thrombosis. It is deemed responsible for about 75% of coronary thrombi leading to heart attacks or death and about 90% of thrombosed carotid plaques causing ischaemic stroke. Only plaque with very thin fibrous caps is at risk of rupture and even just a small lesion is life-threatening. These plaques are essentially unstable because of a deficiency of connective tissue in their matrix. Even in the presence of widespread arterial disease, rarely more than a few plaques appear to be at risk of rupture at any given moment.[134] One group

of researchers observed: 'It is not clear why some plaques lead to clinical manifestations, whereas many others remain asymptomatic and heal with subsequent fibrosis...'.[135] In one sense arterial plaque is a type of wound on the blood vessel wall and vulnerable plaque can be viewed as a wound that is either not healing appropriately or in the early stages of healing (fibrosis).

In two placebo-controlled clinical trials, TTF stabilised low-density carotid[136] and femoral artery plaques.[137] The dose used in both trials was 180 mg/day for 12 months. These clinical outcomes were assessed by significant and marked increases in the ultrasound echogenicity of plaques compared with placebo (p<0.05). For the patients with carotid lesions, symptomatic cerebral events were observed in 6.5% of patients taking TTF compared with 11% of controls (p<0.05) and positive magnetic resonance images (indicating cerebral ischaemic lesions) were 7% in the herbal group, versus 17% for the control group (p<0.05). Arterial plaque which is echolucent (low echogenicity by ultrasound) has a limited connective tissue component and the plaque is weaker and prone to ulceration, rupture and embolisation. This is not quite the same as vulnerable coronary artery plaque, but shares many similarities.

On the basis of these findings it would be interesting to examine the impact of the long-term intake of gotu kola on health outcomes in patients with coronary artery disease.

Wounds, ulcers, and other skin and epithelial disorders

Early publications comprise around 30 mostly small, uncontrolled, open label clinical trials or case observation studies, dating from the late 1950s. These papers variously refer to the use of 'asiaticoside' or a proprietary triterpenoid isolate product, which were probably identical and represent an early version of TECA. The TECA was typically administered by intramuscular (and sometimes intralesional) injection and was often applied topically as well. Although injection was used, the good oral bioavailability of the gotu kola triterpenoids, and the fact that typical oral doses tend to be much higher than the injected doses used, suggest that these early data still have clinical relevance to the oral use of the herb. Conditions with favourable outcomes included bladder ulcers,[138] corneal lesions,[139] episiotomies[140] and other postsurgical lesions,[141] leg ulcers,[142] skin grafts,[143] skin ulcers[144] and traumatic injury.[145] Not all studies yielded positive outcomes.[146,147] A few of the larger, less dated and/or interesting studies are featured below.

Following a positive series of published case reports[148] and their experience with a burn patient who demonstrated a substantial reduction in hypertrophic scars, a group of Canadian clinicians conducted a clinical investigation of TECA as an antikeloid agent.[149] Their first clinical evaluations involved the injectable form, but later they were able to report on 227 patients with keloids or hypertrophic scars who were treated with the oral form of TECA (60 to 90 mg/day, but up to 150 mg/day in stubborn cases). In an open label trial, 116 of 139 patients were found to respond after 2 to 18 months, either by relief of symptoms or by a gradual disappearance of inflammation. These positive results remained after the cessation of therapy. In most cases the treatment was started on well-established, non-responsive lesions, some of many years' duration. A small, concurrent double blind study demonstrated a significant benefit over placebo ($p<0.05$). The authors also studied the preventative action of TECA in 88 patients undergoing surgical scar revision, with treatment started a few weeks prior to surgery and maintained for 3 months after. Improvement was noted in 79% of patients, but there was no comparative control group to account for the benefit of surgery alone.

In a recent clinical trial conducted in Thailand, 200 patients with diabetic foot ulcer were randomised to receive gotu kola extract or placebo.[150] General symptoms, wound characteristics, wound size and wound depths were examined at days 7, 14 and 21. Wound contraction was determined by the decrease in the volume of the wound. Twenty cases dropped out from the study and 10 cases were terminated before the end of treatment because termination criteria were met. (Termination criteria included patient refusal, wound infection, delayed primary sutured wound and secondary healing wound.) Results for the 170 patients who completed the trial were analysed.

By the end of each week, wound contraction was significantly better in the group treated with gotu kola compared with those treated with placebo ($p\le0.001$). The trend to good wound contraction occurred earlier for the herb group than in the placebo group: for example, by day 7, 28.5% of patients receiving gotu kola had good wound contraction, compared with 12.8% in the placebo group; by day 14, the results for good contraction were 38.1% and 18.6% for herbal and placebo treatment, respectively. More granulation tissue formed in the placebo group than the herb group, and the difference between the groups was significant at days 7, 14, and 21 ($p<0.001$). There were no systemic side effects reported and there was no significant difference in wound infection between the two groups. The dose used was unclear, with the capsules variously described as containing '50 mg of extracted asiaticoside' and '50 mg freeze dry lyophilized extract'. The trial author disclosed the dose in a personal communication (March 2011) as 300 mg/day of extract, corresponding to 11.2 g of fresh leaf.

There is some suggestion from case reports in the 1970s that gotu kola might assist liver pathologies. In one study, 30 patients with clinical hepatic cirrhosis (mainly due to bilharzia) and previous splenectomy were given TECA (20 mg/day, im) for 55 days.[151] The nodularity and firm consistency of the liver decreased markedly in all the cases and biopsy revealed a substantial reduction in collagen fibres in both the fine and medium portal tracts. Serum alkaline phosphatase and glycoproteins were also reduced. In a second study, ongoing administration of TECA (90 to 150 mg/day, presumably oral) resulted in improvement in 5 of 12 patients with recently diagnosed alcoholic cirrhosis or chronic liver disease.[152] Benefits were mainly observed in the patients with alcoholic cirrhosis, where biopsy revealed reduced sclerosis or steatosis.

Gotu kola might have value in obstetrics according to studies from the 1960s. Results for 131 cases of episiotomies treated with TECA (25 mg/day, im on the second, fourth and sixth days after surgery) from an open label trial demonstrated improved healing and reduced symptoms in 106 cases compared with other (unspecified) cases treated by different means.[153] Clinical observation of 114 patients with perineal lesions (especially following episiotomy) found injected TECA (with concurrent topical use in some cases) accelerated healing, resulting in reduced hospital stays.[140] Accelerated healing of perineal tears was found in another study.[154]

Some novel uses of gotu kola preparations have also been investigated. Open trials have demonstrated the benefit of topical madecassoside and either intramuscular madecassoside or asiaticoside in patients with previously non-healing wounds or skin ulcers.[155,156] In a prospective, open clinical trial, 30 patients with active leprosy were given 500 mg powdered gotu kola (for 12 months), 60 mg asiaticoside (for 6 months) or dapsone three times per day.[157] Improvement in leprosy ulcers was similar in all groups. Intramuscular (20 mg/day) and/or topical application of TECA in 90 patients with perforating leg ulcers due to leprosy were compared against placebo, and both treatments were found to be significantly superior at healing the ulcers ($p<0.01$).[158] A combination of dapsone, hydnocarpic acid (from *Hydnocarpus wightiana*) and isolated asiaticoside (50 mg/day) for 6 to 11 months in 10 patients with active leprosy was just as effective, but less toxic, than standard multidrug treatments.[159]

The value of gotu kola compounds in the connective tissue disorder scleroderma has been assessed. An open trial involving 13 women with scleroderma and using either 20 or 60 mg/day TECA (im) observed improvement of symptoms in 11.[160] TECA 30 mg/day (oral), sometimes with topical TECA ointment, improved local and systemic scleroderma in the majority of 54 patients investigated in another open trial.[161] Benefits were also seen in another seven patients with scleroderma (TECA, 30 to 60 mg/day, oral),[162] but a review of 15 cases in children found little benefit from current treatments, including asiaticoside (probably TECA).[163]

Some of the early studies on skin disorders also focused on topical application. Topical application of a cream of gotu kola cleared psoriasis lesions in five and improved the remaining two of seven patients in one case series.[164] A cream containing 1% of an extract of gotu kola completely healed previously non-healing, chronic, infected skin ulcers in 17 out of 22 patients after 3 weeks in an open trial.[165] One double blind trial in 18 patients failed to find that a 2% TECA powder had any better effect than placebo on healing after skin graft removal.[143]

In recently published studies there has been a further focus on the topical use of gotu kola compounds, probably thereby underestimating the unique value of the internal use of the herb. In a preliminary open trial, 12 healthy volunteers had a small wound induced on their forearms and then 0.3% madecassoside combined with copper, zinc and manganese was applied daily for 22 days.[166] The researchers concluded that inflammation was resolved more quickly, epidermal regrowth was more rapid, and there was less scarring, apparently compared with no treatment. An ointment containing extracts of gotu kola, *Viola tricolor* and *Mahonia aquifolium* was not superior to a base cream in a randomised double blind, vehicle-controlled, half-side comparison in 88 patients with mild-to-moderate atopic dermatitis.[167]

Some of the topical trials are more cosmetic in nature. One early double blind trial involving 80 pregnant women investigated the effects of a topical cream containing gotu kola, vitamin E and collagen-elastin hydrolysate compared with placebo at preventing striae gravidarum (stretch marks).[168] The cream was applied once per day. After 12 weeks, the group applying the active cream developed significantly fewer striae than the placebo group.

In a double blind, randomised clinical trial, a gel containing gotu kola extract, *Rosmarinus officinalis* extract, tetrahydrocurcumin, and dimethylaminoethanol was compared with placebo in 28 women.[169] Each woman treated half their face with the gel or placebo for 4 weeks. At the end of this time, skin was significantly softer on the gel-treated skin compared with placebo, as rated both objectively and subjectively. Three women left the trial due to mild skin irritation. A cream with 0.1% asiaticoside applied around the eyes of 27 women for 12 weeks in an open trial was associated with improvement or elimination of wrinkles in 18.[170]

A 6-month randomised, double blind study was conducted on photo-aged (sun-damaged) skin in 20 female volunteers to assess the impact of a topical treatment containing 5% vitamin C and 0.1% madecassoside.[171] There was a significant improvement in the clinical score for deep and superficial wrinkles, suppleness, firmness, roughness and skin hydration. These results were corroborated by objective tests. The reappearance of a normally structured, 'young' elastic fibre network was observed.

Nervous system and adaptogenic effects

A single dose of 12 g of crude gotu kola was more effective than placebo at reducing the acoustic startle response in 40 healthy adults in one double blind, placebo-controlled, randomised trial.[172] An uncontrolled trial observed that a 70% ethanolic extract of gotu kola (500 mg/day corresponding to about 4.5 g of starting herb) over 2 months significantly improved measures of stress, anxiety, adjustment, depression and attention (all $p<0.01$ compared with baseline).[173] Results after 2 months were substantially better than after 1 month.

An uncontrolled trial used gotu kola to treat 33 volunteers with generalised anxiety disorder.[173] They received gotu kola extract (about 9 g/day dried herb equivalent) for 60 days. Participants were initially assessed for mental status using the Brief Psychiatric Rating Scale. Results using self-assessment questionnaires revealed significant improvements ($p<0.01$) from baseline in anxiety, stress, depression, adjustment and attention at day 30 and day 60.

Early studies focusing on cognitive function yielded conflicting results. A daily 500 mg tablet of gotu kola herb for 12 weeks significantly improved mental function and behaviour in 30 intellectually impaired children in a placebo-controlled trial.[174] However, a double blind, placebo-controlled trial using the same tablet daily for 1 year observed no effect on the mental ability of children with normal baseline intelligence.[175]

A later trial was more positive. Twenty-eight healthy volunteers with a mean age of 65 years were randomly divided into four groups.[176] One group received a placebo and the others were given respectively 250, 500 and 750 mg/day of a gotu kola extract for 2 months. The gotu kola extract was standardised for total phenolic content and also contained around 5% asiaticoside and asiatic acid. Assessment using a battery of cognitive performance tests was undertaken 1 h after the first dose (for acute effects) and after 1 and 2 months (for chronic effects).

For the acute effect (single dose) assessment, only the highest dose of gotu kola demonstrated a significant effect above placebo for just two of the nine tests used. These were the reaction time of spatial memory and the percentage accuracy of numeric working memory. Based on what is known about these tests, the authors suggested that these acute effects of gotu kola might partly occur via the modulation of dopamine and norepinephrine in the prefrontal cortex, together with the modulation of acetylcholine and serotonin in the hippocampus.

The repeated administration of gotu kola for a further 2 months also showed the same significant increases in spatial memory reaction time and percentage accuracy of numeric working memory. In addition, significant improvements were seen above placebo for choice reaction time, numeric working memory reaction time, accuracy of word recognition and accuracy of picture recognition. These effects were most consistently demonstrated at the highest dose of gotu kola. There was no significant effect on simple reaction time, the digit vigilance test, the accuracy of spatial memory, word recognition reaction time and picture recognition reaction time. The above effects were interpreted by the authors as gotu kola enhancing working memory. The extract not only improved cognitive performance, but also anxiety: the highest dose increased calmness and alertness after both 1 and 2 months of treatment.

When gotu kola powder (dosage not specified) was administered to 43 healthy but impoverished East Indian adults for 6 months, it elevated erythrocytes and haemoglobin and decreased blood urea nitrogen in a low-quality placebo-controlled trial.[177,178] Gotu kola extract at 250, 500 and 750 mg/day significantly improved physical strength and fitness measured by the 30-second chair stand test in 80 healthy older volunteers (average age around 65 years). The two higher doses also improved the physical subscale of a quality of life scale (SF-36). This was a placebo-controlled, randomised, double blind trial and implies an adaptogenic activity for the herb.[179]

Other conditions

An uncontrolled study examined the effect of 60 mg/day oral TECA and 20 mg three times per week (im) in 64 patients with gastric and duodenal ulcers.[180] After 10 weeks, all but two patients had healed completely (and the majority had healed after 6 weeks). In an open randomised trial, patients who had extracts of gotu kola and *Punica granatum* (pomegranate) applied to periodontal pockets experienced significantly better healing than those who received only standard medical care.[181] This confirmed the preliminary results of an earlier study using the same extracts.[182]

Toxicology and other safety data

Toxicology

Gotu kola has been consumed as a leafy vegetable, particularly in Bangladesh, Thailand, Indonesia (West Java), Sri Lanka and South Africa,[183–185] and appears to have no harmful effect when used as a food.[186] The leaf and stolon are eaten raw and cooked.[187]

Acute toxicity testing indicated a low toxicity following oral administration to rats (LD$_{50}$ >675 mg/kg of gotu kola extract, equivalent to >4 g/kg dried leaf). Chronic administration of 150 mg/kg/day of extract (equivalent to 0.9 g/kg dried leaf) for a period of 30 days did not produce any adverse effects.[188] Mice receiving up to 1 g/kg of gotu kola extract (2.5 g/kg dried plant) by mouth did not exhibit adverse effects.[55] Aqueous ethanol extract of gotu kola entire plant

demonstrated a maximum tolerated dose value of 250 mg/kg after ip injection in mice.[189] Subcutaneous injection of 40 to 50 mg/kg of asiaticoside was toxic to mice and rabbits, while 20 to 250 mg/kg resulted in increased bleeding time. An oral dose of 1 g/kg was well tolerated.[190]

The local toxicity of asiaticoside was investigated by the measurement of skin respiration and histological analysis. (The death of a cell is accompanied by loss of respiratory activity.) Compared with other therapeutic agents, the toxicity of asiaticoside was not excessive and was comparable to that of many common antibiotics. Histological effects on guinea-pig skin indicated that moderate concentrations of asiaticoside produced swollen, abnormally staining cells. Higher concentrations resulted in necrotic cultures, showing signs of 'thickening' of the epidermis, even though the cells had mostly disintegrated. This may have been due to the cells becoming rapidly keratinised. Although fairly high concentrations of asiaticoside were required to produce this effect, it occurred in vivo (5 mg, sc) as well as in vitro.[35]

An ethanol extract of gotu kola exhibited mutagenic activity to strain TA98 (Salmonella/microsome test) only in the presence of S9 mix.[191] A water extract of gotu kola was not toxic towards TA98 and TA100 with or without addition of S9 mix at the tested concentration (5 mg/plate). Gotu kola weakly inhibited the mutagenicity of the indirect mutagen IQ (2-amino-3-methylimidazo[4,5-f]quinoline).[192] In another experiment, gotu kola water extract (1 mL of a 1:5 decoction) showed mutagenic activity in strain TA 98 with metabolic activation only.[193] Gotu kola methanol extract induced abnormal metaphases and increased chromosome aberrations in the *Vicia faba* root meristem assay.[194]

Asiaticoside was found to be a weak tumour promoter in the hairless mouse epidermis model and was very weakly carcinogenic to the dermis after topical application.[195]

Contraindications

Gotu kola is contraindicated in cases of known allergy.

Special warnings and precautions

None suggested.

Interactions

No clinically relevant interactions have been found. In an in vivo study investigating wound healing with drugs, the anti-inflammatory drugs dexamethasone and phenylbutazone individually combined with asiaticoside caused a reduction in the tensile strength (and hence therapeutic effect) produced by asiaticoside alone.[28] In this study the test substances were administered by intramuscular injection (asiaticoside is a saponin and has surfactant activity), so it is not known if the observed results extrapolate to the topical use of asiaticoside or oral use of gotu kola in humans.

In open trials, asiaticoside has been used topically in combination with an antibiotic and corticosteroid[196] and was well tolerated.[197]

Use in pregnancy and lactation

Category B1 – no increase in frequency of malformation or other harmful effects on the fetus from limited use in women. No evidence of increased fetal damage in animal studies.

Gotu kola has been traditionally used in Bengal as a contraceptive agent. A reduction in conception rate was observed in female mice fed gotu kola (juice of whole plant, equivalent to 20 to 80g fresh whole plant per kg) by gavage. Two sets of animals received the herb for 14 days (7 days before and 7 days during cohabitation) and 21 days (7 days before and 14 days during cohabitation). In the first set, sterile mating occurred for 50% to 60% of animals versus 15% in the controls, and for the second set 50% to 55% versus 20%. An isolated triterpenoid glycoside (40 to 120mg/kg) and a compound derived from it also demonstrated antifertility activity. In all treatment groups there was no significant decrease in the number of young per litter and birth weight of the young were normal. The authors noted that the isolated glycoside and the compound derived from it caused a consistent reduction of fertility.[198] These were very high doses, well above those normally used in clinical practice. Moreover, an antifertility effect does not imply harm during pregnancy.

Antifertility activity was also demonstrated in vivo in an early study for gotu kola (part undefined). Teratological effects have been studied in the rabbit and found to be negative for that animal.[149]

Gotu kola is compatible with breastfeeding.

Effects on ability to drive and use machines

No adverse effects expected.

Side effects

As with all herbs rich in saponins, oral use may cause irritation of the gastric mucous membranes and reflux.

Cases of allergic contact dermatitis have been reported from the use of gotu kola, TTF and asiaticoside, but they are considered to be low-risk treatments.[199–206] Both the extract and the triterpene constituents are weak sensitisers,[149] although asiaticoside has been classified as a contact allergen.[207] Patch tests in many cases confirmed that gotu kola or its constituents were responsible,[199,200,203,204] although in some cases other constituents in the preparations were also responsible (such as propylene glycol,[202] geraniol, lavender essence and neomycin[201]).

Traditional sources indicate that gotu kola may produce photosensitisation when used in tropical areas, although whether from use by oral or topical application is not indicated.[5,208] Occasional gastrointestinal intolerance has been observed.[149] A review of the use of TTF for the treatment of chronic venous insufficiency indicated that it was safe and well tolerated. Most trials used dosage of TTF in the range of 60 to 120mg/day.[80]

Three cases of idiosyncratic hepatotoxicity have been reported from Argentina in association with extracts of gotu kola, including at least one that was clearly triggered by rechallenge.[209] However, no other such cases are on record and the identity of the herb was not confirmed in these cases. One case of night-eating syndrome was attributed to use of a 70% ethanolic tincture of gotu kola, possibly with other herbs.[210]

Overdosage

There are no reliable reports of overdose with gotu kola.

An early case (prior to 1896) is recorded concerning a 'Dr Boiteau who, in treating himself, progressively increased the dose and found that after two months the drug had produced all the effects of a violent, cumulative poison. ... the plant, properly prepared and administered, is a powerful stimulant of the circulatory system, its action chiefly affecting the vessels of the skin and mucous membrane'.[211] Traditional sources writing in the early to mid-20th century indicate that the plant can be a stupefying narcotic in large doses and in some cases produces headache or vertigo with a tendency to coma.[207]

Safety in children

Adverse effects are generally not expected. Gotu kola dried herb has been assessed in a clinical trial in India as a mental tonic for mentally disabled children.[173] Gotu kola is used in leaf concentrate meals, which are prepared as porridge for preschool children in Sri Lanka to combat nutritional deficiencies.[212] (Although the leaf composition varies with location, fresh gotu kola leaves typically contain 2% protein, 7mg/100g of vitamin C, 0.09mg/100g of vitamin B1 and 5.6mg/100g of iron.)[213]

However, one case of gotu kola-induced hepatotoxicity in a child has been recently reported.[214]

Regulatory status in selected countries

Gotu kola is official in the *Pharmacopoeia of the People's Republic of China* 1997. The usual adult dosage, typically administered in the form of a decoction, is listed as 15 to 30g, or 30 to 60g of the fresh herb.

Gotu kola for external use is included on the General Sale List in the UK. It was not included in the Commission E assessment. Gotu kola is official in the *British Pharmacopoeia* 2011 and the *European Pharmacopoeia* 2011.

Gotu kola does not have GRAS status in the USA. However, it is freely available as a 'dietary supplement' in the USA under DSHEA legislation (Dietary Supplement Health and Education Act of 1994).

Gotu kola is not included in Part 4 of Schedule 4 of the Therapeutic Goods Regulations and is freely available for sale in Australia.

References

1. Nadkarni AK, Nadkarni KM. *Indian Materia Medica*. Bombay: Popular Prakashan; 1976. pp. 662–666.

2. Grieve M. *A Modern Herbal*, vol 1. New York: Dover Publications; 1971.

3. Sharma PV. *Dravyaguna-vijnana*. Varanasi: Chaukambha Bharati Academy; 2003. pp. 3–6.

4. Chen JK, Chen TT. *Chinese Medical Herbology and Pharmacology*. CA: Art of Medicine Press; 2004. pp. 147–148.

5. British Herbal Medicine Association Scientific Committee. *British Herbal Pharmacopoeia*. Bournemouth: BHMA; 1983.

6. Felter HW, Lloyd JU. *King's American Dispensatory*. ed 18, rev 3, 1905. Portland: reprinted Eclectic Medical Publications; 1983.

7. Farnsworth NR, Bunyapraphatsara N, eds. *Thai Medicinal Plants*. Bangkok: Medicinal Plant Information Center; 1992.

8. Dharma AP. *Indonesian Medicinal Plants*. Jakarta: Balai Pustaka; 1987.

9. Cambie RC, Ash J. *Fijian Medicinal Plants*. Australia: CSIRO; 1994.

10. van Wyk B-E, van Oudtshoorn B, Gericke N. *Medicinal Plants of South Africa*. Arcadia: Briza Publications; 1997.

11. Applequst W. *The Identification of Medicinal Plants: A Handbook of the Morphology of Botanicals in Commerce*. St Louis: Missouri Botanical Garden Press; 2006. pp. 45–46.

12. Tang W, Eisenbrand G. *Chinese Drugs of Plant Origin*. Berlin: Springer-Verlag; 1992. pp. 273–275.

13. Brinkhaus B, Linder M, Schuppan D, et al. *Phytomedicine*. 2000;7(5):427–448.

14. Zainol NA, Voo SC, Sarmidi MR, et al. *Malaysian J Anal Sci*. 2008;12(2): 322–327.

15. May A. *Eur J Pharmacol*. 1968;4(3): 331–339.

16. Lu L, Ying K, Wei S, et al. *Br J Dermatol*. 2004;151(3):571–578.

17. Lu L, Ying K, Wei S, et al. *Int J Dermatol*. 2004;43(11):801–807.

18. Marquart FX, Bellon G, Gillery P, et al. *Connect Tissue Res*. 1990;24:107–120.

19. Tenni R, Zanaboni G, De Agostini MP, et al. *Ital J Biochem*. 1988;37:69–77.

20. Bonte F, Dumas M, Chaudagne C, et al. *Ann Pharm Fr*. 1995;53(1):38–42.

21. Bonte F, Dumas M, Chaudagne C, et al. *Planta Med*. 1994;60(2):133–135.

22. Lee J, Jung E, Kim Y, et al. *Planta Med*. 2006;72(4):324–328.

23. Qi SH, Xie JL, Pan S, et al. *Clin Exp Dermatol*. 2008;33(2):171–175.

24. Poizot A, Dumez D. *C R Acad Sci*. 1978;286:789–792.

25. Suguna L, Sivakumar P, Chandrakasan G. *Indian J Exp Biol*. 1996;34(12):1208–1211.

26. Shukla A, Rasik AM, Jain GK, et al. *J Ethnopharmacol*. 1999;65:1–11.

27. Shetty BS, Udupa SL, Udupa AL, Somayaji SN. *Int J Low Extrem Wounds*. 2006;5(3):137–143.

28. Velasco M, Romero E. *Curr Ther Res Clin Exp*. 1976;19(1):121–125.

29. Hartog A, Smith HF, van der Kraan PM, et al. *Exp Biol Med (Maywood)*. 2009;234(6):617–623.

30. Tincani GP, Riva PC, Baldini E. *G Ital Dermatol*. 1963;104:429–440.

31. Sunilkumar Parameshwaraiah S, Shivakumar HG. *Indian J Exp Biol*. 1998;36(6):569–572.

32. Maquart FX, Chastang F, Simeon A, et al. *Eur J Dermatol*. 1996;9(4):289–296.

33. Shukla A, Rasik AM, Dhawan BN. *Phytother Res*. 1999;13(1):50–54.

34. Ju-Lin X, Shao-Hai Q, Tian-Zeng L, et al. *J Cutan Pathol*. 2009;36(2):234–239.

35. Lawrence JC. *Eur J Pharmacol*. 1967;1:414–424.

36. Kimura Y, Sumiyoshi M, Samukawa K, et al. *Eur J Pharmacol*. 2008;584 (2–3):415–423.

37. Liu M, Dai Y, Li Y, et al. *Planta Med*. 2008;74(8):809–815.

38. Cheng CL, Guo JS, Luk J, Koo MWL. *Life Sci*. 2004;74:2237–2249.

39. Cheng CL, Koo MW. *Life Sci*. 2000;67(21):2647–2653.

40. Sairam K, Rao CV, Goel RK. *Indian J Exp Biol*. 2001;39(2):137–142.

41. Dong MS, Jung SH, Kim HJ, et al. *Arch Pharm Res*. 2004;27:512–517.

42. Wojcikowski K, Wohlmuth H, Johnson DW, et al. *Nephrology (Carlton)*. 2009;14(1):70–79.

43. Qi S, Xie J, Li T. *Zhonghua Shao Shang Za Zhi*. 2000;16(1):53–56.

44. Zhang T, Rong XZ, Yang RH, et al. *Nan Fang Yi Ke Da Xue Xue Bao*. 2006;26(1):67–70. [In Chinese].

45. Ming ZJ, Liu SZ, Cao L. *Zhongguo Zhong Xi Yi Jie He Za Zhi*. 2004;24(8):731–734. [In Chinese].

46. Yun KJ, Kim JY, Kim JB, et al. *Int Immunopharmacol*. 2008;8:431–441.

47. Won JH, Shin JS, Park HJ, et al. *Planta Med*. 2010;76(3):251–257.

48. Vogel HG, De Souza N, D'Sa A. *Acta Therapeutica*. 1990;16:285–298.

49. Somchit MN, Sulaiman MR, Zuraini A, et al. *Indian J Pharmacol*. 2004;36(6): 377–380.

50. Li H, Gong X, Zhang L, et al. *Phytomedicine*. 2009;16(6–7):538–546.

51. Liu M, Dai Y, Yao X, et al. *Int Immunopharmacol*. 2008;8(11): 1561–1566.

52. Caballero-George C, Vanderheyde PM, Okamoto Y, et al. *Phytother Res*. 2004;18:729–736.

53. Wijeweera P, Arnason JT, Koszycki D, et al. *Phytomedicine*. 2006;13:668–676.

54. Chen SW, Wang WJ, Li WJ, et al. *Pharmacol Biochem Behav*. 2006;85:339–344.

55. Sakina MR, Dandiya PC. *Fitoterapia*. 1990;61:291–296.

56. Diwan PV, Karwande I, Singh AK. *Fitoterapia*. 1991;3:253–257.

57. Liang X, Huang YN, Chen SW, et al. *Pharmacol Biochem Behav*. 2008;89: 444–449.

58. Nalini K, Aroor AR, Karanth KS, et al. *Fitoterapia*. 1992;63(3):232–237.

59. Xu Y, Cao Z, Khan I, et al. *J Alzheimers Dis*. 2008;13:341–349.

60. Mook-Jung I, Shin JE, Yun SH, et al. *J Neurosci Res*. 1999;58(3):417–425.

61. Veerendra Kumar MH, Cupta YK. *Clin Exp Pharmacol Physiol*. 2003;30(5–6):336–342.

62. Dhanasekaran M, Holcomb LA, Hitt AR, et al. *Phytother Res*. 2009;23(1):14–19.

63. Lee MK, Kim SR, Sung SH, et al. *Res Commun Mol Pathol Pharmacol*. 2000;108(1–2):75–86.

64. Ramanathan M, Sivakumar S, Anandvijayakumar PR, et al. *Indian J Exp Biol*. 2007;45(5):425–431.

65. Krishnamurthy RG, Senut MC, Zemke D, et al. *J Neurosci Res*. 2009;87(11): 2541–2550.

66. Haleagrahara N, Ponnusamy K. *J Toxicol Sci*. 2010;35(1):41–47.

67. Veerendra Kumar MH, Gupta YK. *J Ethnopharmacol*. 2002;79(2):253–260.

68. Subathra M, Shila S, Devi MA, et al. *Exp Gerontol*. 2005;40(8–9):707–715.

69. Shinomol GK, Muralidhara *Phytomedicine*. 2008;15(11):971–984.

70. Shinomol GK, Muralidhara *Neurotoxicology*. 2008;29(6):948–957.

71. Shinomol GK, Ravikumar H, Muralidhara *Phytother Res*. 2010;24(6):885–892.

72. Soumyanath A, Zhong YP, Gold SA, et al. *J Pharm Pharmacol*. 2005;57(9):1221–1229.

73. Mohandas Rao KG, Muddanna Rao S, Gurumadhva Rao S. *Evid Based Complement Altern Med*. 2006;3(3): 349–357.

74. Mohandas Rao KG, Muddanna Rao S, Gurumadhva Rao S. *Evid Based Complement Altern Med*. 2009;6(2): 203–210.

75. Gadahad MR, Rao M, Rao G. *J Chin Med Assoc*. 2008;71(1):6–13.

76. Rao MKG, Rao MS, Rao GS. *Neuroanatomy*. 2005;4:18–23.

77. Rao SB, Chetana M, Uma Devi P. *Physiol Behav*. 2005;86:449–457.

78. Gupta YK, Veerendra Kumar MH, Srivastava AK. *Pharmacol Biochem Behav*. 2003;74(3):579–585.

79. Vattanajun A, Watanabe H, Tantisira MH, et al. *J Med Assoc Thai*. 2005;88(suppl 3): S131–S140.

80. Incandela L, Cesarone MR, Cacchio M, et al. *Angiology*. 2001;52(suppl 2): S9–S13.

81. Cospite M, Ferrara F, Milio G, et al. *Giorn Ital Angiol*. 1984;4(3):200–205.

82. Arpaia MR, Ferrone R, Amitrano M, et al. *Int J Clin Pharmacol Res*. 1990;10(4): 229–233.

83. Belcaro GV, Grimaldi R, Guidi G. *Angiology*. 1990;41(7):533–540.

84. Montecchio GP, Samaden A, Carbone S. *Haematologica*. 1991;76(3):256–259.

85. Pragada RR, Veeravalli KK, Chowdary KP, et al. *J Ethnopharmacol*. 2004;93(1): 105–108.

86. Bian GX, Li GG, Yang Y, et al. *Biol Pharm bull*. 2008;31(3):458–463.

87. Li GG, Bian GX, Ren JP, et al. *Yao Xue Xue Bao*. 2007;42(5):475–480.

88. Gnanapragasam A, Yogeeta S, Subhashini R, et al. *Mol Cell Biochem*. 2007;294(1–2): 55–63.

89. Gnanapragasam A, Ebenezar KK, Sathish V, et al. *Life Sci*. 2004;76(5):585–597.

90. Zheng MS. *J Trad Chin Med*. 1989;9: 113–116.

91. Yoosook C, Bunyapraphatsara N, Boonyakiat Y, et al. *Phytomedicine*. 2000;6(6):411–419.

92. Herbert D, Paramsivan CN, Prabhakar R, et al. *Indian J Leprosy*. 1994;66:65–68.

93. Newton SM, Lau C, Gurcha SS, et al. *J Ethnopharmacol*. 2002;79:57–67.

94. Medda S, Das N, Mahato SB, et al. *Indian J Biochem Biophys*. 1995;32(3):147–151.

95. Chakraborty T, Sinha Babu SP, Sukul NC. *Fitoterapia*. 1995;57(2):110–112.

96. Park BC, Bosire KO, Lee ES, et al. *Cancer Lett*. 2005;218(1):81–90.

97. Yoshida M, Fuchigami M, Nagao T, et al. *Biol Pharm Bull*. 2005;28(1):173–175.

98. Tang XL, Yang XY, Jung HJ, et al. *Biol Pharm Bull*. 2009;32(8):1399–1405.

99. Babykutty S, Padikkala J, Sathiadevan PP, et al. *Afr J Tradit Complement Altern Med*. 2008;6(1):9–16.

100. Huang YH, Zhang SH, Zhen RX, et al. *Ai Zheng*. 2004;23(12):1599–1604. [In Chinese].

101. Babu TD, Kuttan G, Padikkala J. *J Ethnopharmacol*. 1995;48(1):53–57.

102. Bunpo P, Kataoka K, Arimochi H, et al. *Food Chem Toxicol*. 2004;42(12): 1987–1997.

103. Punturee K, Wild CP, Kasinrerk W, et al. *Asian Pac J Cancer Prev*. 2005;6(3): 396–400.

104. Patil JS, Nagavi BG, Ramesh M, et al. *Ind Drugs*. 1998;38:711–714.

105. Jayathirtha MG, Mishra SH. *Phytomedicine*. 2004;11(4):361–365.

106. Chatterjee TK, Chakraborty A, Pathak M, et al. *Indian J Exp Biol*. 1992;30(10): 889–891.

107. Sarma DNK, Khosa RL. *Phytother Res*. 1996;10(2):181–183.

108. Sarma DNK, Khosa RL, Chansauria JPN, et al. *Phytother Res*. 1995;9(8):589–590.

109. Gupta R, Flora SJ. *J Appl Toxicol*. 2006;26(3):213–222.

110. Flora SJ, Gupta R. *Phytother Res*. 2007;21(10):980–988.

111. Shobi V, Goel HC. *Physiol Behav*. 2001;73(1–2):19–23.

112. Sharma J, Sharma R. *Phytother Res*. 2002;16(8):785–786.

113. Sharma J, Sharma R. *Phytother Res*. 2005;19(7):605–611.

114. Zhang L, Li HZ, Gong X, et al. *Phytomedicine*. 2010;17(10):811–819.

115. Chasseaud LF, Fry BJ, Hawkins DR, et al. *Arzneimittelforschung*. 1971;21(9): 1379–1384.

116. Zheng XC, Wang SH. *J Chromatogr B Analyt Technol Biomed Life Sci*. 2009;877(5–6):477–481.

117. Rush WR, Murray GR, Graham DJ. *Eur J Drug Metab Pharmacokinet*. 1993;18(4):323–326.

118. Grimaldi R, De Ponti F, D'Angelo L, et al. *J Ethnopharmacol*. 1990;8:235–241.

119. Incandela L, Cesarone MR, Cachio M, et al. *Angiology*. 2001;52(10 suppl 2): S61–S67.

120. Cesarone MR, Belcaro G, Rulo A, et al. *Angiology*. 2001;52(suppl 1–2):S45–S48.

121. Pointel JP, Boccalon H, Cloarec M, et al. *Angiology*. 1987;38(1 pt 1):46–50.

122. Belcaro G, Laurora G, Cesarone MR, et al. *Curr Ther Res*. 1989;46(6):1015–1026.

123. Cesarone MR, Laurora G, De Sanctis MT, et al. *Minerva Cardioangiol*. 1994;42(6):299–304.

124. De Sanctis MT, Belcaro G, Incandela L, et al. *Angiology*. 2001;52(10 suppl 2): S55–S59.

125. Belcaro GV, Rulo A, Grimaldi R. *Angiology*. 1990;41(1):12–18.

126. Monteverde A, Occhipinti P, Rossi F, et al. *Acta Ther*. 1987;13:629–636.

127. Cesarone MR, Belcaro G, De Sanctis MT, et al. *Angiology*. 2001;52(suppl 2):S15–S18.

128. Lim CS, Davies AH. *Br J Surg*. 2009;96(11):1231–1242.

129. Naoum JJ, Hunter GC. *Vascular*. 2007;15(5):242–249.

130. Incandela L, Belcaro G, Cesarone MR, et al. *Angiology*. 2001;52(suppl 2):S27–S31.

131. Cesarone MR, Incandela L, De Sanctis MT, et al. *Angiology*. 2001;52(suppl 1–2): S49–S54.

132. Cesarone MR, Incandela L, De Sanctis MT, et al. *Angiology*. 2001;52(suppl 1–2): S33–S37.

133. Guarerio F, Sansonetti G, Donzelli R, et al. *Giorn Ital Angiol*. 1986;6(1):46–52.

134. Thim T, Hagensen MK, Bentzon JF, et al. *J Intern Med*. 2008;263(5):506–516.

135. Schoenhagen P, Tuzcu EM, Ellis SG. *Circulation*. 2002;106(7):760–762.

136. Cesarone MR, Belcaro G, Nicolaides AN, et al. *Angiology*. 2001;52(suppl 2): S19–S25.

137. Incandela L, Belcaro G, Nicolaides AN, et al. *Angiology*. 2001;52(suppl 2): S69–S73.

138. Etrebi A, Ibrahim A, Zaki K. *J Egypt Med Assoc*. 1975;58(5–6):324–327.

139. Peyresblanques J. *Bull Soc Ophtalmol Fr*. 1959;8:771–781.

140. Baudon-Glanddier B. *Gaz Med Fr*. 1963;70:2463–2464.

141. Sevin P. *Progr Med (Paris)*. 1962;90: 23–24.

142. Huriez CL. *Lille Med*. 1972;3(suppl. 17): 574–579.

143. O'Keeffe P. *Br J Plast Surg*. 1974;27(2):194–195.

144. Balina LM, Cardama JE, Gatti JC, et al. *Dia Med*. 1961;33:1693–1696.

145. Stassen P. *Rev Med Liege*. 1964;19: 305–308.

146. Mayall RC, Mayall AC, Bertolotti JG, et al. *Rev Bras Med*. 1975;32:26–29.

147. Mekkawi MF. *Bull Ophthalmol Soc Egypt*. 1975;68:77–79.

148. El-Hefnawi H. *Dermatologica*. 1962;125:387–392.

149. Bosse JP, Papillon J, Frenette G, et al. *Ann Plast Surg*. 1979;3(1):13–21.

150. Paocharoen V. *J Med Assoc Thai*. 2010;93(7):S166–S170.

151. El-Zawahry MD, Khalil AM, El-Banna MH. *Bull Soc Int Chir*. 1975;34(4):296–297.

152. Darnis F, Orcel L, de Saint-Maur PP, et al. *Sem Hop*. 1979;55(37–38):1749–1750.

153. Castellani L, Gillet JY, Lavernhe G, et al. *Bull Fed Soc Gynecol Obstet Lang Fr*. 1966;18(2):184–186.

154. Torre MP, Donnadieu JM, Braditch JL. *Clinique (Paris)*. 1963;58:203–206.

155. Kiesewetter H. *Wien Med Wochenschr*. 1964;114:124–126. [In German].

156. Wolfram ST. *Wien Med Wochenschr*. 1965;115:439–442. [In German].

157. Chakrabarty T, Deshmukh S. *Sci Culture*. 1976;11:573.

158. Nebout M. *Bull Soc Pathol Exot Filiales*. 1974;67:471–478. [In French].

159. Chaudhury S, Hazra S, Podder GC, et al. *Indian J Dermatol*. 1987;32(3):63–67.

160. Sasaki S, Shinkai H, Akashi Y, et al. *Jap J Clin Derm*. 1971;25(6):585–593.

161. Guseva NG, Starovoitova MN, Mach ES. *Ter Arkh*. 1998;70(5):58–61. [In Russian].

162. Szczepanski A, Dabrowska H, Blaszczyk M. *Przegl Dermatol*. 1974;61(5):701–703.

163. Frati Munari AC, Culebro Nieves G, Velazquez E, et al. *Bol Med Hosp Infant Mex*. 1979;36(2):201–214.

164. Natarajan S, Paily PP. *Indian J Dermatol*. 1973;18(4):82–85.

165. Kosalwatna S, Shaipanich C, Bhanganada K. *Siriraj Hosp Gaz*. 1988;40(6):455–461.

166. Rougier A, Humbert F. *J Am Acad Dermatol*. 2008;58(2 suppl 2): AB144. Abstract P3109.

167. Klövekorn W, Tepe A, Danesch U. *Int J Clin Pharmacol Ther*. 2007;45(11): 583–591.

168. Mallol J, Belda MA, Costa D, et al. *Int J Cos Sci*. 1991;13:51–57.

169. Sommerfeld B. *Phytomedicine*. 2007;14:711–715.

170. Lee J, Jung E, Lee H, et al. *Int J Cos Sci*. 2008;30(3):167–173.

171. Haftek M, Mac-Mary S, Le Bitoux MA, et al. *Exp Dermatol*. 2008;17(11):946–952.

172. Bradwejn J, Zhou Y, Koszychki D, et al. *J Clin Psychopharmacol*. 2000;20:680–684.

173. Jana U, Sur TK, Maity LN, et al. *Nepal Med Coll J*. 2010;12(1):8–11.

174. Appa Rao MVR, Srinivasan K, Koteswara Rao T. *J Res Indian Med*. 1973;8(4):9–15.

175. Kuppurajan K, Srinivasan K, Janaki K. *J Res Indian Med*. 1978;13(1):37–41.

176. Wattanathorn J, Mator L, Muchimapura S, et al. *J Ethnopharmacol*. 2008;116(2):325–332.

177. Appa Rao MVR, Usha SP, Rajagopalan SS, et al. *J Res Indian Med*. 1967;2:79–85.

178. Appa Rao MVR, Rajapopalan SS, Srinivasan VR, et al. *Nagarjun*. 1969;12:33–41.

179. Mato L, Wattanathorn J, Muchimapura S, et al. *Evid Based Complement Altern Med*, 2009. At <http://ecam.oxfordjournals.org/cgi/reprint/nep177v1>. Accessed 6.7.10.

180. Rhee J, Choi KW. *Korean J Gastroenterol*. 1981;13(1):35–40.

181. Sastravaha G, Gassmann G, Sangtherapitikul P, et al. *J Int Acad Periodontol*. 2005;7(3):70–79.

182. Sastravaha G, Yotnuengnit P, Booncong P, et al. *J Int Acad Periodontol*. 2003;5(4):106–115.

183. Bagchi CD, Puri HS. *Herba Hung*. 1988;27(2–3):137–140.

184. Dharma AP. *Indonesian Medicinal Plants*. Jakarta: Balai Pustaka; 1987. pp. 24–25.

185. van Wyk B-E, Gericke N. *People's Plants: A Guide to Useful Plants of Southern Africa*. Arcadia: Briza Publications; 2000. pp. 68, 142.

186. Rattanapanone V, Sanpitak N, Phornphibul B. *Chiang Mai Med Bull*. 1971;10:17–23.

187. Kays SJ, Silva Dias JC. *Econ Bot*. 1995;49(2):115–152.

188. dede Lucia R, Sertie JAA. *Fitoterapia*. 1997;68(5):413–416.

189. Dhar ML, Dhar MM, Dhawan BN, et al. *Indian J Exp Biol*. 1968;6(4):232–247.

190. Boiteau P, Ratsimamanga AR. *Therapie*. 1956;11:125–149.

191. Ieamworapong C, Kangsadalumpai K, Rojanapo W. *Environ Mol Mutagen*. 1989;14(suppl 15):93.

192. Yen GC, Chen HY, Peng HH. *Food Chem Toxicol*. 2001;39:1045–1053.

193. Rivera IG, Martins MT, Sanchez PS, et al. *Environ Toxicol Water Qual*. 1996;9(2):87–93.

194. Gopalan HNB, Wairimu AN. *Environ Mol Mutagen*. 1989;14(suppl 15):73.

195. Laerum OD, Iversen OH. *Cancer Res*. 1972;32(7):1463–1468.

196. Kartnig T. *Herb Spice Med Plant*. 1988;3:145–173.

197. Hadida E, Sayag J, Bonerandi JJ, et al. *Bull Soc Fr Dermatol Syphiligr*. 1970;77(4):522–525.

198. Dutta T, Basu UP. *Indian J Exp Biol*. 1968;6:181–182.

199. Hausen BM. *Contact Dermatitis*. 1993;29(4):175–179.

200. Danese P, Carnevali C, Bertazzoni MG. *Contact Dermatitis*. 1994;31(3):201.

201. Santucci B, Picardo M, Cristaudo A. *Contact Dermatitis*. 1985;13(1):39.

202. Izu R, Aguirre A, Gil N, et al. *Contact Dermatitis*. 1992;26(3):192–193.

203. Eun HC, Lee AY. *Contact Dermatitis*. 1985;13(5):310–313.

204. Huriez C, Martin P. G *Ital Dermatol Minerva Dermatol*. 1969;44(9):463–464.

205. Gonzalo Garijo MA, Revenga Arranz F, Bobadilla Gonzalez P. *Allergol Immunopathol*. 1996;24(3):132–134.

206. Vena GA, Angelini GA. *Contact Dermatitis*. 1986;15(2):108–109.

207. Goossens A, Beck MH, Haneke E, et al. *Contact Dermatitis*. 1999;40:112–113.

208. Chopra RN, Chopra IC, Handa KL, et al. *Chopra's Indigenous Drugs of India*, 2nd ed., 1958. Calcutta: reprinted Academic Publishers; 1982. pp. 351–353.

209. Jorge OA, Jorge AD. *Rev Esp Enferm Dig*. 2005;97(2):115–124.

210. O'Brien B. *Ir Med J*. 2005;98(10):250–251.

211. Chopra RN, Badhwar RL, Ghosh S. *Poisonous Plants of India*, vol I. New Delhi: Indian Council of Agricultural Research; 1965. pp. 433–434.

212. Cox DN, Rajasuriya S, Soysa PE, et al. *Int J Food Sci Nutr*. 1993;44:123–132.

213. Peiris KHS, Kays SJ. *Hort Tech*. 1996;6(1):13–18.

214. Dantuluri S, North-Lewis P, Karthik SV. *Dig Liver Dis*. 2011;43(6):500.

Hawthorn

(*Crataegus spp.*)

Synonyms

Crataegi (Lat), Weißdorn (Ger), aubépine (Fr), biancospino (Ital), alm. hvidtjørn (Dan).

What is it?

The leaf, flower and berry of several species of hawthorn are used medicinally, most often: *Crataegus laevigata* (Poiret) DC (synonyms: *C. oxyacantha* auct. non L, *C. oxyacanthoides* Thuill.) and *C. monogyna* Jacq. The Greek meaning of *Crataegus oxyacantha* refers to hard (wood) and sharp thorns. References to hawthorn are extensive throughout history and the shrub has been utilised in many ways including for wood, cultivation as a hedge and for flavouring of liquor by the berries. Although the berries were traditionally used as medicine, modern research has tended to focus on preparations from the leaves or leaves and flowers.

The first use of hawthorn in cardiac therapy is attributed to Dr Green, an Irish doctor who used a tincture of the fresh berries. With the increasing incidence of heart disease in the Western world at the time, its use rapidly spread to other countries, notably France, the United States, England and Germany. In Western herbal medicine hawthorn is now considered to be the most significant herb for ischaemic and congestive heart disease and there is considerable objective evidence to support its status.

Effects

Increases force of myocardial contraction, increases coronary blood flow, reduces myocardial oxygen demand, protects against myocardial damage, hypotensive, improves heart rate variability, antiarrhythmic.

Traditional view

Hawthorn berries have been traditionally used to treat cardiovascular problems (including hypertension with myocardial weakness, angina pectoris and tachycardia) and other circulatory disorders (atherosclerosis, Buerger's disease). The flowers and berries were also used as an astringent for sore throats and as a diuretic for kidney problems and dropsy.[1,2] The fruit and bark were used by the Eclectics as a heart remedy for indications such as pain, praecordial oppression, dyspnoea, cardiac hypertrophy, valvular insufficiency and anaemia.[3] The fruit of other *Crataegus* species (*C. pinnatifida*, *C. cuneata*) have been used in traditional Chinese medicine to improve digestion, stimulate circulation and remove blood stasis.[4]

Summary of actions

Cardiotonic (mild), cardioprotective, antioxidant, collagen stabilising, mild astringent, hypotensive (mild), antiarrhythmic.

Can be used for

Indications established by clinical trials

Congestive heart disease due to ischaemia, hypertension or other causes (particularly corresponding to NYHA stages I and II, good evidence), mild hypertension (moderate evidence for a mild effect); topically for acne (uncontrolled trial); anxiety (in combination).

Traditional therapeutic uses

As a treatment for mild heart conditions (angina pectoris, coronary artery disease, cardiac arrhythmias, myocardial weakness) and to assist prevention of arterial degeneration caused by atherosclerosis.

May also be used for

Extrapolations from pharmacological studies

Antioxidant activity; co-factor for vitamin C intake; stabilisation of connective tissue tone; for hyperlipidaemia (especially the berries).

Other applications

Cosmetic and hair care products for antiseborrhoeic and anti-inflammatory activities and to increase hydration and elasticity of the skin.[5]

Preparations

Dried or fresh leaf, flower or fruit for infusion or decoction, liquid extract and tablets or capsules for internal use. Decoction or extract for topical use.

Dosage

- 1.5 to 3.5 g/day of dried flower, leaf or berry, as infusion or decoction
- Hawthorn tablets or capsules (for example containing 1 g leaves and flowers, standardised to 15 to 20 mg oligomeric procyanidins and 6 to 7 mg flavonoids) three to four per day or more
- 3 to 6 mL/day of 1:2 liquid extract of hawthorn leaf, 3 to 7 mL/day of 1:2 liquid extract of hawthorn berry, 7.5 to 15 mL/day of 1:5 tincture of hawthorn leaf, 7.5 to 17.5 mL/day of 1:5 tincture of hawthorn berry. Higher doses than these may be necessary for hypertension
- Concentrated extracts (3:1 or 5:1), typically from the leaves and flowers and standardised to various levels of flavonoid and/or oligomeric procyanidin (OPC) content are also available in solid dosage form. These have been used in clinical trials, with doses (of extract) ranging from 160 to 1800 mg/day (see Table 1).

Duration of use

There is no restriction on the long-term use of hawthorn and it should be prescribed over a period of at least 2 months if used to treat heart conditions.

Summary assessment of safety

No adverse effects from ingestion of hawthorn are expected. Hawthorn may act in synergy with digitalis glycosides and beta-blockers. However, no specific interactions with the pharmacokinetics of digoxin were identified in human subjects and adverse effects are not generally anticipated. Modification of drug dosage may be required, but is unlikely.

Technical data

Botany

Hawthorn, a member of the Rosaceae (rose) family, is a deciduous, thorny shrub or small tree up to 10 m tall. The leaves are broader than long and have three to five lobes. The white flowers, with their red anthers, are arranged in groups of five to ten at the apex of small branches. The dark red,

false fruits are oval and contain a small kernel which is the true fruit.[6,7]

Note: There has been confusion and debate over the nomenclature of *Crataegus*. species It was suggested in 1975 that the name C. *oxyacantha* L. should be rejected since it is a source of confusion[8] and C. *laevigata* used in preference.[9] In addition, extensive hybridisation has occurred between C. *monogyna* and C. *laevigata*.[10–12] Where a research publication refers to the use of 'C. *oxyacantha*', this has generally been described in this monograph as pertaining to C. *laevigata*.

Adulteration

No adulterants known.

Key constituents

- Oligomeric procyanidins (OPCs), mainly procyanidin B-2.[13] The monomers epicatechin and catechin are also present and are generally included in chemical tests for OPC levels.
- Flavonoids, including quercetin glycosides (hyperoside, rutin) and particularly flavone C-glycosides (vitexin and related compounds).[13] The minor flavonoids in C. *laevigata* and C. *monogyna* show differences that enable their differentiation.[14]
- Amines, catechols, carboxylic and triterpene acids (crataegus acids, especially in the berries).[15]

The flowers contain the highest levels of flavonoids and the leaves contain the highest levels of OPCs. The key constituents of *Crataegus monogyna*, with variations with plant part and time of harvest, are outlined below.[16]

	OPC %	Major flavonoids %
Leaves with flowers (average of seven samples)	2.50	0.92
Flowers (average of four samples)	2.67	1.31
Leaves (spring, flowers open)	3.02	0.53
Leaves (summer, berries green)	2.71	0.74
Leaves (autumn, berries ripe)	2.06	0.76
Berries (summer, green)	3.18	0.15
Berries (autumn, ripe)	1.74	0.13

The relative astringency of an OPC increases with its degree of polymerisation. OPCs from *Crataegus oxyacantha* (*laevigata*) berries, with an average number of monomers of four, have an astringency relative to tannic acid of 0.73.[17] While the stability of flavonoids in C. *oxyacantha* (*laevigata*) tinctures was good, OPCs demonstrated relatively poor stability in this dosage form.[18]

Procyanidin B-2

	R[1]	R[2]	R[3]
Quercetin	OH	H	OH
Hyperoside	O-β-galactosyl	H	OH
Vitexin	H	glucosyl	H

Flavonoids

Pharmacodynamics

The therapeutic value of hawthorn may extend beyond its cardiovascular applications, largely due to the significant OPC content. Although most of the research is not specifically on the OPCs found in hawthorn, it is likely that the hawthorn OPCs will share many of the described pharmacological properties for this class of compounds. In 1966 the French scientist Masquelier and his co-workers analysed the bark of several conifers from Quebec. Some species, especially *Tsuga canadensis* (previously known as *Pinus canadensis*), were rich in OPCs. However, Masquelier's interest in this tree was based on the accounts of the French explorer Jacques Cartier.[19] During the winter of 1534 Cartier's group in Canada was afflicted by scurvy, which was cured on the advice of a native who directed that the sailors use a decoction of the bark and leaves of the 'Anneda' tree. The liquid was consumed and the solid residue applied as a poultice to the swollen joints. On the basis of Cartier's description, Masquelier postulated that 'Anneda' was *Tsuga canadensis*. He further speculated that the leaves provided a source of ascorbic acid and the bark, by providing OPCs, acted as a vitamin C synergist (perhaps in a similar manner to the chemically related flavonoids).

Masquelier's original interest in OPCs was for their 'vitamin P-like' activity.[20] He later postulated that they may be important in the prevention of atheroma.[21] Since then, pharmacological and clinical studies of OPCs, as either pine bark (especially *Pinus pinaster*) or grape seed (*Vitis vinifera*) extracts, have revealed an impressive variety of therapeutic properties.

Effect on the cardiovascular system

Effect on cardiac contractility and frequency and coronary blood flow

In early research the crataegus acids increased coronary blood flow in vitro and decreased blood pressure in vivo.[22–24] Crataegolic and ursolic acids increased coronary flow in vitro and crataegolic acid was also positively inotropic.[25]

Hawthorn extract exhibited a positive inotropic effect (increasing the contraction amplitude) of cardiac myocytes in vitro, with a relatively small increase in their energy requirements.[26] Hawthorn also prolonged the apparent refractory period in the presence and absence of isoprenaline (a beta-adrenergic agonist), indicating an antiarrhythmic potential.[27] A standardised leaf and flower extract exerted a positive inotropic effect on isolated left ventricular muscle strips from explants from patients with congestive heart failure.[28] Hawthorn reinforced the positive inotropic action of cardiac glycosides without an increase in glycoside toxicity and increased coronary blood flow, even after experimental damage, in vitro.[29]

Two flavonoid fractions of hawthorn were positively inotropic in isolated heart. One fraction had an effect on frequency, being negatively chronotropic (decreasing the heart rate). In isolated hearts, vitexin-2″-O-rhamnoside was positively inotropic and negatively chronotropic at higher doses, while the flavonoid aglycones were inactive.[25]

The main flavonoids of hawthorn (O-glycosides: luteolin-7-glucoside, hyperoside, rutin; and C-glycosides: vitexin, vitexin-2″-O-rhamnoside and monoacetyl vitexin-2″-O-rhamnoside) increased coronary flow, demonstrated slight positive inotropic effects and raised heart rate in isolated hearts. An inhibition of cAMP phosphodiesterase was also observed.[30]

OPC subfractions were more positively inotropic in isolated heart than flavonoid fractions, but had no effect on frequency.[31] In another study, hawthorn OPCs had a mild negative chronotropic effect in isolated heart, but caused a marked increase in contraction and blood flow. Procyanidin dimers were more active than oligomers with 3 to 4 units, and the OPC fraction from hawthorn leaves was more active than that from the berries. In general, the effects of the OPCs are similar to those of flavonoids, but are elicited at lower doses.[25]

Crataegus OPCs increased coronary blood flow in dogs after oral administration.[32] Vitexin-2″-O-rhamnoside increased coronary blood flow by up to 64% after intracoronary administration.[33] Intravenous or intracoronary administration of hawthorn flavonoids increased coronary blood flow, decreased blood pressure and increased heart contractility. No change was observed in heart rate.[34–36]

Hawthorn (C. laevigata) has also been studied in a model of congestive heart failure. A standardised hawthorn leaf and flower extract had no significant effect on the characteristic immunomodulatory response induced by 6 months of pressure overload in a rat model of heart failure.[37] However, the same research group found that the extract at the same doses (1.3, 13 and 130 mg/kg, oral) modified left ventricular remodelling and counteracted myocardial dysfunction in early (4 weeks) pressure overload-induced cardiac hypertrophy in rats,[38] but only exhibited a modest beneficial effect in the long-term (5 months) model.[39]

Cardioprotective activity and effects under hypoxic conditions

The cardioprotective effect of several fractions of standardised hawthorn leaf and flower extract (containing 18.75% OPCs) was investigated in vitro and in vivo. The lipophilic fraction containing flavonoids was as active as the whole extract in inhibiting human neutrophil elastase, but only half as active as a radical scavenger. The water-soluble fraction was weak in both in vitro systems. In contrast, the inhibiting potencies of the OPC-rich (and flavonoid-free) fraction were significantly higher than the extract. Oral administration of the OPC-rich fraction (20 mg/kg/day) to rats afforded similar protection against ischaemia-reperfusion-induced pathologies to treatment with a higher dose of the standardised extract (100 mg/kg/day).[40]

Oral pretreatment with hawthorn extract (2% of diet) to rats for 3 months resulted in myocardial protection, as evidenced by attenuation of levels of lactase dehydrogenase (LDH) release after induced ischaemia and reperfusion in the isolated hearts. This attenuation of LDH by hawthorn pretreatment suggests a preservation of the cell membrane and a protection from myocardial damage.[41] Pretreatment with hawthorn or garlic extract, but particularly the combination of both, resulted in protective effects against isoprenaline-induced heart, liver and pancreas damage in rats.[42] Oral

administration of hawthorn reduced the deleterious metabolic influence of hypoxia on ventricular muscle fibres in rabbits. Hawthorn may protect the sodium pump against anoxia.[43] In early research, administration of hawthorn to volunteers improved the anoxic symptoms produced by inhalation of an 8% oxygen gas mixture[44] and decreased the signs of ischaemia as assessed by an exercise ECG test in patients with ischaemic heart disease.[45]

Administration of the purified flavonoids from hawthorn leaves to rats with myocardial infarction resulted in a smaller necrotic focus and improved revascularisation of finer vessels when compared to controls.[46] Pretreatment with hawthorn (C. laevigata) fresh berry tincture (5 mL/kg/day for 30 days, oral) prevented the increase in lipid peroxidation and the decrease in antioxidant enzymes, increased the rate of ADP-stimulated oxygen intake and protected against pathological changes induced by isoproterenol in the hearts of rats administered this agent.[47] The beneficial effects of hawthorn were observed to extend to cardiac mitochondria in a second similar study (maintenance of mitochondrial antioxidant status, prevention of mitochondrial lipid peroxidation and increased Krebs cycle enzymes).[48]

In one earlier study the water-soluble fraction of hawthorn extract demonstrated a cardioprotective effect on the ischaemic-reperfused heart in vitro (which mimics myocardial infarction). The cardioprotective effect was not accompanied by an increase in coronary flow.[49] In contrast, no cardioprotective effects were seen during ischaemia and reperfusion, and there was even aggravation of arrhythmias, after oral pretreatment of Wistar rats with C. oxyacantha (laevigata) extract (0.5 g/kg/day for 8 weeks, standardised to 2.2% flavonoids).[50] However, pretreatment with a different leaf and flower extract (10 or 100 mg/kg/day, oral for 7 days) improved cardiac function and reduced infarct size in a similar rat model of prolonged ischaemia and reperfusion.[51]

In vitro and in vivo (rats, 100 mg/kg, oral) studies suggested that hawthorn extract protected against ischaemia-reperfusion injury by inhibiting apoptotic pathways, possibly by regulating Akt (an anti-apoptotic kinase) and HIF-1 (hypoxia-inducible factor 1) signalling pathways.[52,53]

Microcirculatory and vasorelaxant activity

Compared with a digoxin preparation, hawthorn extract increased the erythrocyte flow rate in all the vascular networks examined and reduced both leucocyte endothelial adhesion and diapedesis in the venular network in rat mesenteric vessels.[54] Even after removal of tannins, extracts of Crataegus monogyna still potently inhibited ADP-induced human platelet serotonin release and platelet aggregation in vitro.[55] Hawthorn flower extract inhibited thromboxane A2 biosynthesis in vitro.[56]

In early research intravenous administration of a hawthorn extract decreased blood pressure and increased peripheral blood flow to skeletal muscle in vivo.[57,58] In a placebo-controlled, crossover study, the effect of a single dose of 900 mg of a hawthorn leaf and flower extract (3:1, standardised to 2.2% flavonoids) on the cutaneous microcirculation was compared to 0.3 mg medigoxin. Six hours after taking hawthorn, the haematocrit had dropped by a mean of 3.2%, whereas erythrocyte aggregation increased significantly by 19% 3 h after taking the digoxin. No significant changes were recorded for the other measured parameters (plasma viscosity, flow rate in nail bed capillaries, heart rate, blood pressure).[59]

OPCs in hawthorn extract may be responsible for the observed endothelium-dependent nitric oxide-mediated relaxation in isolated rat aorta, possibly via activation of tetraethylammonium-sensitive K^+ channels.[60] A standardised leaf and flower extract induced a concentration-dependent vasodilation of rat aorta and human mammarian artery in vitro, with activity again residing in the OPC fraction.[61] The mechanism involved appeared to be an endothelium-dependent, NO-mediated vasorelaxation, a finding supported yet again by another in vitro study from a different laboratory.[62] Flavonoids and OPCs from hawthorn demonstrated inhibitory activity on angiotensin converting enzyme (ACE) in vitro.[63]

Mechanistic studies

Hawthorn may exert its activity in vitro in a similar way to phosphodiesterase inhibitors, raising cAMP levels in cardiac muscle cells. The total flavonoids from hawthorn were shown to inhibit phosphodiesterase activity in vitro.[26] However, an in vitro study of hawthorn leaf and flower extract suggested it exerted direct positive inotropic effects, implying a pharmacologic mechanism similar to the cAMP-independent positive inotropic action of cardiac glycosides.[28] Hawthorn extract prolonged the effective refractory period in isolated heart compared to four other inotropic drugs (including adrenaline and digoxin), which all shortened it. Thus, hawthorn has a relatively lower risk of causing arrhythmias and may in fact have antiarrhythmic activity.[64] Multi-electrode techniques have demonstrated that hawthorn extract prolonged the action potential duration and delayed recovery of the maximum upstroke velocity of guinea pig papillary muscle.[65] A hawthorn extract demonstrated negative chronotropic effects in a cultured murine cardiomyocyte assay, independent of beta-adrenergic receptor blockade, possibly involving muscarinic receptor activation.[66]

An interesting in vitro study compared the effects of a hawthorn flower, leaf and berry extract against a berry extract (species not specified) using rat cardiomyocytes.[67] Markedly different effects were observed; for example, the former extract resulted in the initiation of robust calcium transits with eventual calcium overload, whereas the latter initiated calcium transits but with no calcium overload. In other words the flower, leaf and berry extract was more potent. Mechanistic explorations suggested that cardiac activity is exerted via the sodium-potassium pump (Na^+/K^+-ATPase). Another in vitro study in cultured cardiomyocytes comparing a berry and a leaf extract of C. laevigata found similar negative chronotropic effects, unrelated to beta-adrenergic receptor blockade.[68]

A hawthorn leaf and flower extract inhibited induced intimal hyperplasia in vitro and in vivo (rats, oral doses), probably by directly inhibiting platelet-derived growth factor-beta.[69] This might have clinical implications in angioplasty-related restenosis. Reduced endothelium-dependent vasodilator responses with increased synthesis of endothelin-1 (ET-1) are characteristics of endothelial dysfunction in heart failure and are predictive of mortality. Hawthorn and grape seed OPCs equipotently inhibited ET-1 synthesis in cultured endothelial cells.[70]

Hypocholesterolaemic activity

Hawthorn berry tincture administered simultaneously to rats fed an atherogenic diet significantly increased the in vitro binding of LDL (low density lipoprotein) to liver plasma membranes, increased bile acid excretion and depressed hepatic cholesterol synthesis.[71] The results of adding hawthorn (2% of diet) to a rabbit diet high in cholesterol suggested that the mechanism by which Chinese hawthorn berry (Crataegus pinnatifida) decreases serum cholesterol involves, at least in part, the inhibition of cholesterol absorption via downregulation of intestinal acyl-CoA-cholesterol acyltransferase (ACAT) activity.[72] Chinese hawthorn berry also inhibited ACAT in Caco-2 (intestinal) cells, largely due to the activity of the triterpenic acids (oleanolic and ursolic acid).[73] Further to this, a berry dichloromethane extract (0.37% of diet) demonstrated a synergistic effect with plant sterols in lowering plasma cholesterol in hamsters fed a high cholesterol diet.[73] The triterpene acids were also quite active in this model at 0.01% of diet.

In contrast, three flavonoids (quercetin, hyperoside and rutin) and chlorogenic acid from Chinese hawthorn berry weakly inhibited HMG-CoA reductase activity in vitro and demonstrated synergy in combination, thereby perhaps suggesting mild statin-like activity.[74] A synergistic activity on lowering cholesterol and triglycerides was also demonstrated in a mouse model after oral doses of 2.85 mg/kg/day of each compound or the combination (see also Chapter 2).

Antioxidant activity

Hawthorn extracts obtained using acetone, methanol and water demonstrated antioxidant activity on hepatic microsomal preparations in vitro. A correlation was demonstrated between the total phenolic content (mainly flavonoids and OPCs) and antioxidant activity for leaf, flower and berry at all stages of herb growth. The most active individual components were (−)-epicatechin and procyanidin B-2.[75] One recent study found that the ethanolic extract of C. monogyna berries possesses more antioxidant activity than the aqueous extract (with catechin and epicatechin mainly responsible for activity),[76] while another on the berry tincture of the same species attributed the greatest antioxidant contribution to epicatechin and hyperoside.[77]

Most of the polyphenolic compounds in hawthorn demonstrated a dose-dependent protection of human LDL from copper-mediated oxidation, and prevented the peroxyl free radical-induced oxidation of alpha-tocopherol. In addition, supplementation of a hawthorn fruit powder (C. pinnatifida) at 2% of diet significantly elevated serum alpha-tocopherol by 18% to 20% in rats fed a 30% polyunsaturated canola oil diet, as compared to the control.[78] In another study, the in vitro inhibition of LDL oxidation was also linked to hawthorn's polyphenols, in particular the dimeric procyanidin B2 and the flavonol glycoside hyperoside. OPCs were more active than the majority of the flavonoids tested.[79]

Chinese research found that the Chinese hawthorn berry (*C. pinnatifida*) was a potent inducer of superoxide dismutase (SOD) activity in mice.[80] Oral doses of aqueous extracts were used and the SOD activity was measured in red blood cells. (SOD is the enzyme which combats the harmful effects of the superoxide radical.) Further to this, a combination of tinctures of mango bark (*Mangifera indica*) and *C. laevigata* berries (5 mg/kg of each, oral) in rats fed a high cholesterol diet not only significantly lowered LDL-cholesterol and raised HDL-cholesterol, but also restored the observed reductions in SOD, catalase, glutathione peroxidase and glutathione induced by the diet.[81]

Other activity

Oral administration of hawthorn tincture to rats for 30 days afforded good protection against abnormal changes in liver function tests after myocardial infarction (alanine aminotransferase, aspartate aminotransferase, LDH and alkaline phosphatase) and in protein-bound carbohydrate alterations (hexose, hexosamine, fucose and sialic acid). These hepatoprotective effects included a reversal of histological changes in the liver.[82]

Induction of epidermal ornithine decarboxylase (ODC) activity, stimulation of hydroperoxide production and increased DNA synthesis are three biochemical effects linked to skin tumour promotion by the tumour promoter 12-O-tetradecanoylphorbol 13-acetate (TPA). Topical application of OPCs to mouse epidermis prior to administration of TPA resulted in inhibition of ODC activity. The inhibition of ODC activity increased with the degree of polymerisation of the OPCs: trimer (procyanidin C-1) > dimer (procyanidin B-2) > monomer (epicatechin).[83] Further to this, an extract of *C. pinnatifida* berries inhibited skin tumour promotion and demonstrated topical anti-inflammatory activity in various models.[84]

An extract from a mixture of *C. monogyna* and *C. laevigata* berries demonstrated moderate activity against Gram-positive bacteria in vitro, with no effect on *Candida albicans*,[85] and flavonoids and OPCs from *C. sinaica* were inhibitory against herpes simplex virus type 1 in vitro.[86]

High doses (100 to 1000 mg/kg, ip) of an extract of *C. monogyna* fruit pulp exhibited CNS depressant and analgesic activities in mice.[87] Pretreatment with hawthorn (*C. laevigata*) extract (100 mg/kg/day for 15 days, oral in rats) reduced brain damage and improved neurological score by reducing oxidative stress in a model of cerebral ischaemia-reperfusion injury.[88]

Flavonoids in a hawthorn leaf extract inhibited alpha-glucosidase in vitro.[89] An aqueous extract of hawthorn leaf (*C. laevigata*) demonstrated a significant dose-dependent decrease of blood glucose levels in streptozotocin-induced diabetic rats (doses were 150 or 300 mg/kg/day, oral for either 1 or 9 days), but had no such effect in normal rats.[90]

A leaf and flower extract of *C. laevigata* demonstrated a range of effects on isolated human neutrophil function that could be interpreted as reflecting anti-inflammatory activity.[91] These included inhibition of release of chemoattractants and cytokines and inhibition of neutrophil oxidative burst. The mixed species berry combination mentioned above at 50, 100 and 200 mg/kg/day (oral) produced a dose-dependent anti-inflammatory effect in the rat paw oedema model.[85] At similar doses it also exhibited a dose-dependent gastroprotective action in a gastric ulcer model in rats.

Hawthorn fruit (as extract equivalent to 0.5, 1.0 and 2.0 g/kg/day of berries, oral) dose-dependently exerted a protective activity in two experimental models of murine colitis.[92] Anti-inflammatory effects were demonstrated in the colon and the authors reflected on the potential value of this herb in patients with inflammatory bowel disease (the equivalent human dose for 2.0 g/day in a mouse is approximately 12 g/day of berries, which is achievable).

An isolate of hawthorn leaf flavonoids (4, 8 and 16 mg/kg/day, oral for 8 days) significantly increased the activity of muscle lipoprotein lipase (LPL) in mice, with a commensurate decrease of activity in adipose tissue.[93] This indicates that hawthorn flavonoids may reduce lipid accumulation in adipose tissue by regulating LPL expression.

A *C. monogyna* fruit extract significantly protected human lymphocytes against gamma irradiation damage in vitro.[94] Radioprotective activity was also demonstrated in vivo for an extract of an Iranian hawthorn species (*C. microphylla* fruit) given to mice (25, 50, 100 and 200 mg/kg, single dose, ip), as assessed by genotoxic changes in bone marrow cells.[95] Following on from this research, the same investigative group gave a single oral dose of 500 mg of this extract to five human volunteers and then subjected their blood samples to a defined level of gamma irradiation.[96] For samples collected 1 h after the hawthorn dose there was a 44% decrease in genotoxic damage in lymphocytes, compared to samples collected beforehand.

Pharmacokinetics

To date there have been no human pharmacokinetic studies of hawthorn. The pharmacokinetics of oral doses of OPCs given to mice have been studied in early research using an isotopic labelling technique.[97] OPCs showed rapid absorption and preferential localisation in tissues rich in glycosaminoglycans. The plasma half-life was about 5 h, indicating a prolonged presence in the bloodstream. In contrast, the flavonoid glycoside rutin showed poor absorption, the bulk of the radioactivity residing with the contents of the digestive tract. This work and that of others reviewed by Middleton[98] suggests that OPCs, or OPC fragments resulting from bacterial activity in the gut, are more bioavailable than some flavonoids.

More recent research, all from China, has mainly focused on the pharmacokinetics of the typical hawthorn flavonoids using a variety of models. Oral administration of a hawthorn fruit extract (*C. pinnatifida*) to rats revealed only significant bioavailability for catechin.[99] Chlorogenic acid, hyperoside and isoquercitrin present in the extract could not be detected in the rat plasma. The same research group found that epicatechin, isoquercitrin and hyperoside exhibited limited permeability using in vitro models of intestinal absorption and confirmed that only epicatechin was detectable as the parent compound after oral administration to rats.[100]

The oral bioavailability of vitexin-2″-O-rhamnoside (VOR) was determined to be only 3.57% in rats.[101] In vitro modelling of intestinal absorption suggested that this molecule exhibits high permeability via passive diffusion, but its absorption is limited by P-glycoprotein acting as an efflux pump.[102]

The pharmacokinetics of VOR and vitexin-4″-O-glucoside (VOG) after a single oral dose of a hawthorn leaf flavonoid isolate (from C. *pinnatifida*) was determined in rats.[103] After a dose of extract containing 83.3 mg/kg of VOG and 342 mg/kg of VOR, the same Tmax of 0.75 h was observed, with Cmax recorded at 4.1 μg/mL and 16.5 μg/mL, respectively. The mean elimination half-lives of VOG and VOR were 2.53 h and 2.32 h, respectively. High levels of tissue distribution of VOG and VOR were observed in liver and kidney, but none was detected in brain tissue. There was no long-term accumulation of VOG and VOR in the rat tissues examined. The total recovery of the dose in 24 hours was 64.91% (0.70% in urine, 64.21% in faeces) for VOG and 89.01% (0.72% in urine, 88.29% in faeces) for VOR. The cumulative VOG and VOR excreted in bile represented 0.58% and 13.38% of the doses, respectively. The authors concluded that VOG and VOR were not efficiently absorbed. (For further details of the pharmacokinetics of flavonoids and OPCs see Chapter 2.)

Clinical trials

Heart disease

The New York Heart Association (NYHA) classifies loss of cardiac output and heart failure: for stage I the patient is symptom-free when at rest and on treatment; stage II patients have loss of capacity with medium effort; for stage III even minor effort results in dyspnoea, with no symptoms at rest; in stage IV symptoms are present when at rest. There have been a number of clinical studies of the effect of hawthorn on heart failure which are summarised in Table 1. Many of these have been subjected to systematic review and meta-analysis, as discussed below.

A 2008 Cochrane review evaluated the information reported in good quality double blind clinical trials comparing hawthorn leaf and flower extract against placebo in patients with chronic heart failure (NYHA Classes I to III).[126] Fourteen clinical trials were found to be of sufficiently high quality to be included in the evidence review.[126] In most of these studies the hawthorn extract was used in conjunction with conventional treatments, including cardiac drugs. Pooling of the results of 10 trials using meta-analysis found that the average maximum cardiac work capacity was significantly higher in the patients receiving hawthorn compared to placebo (p<0.02). The review also found that a measure of cardiac oxygen need (systolic blood pressure × heart rate) was significantly lower. These findings suggest that hawthorn treatment helped the heart muscle tissue to work more efficiently. The capacity of patients to tolerate exercise was increased and symptoms such as shortness of breath and fatigue were significantly improved. Reported side effects were mild and infrequent and there was no suggestion of any adverse interaction with conventional drugs. The authors concluded that there is significant benefit in both symptom control and physiological outcomes from hawthorn extract as an adjunctive treatment for chronic heart failure.

The 13 published trials included in the 2008 Cochrane review are summarised in date order as the first 13 entries in Table 1. Following these, the table includes another eight published clinical studies of hawthorn in chronic heart failure, also in date order. These trials were not included in the Cochrane review because they did not meet the selection criteria. Also it should be noted that the Cochrane review used an earlier interim conference report of the trial by Zick and co-workers. The version of this study included in Table 1 is the final published analysis from 2009.

Other clinical trials in heart failure patients are as follows. The large SPICE (Survival and Prognosis Investigation of Crataegus Extract) study was a randomised, double blind, placebo-controlled study conducted at 156 centres in 13 European countries.[127] In the 2-year clinical trial, 2681 patients with NYHA Class II or III chronic heart failure were given either hawthorn (900 mg/day of a 5:1 leaf and flower extract containing 18.75% OPCs) or a placebo. All of their conventional medications were continued. The trial was designed to assess whether the regular use of hawthorn by cardiac patients could delay or reduce their likelihood of a 'cardiac event', defined in the study as cardiac death (due either to sudden cardiac arrest, death from progressive heart failure or a fatal heart attack), a non-fatal heart attack or hospitalisation due to progressive heart failure.

While the study did show some minor positive findings, it was probably not large enough or long enough to demonstrate any definitive benefit from hawthorn. The rate of heart attacks (fatal and non-fatal) was about the same in the two groups (hawthorn or placebo). There was a difference in sudden cardiac deaths (20 fewer in the hawthorn group) that failed to reach statistical significance, except in the subgroup of patients with milder heart failure (p=0.025), suggesting a reduced risk of dangerous arrhythmias.

One strong conclusion from the SPICE trial is the excellent safety and low side-effect profile of the hawthorn extract. This was despite the fact that the patients were also taking a wide variety of cardiac drugs including beta-blockers, ACE inhibitors, diuretics and digoxin.

In a retrospective analysis of their data (see the entry in Table 1), Zick and co-workers examined the clinical progression of the chronic heart failure patients participating in their placebo-controlled trial.[128] Progression of heart failure occurred in 46.6% of the hawthorn group and 43.3% of the placebo group. However, hawthorn did appear to increase the risk of progression earlier in the trial, and overall for the more severe patients. By their own admission the authors conceded that their study was limited due to the small sample size and the fact that it was a secondary data analysis from a trial designed to measure different outcomes. Such a negative finding was not supported by the larger and longer SPICE study (see above), which in contrast was designed to assess clinical progression as a primary outcome.

The sinus activity of the heart undergoes a natural fluctuation. Short-term fluctuations occur with inhalation and exhalation (sinus arrhythmia) but there are also second-grade

Table 1 Clinical trials of hawthorn in congestive heart failure

First author Year	Total patients	Preparation Daily dose	Study design	Study duration	Congestive heart failure level	Tolerability/safety	Efficacy versus control
Iwamoto M[104] 1981	80	5:1 extract of hawthorn leaves and berries 180 to 270 mg	Double blind, controlled against placebo	6 weeks	NYHA II and III		Overall improvement ($p<0.001$) Subjective symptoms ($p<0.001$) Heart function ($p<0.01$) Dyspnoea ($p<0.01$) Palpitations ($p<0.01$) Cardiac oedema ($p<0.05$) Pulmonary congestion ($p<0.05$)
Hanack T[105] 1983	60	5:1 extract of hawthorn leaves and berries 180 mg	Double blind, randomised, controlled against placebo	3 weeks	NYHA I and II		ECG changes under exertion
O'Connolly M[106] 1986	36	5:1 extract of hawthorn leaves and flowers 180 mg	Double blind, randomised, controlled against placebo	6 weeks	NYHA I and II	No significant adverse effects	Heart rate x systolic BP (blood pressure) Quality of life Anxiety ($p<0.0001$)
O'Connolly M[107] 1987	36	5:1 extract of hawthorn leaves and flowers 180 mg	Double blind, randomised, controlled against placebo	6 weeks	NYHA I and II	No significant adverse effects, 3 patients on hawthorn reported dizziness	Heart rate x systolic BP (at rest and after exercise) ($p<0.001$) Heart rate ($p<0.001$) Systolic BP ($p<0.001$) Diastolic BP ($p<0.001$) Psychological symptoms
Leuchtgens H[108] 1993	30	5:1 extract of hawthorn leaves and flowers 160 mg (containing 30 mg OPCs)	Double blind, randomised, controlled against placebo	8 weeks	NYHA II	No significant adverse effects	Heart rate x systolic BP after exercise ($p<0.05$) Heart rate after exercise
Bodigheimer K[109] 1994	85	3:1 extract of hawthorn leaves and flowers 300 mg (containing 2.2% flavonoids)	Double blind, randomised, controlled against placebo	4 weeks	NYHA II	Well tolerated with only minor side effects observed	*not* Heart rate x systolic BP *not* Exercise tolerance *not* Subjective symptoms
Forster A[110] 1994	72	3:1 extract of hawthorn leaves and flowers 900 mg (containing 2.2% flavonoids)	Double blind, randomised, controlled against placebo	8 weeks	NYHA II	No relevant side effects observed	Exercise tolerance ($p<0.05$) Subjective symptoms ($p<0.01$)
Schmidt U[111] 1994	78	3:1 extract of hawthorn leaves and flowers 600 mg (containing 2.2% flavonoids)	Double blind, randomised, controlled against placebo	8 weeks	NYHA II	No significant adverse effects	Exercise tolerance during bicycle exercise ($p<0.001$) Heart rate ($p<0.01$) Systolic BP ($p<0.05$) Clinical symptoms

Study	N	Treatment	Design	Duration	NYHA class	Tolerability/Safety	Results
Weikl A[112] 1996	136	5:1 extract of hawthorn leaves and flowers 160 mg (containing 30 mg OPCs)	Double blind, randomised, controlled against placebo	8 weeks	NYHA II	Very good tolerability	Heart rate x systolic BP after exercise (p=0.018); Subjective symptoms (quality of life) (p=0.05)
Eichstadt H[113] 2001	40	5:1 extract of hawthorn leaves and flowers 480 mg (containing 90 mg OPCs)	Double blind, randomised, controlled against placebo	4 weeks	NYHA II	Very good tolerability	Left ventricular ejection fraction (LVEF) at rest (p=0.0001) and after exercise (p=0.0002)
Zapfe G[114] 2001	40	5:1 extract of hawthorn leaves and flowers 240 mg (containing 45 mg OPCs)	Double blind, controlled against placebo	12 weeks	NYHA II	Safe and well tolerated on the basis of biochemical and adverse event data	Exercise tolerance (p=0.06); Heart rate x systolic BP
Tauchert M[115] 2002	209	5:1 extract of hawthorn leaves and flowers 1800 mg and 900 mg (containing 18.75 mg OPCs)	Double blind, randomised, 2 doses controlled against placebo	16 weeks	NYHA III	Incidence of adverse effects lowest in the 1800 mg dose group	Maximum workload during bicycle exercise (1800 mg dose only, p=0.013); Subjective symptoms (1800 mg best on all counts, p=0.004)
Zick SM[116] 2009	120	5:1 extract of hawthorn leaves and flowers 900 mg (containing 18.75% OPCs)	Double blind, randomised, controlled against placebo	6 months	NYHA II and III	Significantly more adverse events in the hawthorn group (p=0.02), although most were non-cardiac	*not* Walking distance; *not* Quality of life; Modest improvement in LVEF (p=0.04)
Eichstadt H[117] 1989	20	5:1 extract of hawthorn leaves and flowers 480 mg (containing 90 mg OPCs)	Open label, uncontrolled trial	1 month	NYHA II		Exercise tolerance during bicycle exercise (p<0.05); Subjective symptoms
Weikl A[118] 1992	7	5:1 extract of hawthorn leaves and flowers 240 mg (containing 45 mg OPCs)	Open label, pilot, uncontrolled trial	1 month	NYHA II and III	Good tolerance	LVEF at rest; Complaints List score
Tauchert M[119] 1994	132	3:1 extract of hawthorn leaves and flowers 900 mg (containing 2.2% flavonoids)	Double blind, controlled against 37.5 mg captopril	8 weeks	NYHA II	One captopril patient had to discontinue due to adverse effects; no hawthorn patients withdrew	No significant difference between two treatments on: • heart rate x systolic BP • exercise tolerance. Both groups improved relative to baseline (p<0.001)
Schmidt U[120] 1998 (also reported as Loew D[121])	1476 for efficacy, 3664 for safety	3:1 extract of hawthorn leaves and flowers 900 mg (containing 2.2% flavonoids)	Postmarketing surveillance	8 weeks	NYHA I and II	1.3% of 3664 patients reported adverse reactions: causal relationship confirmed in 0.7%. Included: gastrointestinal, palpitations, headache, dizziness	Heart rate x systolic BP; Diastolic BP; Incidence of arrhythmias; NYHA I patients largely symptom-free

(Continued)

Table 1 (Continued)

First author Year	Total patients	Preparation Daily dose	Study design	Study duration	Congestive heart failure level	Tolerability/safety	Efficacy versus control
Tauchert M[122] 1999	1011	5:1 extract of hawthorn leaves and flowers 900 mg (containing 18.75% OPCs)	Observational	24 weeks	NYHA II	Only 14 adverse reactions were noted. In two cases (abdominal discomfort, facial pain with tachycardia) a possible connection to hawthorn was postulated	Exercise tolerance Heart rate x systolic BP Fatigue and palpitations LVEF Ankle oedema Nocturia
Rietbrook N[123] 2001	88	Standardised extract of fresh hawthorn berries 75 drops	Double blind, controlled against placebo	3 months	NYHA II	Well tolerated	Exercise tolerance QoL (Minnesota score) Dyspnoea-Fatigue Index
Degenring F[124] 2003	143	Extract of fresh hawthorn berries 90 drops (2.25 mL) (containing at least 6.4 mg OPCs)	Double blind, controlled against placebo; intention-to-treat analysis	2 months	NYHA II	The active treatment well tolerated with a high level of patient acceptability	Exercise tolerance (p=0.045) *not* Heart rate x systolic BP *not* Overall assessment *not* Subjective cardiac symptoms
Habs M[125] 2004	952	5:1 extract of hawthorn leaves and flowers at least 450 mg (containing 18.75% OPCs)	Cohort study as add-on to normal treatment (n=588) compared with normal treatment alone (n=364); matched-pairs analysis on 130 patient pairs	2 years	NYHA II		Reduction in other prescriptions for hawthorn group: • ACEs inhibitors (p=0.004) • cardiac glycosides (p=0.001) • diuretics (p=0.061) • beta-blockers (p=0.052) Both groups improved equally clinically, but less marked for hawthorn were: • fatigue (p=0.036) • stress dyspnoea (p=0.02) • palpitations (p=0.048)

variations associated with blood pressure rhythm. With age, diabetes and damage to the heart, this variability of heart rate decreases. Low heart rate variability (HRV) is a risk factor in coronary heart disease and there is a positive correlation between HRV and life-expectancy.[129] The effect of an extract of hawthorn leaves, flowers and berries (containing 45 mg/day flavonoids) was studied in 20 geriatric patients over 6 weeks in a randomised, double blind, placebo-controlled trial.[130] Patients with a coefficient of variation (CV) in heart rate of less than 5% were chosen for the study. Those with frequent ectopic beats and diabetes were excluded and the average age of patients was about 80 years. A small but statistically significant positive effect was seen for the hawthorn group (p<0.01): the CV of heart rate rose steadily over the 6-week treatment period from 1.9% to 2.5% while there was no change in the placebo group. The authors postulated that this effect might become more marked over longer treatment periods. The improvement in HRV was dramatic in some patients given hawthorn.

The same extract was given at the same dose to nine healthy volunteers for 4 weeks in a placebo-controlled trial.[131] At the end of the trial, the heart rate × systolic blood pressure products were significantly lower in the hawthorn group after exercise (p=0.04). Responsiveness to exogenous catecholamines was not altered.

A case study was described of a 64-year-old male patient scheduled for internal defibrillator placement.[132] After the patient was prescribed a combination of oral coenzyme Q10 (100 mg/day), hawthorn extract (450 mg/day) and chelated magnesium (350 mg/day) his symptoms and ventricular function improved and 11 months later he was not yet needing the surgical procedure.

Hawthorn was also beneficial in combination with passionflower. In a randomised, double blind, placebo-controlled study, 40 patients with dyspnoea commensurate with NYHA stage II received either a hawthorn and passionflower extract combination or placebo over 6 weeks. Exercise capacity, measured in terms of a walking test, increased significantly in those patients receiving the herbal preparation (p<0.05). A slight but significant decrease in heart rate at rest and mean diastolic blood pressure during exercise, and a decrease in total plasma cholesterol, were observed in the group receiving the extract.[21] The two groups did not differ significantly in the other tests: maximum exercise capacity measured during a bicycle ergometer test, subjective assessment of breathlessness or blood lactate levels, although the trend favoured the herbal group.

In early studies, patients previously unsuccessfully treated with digoxin alone were compensated for rest and slight stress with relatively low oral doses of the glycoside in combination with hawthorn.[133,134]

Blood pressure

In an early uncontrolled trial, mean systolic pressure fell from 205 mmHg to 148 mmHg and mean diastolic pressure fell from 112 mmHg to 83 mmHg in hypertensive patients receiving hawthorn berry tincture. When treatment was stopped, blood pressures returned to their initial values over a 2-week period. There was only a slight effect on subjects with normal blood pressure.[135] Other clinical studies (see Table 1) sometimes demonstrate that hawthorn extract resulted in a slight reduction in blood pressure in patients with chronic heart failure.

A pilot study investigated the hypotensive potential of hawthorn extract (500 mg/day of a 3:1 extract of leaves and flowers containing 1.8% flavonoids) and magnesium (600 mg/day), individually and in combination, compared to a placebo in a randomised, double blind trial.[136] In all, 36 mildly hypertensive patients completed the 10-week study. Due to the small patient numbers in each group, only the hawthorn group demonstrated any clinical effects, with trends to lowered diastolic blood pressure (p=0.081) and reduced anxiety (p=0.094).

A follow-up randomised, controlled trial was undertaken among outpatients in general practices to investigate the effect of hawthorn on hypertension in patients with type 2 diabetes taking prescribed drugs. Patients (n=79) were randomised 1200 mg/day of the same hawthorn extract as above (n=39) or placebo (n=40) for 16 weeks. Hypotensive drugs were already being used by 71% of the study population, with a mean intake of 4.4 hypoglycaemic and/or hypotensive drugs per patient. After 16 weeks, the hawthorn group showed greater reductions in diastolic blood pressure (baseline: 85.6 mmHg, 95% CI 83.3 to 87.8; outcome: 83.0 mmHg, 95% CI 80.5 to 85.7) than the placebo group (baseline: 84.5 mmHg, 95% CI 82 to 87; outcome: 85.0 mmHg, 95% CI 82.2 to 87.8) (p=0.035). There was no group difference in systolic blood pressure reduction from baseline. No herb-drug interactions were found and minor health complaints were reduced from baseline in both groups.[137]

In a double blind, placebo-controlled clinical trial involving 92 men and women with primary mild hypertension, a hydroalcoholic extract of the leaves and flowers of *Crataegus curvisepala* showed a significant decrease in both systolic and diastolic blood pressures after 3 months (p<0.05).[138]

Interestingly a combination of hawthorn berry extract and camphor has successfully treated orthostatic and chronic hypotension in a number of clinical trials.[139–141] The typical daily doses from the combination are 25 mg of camphor and around 1000 mg of fresh hawthorn berry extract. The same combination also improved low blood pressure and cognitive function in the elderly in a randomised, placebo-controlled, double blind trial.[142]

Other conditions

In an uncontrolled, multicentre trial, 50 patients with and without acne in various stages of development uniformly applied one to two ampoules of liposome-containing hawthorn extract to the most affected areas of the skin each day for at least 30 days. The hawthorn extract demonstrated a general capillary-protective activity which resulted in the reduction or disappearance of capillary congestion. A mild anti-inflammatory activity was demonstrated by a significant reduction in acne and erythema. (The improvement in stratum corneum hydration and roughness of skin and the antiseborrhoeic effect were attributed to the phosphatidylcholine liposomes.)[5]

A combination of hawthorn leaves and flowers extract (300 mg/day), Californian poppy (*Eschscholtzia californica*) extract (80 mg/day) and magnesium (300 mg/day) was assessed against placebo in a 3-month randomised, double blind clinical trial involving 264 patients with mild-to-moderate generalised anxiety (DSM-III-R).[143] Total and somatic Hamilton anxiety scale scores and subjective patient-rated anxiety fell during treatment and were significantly different to placebo (p=0.005, p=0.054 and p=0.005, respectively). Adverse reactions were similar in the treatment and placebo groups.

Toxicology and other safety data

Toxicology

Studies involving excessive dosing of hawthorn flower extract (600 mg/kg/day, undefined extract strength, 4.4% flavonoids) over 30 days in rats showed unremarkable adverse effects.[144]

The acute oral toxicity in undefined animals of hawthorn was 6 g/kg. No target organ toxicity was defined at 100 times the human dose (2.7 mg/kg) of concentrated hawthorn extract. Standard mutagenic and clastogenic tests were also negative.[145] A study in mice demonstrated a high LD_{50} of 13.5 g/kg for an aqueous extract of *C. laevigata*.[90]

Schimmer and co-workers found that an ethanolic extract of Crataegus was weakly mutagenic in the Salmonella test, a finding which they attributed to the quercetin content of the extract.[146] Popp and co-workers found a DNA-damaging potency of commercial Crataegus preparations in human lymphocyte cultures.[147] The active principles were not identified but were probably flavonoids. Several procyanidins with different degrees of polymerisation (dimers, a trimer and a polymer) were found to be non-mutagenic in the Salmonella mutagenesis assay system.[148]

Contraindications

None known.

Special warnings and precautions

Not to be used concomitantly with heart and blood pressure medication unless supervised by a suitably qualified herbal practitioner or physician.

Interactions

Speculation on a harmful interaction with digoxin has not been borne out in any study.[149] A large number of patients, previously unsuccessfully treated with digoxin alone, were compensated for rest and slight stress with relatively low oral doses of the glycoside in combination with hawthorn and without evidence of adverse effects.[133,134] A randomised, crossover trial published in 2003 involving eight healthy volunteers confirmed that standardised hawthorn extract (leaf and flower extract, 900 mg/day) and digoxin may be safely co-administered.[150]

Hawthorn may act in synergy with digitalis, glycosides, beta-blockers and other hypotensive drugs. Modification of drug dosage may be required. There is also a suggestion from one in vitro study that hawthorn may interfere with one specific method of serum digoxin assay (the Digoxin III immunoassay).[151]

Use in pregnancy and lactation

Category B1 – no increase in frequency of malformation or other harmful effects on the fetus from limited use in women. No evidence of increased fetal damage in animal studies.

At a high oral dose of 2.8 g/kg administered from days 1 to 15 of gestation, hawthorn (part undefined) did not have an adverse effect on reproductive outcome in rats. Fetal weights were slightly increased when the herb was administered from days 8 to 15 of gestation. There were no differences in placental weight, the number of resorptions and litter size and no externally visible malformations. The herb was administered as an ethanol extract and the dose administered was the highest possible for which ethanol remained below the teratogenic threshold.[152] Pregnant rats given 56 times the human dose of hawthorn orally did not exhibit any adverse effects.[153] Hawthorn also did not influence embryonic development in vitro.

Hawthorn is compatible with breastfeeding.

Effects on ability to drive and use machines

No adverse effects expected.

Side effects

An assessment has been made of the safety data from all available human studies on hawthorn products, including library and online searches, and data from the WHO Centre for International Drug Monitoring (18 case reports) and manufacturers. A total of 7311 patients had been enrolled in 24 clinical trials, and data from 5577 patients were available for analysis. Overall, 166 adverse events were identified. Most of these adverse events were mild to moderate. The most frequent adverse events were dizziness/vertigo (n=15), gastrointestinal complaints (n=24), headache (n=9), migraine (n=8) and palpitation (n=11). More severe reactions were falls (n=2), gastrointestinal haemorrhage (n=2), circulation failure (n=2) and erythematous rash (n=2). There were no reports of drug interactions.[154] (See also Table 1 and the discussion of the SPICE study for further information regarding side effects during clinical trials.)

One case of a type I hypersensitivity reaction to hawthorn has been reported.[155]

Overdosage

Not known.

Safety in children

No information available but adverse effects are not expected.

Regulatory status in selected countries

Hawthorn berries, leaf and flower are official in the *British Pharmacopoeia* 2011 and the *European Pharmacopoeia* 2011.

Hawthorn leaf with flower is official in the *United States Pharmacopeia–National Formulary* USP31 NF26 2008.

Hawthorn berry, hawthorn leaf and hawthorn flower are covered by null Commission E monographs. The Commission E suggests that, as the efficacy of hawthorn berry, leaf or flower has not been documented, no therapeutic application can be recommended. In contrast, hawthorn leaf with flower is covered by a positive Commission E monograph and can be used to treat decreased cardiac output as described in functional stage II of NYHA.

Hawthorn is now on the UK General Sale List.

Hawthorn does not have GRAS status. However, it is freely available as a 'dietary supplement' in the USA under DSHEA legislation (1994 Dietary Supplement Health and Education Act).

Hawthorn is not included in Part 4 of Schedule 4 of the Therapeutic Goods Act Regulations which lists herbal substances restricted from free sale within Australia.

References

1. Grieve M. *A Modern Herbal*, vol. 1. New York: Dover Publications; 1971. p. 385.
2. British Herbal Medicine Association Scientific Committee. *British Herbal Pharmacopoeia*. Cowling: BHMA; 1983. pp. 74–75.
3. Felter HW, Lloyd JU. *King's American Dispensatory*. ed 18, rev 3, vol 2, 1905. Portland: Reprinted by Eclectic Medical Publications; 1983. p. 1613.
4. Chang HM, But PP. *Pharmacology and Applications of Chinese Materia Medica*, vol. 1. Singapore: World Scientific; 1987. pp. 100–107.
5. Longhi MG, Rocchi P, Gezzi A, et al. *Fitoterapia*. 1984;55(2):87–99.
6. Launert EL. *The Hamlyn Guide to Edible and Medicinal Plants of Britain and Northern Europe*. London: Hamlyn; 1981. p. 76.
7. Chiej R. *The Macdonald Encyclopedia of Medicinal Plants*. London: Macdonald; 1984. Entry no. 99.
8. Byatt JI. *Bot J Linn Soc*. 1974;69:15–21.
9. Mabberley DJ. *The Plant Book*, 2nd ed. Cambridge: Cambridge University Press; 1997. p. 190.
10. Byatt JI. *Watsonia*. 1975;10:253–264.
11. Bevan J. *Watsonia*. 1980;13(2):119–121.
12. Christensen KI. *Acta Univ Upsaliensis Symb Bot Ups*. 1996;31(3):211–220.
13. Wagner H, Bladt S. *Plant Drug Analysis: A Thin Layer Chromatography Atlas*, 2nd ed. Berlin: Springer-Verlag; 1996. p. 198.
14. Prinz S, Ringl A, Heufner A, et al. *Chem Biodivers*. 2007;4(12):2920–2931.
15. Bisset NG, ed. *Herbal Drugs and Phytopharmaceuticals*. Stuttgart: Medpharm Scientific Publishers; 1994.p. 162.
16. Kartnig T, Hiermann A, Azzam S. *Sci Pharm*. 1987;55(2):95–100.
17. Porter LJ, Woodruffe J. *Phytochemistry*. 1984;23(6):1255–1256.
18. Bilia AR, Eterno F, Bergonzi MC, et al. *J Pharm Biomed Anal*. 2007;44(1):70–78.
19. Masquellier J. In: Beal JL, Reinhard E, eds. *Natural Products as Medicinal Agents*. Stuttgart: Hippokrates-Verlag; 1981. pp. 243–256.
20. Michaud J, Masquellier J. *Prod Probl Pharm*. 1973;28(7):499–520.
21. Von Eiff M, Brunner H, Haegeli A, et al. *Acta Therapeut*. 1994;20(1–2):47–66.
22. Ammon HPT, Handel M. *Planta Med*. 1981;43(2):105–120.
23. Ammon HPT, Handel M. *Planta Med*. 1981;43(3):209–239.
24. Ammon HPT, Handel M. *Planta Med*. 1981;43(4):313–322.
25. Occhiuto F, Circosta C, Costa R, et al. *Plantes Med Phytother*. 1986;20(1):52–63.
26. Petkov E, Nikdov N, Uzunov P. *Planta Med*. 1981;43(2):183–186.
27. Popping S, Rose H, Ionescu I, et al. *Arzneimittelforschung*. 1995;45(11):1157–1161.
28. Schwinger RH, Pietsch M, Frank K, et al. *J Cardiovasc Pharmacol*. 2000;35(5):700–707.
29. Trunzler G, Schuler E. *Arzneimittelforschung*. 1962;12:198–202.
30. Schussler M, Holzl J, Fricke U. *Arzneimittelforschung*. 1995;5(8):842–845.
31. Leukel A, Fricke U, Holzl J. *Planta Med*. 1986;52:545–546.
32. Roddewig C, Hensel H. *Arzneimittelforschung*. 1977;27(7):1407–1410.
33. Manalov P, Daleva L. *Farmatsiya (Sofia)*. 1969;19(3):38–44.
34. Manalov P. *Suvrem Med*. 1971;22:20–23.
35. Petrov L, Gagov S, Popova A. *Acta Physiol Pharmacol Bulg*. 1974;2:82–89.
36. Liévre M, Andrieu JL, Baconin A. *Ann Pharm Franc*. 1985;43(5):471–477.
37. Bleske BE, Zineh I, Hwang HS, et al. *Med Sci Monit*. 2007;13(12):BR255–BR258.
38. Hwang HS, Bleske BE, Ghannam MM, et al. *Cardiovasc Drugs Ther*. 2008;22(1):19–28.
39. Hwang HS, Boluyt MO, Converso K, et al. *Pharmacotherapy*. 2009;29(6):639–648.
40. Chatterjee SS, Koch E, Jaggy H, et al. *Arzneimittelforschung*. 1997;47(7):821–825.
41. Al Makdessi S, Sweidan H, Mullner S, et al. *Arzneimittelforschung*. 1996;46(1):25–27.
42. Ciplea AG, Richter KD. *Arzneimittelforschung*. 1988;38(11):1583–1592.
43. Kanno T, Toshihiro S, Yamamoto M. *Jpn Heart J*. 1976;17:512–520.
44. Frank E, Heymanns E. *Arztl Forsch*. 1956;10:248–254.
45. Kandziora J. *MMW*. 1969;111:295–298.
46. Guendjev Z. *Arzneimittelforschung*. 1977;27(8):1576–1579.
47. Jayalakshmi R, Niranjali Devaraj S. *J Pharm Pharmacol*. 2004;56(7):921–926.
48. Jayalakshmi R, Thirupurasundari CJ, Devaraj SN. *Mol Cell Biochem*. 2006;292(1–2):59–67.
49. Nasa Y, Hashizume H, Hoque AN, et al. *Arzneimittelforschung*. 1993;43(9):945–949.
50. Rothfuss MA, Pascht U, Kissling G. *Arzneimittelforschung*. 2001;51(1):24–28.
51. Veveris M, Koch E, Chatterjee SS. *Life Sci*. 2004;74(15):1945–1955.
52. Swaminathan JK, Khan M, Mohan IK, et al. *Phytomedicine*. 2010;17(10):744–752.
53. Jayachandran KS, Khan M, Selvendiran K, et al. *J Cardiovasc Pharmacol*. 2010;56(5):526–531.
54. Ernst F-D, Reuther G, Walper A. *Munch Med Wochenschr*. 1994;136(suppl 1):S57–S59.
55. Rogers KL, Grice ID, Griffiths LR. *Eur J Pharm Sci*. 2000;9(4):355–363.
56. Vibes J, Lasserre B, Gleye J, et al. *Prostagland Leukot Essent Fatty Acids*. 1994;50(4):173–175.
57. Stepka W, Winters AD. *Lloydia*. 1973;36:436.
58. Braasch W, Bienroth W. *Arzneimittelforschung*. 1960;10:127–129.
59. Fischer K, Jung F, Koscielny J, et al. *Munch Med Wochenschr*. 1994;136(suppl 1):S35–S38.
60. Kim SH, Kang KW, Kim KW, Kim ND. *Life Sci*. 2000;67(2):121–131.
61. Brixius K, Willms S, Napp A, et al. *Cardiovasc Drugs Ther*. 2006;20(3):177–184.

62. Anselm E, Socorro VF, Dal-Ros S, et al. *J Cardiovasc Pharmacol.* 2009;53(3):253–260.

63. Lacaille-Dubois MA, Franck U, Wagner H. *Phytomedicine.* 2001;8(1):47–52.

64. Joseph G, Zhao Y, Klaus W. *Arzneimittelforschung.* 1995;45(12):1261–1265.

65. Muller A, Linke W, Zhao Y, et al. *Phytomedicine.* 1996;3(3):257–261.

66. Salehi S, Long SR, Proteau PJ, et al. *Nat Med (Tokyo).* 2009;63(1):1–8.

67. Rodriguez ME, Poindexter BJ, Bick RJ, et al. *J Med Food.* 2008;11(4):680–686.

68. Long SR, Carey RA, Crofoot KM, et al. *Phytomedicine.* 2006;13(9–10):643–650.

69. Furst R, Zirrgiebel U, Totzke F, et al. *Atherosclerosis.* 2010;211(2):409–417.

70. Corder R, Warburton RC, Khan NQ, et al. *Clin Sci (Lond).* 2004;107(5):513–517.

71. Rajendran S, Deepalakshmi PD, Parasakthy K, et al. *Atherosclerosis.* 1996;123(1–2):235–241.

72. Zhang Z, Ho WK, Huang Y, et al. *J Nutr.* 2002;132(1):5–10.

73. Lin Y, Vermeer MA, Trautwein EA. *Evid Based Complement Altern Med.* 2009. [Published online 19 February 2009].

74. Ye XL, Huang WW, Chen Z, et al. *J Agric Food Chem.* 2010;58(5):3132–3138.

75. Bahorun T, Trotin F, Pommery J, et al. *Planta Med.* 1994;60(4):323–328.

76. Bernatoniene J, Masteikova R, Majiene D, et al. *Medicina (Kaunas).* 2008;44(9):706–712.

77. Masteikova R, Muselik J, Bernatoniene J, et al. *Ceska Slov Farm.* 2008;57(1):35–38.

78. Zhang Z, Chang Q, Zhu M, et al. *J Nutr Biochem.* 2001;12(3):144–152.

79. Quettier-Deleu C, Voiselle G, Fruchart JC, et al. *Pharmazie.* 2003;58(8):577–581.

80. Dai Y, Gao CM, Tian QL, et al. *Planta Med.* 1987;53(3):309–310.

81. Akila M, Devaraj H. *Vascul Pharmacol.* 2008;49(4–6):173–177.

82. Thirupurasundari CJ, Jayalakshmi R, Niranjali *J Med Food.* 2005;8(3):400–404.

83. Gali HU, Perchellet EM, Gao XM, et al. *Planta Med.* 1994;60(3):235–239.

84. Kao ES, Wang CJ, Lin WL, et al. *Food Chem Toxicol.* 2007;45(10):1795–1804.

85. Tadic VM, Dobric S, Markovic GM, et al. *J Agric Food Chem.* 2008;56(17):7700–7709.

86. Shahat AA, Cos P, De Bruyne T, et al. *Planta Med.* 2002;68(6):539–541.

87. Can OD, Ozkay UD, Ozturk N, et al. *Pharm Biol.* 2010;48(8):924–931.

88. Elango C, Jayachandaran KS, Devaraj NS. *Int J Dev Neurosci.* 2009;27(8):799–803.

89. Li H, Song F, Xing J, et al. *J Am Soc Mass Spectrom.* 2009;20(8):1496–1503.

90. Jouad H, Lemhadri A, Maghrani M, et al. *J Herb Pharmacother.* 2003;3(2):19–29.

91. Dalli E, Milara J, Cortijo J, et al. *Pharmacol Res.* 2008;57(6):445–450.

92. Fujisawa M, Oguchi K, Yamaura T, et al. *Am J Chin Med.* 2005;33(2):167–180.

93. Fan C, Yan J, Qian Y, et al. *J Pharmacol Sci.* 2006;100(1):51–58.

94. Leskovac A, Joksic G, Jankovic T, et al. *Planta Med.* 2007;73(11):1169–1175.

95. Hosseinimehr SJ, Azadbakht M, Mousavi SM, et al. *J Radiat Res (Tokyo).* 2007;48(1):63–68.

96. Hosseinimehr SJ, Mahmoudzadeh A, Azadbakht M, et al. *Radiat Environ Biophys.* 2009;48(1):95–98.

97. Laparra J, Michaud J, Masquelier J. *Plantes Med Phytother.* 1977;11:133.

98. Middleton Jr. E. *Trends Pharmacol Sci.* 1984;5(8):335–338.

99. Chang Q, Zuo Z, Ho WK, et al. *J Clin Pharmacol.* 2005;45(1):106–112.

100. Zuo Z, Zhang L, Zhou L, et al. *Life Sci.* 2006;79(26):2455–2462.

101. Liang M, Xu W, Zhang W, et al. *Biomed Chromatogr.* 2007;21(4):422–429.

102. Xu YA, Fan G, Gao S, et al. *Drug Dev Ind Pharm.* 2008;34(2):164–170.

103. Ma LY, Liu RH, Xu XD, et al. *Phytomedicine.* 2010;17(8–9):640–645.

104. Iwamoto M, Ishizaki T, Sato T. *Planta Med.* 1981;42(1):1–16.

105. Hanack T, Bruckel MH. *Therapiewoche.* 1983;33:4331–4333.

106. O'Connolly M, Jansen W, Bernhoft G, et al. *Fortschr Med.* 1986;104(42):805–808.

107. O'Connolly M, Bernhoft G, Bartsch G. *Therapiewoche.* 1987;37(38):3587–3600.

108. Leuchtgens H. *Fortschr Med.* 1993;111(20–21):36–38.

109. Bodigheimer K, Chase D. *Munch Med Wochenschr.* 1994;136(suppl 1):S7–S11.

110. Forster A, Forster K, Buhring M, et al. *Munch Med Wochenschr.* 1994;136 (suppl 1):S21–S26.

111. Schmidt U, Kuhn M, Ploch M, et al. *Phytomedicine.* 1994;1:17–24.

112. Weikl A, Assmus KD, Neukum-Schmidt A, et al. *Fortschr Med.* 1996;114(24):291–296.

113. Eichstadt H, Stork T, Mockel M, et al. *Perfusion.* 2001;14(6):212–217.

114. Zapfe G. *Phytomedicine.* 2001;8:262–266.

115. Tauchert M. *Am Heart J.* 2002;143(5):910–915.

116. Zick SM, Vautaw BM, Gillespie B, et al. *Eur J Heart Fail.* 2009;11(10):990–999.

117. Eichstadt H, Bader M, Danne O, et al. *Therapiewoche.* 1989;39:3288–3296.

118. Weikl A, Noh H. *Herz Gefasse.* 1992;12:516–524.

119. Tauchert M, Ploch M, Hubner WD, et al. *Munch Med Wochenschr.* 1994;136(suppl 1):S27–S33.

120. Schmidt U, Albrecht M, Podzuweit H, et al. *Z Phytother.* 1998;19:22–30.

121. Loew D, Albrecht M, Podzuweit *Phytomedicine.* 1996;3(suppl 1):92. Abstract SL-70.

122. Tauchert M, Gildor A, Lipinski J. *Herz.* 1999;24:465–474.

123. Rietbrock N, Hamel M, Hempel B, et al. *Arzneimittelforschung.* 2001;51(10):793–798.

124. Degenring FH, Suter A, Weber M, et al. *Phytomedicine.* 2003;10(5):363–369.

125. Habs M. *Forsch Komplementarmed Klass Naturheilkd.* 2004:36–39.

126. Pittler MH, Guo R, Ernst E. *Cochrane Database Syst Rev.* 2008;1:CD005312.

127. Holubarsch CJ, Colucci WS, Meinertz T, et al. *Eur J Heart Fail.* 2008;10(12):1255–1263.

128. Zick SM, Gillespie B, Aaronson KD. *Eur J Heart Fail.* 2008;10(6):587–593.

129. Kleiger RE, Miller JP, Bigger Jr JT, et al. *Am J Cardiol.* 1987;59(4):256–262.

130. Rudolph HT, Erben C, Buhring M. *International Congress on Phytotherapy.* Munich, Sept 10–13, 1992.

131. Hellenbrecht D, Saller R, Ruckbeil C, et al. *Eur J Pharmacol.* 1990;183(2):525–526.

132. Islam J, Uretsky BF, Sierpina VS. *Explore (NY).* 2006;2(4):339–341.

133. Wolkerstorfer H. *MMW.* 1966;108:438–441.

134. Jaursch U, Landers E, Schmidt R, et al. *Med Welt.* 1969;27:1547–1552.

135. Graham JDP. *Br Med J.* 1939;2(4114):951–953.

136. Walker AF, Marakis G, Morris AP, et al. *Phytother Res.* 2002;16(1):48–54.

137. Walker AF, Marakis G, Simpson E, et al. *Br J Gen Pract.* 2006;56(527):437–443.

138. Asgary S, Naderi GH, Sadeghi M, et al. *Drugs Exp Clin Res.* 2004;30(38843):221–225.

139. Kroll M, Ring C, Gaus W, et al. *Phytomedicine.* 2005;12(6–7):395–402.

140. Belz GG, Butzer R, Gaus W, et al. *Phytomedicine.* 2002;9(7):581–588.

141. Schandry R, Duschek S. *Phytomedicine.* 2008;15(11):914–922.

142. Werner NS, Duschek S, Schandry R. *Phytomedicine.* 2009;16(12):1077–1082.

143. Hanus M, Lafon J, Mathieu M. *Curr Med Res Opin.* 2004;20(1):63–71.

144. Fehri B, Aiache JM, Boukef K, et al. *J Pharm Belg.* 1991;46(3):165–176.

145. Schlegelmilch R, Heywood R. *J Am Coll Toxicol.* 1994;13(2):103–111.

146. Schimmer O, Hafele F, Kruger A. *Mutat Res.* 1988;206(2):201–208.

147. Popp R, Paulini H, Volkl S, et al. *Planta Med.* 1989;55(7):644–645.

148. Yu CL, Swaminathan B. *Food Chem Toxicol.* 1987;25(2):135–140.

149. Miller LG. *Arch Intern Med.* 1998;158(20):2200–2211.

150. Tankanow R, Tamer HR, Streetman DS, et al. *J Clin Pharmacol.* 2003;43(6):637–642.

151. Dasgupta A, Kidd L, Poindexter BJ, et al. *Arch Pathol Lab Med.* 2010;134(8):1188–1192.

152. Yao M, Brown-Woodman PDC, Ritchie H. *Teratology.* 2001;64:320–325.

153. Yao M, Ritchie HE, Brown-Woodman PD. *J Ethnopharmacol.* 2008;118(1):127–132.

154. Daniele C, Mazzanti G, Pittler MH, Ernst E. *Drug Saf.* 2006;29(6):523–535.

155. Steinman HK, Lovell CR, Cronin E. *Contact Dermatitis.* 1984;11(5):321.

Horsechestnut seed

(*Aesculus hippocastanum* L.)

Synonyms

Hippocastani semen (Lat), Robkastaniensamen (Ger), graine de marronier d'Inde, aescule (Fr), eschilo (Ital), hestekastanje (Dan).

What is it?

The horsechestnut tree (*Aesculus hippocastanum* L.) is mainly grown as an ornamental in parks and gardens in Europe, although it is in fact a native of Asia Minor. Horsechestnut seeds and bark have been extensively used in European herbal medicine since the 16th century and a wine based on the flowers was imbibed for neuralgia and arthritis. The flowers and flower buds are now used to make two of the Bach Flower Remedies. However, this monograph will only describe the herbal use of the seed, principally for the improvement of vein health. Unlike true chestnuts, the seeds of the horsechestnut are not edible, although a specially prepared seed meal has been used as fodder. While it is sometimes regarded as a toxic herb, there is no suggestion from published trials that the normal use of the seed causes toxic effects.

Effects

Increases venous tone, improves capillary resistance, decreases capillary permeability, improves circulation by toning veins; decreases oedema resulting from lymphatic congestion or inflammation.

Traditional view

Horsechestnut seed (hereafter referred to as horsechestnut) was traditionally used in the treatment of rheumatism and neuralgia and conditions of venous congestion, particularly with dull, aching pain and fullness. Other major uses include rectal complaints (particularly haemorrhoids, rectal neuralgia and proctitis) and reflex conditions attributed to rectal involvement (including headache, spasmodic asthma, dizziness and disturbed digestion). It was regarded as a remedy for congestion and engorgement. Uneasy and throbbing sensations, with dull aching pain in any part of the body, but especially in the hepatic region, was one specific indication.[1,2]

Summary actions

Venotonic, anti-oedematous, anti-inflammatory.

Can be used for

Indications supported by clinical trials

Chronic venous insufficiency (high level evidence), varicose veins, varicose ulcer, oedema of the lower limbs. Prophylactic use to decrease the incidence of deep venous thrombosis following surgery (low level evidence). Topically for haematoma, contusions, non-penetrating wounds and sports injuries involving oedema (typically in combination).

Traditional therapeutic uses

Venous problems (especially varicose veins, haemorrhoids); rheumatism; neuralgia; rectal complaints; disease states associated with inflammatory congestion.

May also be used for

Extrapolations from pharmacological studies

To improve circulation by improving venous tone (peripheral vascular disorders, slow-healing leg ulcers); disorders where local tissue oedema may be involved (such as carpal tunnel syndrome, Bell's palsy, congestive dysmenorrhoea, trigeminal neuralgia, intervertebral disc lesions, compression neuropathies); conditions requiring treatment in the early phase of inflammation, such as soft tissue injuries, swelling, minor surgery.

Other applications

Skin care products: for normal skin, baby skin, sensitive skin; to tone the skin; as an anti-inflammatory; to treat fragile capillaries, pimples, sunburn or cellulite.[3] Topically for antiageing effects on skin.

Preparations

Decoction of dried or fresh seeds, tincture, liquid extract, capsules and tablets for internal use. Decoction, extract, cream, gel or ointment for topical use.

Dosage

- 1 to 2 g/day of dried seed
- Horsechestnut tablets or capsules (200 mg of 5:1 concentrated extract, standardised to contain 40 to 50 mg beta-escin): two to three tablets/day

- 2 to 6 mL/day of 1:2 liquid extract, 5 to 15 mL/day of 1:5 tincture
- Preparations containing at least 100 mg/day of beta-escin.

Duration of use

There is no suggestion that the long-term use of horsechestnut should be restricted.

Summary assessment of safety

Despite its inclusion in texts on poisonous plants, there is a very low risk associated with the oral or topical administration of horsechestnut seed.[4]

Technical data

Botany

The horsechestnut, a member of the Hippocastanaceae (buckeye family), is a deciduous tree with grey bark that grows to 25 m. The leaves are opposite and palmate with five to seven strongly ribbed leaflets. The flowers are white with yellow to pink spots, contain five petals and are arranged in noticeable panicles up to 30 cm long. The fruit has a leathery, prickly capsule (the conker) and contains one to two brown seeds with large whitish scar.[5,6]

Adulteration

No known adulterants.

Key constituents

- Saponins (3% to 6%), referred to as escin (which is a complex mixture of over 30 individual pentacyclic triterpene diester glycosides).[7] Beta-escin is a subfraction of escin containing only 22-O-acetyl compounds
- Flavonoids, lipids, sterols.[8,9]

Although from a phytochemical perspective escin and beta-escin are not equivalent, in most products and studies the 'escin' being referred to is actually beta-escin.

Pharmacodynamics

Escin (also spelt 'aescin') was a registered drug in Germany and is the active ingredient in a number of preparations used either topically or orally for the treatment of peripheral vascular disease, in particular that related to altered capillary permeability and resistance. (For conditions associated with oedema it is mainly administered by injection see under Clinical trials.)

Venotonic, vascular protective and anti-oedema activity

Most of the pharmacological research on horsechestnut and escin was conducted prior to 2000; hence a 2001 review still has relevance. This review noted research supporting three key pharmacological actions, namely anti-oedematous, anti-inflammatory and venotonic.[10] The review suggested that all of these appear to be due to a basic molecular mechanism: selective vascular permeabilisation, allowing a higher sensitivity of calcium channels (for example) to molecular ions, resulting in increased venous and arterial tone. In a sense the

R¹= OH (aglycone: barringtogenol C)
R¹= H (aglycone: protoaescigenin)
R²= tigloyl, angelicoyl, 2-methylbutyryl, or isobutyryl

Escin (aescin)

Beta-aescin: major glycosides consist of aglycones protoaescigenin or barringtogenol C esterified with tiglic acid, angelic acid, 2-methylbutyric acid or isobutyric acid anti-oedematous effect is a key feature of the anti-inflammatory activity of horsechestnut and underlies much of its value in conditions linked to local inflammation, with associated swelling and pressure on other structures.

The review goes on to state that these sensitising effects to ions and other molecules such as serotonin probably result in enhanced venous contractile activity, leading to the venotonic effect.[10] In fact, escin can be used as a pharmacological tool to assess the sensitivity of vascular tissues to different agonists.

Escin reduced the localised oedema associated with inflammation[11] probably by reducing capillary permeability to water, thereby decreasing exudation into intercellular spaces.[12] It induced contraction of isolated portal vein and stimulated the generation and release of prostaglandin F_2-alpha in vitro. Hence this antiexudative activity of escin may be mediated by prostaglandin F_2-alpha.[13] Escin administered by injection inhibited oedema induced by several agents in rat paw, but was not effective in models representing the late reparative (proliferative) phase of inflammation.[14,15] This suggests it acts more specifically on the initial stages of inflammation. In contrast, a study using carrageenan-induced paw oedema and induced capillary permeability in mice found that escin (2 mg/kg, by injection) was a potent and long-lasting anti-inflammatory agent without immunosuppressive activity.[16] Parenteral administration of escin to rats indicated the antiexudative activity resulted from an influence on the small pores of the capillary wall (through which fluid is exchanged).[17] Tests conducted on adrenalectomised and hypophysectomised animals indicated the normal production of corticosteroids is necessary for the anti-oedema activity. Escin thus mimics and relies upon the activity of corticosteroids[18–20] and it exerts a synergistic anti-inflammatory effect with low doses of glucocorticoids in vivo and in vitro.[21] Oral administration of escin demonstrated antiexudative and anti-inflammatory activity in another in vivo study. The activity occurred in both prophylaxis and treatment and was due to a beneficial effect on permeability and diuresis.[22] Topical application of escin also significantly inhibited exudation in vivo.[23]

Additional studies have examined the endothelial cell protective activity of escin. Human vascular endothelial cells were exposed to cobalt chloride to mimic hypoxia and to *Escherichia coli* lipopolysaccharide to mimic inflammation.[24] Pretreatment with escin prevented both the induced hypoxia and inflammation, as measured by factors such as the expression of vascular cell adhesion molecule 1 and the reduction of platelet endothelial cell adhesion molecule 1. Escin enhanced endothelium-dependent relaxation in rat aortic rings induced by acetylcholine when such relaxation had been reduced by pyrogallol, a generator of the superoxide radical.[25]

The whole extract of the horsechestnut also shares these properties of escin. In fact, some writers suggest that the combination of escin with flavonoids, as found in the natural plant extract, is a superior treatment to escin alone. Horsechestnut extract demonstrated venotonic activity in vitro by inducing the contraction of isolated vein preparations. Perfusion with horsechestnut extract increased the venous pressure of normal veins and, with prior administration, pathological veins.[26] During perfusion in the opposite direction

to blood flow, a clear contractile effect on the valves was obtained. Horsechestnut extract (2.5, 5.0 mg/kg, iv) increased femoral venous pressure and flow, as well as thoracic lymphatic flow, with no change in arterial parameters. A more recent in vitro study found that horsechestnut extract dose-dependently contracted both veins and arteries, with veins being the most sensitive.[27] ADP-induced platelet aggregation was also significantly reduced. Escin (as the sodium salt) in vitro also contracts blood vessels at lower concentrations (rat aorta).[28]

Oral administration of a horsechestnut standardised extract (HCSE, 50 to 400 mg/kg, containing 70% escin) reduced cutaneous capillary hyperpermeability in rodents.[26] It also increased skin capillary resistance in guinea pigs fed a vitamin C-deficient diet, as measured by the petechiae method. The extract (200 to 400 mg/kg) decreased the formation of oedema of lymphatic or inflammatory origin induced in rat hind paw, suppressed plasmatic extravasation and leucocyte migration into the pleural cavity in experimental pleurisy (200 to 400 mg/kg, oral, and 1 to 10 mg/kg, iv), and decreased connective tissue formation in subchronic inflammatory granuloma (400 mg/kg, oral, and 5 to 10 mg/kg, sc).[26]

In a randomised, double blind, placebo-controlled crossover study, the influence of oral doses of horsechestnut on capillary resistance was tested in 12 healthy volunteers. After 7 days of treatment with a high dose of a HSCE (1500 mg/day, corresponding to 300 mg/day escin), capillary resistance was significantly improved (as measured by the petechiae test). There was no effect from the placebo.[29]

Pharmacological and clinical studies indicate that oral administration of horsechestnut extract can improve connective tissue and circulation by toning the veins. In a double blind, placebo-controlled study, a decrease in the vascular capacity (as measured by increased flow) and filtration coefficients was observed in volunteers with healthy circulation treated with HCSE (600 mg/day, containing 100 mg escin).[30,31] The anti-oedematous activity demonstrated by HCSE in chronic venous insufficiency was mainly dependent on the inhibition of proteoglycan degradation and lysosomal enzyme activity, as determined in a human study after administration of 900 mg/day HCSE for 12 days.[32]

The effect of oral HCSE (360 mg/day, containing 90 mg escin) in 14 healthy volunteers on the venous tone of a segment of the lower leg was compared with placebo controls. Horsechestnut resulted in significant reduction of the pressure-dependent vein capacity ($p < 0.02$), which is an indication of reduced deformation of the veins and an increase in venous tone. An intravenous infusion of escin did not result in a noticeable change, suggesting other components of the extract had this activity.[33] However, in a double blind, placebo-controlled trial involving 20 healthy volunteers, 100 mg of HCSE (containing 16% or 70% escin) demonstrated similar venotonic activity on peripheral venous pressure–volume curves to the placebo.[34] This lack of a positive effect may reflect inadequate dosage.

In an uncontrolled trial, the velocity of blood in varicose veins was assessed after patients received HCSE for 12 days. Blood viscosity was significantly lowered and correlated to subjective improvement in 73% of cases.[35] A single dose of

HCSE (600 mg, containing 100 mg escin) prevented or significantly reduced the increase in ankle and foot oedema (p<0.05) in healthy humans during a 15 h air flight. The study was of randomised, double blind design and the oedema was compared with preflight levels.[36]

Gastrointestinal activity

The inhibitory effects of oral doses of the saponin fraction of horsechestnut extract and its principal constituents escins Ia, Ib, IIa and IIb on gastric emptying were investigated in mice. Gastric emptying of a 1.5% carboxymethyl cellulose sodium salt meal was inhibited by 11.1% to 54.2%. Escins Ia to IIb (50 mg/kg) also inhibited gastric emptying of a 40% glucose meal by 21.1% to 23.5% (except for escin Ia), a milk meal by 18.4% to 33.1%, and a 30% ethanol meal by 13.5% to 15.9%.[37] Further studies were conducted to assess the likely mechanism involved. Results suggested a possible involvement of capsaicin-sensitive sensory nerves (CPSN) stimulating the synthesis and/or release of dopamine to release prostaglandins (PGs) via central dopamine-2 receptors.[38,39] Escins Ib and IIb also demonstrated enhanced absorption of magnesium at 12.5 and 25 mg/kg orally in mice, respectively. The mechanism was suggested to involve constitutive nitric oxide synthase (NOS), but not endogenous PGs or the sympathetic nervous system (SNS).[40,41]

Further to these investigations, the effect of oral pretreatment with escins Ia, IIa and IIb on ethanol-induced gastric mucosal lesions, and the roles of CPSN, endogenous NO, sulphydryls, PGs, gastric secretion and the SNS, were studied in rats.[42] Escins Ia to IIb (10 to 50 mg/kg) potently inhibited ethanol-induced gastric mucosal lesions, whereas their hydrolysed products desacylescins I and II showed no effect. Endogenous PGs, NO, capsaicin-sensitive afferent neurons and the SNS all participated in this activity.

Postoperative adhesions form after trauma through complex processes involving injured tissues and the peritoneum. Escin (0.45 to 3.6 mg/kg, iv, as the sodium salt) was administered in different rodent models to investigate its effect on inflammation, gastrointestinal transit and postoperative adhesion formation.[43] It was shown that escin could inhibit acute inflammation and granuloma formation, accelerate gastrointestinal transit, help recover intestinal mobility and attenuate the formation of postoperative adhesions. The authors suggest that escin attenuated adhesion formation by inhibiting inflammation and promoting gastrointestinal transit. However, an invited commentary noted that the design of the study, for example the different animal species used, made the results difficult to interpret.[44] Gastrointestinal transit acceleration from escin was postulated to involve constitutive NOS and the SNS.[33,45]

Antitumour activity

A few studies have examined the antitumour activity of escin, mainly in vitro. For example, beta-escin inhibited proliferation and induced apoptosis in human hepatocellular carcinoma cells by inhibiting STAT-3 (signal transducer and activator of transcription 3).[46] At 1.4 and 2.8 mg/day, for 7 days, ip administration of escin inhibited hepatocellular carcinoma growth in mice.[47] Escin was observed to chemosensitise human cancer cells in vitro through inhibition of NF-kappaB[48] and beta-escin acted synergistically with 5-fluorouracil in human hepatocellular carcinoma cells.[49]

However, some retractions of published work in this area,[50–52] and the fact that escin does not appear to be as active as other similar saponins,[53] together with its limited oral bioavailability as such, all suggest that more attractive antitumour prospects exist elsewhere.

Oral doses of beta-escin do appear to have chemopreventative activity. The chemopreventive activity of dietary beta-escin on azoxymethane-induced colonic aberrant crypt foci (ACF) was evaluated in vivo.[54] Rats were fed diets containing 0%, 0.025% or 0.05% beta-escin for 1 week. Treatment was then continued for 8 weeks after the addition of azoxymethane (15 mg/kg once weekly for 2 weeks). Both the 0.025% and 0.05% diets significantly suppressed total colonic ACF formation, up to around 40% (p<0.001) and 50% (p<0.0001), respectively, compared with the saline control. The same researchers observed that beta-escin induced cancer growth arrest in HT-29 human colon cancer cells at the G1-S phase, which was associated with induction of the cyclin-dependent kinase inhibitor p21.[54]

Dermatological activity

Contraction forces generated by non-muscle cells such as fibroblasts play important roles in determining cell morphology, vasoconstriction and/or wound healing. They can influence the morphology and mechanical properties of the skin, but few agents are known that can help generate such contraction forces. A screen of around 100 plant extracts found that horsechestnut extract induced the strongest contraction force in cultured human fibroblasts.[55,56] A postulated mechanism was the formation of stress fibres accompanied by actin polymerisation.

Further to this, the effect of horsechestnut extract on various kinases involved in contraction force generation in fibroblasts was examined in vitro.[57] Contraction forces induced in fibroblasts by stimuli such as lysophosphatidic acid and thrombin are accompanied by stress fibre formation, regulated by myosin light chain kinase and Rho kinase. Results suggested that horsechestnut extract produced force generation in fibroblasts via direct activation of Rho kinase through Rho protein, preceded by the formation of stress fibres.

Other activity

Horsechestnut extract demonstrated strong active oxygen-scavenging activity and protective activity in vitro against cell damage induced by active oxygen.[58] HCSE (containing 70% escin) inhibited enzymatic and non-enzymatic lipid peroxidation in vitro and counteracted the deleterious effects of free radical oxidative stress in mice and rats (200 to 400 mg/kg, oral, and 25 mg/kg, iv, respectively).[26]

The inhibitory action of plant constituents on the activity of the connective tissue enzymes elastase and hyaluronidase were investigated in vitro. Saponin constituents from horsechestnut showed inhibitory effects on hyaluronidase. The activity was mainly linked to escin and, to a lesser extent, its genin (aglycone).[59]

Triterpene saponins from horsechestnut (escin Ia, Ib, IIa and IIb) exhibited an inhibitory effect on ethanol absorption and a hypoglycaemic activity in the oral glucose tolerance test in rats.[60] Saponins can inhibit absorption of small molecules that rely on transporter systems (see Chapter 2).

Beta-escin (15, 30 and 60 mg/kg/day for 7 days, oral) was given to rats before induced ischaemia/reperfusion.[61] Higher doses significantly decreased neurological deficit (p<0.05). Beta-escin potently inhibited caspase-3 activation and the release of cytochrome c, increasing the expression of Bcl-2 after cerebral ischaemia/reperfusion, supporting an inhibitory effect on apoptosis. Additional research by the same Chinese research group using a similar model of cerebral ischaemia-reperfusion injury identified that beta-escin (sodium salt) downregulated expression of adhesion molecules and subsequent migration of neutrophils[62] and boosted antioxidant activity, while reducing infarct size and neurological deficit.[63] Some years later, different Chinese investigators observed that escin (0.45, 0.9 and 1.8 mg/kg/day for 3 days, iv) given post-ischaemia to mice improved learning and memory responses and reduced hippocampal injury relative to controls.[64]

Beta-escin (1.0 to 6.0 mg/kg/day, ip) exhibited potent anti-allergic activity and reduced airway inflammation in two mouse models.[65] Its activity was comparable or superior to dexamethasone, a standard reference compound.

An isolate from horsechestnut seeds rich in escin (100 mg/kg/day for 5 weeks, oral) decreased leptin by 31.6% (p<0.05) in mice fed a high fat diet.[66]

Pharmacokinetics

High concentrations of escin were measured in skin and muscle tissue underlying the site of topical application of radio-labelled sodium escinate, but low values were measured in internal organs, blood, urine, skin and musculature from other parts of the body. Between 0.5% and 1% of the applied dose was excreted in urine within 24 h of administration. Total elimination (bile and urine) was calculated at 1% to 2.5% of the administered dose. Less than one half of this was excreted as escin, the remainder as metabolites.[67] However, the true availability of escin to skin and muscle tissue may not be as high as reported in this study, since the radioactivity detected may have been carried by metabolites of escin, as well as by escin itself.

Studies indicate that escin is eliminated quickly following intravenous injection, with two-thirds excreted via the bile and one-third by renal elimination.[68] Two studies of the bioavailability of beta-escin following oral doses of various horsechestnut preparations were conducted using healthy volunteers. Validated radioimmunosorbent assay (RIA) was used to determine levels of beta-escin in plasma. One study on two solid-dose preparations in 18 volunteers found a large variation in absorption parameters for beta-escin. Cmax after a dose containing 50 mg escin varied from 0.19 to 45.1 ng/mL, Tmax varied from 0.73 to 8.5 h and the area under the curve (AUC, an assessment of concentration over time) varied from 24.6 to 389 ng/h/mL.[69] The second study, also of two solid-dose preparations (one sustained-release) and using 24 volunteers found more consistent results.

This may have been because a horsechestnut extract containing a defined dose of escin was used, rather than just escin alone. Parameters for the sustained-release tablet were superior. For example, after a dose containing 50 mg escin, Cmax for the sustained-release tablet was 9.81 ± 8.9 ng/mL, Tmax was 2.23 ± 0.9 h and AUC averaged 187.1 ng/h/mL.[70] The half-life for both preparations was about 20 h.

In a steady-state crossover study over 7 days in 18 healthy volunteers, the relative bioavailability of 100 mg beta-escin after oral administration of an immediate release, enteric-coated test formulation of HCSE was evaluated against a sustained-release product.[71] RIA was used for analysis. The two tested products were bioequivalent with Cmax around 16 to 18 ng/mL for the first dose of the day (containing 50 mg beta-escin) and 10 to 11 ng/mL for the second, the difference apparently being due to food intake.

A review of the pharmacokinetic data published for HCSE up to 2000 identified five single- and four multiple-dose bioequivalence studies, including those reviewed above.[72] Considerable variation was observed for the key pharmacokinetic parameters, leading the authors to suggest that these differences might be due to variations in the relative saponin concentrations from batch to batch (since escin is a complex mixture of many individual saponins). Hence the need was expressed for either specific validation of the RIA technique, or the use of an alternative analytical technology, to better understand the pharmacokinetics of this herb.

Since the review, the comparative bioavailability of beta-escin (from HCSE) was evaluated for two test products in two randomised, open label crossover trials using a multiple-dose treatment schedule in 18 healthy volunteers each.[73] A normal and a sustained-release product were compared and shown to have similar bioavailability, as assessed using RIA. Peak serum concentrations were reached approximately 2 to 4 h (Tmax) after dosing of 100 mg of beta-escin and concentration/time profiles and steady-state concentrations were similar for the two formulations in both trials. Average Cmax concentrations ranged from 12 to 18 ng/mL.

Saponins are large molecules containing highly polar groups and their intact bioavailability can be expected to be low after oral doses. This has been confirmed in all the above studies, since the pharmacokinetic parameters indicate absorptions of less than 1% of the administered oral dose of beta-escin. However, saponins can be hydrolysed by intestinal flora, leaving the less polar aglycone or sapogenin available for absorption. These sapogenins, or their hepatic metabolites, may in fact be the main active form of escin following oral doses. More studies are needed to clarify this issue.

Pursuing this line of reasoning, the effect of human intestinal bacterial enzymes on the biotransformation of escin Ia was examined, and structures of biotransformation products were determined in vitro. Escin Ia was incubated with crude enzymes or *Lactobacillus brevis*. Biotransformation products were isolated and structures determined by spectroscopic techniques. Results suggested that escin Ia is indeed a prodrug and was converted by both the enzymes and Lactobacillus. Biotransformation products included isoescin Ia, desacylescin I, 21beta-O-tigloylprotoaescigenin and protoaescigenin. Of these, desacylescin I showed inhibitory action on mouse sarcoma-180 tumour cell growth, hepatic carcinoma H(22) and lung carcinoma in vivo, thereby indicating biological activity.[74]

Clinical trials with escin

There are several early clinical studies where escin was mainly given by injection, for example to treat road accident victims with severe head injury. Here it reduced the dangerous rise in intracranial pressure, leading to a more favourable prognosis at iv doses of 10 to 20 mg/day.[75] Escin has also been effective in the treatment of cerebral oedema following cranial fracture and cranial trauma (with or without retrograde amnesia), cerebral tumours, intracranial aneurysms, cerebral sclerosis, subdural haematoma, encephalitis, meningitis and cerebral abscess.[76] Depending on the severity of the condition, disappearance of cephalgia, vertigo and general discomfort were observed within 3 to 16 days. Cerebral oedema due to acute vasomotor insufficiency was resolved quickly, while in chronic disease remission occurred slowly over a long period of administration.[76] Other trials examined the value of intravenous escin during routine surgery. For example, in a placebo-controlled trial in patients undergoing surgery of the hand, iv administration of escin (20 mg/day) produced a fast reduction in postoperative inflammation and oedema.[77] Oral escin was also used in some trials. For example a dose of 120 mg/day for up to 2 months markedly and significantly (p<0.01) improved symptoms, bleeding and swelling in an early, double blind, placebo-controlled trial involving 80 patients suffering from acute haemorrhoids.[78]

Recent studies on the clinical use of escin are as follows. The impact of escin was examined in patients experiencing cutaneous pruritus to test the traditional Chinese medicine theory that 'wind should be treated by regulating blood disorder, and wind disappears after activating blood'.[79] A total of 51 patients were randomly divided into either an escin-treated group (n=30) or a loratadine-treated group (n=21) in an open label trial. The dose of escin was 300 mg twice daily for 4 weeks and that of loratadine 10 mg four times daily, both higher than average doses. After 4 weeks the effective treatment rate for escin and loratadine were 86.7% and 80%, respectively. No statistically significant difference was noted in total symptom scores, or specific scores of pruritus and lesion shape between the two groups (p>0.05). However, the score for lesion range was lower for the escin group compared with the loratadine group (p<0.05). The conclusion was that escin has a satisfactory effect in treating pruritus caused by 'blood stasis and wind-dryness'. Note that, while this study refers to 'escin' as the treatment, the active agent might well have been HCSE (based on the incorrect attribution in other clinical studies from China of 'escin').

Following on from positive pharmacological studies (see earlier), an open label, controlled pilot trial was conducted in 64 abdominal surgery patients to assess the impact of escin (0.3 mg/kg, iv, immediately after surgery) on intestinal ileus.[43] Times to first bowel sounds, passage of gas and defecation were all significantly less in the escin group, compared with a saline control treatment (p<0.01). Another pilot trial (of similar design, but undertaken by a different research team) in 72 postoperative colorectal cancer patients demonstrated a dose-response effect

for escin (5, 15 and 25 mg, iv) on the above parameters, with the higher doses achieving statistical significance.[80]

A combination of oral escin (1250 mg/day) and the flavonoid derivative troxerutin (2250 mg/day) was assessed against the drug pentoxyphylline (600 mg/day) in 68 patients with inner ear perfusion disturbances.[81] This 6-week, open label, controlled trial found that 23 of the 34 patients receiving the escin-troxerutin combination demonstrated a hearing increase of at least 10 dB, compared with only six of 34 in the drug control group (p<0.05).

The pathological mechanism involved in Bell's palsy, the most common acute facial paralysis, is believed to involve inflammatory oedema and entrapment neuropathy. It has been postulated that the impact of beta-escin on local oedema and effusion suggests it could be a valuable treatment for Bell's palsy.[82]

Topical use

Topical preparations containing escin have been successfully used for a variety of applications: treatment of oedema and haematoma in surgical practice,[83] the prevention and treatment of sports injuries, including acute injuries, blunt injuries (non-penetrating wounds) and oedema.[84–89] It has been used alone, or more typically in combination with heparin, buphenin, diethylamine salicylate (DEAS) or polyunsaturated phosphatidylcholine in venous disorders (inflammation of veins, venous insufficiency, varicose veins);[90–93] in combination with l-thyroxine for the treatment of hypertrophic scars, keloid scars, stretch marks and lymphoedema after mastectomy,[94–96] and in combination with heparin and phospholipids for the treatment of joint and venous diseases,[97,98] anorectal varicose pathologies (particularly in gynaecology and obstetrics),[99–101] postoperative treatment of episiotomies[102] and during oral and periodontal surgery.[103] Details of some more recent, larger and interesting studies follow.

In a randomised, double blind trial, 81 patients with contused traumas following limb injuries received treatment with a 2% escin and 5% salicylate gel or placebo gel for 9 days. Compared with placebo, the mobility of the injured extremity increased significantly in comparison to the uninjured extremity in those treated with the active gel (p<0.02). The circumferences of the lower extremities returned to almost normal (compared with the uninjured leg) in the treatment group, but remained unchanged in the placebo group. The active gel was also superior for reduction in lower leg swelling, subjective complaints and remission frequencies (p<0.05).[104]

A topically applied 2% escin gel was compared with a placebo in experimentally induced haematoma in a randomised, double blind trial. Efficacy was measured over 9 h after a single application of gel. The escin gel significantly reduced tenderness to pressure within 1 h and then at all other time points during the trial.[105]

The effect of topical escin on pain from blunt injuries caused by sports and leisure activities was examined in a double blind, placebo-controlled clinical trial.[106] In all, 126 patients were randomly assigned to one of four groups: three active preparations (containing various amounts of escin, DEAS and sulphated escin) or a placebo. The gel was applied topically at 0, 4 and 8 h after injury and the variable measured was the pressure required at the centre of the lesion to elicit a pain reaction at different time points up to 24h after the injury. There was a significant difference observed for tenderness at 6h (p=0.0001) for all treatment groups compared with placebo, with similar findings after 24h.

In a similar trial, the clinical efficacy and safety of an escin-containing gel was investigated on blunt impact injuries.[107] Participants in various sports competitions were enrolled within 2h of sustaining a strain, sprain or contusion and randomised to one of either two active treatment groups or a placebo group. Topical treatment occurred three times within a period of 8h. The gels contained either 1% or 2% escin, together with 5% DEAS and heparin. A total of 156 patients were evaluated and results demonstrated that the active gels were significantly more effective than placebo at reducing tenderness (p=0.0001 and p=0.0002, respectively). Both active gel preparations produced more rapid pain relief than the placebo, as well as showing good safety and tolerability.

A proprietary escin-containing gel with 1% escin, 1% essential phospholipids and 10 000 IU sodium heparin has been developed for local treatment of venous and microcirculatory problems, sports injuries and varices in pregnancy. A review suggested that the gel is effective and safe, without contraindications or side effects.[108] A series of small, placebo-controlled and somewhat repetitive clinical trials, all from the same research group, have observed benefits on microcirculation and other related parameters and symptoms in patients with venous hypertensive microangiopathy (with ulcers), diabetic microangiopathy and superficial vein thrombosis.[109–115] Patient numbers ranged from 10 to 35 and treatment times varied from a single application to up to 8 weeks.

A few years later the same research team evaluated a similar topical escin plus phospholipids product, but without the heparin, in a series of four open label clinical trials involving patients with chronic venous insufficiency (hypertension). A 2-week trial in 15 patients compared with 15 normal controls found that the gel significantly increased transcutaneous oxygen levels (PO_2) compared with baseline (p<0.05).[116] The three other 2-week trials tested the gel in similar patient numbers. Significant changes (p<0.05) observed relative to baseline included improvements in skin flux (as measured by laser-Doppler flowmetry),[117] plasma free radicals[118] and transcutaneous carbon dioxide (pCO_2).[119]

Clinical trials with horsechestnut

Chronic venous insufficiency

Chronic venous insufficiency (CVI) is an imprecise term frequently referred to and not easily defined. It describes the impairment of venous return, usually from the legs, often with oedema and sometimes with stasis ulcers at the ankle. Other terms used are chronic deep vein incompetence, peripheral venous incompetence and chronic venous hypertension. According to more recent clinical, aetiological, anatomical and pathological elements, chronic venous disease has been classified into seven clinical classes, designated C0–6.[120] These are defined as follows: C0: no visible sign of venous disease; C1: telangiectasia or reticular veins; C2: varicose veins; C3: oedema; C4a: pigmentation or eczema; C4b:

lipodermatosclerosis; C5: healed ulcer; C6: active ulcer. Classes C4 to C6 have been designated as CVI. There have been a substantial number of clinical trials using various versions of HCSE in the management of CVI published over a time span of around 40 years. Most of these are reviewed below.

A meta-analysis of 16 trials was published in 2002.[121] In all, 13 randomised, controlled trials (1051 patients) and three observational studies (10 725 patients) were identified as meeting the inclusion criteria (out of 75 studies located). Inclusion criteria included treatment of CVI with HCSE versus control (placebo or other therapies), duration of at least 20 days, and trials that permitted adequate data extraction. Examined objective outcomes were leg volume, ankle and calf circumference and oedema. Subjective outcomes were pain, sensation of tension, swelling, leg fatigue/heaviness, calf cramp and itching. Random and fixed effect models were used to pool outcomes and adverse events. Such models were applied separately for the randomised trials and the observational studies. Overall, results from the randomised trials indicated that HCSE improved signs and symptoms in patients with CVI. Leg volume was reduced by 46.4mL compared with placebo (95% confidence interval (CI) 11.3 to 81.4) and likelihood of an improvement in leg pain was increased 4.1-fold (95% CI 0.98 to 16.8). Similarly, improvement probabilities were increased 1.5-fold (95% CI 1.2 to 1.9) for oedema and 1.7-fold (95% CI 0.01 to 3.0) for itching. Subjective improvement scores were transformed into a standardised scale before quantifying pooled effects (such as leg heaviness/fatigue and calf cramps). Treatment effects of HCSE were not as evident for these as the objective outcomes. Based on these results, the authors concluded that there is substantial evidence to support the efficacy, routine effectiveness and safety of HCSE in the treatment of CVI.

Subsequent to this analysis came the review from the Cochrane collaboration. This 2006 review was updated in 2010 with no changes to conclusions.[122] Randomised, controlled clinical trials were included if they compared oral HCSE mono-preparations with placebo or a reference therapy in CVI. In all, 31 trials assessing HCSE in CVI were identified, including two unpublished trials, of which 17 met the inclusion criteria. Fourteen trials were excluded: two used topical application, eight assessed HCSE in combination with other active components, and four did not have appropriate clinical endpoints or were in healthy volunteers. Of the 17 trials included in the systematic review, 10 were placebo-controlled, two compared horsechestnut against treatment with compression stockings and placebo, four were controlled against a flavonoid derivative (beta-O-hydroxyethyl-rutoside) and one was controlled against pine bark extract. In all of the trials the extract was standardised to a defined level of escin and all the included trials bar one used a double blind design. Trials were scored for concealment of treatment allocation, where A=clearly concealed, B=unclear if concealed and C=clearly not concealed. Three trials scored A and the remaining 14 trials scored B. Methodological quality was evaluated using the scoring system developed by Jadad that measures the likelihood of bias inherent in a trial.[123] The scale is from 1 to 5, where 5 denotes high quality with a low risk of bias. Nine of the 17 trials scored 4 or 5 and the average Jadad score for all the trials was 3.4. The majority of the included studies assessed clinical outcomes in terms of leg pain, oedema and pruritus. Other endpoints assessed included leg volume and circumference. For example, leg pain was assessed in seven placebo-controlled trials and six of these (543 patients) reported a statistically significant reduction ($p<0.05$) of leg pain using various measurement scales. Three other comparative studies reported no significant difference for horsechestnut extract relative to the reference treatments in terms of leg pain. Leg volume was assessed in seven placebo-controlled trials. Meta-analysis of six of these (502 patients) suggested a significant reduction in leg volume from HCSE versus placebo. One trial indicated that HCSE may be as effective as treatment with compression stockings. Adverse events were mild and infrequent. The evidence presented suggested that HCSE is an efficacious and safe short-term treatment for CVI. However, the authors noted that more and larger long-term trials are needed.

A brief summary follows of most of the clinical trials included in the above two studies.

In a double blind, placebo-controlled trial, 40 patients with leg oedema caused by chronic deep venous incompetence received either HCSE (738 to 824 mg/day, containing 150 mg escin) or placebo over 7 weeks. A significant reduction in average leg volume was observed for the treated group compared with placebo, both before and after an oedema provocation test ($p<0.01$). Leg pressure at rest was decreased (indicating better venous tone) and a pronounced alleviation of symptoms occurred in the treated group.[124]

A randomised, double blind, placebo-controlled trial assessed treatment with HCSE (600 mg/day, containing 100 mg escin) in 20 patients over a 4-week period. There was a significant improvement in volume changes of the foot and ankle ($p<0.001$) compared with the 20 patients treated with placebo. Symptoms such as oedema, pain, fatigue, feeling of tension and itching were also significantly improved ($p<0.05$). There were, however, no changes in venous capacity or calf muscle spasm.[125]

Seventy-four patients with CVI and lower leg oedema participated in a randomised, double blind, placebo-controlled trial. An anti-oedema effect was observed for those treated with HCSE (600 mg/day, containing 100 mg escin) over 8 weeks. Leg volume was reduced, while in the placebo group it increased. The progression of oedema was slowed in the treatment group, as were subjective symptoms.[126] In a randomised, double blind, placebo-controlled, crossover trial involving 20 women with pregnancy-induced varicose veins or CVI, treatment with HCSE (containing 100 mg/day escin) for 4 weeks resulted in significant reduction in leg volume ($p<0.01$).[127] The influence of HCSE (approximately 600 mg/day, containing 100 mg escin) for 4 weeks was tested in a randomised, placebo-controlled trial involving 30 patients with peripheral venous incompetence (CVI). Horsechestnut effected a reduction in leg circumference and improvement in subjective symptoms.[128] In a double blind trial using the same dosage over 20 days involving 30 outpatients suffering from CVI, a significant reduction of leg circumference was demonstrated ($p<0.05$).[129]

One hundred and eighteen patients with varicose veins or CVI were treated for 40 days with 60 mg/day of HCSE (containing 70% escin) or placebo in a double blind trial. Significant improvements in symptoms (oedema, cramps, pain, fatigue, sensation of heaviness) were observed in the treated group ($p<0.05$).[130] The dosage quoted for this trial is a low dose in comparison to the majority of trials conducted. Similar results were observed in a double blind, placebo-controlled, crossover trial (n=233) for patients treated with horsechestnut. Improvements were observed for oedema and pain ($p<0.01$), itchiness, fatigue and sensation of heaviness ($p<0.05$). Calf cramping, however, was not significantly improved.[131]

Treatment with HCSE (600 mg/day, containing 100 mg escin) for 2 weeks was superior to placebo in a trial in 20 pregnant women with oedema due to CVI. Significant reductions in oedema ($p=0.009$) and symptoms such as pain, fatigue and itching ($p<0.05$) were observed in the treatment group, and these patients also showed a greater resistance to oedema provocation. The trial was double blinded and crossover in design.[132]

In a randomised, partially blinded, placebo-controlled, parallel study published in *The Lancet*, 240 patients with CVI participated in a comparison of the efficacy of compression stockings class II with HCSE (600 mg/day, containing 100 mg escin) over 12 weeks. Lower leg volume decreased by a similar amount (43 to 47 mL) for both horsechestnut and compression therapy compared with placebo. A significant reduction in oedema was observed for horsechestnut ($p=0.005$) and compression ($p=0.002$) compared with placebo, and the two therapies were shown to be equivalent. Compression achieved high oedema reductions at the beginning of the study, while horsechestnut gradually decreased oedema volume, reaching a maximum by the end of the trial. (Patients allocated to compression treatment received a diuretic once daily during the first week of the trial to ensure the best possible stocking fit. Class II stockings provide a defined pressure.) Compliance was better for the herbal therapy.[133]

HCSE (720 to 824 mg/day, containing 150 mg escin) and beta-hydroxyethylrutosides (2000 mg/day) both demonstrated an oedema-protective effect in a randomised, double blind trial involving 40 patients with CVI and peripheral venous oedema.[134] In a multicentre, randomised, double blind trial, the comparative efficacy of oxerutins (beta-hydroxyethylrutosides) and HCSE was investigated in 137 postmenopausal patients with grade II CVI. Patients received 600 mg/day of HCSE (containing 100 mg escin), 1000 mg/day of oxerutins for 12 weeks or 1000 mg/day of oxerutins for 4 weeks followed by 500 mg/day (of oxerutins) for 8 weeks. All treatments achieved a mean leg volume reduction of about 100 mL after 12 weeks of treatment, comparable to that achieved by compression therapy. A 6-week follow-up period without treatment indicated that both treatments also exhibited a substantial carry-over effect.[135]

HCSE (600 mg/day, containing 100 mg escin) was compared with a proprietary French maritime pine bark extract (360 mg/day) in an open, controlled, comparative study in 40 patients over 4 weeks. Outcomes assessed were the circumference of lower legs and the subjective symptoms of pain, cramps, nighttime swelling, feeling of heaviness and reddening of the skin.

HCSE moderately (but not statistically significantly) reduced the circumference of the lower limbs and marginally impacted subjective symptoms compared to baseline, but was inferior to pine bark. Both treatments were well tolerated.[136]

A previously unpublished study by Diehm and Schmidt from 2000 was reported by other authors in 2001.[137] This was a 16-week, three-arm, randomised, double blind trial where HCSE (containing 100 mg/day escin) was compared with placebo or compression stockings in 355 patients with CVI. The drop-out rate was high at 69 patients. From intention-to-treat analysis, compression was significantly superior to placebo (p<0.001), whereas HCSE was not (p=0.115). Only in the per-protocol population (286 patients) did HCSE also demonstrate significance against placebo (p=0.018) for this parameter. Subjective symptoms favoured HCSE over compression, but the difference between the two treatments did not reach statistical significance.

Other published studies of interest that were not covered by, or were specifically excluded from, the Cochrane systematic review are discussed below.

HCSE (600 mg/day, containing 100 mg escin, for 3 weeks) significantly reduced subjective symptoms of patients with varicose veins (p<0.001) in a double blind, placebo-controlled trial.[138] The impact of a single dose of HCSE was investigated in a randomised, double blind, placebo-controlled trial involving 22 patients with proven CVI. Three hours after taking 600 mg of horsechestnut extract (containing 100 mg escin), a significant decrease in the capillary filtration coefficient (22%) was observed in the treated group.[139]

In a case observation study involving more than 800 German general practitioners, more than 5000 patients with CVI were treated with HCSE and followed up at regular intervals. All the symptoms investigated (pain, tiredness, tension, swelling in the leg, itching and tendency towards oedema) improved markedly or completely disappeared. Horsechestnut extract was considered an economical, practice-relevant therapeutic tool which, in comparison with compression therapy, had the additional advantage of better compliance.[140] In a postmarketing surveillance study, 1183 patients with CVI received the recommended dosage of HCSE over a 5-month period. A clear reduction in the objective and subjective symptoms was demonstrated.[141]

A proprietary fresh plant extract of horsechestnut seed, available as an oral tincture, tablets and a topical gel was reviewed for its efficacy in CVI and varicose veins.[142] Five clinical trials were reviewed, of which only one was randomised and placebo-controlled. The trial details were as follows. A daily dose of fresh plant tincture containing 39 mg escin was given to 40 patients with CVI in a prospective, uncontrolled, multicentre trial over 4 weeks. In all, 77% of patients demonstrated a clinically relevant therapeutic result in terms of global efficacy, and more than 60% of patients rated the treatment as 'good' to 'very good' for subjective symptoms such as leg swelling and pruritus. Tablets delivering 120 mg/day escin were examined in 60 patients with CVI in a randomised, placebo-controlled, multicentre, double blind trial. The primary outcome was changes in the circumference of the leg measured just above the ankle, and the treatment group achieved a clinically

relevant, statistically significant reduction compared with placebo (p<0.05). A tablet dose containing 100 mg/day escin was assessed in 87 patients with CVI in an open trial design. The primary assessment variable was safety. Fifty-seven of the 87 patients reported 91 adverse events; all were non-serious and only four were judged to be actually from the trial medication. A gel containing 2% escin was evaluated in 71 CVI patients in an open, uncontrolled, multicentre trial over 6 weeks. The primary trial outcome of ankle circumference decreased significantly (p<0.001). The fifth trial assessed tablets (60 mg/day escin) and the gel in 39 patients with varicose veins in an open, uncontrolled trial over 8 weeks. Trial outcomes were both subjective (by a visual analogue scale) and objective (reduction in ankle oedema). A significant improvement in heaviness and pain in the legs and blue discoloration was observed (p<0.0003) and a moderate rating was given by both therapists and patients for efficacy/satisfaction and tolerability.

Chronic venous ulceration

Fifty-four patients with venous leg ulcers were randomly assigned to treatment with HCSE tablets (containing 150 mg/day escin) or placebo in a parallel, triple blind, multicentre trial over 12 weeks.[143] Assessment of ulceration was performed at 0, 4, 8 and 12 weeks using a wound assessment tool and the Alfred/Medseed Wound Imaging System. Primary outcomes measured were the number of healed leg ulcers, the change in wound surface area, depth, volume, pain and exudate. These variables were found not to be statistically significant between the treatment group and placebo. However, HCSE did have a significant effect on the percentage of wound slough over time (p=0.045) and the number of dressing changes at week 12 (p=0.009). Any assessable impact on the primary trial outcomes was limited by the small size of the trial.

The authors also conducted a 12-week cost–benefit analysis using the data from the above trial.[144] The cost of HCSE, dressing materials, travel, staff salaries and infrastructure for each patient was taken into account. HCSE therapy combined with conventional therapy was found to be more cost-effective than conventional therapy alone, with an average saving of AUD 95 in organisational costs and AUD 10 in dressing materials per patient.

Deep vein thrombosis

A controlled trial involving 4176 patients with thrombosis, pulmonary infarction or pulmonary embolism investigated horsechestnut as a prophylactic treatment for thrombosis and embolism arising from surgery over a 3-year period. Patients received an intravenous injection of horsechestnut extract (10 mL/day), strophanthin or digitalis, vitamin B complex and vitamin C or a similar injection without the horsechestnut extract for 4 days prior to surgery and continuing for up to 7 days after the operation. Horsechestnut significantly reduced the incidence of deep venous thrombosis following surgery compared with the control group (pulmonary embolism patients: p<0.01; other patients: p<0.001).[145] It would be valuable to conduct a randomised, controlled trial of oral HCSE to assess its impact on this problem.

Topical use

A gel containing horsechestnut extract and heparin was found to be effective in the treatment of acute and chronic traumas and venopathies in an uncontrolled study. In particular, the gel quickly broke down haematomas.[146] The tolerability and efficacy of a topical horsechestnut preparation were assessed in 15 patients with first- and second-degree CVI. The horsechestnut preparation contained 1.4% triterpene glycosides calculated as escin and was compared with a preparation containing heparin. Efficacy was assessed by the change in circumference of the lower, middle and upper leg and by changes in symptoms. Both treatments were well tolerated and the horsechestnut preparation showed a greater tendency to improvement than heparin.[147]

The effect of topical horsechestnut was investigated for its impact on skin ageing, based on pharmacodynamic studies suggesting the herb increased contraction forces in fibroblasts (see earlier).[55] Clinical testing was carried out in 40 healthy women using a double blind, placebo-controlled design. The gel (containing 3% horsechestnut extract) was applied twice daily to the periphery of the eye for a total of 9 weeks. Outcomes were evaluated by visual scoring by a specialist, based on photo scales. The active gel showed significant wrinkle-smoothing efficacy at the corner of the eye and the lower eyelid compared with placebo ($p<0.05$ and $p<0.001$, depending on the site). Six weeks of treatment was deemed sufficient to have a significant wrinkle-smoothing effect.

Other uses

The impact of HCSE (containing 60 mg/day escin) on sperm quality was assessed against surgery or a control treatment (20 mg of vitamin E, together with 400 mg pentoxyphylline and 50 mg clomiphene) in an open label trial involving 219 patients with varicocele-associated infertility.[148] Both surgery and HCSE were equally effective, and significantly superior to the control treatment, in terms of sperm density ($p<0.05$). However, only surgery was significantly better than the control treatment in terms of sperm motility ($p<0.05$). Patients with mild or moderate disease appeared to respond better to the HCSE treatment. Adverse effects were mild and infrequent.

The addition of HCSE to HIV treatment with indinavir was examined for its effect on delaying indinavir precipitation in urine, thereby preventing indinavir-associated nephrolithiasis. This pilot clinical trial was multicentre, randomised open label and controlled, with four crossover periods each of 4 weeks. One group of patients (n=22) received HCSE during the second and third treatment periods, the second (n=25) received HCSE during the first and fourth treatment periods. The dose used was 50 mg escin every 12 h (from 300 mg of HCSE) in combination with highly active antiretroviral activity (HAART). Thirty patients out of the 47 enrolled completed the study. Urine samples were collected at the end of each 4-week period and tested for indinavir crystallisation. The mean time to crystallisation averaged 14.7 min with HCSE and 9.9 min without (p=0.008). Urine and plasma concentrations of indinavir were unaffected by HCSE and no adverse effects were experienced.[149]

Toxicology and other safety data

Toxicology

The following LD_{50} data have been recorded for horsechestnut extract and its constituents:

Substance	Route, model	LD_{50}	Reference
Horsechestnut seed extract	Oral, mice	990 mg/kg	4
Horsechestnut seed extract	Ooral, rats	2.15 g/kg	4
Horsechestnut seed extract	Oral, guinea pigs	1.12 g/kg	4
Horsechestnut seed extract	Oral, rabbits	1.53 g/kg	4
Horsechestnut seed extract (water-soluble portion)	Oral, chicks	10.6 g/kg	150
Horsechestnut seed extract (water-soluble portion)	Oral, hamsters	10.7 g/kg	150
Horsechestnut dried seed	Oral, chicks	6.5 g/kg	150
Horsechestnut seed extract	ip, mice	342 mg/kg	4
Horsechestnut seed extract	iv, mice	138 mg/kg	4
Horsechestnut seed extract	iv, rats	165 mg/kg	4
Horsechestnut seed extract	iv, guinea pigs	465 mg/kg	4
Horsechestnut seed extract	iv, rabbits	18 mg/kg	4
Escin	iv, mice	9.3 mg/kg	151
Escin	iv, rats	16.8 mg/kg	151
Escin	iv, guinea pigs	9.1 mg/kg	151
Escin	iv, rabbits	5 mg/kg	151
Escin	iv, dogs	Approx. 3 mg/kg	151
Escin	iv, pigs	Approx. 4 mg/kg	151

These data demonstrate that horsechestnut seed extract has low oral toxicity. The substantially higher toxicity after ip or iv administration is probably a reflection of the low oral bioavailability of escin as such and its haemolytic activity.

No toxic effects were observed on the behaviour, growth, food consumption, haematological and biochemical tests or organ histology of rats fed horsechestnut seed extract at doses of 100 to 400 mg/kg/day for 34 weeks. The only toxic effect observed in dogs orally administered the extract (20 to 80 mg/kg/day, 5 days per week) for the same time period was vomiting in the highest dosage group at 8 weeks. This was eliminated by the use of enteric-coated tablets. No toxic effects were observed in rats after daily intravenous injection of 9 mg/kg of extract for 8 weeks. Lesions were primarily observed in the kidneys after administration of acutely toxic oral and intravenous doses.[4]

Oral administration of the sodium salt of escin (10 mg/kg, 70 mg/kg) to rats did not induce fatty degeneration of the liver.[152] Intraperitoneal administration of escin (10 mg/kg) to juvenile male rats did not affect fertility or cause renal toxicity.[153] Toxic effects in rodents following intravenous injection of high doses of escin were due to massive haemolysis. In contrast, continuous administration of escin (1.1 mg/kg/day) for 1 month was associated with minimal haemolysis in rabbits, only detectable by increased erythropoiesis.[10,154] The route of administration was not clearly specified. However, as the dose was one-fifth of the LD_{50} of escin, it was probably administered by injection.

Horsechestnut seed extract demonstrated weak mutagenic activity in the Ames test in vitro. It was suggested that this effect might be due to the flavonoid quercetin.[155] The potential genotoxicity of quercetin has been extensively studied and the results have been interpreted as being not relevant to human intake (see also Chapter 2).[156]

Contraindications

Because of the irritant effect of the saponins, horsechestnut should not be applied to broken or ulcerated skin. Do not use during pregnancy or lactation without professional advice.

Special warnings and precautions

Saponin-containing herbs are best kept to a minimum in patients with pre-existing cholestasis.

Interactions

A case of acute renal insufficiency after therapy with escin and the antibiotic gentamicin has been reported.[157] (It is likely that the escin was administered by injection.) High doses of intravenous escin have been implicated in acute renal failure.[158] (See the Overdosage section below.) Escin is a saponin that can cause haemolysis after injection. The liberated haemoglobin can deposit in the kidneys and cause renal failure. The risk of haemolysis after oral intake of horsechestnut is minimal because of the low absorption of saponins.

In vitro testing found that horsechestnut is quite a weak inhibitor of CYP3A4, which is unlikely to have clinical significance.[159] It was also moderately active at inhibiting P-glycoprotein activity in vitro, a finding of uncertain clinical relevance.

Use in pregnancy and lactation

Category B3 – no increase in frequency of malformation or other harmful effects on the fetus from limited use in women. Evidence of increased fetal damage in animal studies exists, although the relevance to humans is unknown.

Standardised horsechestnut seed extracts have been successfully used in clinical studies[127,132,138,160] to treat venous conditions in pregnant women at dosages of 600 mg/day (containing 100 mg escin) for 2 to 4 weeks. Some of these studies excluded women in the third trimester of pregnancy.[127,132]

Intravenous administration of standardised horsechestnut seed extract (9 and 30 mg/kg/day) to rats (days 6 to 15 gestation) and rabbits (days 6 to 18 gestation) did not result in teratogenicity or embryotoxicity. The same results were demonstrated in rats (100 and 300 mg/kg/day) and rabbits (100 mg/kg/day) after oral administration. Although no teratogenic effects were observed in rabbits orally administered very high doses of extract (300 mg/kg/day), fetal body weights were significantly reduced compared to controls.[4]

Horsechestnut is compatible with breastfeeding but caution should be exercised.

Effects on ability to drive and use machines

No adverse effects expected.

Side effects

A 2002 meta-analysis of adverse reactions found no significant difference between horsechestnut seed extract and placebo.[121] Meta-analysis of three post-marketing surveillance studies, which included 10 725 patients, found an average of 1.51% of patients treated with horsechestnut seed extract reported mild adverse reactions.[121] From 1968 until 1989 nearly 900 million individual doses of one brand of standardised horsechestnut seed extract were prescribed. In that time, only 15 patients reported significant side effects.[161] Fourteen studies in the Cochrane review provided information on adverse events, which were usually mild and frequent. Gastrointestinal symptoms, dizziness, nausea, headache and pruritus were reported as adverse events in six studies. Four studies reported no adverse events and another four studies reported a good tolerability for the herbal treatment. The reviewers concluded that HCSE is a safe and effective treatment option for CVI and, according to available data, the risk/benefit ratio for treatment of CVI is positive.[122]

A case has been reported in Japan where pruritus, jaundice, elevated liver enzymes, liver cholestasis, centrilobular necrosis and mild eosinophilia developed 60 days after intramuscular injection of a product for pathological bone fracture containing horsechestnut extract. Drug-induced hepatic injury was suspected.[162] The product has been in use in Japan since 1967 and only mild side effects such as nausea, vomiting, urticaria and, rarely, spasm and shock have otherwise been reported.[162,163]

A case of occupational asthma was reported where a 57-year-old man employed in the pharmaceutical industry developed bronchial asthma while working with products, including escin. Various tests were performed and other products eliminated, confirming escin as the causative factor. Characteristics of the asthma were suggestive of a non-IgE immunological mechanism, although an irritative mechanism secondary to long-term, low-level exposure could not be ruled out.[164]

Cases of pseudo-lupus (an autoimmune syndrome) after use of a product containing phenopyrazone, horsechestnut extract and cardiac glycosides have been reported.[165] The ingredient or ingredients responsible for this reaction were not established. Urticaria and dyspnoea have been reported after the topical application of escin.[10,166]

As with all saponin-containing herbs, oral use may cause irritation of the gastric mucous membranes and reflux. However, the gastric irritation and reflux can be avoided by the use of enteric-coated preparations. Because of the irritant effect of the saponins, horsechestnut should not be applied to broken or ulcerated skin. Saponins and sapogenins in the bloodstream cause haemolysis but this effect is negligible at the oral doses used.

Overdosage

Very high doses will result in gastrointestinal irritation. If sufficient quantities of escin are absorbed through damaged or irritated gastrointestinal mucous membranes, haemolysis with associated kidney damage could possibly result.

Cases of acute renal failure have been reported which were suspected to have been caused by escin (510 to 540 μg/kg) administered intravenously for postoperative oedema.[153,158] However, in trials designed to assess the effects of intravenous escin on renal function, no signs of impaired renal function developed in patients with normal renal function, and renal function did not worsen in patients with pre-existing renal impairment. Adults received intravenous escin (10 to 25 mg/day) for 3 to 10 days and two children with normal renal function were prescribed 0.2 mg/day for 6 days.[10,153–155]

In the USA, an analysis of 3099 cases of human exposure to plant parts from eight different *Aesculus spp.* from 1985 to 1994 found that no effect or a non-toxic effect was recorded in 76.6% of cases. Most exposures (49.2%) occurred in children aged 0 to 5 years. Analysis of the 1993 to 1994 subset (571 cases) found that no cases of serious toxicity were reported and gastrointestinal symptoms occurred in only 5% of cases.[167]

Safety in children

Poisonings in children due to the ingestion of horsechestnut seeds or infusions made from the leaves and twigs have been reported, including fatalities.[168] However, in an analysis of human exposures to *Aesculus spp.* which included 1527 children aged 0 to 5 years, serious toxicity was not reported and no effect or a non-toxic effect occurred in the majority of cases.[167] Cases of toxicity in children attributed to horsechestnut seed might have actually resulted from ingestion of the seed capsule (pericarp).

Regulatory status in selected countries

A draft monograph of horsechestnut is being prepared for the *European Pharmacopoeia*.[169,170]

Horsechestnut seed is covered by a positive Commission E monograph and can be used to treat symptoms of venous disorders and chronic venous insufficiency, such as pain and a feeling of heaviness in the legs, night cramps, itching and swelling.

Horsechestnut is included in the UK General Sale List. Horsechestnut products have achieved Traditional Herbal Registration in the UK with the traditional indication of relief of symptoms associated with CVI and varicose veins such as tired heavy legs, pain, cramps and swelling.

Horsechestnut does not have GRAS status. However, it is freely available as a 'dietary supplement' in the USA under DSHEA legislation (1994 Dietary Supplement Health and Education Act).

Horsechestnut is not included in Part 4 of Schedule 4 of the Therapeutic Goods Act Regulations of Australia and is freely available for sale.

References

1. Grieve M. *A Modern Herbal*, vol. 1. New York: Dover Publications; 1971. p. 193.
2. Felter HW. *The Eclectic Materia Medica, Pharmacology and Therapeutics*. 1922; Portland: Reprinted by Eclectic Medical Publications; 1983. p. 406.
3. Smeh NJ. *Creating Your Own Cosmetics – Naturally*. Garrisonville: Alliance Publishing; 1995. pp. 83, 134, 136, 139, 141, 142.
4. Liehn HD, Franco PA, Hampel H, et al. *Pan Med*. 1972;14(3):84–91.
5. Launert EL. *The Hamlyn Guide to Edible and Medicinal Plants of Britain and Northern Europe*. London: Hamlyn; 1981. p. 57.
6. Fitter R, Fitter A, Blamey M. *The Wild Flowers of Britain and Northern Europe*, 2nd ed. London: Collins; 1974. p. 36.
7. Hostettmann K, Marston A. *Chemistry and Pharmacology of Natural Products: Saponins*. Cambridge: Cambridge University Press; 1995. p. 318.
8. Wagner H, Bladt S. *Plant Drug Analysis: A Thin Layer Chromatography Atlas*, 2nd ed. Berlin: Springer-Verlag; 1996. p. 308.
9. Leung AY, Foster S. *Encyclopedia of Common Natural Ingredients Used in Food, Drugs and Cosmetics*, 2nd ed. New York: John Wiley; 1996. pp. 304–306.
10. Sirtori CR. *Pharmacol Res*. 2001;44(3): 183–193.
11. Vogel G, Marek ML. *Arzneimittelforschung*. 1962;12:815–825.
12. Vogel G, Marek ML, Oertner R. *Arzneimittelforschung*. 1970;20(5):699–703.
13. Berti F, Omini C, Longiave D. *Prostaglandins*. 1977;14(2):241–249.

14. Lorenz D, Marek ML. *Arzneimittelforschung.* 1960;10:263–272.

15. Vogel G, et al. *Arztl Forsch.* 1965;19:98.

16. Wang T, Fu F, Zhang L, et al. *Pharmacol Rep.* 2009;61(4):697–704.

17. Vogel G, Strocker H. *Arzneimittelforschung.* 1966;16(12):1630–1634.

18. Preziosi P, Manca P. *Folia Endocrinol.* 1964;17:527–555.

19. Preziosi P, Manca P. *Arzneimittelforschung.* 1965;15(4):404–413.

20. Preziosi P, Manca P. *Arzneimittelforschung.* 1965;15(4):413–415.

21. Xin W, Zhang L, Sun F, et al. *Phytomedicine.* 2011;18(4):272–277.

22. Eisenburger R, Hofrichter G, Liehn HD, et al. *Arzneimittelforschung.* 1976;26(5):821–824.

23. Przerwa M, Arnold M. *Arzneimittelforschung.* 1975;25(7):1048–1053.

24. Montopoli M, Froldi G, Comelli M, et al. *Planta Med.* 2007;73(3):285–288.

25. Carrasco OF, Vidrio H. *Vascul Pharmacol.* 2007;47(1):68–73.

26. Guillaume M, Padioleau F. *Arzneimittelforschung.* 1994;44(1):25–35.

27. Felixsson E, Persson IA, Eriksson AC, et al. *Phytother Res.* 2010;24(9):1297–1301.

28. Li X, Chen GP, Li L, et al. *Microvasc Res.* 2010;79(1):63–69.

29. Wienert V. *Int J Angiol.* 1997;6(2):115–117.

30. Pauschinger P, Piechowiak H, Schnizer W, et al. *Med Welt.* 1974;25(14):603–607.

31. Pauschinger P. *Ergebnisse Angiolog.* 1984;30:129–137.

32. Enghofer E, Seibel K, Hammersen F. *Therapiewoche.* 1984;34(27):4130–4144.

33. Ehringer H. *Arzneimittelforschung.* 1968;18(4):432–434.

34. Lochs H, Baumgartner H, Honzatt H. *Arzneimittelforschung.* 1974;24(9):1347–1350.

35. Klemm J. *Munch Med Wochenschr.* 1982;124:579–582.

36. Marshall M, Dormandy JA. *Phlebology.* 1987;2:123–124.

37. Matsuda H, Li Y, Murakami T, et al. *Eur J Pharmacol.* 1999;368(2–3):237–243.

38. Matsuda H, Li Y, Yoshikawa M. *Life Sci.* 2000;67(24):2921–2927.

39. Matsuda H, Li Y, Yoshikawa M. *Life Sci.* 2000;66(3):PL41–PL46.

40. Li Y, Matsuda H, Wen S, et al. *Eur J Pharmacol.* 2000;387(3):337–342.

41. Li Y, Matsuda H, Wen S, et al. *Bioorg Med Chem Lett.* 1999;9(17):2473–2478.

42. Matsuda H, Li Y, Yoshikawa M. *Eur J Pharmacol.* 1999;373(1):63–70.

43. Fu F, Hou Y, Jiang W, et al. *World J Surg.* 2005;29(12):1614–1620.

44. Sayek I. *World J Surg.* 2005;29(12):1621–1622.

45. Matsuda H, Li Y, Yoshikawa M. *Bioorg Med Chem.* 1999;7(8):1737–1741.

46. Tan SM, Li F, Rajendran P, et al. *J Pharmacol Exp Ther.* 2010;334(1):285–293.

47. Zhou XY, Fu FH, Li Z, et al. *Planta Med.* 2009;75(15):1580–1585.

48. Harikumar KB, Sung B, Pandey MK, et al. *Mol Pharmacol.* 2010;77(5):818–827.

49. Ming ZJ, Hu Y, Qiu YH, et al. *Phytomedicine.* 2010;17(8–9):575–580.

50. [No authors listed] *Leuk Lymphoma* 2009;50(6):1061.

51. Niu YP, Wu LM, Jiang YL, et al. *J Pharm Pharmacol.* 2008;60(9):1213–1220.

52. Niu YP, Li LD, Wu LM. *Leuk Lymphoma.* 2008;49(7):1384–1391.

53. Chan PK. *Biochem Pharmacol.* 2007;73(3):341–350.

54. Patlolla JM, Raju J, Swamy MV, et al. *Cancer Ther.* 2006;5(6):1459–1466.

55. Fujimura T, Tsukahara K, Moriwaki S, et al. *J Cosmet Sci.* 2006;57(5):369–376.

56. Fujimura T, Tsukahara K, Moriwaki S, et al. *Int J Cosmet Sci.* 2007;29:140.

57. Fujimara T, Moriwaki S, Hotta M, et al. *Biol Pharm Bull.* 2006;29(6):1075–1081.

58. Masaki H, Sakaki S, Atsumi T, et al. *Biol Pharm Bull.* 1995;18(1):162–166.

59. Facino RM, Carini M, Stefani R, et al. *Arch Pharm.* 1995;328(10):720–724.

60. Yoshikawa M, Murakami T, Matsuda H, et al. *Chem Pharm Bull.* 1996;44(8):1454–1464.

61. Hu XM, Zhang Y, Zeng FD. *Acta Pharmacol Sin.* 2004;25(10):1267–1275.

62. Hu XM, Zhang Y, Zeng FD. *Acta Pharmacol Sin.* 2004;25(7):869–875.

63. Hu XM, Zeng FD. *Yao Xue Xue Bao.* 2004;39(6):419–423.

64. Zhang L, Fu F, Zhang X, et al. *Neurochem Int.* 2010;57(2):119–127.

65. Lindner I, Meier C, Url A, et al. *BMC Immunol.* 2010;11:24.

66. Avci G, Küçükkurt I, Küpeli AE, et al. *Pharm Biol.* 2010;48(3):247–252.

67. Lang W. *Res Exp Med (Berl).* 1977;169(3):175–187.

68. Markwardt F. *Phlebology.* 1996;11:10–15.

69. Schrader E, Schwankl W, Sieder C, et al. *Pharmazie.* 1995;50(9):623–627.

70. Oschmann R, Biber A, Lang F, et al. *Pharmazie.* 1996;51(8):577–581.

71. Kunz K, Lorkowski G, Petersen G, et al. *Arzneimittelforschung.* 1998;48(8):822–825.

72. Loew D, Schroedter A, Schwankl W, et al. *Methods Find Exp Clin Pharmacol.* 2000;22(7):537.

73. Bässler D, Okpanyi S, Schrödter A, et al. *Adv Ther.* 2003;20(5):295–304.

74. Yang XW, Zhao J, Cui JR, Guo W. *Beijing Da Xue Xue Bao.* 2004;36(1):31–35.

75. Put TR. *Munch Med Wochenschr.* 1979;121(31):1019–1022.

76. Heppner F, Ascher WP, Argyropoulos G. *Wien Med Wochenschr.* 1967;117(29):706–709.

77. Wilhelm K, Feldmeier C. *Med Klin.* 1977;72(4):128–134.

78. Pirard J, Gillet P, Guffens M, et al. *Rev Med Liege.* 1976;31(10):343–345.

79. Li FL, Xu R, Zhou R, et al. *Zhong Xi Yi Jie He Xue Bao.* 2004;2(6):426–428.

80. Xie Q, Zong X, Ge B, et al. *World J Surg.* 2009;33(2):348–354.

81. Siegers CP, Syed AS, Tegtmeier M. *Phytomedicine.* 2008;15(3):160–163.

82. Liu J, Li Y, Yuan X, et al. *Med Hypotheses.* 2008;71(5):762–764.

83. Isbary JW. *Z Allgemeinmed.* 1975;51(14):684–686.

84. Rothhaar J, Thiel W. *Med Welt.* 1982;33(27):1006–1010.

85. Crielaard JM, Franchimont P. *Acta Bel Med Phys.* 1986;9(4):287–298.

86. Pabst H, Kleine MW. *Fortschr Med.* 1986;104(3):44–46.

87. Arslanagic I, Brkic N. *Med Arh.* 1982;36(4):205–208.

88. Zuinen C. *Rev Med Liege.* 1976;31(5):169–174.

89. Anonymous *Munch Med Wochenschr.* 1992;134(70):73.

90. Rocco P. *Minerva Med.* 1980;71(29):2071–2078.

91. Scremin S, Piccinni P, Potenza A. *Eur Rev Med Pharmacol Sci.* 1986;8:219–224.

92. Paciaroni E, Marini M. *Policlin.* 1982;89(3):255–264.

93. Pozza E, Menghi R, Pansini GC, et al. *Acta Chir Ital.* 1980;36:157–166.

94. Baruffaldi M, Turchi G. *Gazzetta Med Ital.* 1982;141(5):251–256.

95. Agostini F, Califano L. *Clin Eur.* 1979;18(6):1008–1012.

96. Dini D, Bianchini M, Massa T, et al. *Minerva Med.* 1981;72(35):2319–2322.

97. Tozzi E, Scatena M, Castellacci E. *Clin Ter.* 1981;98(5):517–524.

98. Wojcicki J, Samochowiec L, Lawczynski L, et al. *Arch Immunol Ther Exp (Warsz).* 1976;24(6):807–810.

99. Tolino A. *Minerva Ginecol.* 1979;31(3):169–174.

100. Malin L, Pollinzi V. *G Clin Med.* 1978;59(11):521–529.

101. Nappi R. *Clin Ter.* 1978;86(3):219–223.

102. Lapas K, Todorov I. *Akush Ginekol (Sofiia).* 1987;26(4):88–89.

103. Bertrand GL. *Rev Odontostomatol Midi Fr.* 1981;39(4):211–216.

104. Rothhaar J, Thiel W. *Med Welt.* 1982;33(27):1006–1010.

105. Calabrese C, Preston P. *Planta Med.* 1993;59(5):394–397.

106. Pabst H, Segesser B, Bulitta M, et al. *Int J Sports Med.* 2001;22:430–436.

107. Wetzel D, Menke W, Dieter R, et al. *Br J Sports Med.* 2002;36(3):183–188.

108. Belcaro G, Nicolaides AN, Geroulakos G, et al. *Angiology.* 2001;52(Suppl 3):S1–S4.

109. Incandela L, Belcaro G, Cesarone MR, et al. *Angiology.* 2001;52(Suppl 3):S17–S21.

110. De Sanctis MT, Incandela L, Belcaro G, et al. *Angiology.* 2001;52(Suppl 3):S29–S34.

111. Incandela L, Belcaro G, Cesarone MR, et al. *Angiology*. 2001;52(Suppl 3): S23–S27.

112. Incandela L, Belcaro G, Cesarone MR, et al. *Angiology*. 2001;52(Suppl 3): S35–S41.

113. Cesarone MR, Incandela L, Belcaro G, et al. *Angiology*. 2001;52(Suppl 3): S43–S48.

114. De Sanctis MT, Cesarone MR, Incandela L, et al. *Angiology*. 2001;52(Suppl 3): S57–S62.

115. Incandela L, De Sanctis MT, Cesarone MR, et al. *Angiology*. 2001;52(Suppl 3):S69–S72.

116. Cesarone MR, Belcaro G, Ippolito E, et al. *Angiology*. 2004;55(Suppl 1):S7–S10.

117. Belcaro G, Cesarone MR, Dugall M. *Angiology*. 2004;55(Suppl 1):S1–S5.

118. Ricci A, Ruffini I, Cesarone MR, et al. *Angiology*. 2004;55(Suppl 1):S11–S14.

119. Ruffini I, Belcaro G, Cesarone MR, et al. *Angiology*. 2004;55(Suppl 1):S19–S21.

120. Raffetto JD, Khalil RA. *Phlebology*. 2008;23(2):85–98.

121. Siebert U, Brach M, Sroczynski G, et al. *Int Angiol*. 2002;21(4):305–315.

122. Pittler MH, Ernst E. *Cochrane Database Syst Rev*. 2006(1):CD003230.

123. Jadad AR, Moore A, Carroll D, et al. *Control Clin Trials*. 1996;17:1–12.

124. Diehm C, Vollbrecht D, Amendt K, et al. *Vasa*. 1992;21(2):188–191.

125. Rudofsky G, Neiss A, Otto K, et al. *Phlebol Proktol*. 1986;15:47–54.

126. Lohr E, Garanin G, Jesau P, et al. *Munch Med Wochenschr*. 1986;128(31):579–581.

127. Steiner M, Hillemanns HG. *Munch Med Wochenschr*. 1986;128(31):551–552.

128. Erdlen F. *Med Welt*. 1989;40:994–996.

129. Pilz E. *Med Welt*. 1990;41:1143–1144.

130. Friedrich HC, Vogelsang H, Neiss A. *Z Hautkr*. 1978;53:369–374.

131. Neiss A, Bohm C. *Munch Med Wochenschr*. 1976;118(7):213–216.

132. Steiner M, Hillemanns HG. *Phlebology*. 1990;5:41–44.

133. Diehm C, Trampisch HJ, Lange S, et al. *Lancet*. 1996;347(8997):292–294.

134. Erler M. *Med Welt*. 1991;42:593–596.

135. Rehn R, Unkauf M, Klein P, et al. *Arzneimittelforschung*. 1996;46(5):483–487.

136. Koch R. *Phytother Res*. 2002;16(Suppl 1): S1–S5.

137. Ottillinger B, Greeske K. *BMC Cardiovasc Disorders*. 2001;1:5.

138. Alter H. *Z Allge Med*. 1973;49(27): 1301–1304.

139. Bisler H, Pfeifer R, Kluken N, et al. *Dtsch Med Wochenschr*. 1986;111(35):1321–1329.

140. Greeske K, Pohlmann BK. *Fortschr Med*. 1996;114(15):196–200.

141. Leskow P. *Therapiewoche*. 1996;46: 874–877.

142. Suter A, Bommer S, Rechner J. *Adv Ther*. 2006;23(1):179–190.

143. Leach MJ, Pincombe J, Foster G. *J Wound Care*. 2006;15(4):159–167.

144. Leach MJ, Pincombe J, Foster G. *Ostomy Wound Manage*. 2006;52(4):68–70. [72–4, 76–78].

145. Kronberger L, Gölles J. *Med Klin*. 1969;64:1207–1209.

146. Saffar H. *Therapiewoche*. 1981;31(36):5666–5667.

147. Buchherger, Metzner. *2nd International Congress on Phytomedicine*, Munich, September 11–14, 1996.

148. Fang Y, Zhao L, Yan F, et al. *Phytomedicine*. 2010;17(3–4):192–196.

149. Grases F, Garc a–Gonz lez R, Redondo E, et al. *Clin Ther*. 2004;26(12):2045–2055.

150. Williams M, Olsen JD. *Am J Vet Res*. 1984;45(3):539–542.

151. Blaschek W, ebel S, Hackenthal E, et al. *HagerROM 2002: Hagers Handbuch der Drogen und Arzneistoffe*. Heidelberg: Springer; 2002.

152. Ulicna O, Volmut J, Kupcova V, et al. *Bratisl Lek Listy*. 1993;94(3):158–161.

153. Von Kreybig T, Prechtel K. *Arzneimittelforschung*. 1977;27:1465.

154. Pangiati D. *Boll Chim Farm*. 1992;131(8):320–321.

155. Schimmer O, Kruger A, Paulini H, et al. *Pharmazie*. 1994;49:448–451.

156. Ito N. *Jpn J Cancer Res*. 1992;83(3): 312–313.

157. Voigt E, Junger H. *Anaesthesist*. 1978;27(2):81–83.

158. Hellberg K, Ruschewski W, de Vivie R. *Thoraxchir Vask Chir*. 1975;23(4): 396–399.

159. Hellum BH, Nilsen OG. *Basic Clin Pharmacol Toxicol*. 2008;102(5):466–475.

160. Steiner M. *Phebol Proktol*. 1990;5:41–44.

161. Hitzenberger G. *Wien Med Wochenschr*. 1989;139(17):385–389.

162. Takegoshi K, Tohyama T, Okuda K, et al. *Gastroenterol Jpn*. 1986;21(1):62–65.

163. Mckenna DJ, Jones K, Hughes K, et al. *Botanical Medicines: The Desk Reference for Major Herbal Supplements*, 2nd ed. New York: The Haworth Herbal Press; 2002. p. 688.

164. Munoz X, Culebras M, Cruz MJ, et al. *Ann Allergy Asthma Immunol*. 2006;96(3): 494–496.

165. Grob PJ, Muller–Schoop JW, Hacki MA, et al. *Lancet*. 1975;2(7926):144–148.

166. Escribano MM, Munoz–Bellido FJ, Velazquez E, et al. *Contact Dermatitis*. 1997;37(5):233.

167. Maytunas N, Krenzelok E, Jacobson T, et al. *J Toxicol Clin Toxicol*. 1997;35: 527–528.

168. Hardin JW, Arena JM. *Human Poisoning From Native and Cultivated Plants*. Durham, NC: Duke University Press; 1965. p. 80.

169. [No authors listed]. *Pharmeuropa* 2008;20(3): 477–481.

170. [No authors listed]. *Pharmeuropa* 2008;20(3): 481–483.

Kava

(*Piper methysticum* Forst. f.)

Synonyms

Kava, kava kava, intoxicating pepper (Engl), Piperis methystici rhizoma (Lat), Kawa Pfeffer, Rauschpfeffer (Ger), kawa (Fr), pepe kava (Ital), kavarod (Dan), kava, kawa, kava kava (Polynesian), yaqona (Fiji).

What is it?

Captain James Cook, in the account of his voyage to the South Seas in 1768, first described for the Western world the ceremonial use of an intoxicating drink prepared from the root of *Piper methysticum*, better known as kava. The kava beverage first causes a numbing and astringent effect in the mouth. This is followed by a relaxed, sociable state where fatigue and anxiety are lessened. Eventually a deep restful sleep ensues, from which the user awakens the next morning refreshed and without a hangover. Excessive consumption can lead to dizziness and stupefaction and a syndrome of kava abuse has been described. For this reason, some practitioners were reluctant to use kava therapeutically. However, clinical studies demonstrated the important value of kava as a non-addictive anxiolytic with an efficacy comparable to benzodiazepines.

In November 2001, the German Health Authority (BfArM) announced that it was intending to ban the use of kava because of reported cases linking kava consumption with hepatotoxicity. Despite submissions from manufacturers, therapeutic use of kava was banned in Germany in 2002 and several other countries such as Japan, France, Switzerland; the UK and Canada followed suit. The therapeutic use of kava is still permitted in Australia, provided aqueous extracts or the powdered root are used.

Kava is found and used in nearly all the Pacific islands except New Zealand, New Caledonia and most of the Solomon Islands. Use in Hawaii was once common, but has now practically disappeared.[1] Potent kava beverages are prepared by first chewing or grinding the fresh root to produce a cloudy, milky mash. Saliva breaks down the starch and facilitates the suspension of the resin. Its cultural role in Pacific societies is compared with the role of wine in southern Europe.

Effects

Decreases anxiety and relaxes the body without loss of mental acuity; a mild analgesic with a local anaesthetic effect on mucous membranes; improves sleep and possibly mood.

Traditional view

Apart from its ceremonial use, kava is also regarded as a medicinal herb in the Pacific region. In Fiji, it is used as a diuretic to treat kidney and bladder troubles, for filariasis and as a panacea for a variety of common complaints including coughs, colds and sore throat. A decoction of the pounded roots is reputedly used as a contraceptive by women who have recently given birth.[2,3] In Samoa the root is used to treat gonorrhoea.[2] At one time, kava was used in Hawaii to treat skin disorders,[4] to soothe nerves, induce relaxation and sleep, and to treat general debility, colds and chills.[5] Topical application in Polynesian medicine included skin diseases, leprosy, to prevent suppuration and for vaginal prolapse.[3] In traditional Western herbal medicine, kava was recommended for acute and chronic gonorrhoea, vaginitis (topically), leucorrhoea (topically), nocturnal incontinence (particularly when due to muscular weakness) and other ailments of the genitourinary tract.[6] In addition to these applications, the Eclectics recommended kava for the treatment of neuralgia, toothache, earache, ocular pain, dizziness, despondency, anorexia, dyspepsia, intestinal catarrh, haemorrhoids and renal colic.[7]

Summary actions

Anxiolytic, hypnotic, mild sedative, skeletal muscle relaxant, local anaesthetic, mild analgesic.

Can be used for

Indications supported by clinical trials

Anxiety, nervous tension, restlessness or mild depression of non-psychotic origin; menopausal symptoms; insomnia.

Traditional therapeutic uses

For inflammation and infection of the genitourinary tract in both men and women; pain of muscular and nervous origin; insomnia. Topically for toothache and vaginitis.

May also be used for

Extrapolations from pharmacological studies

Improvement of cognitive performance; relaxation of skeletal muscle suggests benefit in treating conditions associated with skeletal muscle spasm and tension, such as headaches due to neck tension; improvement of baroreflex control of the heart rate in generalised anxiety disorder; to assist in withdrawal from benzodiazepine drugs; pain relief as an analgesic and/or local anaesthetic.

Preparations

Decoction of dried root, aqueous extract or powdered root in tablets for internal use; liquid extract for external use or as an ingredient in ointments and creams.

Dosage

For anxiolytic activity, the following doses are recommended:
- 1.5 to 3g/day of dried root or in decoction
- Standardised preparations containing 100 to 200mg/day of kava lactones prepared from the aqueous extract.

The daily dose should be divided throughout the day. Clinical trials on standardised extracts employed doses at the higher end of this range. For hypnotic activity, the same daily quantity can be taken as a single dose 1h before bed. For the other effects of kava, similar or higher doses may be required.

Where tinctures and fluid extracts are legal to use, equivalent doses to the above can be used, but caution regarding potential liver reactions should be exercised.

Duration of use

Kava has been used for 6 months in a clinical trial at a dose equivalent to 210mg lactones per day without adverse effects. Long-term ingestion of doses equivalent to 400mg or more of kava lactones per day is linked to the development of a scaly skin rash in some users.

Summary assessment of safety

Adverse effects from ingestion of kava are not generally expected when the recommended dosage is observed. Skin reactions and dopamine antagonism have, however, been reported. Kava has also been implicated in several idiosyncratic, rare cases of liver damage in humans. Aqueous extracts of kava root are likely to be safer in this context.

Technical data

Botany

Piper methysticum is a cultigen derived from *P. wichmannii*. It is indigenous from New Guinea to Vanuatu and is a member of the Piperaceae (pepper) family. Kava is a dioecious shrub growing up to 3m in height and is particularly cultivated in Fiji and the western Pacific.[8,9] The plant has pale green to yellowish leaf blades up to 28cm long, with up to 13 veins spreading from the base. The flower spikes are up to 9cm long and are borne in the leaf axils.[2] The rootstock (also referred to as stump) has been erroneously called a rhizome by botanists. Kava has no rhizome. From the pithy rootstock extends a fringe of lateral roots up to 3m long. Rootstock colour varies from white to dark yellow, depending upon the amount of flavokavains present in a lemon-yellow resin. The first inflorescence appears at 2 to 3 years of age.[10]

Adulteration

Instead of a rhizome with the periderm and roots removed, kava may be presented for commerce as an unpeeled rhizome covered with the cork, or with the roots attached.[11] Peelings from the root and stump are also used in commerce but should be regarded as inappropriate.[12]

Key constituents

- Resin containing 6-styryl-4-methoxy-alpha-pyrone derivatives, known as kava pyrones or kava lactones (5% to 9%, depending on geographical location),[13] including kavain (or kawain), dihydrokavain (DHK), methysticin, dihydromethysticin (DHM), yangonin and desmethoxyyangonin[11,14]
- Flavonoids (flavokavains).[15]

Kavain

Dihydrokavain

Methysticin

Pharmacodynamics

Sedative and hypnotic activity

In an early study, kava resin and kava lactones did not interact with GABA (gamma-aminobutyric acid) or benzodiazepine-binding sites in the brain.[16] Later studies, however, did suggest that the kava lactones do have an effect on $GABA_A$ receptor binding.[17] In particular, modulation of brainstem GABAergic mechanisms by a kava lactone mixture and DHK were observed in vitro[18] and several kava lactones enhanced the binding of radiolabelled bicuculline to the $GABA_A$ receptor in vitro, an effect not based upon an interaction with the benzodiazepine receptor.[19] Kava extract was found to be a reversible inhibitor of monoamine oxidase (MAO)-B in intact human platelets, with kavain being the least potent.[20] An investigation of the acute effects of kava extract (250 and 500 mg/kg, oral) in the mouse found that the lower dose did not affect brain neurotransmitter levels, whereas the higher dose significantly reduced dopamine.[21] These results were in agreement with earlier reports.

Kava extracts or purified lactones demonstrated sedative effects and induced sleep in a variety of in vivo experimental models.[22,23] In one study, the total extract of the rootstock was more active than any of the isolated kava lactones.[24] DHK and DHM produced sedation and hypothermia in mice[25] and kava lactones given to rabbits produced EEG (electroencephalogram) changes similar to sedative drugs.[26] Kava resin inhibited experimentally induced hypermotility and conditioned avoidance responses in mice, but the effect was mild compared to antipsychotic drugs. Higher doses of kava caused marked sedation.[27]

Testing of a lactone-free (aqueous) kava extract and kava resin by injection in mice indicated that the major pharmacological effects of reduced motor control and sleep induction are due to components in the resin (the kava lactones).[28] Sedative effects were also observed from the injection of the aqueous extract of kava.[29]

Modifications of EEG patterns observed in an experimental model suggest that kava and kavain induce sleep by acting on the limbic system, in particular the amygdala complex. Hence, sleep may be promoted by a modulation of emotional processes, leading to an effect on the brain that is different to benzodiazepines or tricyclic antidepressants.[30] Investigations in rats using intraperitoneal injection of lactones suggested that changes in the activity of serotonergic neurons could explain the sleep-inducing action.[31]

Kava extract (100 mg/kg providing 50 mg/kg lactones, oral) and Passiflora extract (250 mg/kg, oral) were tested individually and in combination in a controlled pharmacological study on hypermotility and sleeping time in mice. Both of the herbal extracts exerted statistically significant but different sedative effects. Kava reduced the induced hypermotility to a greater extent than Passiflora, while both herbs prolonged barbiturate sleeping time to a similar extent. Pronounced synergism between the two extracts was observed when they were administered simultaneously.[32,33] In an experimental model, high doses of ethanol (1.5 to 3.0 g/kg) potentiated the sedative and hypnotic activity of kava resin (350, 450 and 600 mg/kg, oral) and markedly increased the toxicity.[34]

Kava extract was examined for its effect on the sleep-wake cycle in sleep-disturbed rats. A significant shortening of sleep latency was observed for an oral dose of 300 mg/kg, but with no effect on total waking and non-REM sleep time. Kava did show a significant increase in delta activity during non-REM sleep. The effect of the kava was not antagonised by flumazenil (a benzodiazepine receptor antagonist).[35]

Anxiolytic activity

Studies using isolated hippocampal tissue of guinea pigs suggest that kavain and DHM may have additive actions and could enhance the effects of the anxiolytic serotonin-1A agonist ipsapirone. The activation of NMDA receptors and/or voltage-dependent calcium channels may be involved in the elementary mechanism of action.[36,37] (NMDA receptors are a class of glutamate receptors characterised by affinity for N-methyl-D-aspartate.)

A review examined the effect of kava lactones (mainly kavain) on neurotransmission and voltage-gated ion channels. The findings suggest that kava lactones have a weak sodium antagonistic effect that may contribute to their anti-epileptic properties. They have pronounced L-type calcium channel antagonistic properties and act as positive modulators of the early potassium outward current (possibly important for mood stabilisation). Furthermore, they exhibit additive effects with the serotonin-1A agonist ipsapirone and show a distinct pattern of action on glutamatergic and GABAergic transmission, without affecting long-term potentiation. The authors concluded that the profile of cellular actions exhibited by kava overlap with several synthetic mood stabilisers, particularly lamotrigine.[38]

Kava extract administered intraperitoneally to mice induced behavioural changes in the mirrored chamber avoidance assay and elevated plus-maze assay, consistent with anxiolytic activity. The effective doses to achieve a result in 50% of mice (ED_{50}) for each model were 125 mg/kg and 88 mg/kg, respectively. Kava extract also caused a profound decrease in locomotor activity (ED_{50} 172 mg/kg). Flumazenil, a benzodiazepine receptor antagonist, did not block any effect of kava (as it did with diazepam). The authors suggested that the anxiolytic-like behavioural changes and sedation observed for kava are not mediated through the benzodiazepine-binding site on the $GABA_A$ receptor complex.[39] However, despite this finding, anxiolytic-like behavioural changes for kava extract (120 and 240 mg/kg, oral) were similar to diazepam in the elevated plus maze test in mice.[40]

DHK was found to be the lactone most likely responsible for the anxiolytic activity observed in the Chick Social Separation Stress procedure. Intraperitoneal doses of kava extract attenuated distress vocalisations in a dose-dependent manner. The kava fraction containing the highest concentration of DHK was most active and attenuated distress vocalisations with a potency equivalent to chlordiazepoxide (CDP).[41,42] Kava extract (up to 560 mg/kg, oral) partially substituted for the anxiolytic effects of CDP in rats in a dose-dependent manner, but was less potent than the drug.[43]

In a single-blind study against placebo involving six healthy volunteers, a standardised extract of kava (300 or 600 mg, containing 70% kava lactones) improved cognitive performance and stabilised emotional disposition without causing sedation. EEG measurements indicate that an anxiolytic activity was produced without sedative or hypnotic effects.[44]

Fifty-four healthy volunteers underwent a standardised mental stress task and were then randomised to treatment for 7 days with either kava (120 mg/day) or valerian extracts (600 mg/day), or to a non-placebo control group. After this period they repeated the task. The kava and valerian groups reported feeling under less pressure and their systolic blood pressures were significantly lower, compared to a week earlier (p<0.001 for both groups). Heart rate was reduced in the valerian group but not the kava group, and diastolic blood pressure did not change in either group. There were no significant differences in blood pressure, heart rate or subjective reports of pressure in the control group.[45]

Preliminary findings suggest a beneficial effect of kava on the baroreflex control of heart rate (BRC). Significantly more patients with generalised anxiety disorder exhibited improved BRC following treatment with kava compared to a placebo (p<0.05). There was no effect on respiratory sinus arrhythmia, a measure of the heart rate changes occurring with respiration. Patients in the study were a subgroup of a larger randomised, double blind trial and received kava extract (280 mg/day, standardised to 30% kava lactones) or placebo for 4 weeks.[46]

Anticonvulsant, muscle relaxant and spasmolytic activities

The potential anticonvulsant activity of kavain was investigated in vitro on stimulated synaptosomes and sodium channel receptor sites. Results suggested an interaction of kavain with voltage-dependent sodium and calcium channels, thereby suppressing an induced increase in cytosolic concentrations of sodium and calcium and the release of endogenous glutamate.[47] Further in vitro tests with kavain and its optical isomer indicated that kavain inhibits veratridine-activated sodium channels non-stereospecifically.[48] Kavain potently inhibited the uptake of labelled noradrenaline (norepinephrine) from synaptosomes. This non-selective inhibition may be responsible for or contribute to the psychotropic properties of kava lactones.[49]

Kava lactones have demonstrated anticonvulsant activity in several in vivo experimental models.[50,51] They were up to 10 times more effective than mephenesin against the convulsant effect of strychnine.[44] A mixture of the lactones (similar to that found in the root) demonstrated a synergistic effect against strychnine-induced convulsions. The potency of the mixture was comparable to the most potent lactone (DHM), which was present at only 5%.[22] When injected intravenously, the differences in the anticonvulsant activity of the lactones were only small.[52] The synergistic effect was more marked for oral administration, due to enhanced absorption of the lactone mixture. (Despite these in vivo results, kava has not proven suitable for the treatment of epilepsy in clinical trials.)

Kava extract and lactones have produced relaxation of skeletal muscle in vitro and in vivo.[53,54] Investigations in rats using intraperitoneal injections of lactones suggested that the skeletal muscle relaxant and slightly euphoric actions may be caused by activation of the mesolimbic dopaminergic neurons.[31]

Kava lactones demonstrated a spasmolytic effect in vitro on smooth muscle similar to papaverine.[1] Studies using isolated guinea pig ileum suggest that kavain may exhibit a general inhibitory effect on contractile activity, exerting a non-specific musculotropic effect on the lipid bilayer of the membrane.[55] Kavain also relaxed aortic rings precontracted with phenylephrine in a dose-dependent manner in vitro. In addition, kavain pretreatment attenuated vascular smooth muscle contraction evoked by phenylephrine. Based on additional experimentation, the authors postulated that the effect of kavain on impairing vascular smooth muscle contraction is likely via calcium channel inhibition.[56] Murine airway smooth muscle contraction was inhibited by kavain in vitro using a tracheal ring preparation.[57]

Local anaesthetic and analgesic activities

The kava lactones have potencies similar to cocaine and procaine as local anaesthetics[58] and have demonstrated analgesic activity in several experimental models.[26,59,60] As an analgesic, DHK was superior to aspirin, but considerably less potent than morphine. Combined administration of DHK with aspirin indicated an additive synergism between the two compounds. Caffeine diminished the duration, but not the intensity, of the analgesic effects of DHK and DHM.[47] Kava resin, kava lactones and a lactone-free (aqueous) extract of kava all demonstrated analgesic properties in experimental models when given by injection. The analgesia produced by kava occurs via non-opiate pathways.[48] This was confirmed using an unspecified kava extract (125 mg/kg, ip) in rats, where kava also demonstrated similar activity to morphine (10 mg/kg, ip).[61]

Effects on performance and vision

Ingestion of 500 mL of traditionally prepared kava beverage by one person caused changes in visual function. A reduced near-point of accommodation and convergence, an increase in pupil diameter and disturbance of the ocular muscle balance were noted. Maximum changes occurred 30 to 40 min after taking the kava drink.[62] A controlled study found that acute administration of a single dose of kava (500 mL of a 1:5 decoction) did not significantly affect cognition compared to placebo, although there was a trend to poorer performance. Those receiving kava reported subjective feelings of intoxication (apparent from increased body sway), which peaked approximately 1 h after ingestion, but there was a high degree of individual variation. Three of the twelve volunteers who received kava reported feeling nauseous.[63]

However, another similar study involving 18 people found no effect on reaction time or errors with typical and excessive doses of a traditional cold macerate of root powder.[64] Also, in a double blind study, 40 healthy subjects received standardised kava extract (300 mg, containing 210 mg kava lactones) to assess the effect on performance capability relevant to operating machines and driving. No significant changes were found.[65]

Hence, any adverse effects are likely dose related. In a small acute randomised study, neither a single dose of 30g of kava powder nor 1g/kg produced any significant changes on cognitive function, compared with a control group of non-kava users.[64]

In a double blind, crossover study to study the effect on event-related potentials in a word recognition task, 12 healthy volunteers received the benzodiazepine drug oxazepam (3 days of placebo, 15mg on the day before testing, 75mg on the morning of testing) or standardised kava extract (600mg/day for 5 days, containing 420mg/day kava lactones). While there was a significant decrease in the quality and speed of responses with oxazepam in several psychometric tests, no changes were observed with kava treatment. In a memory test using word recognition, there was a tendency for kava to improve reaction times and correct answers that was not statistically significant, whereas oxazepam significantly slowed reaction times and reduced the number of correct answers. The changes in event-related potentials induced by kava during the word recognition task were quite different to those caused by oxazepam.[66] In another trial using a similar design, 12 healthy men were tested in a visual search paradigm assessed by event-related potentials. Results indicated kava had a positive effect on the allocation of attention and processing capacity, while these were reduced by oxazepam.[67]

In a placebo-controlled, double blind study involving 40 healthy volunteers, the effect of a standardised kava extract (300mg/day for 8 days, containing 210mg/day kava lactones) combined with ethanol (0.05% blood alcohol concentration) on safety-related performance parameters was investigated. No negative effects were caused by the kava. In fact, it tended to counter the adverse effect of alcohol on mental concentration.[68]

In another randomised, placebo-controlled trial, acute administration of a very high dose of kava (1g/kg) combined with alcohol (0.75g/kg) potentiated both the perceived and measured impairment of motor and cognitive function produced by alcohol alone.[69] Since this study used excessive doses of kava, its relevance to normal clinical use must be questioned.

In a randomised, double blind, crossover clinical study, 12 healthy volunteers received single doses of the following: standardised kava extract (containing 120mg kava lactones), diazepam (10mg) or placebo. Neurophysiological and psychophysiological tests were conducted immediately before and 2 and 6h after administration of the preparations in order to compare mental alertness. Results for both test groups (kava, diazepam) differed significantly from the placebo group. Differences were also apparent between diazepam and kava. The increase in beta-activity, specific to benzodiazepines, did not occur with kava. In addition, the action of kava was undiminished 6h after its application. In one of the psychophysiological tests, performance of complex challenges by kava recipients was better than for placebo or diazepam, despite the relaxing properties of kava. An apparently contradictory combination of properties (increased relaxation and increased performance) was thereby confirmed for kava.[70]

The objective of the another study was to evaluate whether simultaneous administration of bromazepam (4.5mg twice daily) and kava extract (containing 120mg of kava lactones, twice daily) would produce an effect on safety-related performance over and above those anticipated by either single treatment.[71] A double blind, randomised, three-way crossover design was used with 18 healthy volunteers. Performance was measured at 0, 1, 2 and 14 days after each treatment, with a 7-day washout between treatment periods. Seven computer-assisted mental performance tests were used to assess cognitive performance: visual orientation, extended concentration, acoustic reaction time, discriminative reaction time, stress tolerance, vigilance and motor coordination. Vigilance, stress tolerance and motor coordination worsened with bromazepam and the combination, but remained unchanged with kava. Overall, bromazepam and the combination produced the most pronounced impairment of well-being (mainly fatigue). The authors concluded that kava extract plus a benzodiazepine is unlikely to produce greater effects on general well-being and the mental performance aspects required for safety than the benzodiazepine alone. Moreover, patients do not appear to be exposed to additional side effects or risks while taking both treatments at the same time. (See also the Interactions section below.)

Anticancer activity

Kava extract (standardised to 70% kava lactones), isolated kava lactones and isolated flavokavains (A, B and C) were assessed for their effect in vitro on human bladder cancer cells. Both the kava extract and flavokavains exhibited strong antiproliferative and apoptotic effects. Kavain was inactive. Flavokavain A (50mg/kg/day for 25 days, oral) was further tested in vivo on mice injected with bladder tumour cells and was found to attenuate tumour growth by 57%.[72] (An aqueous extract of kava will be low in flavokavains.) Follow-up research showed that flavokavain A induced cell-cycle arrest in wild-type *P53* and mutant *P53* bladder cancer cells in vitro.[73] The same research group also found that flavokavain B induced apoptosis in androgen receptor negative, hormone refractory prostate cancer cell lines. Treatment of mice bearing xenograft tumours with flavokavain B (50mg/kg/day, oral) resulted in tumour growth inhibition.[74]

The correlation between age-standardised cancer incidences and kava consumption in the South Pacific (traditional places of kava consumption) was investigated in an epidemiological study. The cancer incidences in countries such as Vanuatu and Fiji, despite high tobacco consumption, were found to be low.[75] Furthermore, later work demonstrated that cancer incidences in those populations were especially lower in men (the main users of kava), despite much higher smoking rates.[76] Data collected found a close inverse relationship between cancer incidence and kava consumption.[75]

Kava has certainly demonstrated chemopreventative activity in mice. At a dose of 10mg/g diet, 30-week kava treatment reduced lung tumour multiplicity by 56% after repeated exposure to carcinogens.[77] Mechanistically, kava inhibited proliferation and enhanced apoptosis in the lung tumours. A study in six healthy New Caledonian kava users found an association with CYP1A2 inhibition. While this lends to the possibility of drug interactions (see later), the authors also pointed out that CYP1A2 is also responsible for the metabolic activation of potent carcinogens such as aflatoxins.[78] Hence, regular kava users may be protected from the carcinogenic effects of certain environmental toxins (see also below).

Other activity

Kava has been traditionally used as an antibacterial agent, especially for urinary tract infections, but in vitro studies have failed to establish any significant antibacterial activity.[79,80] Some kava lactones exhibited potent fungistatic activity against a wide variety of pathogenic fungi, excluding species of *Candida*.[59] It is possible that the reputed effectiveness of kava in bacterial urinary tract infections is for different reasons. The lactones can undergo chemical changes before being excreted in the urine, which might enhance antimicrobial activity.[81,82]

Kava extract, methysticin and DHK protected brain tissue against ischaemic damage in experimental models. The results were similar to those produced by the anticonvulsant compound memantine.[83] Kava extract (100 and 200 mg/kg, oral) inhibited haloperidol-induced catalepsy in rats.[84] DHK was also active at 100 mg/kg. Hence, kava is unlikely to be responsible for central dopaminergic antagonism. Kava resin did not produce physiological tolerance or learned tolerance in mice when administered at a minimally effective daily dose for 7 weeks or 3 weeks respectively. A considerably higher dose caused partial physiological tolerance.[85]

Antithrombotic activity observed for kavain in vitro is likely to be due to inhibition of cyclo-oxygenase (COX), which suppresses the generation of thromboxane A_2.[86] COX-1 and COX-2 inhibition was later reported in vitro for an ethylacetate kava extract and isolated kava lactones. DHK and yangonin showed the strongest inhibitory effect at 100 µg/mL against both enzymes, activity comparable to the anti-inflammatory drugs ibuprofen, naproxen and aspirin.[87]

Five isolated kava lactones from a methanolic extract of kava (desmethoxyyangonin, yangonin, kavain, DHK and methysticin) were tested in TNF-alpha (tumour necrosis factor-alpha) release assays. Results showed significant inhibition of TNF-alpha release by desmethoxyyangonin and yangonin in vitro, with IC_{50} values of 17 µM and 40 µM, respectively. Each isolated kava lactone or kava root powder was given to diabetic mice via ip injection at 10 mg/kg. TNF-alpha production was then stimulated by lipopolysaccharide (LPS). Both the kava powder and individual lactones significantly suppressed TNF-alpha release. DHK showed the strongest inhibitory activity in vivo, but was weakest in vitro.[88] More recently, kavain was found to counter the LPS-stimulated release of TNF-alpha in vitro and in mice (at a dose of 40 mg/kg, ip).[89]

Flavokavains A and B, as well as kavain and DHK, were shown to inhibit NF-kappaB driven reporter gene expression and TNF-alpha-induced binding of NF-kappaB to a consensus response element in vitro. In addition, kavain and flavokavains A and B countered IkappaB (inhibitor of kappa-B) degradation.[90] Using an in vitro luciferase-based assay with a human lung adenocarcinoma cell line, methysticin was identified as

a potent NF-kappaB inhibitor with minimal toxicity.[91] Other kava constituents demonstrated minimal activity. The authors suggested that methysticin might be responsible for kava's chemopreventative efficacy.

Pharmacokinetics

The bioavailability of kava lactones has been investigated using in vitro models. In one model employing filter-immobilised artificial membranes, assembled from phosphatidylcholine in dodecane, the kava lactones were found to be highly mobile.[92] Of the five lactones tested, kavain had intermediate permeability. Kava lactones readily crossed a Caco-2 monolayer in vitro. The apparent permeability of kavain from ethanol extracts was higher than from water extracts or for the isolated compound.[93] Based on an assessment of molecular characteristics and the available in vitro data, kavain was suggested as the best marker of bioavailability for kava extracts.[94]

After oral doses of kava lactones in rats, approximately half the dose of DHK was found in the urine within 48 h, of which around two-thirds was hydroxylated metabolites. Lower amounts of urinary metabolites were recorded for the other major lactones.[82] Kava lactones are more rapidly absorbed when given orally as an extract of the root than when given as single compounds. The bioavailability of lactones is up to three to five times higher for the extract than when given as single substances.[95]

Kava lactones showed a range of uptake rates into brain tissue when administered as single compounds by intraperitoneal injection to mice. However, when crude kava resin was administered the same way, the brain concentrations of two lactones were markedly increased (two to 20 times), while the others remained at the level established for their individual injection.[96]

Kavain (100 mg/kg) was administered orally to rats with and without co-administration of kava extract (256 mg/kg) and effects on drug disposition were monitored. Kavain was rapidly absorbed into the systemic circulation. Greater than 90% of the dose was eliminated within 72 h, chiefly in urine, and no tissue accumulation was observed. Mean bioavailability of kavain following a single oral dose was 50±7%. Co-administration of kava extract caused a tripling of the kavain area-under-the-curve (AUC) (0–8 h) and a doubling of Cmax, showing an increase in oral bioavailability (the kava extract only delivered an extra 22 mg/kg of kavain). However, a 7-day pre-treatment with the kava extract did not affect the pharmacokinetics on kavain taken alone on day 8. The increased bioavailability of kavain was suggested to be due to an inhibition of the cytochrome P450 system rather than P-glycoprotein.[97]

Several of the above findings suggest that kava lactones are more bioactive and bioavailable when administered as the root extract rather than as isolated compounds.

There have also been some limited pharmacokinetic studies in humans. In an early study, urine was collected from five healthy volunteers after an oral dose of 200 mg of kavain.[98] The main metabolites of kavain in urine were hydroxylation products of the aromatic ring. In addition, opening of the lactone ring, hydroxylation of the lactone ring and subsequent dehydration and reduction of the 7,8-double bond were observed, with further degradation also occurring from these steps. The bulk of the kavain dose was excreted as phase II conjugates. However, different metabolites were observed for an aqueous kava extract given to healthy male volunteers.[81] All the main lactones were detected in urine, and the observed metabolic findings included reduction of the 3,4-double bond and/or demethylation. Neither dihydroxylated metabolites nor products from ring opening were found.

A single oral dose of 800 mg of kavain was administered as a self-medication study.[99] Within 1 and 4 h after uptake, the serum concentrations ranged between 40 and 10 ng/mL for kavain, 300 and 125 ng/mL for p-hydroxykavain, 90 and 40 ng/mL for o-desmethyl-hydroxy-5,6-dehydrokavain, and 50 and 30 ng/mL for 5,6-dehydrokavain. The metabolite p-hydroxy-7,8-dihydrokavain was found in urine only. The compound 6-phenyl-3-hexen-2-one was identified as a metabolite of DHK and kavain (as the mercapturic adduct) in the urine of two people given kava extract.[100] Other novel metabolites (as glucuronate and sulphate conjugates) have also been found in urine after ingestion of a kava extract by a human male volunteer.[101]

Clinical trials

Anxiety

Some earlier trials on anxiety used purified kavain, typically at a dose of 400 mg/day. For example, in a placebo-controlled, double blind study of 84 patients with anxiety symptoms, kavain improved vigilance, memory and reaction time.[102] Kavain demonstrated equivalent activity to an antianxiety drug (oxazepam) in a placebo-controlled, double blind trial involving 38 patients with anxiety associated with neurotic disturbances.[103] The treatments proved to be equivalent in the nature and the potency of their anxiolytic action. Both caused progressive improvement in two different anxiety scores over a 4-week period.

Some case reports and open label trials reporting anxiolytic activity for kava have been published. For example, in an open, observational, multicentre study involving 52 outpatients suffering from anxiety of nonpsychotic origin, 81% of patients rated kava treatment as 'very good' or 'good' on a global improvement scale. Symptoms of anxiety, restlessness and tension also showed a pronounced decrease from baseline on a physician-rated scale. Patients received between 200 and 600 mg/day of standardised kava extract (corresponding to 100 to 300 mg/day of kava lactones) for a mean treatment duration of 51 days. Adverse events were rare and mild.[104]

A 37-year-old female outpatient with generalised anxiety disorder, a simple phobia and a specific social phobia was treated with kava extract at 150 mg three times a day (total daily dose was equivalent to 135 mg kava lactones). After 4 weeks, the patient reported her symptoms were improved by 75%, and clinical tests also reflected this improvement. After 6 months, all clinical and self-rated outcome measures were close to normal. No adverse events were encountered by the patient.[105]

In apparently the first published randomised, double blind, placebo-controlled trial assessing kava, a proprietary extract was evaluated as an acute preoperative medication for anxiety in 60 patients undergoing surgery.[106] Following the kava extract (60 mg), anxiety levels were lower compared to the placebo group, with lower requirement for anxiolytic drugs.

In a randomised, placebo-controlled, double blind study involving patients with anxiety not due to psychotic disorders, a standardised kava extract significantly improved measures of anxiety and depression.[107,108] Patients received a standardised kava extract (300 mg/day, containing 210 mg kava lactones) or placebo over a 4-week period. For patients given the kava extract, there was a significant reduction of anxiety as measured using the Hamilton Anxiety Scale (HAMA, for total score, p<0.02). The difference in anxiety between kava and placebo began in the first week and increased during the course of treatment. There were no adverse effects reported for the kava extract.

A standardised extract of kava was compared to the benzodiazepine drugs bromazepam and oxazepam in a randomised, controlled, double blind study. One hundred and seventy-six outpatients were divided into three approximately equal groups. One group received kava extract equivalent to 210 mg/day of kava lactones, the second group received 15 mg of oxazepam per day and the third group received 9 mg of bromazepam. The total HAMA Score was reduced from 27.3 to 15.6 after 6 weeks of kava treatment, compared to 27.3 down to 13.4 for bromazepam and 27.7 down to 16.6 for oxazepam. Statistical analysis showed that kava treatment was equivalent in efficacy to the benzodiazepine drugs. Side effects were higher in the conventional drug groups.[109] These findings were confirmed in a later three-arm study of similar design involving 145 patients. This study also included a 14-week, open, long-term treatment phase immediately after the 6-week double blind study. Anxiety symptoms continued to decline in this open phase with all the treatments, including kava.[110]

Although there were positive outcomes for the use of kava demonstrated in the above controlled trials, none of the trials lasted for more than 6 weeks, the inclusion criteria were insufficiently defined and patient numbers were relatively small. These issues were addressed in a study published in 1997. In a randomised, placebo-controlled, double blind, multicentre study, 100 patients presenting with nervous anxiety, tension and restlessness of non-psychotic origin (DSM-III-R) were followed over a period of 6 months. Patients were randomised to receive either 300 mg/day of a kava extract containing 210 mg of kava lactones (equivalent to about 4 g of dried root) or placebo. Assessment was based on changes in the cumulative HAMA Score in addition to other assessments. Comparison of the pre- and post-therapy HAMA scores revealed a significant (p=0.0015) superiority of the kava treatment against placebo. The difference between the two treatment groups was apparent after 8 weeks (p=0.055). Kava treatment led to a marked reduction in the symptoms of anxiety, together with its physical and psychic manifestations. In addition, the accompanying depressive component was positively influenced by kava. During the study, six adverse events in five patients were reported in the kava group. Four of these were rated by the investigator as not being related to the treatment, two (in both cases stomach upset) were rated as 'possibly related'. Fifteen adverse events from nine patients were reported in the placebo group. Seven patients dropped out under placebo and three under kava (two of these three were due to improvement of symptoms). There was no significant change in biochemical parameters during the study period and the overall tolerability of kava was rated as excellent. The authors concluded that their results support kava as a treatment alternative to tricyclic antidepressants and benzodiazepines in anxiety, with proven long-term efficacy and apparently none of the tolerance problems associated with these drugs.[111,112]

Sixty patients experiencing daily stress and anxiety of a non-clinical nature were enrolled in a randomised, double blind, placebo-controlled trial.[113] After 4 weeks of 400 mg/day of a proprietary kava extract there were significant differences observed for daily stress and anxiety compared to placebo (p<0.001). No side effects were reported.

A number of large postmarketing surveillance studies were also reported in the 1990s. Treatment of 3029 patients with standardised kava extract (800 mg/day, containing 240 mg kava lactones) over a minimum of 4 weeks resulted in improvement of primary symptoms such as nervousness, restlessness and anger. Other indications including sleep disturbances, menopausal complaints, muscle tension and sexual disturbances were also improved. Sixty-nine patients recorded undesirable side effects, including allergic reaction, gastrointestinal complaints, headache or dizziness.[114] At the end of almost 5 weeks of treatment with standardised kava extract, symptoms of nervousness, restlessness and fear were reduced in 1673 patients. Mild adverse effects were experienced in 1.7% of patients.[115] Similar improvement in symptoms and a similar percentage of mild adverse reactions were observed in 4049 patients treated with standardised kava extract (150 mg/day, containing 105 mg kava lactones) for 7 weeks.[116]

Kava has also been shown to exert a therapeutic benefit in situational anxiety. In a randomised, double blind, placebo-controlled trial (n=20), standardised kava extract taken for 1 week significantly reduced anxiety in patients awaiting the results of medical diagnostic tests for suspected breast carcinoma (p<0.05). Fatigue, introverted behaviour, excitability and depression trended lower compared to placebo (p=0.09, p=0.06, p=0.07 and p=0.08, respectively) and alertness was significantly increased (p=0.05) in patients receiving kava extract. The daily dose of kava contained 150 mg of kava lactones and corresponded to approximately 2.5 g of original dried root.[117]

Results from one study suggest a role for kava in facilitating benzodiazepine withdrawal. A standardised kava extract was significantly superior to placebo in the treatment of anxiety disorders of non-psychotic origin in a randomised, double blind trial lasting 5 weeks and involving 40 patients who had

previously been treated with benzodiazepines. During the first treatment week, the dosage of kava extract was increased from 50 to 300 mg/day in the test group and pretreatment with benzodiazepines was tapered off over 2 weeks. These dosage adjustments were then followed by 3 weeks of treatment with kava extract (300 mg/day) or placebo. Outcomes were measured by HAMA scores and a subjective well-being scale (Bf-S). Kava extract was superior to placebo in both scales (p=0.01 and p=0.002, respectively, and was well tolerated.[118]

Kava extract (400 mg/day, containing 120 mg kava lactones) was compared to buspirone (10 mg/day) and opipramol (100 mg/day) for the treatment of generalised anxiety disorder in a three-arm randomised, double blind multicentre clinical trial. The treatment duration was 8 weeks and the trial involved 129 outpatients. Results demonstrated no difference between the safety and efficacy of the three treatments, with the authors concluding that kava was well tolerated and as effective as buspirone and opipramol.[119]

The efficacy and tolerability of 150 mg/day of kava extract (containing 105 mg kava lactones) were investigated in a 4-week, randomised, placebo-controlled, double blind study in 141 patients suffering from neurotic anxiety (according to the DSM-III-R).[120] While the impact of kava on the Anxiety Status Inventory Clinical Global Impressions Scale (CGI) was greater than placebo, these differences did not achieve statistical significance. As noted by the authors, this lack of a significant finding might be due to the lower dose of kava used compared with other published trials. The kava extract was well tolerated, with no influence on liver function tests and only one minor side effect (tiredness).

A later study did show a positive effect from this dose of kava lactones. Fifty patients were treated with a daily dose of 150 mg of kava extract (containing 105 mg kava lactones) during a 4-week treatment period, followed by a 2-week safety observation phase in a double blind, placebo-controlled clinical trial.[121] In the active treatment group, the total HAMA score showed a therapeutically relevant reduction in anxiety versus placebo (more than four points). This was not significant for intention-to-treat analysis, but did reach significant for per-protocol analysis (p=0.03). In the secondary variables studied, the HAMA 'somatic and psychic anxiety' subscales, the Erlangen Anxiety, Tension and Aggression Scale, the brief personality structure scale (KEPS), the adjective checklist (EWL 60-S) and CGI, a trend in favour of kava was detectable. Kava was well tolerated and showed a good safety profile with no adverse events or post-study withdrawal symptoms.

A systematic review of clinical trials involving kava for the treatment of non-psychotic anxiety was undertaken in 2002 on behalf of the Cochrane Collaboration, published in 2003, and updated in 2005. Twelve out of 22 randomised, double blind, placebo-controlled trials involving a total of 700 participants met the inclusion criteria. A meta-analysis of seven trials using the total HAMA score as a common outcome measure suggested a significant reduction in anxiety for patients receiving kava extract compared to those receiving placebo (all seven trials are reviewed in detail in this monograph). The dosage of standardised kava extract prescribed varied from the equivalent of 105 to 210 mg/day of kava lactones and the duration of treatment ranged from 4 to 24 weeks.[122] A systematic review of herbal remedies for anxiety (that essentially reflected the Cochrane analysis for kava) concluded that only kava has been shown beyond reasonable doubt to have anxiolytic effects in humans.[123]

A meta-analysis was performed on six randomised controlled trials that used only the kava acetone-water extract (containing 70% kava lactones) to avoid heterogeneity.[124] This was undertaken as a supplement to the Cochrane meta-analysis. The one trial that used a female-only cohort was excluded to reduce the heterogeneity further.[125] As a result, the effect of kava on anxiety was reduced slightly, but remained significant (p=0.0738 for a continuous outcome, p<0.0001 for a binary outcome). Sub-group analyses were also performed for age and gender. Improvement of symptoms was noted to be better in younger people (95% CI −0.37 to 17.7, p=0.054) and women (95% CI −1.20 to 15.2, p=0.079). The authors concluded that this specific kava extract was effective in patients with non-psychotic anxiety disorders and also suggested, based on their analysis, that higher doses give results that are more positive.[124]

Another 'meta-analysis' of kava in generalised anxiety disorder, according to the DSM-IV) pooled the results of just three placebo-controlled trials, only one of which had been published.[126] The initial dose contained 140 mg/day kava lactones for 1 week, increasing to 280 mg/day for all three trials. Results of the published trial (duration of 4 weeks) showed no significant difference between kava and placebo for 37 patients in terms of a reduction in the HAMA score.[127] Kava showed improvement in low anxiety groups for the Hospital and Anxiety Depression Scale, an effect deemed non-significant with respect to placebo. Improvement was significant (p<0.01) for the Self Assessment of Resilience and Anxiety scale in low anxiety only. Kava treatment was well tolerated. Results for 58 patients were pooled in the meta-analysis according to HAMA scores. Overall, the authors concluded that kava extract was safe yet ineffective for the treatment of generalised anxiety disorder, due to the lack of any statistical significance of the extract over placebo.[126] The two unpublished trials had been discontinued prematurely due to hepatotoxicity concerns; hence, this meta-analysis has severe limitations, especially the low total patient number and the lack of completion of two of the three trials. As such, its relevance to the overall assessment of the clinical efficacy of kava for anxiety is quite minor.

A randomised, double blind, placebo-controlled trial used a novel Internet-based design to determine if: kava was effective for reducing anxiety and valerian was effective for improving sleep quality.[128] After an initial survey, 391 eligible participants were mailed 4 weeks' supply of either kava (delivering 300 mg/day kava lactones) with valerian placebo (n=121), valerian with kava placebo (n=135) or double placebo. Neither study treatment was statistically superior to placebo, as assessed by questionnaires completed by the trial participants. The kava was well tolerated. Since the authors did not independently verify the quality of the US products they used in the trial, results should be interpreted with caution.

A water-soluble extract of kava was found to be effective in treating anxiety and improving mood in people with chronic anxiety. This short-term placebo-controlled, double blind, crossover trial is the first for evaluating the water-soluble extract.[129,130] After 1 week of placebo (pretreatment phase), 41 adults with 1 month or more of elevated generalised anxiety received aqueous kava extract providing 250 mg/day of kava lactones or placebo tablets for 1 week (phase I). Participants then swapped treatments for an additional week (phase II). HAMA scores were found to be reduced by an average of 9.9 points when kava was received during phase I, compared to a reduction of 0.8 for placebo. They reduced by an average of 10.3 points when kava was received during phase II, compared to an increase of 3.3 for placebo. Considering both phases of the trial, the effect of kava in reducing anxiety was highly significant compared to placebo (p<0.0001). The reduction of 11.4 points over placebo on HAMA compared favourably to benzodiazepine efficacy. Significant relative reductions in depression (Montgomery-Asberg Depression Rating Scale) were also evident (p=0.003). No serious adverse effects were observed.

In the first randomised, double blind, placebo-controlled trial using a combination of St John's wort (900 mg/day standardised to 0.3% total hypericins) and kava (aqueous extract delivering 150 mg/day kava lactones) for the treatment of major depressive disorder with co-morbid anxiety, 28 patients were followed over 4 weeks.[131] The trial employed a crossover design. On both intention-to-treat (p=0.047) and completer analyses (p=0.003), the combination effected a significantly greater reduction in self-reported depression on the Beck Depression Inventory over placebo in the first controlled phase. However, in the crossover phase a replication of these effects did not occur. There was no significant impact on anxiety (Beck Anxiety Index) in either phase of the trial.

Insomnia

The efficacy of standardised kava extract was investigated in a placebo-controlled trial with 12 healthy volunteers over 4 days. Placebo was taken for 3 days and followed the next day by three divided doses totalling either 150 mg kava extract (containing 105 mg kava lactones) or 300 mg extract (containing 210 mg kava lactones). With kava administration the time to fall asleep and the light sleep phase were shortened, the deep sleep phase was lengthened, the duration of REM sleep was not influenced and the duration of wakeful phases in sleep EEG recordings was decreased. These effects were viewed as being favourable, especially compared with conventional sedatives such as benzodiazepines and barbiturates, which depress both REM and deep sleep. Kava administration also increased the density of sleep spindles, an effect which was comparable to sedative drugs.[132]

In a pilot, open label study, patients suffering from stress-induced insomnia were treated in each phase of 6 weeks with a daily dose of 120 mg of a kava extract standardised to 30% kava lactones (n=24), then valerian extract at 600 mg (n=19), then the combination of kava and valerian (n=19), with 2-week washout periods between each treatment phase.[133,134] Total stress severity was significantly relieved by the kava and valerian single treatments (p<0.01) as measured in three areas: social, personal and life events. Insomnia was significantly relieved by the combination of kava and valerian (p<0.05)[133] and the individual treatments (p<0.01).[134] On direct questioning, 16 patients (67%) reported no side effects while on kava, versus 10 (53%) for valerian and 10 (53%) for the combination. The 'commonest' such effects were vivid dreams with kava plus valerian (four cases, 21%) and with valerian alone (three cases, 16%), followed by gastric discomfort and dizziness with kava (three cases each, 3%).[133] The dose of kava lactones used in the trial was relatively low and the results are limited by the lack of a placebo group.

A randomised, placebo-controlled, double blind, multicentre clinical trial assessed a kava extract in sleep disturbances associated with anxiety disorders in 61 patients. The dose of kava extract used was 200 mg/day (containing 140 mg kava lactones) over a period of 4 weeks. Statistically significant group differences were demonstrated in favour of the kava group as measured by the sleep questionnaire SF-B sub-scores 'Quality of sleep' and 'Recuperative effect after sleep' (p=0.007 and p=0.018, respectively). Superior therapeutic efficacy was also demonstrated for kava extract over placebo by way of the Bf-S self-rating scale of well-being, the CGI and the HAMA psychic anxiety sub-score (p=0.002).[135]

A 2005 review of medicinal plants for insomnia suggested that kava '… is a well-established hypnotic drug, with a rapid onset of effect, adequate duration of action and minimal morning after-effects.'[136] However, concerns were expressed over hepatotoxicity.

Other conditions

Past and recent clinical trials indicate kava extract and kava lactones (especially DHM) are not suitable for the treatment of epilepsy. Although efficacy was observed in grand mal seizures, the trials were abandoned due to incidence of side effects (mainly skin problems) when used long-term and in high doses. No efficacy was observed with petit mal.[137,138]

A randomised, double blind, placebo-controlled clinical trial was undertaken using a single dose of 300 mg kava extract (containing 90 mg kava lactones) to assess its impact on emotional reactivity and cognitive performance in 25 kava-naive healthy volunteers.[139] The primary measure used was the state-trait-cheerfulness inventory (measuring three concepts of cheerfulness, seriousness and bad mood as both traits and states). The Sperling partial report was used to examine cognitive performance and the Sternberg item recognition task assessed visual attention and short-term

memory processing. These tests were commenced 60 min after kava or placebo intake. Significant differences were found for kava in the Sperling partial report results, with an increase in correct responses (p=0.006) and a decrease in incorrect responses (p=0.009). The Stenberg task also reflected a benefit for kava, with a decreased average reaction time (p<0.001) and an increase in the percentage of correct responses to probed stimulus (p=0.006), indicating superior recognition. Overall, kava was found to improve performance on a visual search paradigm, facilitate word recognition and enhance the speed of access of information from long-term memory. Kava also increased positive affectivity related to exhilaration (p=0.0001), hence the authors postulated that the improved cognition may be secondary to its mood-enhancing properties.[139]

In a randomised, placebo-controlled, double blind trial of 40 patients with neurovegetative symptoms associated with menopause, a standardised kava extract (containing 210 mg kava lactones per day for 8 weeks) produced a significant reduction in anxiety, depression, severity of symptoms and menopausal symptoms (p<0.01). The subjective well-being of patients improved with kava and the herbal treatment was well tolerated.[125]

The effect of kava extract on menopausal anxiety in combination with hormone replacement therapy was assessed in a 6-month, randomised controlled trial.[140,141] A total of 40 women were assigned to four groups. The first two groups comprised women with physiological menopause, and treatment was 50 μg/day of topical oestradiol plus 50 mg/day oral progestogen for 15 days every 3 months, plus either kava extract (100 mg/day, containing 55% kavain) or placebo. The second two groups comprised women with surgically induced menopause and used the same treatment model as above, but without the progestogen. A significant reduction in the HAMA score was observed across all groups; however, the decrease was more significant in the kava groups than in the hormone-only groups (p<0.05).

In a 3-month, open label, controlled study, 68 perimenopausal women were randomly assigned to receive calcium supplementation (n=34, control), calcium plus kava extract at 100 mg/day (n=15) or calcium plus 200 mg/day kava extract (n=19).[142] The kava extract contained 55% kavain. In the control group during the 3 months, anxiety, depression and climacteric symptoms tended to decline, but not significantly. During kava therapy (pooled results for both doses), all of the clinical measures declined significantly from baseline, but only for anxiety was the decline significantly different to the control group (p<0.009). Side effects of nausea and gastric pain were observed in one patient in the control group and six receiving kava.

In an observational, open label trial involving 42 patients with different psychiatric diagnoses receiving neuroleptic drugs, kava extract (100 to 300 mg/day, containing 70% kava lactones) significantly reduced extrapyramidal signs and symptoms (parkinsonism, dystonia and dyskinesia, p<0.001).[143] The concomitant intake of kava extract was well tolerated by the patients.

Toxicology and other safety data

Toxicology

The following LD_{50} data have been recorded for kava extracts and constituents and indicate low acute toxicity:

Substance	Route, model	LD_{50}	Reference
Standardised kava extract (containing 70% kava lactones)	Oral, mice	1.8 g/kg	144
Standardised kava extract (containing 70% kava lactones)	Oral, rats	16 g/kg	144
Standardised kava extract (containing 70% kava lactones)	ip mice	380 mg/kg	144
Standardised kava extract (containing 70% kava lactones)	ip rats	370 mg/kg	144
Kava extract (undefined)	ip rats	250 mg/kg	145
Kava resin	Oral, mice	700 mg/kg	60
Dihydrokavain	Oral, mice	980 mg/kg	144
Dihydromethysticin	Oral, mice	1050 mg/kg	144
Kavain	Oral, mice	1130 mg/kg	144
Methysticin	Oral, mice	> 800 mg/kg	144
Yangonin	Oral, mice	> 1.5 mg/kg	144

In vitro testing on kavain found neurotoxic effects only at high concentrations, but it may adversely affect neuronal recovery.[146] An ethanolic extract of kava and three isolated lactones did not display metabolic toxicity (activation to toxic metabolites) in vitro using human lymphoblastoid cells.[147]

Chronic administration of DHK (50 mg/kg/day, ip) three times a week for 3 months to rats produced no evidence of chronic toxicity. Six single doses to cats also did not produce chronic toxicity in terms of the haematological parameters measured, although a reversible dermopathy occurred.[144]

Wistar rats of both sexes were fed 7.3 or 73 mg/kg of a dried ethanolic kava extract for 3 and 6 months. When the animals were examined for histological changes and changes in body weight, haematological and liver parameters, no signs of toxicity could be found.[148]

An ether extract of kava administered by stomach tube did not affect the fertility of male rats. The dosage was equivalent to 8 g of dry rhizome twice a week for 2.5 months.[149]

A toxicological review concluded that there was insufficient information to support the safety of kava lactones as cosmetic ingredients.[150]

Testing of kava phytochemicals for in vitro mutagenic activity found that, while the lactones were inactive, two flavonoids from the leaf were mutagenic.[151]

Hepatotoxicity

Because of the serious nature of the hepatotoxic events linked to kava usage, attempts have been made to understand the issues and mechanisms involved. However, the relevance of such in vitro or high-dose in vivo studies to what is more than likely to be a rare idiosyncratic immune-mediated attack on the liver is probably questionable. Nonetheless, a review and discussion along these lines is below.

Kava extracts (methanol and acetone root extracts and a methanol leaf extract) demonstrated toxic effects on isolated HepG2 cells and isolated rat liver mitochondria.[152] The authors suggested that the mitochondrial toxicity of kava may explain the adverse hepatic reactions in predisposed patients. Various explanations have been proposed in the literature as to why the traditionally used aqueous preparations might be safer than the European-style solvent-extracted products. In Europe, kava was often manufactured from the root peelings or kava stumps (and even the aerial peelings), which represented a cheap source of kava lactones. A new piperidine alkaloid ($3\alpha,4\alpha$-epoxy-5β-pipermethystine) was isolated from the stem peelings of one cultivar originating from Papua New Guinea (called Isa, and known in Hawaii as PNG). This constituent was present at a concentration of 0.93%, and was absent from the 10 other cultivars tested. Traditionally Isa has been used only occasionally for drinking purposes, since it causes prolonged nausea. In vitro testing has shown that pipermethystine is far more toxic to liver cells than the kava lactones.[153] However, it failed to produce hepatotoxicity in vivo[154] and was absent from German products previously on the market.[155]

Another problem with the above observation as a mechanism behind any hepatotoxic reaction to kava is that it does not explain why the aqueous extract might differ in safety from solvent-based extracts. One research team has suggested that the answer to this may be glutathione, a protective molecule that is only present in water-based extracts of kava.[156]

However, a more plausible explanation has emerged. In order to investigate the key compounds in kava that might be responsible for any liver toxicity, various kava plant parts (root, leaf and stem peelings) were extracted with a range of solvents (hexane, ethyl acetate, n-butanol and water).[157] The cytotoxicity of these different extracts was tested on a human liver cell line (HepG2) using three different tests for toxicity. In general, the assessment of relative toxicity was consistent across the three tests. In terms of plant parts, the root and stem peelings showed comparable toxic effects on the HepG2 cells, which was considerably greater than the toxicity of the leaf. The organic solvent extracts displayed a far greater cytotoxicity than the water extracts for all the parts of kava tested. In fact, the water extracts of all kava plant parts tested exhibited no toxic effects at all. The hexane extract exhibited the strongest toxic effects (hexane was the least polar of the solvents selected).

The implication from these initial tests was that kava contains non-polar constituents that are responsible for cytotoxic effects on HepG2 cells. Such components would be most soluble in hexane and least soluble in water. The researchers then used bioassay-guided fractionation to identify that the main compound responsible for the cytotoxicity was flavokavain B. Flavokavain B is yellow in colour and is a member of the phytochemical class known as chalcones. Flavokavain B was confirmed in a later study as a potent hepatocellular toxin in vitro, as assessed again on HepG2 cells.[158] Replenishment with exogenous glutathione did neutralise its toxic effect.

Four kava lactones failed to inhibit alcohol dehydrogenase in vitro.[159] Hence, hepatotoxic effects from kava are unlikely to be due to this type of interaction with alcohol. However, a review of this topic suggested that other mechanisms could be involved, specifically the influence of alcohol consumption on various CYP enzymes, with resultant changes in kava metabolism.[160]

One review suggested it was possible that the mechanism of hepatotoxicity from kava was due to the metabolism of the kava lactones to electrophilic quinones, which can subsequently react with glutathione and/or modify proteins.[161] Such a theory could be consistent with a rare idiosyncratic reaction, depending on which proteins were modified (see also below).

However, these speculations are all based on in vitro studies. As might be expected, given the widespread human use of kava, in vivo studies show only mild hepatotoxic effects even at very high doses. Feeding kava to rats (31.25, 62.5 and 133 mg/kg diet for 3 months) did not cause liver injury or enhance galactosamine-induced hepatitis.[162] Treatment of rats with an acetone-water kava root extract (100 mg/kg/day for 3 weeks, oral) failed to elicit any significant changes in liver function tests and produced no signs of hepatotoxicity.[154] A traditional aqueous infusion of kava (equivalent to 200 and 500 mg/kg/day of lactones for 2 and 4 weeks) did not exhibit hepatotoxic activity in rats.[163]

In contrast to the above, higher doses of kava extracts have produced some mild hepatotoxic effects in laboratory models. A high oral dose (equivalent to about 380 mg/kg/day of kava lactones, 100 times the normal human dose) of two different kava extracts for 8 days significantly increased liver weights in rats.[164] CYP1A1 mRNA expression was markedly increased, which could possibly lead to metabolic activation of exogenous toxins, thereby representing an hepatotoxic risk. Doses of 0.5 to 2.0 g/kg of a different dried kava extract produced signs of mild liver toxicity.[165] The no observed adverse effect level was 0.25 g/kg.

The kavain metabolite 6-phenyl-3-hexen-2-one was identified as its mercapturic acid adduct in two people who ingested kava.[100] This is a highly reactive intermediate that could possibly account for idiosyncratic hepatotoxicity via binding to proteins or DNA.

(Some of these issues are discussed further in the Side effects section.)

Contraindications

Kava is best not used during lactation without professional advice and is contraindicated in pre-existing liver damage or diseases.

The Commission E listed the following contraindications: pregnancy, nursing and endogenous depression. However, these ensued from a lack of data, rather than from any direct concerns.

Special warnings and precautions

In August 2002, the Australian Therapeutic Goods Act (TGA) advised that kava-containing medicines should carry a label warning that kava has been implicated in serious liver damage and should be taken only under the supervision of a healthcare practitioner for short periods, not exceeding 6 weeks. In August 2003, an expert committee of the TGA determined that only certain forms of kava were suitable for use. Permitted products must be made from a water extract/dispersion or from the whole rhizome and the daily dosage of kava lactones must be limited to 250 mg. Patients prescribed kava should be closely monitored for signs and symptoms of liver damage.

Due to possible dopamine antagonism, kava should be used cautiously in elderly patients, especially those with Parkinson's disease. (See the Side effects section for more information.)

Consideration of pharmacokinetic data and the possibility of a potentiation of the sedative effects of anaesthetics have led to the recommendation that patients taking kava should discontinue use at least 24 h prior to surgery.[166]

Interactions

According to the Commission E, a synergistic effect is possible for substances acting on the central nervous system, such as alcohol, barbiturates and psychopharmacological agents.[167] However, notwithstanding some single case reports, normal therapeutic doses of kava do not appear to dampen alertness, interact with mild alcohol consumption, cause physiological tolerance or interact with benzodiazepines. (See Effects on performance and vision.)

Kava may interact with central dopamine agonists or antagonists and should not be administered to patients taking L-dopa and other medications for Parkinson's disease (see Side effects).

A case of a possible interaction between kava and a benzodiazepine drug (alprazolam) has been reported. The 54-year-old man was hospitalised in a lethargic and disoriented state. His medications included alprazolam, cimetidine and terazosin. He had not consumed alcohol or any of the medications in excess.[168] Another case was reported in 2001 of a potential interaction with the benzodiazepine drug flunitrazepam.[168] In 2006 a case was described as a potential adverse interaction between kava and valerian with paroxetine.[169] Fever, headaches and confusion were the presenting symptoms.

While in vitro findings show some inhibition of cytochrome P450 enzymes by kava and hence a potential for pharmacokinetic interaction with drugs highly metabolised by CYP enzymes, this remains unsubstantiated in humans.[170]

In fact, the information to date on this topic is inconsistent. Two reviews included studies investigating the impact of kava and kava lactones on hepatic cytochrome P450 (CYP) enzymes.[171,172] As noted above, these reviews highlight the conflicting and confusing nature of the data, especially for in vitro investigations. In such circumstances, emphasis should be given to human studies (as it always should). Even the human data are somewhat inconsistent, which may reflect on the ethnic groups and kava preparations tested.

A study in six healthy volunteers (including one woman) from New Caledonia who were regular consumers of traditional aqueous kava extract for more than 6 years used probe drugs to investigate changes in the activities of different CYP isozymes after 30-day abstinence.[78] Results suggested that traditional kava drinking inhibits CYP1A2 (p<0.02), but had no significant impact on CYP2C19, CYP2D6 and CYP3A4. There was a trend towards inhibition of CYP2E1 that failed to reach significance (p=0.16).

Twelve healthy volunteers (including six women) received a commercial kava extract (2000 mg/day, no standardisation claim) for 28 days.[173] The use of probe drug cocktails indicated a significant reduction in CYP2E1 (p=0.009), with no impact on CYP3A4, CYP1A2 and CYP2D6. The same research group confirmed the lack of activity on CYP2D6 using a different kava extract and dose (409 mg/day, containing 225 mg kava lactones).[174] Similarly, no impact on CYP3A4 was confirmed in another study using a kava extract that also delivered 225 mg/day of kava lactones.[175]

Kava extract for 14 days (1227 mg/day, containing 225 mg kava lactones) in 20 healthy volunteers (10 women) had no impact on digoxin pharmacokinetics.[176] This indicates that kava is unlikely to influence the activity of the transporter P-glycoprotein under normal clinical use.

Use in pregnancy and lactation

Category B1-no increase in frequency of malformation or other harmful effects on the fetus from limited use in women. No evidence of increased fetal damage in animal studies.

The Australian Therapeutic Goods Administration (TGA) recommends that kava-containing medicines should not be taken by pregnant women.

In traditional societies in the Pacific Islands, women have less access to and use of kava than men. Hence the interpretation of information from the traditional literature regarding use in pregnancy needs to take into account this lower usage. In addition, these societies held a number of cultural myths relating to kava that affected women.[177,178]

Kava has been used as an abortifacient on Pohnpei (although this has been said to be denied by another source),[179] and in southeast coastal Irian Jaya, although combined with other herbs such as various 'pepper-roots', chillies and Citrus spp.[180] In Hawaii, women avoided any kava use immediately upon becoming pregnant.[181] There are several references to kava leaf used topically to induce miscarriage (Hawaii and Polynesia).[182] Both the rhizome and leaf are used orally as a contraceptive.[2,183] Folk theory suggests that kava use renders women infertile.[182,184] Yet therapeutic use during pregnancy is also noted: to induce an easy labour and to correct displacement of the womb.[5,185]

Synthetic kavain orally administered on days 6 to 17 of gestation (100 and 500 mg/kg, rats; 20 and 200 mg/kg,

rabbits) did not produce teratogenic effects in terms of the fetal parameters measured. No teratogenic effects were seen in the F1 and F2 generations of rats given DHM (50 mg/kg, ip) three times weekly over a period of 3 months.[144]

Kava use is probably compatible with breastfeeding but caution should be used (on the basis of the presence of kava lactones). Women in some areas of New Guinea traditionally drank kava beverage (prepared by grating and maceration) during their pregnancy to promote the flow of milk.[185] The Australian TGA recommends that kava-containing medicines should not be taken by nursing women.

Effects on ability to drive and use machines

No negative influence is expected at normal therapeutic doses. In a randomised, double blind study, 40 healthy volunteers received either 300 mg standardised kava extract (containing 210 mg/day kava lactones) or placebo for 15 days. Kava did not significantly affect performance capability relevant to operating machines and driving.[65] Administration of kava extract (equivalent to 240 mg/day of kava lactones) to volunteers did not affect performance parameters (stress tolerance, vigilance and motor coordination) compared to baseline values.[71] (For further information, see Effects on performance and vision.)

Side effects

Skin reactions

A dry, scaly, pigmented skin condition known as kava dermopathy is a well-known side effect of excessive and chronic use of kava.[186] The cutaneous effects were first reported by members of Captain James Cook's Pacific expeditions. The cause may be related to interference with cholesterol metabolism[187] and is unlikely to occur after normal therapeutic use. It has also been suggested that this rash may be due to a deficiency of one of the B vitamins, but a clinical trial of 100 mg of nicotinamide per day failed to have a significant effect.[188] The rash quickly regresses if kava intake is ceased. A clinical pharmacological evaluation of DHM found that doses of 300 to 800 mg/day produced a scaly skin rash in a high percentage of subjects.[36]

Adverse effects from heavy kava usage in an Australian aboriginal community have been reported.[189] Kava users were more likely to have adverse biochemical and haematological changes and the typical scaly rash. However, the kava consumption was extremely high, more than 310 g per week for 35 of the 39 kava users. Also, it has been questioned whether all the adverse effects reported were only due to kava consumption,[190] since ethanol in large doses can possibly potentiate the toxicity of kava.[66] (A favourable difference in exhibited behaviour between kava and alcohol intoxication has also been noted: stupor or sleep after kava, aggression or fighting after alcohol.[191])

A case of systemic contact-type dermatitis occurred after oral administration of a kava extract.[192] Two cases of a drug-type eruption in sebaceous gland-rich areas induced by 3 weeks of systemic kava administration have also been reported. No other cause for the reaction, including ingestion of conventional medications, could be found. In one of the cases, a diagnostic allergy test revealed significant proliferation of peripheral blood lymphocytes in response to kava extract and the second patient had a strongly positive patch test to kava extract after 24 h. The authors suggest the skin reactions observed from kava ingestion may relate to interference with cholesterol metabolism.[193]

A case of urticaria was documented in a young male from the Solomon Islands who had ingested kava for the first time one evening. He awoke the following morning with an itchy, urticarial rash that disappeared in 24 h. The following week the man consumed kava again, with the same presentation of marked urticaria the following morning. This time resolution took 2 to 3 days. Another case of urticaria was documented in a Vanuatu man who worked at a kava bar. His skin was itchy, flushed and oedematous with some wheals on his arms. He stated that this reaction always developed after he consumed kava. Further discussion with local members who are regular kava drinkers identified this as a well-recognised problem among selected people.[194] A case was described of a 36-year-old woman who developed a generalised rash (diagnosed as delayed-type hypersensitivity) after 3 weeks of taking a kava extract (containing 120 mg/day kava lactones).[195] Dermatomyositis was linked to kava intake for 2 weeks in a 47-year-old woman.[196]

Patients sometimes comment that the condition of their hair is poorer while taking kava (observation of the authors).

Hepatotoxicity reactions and related issues

Perhaps unsurprisingly, the decision by the German health authority BfArM in 2002 to ban kava has been reviewed critically by the German industry and trade associations, as well as European herbal associations. The conclusion is that the existing data on the benefit/risk assessment of kava- and kavain-containing products did not justify their withdrawal.[197–199] The hepatotoxicity cases that were definitively attributable to kava were most likely immunologically mediated idiosyncratic drug reactions (IDRs), rather than a direct toxic effect. Several theories have been postulated, including the type of kava cultivar used in Europe and kava plant part.[200] It is known that 5% to 10% of Caucasians have a CYP2D6 deficiency, unlike Polynesians.[157] This deficiency may contribute to the kava IDR observed in Western countries. Melanesians have a high incidence of CYP2C19 mutations; again, this might play a role in protection from a reaction to kava.[201]

The traditional kava used is prepared from water. Commercial manufacturers have typically used ethanol, acetone and other organic solvents to extract kava. The use of such solvents may alter the safety profile of kava. For example, there has been postulation that glutathione found in aqueous kava extracts may confer hepatoprotection.[202,203] (See also the discussion in the Toxicology section of this monograph, especially concerning flavokavain B and pipermethystine.)

Given the warm humid climates where kava is grown, aflatoxins have also been discussed as a possible cause of hepatotoxicity.[204] However, there is no information on aflatoxin levels in commercial kava products and such speculation does not sit well with the fact that these apparent hepatotoxic reactions are idiosyncratic.

Several reviews have undertaken to examine critically the reports of hepatotoxicity attributed to kava intake. A detailed assessment of individual cases published up to early 2003 concluded:

> On the basis of the current information it cannot be confirmed that all preparations of kava involving all types of raw materials will cause this hepatotoxic reaction. Probable cases, based on our assessment, have only been confirmed for the acetone extracts commonly used in Germany and Switzerland, with the exception of one case report from the intake of an ethanol-based extract, a case where the patient was shown to have an unusual metabolic enzyme pattern and at the same time developed an immunological reaction to kava intake (allergy). The absence of reported cases of hepatotoxicity in the Pacific Islands adds weight to this assertion.

However, since then a few cases have been published linking idiosyncratic hepatotoxicity to the use of traditional aqueous extracts of kava, and a 2008 review concluded that cultivar and/or plant part could be the more important consideration for safety.[205] Nonetheless, the use of organic solvents could further increase the hepatotoxic reaction risk.[206] In 2003, a paper was published that described two cases of liver injury in New Caledonia linked to traditional use of kava.[207] One case may have been due to an interaction between kava and phenobarbital, which is known to cause liver damage. In neither case was the patient rechallenged with kava to confirm that it was responsible. A German tourist apparently developed a serious toxic liver reaction after consumption of kava in traditional Samoan ceremonies while there on a 20-day honeymoon.[208]

A cross-sectional study in Fiji involving 101 participants investigated the potential adverse effects of traditionally prepared (water-extracted) kava. Kava consumers had been using kava for more than 3 months; non-kava consumers had either never consumed kava, discontinued use for 1 year, or had consumed it less than once in 3 months. Venous blood was collected and the results of liver function tests were compared between the two groups. Significantly high serum GGT (gamma-glutamyltransferase) and ALP (alkaline phosphatase) levels were observed in kava consumers. These enzymes showed a strong association with kava consumption and total lifetime consumption. However, there was no association between kava and clinically significant adverse health effects.[209] The liver enzyme elevations probably represent an induction of these enzymes in response to kava, rather than liver damage.[207] This is supported by the results of a health status review of kava users in 1988: plasma levels of GGT were greatly increased in kava users, but no cases of acute liver injury were identified.

A study in a predominantly Tongan population in Hawaii yielded similar findings.[210] GGT was significantly elevated in healthy adult drinkers compared to non-drinkers (65% of the

31 tested versus 26% of 31 controls, p=0.005), as was ALP (23% versus 3%, p=0.053).

However, it does appear that kava-related liver damage is rare in traditional communities. A survey conducted in Samoa in 2002 failed to find one case, even in heavy kava drinkers.[211] A survey from one Arnhem Land community showed only some mild and reversible changes in liver enzymes (probably due to enzyme induction rather than liver damage), with no evidence of reversible liver damage.[212] According to Singh and Singh, in the South Pacific, mainly men drink kava, often habitually and in much larger amounts than used in the West, yet their incidence of liver toxicity is low and similar to that of island women who do not take kava.[213]

An Australian GP recalls that he spent 2 years living in Vanuatu, observing the regular and occasionally heavy kava consumption. Clinical evaluation revealed occasional cases of kava-related dermopathy and presumptive kava-related cerebral damage. At no time during his 2-year stay did he encounter any case of unexplained hepatitis, despite his vigilance, since 20% of the population were hepatitis B carriers.[214] A GP working in Auckland with the Pacific Island community reported a similar lack of hepatotoxicity in frequent traditional kava users.[215]

A small survey of 150 staff and patients at a Vanuatu hospital found that a high frequency of men and women drank kava on a regular basis without any adverse effects.[216] The above all explains why Pacific islanders are perplexed over the European ban on kava. To them it would be the equivalent of banning tea in Vanuatu (*Camellia sinensis* (green tea) intake has been linked to idiosyncratic hepatotoxic reactions). At the time of writing (2012), there have been no reported cases of hepatotoxicity linked to kava in Australia since the 2003 TGA decision to allow only the aqueous extract.

A clinical survey and critical analysis by German authors of 26 suspected cases of kava hepatotoxicity excluded causality in 18 cases.[217] Only one out of the remaining eight patients adhered to the conditions recommended by European regulatory authorities (no more than 120 mg/day of kava lactones and 3 months of continuous therapy). The authors concluded that kava taken as recommended is associated only rarely with hepatotoxicity, whereas excessive doses, prolonged treatment and co-medication with drugs may carry an increased risk.

The validity of the causality evaluation methods applied in kava hepatotoxicity cases has also been questioned. Scales of causality such as the WHO and Naranjo scales, as used by the BfArM, were suggested as inappropriate due to their lack of liver specificity.[218] When the liver-specific Council for International Organisations of Medical Sciences (CIOMS) scale is applied to reported cases for kava, a greatly reduced likelihood of causality is determined, compared with the above scales.[218,219] When two structured quantitative methods of causality were compared, namely the Maria and Victorino and the CIOMS scales, the latter was deemed to be the preferable tool in assessing kava hepatotoxicity.[220] Grades of causality on these scales were much lower than for the regulatory ad hoc judgements.

A strategy has been proposed for the re-introduction of kava into Europe in a way that should minimise the risk of hepatotoxicity. This is principally by generating additional clinical data for an aqueous extract prepared from a noble kava cultivar.[221] A noble cultivar is one that has been consumed traditionally for centuries in the South Pacific and has undergone a continuous process of selection and breeding. This strategy has been elaborated into a six-point plan in a later publication from the same collaboration.[222] The six points are: (1) use of a noble kava cultivar at least 5 years old at the time of harvest; (2) use of only peeled and dried rhizomes and roots; (3) aqueous extraction; (4) dosage limitation of no more than 250 mg/day kava lactones; (5) systematic rigorous future research; and (6) a pan-Pacific quality control system regulating growers and raw material suppliers.

Other reactions

The systematic review and meta-analysis conducted for the Cochrane collaboration noted that adverse events reported in clinical trials were mild, transient and infrequent.[78]

A group of German neurologists described four cases of patients who developed clinical signs suggestive of dopamine antagonism after taking kava. A 28-year-old man who had a history of acute dystonic reactions after taking anxiolytic drugs also developed involuntary neck extension with forceful upward deviation of his eyes 90 min after taking kava for the first time. A 22-year-old woman experienced involuntary oral and lingual dyskinesia, tonic rotation of the head and painful twisting movements of the trunk 4 h after her first dose of kava. A similar reaction was experienced by a 63-year-old woman after taking kava for 4 days and aggravation of Parkinson's disease occurred in a 76-year-old woman. The authors concluded that the sedative effects of kava might result from dopamine antagonistic properties, which is supported by reports of beneficial effects of kava on schizophrenic symptoms.[223]

A case of severe and persistent parkinsonism was reported in a 45-year-old woman with a family history of essential tremor who took a complex product containing kava extract (65 mg/day for 10 days).[224] The patient was also taking manganese (implicated in parkinsonism), but only apparently for 4 days. However, this case and the ones above are difficult to reconcile with the pharmacological study that found kava is unlikely to be responsible for central dopaminergic antagonism[84] and the clinical study that found kava reduced parkinsonism induced by neuroleptic drugs (see above).[143]

Recent research on abuse in Australian aboriginal communities has revealed links between chronic excessive kava use and increased susceptibility to serious infectious disease and the development of neurological abnormalities; pulmonary hypotension; haematuria (suggesting effects on the kidneys); ischaemic heart disease and sudden cardiac death. In addition to the effect on skin, there have been reports of thrombotic effects, liver damage, lowered body mass index, raised total cholesterol (both LDL and HDL elevated) and adverse effects on the eyes and vision.[225] However, many of these effects might also be due to associated heavy alcohol consumption. A case of an acute neurological syndrome linked to heavy kava consumption was reported. The 27-year-old

Australian Aboriginal man presented three times with generalised choreoathetosis secondary to kava bingeing. During the episodes, he had severe choreoathetosis involving his limbs, trunk, neck and facial musculature, with marked athetosis of the tongue. Other possible medical causes were excluded.[226] (See also the Overdosage and abuse section for a fuller discussion of these issues.)

Kava was falsely implicated in health complications in a group of people believed to have consumed a product containing kava at a 'rave' party in Los Angeles on New Year's Eve, 1996. The label of the product included kava as well as two other herbs. Samples tested initially by the Los Angeles Police Department and subsequently by the American Botanical Council showed no kava lactones present. The product was found to contain caffeine and 1,4-butanediol (an industrial solvent which is metabolised to gamma-hydroxybutyrate) which were not listed on the label.[227] (Analysis conducted on behalf of the FDA confirmed the presence of the industrial solvent.) A Californian chiropractor was sentenced in February 1998 after pleading guilty to misbranding the product. The industrial solvent was deliberately substituted because he could not obtain the kava/kavain in time.[228]

A 61-year-old Tongan male presented to emergency with acute urinary retention. He was distressed and complained of pain in the suprapubic region. On questioning it was found that he had come from a kava drinking session (and had consumed 1 L). Full blood counts and other relevant tests were performed, as well as a thorough history taken, and all other possible causes were excluded. The patient recovered after 6 h of catheter insertion. He was discharged after no further difficulties in voiding. The patient recalled that he had experienced similar less severe problems following previous meetings coinciding with large amounts of kava consumption.[229]

Three cases of meningismus after kava ingestion, two of them with local neurological manifestations, were reported in France.[230] The exact amount of kava consumed was not well described and these cases may have reflected overdosage. Symptoms were transient. All three patients were related; hence the kava they used may have been adulterated in some way.

Overdosage and abuse

Excessive kava drinking may cause pupil dilation, reduced light reflexes, photophobia, bloodshot eyes and poor attention to diet.[231] A 37-year-old-man was transported to emergency after the sudden onset of vertigo. He also presented with vomiting and ataxia. All possible causes were excluded. The man admitted to drinking kava tea immediately before the onset of symptoms. Resolution of symptoms occurred between 4 and 6 h. There was no analysis conducted of the tea for the presence of kava or kava lactones.[232]

Kava was introduced from Fiji in late 1981[178] to Aboriginal communities of Northern Australia and rapidly became a substance of abuse, probably because of a lack of ceremonial or traditional restraints controlling its use. Estimates for individual consumption have been as high as 100 times the amount of kava habitually consumed in the Pacific Islands.[233] A survey of three Aboriginal communities in the mid-1980s found the average consumption per drinker was 14 to 53 g/day of kava powder, although a review in the early 1990s suggested consumption may have been as high as 88.3 g/day.[225]

Subsequently, a large amount of information regarding the adverse effects observed from excessive intake of kava in Australian Aboriginal[189,225,232,234] and Fijian communities[235] was documented. Intake most commonly ranged from 100 to 500 g/week,[189,235] but could be as high as 900 g/week.[189] Common adverse reactions included scaly skin, weight loss, watery eyes, headache, decreased blood lymphocytes and an increase in liver enzymes (not due to alcohol consumption).[189,225,232,234–236] Ischaemic cardiac events (including sudden death), chest pain and pulmonary hypertension were noted.[189,225,232,235] There was no impairment in cognitive function and some improvement in psychotic individuals.[232,234] There is also record of three cases of sudden cardiac death in young Aboriginals who drank kava on the evening before an Australian rules football game.[237] However, there is no electrocardiographic or epidemiological evidence to show that sudden deaths are more frequent in kava-using communities than in other Aboriginal communities.[189] A small (and underpowered) case-control study failed to demonstrate an association between kava consumption in an Aboriginal community and ischaemic heart disease.[238]

Some of the findings of a pilot survey[189] and the anecdotal reports from healthcare workers[225] have been questioned.[239–242] The effect of kava abuse on liver enzymes is not conclusive,[239,242] and the involvement of factors other than kava ingestion in the occurrence of the reported adverse events cannot be ruled out.[240–242]

In addition, three case reports arising from abuse of traditionally prepared kava have been documented.[62,226,243] Adverse reactions included visual disturbance,[62] acute neurological syndrome,[225] scaly skin, confusion, hypotonic limbs and elevated GGT (in a non-alcohol drinker).[243] This last finding may have been due to enzyme induction by kava, rather than hepatotoxicity. Liver function changes were measured in users of moderate amounts of aqueous extracts of kava after cessation of kava use. They were found to be reversible and began to return to baseline after 1 to 2 weeks of kava abstinence.[212]

The performance of individuals within an Australian indigenous community intoxicated from kava drinking was compared with a control group. Tests were performed to measure saccade and cognitive impairment after intoxication. The average amount of kava consumed was 205 g per person (approximately 100 times a clinical dose) within a time frame of 14.4 h (8 h before testing). Intoxicated kava drinkers showed ataxia, tremors, sedation, blepharospasm and elevated liver enzymes (GGT and ALP) as well as saccadic dysmetria (an impaired ability to control fast voluntary eye movement from different fixation points), saccadic slowing (a slowing of this voluntary eye movement) and therefore reduced accuracy performing a visual task that only became evident as the task complexity increased. Complex cognitive functions were performed normally. The authors suggested that the saccade abnormalities imply disruption of cerebellar and GABAergic functions.[244]

A case-control study of the association between kava use and pneumonia in northern Aboriginal communities in Australia found no association.[245] Associations between pneumonia and cannabis and alcohol use were significant, suggesting the study was sufficiently powered.

An interview of 12 Tongan-born men living in New Zealand noted some adverse effects associated with chronic kava use, even within a strong cultural context.[246] These were mainly low energy and lack of libido.

Safety in children

The Australian TGA recommends that kava-containing medicines should not be taken by children under 12 years of age.

In Polynesia, kava has been traditionally used in children for general debility, stomach disorders and for fretting.[5]

Regulatory status in selected countries

The regulatory status of kava has changed in many countries due to concerns over hepatotoxicity.

In Australia, kava is subject to control under the Customs Import/Export Legislation. Those intending to import kava must have the appropriate licence and permit(s) to import. In July 1988, the Western Australia government restricted the sale and supply of kava under the Poisons Act 1964 to cultural uses and medical/scientific research. However, the sale of kava as a therapeutic good was not restricted in the other states of Australia. In May 1998, the Northern Territory government restricted the use and sale of kava in order to control the use of kava as a beverage in Australian Aboriginal communities. This did not affect the use of kava as a therapeutic good. In July 2002, the Therapeutic Goods Administration (TGA) initiated a voluntary withdrawal of all over-the-counter complementary medicines containing kava. The listable (automatic registration) status of kava was reviewed in 2003, with the result that kava is now included in Part 4 of Schedule 4 of the Therapeutic Goods Regulations of Australia. Preparations allowed for oral (non-homeopathic) use must be either an aqueous dispersion or an aqueous extract of whole or peeled rhizome or dried whole or peeled rhizome. The following conditions must be adhered to:

- The preparation does not contain, for its recommended daily dose, more than 250 mg of kava lactones
- If the preparation is in the form of a tablet or capsule, the amount of kava lactones does not exceed 125 mg for each tablet or capsule; and if the preparation is in the form of a tea bag, the amount of dried whole or peeled rhizome does not exceed 3 g for each tea bag.
- If the preparation contains more than 25 mg of kava lactones per dose, the label on the goods includes the following warnings (or words to the same effect): not for prolonged use. If symptoms persist, seek advice from a healthcare practitioner. Not recommended for use by pregnant or lactating women. May harm the liver.

In the UK kava was included on the General Sale List, with a maximum single dose of 625 mg. In December 2002 legislation was enacted to prohibit the sale of food consisting of, or containing, kava (Statutory Instrument No. 3169 The Kava-kava in Food (England) Regulations 2002), and to prohibit the sale of any medicinal product which consists of or contains kava (Statutory Instrument No. 3170 The Medicines for Human Use (Kava-kava) (Prohibition) Order 2002).

Kava is covered by a positive Commission E monograph. However, in June 2002 the German Health Authority (BfArM) banned the therapeutic use of kava. This ban was apparently repealed in May 2005, but no kava products have received new licences since then.[247]

In the USA kava does not have GRAS status. However, it is freely available as a 'dietary supplement' under DSHEA legislation (Dietary Supplement Health and Education Act of 1994).

References

1. Singh YN. *J Ethnopharmacol.* 1992;37(1):13–45.
2. Cambie RC, Ash J. *Fijian Medicinal Plants.* Australia: CSIRO; 1994. pp. 239–240.
3. Lebot V, Merlin M, Lindstrom L. *Kava-The Pacific Elixir: The Definitive Guide to its Ethnobotany, History and Chemistry.* New Haven: Yale University Press; 1992. pp. 112–117.
4. Norton SA. *Hawaii Med J.* 1998;57(1):382–386.
5. Titcomb M. *J Polynes Soc.* 1948;57: 105–171.
6. Grieve M. *A Modern Herbal*, vol. 2. New York: Dover Publications; 1971. pp. 454–455.
7. Felter HW, Lloyd JU. *King's American Dispensatory.* 18th ed. rev 3, vol. 2, 1905. Portland: Reprinted by Eclectic Medical Publications; 1983. pp. 1505–1507.
8. Mabberley DJ. *The Plant Book*, 2nd ed. Cambridge: Cambridge University Press; 1997. p. 560.
9. Leung AY, Foster S. *Encyclopedia of Common Natural Ingredients Used in Food, Drugs and Cosmetics*, 2nd ed. New York: John Wiley; 1996. pp. 330–331.
10. Lebot V, Merlin M, Lindstrom L. *Kava-The Pacific Elixir: The Definitive Guide to its Ethnobotany, History and Chemistry.* New Haven: Yale University Press; 1992. pp. 10–13.
11. Pharmaceutical Society of Great Britain. *British Pharmaceutical Codex 1934.* London: The Pharmaceutical Press; 1941. pp. 573–574.
12. Dragull K, Yoshida WY, Tang CS. *Phytochemistry.* 2003;63(2):193–198.
13. Wagner H, Bladt S. *Plant Drug Analysis: A Thin Layer Chromatography Atlas*, 2nd ed. Berlin: Springer-Verlag; 1996. pp. 258–259.
14. Smith RM, Thakrar H, Arowolo TA, et al. *J Chromatogr.* 1984;283:303–308.
15. Lebot V, Merlin M, Lindstrom L. *Kava-The Pacific Elixir: The Definitive Guide to its Ethnobotany, History and Chemistry.* New Haven: Yale University Press; 1992. pp. 68–69.

16. Davies LP, Drew CA, Duffield P, et al. *Pharmacol Toxicol.* 1992;71(2):120–126.

17. Jussofie A, Schmiz A, Hiemke C. *Psychopharmacology (Berl).* 1994;116(4):469–474.

18. Yuan CS, Dey L, Wang A, et al. *Planta Med.* 2002;68(12):1092–1096.

19. Boonen G, Häberlein H. *Planta Med.* 1999;64(6):504–506.

20. Uebelhack R, Franke L, Schewe HJ. *Pharmacopsychiatry.* 1998;31(5):187–192.

21. Serdarevic N, Eckert GP, Müller WE. *Pharmacopsychiatry.* 2001;34(suppl 1):S134–S136.

22. Keller F, Klohs MW. *Lloydia.* 1963;26(1):1–15.

23. Hänsel R, Beiersdorff HV. *Arzneimittelforschung.* 1959;9:581–585.

24. Klohs MW, Keller WF, Williams RE, et al. *J Med Pharm Chem.* 1959;1(1):95–103.

25. Meyer HJ. *Arch Int Pharmacodyn Ther.* 1962;138(3–4):505–535.

26. Kretzschmar R, Teschendorf HJ. *Chemtg Z.* 1974;98:24–28.

27. Duffield PH, Jamieson DD, Duffield AM. *Arch Int Pharmacodyn Ther.* 1989;301:81–90.

28. Jamieson DD, Duffield PH, Cheng D, et al. *Arch Int Pharmacodyn Ther.* 1989;301:66–80.

29. Furgiuele AR, Kinnard WJ, Aceto MD, et al. *J Pharm Sci.* 1965;54:247–252.

30. Holm E, Staedt U, Heep J, et al. *Arzneimittelforschung.* 1991;41(7):673–683.

31. Baum SS, Hill R, Rommelspacher H. *Prog Neuropsychopharmacol Biol Psychiatry.* 1998;22(7):1105–1120.

32. Capasso A, Pinto A. *Acta Therapeut.* 1995;21(2):127–140.

33. Capasso A, Sorrentino L. *Phytomedicine.* 2005;12(1–2):39–45.

34. Jamieson DD, Duffield PH. *Clin Exp Pathol Physiol.* 1990;17:509–514.

35. Shinomiya K, Inoue T, Utsu Y, et al. *Psychopharmacology (Berl).* 2005;180(3):564–569.

36. Walden J, Von Wegerer J, Winter U, et al. *Prog Neuropsychopharmacol Biol Psychiatry.* 1997;21(4):697–706.

37. Walden J, Von Wegerer J, Winter U, et al. *Hum Psychopharmacol.* 1997;12(3):265–270.

38. Grunze H, Langosch J, Schirrmacher K, et al. *Prog Neuropsychopharmacol Biol Psychiatry.* 2001;25(8):1555–1570.

39. Garrett KM, Basmadjian G, Khan IA, et al. *Psychopharmacology (Berl).* 2003;170(1):33–41.

40. Rex A, Morgenstern E, Fink H. *Prog Neuropsychopharmacol Biol Psychiatry.* 2002;26(5):855–860.

41. Feltenstein MW, Lambdin LC, Ganzera M, et al. *Phytother Res.* 2003;17(3):210–216.

42. Smith KK, Dharmaratne HR, Feltenstein MW, et al. *Psychopharmacology (Berl).* 2001;155(1):86–90.

43. Bruner NR, Anderson KG. *Pharmacol Biochem Behav.* 2009;92(2):297–303.

44. Johnson D, Frauendorf A, Stecker K, et al. *TW Neurol Psychiatrie.* 1991;5:349–354.

45. Cropley M, Cave Z, Ellis J, et al. *Phytother Res.* 2002;16(1):23–27.

46. Watkins LL, Connor KM, Davidson JRT. *J Psychopharmacol.* 2001;15(4):283–286.

47. Gleitz J, Friese J, Beile A, et al. *Eur J Pharmacol.* 1996;315(1):89–97.

48. Gleitz J, Gottner N, Ames A, et al. *Planta Med.* 1996;62(6):580–581.

49. Seitz U, Schule A, Gleitz J. *Planta Med.* 1997;63(6):548–549.

50. Kretzschmar R, Meyer HJ, Teschendorf HJ. *Experientia.* 1970;26(3):283–284.

51. Kretzschmar R, Meyer HJ. *Arch Int Pharmacodyn Ther.* 1969;177(2):261–267.

52. Meyer HJ, Kretzschmar R. *Arzneimittelforschung.* 1969;19(4):617–623.

53. Meyer HJ, Kretzschmar R. *Klin Wochenschr.* 1966;44(15):902–903.

54. Singh YN. *J Ethnopharmacol.* 1983;7(3):267–276.

55. Seitz U, Ameri A, Pelzer H, et al. *Planta Med.* 1997;63(4):303–306.

56. Martin HB, McCallum M, Stofer WD, et al. *Planta Med.* 2002;68(9):784–789.

57. Martin HB, Stofer WD, Eichinger MR. *Planta Med.* 2000;66(7):601–606.

58. Meyer HJ, May HU. *Klin Wochenschr.* 1964;42(8):407.

59. Bruggenmann F, Meyer HJ. *Arzneimittelforschung.* 1963;13:407–409.

60. Jamieson DD, Duffield PH. *Clin Exp Pharmacol Physiol.* 1990;17(7):495–507.

61. Sullivan J, Romm J, Reilly M. *Dimens Crit Care Nurs.* 2009;28(3):138–140.

62. Garner LF, Klinger JD. *J Ethnopharmacol.* 1985;13(3):307–311.

63. Prescott J, Jamieson D, Emdur N, et al. *Drug Alcohol Rev.* 1993;12:49–58.

64. Russell P, Bakker D, Singh N. *Bull Psychonomic Soc.* 1987;25:236–237.

65. Herberg KW. *Z Allg Med.* 1991;67:842–846.

66. Munte TF, Heinze HJ, Matzke M, et al. *Neuropsychobiol.* 1993;27(1):46–53.

67. Heinze HJ, Munthe TF, Steitz J, et al. *Pharmacopsychiatry.* 1994;27(6):224–230.

68. Herberg KW. *Blutalkohol.* 1993;30(2):96–105.

69. Foo H, Lemon J. *Drug Alcohol Rev.* 1997;16(2):147–155.

70. Gessner B, Cnota P. *Z Phytother.* 1994;15(1):30–37.

71. Herberg KW. *Z Allg Med.* 1996;72(16):963–977.

72. Zie X, Simoneau AR. *Cancer Res.* 2005;65(8):3479–3486.

73. Tang Y, Simoneau AR, Xie J, et al. *Cancer Prev Res (Phila).* 2008;1(6):439–451.

74. Tang Y, Li X, Liu Z, et al. *Int J Cancer.* 2010;127(8):1758–1768.

75. Steiner GG. *Hawaii Med J.* 2000;59(11):420–422.

76. Agarwal R, Deep G. *Cancer Prev Res (Phila).* 2008;1(6):409–412.

77. Johnson TE, Kassie F, O'Sullivan JG, et al. *Cancer Prev Res (Phila).* 2008;1(6):430–438.

78. Russmann S, Lauterburg BH, Barguil Y, et al. *Clin Pharmacol Ther.* 2005;77(5):453–454.

79. Hänsel R. *Pacific Sci.* 1966;22:293–313.

80. Hänsel R, Weiss D, Schmidt B. *Planta Med.* 1966;14(1):1–9.

81. Duffield AM, Jamieson DD, Lidgard RO, et al. *J Chromatogr.* 1989;475(2):273–281.

82. Rasmussen AK, Scheline RR, Solheim E, et al. *Xenobiotica.* 1979;9(1):1–16.

83. Backhauss C, Krieglstein J. *Eur J Pharmacol.* 1992;215(2–3):265–269.

84. Nöldner M, Chatterjee SS. *Phytomedicine.* 1999;6(4):285–286.

85. Duffield PH, Jamieson D. *Clin Exp Pathol Physiol.* 1991;18(8):571–578.

86. Gleitz J, Beile Z, Wilkens P, et al. *Planta Med.* 1997;63(1):27–30.

87. Wu D, Yu L, Nair MG, et al. *Phytomedicine.* 2002;9(1):41–47.

88. Hashimoto T, Suganuma M, Fujiki H, et al. *Phytomedicine.* 2003;10(4):309–317.

89. Pollastri MP, Whitty A, Merrill JC, et al. *Chem Biol Drug Des.* 2009;74(2):121–128.

90. Folmer F, Blasius R, Morceau F, et al. *Biochem Pharmacol.* 2006;71(8):1206–1218.

91. Shaik AA, Hermanson DL, Xing C. *Bioorg Med Chem Lett.* 2009;19(19):5732–5736.

92. Avdeef A, Strafford M, Block E, et al. *Eur J Pharm Sci.* 2001;14(4):271–280.

93. Matthias A, Blanchfield JT, Penman KG, et al. *J Clin Pharm Ther.* 2007;32(3):233–239.

94. Pade D, Stavchansky S. *Mol Pharm.* 2008;5(4):665–671.

95. Biber A. Internal publications of Dr Willmar Schwabe GmbH & Co; Karlsruhe: 1989.

96. Keledjian J, Duffield PH, Jamieson DD, et al. *J Pharm Sci.* 1988;77(12):1003–1006.

97. Mathews JM, Etheridge AS, Valentine JL, et al. *Drug Metab Dispos.* 2005;33(10):1555–1563.

98. Köppel C, Tenczer J. *J Chromatogr.* 1991;562(1–2):207–211.

99. Tarbah F, Mahler H, Kardel B, et al. *J Chromatogr B Analyt Technol Biomed Life Sci.* 2003;789(1):115–130.

100. Zou L, Harkey MR, Henderson GL. *Planta Med.* 2005;71(2):142–146.

101. Johnson BM, Qiu SX, Zhang S, et al. *Chem Res Toxicol.* 2003;16(6):733–740.

102. Scholing WE, Clausen HD. *Med Klin.* 1977;72(32–33):1301–1306.

103. Lindenberg D, Pitule–Schodel H. *Fortschr Med.* 1990;108(2):49–50. 53–54.

104. Scherer J. *Adv Ther.* 1998;15(2):261–269.

105. Boerner RJ. *Phytother Res.* 2001;15(7):646–647.

106. Bhate H, Gerster G, Gracza E. *Erfahrungsheilkunde.* 1989;38(6):339–345.

107. Kinzler E, Kromer J, Lehmann E. *Arzneimittelforschung*. 1991;41(6):584–588.

108. Lehmann E, Kinzler E, Friedemann J. *Phytomedicine*. 1996;3(2):113–119.

109. Woelk H, Kapoula O, Lehrl S, et al. *Z Allg Med*. 1993;69(10):271–277.

110. Lehrl S, Woelk H. *MMW Fortschr Med*. 2002;144(23):47.

111. Volz HP. *6th Phytotherapy Conference*. Berlin: October 5–7, 1995.

112. Volz HP, Kieser M. *Pharmacopsychiatry*. 1997;30(1):1–5.

113. Singh NN, Ellis CR, Singh YN. *Alt Ther*. 1998;4(2):97–98.

114. Hofmann R, Winter U. *5th Phytotherapy Congress*. Bonn: November 3–5, 1993.

115. Spree MH, Croy HH. *Kassenarzt*. 1992;17(1):44–51.

116. Siegers CP, Honold E, Krall B, et al. *Arztl Forsch*. 1992;39(1):7–11.

117. Neuhaus W, Ghaemi Y, Schmidt T, et al. *Zentralbl Gynakol*. 2000;122(11):561–565.

118. Malsch U, Kieser M. *Psychopharmacology (Berl)*. 2001;157(3):277–283.

119. Boerner RJ, Sommer H, Berger W, et al. *Phytomedicine*. 2003;10(suppl 4):38–49.

120. Gastpar M, Klimm HD. *Phytomedicine*. 2003;10(8):631–639.

121. Geier FP, Konstantinowicz T. *Phytother Res*. 2004;18(4):297–300.

122. Pittler MH, Ernst E. *Cochrane Database Syst Rev*. 2003(1):CD003383.

123. Ernst E. *Phytomedicine*. 2006;13(3):205–208.

124. Witte S, Loew D, Gaus W. *Phytother Res*. 2005;19(3):183–188.

125. Warnecke G. *Fortschr Med*. 1991;109(4):119–122.

126. Connor KM, Payne V, Davidson J. *Int Clin Psychopharmacol*. 2006;21(5):249–253.

127. Connor KM, Davidson JR. *Int Clin Psychopharmacol*. 2002;17(4):185–188.

128. Jacobs BP, Bent S, Tice JA, et al. *Medicine (Baltimore)*. 2005;84(4):197–207.

129. Sarris J, Kavanagh DJ, Byrne G, et al. *Psychopharmacology (Berl)*. 2009;205(3):399–407.

130. Sarris J, Kavanagh DJ, Adams J, et al. *Complement Ther Med*. 2009;17(3):176–178.

131. Sarris J, Kavanagh DJ, Deed G, et al. *Hum Psychopharmacol*. 2009;24(1):41–48.

132. Emser W, Bartylla K. *TW Neurol Psychiatrie*. 1991;5:636–642.

133. Wheatley D. *Hum Psychopharmacol*. 2001;16(4):353–356.

134. Wheatley D. *Phytother Res*. 2001;15(6):549–551.

135. Lehrl S. *J Affect Disord*. 2004;78(2):101–110.

136. Wheatley D. *J Psychopharmacol*. 2005;19(4):414–421.

137. Kretzschmar R. In: Loew D, Rietbrock N, eds. *Phytopharmaka in Forschung Und Klinischer Anwendung*. Darmstadt: Steinkoff Verlag; 1995. pp. 29–38.

138. Hänsel R. *Z Phytother*. 1996;17:180–195.

139. Thompson R, Ruch W, Hasenohrl RU. *Hum Psychopharmacol Clin Exp*. 2004;19(4):243–250.

140. De Leo V, la Marca A, Morgante G, et al. *Maturitas*. 2001;39(2):185–188.

141. De Leo V, La Marca A, Lanzetta D, et al. *Minerva Ginecol*. 2000;52(6):263–267.

142. Cagnacci A, Arangino S, Renzi A, et al. *Maturitas*. 2003;44(2):103–109.

143. Boerner RJ, Klement S. *Wien Med Wochenschr*. 2004;154(21–22):508–510.

144. Hänsel R, Woelk H. *Spektrum Kava-Kava (Arzneimitteltherapie heute: Phytopharmaka; Band 6)*. Basel: Aesopus Verlag; 1994. pp. 40–41.

145. Edwards J, Wang M, Pecore N, et al. *FASEB J*. 1998;12:A464.

146. Mulholland PJ, Prendergast MA. *Brain Res*. 2002;945(1):106–113.

147. Zou L, Harkey MR, Henderson GL, et al. *Planta Med*. 2004;70(4):289–292.

148. Sorrentino L, Capasso A, Schmidt M. *Phytomedicine*. 2006;13(8):542–549.

149. Van Dam-Bakker AWI, de Groot AP, Luyken R. *Trop Geogr Med*. 1958;10:68–70.

150. Robinson V, Bergfeld WF, Belsito DV, et al. *Int J Toxicol*. 2009;28(6 suppl):175S–188S.

151. Jhoo JW, Ang CY, Heinze TM, et al. *J Food Sci*. 2007;72(2):C120–C125.

152. Lüde S, Török M, Dieterle S, et al. *Phytomedicine*. 2008;15(1–2):120–131.

153. Nerurkar PV, Dragull K, Tang CS. *Toxicol Sci*. 2004;79(1):106–111.

154. Lim ST, Dragull K, Tang CS, et al. *Toxicol Sci*. 2007;97(1):214–221.

155. Lechtenberg M, Quandt B, Schmidt M, et al. *Pharmazie*. 2008;63(1):71–74.

156. Whitton PA, Lau A, Salisbury A, et al. *Phytochemistry*. 2003;64(3):673–679.

157. Jhoo JW, Freeman JP, Heinze TM, et al. *J Agric Food Chem*. 2006;54(8):3157–3162.

158. Zhou P, Gross S, Liu JH, et al. *FASEB J*. 2010;24(12):4722–4732.

159. Anke J, Fu S, Ramzan I. *Phytomedicine*. 2006;13(3):192–195.

160. Li XZ, Ramzan I. *Phytother Res*. 2010;24(4):475–480.

161. Dietz BM, Bolton JL. *Chem Biol Interact*. 2011;192(1–2):72–80.

162. DiSilvestro RA, Zhang W, DiSilvestro DJ. *Food Chem Toxicol*. 2007;45(7):1293–1300.

163. Singh YN, Devkota AK. *Planta Med*. 2003;69(6):496–499.

164. Yamazaki Y, Hashida H, Arita A, et al. *Food Chem Toxicol*. 2008;46(12):3732–3738.

165. Clayton NP, Yoshizawa K, Kissling GE, et al. *Exp Toxicol Pathol*. 2007;58(4):223–236.

166. Ang-Lee MK, Moss J, Yuan CS. *JAMA*. 2001;286(2):208–216.

167. German Federal Minister of Justice. *German Commission E for Human Medicine Monograph*. Bundes-Anzeiger (German Federal Gazette) no. 101, dated 01.06.1990.

168. Almeida JC, Grimsley EW. *Ann Intern Med*. 1996;125(11):940–941.

169. Rubin D, McGovern B, Kopelman RI. *Am J Med*. 2006;119(6):482–483.

170. Singh YN. *J Ethnopharmacol*. 2005;100(1–2):108–113.

171. Fu PP, Xia Q, Guo L, et al. *J Environ Sci Health C Environ Carcinog Ecotoxicol Rev*. 2008;26(1):89–112.

172. Shord SS, Shah K, Lukose A. *Integr Cancer Ther*. 2009;8(3):208–227.

173. Gurley BJ, Gardner SF, Hubbard MA, et al. *Clin Pharmacol Ther*. 2005;77(5):415–426.

174. Gurley BJ, Swain A, Hubbard MA, et al. *Mol Nutr Food Res*. 2008;52(7):755–763.

175. Gurley BJ, Swain A, Hubbard MA, et al. *Clin Pharmacol Ther*. 2008;83(1):61–69.

176. Gurley BJ, Swain A, Barone GW, et al. *Drug Metab Dispos*. 2007;35(2):240–245.

177. Lebot V, Merlin M, Lindstrom L. *Kava-The Pacific Elixir: The Definitive Guide to its Ethnobotany, History and Chemistry*. New Haven: Yale University Press; 1992. pp. 119–174.

178. Alexander K. *Kava in the North. A Study of Kava in Arnhem Land Aboriginal Communities*. : Casuarina, Australian National University North Australia Research Unit; 1985. p. 9.

179. Riesenberg SH. *The Native Polity of Ponape*. Washington: Smithsonian Institution Press; 1968. p. 103.

180. Serpenti LM. *Cultivators in the Swamps: Social Structure and Horticulture in a New Guinea Society (Frederik-Hendrik Island West New Guinea)*. Assen: Van Gorcum; 1965. p 145.

181. Gutmanis J. 1976. Cited in: McKenna DJ, Jones K, Hughes K, et al. *Botanical Medicines: The Desk Reference for Major Herbal Supplements*. 2nd ed. New York: Haworth Herbal Press; 2002. p. 720.

182. Lebot V, Merlin M, Lindstrom L. *Kava-The Pacific Elixir: The Definitive Guide to Its Ethnobotany, History and Chemistry*. New Haven: Yale University Press; 1992. pp. 111, 135–136.

183. Lebot V, Merlin M, Lindstrom L. *Kava-The Pacific Elixir: The Definitive Guide to Its Ethnobotany, History and Chemistry*. New Haven: Yale University Press; 1992. p. 114.

184. Steinmetz EF. *Piper Methysticum (Kava-Kawa-Yaqona): Famous Drug Plant of the South Sea Islands*. Amsterdam: E.F. Steinmetz; 1960. p. 43.

185. Steinmetz EF. *Piper Methysticum (Kava-Kawa-Yaqona): Famous Drug Plant of the South Sea Islands*. Amsterdam: E.F. Steinmetz; 1960. p. 31.

186. Suss R, Lehmann P. *Hautarzt.* 1996;47(6):459–461.
187. Norton SA, Ruze P. *J Am Acad Dermatol.* 1994;31(1):89–97.
188. Ruze P. *Lancet.* 1990;335(8703):1442–1445.
189. Mathews JD, Riley MD, Fejo L, et al. *Med J Aust.* 1988;148(11):548–555.
190. Douglas W. *Med J Aust.* 1988;149(6):341–342.
191. Cantor C. *Med J Aust.* 1997;167(10):560.
192. Côté CS, Kor C, Cohen J, et al. *Biochem Biophys Res Commun.* 2004;322(1):147–152.
193. Jappe U, Franke I, Reinhold D, et al. *J Am Acad Dermatol.* 1998;38(1):104–106.
194. Grace R. *J Am Acad Dermatol.* 2005;53(5):906.
195. Schmidt P, Boehncke WH. *Contact Dermatitis.* 2000;42(6):363–364.
196. Guro-Razuman S, Anand P, Hu Q, et al. *J Clin Rheumatol.* 1999;5(6):342–345.
197. Mills SY, Steinhoff B. *Phytomedicine.* 2003;10(2–3):261–262.
198. Denham A, McIntyre M, Whitehouse J. *J Altern Complement Med.* 2002;8(3):237–263.
199. Schulze J, Raasch W, Siegers C. *Phytomedicine.* 2003;10(suppl 4):68–73.
200. Teschke R. *Liver Int.* 2010;30(9):1270–1279.
201. Kaneko A, Lum JK, Yaviong J, et al. *Pharmacogenetics.* 1990;9(5):581–590.
202. Schmidt M. *J Altern Complement Med.* 2003;9(2):183–187.
203. Whitton PA, Lau A, Salisbury A, et al. *Phytochemistry.* 2003;64(3):673–679.
204. Teschke R, Qiu SX, Lebot V. *Dig Liv Dis.* 2011;43(9):676–681.
205. Teschke R, Genthner A, Wolff A. *J Ethnopharmacol.* 2009;123(3):378–384.
206. Teschke R, Schulze J. *JAMA.* 2010;304(19):2174–2176.
207. Russmann S, Barguil Y, Cabalion P, et al. *Eur J Gastroenterol Hepatol.* 2003;15(9):1033–1036.
208. Christl SU, Seifert A, Seeler D. *J Travel Med.* 2009;16(1):55–56.
209. Kumar B, Kaur J. *Clin Chem.* 2007;53 (6 suppl S):A50.
210. Brown AC, Onopa J, Holck P, et al. *Clin Toxicol (Phila).* 2007;45(5):549–556.
211. Tavana G, Stewart P, Snyder S, et al. *HerbalGram.* 2003;59:28–32.
212. Clough AR, Bailie RS, Currie B. *J Toxicol Clin Toxicol.* 2003;41(6):821–829.
213. Singh YN, Singh NN. *CNS Drugs.* 2002;16(11):731–743.
214. Personal communication from Dr Graham Pinn. 15 June, 2002.
215. Personal communication from Dr Fiona McLean. 15 October, 2002.
216. Grace RF. *Pac Health Dialog.* 2003;10(2):41–44.
217. Teschke R, Schwarzenboeck A, Hennermann KH. *Eur J Gastroenterol Hepatol.* 2008;20(12):1182–1193.
218. Teschke R, Wolff A. *Regul Toxicol Pharmacol.* 2011;59(1):1–7.
219. Teschke R, Wolff A. *Dig Liver Dis.* 2009;41(12):891–901.
220. Teschke R, Fuchs J, Bahre R, et al. *J Clin Pharm Ther.* 2010;35(5):545–563.
221. Sarris J, Teschke R, Stough C, et al. *Planta Med.* 2011;77(2):107–110.
222. Teschke R, Sarris J, Lebot V. *Phytomedicine.* 2011;18(2–3):96–103.
223. Schelosky L, Raffauf C, Jendroska K, et al. *J Neurol Neurosurg Psychiatry.* 1995;58(5):639–640.
224. Meseguer E, Taboada R, Sánchez V, et al. *Mov Disord.* 2002;17(1):195–196.
225. D'Abbs P, Burns C. *Report on Inquiry into the Issue of Kava Regulation.* Prepared for the Sessional Committee on the Use and Abuse of Alcohol by the Community, Legislative Assembly of the Northern Territory. Menzies School of Health Research: Darwin; 1997.
226. Spillane PK, Fisher DA, Currie BJ. *Med J Aust.* 1997;167(3):172–173.
227. Blumenthal M. *Natural Pharmacy.* 1997:12–15.
228. Nordenberg T. *FDA Consumer. FDA Investigators' Reports-July/August 1998*, vol. 32, no. 4. Washington, DC: FDA; 1998.
229. Leung N. *Emerg Med Australas.* 2004;16(1):94.
230. Sibon I, Rosier E, Orgogozo JM. *Rev Neurol (Paris).* 2002;158(12):1205–1206.
231. Lebot V, Merlin M, Lindstrom L. *Kava-The Pacific Elixir: The Definitive Guide to Its Ethnobotany, History and Chemistry.* New Haven: Yale University Press; 1992. pp. 59–60.
232. Perez J, Holmes JF. *J Emerg Med.* 2005;28(1):49–51.
233. Cawte J. *Aust NZ J Psychiatry.* 1986;20(1):70–76.
234. Cairney S, Clough AR, Maruff P, et al. *Neuropsychopharmacology.* 2003;28(2):389–396.
235. Kava R. *Pacific Health Dialog.* 2001;8(1):115–118.
236. Clough AR, Jacups SP, Wang Z, et al. *Intern Med J.* 2003;33(8):336–340.
237. Young MC, Fricker PA, Thomson NJ, et al. *Med J Aust.* 1999;170(9):425–428.
238. Clough AR, Wang Z, Bailie RS, et al. *J Epidemiol Community Health.* 2004;58(2):140–141.
239. Markey P. *Proceedings of the 28th Annual Conference of the Public Health Association of Australia.* Perth: 1996. p. 192.
240. Douglas W. *Med J Aust.* 1988;149(6):341–342.
241. Lebot V, Merlin M, Lindstrom L. *Kava-The Pacific Elixir: The Definitive Guide to Its Ethnobotany, History and Chemistry.* New Haven: Yale University Press; 1992. p. 201.
242. Mathews JD, Riley MD. *Med J Aust.* 1988;149(6):342.
243. Chanwai GL. *Emerg Med.* 2000;12(2):142–145.
244. Cairney S, Maruff P, Clough AR, et al. *Hum Psychopharmacol.* 2003;18(7):525–533.
245. Clough AR, Wang Z, Bailie RS, et al. *Epidemiol Infect.* 2003;131(1):627–635.
246. Nosa V, Ofanoa M. *Pac Health Dialog.* 2009;15(1):96–102.
247. Blumenthal M. *HerbalGram.* 2005;67:21–22.

(Glycyrrhiza glabra L.)

Synonyms

Liquiritia officinalis (botanical synonym), liquorice, sweet root (Engl), Liquiritiae radix, Radix glycyrrhizae (Lat), Subholzwurzel, Lakritzenwurzel (Ger), réglisse, bois doux (Fr), liquirizia (Ital), Lakrids (Dan), yashimadhu (Sanskrit), gancao (Chin), kanzo (Jap), kamcho (Kor).

What is it?

Licorice is one of the herbs widely used by Western herbal clinicians and is also a major herb of the Chinese, Kampo and Ayurvedic traditions. It has a long history, being used by the ancient Chinese, Egyptians and Greeks. The generic name *Glycyrrhiza* is derived from the Greek meaning 'sweet root' and it is the dried root and stolons that are the parts used medicinally. The sweet taste of licorice root is due to the presence of glycyrrhizin, an intensely sweet saponin. Licorice is also used extensively in food (especially confectionery) and tobacco products. Monographs in the *British Pharmacopoeia* (BP)[1] and the *Pharmacopoeia of the People's Republic of China*[2] allow for the use of any of three closely related species: *Glycyrrhiza glabra*, *G. uralensis* or *G. inflata*. Although they are regarded as being medicinally interchangeable, minor constituents such as the phenolics differ between these species.

Since the 1950s, scientific investigation into the pharmacological properties of licorice and glycyrrhizin has revealed a wide variety of activities that have resulted in the development of a major anti-ulcer drug in the 1980s and, more recently, an antiviral treatment for chronic hepatitis. Research on licorice and a number of its phytochemical constituents continues in a wide variety of fields. Licorice use also has well-documented side effects, and, while the informed use of licorice is a powerful aspect of phytotherapy, a full understanding of these is necessary for its safe and effective use.

Effects

Eases inflammation and tissue damage in the upper digestive tract; potentiates the anti-inflammatory effect of glucocorticoids; supports the adrenal cortex; mimics aldosterone (by potentiation of cortisol); facilitates movement of mucus from the respiratory tract and soothes cough; protects the liver; may assist with weight loss; affects levels of some sex hormones. Several of these effects are mediated by the interaction of glycyrrhizin metabolites with the cortisol regulatory enzyme 11-beta-hydroxysteroid dehydrogenase (11-beta-HSD).

Traditional view

Licorice has been utilised extensively for the treatment of cough, consumption, chest complaints (especially bronchitis) and as a soothing ingredient in cough medicines.[3] The Eclectics used it to reduce irritation of the mucous surfaces of the urinary, respiratory and digestive tracts.[4] Licorice was also highly regarded for chronic gastritis, peptic ulcer and adrenocortical insufficiency (specifically Addison's disease).[5] In traditional Chinese medicine, licorice tonifies the *Spleen*, benefits the *Qi*, moistens the *Lungs* and stops coughing, clears *Heat* and detoxifies *Fire Poison* (boils, sore throat) and soothes spasms. It moderates and harmonises the characteristics of other herbs and is also employed as an antidote for a variety of toxic substances.[6] In Ayurvedic medicine, licorice is used as a tonic and to treat eye diseases, throat infections, peptic ulcer, catarrh of the genitourinary tract, constipation and arthritis.[7,8]

Summary actions

Anti-inflammatory, mucoprotective, adrenal tonic, expectorant, demulcent, mild laxative, anticariogenic, antiviral, antitussive, hepatoprotective, spasmolytic.

Can be used for

Indications supported by clinical trials

Indications supported by trials using glycyrrhizin, carbenoxolone or deglycyrrhizinised (deglycyrrhizinated, deglycyrrhinised, deglycyrrhized) licorice: gastric and duodenal ulceration, functional dyspepsia, insulin resistance, topical use for recurrent mouth ulcers (generally uncontrolled trials lacking modern rigour).

Indications supported by trials using intravenous glycyrrhizin: viral hepatitis, oral lichen planus.

Indications supported by trials using licorice: gastric and duodenal ulceration, polycystic ovary syndrome and hyperprolactinaemia (uncontrolled trials in combination), recurrent mouth ulcers (topically), menopausal symptoms, post-operative sore throat (as a gargle), weight loss, possible value in patients with HIV/AIDS (preliminary data).

Traditional therapeutic uses

Bronchitis, cough; peptic ulcer, gastritis; adrenal insufficiency, Addison's disease; urinary tract inflammation.

May also be used for

Extrapolations from pharmacological studies

Treatment of corticosteroid dependency (to aid the withdrawal of corticosteroid drugs) and to extend the pharmacological effects of steroid drugs; hyperkalaemia (resulting from low aldosterone) associated with type 2 diabetes; inflammatory conditions, such as rheumatoid arthritis and allergic states; as an antitussive; to protect against ulcer-forming medications; for liver damage and as a hepatoprotective agent; to reduce the complications of long-standing diabetes mellitus by inhibiting aldose reductase; as a neuroprotective agent; for depression; prevention of carcinogenesis; respiratory viral infections and Epstein–Barr viral infection; to prevent bacterial adherence in bladder infections; topical use as an antiviral and anti-inflammatory agent; effects from 11-beta-HSD1 inhibition including osteopenia, glaucoma and metabolic syndrome.

Other applications

As a flavouring agent to disguise the taste of nauseating medicines and senna extract; as a component of cough lozenges; as an absorbent excipient in pill manufacture;[9] as a solubilising agent for aqueous extracts of herb mixtures; glycyrrhizin is used in drug manufacture to enhance drug absorption.[10]

Preparations

Dried root as a decoction, liquid extract, tablet or capsule for internal use. Decoction or liquid extract for external use or as an ingredient in a mouthwash, gargle, cream or ointment. Glycyrrhizin for intravenous use is used in some countries.

Dosage

Typical adult dosage ranges are:
- 3 to 12 g/day of dried root and stolon or by decoction or infusion
- 2 to 6 mL/day of a 1:1 liquid extract
- 1.5 to 4.5 mL/day of a 1:1 high glycyrrhizin liquid extract or its equivalent in tablet or capsule form
- 1.2 to 4.8 mL/day of deglycyrrhizinised licorice extract BP or its equivalent as a dry extract.

The Commission E indicates that, when licorice is used as a flavouring component, a maximum daily dosage of less than 100 mg glycyrrhizin is acceptable.[11]

Duration of use

Higher doses of licorice should not be consumed long term. The Commission E advises that licorice should not be taken for longer than 6 to 8 weeks without professional supervision.[11] (This relatively short time restriction is probably related to the high dose of licorice recommended by the Commission E: 5 to 15 g of root, equivalent to 200 to 600 mg of glycyrrhizin. For dosages at the lower end of the range recommended above, licorice can be administered for a longer time period without risk of side effects.)

Safety assessment of safety

Since higher doses can cause an aldosterone-like side effect, licorice must be taken within the recommended therapeutic range. Careful assessment of the patient's blood pressure and other medications is required before prescribing licorice. A high potassium and low sodium intake will minimise the risk of this adverse reaction. Use of high doses of licorice should not be recommended in conjunction with digoxin and potassium-losing drugs such as laxatives and thiazide diuretics.

Technical data

Botany

Glycyrrhiza glabra is a member of the Fabaceae (Leguminosae or pea) family, the Faboideae subfamily and the tribe Galegeae (as is the genus *Astragalus*).[12] It is a perennial herb, up to 150 cm tall, with a thick rhizome of dark, reddish-brown colour outside and yellowish inside, from which its stolons and roots arise. Leaves are compound, imparipinnate, 5 to 14 cm long with 11 to 17 leaflets that are ovate, oblong-lanceolate or elliptical in shape. Flowers are zygomorphic, of pea flower structure, in densely flowered racemes: petals purple, calyx glandular and five-toothed. Fruit is a flat legume (pod), up to 35 mm long.[13]

Adulteration

Supplies of licorice from the Far East are likely to contain quantities of *Glycyrrhiza uralensis*, the favoured licorice in Chinese medicine. However, this species is at least comparable in effect and the two species are regarded as medicinally interchangeable.

Taverniera cuneifolia is a wild relative of *G. glabra*. Both species contain the triterpenoid saponin glycyrrhizin and display other phytochemical similarities, making *T. cuneifolia* a potential licorice substitute.[14]

Key constituents

- Triterpenoid saponins: primarily the sweet tasting glycyrrhizin (GL),[15] which is a mixture of the potassium and calcium salts of glycyrrhizic acid (glycyrrhizinic acid);[16] other saponins are also present.[17] The concentration of glycyrrhizin in the root depends on the source and the method of assay[18] and is typically 2% to 6%.[19,20]
- Glycyrrhetic acid (glycyrrhetinic acid, 18-beta-glycyrrhetinic acid, GA), the aglycone of glycyrrhizic acid

Glycyrrhizic acid

	R
Liquiritigenin	H
Liquiritin	glucosyl

(and hence of glycyrrhizin) is also present in the root (0.5% to 0.9%).[21]

- A wide range of flavonoids (1% to 1.5%) that impart a yellow colour to the root: flavanones (including various liquiritigenin glycosides such as liquiritin and rhamnoliquiritin),[15,22] chalcones (including isoliquiritin) and isoflavonoids (including glabridin, glabrone and formononetin).[22,23]
- Other compounds include sterols, coumarins, fatty acids (C_2 to C_{16}), phenolics and arabinogalactans.[17,22]

The *British Pharmacopoeia* requires licorice to contain no less than 4% glycyrrhizic acid.

Much of the literature uses the terms glycyrrhizin and glycyrrhizic acid synonymously.

Pharmacodynamics

The immunostimulating, antiviral, antitumour, anti-inflammatory, hepatoprotective and choleretic activity of licorice could possibly be interpreted as correlated to the induction of the glutathione-dependent adenosylmethionine transferase and resultant methylation processes, such as those of viral and human DNA and RNA.[24] However, given the chemical complexity of the herb, other underlying mechanisms probably also apply for these specific actions.

Anti-ulcer activity

In the late 1940s a Dutch doctor named Revers noticed that patients with gastric ulcers were being cured by high doses of a licorice extract dispensed by a local pharmacist. Revers conducted a clinical trial on licorice and found it to be effective, but he also observed a significant incidence of side effects, mainly fluid retention and hypertension.[25] Revers' study led

to the investigation of glycyrrhizin (GL) and glycyrrhetinic acid (GA) as the constituents responsible for ulcer healing and it was found that these compounds, especially GA, also exhibited significant local anti-inflammatory activity. However, the relatively poor water solubility of GA prohibited the use of high doses in pharmacological experiments, so English scientists developed a semisynthetic derivative and named it carbenoxolone. Although carbenoxolone was developed with a view to its anti-inflammatory properties, it was soon discovered that it was very effective at healing gastric ulcers and it became the major anti-ulcer drug of the 1960s. It was also shown to heal duodenal ulcers, although this application was more controversial. Unfortunately, carbenoxolone also caused the same side effects as licorice and GL, and its use rapidly diminished when cimetidine, the first of the acid inhibitors, became available.

Some investigators were not satisfied that the anti-ulcer activity of licorice was entirely due to GL. Moreover, GL was responsible for the undesired side effects. This led to the investigation of deglycyrrhinised licorice (DGL), which ironically was a by-product of the manufacture of carbenoxolone. DGL has been shown to be an effective treatment for both gastric and duodenal ulcers, although its use has always been controversial in medical circles. If GL and carbenoxolone increase gastric mucosal resistance, what are the factors in DGL that also confer ulcer-healing properties? Is DGL effective? These questions were the subject of much debate in the 1970s. In fact, DGL is not completely free of GL: it is typically a concentrated extract of licorice (a soft extract) with a GL content not exceeding 3%.[26] It also contains a high level of flavonoids.

Carbenoxolone is chemically and pharmacologically similar to GL and most of the effects attributed to carbenoxolone also apply to GL. It was the first successful modern drug for

721

the treatment of gastric ulcers and acts by restoring gastric physiology to normal.[27] It improves the protective qualities of the gastric mucosal barrier[27] and research suggests that these effects may involve the mediation of prostaglandins,[28] specifically the inhibition of 15-hydroxyprostaglandin dehydrogenase and delta-13-prostaglandin reductase. Thus, licorice-derived compounds have the effect of raising the local concentration of those prostaglandins that promote mucus secretion and cell proliferation in the stomach, leading to healing of ulcers.[29] Carbenoxolone was also effective for the treatment of duodenal ulcers,[27] but there was debate as to whether this was a local or a systemic effect.

The use of carbenoxolone was largely supplanted by modern acid-inhibiting drugs initially, and more recently by antibiotics combined with proton pump inhibitor therapy. However, given its properties, licorice might still have a role in the healing of peptic ulcers.

In early animal studies DGL prevented ulcer development,[30] inhibited gastric acid secretion[31] and protected the gastric mucosa against damage from aspirin and bile.[32] Licorice and licorice derivatives protected against gastric ulcer induced by aspirin[33] or ibuprofen[34] in rats. DGL and GA also reduced the number and size of ulcers.[34] Licorice (500 mg/kg) was effective in preventing gastric mucosal damage by ethanol in rats. It affected surface mucin production, which was increased to 146% of the control value with pretreatment.[35]

Japanese workers have demonstrated a number of effects for Fm100, a semi-purified methanolic extract of licorice that contains about 19% GL and 13% flavonoids.[36] As might be expected, Fm100 has marked anti-ulcer activity.[37-39] More surprisingly, both Fm100 and an aqueous extract of licorice were found to directly stimulate exocrine secretion from the pancreas, but this effect was not due to GL or flavonoids.[32] However, total enzyme release from the pancreas was not increased. The authors found a correlation between the gastric antisecretory activity and the pancreatic stimulation, which implies that an unidentified constituent may be responsible for both effects.[36] A study in healthy volunteers showed that Fm100 increased both plasma secretin concentration and pancreatic bicarbonate output.[40] Fm100 also increased the content of endogenous prostaglandins in the gastric mucosa. The ability to release endogenous secretin in humans as well as animals may contribute to the anti-ulcer effect.[41]

The bacterium *Helicobacter pylori* was first isolated in 1982 by the Australian researchers, Marshall and Warren, and was found to be a cause of acute and chronic gastritis, peptic ulcer disease and gastric adenocarcinoma. The therapeutic management of peptic ulcer disease has fundamentally changed since this discovery, from the use of acid inhibiting drugs to a triple therapy regime consisting of a proton-pump inhibitor drug and two antibiotics for 7 to 14 days.[42] Since 2000, a non-invasive rapid urease breath test has been available to detect (with 80% to 90% sensitivity) the presence of *H. pylori*, now believed to be the cause of more than 90% of duodenal ulcers and up to 80% of gastric ulcers. A positive test for the bacterium allows for the quick instigation of treatment to prevent gastric ulcer formation.[43]

The discovery of *H. pylori* offers an alternative/additional explanation for the role of licorice in peptic ulcers. In vitro studies of GL, GA and flavonoids from *Glycyrrhiza spp.* show potent inhibition of growth of 29 strains of *H. pylori*.[44-48] *G. glabra* extract and polysaccharides have also been found to significantly inhibit the adhesion of *H. pylori* to human stomach tissue in vitro.[49,50] Antibiotic drug resistance is emerging as a major factor affecting treatment outcome in *H. pylori* infections, and researchers are now looking at plant substances, including licorice, to use in combination with drugs to treat gastrointestinal infections.[51-54]

In more recent research, the anti-ulcer activity of licorice has been reaffirmed. Licorice-derived compounds promoted mucus secretion by increasing prostaglandin concentrations in the gastrointestinal tract, prolonging the lifespan of surface cells of the stomach. They also exerted an antipepsin effect.[35]

A study of indomethacin-induced ulceration in the rat stomach found that famotidine (a proton pump inhibitor) in combination with an aqueous licorice extract exhibited higher anti-ulcer activity than either agent alone.[55] Another study compared the activity of *G. glabra* with omeprazole and misoprostol for the treatment of aspirin-induced gastric ulcers in rats and found no significant difference between treatments.[56] A standardised deglycyrrhizinised extract of *G. glabra* (12.5, 25 and 50 mg/kg, oral) demonstrated anti-ulcerogenic and antioxidant properties in indomethacin-induced gastric mucosal injury in rats.[57]

Preparations containing multiple herbal extracts have been researched in the context of gastrointestinal ulcers. STW 5 (a commercial herbal preparation containing licorice) was anti-ulcerogenic in vivo and inhibited secondary hyperacidity more efficiently than did commercial antacid preparations in mild, indomethacin-induced hyperacidity in rats.[58]

Anti-inflammatory activity

In the 1950s, GA and GL were investigated as anti-inflammatory agents because of their ulcer-healing properties. Anti-inflammatory effects were demonstrated in a number of animal models.[59-61] The mechanism is not fully understood and GA and GL have no intrinsic glucocorticoid action, although they do potentiate the action of cortisol and hydrocortisone, at least in part by inhibiting their metabolism as detailed below. Also, oral doses of GL were anti-inflammatory in adrenalectomised rats, implying an intrinsic anti-inflammatory activity.[62] GA was found to have anti-inflammatory activity similar to hydrocortisone in experimental arthritis in normal rats.[61] These studies led to the use in France of GA and licorice for the treatment of rheumatoid arthritis.[63] The fact that GA uncouples oxidative phosphorylation aroused speculation that this was responsible for its anti-inflammatory activity,[64,65] but this particular mechanism is no longer current in the understanding of anti-inflammatory effects.[66]

More recently, several possible mechanisms behind the anti-inflammatory activity have been proposed. GL has been shown to inhibit thrombin[67] and the generation of reactive oxygen species by neutrophils.[68] An animal study demonstrated moderate anti-inflammatory activity for oral doses of GA but, unlike many other anti-inflammatory agents, GA did not inhibit prostaglandin synthesis.[69] It was proposed that GA may inhibit the migration of white cells into sites of inflammation.[69] While in vitro studies have shown that GL inhibits prostaglandin production and phospholipase A_2,[70] the human significance of these findings can be questioned since GL is converted to GA in vivo after oral doses.[71] Subsequent research has identified the flavonoids as possible inhibitors of prostaglandin production (see below), although bioavailability factors are also an issue here in terms of human significance.

Reactive oxygen species, known to be potent mediators of tissue inflammation, have been shown to be inhibited by GL and glabridin in vitro.[72,73] Another in vitro study was used to examine the effects of licorice root and its constituents, GL, glabridin and isoliquiritigenin on the proinflammatory pathways controlled by cyclo-oxygenase (COX) and 5-lipoxygenase (5-LOX). Licorice root and glabridin were found to inhibit the production of proinflammatory mediators arising from both the COX pathway (PGE_2, thromboxane B_2) and the 5-LOX pathway (leukotriene B_4). Isoliquiritigenin inhibited only the COX pathway, while GL failed to inhibit the formation of products of either pathway in this study (in contrast to earlier studies above).[74]

The chemokine eotaxin-1 is involved in the recruitment of eosinophils to antigen-induced inflammation in asthmatic airways. Five flavonoids (including liquiritin, liquiritigenin and isoliquiritigenin) isolated from G. uralensis were shown to inhibit eotaxin-1 secretion in cultured lung fibroblasts.[75]

A study found both aqueous licorice extract and GA via intramuscular injection produced an anti-inflammatory action similar to diclofenac sodium (10 mg/kg) using the carrageenan-induced paw oedema rat model.[76] GL (10 mg/kg, ip) attenuated the development of carrageenan-induced lung injury in mice.[77] Inhibition of NF-kappaB and STAT-3 activation were possible mechanisms involved.

Topical anti-inflammatory activity

In early studies GA caused considerable interest as a topical treatment for inflammatory skin disorders.[78] However, there were a number of negative findings, possibly due to inactive isomers of GA being produced by incorrect extraction procedures.[79] Anti-inflammatory activity was demonstrated on guinea pig skin for a licorice extract liniment, which had similar activity to a 0.5% prednisolone preparation.[80] In the skin vasoconstrictor assay, GA potentiated the action of hydrocortisone on human skin.[81] GA is only present in low levels in licorice; it is mainly formed from GL after oral ingestion, therefore this particular research may be not be relevant to the topical use of licorice.

Using the conjunctival inflammation method for the quantitative evaluation of topically applied anti-inflammatory agents, a 5% solution of GL demonstrated comparable anti-inflammatory activity to a 1% solution of the steroidal anti-inflammatory drug dexamethasone.[82] Topical application of licochalcone A demonstrated anti-inflammatory activity in experimentally induced mouse ear oedema.[83]

Influence on steroid metabolism

There is no doubt that GL and GA exert a powerful influence on human steroid hormone function. However, their intrinsic glucocorticoid, mineralocorticoid and oestrogenic activities are low.[64–66,69,78–80,84–87] There is instead strong evidence to suggest that GA and GL act by altering the way that certain steroid hormones are metabolised.

In an early clinical study it was found that GL inhibited the metabolism of corticosteroids and thereby potentiated the effect of cortisone and ACTH (adrenocorticotropic hormone).[88] In vitro studies on rat liver preparations have shown that both GA and GL inhibit 5-beta-reductase, thereby probably inhibiting the breakdown of corticosteroids by the liver.[89] While GL has been shown to increase the anti-inflammatory action of cortisol,[90] it also antagonised some of its less desirable effects such as its antigranulomatous action[91] and its suppressive effect on ACTH synthesis and secretion and on adrenal weight.[92]

In a follow-up clinical study, oral administration of GL (150 to 300 mg/day) blocked the effect of the glucocorticoid dexamethasone in lowering the amount of urinary metabolites of cortisol resulting from pituitary (ACTH) inhibition.[92] These findings have important clinical significance for the use of licorice to aid the withdrawal of steroidal anti-inflammatory drugs and as an adrenal restorative herb.

GA also antagonises some of the effects of exogenously administered oestrogen, but has no action on the effects of natural levels of oestrogen.[93]

The aldosterone-like activity of licorice and carbenoxolone are well documented and these effects can also be produced by both GA and GL.[94] Research has shown that the site of action is in the kidney and this curious effect of licorice has proven to be a valuable tool in increasing understanding of kidney physiology. Briefly put, GA inhibits the enzyme (see below) that inactivates cortisol (to cortisone), leading to a higher level than normal of cortisol in the kidney. This in turn activates type 1 mineralocorticoid receptors to cause potassium loss and sodium retention.[95,96] The fact that licorice or GA potentiates the effect of cortisol, and not aldosterone, to cause sodium and fluid retention would explain why cortisone and licorice can control sodium balance in Addison's disease without the need for a mineralocorticoid.[97]

The enzyme type 2 11-beta-hydroxysteroid dehydrogenase (11-beta-HSD2) converts cortisol, the active form, into its inactive metabolites. Oral doses of GL to rats, and GA in vitro, inhibited 11-beta-HSD2 activity and decreased its production. This led to significantly increased levels of cortisol and thereby greater stimulation of the glucocorticoid receptor as well as a mineralocorticoid effect in the kidney. As further confirmation of this mechanism, pure GA (500 mg/day) administered orally to 10 healthy, normotensive young volunteers resulted in an elevated urinary excretion of free cortisol and unchanged plasma cortisol levels in the presence of markedly decreased levels of both plasma cortisone and urinary free cortisone.[98]

Licorice metabolites can also inhibit the type 1 isoform of 11-beta-HSD. Specifically, 18-alpha-GA selectively inhibited 11-beta-HSD1, but not 11-beta-HSD2 in transfected cells.[99] In contrast, 18-beta-GA preferentially inhibited 11-beta-HSD2. Both metabolites of GA have been detected in human plasma after GL intake (as the ammonium salt).[100]

Licorice in vitro inhibits corticoid, progesterone and prostaglandin dehydrogenases. The mechanism for conferring cellular specificity on mineralocorticoid action thus appears to share a common ancestor with a mechanism for regulating prostaglandin action.[101] Licorice also inhibits 3-alpha, 20-beta-hydroxysteroid dehydrogenase, an enzyme derived from a certain species of bacteria which is homologous to both 11-beta-HSD and 15-hydroxyprostaglandin dehydrogenase. (These enzymes diverged at least 2 billion years ago from a common ancestor. It is therefore likely that other oxidoreductases will be inhibited by licorice-derived compounds.)[29]

No difference in blood levels of GA was observed between patients with and without licorice-induced pseudoaldosteronism. Further testing suggested that licorice-induced pseudoaldosteronism is due to an increased concentration of 3-beta-D-(monoglucuronyl)-18-beta-GA (another metabolite of GL), but not GA itself.[102] This liver metabolite of GA is probably the active form of GL in the bloodstream with aldosterone-like activity. The mechanism behind the mineralocorticoid activity of licorice in humans was further evaluated in six male volunteers who received 7 g/day of a licorice preparation (containing 500 mg/day of GL) for 7 days. Pseudoaldosteronism was evident during the treatment as expressed by increased body weight, suppression of plasma renin activity and plasma aldosterone and reduced serum potassium. The study concluded that pseudoaldosteronism is initially related to decreased activity of 11-beta-HSD2, but afterwards also to a direct effect of licorice derivatives on mineralocorticoid receptors in some cases. In other cases, the effect on the enzyme is prevailing, probably as a result of individual factors.[103]

A study examined the effect of confectionery licorice 100 g/day (150 mg GA) for 4 weeks on serum dehydroepiandrostenedione sulphate (DHEAS) in 15 women and 21 men (healthy or suffering from essential hypertension). Researchers observed a moderate but significant decrease in serum DHEAS in men (p=0.002) and a non-significant increase in women following ingestion of these doses of licorice over a 4-week period. The serum concentrations of DHEAS differed between the genders (p=0.03). Serum testosterone levels and urinary androgen excretion showed no significant change. It was concluded that licorice primarily affects cortisol metabolism, whereas androgens are only marginally affected. Gender may influence the action of licorice, but pre-existing hypertension did not appear to have an influence.[104] (See also under Side effects for a further review of the impact of licorice on serum testosterone.)

Immunomodulatory activity

Beta-GA demonstrated potent inhibition of the classic complement pathway in vitro, but exerted no activity towards the alternative pathway. This anticomplementary activity was dependent on conformation, since the alpha-form of the compound was not active. GA acted at the level of the complement component C2.[105]

The daily consecutive oral administration of G. uralensis decoction at dose of 2 g/kg/day to mice countered the carrageenan-induced decrease in immune complex clearance. However, oral administration to normal mice did not reduce immune complex clearance. This effect of licorice decoction could not be explained by the action of GL.[106] Licorice

(50 mg/kg/day, oral) and GA (5 mg/kg/day, ip) helped the recovery of total leucocyte count, lymphocyte count and cellular immunity in irradiated mice.[107]

An in vivo study investigated the immunomodulatory activity of the licorice flavonoid liquiritigenin and its glycoside liquiritin against disseminated candidiasis. Mice treated intraperitoneally with liquiritigenin before intravenous challenge with live Candida albicans cells had a longer mean survival time than untreated mice (p<0.05), whereas mice treated with the glycoside liquiritin did not (illustrating the common requirement for glycosides to be activated through intestinal hydrolysis). Treatment with liquiritigenin favoured the production of interferon-gamma and interleukin (IL)-2 over IL-4 and IL-10, and results suggested that liquiritigenin protected mice against disseminated candidiasis by activating CD4 and Th1 immune responses.[108]

Chemopreventative and antitumour activities

Tumour promotion is considered to be an important factor in the chemical induction of cancers. GA but not GL exhibits a significant and specific antitumour-promoting activity[109,110] by inhibiting the binding of tumour promoters to test cells.[111] The mechanism may involve inhibition of protein kinase C.[112]

GA inhibited the growth of cultured mouse melanoma cells but was cytostatic and not cytotoxic.[113] It also induced phenotypic reversion: that is, the cancer cell becomes more like a normal cell.[113] GA inhibited ear oedema and ornithine decarboxylase activity induced by croton oil in mice. It also protected rapid DNA damage and decreased the experimentally induced, unscheduled DNA synthesis, which demonstrates a potential chemopreventive activity. (Although not stated, it is likely that GA was administered by injection.)[114] Oral administration of 1% aqueous extract of licorice to mice protected against lung and forestomach tumorigenesis induced by chemical carcinogens.[115] Chronic oral feeding of GL to mice also resulted in substantial protection against skin tumorigenesis.[116] Topical application of GA decreased skin tumour-initiating and promoting activities in mice.[117]

Licorice extract showed antimutagenic activity against ethylmethanesulphonate and ribose-lysine in the Salmonella/microsome reversion assay.[118] It also decreased the mutation frequencies induced by a series of well-known mutagens and carcinogens in vitro over a range of concentrations well below the toxic level.[119] GA inhibited mutagenicity in the Salmonella assay.

In vitro studies suggest that licorice may exert chemopreventative and antitumour activities via a range of mechanisms, including protecting against carcinogen-induced DNA damage. GA is an inhibitor of COX, LOX and protein kinase C and downregulates the epidermal growth factor receptor, while licorice polyphenols can induce apoptosis in tumour cells.[72] Isoliquiritigenin has shown both oestrogenic and antiproliferative activities in hormone sensitive MCF7 breast cancer cells in vitro.[120] These seemingly paradoxical in vitro findings are difficult to translate to a clinical setting, and both level and duration of exposure may determine any in vivo effects. Licochalcone A has been shown to potentiate chemotherapeutic agents such as paclitaxel and vinblastine.[121] Isoliquiritigenin inhibited cell proliferation and induced cell arrest in prostate cancer cells in vitro.[122] A novel polyphenol isolated from licorice induced apoptosis, cell arrest and the phosphorylation of the anti-apoptotic protein Bcl-2 in breast and prostate tumour cells in a manner similar to paclitaxel.[123] Isoliquiritigenin (300 mg/kg) reduced the incidence of induced colon and lung tumours in mice.[124] The same compound suppressed growth and induced apotosis in human and mouse colon cells in vitro and inhibited the induction of preneoplastic lesions in the rat colon in vivo.[125]

Human LNCaP prostate cancer cells exposed to licorice or the constituent licochalcone A demonstrated induced caspase-dependant and autophagy-related cell death in vitro.[126] A G. glabra root 50% ethanolic extract inhibited angiogenic and proliferative effects mediated by vascular endothelial growth factor both in vitro and in vivo (using the chorioallantoic membrane assay).[127] Licochalcone A was cytotoxic against gastric cancer cells; the mechanism of action involved cell cycle arrest and apoptosis.[128]

Colorectal cancer remains a leading cause of death. One promising chemopreventative strategy is to target cyclo-oxygenase 2 (COX-2) which promotes disease progression via PGE_2. COX-2 inhibition can be achieved with NSAIDs or selective COX-2 inhibitors, but these have potentially serious adverse side effects. It has been demonstrated that the expression of 11-beta-HSD2 correlates with COX-2 expression and activity, and increased human colonic and mouse intestinal adenomas. In addition, the same study found that, when 11-beta-HSD was inhibited with GA (or the gene silenced), COX-2 mediated PGE_2 production in tumours was reduced and adenoma formation, tumour growth and metastasis were prevented in mice.[129] Doses used were 1 to 30 mg/kg/day of GA by intraperitoneal injection.

Hepatoprotective activity

In early research it was proposed that GL was only active by injection as a protective agent for the liver.[130] However, in vitro studies on hepatocytes have shown that both GL and GA, the oral metabolite of GL, are equally hepatoprotective.[131,132] The clinical significance of oral doses of GL or licorice in liver disease remains to be established. (See Clinical trials section for studies on injected GL.)

Oral administration of licorice root (1 g/kg) or GL (23 mg/kg) activated glucuronidation in a study investigating the metabolism of paracetamol (acetaminophen). This result suggests that licorice may influence the detoxification of drugs in rat liver.[133] Very high oral doses of licorice or GL induced cytochrome P450-dependent enzyme (CYP) activities in mice.[134]

In an experimental hepatotoxicity model, oral administration of GA reduced the increase in serum transaminase activities, whereas GL did not. In vitro studies suggest that the potency of the hepatoprotective compounds parallels their absorption by hepatocytes.[135]

GA has been shown to protect a human hepatoma cell line (HepG2) against aflatoxin B1-induced cytotoxicity in vitro. Pretreatment with GA increased the activity of detoxifying enzymes glutathione-S-transferase and CYP1A1 (but not CYP1A2), suggesting that GA may inhibit the metabolic activation of aflatoxin B1, a critical aspect of the carcinogenicity of this substance.[136]

Carbon tetrachloride (CCl_4) is a potent hepatotoxin that causes peroxidative damage. A study in CCl_4-treated rats demonstrated that co-administration of G. glabra almost normalised the decreased activity of antioxidant defences including superoxide dismutase, catalase, glutathione peroxidase and glutathione, thereby attenuating the hepatotoxic effect of CCl_4.[137] Another study evaluated the effect of GL (intraperitoneally) in a mouse model of CCl_4-induced liver injury. Results showed that GL protected against injury, likely as a result of the induction of haem-oxygenase-1 and downregulation of proinflammatory mediators including COX-2 and nitric oxide.[138] These results suggest a possible activation of the Nrf2/ARE cellular protective pathway.

Non-alcoholic fatty liver disease (NAFLD) is a common liver pathology that appears to be increasing in prevalence. It is believed free fatty acid-induced lipotoxicity plays a crucial role in the pathogenesis of NAFLD. GL's well-documented pharmacological properties such as anti-inflammatory, antioxidant and immune modulating may be relevant to NAFLD. In an in vitro model of NAFLD (using the human hepatocyte cell line HepG2) GA prevented free fatty acid-induced lipid accumulation and cell apoptosis.[139]

Antiviral activity

A 2008 review noted that randomised controlled trials have clearly demonstrated that intravenous treatment with GL can reduce hepatocellular damage from chronic hepatitis B and C. Animal studies have demonstrated antiviral activity against herpes simplex, encephalitis and influenza A virus and in vitro studies have demonstrated antiviral activity against human immunodeficiency virus (HIV), SARS, arboviruses and vaccinia virus.[140] Several antiviral mechanisms have been documented, including induction of interferon-gamma by T cells, inhibition of viral uptake and reduced viral latency.

Early research observed that GL but not GA inhibited virus growth and in some instances inactivated virus particles. GL was particularly active against herpes simplex virus (HSV),[141,142] varicella-zoster virus,[143] human herpesvirus[144,145] and HIV.[146,147] GL also induced interferon production in vivo and in vitro, but GA was found to have only weak activity.[148] Indigenous GL (isolated from licorice) was a more potent antiviral agent than licorice and synthetic GL (ammonium salt of GA) for Japanese encephalitis virus in vitro.[149] Intraperitoneal administration of GL reduced morbidity and mortality of mice infected with lethal doses of influenza virus.[150]

In vitro studies have indicated that the antiviral agent idoxuridine penetrates skin more effectively when incorporated in a GL gel than a commercial idoxuridine ointment.[151] Isoliquiritigenin and glycycoumarin from G. glabra have been shown in vitro to specifically inhibit hepatitis C virus replication.[152]

In contrast with early research suggesting that GA lacked significant antiviral activity, researchers in Taiwan and Russia have demonstrated that not only is GA active against

Epstein–Barr virus (EBV) in vitro by interfering with an early step of the EBV replication cycle, it is 7.5 times more active than GL at inhibiting viral growth in infected cells.[153] Since the target of most conventional antiviral drugs is the virus-encoded enzyme DNA polymerase, involved in producing viral copies, GL and GA represent a new class of anti-EBV agents with a different mode of action.[154]

GL has also been found to protect human lung cells from influenza A virus in vitro. The antiviral activity appeared to be mediated by an interaction with the cell membrane, which reduced virus uptake.[155] GL demonstrated inhibition of HIV replication in cultures of peripheral blood mononuclear cells from HIV-infected patients by inducing the production of beta chemokines in the non-syncytium inducing variant of the virus.[156] Other authors have reported an inhibitory effect of GL on the neutrophil-dependent increase of HIV replication in macrophages.[157,158] GL is also reported to lower membrane fluidity, which suppresses HIV infection, as cell entry of enveloped viruses requires a wide fusion pore mechanism.[159] GL also inhibited replication of the SARS-associated coronavirus in vitro.[160]

Antimicrobial activity

The following isoflavonoids and related substances isolated from licorice have demonstrated significant antimicrobial activity in vitro in early research: hispaglabridin A, hispaglabridin B, 4'-O-methylglabridin, glabridin, glabrol, 3-hydroxyglabrol.[161] Licochalcone A inhibited the growth of both chloroquine-susceptible and chloroquine-resistant *Plasmodium falciparum* strains in vitro and protected mice from *P. yoelii* infection when administered either orally or intraperitoneally for 3 to 6 days.[162] Licochalcone A also inhibited the growth of *Leishmania major* and *L. donovani* promastigotes and amastigotes at concentrations that are non-toxic to host cells.[163]

Neither licorice nor GL promoted growth of *Streptococcus mutans* or induced plaque formation (measured by adherence of *S. mutans* to the surface) in vitro. In the presence of sucrose, GL did not affect bacterial growth, but plaque formation was markedly inhibited. GL at 0.5% to 1% caused almost complete inhibition.[164]

An extract from *G. uralensis* eliminated *Streptococcus mutans* and other common bacteria responsible for dental cavity forming acids. The licorice extract did not kill bacteria necessary for good oral hygiene. The extract is apparently being developed into a confectionery to prevent susceptible patients from forming dental cavities, with promising results.[165,166]

GA (30 mg/kg) administered subcutaneously to interleukin-deficient mice infected with *Porphyromonas gingivalis* resulted in a dramatic reduction of infection-induced bone loss, both when administered prophylactically and therapeutically. These findings suggest that GA might inhibit periodontitis in a glucocorticoid-independent manner, via inactivation of NF-kappaB.[167]

The phenolic licorice constituents glicophenone and glicoisoflavone, licochalcone A and isoflavones have been shown be antibacterial against methicillin-resistant *Staphylococcus aureus* (MRSA) in vitro.[168]

(See also the studies on *H. pylori* under Anti-ulcer activity.)

Cognitive function and neuroprotection

Licorice aqueous extract (150 mg/kg/day for 7 days, oral) has been shown to enhance memory and learning in mice. Researchers suggested both the anti-inflammatory and antioxidant properties of licorice may be contributing to the effect, as the dose reversed the amnesic effect induced by diazepam and scopolamine.[169] Cognitive function and cholinesterase activity were investigated in a study of glabridin (1, 2 and 4 mg/kg, ip) in mice for 3 days. Brain cholinesterase activity was reduced, suggesting glabridin might be a useful therapy for memory improvement.[170] Enhancement of spatial memory retention in rats orally treated with licorice extract (5 mg/mL of GL in daily water intake) occurred up to 4 weeks after treatment.[171]

The antioxidant activity of licorice components has been the subject of a number of in vitro and in vivo studies aiming to investigate their neuroprotective effect. GA and 18-beta-GA were neuroprotective in PC12 cells subjected to glucose deprivation and 6-hydroxydopamine-induced cytotoxicity in vitro.[172] Inhibition of NF-kappaB was associated with neuroprotective effects of GA in vitro on glutamate-induced excitotoxicity in primary neurons.[173] GL (16.8 mg/kg, ip) has also demonstrated neuroprotective effects in the 1-methyl-4-phenyl-1,2,3,6-tetrahydropyridine mouse model of Parkinson's disease.[174] Glabridin (25 mg/kg, ip), a licorice flavonoid, exerted a neuroprotective effect via modulation of multiple pathways associated with apoptosis in cerebral injury induced by middle artery occlusion in rats.[175] Isoliquiritigenin, another licorice flavonoid, has exhibited a neuroprotective role in cocaine-induced neuronal toxicity in rats.[176,177] Treatment with GL (10 mg/kg, ip) has also been shown in animal studies to reduce the development of inflammation and tissue injury associated with spinal cord trauma.[178]

The role of the complement system in neurodegenerative disorders such as Alzheimer's disease, multiple sclerosis, myasthenia gravis, Parkinson's disease, traumatic brain injury and spinal cord injury are well documented. GA and GL from *G. glabra* were found to have complement inhibitory potential in vitro, as both induced conformational changes in C3 (see also under Immunomodulatory activity).[179]

Antidepressant activity

The flavonoid liquiritin (10 to 40 mg/kg, oral) has been studied in a rat model for its effect in chronic, variable stress-induced depression. An antidepressant-like effect was found, which may be related to the observed prevention of oxidative stress, as demonstrated by an increase in SOD (superoxide dismutase) activity, inhibition of lipid peroxidation and reduced production of MDA, whereas fluoxetine did not exert these effects.[180] In another study, an extract of *G. glabra* (75, 150 or 300 mg/kg, oral) was administered for 7 days to two groups of Swiss male albino mice to investigate the antidepressant effects using the forced swim and tail suspension tests. At the 150 mg/kg dose there appeared to be a significant antidepressant-like effect comparable with imipramine (15 mg/kg, ip) and fluoxetine (20 mg/kg, ip). The effect appeared to be mediated by brain noradrenaline (norepinephrine) and dopamine increases, but not by serotonin, leading the investigators to conclude that licorice extract may have a monoamine oxidase inhibiting effect.[181]

Dyslipidaemia and insulin resistance

In early research, six constituents isolated from licorice demonstrated potent antioxidant activity toward LDL-cholesterol in vitro. The constituents were four isoflavans (including glabridin, which was the most abundant and most potent antioxidant) and two chalcones. The isoflavone formononetin was inactive.[182]

Both licorice extract and glabridin protected LDL-cholesterol against peroxidation in vitro and ex vivo in humans and in atherosclerotic apolipoprotein E-deficient mice. In the ex vivo study, LDL-cholesterol isolated from the plasma of 10 normolipidaemic subjects orally supplemented for 2 weeks with 100 mg/day of licorice (presumably as an extract dose) was more resistant to oxidation than LDL-cholesterol isolated before licorice administration.[183]

Several animal studies support the use of licorice as a lipid-lowering agent, potentially reducing the risk of cardiovascular disease. The antidyslipidaemic activity of an ethanolic extract of *G. glabra* root was investigated in the high fructose diet dyslipidaemic hamster model. Compared with controls, animals administered 100 mg/kg (oral) of a 95% ethanolic licorice extract for 30 days showed significant reductions in total cholesterol, triglycerides and LDL- and VLDL-cholesterol.[184] A later study by the same group using the same model suggested downregulation of hepatic HMG-CoA reductase was one possible mechanism.[185]

G. glabra root (5 and 10g% in diet) had previously been investigated for its hypocholesterolaemic and antioxidant effects in hypercholesterolaemic albino rats. Four weeks administration of licorice resulted in a significant reduction in hepatic total lipids, total cholesterol, triglycerides, LDL- and VLDL-cholesterol. There was also an increase in HDL-cholesterol, accelerated faecal cholesterol, neutral sterol and bile acid excretion, and increased hepatic HMG-CoA reductase activity (in contrast to the above study) and bile acid production, along with reduced hepatic lipid peroxidation and increased SOD and catalase activities.[186]

Another in vivo investigation found oral administration of GA (100 mg/kg) to high-fat diet-induced obese rats for 28 days resulted in a significant reduction in blood glucose, an improvement in insulin resistance ($p<0.05$), decreased triglycerides and increased HDL-cholesterol ($p<0.05$), together with reduced free fatty acids, total cholesterol, LDL-cholesterol and tissue lipid deposition ($p<0.01$).[187] Previous studies indicated that GA could act as a peroxisome proliferator-activated receptor agonist and thus restore lipoprotein lipase (LPL) expression in the insulin resistant state. GA may therefore exert its dyslipidaemic action by selectively inducing LPL expression in non-hepatic tissues, and may also be associated with a decrease in tissue lipid deposition.[188,189]

The effect of licorice flavonoid oil (LFO) was studied in five groups of obese, diabetic mice fed a high-fat diet containing 0 (control), 0.5%, 1% or 2% LFO or 0.5% conjugated linoleic acid for 4 weeks. Body weight gain and abdominal adipose tissue weight were suppressed ($p<0.05$) in animals fed the 2% LFO diet. Blood glucose was also reduced ($p<0.05$)

by all diets containing LFO. These results indicate that LFO can reduce abdominal fat accumulation and has hypoglycaemic effects.[190] Another study found that LFO at similar doses could reduce abdominal fat accumulation and body weight gain in high-fat diet-induced obese mice.[191] (See also in the Clinical trials section for a discussion of effects on 11-beta-HSD1 and body fat loss.)

Anti-allergic activity

In early research, GA demonstrated a strong, dose-dependent inhibitory effect on histamine synthesis and release in cultured mast cells. It also inhibited the transdifferentiation of the cells.[192]

Licorice has been traditionally used to treat inflammatory and allergic conditions. Isolated constituents have been evaluated in vitro and in vivo for their inhibition of IgE production and in assays of anti-scratching behaviour. Liquiritigenin and 18-beta-GA potently inhibited IgE-induced degranulation in a mast cell model and also inhibited the passive cutaneous anaphylactic reaction as well as the scratch behaviour in mice (at oral doses of 10 and 50 mg/kg). These results suggest that licorice may be useful in the treatment of allergic asthma and dermatitis.[193]

GL was also evaluated in a mouse model of asthma, administered orally in doses of 2.5 to 20 mg/kg to sensitised mice challenged with ovalbumin. It significantly inhibited ovalbumin-induced airway constriction, lung inflammation and eosinophil infiltration. GL also reduced IgE ovalbumin specific levels ($p<0.01$) and prevented the reduction of total IgG2a ($p<0.01$) in the serum, with no effect on serum cortisol.[194]

Antitussive activity

Early research found that oral doses of GA exerted an antitussive effect similar to codeine.[195] The antitussive effects of licorice and its components have been demonstrated in several animal studies. For example, liquiritin apioside and liquiritigenin at oral doses of 30 mg/kg in guinea pigs caused a significant reduction in capsaicin-induced cough 1 h post-administration, while liquiritin apioside, liquiritin and liquiritigenin reduced cough by more than 40% 4 h post-administration.[196] Tracheal relaxation was shown in guinea pig models to be induced by the licorice flavonoid isoliquiritigenin.[197]

Other activity

Carbenoxolone enhanced the defence mechanism of the bladder[198] and inhibited bacterial adherence to the injured urothelium.[199]

In Chinese medicine, licorice is considered to have an antitoxic activity and a protective effect of GL against saponin toxicity has been demonstrated.[200]

Liquiritin, the glycoside mainly present in licorice root, was inactive as a spasmolytic.[201] However, on hydrolysis, which occurs with the application of heat, it is converted to isoliquiritigenin which exerted strong spasmolytic activity.[201]

Isoliquiritigenin inhibited platelet aggregation in vitro, with activity comparable to that of aspirin. It also showed antiplatelet activity in vivo. Isoliquiritigenin appears to be the only aldose reductase inhibitor with a significant antiplatelet activity, which may be of benefit in prophylaxis of diabetic complications.[202] Oral administration of licorice extract (7.5 mg/kg/day for 7 days) dramatically reduced sorbitol levels in red blood cells of diabetic rats without affecting blood glucose levels significantly. Licorice therefore inhibits aldose reductase after oral doses.[203,204] Later in vitro research using rat lens aldose reductase identified semilicoisoflavone as the most potent phytochemical inhibitor of this enzyme in licorice.[205] Oral administration of licorice reduced hyperphagia and polydipsia in diabetic mice compared with controls. There was no effect observed on hyperglycaemia or hypoinsulinaemia.[206]

Licorice extract, administered by mouth or intravenous injection, exerted choleretic activity in rats.[207]

The GL metabolites 18-alpha-GA and 18-beta-GA are cellular gap junction inhibitors in vitro.[208,209] Gap junctions play an important role in intercellular communication and regulation. However, the pharmacological and safety implications of this property are not well understood.

Proposed treatment strategies for acute respiratory distress syndrome include suppressing platelet responses thought to be responsible for the onset of rapid shock caused by severe sepsis. GL injection (200 mg/kg) in a mouse model suppressed platelet responses and delayed death caused by sepsis.[210]

GL has been shown to enhance the percutaneous absorption of diclofenac sodium in sodium carboxymethylcellulose gel on abdominal rat skin.[211]

A licorice beverage extract was shown to mildly increase intestinal iron absorption in an animal model, and the investigators suggested that it might be recommended as a preventive agent for iron deficiency anaemia or to increase the absorption of supplemental iron.[212]

Pharmacokinetics

From early studies in rats, it was found that the intestinal absorption of GA was greater than that of GL. Furthermore, the absorption of GA was higher in the small intestine than in the large intestine. Although GL was poorly absorbable, both GL and GA were detected in rat plasma after oral administration of GL, suggesting that GL might be absorbed in both parent and metabolite forms, although their bioavailabilities were low.[213]

In vitro studies using rat liver homogenate indicate GL is first hydrolysed to 18-beta-GA mono-beta-D-glucuronide. The latter is then successively slowly hydrolysed to GA.[214] This suggests that even if GL is absorbed after oral ingestion it is still broken down by the liver.

Recent studies have contributed to the growing understanding of the pharmacokinetics of GL and GA in humans. These are summarised below. For a comprehensive review, the reader is referred to Ploeger and colleagues.[215]

Overall, results suggest that in humans GL in licorice is almost entirely hydrolysed by bacterial enzymes in the intestine to the aglycone GA, which is readily absorbed. In plasma, GA is extensively bound to albumin. Hepatic metabolism produces conjugates of GA, which are secreted into the bile and released back into the intestine, where they can be hydrolysed to again release GA. These GA conjugates resemble GL and

may have been misinterpreted as the latter in early studies. GA thus undergoes enterohepatic cycling with slow plasma clearance as a result. Urinary excretion is negligible.

In the intestine, GL is hydrolysed to GA by beta-glucuronidases produced by commensal bacteria. It appears that only certain bacteria (including certain *Eubacterium*, *Ruminococcus*, *Clostridium* and *Streptococcus* strains) produce the right type of enzyme required for this hydrolysis, while more common beta-glucuronidases (such as those produced by *Escherichia coli*) are not active.[71,216–218]

Hence, GL has poor oral bioavailability as such due to its being extensively hydrolysed in the intestine. In healthy volunteers given oral doses of 100 to 800 mg, no unchanged compound was detected in plasma; GA was instead found.[219–221]

In contrast, orally administered GA appears to be almost completely absorbed in both humans and rats at doses up to at least 20 to 25 mg/kg, indicating that at such levels GA liberated in the intestine has high bioavailability.[222,223] However, the bioavailability of GA was reduced to 14% in rats given a high oral dose (200 mg/kg) of GL, suggesting a limited capacity of either intestinal hydrolysis of GL or the absorption of the newly formed GA (or a combination or both).[224]

There is evidence that licorice extracts provide for lower bioavailability of GA compared with pure GL, presumably due to the impact of other constituents present in the extract. This may explain the more frequent side effects that appear to result from chronic GL administration compared with aqueous licorice extracts.[224,225]

Once absorbed, GA binds extensively to plasma albumin in both humans and rats; this binding can become saturated with high plasma concentrations.[226,227] Time to peak plasma level (Tmax) for GA following oral intake of GL is 8 to 12 h in humans, consistent with the delay resulting from intestinal hydrolysis.[225,228] An oral dose of 130 mg/day GA for 5 days resulted in peak plasma concentrations ranging from 1.1 to 1.8 mg/L.[229] The half-life of GA has been measured at 23.6 h, with the metabolite still detectable in plasma 219 hours after the last dose.[230]

In support of the research cited above, intravenously administered GL is metabolised in the liver to GA-3-mono-glucuronide, which was found to be excreted with bile into the intestine where it was further metabolised by bacterial enzymes to GA, which can then be reabsorbed.[231] In the rat, other hepatic conjugates of GA have been identified (glucuronides and a sulphate).[232]

Enterohepatic cycling of GA metabolites has been demonstrated in the rat and is assumed to also occur in humans.[215] In a human pharmacokinetic model developed for GL, and a related pharmacokinetic study in 16 volunteers, a second plasma concentration peak for GA was attributed to enterohepatic cycling. It is assumed that GA metabolites are secreted into bile and stored in the gallbladder until release occurs. Once in the intestine, bacterial beta-glucuronidases can again release GA, leading to the second peak in plasma concentration (about 20 h post dosage).[233] The degree to which enterohepatic cycling occurs is likely to be variable and dependent on gastrointestinal transit time.[215]

Plasma clearance of intravenous GL was significantly decreased in patients with chronic hepatitis C and liver cirrhosis,[234] and a similar effect on the clearance of GA following oral administration of licorice is to be expected. Urinary excretion of GA is very low (2% or less).[222,235]

Results from earlier studies in volunteers given oral GL suggest that after multiple doses of 1.5 g/day GL, 11-beta-HSD might be constantly inhibited, whereas at doses of 500 mg/day or less such an inhibition might occur only transiently.[236] Maximum levels of GA of 6.3 mg/L were reached 2 to 4 h after ingestion of 500 mg GA in 10 healthy young volunteers. Twenty-four hours after ingestion GA levels could still be detected in seven people.[237]

Clinical trials

Gastric and duodenal ulcer and functional dyspepsia

Clinical trials investigating licorice and licorice derivatives for ulcer disease fall into four categories in terms of the substances tested: licorice extract, deglycyrrhizinised licorice (DGL), DGL combined with other agents, and analogues of GL (such as carbenoxolone and enoxolone). Many of these trials were conducted more than 30 years ago and several have been criticised for poor design or small numbers, yet practitioners of herbal medicine report reduction of symptoms in patients with ulcer disease using licorice products.[238,239]

Despite showing early promise, there were several trials on DGL that gave negative findings,[240–242] although some of these may have been due to poor product formulation.[243] Subsequently, in well-controlled clinical trials DGL was shown to be as effective in healing gastric and duodenal ulcers as carbenoxolone, cimetidine and ranitidine.[244–246] DGL was widely used in the UK, in combination with conventional antacids, which may have also contributed to the observed clinical effects.[243]

More recently, a proprietary DGL product at 150 mg/day was tested in patients with functional dyspepsia in a 30-day, randomised, double blind, placebo-controlled trial.[247] Compared with placebo, the DGL group demonstrated a significant decrease ($p \leq 0.05$) in various symptom scores on days 15 and 30.

Revers successfully treated patients with peptic ulcer using about 7 g/day of licorice juice, but he also found that about 70% of his patients developed oedema.[248–250] The curative effects of licorice extract on peptic ulcer and the unfortunate side effects were confirmed by many other workers, some using up to 40 g/day of licorice extract.[251–253] Side effects could be countered by a low sodium diet,[254,255] but daily doses of 40 g still caused side effects even with restricted sodium intake.[256] Unfortunately, the quantities of GL corresponding to these doses of licorice were not assayed and variations in GL content could explain discrepancies as to what was a safe dose of extract.

Dyslipidaemia

A 9-month, random-order, double blind, placebo-controlled trial was conducted in 19 healthy volunteers (30 to 70 years) to investigate the effect of an isoflavone antioxidant, glabridin (60 mg/day) from licorice root, on LDL oxidation. Results indicated that glabridin had a protective effect on LDL oxidation and reduced oxidative stress levels by 20% ($p < 0.05$), and thus may attenuate atherosclerosis.[257]

An ethanolic extract of licorice root rich in flavonoids and GL-free at 100 mg/day for 1 month moderately reduced hypercholesterolaemic patients' plasma LDL-cholesterol by 9%, triglycerides by 14% and improved the resistance of LDL to three major atherogenic modifications (including oxidation, by 55%).[258] The trial was a small crossover design against placebo in 12 patients.

Insulin resistance

One trial suggested that licorice might have the potential to improve insulin sensitivity based on its 11-beta-HSD inhibitory activity. Lowering intracellular cortisol enhances insulin sensitivity in type 2 diabetes, obesity and hyperlipidaemia. The study in question investigated the effects of carbenoxolone (a non-selective 11-beta-HSD inhibitor and synthetic derivative of GA) on insulin sensitivity in healthy men and lean male patients with type 2 diabetes. Carbenoxolone (100 mg every 8 h, orally for 7 days) significantly reduced the rate of glucose production during hyperglucagonaemia in diabetic patients as a result of reduced glycogenolysis. As expected, it also caused an increase in blood pressure and a lowering of serum potassium. Total cholesterol decreased in the healthy volunteers ($p < 0.01$), but there was no effect on serum lipids or cholesterol in diabetic patients.[259]

Other consequences of 11-beta-HSD1 inhibition

As noted in the Pharmacology section, GL metabolites inhibit 11-beta-HSD. This enzyme is involved in peripheral cortisol metabolism; 11-beta-HSD1 mainly converts inactive cortisone into active cortisol, whereas 11-beta-HSD2 only inactivates cortisol into cortisone. Inhibition of 11-beta-HSD1 is now understood to offer significant therapeutic opportunities and agents that inhibit this enzyme are being investigated as treatments for metabolic syndrome, type 2 diabetes, glaucoma and osteoporosis.[260]

Recent studies have revealed an association of elevated 11-beta-HSD1-dependent glucocorticoid activation with insulin and leptin resistance, visceral obesity (see also under Weight loss in this section), dyslipidaemia, type 2 diabetes and cardiovascular complications. Based on animal models, abnormal hepatic 11-beta-HSD1 activity seems to play an important role in insulin resistance.[99,261] Activity of 11-beta-HSD1 is upregulated in the subcutaneous fat and livers of postmenopausal women and may cause a shift in adipose distribution from glutofemoral to abdominal deposits.[262]

Clinical trials on the GL analogue carbenoxolone suggest that 11-beta-HSD1 inhibition by licorice could have further novel clinical consequences. Ingestion of carbenoxolone (300 mg/day) by eight normal volunteers for 7 days resulted in a significant decrease in markers of bone resorption, with no overall change in bone formation markers.[263] Oral doses of carbenoxolone (300 mg/day) have also resulted in significant reductions in intraocular pressure in both healthy volunteers and patients with glaucoma.[264] These studies suggest potential clinical applications for licorice in both osteopenia and glaucoma that require further investigation. For the latter condition, licorice might even be clinically relevant after topical application to the eye (of a sterile, alcohol-free preparation).

Addison's disease

A craving for licorice sweets was found in 25% of patients with Addison's disease, a phenomenon known as 'glycyrrhizophilia'.[265] Dutch workers in the early 1950s found that licorice extract alone had a dramatic effect in maintaining electrolyte equilibrium in patients with Addison's disease. If adrenal cortex function was severely impaired, licorice alone was not a suitable treatment. However, a synergistic action was demonstrated for licorice and cortisone prescribed together.[266]

Topical application

In a pilot trial, 40 volunteers brushed their teeth twice daily with toothpaste containing 0.05% and 0.25% GL or a control toothpaste for 6 weeks. The GL toothpastes did not induce significant changes in plaque, gingival or bleeding parameters compared with controls. The authors noted that the lack of efficacy may have been due to an insufficient GL concentration or chemical incompatibility with the toothpaste itself.[267] An open, controlled clinical trial was conducted in 21 dental students, using a split-mouth technique for GL application. After 3 days, a reduction in plaque was detected in the experimental sides relative to the control sides of students' mouths.[268] However, a licorice starch gel (6g, containing 2.5% licorice extract three times per day for 2 weeks) had no impact on oral plaque in a randomised, crossover trial in 16 healthy volunteers.[269]

A carbenoxolone mouthwash was used in a double blind, crossover trial for the treatment of recurrent aphthous ulcers. The mouthwash significantly reduced the average number of ulcers per day, the formation of new ulcers and the discomfort associated with the lesions.[270] Twenty patients with mouth (aphthous) ulcers were treated with DGL for 2 weeks in an uncontrolled trial. Fifteen of the patients experienced improvement within 1 day, followed by complete healing of the ulcers by the third day.[271]

A randomised, double blind clinical trial of an intraoral adhesive patch medicated with licorice extract (used during waking, 16h/day) or placebo was conducted in two groups (n=23) of patients with recurrent aphthous ulcers. Ulcer size in the active group was significantly smaller (p<0.05) on the eighth day and pre-stimulus pain was reported as zero by 81% of the treatment group (p<0.01).[272,273] An open label trial in 15 patients with recurrent aphthous stomatitis/ulcer observed a reduction in pain and inflammation after use of a licorice bioadhesive oral hydrogel patch for 5 consecutive days.[274]

An ointment containing crude licorice powder gave good results for the treatment of chronic eczema.[275] Appreciable activity without side effects was demonstrated for topical application of licorice extract in patients with melasma (increased melanin pigmentation).[276] A 2% licorice topical gel was more effective than a 1% gel in a double blind, clinical trial in 60 patients with atopic dermatitis.[277] After 2 weeks, scores for erythema, oedema and itching were significantly reduced (p<0.05).

The efficacy of a formulation incorporating the antiviral drug idoxuridine (0.2%) in a GL gel was tested on patients suffering from herpes of the lips and nose. The preparation was significantly more effective than a 0.5% idoxuridine ointment in reducing the healing time and providing almost instantaneous pain relief. The higher efficacy of the preparation is believed to be due to the anti-inflammatory and antiviral activities of GL, combined with enhanced skin penetration of the idoxuridine.[278] Carbenoxolone cream showed some beneficial effect (although not significant) compared with placebo in the treatment of initial and recurrent herpes genitalis under double blind conditions.[279]

Some patients experience a sore throat after orotracheal intubation as part of general anaesthesia. The efficacy of a licorice gargle for the prevention of post-operative sore throat was evaluated in a randomised, single blind study. Patients gargled with a 1:60 decoction of G. glabra root powder or water (control) for 30 seconds, 5 minutes before the induction of anaesthesia. Those using the licorice experienced less post-extubation cough and a reduction in the incidence of post-operative sore throat at rest and on swallowing at all time points (0, 2, 4, 24h post-operatively). Severity of post-operative sore throat was also reduced at rest and on swallowing for all time points with licorice use, except for at rest at 24h.[280]

Polycystic ovary syndrome

Eight infertile, hyperandrogenic and oligomenorrhoeic women were investigated for the lowering of serum testosterone levels and the induction of regular ovulation by a formulation comprising *Paeonia lactiflora* and licorice (G. uralensis) in an uncontrolled trial.[281] The combination was prescribed for 2 to 8 weeks at doses of 5 to 10g/day. After the treatment period, serum testosterone levels had normalised in seven patients and six patients were ovulating regularly. Two of these six patients subsequently became pregnant. A later pharmacological study found that paeoniflorin (from Paeonia) and GA significantly decreased testosterone production from ovaries.[282]

A subsequent study specifically examined the effect of this Paeonia-licorice combination in polycystic ovary syndrome (PCOS). Thirty-four Japanese women with PCOS were treated daily with 7.5g of the combination for 24 weeks in an uncontrolled trial.[283] Serum testosterone and free testosterone levels were significantly decreased after 4 weeks. However, after 12 weeks testosterone was only lower in the patients who became pregnant. After 24 weeks the LH to FSH ratio was significantly lower.

A later clinical study investigated the effect of licorice combined with spironolactone (an aldosterone and androgen receptor antagonist often used in the management of PCOS) or spironolactone alone in 32 hirsute women (21 to 28 years) with PCOS. One group received spironolactone 100mg plus 3.5g of licorice (265mg/day GA), the other group received only spironolactone 100mg. Results showed systolic blood pressure decreased significantly at days 30 and 60 in women taking spironolactone, but not in the group taking spironolactone plus licorice. Diastolic blood pressure did not change in either group. In the spironolactone only group, 20% of patients reported fatigue, orthostatic symptoms and polyuria, while women taking licorice plus spironolactone did not describe these symptoms. Plasma renin activity and aldosterone were increased in the spironolactone only group, but there were no changes in SHBG (sex hormone binding globulin) in either group. Plasma cortisol increased in both groups after 30 and 60 days. Metrorrhagia was noted to be significantly lower in the licorice plus spironolactone patients. This particular beneficial response is not clearly understood, but it is postulated that glabridin and glabrene in licorice have oestrogen-modulating activity. The researchers concluded the addition of licorice to spironolactone has therapeutic value in women with androgen excess, as the two agents appear to have opposing effects on mineralocorticoid mechanisms and a synergistic effect on androgen excess.[284]

Hyperprolactinaemia

Some herbal medicines have been used traditionally for hyperprolactinaemia.[285] Risperidone is an antipsychotic drug used in the management of schizophrenia and bipolar disorder. A side effect of risperidone and other dopamine D2 receptor antagonists is an increase in prolactin levels, which often results in the discontinuation of the drug. Elevated prolactin levels can cause disruption to the menstrual cycle, galactorrhoea and sexual impairment. The dopamine-agonist drug bromocriptine may be prescribed to relieve these side effects, but often aggravates the psychosis and may cause abnormal involuntary movements (tardive dyskinesia).

A crossover study compared the above Paeonia-licorice combination with bromocriptine in women (n=20) with schizophrenia on risperidone treatment who had hyperprolactinaemia (>50 μg/L) and were experiencing oligomenorrhoea or amenorrhoea. Patients were randomised to additional treatment with either Paeonia-licorice (45 g/day, equivalent to 15 g licorice and 30 g/day Paeonia) followed by bromocriptine (5 mg/day) or bromocriptine followed by the herbal combination at the same dose for 4 weeks each, with a 4-week washout period between the two treatment phases. The Paeonia-licorice treatment produced a significant decrease in serum prolactin, similar to that resulting from bromocriptine, without exacerbating psychosis or altering other hormones. Patients on the herbal treatment showed reduced adverse effects associated with hyperprolactinaemia compared with the drug treatment group (56% versus 17%, p=0.037).[286]

Hyperkalaemia

Patients with endstage renal disease often have severe hyperkalaemia (serum potassium >6 mmol/L). Because GA inhibits 11-beta-HSD2 it can increase cortisol availability at the mineralocorticoid receptor and thus has the potential to lower serum potassium. In a 6-month prospective, placebo-controlled crossover study, 10 haemodialysis patients were randomly assigned to receive oral GA (500 mg/day) or placebo. Treatment with GA significantly lowered serum potassium concentrations (p<0.01).[287]

In an earlier study involving eight patients, GL (150 mg/day) was observed to be a safe treatment for hyperkalaemia due to selective hypoaldosteronism in diabetes mellitus. The mean serum potassium concentration decreased

significantly after the addition of GL to therapy.[288] The dose of GL used in this study correlates to about 3 to 4 g/day of licorice. This study also demonstrates the potential danger of even normal doses of licorice to cause hypokalaemia where potassium intake is compromised, since elevated potassium levels were reduced.

HIV/AIDS

One hundred and twelve HIV patients (72 of whom had AIDS) received oral doses of 120 mg of Glyke for 3 to 6 months in an uncontrolled study. (Glyke is a patent preparation made from G. uralensis by the Chinese Academy of Traditional Medicine.) The total effective rate was 46.4%; 30% of patients improved immunologically (as measured by the T4:T8 ratio and T4 counts). Three patients showed seronegative conversion after treatment, but tests confirmed the virus was still present.[289]

A group of 16 asymptomatic HIV-positive haemophiliacs were treated with daily oral doses of GL ranging from 150 to 225 mg for 3 to 7 years in an open study.[290] There was no change in the treated group, whereas untreated controls showed decreases in T lymphocyte counts. A follow-up study revealed similar results.[291] Results of a clinical trial in which GL was administered intravenously to haemophiliacs with AIDS suggests that GL might inhibit HIV-1 replication in vivo.[292]

Viral hepatitis

Intravenous administration of GL has been beneficial in the treatment of chronic viral hepatitis.[293] In Japan, a preparation of GL, cysteine and glycine known as SNMC is administered by injection for the treatment of acute hepatitis, chronic hepatitis (including hepatitis C) and subacute hepatic failure due to viral hepatitis.[294–298]

Chronic hepatitis C (HCV) is a progressive liver disease that often evolves to cirrhosis, liver failure or hepatocellular carcinoma. Alpha-interferon is used as a treatment to clear the viral load and has a success rate of 20% to 40% in patients without cirrhosis, and less than 20% in those with cirrhosis. As noted above, in Japan GL has been used intravenously for the treatment of chronic hepatitis for over 30 years. In clinical trials, improvements in serum aminotransferases and liver histology have been clearly demonstrated. Retrospective studies are now showing the long-term use of GL prevents hepatocellular carcinoma in patients with chronic hepatitis C.[299]

For example, in a double blind, randomised, placebo-controlled trial, 57 HCV patients (non-responders or unlikely to respond to interferon therapy) were randomised to receive 80 to 240 mg/kg intravenous GL or placebo three times weekly for 4 weeks, with a 4-week follow-up period. Within 2 days, GL treatment (any dose) caused a 15% drop in serum ALT (p<0.02) and after 4 weeks the mean decrease in ALT levels was 26% across the three GL groups, compared with a 6% reduction in the placebo group. ALT levels were normalised in 10% of patients and a clear dose–response effect was evident. The effect on ALT ceased after treatment was stopped and a change in viral clearance was not demonstrated. No major side effects were reported and the treatment was well tolerated.[300]

A further study demonstrated that patients treated six times/week rather than three times/week experienced more benefit.[301]

Combined ursodeoxycholic acid and GL therapy has been shown in a randomised, controlled trial in 170 patients to be safe and effective in improving liver-specific enzyme levels, and an alternative to interferon in chronic HCV, especially in patients who are interferon resistant.[302]

Stronger neo-minophagen C (SNMC) was trialled in China in 194 patients with chronic hepatitis B (ALT >80 IU/L) who received the intravenous therapy (40 mL or 100 mL/day) for 4 weeks followed by oral GL for another 4 weeks. The primary outcome, a reduction of ALT to 60 IU/L or less, was achieved in 74% to 79% of both groups, and normalisation of ALT levels (<40 IU/L) was seen in 57% and 58%, respectively. Hence no dose response was observed.[303] In one double blind, multicentre study, SNMC (40 mL/day for 4 weeks) caused ALT levels to decrease at a greater rate compared with placebo (p<0.001), while another study found SNMC (100 mL/day for 8 weeks) improved liver histology as well as serum ALT values.

Intravenous GL has also been clinically trialled in patients with acute sporadic hepatitis E and found to be well-tolerated and beneficial for reducing AST and ALT levels by 94% and 97%, respectively.[304]

A small clinical trial compared the efficacy of GL suppositories with intravenous GL in patients with chronic hepatitis C. Suppositories containing 300 mg GL ammonium salt and 60 mg sodium capric acid were administered rectally for 12 weeks. The two routes of administration were equally effective in reducing serum ALT levels and no serious adverse reactions were seen.[305]

Lichen planus is an inflammatory disease characterised by lymphocytic hyperkeratosis of the mucous membranes commonly in the mouth. Chronic hepatitis C (HCV) patients are often affected by this intractable and painful condition. An intravenous dose of 40 mL (0.2% solution) of GL was given daily for 4 weeks to 17 HCV patients with oral lichen planus, routine dental care was used as the control. Six of the nine patients given GL improved clinically (reduced redness, fewer white papules and less erosion to the mucous membrane), while only one of four controls improved with dental care alone.[306]

Hepatocellular carcinoma (HCC) is a common malignancy and, despite early detection, the mortality rate remains high. Secondary prevention of HCC by actively treating chronic liver disease can reduce mortality, and intravenous GL is one of several therapies available.[307]

The mechanism by which HCV infection causes hepatocellular cancer is not fully understood, but necro-inflammatory changes in HCV appear to accelerate the development of liver cirrhosis and, ultimately, HCC in some cases. Clinical data suggest that long-term treatment with SNMC can prevent the development of HCC in patients with chronic hepatitis.

Patients receiving long-term SNMC treatment had a lower risk of developing liver cirrhosis after 13 years compared with controls (28% risk versus 40% risk, p<0.002), and the risk of developing HCC was also reduced in 84 patients on long-term treatment compared with controls (13% risk versus 25% risk after 15 years, p<0.002).[308] A meta-analysis of individual data

from 1093 Japanese patients with chronic hepatitis C (non-responders to interferon therapy) found that treatment with SNMC reduced the risk of developing HCC (relative risk 0.52, p=0.10).[309]

Another retrospective study found that intravenous GL treatment significantly decreased the incidence of HCC in 1249 patients with chronic active interferon-resistant HCV infection. In patients with high ALT values (twice or more the upper limit of normal), treatment with GL decreased the rate of hepatocarcinogenesis (hazard ratio 0.49, 95% CI 0.27 to 0.86, p=0.014).[310]

Weight loss

A commercial licorice preparation was studied in terms of its effects on body fat mass (BFM) in healthy volunteers (seven men, 22 to 26 years, and eight women, 21 to 26 years). Participants consumed 3.5 g/day of the preparation for 2 months. Results showed that aldosterone and plasma renin activity were suppressed, body mass index (BMI) did not alter, extracellular water increased while BFM was significantly reduced (p<0.02 for both sexes). These findings suggest that licorice can reduce fat by inhibiting 11-beta-HSD1 in fat cells.[311]

Another study evaluated the activity of topical application of 2.5% GA or placebo on the dominant thigh of 18 healthy women with a normal BMI, aged 20 to 33 years. Thigh circumference and thickness were measured by ultrasound, at baseline and after 1 month. The treatment group (n=9) showed a significant reduction in circumference and thickness of superficial fat layers of the treated thigh compared with the untreated thigh and the placebo group (n=9). Blood pressure, plasma renin activity, aldosterone and cortisol remained unchanged during treatment.[312]

Licorice flavonoid oil (LFO) contains hydrophobic licorice flavonoids in medium-chain triglycerides (see also below). In a placebo-controlled, double blind, 12-week study in 103 overweight participants (BMI 24 to 30), LFO (300 mg/day) was shown to prevent weight gain. While body weight increased in the placebo group over the course of the study, it was maintained in the treatment group, resulting in significant differences between the two groups (p<0.05). Measurements indicated that the difference in body weight between the groups was due to differences in body fat. No clinically significant adverse events occurred during the trial period. The safety of the preparation was further demonstrated in a 4-week safety study in which 1800 mg/day did not produce clinically significant adverse event in 40 people.[313]

Less striking results were produced in another randomised, double blind, placebo-controlled study of LFO carried out by the same Japanese researchers. This study assessed effects on total body fat, visceral fat, body weight and BMI in 84 overweight men and women (40 to 60 years, BMI 24 to 30). The LFO consisted of 30% licorice root ethanolic extract mixed with 70% medium-chain triglycerides and contained 1% glabridin, but only 0.005% GL. Participants were assigned to one of four groups, receiving 300 mg/day (n=20), 600 mg/day (n=21), 900 mg/day (n=21) of LFO or placebo (n=19). Only the high dose resulted in modest but significant changes in body weight and BMI (p<0.05). Body weight was reduced by less than 1 kg and BMI by less than 1 after 4 and 8 weeks in the high-dose group only.[314] The authors did not provide a statistical comparison of the different groups, giving rise to the assumption that no statistically significant differences were observed between groups.

Other conditions

The successful treatment of chronic fatigue syndrome (CFS) by licorice has been reported in a case study. Although the pathogenesis of CFS is unknown, symptoms (such as hypocortisolism) may reflect a mild glucocorticoid insufficiency in patients who fail to show the symptoms of classic Addison's disease and hence may respond to treatment with licorice.[315]

Ingestion of a commercial licorice preparation, calculated at 3 g/day of GL, ameliorated postural hypotension caused by diabetic autonomic neuropathy in a 63-year-old patient with type 2 diabetes.[316]

A controlled clinical trial was performed in menopausal women (last menstrual period between 1 and 5 years ago) who were seeking treatment for hot flushes. The women were randomly allocated to treatment with licorice taken three times daily or hormone treatment (0.312 mg conjugated oestrogen and 2.5 mg medroxyprogesterone daily). Hot flushes were assessed using the Kupperman index. Results showed no significant differences between the two groups (p>0.05), leading the researchers to suggest that licorice has equivalent effect to the hormones in reducing hot flushes and could be used as an alternative.[317] However, placebo-controlled trials are necessary to support this assertion.

Results of a study suggest that licorice can increase serum levels of parathyroid hormone (PTH) and calcium and may have an effect on calcium metabolism. Nine healthy women (22 to 26 years) in the luteal phase of their menstrual cycle were given 3.5 g of licorice (7.6% w/w GL) for 2 months. PTH, vitamin D and urinary calcium increased significantly after 8 weeks of treatment; blood pressure and cortisol were unchanged. All values returned to pre-treatment levels within 4 weeks of discontinuing licorice.[318]

A randomised, double blind, placebo-controlled trial examined the clinical effects of intravenous GL (200 mg/day) in patients (n=67) who had undergone hepatobiliary surgery. Results showed that liver function was significantly better in the treated group compared with the untreated group of 32 patients (p<0.05).[319]

Toxicology and other safety data

Toxicology

A review of the safety of GL derivatives noted that the acute intraperitoneal LD_{50} for GA in mice was 308 mg/kg and the oral LD_{50} was greater than 610 mg/kg.[320] Little short-term, subchronic or chronic toxicity was seen in rats given salts of GL. Genotoxic and carcinogenic effects have not been observed for GL derivatives.[320]

Oral doses of 100, 250 and 500 mg/kg licorice extract in rats showed a strong dose-dependent suppression of the adrenal-pituitary axis, with significant decreases in the concentration of cortisol, ACTH, aldosterone and potassium, as well as stimulation of renin production with an increase in sodium.[321]

Long-term administration of GL to mice did not induce tumours.[322] Oral consumption of GA by rats (0.1 to 1.0 mg/mL) caused an increase in right atrial pressure and thickening of the pulmonary vessels, suggesting pulmonary hypertension.[323]

At doses of 100 to 1000 mg/kg/day (intragastric route, for a 1-year period) no significant changes were observed in rats. Dogs given the highest dose displayed decreased body weight gain and increased transaminase levels. The maximum tolerated dose is 300 mg/kg/day for dogs.[324]

As noted in the Pharmacokinetics section, after their metabolism GA conjugates are excreted in the bile and undergo enterohepatic recycling. The transit rate of gastrointestinal contents through the small and large intestines predominantly determines to what extent these GA conjugates will be reabsorbed. This parameter, which can be estimated non-invasively, may serve as a useful risk estimator for GL-induced adverse effects, because, in individuals with prolonged gastrointestinal transit times, GA might accumulate after repeated intake.[325]

In pharmacokinetic studies, significantly lower GL and GA plasma levels were found in rats and humans treated with aqueous licorice root extract compared with levels obtained for the equivalent amount of pure GL. This was attributed to the interaction during intestinal absorption between GL and the several components in the whole root extract.[225] Furthermore, the whole root extract demonstrates a significant choleretic effect. As bile is involved in GA excretion, this effect might be expected to further lower GA plasma levels after administration of the whole root.[326] Hence, toxicology differences can be expected between pure GL and the equivalent dose of GL administered as a licorice extract.

Licorice flavonoid oil (LFO) is used as a functional food ingredient in Japan. A genotoxicity study conducted in rats receiving up to 5000 mg/kg/day concluded that LFO consumption is unlikely to be a genotoxic hazard in humans.[327] Another study, designed to assess the safety of LFO in healthy humans in a placebo-controlled, single blind trial, found that LFO was safe when administered once daily up to 1200 mg/day.[328]

Contraindications

Contraindications for licorice listed by the Commission E include cholestatic liver disorders, liver cirrhosis, hypertension, hypokalaemia, severe kidney insufficiency and pregnancy.[329] Licorice is also contraindicated if there is oedema or congestive heart failure. Licorice is contraindicated in conjunction with potassium-depleting diuretic drugs and high doses should not be prescribed in conjunction with digoxin and laxatives that deplete potassium.

The hypokalaemic effects may be particularly serious for patients with anorexia nervosa who exhibit additional causes of lowered potassium levels, and permanent renal damage has been reported in one such case where high levels of licorice were consumed.[330]

Because of the potential irritant effect of the saponins, licorice should not be applied to broken or ulcerated skin.

Special warnings and precautions

Patients who are prescribed licorice preparations high in GL for prolonged periods should be placed on a high potassium and low sodium diet. They should be closely monitored for blood pressure increases and weight gain. Hypokalaemia is the earliest clinical indication and can occur at relatively low doses, as noted previously.

Special precautions should be taken with elderly patients and patients with hypertension or cardiac, renal or hepatic disease. They should not receive licorice preparations high in GL for prolonged periods and should be closely monitored if prescribed licorice preparations containing GL.

The Commission E advises that (at the high doses of 5 to 15g used in Germany) licorice should not be taken for longer than 6 to 8 weeks without professional supervision.

Avoid high and prolonged doses in pregnancy and lactation.

Interactions

Diuretics and laxatives are among a range of important drugs that deplete the body of potassium. Licorice should therefore not be taken together with these drugs if they are being used long term. There is one case report of hypokalaemic crisis with neuromuscular paralysis in a woman taking excessive doses of the diuretic furosemide along with high licorice consumption.[331] Since the toxicity of digoxin and other cardiac glycosides is enhanced by low serum potassium levels, licorice should be prescribed cautiously in conjunction with this drug.[332] A case of aggravated congestive heart failure caused by digoxin toxicity has been reported in an elderly man who also took a Chinese herbal laxative containing licorice (400mg) and rhubarb (1600mg), three times a day for 7 days. The patient, who had mitral regurgitation with atrial fibrillation, was being treated with furosemide (80mg) and digoxin (25mg). Blood tests indicated elevated digoxin and lowered potassium levels.[333]

A randomised, open, crossover trial in 10 healthy volunteers investigated the combination of a licorice confectionery (32g/day containing 42mg GL) with 25mg/day hydrochlorothiazide.[334] During the licorice phase there were no significant changes in any parameters. However, during the licorice-diuretic phase, plasma potassium decreased by 0.32mmol/L(p=0.0015),plasmareninactivityincreasedby1.6µg/L/h (p=0.0064) and body weight decreased by 0.9kg (p=0.0065). Two participants became hypokalaemic during the combined phase within the first week.

There is a small theoretical risk that licorice may counteract the contraceptive pill and long-term use of high doses of licorice is best avoided in this circumstance. The intake of licorice may also exaggerate the effects of a high salt diet.

The pharmacokinetics of prednisolone with or without pretreatment with oral GL (four doses of 50mg) was investigated in six healthy men. Results suggest that oral administration of GL increases plasma prednisolone concentrations and influences its pharmacokinetics by inhibiting its metabolism,

but not by affecting its distribution. Licorice can thereby influence the pharmacological effects of prednisolone,[335,336] but also might be an aid to patients needing to reduce or withdraw their prednisolone treatment, mainly because of its potential to support the adrenal glands.

The pharmacokinetics of methotrexate (an immunosuppressant drug with a narrow therapeutic window) has been found to be significantly affected by GL and licorice in vivo. Rats receiving an oral dose of methotrexate with GL or licorice decoction in different oral dose regimens exhibited significant increases in the bioavailability (measured as the area under the time-concentration curve) and mean residence time of methotrexate. Although it is unclear how these findings translate to humans, the authors suggested that methotrexate and licorice should be co-administered with caution.[337]

Other in vivo experiments found possible interactions of licorice with verapamil in rabbits (decreased drug activity),[338] with lidocaine in rats (decreased drug activity)[339] and with warfarin in rats (decreased drug activity).[340]

An in vitro study found that glabridin inactivated the drug metabolising cytochrome P450 (CYP) enzymes 3A4, 2B6 and 2C9 in a time- and concentration-dependent manner, whereas CYP2D6 and 2E1 were virtually unaffected.[341] These findings suggest that licorice might interact with drugs that are metabolised by certain CYP enzymes, but in vitro data of this nature are not clinically meaningful without supporting in vivo evidence.

(See also Appendix C for a summary of potential herb–drug interactions with licorice and clinically relevant recommendations.)

Use in pregnancy and lactation

Category C-has caused, or may be suspected of causing, harmful effects on the fetus or neonate without causing malformations. Studies indicate that heavy licorice consumption (as a confectionery) was associated with an increased incidence of preterm delivery and other adverse outcomes.

An epidemiological study involving 1049 Finnish women and their healthy babies published in 1998 observed that heavy GL exposure (500mg/week or greater) during pregnancy did not significantly affect birth weight or maternal blood pressure, but was significantly associated with lower gestational age. Consumption of this level of GL shortened the mean duration of gestation by 2.5 days.[342] A follow-up study in 2000 to 2001 with 95 Finnish women who delivered preterm babies noted that heavy GL consumption was associated with a more than 2-fold increased risk of preterm (<37 weeks) delivery. The association was stronger when only the 40 births classified as early preterm delivery (<34 weeks) were included. The authors suggest that heavy GL exposure may be a novel marker for preterm delivery.[343]

A study was undertaken to determine whether prenatal exposure to GL in licorice exerted detrimental effects on cognitive performance in 321 healthy Finnish children aged on average 8.1 years and born in 1998 at 35 to 42 weeks' gestation. The comparison group had a GL maternal exposure of none to 249mg/week, whereas the high exposure group was ≥500mg/week. The findings appeared to be dose related; the high exposure group demonstrated deficiencies in verbal and visuospacial abilities, narrative memory, increases in externalising symptoms and for attention, rule breaking and aggressive behaviour. The authors concluded the data are comparable with fetal programming by overexposure to glucocorticoids and warned against a high intake of licorice during pregnancy.[344]

A further follow-up study by the same group in the same children found higher salivary cortisol levels in those exposed to higher levels of licorice in utero.[345] These findings lend support to a prenatal programming of the hypothalamic-pituitary-adrenal axis by overexposure to glucocorticoids as a result of inhibition of placental 11-beta-HSD2 by licorice metabolites.

European authorities advise that licorice generally is contraindicated in pregnancy, and the above highlights concerns about its link between prematurity and the health of the newborn. However, doses up to 3g/day of root are likely to be safe for short periods.

For other reasons that are referred to in this monograph women with, or prone to, hypertension in pregnancy (preeclampsia) should avoid licorice. Specifically, 11-beta-HSD activity was significantly lower in the placentas of pre-eclamptic patients and cortisol levels in umbilical cord blood were higher.[346] This was accompanied by a decrease in fetal weight.

An ethanolic extract of licorice root (250mg/kg) did not demonstrate any significant anti-implantation activity when administered orally to female rats.[347] A review noted no adverse effects during pregnancy for salts of GL given to a variety of animals, except for a dose-dependent increase in sternebral variants in rats.[320]

Licorice is compatible with breastfeeding.

Effects on ability to drive and use machines

No adverse effects expected.

Side effects

Chronic use of licorice can lead to an 'apparent mineralocorticoid excess' syndrome with sodium and water retention, potassium loss and suppression of the renin-angiotensin-aldosterone system. As noted earlier, this is thought to follow inactivation of 11-beta-HSD2 and the binding of cortisol to mineralocorticoid receptors in the kidneys. In addition to clinical consequences, such as raised blood pressure and oedema,[348] there are reversible effects on angiotensin I and the renin-aldosterone axis from chronic use.[349] There are early reports of severe hypertension, heart enlargement and congestive heart failure in individuals consuming licorice confectionery (up to 100g/day) for extended periods of time. Symptoms disappeared after cessation of licorice ingestion.[350–352]

Long-term high consumption of licorice with consequent hypokalaemia has also been associated with embolism.[353] Licorice-induced pseudoaldosteronism has also been linked to a hypokalaemic myopathy and ECG findings suggesting dilated cardiomyopathy.[354] Pseudoaldosteronism induced by GL was reported in five women (mean age 77.8 years) admitted to hospital suffering hypertension, severe hypokalaemia (mean potassium 1.66mEq/L), low plasma aldosterone levels, suppressed plasma renin activity and progressive muscle weakness with elevated creatine phosphokinase. One patient developed cardiac dysfunction. Three of the patients had been receiving Chinese medicines containing licorice, one was taking GL and one had received both. After ceasing these medications and being treated with oral and intravenous potassium, clinical symptoms resolved and serum potassium normalised in 12 days.[355]

Another case report of pseudoaldosteronism described a 79-year-old patient taking Shakuyaku-kanzo-to (a Japanese herbal formulation used to treat cramps derived from *Paeonia lactiflora* and *G. uralensis*). The patient presented with fatigue, numbness of the hands, weakness of lower limbs, hypokalaemia (1.7mEq/L), ECG abnormalities, rhabdomyolysis, myopathy, metabolic acidosis with respiratory compensation, hypertension, hyperglycaemia, suppressed plasma renal activity, decreased aldosterone levels and increased urinary cortisol. She responded to treatment with spironolactone and potassium and discontinuation of the herbal preparation.[356]

There is an argument that the effect of licorice can be selective on sodium retention with no impact on blood pressure itself. For example, a case is reported of generalised oedema without any increase in blood pressure, with biochemical and hormonal features of apparent mineralocorticoid excess, in a young woman who had been ingesting substantial amounts of licorice for several years.[357]

However, one clinical study observed that licorice significantly raised the blood pressure of volunteers, even with amounts as low as 50g of licorice confectionery (75mg GA) consumed daily for 2 weeks. A linear dose–response relationship was observed and the degree of individual response to licorice consumption followed the normal distribution curve.[358] However, it should be noted that the mean rise in systolic blood pressure after 4 weeks of 75mg/day GA was quite small, being 1.9mmHg.

A literature review published in 1993 indicated there was indeed individual variation in susceptibility to GL. Regular daily intake of 100mg GL produced adverse effects, but there were no adverse effects documented for consumption below this value. Most individuals who consumed 400mg/day GL experienced adverse effects. The authors considered that a regular intake of 100mg/day of GL is the lowest observed adverse effect level and, using a safety factor of 10, a daily intake of 10mg GL would represent a safe dose for most healthy adults.[359] This is a very conservative estimate, and it is clear that many people regularly consume GL at much higher levels without experiencing adverse effects. This finding is supported by a later study in 39 women that suggested a no-effect level of 2mg/kg for GL.[360]

Graded daily doses of dried, aqueous extract of licorice root (containing 108, 217, 380 and 814mg of GL) were administered to four groups (with group 1 receiving the lowest dose and group 4 the highest) of six healthy volunteers of both sexes for 4 weeks in an early study. No significant effects occurred in groups 1 and 2. After 2 weeks, side effects leading to withdrawal from the protocol occurred in one woman in group 3 (headache), a man with a family history of hypertension in group 4 (arterial hypertension) and a woman also taking an oral contraceptive in group 4 (hypertension, hypokalaemia and peripheral oedema). In group 4, a transient reduction in serum potassium and an increase in body weight were found after 1 and 2 weeks, respectively. A depression of plasma renin activity occurred only in groups 3 and 4. Hence, in healthy volunteers only the highest doses of licorice led to side effects. These were favoured by subclinical disease or the oral contraceptive and were less common and pronounced than previously reported after the intake of GL, either taken as such or as a flavouring agent in confectionery products.[361]

A clinical trial published in 2003 concluded that patients with essential hypertension are more sensitive to the inhibition of 11-beta-HSD by licorice than normotensive patients, and that this inhibition caused more clinical symptoms in women than in men. Participants consumed 100g/day of licorice for 4 weeks, corresponding to a daily intake of 150mg GL.[362]

Further to this, however, patients with essential hypertension (eight men and three women, mean age 40.7 years) and a healthy control group (13 men and 12 women, mean age 31.2 years) consumed 100g of confectionery licorice (150mg/day GA) for 4 weeks. Results demonstrated that licorice-induced inhibition of aldosterone differed between the sexes (<0.02) with men being more reactive than women, but not between patients with essential hypertension and healthy patients.[363] A lack of difference in sensitivity to GA between normotensive and hypertensive individuals was also confirmed in another study.[364]

A study in 20 healthy volunteers found that potential sensitivity to the side effects of GA (as assessed by cortisol metabolites) was more marked in salt-sensitive individuals.[365] This implies that sodium restriction will help mitigate the side effects of licorice. However, results of another study in 30 people with previously documented licorice-induced hypertension suggest defects in the 11-beta-HSD2 gene are unlikely to cause an increased sensitivity to this phenomenon.[366]

Inhibition of 11-beta-HSD in susceptible individuals has been associated with the rare cases of hypertensive encephalopathy following regular daily intake of doses of licorice as a confectionery equating to around 100mg/day of GL.[367] There are also case reports of rhabdomyolysis, resulting in acute renal failure and deposition of calcium into damaged skeletal and cardiac muscles associated with licorice ingestion.[368,369]

A study in the *New England Journal of Medicine* (*NEJM*) published in October 1999 reported that serum testosterone was reduced by 35% after 4 days of licorice consumption in seven men. The administered dose was 7g/day of a licorice preparation containing 500mg of GL (since good-quality licorice contains about 4% GL, this high dose corresponds to around 12.5g/day of licorice root).[370] During the period of licorice administration there was a substantial and significant drop in the men's serum testosterone and a (smaller) significant increase in 17-hydroxyprogesterone (p<0.001). Serum androstenedione was also raised, but the difference did not achieve statistical significance, probably because of the small size of the experimental group.

The authors concluded that these results demonstrate that licorice metabolites inhibit both 17-beta-hydroxysteroid dehydrogenase and 17,20-lyase. They suggested that men with decreased libido or other sexual dysfunction, as well as

those with hypertension, should be questioned about their intake of licorice sweet.

Two unsuccessful attempts at replicating these results were made by another research team using the same dose of GL. A non-significant decrease in testosterone concentration was observed in both studies. These authors disagreed with the recommendation from the *NEJM* study that men with low libido should avoid licorice consumption.[371]

Later a team from Iran investigated the effect of licorice root extract in 20 healthy male volunteers. The men took 1.3g of dried extract (containing around 400 to 500mg GL) daily for 10 days. Blood samples were collected before the study and then for 20 days to measure testosterone levels.[372] A significant (p<0.05) decrease in serum testosterone levels of again around 35% after 10 days of licorice consumption was observed. The effect on testosterone was believed to relate to interference of GL metabolites with 17-beta-hydroxysteroid dehydrogenase, the enzyme that catalyses conversion of androstenedione to testosterone. However, the doses used were again high.

A case was reported in 2001 of a woman diagnosed with adenocarcinoma of the endometrium 'whose history was notable for extensive use of supplemental phytoestrogens'. Herbs included chaste tree, dong quai, black cohosh and licorice.[373] No causality was demonstrated.

Five case reports have linked high-dose licorice ingestion to transient loss of vision; this was assumed to be a result of vasospasm, possibly secondary to 11-beta-HSD inhibition.[374,375]

Overdosage

Six male volunteers took daily 7g of a commercial preparation of licorice for 7 days, corresponding to an intake of 500mg/day of GL. Pseudoaldosteronism was evident during the treatment, with an increase of body weight, suppression of plasma renin activity and plasma aldosterone and reduction of serum potassium.[370]

Excessive consumption of licorice confectionery has been shown to lead to transient visual loss. It is believed that licorice derivatives can cause retinal or occipital vasospasm, giving rise to transient monocular or binocular visual loss/aberrations.[375]

Consumption of 300 to 400g/day of licorice confectionery induced reversible growth retardation in a child with Addison's disease.[376]

Safety in children

As children often like licorice confectionery, care should be taken not to expose them to high levels. The use of licorice as a flavouring in herbal tinctures and extracts should be moderate.

Regulatory status in selected countries

Licorice is official in the *Pharmacopoeia of the People's Republic of China* 2010. The typical adult dosage, usually administered in the form of a decoction, is listed as 1.5 to 9g.

Licorice is included on the General Sale List. It is covered by a positive German Commission E monograph with the average daily dosage prescribed as 5 to 15 g of root, equivalent to 200 to 600 mg of glycyrrhizin or equivalent preparations. Licorice is official in the *European Pharmacopoeia* 7.2.

Licorice does have GRAS status. It is also freely available as a 'dietary supplement' in the USA under DSHEA legislation (Dietary Supplement Health and Education Act of 1994). Licorice is official in the *United States Pharmacopeia-National Formulary* (USP 34–NF 29, 2011).

Licorice is not included in Part 4 of Schedule 4 of the Therapeutic Goods Regulations in Australia and is freely available for sale.

References

1. *British Pharmacopoeia*. London: The Stationery Office; 2010.
2. *Pharmacopoeia of the People's Republic of China*. Beijing: People's Medical Publishing House; 2005.
3. Grieve M. *A Modern Herbal*, vol. 2. New York: Dover Publications; 1971. pp.487–492.
4. Felter HW, Lloyd JU. *King's American Dispensatory*. ed 18, rev 3, vol. 2, 1905. Portland: Reprinted by Eclectic Medical Publications; 1983. pp. 946–948.
5. British Herbal Medicine Association Scientific Committee. *British Herbal Pharmacopoeia*. Cowling: BHMA; 1983. pp. 104–105.
6. Bensky D, Gamble A. *Chinese Herbal Medicine Materia Medica*. Seattle: Eastland Press; 1986. pp. 463–466.
7. Swami Prakashananda Ayurveda Research Centre. *Selected Medicinal Plants Of India*. Bombay: Chemexcil; 1992. pp. 171–173.
8. Chopra RN, Chopra IC, Handa KL, et al. *Chopra's Indigenous Drugs Of India*. ed 2, 1958. Calcutta: Reprinted by Academic Publishers; 1982. pp. 183–187.
9. Pharmaceutical Society of Great Britain. *British Pharmaceutical Codex 1934*. London: Pharmaceutical Press; 1941. pp. 487–488.
10. Kang MJ, Cho JY, Shim BH. *J Med Plant Res*. 2009;3(13):1204–1211.
11. German Federal Minister of Justice. *German Commission E for Human Medicine Monograph*. Bundes-Anzeiger (German Federal Gazette), no. 90, dated 15.05.1985, no. 50, dated 13.03.1990, no. 74, dated 19.04.1991 and no. 178, dated 21.09.1991
12. USDA, ARS, National Genetic Resources Program. (n.d.). Germplasm Resources Information Network-(GRIN) [Online Database], from <http://www.ars-grin.gov/cgi-bin/npgs/html/taxon.pl?17820>. Accessed 25.02.11.
13. *Flora of China*. (n.d.). vol. 10, p. 510, from <http://www.efloras.org/florataxon.aspx?flora_id=2&taxon_id=242323657>. Accessed 25.02.11.
14. Zore GB, Winston UB, Surwase BS, et al. *Phytomedicine*. 2008;15(4):292–300.
15. Wagner H, Bladt S. *Plant Drug Analysis: A Thin Layer Chromatography Atlas*, 2nd ed. Berlin: Springer-Verlag; 1996. p. 308.
16. Hostettmann K, Marston A. *Chemistry and Pharmacology of Natural Products: Saponins*. Cambridge: Cambridge University Press; 1995. pp. 312–318.
17. Bisset NG, ed. *Herbal Drugs and Phytopharmaceuticals*. Stuttgart: Medpharm Scientific Publishers; 1994. p. 302.
18. De Smet PAGM, editor. *Adverse Effects of Herbal Drugs*, vol. 3. Berlin: Springer-Verlag; 1997. p. 67.
19. Sticher O, Soldati F. *Pharm Acta Helv*. 1978;53(2):46–52.
20. Takino Y, Koshioka M, Shiokawa M, et al. *Planta Med*. 1979;36:74–78.
21. Killacky J, Ross MS, Turner TD, et al. *Planta Med*. 1976;30(4):310–316.
22. Asl MN, Hosseinzadeh H. *Phytotherapy Res*. 2008;22:709–724.
23. British Herbal Medicine Association *British Herbal Compendium*, vol. 1. Bournemouth: BHMA; 1992. pp. 145–148.
24. Bielenberg J. *Z Phytother*. 1998;19:197–208.
25. Doll R, Hill ID, Hutton C, et al. *Lancet*. 1962:793–796.
26. Anonymous. *Br Med J*. 1(5689);1970:159–160.
27. Jones FA, Langman MJS, Mann RD, eds. *Peptic Ulcer Healing: Recent Studies on Carbenoxolone*. Lancaster: MTP Press; 1978. p. 1.
28. Wan BY, Gottfried S. *J Pharm Pharmacol*. 1985;37(10):739–741.
29. Baker ME. *Steroids*. 1994;59(2):136–141.
30. Andersson S, Barany F, Caboclo JL, et al. *Scand J Gastroenterol*. 1971;6(8):683–686.
31. Hakanson R, Liedberg G, Oscarson J, et al. *Experientia*. 1973;29(5):570–571.
32. Russell RI, Morgan RJ, Nelson LM, *Scand J Gastroenterol*. 1984;92(suppl):97–100.
33. Dehpour AR, Zolfaghari ME, Samadian T, et al. *J Pharm Pharmacol*. 1994;46(2):148–149.
34. Dehpour AR, Zolfaghari ME, Samadian T, et al. *Int J Pharm*. 1995;119(2):133–138.
35. Goso Y, Ogata Y, Ishihara K, et al. *Comp Biochem Physiol C Pharmacol Toxicol Endocrinol*. 1996;113(1):17–21.
36. Ishii Y, Terada M, *Jpn J. Pharmacol*. 1979;29(4):664–666.
37. Takagi K, Ishii Y. *Arzneimittelforschung*. 1967;17(12):1544–1547.
38. Ishii Y. *Arzneimittelforschung*. 1968;18:53–56.
39. Takagi K, Okabe S, Kawashima K, et al. *Jpn J Pharmacol*. 1971;21(6):832–833.
40. Shiratori K, Watanabe S, Takeuchi T. *Pancreas*. 1986;1(6):483–487.
41. Takeuchi T, Shiratori K, Watanabe S, et al. *J Clin Gastroenterol*. 1991;13 (suppl 1):S83–S87.
42. Ahmed N. *Ann Clin Microbiol Antimicrob*. 2005;4:17.
43. Hahn M, Fennert MB, Corless CL, et al. *J Gastrointest Endosc*. 2000;52(1):20–26.
44. Chung JG. *J Drug Chem Toxicol*. 1998;21(3):355–370.
45. Kim DH, Hong SW, Kim BT, et al. *Arch Pharmacol Res*. 2000;23(2):172–177.
46. Fukai T, Marumo A, Kaitou K, et al. *Life Sci*. 2002;71(12):1449–1463.
47. Krausse R, Bielenberg J, Blaschek W, et al. *J Antimicrob Chemother*. 2004;54(1):243–246.
48. Krausse R, Bielenberg J, Blaschek W. *Planta Med*. 2007;73(9):P104.
49. Wittschier N, Faller G, Hensel A. *J Ethnopharmacol*. 2009;125(2):218–223.
50. Wittschier N, Faller G, Beikler *Planta Med*. 2006;72(11):238.
51. O'Mahony R, Al-Khtheeri H, Weerasekera D, et al. *World J Gastroenterol*. 2005;11(47):7499–7507.
52. Kamiji MM, De Oliveira RB. *Eur J Gastroenterol Hepatol*. 2005;17(9):973–981.
53. Weerasekera D, Fernando N, Bogahawatta L, et al. *J Natl Sci Found Sri Lanka*. 2008;36(1):91–94.
54. Nariman F, Eftekhar F, Habibi Z, et al. *Iranian J Basic Med Sci*. 2009;12(2):105–111.
55. Aly AM, Al–ALousi L, Salem HA. *AAPS PharmSciTech*. 2005;6(1):E74–E82.
56. Sancar M, Hantash T, Okuyan B. *Afr J Pharm Pharmacol*. 2009;3(12):615–620.
57. Mukherjee M, Bhaskaran N, Srinath R, et al. *Indian J Exp Biol*. 2010;48(3):269–274.
58. Khayyal MT, Seif-El-Nasr M, El-Ghazaaly MA, et al. *Phytomedicine*. 2006;13:56–66.
59. Finney RSH, Somers GF, Wilkinson JH. *J Pharm Pharmacol*. 1958;10:687–695.
60. Finney RSH, Somers CF. *J Pharm Pharmacol*. 1958;10:613–620.
61. Tangri KK, Seth PK, Parmar SS, et al. *Biochem Pharmacol*. 1965;14(8):1277–1281.
62. Gujral ML, Sareen K, Phukan DP, et al. *Indian J Med Sci*. 1961;15:624–629.
63. Trease GE, Evans WC. *Pharmacognosy*, 13th ed. London: Baillière Tindall; 1983. p. 493.

64. Whitehouse MW, Haslam JM. *Nature.* 1962;196(4861):1323–1324.
65. Whitehouse MW, Dean PD, Halsall TG. *J Pharm Pharmacol.* 1967;19(8):533–544.
66. Crossland J. *Lewis's Pharmacology,* 5th ed. London: Churchill Livingstone; 1980.
67. Francischetti IM, Monteiro RQ, Guimaraes JA, et al. *Biochem Biophys Res Commun.* 1997;235(1):259–263.
68. Akamatsu H, Komura J, Asada Y, et al. *Planta Med.* 1991;57(2):119–121.
69. Capasso F, Mascolo N, Autore G, et al. *J Pharm Pharmacol.* 1983;35(5):332–335.
70. Ohuchi K, Kamada Y, Levine L, et al. *Prostagland Med.* 1981;7:457–463.
71. Hattori M, Sakamoto T, Kobashi K, et al. *Planta Med.* 1983;48(1):38–42.
72. Wang ZY, Nixon DW. *Nutr Cancer.* 2001;39(1):1–11.
73. Kang JS, Yoon YD, Cho IJ. *J Pharmacol Exp Ther.* 2005;312(3):1187–1194.
74. Chandrasekaran CV, Deepak HB, Thiyagarajan P, et al. *Phytomedicine.* 2011;18(4):278–284.
75. Jayaprakasam B, Doddaga S, Wang R. *J Agric Food Chem.* 2009;11(57):820–825.
76. Aly AM, Al-Alousi L, Salem HA. *AAPS Pharmscitech.* 2005;6(1):E72–E82.
77. Menegazzi M, DiPaola R, Mazzon E. *Pharmacol Res.* 2008;58(1):22–31.
78. Evans Q. *Br Med J.* 1956;2(5003):1239.
79. Jorgensen BB. *Acta Derm Venereol.* 1958;38:189–193.
80. Murav'ev IA, Mar'iasis ED, Krasova TG, et al. *Farmakol Toksikol.* 1983;46(1):59–62.
81. Teelucksingh S, Mackie AD, Burt D, et al. *Lancet.* 1990;335(8697):1060–1063.
82. Tanaka H, Hasegawa T, Matsushita M, et al. *Ophthalmic Res.* 1987;19(4):213–220.
83. Shibata S, Inoue H, Iwata S, et al. *Planta Med.* 1991;57(3):221–224.
84. Ohuchi K, Kamada Y, Levine L, et al. *Prostagland Med.* 1981;7(5):457–463.
85. Armanini D, Karbowiak I, Funder JW. *Clin Endocrinol (Oxf).* 1983;19(5):609–612.
86. Takeda R, Miyamori I, Soma R, et al. *J Steroid Biochem.* 1987;27(4–6):845–849.
87. Tamaya T, Sato S, Okada H. *Acta Obstet Gynecol Scand.* 1986;65(8):839–842.
88. Kumagai A, Yano S, Otomo M, et al. *Endocrinol Jpn.* 1957;4(1):17–27.
89. Tamura Y. *Folia Endocrinol Jpn.* 1975;51:589–600.
90. Suzuki H, Ohta Y, Takino T, et al. *Asian Med J.* 1984;26:423–438.
91. Kumagai A, Yano S, Takeuchi K, et al. *Endocrinology.* 1964;74:145–148.
92. Kumagai A, Asanuma Y, Yano S, et al. *Endocrinol Jpn.* 1966;13(3):234–244.
93. Kraus SD, Kaminskis A. *Exp Med Surg.* 1969;27(4):411–420.
94. Takeda R, Morimoto S, Uchida K, et al. *Endocrinol Jpn.* 1979;26(5):541–547.
95. Stewart PM, Wallace AM. *Lancet.* 1987;2(8563):821–824.
96. Edwards CR, Stewart PM, Burt D, et al. *Lancet.* 1988;2(8618):986–989.
97. Pelser HE, Willebrands AF, Frenkel M, et al. *Metabolism.* 1953;2:322–334.
98. MacKenzie MA, Hoefnagels WH, Jansen RW, et al. *J Clin Endocrinol Metab.* 1990;70(6):1637–1643.
99. Classen-Houben D, Schuster D, Da Cunha T, et al. *J Steroid Biochem Mol Biol.* 2009;113(3–5):248–252.
100. Zou Q, Wei P, Li J, et al. *Biomed Chromatogr.* 2009;23(1):54–62.
101. Baker ME, Fanestil DD. *Mol Cell Endocrinol.* 1991;78(1–2):C99–C102.
102. Kato H, Kanaoka M, Yano S, et al. *J Clin Endocrinol Metab.* 1995;80(6):1929–1933.
103. Armanini D, Lewicka S, Pratesi C, et al. *J Endocrinol Invest.* 1996;19(10):1387–1389.
104. Sigurjonsdottir HA, Axelson M, Johannsson G, et al. *Horm Res.* 2006;65(2):106–110.
105. Kroes BH, Beukelman CJ, Van Den Berg AJ, et al. *Immunology.* 1997;90(1):115–120.
106. Matsumoto T, Tanaka M, Yamada H, et al. *J Ethnopharmacol.* 1996;53(1):1–4.
107. Lin IH, Hau DM, Chen KT, et al. *Chin Med J (Engl).* 1996;109(2):138–142.
108. Lee JY, Lee JH, Park JH, et al. *Int Immunopharmacol.* 2009;9(5):632–638.
109. Okamoto H, Yoshida D, Saito Y, et al. *Cancer Lett.* 1983;21(1):29–35.
110. Okamoto H, Yoshida D, Mizusaki S. *Cancer Lett.* 1983;19(1):47–53.
111. Kitagawa K, Nishino H, Iwashima A. *Oncology.* 1986;43(2):127–130.
112. O'Brian CA, Ward NE, Vogel VG. *Cancer Lett.* 1990;49(1):9–12.
113. Abe H, Ohya N, Yamamoto KF, et al. *Eur J Cancer Clin Oncol.* 1987;23(10):1549–1555.
114. Chen X, Han R. *Chin Med Sci J.* 1995;10(1):16–19.
115. Wang ZY, Agarwal R, Khan WA, et al. *Carcinogenesis.* 1992;13(8):1491–1494.
116. Agarwal R, Wang ZY, Mukhtar H. *Nutr Cancer.* 1991;15(3–4):187–193.
117. Wang ZY, Agarwal R, Zhou ZC, et al. *Carcinogenesis.* 1991;12(2):187–192.
118. Zani F, Cuzzoni MT, Daglia M, et al. *Planta Med.* 1993;59(6):502–507.
119. Hrelia P, Fimognari C, Maffei F, et al. *Phytother Res.* 1996;10:S101–S103.
120. Maggiolini M, Statti G, Vivacqua A, et al. *J Steroid Biochem Mol Biol.* 2002;82(4–5):315–322.
121. Rafi MM, et al. *Anticancer Res.* 2000;2(4):2653–2658.
122. Kanazawa M, Satomi Y, Mizutani Y, et al. *Eur Urol.* 2003;43(5):580–586.
123. Rafi MM, Vastano BC, Zhu CT, et al. *J Agric Food Chem.* 2002;50(4):677–684.
124. ChinY W, Jung HA, Liu Y, et al. *J Agric Food Chem.* 2007;55(12):4691–4697.
125. Takahashi T, Takasuka N, Iigo M, et al. *Cancer Sci.* 2004;95(5):448–453.
126. Yo YT, Shieh GS, Hsu KF, et al. *J Agric Food Chem.* 2009;57(18):8266–8273.
127. Sheela ML, Ramakrishna MK, Salimath BP. *Int Immunopharmacol.* 2006;6(3):494–498.
128. Xiao XY, Hao M, Yang XY, et al. *Oncology Stat.* 2011;302(1):69–75.
129. Zhang MZ, Xu J, Yao B. *J Clin Invest* 119(4): 876–885, 200.
130. Hikino H. In: Farnsworth NR, ed. *Economic and Medicinal Plant Research,* vol. 1. London: Academic Press; 1985. p. 58.
131. Kiso Y, Tohkin M, Hikino H. *Planta Med.* 1983;49(4):222–225.
132. Kiso Y, Tohkin M, Hikino H, et al. *Planta Med.* 1984;50(4):298–302.
133. Moon A, Kim SH. *Planta Med.* 1997;63(2):115–119.
134. Paolini M, Pozzetti L, Sapone A, et al. *Life Sci.* 1998;62(6):571–582.
135. Nose M, Ito M, Kamimura K, et al. *Planta Med.* 1994;60(2):136–139.
136. Chan H, Chan C, Ho J. *Toxicology.* 2003;188(2–3):211–217.
137. Rajesh MG, Latha MS. *Indian J Pharmacology.* 2004;6(5):278–284.
138. Lee CH, Park SW, Kim YS, et al. *Biol Pharm Bull.* 2007;30(10):1898–1904.
139. Wu X, Zhang L, Gurley E, et al. *Hepatology.* 2008;47(6):1905–1915.
140. Fiore C, Eisenhut M, Krausse R, et al. *Phytother Res.* 2008;22(2):141–148.
141. Pompei R, Flore O, Marccialis MA, et al. *Nature.* 1979;281(5733):689–690.
142. Pompei R, Pani A, Flore O, et al. *Experientia.* 1980;36(3):304.
143. Baba M, Shigeta S. *Antiviral Res.* 1987;7(2):99–107.
144. Lojda Z, Maratka Z. *Hepatogasterenterology.* 1982;29:88–89.
145. Cermelli C, Portolani B, Colombari B, et al. *Phytother Res.* 1996;10:S27–S28.
146. Nakashima H, Matsui T, Yoshida O, et al. *Jpn J Cancer Res.* 1987;78(8):767–771.
147. Ito M, Nakashima H, Baba M, et al. *Antiviral Res.* 1987;7:127–137.
148. Abe N, Ebina T, Ishida N. *Microbiol Immunol.* 1982;26(6):535–539.
149. Badam L. *J Commun Dis.* 1997;29(2):91–99.
150. Utsunomiya T, Kobayashi M, Pollard RB, et al. *Antimicrob Agents Chemother.* 1997;41(3):551–556.
151. Touitou E, Segal R, Pisanty S, et al. *Drug Des Deliv.* 1988;3(3):267–272.
152. Sekine-Osajima Y, Sakamoto N, Nakagawa M, et al. *Hepatol Res.* 2009;39(1):60–69.
153. Lin JC, Cherng JM, Hung MS, et al. *Antiviral Res.* 2008;79(1):6–11.
154. Bone K. *MediHerb e-Monitor.* 2009;25:2.
155. Wolkerstorfer A, Kurz H, Bachhofner N, et al. *Antiviral Res.* 2009;83(2):171–178.
156. Sasaki H, Takei M, Kobayashi M, et al. *J Immunopathol.* 2002;70(4):229–236.
157. Yoshida T, Kobayashi M, Li XD. *Immunol Cell Biol.* 2009;87(7):554–558.

158. Yoshida T, Kobayashi M, Matsumoto H. *J Immunol*. 2006;176:S94.

159. Harada S. *Biochem J*. 2005;392(1):191–199.

160. Cinatl J, Morgenstern B, Chandra P. *Lancet*. 2003;361(9374):2045–2046.

161. Mitscher LA, Park YH, Clark D, et al. *J Nat Prod*. 1980;43(2):259–269.

162. Chen M, Theander TG, Christensen SB, et al. *Antimicrob Agents Chemother*. 1994;38(7):1470–1475.

163. Chen M, Christensen SB, Blom J, et al. *Antimicrob Agents Chemother*. 1993;37(12):2550–2556.

164. Segal R, Pisanty S, Wormser R, et al. *J Pharm Sci*. 1985;74(1):79–81.

165. Peters MC, Tallman JA, Braun TM, Jacobson JJ. *Eur Arch Paediatr Dent*. 2010;11(6):274–278.

166. Hu CH, He J, Eckert R, et al. *Int J Oral Sci*. 2011;3(1):13–20.

167. Sasaki H, Suzuki N, Aishwaimi E, et al. *J Peridontal Res*. 2010;45(6):757–763.

168. Hatano T, Aga Y, Shintani Y, et al. *Phytochemistry*. 2000;55(8):959–963.

169. Dhingra D, Parle M, Kulkarni SK. *J Ethnopharmacol*. 2004;91(2–3):361–365.

170. Cui YM, Ao MZ, Yu LJ. *Planta Med*. 2008;74(4):377–380.

171. Sharifzadeh M, Shamsa F, Shiran S, et al. *Planta Med*. 2008;74(5):485.

172. Kao TC, Shyu MH, Yen GC. *J Agric Food Chem*. 2009;57(2):754–761.

173. Cherng JM, Lin HJ, Hung MS, et al. *Eur J Pharmacol*. 2006;547(1–3):10–21.

174. Kim DE, Park SE, Han JH. *J Neurol*. 2008;255(suppl 2):1–235. Abstract P665.

175. Yu XQ, Xue CC, Zhou ZW, et al. *Life Sci*. 2008;82(1–2):68–78.

176. Jeong JP, Buono RJ, Han BG, et al. *J Proteome Res*. 2008;7(12):5094–5102.

177. Zhan C, Yang J. *Pharmacol Res*. 2006;53(3):303–309.

178. Genovese T, Menegazzi M, Mazzon E. *J Shock*. 2009;31(4):367–375.

179. Kulkarni A, Kellaway L, Kotwal G. *Ann NY Acad Sci*. 2005;1056:413–429.

180. Zhao ZY, Wang WX, Guo HZ, et al. *J Behav Brain Res*. 2008;194(1):108–113.

181. Dhingra D, Amandeep S. *Prog Neuropsychopharmacol Biol Psychiatry*. 2006;30(3):449–454.

182. Vaya J, Belinky PA, Aviram M. *Free Radic Biol Med*. 1997;23(2):302–313.

183. Fuhrman B, Buch S, Vaya J, et al. *Am J Clin Nutr*. 1997;66(2):267–275.

184. Maurya SK, Raj K, Srivastava A. *Indian J Clin Biochem*. 2009;24(4):404–409.

185. Maurya SK, Srivastava AK. *Prague Med Rep*. 2011;112(1):29–37.

186. Visavadiya NP, Narasimhacharya AVRL. *Mol Nutr Food Res*. 2005;50(11):1080–1086.

187. Eu CHA, Lim WAY, Ton SO, et al. *Lipids Health Dis*. 2010;9:81–92.

188. Lim WAY, Chia YY, Liong SY, et al. *Lipids Health Dis*. 2009;8:31.

189. Fuhrman B, Volkova N, Kaplan M, et al. *Nutrition*. 2002;18(3):268–273.

190. Nakagawa K, Kishida H, Arai N, et al. *Biol Pharm Bull*. 2004;27(11):1775–1778.

191. Aoki F, Honda S, Kishida H, et al. *Biosci Biotechnol Biochem*. 2007;71(1):206–214.

192. Lee YM, Kim YC, Kim HM. *Arch Pharmacol Res*. 1996;19(1):36–40.

193. Shin YW, Bae EA, Lee SH. *Planta Med*. 2007;73(3):257–261.

194. Ram A, Mabalirajan U, Das M. *Int Immunopharmacol*. 2006;6(9):1468–1477.

195. Anderson DM, Smith WG. *J Pharm Pharmacol*. 1961;13:396–404.

196. Kamei J, Saitoh A, Asano T, et al. *Eur J Pharmacol*. 2005;507(1–3):163–168.

197. Lui B, Yang J, Wen QS. *Acta Pharmacol Sin*. 2006;27:156.

198. Mooreville M, Fritz RW, Mulholland SG. *J Urol*. 1983;130(3):607–609.

199. Pantazopoulos D, Legakis N, Antonakopoulos G, et al. *Br J Urol*. 1987;59(5):423–426.

200. Segal R, Milo–Goldzweig I, Kaplan G, et al. *Biochem Pharmacol*. 1977;26(7):643–645.

201. Wagner H. In: Swain T, Harborne JB, Van Sumere CF, eds. *Biochemistry of Plant Phenolics*. New York: Plenum Press; 1979. pp. 604–605.

202. Tawata M, Aida K, Noguchi T, et al. *Eur J Pharmacol*. 1992;212(1):87–92.

203. Zhou Y, Zhang J. *Chung Kuo Chung Yao Tsa Chih*. 1990;15(7):433–435.

204. Zhou YP, Zhang JQ. *Chin Med J (Engl)*. 1989;102(3):203–206.

205. Lee YS, Kim SH, Jung SH, et al. *Biol Pharm Bull*. 2010;33(5):917–921.

206. Swanston-Flatt SK, Day C, Bailey CJ, et al. *Diabetologia*. 1990;33(8):462–464.

207. Raggi MA, Bugamelli F, Nobile L, et al. *Boll Chim Farm*. 1995;134(11):634–638.

208. Chaytor AT, Marsh WL, Hutcheson IR, Griffith TM. *Endothelium*. 2000;7(4):265–278.

209. Taylor HJ, Chaytor AT, Evans WH, Griffith TM. *Br J Pharmacol*. 1998;125(1):1–3.

210. Yu ZQ, Ohtaki Y, Kai KZ, et al. *Int Immunopharmacol*. 2005;5(3):571–580.

211. Nokhodchi A, Nazemiyeh H, Ghafourin T. *Farmaco*. 2003;57(11):883–888.

212. el-Shobaki FA, Saleh ZA, Saleh N. *Z Ernahrungswiss*. 1990;29(4):264–269.

213. Wang Z, Kurosaki Y, Nakayama T, et al. *Biol Pharma Bull*. 1994;17(10):1399–1403.

214. Akao T, Akao T, Hattori M, et al. *Biochem Pharmacol*. 1991;41(6–7):1025–1029.

215. Ploeger B, Mensinga T, Sips A, et al. *Drug Metab Rev*. 2001;33(2):125–147.

216. Akao T, Akao T, Kobashi K. *Chem Pharm Bull*. 1987;35(2):705–710.

217. Hattori M, Sakamoto T, Yamagishi T, et al. *Chem Pharm Bull*. 1985;33(1):210–217.

218. Kim DH, Lee SW, Han MJ. *Biol Pharm Bull*. 1999;22:320–322.

219. Yamamura Y, Kawakami J, Santa T, et al. *J Pharm Sci*. 1992;81(10):1042–1046.

220. Groot de G, Koops R, Hogendoorn EA, et al. *J Chromatogr*. 1988;456(1):71–81.

221. Gunnarsdottir S, Johannesson T. *Pharmacol Toxicol*. 1997;81(6):300–302.

222. Krahenbuhl S, Hasler F, Frey BM, et al. *J Clin Endocrinol Metab*. 1994;78(3):581–585.

223. Parke DV, Pollock S, Williams RT. *J Pharm Pharmacol*. 1963;15:500–506.

224. Wang Z, Nishioka M, Kurosaki Y, et al. *Biol Pharm Bull*. 1995;18(9):1238–1241.

225. Cantelli-Forti G, Maffei F, Hrelia P, et al. *Environ Health Perspect*. 1994;102(suppl 9):65–68.

226. Ishida S, Sakiya Y, Ichikawa T, et al. *Chem Pharm Bull*. 1989;37(9):2509–2513.

227. Ishida S, Sakiya Y, Ichikawa T, et al. *Chem Pharm Bull*. 1989;37(1):226–228.

228. Takeda S, Ono H, Wakui Y, et al. *J Chromatogr B*. 1990;530(2):447–451.

229. Ploeger BA, Mensinga T, Sips AJAM, et al. *Toxicol Appl Pharmacol*. 2001;170(1):46–55.

230. Cosmetic Ingredient Review Panel. *Int J Toxicol*. 2007;26(suppl. 2):79–112.

231. Akao T, Akao T, Hattori M, et al. *Biochem Pharmacol*. 1991;41:1025–1029.

232. Iveson P, Lindup WE, Parke DV, et al. *Xenobiotica*. 1971;1:79–95.

233. Ploeger B, Mensinga T, Sips A, et al. *Pharm Res*. 2000;17(12):1516–1525.

234. van Rossum TG, Vulto AG, Hop WC, et al. *Clin Ther*. 1999;21:2080–2090.

235. Terasawa K, Bandoh M, Tosa H, et al. *J Pharmacobio–Dyn*. 1986;9:95–100.

236. Krahenbuhl S, Hasler F, Frey BM, et al. *J Clin Endocrinol Metab*. 1994;78(3):581–585.

237. Heilmann P, Heide J, Schoneshofer M. *Eur J Clin Chem Clin Biochem*. 1997;35(7):539–543.

238. Kaczor T. *Nat Med J*. 2009;1(3):1–4.

239. Ryan SW. *Altern Ther Health Med*. 2005;11(5):26–29.

240. Anonymous. *Br Med J*. 1971;3(773):501–503.

241. Feldman H, Gilat T. *Gut*. 1971;12(6):449–451.

242. Bardhan KD, Cumberland DC, Dixon RA, et al. *Gut*. 1978;19(9):779–782.

243. Glick L. *Lancet*. 1982;2(8302):817.

244. Larkworthy W, Holgate PF. *Practitioner*. 1975;215(1290):787–792.

245. Gutz HJ, Berndt H, Jackson D. *Practitioner*. 1979;222(1332):849–853.

246. Morgan AG, McAdam WA, Pacsoo C, et al. *Gut*. 1982;23(6):545–551.

247. Raveendra KR, Jayachandra Srinivasa V, et al. *Evid Based Complement Altern Med*. 2012 [216970].

248. Revers FE. *Ned Tijdschr Geneeskd*. 1946;90:135–137.

249. Revers FE. *Ned Tijdschr Geneeskd*. 1948;92:2968–2973.

250. Revers FE. *Ned Tijdschr Geneeskd.* 1948;92:3567–3569.

251. Schulze E, Franke R. *Dtsch Med Wochenschr.* 1951;76:988–990.

252. Argelander H. *Arztl Wochenschr.* 1952;7:35.

253. Hensel O. *Pharmazie.* 1955;10:60.

254. Wilde G. *Arztl Wochenschr.* 1952;7: 1058–1061.

255. Schulze E, Franke R, Keller N. *Dtsch Med Wochenschr.* 1954;79:716–719.

256. Klimpel W, Finkenauer H. *Therapiewoche.* 1952;2:520–523.

257. Carmeli E, Fogelman Y. *Toxicol Ind Health.* 2009;25(4–5):321–324.

258. Fuhrman B, Volkova N, Kaplan M, et al. *Nutrition.* 2002;18(3):268–273.

259. Andrew RC, Rooyackers O, Walker BR. *J Clin Endocrinol Metab.* 2003;88(1): 285–291.

260. Cooper MS, Stewart PM. *J Clin Endocrinol Metab.* 2009;94(12):4645–4654.

261. Staab CA, Maser E. *J Steroid Biochem Mol Biol.* 2010;119(1–2):56–72.

262. Andersson T, Simonyte K, Andrew R, et al. *PLoS One.* 2009;4(12):e8475.

263. Cooper MS, Walker EA, Bland R, et al. *Bone.* 2000;27(3):375–381.

264. Rauz S, Cheung CM, Wood PJ, et al. *QJM.* 2003;96(7):481–490.

265. Knowles JP. *Proc R Soc Med.* 1958;51:178.

266. Borst JGG, de Vries LA, Holt SP, et al. *Lancet.* 1953:657–663.

267. Goultschin J, Palmon S, Shapira L, et al. *J Clin Periodontol.* 1991;18(3):210–212.

268. Steinberg D, Sgan–Cohen HD, Stabholz A, et al. *Isr J Dent Sci.* 1989;2(3):153–157.

269. Söderling E, Karjalainen S, Lille M, et al. *Clin Oral Investig.* 2006;10(2):108–113.

270. Poswillo D, Partridge M. *Br Dent J.* 1984;157(2):55–57.

271. Das SK, Das V, Gulati AK, et al. *J Assoc Physicians Ind.* 1989;37(10):647.

272. Martin MD, Sherman J, van der Ven P, et al. *J Gen Dent.* 2008;56(2):211–224.

273. Burgess JA, van der Ven PF, Martin M, et al. *J Contemp Dent Pract.* 2008;9(3): 88–98.

274. Moghadamnia AA, Motallebnejad M, Khanian M. *Phytother Res.* 2009;23(2):246–250.

275. Loewy E. *Ars Medici.* 1956;46(1):483.

276. Iurassich S, Bianco P, Rossi E. *Chron Dermatol.* 1996;6(5):653–658.

277. Saeedi M, Morteza-Semnani K, Ghoreishi MR. *J Dermatolog Treat.* 2003;14(3): 153–157.

278. Segal R, Pisanty S. *J Clin Pharm Ther.* 1987;12(3):165–175.

279. Csonka GW, Tyrrell DA. *Br J Vener Dis.* 1984;60(3):178–181.

280. Agarwal A, Gupta D, Yadav G, et al. *Anesth Analg.* 2009;109(1):77–81.

281. Yaginuma T, Izumi R, Yasui H, et al. *Nippon Sanka Fujinka Gakkai Zasshi.* 1982;34(7):939–944.

282. Takeuchi T, Nishii O, Okamura T, et al. *Am J Chin Med.* 1991;19(1):73–78.

283. Takahashi K, Kitao M. *Int J Fertil Menopausal Stud.* 1994;39(2):69–76.

284. Armanini D, Castello R, Scaroni C, et al. *Eur J Obstet Gynecol Reprod Biol.* 2007;131(1):61–67.

285. Hasani-Ranjbar S, Vahidi H, Taslimi S, et al. *Int J Pharmacol.* 2010;6(5):691–695.

286. Yuan HN, Wang CY, Sze CW, et al. *J Clin Psychopharmacol.* 2008;28(3):264–270.

287. Farese S, Kruse A, Pasch A, et al. *Kidney Int.* 2009;76:877–884.

288. Murakami T, Uchikawa T. *Life Sci.* 1993;53(5):PL63–PL68.

289. Lu W. *Int Conf AIDS.* August 7–12 1994;10(2):214. Abstract no. PB0868.

290. Ikegami N, Akatani K, Imai M, et al. *Int Conf AIDS.* June 6–11 1993;9(1):234. Abstract no. PO-A25-0596.

291. Kinoshita S, Tsujino G, Yoshioka K, et al. *Int Conf AIDS.* August 7–12 1994;10(1):222. Abstract no. PB0317.

292. Hattori T, Ikematsu S, Koito A, et al. *Antiviral Res.* 1989;11(5–6):255–261.

293. Eisenburg J. *Fortschr Med.* 1992;110(21):395–398.

294. Fujisawa K, Watanabe Y, Kimura K. *Asian Med J.* 1980;23(10):745–756.

295. Matsunami H, Lynch SV, Balderson GA, et al. *Am J Gastroenterol.* 1993;88(1): 152–153.

296. Arase Y, Ikeda K, Murashima N, et al. *Cancer.* 1997;79(8):1494–1500.

297. Acharya SK, Dasarathy S, Tandon A, et al. *Indian J Med Res.* 1993;98:69–74.

298. Iino S, Tango T, Matsushima T, et al. *Hepatology Res.* 2001;19(1):31–40.

299. van Rossum TG, Vulto AG, DeMan RA. *Aliment Pharmacol Ther.* 1998;12(3): 199–205.

300. Van Rossum TGJ, Vulto AG, Hop WCJ, et al. *J Gastroenterol Hepatol.* 1999;14(11):1093–1099.

301. Van Rossum TGJ, Vulto AG, Hop WCP, et al. *Am J Gastroenterol.* 2001;96(8):2432–2437.

302. Tsubota A, Kumada H, Arase Y, et al. *Eur J Gastroenterol Hepatol.* 1999;11(10): 1077–1083.

303. Zhang LX, Wang B. *Hepatol Res.* 2002;24(3):220–227.

304. Tandon A, Tandon BN, Bhujwala RA. *Hepatol Res.* 2002;23(1):55–61.

305. Fujioka T, Kondou T, Fukuhara A, et al. *Hepatol Res.* 2003;26(1):10–14.

306. Da Nagao Y, Sata M, Suzuki H, et al. *J Gastroenterol.* 1996;31(5):691–695.

307. Song H, Hwang S. *Korean J Gastroenterol.* 2007;49(4):201–208.

308. Kumada H. *Oncology.* 2002;62(1):94–100.

309. Hansen BE, Ikeda K, Veldt BJ, et al. *J Hepatol.* 2003;38(suppl 2):143–144. Abstract 493.

310. Ikeda K, Arase Y, Kobayashi M, et al. *Dig Dis Sci.* 2006;51(3):603–609.

311. Armanini D, De Palo CB, Mattarello MJ. *J Endocrinol Invest.* 2003;26(7):646–650.

312. Armanini D, Nacamulli D, Francini-Pesenti F, et al. *Steroids.* 2005;70(8):538–542.

313. Tominaga Y, Mae T, Kitano M. *J Health Sci.* 2006;52(6):672–683.

314. Tominaga Y, Nakagawa K, Tatsumasa M, et al. *Obes Res Clin Pract.* 2009;3:169–178.

315. Baschetti R. *NZ Med J.* 1995;108(1002):259.

316. Basso A, Dalla Paola L, Erle G, et al. *Diabetes Care.* 1994;17(11):1356.

317. Menati L, Siahpoosh A, Tadayon M. *Sci Med J.* 2010;9(2):157–167. [In Arabic].

318. Mattarello M, Benedini S, Fiore C, et al. *Steroids.* 2006;71:403–408.

319. Song F, Huang S, Li D. *Lingnan Modern Clinics Surg.* 2007;3.

320. Cosmetic Ingredient Review Expert Panel. *Int J Toxicol.* 2007;26(suppl 2):79–112.

321. Al–Qarawi AA, Abdel-Rahman HA, Ali BH, et al. *Food Chem Toxicol.* 2002;40(10):1525–1527.

322. Kobuke K, Inai K, Nambu S, et al. *Food Chem Toxicol.* 1985;23:979–983.

323. Ruszymah BH, Nabishah BM, Aminuddin S, et al. *Clin Exp Hypertens.* 1995;17(3):575–591.

324. Kelloff GJ, Crowell JA, Boone CW, et al. *J Cell Biochem Suppl.* 1994;20:166–175.

325. Ploeger B, Mensinga T, Sips A, et al. *Drug Metab Rev.* 2001;33(2):125–147.

326. Cantelli-Forti G, Raggi MA, Bugamelli F, et al. *Pharmacol Res.* 1997;35(5):463–470.

327. Nakagawa K, Hidaka T, Asakura M, et al. *Food Chem Toxicol.* 2008;46(7):2525–2532.

328. Aoki F, Nakagawa K, Kitano M, et al. *Nutrition.* 2007;26(3):209–218.

329. Blumenthal M, ed. *The Complete German Commission E Monographs: Therapeutic Guide to Herbal Medicines.* Austin: American Botanical Council; 1998.

330. Ishikawa S, Kato M, Tokuda T, et al. *Int J Eat Disord.* 1999;26(1):111–114.

331. Famularo G, Corsi FM, Giacanelli M. *Acad Emerg Med.* 1999;6(9):960–964.

332. MIMS Australia Pty Ltd. *E-MIMS.* Version 4.00.0457, 2000.

333. Harada T, Ohtaki E, Misu K, et al. *Cardiology.* 2002;98(4):218.

334. Hukkanen J, Ukkola O, Savolainen MJ. *Blood Press.* 2009;18(4):192–195.

335. Chen MF, Shimada F, Kato H, et al. *Endocrinol Jpn.* 1991;38(2):167–174.

336. Chen MF, Shimada F, Kato H, et al. *Endocrinol Jpn.* 1990;37(3):331–341.

337. Lin SP, Tsai SY, Hou YC, et al. *J Agric Food Chem.* 2009;11(57):1854–1859.

338. Al-Deeb ID, Arafat TA, Irshaid YM. *Drug Metab Lett.* 2010;4(3):173–179.

339. Tang J, Song X, Zhu M, Zhang J. *Phytother Res.* 2009;23(5):603–607.

340. Mu Y, Zhang J, Zhang S, et al. *J Pharmacol Exp Ther.* 2006;316(3):1369–1377.

341. Kent UM, Aviram M, Rosenblat M, et al. *Drug Metab Dispos.* 2002;30(6):709–715.

342. Strandberg TE, Jarvenpaa AL, Vanhanen H, et al. *Am J Epidemiol*. 2001;153(11):1085–1088.

343. Strandberg TE, Andersson S, Jarvenpaa AL, et al. *Am J Epidemiol*. 2002;156(9):803–805.

344. Raikkanen K, Pesonen A, Heinonen K, et al. *Am J Epidemiol*. 2009;170(9):1137–1146.

345. Räikkönen K, Seckl JR, Heinonen K, et al. *Psychoneuroendocrinology*. 2010;35(10):1587–1593.

346. McCalla CO, Nacharaju VL, Muneyyirci-Delale O, et al. *Steroids*. 1998;63(10): 511–515.

347. Sharma BB, Varshney MD, Gupta DN, et al. *Int J Crude Drug Res*. 1983;21(4):183–187.

348. Olukoga A, Donaldson D. *J R Soc Health*. 2000;120(2):83–89.

349. Megia A, Herranz L, Martin-Almendra MA, et al. *Nephron*. 1993;65(2):329–330.

350. Chamberlain TJ. *JAMA*. 1970;213(8):1343.

351. Koster M, David GK. *N Engl J Med*. 1968;278(25):1381–1383.

352. Conn JW, Rovner DR, Cohen EL. *JAMA*. 1968;205(7):492–496.

353. Lozano P, Flores D, Martinez S, et al. *J Cardiovasc Surg (Torino)*. 2000;41(4): 631–632.

354. Hasegawa J, Suyama Y, Kinugawa T, et al. *Cardiovasc Drugs Ther*. 1998;12(6): 599–600.

355. Yamamoto T, Hatanaka M, Matsuda J, et al. *Nippon Jinzo Gakkai Shi*. 2010;52(1):80–85.

356. Kinoshita H, Okabayashi M, Kaneko M, et al. *J Altern Complement Med*. 2009;15(4):439–443.

357. Negro A, Rossi E, Regolisti G, et al. *Ann Ital Med Int*. 2000;15(4):296–300.

358. Sigurjonsdottir HA, Franzson L, Manhem K, et al. *J Hum Hypertens*. 2001;15(8):549–552.

359. Stormer FC, Reistad R, Alexander J. *Food Chem Toxicol*. 1993;31(4):303–312.

360. van Gelderen CE, Bijlsma JA, van Dokkum W, Savelkoul TJ. *Hum Exp Toxicol*. 2000;19(8):434–439.

361. Bernardi M, D'Intino PE, Trevisani F, et al. *Life Sci*. 1994;55(11):863–872.

362. Sigurjonsdottir HA, Manhem K, Axelson M, et al. *J Hum Hypertens*. 2003;17(2):125–131.

363. Sigurjonsdottir HA, Axelson M, Johannsson G, et al. *Blood Press*. 2006;15(3):169–172.

364. van Uum SH, Walker BR, Hermus AR, et al. *Clin Sci (Lond)*. 2002;102(2): 203–211.

365. Ferrari P, Sansonnens A, Dick B, Frey FJ. *Hypertension*. 2001;38(6):1330–1336.

366. Miettinen HE, Piippo K, Hannila-Handelberg T, et al. *Ann Med*. 2010;42(6):465–474.

367. Russo S, Mastropasqua M, Mosetti MA, et al. *Am J Nephrol*. 2000;20(2):145–148.

368. Firenzuoli F, Gori L. *Recenti Prog Med*. 2002;93(9):482–483.

369. Saito T, Tsuboi Y, Fujisawa G, et al. *Nippon Jinzo Gakkai Shi*. 1994;36(11): 1308–1314.

370. Armanini D, Bonanni G, Palermo M. *N Engl J Med*. 1999;341(15):1158.

371. Josephs RA, Guinn JS, Harper ML, et al. *Lancet*. 2001;358(9293):1613–1614.

372. Mosaddegh M, Naghibi F, Abbasi PR, et al. *J Pharm Pharmacol*. 2003;55(suppl):87–88.

373. Johnson EB, Muto MC, Yanushpolsky EH, et al. *Obstet Gynecol*. 2001;98 (5 Pt 2):947–950.

374. Fraunfelder FW. *Am J Ophthalmol*. 2004;138(4):639–647.

375. Dobbins KR, Saul RF. *J Neuroophthalmol*. 2000;20(1):38–41.

376. Doeker BM, Andler W. *Horm Res*. 1999;52(5):253–255.

Meadowsweet

(Filipendula ulmaria L.)

Synonyms

Spiraea ulmaria L. (botanical synonym), Filipendula, queen of the meadow (Engl), Spiraeae flos, flores Ulmariae (Lat), Mädesüssblüten, Spierblumen (Ger), fleur d'ulmaire, reine des prés, ulmaire (Fr), ulmaria (Ital), almindelig mjødurt (Dan).

What is it?

Meadowsweet was one of three herbs held most sacred by the Druids. It was one of 50 ingredients in a drink called 'Save', mentioned by Chaucer in his *Knight's Tale* in the 14th century. It was then known as medwort or meadwort, the mead or honey-wine herb, and the flowers were often ingredients of wine or beers.

Meadowsweet played an important role in the development of the drug aspirin. In 1839 salicylic acid was first isolated from the flowerbuds. It was later synthesised and became an important drug in the 19th century. Unfortunately, unlike the herb, salicylic acid caused so much gastric discomfort and nausea in users that the pain was preferable to the cure. In an effort to overcome this problem, the drug acetylsalicylic acid was developed and named aspirin, from the combination of 'a' for 'acetyl' and 'spirin' from 'Spirae', the generic name of the plant at that time. (See also the willow bark monograph.)

Effects

Reduces excess stomach acidity; protects and heals the mucosa of the upper gastrointestinal tract; reduces fever; anti-inflammatory for joint and rheumatic pain; thins the blood; protects the cells of the cervix and vagina.

Traditional view

Meadowsweet is used to treat conditions of the upper gastrointestinal tract associated with flatulence and hyperacidity, including indigestion, gastric reflux, gastric ulceration and foul breath.[1] Its astringent property is valuable for the treatment of diarrhoea,[2] and it is almost a specific for children's diarrhoea.[3] It has also been used in the treatment of arthritis and rheumatism, oedema, cellulitis, liver disorders, kidney disorders, cystitis, urinary stones and red sandy deposits in the urine with an oily film on the surface.[1] King reported it effective in passive haemorrhage, menorrhagia and leucorrhoea, and as a tonic in cases of debility and convalescence from diarrhoea.[2]

The leaves were also traditionally used to ease cramps and to promote sweating and as a diuretic. Wizenman considered it good for fevers and Künzle recommended it for puerperal fever.[4]

Summary actions

Anti-ulcerogenic, antacid, anti-inflammatory, possibly diuretic, mild urinary antiseptic, astringent.

Can be used for

Indications supported by clinical trials

Cervical dysplasia, acne (topical application, uncontrolled trials).

Traditional therapeutic uses

Disorders of the upper digestive tract associated with flatulence and hyperactivity (indigestion, gastric reflux, gastric ulcers), diarrhoea (particularly in children), urinary disorders (cystitis, kidney stones), gout and rheumatic disease, fevers.

May also be used for

Extrapolations from pharmacological studies

Gastric disorders requiring repair or protection of the gastric mucosa (ulceration, gastritis); as an antithrombotic agent; as a topical antibacterial agent to aid wound healing; topically to protect and repair the mucosa of the vagina and cervix.

Other applications

Included as a food additive in many herb beers and wines.[3]

Preparations

Dried flowers and herb as a powder, decoction, tincture and fluid extract for internal use. Decoction or extract for topical use.

Dosage

Typical adult dosage ranges are:

- 12 to 18g/day of dried aerial parts or by infusion
- 4.5 to 18mL/day of a 1:1 liquid extract

- 3 to 6 mL/day of a 1:2 liquid extract or equivalent in tablet or capsule form
- 6 to 12 mL/day of a 1:5 tincture.

Duration of use

May be taken long term for most applications.

Summary assessment of safety

No significant adverse effects from the ingestion of meadowsweet are expected; however, caution should be observed in cases of salicylate sensitivity and in patients taking warfarin.

Technical data

Botany

Filipendula ulmaria, a member of the Rosaceae (rose) family, is a perennial herb up to 120 cm tall, with long petioled leaves up to 65 cm long and composed of two to five pairs of 8 cm-long ovate leaflets with double-toothed margins and a tomentose underside. The small creamy white flowers are arranged in dense, many flowered, cymose panicles with many protruding stamens.[5]

Key constituents

- Flavonoids (3% to 5%) consisting primarily of rutin and other glycosides of quercetin; kaempferol glycosides[6,7]
- Hydrolysable tannins (10% to 15%), the major one being rugosin-D[6,8]
- Phenolic glycosides, including spiraein (salicylaldehyde primeveroside) in the flowers, monotropitin (methylsalicylate primeveroside) in the flowers and leaves, and isosalicin, a glucoside of salicyl alcohol[6]
- Essential oil (0.2% from the flowers) containing salicylaldehyde (75%), phenylethyl alcohol (3%), benzyl alcohol (2%), methylsalicylate (1.3%) and others.[6]

	R
Spiraein	CHO
Monotropitin	COOCH$_3$

Salicylaldehyde

Adulteration

Confusion with *Filipendula hexapetala* and *Sambucus nigra* (elderflower) has occurred.[9,10]

Pharmacodynamics

Anti-ulcerogenic activity

Orally administered decoctions (1:10, 1:20) of the flowers of meadowsweet (at doses of 5.0 or 25 mL/kg, respectively) reduced the ulcerogenic effect of procedures (such as ligation of the pylorus in rats) and decreased the formation of experimental lesions of the glandular part of the stomach after reserpine injections in rats and mice and phenylbutazone injections in rats. The decoctions were also effective in preventing acetylsalicylic acid-induced lesions of the stomach in rats and promoted healing of the stomach lesions induced by ethanol in rats.[11] However, the decoction did not protect rats from the ulcerogenic action of cinchophen and increased the bronchospastic and ulcerogenic properties of histamine in guinea pigs.[11] (Cinchophen increases gastric secretion and reduces gastric mucosal microcirculation.)[12]

Alcohol extracts and water decoctions of the flowers decreased the development of experimental erosion and ulcers in vivo when administered in high doses by injection or orally.[13]

Immunomodulatory activity

An in vitro study demonstrated that the ethyl acetate extract of the flowers strongly inhibited the classical pathway of complement activation. The observed inhibitory action could not be attributed to the presence of salicylates, flavonoids or tannins.[14] In the same model, strong inhibitory activity was also observed using methanol extracts of herb and flower. Further testing indicated that only the ethyl acetate extract of the flowers retained this activity, indicating that complement inhibitory activity could be attributed to compounds other than tannins.

Except for the light-petroleum extract, all fractions (ethyl acetate, diethyl ether, methanol and freeze-dried aqueous extracts of flowers and of herb) inhibited the production of reactive oxygen species by human polymorphonuclear leucocytes in vitro. The inhibitory activity and the total flavonoid content of fractions did not correlate, suggesting that other constituents may be involved in the immunomodulatory activity. The authors suggested that this activity may explain the use of meadowsweet preparations in inflammatory diseases.[15]

Meadowsweet extract administered intragastrically in doses from 10 to 500 mg/kg stimulated both inductive and productive phases of humoral immunity in mice. The extract also exhibited a pronounced anti-inflammatory effect, which was manifested by a decrease in the synthesis of interleukin-2 by splenocytes and suppression of proinflammatory cytokines in a delayed-type hypersensitivity model.[16]

Antimicrobial activity

In vitro studies have demonstrated weak antimicrobial activity for extracts from the rhizomes, leaves, flowers and upper stems against *Staphylococcus aureus haemolyticus, Streptococcus pyogenes haemolyticus, Escherichia coli, Shigella flexneri, Klebsiella pneumoniae* and *Bacillus subtilis* when tested at 5% concentration in the culture medium.[17] Another study suggested that water extracts of various parts of meadowsweet showed antibacterial activity in vitro and can possibly be used on wounds.[18] The test concentrations used in both studies were relatively high, which casts doubt on their clinical significance.

The essential oil of meadowsweet showed a marked growth-inhibitory activity against a range of bacteria and fungi. There appeared to be a pronounced synergy between key components.[19] However, given the low quantity of essential oil in meadowsweet, this finding is likely to be of little clinical relevance to the herbal extract.

Other activity

Both in vivo (oral doses) and in vitro studies have demonstrated that extracts of the flowers and seeds show fibrinolytic and anticoagulant activity.[20] This action was thought to be due to a heparin-like anticoagulant found in the flowers.[21] These findings need to be confirmed in current models.

In an investigation of 42 Rosaceae species, only species from the Rosoideae sub-family including meadowsweet exhibited high tannin content and elastase-inhibiting activity.[22]

Local administration of a decoction of the flowers resulted in a 39% drop in the frequency of squamous cell carcinoma of the cervix and vagina induced in mice by carcinogen administration.[23] A 40% ethanolic extract of meadowsweet flowers showed marked cytotoxic activity in vitro against human lymphoblastoid Raji cells at concentrations of 10 and 50 μg/mL.[24] Oral administration of a flower decoction demonstrated anticancer activity in various cancer models in mice and rats, but was only chemopreventative for cervical and vaginal carcinogenesis after local application in mice.[25]

A study of neurotropic properties demonstrated a moderate inhibitory effect on CNS activity.[26] Ethanol extracts and water decoctions of the flowers depressed the CNS in vivo, as exhibited by decreased motor activity and rectal temperature, induced myorelaxation and increased effects of narcotic toxins. Preparations also decreased vascular permeability.[14]

Meadowsweet extracted with 70% ethanol (100 mg/g orally for 5 days) exhibited hepatoprotective activity during CCL_4-induced toxic hepatitis in rats.[27,28] The ethyl acetate fraction was most active.[27]

A dried aqueous extract of meadowsweet leaf demonstrated a very modest inhibition of cyclo-oxygenase in vitro, but was rather better at inhibiting platelet activating factor-induced exocytosis in neutrophils at 0.25 mg/mL concentration.[29]

Pharmacokinetics

No data available.

Clinical trials

Cervical dysplasia

In 48 cases of cervical dysplasia treated with an ointment containing meadowsweet, a positive result was recorded in 32 patients and complete remission in 25 cases. No recurrence was observed in 10 patients within 12 months of the complete cure.[23]

An extract described as purified from meadowsweet and rich in phenolic acids reduced skin lipid production in 71% of healthy volunteers after 28 days of twice-daily topical application at 4% concentration in an open label pilot study. The number of acne blemishes and inflammatory lesions were each reduced by 10%.[30]

Toxicology and other safety data

Toxicology

Animal studies on the flowers and the alcoholic and aqueous extracts have suggested that meadowsweet is without toxic hepatic effects.[31] LD_{50} values for an ethanolic extract or decoction ranged from 535 to 1770 mg/kg when administered intraperitoneally to male or female mice.[13]

Contraindications

Meadowsweet should not be used during pregnancy or lactation without professional advice.

Special warnings and precautions

The use of tannins can be inappropriate in constipation, iron deficiency anaemia and malnutrition. Because of the tannin content of this herb, long-term use of high doses should be avoided. Use cautiously in highly inflamed or ulcerated conditions of the gastrointestinal tract.

Meadowsweet contains salicylates and should be avoided or used with caution in patients with salicylate sensitivity or glucose-6-phosphate dehydrogenase deficiency (in this condition salicylic acid can cause haemolytic anaemia).

Meadowsweet should be used with caution in patients with bleeding disorders, as anticoagulant activity for extracts of the flowers and seeds have been demonstrated in vitro and in vivo after oral administration.[20]

Interactions

None known. Given the experimental anticoagulant effect for the flowers, the flowering herb should be used with caution if patients are taking anticoagulant drugs, although no adverse effects are expected.

Tannins can bind metal ions, thiamine and alkaloids and reduce their absorption. Meadowsweet should be consumed at least 2 h away from oral thiamine, mineral supplements, such as iron and alkaloid-containing drugs.

Use in pregnancy and lactation

Category B3-no increase in frequency of malformation or other harmful effects on the fetus from limited use in women. Evidence of increased fetal damage in animal studies exists, although the relevance to humans is unknown.

An aqueous infusion (1:20) of meadowsweet flowers increased the tone and force of contraction of smooth muscle from sections of the uterine horns of rats, guinea pigs and cats in vitro.[26]

Fetal toxicity, measured as the number of resorptions, deaths and malformations, was 46.1% in pregnant rats subcutaneously administered salicylaldehyde (400 mg/kg) on day 11 of gestation compared with 2.7% in the control group.[27] This dose of salicylaldehyde is considerably higher than the amount contained in a therapeutic dose of meadowsweet and the study is unlikely to be relevant to the therapeutic use of meadowsweet.

Meadowsweet is compatible with breastfeeding but caution should be exercised. Salicylates excreted in breast milk have been reported to cause macular rashes in breast-fed babies.

Effects on ability to drive and use machines

No adverse effects expected.

Side effects

None known.

Overdosage

No effects known.

Safety in children

Clinicians should be aware of the possibility of Reye's syndrome, an acute sepsis-like illness encountered exclusively in children below 15 years of age. The cause is unknown, although viral agents and drugs, especially salicylate derivatives, have been implicated.[28] However, it is unknown if the salicylates in meadowsweet are capable of causing this reaction.

Regulatory status in selected countries

Meadowsweet is covered by a positive Commission E monograph and has the following application:

- Supportive treatment for chills, colds, etc.
- Externally: rheumatic conditions affecting muscles and joints, blunt traumas such as contusions, strains, sprains, bruises, haematomas, etc.

Meadowsweet is on the UK General Sale list.

Meadowsweet does not have GRAS status. However, it is freely available as a 'dietary supplement' in the USA under DSHEA legislation (1994 Dietary Supplement Health and Education Act).

Meadowsweet is not included in Part 4 of Schedule 4 of the Therapeutic Goods Act Regulations of Australia and is freely available for sale.

References

1. Bartram T. *Encyclopaedia of Herbal Medicine*, 1st ed. Dorset: Grace Publishers; 1995. p. 287.
2. Felter HW, Lloyd JU. *King's American Dispensatory*. ed 18, rev 3, vol 2, 1905. Reprinted Portland: Eclectic Medical Publications; 1983. p. 1809.
3. Grieve M. *A Modern Herbal*, vol. 1. New York: Dover Publications; 1971. pp. 524–525.
4. Madaus G. *Lehrbuch der Biologischen Heilmettel, Band III und Register*. Hildesheim: Georg Olms Verlag; 1976. pp. 2592–2596.
5. Launert EL. *The Hamlyn Guide to Edible and Medicinal Plants of Britain and Northern Europe*. London: Hamlyn Publishing Group; 1981. p. 66.
6. British Herbal Medicine Association. *British Herbal Compendium*, vol. 1. Dorset: BHMA; 1992. p. 158.
7. Wagner H, Bladt S. *Plant Drug Analysis: A Thin Layer Chromatography Atlas*, 2nd ed. Berlin: Springer-Verlag; 1996. p. 199.
8. Fecka I. *Phytochem Anal*. 2009;20(3): 177–190.
9. Bisset NG, ed. *Herbal Drugs and Phytopharmaceuticals: A Handbook for Practice on a Scientific Basis*. Stuttgart: Medpharm Scientific Publishers; 1994. pp. 480–482.
10. Blaschek W, Ebel S, Hackenthal E, et al. *HagerROM 2002, Hagers Handbuch der Drogen und Arzneistoffe*. Heidelberg: Springer; 2002.
11. Barnaulov OD, Denisenko PP. *Farmakol Toksikol*. 1980;43(6):700–705.
12. Nagamachi Y, Nishida Y, Akiyama N. *Gastroenterol Jpn*. 1979;14(2): 95–102.
13. Barnaulov OD, Kumkov AV, Khalikova NA, et al. *Rastitel Nye Resursy*. 1977;13(4):661–669.
14. Halkes SBA, Beukelman CJ, Kroes BH, et al. *Pharm Pharmacol Lett*. 1997; 7(2–3):79–82.
15. Halkes SBA, Beukelman CJ, Kroes BH, et al. *Phytother Res*. 1997;11:518–520.
16. Churin AA, Masnaia NV, Sherstoboev EIu, et al. *Eksp Klin Farmakol*. 2008;71(5):32–36.
17. Csedo K, Monea M, Sabau M, et al. *Planta Med*. 1993;59(suppl 7):A675.
18. Kallman S. *Svensk Bot Tidskr*. 1994;88(2):97–101.
19. Radulovic N, Misic M, Aleksic J, et al. *Fitoterapia*. 2007;78(7–8):565–570.
20. Liapina LA, Koval'chuk GA. *Izv Akad Nauk Ser Biol*. 1993;4:625–628.
21. Kudryashov BA, Lyapina LA, Kondashevskaya VM, et al. *Vestn Moskovskogo Universiteta Seriya Xvi Biologiya*. 1994;3:15–17.
22. Lamaison JL, Carnat A, Petitjean–Freytet C. *Ann Pharm Fr*. 1990;48(6):335–340.
23. Peresun'ko AP, Bespalov VG, Limarenko AI, et al. *Vopr Onkol*. 1993;39(7–12): 291–295.
24. Spiridonov NA, Konovalov DA, Arkhipov VV. *Phytother Res*. 2005;19(5):428–432.
25. Bespalov VG, Limarenko AY, Voitenkov BL. *Khim Farm Zh*. 1992;26:59–61, through *Chem Abstr* 116: 227822, 1992.

26. Lymarenko AY, Barnaulov OD, Yanutsh AY, et al. *Farmatsevtychnyi Zh.* 1984;4:57–59.

27. Shilova IV, Zhavoronok TV, Souslov NI, et al. *Bull Exp Bio Med.* 2008;146(1):49–51.

28. Shilova IV, Zhavoronok TV, Souslov NI, et al. *Bull Exp Bio Med.* 2006;142(2):216–218.

29. Tunon H, Olavsdotter C, Bohlin L. *J Ethnopharmacol.* 1995;48(1):61–76.

30. Lenaers C, Brunet D, Ladegaillerie K, et al. *Int J Cosmet Sci.* 2007;29(2):143–144.

31. Barnaulov OD, Boldina IG, Galushko VV, et al. *Rastitel Nye Resursy.* 1979;15(3):399–407.

32. Barnaulov OD, Bukreeva TB, Kokarev AA, et al. *Rastitel Nye Resursy.* 1978;14:573–579.

33. Saito H, Yokoyama A, Takeno S, et al. *Res Commun Chem Pathol Pharmacol.* 1982;38(2):209–220.

34. Isselbacher KJ, Podolsky DK. In: Harrison TR, Fauci AS, eds. *Harrison's Principles of Internal Medicine,* 14th ed. New York: McGraw-Hill; 1998.

Melilotus

(*Melilotus officinalis* L.)

Synonyms

Sweet clover, melilot (Engl), Meliloti herba (Lat), Gelber Steinklee, Honigklee (Ger), couronne royale (Fr), meliloto (Ital), mark-stenkløver (Dan).

What is it?

When in flower *Melilotus officinalis* has a characteristic fragrant odour (similar to newly mown hay) that intensifies upon drying. This is due to the formation of coumarin (benzo(a) pyrone). As a consequence the flowers have been used to perfume snuff and pipe tobacco and to give an aromatic quality to tisanes and herbal medicines.

In Europe, Melilotus is regarded as an important and safe herb for the circulatory system, particularly the venous and lymphatic circulation. Over the past 50 years coumarin, its major constituent, has been responsible for some important pharmacological advances. Most notably, the discovery of dicoumarol (a bacterial metabolite of coumarin) in spoiled Melilotus hay resulted in the development of modern anticoagulant drugs such as warfarin.

Effects

Reduces inflammatory and congestive oedema by breaking down accumulated protein; increases venous return and improves lymph flow.

Traditional view

Melilotus was much esteemed in medicine as an emollient and digestive[1] and the Eclectics favoured its use in neuralgic conditions.[2] It was recommended for many external applications including the juice or infusion as an eyewash and plasters and ointments for abdominal and rheumatic pains and for application to veins and ulcers.[1]

Summary actions

Antio-edematous, anti-inflammatory, possibly antitumour, possibly immune enhancing.

Can be used for

Indications supported by clinical trials

Clinical indications supported by Melilotus trials: postsurgical bruising.

Clinical indications supported by Melilotus/coumarin with rutin trials: lymphoedema; venous insufficiency, haemorrhoids, varicose veins; episiotomy, post-traumatic inflammation.

Clinical indications supported by coumarin trials: filarial lymphoedema and elephantiasis; cancer (malignant melanoma, renal cell carcinoma, prostatic carcinoma), particularly to prevent recurrence or metastases.

Traditional therapeutic uses

Internally to relieve flatulence, colic and diarrhoea. For neuralgia affecting many areas (headaches, ovarian, stomach) and particularly for conditions marked by pain with cold, soreness or tenderness; externally for ulcers, veins, abdominal and rheumatic pains.[1,2]

May also be used for

Extrapolations from pharmacological studies

High-protein oedemas including burns; thrombophlebitis; to reduce vascular damage such as endothelaemia, for the prevention of ischaemic heart disease; for conditions requiring enhanced peripheral blood mononuclear cell activity.

Other possible applications

Coumarin has also been used to treat brucellosis in humans and other chronic infections including mononucleosis, mycoplasmosis, toxoplasmosis, Q fever and psittacosis.[3] This may reflect on immune-enhancing activity.

The dried plant has been used to scent linen and protect it from moths and used to scent snuff and smoking tobacco.[1] Melilotus has been included in oral preparations to reduce cellulite but its efficacy is unproven.

Preparations

Dried or fresh aerial parts for infusion, liquid extract or tincture for internal or external use.

Dosage

The therapeutic dose of coumarin has been established at around 1 mg/kg per day,[4] although higher doses have been recommended.[5] This probably corresponds to about 10 mL/ day of a Melilotus 1:2 extract or 25 mL/day of a 1:5 tincture, which for best results can be divided into several doses taken at regular intervals throughout the day. However, lower doses than these have been used in clinical trials.

Melilotus is best used in combination with herbs having a vitamin P-like activity such as horsechestnut, hawthorn flower, lime flowers and other herbs containing flavone glycosides.

Duration of use

May be used in the long term if prescribed within the recommended therapeutic range.

Summary assessment of safety

No adverse effects from ingestion of Melilotus are expected when consumed within the recommended dosage. Coumarin use has been associated with idiosyncratic hepatotoxicity.

Technical data

Botany

Melilotus officinalis is a member of the Leguminosae (Fabaceae, pea) family and of the subfamily Papilionoideae.[6] It is a trailing to erect branched herb reaching up to 120 cm tall. The leaves consist of three oblong-elliptic leaflets, 1.5 to 3 cm long with finely toothed margins. The flowers are borne in slender racemes, are yellow and up to 6 mm long. The fruit is a pod containing greenish seeds.[7,8]

Key constituents

- Coumarin (0.2% to 0.45%) and its precursor melilotoside and the substituted coumarins umbelliferone and scopoletin[9]
- Flavonoids, caffeic acid and derivatives.[9]

Coumarin   Melilotoside

Pharmacodynamics

Historical background

'Sweet clover disease' was a bleeding disorder first noted in cattle fed spoiled Melilotus. Although it was originally described in the 1920s, it was not until 1941 that the causative factor was identified as dicoumarol.[10] Dicoumarol is formed from coumarin by bacterial action in damaged hay and was subsequently developed as the first oral anticoagulant. However, its anticoagulant action was slow in onset and difficult to terminate and this led to the development of synthetic analogues, the most widely used of which is warfarin. Properly dried Melilotus does not contain dicoumarol and has no anticoagulant activity under normal circumstances. Coumarin has an anticoagulant activity that is 1000 times less than dicoumarol because it lacks a 4-hydroxy group.[11] However, one case of excessive bleeding due to a large consumption of coumarin-containing herbs has been recorded,[12] but the possibility exists that the herbs were not properly dried and contained some dicoumarol. Other factors also contributed to the anticoagulant effect.[12]

In the 1960s research conducted in Germany demonstrated the beneficial effects of a Melilotus extract on circulatory problems. This led to the development of a synthetic drug consisting of coumarin and a rutin derivative (troxerutin). Several other research groups followed up this work, including workers at Flinders University in Adelaide. The Australian scientists discovered the potential value of coumarin for the treatment of lymphoedema and elephantiasis, disorders that affect more than 140 million people. Large-scale clinical trials were conducted in China and India.

Most of the research was conducted on isolated coumarin or a mixture of coumarin and troxerutin (a flavone glycoside). Since Melilotus contains coumarin and flavone glycosides, this research can probably be extrapolated to the use of the herb. The other coumarin-related compounds in Melilotus also appear to have an activity similar to coumarin.[13]

Pharmacodynamics of coumarin

Anti-oedema and anti-inflammatory activities

Coumarin possesses unique anti-oedema and anti-inflammatory activities[5] that make it particularly effective for the treatment of high-protein oedemas, such as burn injury and lymphoedema.[14,15] It enhances the breakdown by macrophages of protein accumulated in the extracellular spaces.[5] Coumarin also has other important actions on the vascular system. It causes constriction of the precapillary sphincters and dilation of arteriovenous junctions,[16] which can result in an improved blood flow to injured tissue. Thoracic duct and lymph flow are increased by coumarin,[17] hence it aids lymphatic drainage.

Intraperitoneal injection of 1 mL/100 g of a hydroethanolic extract of Melilotus in rabbits just before intramuscular injection of turpentine, which normally induces systemic inflammation, led to a significant inhibition of this process. The effect was similar to that seen with hydrocortisone (125 mg/kg) or pure coumarin (25 mg/kg) injections.[18] Specifically, Melilotus and the control substances inhibited excessive phagocytosis and decreased nitric oxide production and excessive leucocyte counts.

Coumarin improves the course of experimental thrombophlebitis,[19] reduces postoperative oedema[20] and improves venous return.[21] Coumarin slows the onset of blood coagulation, but this is *not* an anticoagulant effect since bleeding and prothrombin times are not changed.[22]

Coumarin and 7-hydroxycoumarin successfully corrected lymphoedema in an experimental model (p<0.01). These compounds may activate the production of proteinases by mononuclear phagocytes.[23] (7-Hydroxycoumarin, also known as umbelliferone, the major human metabolite of coumarin, may be the active form of the drug.)[24]

The administration of coumarin in lymphoedema stimulates macrophage activity and numbers. The reasons for stimulation are uncertain but alterations in the fine structure of the proteins and complement that renders these more attractive for phagocytosis seem the most likely. The end result is a rapid, enhanced break-up of excess interstitial protein and the removal of the osmotically attracted fluid, together with a more gradual removal of the deposits of fibrotic tissue by the non-stimulated macrophage. Clinically, this manifests itself as a softening of the tissues, a reduction in circumference of the lymphoedematous extremity, a return to normal tissue remodelling processes and a range of subjective improvements for the patient.[25]

Cardiovascular activity

Endothelaemia, the presence of vascular endothelial cells in the blood, is an indicator of vascular damage.[26] Low doses of coumarin reduce the endothelaemia caused by various chemicals, as does aspirin.[26] This effect may be partly responsible for the beneficial effect of low-dose aspirin on the course of ischaemic heart disease. Given that coumarin also inhibits prostaglandin formation in a similar manner to aspirin,[27] and has a favourable effect on myocardial ischaemia,[13] it may also prove useful in the management of ischaemic heart disease.

Immunomodulatory and anticancer activity

Both HLA-DR and HLA-DQ antigen expression by peripheral blood mononuclear cells were enhanced in vitro over controls after 48 h of exposure to coumarin. Enhanced expression is consistent with an activated state. This supports the hypothesis that coumarin acts, at least in part, through immune augmentation. Coumarin therapy resulted in augmented HLA-DR antigen expression by peripheral blood monocytes in cancer patients.[28]

The action of coumarin is dose dependent and a doubling of the dose can produce inhibition instead of activation of cellular immunity. As well as acting in low doses through the cellular immune system and the macrophages, coumarin appears to act by inhibiting oncogene activity, while high doses have a direct action on the tumour.[29]

Coumarin has exhibited anticancer properties in vitro against multiple cancer cell lines.[30] Several in vitro studies assessed the effect of coumarin and its natural and synthetic metabolites against malignant melanoma cells. Coumarin exhibited similar or slightly lower activity than synthetic variants in these studies.[31,32]

Coumarin inhibited the hepatic carcinogenicity of aflatoxin B_1 in rats by inducing various enzymes that break down the toxin.[33]

Pharmacokinetics

The pharmacokinetics of coumarin are well studied. Human metabolism of coumarin is unique[34] and results in quick conversion of coumarin to umbelliferone.[35] Umbelliferone (7-hydroxycoumarin) does not possess all the activities of coumarin,[36] implying that best results from coumarin therapy are obtained with frequent dosing or slow-release preparations, especially for acute treatment. In a crossover study with a healthy volunteer, grapefruit juice given at the high dose of 1 L with coumarin (10 mg) retarded the appearance of umbelliferone.[37]

Clinical trials with coumarin

Most clinical trials were conducted using oral doses of a combination of coumarin and troxerutin. These trials have shown beneficial effects in haemorrhoids,[38] acute pancreatitis[39] and the complications of varicose veins, particularly varicose ulcers, oedema and subjective symptoms.[16] A beneficial effect from oral doses in the postoperative treatment of episiotomy was demonstrated in a double blind trial.[4] This study would also indicate the value of coumarin and troxerutin for the general treatment of post-traumatic inflammation. A similar preparation was effective in the treatment of long-standing lymphoedema. After more than 24 months all patients experienced subjective improvement and 53% also showed objective improvement.[40]

Lymphoedema

Benzopyrones, including coumarin and oxerutins, have been used in high doses in many clinical trials investigating a variety of high-protein oedemas. The results of four such trials (lymphoedema from many causes in Australia and filaritic lymphoedema and elephantiasis in India and China) are summarised here, although a recent meta-analysis concluded that not enough data were available from these and other trials to draw any conclusion about the efficacy of coumarin, alone or combined with flavonoids, for treating patients with lymphoedema.[41]

Coumarin (400 mg/day) was administered over 6 months to patients in the Australian trial and for 1 to 2 years in India. In China, oxerutin (3 g/day) was administered for 6 months. The drugs reduced these conditions much more slowly than adequate physical therapy, but did reduce them. About half the excess volume was removed over 6 months in the Australian trials. In India and China similar rates were achieved with lymphoedema, but elephantiasis reduced at a slower rate. The benzopyrones convert a slowly worsening condition into a slowly improving one. In these trials, compression garments were not necessary. The agents considerably reduce the number of attacks of secondary acute infection, reduce the deformities of elephantiasis and improve patients' comfort and mobility. Taken orally or topically, they have very low toxicities and only few, minor side effects. They act by increasing the numbers of macrophages and their normal proteolysis.[42]

In addition to the trials described above, a randomised, double blind, placebo-controlled trial investigated the use of coumarin (400 mg/day) and diethylcarbamazine (6 mg/kg/day) on patients with filaritic lymphoedema and elephantiasis over 2 years. In 169 patients there were significant reductions (p<0.01) in the amount of oedema for the patients taking coumarin. The excess limb volumes were reduced from 40% to 25%. A similar but less significant improvement (p<0.05) was found for circumference measurements. The rate of reduction was increased when the initial amount of oedema was greater. There were no significant reductions from the use of diethylcarbamazine.[43]

Cancer

Activity of coumarin in cancer is believed to be due to enhanced cellular immunity.[3] Coumarin (50 mg/day) was evaluated in a multicentre, prospectively randomised, double blind, placebo-controlled trial to prevent early recurrence of malignant melanoma TNM stage IB and stage II. Intake began in 1984 and was stopped prematurely in 1987. There were two recurrences in 13 treated patients and 10 in 14 controls, which was significant (p=0.01). The sites of the metastases differed in each group, being local and in bone in the treated group and in lymph nodes, skin and lung in the control group. No toxic effects were observed with coumarin treatment.[44] On subsequent publication in 1994, there were four recurrences in the coumarin-treated group and 10 recurrences in the placebo group.[29]

Twenty-two patients with advanced melanoma received coumarin (100 mg/day) for 14 days; on day 15 cimetidine (1200 mg/day) was added. Both treatments were continued until progression of disease. No response was observed in 19 patients, two patients with a low tumour burden achieved a partial response and a third of patients showed a minor response. No toxicity was observed.[45] Earlier it was observed that the combination of coumarin and cimetidine yielded objective tumour regression in patients with metastatic renal cell carcinoma and malignant melanoma. Coumarin appears to have direct effects on tumour cells as well as immunomodulatory activity, while cimetidine appears to be immunomodulatory.[12]

Patients with advanced malignancies received coumarin (100 mg/day) for 14 days; on day 15 cimetidine (1200 mg/day) was added. The following laboratory tests were performed at pretreatment and at 2, 4 and 8 weeks on therapy: monoclonal antibody labelling techniques to monitor peripheral blood lymphocytes and natural killer (NK) cell and monocyte phenotypes. There were no alterations in T cells, helper/inducer T cells, cytotoxic/suppressor T cells, B cells, Ia+ lymphocytes or NK cells. An increase was, however, noted after 2 weeks in the percentage of monocytes and the percentage of DR+ monocytes and this occurred in the presence of coumarin alone, before the addition of cimetidine.[46] The same design was used in an earlier pilot study involving 45 patients with metastatic renal cell carcinoma. Objective responses (greater than or equal to 50% reduction in measurable disease) occurred in 14 of 42 evaluable patients, with three complete responses and 11 partial responses. There was no toxicity observed amongst these patients.[47]

The same design was used in a phase I trial of 54 patients with advanced malignancies, 37 having renal cell carcinoma. The dose of coumarin was escalated (400 to 7000 mg/day) while the cimetidine dose was held constant. Responses occurred over a wide range of doses (600 to 5000 mg/day), giving no hint of a dose–response relationship. Objective tumour regressions were observed in six patients.[48] Preliminary results of multicentre clinical trials of metastatic prostatic carcinoma patients treated with coumarin (1 g/day) suggest that patients with normal performance status and small tumour volumes are the most likely to respond.[49] A preliminary trial of 3 g/day in patients with advanced prostate cancer showed minimal benefit, except in one patient.[50]

Clinical trials with Melilotus

An extract of Melilotus standardised to 1% coumarin at a dose of 300 mg/day for 7 days after cosmetic surgery was as effective as oral dexamethasone at controlling eyelid and paranasal oedema.[51] The study was randomised and double blind. Melilotus extract was superior to dexamethasone at relieving postsurgical bruising and was significantly superior to placebo for improving both bruising and oedema after surgery.

In an uncontrolled trial, 76 patients with lymphoedema of the lower limbs at the IId stage of surgical classification received the following preparation at the indicated oral dosage for 6 to 8 months: Melilotus extract (40 mg/day), Ginkgo extract (40 mg/day) and coumarin (60 mg/day). The preparation induced a very significant improvement in lymphoedema (centimetre aspect) both in functional symptoms (pain and heaviness in affected limbs) and physical signs (oedema, episodes of infection). Tolerance was good and improvement was observed from the third month of treatment.[52]

Many trials have been conducted using a proprietary preparation containing Melilotus and rutin. In an uncontrolled trial on 385 patients with venous insufficiency, oral administration of the preparation (600 mg/day Melilotus extract) over 45 days resulted in 90% improvement. Marked reduction of oedema in both legs was also noted. (In some acute cases, intramuscular injections were also given for approximately 1 week.)[53] Twenty-five pregnant women received a Melilotus/rutin preparation containing 400 mg of Melilotus extract and 150 mg of rutin per day for at least 20 days in an uncontrolled trial. Symptoms such as heavy legs disappeared completely in 68% of cases.[54]

Toxicology and other safety data

Toxicology

Coumarin (0.8 and 1.71 mmol/kg) produced dose-related acute hepatic necrosis in rats.[55] In contrast, none of the coumarin derivatives examined produced either hepatic necrosis or elevated plasma transaminase activities. A no-effect dose of 8 mg/kg coumarin was established.[56] The rat is particularly sensitive to hepatotoxic effects from coumarin.[57]

Although some early chronic toxicology research with high doses implicated coumarin as a carcinogen,[58] subsequent work has demonstrated a low toxicity and absence of carcinogenicity,[59] absence of teratogenicity[60] and even an anticarcinogenic effect.[61] Tumour formation in the rat appears due to chronic hepatotoxicity with sustained regenerative hyperplasia.[57] An oral dose of 200 mg/kg of coumarin increased the incidence of alveolar/bronchiolar adenomas and carcinomas in mice in a chronic bioassay.[62] Acute administration caused selective lung cell injury in mice.

Rodents produce toxic metabolites of coumarin that are not found in humans, thus such studies are of highly dubious relevance to human safety. Induction or high genetic activity of CYP2E1 in the liver and deficiency of glutathione, important to excretion of coumarin, could increase the toxicity of coumarin. Coumarin does not appear to be genotoxic or carcinogenic in humans.[63]

Contraindications

Avoid Melilotus in patients with impaired liver function or elevated liver enzymes.

Special warnings and precautions

Watch for hepatotoxicity.

Contrary to popular writings, properly dried Melilotus does not have anticoagulant activity. One case report linked a haemorrhagic diathesis to a herbal tea intake, which included coumarin-containing herbs such as Melilotus.[12] However, there were many confounding factors in this case. In contrast, a double blind, comparative study in 41 patients suffering from chronic venous insufficiency found that an oral coumarin/troxerutin preparation over 6 weeks did not cause anticoagulant effects.[64] There were no significant changes in coagulation, clotting factors or fibrinolysis over the treatment period.

Interactions

Caution is advised when prescribing Melilotus with warfarin and aspirin.[65]

Use in pregnancy and lactation

Category B2-no increase in frequency of malformation or other harmful effects on the fetus from limited use in women. Animal studies are largely lacking.

No adverse effects are expected with lactation.

Effects on ability to drive and use machines

No adverse effects are expected.

Side effects

There are no data available for Melilotus.

The European Food Safety Authority has set a maximum tolerated daily intake (TDI) for coumarin of 0.1 mg/kg/day.[66] The main concern is that long-term use of high-coumarin supplements or foods could lead to liver problems. Use of *Cinnamomum cassia* (cassia) to treat diabetes was the main provocation of this policy and not Melilotus or other coumarin-based products.

Treatment of 2173 patients with cancer or chronic infections with coumarin (25 to 2000 mg/day, mostly exceeding the European TDI) in a clinical trial resulted in the incidence of hepatotoxicity in eight patients.[67] The authors suggested that this hepatitis was probably a form of idiosyncratic hepatotoxicity and may have been immune in origin. An overview of trials of coumarin for lymphoedema patients found a 0.3% incidence of elevated serum liver enzymes.[68]

In the phase I trial outlined above, in which the dose of coumarin was escalated (400 to 7000 mg/day) in combination with cimetidine, renal cell carcinoma patients experienced a few, mild symptomatic side effects (insomnia, nausea, vomiting, diarrhoea, dizziness). Of the 44 patients, two withdrew because of these side effects. In most patients, side effects abated spontaneously with continuation of therapy. No significant haematological or renal toxicity occurred. Mild hepatotoxicity occurred in only one patient and was manifested as asymptomatic abnormal elevations of serum hepatic transaminases, which were reversible upon interruption of therapy.[48]

Overdosage

No acute toxic effects in humans have reported for Melilotus.

Regulatory status in selected countries

Melilotus is covered by a positive Commission E monograph with the following internal applications:

- Disorders arising from chronic venous insufficiency, such as pains and heaviness in the legs, night cramps in the legs, itching and swellings
- In supportive treatment of thrombophlebitis, post-thrombotic syndrome, haemorrhoids and lymphatic congestion.

I can be used for the following external applications:

- Contusions, sprains and superficial effusion of blood.

Melilotus is not on the UK General Sale List.

Melilotus does not have GRAS status. However, it is freely available as a 'dietary supplement' in the USA under DSHEA legislation (1994 Dietary Supplement Health and Education Act).

Melilotus is not included in Part 4 of Schedule 4 of the Therapeutic Goods Act Regulations of Australia. Coumarin is listed in the SUSDP (Standard for the Uniform Scheduling of Drugs and Poisons) with a Schedule 4 rating. Such substances are available from a pharmacist on presentation of a prescription by a medical practitioner (doctor, dentist or veterinarian). This restriction also now applies to Melilotus because of its coumarin content.

References

1. Grieve M. *A Modern Herbal*, vol. 2. New York: Dover Publications; 1971. p. 527.
2. Felter HW, Lloyd JU. *King's American Dispensatory*. 18th ed, rev 3, vol 2, 1905. Portland, Reprinted by Eclectic Medical Publications; 1983. p. 1251.
3. Egan D, O'Kennedy R, Moran E, et al. *Drug Metab Rev*. 1990;53(suppl):209–218.
4. Pethö A. *Arzneimittelforschung*. 1981;31:1303–1307.
5. Piller NB. *Arzneimittelforschung*. 1977;27(6):1135–1138.
6. Mabberley DJ. *The Plant Book*, 2nd ed. Cambridge: Cambridge University Press; 1997. pp. 396–397, 468.
7. Launert EL. *The Hamlyn Guide to Edible and Medicinal Plants of Britain and Northern Europe*. London: Hamlyn; 1981. p. 62.
8. Chiej R. *The Macdonald Encyclopedia of Medicinal Plants*. London: Macdonald; 1984. Entry no. 192.
9. Wagner H, Bladt S. *Plant Drug Analysis: A Thin Layer Chromatography Atlas*, 2nd ed. Berlin: Springer-Verlag; 1996. p. 127.
10. Stahmann MA, Huebner CF, Link KP. *J Biol Chem*. 1941;138:513–527.
11. Sione TO. *J Pharm Sci*. 1964;53:231–264.
12. Hogan RP. *JAMA*. 1983;249(19):2679–2680.
13. Kovách AG, Hamar J, Dora O, et al. *Arzneimittelforschung*. 1970;20(11 suppl 11A):1630.
14. Casley-Smith JR, Foldi-Borcsok E, Foldi M. *Br J Exp Pathol*. 1974;55(1):88–93.
15. Piller NB. *Br J Exp Pathol*. 1975;56(1):83–91.
16. Casley-Smith JR. *Folia Angiol*. 1976;24:7–22.
17. Bartós V, Brzék V. *Med Klin*. 1970;65(39):1701–1703.
18. Plesca-Manea L, Parvu AE, Parvu M, et al. *Phytother Res*. 2002;16:316–319.
19. Piukovich I, Zoltan OT, Traub A, et al. *Arzneimittelforschung*. 1966;16(1):94–95.
20. Hopf G, Kaeffmann HJ, Pekker I, et al. *Arzneimittelforschung*. 1971;21(6):854–855.
21. Aso K, Hishida Y. *Arztl Prax*. 1965;17:2463.
22. Shimamoto K, Takaori S. *Arzneimittelforschung*. 1965;15(8):897–899.
23. Knight KR, Khazanchi RK, Pedersen WC, et al. *Clin Sci*. 1989;77(1):69–76.
24. Marshall ME, Mohler JL, Edmonds K, et al. *J Cancer Res Clin Oncol*. 1994;120(suppl):S39–S42.
25. Piller NB. *Arch Histol Cytol*. 1990;53(suppl):209–218.
26. Hladovec J. *Arzneimittelforschung*. 1977;27(5):1073–1076.
27. Lee RE, Bykadi G, Ritschel WA. *Arzneimittelforschung*. 1981;31(4):640–642.
28. Marshall ME, Rhoades JL, Mattingly C, et al. *Mol Biother*. 1991;3(4):204–206.
29. Thornes D, Daly L, Lynch G, et al. *J Cancer Res Clin Oncol*. 1994;120(suppl):S32–S34.
30. Lacy A, O'Kennedy R. *Curr Pharm Des*. 2004;10(30):3797–3811.
31. Jimenez-Orozco FA, Molina-Guarneros JA, Mendozz-Patiño N, et al. *Melanoma Res*. 1999;9:243–247.
32. Finn GJ, Creaven B, Egan DA. *Melanoma Res*. 2001;11:461–467.
33. Kelly VP, Ellis EM, Manson MM, et al. *Cancer Res*. 2000;60:957–969.
34. Shilling WH, Crampton RF, Longland RC. *Nature*. 1969;221(5181):664–665.
35. Ritschel WA, Brady ME, Tan HSI, et al. *Int J Clin Pharmacol Biopharm*. 1979;17(3):99–103.
36. Hardt TJ, Ritschel WA. *Arzneimittelforschung*. 1983;33(12):1662–1666.
37. Runkel M, Tegtmeier M, Legrum W. *Eur J Clin Pharmacol*. 1996;50(3):225–230.
38. Florian A. *Med Mschr*. 1972;26(3):135–136.
39. Vida S. *Therapiewoche*. 1977;27:5476–5483.
40. Piller NB, Clodius L. *Lymphology*. 1976;9(4):127–132.
41. Badger C, Preston N, Seers K, Mortimer P. *Cochrane Database Syst Rev*. 2004;2:CD003140.
42. Casley-Smith JR, Casley-Smith JR. *Australas J Dermatol*. 1992;33(2):69–74.
43. Jamal S, Casley-Smith JR, Casley-Smith JR. *Ann Trop Med Parasitol*. 1989;83(3):287–290.
44. Thornes D, Daly L, Lynch G, et al. *Eur J Surg Oncol*. 1989;15(5):431–435.
45. Marshall ME, Butler K, Cantrell J, et al. *Cancer Chemother Pharmacol*. 1989;24(1):65–66.
46. Marshall ME, Riley LK, Rhoades J, et al. *J Biol Response Mod*. 1989;8(1):62–69.
47. Marshall ME, Mendelsohn L, Butler K, et al. *J Clin Oncol*. 1987;5(6):862–866.
48. Marshall ME, Butler K, Fried A. *Mol Biother*. 1991;3(3):170–178.
49. Mohler JL, Williams BT, Thompson IM, et al. *J Cancer Res Clin Oncol*. 1994;120(suppl):S35–S38.
50. Mohler JL, Gomella LG, Crawford ED, et al. *Prostate*. 1992;20:123–131.
51. Xu FZ, Zeng W, Mao XH, Gan GK. *Aesth Plast Surg*. 2008;32:599–603.
52. Vettorello G, Cerrata G, Derwish A, et al. *Minerva Cardioangiol*. 1996;44(9):447–455.
53. Babilliot J. *Gaz Med Fr*. 1980;87:3242–3246.
54. Leng JJ, Heugas-Darraspen JP, Fernon MJ. *Bordeaux Med*. 1974;7:2755–2756.
55. Lake BG, Evans JG, Lewis DFV, et al. *Food Chem Toxicol*. 1994;32(4):357–363.
56. Preuss-Ueberschar C, Ueberschar S. *Arzneimittelforschung*. 1988;38(9):1318–1326.
57. Lake BG, Grasso P. *Fundam Appl Toxicol*. 1996;34(1):105–117.
58. Bar F, Griepentrog F. *Med Ernähr*. 1967;8:244–251.
59. Cohen AJ. *Food Cosmet Toxicol*. 1979;17(3):277–289.
60. Grote W, Sudeck M. *Arzneimittelforschung*. 1973;23(9):1319–1320.
61. Wattenberg LW, Lam LKT, Fladmore AV. *Cancer Res*. 1979;39(5):1651–1654.
62. Born SL, Fix AS, Caudill D, et al. *Toxicol Appl Pharmacol*. 1998;151(1):45–56.
63. Felter SP, Vassallo JD, Carlton BD, et al. *Food Chem Toxicol*. 2006;44:462–475.
64. Kostering VH, Bandura B, Merten HA, et al. *Arzneimittelforschung*. 1985;35(2):1303–1306.
65. Harder S, Thurmann P. *Clin Pharmacokinet*. 1996;30(6):415–444.
66. Bundesinstitute für Risikobewertung. *Health Assessment* 044/2006, 18 Aug 2006.
67. Cox D, O'Kennedy R, Thornes RD. *Hum Toxicol*. 1989;8(6):501–506.
68. Casley-Smith JR. *Int Angiol*. 1999;18:31–41.

Myrrh

(*Commiphora molmol* Engl.)

Synonyms

Balsamodendron myrrha (Nees) Engl., *C. myrrha* (Nees) Engl. var. *molmol* Eng., vola or samudraguggul (Indian), Mo Yao (Chin).

What is it?

The name 'myrrh' is probably derived from the Arabic or Hebrew word 'mur', which means bitter. Myrrh (Arabian or Somali myrrh) is an oleo-gum resin, obtained from the stem of various species of *Commiphora* (Burseraceae) growing in north-east Africa and Arabia. Texts have traditionally given the principal source as *C. molmol* but the chief source today is probably *C. myrrha* (Nees) Engl. (*C. myrrha* Holmes).[1]

Almost all members of the Burseraceae possess oleoresin canals in the phloem and resin exudes spontaneously when cracks and fissures form in the bark. This yellowish-white viscous fluid soon hardens in the ambient heat to reddish-brown crystalline masses. In some cases incisions are made in the bark to encourage resin production.[1]

Myrrh has been used as a medicinal herb for thousands of years. It is mentioned several times in the Bible in writings as old as Psalms and the Song of Solomon and of course it is well known as one of the three gifts that the Magi brought to Jesus Christ.[2] Despite this ancient record of use, clinical trials on myrrh were lacking until recently when a group of Egyptian scientists examined its value in the treatment of fascioliasis (liver fluke).[3,4] Since then a number of other clinical studies have been published suggesting that the clinical use of myrrh represents a significant advance in the herbal treatment of parasites. What is particularly interesting is myrrh seems to be active against parasites that infest deeper into the body than the gut, such as in the liver and bladder (the latter in the case of schistosomiasis).

Effects

Controls infections and promotes healing and local immunity when applied topically. Internally has antiparasitic activity, possibly by stimulating the immune response against parasites.

Traditional view

Myrrh has been used in all the great traditions of herbal medicine.

In the lands of its origin, in East Africa and the Middle East, it has long been used for respiratory infections, as a digestive aid, as a wound healing remedy and as an anthelmintic.[5] Galen also mentioned myrrh as a treatment for intestinal helminths.[6]

Traditional Western herbal uses include:

- mouth ulcers, pharyngitis, gingivitis, laryngitis, respiratory catarrh, the common cold, chronic catarrh, bronchitis, excessive mucus secretion and boils[7,8]
- chronic gastritis, atonic dyspepsia; amenorrhoea and female reproductive tract disorders accompanied by a dragging sensation and leucorrhoea[8]
- topically for damaged gums, wounds, abrasions, poorly healing skin ulcers and sinusitis.[7–9]

Uses and properties from traditional Chinese medicine (TCM) include:

- invigoration of the *blood*, dispersing *congealed blood*, reducing swelling and alleviating pain, thus used to treat trauma, sores, boils, swelling, abdominal masses or pain, chest pain and amenorrhoea[10]
- topically for chronic, poorly healing sores.[10]

Traditional Ayurvedic uses include:

- dyspepsia, chlorosis (hypochromic anaemia), amenorrhoea, uterine disorders, menstrual disorders in young girls, chronic bronchitis and tuberculosis[11]
- as a mouthwash for mouth ulcers and sore throat.[11]

In modern Western herbal use, myrrh (as noted above) has been largely relegated to a topical agent, especially for the mouth, gums and throat. Hence the rediscovery of the antiparasitic properties of myrrh places this herb into a completely new perspective. Rediscovery is the appropriate term, since apart from its traditional use in the Middle East, the US Eclectic text *King's Dispensatory*[12] mentions its use as a vermifuge and Maude Grieve also makes mention of the same use.[13]

Summary actions

Astringent, antimicrobial, antiparasitic, anti-inflammatory, vulnerary.

Can be used for

Indications supported by clinical trials

For parasitic infestations, especially fascioliasis and schistosomiasis, when conventional treatments are ineffective or inappropriate (open label trials, mixed results).

Traditional therapeutic uses

Chronic bronchitis, the common cold, chronic catarrh; inflammation of the mouth and throat; gastritis, dyspepsia and topical treatment for inflammations of the mouth and throat, skin inflammation, wounds and abrasions.

In Germany the use of myrrh topically to treat mild inflammation of the oral and pharyngeal mucosa was supported by the Commission E.[14] ESCOP recommends myrrh for the topical treatment of gingivitis, stomatitis (mouth ulcers), minor skin inflammation, minor wounds and abrasions and as a supportive treatment for pharyngitis and tonsillitis.[15]

May also be used for

Extrapolation from pharmacological studies

Myrrh may have value as an anti-inflammatory agent. However, long-term internal use increases the risk of an allergic reaction.

Other applications

The molluscicidal activity may be relevant for the control of snails as vectors for *Schistosoma* species and other parasites.

Preparations

Myrrh is typically used as a 1:5 tincture in 90% alcohol. This is diluted with water for topical application or as a gargle. However, the clinical trials of antiparasitic activity typically used a concentrated soft extract (closely resembling the oleoresin) in capsule form that allowed the convenient use of higher doses.

Dosage

The typical adult dose is 1.5 to 4.5 mL/day of the 90% ethanol 1:5 tincture for most of the clinical indications described above.

However, higher doses for short periods (3 to 6 days) are required for antiparasitic effects. For example, the 600 mg dose of the myrrh extract typically used in the trials probably corresponds to about 2 to 3 g of crude resin or 10 to 15 mL of 1:5 tincture.

Duration of use

Myrrh should not be ingested for prolonged periods (more than a few weeks at a time) because of its potential to cause allergic contact dermatitis and other allergic reactions.

Summary assessment of safety

Except in cases of allergy in susceptible patients, myrrh is a safe herb.

Technical data

Botany

The myrrh-producing *Commiphora* species are shrubs or small trees with large, sharply pointed thorns on the stem. The unequal ternate leaves are alternate and the small flowers are arranged in terminal panicles. When damaged, the schizogenous resin ducts yield the product known as myrrh.[16]

Adulteration

Authorative texts and pharmacopoeias define medicinal myrrh as *Commiphora molmol* and/or other *Commiphora* species.[9,15,17–19] The German Commission E regarded these other species as those with comparable chemical composition to *C. molmol*.[14] Other species of Commiphora may be used if their chemical composition compares favourably with that specified in the *German Pharmacopoeia* (DAB 10).[20] Such other possible acceptable species in addition to *C. myrrha* could include *C. abyssinica* (Berg) Engl. (*C. madagascariensis* Jacq.) and *C. schimperi* (Berg) Engl.[9,20]

In terms of adulteration, small stones may be present and gum arabic has been found as an adulterant. Products from many other species of Commiphora are probably occasionally passed off as myrrh. Adulterants of plant origin include *C. mukul* Hook. (Engl.), *C. erythraea* (Ehrenb.) Engl., *C. agallocha* (Roxb.) Engl., *C. ugogensis* Engl.,[16,18] *C. sphaerocarpa* Chiov., *C. holtziana* Engl. and *C. kataf* (Forssk.) Engl.[21]

Key constituents

Myrrh contains an essential oil (2% to 10%), which largely comprises sesquiterpenes; an alcohol-soluble resin (25% to 40%) containing commiphoric acids; and a water-soluble gum (30% to 60%).[22,23]

Pharmacodynamics

Antiparasitic activity

Studies on mice demonstrated that a myrrh extract at an oral dose of 500 mg/kg for 5 days,[24] or at a dose of 600 mg/kg for 3 days,[25] had a schistosomicidal effect against the different maturation stages of *Schistosoma mansoni*. This organism causes bilharzia. In addition, the livers of mice treated with myrrh extract (500 mg/kg, oral) for 8 weeks after infection with schistosoma showed a marked reduction in degenerative changes.[26] Myrrh has also demonstrated activity against *S. mansoni* worms in vitro.[27] A study in mice found that myrrh extract (500 mg/kg/day for 5 days, oral) exerted a valuable schistosomicidal effect against different stages of the parasite.[28]

Not all studies have been positive. There is one reported study where myrrh failed to exhibit any significant antiparasitic activity in mice and hamsters infected with *S. mansoni*,[29] and another negative study in hamsters for the same parasite.[30]

An oral dose of myrrh extract (20 mg/day for six consecutive days) induced eradication of *Fasciola gigantica* worms in experimentally infected rabbits, with an associated increase in IgG production.[31] In contrast, myrrh extract (10 mg/kg/day for 6 days, oral) exerted only a modest effect against fascioliasis in sheep.[32]

Myrrh extract (10 mg/bird, oral) significantly reduced experimental coccidiosis (due to *Eimeria* species) in chickens[33] and in domestic rabbits (dose 500 mg/kg, oral).[34] Treatment of rats infected with *Giardia lamblia* indicated that myrrh extract was capable of completely reducing parasite loads in intestinal and faecal samples.[35] It appeared to exert a direct toxic effect on the giardia trophozoite.

Molluscicidal activity

Snails act as vectors for *S. mansoni*, hence molluscicidal activity can play a role in the prevention of bilharzia (schistosomiasis). The molluscicidal properties of the oil extract of myrrh were tested against the Egyptian snail species *Biomphalaria alexandrina*, *Bulinus truncatus* and *Limnaea cailliaudi*.[36] The impact of the extract on the egg clutches of *B. alexandrina* and *L. cailliaudi* was also evaluated. Snails and their eggs were exposed for 24 and 48 h at 22 to 26°C to various concentrations of the extract. Results showed different susceptibilities. *B. alexandrina* exhibited higher LD_{50} and LD_{90} concentrations (155 and 195 ppm, respectively) than *B. truncatus* (50, 95 ppm) and *L. cailliaudi* (50, 85 ppm) after 24 h exposure. Myrrh also inhibited the spreading of *S. mansoni* eggs from infected snails at a concentration of one part per million (ppm).[37]

The effect of exposing *B. alexandrina* to a sub-lethal dose (LD_{10} and LD_{20}) of myrrh on its susceptibility to infection with *S. mansoni* has also been determined.[38] Starting 3 weeks post exposure, cercarial shedding was monitored. No shedding of cercariae was observed from snails treated with the LD_{20} dose. The study revealed that sub-lethal exposure to myrrh decreased the compatibility of *B. alexandrina* to *S. mansoni* infection, thus playing an important role in the control of schistosomiasis.

Insecticidal activity

Myrrh has been shown in vitro to be toxic to the fowl tick *Argas persicus*[39] and was larvicidal against the *Culex pipiens* and *Aedes caspius* mosquitoes.[40,41]

Anti-inflammatory and analgesic activity

A petroleum ether extract of myrrh (500 mg/kg, oral) produced significant anti-inflammatory activity in carrageenan-induced inflammation and cotton pellet granuloma models.

Antipyretic activity was also observed in vivo.[42] Myrrh demonstrated significant anti-inflammatory activity in the following experimental models: xylene-induced ear oedema (400 mg/kg, pretreatment by injection) and cotton pellet granuloma (400 mg/kg, oral).[43]

An analgesic activity was demonstrated after oral administration of myrrh in vivo. The active analgesic compounds were identified as two sesquiterpenes, particularly furanoeudesma-1,3-diene. This compound was shown to bind to opioid receptors in isolated brain membrane. Naloxone, an opioid antagonist, completely inhibited the analgesic effect of this compound by injection. Furanoeudesma-1,3-diene exhibited structural similarities with two opioid agonists (morphiceptin and DPDPE).[44,45]

Using the model of formalin-induced paw oedema in mice, an 85% ethanolic extract of myrrh (100 mg/kg, oral) exerted significant anti-inflammatory activity.[46] The extract also exhibited significant analgesic activity at the same dose in one model, but not in another. The petroleum ether fraction of the extract possessed the highest activity.

Other activity

A sesquiterpene fraction from myrrh (a mixture of furanodiene-6-one and methoxyfuranoguaia-9-ene-8-one) demonstrated local anaesthetic activity in vivo and showed antibacterial and antifungal activity in vitro against standard pathogenic strains of *Escherichia coli*, *Staphylococcus aureus*, *Pseudomonas aeruginosa* and *Candida albicans*, with minimum inhibitory concentrations ranging from 0.18 to 2.8 μg/mL.[47]

Myrrh increased glucose tolerance in rats under both normal and diabetic conditions.[48] Two furanosesquiterpenes isolated from myrrh exhibited hypoglycaemic activity in an experimental model of diabetes.[49]

Oral pretreatment with an aqueous suspension of myrrh (250 to 1000 mg/kg) protected against the ulcerogenic effects of several necrotising agents in rats, including ethanol and indomethacin. The protective effect of myrrh was attributed to its effect on mucus production and an increase in nucleic acid and non-protein sulphydryl concentrations, which appeared to be mediated through free radical-scavenging, thyroid-stimulating and prostaglandin-inducing properties.[50]

Treatment with a myrrh extract (250 and 500 mg/kg/day) was found to have an anticarcinogenic effect in mice for solid tumours induced by Ehrlich carcinoma cells. The activity was comparable to the standard cytotoxic drug cyclophosphamide and was more pronounced after 25 days compared with 50 days of treatment.[51,52] Another study in mice found that pretreatment with myrrh did not alter the biochemical and cytological effects of cyclophosphamide and did not show any additive effect.[53]

Both an extract and a fraction of myrrh stimulated phagocytosis in vivo after intraperitoneal injection.[54] Myrrh (500 mg/kg/day, oral) enhanced white blood cell counts in rats both before and after gastric or skin damage.[55]

Myrrh exhibited significant antiplatelet activity in mice at an oral dose of 100 mg/kg.[56]

Pharmacokinetics

No data available.

Veterinary studies

Myrrh has been tested in uncontrolled field trials for the treatment of various parasitic infestations in sheep. In sheep naturally infected with fascioliasis, doses of 300 to 600 mg of extract were administered for 1 to 3 days.[57] A total dose of 900 to 1200 mg of extract gave a complete cure rate as assessed by stool or physical examination.

Fifteen sheep naturally infected with *Dicrocoelium dendriticum* (as proven parasitologically) were successfully and safely treated with myrrh extract (600 mg/day on an empty stomach an hour before eating for 4 successive days).[58] Cure (100%) was achieved as determined by stool analysis for 7 days and macroscopically by lack of detection of any adult worms.

In sheep infected naturally with *Moniezia expansa*, a total dose of 3600 mg of myrrh extract (as 900 mg/day for 4 days) or 4800 mg (as 600 mg/day of extract for 8 days) gave 100% cure rates.[59] Response rates were assessed by microscopic and macroscopic stool examination.

Clinical studies

All the studies cited below are open label studies. However, it can be reasonably inferred that a marked placebo effect in parasitic infestation is unlikely and that a true therapeutic effect was observed for myrrh in the positive trials. On the other hand, the use of a treated infested control group would have been preferable to validate the clinical assessment methods used in the trials. The mode of action of myrrh has not been established. Rather than exerting a direct antiparasitic effect, it could act by stimulating the patient's natural immunity against parasites. All of the clinical studies, and indeed most of the experimental and veterinary studies of antiparasitic activity, have tested a commercial oleoresin extract derived from myrrh.

Fascioliasis

An open label pilot study examined the action of myrrh in seven patients with fascioliasis (infection with *Fasciola hepatica*).[3] The treatment (a formulation consisting of eight parts of resin and 3.5 parts of volatile oil, all extracted from myrrh) was given at a dose of 12 mg/kg/day for 7 consecutive days in the morning on an empty stomach. Patients were followed for 3 months. The therapy proved to be effective, with pronounced improvement of the general condition of patients and amelioration of all symptoms and signs. A dramatic drop in egg count was detected at the end of treatment. High eosinophilic counts, elevated liver enzymes and fasciola antibody titres returned to nearly normal. No signs of toxicity or adverse effects were observed and the authors concluded that the formulation of myrrh was safe, well tolerated and effective for treating fascioliasis.

In an open label, controlled study, 68 patients were included: 30 with fasciola infection, 20 infected with other parasites, but not fasciola (infected control group), and 18

individuals who were parasite-free (normal control group).[60] Stool samples were evaluated for egg counts. Circulating fasciola antigens (CFAgs) and the anti-fasciola IgG4 isotype were also evaluated. Complete blood count, liver function tests and abdominal ultrasonography were performed for all fasciola-infected patients. Patients with fascioliasis received myrrh extract at a dose of 10 mg/kg, 1 hour before breakfast for 6 consecutive days. The level of CFAgs correlated positively with signs of cure-parasitologically, clinically or ultrasonographically. Myrrh extract was found to have a high therapeutic efficacy (100% cure rate) on fascioliasis without remarkable side effects.

To determine their role in the immunopathogenesis of fascioliasis in the context of treatment with myrrh, a study was designed to evaluate total IgE and the in vitro production of IL-1beta and IL-4 by peripheral blood mononuclear cells.[61] A total of 35 patients with chronic fascioliasis with an age range from 9 to 45 years were included in the trial. In addition, 10 healthy people with matched age and sex served as controls. Serum IgE and in vitro IL-1 and IL-4 were estimated by enzyme immunoassay (ELISA) before and 3 months after therapy. Compared with controls, results revealed significant elevation of IL-1beta in patients before treatment ($p<0.001$), but this decreased significantly after therapy ($p<0.001$) to reach the control level ($p=0.16$). In contrast, IL-4 was significantly lower than controls before therapy ($p=0.04$) and increased significantly after treatment ($p<0.001$) to reach control levels ($p=0.59$). Total IgE was significantly elevated in patients before treatment ($p<0.001$) and it decreased significantly with treatment ($p<0.001$), although it remained significantly higher than the control level. The authors concluded that myrrh is an effective fasciolicidal treatment. IL-1 may be involved in disease immunopathogenesis and depressed IL-4 may be a phenomenon of parasite immune suppression.

A field trial was conducted in Egypt to assess the efficacy and safety of a myrrh extract (1200 mg/day for 6 consecutive days) for the treatment of human fascioliasis.[62] Evaluation of 1019 individuals revealed the presence of fascioliasis in 17. Cure rates in these patients were 88.2% and 94.1%, respectively, at 2 and 3 months following treatment.

A total of 21 children with fascioliasis (eight boys and 13 girls) with a mean age of 10.4 years and eight children infected with *Schistosoma mansoni* (six boys and two girls) with a mean age of 11.4 years were treated with a myrrh extract in an open label trial.[63] Also, 10 healthy matched children acted as controls. Diagnosis was based on the detection of *Fasciola hepatica* or *Schistosoma mansoni* eggs in stool samples. Myrrh extract was given as 10 mg/kg/day 1 hour before breakfast for 3 consecutive days in schistosomiasis and for 6 days in fascioliasis. The cure rate was 90.9% in fascioliasis and 100% in schistosomiasis at 4 weeks' post-treatment. After a second course of treatment, those fasciola patients who remained positive were cured. Total IgE was significantly higher in fasciola and schistosoma patients before treatment compared with controls ($p<0.001$ and 0.005, respectively) and decreased significantly with therapy ($p=0.001$ and 0.036). There were also favourable and significant shifts in IL-1beta, IL-5 and IL-4.

A total of 60 patients with fascioliasis (n=15), schistosomiasis (n=40) and heterophyiasis (n=5) were treated with myrrh extract at 10 mg/kg/day for 6 consecutive days an hour before breakfast in an open label study.[64] Results showed a significant improvement in symptoms with minimal side effects and cure rates for each parasite in excess of 90% after 3 months.

Schistosomiasis

As well as the trials described above, other studies conducted in Egypt have investigated the activity of myrrh extract in schistosomiasis. An open label trial was conducted in 204 patients suffering from this infestation.[65] Myrrh extract was given at a dose of 10 mg/kg for 3 days and found to effect a cure rate of 91.7%. Retreatment of the non-responsive cases with the same dose for 6 days increased the overall cure rate to 98%. Myrrh was observed to be well tolerated and side effects were mild and transient. Twenty people provided biopsy specimens 6 months later and none of them showed living ova.

Among 1019 individuals parasitologically examined in an open label field trial, the prevalence of S. haematobium and S. mansoni were 4.2% and 2.4% respectively.[66] Most of the patients with haematobiasis and mansoniasis were <15 years (56.4% and 53.8%) and male (56.4% and 53.8%). All cases were treated with myrrh extract as two capsules (600 mg) on an empty stomach an hour before breakfast for 6 consecutive days and were followed up clinically and parasitologically by urine and stool analysis. Parasitological cure rates after 3 months were 97.4% and 96.2% for the S. haematobium and S. mansoni cases, respectively, without any major side effects. Patients not completely responding to a single course of treatment showed a marked reduction of egg levels. A similar dosage protocol proved to be safe and effective for the eradication of S. haematobium in patients recruited from an Egyptian village.[67]

A more recent trial was again an open label design, but with the important inclusion of randomisation and an active control group. The results for myrrh were less impressive than the above, but the trial dosage used was either lower or for less time than in previous clinical evaluations (being 600 mg/day for 3 consecutive days). One hundred and four individuals infected with Schistosoma mansoni were randomised in two groups, one for myrrh and the second for praziquantel.[68] Treatment, whether myrrh or praziquantel, was given twice, with a 3-week interval in between. The cure rate with myrrh was very low, 15.6% after the first treatment, and 8.9% after the second treatment. Egg reduction amongst uncured patients was also very low, being 17.2% after the first treatment and 28% after the second treatment. The praziquantel cure rates were 73.7% and 76.3% and individuals still passing S. mansoni ova after praziquantel treatment showed a substantial reduction in geometric mean egg counts (84% and 88.2% after the first and second treatments, respectively). Similarly, another trial comparing myrrh with praziquantel found low cure rates for myrrh (around 9%), but again a lower dose than that used in previous trials was employed (300 mg/day of extract for only 3 days).[69]

However, a myrrh extract at the recommended dose of 600 mg for 6 consecutive days exerted a modest cure rate in 27 patients with schistosomiasis and a zero cure rate in 16 patients with fascioliasis in an open label trial.[70]

Other parasitic infestations

Dicrocoelium dendriticum is a problem animal and human parasite in the Middle East. Myrrh extract (600 mg/day before breakfast for 6 successive days) effectively treated infestation with this parasite in 18 patients in an open label trial.[58]

Another parasite commonly found in Egypt is Heterophyes heterophyes. In addition to the trial mentioned above, myrrh extract (600 mg/day before breakfast for 9 consecutive days) eradicated the parasite in 47 of 50 patients with clinically and parasitologically proven infestation in an open label trial.[71] Another course was given to the three patients who were still positive, but only two of them responded.

Myrrh has also been investigated in the treatment of human hymenolepiosis. In 51 cases of infestation with Hymenolepis nana and two cases of H. diminuta the extract was given at a dose of 10 mg/kg/day for 9 consecutive days 1 hour before breakfast.[72] High cure rates based on parasite testing (>90%) were confirmed in this open label trial for the patients who completed the course of treatment.

Oral use of myrrh extract (600 mg/day for 6 to 8 days) was evaluated in 13 women with metronidazole-resistant trichomoniasis (Trichomonas vaginalis) in an open label trial.[73] Successful treatment occurred in 11 patients.

Sixty cryptosporidiosis patients (aged from a few months to 10 years) were divided into three groups and received either myrrh extract (10 mg/kg for 2 weeks), the drug paromomycin (500 mg four times a day for 2 weeks) or a combination of the two treatments.[74] All treatment groups demonstrated reduced oocyst counts and symptomatic improvement over 4 weeks, but the combination was the most effective at improving symptoms.

Toxicology and other safety data

Toxicology

The LD_{50} for oil of myrrh was determined as 1.65 g/kg in rats.[75] Doses of an ethanolic extract administered by mouth at 1.0 g/kg to male Wistar rats for 2 weeks led to depression, jaundice, ruffled hair, hepatonephropathy, haemorrhagic myositis and death, accompanied by increases in serum ALP and ALT activities, bilirubin, cholesterol and creatinine concentrations, decreases in total protein and albumin levels, and macrocytic anaemia and leucopenia.[76] In acute toxicity testing, myrrh oleo-gum resin exhibited no visible signs of toxicity, and no mortality was observed at doses up to 3 g/kg in mice. A decrease in locomotor activity was however noticed at this dose. In chronic oral testing (100 mg/kg/day, 90 days) there was no significant difference in mortality compared with controls. Assessment at the end of treatment revealed a significant increase in the weights of testes, caudae epididymides and seminal vesicles and in red blood count and haemoglobin levels.[77]

Death occurred after consumption of between 5 g and 16 g crude resin/kg/day in goats. Enterohepatonephrotoxicity was accompanied by anaemia, leucopenia, increases in serum ALP activity and concentrations of bilirubin, cholesterol, triglycerides and creatinine, and decreases in total protein and albumin. An oral dose of 0.25 g crude resin/kg/day was not toxic.[78]

Adult male albino rats received either a weekly oral dose of the antiparasitic agent praziquantel (1500 mg/kg) for 6 weeks or a daily dose of myrrh extract (500 mg/kg) for the same period.[79] Praziquantel induced significant increases in hepatic enzymes (AST and ALT), bilirubin, hepatic necrosis and chromosomal aberrations. In contrast, the myrrh extract induced a non-significant increase in AST, ALT and bilirubin without significantly damaging hepatic tissue or chromosomes compared with controls.

Contraindications

Known allergy. According to traditional Chinese medicine myrrh is contraindicated in pregnancy and in cases of excessive uterine bleeding.[10]

Special warnings and precautions

Depending on the level of dilution of the tincture, a transient burning sensation on the skin or mucous membranes may be experienced from the topical application of myrrh. Myrrh should not be ingested for prolonged periods (more than a few weeks at a time) because of the potential for allergic contact dermatitis and other allergic reactions.

Interactions

One case has been reported from Saudi Arabia of an antagonism of the anticoagulant effect of warfarin.[80]

Use in pregnancy and lactation

Category B1-no evidence of an increase in frequency of malformation or other harmful effects on the fetus from limited use in women. No evidence of increased fetal damage in animal studies.

Administration of a combination of resin and essential oil extracted from myrrh to pregnant rats (50 to 200 mg/kg from days 6 to 15) caused no abnormalities in the fetal skeleton.[81]

As noted above, according to traditional Chinese medicine myrrh is contraindicated in pregnancy and in cases of excessive uterine bleeding.[10]

Myrrh is compatible with breastfeeding, but caution should be observed due to the potential for allergy.

Effects on ability to drive and use machines

No adverse effects are expected.

Side effects

Contact allergy has been reported for the use of myrrh by topical application.[82–85] Continued topical use of essential oils, including those of myrrh, was associated with a deterioration of symptoms in a study on children with atopic eczema, suggesting a possible build-up of contact sensitivity.[86]

Two cases of allergy due to oral administration of myrrh have been reported in the accessed traditional Chinese medicine literature. In both cases, the patients received a formulation containing myrrh, which was subsequently identified as the allergen.[87]

Overdosage

No incidents found in the published literature.

Safety in children

Clinical trials of myrrh have been conducted in children without marked adverse events.

Regulatory status in selected countries

In the UK myrrh is included on the General Sale List. It is covered by a positive German Commission E monograph and in Europe by an ESCOP monograph.

In the USA myrrh does not have GRAS status. However, it is freely available as a 'dietary supplement' in the USA under DSHEA legislation (Dietary Supplement Health and Education Act of 1994).

Myrrh is official in the *United States Pharmacopeia–National Formulary* (USP 31-NF 26, 2007).

In Australia myrrh is not included in Part 4 of Schedule 4 of the Therapeutic Goods Regulations and is freely available for sale.

References

1. Evans WC. *Trease and Evans' Pharmacognosy*, 14th ed. London: WB Saunders; 1996. p. 289.
2. Nabataean Trade Items. Nabataea.Net, CanBooks; 2002.
3. Massoud A, El Sisi S, Salama O, et al. *Am J Trop Med Hyg*. 2001;65(2):96–99.
4. Massoud A, Salama O, Bennet J. *Parasitol Int*. 1998;47:125.
5. Ghazanfar SA. *Handbook of Arabian Medicinal Plants*. Boca Raton, Florida: CRC Press; 1994.
6. Jirsa F, Winiwarter V. *Wien Klin Wochenschr*. 2010;122(3):14–18.
7. British Herbal Medicine Association Scientific Committee. *British Herbal Pharmacopoeia*. Bournemouth: BHMA; 1983.
8. Felter HW. *The Eclectic Materia Medica, Pharmacology and Therapeutics*, 1922, Portland, reprinted Eclectic Medical Publications, 1983.

9. British Herbal Medicine Association. *British Herbal Compendium*. Bournemouth: BHM; 1992.

10. Bensky D, Gamble A. *Chinese Herbal Medicine Materia Medica*. Seattle: Eastland Press; 1986.

11. Chopra RN, Chopra IC, Handa KL, et al. *Chopra's Indigenous Drugs of India*, ed 2, 1958, Calcutta, reprinted Academic Publishers, 1982.

12. Felter HW, Lloyd JU. *King's American Dispensatory*, ed 18, rev 3. First published 1905, Portland, reprinted Eclectic Medical Publications, 1983, pp. 1298–1301.

13. Grieve M. *A Modern Herbal*, vol. 2. New York: Dover Publications; 1971. pp. 571–572.

14. Blumenthal M, ed. *The Complete German Commission E Monographs: Therapeutic Guide to Herbal Medicines*. Austin: American Botanical Council; 1998.

15. Scientific Committee of ESCOP (European Scientific Cooperative on Phytotherapy). *ESCOP Monographs: Myrrha*. European Scientific Cooperative on Phytotherapy, ESCOP Secretariat, UK, October 1999.

16. Bisset NG, ed. *Herbal Drugs and Phytopharmaceuticals*. Stuttgart: Medpharm Scientific Publishers; 1994. p. 345.

17. *British Pharmacopoeia*. 2007; CD–ROM.

18. *European Pharmacopoeia*, ed 5.3, 2006. <http://www.agemed.es/profHumana/farmacopea/docs/index_5–3edic.pdf>.

19. *The United States Pharmacopeia. The National Formulary*. USP31–NF26, 2007 CD-ROM.

20. Blaschek W, Ebel S, Hackenthal E, et al. *HagerROM Hagers Handbuch der Drogen und Arzneistoffe*. Heidelberg: Springer; 2002.

21. Dekebo A, Dagne E, Sterner O. *Fitoterapia*. 2002;73(1):48–55.

22. Mills S, Bone K. *The Essential Guide to Herbal Safety*. USA: Churchill Livingstone; 2005. p. 514.

23. Hanuš LO, Řezanka T, Dembitsky VM, et al. *Biomed Papers*. 2005;149(1):3–28.

24. Massoud AM, El Ebiary FH, Abou-Gamra MM, et al. *J Egypt Soc Parasitol*. 2004;34(3 suppl):1051–1076.

25. Hamed MA, Hetta MH. *Mem Inst Oswaldo Cruz*. 2005;100:771–778.

26. Massoud AM, El Ebiary FH, Abd El Salam NF. *J Egypt Soc Parasitol*. 2004;34(1):1–21.

27. Hassan M, El-Motaiem M, Afify H, et al. *J Egypt Soc Parasitol*. 2003;33(3):999–1008.

28. Massoud AM, El Ebiary FH, Ibrahim SH, et al. *J Egypt Soc Parasitol*. 2010;40(1):245–258.

29. Botros S, William S, Ebeid F, et al. *Am J Trop Med Hyg*. 2004;71(2):206–210.

30. Ramzy F, Mahmoud S, William S. *Pharm Biol*. 2010;48(7):775–779.

31. Mahmoud MS, Dobal SA, Soliman K. *Res J Parasitol*. 2008;3:40–49.

32. Botros SS, El-Lakkany NM, Badawy AA, et al. *Ann Trop Med Parasitol*. 2009;103(7):605–616.

33. Massoud A, El Khateeb RM, Kutkat MA. *J Egypt Soc Parasitol*. 2010;40(3):751–758.

34. Baghdadi HB, Al-Mathal EM. *J Egypt Soc Parasitol*. 2010;40(3):653–668.

35. Fathy FM. *J Egypt Soc Parasitol*. 2011;41(1):155–177.

36. Allam AF, el-Sayad MH, Khalil SS. *J Egypt Soc Parasitol*. 2001;31(3):683–690.

37. Massoud AM, Habib FS. *J Egypt Soc Parasitol*. 2003;33(2):585–596.

38. Massoud A, Metwally DM, Khalifa KE, et al. *J Egypt Soc Parasitol*. 2004;34(3):995–1008.

39. Massoud AM, Kutkat MA, Abdel Shafy S, et al. *J Egypt Soc Parasitol*. 2005;35(2):667–686.

40. Massoud AM, Labib IM, Rady M. *J Egypt Soc Parasitol*. 2001;31(2):517–529.

41. Massoud AM, Labib IM. *J Egypt Soc Parasitol*. 2000;30(1):101–115.

42. Tariq M, Ageel AM, Al-Yahya MA, et al. *Agents Actions*. 1986;17(3–4):381–382.

43. Atta AH, Alkofahi A. *J Ethnopharmacol*. 1998;60:117–124.

44. Dolara P, Luceri C, Ghelardini C, et al. *Nature*. 1996;379(6560):29.

45. Dolara P, Moneti G, Pieraccini H, et al. *Phytother Res*. 1996;10(suppl 1):S81–S83.

46. Su S, Wang T, Duan JA, et al. *J Ethnopharmacol*. 2011;134(2):251–258.

47. Dolara P, Corte B, Ghelardini C, et al. *Planta Med*. 2000;66(4):356–358.

48. Al-Awadi FM, Gumaa KA. *Acta Diabetol Lat*. 1987;24(1):37–41.

49. Ubillas RP, Mendez CD, Jolad SD, et al. *Planta Med*. 1999;65(8):778–779.

50. al-Harbi MM, Qureshi S, Raza M, et al. *J Ethnopharmacol*. 1997;55(2):141–150.

51. al-Harbi MM, Qureshi S, Raza M, et al. *Chemotherapy*. 1994;40(5):337–347.

52. Qureshi S, al-Harbi MM, Ahmed MM, et al. *Cancer Chemother Pharmacol*. 1993;33(2):130–138.

53. al-Harbi MM, Qureshi S, Ahmed MM, et al. *Am J Chin Med*. 1994;22(1):77–82.

54. Delaveau P, Lallouette P, Tessier AM. *Planta Med*. 1980;40(1):49–54.

55. Haffor AS. *J Immunotoxicol*. 2010;7(1):68–75.

56. Olajide OA. *Phytother Res*. 1999;13(3):231–232.

57. Haridy FM, El Garhy MF, Morsy TA. *J Egypt Soc Parasitol*. 2003;33(3):917–924.

58. Al-Mathal EM, Fouad MA. *J Egypt Soc Parasitol*. 2004;34(2):713–720.

59. Haridy FM, Dawoud HA, Morsy TA. *J Egypt Soc Parasitol*. 2004;34(3):775–782.

60. Hegab MH, Hassan RM. *Egypt Soc Parasitol*. 2003;33(2):561–570.

61. Massoud AM, El-Kholy NM, El-Shennawy FA, et al. *J Egypt Soc Parasitol*. 2004;34(1):315–332.

62. Abo-Madyan AA, Morsy TA, Motawea SM, et al. *J Egypt Soc Parasitol*. 2004;34(3):807–818.

63. Soliman OE, El-Arman M, Abdul-Samie ER, et al. *J Egypt Soc Parasitol*. 2004;34(3):941–966.

64. Massoud AM, El-Sherbini ET, Mos N, et al. *J Egypt Soc Parasitol*. 2010;40(1):119–134.

65. Sheir Z, Nasr AA, Massoud A, et al. *Am J Trop Med Hyg*. 2001;65(6):700–704.

66. Abo-Madyan AA, Morsy TA, Motawea SM. *J Egypt Soc Parasitol*. 2004;34(2):423–446.

67. El Baz MA, Morsy TA, El Bandary MM, et al. *J Egypt Soc Parasitol*. 2003;33(3):761–776.

68. Barakat R, Elmorshedy H, Fenwick A. *Am J Trop Med Hyg*. 2005;73(2):365–367.

69. Botros S, Sayed H, El-Dusoki H, et al. *Am J Trop Med Hyg*. 2005;72(2):119–123.

70. Osman MM, El-Taweel HA, Shehab AY, et al. *East Mediterr Health J*. 2010;16(9):932–936.

71. Massoud AM, El-Shazly AM, Morsy TA. *J Egypt Soc Parasitol*. 2007;37(2):395–410.

72. Massoud AM, Shazly AM, Shahat SA, et al. *J Egypt Soc Parasitol*. 2007;37(3):863–876.

73. El-Sherbini GT, El Gozamy BR, Abdel-Hady NM, et al. *J Egypt Soc Parasitol*. 2009;39(1):47–58.

74. Massoud AM, Hafez AO, Abdel-Gawad AG, et al. *J Egypt Soc Parasitol*. 2008;38(2):399–418.

75. Opdyke DLJ. *Food Cosmet Toxicol*. 1976;14:621.

76. Omer SA, Adam SE, Khalid HE. *Vet Hum Toxicol*. 1999;41(4):193–196.

77. Rao RM, Khan ZA, Shah AH. *J Ethnopharmacol*. 2001;76(2):151–154.

78. Omer SA, Adam SE. *Vet Hum Toxicol*. 1999;41(5):299–301.

79. Omar A, Elmesallamy Gel S, Eassa S. *J Egypt Soc Parasitol*. 2005;35(1):313–329.

80. Al Faraj S. *Ann Trop Med Parasitol*. 2005;99(2):219–220.

81. Massoud AM, El-Ashmawy IM, Hemeda SA, et al. *Alex J Pharm Sci*. 2000;14(1):61–68.

82. Lee TY, Lam TH. *Contact Dermatitis*. 1993;29(5):279.

83. Al-Suwaidan SN, Gad el Rab MO, Al-Fakhiry S, et al. *Contact Dermatitis*. 1998;39(3):137.

84. Gallo R, Rivara G, Cattarini G, et al. *Contact Dermatitis*. 1999;41(4):230–231.

85. Lee TY, Lam TH. *Contact Dermatitis*. 1993;28(2):89–90.

86. Anderson C, Lis-Balchin M, Kirk-Smith M. *Phytother Res*. 2000;14(6):452–456.

87. Bian HZ, Pan MS. *Bull Chin Materia Med*. 1987;12(9):565.

(Urtica dioica L., Urtica urens L.)

Synonyms

Nettles, stinging nettle (Engl), *Urtica herba, Urtica radix* (Lat), Brennesselkraut, Haarnesselkraut, Brennesselwurzel, Haarnesselwurzel (Ger), herbe d'ortie, racine d'ortie (Fr), ortica (Ital), brændenælde (Dan).

Urtica dioica: stinging nettle, common nettle (Engl), Grosse Brennessel (Ger), grande ortie (Fr).

Urtica urens: small nettle (Engl), Kleine Brennessel (Ger), ortie bûrlante, petite ortie (Fr).

What is it?

Nettle is generally regarded as a weed. It grows throughout the temperate regions of the world, particularly on nitrate-rich soil in waste places. The plant has been used extensively throughout history for a variety of applications and possesses very fine, sharp stinging hairs. It provided a source of fibre before the general introduction of flax and has an old reputation as a spring vegetable, the young shoots being cooked and eaten like spinach (and as a remedy for scurvy). The leaf was used as livestock fodder and the oil from nettle seed was employed as burning oil in Egypt. Nettle is currently a commercial source of chlorophyll. The leaf, root and seeds are all used medicinally. The *British Herbal Compendium* recommends nettle leaf should comprise the dried leaf or aerial parts, collected during the flowering period.[1] Nettle root includes the root and rhizome and is mainly indicated for benign prostatic hyperplasia.

Effects

- Nettle leaf: decreases inflammation; assists eliminative function
- Nettle root: inhibits cellular proliferation in benign prostatic hyperplastic tissue; inhibits binding activity of sex hormone-binding globulin.

Traditional view

Nettle leaf was traditionally regarded as a blood purifier, a styptic (stops bleeding) and a stimulating tonic and diuretic. It was used to treat diarrhoea, dysentery, discharges, chronic diseases of the colon and chronic skin eruptions. (The Eclectics used both leaf and root for these applications.)[2,3] A syrup made from the juice of root or leaves was said to relieve bronchial and asthmatic troubles. Nettle infusion or fresh plant tincture has been applied topically for nosebleed, as a lotion for burns, as an astringent gargle and as a hair lotion. The beating of nettle leaves on afflicted joints was considered a remedy for arthritis, chronic rheumatism and loss of muscular power and is based on the principle of counter-irritation.[2] A poultice was also used to relieve gout, sciatica or joint pain.[4] The seeds were utilised in cases of consumption and goitre and combined with flowers for ague.[2,3] *U. urens* was considered very efficient in uterine haemorrhage and reputedly eased urethral and bladder irritation and had galactagogue activity.[3] Oral intake of nettle leaf was used to treat eczema, nettle rash and other skin conditions.[5]

Summary actions

- Nettle leaf: antirheumatic, antiallergic, depurative, styptic (haemostatic), counter-irritant (topically, fresh leaves)
- Nettle root: antiprostatic.

Can be used for

Indications supported by clinical trials

- Nettle leaf: allergic rhinitis, oral and topical use for relief of osteoarthritis
- Nettle root: improvement of urological symptoms in benign prostatic hyperplasia (BPH).

Traditional therapeutic uses

- Nettle leaf or root: diarrhoea, dysentery, internal bleeding, chronic diseases of the colon, chronic skin eruptions, bladder irritations, bronchial or asthmatic conditions
- Nettle leaf: topically for burns, wounds, nosebleeds, inflammation of the mouth or throat, joint pain (via the stinging of the skin around the joint); orally for skin rashes.

May also be used for

Extrapolations from pharmacological studies

- Nettle leaf: as an anti-inflammatory with broad activity including inhibition of cytokines.

Other applications

Nettle leaf can be applied topically for treatment of insect bites in combination with other herbs. It may also provide a source of absorbable silica. The silicon in nettle is more rapidly extracted than from horsetail (*Equisetum arvense*). A 1:100 decoction of the dried leaves simmered for 30 minutes yielded about 5 mg of soluble amount of silicon for every 1 g of nettle used. This is about half the amount of silicon obtained from the same quantity of horsetail decocted for 3 h.[6]

Preparations

Liquid and solid dosage forms as normal.

Dosage

- 8 to 12 g/day of dried herb; 4 to 6 g/day of dried root
- Nettle herb: 3 to 6 mL/day of 1:2 liquid extract, 7 to 14 mL/day of 1:5 tincture
- Nettle root: 4 to 9 mL/day of 1:2 liquid extract.
  Doses mainly used in clinical trials are as follows:
- Nettle root and BPH: 600 to 1200 mg/day of a 5:1 extract (3 to 6 g/day)
- Nettle leaf and arthritis: extract equivalent to about 9 g/day.

Duration of use

No restriction on long-term use.

Summary assessment of safety

Except in rare cases of contact allergy following topical use of the leaf in susceptible patients, nettle is a safe herb.

Technical data

Botany

Nettle is a member of the Urticaceae family. *Urtica dioica* is a perennial herb, 25 to 150 cm in height and covered all over with brittle stinging hairs. The leaves are opposite, 3.5 to 8.5 cm long, ovate from a usually heart-shaped base with toothed margins. The small flowers are green, unisexual and arranged in axillary inflorescences up to 10 cm long. The fruit is an achene (1 to 1.25 mm long), enclosed by large perianth segments. *Urtica urens* can be distinguished by its annual habit, smaller size, smaller leaves[7] and is monoecious (containing male and female flowers in separate clusters).[8] The root and rhizome are long, creeping and yellowish in colour.[9]

Adulteration

A woman showing the symptoms of atropine poisoning after drinking nettle leaf tea was found to have consumed a tea mixture containing belladonna (*Atropa belladonna*) among other contaminants.[10] However, this type of adulteration is likely to be rare. *Lamium album* (the white deadnettle) is noted as a potential adulterant.[11]

Key constituents

Nettle leaf

- Flavonol glycosides (especially rutin), sterols, scopoletin (isolated from the flowers),[12] chlorophyll, carotenoids, vitamins (including C, B group, K_1), minerals, plant phenolic acids (especially chlorogenic and 2-O-caffeoylmalic acids).[13] The stinging hairs contain amines, including histamine, serotonin[14] and acetylcholine.[15] The vitamin K content may be responsible for the styptic action associated with nettle leaf[16]
- Nettle leaf is also a rich source of silicon. Much of this silicon occurs in the stinging hairs, which are effectively fine silica glass needles.[6] The leaf also contains low levels of nitrate, which vary according to its habitat.[17]

Nettle root

- Sterols and steryl glycosides (including sitosterol),[18] lignans (including (–)-secoisolariciresinol),[19] a small, single-chain lectin (UDA, *Urtica dioica* agglutinin)[20]
- Phenylpropanes, polyphenols, polysaccharides[21]
- The coumarin scopoletin.[22]

Pharmacodynamics

Nettle root and benign prostatic hyperplasia

There have been several studies attempting to understand the potential mechanism of action of nettle root in BPH. The picture is still unclear and there have been relatively few studies published on this topic since 1999.

Several lignans from nettle root including secoisolariciresinol reduced the binding activity of human sex hormone-binding globulin (SHBG) in vitro.[23] Additionally the lignans from nettle root (except (–)-pinoresinol) demonstrated a direct binding affinity for SHBG in vitro. The affinity of (–)-3,4-divanillyltetrahydrofuran was particularly high. Metabolites of secoisolariciresinol (enterodiol, enterolactone) also displayed binding affinities for SHBG and a relatively higher binding affinity was observed for the metabolite of (–)-3,4-divanillyltetrahydrofuran (enterofuran).[19] Results from assays using a number of lignans, including those found in nettle root, suggest they may also competitively inhibit the interaction between SHBG and 5-alpha-dihydrotestosterone (DHA).[24] An aqueous extract of nettle root demonstrated dose-dependent (0.6 to 10 mg/mL) inhibition of SHBG binding with its receptor on human prostatic membranes. The alcoholic extract (70% ethanol), *Urtica dioica* agglutinin (UDA) and stigmasta-4-en-3-one were all inactive.[25] Other studies indicated that nettle root extract (20% methanol) inhibited the binding capacity of SHBG after preincubation with human serum.[26]

Morphological studies of BPH cells were performed in 31 patients treated orally with nettle root extract (1200 mg/day of 5:1 extract) for 20 weeks. Relevant changes were observed in the nucleus and cytoplasm of prostate cells harvested at the end of treatment, which may be due to an inhibition of the binding capacity of SHBG.[27] (See also under Clinical trials for studies examining the clinical impact of nettle root on SHBG binding activity.)

Five subfractions of an aqueous methanol extract of nettle root inhibited cellular proliferation of BPH tissue in concentrations ranging from 10 to 1500 μg/mL.[28] A reduction in cellular proliferation of BPH tissue was observed ex vivo after treatment of patients with an aqueous-methanolic nettle root extract.[29] Five differently prepared nettle root extracts were tested in experimentally induced BPH in mice. The methanolic extract was the most effective and demonstrated significant inhibition of prostate growth compared with controls (51%, p<0.003). The aqueous extract also inhibited growth, although not significantly. There was no correlation between the amounts of sitosterol and scopoletin and the growth-inhibiting effect.[30] After 100 days of oral treatment with 90 mg/kg nettle root extract (5:1), an average decrease of 30% in prostatic volume and a slight lowering of plasma testosterone was observed in animals suffering from BPH.[31]

The 20% methanolic extract of nettle root (160 mg/kg/day for 28 days, oral) inhibited prostate growth by 57% in a mouse model of BPH.[32] The active fraction was found to contain proteins and polysaccharides (as assessed using oral doses). UDA and secoisolariciresinol were inactive and even stimulated prostate growth.

Nettle root (either as the petroleum ether or ethanolic extract, 10 to 50 mg/kg, oral) ameliorated the effect of testosterone on inducing prostatic hyperplasia in rats.[33] The extracts also demonstrated weak 5-alpha-reductase inhibitory activity in vitro. The authors suggested that the beta-sitosterol and scopoletin present in the extracts can be considered clinically relevant biomolecules in the context of treating BPH.

A decrease in biological activity was observed for prostate cells removed from 33 BPH patients given 1200 mg of 5:1 nettle root extract for 20 weeks. The morphological changes were associated with a decrease in secretory granules.[34] Ultrastructural changes in smooth muscle cells of BPH tissue were also observed before and after therapy with nettle root extract.[35]

Organic solvent extracts of nettle root (0.1 mg/mL) caused an inhibition (27% to 82%) of Na^+,K^+-ATPase from BPH tissue. Hydrophobic constituents of the root, especially stigmasta-4-en-3-one, also inhibited this enzyme,[36] which is believed to be responsible for androgen control (as an androgen receptor).[37]

Pygeum extract (0.1 mg/mL) was shown to be a mild inhibitor of 5-alpha-reductase (which converts testosterone into DHT in vitro), but nettle root (>12 mg/mL) was only a very weak inhibitor. The combined Pygeum/nettle root extract had an activity similar to the nettle root. Both extracts also inhibited aromatase, which converts testosterone into oestradiol.[38] Another in vitro study found that inhibitory effects on aromatase were only detected after the separation of a methanolic extract of nettle root into its constituents. Weak-to-moderate activity was observed for some of the isolated compounds including secoisolariciresinol, oleanolic acid, ursolic acid and 13-hydroxy-9,11-octadecadienoic acid.[39] In contrast, an aqueous-ethanolic nettle root extract did inhibit aromatase in vitro in another study. Suggested active

constituents included fatty acids and 9-hydroxy-10,12-octadecadienoic acid. Although nettle extracts are weak inhibitors of aromatase compared with synthetic preparations, a pharmacological effect might be achievable through the lipophilic nettle compounds concentrating in fatty tissues, where androgens are aromatised.[40,41] Evaluation of the combined activity of nettle root and saw palmetto extracts indicated that they each inhibited aromatase by a different mechanism.[42,43]

In support of a finding noted above, nettle root extract at concentrations up to 0.5 mg/mL did not inhibit 5-alpha-reductase in vitro or the binding of dihydrotestosterone to the rat prostatic androgen receptor. It also did not inhibit testosterone- or dihydrotestosterone-stimulated prostate growth in castrated rats.[44] A mild inhibition of DHT binding to cytosolic androgen receptors in the prostate has been observed in vitro.[26]

Nettle root extract demonstrated a specific and dose-dependent inhibition of human leucocyte elastase (HLE) in vitro.[45] (The presence of the proteolytic enzyme HLE in seminal plasma is an important marker in clinically silent genitourinary tract infection/inflammation.[46]) The root extract inhibited the alternative and the classic complement pathways in vitro with a half maximum inhibition concentration of <50 μg/mL.[47]

Fluorescence measurements indicated that a specific reaction occurred in BPH tissue after administration of nettle root extract both in vitro and in vivo.[48] This phenomenon may have been due to the presence of the fluorescent compound scopoletin and is of uncertain relevance, but does indicate that phytochemicals in nettle root are bioavailable to the prostate.[22]

Nettle root (20% methanolic extract), and the polysaccharide fraction from this extract, have also demonstrated anti-proliferative activity on human prostatic epithelial and stromal cancer cells in vitro.[49,50]

Anti-inflammatory activity (nettle leaf)

In order to understand the anti-inflammatory potential of nettle leaf, a group of German scientists carried out a series of in vitro tests. In the first study, the effect of a nettle leaf extract on biosynthesis of arachidonic acid metabolites was evaluated in vitro. The nettle leaf extract and caffeoyl malic acid (the major phenolic component of the extract) showed partial, concentration-dependent inhibition of both cyclo-oxygenase - and 5-lipoxygenase-derived reactions.[51]

In the second published series of experiments, the effects of a nettle leaf extract and possible active components on the in vitro release of pro-inflammatory cytokines were examined after lipopolysaccharide (LPS) stimulation of whole blood samples taken from healthy human volunteers. In this assay system, LPS stimulation causes an increase of tumour necrosis factor-alpha (TNF-alpha) and interleukin-1beta (IL-1beta) secretion. Nettle leaf extract significantly reduced this release of cytokines in a concentration-dependent manner and also independently stimulated the secretion of interleukin-6 (IL-6). Since IL-6 acts antagonistically to IL-1beta in decreasing prostaglandin E_2 synthesis and also induces inhibitors of proteinases, this finding might also reflect an anti-inflammatory result. Phenolic acid derivatives and flavonoids showed no activity in this assay.[52]

Conflicting results have been reported using the carrageenan rat paw oedema model of inflammation. No activity was detected using an ethanolic extract of nettle.[53] Prolonged activity for 22h (with similar efficacy to indomethacin) began 5h after the oral administration of the crude polysaccharide fraction of nettle. Some polysaccharides isolated from nettle stimulated T-lymphocytes in vitro, others influenced the complement system or triggered the release of TNF-alpha.[54]

Twenty healthy volunteers ingested 1.34g/day of a nettle leaf extract for 21 days in an open label study. This dose was probably equivalent to about 10g/day of dried nettle leaf. Although the nettle leaf had no effect on basal levels of cytokines, it did significantly decrease the release of TNF-alpha and IL-1beta after LPS stimulation ex vivo. However, an increase in IL-6 was not observed after oral ingestion, confirming that in vitro results are not necessarily translatable into clinical findings. This is probably because some compounds in the plant exhibit poor bioavailability after oral doses.[55] The inhibition of these cytokines offers a possible approach for inhibiting joint and bone destruction, thereby slowing the progression of the disease.

Other related anti-inflammatory mechanisms have been subsequently investigated. A 95% propanolic nettle leaf extract and the constituent 13-hydroxyoctadecatrienic acid were both shown to decrease matrix metalloproteinase (MMP) expression in vitro.[56] MMP is primarily mediated by IL-1beta and TNF-alpha and is responsible for the extracellular matrix degradation in inflammatory disorders such as rheumatoid arthritis and osteoarthritis. Both the nettle and 13-hydroxyoctadecatrienic acid significantly inhibited IL-1beta-induced MMP in human chondrocytes. A 50% ethanolic extract of nettle leaf has also been shown to inhibit NF-kappaB in vitro.[57]

The 95% propanolic extract suppressed the maturation of human myeloid dendritic cells in vitro.[58] Dendritic cells are antigen presenting and therefore suppression of these cells could lead to a reduced induction of the primary T cell responses that mediate inflammation in rheumatoid arthritis. A marked reduction of TNF-alpha release was also noted.

The long-term use of the propanolic extract reduced the induction of colitis in vivo.[59] Mice were given dextran sodium sulphate to induce colitis and either nettle extract (5mg/mL in drinking water) or water. Treated animals consistently showed significant clinical and histological improvements, with lower faecal IL-1beta and mucosal TNF-alpha concentrations.

An ethanolic extract of Urtica urens (300mg/kg, ip) demonstrated anti-inflammatory activity in rats (carrageenan-induced oedema) and significant antinociceptive activity in mice in some models.[60] Chlorogenic acid was a major component of the extract (67%).

Nettle leaf urticaria

A study involving six people up to 12h after nettle contact suggested that part of the immediate reaction to nettle stings is due to histamine introduced by the nettle. However, the persistence of the stinging sensation might be due to the presence of substances in nettle fluid directly toxic to nerves or capable of secondary release of other mediators.[61] Acetylcholine is present in the hairs and contributes to the stinging reaction. The sting produced by the hairs can be imitated by the intradermal injection of a mixture of acetylcholine and histamine, but not by either agent given separately. The high concentration of acetylcholine in nettle hairs may be comparable to that in stores of cholinergic nerve endings in animals. Extracts of acetone-dried nettle leaf powder catalysed the synthesis of acetylcholine in vitro, indicating the presence of choline acetyltransferase. Synthesis of acetylcholine is not restricted to the younger leaves and continues in older plants.[15]

In another study, nettle hairs and whole plant extract were found to contain high levels of leukotrienes (LTB_4, LTC_4) as well as histamine. Nettle hairs therefore could resemble insect venoms and cutaneous mast cells with regard to their spectrum of mediators.[62] In addition, a phospholipid isolated from nettle leaf that induced rabbit platelet aggregation was identified as platelet-activating factor (PAF). Hence the urtication caused by nettle could be partly due to the presence of PAF.[63]

An in vitro study using mouse skin samples concluded that the mechanism of action in nettle leaf urticaria is mechanical as well as biochemical.[64] Impalement of silica glass spicules into the skin likely accounts for the mechanical irritation.

Glycaemic control (nettle leaf)

Pharmacological research has demonstrated conflicting results for nettle leaf in terms of glycaemic control and its activity remains uncertain. Most of the positive studies relied on administration by injection.

An infusion of nettle leaf administered via the diet to experimentally induced diabetic mice aggravated the diabetic condition, as measured by parameters of glucose homeostasis. It did not affect these parameters in normal mice.[65] An aqueous decoction of nettle leaf or aqueous ethanol extract of nettle leaf orally administered 2h prior to glucose load showed a hyperglycaemic activity in normal mice. The dose was equivalent to 25g/kg herb.[66] In another in vivo study, the effect of nettle leaf on induced hyperglycaemia (oral glucose tolerance test) and alloxan-induced diabetic rats was investigated.[67] An aqueous extract (250mg/kg, oral) administered to normal rats 30 minutes before glucose loading resulted in an average glycaemic reduction of 33% compared with controls. Intestinal glucose absorption in situ in a perfused rat jejunum segment showed a significant reduction (11.11 ± 0.75mg versus 8.05 ± 0.68mg) over 2h. However, oral administration of the nettle extract (500mg/kg) failed to modify blood glucose levels in alloxan-induced diabetic rats.

An active fraction (F1) from an aqueous extract of nettle leaf caused a marked increase in insulin secretion from Langerhans' islets in vitro.[68] The fraction was also found to increase blood insulin levels and decrease blood glucose in normal and streptozotocin-induced diabetic rats after ip administration. Another fraction of the aqueous extract (UD-1) did not stimulate insulin release in vitro, but significantly enhanced glucose uptake by myoblasts.[69] The possible active agent was an insulin mimetic cyclic peptide.

Several subsequent in vivo studies have demonstrated a positive activity for hydroalcoholic nettle extracts in rat diabetic models after ip injection, including beta cell preservation,[70] neuroprotective effects[71,72] and hepatoprotective activity.[73] However, no protective effect on the kidneys was demonstrated.[74]

Of four medicinal plants from Morocco tested for hypoglycaemic activity in streptozotocin-induced diabetic rats at 400 mg/L of aqueous extract in drinking water, nettle leaf showed the lowest activity.[75] In contrast nettle extract was the most active after ip injection.

Antioxidant and hepatic activities (nettle leaf)

An in vitro study demonstrated antioxidant activity for an aqueous extract of nettle leaf.[76] Amounts of 50, 100 and 250 µg demonstrated 39%, 66% and 98% inhibition of linoleic acid emulsion peroxidation, respectively. This was compared with alpha-tocopherol (100 µg), which produced only 30% inhibition. At the same amounts, nettle also exhibited effective reducing power, superoxide anion radical and hydrogen peroxide scavenging activity and metal chelating ability.

In a forced swimming test, both nettle (1% w/w dried leaf in food) and exercise were found to reduce free radical concentrations in the rat brain.[77] It was suggested that nettle was an effective antioxidant capable of prolonging cerebral cell survival. Another in vivo experiment suggested a potential activity of oral doses of nettle for the prevention of oxidative stress in muscle tissue, as assessed in rats.[78]

An 80% ethanolic extract of nettle (50 and 100 mg/kg/day for 14 days, oral) was investigated for its effects on various liver parameters including phase I and phase II enzymes, antioxidant enzymes, lactate dehydrogenase, lipid peroxidation and sulphydryl groups in mice.[79] The extract significantly lowered the activity of cytochrome P450, lactate dehydrogenase, NADPH-cytochrome P450 reductase, total sulphydryl groups, non-protein sulphydryl groups and protein-bound sulphydryl groups. It also considerably increased cytochrome b5, NADH-cytochrome b5 reductase, glutathione S-transferase, DT-diaphorase, glutathione peroxidase, glutathione reductase, superoxide dismutase (SOD) and catalase in the liver. The extract was also effective in inducing glutathione S-transferase, DT-diaphorase, SOD and catalase activity in the forestomach, and SOD and catalase activity in the lung at both doses. Hence the extract induced both phase II and antioxidant enzymes. Follow-up research using the same doses and model found that activity of the phase I enzyme aniline 4-hydroxylase was increased in the livers of mice.[80]

Cardiovascular activity

Nettle is a popular antihypertensive treatment in Morocco and several in vitro and in vivo studies have sought to understand the potential mechanisms behind this use.[81–83] In one in vitro study, a nettle root extract fraction demonstrated vasorelaxant properties in rat aorta (via the release of endothelial nitric oxide and the opening of potassium channels) and exerted a negative inotropic action in guinea pig atria.[81] The same fraction also demonstrated a transient hypotensive activity in rats after iv injection. An in vivo study in rats compared the effects of continuous intravenous perfusion (1.25 h) of an aqueous extract of aerial parts (4 mg/kg/h or 24 mg/kg/h) with furosemide (2 mg/kg/h).[82] Dose-dependent hypotensive and diuretic effects were demonstrated. However, the higher dose of nettle appeared to produce a toxic effect, as blood pressure did not normalise during the recovery period.

Nettle leaf has been shown to inhibit platelet aggregation in vitro.[84–86] In one study, flavonoids isolated from the plant produced a significant effect on thrombin-, ADP-, collagen- and adrenaline (epinephrine)- induced platelet aggregation.[86] Aqueous nettle leaf extract (150 mg/kg/day for 30 days, oral) also demonstrated hypocholesterolaemic activity in rats fed a high fat diet, decreasing total and LDL-cholesterol and thereby improving the LDL/HDL-cholesterol ratio and plasma total apoB.[87] These findings were confirmed in hypercholesterolaemic rats for a nettle leaf extract at oral doses of 100 and 300 mg/kg.[88] In another study the 90% ethanolic extract of nettle leaf (100 mg/kg, oral) decreased LDL-cholesterol, whereas the aqueous extract (100 mg/kg, oral) increased HDL-cholesterol in mice fed a cholesterol-rich diet.[89]

Other activity

UDA, a lectin isolated from nettle root, demonstrated potent inhibition of chitin-containing fungal growth in vitro (*Trichoderma hamatum*, *Phycomyces blakesleeanus*, *Botrytis cinerea*) and exhibited binding specificity toward chitin. The antifungal activity of UDA differs from the action of chitinases and it acts synergistically with these in inhibiting fungal growth.[90,91] This activity of UDA may be applicable to topical application. UDA has also demonstrated antiviral,[92,93] cytotoxic,[94] immunomodulatory and mitogenic[95,96] and anticancer activities,[97,98] mainly in vitro. However, such activities are uncertain for normal oral doses of nettle root preparations due to the poor bioavailability of UDA (see the Pharmacokinetics section).

An aqueous alkaline extract of nettle leaf demonstrated antibacterial activity in vitro. It depressed the growth of staphylococci (500 µg/mL), Sporozoa (62.5 µg/mL)[99] and inhibited the protease activity of botulinum neurotoxin type A.[100] In another in vitro study, the aqueous extract of nettle leaves (250 µg/disc) demonstrated activity against *Pseudomonas aeruginosa*, *Escherichia coli*, *Proteus mirabilis*, *Citrobacter koseri*, *Staphylococcus aureus*, *Streptococcus pneumoniae*, *Enterobacter aerogenes*, *Micrococcus luteus*, *Staphylococcus epidermidis* and *Candida albicans*.[76]

Three flavonoid glycosides isolated from nettle leaf, namely quercetin-3-O-rutinoside, kaempherol-3-O-rutinoside and isorhamnetin-3-O-glucoside, showed immunostimulatory activity on neutrophils in vitro.[101]

No significant diuretic effect was observed in rats after oral treatment with nettle leaf extract (1 g/kg) during a 2 h observation period, but urinary (and potassium ion) excretion increased after intraperitoneal injection (500 mg/kg).[53] However, 45 mL/day of nettle leaf juice did exert an apparent diuretic activity in an early open label clinical trial.[102]

An aqueous-ethanolic extract of nettle leaf demonstrated in vitro inhibition of several key inflammatory events related to seasonal allergies, including activity against the histamine-1 receptor and inhibition of mast cell tryptase.[103]

Pharmacokinetics

Oral administration of radiolabelled UDA indicated excretion occurred via the gut and kidneys.[104] Following oral administration of 20 mg UDA to volunteers and patients, it was excreted with the faeces (30% to 50%) and via urine (<1%).[105] This indicates that the bioavailability of UDA is low, with a significant proportion excreted unchanged from the digestive tract.

Clinical trials

Benign prostatic hyperplasia

In a number of uncontrolled clinical trials conducted from 1979 to 2004, nettle root extract demonstrated improvement of urological symptomatology in BPH patients. Since these have been comprehensively reviewed elsewhere,[106,107] only some key studies are discussed below. The dosage ranged from 600 to 1200 mg/day of nettle root extract (5:1) over 3 weeks to 20 months.[108–117] In a large multicentre observational trial conducted in 4051 patients with BPH at various stages, a reduction in nocturia (by 50%) was observed after 8 to 9 weeks.[111] In another similar multicentre trial, results for 4396 patients indicated improvement in 78% of patients after 3 months and in 91% of patients after 6 months. Urinary frequency and mean urinary flow were significantly improved. Patients received 1200 mg of nettle root extract (5:1) daily for 3 months and 500 mg/day for the remaining period.[112]

In an uncontrolled study involving 253 patients who received nettle root extract (1200 mg/day (5:1) for 12 weeks), significant decreases (p<0.05) in SHBG, oestradiol and oestrone, as well as decreases in prostate volume and residual urine, were observed.[116] Long-term treatment over 8 to 10 years of 226 BPH patients found that therapy with nettle root extract could maintain more than 50% of patients without the need for surgery. Using this long-term treatment, the typical enlargement of the prostate was not evident.[118]

Zinc, calcium and sodium levels in prostatic secretions from patients with BPH were investigated in a randomised, controlled, open trial. The treated group comprised 20 patients who received 1800 mg of nettle root extract (5:1) daily for 7 days. Both treated and control patients had samples taken on the first day (prior to treatment) and the seventh day. The 7-day specimens from treated patients revealed a significant drop in the zinc level, and a correlation was found to exist between the zinc and calcium levels. No difference was observed between the first-day and seventh-day samples in the control group. The authors concluded that nettle root extract may alter the zinc-testosterone metabolism and lower zinc secretion in adenomatous tissue.[119]

Liquid preparations of nettle root have also been successfully assessed in uncontrolled trials.[120,121] Sixty-seven patients experienced a reduction of nocturnal micturition frequency after 6 months of treatment with nettle root tincture (5 mL of 1:5 per day). In those with a mild condition, symptoms could be relieved within about 3 weeks.[121]

Given that there is a significant placebo effect in BPH, more relevant are the controlled trials using a placebo or active treatment. These are reviewed below.

Nettle root extract (1200 mg (5:1) per day) demonstrated a significant decrease in urinary frequency (p<0.05) and serum levels of SHBG in a double blind, placebo-controlled trial with 40 BPH patients.[122] In a placebo-controlled clinical trial involving 79 BPH patients, nettle root extract (600 mg/day (5:1) for 6 to 8 weeks) was superior to placebo in all parameters measured (urinary flow, urinary volume, residual urine).[123] In a similar trial design, 50 patients (BPH stages I and II) treated with nettle root extract (600 mg/day (5:1) for 9 weeks) demonstrated a significant decrease in SHBG (p<0.0005) and significant improvements in micturition volume and maximum urinary flow. There was also an improvement in average flow for the herbal group.[124]

A randomised, double blind, placebo-controlled, partial crossover comparative trial of nettle root for the treatment of lower urinary symptoms (LUTS) secondary to BPH was completed in 558 men.[125] At the end of the 6-month trial, 81% of patients in the active treatment group reported improvements in LUTS compared with 16% in the placebo group (p<0.001). The International Prostate Symptom Score (IPSS) dropped from 19.8 to 11.8 in the nettle group and from 19.2 to 17.7 for the placebo group (p=0.002). Peak flow rate improved by 8.2 mL/s for treated patients and 3.4 mL/s for the placebo recipients (p<0.05). Post-void residual urine volume (PVR) decreased from 73 to 36 mL in the nettle group (versus no appreciable change in the placebo group, p<0.001), while prostaespecific antigen and testosterone remained the same in both groups. There was a small non-significant decrease in prostate size for the herbal group only. The dose used was 360 mg/day of an unspecified nettle extract.

In a randomised, 12-month double blind, placebo-controlled, multicentre trial involving 246 patients with BPH, nettle root (459 mg/day extract, about 5 g of root) was shown to be a safe and effective treatment.[126] The nettle group reported a significant decrease in IPSS compared with placebo (p<0.02), although the difference in the reduction between the two groups was small. There was less irritation and infection and fewer side effects than placebo; however, peak flow and PVR were not statistically altered relative to the placebo treatment.

Combination therapy for BPH

In an uncontrolled, prospective, multicentre observational study, the efficacy and tolerability of combined nettle root and saw palmetto extract in 2080 patients with BPH stage I–II were rated as 'very good' or 'good' by physicians. An improvement in pathological findings and in obstructive and irritative symptoms was observed: for example, urinary flow rate and voided volume increased by 30% and nocturia was halved. Fifteen patients (0.7%) were suspected of developing mild side effects.[127] Other uncontrolled studies of combinations with nettle root have been reviewed elsewhere.[107]

In a placebo-controlled clinical trial, 40 patients with BPH were treated with a nettle and saw palmetto extract combination (240 mg/day of 10:1 extract of nettle root, 320 mg/day liposterolic extract of saw palmetto) or placebo over 24 weeks. Significant improvement was observed in the herbal treatment group, with peak flow up by 23% compared to 4%

in placebo (p<0.05) and IPSS down by 40% compared to 7% (p<0.05). PVR was also better compared to placebo (−33% versus −13%). A curious aspect of this study was the marked placebo effect that developed in a 24-week unblinded phase following the placebo phase. Nonetheless, active treatment remained significantly better than placebo.[128]

In a randomised, double blind, multicentre clinical trial, the efficacy of the above combined nettle and saw palmetto extracts was compared with the drug finasteride in the treatment of BPH stages I–II. Five hundred and sixteen patients completed a 48-week treatment with the herbal combination or finasteride (5 mg/day).[129,130] Both treatments significantly improved urinary flow and IPSS and there was no significant difference between them. Fewer adverse events were reported for the herbal combination, especially in terms of diminished ejaculation volume, erectile dysfunction and headache. Economic evaluation revealed that the herbal treatment was also more cost-effective.[129]

The efficacy and tolerability of the same combination of saw palmetto and nettle root was investigated in elderly, male patients suffering from LUTS caused by BPH in a prospective multicentre trial.[131] A total of 257 patients (129 and 128, respectively) were randomised to treatment with the herbal combination or placebo (127 and 126 were evaluable for efficacy). Following a single-blind placebo run-in phase of 2 weeks, the patients received the study medication under double blind conditions over a period of 24 weeks. The double blind treatment was followed by an open label period of 24 weeks during which all patients were administered the active treatment. Patients treated with the saw palmetto/nettle root combination exhibited a higher reduction in IPSS after the 24 weeks of double blind treatment than patients in the placebo group (6 points versus 4 points; p=0.003). This applied to obstructive as well as irritative symptoms, and in patients with moderate or severe symptoms at baseline. The patients originally randomised to placebo showed a marked improvement in LUTS (as measured by the IPSS) after being switched to the herbal combination during the open period (p=0.01). The tolerability of the herbal combination was comparable with the placebo.

In a long-term, open label follow-up of the patients involved in this trial, 219 patients received the herbal combination for another 48 weeks, resulting in a total observation period of 96 weeks.[132] Between baseline and week 96, IPSS was reduced by 53%, peak and average urinary flow both increased by 19% and residual volume decreased by 44%. During the follow-up 61 adverse events were reported, corresponding to one event in each 1181 days of treatment.

The same combination of saw palmetto and nettle root reduced the subjective symptoms of BPH to an extent comparable to the well-researched alpha1-adrenoceptor antagonist drug tamsulosin.[133] The two treatments were administered in a prospective, randomised, double blind, double-dummy, multicentre trial to patients suffering from BPH and not requiring surgery. Tamsulosin was administered at the full therapeutic dose of 0.4 mg/day. After a single blind, placebo run-in phase of 2 weeks, patients who were still eligible were randomised to double blind treatment lasting 60 weeks. By week 60 the change from baseline in IPSS was similar for both treatments.

Although treatment with tamsulosin led to larger improvements in maximum and average urinary flow than the herbal combination, both treatments produced clinically relevant, beneficial effects for many of the urodynamic parameters assessed. A reduction in prostatic volume was not observed for either treatment. Fewer adverse events were reported for the herbal combination (one adverse event in 1514 treatment days) than for tamsulosin (one adverse event in 1164 treatment days).

In a randomised, double blind clinical trial, 134 patients received either two capsules of a nettle/Pygeum preparation (each capsule containing 300 mg of nettle root extract (5:1) and 25 mg of Pygeum bark extract (200:1)) or two capsules containing half this dosage, twice daily for 8 weeks. The lower dosage was found to be effective, since urinary flow, nocturia and residual volume improved equally with both. However, the lack of a placebo control makes this conclusion tenuous. Five patients reported adverse effects.[134] In a randomised, double blind clinical trial involving 63 patients, a nettle/Pygeum combination (one capsule: 300 mg of nettle root extract (5:1) and 25 mg of Pygeum bark extract (200:1)) was therapeutically superior to Pygeum extract alone, particularly in reducing urine flow and residual urine volume. The two preparations were equally effective in the control of nocturia. Both treatments were equally well tolerated.[135] However, a small double blind, randomised, placebo-controlled clinical trial of the same preparation in 49 men failed to show statistically significant results after 6 months of treatment.[136] Changes in IPSS (21.6% reduction in the herbal group as compared to 19.7% for placebo), quality of life index (9.26% versus 5.98%), rectal examination and maximum urinary flow rate (17.2% versus 13.3%) were similar in both groups.

In a prospective, randomised, open trial, 143 patients with bacterial prostatitis received either a 14-day course of 600 mg/day prulifloxacin combined with a natural combination, or the antibiotic alone.[137] The natural combination contained saw palmetto (160 mg/day extract, 30% fatty acids and sterols), nettle root (120 mg/day extract, 0.4% beta-sitosterol), quercitin (100 mg/day) and turmeric (200 mg/day extract, 95% curcumin). Compared with prulifloxacin alone, combined therapy resulted in significantly better symptom relief at both the 1-month and 6-month visits (p<0.001), as assessed by IPSS and the Chronic Prostatitis Symptom Index. However, it has been pointed out that prulifloxacin is still an investigational treatment for this condition.[138]

Arthritis

A case was reported of a man with osteoarthritis and joint narrowing in the left hip who self-prescribed the application of nettle to the region after NSAID therapy did not ease the pain. Counter-irritation with fresh nettle leaves over several weeks produced a remarkable improvement and reduction of pain, to the extent he was able to decrease the application of nettle to once every few days.[139]

Following a positive case series in 18 people self-treating with nettle sting,[140] a randomised, controlled, double blind, crossover study in 27 patients with osteoarthritic pain at the base of the thumb or index finger was undertaken.[141] Patients applied fresh stinging nettle leaf daily for 1 week to the painful area. The effect of this treatment was compared with that of a placebo (white deadnettle leaf, *Lamium album*). Treatment was for 1 week with a 5-week washout period before the second treatment phase of 1 week. Reductions on both a visual analogue scale (pain) and health assessment questionnaire (disability) were significantly greater for nettle than placebo (p=0.026 and p=0.0027, respectively). The localised rash or slight itching from the nettle sting was acceptable to 23 of the 27 patients.

In a pilot, single blind, placebo-controlled study, 42 patients with chronic knee pain and a presumptive diagnosis of osteoarthritis received either topical treatment (nettle sting) with *Urtica dioica* leaf or a placebo leaf (*Urtica galeopsifolia*) for 1 week.[142] Nettle leaf was not superior to the placebo in terms of the WOMAC symptom score. However, the placebo treatment was probably active, as a stinging effect was noted from it.

The effect of a cream containing 13.3% of an extract of stinging nettle leaf was evaluated in 23 patients with osteoarthritis in an open label trial.[143] There was a mean reduction of 4.2 in the WOMAC score from a baseline of 17.2. Mild side effects were seen in two patients and many trial participants requested a continuance of the treatment at the completion of the study. However, the lack of a placebo control limits the conclusions that can be made from this study.

All trials of the oral use of nettle leaf extracts in arthritis have not used a blinded placebo control, hence results must be regarded as preliminary. In an open, multicentre, comparative trial with NSAID therapy, oral doses of 1340 mg/day of nettle leaf extract (about 10 g of leaf) exhibited comparable efficacy in terms of a reduction in pain and improvement of motility, with a very good tolerability. The trial was conducted over 3 weeks in 219 patients with rheumatic articular complaints.[144] Thirty-seven patients with acute arthritis completed an open, randomised trial comparing the effects of a combination of nettle leaf (50 g/day stewed fresh young leaf) with 50 mg/day diclofenac against 200 mg/day diclofenac over 2 weeks. C-reactive protein and total joint scores improved significantly in both groups, with a median score change of about 70% relative to the initial value. The authors concluded that stewed nettle leaf may enhance the antirheumatic effectiveness of NSAIDs. (A 50 mg daily dose of diclofenac is below a therapeutic level.)[145]

In an open pilot study, patients suffering from painful osteoarthritis and arthritis of the knee achieved a reduction in NSAID use of 50% by consuming a proprietary nettle leaf preparation (1.34 g per day of an 8 to 10:1 extract).[146] A multicentre, uncontrolled, postmarketing surveillance study was undertaken over a 3-week period to research the safety and efficacy of a nettle leaf preparation in 8,955 patients with arthritis (7,935 had osteoarthritis, the remainder suffered from rheumatoid arthritis).[147] Results from a 12-point self-rating scale indicated that 82% of patients felt that the treatment had relieved their symptoms. In addition, 38% could have their NSAID therapy reduced and 26% no longer required NSAID therapy. Only 1.2% of patients showed minor side effects, such as unspecified gastrointestinal problems. A 12-month post-marketing surveillance study involving 819 patients with osteoarthritis of the knee observed only minor adverse events in 3% and a reduction in clinical symptoms by 61% after 1.34 g/day of an 8:1 to 10:1 nettle leaf extract.[148]

In an open label study, 20 patients with acute exacerbation of osteoarthritis of the knee or hip received 290 to 435 mg/day of a 95% propanolic extract of nettle leaf (19:1 to 33:1) for 12 weeks.[149] In all, 17 patients completed the study and reported considerable symptom improvements. Release of some inflammatory cytokines was reduced compared with baseline. A second open study in 763 osteoarthritis patients, using the same extract and dosage range over 6 months, observed significant reductions in symptoms and NSAID use.[150]

Other conditions

In a randomised, double blind, placebo-controlled clinical trial, the efficacy of a homeopathic combination gel (homeopathic mother tinctures of nettle, Echinacea, *Ledum palustre* and witchhazel extract) was compared with placebo in the treatment of insect bites. Although the homeopathic gel reduced erythema development (p=0.098), there was no difference for itch relief, even though a reduction in erythema may reduce itching.[151]

Sixty-nine volunteers completed a randomised, double blind, placebo-controlled study investigating the effect of a freeze-dried preparation of nettle leaf on allergic rhinitis. Volunteers were advised to take two capsules of nettle (300 mg/capsule) or placebo at the onset of symptoms. Assessment was based on daily symptom diaries and global response recorded after 1 week of therapy. In the global assessment, participants were asked to compare the medicines with previous medications and whether they would buy the medicine for future use. Nettle was rated higher than placebo in the global assessments, but was only slightly higher in the diary data.[152]

A German study found that intake of nettle and dandelion juices improved skin parameters in healthy women.[153] Both active and control groups used a moisturising cream, but only the active group took the herbal juices. Skin hydration improved significantly after 6 weeks in the experimental group (p<0.05). Elasticity was also significantly improved compared with the control group. After 6 weeks of treatment, volunteers in the active group rated their skin condition as significantly improved, whereas there was little change for the control group.

In an open label study, an expressed juice of nettle leaf (10 to 20 mL/day) was administered for 12 weeks to 114 patients (81 women, 33 men, median age 55 years) for the European indications (see under Regulatory status) of irrigation of the urinary tract (and thereby prevention of kidney gravel) and as a supportive therapy for rheumatic complaints.[154] Physician-rated symptoms were significantly improved for both indications at 6 weeks (30% and 55%, respectively) and at 12 weeks (65% and 50%, respectively), and patients' ratings reflected similar improvements. A strong increase in urinary flow was noted by the patients, as were marked decreases in urinary pain and burning, dysuria, and joint stiffness and pain. The treatment was well tolerated, but the lack of a placebo group limits the usefulness of these findings.

Toxicology and other safety data

Toxicology

The LD$_{50}$ values for nettle leaf infusion and nettle leaf decoction administered intravenously to mice were 1.92 g/kg and 1.72 g/kg, respectively. The LD$_{50}$ in chronic experiments with rats given nettle leaf infusion by gavage was 1.31 g/kg.[155] An aqueous extract of nettle leaf had an LD$_{50}$ of 3.5 g/kg after ip administration to mice.[67]

Nettle leaf did not demonstrate any antifertility activity when administered orally to rats.[156] Nettle leaf tea demonstrated weak genotoxic activity in a somatic assay. Quercetin and rutin also exhibited weak activity.[157]

Contraindications

Patients who are allergic to nettle stings should not apply the fresh or unprocessed dried leaves topically.

Special warnings and precautions

The use of nettle root for benign prostatic hyperplasia should occur under professional supervision and include monitoring of the state of the prostate.[158]

Interactions

None known.

Use in pregnancy and lactation

Category B2-no increase in frequency of malformation or other harmful effects on the fetus from limited use in women. Animal studies are lacking.

The lignans in nettle root, as well as their intestinal transformation products (enterodiol and enterolactone), are known to bind to SHBG in vitro.[159] The affinity of (−)-3,4-divanillyltetrahydrofuran was notably high.[19] This may provide a mechanism for the claimed benefit of nettle root in BPH, but is not thought to pose a risk in pregnancy. An ethanol extract of nettle aerial parts (250 mg/kg) did not demonstrate any significant anti-implantation activity when administered orally to female rats.[160]

Both nettle leaf and root are compatible with breastfeeding.

Effects on ability to drive and use machines

No negative influence is expected.

Side effects

Nettle stings are largely due to the histamine and serotonin introduced by the nettle hair (each contains 6.1 ng and 33.25 pg, respectively). However, the persistence of the stinging sensation suggests the presence of substances in nettle fluid directly toxic to nerves or capable of inducing the secondary release of other mediators (see the earlier discussion of such factors).[161] The result is an urticaria that generally, but not always, passes quickly. No such reaction is expected from ingesting the extracted leaf.

Both an immediate and delayed hypersensitivity reaction was exhibited in a child after falling into a nettle patch.[162] A man who had developed a contact dermatitis after treating his eczema with a poultice of herbs including chamomile also manifested a diffuse oedematous gingivostomatitis. He regularly drank nettle tea. This reaction was believed to be an allergic contact reaction to the chamomile and also the nettle (and not an irritant reaction).[163] Generalised urticaria has been noted in a neonate after the breastfeeding mother applied a nettle leaf decoction onto her nipples.[164] However, nettle leaf has been noted to have relatively low allergenic potential.[165]

In one multicentre trial of the effect of nettle root in 4051 BPH patients, mild side effects affecting the gastrointestinal tract were experienced in 0.7% of cases.[166] (See also the Clinical trials section for further information on adverse reactions.)

A case of hypoglycaemia was noted in a 78-year-old diabetic man taking a complex herbal formulation for BPH that included nettle leaf and root.[167] Gynaecomastia in a man and hyperoestrogenism in a woman were associated with the regular consumption of nettle tea (presumably leaf, although the authors discuss the properties of nettle root in their implication of causality).[168]

Overdosage

No incidents found in the published literature.

Safety in children

No information available, but adverse effects are not expected.

Regulatory status in selected countries

Nettle is listed in the *United States Pharmacopeia–National Formulary* (USP34–NF 29, 2011).

Nettle leaf is covered by a positive Commission E monograph and has the following applications:

- Internally and externally: only as supportive treatment for rheumatic complaints
- Internally: for irrigation in inflammation of the urinary tract and in the prevention and treatment of kidney gravel. The following warning is advised: in irrigation therapy, care must be taken to ensure an abundant fluid intake.

Nettle root may be used for difficulties in urination associated with stages I and II prostate adenoma. The following warning is advised: this remedy only improves the problems associated with an enlarged prostate without reducing the actual enlargement itself. A doctor should be consulted at regular intervals.

Nettle is on the UK General Sale List.

Nettle does not have GRAS status. However, it is freely available as a 'dietary supplement' in the USA under DSHEA legislation (1994 Dietary Supplement Health and Education Act). Nettle has been present in over-the-counter digestive aid drug products. The FDA, however, advises that: 'based on evidence currently available, there is inadequate data to establish general recognition of the safety and effectiveness of these ingredients for the specified uses'.

Nettle is not included in Part 4 of Schedule 4 of the Therapeutic Goods Act Regulations of Australia and is freely available for sale.

References

1. British Herbal Medicine Association. *British Herbal Compendium*, vol. 1. Bournemouth: BHMA; 1992. pp. 166–167.

2. Grieve M. *A Modern Herbal*, vol. 2. New York: Dover Publications; 1971. pp. 574–579.

3. Felter HW, Lloyd JU. *King's American Dispensatory*. 18th ed. rev 3, vol. 2. 1905. Portland: Reprinted by Eclectic Medical Publications; 1983. pp. 2032–2034.

4. Sales H. *Culpeper's Complete Herbal and English Physician*. Reproduced from an original edition published in 1826. Bath: Pitman Press; 1981. p. 106.

5. British Herbal Medicine Association Scientific Committee. *British Herbal Pharmacopoeia*. Cowling: BHMA; 1983. pp. 224–225.

6. Piekos R, Paslawaska S. *Planta Med*. 1976;30(4):331–336.

7. Launert EL. *The Hamlyn Guide to Edible and Medicinal Plants of Britain and Northern Europe*. London: Hamlyn; 1981. p. 118.

8. Chiej R. *The Macdonald Encyclopedia of Medicinal Plants*. London: Macdonald; 1984. Entry no. 319.

9. Bruneton J. *Pharmacognosy, Phytochemistry, Medicinal Plants*. Paris: Lavoisier Publishing; 1995. pp. 603–605.

10. Scholz H, Kascha S, Zingerle H. *Fortschr Med*. 1980;98(39):1525–1526.

11. Wichtl M, ed. Brinckmann JA, Lindenmaier MP (translators). *Herbal Drugs and Phytopharmaceuticals*. 3rd ed. Boca Raton: CRC; 2004. p. 619.

12. Chaurasia N, Wichtl M. *Planta Med*. 1987;53(5):432–433.

13. Pinelli P, Ieri F, Vignolini P, et al. *J Agric Food Chem*. 2008;56(19):9127–9132.

14. Lutomski J, Speichert H. *Pharm Unserer Zeit*. 1983;12(6):181–186.

15. Barlow RB, Dixon RO. *Biochem J*. 1973;132(1):15–18.

16. Sapronova NN, Grinkevich NI, Orlova LP, et al. *Rastitel Nye Resursy*. 1989;25(2):243–247.

17. Szabo Z, Boddi K, Mark L, et al. *J Agric Food Chem*. 2006;54(12):4082–4086.

18. Chaurasia N, Wichtl M. *J Nat Prod*. 1987;50(5):881–885.

19. Schottner M, Gansser D, Spiteller G. *Planta Med*. 1997;63(6):529–532.

20. Peumans WJ, De Ley M, Broekaert WF. *FEBS Lett*. 1984;177(1):99–103.

21. Bisset NG, ed. *Herbal Drugs and Phytopharmaceuticals*. Stuttgart: Medpharm Scientific Publishers; 1994. pp. 508–509.

22. Schilcher H. *Phytotherapie in der Urologie*. Stuttgart: Hippokrates; 1992. pp. 84–88.

23. Gansser D, Spiteller G. *Z Naturforsch [C]*. 1995;50(1–2):98–104.

24. Schottner M, Spiteller G, Gansser D. *J Nat Prod*. 1998;61(1):119–121.

25. Hryb DJ, Khan MS, Romas NA, et al. *Planta Med*. 1995;61(1):31–32.

26. Schmidt K. *Fortschr Med*. 1983;101(15):713–716.

27. Ziegler H. *Fortschr Med*. 1982;100(39):1832–1834.

28. Enderle-Schmidt U, Gutschank WM, Aumuller G. In: Bauer HW, ed. *Benigne Prostatahyperplasie II*. München: Zuckschwerdt; 1988. pp. 56–61.

29. Rausch U, Aumuller G, Eicheler W, et al. In: Rutishauser G, ed. *Benigne Prostatahyperplasie III*. München: Zuckschwerdt; 1992. pp. 117–124.

30. Lichius JJ, Muth C. *Planta Med*. 1997;63(4):307–310.

31. Daube G. In: Bauer HW, ed. *Benigne Prostatahyperplasie II*. München: Zuckschwerdt; 1988. pp. 63–66.

32. Lichius JJ, Renneberg H, Blaschek W, et al. *Planta Med*. 1999;65(7):666–668.

33. Nahata A, Dixit VK. *Andrologia*. 2011 [Epub ahead of print].

34. Ziegler H. *Fortschr Med*. 1983;101(45):2112–2114.

35. Oberholzer M, Schambock A, Rugendorff EW, et al. In: Bauer HW, ed. *Benigne Prostatahyperplasie*. München: Zuckschwerdt; 1986. pp. 13–17.

36. Hirano T, Homma M, Oka K. *Planta Med*. 1994;60(1):30–33.

37. Farnsworth WE. *Med Hypotheses*. 1993;41(4):358–362.

38. Hartmann RW, Mark M, Soldati F. *Phytomedicine*. 1996;3(2):121–128.

39. Gansser D, Spiteller G. *Planta Med*. 1995;61(2):138–140.

40. Koch E. In: Loew D, Rietbrock N, eds. *Phytopharmaka in Forschung und klinischer Anwendung*. Darmstadt: Steinkopff Verlag; 1995. p. 69.

41. Kraus R, Spiteller G, Bartsch W. *Liebigs Ann Chem*. 1991;4:335–339.

42. Koch E, Biber A. *Urologe B*. 1994;34: 90–95.

43. Koch E, Biber A. In: Loew D, Rietbrock N, eds. *Phytopharmaka in Forschung und Klinischer Anwendung*. Darmstadt: Steinkopff Verlag; 1995. p. 69.

44. Rhodes L, Primka RL, Berman C, et al. *Prostate*. 1993;22(1):43–51.

45. Koch E, Jaggy H, Chatterjee SS. *Naunyn Schmiedebergs Arch Pharmacol*. 1995;351:R57.

46. Wolff H, Bezold G, Zebhauser M, et al. *J Androl*. 1991;12(5):331–334.

47. Koch E. In: Loew D, Rietbrock N, eds. *Phytopharmaka in Forschung und Klinischer Anwendung*. Darmstadt: Steinkopff Verlag; 1995. p. 70.

48. Dunzendorfer U. *Z Phytother*. 1984;5: 800–804.

49. Konrad L, Muller HH, Lenz C, et al. *Planta Med*. 2000;66(1):44–47.

50. Lichius JJ, Lenz C, Lindemann P, et al. *Pharmazie*. 1999;54(10):768–771.

51. Obertreis B, Giller K, Teucher T, et al. *Arzneim-Forsch*. 1996;46(1):52–56.

52. Obertreis B, Ruttkowski T, Teucher T, et al. *Arzneimittelforschung*. 1996;46(4): 389–394.

53. Tita B, Faccendini P, Bello U, et al. *Pharmacol Res*. 1993;27(suppl 1):21–22.

54. Wagner H, Willer F, Samtleben R, et al. *Phytomedicine*. 1994;1:213–224.

55. Teucher T, Obertreis B, Ruttkowski T, et al. *Arzneimittelforschung*. 1996;46(9): 906–910.

56. Schulze-Tanzil G, de SP, Behnke B, et al. *Histol Histopathol*. 2002;17(2):477–485.

57. Riehemann K, Behnke B, Schulze-Osthoff K. *FEBS Lett*. 1999;442(1):89–94.

58. Broer J, Behnke B. *J Rheumatol*. 2002;29(4):659–666.

59. Konrad A, Mahler M, Arni S, et al. *Int J Colorectal Dis*. 2005;20(1):9–17.

60. Marrassini C, Acevedo C, Mino J, et al. *Phytother Res*. 2010;24(12): 1807–1812.

61. Oliver F, Amon EU, Breathnach A, et al. *Clin Exp Dermatol*. 1991;16(1):1–7.

62. Czarnetzki BM, Thiele T, Rosenbach T. *Int Arch Allergy Appl Immunol*. 1990;91(1):43–46.

63. Antonopoulou S, Demopoulos CA, Andrikopoulos NK. *J Agric Food Chem*. 1996;44(10):3052–3056.

64. Cummings AJ, Olsen M. *Wilderness Environ Med*. 2011;22(2):136–139.

65. Swanston-Flatt SK, Day C, Flatt PR, et al. *Diabetes Res*. 1989;10(2):69–73.

66. Neef H, Declercq P, Laekeman G. *Phytother Res*. 1995;9(1):45–48.

67. Bnouham M, Merhfour FZ, Ziyyat A, et al. *Fitoterapia*. 2003;74(7–8):677–681.
68. Farzami B, Ahmadvand D, Vardasbi S, et al. *J Ethnopharmacol*. 2003;89(1):47–53.
69. Domola MS, Vu V, Robson-Doucette CA, et al. *Phytother Res*. 2010;24(suppl 2):S175–S182.
70. Golalipour MJ, Khori V. *Pak J Biol Sci*. 2007;10(8):1200–1204.
71. Fazeli SA, Gharravi AM, Ghafari S, et al. *Folia Morphol (Warsz)*. 2008;67(3):196–204.
72. Jahanshahi M, Golalipour MJ, Afshar M. *Folia Morphol (Warsz)*. 2009;68(2):93–97.
73. Golalipour MJ, Ghafari S, Afshar M. *Turk J Gastroenterol*. 2010;21(3):262–269.
74. Golalipour MJ, Gharravi AM, Ghafari S, et al. *Pak J Biol Sci*. 2007;10(21):3875–3879.
75. Bnouham M, Merhfour FZ, Ziyyat A, et al. *Hum Exp Toxicol*. 2010;29(10):865–871.
76. Gulcin I, Kufrevioglu OI, Oktay M, et al. *J Ethnopharmacol*. 2004;90(2–3):205–215.
77. Toldy A, Stadler K, Sasvari M, et al. *Brain Res Bull*. 2005;65(6):487–493.
78. Cetinus E, Kilinc M, Inanc F, et al. *Tohoku J Exp Med*. 2004;203(3):215–221.
79. Ozen T, Korkmaz H. *Phytomedicine*. 2003;10(5):405–415.
80. Ozen T, Korkmaz H. *Acta Pol Pharm*. 2009;66(3):305–309.
81. Testai L, Chericoni S, Calderone V, et al. *J Ethnopharmacol*. 2002;81(1):105–109.
82. Tahri A, Yamani S, Legssyer A, et al. *J Ethnopharmacol*. 2000;73(1–2):95–100.
83. Legssyer A, Ziyyat A, Mekhfi H, et al. *Phytother Res*. 2002;16(6):503–507.
84. Pierre S, Crosbie L, Duttaroy AK. *Platelets*. 2005;16(8):469–473.
85. Mekhfi H, El Haouari M, Legssyer A, et al. *J Ethnopharmacol*. 2004;94(2–3):317–322.
86. El Haouari M, Bnouham M, Bendahou M, et al. *Phytother Res*. 2006;20(7):568–572.
87. Daher CF, Baroody KG, Baroody GM. *Fitoterapia*. 2006;77(3):183–188.
88. Nassiri-Asl M, Zamansoltani F, Abbasi E, et al. *Zhong Xi Yi Jie He Xue Bao*. 2009;7(5):428–433.
89. Avci G, Kupeli E, Eryavuz A, et al. *J Ethnopharmacol*. 2006;107(3):418–423.
90. Van Parijs J, Broekaert WF, Peumans WJ, et al. *Arch Int Physiol Biochim*. 1988;96(1):31.
91. Broekaert WF, Van Parijs J, Leyns F, et al. *Science*. 1989;245(4922):1100–1102.
92. Balzarini J, Neyts J, Schols D, et al. *Antiviral Res*. 1992;18(2):191–207.
93. Balzarini J, Van Laethem K, Hatse S, et al. *J Biol Chem*. 2005;280(49):41005–41014.
94. Wagner H, Willer F. In: Bauer HW, ed. *Benigne Prostatahyperplasie II*. München: Zuckschwerdt; 1988. pp. 51–54.
95. Musette P, Galelli A, Chabre H, et al. *Eur J Immunol*. 1996;26(8):1707–1711.
96. Koch E. In: Loew D, Rietbrock N, eds. *Phytopharmaka in Forschung und klinischer Anwendung*. Darmstadt: Steinkopff Verlag; 1995. p. 71.
97. Wagner H, Geiger WN, Boos G, et al. *Phytomedicine*. 1995;4:287–290.
98. Suh N, Luyengi L, Fong HH, et al. *Anticancer Res*. 1995;15(2):233–239.
99. Lezhneva LP, Murav'ev IA, Cherevatyi VS. *Rastilel Nye–Resursy*. 1986;22(2):255–257.
100. Gul N, Ahmed SA, Smith LA. *Basic Clin Pharmacol Toxicol*. 2004;95(5):215–219.
101. Akbay P, Basaran AA, Undeger U, et al. *Phytother Res*. 2003;17(1):34–37.
102. Kirchhoff HW. *Z Phytother*. 1983;4:621–626.
103. Roschek Jr B, Fink RC, McMichael M, et al. *Phytother Res*. 2009;23(7):920–926.
104. Geiger WN, Haak C, Wagner H. *2nd International Congress on Phytomedicine*. Munich: September 11–14, 1996.
105. Samtleben R, Boos G, Wagner H. *2nd International Congress on Phytomedicine*. Munich: September 11–14, 1996.
106. Chrubasik JE, Roufogalis BD, Wagner H, et al. *Phytomedicine*. 2007;14(7–8):568–579.
107. Upton R, ed. *Stinging Nettle Root: Urtica dioica L.* USA: AHP; 2010.
108. Barsom S, Bettermann AA. *Z Allg Med*. 1979;55(33):1947–1950.
109. Djulepa J. *Arztl Praxis*. 1982;63:2199–2202.
110. Tosch U. *Euromed*. 1983;6:1–3.
111. Stahl HP. *Z Allg Med*. 1984;60(3):128–132.
112. Friesen A. In: Bauer HW, ed. *Benigne Prostatahyperplasie II*. München: Zuckschwerdt; 1988. pp. 121–130.
113. Feiber H. In: Bauer HW, ed. *Benigne Prostatahyperplasie II*. München: Zuckschwerdt; 1988. pp. 75–82.
114. Romics I. *Int Urol Nephrol*. 1987;19(3):293–297.
115. Maar K. *Fortschr Med*. 1987;105(1):50–52.
116. Bauer HW, Sudhoff F, Dressler S. In: Bauer HW, ed. *Benigne Prostatahyperplasie II*. München: Zuckschwerdt; 1988. pp. 44–49.
117. Vandierendounck EJ, Burkhardt P. *Therapiewoche Schweiz*. 1986;2:892–895.
118. Ziegler H. *6th Phytotherapy Conference*. Berlin: October 5–7, 1995.
119. Romics I, Bach D. *Int Urol Nephrol*. 1991;23(1):45–49.
120. Goetz P. *Z Phytother*. 1989;10:175–178.
121. Belaiche P, Lievoux O. *Phytother Res*. 1991;5:267–269.
122. Fischer M, Wilbert D. In: Rutishauser G, ed. *Benigne Prostatahyperplasie III*. München: Zuckschwerdt; 1992. pp. 79–84.
123. Dathe G, Schmid H. *Urologe B*. 1987;27:223–226.
124. Vontobel HP, Herzog R, Rutishauser G, et al. *Urologe A*. 1985;24(1):49–51.
125. Safarinejad MR. *J Herb Pharmacother*. 2005;5(4):1–11.
126. Schneider T, Rubben H. *Urologe A*. 2004;43(3):302–306.
127. Schneider HJ, Honold E, Masuhr T. *Fortschr Med*. 1995;113(3):37–40.
128. Metzker H, Kieser M, Holscher U. *Urologe B*. 1996;36(4):292–300.
129. Sokeland J, Albrecht J. *Urologe A*. 1997;36(4):327–333.
130. Sokeland J. *BJU Int*. 2000;86(4):439–442.
131. Lopatkin N, Sivkov A, Walther C, et al. *World J Urol*. 2005;23(2):139–146.
132. Lopatkin N, Sivkov A, Schlafke S, et al. *Int Urol Nephrol*. 2007;39(4):1137–1146.
133. Engelmann U, Walther C, Bondarenko B, et al. *Arzneimittelforschung*. 2006;56(3):222–229.
134. Krzeski T, Kazon M, Borkowski A, et al. *Clin Ther*. 1993;15(6):1011–1020.
135. Montanari E, Mandressi A, Magri V, et al. *Informierte Arzt*. 1991;6A:593–598.
136. Melo EA, Bertero EB, Rios LA, et al. *Int Braz J Urol*. 2002;28(5):418–425.
137. Cai T, Mazzoli S, Bechi A, et al. *Int J Antimicrob Agents*. 2009;33(6):549–553.
138. Giannarini G, Autorino R. *Int J Antimicrob Agents*. 2009;34(3):283–284.
139. Randall CF. *Br J Gen Pract*. 1994;44(388):533–534.
140. Randall C, Meethan K, Randall H, et al. *Comp Ther Med*. 1999;7(3):126–131.
141. Randall C, Randall H, Dobbs F, et al. *J R Soc Med*. 2000;93:305–309.
142. Randall C, Dickens A, White A, et al. *Complement Ther Med*. 2008;16(2):66–72.
143. Rayburn K, Fleischbein E, Song J, et al. *Altern Ther Health Med*. 2009;15(4):60–61.
144. Sommer RG, Sinner B. *Therapiewoche*. 1996;46(1):44–49.
145. Chrubasik S, Enderlein W, Bauer R, et al. *Phytomedicine*. 1997;4(2):105–108.
146. Ramm S, Hansen C. *Therapiewoche*. 1996;28:3–6.
147. Buck G. *Z Phytother*. 1998;19(4):216.
148. Wolf F. *Kassenarzt*. 1998;44:52–54.
149. Wolf F, Gulbin K, Mlelke F. *Der Kassenarzt*. 2001;16:42–47.
150. Hubbe M. *Der Kassenarzt*. 2002;16:32–38.
151. Hill N, Stam C, Van Haselen RA. *Pharm World Sci*. 1996;18(1):35–41.
152. Mittman P. *Planta Med*. 1990;56(1):44–47.
153. Schmid D, Lang A, Allgauer T, et al. *Akt Dermatol*. 2001;27:25–29.
154. Wegnener T. *Z Phytother*. 2009;30:243–248.
155. Baraibar C, Broncano FJ, Lazaro-Carrasco MJ, et al. *An Bromatol*. 1984;35(1):99–103.
156. Sharma BB, Varshney MD, Gupta DN, et al. *Int J Crude Drug Res*. 1983;21(4):183–187.
157. Graf U, Moraga AA, Castro R, et al. *Food Chem Toxicol*. 1994;32(5):423–430.
158. Blumenthal M, ed. *The Complete German Commission E Monographs: Therapeutic*

Guide to Herbal Medicines. Austin: American Botanical Council; 1998. pp. 216–217.

159. Gansser D, Spiteller G. *Z Naturforsch [C]*. 1995;50(1–2):98–104.

160. Sharma BB, Varshney MD, Gupta DN, et al. *Int J Crude Drug Res*. 1983;21(4):183–187.

161. Oliver F, Amon EU, Breathnach A, et al. *Clin Exp Dermatol*. 1991;16(1):1–7.

162. Edwards Jr EK, Edwards Sr. EK. *Contact Dermatitis*. 1992;27(4):264–265.

163. Bossuyt L, Dooms-Goossens A. *Contact Dermatitis*. 1994;31(2):131–132.

164. Uslu S, Bulbul A, Diler B, et al. *Eur J Pediatr*. 2011;170(3):401–403.

165. Vega-Maray AM, Fernandez-Gonzalez D, Valencia-Barrera R, et al. *Ann Allergy Asthma Immunol*. 2006;97(3):343–349.

166. Geiger WN, Haak C, Wagner H. *2nd International Congress on Phytomedicine*. Munich: September 11–14, 1996.

167. Edgcumbe DP, McAuley D. *Eur J Emerg Med*. 2008;15(4):236–237.

168. Sahin M, Yilmaz H, Gursoy A, et al. *N Z Med J*. 2007;120(1265):U2803.

Pau d'Arco

(*Tabebuia spp.* Gomes ex DC.)

Synonyms

Lapacho (Engl, Span), ipe roxo, peuva, taheebo, lapacho (Sth Amer), *Handroanthus spp.*

What is it?

Pau d'arco has been utilised as a medicine for at least 1000 years by the Brazilian Indians, from where its use gradually spread to other parts of South America. These large timber trees with spectacular tubular flowers originate mostly in Brazil and Argentina, although they are widely planted throughout the South American tropics. They are renowned for their durable timber and resistance to insect and fungal attack. The most widely used species in Western countries are *Tabebuia impetiginosa* (*T. avellanedae, Handroanthus impetiginosus*) and *T. ipe*. Other species used include *Tabebuia rosea* (*T. pentaphylla*), *T. chrysantha* (*H. chrysanthus*), *T. cassinoides* and *T. serratifolia*.

Pau d'arco was first used in Western medicine in Sao Paulo, Brazil, in 1960 where physicians prescribed decoctions of the inner bark for terminal cancer patients at the Santo Andre hospital. According to reports, most patients showed no symptoms after 30 days of commencing treatment. Subsequently, the hospital also used the unapproved medicine for viral-linked diseases, including leukaemia. One of the doctors, Professor Accorsi, stated that pau d'arco eliminated the pain (of cancer) and increased the amount of red blood cells. Knowledge of the herb became more widespread following a number of 'miraculous' cancer cures, including three successful leukaemia treatments by Dr Ruiz at the Concepcion hospital.

Dr Theodore Meyer, a leading South American botanist born in Argentina, was the first scientist on record to analyse pau d'arco's chemical composition, discovering xyloidone, an antimicrobial and virucidal agent. Meyer supplied medicinal plants, including pau d'arco, to pharmaceutical companies but is also credited with beginning the effort to save the tree from decline. At one time pau d'arco attained almost fad status in the West, particularly as an antifungal agent in chronic candidiasis. While its use has faded as other treatments have become available, it is still valued for several applications, including fungal infections and weakened immunity. Few side effects have been recorded despite its widespread usage (often self-administered) and the potential toxicity of its active components.

The inner bark is the main part of the tree used in medicine, but the wood contains the same constituents, to a lesser or greater degree, depending on the species of tree.

Effects

Cytotoxic (via induction of cellular and immune factors); active against certain species of parasites, antimicrobial; immune enhancing.

Traditional view

The Incas used pau d'arco to cure many diseases, including even degenerative disorders. The Brazilian Indians utilised the bark as a poultice or decoction for treating skin diseases such as eczema, psoriasis, fungal infections and skin cancers. A tea from the bark is used as a blood purifier, while the inner bark has been favoured for dysentery, fever, sore throat, wounds, snakebites and carcinomas.[1]

Inhabitants of the Rio Vaupés believe the decoction of the bark of *T. insignis* var. *monophylla* to be an excellent treatment for stomach ulcers. The Tikunas use *T. neochrysantha* to treat malaria, chronic anaemia and ulcers. The bark of *T. obscura* is used as an antirheumatic by the Boras of Peru.[2]

Summary actions

Immune enhancing, antitumour, antimicrobial, antiparasitic, depurative.

Can be used for

Indications supported by clinical trials

Clinical trials using lapachol: carcinoma and leukaemia, used as an adjuvant complementary therapy in cancer (all studies uncontrolled and weak evidence).

Traditional therapeutic uses

Internally for dysentery, fever, malaria, sore throat, wounds, carcinomas, stomach ulcers, anaemia, degenerative disorders and as a depurative and antirheumatic. Topically for skin diseases, fungal infections, skin cancers.

May also be used for

Extrapolations from pharmacological studies

As an adjunctive treatment for bacterial, fungal and protozoal infections; to enhance immune function. Topical application for fungal infections, scabies, ulcers and wounds.

Preparations

Decoction of dried inner bark or liquid extract, tincture, tablets or capsules for internal use; decoction of dried inner bark or liquid extract for external use.

Dosage

1.5 to 3.5 g/day or 3 to 7 mL/day of a 1:2 extract in 45% ethanol or equivalent doses in tincture, tablet or capsule form.

In adjuvant therapy for cancer, pau d'arco is often administered in higher doses both as an ethanolic extract and as a decoction. Alcohol is a better solvent than water for the naphthoquinones. For a decoction, simmer 10 g of bark in 600 mL of water for 15 minutes. Strain and drink throughout the day.

Duration of use

May be used long term if prescribed within the recommended therapeutic range.

Summary assessment of safety

No adverse effects from ingestion of pau d'arco are expected when consumed within the recommended dosage. It is contraindicated in pregnancy.

Technical data

Botany

Pau d'arco refers to several trees in the Bignoniaceae (jacaranda) family which are indigenous to South America. They belong to the genera Tabebuia (100 species) and Tecoma (13 species). Pau d'arco is a tropical tree growing up to 38 m high, with opposite, long-petiolate leaves with entire or toothed leaflets. The flower is large in terminal cymes or panicles, with tubular or campanulate calyx, four stamens, corolla tube ampiate. The capsule is slender-cylindrical and the seeds are broadly winged.[2–4]

Species identification is determined by leaf configuration and flower colour; the red, violet and pink flowering species are preferred as medicines while the yellow flower species are considered inferior (but see below under Adulteration).[5]

The large Tabebuia genus was subdivided into several genera in 2007, including Handroanthus.

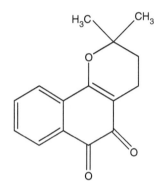

Lapachol

beta-Lapachone

Adulteration

As noted above, 'pau d'arco' is a common name in South America referring to trees of the Tabebuia (Handroanthus) and Tecoma genera. Throughout the Amazon a number of species of Tabebuia are used medicinally. The Western preference for *Tabebuia avellanedae* originates from the Brazilian clinical investigations in the late 1960s from which the 'purple' species were suggested to be superior to the yellow-flowered pau d'arco. However there is evidence to suggest that the yellow-flowered *T. serratifolia* (*H. serratifolius*) is used for similar therapeutic purposes by natives in other parts of South America.[6]

Traditional Brazilian sources indicate that side effects may occur from ingestion of the bark of the following yellow-flowered pau d'arco plants: *T. umbellata* (such as swelling, burning, vomiting) and *T. pedicellata*.[7]

Exploitation of *Tabebuia impetiginosa* has been to such an extent (for timber) that a 1994 article noted significant population declines in Brazil and at a local level in Argentina.[8] In the 1997 review of the application of the 1994 CITES (Convention on International Trade in Endangered Species of Wild Fauna and Flora) listing criteria to timber species, there was insufficient information available on *Tabebuia impetiginosa* to recommend its inclusion.

In recent times the outer bark of pau d'arco has become a very common substitute for the inner bark. It generally lacks significant levels of key naphthoquinones.

Key constituents

Tabebuia impetiginosa

- Naphthoquinones of the 1,4 type (including lapachol, beta-lapachone, xyloidone, deoxylapachol, alpha-lapachone and dehydro-alpha-lapachone);[1,9] several of these, as well as other compounds in the herb, can be further classified as naphthofurandiones (or furonaphthoquinones), which are naphthoquinones with a furan ring attached to the carbons at the 2 and 3 positions[10–13]
- Anthraquinones (which rarely occur in other plants containing naphthoquinones)[1,9]
- Benzoic acid derivatives, benzaldehyde derivatives, iridoids, coumarins, flavonoids and carnosol.

A 1994 review of pau d'arco products on the Canadian market found no or low levels of lapachol in all of the products. In contrast, two Brazilian products contained relatively high amounts of lapachol.[14] While poor quality of products is probably one reason for this finding, levels of lapachol also depend on whether the inner bark or the wood is used. Typical levels of total naphthoquinones expressed as 'lapachol' are 1 to 2% for the inner bark, but lapachol itself is likely to be only a minor constituent of this plant part.

Pharmacodynamics

Lapachol was originally identified as the 'signature' compound in pau d'arco and much of the earlier pharmacological research was focused on it.[15] More recently, its significance has been questioned. In particular, beta-lapachone possesses marked antimicrobial and antitumour activities and has been the main focus of current research.

Quinones form an important component of the electron-transport system in plants and mammals. Ubiquinol, the reduced form of co-enzyme Q_{10}, and menaquinone (a vitamin K) have significant antioxidant properties and play a major role in protecting cells from free radical damage. Redox reactions are inherent features of quinones and are recognised as 'the basis for their functional roles and cytotoxic and chemotherapeutic actions'.[16]

Antitumour and immune-enhancing activity

Lapachol and pau d'arco extracts

Following the clinical use of pau d'arco for cancer in Brazilian hospitals, studies in 1968 first identified lapachol as an antitumour agent. In vivo tests showed lapachol to have significant activity against Walker 256 carcinosarcoma, particularly following twice daily oral administration.[17] This result was confirmed in studies by De Santana and co-workers, who found lapachol inhibited Yoshida's sarcoma (82%) and Walker 256 carcinosarcoma (50%) at a dose of 100 mg/kg. Beta-lapachone also inhibited Yoshida's sarcoma (16%) and Walker 256 carcinosarcoma (33.5%) at a dose of 7 mg/kg. However, alpha-lapachone and xyloidone showed no inhibition of Walker 256 carcinosarcoma at a dose of 200 mg/kg.[18] Lapachol was compared with lawsone, another 1,4

naphthoquinone, and found to have stronger growth inhibitory effects than the latter compound, especially against Yoshida's sarcoma.[19] Aqueous extracts of pau d'arco also inhibited Walker carcinoma (44%) when administered by injection to rats.

Lapachol was also shown to be active against Murphy-Sturm lymphosarcoma, but was inactive in the mice neoplasias sarcoma 180, adenocarcinoma 775, Lewis lung carcinoma, lymphocytic leukaemia P-388 and leukaemia L1210. However, in confirmation of previous results, it was found to be active against Walker 256 with a therapeutic index of 6.[20] Under different experimental conditions, twelve 1,4 naphthoquinones prolonged the life of mice bearing ascitic sarcoma 180 tumours. Statistical analysis revealed a link between the redox potentials of various compounds and their antitumour activity.[21] Later studies evaluated in vitro inhibitory effects of 1,4 naphthoquinones on beef heart mitochondrial succinoxidase and NADH-oxidase enzyme systems and found a strong relationship between succinoxidase inhibition, redox potential and antitumour activity. However, NADH-oxidase inhibition per se did not appear to influence the incidence of tumours.[22]

Lapachol has demonstrated additional antitumour activity in vitro as well as in vivo.[23] Lapachol and other naphthoquinones showed growth inhibitory activity on KB cells.[24] It demonstrated significant dose-dependent inhibition of four human melanoma cell lines and a human renal cell carcinoma line, though only after continual exposure.[25]

In the 1960s lapachol was positively identified as an uncoupling agent of mitochondrial respiration that mimics the behaviour of the classic uncoupling agent 2,4-dinitrophenol. This phenomenon occurs because of the structural similarity between lapachol and the endogenous hydroxyquinone, with which it competes for a position in the respiratory chain. According to this hypothesis, lapachol exposes a mitochondrial thiol group occupying a pivotal position between the respiration cycles.[26] This mechanism might explain its cytotoxic activity.

However, other mechanisms may apply. Studies with quinone anticancer agents, including lapachol, used microsomal systems in normal and malignant tissues and found that quinones are converted intracellularly to site-specific free radical intermediaries producing cytotoxic activity. These bind to DNA or RNA, resulting in chromosomal damage, and also have potential to generate superoxide or hydroxyl radicals.[27] Lapachol also inhibits de novo pyrimidine synthesis by inhibiting dihydro-orotate, resulting in depletion of nucleotide pools. Depletion of uridine triphosphate and cytidine triphosphate in hepatoma cells leads to their death. Hence lapachol might be combined with other antipyrimidines in tumour chemotherapy.[28] Vitamin K3 and other quinones, including lapachol, were also found to alter the affinity of receptors for epidermal growth factor, a potent mitogen capable of stimulating growth of human fibroblasts and other cells.[29]

Another potential mechanism behind lapachol's cytotoxicity may be inhibition of glyoxalase I, which may lead to a lethal build-up of alpha-ketoaldehydes. In vitro studies showed lapachol to be a linear competitive inhibitor of yeast glyoxalase I.[30,31] Later studies examined glyoxalase inhibition in terms of tumour cell selectivity. However, it was found that lapachol was far less inhibitory of tumour than normal cells.[32] Lapachol was also found to be an inhibitor of ribonucleotide reductase, an enzyme involved in DNA replication that occurs at much higher levels in malignant cells than in non-proliferating cells.[33]

The effect of lapachol on metastasis was tested in vitro using HeLa cells.[34] At 400 µg/mL lapachol was found to induce alterations in the protein profile and inhibit the invasiveness of HeLa cells in the chick chorioallantoic membrane model. The authors concluded that lapachol has potential in fighting metastasis.

Pau d'arco extracts and other components have also demonstrated antitumour effects in vivo (see above and below). A methanolic extract of the inner bark of *T. avellanedae* reduced the number of papillomas in mice with induced skin carcinogenesis.[23] An alcoholic extract of stem bark from *Tabebuia cassinoides* showed slight, reproducible activity against leukaemia P-388 in vivo. Further investigations identified the active constituents as three previously unknown furonaphthoquinones.[35] In a separate study, two furonaphthoquinones from *T. impetiginosa* cell cultures showed significant dose-dependent antitumour activity.[36]

The antiproliferative activity of an aqueous extract of *T. avellanedae* extract (1.5 mg/mL) against oestrogen receptor positive MCF-7 human breast cancer cells was investigated in vitro.[37] The observed inhibition of cell growth correlated with downregulated cell cycle regulatory and oestrogen-responsive genes and upregulated apoptosis-specific genes.

Treatment with *T. avellanedae* extract (30 to 500 mg/kg) and beta-lapachone (1 to 5 mg/kg) reversed the myelosuppression observed in Ehrlich ascites tumour-bearing mice and prolonged their lifespan.[38] However, beta-lapachone was absent from the herbal extract tested.

Beta-lapachone

Following the somewhat disappointing (in terms of side effects) initial human trials using lapachol in cancer patients (see later), research interest switched to beta-lapachone. As for lapachol, most investigations have focused on determining its mechanisms of action via in vitro studies.

Studies conducted at Harvard Medical School showed that beta-lapachone can sensitise X-ray-resistant human melanoma cell lines when administered following X-radiation. The mechanism was thought to involve the inactivation of eukaryotic topoisomerase I, which is involved in DNA repair mechanisms following X-ray damage. Lapachol and other related compounds were inactive in this model.[39]

Beta-lapachone at a concentration of 5 µM was found to induce apoptosis in the hepatoma HG2 cell line through induction of Bax and activation of caspase.[40] This was evidenced by the formation of apoptotic bodies and DNA fragmentation. Induced apoptosis was associated with proteolytic activation of caspase-3 and -9 and degradation of poly (ADP-ribose) polymerase (PARP), a main regulator of the DNA damage response pathway. Over 48 h beta-lapachone caused an 82% inhibition of cell growth compared with the control.

Apoptosis also resulted from micromolar concentrations of beta-lapachone in the human bladder carcinoma cell line T24 in vitro. As well as causing downregulation of Bcl-2 expression, treatment of T24 cells with beta-lapachone resulted in upregulation of Bax expression. Apoptosis was again associated with activation of caspase-3 and -9 and degradation of PARP.[41] These apoptosis events were replicated in vitro for beta-lapachone for models of prostate,[42–44] breast[45,46] and colon cancer.[47] Bcl-2 are apoptosis regulator proteins of which Bax is a key member.

Additional suggested apoptosis mechanisms from other in vitro studies include inactivation of nuclear factor kappa-B (NF-kappaB),[47] p53 phosphorylation induction[44] and downregulation of retinoblastoma protein (pRB) phosphorylation, as well as enhanced binding of pRB and transcription factor E2F-1.[43] One trigger factor for apoptosis was reported to be DNA damage, resulting in induction of cyclin-dependent kinase inhibitors and subsequent stimulation of caspase activation.[48] Telomerase inhibition was also noted.[42,49]

Cell death induced by beta-lapachone is further suggested to be a combination of both necrotic cell death[50,51] and apoptosis.[51,52] The main mechanism involved is postulated to be via the enzyme NADPH:quinone oxidoreductase-1 (NQO1) and resultant changes in intracellular calcium levels.[51,53] A review of the in vitro laboratory data proposed that NQO1 'bioactivates' beta-lapachone, creating a futile cycling between the parent quinone and hydroquinone forms that generates reactive oxygen species (ROS). These ROS contribute towards toxicity to cancer cells (many tumour cells are found to over-express NQO1),[51,54,55] and also result in DNA damage and release of intracellular calcium. As the cell focuses to repair DNA, PARP-1 is activated and eventually hyperactivated. This in turn creates a depletion of the cellular nucleotides NAD$^+$ and ATP (which inactivate energy-dependent DNA repair processes) and progresses to mu-calpain[56] and endonuclease activation, leading to cell death. Calpain is a calcium-dependent protease[46] and its activation is reported to cause cell death independent of caspase.[57]

The anti-angiogenic effect of beta-lapachone on endothelial cells was investigated in vitro.[58] Exogenous NO (nitric oxide) protected against cell death from beta-lapachone but not against its anti-angiogenic affect, leading the authors to suggest a potential role for beta-lapachone as an anti-angiogenic agent. Beta-lapachone dose-dependently reduced cell viability and migration of two human hepatocarcinoma cell lines, thereby potentially inhibiting their progression and metastasis.[59]

Although many proposed anticancer agents (including beta-lapachone) induce apoptosis, such pathways are often deficient in cancer cells. One way to bypass defective apoptotic pathways is to induce necrotic cell death. As mentioned above, it was demonstrated in vitro that beta-lapachone can induce selective necrotic cell death in cancer cells.[60] Furthermore, after treatment of human xenograft tumours with beta-lapachone in mice (60 mg/kg, ip), PARP-1 activation occurred as a necessary step in the induction of necrosis.

In addition to the earlier work on X-ray sensitisation, beta-lapachone was shown to act synergistically with ionising radiation to kill cancer cells.[61–63] This was confirmed in DU-145 human prostate cancer cell lines.[61] Results indicated that two distinct mechanisms were involved: radiation sensitises cells to beta-lapachone by upregulating NQO1 and beta-lapachone sensitises cells to radiation by inhibiting sublethal radiation damage repair. Beta-lapachone was only effective when it was given after irradiation.[61,63]

The addition of heat was found to upregulate NQO1 in the human lung cancer cell line A549 in vitro. This heat-induced upregulation enhanced the anticancer activity of beta-lapachone. In vivo testing in mice also found heat increased the anticancer action of beta-lapachone (40 mg/kg, ip). The mouse tumour was heated to 42°C for 1 h every other day for four times after beta-lapachone injection.[64]

The in vitro combination of beta-lapachone and taxol was shown to synergistically induce death of cultured breast, prostate, melanoma, lung, colon and pancreatic cancer cells. Taxol must be added either simultaneously or after the beta-lapachone. This was also verified in vivo for xenograft models of human ovarian and prostate cancers in mice. The authors hypothesised that the agents act at different cycle cell checkpoints.[65] Drug-resistant (dexamethasone, melphalan, doxorubicin and mitoxandrone) multiple myeloma cell lines were tested in vitro for any activity of beta-lapachone at concentrations of 4 to 8 μM. Beta-lapachone showed significant toxicity and induced typical apoptosis events such as caspase-3 activation and PARP cleavage.[66,67] A combination of genistein and beta-lapachone in vitro exhibited improved rates of cell death in the human prostate cancer cell lines PC3 and LNCaP compared with either treatment alone. Beta-lapachone was reported to act at G1 and S phase checkpoints, while genistein induced cell cycle arrest at the G2-M stage.[68] Paclitaxel and beta-lapachone synergistically induced apoptosis in human retinoblastoma Y79 cells by downregulating levels of the protein kinase phospho-Akt[69] and cisplatin enhanced the anticancer effect of beta-lapachone by upregulating NQO1.[70]

Antiparasitic activity

Pau d'arco and some of its constituents, including lapachol, are active against various tropical parasites. Wendel carried out original work on naphthoquinones and malarial parasites in ducks, concluding the compounds inhibit oxygen uptake of parasitised cells at more than 100 times the concentration required to inhibit respiration in normal cells.[71] Further studies confirmed these results and proposed that lapachol and other naphthoquinones act like cyanide in inhibiting the main respiration pathway, but leaving certain secondary and minor respiratory processes untouched. The authors concluded that naphthoquinones act below cytochrome c and above cytochrome b in the main chain of respiratory enzymes.[72] Willard suggests respiratory inhibition may apply to the more general antimicrobial actions of lapachol and its chemical relatives.[9] Naphthoquinones tested against drug-resistant strains of Plasmodium falciparum were superior to the

controls chloroquine and quinine. Eight compounds related to lapachol, all isolated from plants in the Bignoniaceae family, showed this activity. However, despite its reputed antimalarial action, lapachol showed borderline activity only.[73]

Lapachol has been used as a chemoprophylactic against Schistosoma mansoni (a tropical fluke) cercarial penetration and infection. Studies by Austin showed that 0.9% lapachol in the diet of mice reduced infections by 97% after 3 days' feeding. The study further demonstrated that lapachol is secreted onto the skin where it forms a barrier to penetration.[74] Lapachol and other naphthoquinones derived from lapachol were also shown to work as topical applications.[75] Strong molluscicidal activity was shown by lapachol against the adult snail Biomphalaria glabrata, which is a vector for the parasite, as well as significant toxicity against snail egg masses.[76] In a later study, potassium salts of lapachol and isolapachol both showed significant molluscicidal activity as well as activity against Schistosoma mansoni cercariae.[77]

Lapachol, and lapachol analogues isolapachol and dihydrolapachol, showed significant activity against Leishmaniasis amazonensis and L. braziliensis in vitro. Isolapachol acetate was the most active and also displayed activity in vivo when assayed.[78] Leishmanicidal activity was also demonstrated in vitro against the intracellular amistigote L. (Vianna) braziliensis (LVb) by lapachol (0.0125 to 4.0 mg/mL). However, lapachol treatment at an oral dose of 300 mg/kg/day for 42 days did not prevent the development of LVb-induced lesions in hamsters.[79]

Trypanosoma cruzi is a parasite responsible for American trypanosomiasis or Chagas' disease, which is particularly common in Brazil.[80] Lapachol and several of its derivatives are toxic to T. cruzi in vitro but the toxic effect is nullified in the presence of blood. Hence, in vivo tests do not confirm the in vitro studies. However, a synthetic beta-lapachone derivative, allyl-beta-lapachone, is not inactivated by blood and retains potent suppressive activity on trypomastigote infectivity.[81,82]

Antibacterial and antifungal activity

De Lima and co-workers in the 1950s first demonstrated antibacterial activity for lapachol, alpha and beta-lapachone and xyloidone, as well as antifungal activity for alpha- and beta-lapachone and xyloidone. Naphthoquinones from pau d'arco, especially xyloidone, were effective against Candida albicans and Trichophyton, the fungus responsible for ringworm.[19] Pau d'arco tea is used as a topical application (via tampon) for vaginal candidiasis and taken internally for systemic infections.[1] The wide range of organisms that are susceptible to compounds from pau d'arco are summarised by Willard.[9] These include pathogenic species of Brucella, Staphylococcus and Candida.

In more recent studies, aqueous extracts of T. heptaphylla and T. impetiginosa showed no antibacterial activity against Pseudomonas aeruginosa for in vitro studies.[83] In a separate study, T. impetiginosa extract inhibited a penicillin-resistant strain of Staphylococcus aureus but was inactive against Escherichia coli and Aspergillus niger.[84]

Activity of *T. avellanedae* extract was examined against methicillin resistant *Staph. aureus* (MRSA). The hexane and chloroform fractions of the inner bark of the plant demonstrated antibacterial activity against all the *S. aureus* strains tested in vitro. The two main naphthoquinones that demonstrated this inhibitory effect were alpha-lapachone and alpha-xyloidone II, contained in the hexane fraction (minimum inhibitory concentration (MIC) 125 mg/L). The ethanolic extract (MIC 125 to 250 mg/L) was more active than the hexane and chloroform extracts (≥250 mg/L), which may be a result of synergy between compounds within the ethanolic extract.[85]

Beta-lapachone, 3-hydroxy-beta-N-lapachone and alpha-lapachone from *T. avellanedae* were tested in vitro and for activity against MRSA. In vivo testing was performed to assess for dermal irritation in rabbits. Results demonstrated that all compounds had antibacterial activity, but were not bactericidal (that is there was inhibition of growth, but no killing of bacteria). MIC concentrations were 8, 4 to 8 and 64 to 128 μg/mL respectively for the test compounds. No dermal irritation was observed and the authors suggested the possible use of these compounds as topical antibacterial agents.[86]

T. impetiginosa inner bark extract was examined for its activity against *Helicobacter pylori* in vitro. The activities of the isolated compounds 2-(hydroxymethyl) anthraquinone, anthraquinone-2-carboxylic acid and lapachol from the extract were compared with amoxicillin, metronidazole and tetracycline antibiotics (current pharmaceutical treatments against *H. pylori*). Results were measured by the paper disc diffusion method and MIC. Lapachol and anthraquinone-2-carboxylic acid showed moderate inhibitory activity at 0.1 mg/disc, equivalent to metronidazole. At the dose 0.005 mg/disc, 2-(hydroxymethyl) anthraquinone showed moderate activity while amoxicillin and tetracycline were still potent. In the MIC bioassay, all isolated compounds were more active than metronidazole, but less active than the other two antibiotics.[87]

In another study anthraquinone-2-carboxylic acid and lapachol were tested on 10 human intestinal bacteria in vitro using the same methods as above. The former compound showed strong activity against *Clostridium paraputrificum*, greater than lapachol (1 μg/disk compared with 100 μg/disk). However, both compounds showed only weak activity (100 μg/disk) against *Clostridium perfringens* and *Escherichia coli*. None of the other bacteria tested was inhibited.[88]

Campos-Takaki and co-workers studied the influence of culture medium composition on the antifungal activity of lapachol and beta-lapachone from *T. avellanedae* and four synthetic hydroxy-naphthoquinones. Lapachol demonstrated some activity against Candida and Cryptococcus fungi, contradicting previous results obtained by De Lima.[19] Of the six compounds tested, beta-lapachone and two synthetic naphthoquinones showed the best overall activity.[89] French workers also found beta-lapachone was more efficient than lapachol at inhibiting both bacteria and fungi. The antibacterial action showed a narrow spectrum, consisting mainly of Gram-positive strains and the Gram-negative Brucella. Beta-lapachone was more effective as an antifungal agent than ketoconazole, the standard used. The

mechanism behind the antimicrobial action may involve uncoupling of oxidative phosphorylation or electron transfer inhibition.[90]

Following this work, the antifungal activity of *T. avellanedae* bark extract was tested in vitro against 11 different fungal strains.[91] The powdered air-dried plant material was extracted with water, dichloromethane and methanol. The dichloromethane extract, both 5 and 10 mg/disk, showed the highest activity, inhibiting growth from 10 out of 11 fungal species including *Aspergillus fumigatus*, *Cryptococcus neoformans*, *Microsporum gypseum*, *Penicillium purpurogenum*, *Saccharomyces cerevisiae*, *Trichophyton mentagrophytes* and *Candida albicans*. Both the water and methanol extracts (again at 5 and 10 mg/disk) inhibited the fungal growth of four strains: *Cryptococcus neoformans*, *Microsporum gypseum*, *Penicillium purpurogenum* and *Trichophyton mentagrophytes*.

Antiviral activity

Studies in 1975 by Linhares and De Santa showed that lapachol inhibited a number of viral strains in vitro including human herpes virus types I and II.[9] In separate studies, beta-lapachone was shown to be a potent inhibitor of reverse transcriptase from the retroviruses avian myeloblastosis virus and Rauscher murine leukaemia virus. It also inhibited eukaryotic DNA-dependent DNA polymerase. It is possible other retroviruses such as HIV are also susceptible.[92]

In 1983, Lagrota and co-workers tested lapachol for activity against a range of viruses in vitro. Lapachol demonstrated significant inhibition of poliovirus and vesicular stomatitis virus. It also significantly inhibited haemagglutinating titres of influenza viral strains.[93] Three years later, the same team found several 1,4-naphthoquinone derivatives to be inactive against various viral cell cultures, while 1,2-naphthoquinone derivatives inhibited echovirus.[94] Only one of these, beta-norlapachone, was a natural compound. However, the antiviral action could only be shown in vitro and no virucidal action against viral particles was observed. The authors suggest this antiviral action occurs through either interferon production or enzyme inhibition.[95,96]

Extracts of the inner bark of *T. avellanedae* were found to inhibit induction of Epstein-Barr virus (EBV)-associated early antigen in EBV genome-carrying human lymphoblastic cell lines. The aqueous extract was found to be less active than the methanolic extract, while lapachol caused viral inhibition at the lowest concentration.[23]

Anticoagulant and antiplatelet activity

Lapachol and related naphthoquinones are known to be anticoagulants in rats and humans. Using animal models, Pruesch and Suttie found the anticoagulant activity occurred as a result of potent inhibition of vitamin K quinone and epoxide reductases. This action of lapachol appears similar to that of 4-hydroxy-coumarin anticoagulants: they bind to the oxidised form of the vitamin K reductases.[97] Further studies by Preusch on rat liver microsomes showed that lapachol inhibits another enzyme linked to blood coagulation.[98] Some writers link this anticoagulant activity to the anticancer applications of pau d'arco.

A more recent study examined the in vitro effects of various extract fractions of *T. impetiginosa* inner bark on platelet aggregation and vascular smooth muscle cell proliferation. Washed rabbit platelets and cultured rat aortic vascular smooth muscle cells were used. All fractions showed marked and selective dose-dependent inhibition of platelet aggregation induced by arachidonic acid (AA) and collagen. They significantly suppressed AA liberation induced by collagen in platelets and potently inhibited cell proliferation and DNA synthesis induced by platelet-derived growth factor.[99]

Other activity

An ethanolic extract of *T. avellanedae* exhibited antidepressant activity in two experimental models in mice (active oral doses 100 mg/kg or 10 to 300 mg/kg depending on the model).[100] The extract was additive with drugs such as fluoxetine and bupropion, suggesting that its mechanism of action involves the monoaminergic system.

Lapachol has been found to have anti-ulcerogenic activity in experimental models.[101] Such activity was also demonstrated for *T. avellanedae* extract.[102] Lapachol has demonstrated anti-inflammatory effects, producing significant inhibition of carrageenan-induced paw oedema comparable to phenylbutazone in vivo.[103] *T. avellanedae* extract reduced AA-induced mouse ear oedema (100 mg/kg, oral).[104]

An ethanolic extract of *Tabebuia chrysotricha*, and lapachol isolated from this species, showed significant analgesic activity in vivo.[105] Topical application of a lapachol gel reduced the increase in hind-paw volume induced by carrageenan injection in rats and demonstrated analgesic activity in mice.[106]

Lapachol has been found to possess both oestrogenic and anti-oestrogenic activity in mice. Lapachol from *Tectona grandis* demonstrated significant uterotrophic effects following intramuscular injection, although its oestrogenic activity was weak. Administration postcoitum resulted in inhibition of pregnancy and embryo resorption.[107]

T. impetiginosa compounds, as well as some synthetic analogues, were tested in vitro for their antipsoriatic activity. They were evaluated against the growth of the human keratinocyte cell line HaCaT. Beta-lapachone was shown to have comparable activity to the antipsoriatic drug anthralin, with an IC_{50} value of 0.7 µM. Plasma membrane damage was evidenced by lactate dehydrogenase leakage into the cell medium.[108] Beta-lapachone demonstrated in vitro proliferation of cells involved in healing such as fibroblasts and accelerated wound healing after topical application in vivo.[109]

Wagner and co-workers proposed that lapachol and other naphthoquinones such as furonaphthoquinones exert cytotoxic or immunosuppressive effects, while in low concentrations they have immunostimulating properties.[110] They concluded the cytotoxic effect of the extracts may arise by induction of cellular and immune factors. Later in vitro investigations of compounds isolated from *T. impetiginosa* confirmed dose-dependent immune-modulating effects on human granulocytes and lymphocytes.[111]

The effects of beta-lapachone on lipopolysaccharide-(LPS)-induced responses in rat alveolar macrophages and its resultant anti-inflammatory effect were examined.[112] Beta-lapachone inhibited the nitrite production increase and nitric oxide synthase expression elicited in LPS-treated macrophages in vitro. It also inhibited production of tumour necrosis factor-alpha and NF-kappaB induced by LPS. Beta-lapachone was found to protect lung tissue against oedema in vivo and overall reduce mortality.

Pharmacokinetics

No pharmacokinetic data are available for pau d'arco. Studies with lapachol in humans indicated that intestinal absorption was considerably less than that determined for the rat.[113]

Bioavailability was reported to be low for isolated beta-lapachone. Complexation with beta-cyclodextrin was found to greatly improve its solubility and bioavailability.[114] However, beta-lapachone may be more bioavailable in the natural plant matrix than in its isolated form.

Clinical trials

Although pau d'arco contains potentially toxic active components that can generate free radicals and interfere with mitochondrial respiration and blood coagulation, there is no evidence that the long-term use of the inner bark is unsafe, provided certain precautions are observed (the dosage should not be too high).

However, it also follows that the therapeutic effects of the inner bark are likely to be mild, and the herb should not be relied upon as a sole treatment for cancer or infections. One qualification of this is the immune-enhancing potential of pau d'arco, which could eventually lead to a re-evaluation of its therapeutic potential. This property requires more investigation in well-designed clinical studies.

Cancer

A phase I clinical trial of lapachol was initiated in 1967 at the Baltimore Cancer Research Center. The trial involved 21 leukaemia patients, each of whom was initially given capsules containing 0.25 or 0.5 g lapachol and later switched to a syrup formulation. The trial was stopped prematurely because prolonged prothrombin times (that is, potential anticoagulation effects) were observed at the high oral doses required to test for antitumour activity. The high oral doses also resulted in nausea and vomiting, while measurements of plasma lapachol showed intestinal absorption of lapachol to be considerably less than previously determined for rats.[113] However, lapachol may be much better absorbed from its natural plant matrix.

In a later study, prescription of lapachol (daily dose 20 to 30 mg/kg) caused shrinkage of tumours and reduction in pain for nine cancer patients partaking in a small clinical trial. Three patients ceased the treatment due to experiences of nausea and vomiting, the other patients had no significant side effects. Three patients had complete remissions.[115]

Toxicology and other safety data

Toxicology

Despite the widespread use of pau d'arco preparations, often for lengthy periods, there is no apparent evidence of toxicity in humans. Some toxicity studies have been carried out on isolated constituents. De Santana and co-workers reported intraperitoneal LD_{50} values in white mice at 1600 mg/kg for lapachol, 600 mg/kg for xyloidone and 80 mg/kg for beta-lapachone.[15] Lapachol had a relatively high therapeutic index of nearly 20. In 1970 the toxic effects of lapachol were studied in rodents and other animals. The LD_{50} for mice was 621 mg/kg and for albino rats >2.4 g/kg. The following signs of toxicity were recorded: moderate-to-severe anaemia, reticulocytosis, normoblastosis, transient thrombocytosis and leucocytosis and elevated serum alkaline phosphatase activity and prothrombin times.[116]

The LD_{50} data for pau d'arco constituents are summarised below and include the above studies.

Substance	Route, model	LD_{50}	Reference
Lapachol	Oral, mice	621 mg/kg	116
Lapachol	Oral, male mice	487 mg/kg	116
Lapachol	Oral, female mice	792 mg/kg	116
Lapachol	Oral, rats	>2.4 g/kg	116
Lapachol	ip, mice	400 mg/kg	117
Lapachol	ip, mice	1.6 g/kg	118
Xyloidone	ip, mice	600 mg/kg	118
Beta-lapachone	ip, mice	80 mg/kg	118

No lethal effect was observed in dogs given daily oral doses of 0.25 to 2 g/kg of lapachol, 6 days per week for 4 weeks. Monkeys were treated on the same schedule (at doses of 0.625 to 1 g/kg) and death occurred after six doses of 0.5 g/kg and after five doses of 1 g/kg. Severe anaemia, elevated alkaline phosphatase activity and other blood changes also occurred in dogs and monkeys. Haemorrhage was not observed and clotting times in dogs remained normal even though prothrombin times were elevated.[116]

Information provided to the Brazilian Ministry of Health in 1967 indicated that purple pau d'arco had 'no toxicity'.[119] Studies conducted 2 years later confirmed a low toxicity for *T. avellanedae* extracts in rats.[120] It was not possible to measure the LD_{50} due to the lack of mice deaths, even at the high concentration of inner bark aqueous extract administered (1 to 5 g/kg, oral).[121] No toxic effect was observed from an ethanol extract of the inner bark of *T. serratifolia* (1 g/kg, oral, or 100 mg/kg, iv).[7]

A study investigating the mutagenicity of naphthoquinones using the Ames test found lapachol was not mutagenic towards any of the tested strains.[122] However, when male Wistar rats were given single oral doses of lapachol (122, 244 and 365 mg/kg), the highest dose produced a significant increase in the frequency of micronucleated polychromatic erythrocytes and chromosomal aberrations in bone marrow cells, indicating potential clastogenic effects.[123]

Adult male Wistar rats were treated orally with 100 mg/kg lapachol for 5 days.[124] Analysis 3 or 14 days later found that lapachol at 3 days post-treatment significantly reduced seminal vesicle weight. No other significant changes were observed. Male and female Wistar rats were given beta-lapachone (40, 80 and 160 mg/kg, ip) for 21 days.[125] All doses promoted significant increases in white cell count, liver enzymes, bilirubin and alkaline phosphatase. The highest dose resulted in abnormal spleen histology, but there were no changes in liver structure.

Contraindications

Pau d'arco is contraindicated in pregnancy.

Special warnings and precautions

Patients on anticoagulant therapy should be prescribed pau d'arco with caution due to the warfarin-like action of naphthoquinones at high doses.

Although pau d'arco contains constituents that can generate free radicals and interfere with mitochondrial respiration and blood coagulation, there is no evidence that the pau d'arco will cause adverse effects if taken within the recommended dosage and guidelines. The therapeutic effects of pau d'arco are likely to be mild and it should not be relied upon as a sole treatment for cancer or infections.

Caution is advised for women wishing to conceive. Do not use pau d'arco during lactation except under professional advice.

Interactions

Although there is no evidence that pau d'arco (as opposed to lapachol) has any effect on blood coagulation, it should only be cautiously combined with anticoagulant drugs and under professional supervision. High doses of lapachol have caused prolonged prothrombin time in patients (see under Side effects).

Use in pregnancy and lactation

Category D – has caused or is associated with a substantial risk of causing fetal malformation or irreversible damage.

Decoction of *Tabebuia heptaphylla* (in formulations) is recommended for inducing abortion in Argentinean folk medicine, although it is possible that other plants in the formula are the abortifacients.[119] Yellow-flowered *Tabebuia argentea* (*T. aurea*) is part of a formula used by indigenous people of Paraguay to induce abortion. Other plants in the formula include rue (*Ruta graveolens*) and caroa (*Jacaranda mimosifolia*). The part of the Tabebuia used was not defined.[7,126]

The results of animal studies investigating the effect of lapachol on reproduction are summarised below. As can be seen, results are conflicting.

Lapachol administration, route and pregnancy model	Day administered	Results	Ref.
10 mg (approx. 56 mg/kg), oral, rats	Day 8 to 12	99.2% fetal mortality rate	127
20 mg (approx. 112 mg/kg), oral, rats	Day 8 to 12	100% fetal mortality rate	128
100 mg/kg, oral, rats	Day 17 to 20	No effect on implantation or resorption Fetal growth retardation occurred	129
100 mg/kg, oral, rats	Day 1 to 5	100% fetal resorption	130
100 mg/kg, oral, rats	Day 7 to 12	78.7% fetal resorption Fetal malformation observed at day 21 (5.8% exophthalmia, 11.6% leporine lip)	130
100 mg/kg, oral, rats	Day 14 to 19	No fetal resorption	130
20 mg/kg, im, mice	Day 1 to 7	100% inhibition of pregnancy	131
20 mg/kg, im, mice	Day 1 to 3	71.2% inhibition of pregnancy	131
20 mg/kg, im, mice	Day 4 to 6	84.5% inhibition of pregnancy	129
100 to 200 mg/kg, oral, rats	Day 3 to 5	No effect on implantation or resorption	132,133
100 mg/kg, oral, rats	Day 1 to 5	No effect on embryonic development	133,134

Beta-lapachone (40, 80 and 160 mg/kg, ip) was administered to pregnant female Wistar rats on days 7 to 12 of gestation.[125] Significant fetal toxicity and resorption was observed at all doses, together with a range of malformations.

Pau d'arco is compatible with breastfeeding but best used with caution.

Effects on ability to drive and use machines

No adverse effects expected.

Side effects

A case was reported of hepatic failure in a man who was self-treating mild multiple sclerosis with zinc, skullcap tablets and pau d'arco tablets. The authors postulated that the skullcap tablets were adulterated, possibly with *Teucrium* species.[135]

Adverse effects were recorded in patients taking high doses of lapachol during an uncontrolled clinical trial. No toxicity was observed at oral doses below 1.5 g. Above this dosage, nausea and vomiting were usual, although the unpalatable nature of the formulation may have contributed. Liver function tests were normal. At doses above 2 g/day prothrombin time was often markedly prolonged and required correction with parenteral vitamin K. The results of other tests for clotting were normal.[113] This is a high dose of lapachol and there is no evidence to suggest that pau d'arco would cause similar effects at its recommended dosage.

Allergic contact dermatitis caused by exposure to lapachol and other naphthoquinones has been reported in woodworkers.[136,137] Occupational exposure to *Tabebuia spp.* dust was reported to cause asthma in a worker in Brazil. After removal from exposure to the herb, serial lung function measurements showed sustained improvement. Skin prick tests were positive and specific bronchial challenge showed a late asthmatic reaction.[138]

Overdosage

No incidents found in published literature. Information provided to the Brazilian Ministry of Health in 1967 indicated that patients taking an extract of purple pau d'arco in a high dose 'will feel a slight irritation, a sort of itchiness, although it is of no consequence … A person can take 5 g/kg (of extract) daily with no damage'.[119] (Although not defined, it is possible that these were aqueous extracts.)

Safety in children

Information provided to the Brazilian Ministry of Health in 1967 indicated that purple pau d'arco was suitable to administer to children.[119]

Regulatory status in selected countries

Pau d'arco is not covered by a Commission E monograph and it is not on the UK General Sale List.

Pau d'arco does not have GRAS status. However, it is freely available as a 'dietary supplement' in the USA under DSHEA legislation (1994 Dietary Supplement Health and Education Act).

Pau d'arco is not included in Part 4 of Schedule 4 of the Therapeutic Goods Act Regulations of Australia and is freely available for sale.

References

1. Oswald EH. *Br J Phytother.* 1993/1994;3(3):112–117.

2. Evans Schultes R, Raffauf RF. *The Healing Forest: Medicinal and Toxic Plants of The Northwest Amazonia.* Portland: Dioscorides Press; 1990. pp. 107–108.

3. Mabberley DJ. *The Plant Book*, 2nd ed Cambridge: Cambridge University Press; 1997. pp. 696, 702.

4. Willard T. *Textbook of Advanced Herbology.* Calgary: Wild Rose College of Natural Healing; 1992. pp. 198–203.

5. Pederson M. *Nutritional Herbology.* Utah: Pederson Publishing; 1987. p. 206.

6. Jones K. *Pau d'Arco: Immune Power from the Rain Forest.* Vermont: Healing Arts Press; 1995. pp. 4, 33–34, 45–46.

7. Jones K. *Pau d'Arco: Immune Power from the Rain Forest.* Vermont: Healing Arts Press; 1995. p. 98.

8. Annex 2. *Profiles of Tree Species: The Americas.* Available from UNEP–WCMC website: <www.unep-wcmc.org/>. Accessed June 2003.

9. Willard T. In: Pizzorno JE, Murray MT, eds. *A Textbook of Natural Medicine*, vol. 1. Seattle: John Bastyr College Publications; 1987. [V:Tabeb–1–8].

10. Girard M, Kindack D, Dawson BA, et al. *J Nat Prod.* 1988;51(5):1023–1024.

11. Wagner H, Kreher B, Lotter H, et al. *Helv Chim Acta.* 1989;72:659–667.

12. Fujimoto Y, Eguchi T, Murasaki C, et al. *J Chem Soc Perkin Trans.* 1991;1:2323–2327.

13. Steinert J, Khalaf H, Rimpler M. *J Chromatogr A.* 1995;693:281–287.

14. Awang DVC, Dawson BA, Ethier JC, et al. *J Herbs Spices Med Plants.* 1994;2:27–43.

15. Houghton PJ, Kahdra J, Theobald AE. *J Pharm Pharmacol.* 1992;44(suppl):S1081.

16. Cadenas E, Hochstein P. *Adv Enzymol Relat Areas Mol Biol.* 1992;65:97–146.

17. Rao KV, McBride TJ, Oleson JJ. *Cancer Res.* 1968;28:1952–1954.

18. De Santana CF, De Lima OG, D'Albuquerque IL, et al. *Rev Inst Antibiot (Recife).* 1968;8(1–2):89–94.

19. De Lima OG, De Barros Coelho JS, D'Albuquerque IL, et al. *Rev Inst Antibiot (Recife).* 1971;11(1):21–26.

20. Da Consolacao M, Linardi F, De Oliveira MM, et al. *J Med Chem.* 1975;18(11):1159–1161.

21. Hodnett E, Wongwiechintana C, Dun III WJ, et al. *J Med Chem.* 1983;26(4):570–574.

22. Pisani DE, Elliott AJ, Hinman DR, et al. *Biochem Pharmacol.* 1986;35(21):3791–3798.

23. Ueda S, Tokuda H. *Planta Med.* 1990;56:669–670.

24. Favaro OCN, De Oliveira MM, Rossini MAA, et al. *An Acad Bras Cienc.* 1990;62(3):217–224.

25. Houghton PJ, Photiou A, Uddin S, et al. *Planta Med.* 1994;60(5):430–433.

26. Hadler H, Moreau T. *J Antibiot.* 1969;22(11):513–520.

27. Bachur NR, Gordon SL, Gee MV. *Cancer Res.* 1978;38:1745–1750.

28. Keppler D, Fauler J, Gasser T, et al. *Adv Enzyme Regul.* 1985;23:61–79.

29. Shoyab M, Todaro G. *J Biol Chem.* 1980;255(18):8735–8739.

30. Douglas KT, Nadvi IN, Thakrar N. *IRCS Med Sci.* 1982;10:683.

31. Douglas KT, Gohel DI, Nadvi IN, et al. *Biochim Biophys Acta.* 1985;829(1):109–118.

32. Douglas KT, Keyworth LTA. *Med Sci Res.* 1994;22:641–642.

33. Smith S, Douglas K. *IRCS Med Sci.* 1986;14:541–542.

34. Balassiano IT, De Paulo SA, Henriques Silva N, et al. *Oncol Rep.* 2005;13(2):329–333.

35. Rao MM, Kingston DGI. *J Nat Prod.* 1982;45:600–604.

36. Ueda S, Umemura T, Dohguchi K, et al. *Phytochemistry.* 1994;36(2):323–325.

37. Mukherjee B, Telang N, Wong GY. *Int J Mol Med.* 2009;24(2):253–260.

38. Queiroz ML, Valadares MC, Torello CO, et al. *J Ethnopharmacol.* 2008;117(2):228–235.

39. Boothman DA, Trask DK, Pardee AB. *Cancer Res.* 1989;49(3):605–612.

40. Woo HJ, Park KY, Rhu CH, et al. *J Med Food.* 2006;9(2):161–168.

41. Lee JI, Choi DY, Chung HS, et al. *Exp Oncol.* 2006;28(1):30–35.

42. Lee JH, Cheong J, Park YM, Choi YH. *Pharmacol Res.* 2005;51(6):553–560.

43. Choi YH, Kang HS, Yoo MA. *J Biochem Mol Biol.* 2003;36(2):223–229.

44. Choi YH, Kim MJ, Lee SY, et al. *Int J Oncol.* 2002;21(6):1293–1299.

45. Pink JJ, Wuerzberger–Davis S, Tagliarino C, et al. *Exp Cell Res.* 2000;255(2):144–155.

46. Pink JJ, Planchon SM, Tagliarino C, et al. *J Biol Chem.* 2000;275(8):5416–5424.

47. Choi BT, Cheong J, Choi YH. *Anticancer Drugs.* 2003;14(10):845–850.

48. Doo MJ, Chang YH, Chen KK, et al. *Mol Pharmacol.* 2001;59(4):784–794.

49. Woo HJ, Choi YH. *Int J Oncol.* 2005;26(4):1017–1023.

50. Liu TJ, Lin SY, Chau YP. *Toxicol Appl Pharmacol.* 2002;182(2):116–125.

51. Bentle MS, Bey EA, Dong Y, et al. *J Mol Histol.* 2006;37(5–7):203–218.

52. Li YZ, Li CJ, Pinto AV, Pardee AB. *Mol Med.* 1999;5(4):232–239.

53. Tagliarino C, Pink JJ, Dubyak GR, et al. *J Biol Chem.* 2001;276(22):19150–19159.

54. Pardee AB, Li YZ, Li CJ. *Curr Cancer Drug Targets.* 2002;2(3):227–242.

55. Fernandez Villamil S, Stoppani AO, Dubin M. *Methods Enzymol.* 2004;378:67–87.

56. Tagliarino C, Pink JJ, Reinicke KE, et al. *Cancer Biol Ther.* 2003;2(2):141–152.

57. Guicciardi ME, Gores GJ. *Cancer Biol Ther.* 2003;2(2):153–154.

58. Kung HN, Chien CL, Chau GY, et al. *J Cell Physiol.* 2007;211:522–532.

59. Kim SO, Kwon JI, Jeong YK, et al. *Biosci Biotechnol Biochem.* 2007;71(9):2169–2176.

60. Sun X, Li Y, Li W, et al. *Cell Cycle.* 2006;5(17):2029–2035.

61. Suzuki M, Amano M, Choi J, et al. *Radiat Res.* 2006;16(5):525–531.

62. Park HJ, Ahn KJ, Ahn SD, et al. *Int J Radiat Oncol Biol Phys.* 2005;61(1):212–219.

63. Miyamoto S, Huang TT, Wuerzberger-Davis S, et al. *Ann N Y Acad Sci.* 2000;922:274–292.

64. Park HJ, Choi EK, Choi J, et al. *Clin Cancer Res.* 2005;11:8866–8871.

65. Li CJ, Li YZ, Pinto AV, Pardee AB. *Proc Natl Acad Sci USA.* 1999;96(23):13369–13374.

66. Gupta D, Podar K, Tai YT, et al. *Exp Hematol.* 2002;30(7):711–720.

67. Li Y, Li CJ, Yu D, Pardee AB. *Mol Med.* 2000;6(12):1008–1015.

68. Kumi-Diaka J. *Biol Cell.* 2002;94(1):37–44.

69. D'Anneo A, Augello G, Santulli A, et al. *J Cell Physiol.* 2010;222(2):433–443.

70. Terai K, Dong GZ, Oh ET, et al. *Anticancer Drugs.* 2009;20(10):901–909.

71. Wendel WB. *Fed Proc.* 1946;5:406–407.

72. Ball E, Anfinsen CB, Cooper O. *J Biol Chem.* 1947;168:257–270.

73. Carvalho LH, Rocha EM, Raslan DS, et al. *Braz J Med Biol Res.* 1988;21(3):485–487.

74. Austin F. *Am J Trop Med Hyg.* 1974;23(3):412–419.

75. Pinto AV, Pinto MD, Gilbert B, et al. *Trans R Soc Trop Med Hyg.* 1977;71(2):133–135.

76. Dos Santos AF, Ferraz PA, Pinto AV, et al. *Int J Parasitol.* 2000;30(11):1199–1202.

77. Lima NM, dos Santos AF, Porfirio Z, et al. *Acta Trop.* 2002;83(1):43–47.

78. Lima NM, Correia CS, Leon LL, et al. *Mem Inst Oswaldo Cruz.* 2004;99(7):757–761.

79. Teixeira MJ, de Almeida YM, Viana JR, et al. *Phytother Res.* 2001;15(1):44–48.

80. Chiari E, De Oliveira AB, Raslan DS, et al. *Trans R Soc Trop Med Hyg.* 1991;85(3):372–374.

81. Lopes JN, Cruz FS, Docampo R, et al. *Ann Trop Med Parasitol.* 1978;72(6):523–531.

82. Sepulveda-Boza S, Cassels B. *Planta Med.* 1996;62:98–105.

83. Perez C, Anesini C. *Fitoterapia.* 1994;65(2):169–172.

84. Anesini C, Perez C. *J Ethnopharmacol.* 1993;39(2):119–128.

85. Machado TB, Pinto AV, Pinto MC, et al. *Int J Antimicrob Agents*. 2003;21(3): 279–284.

86. Pereira EM, Machado Tde B, Leal IC, et al. *Ann Clin Microbiol Antimicrob*. 2006;5:5.

87. Park BS, Lee HK, Lee SE, et al. *J Ethnopharmacol*. 2006;105(1–2):255–262.

88. Park BS, Kim JR, Lee SE, et al. *J Agric Food Chem*. 2005;53(4):1152–1157.

89. Campos-Takaki G, Steiman R, Seigile-Murandi F, et al. *Rev Latinoam Microbiol*. 1992;23(2):106–111.

90. Guiraud P, Steiman R, Campos-Takaki GM, et al. *Planta Med*. 1994;60(4): 373–374.

91. Portillo A, Vila R, Freixa B, et al. *J Ethnopharmacol*. 2001;76:93–98.

92. Schuerch AR, Wehrli W. *Eur J Biochem*. 1978;84(1):197–205.

93. Do Carmo Lagrota MM, Wigg MD, Pereira LOB, et al. *Rev Latinoam Microbiol*. 1983;14(1):21–26.

94. Preusch PC, Hazelett SE, Lemasters KK. *Arch Biochem Biophys*. 1989;269(1):18–24.

95. Do Carmo Lagrota MM, Wigg MD, Aguiar ANS, et al. *Rev Latinoam Microbiol*. 1986;28:221–225.

96. Pinto AV, Pinto M, de C, Lagrota MH, et al. *Rev Latinoam Microbiol*. 1987;29(1):15–20.

97. Preusch PC, Suttie JW. *Arch Biochem Biophys*. 1984;234(2):405–412.

98. Preusch PC. *Biochem Biophys Res Commun*. 1986;137(2):781–787.

99. Son DJ, Lim Y, Park YH, et al. *J Ethnopharmacol*. 2006;108(1): 148–151.

100. Freitas AE, Budni J, Lobato KR, et al. *Prog Neuropsychopharmacol Biol Psychiatry*. 2010;34(2):335–343.

101. Goel RK, Pathak NK, Biswas M, et al. *J Pharm Pharmacol*. 1987;39(2): 138–140.

102. Twardowschy A, Freitas CS, Baggio CH, et al. *J Ethnopharmacol*. 2008;118(3): 455–459.

103. De Almeida ER, Da Silva Filho AA, Dos Santos ER, et al. *J Ethnopharmacol*. 1990;29(2):239–241.

104. Byeon SE, Chung JY, Lee YG, et al. *J Ethnopharmacol*. 2008;119(1):145–152.

105. Grazziotin JD, Schapoval EE, Chaves CG, et al. *J Ethnopharmacol*. 1992;36(3): 249–251.

106. Lira AA, Sester EA, Carvalho AL, et al. *AAPS PharmSciTech*. 2008;9(1):163–168.

107. Sareen V, Jain S, Narula A. *Phytother Res*. 1995;9:139–141.

108. Muller K, Sellmer A, Wiegrebe W. *J Nat Prod*. 1999;62(8):1134–1136.

109. Kung HN, Yang MJ, Chang CF, et al. *Am J Physiol Cell Physiol*. 2008;295(4): C931–C943.

110. Wagner H, Knaus U. *Planta Med*. 1986;52:550A. (P99).

111. Kreher B, Lotter H, Cordell GA, et al. *Planta Med*. 1988;54(6):562–563.

112. Tzeng HP, Ho FM, Chao KF, et al. *Am J Respir Crit Care Med*. 2003;168(1):85–91.

113. Block JB, Serpick AA, Miller W, et al. *Cancer Chemother Rep 2*.1974;4(4):27–28.

114. Nasongkla N, Wiedman AF, Bruening A, et al. *Pharm Res*. 2003;20(10):1626–1633.

115. De Santana CF, Pessoalins LJ, Asfora JJ, et al. *Rev Inst Antibiot (Recife)*. 1980/1981;20:61.

116. Morrison RK, Brown DE, Oleson JJ, et al. *Toxicol Appl Pharmacol*. 1970;17(1):1–11.

117. Schuerch AR, Wehrli W. *Eur J Biochem*. 1978;84(1):197–205.

118. de Santana CF, de Lima OG, d'Albuquerque IL, et al. *Rev Inst Antibiot (Recife)*. 1968;8(1–2):89–94.

119. Jones K. *Pau d'Arco: Immune Power from the Rain Forest*. Vermont: Healing Arts Press; 1995. p. 99.

120. Oga S, Sekina T. *Rev Fac Farm Bioquim Univ Sao Paulo*. 1969;7(1):47–53.

121. Miranda FG, Vilar JC, Alves IA, et al. *BMC Pharmacol*. 2001;1(1):6.

122. Hakura A, Mochida H, Tsutsui Y, et al. *Chem Res Toxicol*. 1994;7(4):559–567.

123. Maistro EL, Fernandes DM, Pereira FM, et al. *Planta Med*. 2010;76(9):858–862.

124. E Sá deC daS R, Guerra Mde O. *Phytother Res*. 2007;21(7):658–662.

125. De Almeida ER, Lucena FRS, Silva CVNS, et al. *Phytother Res*. 2009;23(9): 1276–1280.

126. Arenas P, Moreno Azorero R. *Econ Bot*. 1977;31(3):298–301.

127. Guerra MO, Mazoni AS, Brandao MA, et al. *Braz J Biol*. 2001;61(1):171–174.

128. Guerra MO, Mazoni AS, Brandao MA, et al. *Contraception*. 1999;60(5):305–307.

129. Felicio AC, Chang CV, Brandao MA, et al. *Contraception*. 2002;66(4):289–293.

130. de Almeida RE, de Mello AC, de Santana FC, et al. *Rev Port Farm*. 1988;38:21–23.

131. Sareen V, Jain S, Narula A. *Phytother Res*. 1995;9:139–141.

132. Almeida ME, Brandao MA, Guerra MO, et al. 1999. Cited in Felicio AC, Chang CV, Brandao MA et al. *Contraception* 2002;66(4):289–293.

133. Guerra M. Personal communication, February 2003.

134. Souza ER, Guerra MO, Peters VM. Cited in Felicio AC, Chang CV, Brandao MA et al. *Contraception* 2002;66(4):289–293.

135. Hullar TE, Sapers BL, Ridker PM, et al. *Am J Med*. 1999;106(2):267–268.

136. Estlander T, Jolanki R, Alanko K, et al. *Contact Dermatitis*. 2001;44(4):213–217.

137. Schulz KH, Garbe I, Hausen BM, et al. *Arch Dermatol Res*. 1977;258(1):41–52.

138. Algranti E, Mendonca EM, Ali SA, et al. *J Investig Allergol Clin Immunol*. 2005;15(1):81–83.

Peppermint

(Mentha x piperita L.)

Synonyms

Pfefferminze, Katzenkraut (Ger), menthe anglaise, menthe poivrée, feuilles de menthe (Fr), menta prima (Ital), pebermynte (Dan).

What is it?

The mints, including peppermint, are amongst the oldest European herbs used for both culinary and medicinal purposes. The Greeks and Romans crowned themselves with peppermint at their feasts and adorned their tables with its sprays. Their cooks flavoured both their sauces and their wines with its essence. Peppermint was cultivated by the Egyptians and is mentioned in the Icelandic pharmacopoeias of the 13th century, but only came into general use in the medicine of western Europe in the 18th century. Mints are used in both home remedies and pharmaceutical preparations to relieve the stomach of intestinal gas associated with the consumption of certain foods; hence the many different varieties of after-dinner mints. Menthol, a major compound in peppermint, has been used as an inhalant for upper respiratory ailments and as an ingredient in many liniments and rubs for sore muscles. Recently, peppermint oil has been established as an evidence-based treatment for irritable bowel syndrome (IBS) symptoms.

Effects

Gastrointestinal spasmolytic; carminative; increases bile production; reduces cough frequency; local anaesthetic; antimicrobial; activates the TRPM8 ion channel in cold-sensitive sensory neurons; regulates body temperature during fever.

Traditional view

Peppermint was used to treat flatulent colic, digestive pain, cramps and spasms of the stomach, dyspepsia, nausea and vomiting, morning sickness and dysmenorrhoea. As an inhalant it was used to relieve the cough of bronchitis and pneumonia and to induce perspiration in the early phase of a cold. The bruised fresh herb was applied over the bowel to allay a sick stomach and the same kind of application was also used to relieve headaches.[1,2] An infusion of peppermint in combination with wood betony and caraway was used in the treatment of nervous disorders and hysteria and in combination with elder flowers, yarrow or boneset for the treatment of colds and mild cases of influenza.[3]

Summary actions

Spasmolytic, carminative, cholagogue, antiemetic, antitussive, antimicrobial, diaphoretic. Locally: antiseptic, analgesic, antipruritic.

Can be used for

Indications supported by clinical trials

Indications supported by trials using menthol: to reduce airway hyper-responsiveness in asthma (by inhalation).

Indications supported by trials using peppermint oil: symptoms of IBS (good evidence); postoperative nausea; bacterial lung infection (by inhalation); topically as an analgesic for headaches and postherpetic neuralgia.

Indications supported by trials using a combination of peppermint oil and caraway oil: non-ulcer dyspepsia.

Indications supported by trials using peppermint leaf in combination with other herbs: for the treatment of dyspepsia.

Traditional therapeutic uses

Digestive disorders (dyspepsia, flatulence, colic, cramps, vomiting, nausea); inhalation and oral doses for respiratory disorders (bronchitis, cough, colds, influenza); headaches (topically) and nervous disorders.

May also be used for

Extrapolations from pharmacological studies

Reduction in pain sensitivity by activating the endogenous opiate system and TRPM8 ion channels; countering increased bronchial secretion and inhibition of cough; reduction of dental plaque by topical application; antiviral effects by topical application; acceleration of gastric emptying time.

Other applications

Peppermint leaf and oil are widely used as flavourings in medicinal teas, cough preparations, food products and beverages.[4] Peppermint leaf has also been used as a carminative in antacid products.[5]

Preparations

As with all essential oil-containing herbs, use of the fresh plant or carefully dried herb is advised. Keep covered if infusing the herb to retain the essential oil.

Dried leaf as an infusion, liquid extract, tincture or essential oil for internal use. The essential oil dissolved in alcohol works well for topical use.

Dosage

- 6 to 9 g/day of the dried leaf or as infusion
- 1.5 to 4 mL/day of 1:2 liquid extract, 3.5 to 11 mL/day of 1:5 tincture, or equivalent doses in other dosage forms
- 0.6 to 1.8 mL/day of the essential oil.

Duration of use

May be taken long term for most applications.

Summary assessment of safety

No significant adverse effects from the ingestion of peppermint leaf are expected, but higher doses of the essential oil can produce a variety of adverse reactions including skin rashes, headaches, bradycardia, muscle tremor, heartburn and ataxia. The oil and herb can rarely cause contact dermatitis and large quantities of the oil in the stomach will predispose to gastric reflux and heartburn (as might be expected from its carminative properties).

Technical data

Botany

Mentha × piperita, a member of the Labiatae (Lamiaceae, mint) family, is a perennial plant approximately 50 cm in height with quadrangular stems terminated with a flower spike consisting of numerous congested whorls. The leaves have very short petioles, are opposed, ovate-lanceolate from a wedge shape to an almost heart-shaped base. They have a venation that gives them a rough-textured appearance, are dark green on the upper surface and slightly paler on the lower. The pinkish mauve flowers are tubular with four lobes, one of which is normally larger than the others, contained within a calyx with five pointed lobes. The fruits are dark, four-sectioned, glossy ovoid cremocarps. The plant is always sterile and has a pungent peppermint scent.[6,7] Peppermint is a hybrid species from two parents: Mentha spicata (spearmint) and Mentha aquatica (water mint).[8]

Adulteration

Although many Mentha species are also used, notably Mentha arvensis and M. spicata, the cultivation of most peppermint makes confusion rare. Peppermint oil is liable to augmentation with extra menthol, synthetic or natural menthofuran and menthyl acetate.

Adulteration with Mentha pulegium (pennyroyal) may occur from wildcrafting.[9]

Key constituents

- Essential oil (0.5% to 4%), consisting predominantly of menthol (35% to 45%) and (−)-menthone (10% to 30%)[10]
- Flavonoids, tannins (6% to 12%), triterpenes and bitter substances.[11]

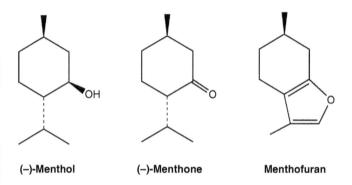

(−)-Menthol   (−)-Menthone   Menthofuran

The *European Pharmacopoeia* recommends that whole peppermint leaf contain not less than 12 mL/kg and the cut leaf not less than 9 mL/kg of essential oil.[12] Peppermint oil is obtained by steam distillation from the fresh aerial parts of flowering Mentha × piperita.[13]

Pharmacodynamics

Gastrointestinal effects

The in vitro effects of peppermint oil on the gastrointestinal smooth muscle of guinea pigs and rabbits resemble those of calcium antagonist drugs. Peppermint oil markedly attenuated contractile responses in guinea pig taenia coli to acetylcholine, histamine, serotonin and substance P. It also reduced contractions evoked by potassium depolarisation and inhibited potential-dependent calcium currents in rabbit jejunum smooth muscle cells in a dose-dependent manner.[14] Intravenous administration of an aqueous solution of peppermint oil reduced morphine-induced spasm in Oddi's sphincter in guinea pigs.[15]

Peppermint leaf extract demonstrated spasmolytic activity on acetylcholine-, carbachol- and histamine-induced contractions in isolated guinea pig ileum.[16,17] An aqueous solution of flavonoids isolated from peppermint inhibited barium chloride-induced contractions in a similar model.[18]

The intraluminal (topical) administration of peppermint oil to the sigmoid colon of five normal people produced increased intraluminal pressure, abdominal cramps and the urge to defecate and micturate, which suggested a widespread stimulation of smooth muscle.[19] This might reflect a local irritant effect of the peppermint oil, since in other studies examining the impact of peppermint oil on colonic spasm during colonoscopy the opposite effect was observed. For example, peppermint oil injected along the biopsy channel of the colonoscope in 20 patients relieved colonic spasm within 30 s, allowing easier passage of the instrument or assisting in polypectomy. Due to the potential irritant action of peppermint oil, a diluted suspension is often used with equally good effects.[20] The direct administration of 15 drops of peppermint oil in 30 mL of water into the stomachs of 27 volunteers caused relaxation of the lower oesophageal sphincter and equalisation of intragastric and intra-oesophageal pressures (carminative activity). Reflux occurred in 25 out of 27 patients within 1 to 7 min of administration. The sphincter relaxation lasted approximately 30 s and was terminated by an oesophageal peristaltic wave.[21]

Since the above research, several clinical trials have demonstrated that intraluminal administration of peppermint oil reduces gastric and colonic spasm, and is safe and useful for upper gastrointestinal endoscopy, colonoscopy and double contrast barium enema examination (DCBE). A prospective, case-controlled study evaluated the efficacy of orally administered peppermint oil (10 mL of a 1.6% emulsified solution) as an antispasmodic for DCBE. Oral peppermint oil emulsification reduced spasm of the oesophagus, lower stomach and duodenal bulb and improved the diagnostic quality of the procedure, without requiring injection of an antispasmodic drug.[22] The efficacy of topical peppermint oil in producing duodenal relaxation has also been demonstrated in endoscopic retrograde cholangiopancreatography.[23] Clinical studies indicate that the duration of the spasmolytic action of peppermint oil is limited to approximately 20 min.[24]

The above effects were confirmed in a large study where 409 patients received about 200 mL of an oil-in-water emulsion containing 8 mL/L of peppermint oil and 0.2 mL/L of Tween 80 via a colonoscope using a hand pump.[25] A spasmolytic action was seen in 88.5% of treated patients versus 33.3% of 36 controls (p<0.0001). Onset was in seconds and the spasmolytic effect lasted for at least 20 min, although the efficacy was significantly lower in patients with IBS.

Results from a randomised, double blind, controlled trial in 100 patients found that intraluminal administration of a peppermint oil solution had superior efficacy and fewer side effects than injection of hyoscine-N-butylbromide during upper endoscopy, in terms of reducing hyperperistalsis in the stomach.[26] A pilot study in 10 healthy men found that peppermint oil (0.64 mL) combined with a test meal accelerated only the early stages of gastric emptying.[27] An earlier study found peppermint oil accelerated gastric emptying rate in both dyspeptic patients and controls. The gastric emptying rate of dyspeptic patients became comparable with age-matched controls after administration of 0.2 mL peppermint oil in 25 mL of water (p<0.001).[28]

Development of symptoms in functional gastrointestinal disorders is frequently preceded by acute gastrointestinal infections and linked to visceral hyperalgesia. Administration of a peppermint and caraway oil preparation reduced experimentally induced visceral hyperalgesia in rats.[29] The effects of enteric-coated and non-enteric-coated preparations each containing 90 mg peppermint oil and 50 mg caraway oil were studied on gastroduodenal motility in six healthy volunteers.[30] Both preparations caused smooth muscle relaxation, with the effect of the enteric-coated preparation being relatively delayed. Each oil, tested separately by intraduodenal application to healthy volunteers, was found to contribute to this activity.[31] Further testing in healthy volunteers (90 mg peppermint oil, 50 mg caraway oil) found that both oils relaxed the gallbladder, but only peppermint oil slowed orocaecal transit time.[32] Neither oil in these quantities influenced gastric emptying time.

Peppermint aqueous extract (infusion) and isolated flavonoids given to rats by injection increased bile acid production.[18] A single oral dose of peppermint oil (0.83 mL/kg) to rats resulted in a 70% increase in bile flow.[33]

Peppermint oil in the intestinal lumen at concentrations varying from 1 to 5 mg/mL inhibited enterocyte glucose uptake via a direct action at the brush border membrane in vitro. This was thought to be due to changes in the charge on tight junctions between cells and to an inhibition of sodium-linked active transport. The standard bolus dose of peppermint oil for humans is about 400 mg and this could achieve a local concentration within the tested range in the intestinal lumen during the fasting state.[34] An ethanolic extract of peppermint leaf demonstrated antiulcerogenic activity after oral doses when given to rats pre-treated with indomethacin.[35]

Antimicrobial and antiparasitic activity

Peppermint oil has shown significant antibacterial and antifungal effects in several studies.[36–38] Samples of 18 different commercial peppermint oils were tested for antibacterial activity against 25 different species of bacteria and 20 different strains of *Listeria monocytogenes* isolated from different food sources. Antifungal activity was also assessed against *Aspergillus niger*, *Aspergillus ochraceus* and *Fusarium culmorum*. The chemical composition of the oils varied, with menthone ranging from 16.7% to 31.4%, menthol 32.1% to 49% and menthofuran 5.1% to 12%. Growth of most of the species of bacteria tested, with the exception of *Acaligenes faecalis*, *Flavobacterium suaveolens*, *Leuconostoc cremoris*, *Pseudomonas aeruginosa* and *Streptococcus faecalis*, was inhibited by some of the peppermint oils, with nine species being inhibited by all the oils. All strains of *Listeria monocytogenes* were inhibited by some peppermint oils, nine strains by all of the oils and one strain by only three of the oils. The three filamentous fungi were inhibited by all peppermint oils, but three oils showed a low activity against *Fusarium culmorum*. The oils showing the most potent antibacterial activity were amongst the most ineffectual oils against one of the fungal species, and there appeared to be an inverse relationship between antibacterial and antifungal activity.[36] Another study found that peppermint oil (0.1%) was more inhibitory towards Gram-negative than Gram-positive bacteria.[39]

Peppermint oil has demonstrated moderate antimicrobial activity towards *Candida albicans* in vitro. Moderate activity was defined as a MIC (minimum inhibitory concentration) value of between 0.6 and 1.5 mg/mL. (MIC is the lowest concentration of substance needed to prevent the growth of a bacterial or fungal suspension.) The MIC of essential oil of peppermint distilled from fresh leaf in Brazil was measured at 0.6 mg/mL. The ethanol extract was inactive (defined as having a MIC higher than 2 mg/mL). By comparison, the antibiotic drug nystatin had value of 0.05 mg/mL.[40] In Yugoslavia, similar results were obtained (MIC 0.8 mg/mL), which was stronger than the antifungal drug bifonazole (2 mg/mL). Peppermint oil was also active against other pathogenic fungi, especially *Trichophyton tonsurans* (0.4 mg/mL).[41]

In Turkey, a research team tested four peppermint oils (one from Turkey, two from the USA, one from India) for in vitro antimicrobial activity against pathogenic bacteria. Variation in activity was observed between the oils. The best activity was against *Listeria monocytogenes* with MIC values for three of the oils ranging from 0.16 to 0.6 mg/mL. *Staphylococcus aureus* was inhibited by two oils (MIC 0.6 mg/mL). The activity towards *Candida albicans* was similar to that reported above (MIC 0.3 to 0.6 mg/mL for the four oils), and was weaker than the antifungal drug ketoconazole (MIC 0.1 mg/mL). In terms of components, menthol demonstrated stronger antimicrobial activity than menthone.[42] Of several Mexican traditional herbs tested, an aqueous extract of peppermint effected relatively good inhibition of the growth of *Helicobacter pylori*.[43]

Peppermint oil inhibited the replication of a plasmid of *Escherichia coli* by 37.5% in vitro. (Plasmids are DNA molecules that are self-replicating and transferable from one organism to another.) Menthol also had antiplasmid activity, with a concentration of 0.325 mg/mL approximating 100% plasmid elimination. An additive antibacterial activity against the *E. coli* strain was observed from the combination of either peppermint oil or menthol with oxytetracycline.[44]

Peppermint essential oil showed better activity than chlorhexidine against the cariogenic organisms *Streptococcus mutans* and *S. pyogenes* in vitro using antibacterial and biofilm models.[45] A peppermint essential oil toothpaste was more effective than chlorhexidine in controlling supragingival dental plaque.

Of a range of extracts and fractions of peppermint, the dichloromethane fraction showed the best in vitro inhibition of *Giardia lamblia*.[46] However, peppermint essential oil was less active in vitro against Giardia than several other oils containing phenolic compounds.[47]

Peppermint oil demonstrated a virucidal activity on herpes simplex virus type 1 (HSV-1) and type 2 (HSV-2) in vitro. The effect was similar to that previously documented for tea tree oil. The oil affected the virus before its adsorption onto the cell, but not after penetration, indicating that it had a direct virucidal action. It was also active against an acyclovir-resistant strain of HSV-1.[48] Aqueous extracts from peppermint, sage and lemon balm displayed strong anti-HIV activity in vitro and ex vivo, acting directly on the virion before entry into the cell.[49] These observed antiviral activities would be most relevant to topical use.

Respiratory effects

Volatile aromatics such as menthol exhibit a surfactant-like effect in vitro. In vivo, menthol decreased the surface tension between water and air and therefore improved lung compliance values.[50] Oral administration of a fraction obtained from an aqueous ethanolic extract of peppermint inhibited nasal symptoms, sneezing and nasal rubbing induced by antigen challenge in sensitised rats in an experimental model of allergic rhinitis.[51] Menthol inhalation produced a significant reduction in cough frequency and an increase in cough latency in guinea pigs challenged with aerosolised citric acid for 2 min, demonstrating the efficacy of menthol as an antitussive in chemically induced cough.[52]

In studies on healthy volunteers (inhalation of menthol vapour)[53,54] and those with nasal congestion associated with common cold infection (oral administration of a menthol lozenge),[55] menthol brought about a change in the nasal sensation of airflow, with a subjective sensation of nasal decongestion. However, it had no effect on the nasal resistance to airflow. This finding is due to a significant pharmacological action on nasal sensory nerve endings and is unrelated to the peppermint smell.[56] These findings were confirmed in a study involving 18 healthy volunteers who inhaled menthol vapour and rated their subjective impression of nasal potency.[57] Objective measurements included the septal mucosal temperature within the nasal valve area and nasal airflow. While 16 of the 18 volunteers reported a subjective improvement of nasal breathing after menthol inhalation, there were no significant changes in measured nasal airflow and mucosal temperature. These results support the hypothesis that menthol leads to a direct stimulation of mucosal cold receptors creating a subjective feeling of clear and wide nasal passages, but without any objective change in nasal airflow.

The transient receptor potential (TRP) channel melastatin 8 (TRPM8) is a non-selective cation channel on primary afferent nerve fibres activated by noxious and innocuous cool temperatures.[58] TRPM8 is the predominant thermoceptor for cellular and behavioural responses to cold temperatures. It is now recognised that TRPM8 is also activated by compounds evoking cooling sensations such as menthol. The above effects on nasal sensations are probably mediated by TRPM8 stimulation by menthol. See also below.

The spasmolytic and secretolytic effects of an ointment containing menthol, camphor and essential oils were tested in animals. Acetylcholine-induced bronchospasm was reduced by 50% when the ointment was insufflated through the respiratory tract, whereas the epicutaneous application of the ointment produced only a slight reduction. Significant secretolytic effects were demonstrated after insufflation and topical administration.[59] Using magnetic resonance imaging, the secretory response to essential oil inhalation was assessed in vivo in rats.[60] Scotch pine and rosemary oils increased tracheal respiratory secretions, but peppermint oil had no effect. Peppermint oil (100 and 300 μg/mL) exhibited spasmolytic activity on rat trachea in vitro via mechanisms involving prostaglandins and nitric oxide synthase.[61]

Analgesic effects

An ethanolic extract of peppermint produced dose-dependent central and peripheral analgesic effects in vivo when administered orally or via injection at relatively high doses (200 to 400 mg/kg) to mice.[62]

Topical application of menthol (1% to 30% concentration in ethanol) showed a major antinociceptive activity in the early phase of the pain response using the formalin test in mice. Menthol-induced analgesia was blocked by naloxone and potentiated by bestatin. Menthol also produced antinociceptive effects in the hot plate test of mice and hind paw pressure test in rats, but did not inhibit carrageenan-induced paw oedema in rats and synthesis of prostaglandin E_2 in vitro. These results suggest that menthol produces antinociceptive effects by activation of the endogenous opioid system and/or partially by local anaesthetic actions, but without anti-inflammatory effects.[63] (However, an anti-inflammatory effect was seen in one study; see below.)

The long-lasting cooling effect produced by the topical application of peppermint oil is caused by a steric alteration of the calcium channels of cold receptors.[64,65] In a double blind, crossover study in 15 healthy volunteers, the analgesic activity of peppermint oil was differentiated from the physical effect resulting from heat of evaporation and appeared to be based on central inhibitory effects mediated by cold-sensitive A delta nerve fibres.[66] Further experimental studies indicate that this central analgesic activity of menthol could occur via activation of the kappa opioid system.[67]

A role for TRPM8 in nociceptive pathways has been described. This led a team of researchers to investigate the role of this ion channel in colonic sensory pathways as a possible explanation for the value of peppermint oil in IBS.[68] TRPM8 was present on a select population of colonic high threshold sensory neurons, which may also co-express pain-sensing (TRPV1) and mechanosensory (TRPA1) receptors. TRPM8 activation couples to these to inhibit their downstream actions, thereby potentially relieving sensations of pain and fullness in IBS patients.

Radioprotective activity

Aqueous extract of peppermint leaf (1 g/kg) given orally to mice prior to exposure to gamma radiation provided a protective effect. In comparison with control animals, administration of peppermint increased spleen weight, improved haematological parameters, protected intestinal mucosa, provided antioxidant activity and protected against chromosomal damage in bone marrow.[69–71] Enhanced survival and improved haematological parameters were also observed in separate experiments after oral administration of peppermint essential oil (0.04 mL per animal).[72] Peppermint leaf extract (1 g/kg/day for 3 days, oral) before radiation exposure protected against testicular damage in mice.[73] These and other studies were the subject of a 2010 review of the radioprotective properties of peppermint.[74]

Other effects

Peppermint oil induced a significant increase in the skin blood flow of capillaries of the forehead in healthy subjects and migraine patients after local application, as measured by laser Doppler flowmetry.[75]

A methanolic extract of peppermint exhibited neuroprotective and MAO-A (monoamine oxidase A) inhibiting activities in vitro.[76]

A dried aqueous extract of peppermint containing approximately 3.3% flavonoids, 18.4% tannins and 1.2% essential oil produced an initial excitatory effect followed by a mild sedative action on mice at a dose of 1000 mg/kg. The initial excitation was thought to be due to a stimulation of the sensorial system. The same extract also showed a mild diuretic activity.[77]

An ethanolic extract of peppermint demonstrated anti-inflammatory activity in rodent models of acute and chronic inflammation. The extract was administered by injection in the former model and by oral route in the latter at doses of 200 to 400 mg/kg.[62]

Daily consumption of peppermint tea (20 g/L) instead of drinking water decreased total testosterone levels and spermatogenesis in male rats, compared with a control group. Follicle stimulating hormone and luteinising hormone levels were increased.[78]

Antitumour and antigenotoxic activity was demonstrated for oral administration of peppermint (water extract, 1 g/kg) given subsequent to an initiating dose of benzo(a)pyrene in newborn mice. Antioxidant effects may have contributed to this demonstrated activity.[79] Dietary additions of menthol and limonene resulted in a significant inhibition of DMBA-initiated rat mammary tumours.[80]

The action of peppermint tea (2%, w/v) as drinking water for 4 weeks on hepatic drug metabolising enzymes was investigated in rats. The activities of cytochrome P450 1A2 and 2E were significantly decreased.[81] Single oral doses of menthol (468 mg/kg) or cineole (262 mg/kg) inhibited HMG-CoA reductase activity in rats by up to 70%. The effect was specific and not due to generalised hepatotoxicity.[82,83]

The addition of dried peppermint leaf at 5% to feed did not significantly affect dry matter intake, nutrient digestibility, ruminal fermentation or milk production in early lactating dairy cows. Compared with cows on a control feed, there was no difference in milk composition, except for the milk fat content. There was a tendency for the milk fat content to be lower in the cows receiving peppermint.[84] Peppermint ingestion by late lactating cows led to decreased nutrient digestibility, which may have been due to a difference in the passage rate of the feed. (The passage rate of feed in early lactating cows is higher than that in late lactating cows.)[84,85]

Pharmacokinetics

Peppermint oil was relatively rapidly absorbed after oral administration to rats and eliminated mainly via the bile. The major biliary metabolite is menthol glucuronide, which undergoes enterohepatic circulation. Urinary metabolites included a series of mono- and dihydroxymenthols and carboxylic acids, some of which were excreted in part as glucuronic acid conjugates.[86] Pharmacokinetic studies in healthy volunteers demonstrate that peppermint oil in normal capsules gives higher peak excretion levels of menthol (as glucuronide) than enteric-coated capsules. Peppermint oil is mainly absorbed in the upper gastrointestinal tract unless enterically coated, and hence should be taken in this form for effects in the lower gastrointestinal tract.[24,87]

Clinical trials

Gallstones

In a controlled, double blind trial, the addition of menthol to ursodeoxycholic acid significantly reduced the size of gallstones by assisting in their dissolution, and lowered the incidence of stone calcification.[88] A proprietary choleretic product containing menthol 32%, pinene 17%, menthone 6%, borneol 5%, camphene 5% and cineole 2% dissolved in olive oil (hence with a similar profile to peppermint oil) significantly lowered the cholesterol saturation index of human bile. Twenty-four patients with radiolucent gallstones were given two capsules three times daily for periods in excess of 6 months in an uncontrolled study. At 6 months the gallstones had disappeared in two patients and were significantly fewer or smaller in a further three patients. The stones in the remaining 19 patients were unchanged, but one of these showed evidence of a reduction in size after 1 year.[89]

Irritable bowel syndrome

There is high level clinical evidence that enteric-coated peppermint oil can alleviate symptoms of IBS. A review published in 2005 found 16 clinical trials dating from 1979 to 1997.[90] All but two were randomised and double blind in design (the others were open label studies). Of the randomised, double blind trials, nine were also crossover. Twelve trials were placebo-controlled, and three utilised anticholinergic drugs for comparison. One trial investigated recurrent abdominal pain in children, and was included in the review due to the spasmodic nature of this condition. In total, 651 patients were enrolled. Eight of the 12 placebo-controlled trials showed statistically significant effects for administration of peppermint oil. Overall, the results indicate that peppermint oil administered orally in an enteric-coated form is a safe and efficacious symptomatic short-term treatment. Peppermint oil reduced global symptoms and pain. In 11 of the 16 studies the efficacy was assessed by a daily patient rating of a set of or selected symptoms (e.g. abdominal pain, distension, flatulence, stool frequency, stool quality, urgency, bloating, frequency of attacks and severity of attacks). To allow for comparison of results, 'overall success' (overall benefit, global improvement, overall assessment) was calculated where possible in the review process. Such average response rates were 58% for peppermint oil and 29% for placebo. No differences were observed in the three comparative trials against smooth muscle relaxant drugs, suggesting a similar efficacy between peppermint oil and the anticholinergics. Thirteen of the 16 trials used a defined peppermint oil preparation with enteric coating. (Peppermint oil capsules are usually enteric coated to prevent the side effect of gastric reflux and to deliver the dose further down the gastrointestinal tract.) Dosage was one to two capsules, three times a day, with each capsule containing between 182 and 200 mg of peppermint oil. Treatment duration was usually 2 to 4 weeks. Mild and transient adverse effects were observed: heartburn, anal burning or discomfort for peppermint oil, dry mouth and blurred vision for the anticholinergics.[90] An earlier meta-analysis that assessed five of these trials (1979 to 1991) found a significant (p<0.001) global improvement of IBS symptoms in patients treated with peppermint oil compared with placebo, but did note methodological flaws.[91]

Trials of peppermint oil in IBS published since 1997 add further weight to the positive findings of the 2005 review. In a randomised, double blind trial, 42 children with IBS (aged 8 to 17 years) received enteric-coated peppermint oil capsules (270 to 540 mg/day) or placebo.[92] After 2 weeks, 75% of the children in the peppermint oil group experienced reduced pain severity compared with 43% for placebo. An Italian study assessed the impact of enteric-coated peppermint oil (1590 mg/day) or placebo for 3 months in 178 patients with IBS.[93] Using a double blind, placebo-controlled design there was a significant advantage observed for peppermint oil over placebo in terms of overall symptoms, with 80% improved versus 36%, respectively (p<0.02). Another Italian study over 4 weeks used a similar design in a trial involving 57 patients with IBS.[94] Symptoms evaluated included abdominal bloating, abdominal pain, diarrhoea, constipation and passage of gas or mucus. By the end of the trial, 75% of patients taking peppermint oil achieved a >50% reduction in symptom score, compared with 39% in the placebo group (p<0.009). Only the herbal group exhibited a significant overall reduction in symptom score compared with baseline (p<0.01). A randomised, double blind Iranian trial over 8 weeks assessed 540 mg/day of enteric-coated peppermint oil or placebo in 90 patients with IBS.[95] There was a significant difference favouring peppermint oil in terms of the number of pain-free patients (p<0.001) by the end of the trial.

A systematic review and meta-analysis identified and combined four high-quality trials of peppermint oil (average Jadad score 4.25) and found that it was more effective than fibre or conventional antispasmodic drugs in relieving symptoms of IBS.[96] Compared with placebo, the relative risk of persistent symptoms after peppermint oil use was 0.43 (confidence interval 0.32 to 0.59). This meta-analysis included the two Italian trials[93,94] discussed above and two earlier trials.

Treatment with enteric-coated peppermint oil (540 mg/day for 20 days) is said to have reduced small-intestinal overgrowth in one patient with IBS and improved symptoms,[97] although the method used to assess efficacy (breath hydrogen excretion) has been questioned.[98]

The spasmolytic activity of peppermint oil on the gastrointestinal tract has been demonstrated in a number of studies in patients undergoing diagnostic procedures (see Gastrointestinal effects under Pharmacodynamics for more details).

Other gastrointestinal disorders

Fifty-four patients with non-ulcer dyspepsia were given one enteric-coated capsule containing 90 mg of peppermint oil and 50 mg of caraway oil three times a day in a double blind, placebo-controlled, multicentre trial. After 4 weeks of treatment the intensity of pain (p=0.015) and global clinical impression score (p=0.008) were significantly improved for the active group compared with the placebo group. Before treatment commenced, all active patients reported moderate to severe pain, but by the end of the study 63.2% were pain free and

26.3% reported a reduction of their pain.[99] The same preparation at the same dose was found to have comparable efficacy to the drug cisapride in a randomised, double blind trial conducted over 4 weeks in 118 patients with functional dyspepsia.[100] Another trial in 223 patients with non-ulcer dyspepsia established the superiority of the enteric-coated capsule delivery over a normal acid-soluble capsule in terms of reduced side effects, although both preparations exhibited somewhat comparable efficacy when the differing dosage used is taken into account.[101] The enteric-coated peppermint and caraway oil combination was tested against placebo at two capsules per day for 28 days in 96 patients with functional dyspepsia in a randomised, double blind trial.[102] There were significant reductions in a variety of typical symptoms for the active group compared with placebo. The herbal treatment was well tolerated.

In two randomised, double blind trials, a tablet containing fennel fruit, peppermint, caraway and gentian was evaluated in patients with idiopathic dyspepsia. The tablets reduced both acute and chronic symptoms.[103] A liquid herbal formula (25 drops three times daily) containing, in increasing proportions, wormwood, caraway, fennel and peppermint was found to be superior to the spasmolytic drug metoclopramide in terms of relief of symptoms such as pain, nausea, belching and heartburn in a randomised, double blind clinical trial of the treatment of dyspepsia (p=0.02).[104] In another placebo-controlled, randomised, double blind clinical trial, 70 patients with marked chronic digestive problems such as flatulence or bloating were treated with either a herbal formula containing caraway, fennel, peppermint and gentian in tablet form or a placebo over a 14-day period. Analysis of the trial results established a significant improvement in the gastrointestinal complaint scores of the group receiving herbal tablets compared with the placebo group (p<0.05). Ultrasound results evaluating the amount of gas present in the bowel also demonstrated a significant benefit from the herbal formula (p<0.05).[105]

A proprietary formulation containing *Iberis amara*, chamomile, peppermint, caraway, licorice and other herbs was assessed in the treatment of functional dyspepsia using a randomised, double blind, placebo-controlled design involving 120 patients.[106] After 8 weeks 43.3% of patients on the herbal treatment versus 3.3% on placebo reported complete relief of symptoms (p<0.001). There have been other positive trials in functional dyspepsia for this and a similar formulation.[107,108]

Diffuse oesophageal spasm (DOS) is a rare condition that results in simultaneous oesophageal contractions, leading to symptoms of chest pain and dysphagia. Diagnosis can be controversial. In an open label pilot study in eight patients with DOS, five drops of peppermint oil in 10 mL of water completely eliminated simultaneous oesophageal contractions in all patients (p<0.01).[109] The number of multiphasic, spontaneous and missed contractions also improved. Two of the eight patients had chest pain that resolved after the peppermint oil.

Headache

The topical application of peppermint oil in an ethanol solution has proven to be a well-tolerated and cost-effective treatment for tension headache. In a randomised, placebo-controlled, double blind, crossover study, 10% of peppermint oil (in 90% ethanol solution) was compared with paracetamol (1 g) and placebo in the treatment of 164 chronic tension headaches in 41 patients of both sexes. Headache episodes were treated with the following: placebo capsule and peppermint oil, paracetamol (acetaminophen) and placebo solution, paracetamol and peppermint oil, or placebo capsule and placebo solution. Peppermint oil solution was spread across the forehead and temples and the application was repeated after 15 and 30 min. The oil solution significantly reduced headache intensity after 15 min compared with placebo (p<0.01). Paracetamol was effective relative to placebo (p<0.01), but did not differ significantly from treatment with peppermint oil. The simultaneous administration of the peppermint oil solution with paracetamol produced an additive effect (p<0.001). The authors concluded that peppermint oil was an acceptable and cost-effective alternative to oral analgesics in the treatment of tension headache.[110] This peppermint oil preparation was also evaluated against 1 g of aspirin (acetylsalicylic acid). Forty-four patients with episodic tension-type headache treated four headache attacks each in a randomised, double blind study with a double-dummy design: peppermint oil + placebo, peppermint oil + aspirin, placebo oil + aspirin or placebo oil + placebo. Application of peppermint oil resulted in a highly significant reduction in pain intensity compared with placebo and with similar efficacy to aspirin. The combination of peppermint oil and aspirin was significantly superior to either single preparation and a significant reduction in headache-induced general incapacity was observed only for the combination.[111]

In a randomised, double blind, placebo-controlled crossover study, the effects of topical application of peppermint and/or eucalyptus oil preparations on headache parameters were investigated in 32 healthy men. The combination of peppermint oil, eucalyptus oil and ethanol increased cognitive performance while exerting muscle-relaxing and mentally relaxing effects, but had no significant influence on pain sensitivity. In contrast, the peppermint oil and ethanol preparation produced a significant analgesic effect, with reduction in sensitivity to headache (p<0.01 for experimental ischaemia, p<0.001 for experimental heat stimuli). These pharmacological and clinical results indicate that peppermint oil has both central and peripheral activity.[112,113]

The topical application of a 10% menthol solution in ethanol as an abortive treatment of migraine headache without aura was studied in a randomised, double blind, placebo-controlled, crossover study.[114] The intention-to-treat population consisted of 35 patients (28 women, seven men) with 118 migraine attacks. Menthol solution applied to the forehead and temples was statistically superior to the placebo on 2-h pain free (p=0.001), 2-h pain relief (p<0.001) and sustained pain free and pain relief endpoints (p=0.008). It was also superior in terms of relief of nausea and/or vomiting and phonophobia and/or photophobia (p=0.02). No significant difference was seen between adverse effects in the treatment and placebo groups (p=0.13).

Respiratory conditions

Peppermint oil in the form of an inhalation (20-minute heat evaporation into the patient's room daily for a period of 2 months) was used to supplement multidrug therapy for pulmonary tuberculosis in Russia. Positive results were observed: reductions of bacterial infection by 26.8% and 58.5% occurred with doses of 0.01 mL/m³ and 0.005 mL/m³, respectively. This was followed by earlier onset of positive X-ray changes in the lung.[115]

The impact of inhaled menthol on asthma was studied in a placebo-controlled trial involving 23 patients. The menthol vapour did not produce acute bronchodilatory effects, but long-term inhalation over 4 weeks produced an improvement of airway hyper-responsiveness without altering the magnitude of airflow limitation. There was decreased diurnal variation in peak expiratory flow rate (p<0.05), a parameter that reflects airway hyper-responsiveness, but no significant effects on the forced expiratory volume in 1 sec. The number of metered dose inhalations of bronchodilator drugs were also significantly reduced in the menthol group (p<0.01).[116]

Other conditions

Topical application of peppermint oil (containing 10% menthol) provided an analgesic effect in a woman with postherpetic neuralgia whose pain had been resistant to standard therapies.[117]

The incidence of postoperative nausea in gynaecological patients was significantly reduced (p=0.02) in the group that inhaled peppermint oil in a placebo-controlled trial involving 18 patients.[118] However, a comparison between inhalation of peppermint oil, isopropyl alcohol and a saline placebo in 33 patients with postoperative nausea found good and equal efficacy for all three interventions.[119]

A study in 196 mothers was conducted to assess the efficacy of peppermint water in the prevention of nipple cracks during breastfeeding compared with the application of expressed breast milk.[120] The peppermint water was significantly more effective at preventing nipple pain and damage (p<0.01). A follow-up study compared a peppermint gel, lanolin ointment and a placebo gel in a 14-day randomised, double blind trial involving 216 primiparous, breastfeeding mothers.[121] The peppermint gel was superior to both the lanolin and placebo in terms of preventing nipple crack.

Inhalation of peppermint during acute exercise had no significant influence on pulmonary function and physical performance in a randomised, controlled clinical trial involving 36 women soccer players.[122] However, when 144 volunteers were randomly assigned to inhalation of peppermint, ylang-ylang or no aroma, peppermint was found to enhance memory and alertness, whereas ylang-ylang decreased these parameters.[123] Other clinical studies have also shown that inhalation of peppermint aroma can improve cognitive function and alertness.[124]

Toxicology and other safety data

Toxicology

Oral administration of a 4.2:1 peppermint concentrate (4g/kg) did not result in any macroscopic signs of toxicity or death in mice over a 7-day period.[77] Peppermint infusion (20g/L)

provided as drinking water for 30 days did not produce nephrotoxicity in rats. Only minimal hepatic degeneration was observed.[125,126]

Chronic oral administration of peppermint oil (83μL/kg/day for 28 days) to rats resulted in a 45% increase in alkaline phosphatase. No other change in liver enzyme activity was found.[33] The oral LD$_{50}$ of peppermint oil has been measured at 2.4g/kg in mice and 4.4g/kg in rats.[127] Histopathological changes, consisting of cyst-like spaces scattered in the white matter of the cerebellum and nephropathy were seen in male rats given a daily oral dose of 100mg/kg of peppermint oil for 90 days. No other signs of encephalopathy were observed. Nephropathy was also seen in the male rats in the highest dose group. No adverse effects were seen at doses below 40mg/kg.[128] Peppermint oil containing 1% to 2% pulegone was administered to rats (20 to 500mg/kg/day) for 5 weeks. The rats exhibited no adverse effects on general health, behaviour nor body weight, and haematological and urinary parameters were normal. Histological examination revealed no specific pathological lesions.[129] Repeated intradermal dosing with peppermint oil produced moderate and severe reactions in rabbits, although peppermint oil did not appear to be phototoxic.[127]

The acute oral LD$_{50}$ of menthol was reported to be 3.3g/kg in the rat and 0.8 to 1g/kg in the cat.[127,130] The estimated lethal dose for menthol in humans may be as low as 2g but there are reports of individuals surviving doses as high as 9g.[131]

Menthone at dose levels in rats of 200, 400 and 800mg/kg/day for 28 days led to a dose-dependent decrease in creatinine and increases in alkaline phosphatase and bilirubin. The no-effect level for menthone in this study was lower than 200mg/kg/day.[132]

Peppermint infusion did not show significant genotoxicity in the somatic mutation and recombination test in *Drosophila melanogaster*.[133] However, peppermint oil induced mutations in a dose-independent manner in this test.[134]

Contraindications

Patients with oesophageal reflux symptoms should eliminate high doses of agents that decrease lower oesophageal sphincter pressure, including peppermint.[135]

The Commission E suggests that peppermint oil is contraindicated for internal use in occlusion of the gallbladder passages, cholecystitis and severe liver disease.

Peppermint oil should not be applied to the facial areas and chest of babies and small children, and especially not around the nose.[136]

Special warnings and precautions

Use with care in patients with salicylate sensitivity and aspirin-induced asthma. Care should be taken in patients with gallstones.[11] Oral intake of peppermint oil should be used with caution in patients with pre-existing heartburn. Enteric-coated capsules may produce anal burning in patients with diarrhoea, due to excreted peppermint oil.[130]

Interactions

Peppermint tea reduced the absorption of iron by 84% from a bread meal (compared with a water control) in adult volunteers. The inhibition was dose-dependent and related to its tannin content. Inhibition by black tea was 79% to 94%.[137] This indicates a potential interaction for concomitant administration of peppermint during iron intake. In anaemia and cases where iron supplementation is required, peppermint should not be taken simultaneously with meals or iron supplements.

There is evidence that topical use of menthol could enhance penetration of other agents. This could affect the use of other topical ingredients that have a safety assessment based on their relative lack of absorption.[127] Peppermint oil also slows intestinal transit in healthy volunteers;[32,138] this may slow the absorption rate or increase the total absorption of other drugs.

Peppermint oil (600 mg) increased the oral bioavailability of the calcium channel blocking drug felodipine and simvastatin in healthy volunteers. However, the increase was not as great as that produced by administration of grapefruit juice.[139] A case of suspected interaction between the high intake of menthol cough drops and warfarin (reduced activity) has been described.[140]

Use in pregnancy and lactation

Category B2 – no increase in frequency of malformation or other harmful effects on the fetus from limited use in women. Animal studies are largely lacking.

A tea consisting of peppermint, *Urtica dioica*, *Glycyrrhiza glabra*, *Helichrysum arenarium* and a species of Rosa did not affect postnatal development or demonstrate embryotoxicity or teratogenicity when administered to rats.[141]

Teratogenic effects were not observed in mice, rats, hamsters and rabbits for menthol tested at maximum oral doses of 190, 220, 400 and 430 mg/kg/day, respectively.[142]

Peppermint is compatible with breastfeeding but caution should be used. While the leaf probably is compatible with breastfeeding, use of the oil should be discouraged. Caution should be exercised because there is the view that use of peppermint may dry up milk secretions. However, this was not observed in lactating dairy cows (see earlier in this monograph).

Effects on ability to drive and use machines

No adverse effects expected.

Side effects

Allergic reactions to peppermint leaf appear to be rare or of a relatively minor nature. In fact, most adverse reactions relate to the use of the oil or pure menthol. Reports of gastrointestinal irritation or aggravation of gastrointestinal complaints including stomatitis, severe oesophagitis, gastritis, unexplained diarrhoea and pancreatitis have been associated with the use of peppermint preparations, including confectionery.[131] It has been reported from hospitals in a particular area of Turkey that daily consumption of four cups of tea made from peppermint or *Mentha spicata* has resulted in reduced libido in men.[78]

Peppermint oil use has been associated with mucosal ulcerations.[143,144] These are consistent with the development of a buccal contact sensitivity reaction to peppermint or menthol.[145,146] Three constituents of peppermint oil, alphapinene, limonene and phellandrene, also found in turpentine oil, are thought to be the primary sensitising agents.[147] Cases of allergic contact sensitivity have been reported for peppermint oil and the tea.[148,149]

Skin rashes, headache, bradycardia, muscle tremor, heartburn and ataxia are rarely reported side effects associated with enteric-coated capsules of peppermint oil.[131,150] The use of non-enteric-coated oil preparations occasionally causes heartburn, especially in persons suffering from reflux oesophagitis.[87,150] Enteric-coated capsules may produce anal burning in patients with diarrhoea due to excreted peppermint oil.

Mild dermatological reactions on the skin and mucous membranes have been described, and neat peppermint oil can produce chemical burns.[131]

Menthol can cause jaundice in newborn babies. This has been linked to glucose-6-phosphate dehydrogenase deficiency in some cases.[151] A case of exacerbation of urticaria and asthma after ingestion of menthol-containing lozenges has been reported.[152]

Menthol inhalations can also cause breathlessness and laryngeal spasm in susceptible individuals.[153] Nasal preparations containing menthol may cause spasm of the glottis in young children. Bradycardia has been reported in a patient addicted to menthol cigarettes, and fibrillation has been associated with the excessive consumption of peppermint-flavoured confectionery.[131]

High doses of tannins can lead to excessive astringency on mucous membranes, which has an irritating effect.

Overdosage

Bradycardia has been reported in a patient addicted to menthol cigarettes[154] and fibrillation has been associated with the excessive consumption of peppermint-flavoured confectionery (up to 225 g/day).[155]

Excessive inhalation of mentholated products has caused reversible, undesirable effects, such as nausea, anorexia, cardiac problems, ataxia and other CNS problems, probably due to the presence of volatile menthol.

No cases of overdosage are documented for peppermint leaf.

Safety in children

Direct application of peppermint oil preparations to the nasal area or chest of babies and small children must be avoided because of the risk of laryngeal and bronchial spasms. No adverse effects are expected from use of peppermint leaf.

Regulatory status in selected countries

Both peppermint leaf and peppermint oil are official in the *European Pharmacopoeia* (2011), the *British Pharmacopoeia* (2011) and the *United States Pharmacopeia-National Formulary* (USP 34-NF 29 2011).

Peppermint leaf and peppermint oil are covered by positive Commission E monographs and can be used for the following applications.

Peppermint leaf:

* Cramp-like complaints in the gastrointestinal tract and the gallbladder and biliary tract.

Peppermint oil:

* Internal: spastic discomfort of the upper gastrointestinal tract and bile ducts, irritable colon, catarrh of the respiratory tract, inflammation of the oral mucosa
* External: myalgia and neuralgia.

Peppermint is on the UK General Sale List. A peppermint oil product in aqueous solution has achieved Traditional Herbal Registration in the UK with the traditional indication of symptomatic relief of minor digestive complaints such as dyspepsia, flatulence and stomach cramps.

Peppermint, peppermint oil and menthol have GRAS status. Peppermint is also freely available as a 'dietary supplement' in the USA under DSHEA legislation (1994 Dietary Supplement Health and Education Act). Peppermint has been present in OTC (over-the-counter) digestive aid drug products. Peppermint oil has been present in OTC nasal decongestant drug products (mouthwash), expectorant drug products, digestive aid drug products, insect bite and sting drug products and astringent drug products. The FDA, however, advises that: 'based on evidence currently available, there is inadequate data to establish general recognition of the safety and effectiveness of these ingredients for the specified uses'.

Peppermint and peppermint oil are not included in Part 4 of Schedule 4 of the Therapeutic Goods Act Regulations of Australia and are freely available for sale.

References

1. Felter HW, Lloyd JU. *King's American Dispensatory*. 18th ed. rev 3, vol. 1. 1905. Portland: reprinted by Eclectic Medical Publications; 1983. pp. 1254–1255.
2. British Herbal Medicine Association Scientific Committee. *British Herbal Pharmacopoeia*. Cowling: BHMA; 1983. p. 142.
3. Grieve M. *A Modern Herbal*, vol. 2. New York: Dover Publications; 1971. pp. 537–543.
4. Leung AY, Foster S. *Encyclopedia of Common Natural Ingredients Used in Food, Drugs and Cosmetics*, 2nd ed New York: John Wiley; 1996. pp. 368–372.
5. Robson NJ. *Anaesthesia*. 1987;42(7): 776–777.
6. Chiej R. *The Macdonald Encyclopedia of Medicinal Plants*. London: Macdonald; 1984. Entry no. 195.
7. Launert EL. *The Hamlyn Guide to Edible and Medicinal Plants of Britain and Northern Europe*. London: Hamlyn; 1981. p. 156.
8. Evans WC. *Trease and Evans' Pharmacognosy*, 14th ed. London: WB Saunders; 1996. pp. 259–261.
9. Blaschek W, Ebel S, Hackenthal E, et al. *HagerROM 2002: Hagers Handbuch Der Drogen und Arzneistoffe*. Heidelberg: Springer; 2002.
10. Wagner H, Bladt S. *Plant Drug Analysis: A Thin Layer Chromatography Atlas*, 2nd ed Berlin: Springer-Verlag; 1996. p. 156.
11. Bisset NG, ed. *Herbal Drugs and Phytopharmaceuticals*. Stuttgart: Medpharm Scientific; 1994. pp. 336–338.
12. *European Pharmacopoeia*, 3rd ed. Strasbourg: European Department for the Quality of Medicines within the Council of Europe; 1996. p. 1298.
13. *European Pharmacopoeia*, 3rd ed. Strasbourg: European Department for the Quality of Medicines within the Council of Europe; 1996. p. 1299.
14. Hills JM, Aaronson PI. *Gastroenterology*. 1991;101(1):55–65.
15. Giachetti D, Taddei E, Taddei I. *Planta Med*. 1988;54(5):389–392.
16. Forster HB, Niklas H, Lutz S. *Planta Med*. 1980;40(4):309–319.
17. Forster H. *Z Allg Med*. 1983;59(24): 1327–1333.
18. Lallement-Guilbert N, Bezanger-Bearuquesne L. *Plant Med Phytother*. 1970;4:92–107.
19. Rogers J, Tay HH, Misiewicz JJ. *Lancet*. 1988;2(8602):99.
20. Leicester RJ, Hunt RH. *Lancet*. 1982;2(8305):989.
21. Sigmund CJ, McNally EF. *Gastroenterology*. 1969;56(1):13–18.
22. Mizuno S, Kato K, Ono Y, et al. *J Gastroenterol Hepatol*. 2006;21(8): 1297–1301.
23. Yamamoto N, Nakai Y, Sasahira N, et al. *J Gastroenterol Hepatol*. 2006;21(9): 1394–1398.
24. Grigoleit HG, Grigoleit P. *Phytomedicine*. 2005;12(8):607–611.
25. Asao T, Mochiki E, Suzuki H, et al. *Gastrointest Endosc*. 2001;53(2): 172–177.
26. Hiki N, Kurosaka H, Tatsutomi Y, et al. *Gastrointest Endosc*. 2003;57(4):475–482.
27. Inamori M, Akiyama T, Akimoto K, et al. *J Gastroenterol*. 2007;42(7):539–542.
28. Dalvi SS, Nadkarni PM, Pardesi R, et al. *Indian J Physiol Pharmacol*. 1991;35(3): 212–214.
29. Holtmann G, Adam B, Liebregts T, et al. *Gastroenterology*. 2004;126(4 suppl 2):A640.
30. Micklefield GH, Creving I, May B. *Phytother Res*. 2000;14(1):20–23.
31. Micklefield G, Jung O, Greving I, et al. *Phytother Res*. 2003;17(2):135–140.
32. Goerg KJ, Spilker T. *Aliment Pharmacol Ther*. 2003;17(3):445–451.
33. Vo LT, Chan D, King RG. *Clin Exp Pharmacol Physiol*. 2003;30(10):799–804.
34. Beesley A, Hardcastle J, Hardcastle PT, et al. *Gut*. 1996;39(2):214–219.
35. Kayyal MT, El-Ghazaly MA, Kenawy SA, et al. *Arzneimittelforschung/Drug Res*. 2001;51:545–553.
36. Lis-Balchin M, Deans SG, Hart S. *Med Sci Res*. 1997;25:151–152.
37. El-Naghy MA, Maghazy SN, Fadl-Allah EM, et al. *Zentralbl Mikrobiol*. 1992;147(3–4):214–220.
38. Maiti D, Kole CR, Sen C. *Pfl Krankh*. 1985;92(1):64–68.
39. Shapiro S, Meier A, Guggenheim B. *Oral Microbiol Immunol*. 1994;9:202–208.
40. Duarte MC, Figueira GM, Sartoratto A, et al. *J Ethnopharmacol*. 2005;97(2): 305–311.
41. Mimica-Dukic N, Bozin B, Sokovic M, et al. *Planta Med*. 2003;69(5):413–419.
42. Iscan G, Kirimer N, Kurkcuoglu M, et al. *J Agric Food Chem*. 2002;50 (14):3943–3946.
43. Castillo-Juárez I, González V, Jaime-Aguilar H, et al. *J Ethnopharmacol*. 2009;122(2):402–405.
44. Schelz Z, Molnar J, Hohmann J. *Fitoterapia*. 2006;77(4):279–285.
45. Shayegh S, Rasooli I, Taghizadeh M, et al. *Nat Prod Res*. 2008;22(5):428–439.

46. Vidal F, Vidal JC, Gadelha AP, et al. *Exp Parasitol*. 2007;115(1):25–31.

47. Machado M, Sousa C, Salgueiro L, et al. *Nat Prod Commun*. 2010;5(1):137–141.

48. Schuhmacher A, Reichling J, Schnitzler P. *Phytomedicine*. 2003;10(6–7):504–510.

49. Geuenich S, Goffinet C, Venzke S, et al. *Retrovirology*. 2008;5:27.

50. Zanker KS, Tolle W, Blumel G, et al. *Respiration*. 1980;39(3):150–157.

51. Inoue T, Sugimoto Y, Masuda H, et al. *Biol Pharm Bull*. 2001;24(1):92–95.

52. Laude EA, Morice AH, Grattan TJ. *Pulmon Pharmacol*. 1994;7(3):179–184.

53. Eccles R, Jones AS. *J Laryngol Otol*. 1983;97(8):705–709.

54. Burrow A, Eccles R, Jones AS. *Acta Otolaryngol*. 1983;96(1–2):157–161.

55. Eccles R, Jawad MS, Morris S. *J Pharm Pharmacol*. 1990;42(9):652–654.

56. Eccles R, Griffiths DH, Newton CG, et al. *Clin Otolaryngol*. 1988;13(1):25–29.

57. Lindemann J, Tsakiropoulou E, Scheithauer MO, et al. *Am J Rhinol*. 2008;22(4): 402–405.

58. Knowlton WM, McKemy DD. *Curr Pharm Biotechnol*. 2011;12(1):68–77.

59. Rai MK, Upadhyay S. *Arzneimittelforschung*. 1981;31(1):82–86.

60. Nicolato E, Boschi F, Marzola P, et al. *J Ethnopharmacol*. 2009;124(3):630–634.

61. de Sousa AA, Soares PM, de Almeida AN, et al. *J Ethnopharmacol*. 2010;130(2): 433–436.

62. Atta AH, Alkofahi A. *J Ethnopharmacol*. 1998;60(2):117–124.

63. Taniguchi Y, Deguchi Y, Saita M, et al. *Nippon Yakurigaku Zasshi*. 1994;104(6):433–446.

64. Watson HR, Hems R, Rowsell DG, et al. *J Soc Cosmet Chem*. 1978;29(4):185–200.

65. Eccles R. *J Pharm Pharmacol*. 1994;46:618–630.

66. Bromm B, Scharein E, Darsow U, et al. *Neurosci Lett*. 1995;187:157–160.

67. Galeotti N, Di Cesare Mannelli L, Mazzanti G, et al. *Neurosci Lett*. 2002;322(3):145–148.

68. Harrington AM, Hughes PA, Martin CM, et al. *Pain*. 2011;152(7):1459–1468.

69. Samarth RM, Kumar A. *J Radiat Res*. 2003;44(2):101–109.

70. Samarth RM, Kumar A. *Indian J Exp Biol*. 2003;41(3):229–237.

71. Samarth RM, Saini MR, Maharwal J, et al. *Indian J Exp Biol*. 2002;40(11): 1245–1249.

72. Samarth RM, Goyal PK, Kumar A. *Phytother Res*. 2004;18(7):546–550.

73. Samarth RM, Samarth M. *Basic Clin Pharmacol Toxicol*. 2009;104(4):329–334.

74. Baliga MS, Rao S. *J Cancer Res Ther*. 2010;6(3):255–262.

75. Gobel H, Dworschak M, Ardabili S, et al. *The 7th International Headache Congress*. Toronto; September 16–20, 1995.

76. Lopez V, Martin S, Gomez-Serranillos MP, et al. *Phytother Res*. 2010;24(6):869–874.

77. Della Loggia R, Tubaro A. *Fitoterapia*. 1990;61(3):215–221.

78. Akdogan M, Ozguner M, Kocak A, et al. *Urology*. 2004;64(2):394–398.

79. Samarth RM, Panwar M, Kumar A. *Environ Mol Mutagen*. 2006;47(3): 192–198.

80. Russin WA, Hoesly JD, Elson CE, et al. *Carcinogenesis*. 1989;10(11):2161–2164.

81. Maliakal PP, Wanwimolruk S. *J Pharm Pharmacol*. 2001;53(10):1323–1329.

82. Clegg RJ, Middleton B, Bell GD, et al. *J Biol Chem*. 1982;257(5):2294–2299.

83. Clegg RJ, Middleton B, Bell GD, et al. *Biochem Pharmacol*. 1980;29(15): 2125–2128.

84. Hosoda K, Matsuyama H, Park WY, et al. *Anim Sci J*. 2006;77(5):503–509.

85. Hosoda K, Nishida T, Park WY, et al. *Asian Australas J Anim Sci*. 2005;18 (12):1721–1726.

86. Grigoleit HG, Grigoleit P. *Phytomedicine*. 2005;12(8):612–616.

87. Somerville KW, Richmond CR, Bell GD. *Br J Clin Pharmacol*. 1984;18:638–640.

88. Leuschner M, Leuschner U, Lazarovici D, et al. *Gut*. 1988;29(4):428–432.

89. Bell CD, Doran J, Middleton A, et al. *Br J Clin Pharmacol*. 1978;6(5):454P.

90. Grigoleit HG, Grigoleit P. *Phytomedicine*. 2005;12(8):601–606.

91. Pittler MH, Ernst E. *Am J Gastroenterol*. 1998;93(7):1131–1135.

92. Kline RM, Kline JJ, Di Palma J, et al. *J Pediatr*. 2001;138(1):125–128.

93. Capanni M, Surrenti E, Biagini MR, et al. *Gazz Med Ital Arch Sci Med*. 2005;164:119–126.

94. Cappello G, Spezzaferro M, Grossi L, et al. *Dig Liver Dis*. 2007;39(6):530–536.

95. Merat S, Khalili S, Mostajabi P, et al. *Dig Dis Sci*. 2010;55(5):1385–1390.

96. Ford AC, Talley NJ, Spiegel BMR, et al. *BMJ*. 2008;337:a2313.

97. Logan AC, Beaulne TM. *Altern Med Rev*. 2002;7(5):410–417.

98. Gaby AR. *Altern Med Rev*. 2003;8(1):3.

99. May B, Kuntz HD, Kieser M, et al. *Arzneimittelforschung*. 1996;46(12):1149–1153.

100. Madisch A, Heydenreich C–J, Wieland V, et al. *Arzneimittelforschung*. 1999;49(11): 925–932.

101. Freise J, Kohler S. *Pharmazie*. 1999;54(3):210–215.

102. May B, Kohler S, Schneider B. *Aliment Pharmacol Ther*. 2000;14(12):1671–1677.

103. Uehleke B, Silberhorn H, Wohling H. *Fortschr Med*. 2002;144(27/28):695.

104. Westphal J, Hörning M, Leonhardt K. *Phytomedicine*. 1996;2(4):285–291.

105. Silberhorn H, Landgrebe N, Wohling D, et al. *6th Phytotherapy Conference*. Berlin: October 5–7, 1995.

106. Madisch A, Holtmann G, Mayr G, et al. *Digestion*. 2004;69(1):45–52.

107. Raedsch R, Hanisch J, Bock P, et al. *Z Gastroenterol*. 2007;45(10):1041–1048.

108. von Arnim U, Peitz U, Vinson B, et al. *Am J Gastroenterol*. 2007;102(6): 1268–1275.

109. Pimentel M, Bonorris GG, Chow EJ, Lin HC. *J Clin Gastroenterol*. 2001;33(1): 27–31.

110. Gobel H, Fresenius J, Heinze A, et al. *Nervenarzt*. 1996;67(8):672–681.

111. Gobel H, Heinze A, Wagner S, et al. *Cephalalgia*. 1999;19(4):452. Abstract VI–G4–2.

112. Gobel H, Schmidt G, Soyka D. *Cephalalgia*. 1994;14(3):228–234.

113. Gobel H, Schmidt G, Dworschak M, et al. *Phytomedicine*. 1995;2(2):93–102.

114. Borhani Haghighi A, Motazedian S, Rezaii R, et al. *Int J Clin Pract*. 2010;64(4): 451–456.

115. Shkurupii VA, Kazarinova NV, Ogirenko AP, et al. *Probl Tuberk*. 2002(4):36–39.

116. Tamaoki J, Chiyotani A, Sakai A, et al. *Respir Med*. 1995;89(7):503–504.

117. Davies SJ, Harding LM, Baranowski AP. *Clin J Pain*. 2002;18(3):200–202.

118. Tate S. *J Adv Nurs*. 1997;26(3): 543–549.

119. Anderson LA, Gross JB. *J Perianesth Nurs*. 2004;19(1):29–35.

120. Sayyah MM, Rashidi MR, Delazar A, et al. *Int Breastfeed J*. 2007;2:7.

121. Melli MS, Rashidi MR, Nokhoodchi A, et al. *Med Sci Monit*. 2007;13(9): CR406–CR411.

122. Pournemati P, Azarbayjani MA, Rezaee MB, et al. *Bratisl Lek Listy*. 2009;110(12):782–787.

123. Moss M, Hewitt S, Moss L, et al. *Int J Neurosci*. 2008;118(1):59–77.

124. Blumenthal M. *The ABC Clinical Guide to Herbs*. USA: American Botanical Council; 2003. pp. 300–308

125. Akdogan M, Kilinc I, Oncu M, et al. *Hum Exp Toxicol*. 2003;22(4):213–219.

126. Akdogan M, Ozguner M, Aydin G, et al. *Hum Exp Toxicol*. 2004;23(1):21–28.

127. Nair B. *Int J Toxicol*. 2001;20(suppl 3): 61–73.

128. Spindler P, Madsen C. *Toxicol Lett*. 1992;62(2–3):215–220.

129. Mengs U, Stotzem CD. *Med Sci Res*. 1989;17:499–500.

130. Opdyke DLJ. *Food Cosmet Toxicol*. 1976;14:471–472.

131. De Smet PAGM, Keller K, Hansel R, eds. *Adverse Effects of Herbal Drugs*, vol. 1. Berlin: Springer-Verlag; 1992. pp. 171–176.

132. Madsen C, Wurtzen G, Carstensen J. *Toxicol Lett*. 1986;32(1–2):147–152.

133. Romero-Jimenez M, Campos-Sanchez J, Analla M, et al. *Mutat Res*. 2005;585 (1–2):147–155.

134. Lazutka JR, Mierauskiene J, Slapsyte G, et al. *Food Chem Toxicol.* 2001;39(5): 485–492.

135. Friedman G. *Gastroenterol Clin North Am.* 1991;20(2):313–324.

136. German Federal Minister of Justice. *German Commission E for Human Medicine Monograph.* Bundes-Anzeiger (German Federal Gazette); no. 50, dated 13.03.1986.

137. Hurrell RF, Reddy M, Cook JD. *Br J Nutr.* 1999;81(4):289–295.

138. Holtmann G, Haag S, Adam B, et al. *Phytomedicine.* 2003;10(suppl 4): 56–57.

139. Dresser GK, Wacher V, Ramtoola Z, et al. *Clin Pharmacol Ther.* 2002;71:P67. Abstract TPII–95.

140. Coderre K, Faria C, Dyer E. *Pharmacotherapy.* 2010;30(1):50e–52e.

141. Ubasheev IO, Lonshakova KS, Matkhanov EI, et al. *Khim Farm Zh.* 1988;22(4): 445–450.

142. Fifty-first Meeting of the Joint FAO/WHO Expert Committee on Food Additives (JECFA). *Safety Evaluation of Certain Food Additives.* WHO Food Additives Series: 42. Geneva: WHO; 1999.

143. Moghadam BK, Gier R, Thurlow T. *Cutis.* 1999;64(2):131–134.

144. Rogers SN, Pahor AL. *Dent Update.* 1995;22(1):36–37.

145. Morton CA, Garioch J, Todd P, et al. *Contact Dermatitis.* 1995;32(5): 281–284.

146. Sainio EL, Kanerva L. *Contact Dermatitis.* 1995;33(2):100–105.

147. Dooms-Goossens A, Degreef H, Holvoet C, et al. *Contact Dermatitis.* 1977;3(6):304–308.

148. Tran A, Pratt M, DeKoven J. *Dermatitis.* 2010;21(2):111–115.

149. Vermaat H, van Meurs T, Rustemeyer T, et al. *Contact Dermatitis.* 2008;58(6): 364–365.

150. Nash P, Gould SR, Barnardo DE. *Br J Clin Pract.* 1986;40(7):292–293.

151. Owa JA. *Acta Paediatr Scand.* 1989;78:848–852.

152. Marlowe KF. *Am J Health Syst Pharm.* 2003;60(16):1657–1659.

153. Lässig W, Graupner I, Leonhardt H, et al. *Z Klin Med.* 1990;45:969–971.

154. Luke E. *Lancet.* 1962;1:110–111.

155. Thomas JG. *Lancet.* 1962;1:222.

Poke root

(*Phytolacca decandra* L.)

Synonyms

Phytolacca americana L. (botanical synonym), poke weed (Engl), Phytolaccae radix (Lat), Kermesbeere (Ger), herbe de la laque (Fr), fitolacca (Ital), kermesbær (Dan).

What is it?

Phytolacca decandra is a striking plant with large leaves, clusters of purple berries often on the same branch with green unripe fruit and flowers still in bloom. It is indigenous to the United States of America with the following common names: poke root, poke weed. The common name derives from the indigenous word *pocon* meaning a plant with red or yellow dye (referring to the juice of the ripe berries). The genus name Phytolacca is from the Greek *phuton* meaning plant and from the Latin *lacca* meaning milky lac. Many parts have been used medicinally, including the berries, leaves and roots. This monograph focuses on the therapeutic use of the dried root, which is toxic in overdose.

The term 'poke weed' occurs extensively in medical literature due to the use of poke weed mitogens (PWM) to investigate cellular immune responses and a poke weed antiviral protein that inhibits viral protein synthesis. These entities are unlikely to be significantly absorbed into the bloodstream after oral doses, except when the gastrointestinal tract is damaged.

Effects

An anti-inflammatory remedy with action on the lymphatic and respiratory systems. Potentially immune stimulating, but caution is required with dosage.

Traditional view

Poke root has been used traditionally for the treatment of inflammatory conditions of the upper respiratory tract (such as laryngitis, tonsillitis), lymphadenitis, mumps and chronic rheumatism. Topically it has been used for the treatment of skin and glandular disorders, such as scabies, tinea, acne, mastitis and mammary abscess.[1] The Eclectic physicians favoured poke root to act upon the skin and the glandular structures, particularly of the mouth, throat or reproductive tract (tonsillitis, ulceration, ovaritis, glandular swellings) and to act markedly on the mammary glands. It was used as an emetic and depurative.[2] Traditional texts record its application in breast cancer (oral use) and topically for uterine cancer.[3]

Radix Phytolaccae, or shang lu in traditional Chinese medicine, refers to *Phytolacca acinosa* or *P. americana*, which has been used to treat oedema, oliguria and ascites and externally for trauma, haemorrhage and pyogenic infections of the skin.[4]

Summary actions

Anti-inflammatory, lymphatic, depurative, immunostimulant, expectorant.

Can be used for

Indications supported by clinical trials

No clinical trials have been conducted using poke root.

Traditional therapeutic uses

As a depurative for skin conditions acting primarily via the lymphatic system; for treatment of inflammatory conditions or infections, especially of the respiratory tract and reproductive systems. Topically for treatment of skin irritation/infection/ infestation and female reproductive system disorders (mastitis, mammary abscess, possibly uterine cancer). This is a valuable herb which must be treated with respect.

Preparations

Only the dried root should be used for making decoctions (the fresh root should not be used). Tincture can also be used for internal or external use.

Dosage

* Up to 0.2 g of dried root per day for adults
* 0.15 to 0.7 mL/day of 1:5 tincture for adults.

Avoid the use of stronger liquid extracts and fresh plant tinctures because of potential toxic effects.

Duration of use

In light of the potential risks, medium-term use of poke root up to 6 months is advised.

Summary assessment of safety

Poke root tinctures may be safely prescribed if the recommended dosage is not exceeded and the contraindications below are observed. Liquid extracts and fresh plant tinctures have the potential to cause poisoning because they are more active and may contain higher levels of PWM.

Technical data

Botany

Poke root, a member of the Phytolaccaceae family, is a herbaceous perennial that grows up to 3 m. The stem divides into two, with the alternate leaves borne on a very short petiole. The flowers, carried on short pedicles, have a bract and no petals but five greenish-white tepals (combined calyx and corolla). The fruit consists of dark, fleshy berries with raised ribs on the surface.[5] The large root is tuberous, with an outer colouring of yellowish-, reddish- or greyish-brown.[6] The plant is striking as its large leaves and beautiful clusters of purple berries often mingle upon the same branch with the green unripe fruit and flowers.[7]

Adulteration

No adulterants known.

Key constituents

* Triterpenoid saponins (phytolac(c)osides, esculentosides and phytolaccasponins) with the main aglycone being phytolaccagenin.[8,9] The nomenclature is inconsistent, with some saponins having two or more names, eg phytolac(c)-oside E = esculentoside A = phytolaccasaponin E
* Sterols; mitogens and antiviral proteins as noted above.[8]

Pharmacodynamics

The immunological activity of poke root is probably due to the presence of traces of lectins such as PWM which, although too large to be substantially absorbed through the gut wall, may interact with gut-associated lymphoid tissue and might even be absorbed in small quantities. In situations of overdosage the saponins may facilitate the bioavailability of the lectins via their detergent activity and their irritating effect on the gastrointestinal mucosa.

Immunological activity

Poke weed mitogen (PWM) is a lectin possessing three distinct biological activities: haemagglutination, leucagglutination and mitogenicity (stimulation of the replication of lymphocytes in vitro).[10] The studies on or using the mitogenic activity of PWM are extensive. Peripheral blood plasmacytosis (increased plasma cells) occurred in children after systemic exposure to PWM from *P. decandra* berries. Such exposure occurred through oral ingestion of large amounts of berries or by contact of fresh cuts and abrasions with the berry juice.[11]

Lymphocyte-stimulating factors (LSFs) were isolated from cultures of murine spleen or thymus cells to which PWM was added. LSFs induced cultured lymphocytes to differentiate into IgM-secreting cells and to proliferate without the addition of mitogen. LSF also stimulated polyclonal

B-cell differentiation into IgM-secreting cells.[12] Extracts of *P. americana* ripe and unripe berries, seeds, pulp, stem, leaf and root demonstrated mitogenic effects in human peripheral blood cells in vitro. While some of the extracts showed mitogenic activity up to dilution of 1:15 000, the most potent root extract was mitogenic at a dilution of 1:1 000 000.[13]

Poke root antiviral protein (PAP, isolated from the leaves and seeds) is a ribosome-inactivating protein that acts on eukaryotic and prokaryotic ribosomes.[14] PAP has potent antiviral activity against many plant and animal viruses in vitro, including HIV,[15] and has demonstrated immunological activity in vivo by injection.[16] Due to its potent antiviral activity and lack of spermicidal effects, PAP is under consideration as a topical anti-HIV agent. Topical administration of a gel containing 0.01% to 1% PAP resulted in moderate-to-marked vaginal irritation in one-third of animals treated.[17] However, it should be noted that poke root probably does not contain significant quantities of PAP.

Anti-inflammatory activity

Crude saponins isolated from poke root exhibited potent inhibitory activity on acute oedema in rats and mice when given by intraperitoneal injection. A 50% inhibition of carrageenan-induced paw oedema in rats was demonstrated at 15 to 30 mg/kg.[18,19]

Pharmacokinetics

No data available.

Clinical trials

No clinical trials have been conducted using poke root.

Toxicology and other safety data

Toxicology

Saline suspensions of poke root extract produced high intraperitoneal lethality in mice, rats and guinea pigs. Large oral doses of liquid extracts markedly impaired liver function, but not kidney function, in rabbits.[20]

An acidic steroidal saponin obtained from poke root had an LD_{50} of 0.065 mg/kg by the intraperitoneal route in mice, indicative of a high toxicity by this route.[21] The following LD_{50} values of a saponin extract of *P. americana* root have been recorded: 181 mg/kg (ip, mice) and 208 mg/kg (ip, rats).[18]

A number of sources state that the root is considered the most toxic part of the plant, although all parts are noted as toxic. Toxicity is said to increase as the plant matures, with the only exception being that the green berries are more toxic than the mature berries. Primary references are not provided.[22-24] However, early animal studies with the berry extract reported that it had milder toxic effects than the root. Poisonings after consumption of the leaves, berries or root have been reported in livestock.[25] Two sheep receiving 20 and 25 g/kg of fresh green leaves of *P. decandra* died 6 h after feeding. The remaining nine became mildly sick but recovered.[26]

Parts of the plant are commonly assumed to be safe to eat when they are prepared properly: that is, when the berries have been cooked or when the young green shoots or leaves have been boiled using two changes of water.[22–24] However, poisonings have still occurred when these precautions have been taken.[22,27,28]

From the literature, it is apparent that there is considerable variability in the toxicity of various Phytolacca preparations. The main toxic components are the saponins, which act as gastrointestinal irritants and probably account for the severe nausea, vomiting and diarrhoea that accompany an overdose.[21,29] The immunological changes that usually accompany poisoning are probably due to the lectins.[21,22] The saponins are not considered to be cardiotoxic.[22] Cardiac effects may be secondary to the increased vagal tone seen with severe gastrointestinal irritation.[30] To date, there have been no studies that correlate toxic effects with levels of particular saponins.

Contraindications

Pregnancy, lactation, lymphocytic leukaemia and gastrointestinal irritation. Poke root should not be used in children.

Special warnings and precautions

The recommended dosage of poke root has been exceeded in some cases (see section on Side effects) due to variation in the potency of the root. Fresh plant tinctures are potentially more unsafe and should not be used. Accurate measurement of a tincture dose is vital to ensure the safe dosage is not exceeded.

Interactions

None known.

Use in pregnancy and lactation

Category D – has caused or is associated with a substantial risk of causing fetal malformation or irreversible damage.

Poke root is contraindicated in pregnancy due to its potential toxicity. Mid-term abortifacient activity has been reported for the seeds (10 mg/kg), roots (20 mg/kg) and leaves (40 mg/kg) of P. acinosa (a species used in traditional Chinese medicine) after intraperitoneal administration to pregnant mice.[31] Abortion in cows has been described as a result of toxicity from the berries.[23] Use of the root as an abortifacient has been reported.[25]

Poke root is used topically in traditional Western medicine to treat mastitis.[1] Breastfeeding infants should not be exposed to poke root applied topically to the breasts, so application to the nipple should be avoided. Otherwise poke root is contraindicated during breastfeeding.

Effects on ability to drive and use machines

None known.

Side effects

As with all herbs rich in saponins, oral use may cause irritation of the gastric mucous membranes and reflux. Individual

responses to the ingestion of poke root plant parts appear to vary greatly and can be independent of the quantity of the plant part consumed.[27] More severe adverse reactions (possibly from mild overdose) include nausea, abdominal pain, haematemesis, diarrhoea, hypotension and tachycardia. A number of adverse events related to the use of poke root have occurred in Australia. These have all been caused by excessive intake.

Topical application of preparations derived from the green plant and root have produced inflammation of the skin.[32] Reddening and irritation of the conjunctivae occurred after instillation of saline suspension of poke root extract into rabbit eyes.[20] Topical application of poke root should be restricted to tinctures and contact with the eyes should be avoided.

Overdosage

Toxic effects will typically result from overdose with poke root. Medical advice should be sought immediately. Intoxication with poke root usually involves an initial burning sensation in the mouth and throat followed a few hours later by nausea, repeated vomiting, salivation, profuse sweating, severe abdominal cramps and watery or bloody diarrhoea. Other symptoms include generalised weakness, headaches, dizziness, hypotension and tachycardia. Urinary incontinence, confusion, unconsciousness and tremors may also occur. The cardiac effects of poke root may be secondary to the increased vagal tone that accompanies the usually severe gastrointestinal colic. The onset of symptoms usually occurs 2 to 4 h after ingestion. Non-fatal cases usually recover within 24 to 48 h with medical treatment.[22–24,33]

Poisonings were widespread in North America during the 19th century, due to overdose of tincture or ingestion of berries or roots mistaken for other vegetables. Fatalities were reported.[25,34] Poisonings have continued into the 20th and 21st centuries from ingestion of the root (sometimes mistakenly) or leaves (fresh and/or cooked) and from drinking tea prepared from the leaf and stem. In one case of poisoning caused by chewing the fresh root, the patient's lymphocyte count increased nearly 4-fold within 1 week of intoxication. A 43-year-old woman experienced overdosage symptoms after she drank one cup of powdered poke root tea, which was prepared as per the label directions (about 1 g/cup of boiling water).[22,30,32,35–38]

As noted earlier, peripheral blood plasmacytosis occurred in children exposed through the oral ingestion of large amounts of berries or by the exposure of fresh cuts and abrasions to berry juice.[11] Large immature basophilic lymphocytes appeared in the peripheral blood of two adults shortly after accidental exposure to a root extract (one through the conjunctiva and the other through a subcutaneous puncture wound).[39] Although described as a 'root extract' in the research paper[39] the latter effect was likely to have been due to exposure to concentrated 'root-derived poke weed mitogen'.[40]

Safety in children

There are no reports of harm in children from consuming poke root as a remedy. However, given the variation in product quality and the risk of overdosage, poke root should not be used in children.

Preschool children are more likely to be poisoned by ingestion of the berries rather than by leaf or root.[24] Up to 10 raw berries can be considered harmless for adults and older children, but may lead to serious poisoning in infants.[41] A few fatal cases of poisoning in children from eating the fruit have been recorded, but it is not clear whether death was caused by the seed or the pulp.[25] Another source suggests that reports of poisoning of children by the berries are not conclusive.[42]

Regulatory status in selected countries

Poke root (*P. acinosa*) is official in the *Pharmacopoeia of the People's Republic of China* (English edition, 2000). It is not covered by a Commission E monograph but it is on the UK General Sale List.

Poke root does not have GRAS status. However, it is freely available as a 'dietary supplement' in the USA under DSHEA legislation (1994 Dietary Supplement Health and Education Act).

Poke root is included in Part 4 of Schedule 4 of the Therapeutic Goods Act Regulations of Australia. This means that OTC (over-the-counter) products containing poke root need to undergo a full evaluation by a committee for quality, safety and efficacy. This restriction regulates the activity of suppliers of OTC products, but does not directly affect practitioners of herbal medicine, who use the tincture as a starting material for individual prescriptions.

References

1. British Herbal Medicine Association Scientific Committee. *British Herbal Pharmacopoeia*. Cowling: BHMA; 1983. pp. 156–157.
2. Felter HW, Lloyd JU. *King's American Dispensatory*, ed 18, 3rd rev, vol. 2, 1905. Portland: Reprinted by Eclectic Medical Publications; 1983. pp. 1471–1475.
3. Grieve M. *A Modern Herbal*, vol. 2. New York: Dover Publications; 1971. pp. 648–649.
4. Chang HM, But PP. *Pharmacology and Applications of Chinese Materia Medica*, vol. 2. Singapore: World Scientific Publishing; 1987. pp. 1131–1134.
5. Chiej R. *The Macdonald Encyclopedia of Medicinal Plants*. London: Macdonald; 1984. Entry no. 229.
6. British Herbal Medicine Association Scientific Committee. *British Herbal Pharmacopoeia*, 4th ed. Bournemouth: BHMA; 1996. pp. 151–152.
7. Osol A, Farrar GE, et al. *The Dispensatory of the United States of America*, 24th ed. Philadelphia: JB Lippincott; 1947. p. 1551.
8. Tang W, Eisenbrand G. *Chinese Drugs of Plant Origin*. Berlin: Springer Verlag; 1992. pp. 763–775.
9. Wang L, Bai L, Nagasawa T, et al. *J Nat Prod*. 2008;71:35–40.
10. Reisfeld RA, Börjeson J, Chessin LN, et al. *Biochem*. 1967;58:2020–2027.
11. Barker BE, Farnes P, LaMarche PH. *Pediatrics*. 1966;38(3):490–493.
12. Basham TY, Toyoshima S, Finkelman F, et al. *Cell Immunol*. 1981;63(1):118–133.
13. Farnes P, Barker BE, Brownhill LE, et al. *Lancet*. 1964;284(7369):1100–1101.
14. Cenini P, Bolognesi A, Stirpe F. *J Protozool*. 1988;35(3):384–387.
15. Tumer NE, Hwang DJ, Bonness M. *Proc Natl Acad Sci USA*. 1997;94(8):3866–3871.
16. Spreafico F, Malfiore C, Moras ML, et al. *Int J Immunopharmacol*. 1983;5(4):335–343.
17. D'Cruz OJ, Waurzyniak B, Uckun FM. *Toxicol Pathol*. 2004;32(2):212–221.
18. Woo WS, Shin KH, Kang SS. *Soul Taehakkyo Saengyak Yonguso Opjukjip*. 1976;15:103–106.
19. Woo WS, Shin KH. *Soul Taehakkyo Saengyak Yonguso Opjukjip*. 1976;15:90–96.
20. Macht DI. *J Am Pharm Assoc Sci Ed*. 1937;26:594–599.
21. Ahmed ZF, Zufall CJ, Jenkins GL. *J Am Pharm Assoc*. 1949;38:443–448.
22. Roberge R, Brader E, Martin ML, et al. *Ann Emerg Med*. 1986;15(4):470–473.
23. De Smet PAGN, Keller K, Hansel R, editors. *Adverse Effects of Herbal Drugs*, vol. 2. Berlin: Springer-Verlag; 1993. pp. 253–261.
24. Mack RB. *North Carolina Med J*. 1982;43(5):365.
25. Watt JM, Breyer-Brandwijk MG. *The Medicinal and Poisonous Plants of Southern and Eastern Africa: Being an Account of Their Medicinal and Other Uses, Chemical Composition, Pharmacological Effects and Toxicology in Man and Animal*, 2nd ed. Edinburgh: Livingstone; 1962. pp. 834–836.
26. Ecco R, de Barros CSL, Irigoyen LF. *Cienc Rural*. 2001;31(2):319–322.
27. Edwards N, Rodgers GC. *Vet Hum Toxicol*. 1982;24(suppl):135–137.
28. [No authors listed]. *MMWR Morb Mortal Wkly Rep*. 1981;30(6):65–67.
29. Woo WS, Kang SS, Wagner H, et al. *Planta Med*. 1978;34:87–92.
30. Hamilton RJ, Shih RD, Hoffman RS. *Vet Human Toxicol*. 1995;37(1):66–67.
31. Yeung HW, Feng Z, Li WW, et al. *J Ethnopharmacol*. 1987;21(1):31–35.
32. Mitchell J, Rook A. *Botanical Dermatology: Plants and Plant Products Injurious to the Skin*. Vancouver: Greengrass; 1979. p. 513.
33. Kell SO. *Vet Hum Toxicol*. 1982;24(suppl):138.
34. Lewis WH, Smith PR. *JAMA*. 1979;242(25):2759–2760.
35. Brooker J, Obar C, Courtemanche L. *J Toxicol Clin Toxicol*. 2001;39(5):549–550.
36. Jaeckle KA, Freemon FR. *South Med J*. 1981;74(5):639–640.
37. Stein ZLG. *Am J Hosp Pharm*. 1979;36:1303.
38. Lawrence RA. *Vet Hum Toxicol*. 1990;32(4):369.
39. Barker BE, Farnes P, Fanger H. *Lancet*. 1965;285(7377):170.
40. Wimer BM, Mann PL. *Cancer Biother Radiopharm*. 2002;17(5):569–597.
41. Frohne D, Pfander HJ. *A Colour Atlas of Poisonous Plants: A Handbook for Pharmacists, Doctors, Toxicologists, and Biologists*. Translated from the 2nd German edition by NG Bisset. London: Wolfe Publishing; 1984. pp. 166–167.
42. Kingsbury JM. *Poisonous Plants for the United States and Canada*. Englewood Cliffs: Prentice Hall; 1964. pp. 225–227.

Rehmannia

(*Rehmannia glutinosa* (Gaertn.) Libosch.)

Synonyms

Glutinous Rehmannia, Chinese foxglove (Engl), Rehmanniae radix (Lat), di huang (Chin), shojio (Jap), saengjihwang (Kor).

What is it?

The roots of *Rehmannia glutinosa* (Gaertn.) Libosch., *R. glutinosa* var. *hueichingensis* (Chao et Schih) Hsiae., *R. glutinosa* var. *purpurea* Makino or *R. glutinosa* var. *lutea* Makino have been used extensively in traditional Chinese medicine (TCM). Rehmannia can be used fresh, dried or after processing (curing), and has various Chinese names depending on its form: shen di huang (uncured), shu di hung (cured).

Effects

Anti-inflammatory in autoimmune disease and allergies and supports the adrenal cortex; may protect against the suppressive effects of corticosteroid therapy and chemotherapy.

Traditional view

Uncured Rehmannia is described as sweet, slightly bitter and cold; cured Rehmannia is sweet and slightly warm. The former clears *Heat* and cools the *Blood* (used in *Warm*-febrile diseases causing high fever, thirst and a scarlet tongue, haemorrhage due to *Heat* entering the *Blood* level), nourishes *Yin* and *Blood* and generates *Fluids* (used in some cases of dry mouth, low-grade fever, constipation), cools the upward blazing of *Heart Fire* (mouth sores, insomnia, low-grade fevers, constipation) and is used for *Wasting* and *Thirsting* syndrome (that probably included diabetes).[1]

Summary actions (uncured Rehmannia)

Antipyretic, adrenal trophorestorative, antihaemorrhagic, anti-inflammatory, mild laxative.

Can be used for

Indications supported by clinical trials

Although thorough clinical trial data on Rehmannia are lacking, the following conditions have been successfully treated in Chinese studies: rheumatoid arthritis, asthma, urticaria and chronic nephritis.

Traditional therapeutic use

- Uncured Rehmannia: antipyretic, haemostatic and removes latent heat from the blood; used for skin rashes, diabetes, low-grade fevers and bleeding.
- Cured Rehmannia: regulates menstruation and promotes blood production; used for anaemia, dizziness, weakness, tinnitus; amenorrhoea and metrorrhagia.

May also be used for

Extrapolations from pharmacological studies

To prevent the suppressive effects of corticosteroid drugs on endogenous levels of corticosteroids. Rehmannia gives support to adrenal function but, unlike licorice, is not hypertensive. A useful review paper of the pharmacological research has been published.[2]

Preparations

Dried or fresh root, decoction and liquid extract, tincture, tablet or capsule for internal use.

To prepare cured Rehmannia, fresh roots are washed in millet wine, steamed and dried with resteaming and redrying several times.

Dosage

- 10 to 30 g/day of the dried (uncured) root in decoction
- 4 to 12 mL/day of the 1:2 liquid extract or equivalent doses as tincture, tablet or capsule.

Duration of use

May be used long term.

Summary assessment of safety

No adverse effects are expected.

Technical data

Botany

Rehmannia glutinosa was classified as a member of the Scrophulariaceae (foxglove) family but is now provisionally assigned to the Orobanchaceae family. It is a hairy perennial herb growing to 40 cm. The plant bears light reddish-purple tubular flowers and has a thick orange tuberous root approximately 3 to 6 cm in diameter.[3]

Adulteration

No information available.

Key constituents

- Iridoid glycosides, including aucubin, catalpol (0.3% to 0.5%), ajugol, rehmanniosides A to D,[4] jioglutosides and rehmaglutins A to D[5]
- Other glycosides, including the phenethyl alcohol glycosides (jionosides).[6]

Pharmacodynamics

Immune and adrenal cortex function

Uncured Rehmannia inhibited the metabolism of cortisol by hepatocytes in vitro. Simultaneous administration of exogenous adrenocortical hormones resulted in cortisol levels remaining close to normal. The authors believed the mechanism to be a competitive effect at the hepatocellular receptor that affected the uptake of corticosteroid hormone, thereby slowing the catabolism of cortisol.[7]

In a model designed for assessing effects in adrenal depletion, oral administration of uncured Rehmannia (3 g/kg) for 2 weeks to rabbits chronically treated with the glucocorticoid dexamethasone significantly raised serum corticosterone levels (p<0.001). Continuation of treatment resulted in further increases. Rehmannia treatment also prevented or reversed morphological changes in the pituitary and adrenal cortex, appearing to antagonise the suppressive effect of glucocorticoids on the hypothalamic-pituitary-adrenal (HPA) axis.[8] Such inhibition of the negative feedback of glucocorticoids on the HPA axis by Rehmannia could explain a trophic effect on the adrenal cortex.[9]

Oral administration of Rehmannia enhanced experimentally induced alkaline phosphatase activity of splenocytes in thyroxine-treated mice. Juice of fresh Rehmannia was stronger than that of decoction of dried Rehmannia. This preparation also enhanced experimentally induced splenocyte mitogenesis.[10]

Jioglutoside A

Catalpol

gal = beta-D-galactopyranose

Jionoside A$_1$

Oral administration (10 to 500 mg/kg) of several fractions from the ethanol extract of Rehmannia suppressed the induction of haemolytic plaque-forming cells in mice. Further fractionation yielded the following immunosuppressive phenolic glycosides: jionoside A[1], jionoside B[1], acetoside, isoacetoside, purpureaside C, cistanoside A and cistanoside F.[6]

Oral administration of cured Rehmannia to mice abolished the suppressive effects of cyclophosphamide and dexamethasone on immunity. Parameters measured included spleen and thymus indices, serum haemolysin, lymphocyte transformation rate, phagocytic activity of peritoneal macrophages and numbers of peritoneal T lymphocytes.[11]

Oral administration of a herbal preparation containing Rehmannia demonstrated protective effects on haematopoiesis, immunity, heart, liver and kidney functions during chemotherapy in tumour-bearing mice.[12]

Pretreatment with injection of a water extract of *Rehmannia glutinosa* var. *purpurea* inhibited fatal shock caused by an experimentally induced systemic allergic reaction. In this test model Rehmannia inhibited plasma histamine levels. By the same route, Rehmannia also inhibited an IgE-dependent skin (allergic) reaction, suggesting antiallergic activity.[13]

Neuroprotective activity

Among four herbs used in TCM for dementia, Rehmannia was found to induce the gene expression of glial cell line-derived neurotrophic factor (GDNF) in vitro.[14] GDNF is a growth factor that promotes survival of various CNS neurons. Most of the interest in neuroprotective activity has focused on catalpol, isolated from the herb. Catalpol has demonstrated neuroprotective activity across a range of in vitro models including oxidative stress,[15] ischaemia,[16] various neurotoxins[17–19] and even beta-amyloid.[20] The neuroprotective activity of catalpol has also been reflected in vivo, albeit following injection of the iridoid glycoside.[19,21]

Antidiabetic activity

Uncured Rehmannia by oral route reduced the pathology of diabetic nephropathy in an animal model. Treatment with Rehmannia resulted in a decrease in the accumulation of advanced glycation endproducts, possibly due to a reduction in oxidative stress.[22] A high dose of aqueous-ethanol extract of Rehmannia (by intragastric route) improved experimentally induced diabetic complications, including retinopathy[23] and diabetic foot ulcers[24] in rats.

The effect of Rehmannia individually and in combination with metformin was investigated in streptozotocin-induced diabetic rats.[25] Rehmannia at 200 mg/kg (oral doses) did not reduce blood sugar, but plasma C-reactive protein was significantly lowered compared with diabetic controls (p<0.05) and the metformin-treated group (p<0.05), suggesting an anti-inflammatory activity for the herb in this context.

Other activity

Steamed Rehmannia was found in a dose dependent manner to reduce symptoms of unpredictable mild stress in mice, including aggravated gastric ulceration and altered liver enzymes and metabolites.[26]

An in vitro study has found that three compounds of Rehmannia (acetylacteoside, jionoside C and jionoside D) demonstrated aldose reductase inhibitory activity.[27]

Orally administered cured Rehmannia demonstrated improvement in haemorrheology in arthritic and thrombotic rats.[28]

Ethanol extract of cured Rehmannia increased erythrocyte deformability and erythrocyte ATP contents, reduced erythrocyte aggregation and promoted activity of the fibrinolytic system in vivo. Extracts of uncured Rehmannia had weak or no activity.[29] Oral administration of Rehmannia inhibited aspirin-induced blood clotting in mice. The action of the juice of fresh Rehmannia was stronger than that of decoction of dried Rehmannia.[10]

In an animal model, cured Rehmannia (by oral route) prevented osteoporotic bone loss induced by ovariectomy. Rehmannia alleviated the decrease in the trabecular bone mineral density and increased cortical bone thickness and trabeculation of the bone marrow spaces.[30]

Oral administration of a water extract of cured Rehmannia reduced renal defects in rats with ischaemia-reperfusion induced acute renal failure.[31] Reduced expression of angiotensin II and AT(1) receptor and regulation of tumour growth factor (TGF)-beta1 and type IV collagen expression has been suggested after similar studies.[32]

Uncured Rehmannia had a protective effect on experimentally induced cytotoxicity in cardiac muscle cells in vitro.[33]

Intraperitoneal administration of a polysaccharide isolated from Rehmannia to mice bearing sarcoma improved production of the suppressor T-lymphocyte subset.[34] Two acidic polysaccharides isolated from raw Rehmannia showed remarkable reticuloendothelial system-potentiating activity in a carbon clearance test.[35] A hot water extract of Rehmannia containing polysaccharides inhibited the proliferation of hepatocellular carcinoma cells in vitro. Rehmannia also stimulated apoptosis.[36] Although polysaccharides may show considerable immune-enhancing activity in vitro or by injection, this activity may not be relevant to the oral use of Rehmannia.

Pharmacokinetics

No data available.

Clinical trials

Uncured Rehmannia has produced therapeutic effects in uncontrolled trials involving patients with rheumatoid arthritis, asthma and urticaria.[37]

Oral administration of a herbal preparation including Rehmannia and Astragalus demonstrated therapeutic effects on chronic nephritis. Significant improvement was observed in 91% of patients in the treatment group, compared with 67% in the control group (p<0.001). The preparation also demonstrated antiallergic effects and promotion and modulation of immunity.[38] The design of this clinical research was not rigorous and results should be interpreted with caution.

Toxicology and other safety data

Toxicology

The mutagenic potential of Rehmannia was tested with the Ames test and in vivo. Uncured Rehmannia showed no mutagenic activity, whereas cured Rehmannia was mutagenic in the in vivo mammalian (mice) assay when given by intraperitoneal injection (2 to 4g/kg).[39]

Oral administration of Rehmannia tended to increase the levels of urea nitrogen, creatinine, methylguanidine and guanidinosuccinic acid in rats with renal failure.[40]

Intragastric administration of either Rehmannia decoction or an alcohol extract at a dose of 60g/kg/day for 3 days did not cause adverse reactions in mice observed for 1 week. Rats were administered the same preparations by the same route at a dose of 18g/kg and observed for 1.5 months. There were no significant changes in behaviour, body weight, serum non-protein nitrogen or hepatic or renal tissues.[41]

A Chinese herbal formula (Man-Shen-Ling) containing Rehmannia did not exhibit toxic, mutagenic, teratogenic or carcinogenic effects in acute and chronic toxicity tests in animal models.[38]

Contraindications

None known.

Special warnings and precautions

Cured Rehmannia may be unsuitable for gluten intolerant patients due to its treatment with millet wine.

Interactions

None known.

Use in pregnancy and lactation

Category B3 – no increase in frequency of malformation or other harmful effects on the fetus from limited use in women. Evidence of increased fetal damage in animal studies exists, although the relevance to humans is unknown.

Subcutaneous administration of Rehmannia aqueous extract (0.1 to 0.4mL/day) for 5 days decreased litter numbers in mice. This antifertility effect was not associated with systemic toxicity or interruption of the oestrus cycle.

In TCM, uncured Rehmannia is contraindicated in pregnant women with deficient blood, deficient spleen or deficient stomach.[42]

Rehmannia is compatible with breastfeeding.

Effects on ability to drive and use machines

No adverse effects anticipated.

Side effects

In a small open trial involving patients with rheumatoid arthritis, intermittent treatment with Rehmannia decoction elicited mild oedema in a minority of patients.[35]

Based on clinical trials in China, a minority of patients may develop diarrhoea, abdominal pain, dizziness, fatigue and palpitations that disappear spontaneously within a few days.[37] Excessive doses can cause diarrhoea.

Two cases of liver toxicity[43,44] (one fatal) and two cases of elevated serum levels of a liver enzyme[45] were reported after the ingestion of preparations containing Rehmannia used for the treatment of skin conditions. However, these formulations contained eight or more different Chinese herbs and the herb or herbs responsible have not been identified. The adverse reactions were not conclusively ascribed to the treatment with Chinese herbs in all cases.[46]

Overdosage

No incidents found in published literature.

Safety in children

No adverse effects expected at usual doses.

Regulatory status in selected countries

Rehmannia was official in the *Pharmacopoeia of the People's Republic of China* (English edition, 1997).

Rehmannia is not covered by a Commission E monograph and is not on the UK General Sale List.

Rehmannia does not have GRAS status. However, it is freely available as a 'dietary supplement' in the USA under DSHEA legislation (1994 Dietary Supplement Health and Education Act).

Rehmannia is not included in Part 4 of Schedule 4 of the Therapeutic Goods Act Regulations of Australia and is freely available for sale.

References

1. Bensky D, Clavey S, Stoger E. *Chinese Herbal Medicine Materia Medica*, 3rd ed. Seattle: Eastland Press; 2004. pp. 120–123.
2. Zhang RX, Li MX, Jia ZP. *J Ethnopharmacol.* 2008;117(2):199–214.
3. World Health Organization. *Medicinal Plants in China.* Manila: Regional Office for the Western Pacific, World Health Organization; 1989. p. 247.
4. Wagner H, Bladt S. *Plant Drug Analysis: A Thin Layer Chromatography Atlas*, Berlin: Springer-Verlag; 1996. p. 76.
5. Tang W, Eisenbrand G. *Chinese Drugs of Plant Origin.* Berlin: Springer Verlag; 1992. pp. 849–852.
6. Sasaki H, Nishimura H, Morota T, et al. *Planta Med.* 1989;55:458–462.
7. Zhang LL. *Acta Acad Med Primae Shanghai.* 1980;7(1):37–42.
8. Zha LL, Shen ZY, Zhang XF, et al. *Chin J Integr Trad West Med.* 1988;8(2):95–97.
9. Chen JK, Chen TT, Crampton L. *Chinese Medical Herbology and*

9. *Pharmacology*. California: Art of Medicine Press; 2004.

10. Liang A, Xue B, Wang J, et al. *Zhongguo Zhong Yao Za Zhi*. 1999;24(11):663–666. 702.

11. Li P, Shi XH, Wang FL. *Chin J Immunol*. 1987;3(5):296–298. 320.

12. Xu JP. *Chung Kuo Chung Hsi I Chieh Ho Tsa Chih*. 1992;12(12):734–737. 709–710.

13. Kim H, Lee E, Lee S, et al. *Int J Immunopharmacol*. 1998;20(4–5):231–240.

14. Yu H, Oh-Hashi K, Tanaka T, et al. *Pharmacol Res*. 2006;54(1):39–45.

15. Bi J, Jiang B, Liu JH, et al. *Neurosci Lett*. 2008;442(3):224–227.

16. Li Y, Bao Y, Jiang B, et al. *Int J Dev Neurosci*. 2008;26(3–4):309–317.

17. Bi J, Wang XB, Chen L, et al. *Toxicol In Vitro*. 2008;22(8):1883–1889.

18. Jiang B, Zhang H, Bi J, et al. *Neurol Res*. 2008;30(6):639–644.

19. Zhang XL, Jiang B, Li ZB, et al. *Pharmacol Biochem Behav*. 2007;88(1):64–72.

20. Jiang B, Du J, Liu JH, et al. *Brain Res*. 2008;1188:139–147.

21. Zhang XL, An LJ, Bao YM, et al. *Food Chem Toxicol*. 2008;46(8):2888–28894.

22. Yokozawa T, Kim HY, Yamabe N. *Am J Chin Med*. 2004;32(6):829–839.

23. Zhang Y, Dai DZ. *Drug Dev Res*. 2005;66(3):238.

24. Lau TW, Lam FF, Lau KM, et al. *J Ethnopharmacol*. 2009;123(1):155–162.

25. Waisundara VY, Huang M, Hsu A, et al. *Am J Chin Med*. 2008;36(6):1083–1104.

26. Zhang D, Wen XS, Wang XY, et al. *J Ethnopharmacol*. 2009;123(1):55–60.

27. Nishimura H, Yamaguchi T, Sasaki H, et al. *Planta Med*. 1990;56:684.

28. Kubo M, Asano T, Shiomoto H, et al. *Biol Pharm Bull*. 1994;17(9):1282–1286.

29. Kubo M, Asano T, Matsuda H, et al. *Yakugaku Zasshi*. 1996;116(2):158–168.

30. Oh KO, Kim SW, Kim JY, et al. *Clin Chim Acta*. 2003;334(1–2):185–195.

31. Kang DG, Sohn EJ, Moon MK, et al. *Biol Pharm Bull*. 2005;28(9):1662–1667.

32. Lee BC, Choi JB, Cho HJ, Kim YS. *J Ethnopharmacol*. 2009;122(1):131–135.

33. Chae HJ, Kim HR, Kim DS, et al. *Life Sci*. 2005;76(18):2027–2042.

34. Chen LZ, Feng XW, Zhou JH. *Chung Kuo Yao Li Hsueh Pao*. 1995;16(4):337–340.

35. Tomoda MI, Miyamoto H, Shimizu N, et al. *Biol Pharm Bull*. 1994;17(11):1456–1459.

36. Chao JC, Chiang SW, Wang CC, et al. *World J Gastroenterol*. 2006;12(28): 4478–4484.

37. Hu CS. *Chin Med J*. 1965;51:290.

38. Su ZZ, He YY, Chen G. *Chung Kuo Chung Hsi I Chieh Ho Tsa Chih*. 1993;13(5):259–260. 269–272.

39. Yin XJ, Liu DX, Wang HC, et al. *Mutat Res*. 1991;260(1):73–82.

40. Yokozawa T, Fujioka K, Oura H, et al. *Phytother Res*. 1995;9(1):1–5.

41. Chang HM, But PP. *Pharmacology and Applications of Chinese Materia Medica*, vol. 1. Singapore: World Scientific; 1987. p. 465.

42. Bensky D, Gamble A. *Chinese Herbal Medicine Materia Medica*. Seattle: Eastland Press; 1986. pp. 95–97.

43. Perharic-Walton L, Murray V. *Lancet*. 1992;340(8820):674.

44. Kane JA, Kane SP, Jain S. *Gut*. 1995;36(1):146–147.

45. Sheehan MP, Atherton DJ. *Br J Dermatol*. 1994;130(4):488–493.

46. Rustin M, Atherton D. *Lancet*. 1992;340(8820):673–674.

47. Matsui AS, Rogers J, Woo YK, et al. *Med Pharmacol Exp*. 1967;16:414–424.

(*Serenoa repens* (Bartram) Small)

Synonyms

Serenoa serrulata (Michaux) Nutall ex Schultes, *Sabal serrulata* R. et Sch. (botanical synonyms), sabal (Engl), Sabal fructus (Lat), Zwegpalme, Sabalfrüchte (Ger), palmier de l'Amérique du Nord (Fr), savpalme (Dan).

What is it?

Saw palmetto has traditionally been associated with therapy for the prostate gland. Earlier last century, entries could be found in many pharmacopoeias testifying to its use for benign prostatic hyperplasia (BPH). The petiole has a sharp spiny edge that can cut the clothing or legs of those unfortunate enough to come in contact with it, hence the common name of saw palmetto (literally a small saw-like palm). The fruit, a one-seeded dark brown to black drupe (known as the berry), is the part used in medicine. In recent times a more sophisticated pharmaceutical form of saw palmetto has been developed, known as the liposterolic extract (containing lipids and sterols). This liposterolic extract (LESP) has been the subject of many clinical trials. Although these trials have resulted in increased use of the liposterolic extract, especially in Europe where it is widely prescribed by medical practitioners for BPH, the strong traditional use information suggests that the use of galenical forms of saw palmetto, such as extracts and tinctures, should not be discounted.

Effects

Reduces inflammation and oedema; reduces smooth muscle spasm; decreases androgen activity.

Traditional view

The dried berries, liquid extract or pressed oil of saw palmetto were used for respiratory complaints, particularly those accompanied by chronic catarrh, and conditions of the genitourinary tract, especially to reduce irritation (for all forms of cystitis) and for prostatic hyperplasia. It was considered to build tissues.[1,2]

The Eclectics used saw palmetto for upper and lower respiratory problems, atrophy of the breast, ovaries and testes and for BPH. It was described as the 'old man's friend' and, with amazing accuracy, as 'a remedy for prostatic irritation and relaxation of tissue (rather) than for a hypertrophied prostate'. It was also used for inflamed gonads in the male or female and as an aphrodisiac. One interesting application was uterine hypertrophy.[3]

Summary actions

Anti-inflammatory, endocrine agent, spasmolytic, antiandrogenic.

Can be used for

Indications supported by clinical trials

Mild-to-moderate BPH (mixed evidence); including in combination productions (more consistent evidence); assisting recovery from surgery for BPH; male pattern baldness.

Traditional therapeutic uses

Inflammation of the respiratory tract; inflammation of the genitourinary tract, especially cystitis, prostatic hyperplasia; atrophy of sexual tissues; as an aphrodisiac.

May also be used for

Extrapolations from pharmacological studies

Non-infectious prostatitis; reduction of prostatic inflammation and oedema.

Other applications

As a topical application for male pattern baldness and scalp problems.

Preparations

Decoction of dried berries, tablets, capsules or liquid extract for internal use.

The liposterolic extract is mentioned often in this monograph. According to the German Commission E, this can be prepared by extraction of dried saw palmetto berries with either hexane or 90% ethanol. Extracts prepared using supercritical carbon dioxide are also suitable. The hexane extract has probably been the subject of more clinical trials than the other preparations.

The liposterolic extract contains 85% to 95% fatty acids (including a relatively high percentage of free fatty acids, FFAs) and 0.2% to 0.4% total sterols (with 0.1% to 0.3% beta-sitosterol). Flavonoids are unlikely to be present, except in the extract prepared using 90% ethanol.

Dosage

The typically accepted dose is 160 mg twice a day or 320 mg once a day of the liposterolic extract. This extract is about an 8:1 to 10:1 concentrate compared to the original dried berries. Hence this dose corresponds to about 1.5 to 3 g of dried berries per day. Otherwise, around 2 to 5 mL/day of a 1:2 extract prepared using 45% to 90% ethanol can be used, or the equivalent in other dosage forms (for example, 5 to 12.5 mg/day of a 1:5 tincture). The higher ethanol percentages will better extract the liposterolic components. Saw palmetto combines well with pumpkin seed oil or extract, and with extract of nettle root (see the nettle monograph).

Duration of use

No restriction on long-term use in fact prolonged usage (months or years) is generally necessary for best clinical results.

Summary assessment of safety

No adverse effects are expected if used as recommended.

Technical data

Botany

Serenoa repens, a member of the Palmae (palm) family, is a small shrub native to the south-eastern region of North America.[4,5] The leaves are palmate, without continuing rib, divided into lance-shaped linear-lanceolate leaflets, the petioles armed with spiny teeth. The inflorescence is many-branched, less than 1 m, with white flowers. The fruit is a prominent olive-like mesocarp, 16 to 25 mm long, with a single large oblong seed.[5]

Adulteration

No adulterants known for the dried herb. The liposterolic extract is susceptible to adulteration from other plant-derived fatty oils, for example palm or olive oil. Apparently such adulteration has occurred (see below under Key constituents).

Key constituents

- Lipid content: free fatty acids (including lauric, myristic, palmitic and oleic acids) together with triglycerides, diglycerides and monoglycerides, phytosterols (mainly beta-sitosterol) and fatty alcohols[6]
- A particularly active lipase which splits the triglycerides into free fatty acids during ripening and drying[6]
- Flavonoids and polysaccharides.[6]

The action of the lipase gives the fruit its characteristic rancid odour and taste due to the formation of free fatty acids. This 'rancidity' can cause digestive upsets in some people.

Methyl and ethyl esters of fatty acids also form in the fruit and contribute to the characteristic aroma.[6]

A 2002 survey of six saw palmetto products on the Canadian market found that, based on expected fatty acid content, 'actual' dosages were within a range of −97% to 140% of stated dosages, with three products containing less than 20% of the stated dosages.[7] However, these three 'low' products might have contained just the dried herb, as the authors based the 'actual' dose on the expected fatty acid content of the liposterolic extract, not the dried herb. This study highlights the often-encountered confusion over herbal dosage, where, for example, the statement '320 mg of saw palmetto' on a label could mean 320 mg of the dried herb, 320 mg of the liposterolic extract, or even 320 mg of an undefined extract.

In a better-designed subsequent study, the chemical variation of various liposterolic extract of saw palmetto (LESP) brands was investigated using liquid and gas chromatography.[8] Considerable differences in the free fatty acid (FFA) and glyceride contents were found. The FFA content varied from 81% to 41% and the glyceride content ranged from 7% to 52%. In general, there was an inverse relationship between the two, implying that the low FFA products might have been adulterated with other vegetable oils. The authors noted that such a wide variation in chemical content could impact significantly on clinical outcomes. However, this study analysed products, and in some cases the vegetable oil could have been intentionally added as a carrier during the soft gel capsule manufacturing process.

Pharmacodynamics

BPH is a slow, progressive enlargement of the fibromuscular and epithelial structures (due to the proliferation of stromal and epithelial cells) within the periurethral area of the prostate gland. This can eventually narrow the urethra, impeding the flow of urine. However, there is no direct correlation between histological and macroscopic BPH and lower urinary tract symptoms (LUTS). Histological evidence of BPH is found in more than 50% of men aged 60, and this increases to 90% at age 85. Yet of men with histological changes, only 50% will have clinical enlargement of the prostate or macroscopic changes, and of these individuals only 50% will develop LUTS. Symptoms can be due to obstruction or irritation or both. The clinical course of BPH is variable. Not every man with symptomatic BPH worsens clinically with time and symptom severity does not correlate well with prostate size or urinary outlet obstruction.[9,10] Although BPH is a common problem, the pathogenesis of the disease is poorly understood. Many factors are thought to be involved including sex hormones, stem cells, growth factors, insulin and prolactin. Irritation and associated spasm of smooth muscle tissue, inflammation and oedema may also contribute to the development of symptoms.

The recent understanding of BPH downplays androgens, both testosterone and dihydrotestosterone, as aetiological agents.[11] Their role is said to be permissive. However, a higher oestrogen/testosterone ratio could be a causative hormonal factor: increased peripheral conversion of testosterone to oestradiol by aromatase could be at play. Chronic inflammation is also a common finding. In fact, one theory has proposed that BPH is an immune-mediated inflammatory disease caused either by infection or autoimmunity (more likely the latter).[12] There is a strong link between chronic prostatitis and BPH.[13]

Another theory proposes that higher circulating insulin stimulates prostate growth.[10,14] Multiple experimental, clinical and epidemiological studies have demonstrated the link between either hyperinsulinaemia, elevated fasting blood glucose or type 2 diabetes and prostate enlargement and LUTS.[14,15] An association with obesity has also been observed.[16] The sympathetic overactivity linked to obesity, metabolic syndrome and hypertension may increase the risk of LUTS.[17]

In the context of these developments, attempts have been made to understand the pharmacological influence of saw palmetto extracts on some of the various pathogenic factors implicated in BPH.

Inhibition of 5-alpha-reductase

Testosterone is the major circulating androgen in humans. Most of the testosterone circulating in the bloodstream is bound to sex hormone-binding globulin (SHBG). The remaining unbound or free testosterone exerts the biological effects. Synthesis of SHBG is controlled by the ratio of oestradiol to testosterone. In many androgen target tissues, including the prostate, testosterone is converted by the enzyme 5-alpha-reductase into 5-alpha-dihydrotestosterone (DHT), which is about five times more potent than testosterone. There are two isoforms of 5-alpha-reductase (5-AR): type I and type II. Studies suggest that type 2 is mainly found in the prostate gland.

Inhibitors of 5-AR, such as the drug finasteride, block the conversion of testosterone to DHT and have been found to reduce the size of the prostate, leading to an increase in peak urinary flow rate and a reduction in LUTS.[18] In various reviews, much is often made of the observation that saw palmetto extracts also appear to inhibit 5-AR. This, together with inhibition of androgen binding, is often given as an explanation for the pharmacological activity of saw palmetto in BPH.

In 1984 it was shown that LESP (see above in the Preparations section) inhibited the 5-AR-mediated intracellular conversion of testosterone to DHT in vitro using human foreskin fibroblasts.[19] Inhibition of 5-AR was also demonstrated in vitro using genital fibroblasts for an alcoholic extract.[20] Furthermore, in vitro studies using a eukaryotic (baculovirus-directed insect cell) expression system found that LESP inhibited the activity of both isoenzymes of 5-AR, whereas finasteride selectively inhibited type 2.[21,22] Finasteride is a competitive inhibitor, whereas LESP displayed non-competitive inhibition of the type I isoenzyme and uncompetitive inhibition of the type II isoenzyme.[23] These observations suggest that the lipid components of LESP might be responsible for the inhibitory effect by modulating the membrane environment of 5-AR. Subsequent in vitro studies using epithelial and stromal cells from human BPH confirmed that the inhibitory activity was mainly due to the FFAs found in LESP.[24,25]

However, in one study the relative in vitro inhibitory effects of various saw palmetto extracts on 5-AR activity were measured to be 5600 to 40 000 times weaker than finasteride.[26] Since, LESP is usually administered at about 100 times the dose of finasteride, this suggests its clinical potency is about 60 times weaker in terms of 5-AR inhibition.

LESP at $10\,\mu g/mL$ was incubated with cell cultures of fibroblast and epithelial cells from the prostate, epididymis testes, kidney, skin and breast.[27] There were changes in the morphology of the prostate cells, including accumulation of lipid in the cytoplasm and damage to the nuclear mitochondrial membranes. No similar changes were observed in the other cells. LESP inhibited 5-AR types I and II in prostate cells, but the other cells exhibited no such inhibition of 5-AR. These results indicate a selectivity of LESP for prostate cells.

Several studies have further investigated the in vitro activities of fatty acids found in LESP on 5-AR. Using the eukaryotic (baculovirus-directed insect cell) expression system, IC_{50} values were determined at $4\,\mu g/mL$ for myristic acid and $19\,\mu g/mL$ for lauric acid on the type II isozymes of 5-AR.[28] Long unsaturated fatty acids (oleic and linolenic) were much less active. In contrast, IC_{50} values for 5-AR inhibition in rat liver microsomes were 54 and $66\,\mu g/mL$ for oleic and lauric acids, respectively.[29] Using the same model, the IC_{50} ranged from 42 to $68\,\mu g/mL$ for linoleic, oleic, myristic and lauric acids, and was $101\,\mu g/mL$ for LESP.[30]

In a reflection of earlier work that compared different extracts, the testing of a range of commercial LESPs (including different batches of the same extract) found a wide variation in the inhibition of 5-AR activity using prostatic co-cultured epithelial and fibroblast cells.[31] While extracts tested were able to inhibit both isoforms of 5-AR, the relative potencies varied by a factor of 24 for type I and 237 for type II inhibition. The lowest observed IC_{50} for type II inhibition was around $4\,\mu g/mL$ of extract. The authors suggested this variability indicates the potential for a wide diversity of clinical activity for these different extracts of saw palmetto.

A novel LESP (extraction methodology not defined) demonstrated relatively good inhibition of 5-AR type II in transfected human embryonic kidney cells (IC_{50} $2.9\,\mu g/mL$).[32] However, while the authors state that this bioactivity 'corresponds favourably … to the established prescription drug … finasteride', in fact the IC_{50} in the same model for finasteride was found to be 3.2 nM (or about $0.0012\,\mu g/mL$), around 2000 times lower on a weight for weight basis. While this difference is not as high as the 5600 to 40 000 ratios observed in an earlier comparative study,[26] it still indicates that saw palmetto is a relatively weak 5-AR inhibitor.

LESP at $10\,\mu g/mL$ (the apparent calculated plasma concentration in a patient receiving the recommended therapeutic dosage; see later under Pharmacokinetics) inhibited both isozymes of 5-AR in vitro using the co-culture model of BPH, without influencing the secretion of prostate-specific antigen (PSA) by epithelial cells (even after stimulation with testosterone).[33] This outcome was also demonstrated in a culture of human prostate cancer cells.[34] The molecular mechanisms behind this novel finding were also elucidated.[34] The authors of both studies noted that, unlike finasteride, LESP can inhibit 5-AR in vitro without inhibiting PSA secretion. The clinical extrapolation from this finding is that LESP does not lower PSA and hence interfere with its value as a cancer biomarker. However, while it has been observed that finasteride lowers PSA clinically and LESP does not (see later under Clinical trials), this observation could equally be explained by the lower clinical potency of LESP as a 5-AR inhibitor (since it does not reduce prostate size like finasteride).

In castrated rats stimulated with testosterone or DHT, finasteride but not LESP inhibited testosterone-stimulated prostate growth, while neither inhibited DHT-stimulated growth.[26] LESP (300 mg/kg/day for 12 or 24 weeks, oral) reduced the concentration of DHT in the prostate in transgenic mice with prostate cancer.[35] There was a significant increase in apoptosis and a decrease in tumour grade and incidence. A lower dose (50 mg/kg) was ineffective.

In one 7-day human trial, only finasteride (5 mg/day) and not LESP (320 mg/day) nor placebo decreased serum DHT in men.[26] This finding was confirmed in a larger double blind, randomised study in 32 healthy male volunteers; normal doses of LESP (320 mg/day) had no effect above placebo on serum DHT levels.[36] But there could be an effect within prostate tissue. A German group studied 18 patients in a randomised, placebo-controlled, double blind trial. Patients with BPH received six times the normal dose of LESP (eight cases) or placebo (10 cases) daily for 3 months. Following prostatectomy, prostatic epithelia and stroma were examined for enzyme activities. While these high doses of LESP caused some moderate biochemical changes, including a small reduction in 5-AR activity in prostatic epithelium, the authors volunteered that the significance of their results in understanding the effects of LESP in BPH were uncertain.[37]

In a 3-month open label, controlled trial, 25 symptomatic BPH patients were randomised to 320 mg/day LESP or no treatment.[38] Following suprapubic prostatectomy, statistically significant reductions were observed for DHT (down 68%, p<0.001) and epidermal growth factor (down 67%, p<0.01) in the prostatic tissue from the LESP-treated men, mainly in the periurethral region. Testosterone was correspondingly increased (up 66%, p<0.001), but prostate size was largely unaffected.

Another trial used biopsy cores for in situ quantification of prostatic androgens and compared LESP with finasteride.[39] Prostate levels of testosterone and DHT were measured in 5 to 10 mg biopsy specimens (18-gauge needle cores) in three groups of men with symptomatic BPH: 15 men receiving chronic finasteride therapy versus seven untreated controls; four men undergoing prostate adenomectomy to determine sampling variability (10 specimens each); and 40 men participating in a 6-month randomised trial of LESP (320 mg/day) versus placebo, before and after treatment. Prostatic tissue DHT levels were found to be several times higher than the levels of testosterone (5 versus 1.5 ng/g), that ratio becoming reversed (1.05 versus 3.63 ng/g) with chronic finasteride therapy. The finasteride effect was statistically significant for both androgens (p<0.01), and little overlap of individual values between finasteride-treated and control patients was seen. In the randomised trial, tissue DHT levels were reduced by 32% from 6.49 to 4.40 ng/g in the LESP group (p<0.005), with no significant change in the placebo group. Prostatic testosterone levels exhibited no significant change after LESP treatment.

Based on all the above findings, it can be concluded that while LESP is probably a significant inhibitor of the 5-AR type II isozymes in men with BPH, its clinical activity is relatively modest compared with finasteride, even in the best-case scenario for the most active forms of this extract. Hence, inhibition of 5-AR is likely to be only one factor behind the clinical effect of LESP in patients with BPH/LUTS, and certainly does not fully explain its therapeutic activity in this condition.

Spasmolytic activity

Antiadrenergic agents are used in BPH to decrease dynamically caused obstruction associated with increased smooth muscle tone in the bladder trigone and membranous urethra of the prostate. In particular, the selective alpha1-blockers are clinically preferred and include terazosin, doxazosin, tamsulosin and alfuzosin. Prazosin is also used. This has stimulated an interest among researchers as to whether saw palmetto extracts might act in a similar way.

An ethanolic LESP and a saponifiable extract produced a spasmolytic effect on isolated rat uterus, bladder and aorta in vitro.[40] This effect appeared to be related to an inhibition of calcium influx and intracellular effects. Follow-up research suggested that cyclic AMP may be a possible mediator, together with the involvement of protein synthesis.[41] Additional in vitro research on the above LESP found spasmolytic effects that were attributed to alpha-adrenoceptor and calcium channel blocking activities.[42]

Preparations of beta-sitosterol and extracts of nettle root, medicinal pumpkin seed and saw palmetto were tested for their in vitro ability to inhibit tamsulosin binding to human prostatic alpha1-adrenoceptors (A1A receptors) and prazosin binding to cloned human A1A and alpha1B-adrenoceptors.[43] Only saw palmetto (several extracts) potently and non-competitively inhibited A1A in vitro. The in vitro binding affinities for A1A, muscarinic and purinergic receptors in the rat prostate and bladder were measured by radioligand binding assays for saw palmetto.[44] LESP inhibited specific binding of prazosin and N-methylscopolamine (NMS) in the rat prostate and bladder. The binding activity of LESP for muscarinic receptors was four times greater than that for A1A receptors. This in vitro activity (including also binding to calcium channel antagonist receptors) was subsequently identified by the same research centre as due to the FFAs, specifically oleic, lauric, myristic and linoleic acids.[29,30]

In contrast, a different research group found that saw palmetto ethanolic extracts (45% and 70% ethanol) caused contraction of the rat prostate gland consistent with sympathomimetic activity and identified tyramine as the responsible agent.[45] However, tyramine is likely to be inactivated by the gastrointestinal tract on oral ingestion, especially at the low doses involved (one saw palmetto 1:2 extract tested had a recommended dose of 2 to 4 mL/day and contained about 4 mg/mL tyramine.) Nonetheless, it does imply the theoretical possibility of an interaction of saw palmetto with monoamine oxidase inhibitor drugs, as noted by the authors.

LESP (12, 20 and 60 mg/day, intraduodenal) alleviated urodynamic symptoms in a model of hyperactive bladder in spontaneous hypertensive rats by increasing bladder capacity and subsequently prolonging the micturition interval.[46] A repeated oral dose of 6 mg/kg in the same rat breed decreased voiding frequency under normal conditions. Rats given LESP (6 and 60 mg/kg/day, orally for 4 weeks) exhibited a significant increase in prostate binding sites for prazosin and a significant decrease in bladder binding sites for NMS.[44] The exact meaning of these findings is not clear.

In a placebo-controlled, double blind, four-way, crossover study, 12 healthy young men received three different LESPs (320 mg/day) or placebo for 8 days each.[47] Although the saw palmetto extracts caused minor reductions in supine blood pressure, they did not affect blood pressure during orthostatic stress testing nor influence plasma catecholamines. Plasma samples taken from the men did not demonstrate an influence on A1A receptors using radioligand binding assays. (This assay methodology does exhibit sensitivity to the drugs tamsulosin and terazosin.) The authors proposed the clinical effects of LESP are unlikely to result from A1A receptor antagonism. However, while this conclusion may be valid, animal experiments do suggest that LESP can influence bladder function in a way that would be beneficial in LUTS.

Inhibition of androgen binding and antiandrogenic activity

Androgens exert their effects by binding to an intracellular cytoplasmic receptor, forming a hormone-receptor complex that is transferred to the cell nucleus, binds to DNA and can activate and modulate protein transcription. Androgen potency is determined by their binding affinity to the receptor. Hence, another important component of the mechanism of LESP might be an inhibitory effect on the binding of DHT to androgen receptors in the cytosolic component of prostate cells.

This inhibitory effect was demonstrated for LESP prepared using n-hexane in two in vitro models,[9,48] but not for an ethanolic LESP.[10] Subsequent in vitro research found that LESP inhibited testosterone and DHT binding in several tissue specimens, including vaginal skin and prepuce.[49] However, a later study found that LESP did not inhibit the binding of DHT to the rat prostatic androgen receptor at LESP concentrations up to 100 µg/mL.[16]

The effects of LESP on two prostatic cancer cell lines differing in androgen responsiveness were investigated.[50] LESP had a proliferative effect on androgen-responsive cells at lower concentrations ($\leq$10 µg/mL) and a cytotoxic effect at higher concentrations ($\geq$25 µg/mL). At 25 µg/mL, LESP antagonised androgen-stimulated cell growth. In cells unresponsive to androgen stimulation, LESP had a concentration-dependent antiproliferative action. When these cells were co-transfected with wild-type androgen receptors, LESP inhibited androgen-induced effects. The authors concluded that their findings support an antiandrogenic action of LESP. This antiandrogenic activity was supported for LESP in several animal models.[51,52] For example, a hypercritical carbon dioxide extract (300 mg/rat, oral) antagonised the effect of testosterone on prostate size in castrated rats.[52]

Other hormonal activity

Prolactin may stimulate prostate growth, although its role in BPH is controversial.[53] Addition of LESP at concentrations ranging from 1 to 10 µg/mL to Chinese hamster ovary cells completely inhibited prolactin signal transduction pathways, implying that the extract may inhibit prolactin-induced prostate growth.[54] The authors suggested that LESP might also be useful for other diseases implicating prolactin. (See also under 'Activity in BPH or its experimental models'.)

Early in vivo experiments indicated that saw palmetto had oestrogenic activity.[55] However, subsequent evidence implies that LESP in fact has anti-oestrogenic activity in patients with BPH.[56] In a double blind, placebo-controlled study, 35 patients received either LESP at 320 mg/day (18 cases) or placebo (17 cases) for 3 months. Following prostatectomy, steroid receptors were evaluated in the nuclear and cytosolic fractions of prostate cells. Oestrogen receptors in the nuclear fraction were significantly lower in the group receiving LESP, as determined by three different tests. Single-point assay found that androgen receptors in the nuclear fraction were also reduced by treatment with LESP. These results indicate that LESP exerted an anti-oestrogenic effect, possibly by competitively blocking translocation of cytosolic oestrogen receptors to the nucleus. It may even be that the inactivation of androgen receptors is secondary to oestrogen blockade and this anti-oestrogenic effect may potentiate other actions of LESP.

Twenty men with BPH were treated with 320 mg/day of LESP for 30 days.[57] No changes in plasma levels of testosterone, follicle-stimulating hormone and luteinizing hormone occurred as a result of treatment. A combination of LESP and astaxanthin demonstrated a significant dose-dependent reduction in serum oestrogen levels in an uncontrolled study in 42 healthy men.[58]

Basic fibroblast growth factor (bFGF) and epidermal growth factor (EGF) are two other mediators possibly involved in the pathogenesis of BPH. LESP did not affect basal prostate cell proliferation, with the exception of two prostate specimens, for which a significant inhibition of basal proliferation was observed with the highest concentration (30 µg/mL).[59] In contrast, LESP inhibited bFGF-induced proliferation of human prostate cell cultures; this effect was significant at 30 µg/mL. Unsaturated FFAs from LESP markedly inhibited the bFGF-induced cell proliferation down to the basal value. Lupenone, hexacosanol and the unsaponified fraction of LESP also inhibited bFGF-induced cell proliferation, whereas a minimal effect on basal cell proliferation was noted. A less pronounced inhibition of EGF-induced proliferation was also observed for LESP. A clinical study cited previously found that LESP (320 mg/day) inhibited EGF in the prostate tissue of men with BPH.[38]

Anti-inflammatory activity

As a result of secretory stagnation, BPH is associated with congestion and non-infectious prostatitis, as evidenced by white cell infiltration of the prostate. For this reason, agents with anti-inflammatory and oedema-protective activities may improve the clinical picture of BPH.

French scientists have reported on the anti-oedematous activity of LESP.[25,60] Various experimental models were used to test the influence of LESP on cutaneous permeability. Interestingly, an antagonistic effect of the extract was observed whenever histamine was involved, either directly through injection or indirectly via mast cell degranulation. An oral dose of 5 to 10 mL/kg produced a significant effect. However, this is a very high dose. LESP showed no action on serotonin- or bradykinin-induced weals in rats. Since the anti-oedematous effect was also demonstrable in adrenalectomised rats, the participation of glucocorticoids is definitely excluded. Adult male rats received either tocopherol (the LESP vehicle) or LESP (50 and 100 mg/kg orally every second day for 90 days).[61] A dose-dependent, significant decrease in mast cell accumulation and a provocation of epithelial atrophy was observed within the central area of the rat ventral prostate. The authors noted that since prostatic mast cell degranulation can induce smooth muscle contraction in that gland, these findings could have implications for the activity of LESP in BPH.

A pronounced anti-oedematous effect was observed for oral doses of an alcoholic extract of saw palmetto in carrageenan-induced oedema of rat paw.[62] A water-based preparation had no effect, and polysaccharides, beta-sitosterol derivatives and flavonoids were not responsible for the anti-inflammatory outcome. Another group of scientists reported on the isolation of an acidic polysaccharide with anti-inflammatory activity (after intravenous injection) from a water-based extract of saw palmetto.[63,64] Since this polysaccharide could be expected to have poor oral bioavailability and would not occur in LESP, the clinical significance of this finding is doubtful.

The most important proinflammatory metabolites of arachidonic acid are prostaglandins and leukotrienes and their production is respectively mediated by the enzymes cyclo-oxygenase (COX) and 5-lipoxygenase (5-LOX). LESP prepared by supercritical liquid extraction with carbon dioxide was found in vitro to be a dual inhibitor of COX (IC$_{50}$ 28.1 μg/mL) and 5-LOX (IC$_{50}$ 18 μg/mL).[65] Activity was found to reside in the acidic lipophilic fraction; fatty alcohols and sterols were inactive. It is possible that this inhibition of the arachidonic acid cascade causes the observed anti-oedematous effect of LESP. The potent in vitro inhibition of the production of 5-LOX metabolites (especially leukotriene B$_4$) by LESP has been confirmed in another study using human neutrophils.[66]

After stimulation of peritoneal rat macrophages with lipopolysaccharide, an undefined saw palmetto extract inhibited the expression of the inflammatory enzymes COX, 5-LOX and inducible nitric oxide synthase.[67] At an oral dose of 28.5 mg/kg it also inhibited prostate inflammation induced in rats by partial bladder outlet obstruction.

In an open clinical trial of 29 men with BPH, 12 took LESP (320 mg/day) for 3 months, while 17 controls received no treatment prior to surgical treatment for their condition.[68] Assessment of surgically obtained samples revealed significantly lower levels of IL-1 and TNF-alpha in the prostate tissue of the men who took LESP compared with controls (p<0.006). This trial strongly supports a real-world reduction in inflammatory cytokines associated with the pathogenesis of BPH by the use of saw palmetto.

Activity in BPH or its experimental models

High oral doses of LESP (300 mg/day for 12 days) inhibited prostatic growth in castrated mice given testosterone, and 200 mg/day for 6 days achieved a similar outcome in a rat model.[51] The increase of prostate weight induced by oestradiol/testosterone treatment in castrated rats was countered by oral administration of LESP at 50 mg/kg/day.[69] This is a model that exhibits both prostatic inflammation and hyperplasia. In contrast, high oral doses of LESP (180 mg/day and 1800 mg/day) did not influence prostatic growth induced by testosterone and DHT in castrated rats in another study.[26]

One model of BPH uses transplants of human prostate tissue into hairless mice. Growth of this tissue is then stimulated by the administration of DHT and oestradiol. Using this model, high oral doses of LESP (6 mL/kg) were observed to reverse the hormonal stimulation of prostate growth.[70]

Using an in vivo model of rat prostate hyperplasia induced by hyperprolactinaemia, LESP (320 mg/kg, oral) but not finasteride (5 mg/kg, oral) countered the hyperplastic effect of prolactin in the lateral prostate in castrated rats treated with DHT.[71]

The rate of apoptosis and cell proliferation was compared in normal human prostate tissue (from organ donors) and tissue samples from patients with BPH either treated with LESP (320 mg/day) or not.[72] There were 10 tissue samples in each group. No difference was observed between the mean proliferative index and the mean apoptotic index in the epithelium or stroma of the normal prostate samples. In contrast, proliferation exceeded apoptosis in the untreated BPH tissue samples, and the proliferative index was significantly higher than in the normal prostate. BPH tissue samples from the men treated with LESP reversed this apoptosis/proliferation ratio. In fact, a significantly higher apoptotic index and a significantly lower proliferative index were measured. The differences in these indexes resulting from LESP treatment were quite marked. The authors concluded that LESP induces apoptosis and inhibits cell proliferation at normal clinical doses in the prostates of men with BPH, and that these observations could explain its clinical benefit for this disorder. An increase in the apoptotic index in prostate tissue is also supported by in vitro work cited previously.[27]

In an open label pilot study, patients with BPH preceding surgery were randomised to be followed without any treatment for 3 weeks (control group) or received LESP (320 mg/day) for a 3-month period.[73] Surgery was ultimately performed in 17 controls and 12 patients by using transurethral prostate resection or retropubic adenomectomy. The Bax/Bcl-2 ratio, which is an apoptotic index, was significantly increased in the prostatic tissue of treated patients, as was evidence of increased caspase 3 activity in the prostate.

Antitumour activity

Several studies have investigated the effect of saw palmetto extracts on various prostate cancer cell lines in vitro. Generally, increased apoptosis and growth inhibition have been observed, either for LESP[74–78] or aqueous-ethanolic extracts.[79–81] The ethanolic extract has also demonstrated STAT3 (signal transducer and activator of transcription 3) signalling inactivation,[80] including in human multiple myeloma cell cultures.[82] However, the 70% ethanolic extract was relatively weak at inhibiting the growth of three prostate cancer cell lines compared with other herbs,[83] and one study found that LESP was not able to induce apoptosis or cell cycle arrest in two prostate cancer cell lines, although it did inhibit cell growth.[84]

Some in vivo studies have also been undertaken using either tumour xenograft or transgenic models. Saw palmetto 70% ethanolic extract (10 mg/kg, oral) inhibited the growth of xenografts in immunodeficient mice injected with prostate cancer cells.[80] Serum levels of PSA were reduced by approximately 66%. As cited previously, LESP increased apoptosis and decreased tumour grade and incidence in transgenic mice with prostate cancer.[35]

Studies are ongoing and the clinical significance of the above work is not known. However, it does appear on current information that saw palmetto use will not prevent prostate cancer. To evaluate whether saw palmetto intake was associated with a reduced risk of prostate cancer, a prospective cohort study of 35 171 men aged 50 to 76 years in western Washington State, USA, was undertaken.[85] Participants completed questionnaires between 2000 and 2002 on frequency of use of saw palmetto or saw palmetto-containing combination products over the previous 10 years, in addition to other information on supplement intake, medical history and demographics. Men were followed through to December 2003 (mean of 2.3 years of follow-up), during which time 580 developed prostate cancers. Ten per cent of the cohort used saw palmetto at least once per week for a year in the 10 years before baseline. No association was found between this level of use of saw palmetto and risk of prostate cancer development (hazard ratio 0.95; 95% CI 0.74 to 1.23) or with increasing frequency or duration of use. Certainly, the use of saw palmetto did not apparently increase the risk of prostate cancer. Whether LESP, which is probably more active than many of the products also included in the survey, will affect prostate cancer risk remains to be studied.

Other activity

A form of LESP stimulated macrophage phagocytosis in vitro, as well as human natural killer (NK) cell synthesis of interferon-gamma.[86] However, relatively high concentrations were used (up to 1.28 mg/mL).

Saw palmetto (dosage and extract not defined) had no influence on platelet function after administration to 10 healthy volunteers for 2 weeks.[87]

Pharmacokinetics

A study carried out on rats given oral doses of LESP supplemented with ^{14}C-labelled oleic or lauric acids or beta-sitosterol demonstrated that radioactivity uptake in prostatic tissue was highest after administration of LESP supplemented with ^{14}C-labelled oleic acid.[88] This uptake was clearly demonstrated in a rat with experimentally induced BPH. Interestingly, uptake of radioactivity in the prostate was greater than for other organs.

Human pharmacokinetic data on LESP can be gleaned from a bioequivalence study on two different dosage forms.[89] Twelve healthy men each received a single oral dose of 320 mg

of LESP. Since LESP is a complex mixture of several components, one component was chosen for the study. This component was not identified, but was defined by a validated HPLC method and referred to as 'Serenoa repens second component'. Based on analysis of this component, a mean peak plasma concentration of 2.6 μg/mL was reached after 1.5 h. The mean elimination half-life was 1.9 h. Given this half-life, administration of LESP twice daily is probably preferable, although at least two clinical trials have found that 320 mg once daily appears to be as effective as 160 mg twice daily for BPH symptoms.[90,91]

Clinical trials

Saw palmetto has been used for the treatment of BPH for at least 100 years. The modern clinical evidence supporting the efficacy of its liposterolic extract for this disorder is reasonably good, especially in combination, despite the finding of a 2009 systematic review. While the evidence is controversial, it is considered sufficient to justify the use of this plant for the treatment of mild-to-moderate BPH in circumstances where conventional therapy is either not wanted or inadvisable. In particular, LESP appears to work well in combination with nettle root. The safety profile of this herbal preparation is very good.

Benign prostatic hyperplasia

The Fifth International Consultation on BPH in 2000 set the basic criteria for assessing the pharmacological treatment of BPH.[92] All clinical trials were expected to be randomised, placebo-controlled and double blind and to include a follow-up period of at least 1 year. All trials should assess several independent parameters for treatment outcome and should include an analysis of the tolerability of the treatment. Several clinical trials of LESP in BPH have completely satisfied these criteria.

A 2009 systematic review and meta-analysis of clinical trials involving saw palmetto (and particularly various forms of LESP) in the treatment of BPH was published on behalf of the Cochrane Collaboration.[93] Trials were eligible if they randomised men with symptomatic BPH to receive saw palmetto (alone or in combination) for at least 4 weeks in comparison with placebo or other interventions. Overall, 5222 patients from 30 randomised trials lasting from 4 to 60 weeks were assessed. Meta-analysis of nine trials for nocturia found saw palmetto (as the sole treatment) was significantly better than placebo, with an improvement of 0.78 fewer nocturnal visits (p<0.05). However, when the five larger trials (740 patients) were included in a meta-analysis a smaller improvement in nocturia was calculated that did not achieve significance. Using the subjective 8-question International Prostate Symptom Score (IPSS) as the outcome, meta-analysis of just two trials found saw palmetto was no better than placebo. Saw palmetto (as the sole treatment) was also not superior to placebo in terms of peak urine flow (meta-analysis of 10 trials) or reducing prostate size (results from three trials). However, it was superior to placebo on patient self-rating (meta-analysis of five trials, p=0.01) and clinician assessment (meta-analysis of three trials, p=0.015). Despite some of these positive outcomes, and the fact that the authors' analysis of trial data concluded that saw palmetto as a sole treatment was equivalent to the standard BPH drugs finasteride (one trial) and tamsulosin (two trials), they concluded that saw palmetto was not more effective than placebo for the treatment of urinary symptoms consistent with BPH.

A large influence of this outcome was the US-government-funded trial of Bent and colleagues published in 2006 in the *New England Journal of Medicine* (*NEJM*).[94] This was a well-designed and conducted double blind, randomised, placebo-controlled trial in 225 men with BPH that found LESP (160 mg twice a day) for 1 year was not superior to placebo in terms of changes in a US version of the IPSS, maximal urinary flow rate, prostate size, residual volume after voiding or PSA levels.

As noted in the accompanying editorial,[95] a limitation of this study is that Bent and colleagues tested a specific preparation of saw palmetto, leaving open the possibility that a different preparation might have been effective. Specifically, they tested a US LESP product, whereas most of the positive earlier trials were on European products, especially a hexane extracted LESP. While they went to great lengths to authenticate the LESP used, this validation was based largely on the determination of total fatty acids. As noted above, the more active versions of LESP have higher levels FFAs, which will also reflect on their being free of adulteration with other plant-derived fatty oils.[8] A lower level of FFAs in LESP will also reflect on less pharmacological activity, such as inhibition of 5-AR in vitro.[31] It is clear from the information provided that FFAs were not determined in the LESP product used in the *NEJM* study.

A reviewer's feedback commentary on the Cochrane analysis noted the same issue: that variability in the quality of the saw palmetto products used in clinical trials might have concealed a true benefit in BPH and undermined the authors' conclusions.[93]

Earlier systematic reviews have drawn more positive conclusions regarding the efficacy of LESP in BPH. They have essentially drawn on the same data as the Cochrane review, apart from the *NEJM* trial. In 2004, an updated meta-analysis of 14 randomised clinical trials and three open label trials involving 4280 patients found a significant improvement in peak flow rate and a reduction in nocturia above placebo, together with a five-point reduction in the IPSS.[96] Four of the randomised trials compared LESP with other drugs including finasteride and tamsulosin. The mean placebo effect on peak urinary flow rate was an increase of 1.20 mL/sec. The estimated effect of LESP was a further increase above placebo of 1.02 mL/sec (p=0.042), which means that the herbal treatment was associated with an overall increase in peak urinary flow of 2.22 mL/sec. This represents a clinically significant 15% to 20% increase. Effects on nocturia were less striking, due to the influence of one large study involving 396 patients that showed no difference to placebo treatment. Placebo was associated with a reduction in the mean number of nocturnal voids of 0.63 and there was a further reduction attributable to LESP of 0.38 (p<0.001). Hence the use of saw palmetto was associated with an average reduction from baseline of one event per night in terms of nocturnal voiding, which is clinically significant. Results were not significantly altered if the three open trials considered in this analysis were excluded. The authors included data from at least four unpublished trials to remove concerns about publication bias. It was concluded that LESP is extremely safe, with a very low rate of any adverse effects. To address concerns over product variability, this meta-analysis and the 2000 publication that it updated[97] included only LESP from just one supplier (a hexane extract).

Apart from the *NEJM* study, the better conducted more recent trials on LESP have compared its efficacy in BPH with standard drug treatments, rather than placebo. These, together with some key earlier trials, are summarised in Table 1.

Although results from these trials were covered in the Cochrane review, their significance was not emphasised, as noted in the feedback reviewer's comments.[93] As shown in the table, results from these trials demonstrate that LESP is generally just as efficacious as standard drug treatments, and perhaps superior in some circumstances.

A significant comparative trial is the large-scale comparison with finasteride.[98] Patients were recruited from a number of urology centres in nine European countries and the study was the largest international comparative trial for the treatment of BPH. The trial data clearly support the therapeutic value of LESP in BPH. However, this study did have some problems with its design. Most notable of these were the absence of a placebo group or placebo run-in period (which would have afforded a three-way comparison) and the insufficient duration of the trial (minimum 1 year). This latter point is particularly relevant to comparisons using finasteride, since this agent can show increasing efficacy up to 1 year after initiation of therapy.[103]

One important outcome of the study was the observation that LESP does not significantly influence prostate volume or serum PSA, whereas finasteride does. This is clear and significant clinical evidence that LESP does not act as a strong 5-AR inhibitor (although other evidence discussed above supports LESP as moderately active against type II intraprostatic 5-AR). Since PSA is used as a screening test for prostate cancer and 5-AR inhibitors can decrease PSA, there is a concern that these agents could mask the detection of prostate cancer. On the basis of the data provided by this large trial, it can be confidently concluded that this concern would not apply to LESP. This is particularly reassuring, since LESP is often self-prescribed and an investigating urologist may be unaware of its use by a particular patient.

The large comparison with tamsulosin was a French study known as the PERMAL study, published in 2002.[90] Over 1 year in 704 patients the two treatments were found to be equivalent for BPH. A subset analysis published in 2004 examined results for patients with severe LUTS of BPH.[102] Severe LUTS was defined as an IPSS greater than 19. Analysis was performed on 124 patients with severe LUTS (59 receiving LESP (320 mg/day) and 65 receiving tamsulosin). After 12 months, IPSS had decreased by 7.8 with saw palmetto and 5.8 with tamsulosin (p=0.051). The irritative symptoms subscore improved significantly more (p=0.049) with saw palmetto (−2.9 versus −1.9 with tamsulosin). The superiority of LESP in reducing irritative symptoms appeared at month 3 and was maintained up to month 12 (p=0.03).

Table 1 Key comparative clinical trials of LESP

Reference	Year	Daily dose of LESP	Trial design	Comparative treatment and daily dose	Relative results	LESP	Drug	Relative tolerability
Carraro et al[98]	1996	320 mg	Double blind, over 26 weeks on 1098 patients with moderate BPH	Finasteride 5 mg (5-alpha-reductase inhibitor)	IPSS	−37%	−39%	LESP showed a small advantage over finasteride in a sexual function score[**] and gave rise to fewer complaints of decreased libido and impotence
					Quality of life (improvement)	+38%	+41%	
					Peak flow rate	+25%	+30%[*]	
					Prostate volume	−6%	−18%[**]	
					PSA	No change	−41%[**]	
Grasso et al[99]	1995	320 mg	Double blind over 3 weeks on 63 patients	Alfuzosin 7.5 mg (alpha1-blocker)	Boyarsky score	−26.9%	−38.8%[*]	Both treatments were well tolerated
					Obstructive score	−23.1%	−37.8%[*]	
					Peak flow responders	48.4%	71.8%	
					No significant difference between mean PVR, peak urinary flow and between the two groups			
Adriazola Semino et al[100]	1992	320 mg	Double blind over 12 weeks on 41 patients	Prazosin 4 mg (alpha1-blocker)	Improvements in urinary frequency, mean urinary flow rate and PVR slightly favoured prazosin. No statistical analysis was conducted			NA
Hizli and Uygur[101]	2007	320 mg	Open, over 6 months on 60 men with moderate BPH	Tamsulosin 0.4 mg (alpha1-blocker) or LESP + tamsulosin	IPSS	−28%	−34%	Combination therapy no better than either agent alone. No adverse effects in LESP alone group, 11 in tamsulosin group had problems.
					Qmax	+34%	+35%	
					PVR	−42%	−36%	
					Pr vol	−2%	−3%	
Debruyne, et al.[90]	2002	320 mg	Double blind, over 1 year, on 704 men with moderate BPH	Tamsulosin 0.4 mg (alpha1-blocker)	IPSS	−29%	−29%	No difference in erectile function between groups. Much more ejaculatory dysfunction with tamsulosin. Other adverse effects no different and minor
					Qmax	+17%	+16%	
					Pr vol	+2%	−1%	
Debruyne, et al.[102]	2004	320 mg	Double blind, over 1 year, on 124 men with severe BPH	Tamsulosin 0.4 mg (alpha1-blocker)	IPSS	−35%	−25%	Both agents were similarly well tolerated
					Qmax	+11%	+17%	

PVR = postvoid residual; NA = not assessed; IPSS = International Prostate Symptom Score; PSA = prostate-specific antigen.
[*]p<0.05.
[**]p<0.001.

One interesting study cited earlier compared two dosage forms of LESP in 132 patients with BPH over 1 year.[91] The interest comes from the observation that both dosage forms strikingly and progressively reduced average IPSS from around 17 at the start of the trial to around 7 after 1 year. This would be a very unusual placebo effect if it was still actively reducing symptoms even after 9 months of use. Similar sustained and progressive IPSS improvement over 2 years was observed for a later uncontrolled study in 120 men with mild or moderate LUTS due to BPH taking LESP (320 mg/day).[104]

The TRIUMPH study recorded the treatment and outcomes of 2351 newly presenting LUTS/BPH patients in six European countries over a 1-year follow-up period.[105] At each visit the clinician recorded the treatment, co-morbidities, complications and drugs prescribed, and the patient completed an IPSS questionnaire. The results were analysed using change in IPSS as the primary outcome measure. Over the study period 74.9% of patients were prescribed medication, the majority (83% of those medicated) were prescribed only a single treatment. Significant improvements were seen in 43% of patients on phytotherapy with saw palmetto or *Pygeum africanum*, compared with 57% of those on finasteride and 68% on alpha-blockers. All treatments showed some improvement over watchful waiting for most patients over the study period: the alpha-blockers were found to be the most effective. The average IPSS reductions were 1.4 points for watchful waiting, around three points for each herbal treatment and around six points for the alpha-blockers.

LESP may have a preventative role in BPH. A prospective, multicentre study was designed to determine the effect of treatment with LESP on the progression of mild symptoms of bladder outlet obstruction (defined as an IPSS of less than 8) secondary to BPH, compared with watchful waiting.[106] Treatment with LESP reduced the incidence of clinical disease progression, and the effect was noticed as early as 6 months. At the end of 24 months, the rate of progression was 16% in the LESP group, compared to 24% in the watchful waiting group. This difference was significant ($p<0.05$). LESP also improved urinary symptoms, quality of life scores and urinary flow rates. It was administered for 2 years at a dose of 320 mg/day. The relevance of this study would have been improved by the inclusion of a treated or placebo control group, with appropriate randomisation.

Saw palmetto has demonstrated good clinical results in trials when used in combination with other agents. In particular, trials of LESP in conjunction with nettle root extract have been consistently positive. (These trials are reviewed in the nettle monograph).

Chronic prostatitis

Given the co-morbidity between BPH and chronic prostatitis (CP), it is not surprising that LESP has been investigated clinically for the latter. A study was undertaken to assess the efficacy of saw palmetto or finasteride in men with category III chronic prostatitis/chronic pelvic pain syndrome (CP/CPPS).[107] This category denotes non-bacterial prostatitis. Patients (n=64) were randomised to finasteride (5 mg/day) or LESP (320 mg/day) for 1 year using an open label study design.

There were 61, 57 and 56 patients available for evaluation at 3, 6 and 12 months, respectively. At 1 year the mean total NIH Chronic Prostatitis Symptom Index (CPSI) score decreased from 23.9 to 18.1 in the finasteride group ($p<0.003$) and from only 24.7 to 24.6 in the saw palmetto group ($p=0.41$). The authors concluded that the patients treated with saw palmetto had no appreciable long-term improvement.

Other uncontrolled trials have demonstrated some clinical benefit for LESP in both bacterial and non-bacterial prostatitis, although the lack of a placebo group impairs the clinical relevance of such data.[108,109] Saw palmetto as LESP has also been used as a part of a complex regime for bacterial and non-bacterial prostatitis including antibiotics and alpha-blockers, with positive results.[110,111] However, it is difficult to ascertain what role the herbal extract played in patients' recoveries.

In an interesting trial, 102 men with category IIIa CP/CPPS were randomised to receive LESP (320 mg/day) or LESP plus lycopene and selenium for 8 weeks.[112] The mean CPSI score decreased significantly ($p<0.001$) in both groups, but was greater for the combination.

Prostate surgery

One intriguing application from clinical trials is the potential role of LESP in reducing complications following transurethral resection of the prostate (TURP).[113] In an open label, controlled Italian study, patients were randomly assigned to receive either 320 mg/day of LESP or no additional treatment for at least 8 weeks before the TURP procedure. Out of 108 enrolled patients, 88 were evaluated at the end of the trial. In the treated group, perioperative bleeding was significantly lower than controls (124 mL versus 287 mL) and the need for transfusion was substantially reduced. In addition, for the saw palmetto group the duration of postoperative catheterisation was considerably lower (3 days versus 5 days for controls) and haematological findings (red cell count, haemoglobin and haematocrit) were more favourable. The authors concluded that pretreatment with saw palmetto before TURP improves the efficacy of the procedure and reduces the risk of complications.

A later Italian study of similar design included 144 patients who were candidates for either TURP or open prostatectomy.[114] In the group receiving 320 mg/day of LESP, the duration of surgery was shorter than for the control group (59.8 min versus 77.6 min, $p<0.001$), no intraoperative complications were observed (0% versus 15%, $p=0.001$) and transfusion needs were remarkably lower (0% versus 38.3%, $p<0.001$). The postoperative course was more favourable after LESP pretreatment, with a shorter duration of catheterisation (65 h versus 92 h, $p<0.001$) and length of hospitalisation (5.9 days versus 7.9 days, $p<0.001$).

Another study compared the effects of the 5-AR inhibitor dutasteride (5 mg/day) with LESP (160 mg/day) in men about to undergo TURP.[115] The treatments were given for 5 weeks and compared with an untreated control group. Neither treatment influenced blood loss during or after surgery. However, this was a Turkish study that used a local LESP product, so product quality might have been an issue, as per the discussions elsewhere in this monograph.

Androgenic alopecia and scalp problems

Given the influence of LESP on 5-AR activity, it follows that it might have value in the treatment of male pattern baldness (MPB). A group of scientists decided to test the effect of oral intake of LESP on MPB in a pilot study involving 19 men between the ages of 23 and 64 under double blind conditions.[116] The product tested also contained beta-sitosterol (110 mg/day) and nutrients; the dose of LESP used was 400 mg/day. The blinded investigative staff rated 60% of the volunteers receiving active treatment as improved, compared to only 11% for the placebo group. Self-assessment by volunteers showed a similar but less striking trend.

Two studies involving topical use have only been published as conference proceedings and were summarised in a brief review.[117] In a study involving 34 men and 28 women, saw palmetto applied topically for 3 months in a lotion and shampoo base led to a 35% increase in hair density and a 67% sebum reduction, as assessed using standard objective techniques. Addition of 0.5% saw palmetto (possibly LESP) and taurine to a 0.5% ketoconazole shampoo gave better results than ketoconazole alone (at 1.0%) in patients with dandruff and seborrhoeic dermatitis.

Toxicology and other safety data

Toxicology

Published toxicological data on saw palmetto and LESP is limited. Brine shrimp lethality directed fractionation of an ethanolic LESP led to the isolation of two monoacylglycerides.[118] These compounds showed moderate biological activities in the brine shrimp lethality test and against renal and pancreatic human tumour cells in vitro; borderline cytotoxicity was exhibited against human prostatic cells.

The company Madaus has released toxicological data on its ethanolic LESP.[119] The LD_{50} in the rat, mouse and guinea pig is greater than 10 g/kg. High doses given to rats over 6 weeks (360 times the human therapeutic dose of about 5 mg/kg) did not cause adverse haematological, histological or biochemical changes. A long-term study over 6 months in rats at 80 times the human dose again found no negative influences. The same dose administered to rats had no influence on fertility.

LESP as the hexane extract did not produce any indications of liver toxicity when given to rats for up to 4 weeks at oral doses of 9.14 or 22.86 mg/kg/day.[120]

A poorly characterised liposterolic extract fed to mice for 6 weeks failed to show any genotoxic effects.[121]

Contraindications

None known.

Special warnings and precautions

Prostate cancer should be excluded before patients receive saw palmetto treatment as the herb treatment may mask the symptoms of this disease (but will not alter PSA readings). Exercise caution for concurrent use with warfarin.

Interactions

LESP at relatively high concentrations inhibited CYP3A4, 2D6 and 2C9 in vitro.[122] However, using alprazolam, midazolam, caffeine, chlorzoxazone, desbrisoquine and dextromorphan as probe drugs, two clinical studies found that LESP (320 mg/day) for 14 or 28 days exerted no significant influence on CYP3A4, CYP1A2, CYP2D6 and CYP2E1 in healthy volunteers.[123,124]

A 61-year-old man had long been treated with warfarin and simvastatin. His INR values had been stable at around 2.4. Due to micturition difficulties he started to take a saw palmetto, pumpkin seed and vitamin E preparation, five tablets daily. After 6 days' treatment his INR increased to 3.4. The herbal product was discontinued and 1 week later the INR returned to its previous level.[125]

Use in pregnancy and lactation

Category B2 – no increase in frequency of malformation or other harmful effects on the fetus from limited use in women. Animal studies are lacking. However, saw palmetto treatment is unlikely to be indicated for a pregnant women.

Saw palmetto is probably compatible with breastfeeding.

Addition of liposterolic extract at concentrations ranging from 1 to 10 µg/mL to Chinese hamster ovary cells completely inhibited the effects of prolactin, suggesting that saw palmetto may inhibit prolactin-induced hormonal effects.[54] However, the relevance of this research to normal human use is unclear.

Effects on ability to drive and use machines

No adverse effects are expected.

Side effects

Saw palmetto is well tolerated by most patients and causes relatively few side effects. Most side effects are minor gastrointestinal problems such as nausea, which are usually resolved when the herb is taken with meals.

The large comparative study of Carraro and co-workers[98] found that gastrointestinal complaints were the most frequently reported adverse events with both therapies and tended to occur more frequently with finasteride. As might be expected, decreased libido and impotence were also more common with finasteride treatment. Two deaths occurred during the trial (one in each group) and three serious adverse events occurred (two with saw palmetto, one with finasteride). None of these was deemed to be related to treatment. PSA was not changed by saw palmetto treatment, indicating that the herb is unlikely to interfere with the diagnostic value of this test.

The German Commission E lists stomach upsets as the only side effect from treatment with saw palmetto liposterolic extract.[126]

A 2009 systematic review assessed all available human safety data for saw palmetto monopreparations up to early 2008.[127] Systematic literature searches were conducted in five electronic databases, reference lists and departmental files were checked for further relevant publications. Information was requested from spontaneous reporting schemes of the WHO and national safety bodies. Twenty-four manufacturers/distributors of saw palmetto products and four herbalist organisations were contacted for additional information. Forty articles (26 randomised controlled trials, four non-randomised controlled trials, six uncontrolled trials and four case reports/series) were included. They suggest that adverse events associated with the use of saw palmetto are mild and similar to those with placebo. The most frequently reported adverse events were abdominal pain, diarrhoea, nausea, fatigue, headache, decreased libido and rhinitis. More serious adverse events, such as death and cerebral haemorrhage, are reported in isolated case reports and data from spontaneous reporting schemes, but causality was questionable.

A review of the data from three large clinical trials of the hexane extract of LESP that included 2511 patients found it had no negative impact on male sexual function.[128]

Intraoperative floppy-iris syndrome (IFIS) has been associated with many A1A receptor antagonist drugs including tamsulosin.[129] Their probable mode of action in causing IFIS is a direct inhibition of the A1 receptors in the smooth muscle of the iris, which leads to a loss of iris tone. This can result in poor iris dilation and complications during cataract surgery (IFIS).

Two surgeons have reported IFIS in two patients taking saw palmetto for BPH who were undergoing cataract surgery.[129] The first patient had used saw palmetto for 2 years and the other for 5 years, and neither patient reported taking conventional drugs for their BPH. Both patients experienced good outcomes following their surgery. No information regarding the saw palmetto dose and preparation was provided.

Analysis of 899 eyes of 660 patients undergoing routine cataract surgery found a strong association of IFIS with tamsulosin use (p<0.001).[130] Saw palmetto showed a slight, nonsignificant trend, indicating that current or past use may be associated with IFIS.

As a precaution, patients taking saw palmetto should be advised to temporarily stop their herbal treatment 10 days before cataract surgery in order to minimise the potential for the mild complications described above.

One case of haemorrhage during surgery, which was associated with intake of saw palmetto extract, has been reported.[131] A case has also been described of haematuria and coagulopathy (INR of 4.0) in a patient using saw palmetto.[132] The 79-year-old man had been taking 320mg/day LESP for 4 years, but had recently increased the dose to 1000mg/day. He was also taking aspirin and clopidogrel. However, these reports contrast with clinical trials demonstrating reduced blood loss in BPH patients undergoing surgery (see above).

A case of protracted cholestatic hepatitis after the use of a herbal and nutritional preparation has been reported. The herbal preparation contained saw palmetto, hydrangea, *Pygeum africanum*, *Panax ginseng*, zinc picolinate, pyridoxine, alanine, glutamic acid, bee pollen and silica.[133] The ingredient causing the adverse reaction was not identified. Use of saw palmetto (900mg/day of a dried extract that was not LESP, together with 660mg of berry powder) for a few days was associated with acute liver damage.[134] The product was discontinued and all symptoms disappeared without residual harm to the patient. A causal association is unlikely, given the brief exposure to the product.

Two cases of acute pancreatitis associated with intake of LESP have been reported.[135,136] One report suggested rechallenge with saw palmetto caused a recurrence of symptoms.[136] The fatty nature of LESP could be a possible cause of this reaction, although the exact nature of the products involved was not provided.

A case of contact sensitivity following the topical use of saw palmetto was reported in a 24-year-old woman with androgenic alopecia.[137]

Exposure of human sperm samples to a relatively high concentration of LESP (900μg/mL) in vitro had no impact on kinematic parameters.[138] However, motility was impaired after 48h of exposure to 9mg/mL LESP. Even assuming a high bioavailability for LESP and efficient transport to the testes, this still represents an exposure of around 1000 times the normal human dose. Zona-free hamster oocytes incubated with LESP in vitro at the same high concentrations exhibited no change in their viability.[139] Such studies are unlikely to have any clinical relevance (see also the discussion of this issue in Chapter 5).

Overdosage

No incidents found in the published literature.

Safety in children

No information available, but adverse effects are not anticipated.

Regulatory status in selected countries

Saw palmetto is official in the *United States Pharmacopeia-National Formulary* (USP34–NF 29 2011).

Saw palmetto is covered by a positive Commission E monograph and has the following application: urination problems in benign prostatic hyperplasia stages I and II.

Saw palmetto is on the UK General Sale List. Saw palmetto products have achieved Traditional Herbal Registration in the UK with the traditional indication of relief of symptoms of urinary discomfort in men who have BPH. Prior to treatment, other serious conditions should have been ruled out by a doctor.

Saw palmetto does not have GRAS status. However, it is freely available as a 'dietary supplement' in the USA under DSHEA legislation (1994 Dietary Supplement Health and Education Act). Saw palmetto has been present in OTC (over-the-counter) drug products to relieve the symptoms of BPH. The FDA, however, advises that: 'based on evidence currently available, there is inadequate data to establish general recognition of the safety and effectiveness of these ingredients for the specified uses, and … there is no definitive evidence that any drug product offered for the relief of the symptoms of benign prostatic hypertrophy would alter the obstructive or inflammatory signs and symptoms of this condition'.

Saw palmetto is not included in Part 4 of Schedule 4 of the Therapeutic Goods Act Regulations of Australia and is freely available for sale.

References

1. Grieve M. *A Modern Herbal*, vol. 2. New York: Dover Publications; 1971. pp. 719–720.

2. British Herbal Medicine Association Scientific Committee. *British Herbal Pharmacopoeia*. Cowling: BHMA; 1983. pp. 196–197.

3. Felter HW, Lloyd JU. *King's American Dispensatory*. ed18, rev 3, vol. 2, 1905. Portland: Reprinted by Eclectic Medical Publications; 1983. pp. 1750–1752.

4. Mabberley DJ. *The Plant Book*, 2nd ed Cambridge: Cambridge University Press; 1997. p. 657.

5. Leung AY, Foster S. *Encyclopedia of Common Natural Ingredients Used in Food, Drugs and Cosmetics*, 2nd ed New York: John Wiley; 1996. p. 467.

6. Bombardelli E, Morazzoni P. *Fitoterapia*. 1997;68(2):99–113.

7. Feifer AH, Fleshner NE, Klotz L. *J Urol*. 2002;168(1):150–154.

8. Habib FK, Wyllie MG. *Prostate Cancer Prostatic Dis*. 2004;7(3):195–200.

9. Tenover JS. *Endocrinol Metab Clin North Am*. 1991;20(4):893–909.

10. Bushman W. *Urol Clin North Am*. 2009;36(4):403–415.

11. Roehrbornb CG. *Int J Impot Res*. 2008;20(suppl 3):S11–S18.

12. Kramer G, Mitteregger D, Marberger M. *Eur Urol*. 2007;51(5):1202–1216.

13. Sciarra A, Mariotti G, Salciccia S, et al. *J Steroid Biochem Mol Biol*. 2008; 108(3–5):254–260.

14. Vikram A, Jena G, Ramarao P. *Eur J Pharmacol*. 2010;641(2–3):75–81.

15. Moul S, McVary KT. *Curr Opin Urol*. 2010;20(1):7–12.

16. Sarma AV, Parsons JK, McVary K, et al. *J Urol*. 2009;182(6 suppl):S32–S37.

17. Parsons JK, Sarma AV, McVary K, et al. *J Urol*. 2009;182(6 suppl):S27–S31.

18. Farmer A, Nobel J. *Br Med J*. 1997;314(7089):1215–1216.

19. Sultan C, Terraza A, Devillier C, et al. *J Steroid Biochem*. 1984;20(1):515–519.

20. Düker EM, Kopanski L, Schweikert HU. *Planta Med*. 1989;55:587.

21. Delos S, Iehle C, Martin P-M, et al. *J Steroid Biochem Mol Biol*. 1994;48(4):347–352.

22. Delos S, Carsol JL, Ghazararossian E, et al. *J Steroid Biochem Mol Biol*. 1995;55(34):375–383.

23. Iehle C, Delos S, Guirou O, et al. *J Steroid Biochem Mol Biol*. 1995;54(5–6):273–279.

24. Niederprüm HJ, Schweikert HU, Zanker KS. *Phytomedicine*. 1994;1:127–133.

25. Weisser H, Tunn S, Behnke B, et al. *Prostate*. 1996;28(5):300–306.

26. Rhodes L, Primka RL, Berman C, et al. *Prostate*. 1993;22(1):43–51.

27. Bayne CW, Ross M, Donnelly F, Habib FK. *J Urol*. 2000;164(3 Pt1):876–881.

28. Raynaud JP, Cousse H, Martin PM. *J Steroid Biochem Mol Biol*. 2002;82 (2–3):233–239.

29. Abe M, Ito Y, Suzuki A, et al. *Anal Sci*. 2009;25(4):553–557.

30. Abe M, Ito Y, Oyunzul L, et al. *Biol Pharm Bull*. 2009;32(4):646–650.

31. Scaglione F, Lucini V, Pannacci M, et al. *Pharmacology*. 2008;82(4):270–275.

32. Pais P. *Adv Ther*. 2010;27(8):555–563.

33. Bayne CW, Donnelly F, Ross M, Habib FK. *Prostate*. 1999;40(4):232–241.

34. Habib FK, Ross M, Ho CK, et al. *Int J Cancer*. 2005;114(2):190–194.

35. Wadsworth TL, Worstell TR, Greenberg NM, Roselli CE. *Prostate*. 2007;67(6):661–673.

36. Strauch G, Perles P, Vergult G, et al. *Eur Urol*. 1994;26(3):247–252.

37. Weisser H, Behnke B, Helpap B, et al. *Eur Urol*. 1997;31(1):97–101.

38. Di Silverio F, Monti S, Sciarra A, et al. *Prostate*. 1998;37(2):77–83.

39. Marks LS, Hess DL, Dorey FJ, et al. *Urology*. 2001;57(5):999–1005.

40. Gutierrez M, Garcia de Boto MJ, Cantabrana B, et al. *Gen Pharmacol*. 1996;27(1):171–176.

41. Gutierrez M, Hidalgo A, Cantabrana B. *Planta Med*. 1996;62(6):507–511.

42. Odenthal KP. *Phytother Res*. 1996;10(suppl):S141–S143.

43. Goepel M, Hecker U, Krege S, et al. *Prostate*. 1999;38(3):208–215.

44. Suzuki M, Oki T, Sugiyama T, et al. *Urology*. 2007;69(6):1216–1220.

45. Chua T, Simpson JS, Ventura S. *Prostate*. 2011;71(1):71–80.

46. Oki T, Suzuki M, Nishioka Y, et al. *J Urol*. 2005;173(4):1395–1399.

47. Goepel M, Dinh L, Mitchell A, et al. *Prostate*. 2001;46(3):226–232.

48. Carilla E, Briley M, Fauran F, et al. *J Steroid Biochem*. 1984;20(1):521–523.

49. El Sheikh MM, Dakkak MR, Saddique A. *Acta Obstet Gynecol Scand*. 1988;67(5):397–399.

50. Ravenna L, Di Silverio F, Russo MA, et al. *Prostate*. 1996;29(4):219–230.

51. Stenger A, Tarayre JP, Carilla E, et al. *Gaz Med Fr*. 1982;89(17):2041–2048.

52. Cristoni A, Morazzoni P, Bombardelli E. *Fitoterapia*. 1997;68(4):355–358.

53. Buck AC. *J Urol*. 2004;172(5 Pt 1): 1792–1799.

54. Vacher P, Prevarskaya N, Skryma R, et al. *J Biomed Sci*. 1995;2(4):357–365.

55. Elghamry MI, Hansel R. *Experientia*. 1969;25(8):828–829.

56. Di Silverio F, D'Eramo G, Lubrano C, et al. *Eur Urol*. 1992;21(4):309–314.

57. Casarosa C, Cosci di Coscio M, Fratta M. *Clin Ther*. 1988;10(5):585–588.

58. Angwafor III F, Anderson ML. *J Int Soc Sports Nutr*. 2008;5:12.

59. Paubert–Braquet M, Cousse H, Raynaud JP, et al. *Eur Urol*. 1998;33(3):340–347.

60. Tarayre JP, Delhon A, Lauressergues H, et al. *Ann Pharm Fr*. 1983;41(6):559–570.

61. Mitropoulos D, Hyroudi A, Zervas A, et al. *World J Urol*. 2002;19(6):457–461.

62. Hiermann A. *Arch Pharm*. 1989;322(2):111–114.

63. Wagner H, Flachsbarth H. *Planta Med*. 1981;41(3):244–251.

64. Wagner H, Flachsbarth H, Vogel G. *Planta Med*. 1981;41(3):252–258.

65. Breu W, Hagenlocher M, Redl K, et al. *Arzneimittelforschung*. 1992;42(4):547–551.

66. Paubert-Braquet M, Mencia Huerta J-M, Cousse H, et al. *Prostagland Leukot Essent Fatty Acids*. 1997;57(3):299–304.

67. Bonvissuto G, Minutoli L, Morgia G, et al. *Urology*. 2011;77(1):248.e9–248.e16.

68. Vela Navarrete R, Garcia Cardoso JV, Barat A, et al. *Eur Urol*. 2003;44:549–555.

69. Paubert-Braquet M, Richardson FO, Servent-Saez N, et al. *Pharmacol Res*. 1996;34(3–4):171–179.

70. Otto U, Wagner B, Becker H, et al. *Urol Int*. 1992;48:167–170.

71. Van Coppenolle F, Le Bourhis X, Carpentier F, et al. *Prostate*. 2000;43(1):49–58.

72. Vacherot F, Azzouz M, Gil-Diez-De-Medina S, Colombel M, et al. *Prostate*. 2000;45(3):259–266.

73. Vela-Navarrete R, Escribano-Burgos M, Farré AL, et al. *J Urol*. 2005;173(2):507–510.

74. Ishii K, Usui S, Sugimura Y, et al. *Biol Pharm Bull*. 2001;24(2):188–190.

75. Iguchi K, Okumura N, Usui S, et al. *Prostate*. 2001;47(1):59–65.

76. Goldmann WH, Sharma AL, Currier SJ, et al. *Cell Biol Int*. 2001;25(11):1117–1124.

77. Petrangeli E, Lenti L, Buchetti B, et al. *J Cell Physiol*. 2009;219(1):69–76.

78. Baron A, Mancini M, Caldwell E, et al. *BJU Int*. 2009;103(9):1275–1283.

79. Hostanska K, Suter A, Melzer J, Saller R. *Anticancer Res*. 2007;27(2):873–881.

80. Yang Y, Ikezoe T, Zheng Z, et al. *Int J Oncol*. 2007;31(3):593–600.

81. Scholtysek C, Krukiewicz AA, Alonso JL, et al. *Biochem Biophys Res Commun*. 2009;379(3):795–798.

82. Che Y, Hou S, Kang Z, Lin Q. *Oncol Rep*. 2009;22(2):377–383.

83. Adams LS, Seeram NP, Hardy ML, et al. *Evid Based Complement Altern Med*. 2006;3(1):117–124.

84. Hill B, Kyprianou N. *Prostate*. 2004;61(1):73–80.

85. Bonnar-Pizzorno RM, Littman AJ, Kestin M, White E. *Nutr Cancer*. 2006;55(1):21–27.

86. Groom SN, Johns T, Oldfield PR. *J Med Food*. 2007;10(1):73–79.

87. Beckert BW, Concannon MJ, Henry SL, et al. *Plast Reconstr Surg*. 2007;120(7):2044–2050.

88. Chevalier G, Benard P, Cousse H, et al. *Eur J Drug Metab Pharmacokinet*. 1997;22(1):73–83.

89. De Bernardi Di Valserra M, Tripodi AS, Contos S, et al. *Acta Toxicol Ther*. 1994;15(1):21–39.

90. Debruyne F, Koch G, Boyle P, et al. *Eur Urol*. 2002;41:497–507.

91. Braeckman J, Bruhwyler J, Vandekerckhove K, Géczy J. *Phytother Res*. 1997;11:558–563.

92. *5th International Consultations of BPH*. Paris: Recommendations of the International Scientific Committee; 2000.

93. Tacklind J, MacDonald R, Rutks I, Wilt TJ. *Cochrane Database Syst Rev*. 2009;2:CD001423.

94. Bent S, Kane C, Shinohara K, et al. *N Engl J Med*. 2006;354(6):557–566.

95. DiPaola RS, Morton RA. *N Engl J Med*. 2006;354(6):632–634.

96. Boyle P, Robertson C, Lowe F, et al. *BJU Int*. 2004;93(6):751–756.

97. Boyle P, Robertson C, Lowe F, Roehrborn C. *Urology*. 2000;55(4):533–539.

98. Carraro J-C, Raynaud J-P, Koch G, et al. *Prostate*. 1996;29(4):231–240.

99. Grasso M, Montesano A, Buonaguidi A, et al. *Arch Esp Urol*. 1995;48(1):97–103.

100. Adriazola Semino M, Lozano Ortega JL, Garcia Cobo E, et al. *Arch Esp Urol*. 1992;45(3):211–213.

101. Hizli F, Uygur MC. *Int Urol Nephrol*. 2007;39(3):879–886.

102. Debruyne F, Boyle P, Calais Da Silva F, et al. *Eur Urol*. 2004;45(6):773–780.

103. Denis LJ. *Prostate*. 1996;29:241–242.

104. Sinescu I, Geavlete P, Multescu R, et al. *Urol Int*. 2011;86(3):284–289.

105. Hutchison A, Farmer R, Verhamme K, et al. *Eur Urol*. 2007;51(1):207–216.

106. Djavan B, Fong YK, Chaudry A, et al. *World J Urol*. 2005;23(4):253–256.

107. Kaplan SA, Volpe MA, Te AE. *J Urol*. 2004;171(1):284–288.

108. Wu T, Zhang X, Wu R, Liu X. *Zhonghua Nan Ke Xue*. 2004;10(5):337–339. [Article in Chinese].

109. Lopatkin NA, Apolikhin OI, Sivkov AV, et al. *Urologiia*. 2007;5:3–7. [Article in Russian].

110. Magri V, Trinchieri A, Montanari E, et al. *Arch Ital Urol Androl*. 2007;79(2):84–92.

111. Magri V, Trinchieri A, Pozzi G, et al. *Int J Antimicrob Agents*. 2007;29(5):549–556.

112. Morgia G, Mucciardi G, Galì A, et al. *Urol Int*. 2010;84(4):400–406.

113. Pecoraro S, Annecchiarico A, Gambardella MC, et al. *Minerva Urol Nefrol*. 2004;56(1):73–78.

114. Anceschi R, Bisi M, Ghidini N, et al. *Minerva Urol Nefrol*. 2010;62(3):219–223.

115. Tuncel A, Ener K, Han O, et al. *Scand J Urol Nephrol*. 2009;43(5):377–382.

116. Prager N, Bickett R, French N, et al. *J Altern Complement Med*. 2002;8(2):143–152.

117. Murugusundram S. *J Cutan Aesthet Surg*. 2009;2(1):31–32.

118. Kondás J, Philipp V, Diószeghy G. *Orv Hetil*. 1997;138(7):419–421.

119. Prosta Urgenin® Uno, Zur Behandlung der BPH. Koln: Madaus AG; 1996. p. 33.

120. Singh YN, Devkota AK, Sneeden DC, et al. *Phytomedicine*. 2007;14(2–3):204–208.

121. Trinachartvanit W, Francis BM, Rayburn AL. *Environ Toxicol Pharmacol*. 2009;27:149–154.

122. Yale SH, Glurich I. *J Altern Complement Med*. 2005;11(3):433–439.

123. Markowitz JS, Donovan JL, Devane CL, et al. *Clin Pharmacol Ther*. 2003;74(6):536–542.

124. Gurley BJ, Gardner SF, Hubbard MA, et al. *Clin Pharmacol Ther*. 2004;76(5):428–440.

125. Yue Q-Y, Jansson K. *J Am Geriatr Soc*. 2001;310(4):838.

126. Blumenthal M, ed. *The Complete German Commission E Monographs: Therapeutic Guide to Herbal Medicines*. Austin: American Botanical Council; 1998. p. 201.

127. Agbabiaka TB, Pittler MH, Wider B, Ernst E. *Drug Saf*. 2009;32(8):637–647.

128. Zlotta AR, Teillac P, Raynaud JP, Schulman CC. *Eur Urol*. 2005;48(2):269–276.

129. Yeu E, Grostern R. *J Cataract Refract Surg*. 2007;33(5):927–928.

130. Neff KD, Sandoval HP, Fernández de Castro LE, et al. *Ophthalmology*. 2009;116(4):658–663.

131. Cheema P, El-Mefty O, Jazieh AR. *J Intern Med*. 2001;250(2):167–169.

132. Villanueva S, González J. *Bol Asoc Med PR*. 2009;101(3):48–50.

133. Hamid S, Bojter S, Vierling J. *Ann Intern Med*. 1997;127(2):169–170.

134. Lapi F, Gallo E, Giocaliere E, et al. *Br J Clin Pharmacol*. 2010;69(5):558–560.

135. Wargo KA, Allman E, Ibrahim F. *South Med J*. 2010;103(7):683–685.

136. Jibrin I, Erinle A, Saidi A, Aliyu ZY. *South Med J*. 2006;99(6):611–612.

137. Sinclair RD, Mallari RS, Tate B. *Australas J Dermatol*. 2002;43(4):311–312.

138. Ondrizek RR, Chan PJ, Patton WC, King A. *J Assist Reprod Genet*. 1999;16(2):87–91.

139. Ondrizek RR, Chan PJ, Patton WC, King A. *Fertil Steril*. 1999;71(3):517–522.

(*Eleutherococcus senticosus* (Rupr. & Maxim.) Maxim.)

Synonyms

Acanthopanax senticosus (botanical synonym), Eleutherococcus (Engl), Eleutherococci radix (Lat), Taigawurzel (Ger), Éleuthérocoque (Fr), Wu Jia Pi, Cu Wu Jia (Chin), Gokahi (Jap), Ogap'I (Kor), Russisk rod (Dan), Eleuterokokka (Russ).

What is it?

For reasons more related to marketing than botany, the root of *Eleutherococcus senticosus* is often known in the West as Siberian ginseng. Although the use of Eleutherococcus is important to traditional Chinese medicine (where it is known by its synonym *Acanthopanax senticosus*), its potential as an adaptogen was demonstrated more recently.

The work of Russian scientists from the 1950s onwards lead to the inclusion of Eleutherococcus in the *Soviet Pharmacopoeia*, and by 1976 it was estimated that more than 3 million people were using the extract regularly. It was used by Russian athletes to prepare for the Olympics games in the late 1970s and early 1980s, and was included in the Russian space programme for cosmonauts in 1977. It was, however, not known in Russian folk medicine.

A survey conducted in the early 1980s of products sold as 'Siberian ginseng' in the USA revealed that many products were not authentic, being derived from related species or adulterants.[1] The problem may have originated from companies importing 'Jia pi' and not distinguishing between the various forms, which include species of Eleutherococcus and species of Periploca.[2]

Effects

Helps restore mental and physical capacity, especially in exhaustion and when convalescing from fatigue;[3] assists the body to counteract and adapt to stress of many origins; restores and strengthens the body's immune response.

Traditional view

In Chinese Medicine the root barks of several species of Eleutherococcus (including *E. senticosus*, *E. gracilistylus* and *E. sessiliflorus*) are used to expel *Wind Dampness*, to strengthen the sinews and bones, transform *Dampness* and reduce swelling. It is especially useful when the smooth flow of *Qi* and *Blood* is obstructed, and is particularly used for treating the elderly. These properties mean that it is used to treat oedema, joint pain, muscular spasm, difficult urination

and, in combination with other herbs, to assist muscular development in children.[4] It has *Spleen* invigorative, *Kidney* tonifying and tranquillising actions, and is also used for back pain, insomnia and anorexia.[5]

Summary actions

Adaptogen, mild stimulant, immunomodulator, tonic.

Can be used for

Indications supported by clinical trials

To improve mental and physical performance or minimise the effects of stress in people subject to chronic illness or to environmental or occupational stress (generally open label trials); to enhance immune function, especially natural killer cells and T-helper cells; adjuvant treatment in dysentery; cancer (especially to improve immune function and decrease side effects from conventional therapy); and convalescence after antibiotic therapy.

Eleutherococcus can be taken on a long-term basis to minimise the incidence of acute infections and to improve well-being, (low quality trials).

Traditional therapeutic uses

Oedema, joint pain, muscular spasm, difficult urination. Used as a tonic, particularly in the elderly,[6] and to treat fatigue, stress and lowered immunity.

May also be used for

Extrapolations from pharmacological studies

To treat the effects of prolonged stress or overwork such as exhaustion, chronic fatigue syndrome, irritability, insomnia and mild depression; to assist recovery from acute or chronic diseases, trauma, surgery and other stressful episodes.

Preparations

Dried root for decoction; fluid extract, tablets, capsules or powdered root for internal use.

Dosage

Adult doses used in most studies were in the range of 1 to 4 g/day, which corresponds to 2 to 8 mL/day of a 1:2 extract or Eleutherococcus tablets (for example 1.25 g, standardised to contain 0.7 mg eleutheroside E), one to three times per day.

Maintenance doses for healthy individuals can be toward the lower end of the dosage range, but higher doses should be used for the treatment of illnesses and for high stress situations. Single applications of the highest doses may be appropriate where a rapid response to tension or stress is required.[7]

Duration of use

The recommended regime in healthy people or the elderly or long-term infirm[6] is for a course of 6 weeks followed by a 2-week break. This regime can be repeated for as long as is necessary. For the treatment of specific illnesses, continuous use is preferable. Because of their favourable effect in conserving energy during stress, adaptogens in fact work best with long-term use.

However, the Commission E and *British Herbal Compendium* take a more cautious stance, recommending the following:

- Generally no longer than 3 months. Use again at a later time[8]
- Eleutherococcus should not be taken continuously for long periods. Occasional use or courses of 1 month followed by a 2-month interval are preferable.[9]

However, there appears to be little reason or evidence to support this dosage approach, which may in fact be contrary to achieving optimum benefit from this adaptogenic herb, as supported by some of the Russian research.

Summary assessment of safety

No adverse effects are expected if used as recommended. It is advisable to discontinue use of high doses during acute infections, unless used in conjunction with powerful antimicrobial therapy or in a formulation with proven efficacy.

Technical data

Botany

Eleutherococcus senticosus, a member of the Araliaceae (ginseng, ivy) family, is a hardy, wild shrub that grows abundantly in parts of the Soviet Far East, Korea, China and Japan, north of latitude 38. It usually grows to about 2 m, with grey-brown coloured branches covered with thin, downward-pointing spikes. The bright green leaves (12 to 15 cm long) are divided into three to five leaflets. It produces three types of flowers (male, female, bisexual) which are branched together in umbrella-shaped clusters. The flowers vary in colour, depending on type: light violet or yellow. The fruits are oval and berry-like. The rhizome lies shallow in the ground and is 1.5 cm in diameter. The roots are long, woody and pliable, spreading beneath the surface in massive webs and thickets.[10]

Key constituents

- Lignans and phenylpropanoids known as eleutherosides (0.1%),[11] notably eleutherosides E (syringaresinol diglucoside) and B (syringin); also B_4 (sesamin), D (an optical isomer of E), and several others
- Triterpenoid saponins (glycosides of protoprimulagenin A)[12]
- Glycans (eleutherans A, B, C, D, E, F and G).[13]

The source of Eleutherococcus is likely to be important to its activity: a chromatographic study of Eleutherococcus roots[14] indicated that Russian and Korean Eleutherococcus samples are chemically different to Chinese Eleutherococcus and contain higher levels of eleutheroside E. The eleutherosides are not unique to Eleutherococcus, although eleutherosides D and E are not common and are probably pharmacologically important. The eleutherosides are quite different from the triterpenoid saponins found in Panax (the ginsenosides).

Eleutheroside B

Eleutheroside D

Pharmacodynamics

In the 1950s, Russian scientists became interested in agents that could improve general health and performance under stress. In their systematic search for a cheaper and more abundant alternative to *Panax ginseng* they found Eleutherococcus an almost ideal herbal 'adaptogen'. This term was first coined by Lazarev and was elaborated by Brekhman[15] who defined an adaptogen as a substance that can effect a non-specific increase in the resistance of an organism to noxious influences. In principle an adaptogen has the following properties:

- It is non-toxic and relatively free from side effects
- It is non-specific, i.e. it can increase resistance to a wide range of physical, chemical and biological stressors
- It may have a normalising action irrespective of whether the stress-driven pathological state is hypo- or hyperfunctional.

Modern developments of the adaptogenic concept focus on the role of these remedies on the hypothalamic-pituitary-adrenal axis in the stress response; short-term stimulation of the adreno sympathetic system has also been identified for this group of remedies, including Eleuterocccus.[6]

Since much of the original research on Eleutherococcus is from the early Russian work, this monograph has drawn from several English language reviews. The rigour of this work is sometimes uncertain, and it has been important to check its inferences with new research. This has sometimes cast doubt on the original findings.

The observed activity of Eleutherococcus may be due to the combined effect of all its constituents, discovered or otherwise.[16] In contrast to isolated eleutherosides B and E and the re-mixed eleutherosides B and E, in one study only the whole ethanolic fluid extract of *Eleutherococcus senticosus* was able to induce and enhance interleukin-1 and interleukin-6, but not interleukin-2, production in vitro.[17] In contrast, another study concluded that eleutheroside E was particularly responsible for increasing resistance to stress and fatigue.[18]

Several polysaccharides found in the root when administered by injection, such as the glycans mentioned above, have demonstrated immunostimulant[19] and hypoglycaemic[13] effects. However the importance of these types of compounds to the oral activity of Eleutherococcus is questionable, and the exact mechanism of action of Eleutherococcus and the significance of each of its various constituents is not yet fully understood.

Adaptation to stress

Published animal studies, mostly conducted in the Far East and Eastern Europe, consistently demonstrate the adaptogenic effect of Eleutherococcus under a wide variety of stressful conditions. In his original work with mice, Brekhman found that Eleutherococcus increased stamina by up to 70%.[20] Severely stressed rats show enlarged adrenal glands, reduced thymus and spleen size and damage to the gastric mucosa.[21] Eleutherococcus significantly reduced this adrenal hypertrophy and adrenal ascorbic acid depletion.[15] These and other effects suggested that Eleutherococcus modified the physiological response to stressors (general adaptation syndrome) to help the organism better to withstand prolonged stress.

Additional research found that Eleutherococcus could increase the resistance of animals to stressors such as heat, cold, immobilisation, trauma, surgery, blood loss, increased or decreased barometric pressure, narcotics, toxins and bacteria.[22,23] Eleutherococcus also appears to exert an immune-enhancing action in immune-compromised mice.[24]

Oral administration of water extract of Eleutherococcus and its components, eleutheroside B and eleutheroside E demonstrated protective effects on behavioural, functional and biochemical changes in mice subjected to acute or chronic stress (exhaustion).[25] Oral administration of this extract (500 mg/kg per day) for 7 weeks led to improvements in learning and memory in the active avoidance rat model.[26]

Addition of an aqueous extract of Eleutherococcus (0.1 mg/mL) caused significant liberation of adrenocorticotropic hormone (ACTH) and luteinising hormone from isolated rat pituitary glands in vitro. In vivo experiments indicate that a single intraperitoneal dose of standardised aqueous extract (3 mg/mL) enhanced the liberation of corticosterone, while subchronic administration (3 mg/mL, ip, or 500 mg/kg, oral) did not alter ACTH or corticosterone levels, body or organ weight after 7 weeks. However, elevations of corticosterone serum levels induced by mild stress were significantly suppressed in animals treated either subchronically by oral administration or by intraperitoneal injection of standardised Eleutherococcus extract.[27]

Some studies have shown stimulant rather than adaptogenic effects. An American investigation of the adaptogenic effects of Eleutherococcus in stressed mice did not confirm improved stamina, and instead demonstrated aggressive behaviour for mice given unlimited quantities of the root.[28] Rats given Eleutherococcus show increased brain levels of noradrenaline (norepinephrine) and serotonin and adrenal levels of adrenaline (epinephrine), which may explain the increased aggressive behaviour observed above.[29]

Eleutherococcus may exert some of its effects by inducing enzyme activity. It inhibited metabolism of the sedative hexobarbitol in mice to produce a longer sleep period.[30] In one study, the stress of swimming for 15 minutes inhibited RNA polymerase in the liver and skeletal muscle of rats; prior injection of eleutherosides delayed the RNA polymerase inhibition and accelerated its restoration during rest.[31] Another study suggested that the effects of swimming stress in inhibiting NK activity and corticosterone could be countered by eleutheroside E.[32]

Experiments conducted in stressed BALB/c mice using oral doses (30, 90 and 180 mg/kg) of a proprietary combination of extracts from *Eleutherococcus senticosus*, *Schisandra chinensis* and *Rhodiola rosea* found increased endurance.[33] In addition, repeated administration of the adaptogen formulation dose-dependently increased basal serum levels of the heat shock protein Hsp72, which was even stronger than the effect of stress on this measure. Based on their findings, the authors suggested that the increased tolerance to stress induced by adaptogens is associated with stimulation of Hsp72 production and release into the systemic circulation. Hsp72 is a known mediator of the stress response involved in protein maintenance and repair. This finding implies that adaptogens could be acting as hormetic agents.

Resistance to radiation and chemical carcinogens

The independent application of Eleutherococcus extract (given orally and prophylactically, 5 g/kg) and a chemical radioprotector (adeturone) demonstrated a favourable effect on rats subjected to radiation injury. This favourable effect was only demonstrated on the course of the recovery processes. The two agents mutually potentiated each other and provided a high degree of protection.[34]

Eleutherococcus given to mice by injection prior to radiation treatment improved self-repair rather than exerting a direct protective effect. This further supports the concept of its non-specific activity.[34] Up to 80% of mice given Eleutherococcus beforehand survived a lethal dose of radiation. When Eleutherococcus was administered as late as 12 hours after irradiation the survival rate was 30%.[35] The stimulation of red blood cell production by the spleen was considered to be responsible for this sustained effect.[32] An in vitro study using isolated mammalian cells exposed to gamma radiation found that *Panax ginseng* increased their resistance to irradiation whereas Eleutherococcus did not.[36] The above studies suggest that Panax confers a direct resistance to cells by altering cell physiology, whereas the improved survival from Eleutherococcus is via an indirect action on the whole organism.

In their early seminal review of Eleutherococcus, Brekhman and Dardymov found that it inhibited both spontaneous malignant tumours and those induced by a number of carcinogens. Evidence was obtained of a decreased transplantability of tumours in mice and an inhibition of metastases occurred in some cases.[15] An earlier study indicated a decreased incidence of lung cancer in mice when Eleutherococcus was given for several weeks with or after the administration of a carcinogenic agent.[37] Further in vitro research found that components of Eleutherococcus exerted an antiproliferative action upon murine cancer cells; the effect of some cytotoxic drugs was also potentiated by Eleutherococcus, thereby reducing the amount of drug needed.[38] Eleutherococcus lowered the occurrence of chromosomal mutations and increased the survival rate of plants exposed to mutagens.[39]

Immune effects

Resistance to bacterial infection is increased in mice and rabbits by prior dosing with Eleutherococcus. However, simultaneous administration with the infecting organism increased the severity of the disease.[40] This work and clinical experience in Russia have led to the notion that use of Eleutherococcus should be discontinued during acute infections, although it has been used in combination for such conditions.[41] Antiviral immunity is also stimulated in vivo and in vitro by prior administration of Eleutherococcus.[42] Preparations of Eleutherococcus were analysed and found in vitro to selectively inhibit COX-2 enzymes and lipid peroxidation which are elevated in inflamed or cancerous conditions.[43]

Normalising actions

Brekhman and Dardymov demonstrated that Eleutherococcus impeded both hypertrophy and atrophy of the adrenal and thyroid glands, reduced blood sugar level in hyperglycaemia and increased it in hypoglycaemia. A normalising action was also observed in both leucopenia and leucocytosis.[15]

Cardiovascular effects

Eleutherococcus countered the effects of cerebral ischaemia in rats,[44] and in other studies increased their resistance to coagulant drugs.[45] Rats recovering from heart damage demonstrated increased repair of heart muscle: Eleutherococcus was found to increase the number of mitochondria in the cardiac muscle, resulting in better oxygen metabolism and increased conversion of fat into glycogen for energy.[46]

Other activity

Eleutherococcus displayed a marked benefit in diabetic rats by increasing insulin and lowering glucagon.[47] The eleutherosides had an insulin-like activity in diabetic rats[48] and the eleutherans are hypoglycaemic.[13] There is some evidence of hypoglycaemic effects in healthy adults,[49] but no such benefits have been observed in diabetes patients.[50]

Eleutherococcus has demonstrated anabolic effects, with improved egg weight and yield in hens, increased reproductive capacity in bulls, and weight gain in growing rabbits[51] and in rats.[52] It is claimed to have a gonadotropic effect in young male mice, with 1 g of root (by intraperitoneal injection) being equivalent to 6 mg of testosterone (by intramuscular injection).[53] However, components of an Eleutherococcus extract only demonstrated a modest affinity for steroid receptor sites in an in vitro study.[54]

An antitoxic effect has been demonstrated in vivo for the simultaneous administration of drugs and toxins with Eleutherococcus.[55]

Pharmacokinetics

Early studies with intraperitoneal injections of eleutheroside B in rats suggested a short half-life in the blood, with some accumulation in the adrenal glands and elimination mostly through the urine.[3]

Clinical trials

Effect on healthy or stressed individuals

Studies (mostly from Russia) of Eleutherococcus in individuals without pathology have indicated an increased capacity to adapt to changed environmental and working conditions. In healthy humans, Eleutherococcus improved short-term memory and light and colour perception.[56,57] The herb has been reported as improving the performance and stamina of explorers, sailors, deep sea divers, mine and mountain rescue workers, truck drivers, pilots, factory workers and even cosmonauts in open label trials and case observations.[58] Improved mental and physical output is noted, for example proofreaders were quicker and made fewer errors, cognitive performance increased in the elderly,[59] and labourers improved work capacity.[60]

In a double blind study of 1000 workers in a Siberian factory who received Eleutherococcus daily for 30 days, a 40% reduction in lost work days and a 50% reduction in general illness over a 1-year period was reported.[61] A Japanese single blind crossover study with six adolescent male athletes demonstrated that Eleutherococcus improved maximal work capacity by 23.3% in male athletes compared with a 7.5% increase in the placebo group.[62] In another study on athletes, Eleutherococcus also improved the strength of larger muscles, but its effect was weaker than Panax.[63]

The results of a study comparing Eleutherococcus (4 g/day), Panax (2 g/day) and placebo on endurance athletes showed that over 6 weeks there was no effect on immune cell markers, but in the Eleutherococcus group (not Panax) the testosterone/cortisol ratio decreased by almost 30% (mostly due to increased cortisol). The authors suggest this is consistent with animal research suggesting a threshold of stress below which Eleutherococcus increases the stress response and above which it decreases the stress response.[64] They went on to propose that Eleutherococcus may competitively engage stress hormone receptors that function to mobilise energy reserves in activity.[65] This again implies hormetic activity for the herb.

In healthy people exposed to heat stress, Eleutherococcus caused faster activation and greater intensity of perspiration.[66] In a study on 225 volunteers to assess microvascular reactions in the skin from UV light and after application of low pressure cupping, Eleutherococcus taken over 30 days showed significant benefits over placebo.[67]

Due to such reports and its local reputation, Eleutherococcus was widely used in Russia by track and field athletes, gymnasts and weight lifters.[68,69] There is, however, some modern contention about the reliability of some of the earlier studies and the effects of Eleutherococcus on athletes are not judged strong enough for it to be a banned drug. A review of the available evidence found serious methodological flaws in the earlier papers and a trend in more rigorous studies to find no effect on endurance.[70] For example, in a rigorous randomised, double blind crossover study of endurance cyclists, supplementation with 1.2 g Eleutherococcus extract for 7 days did not alter cycling performance.[71] Twenty highly trained distance runners randomly assigned in matched pairs participated in an 8-week double blind study during which they completed five trials of a 10-minute treadmill run at their 10 km race pace and a maximal treadmill test. Following a baseline trial, participants consumed Eleutherococcus extract or placebo daily for 6 weeks. Data from the measured parameters (including heart rate, respiratory parameters and serum lactate) did not support an ergogenic effect of Eleutherococcus supplementation for submaximal and maximal aerobic exercise tasks.[72]

There is some support for a role for Eleutherococcus in supporting immune function, elaborated further in the next section. A placebo-controlled study of the effect of an *Eleutherococcus senticosus* extract on quantitative flow cytometric measures of cellular immune status in 36 healthy volunteers showed that over 6 months there was a significant increase in the activity and number of immunocompetent cells, notably helper T lymphocytes and natural killer (NK) cells.[73] In another study 50 healthy volunteers were given either Echinacea fresh plant tincture or a liquid preparation containing Eleutherococcus (about 2 to 3 g/day of root) for 30 days. Changes in the Eleutherococcus group were observed for cellular defence and physical fitness, together with significantly decreased total cholesterol (14%), LDL-cholesterol (23%), triglycerides (23%) and glucose levels (11%) (p<0.001).[74]

Nine recreationally trained college male students participated in a small randomised, double blind, crossover trial conducted in Taiwan. Eleutherococcus root and rhizome extract (equivalent to 3.2 g/day) or placebo was taken for 8 weeks, with a washout period of 4 weeks. Participants cycled on a cycle ergometer at 75% of peak oxygen uptake (VO$_2$ peak) until exhaustion (endurance time). Eleutherococcus increased VO2 peak by 12% and endurance time by 23% from baseline. This response was statistically significant compared with placebo (VO$_2$ peak and endurance time increased by 3% and 6% from baseline, respectively). Taking Eleutherococcus for 8 weeks allowed participants to tolerate a greater cardiac work load. Plasma free fatty acids were increased and glucose was decreased. These alterations, combined with the significant decrease in respiratory exchange ratio, suggest a shift in metabolism from carbohydrate to fat (thus sparing muscle glycogen).[75]

Effect on unwell individuals

Administration of Eleutherococcus has shown beneficial effects in a wide range of functional and pathological disorders in open label trials and case observation studies. It has been used in both China and Russia to treat diseases of the heart, kidneys and nervous system. It is likely that Eleutherococcus exerts its beneficial effects by improving the overall health of the patient, rather than by any direct effect on the pathological process.

The results of a postmarketing surveillance study of 160 patients using an Eleutherococcus preparation demonstrated a beneficial effect on antibiotic-induced diarrhoea in convalescence, leading to its recommendation as an adjuvant treatment in convalescence after antibiotic therapy to prevent or to clear gastrointestinal complications.[76]

Several studies have looked at the effect of Eleutherococcus on immunological activity. In a double blind, placebo-controlled study involving 93 patients, 75% taking Eleutherococcus dry extract for 6 months (equivalent to 2 g/day) reported an improvement in the duration, severity and frequency of recurrent herpes simplex type II infections, compared with 34% in the placebo group.[77] Studies with cancer patients given Eleutherococcus while undergoing antitumour treatment demonstrated enhanced innate immunity,[78] and it also minimised the side effects from radiation, chemotherapy and surgery, and improved healing, well-being and survival time.[79] Twenty eight patients with stage III-IV epithelial ovarian cancer were given 270 mg/day of a proprietary combination of dried ethanol/water extracts of *Leuzea carthamoides*, *Rhodiola rosea*, *Eleutherococcus senticosus* and *Schisandra chinensis* for 4 weeks following chemotherapy. Results suggested that the combination may boost suppressed immunity.[80]

Reviews of earlier clinical studies have suggested improved general well-being in a wide range of patients with both mild health disturbances and more serious illness; there was added improvements reported in cardiovascular functions in atherosclerotic patients and those with rheumatic heart lesions, in lung capacity in patients with chronic bronchitis, pneumoconiosis and pneumonia, and in blood pressure in both hypertensive and hypotensive patients.[81] Hypotensive children demonstrated a significant rise of blood pressure and peripheral resistance when given Eleutherococcus.[82] Children with dysentery responded faster to medical treatment when Eleutherococcus was added.[83]

A randomised placebo-controlled trial in patients with substantial fatigue for at least 6 months with no identifiable cause was conducted in Iowa. After 2 months there were no significant differences in fatigue relief between placebo or Eleutherococcus (extract corresponding to 2 to 4 g/day of root) among the 76 patients who completed the study. However, in a subset of 45 patients with less severe fatigue there was a significant difference in favour of the herb, suggesting that it may be more efficacious for mild-to-moderate fatigue.[84] A double blind, placebo-controlled, parallel-group clinical study on Kan Jang (a combination of *Andrographis paniculata* and *Eleutherococcus senticosus*) showed positive effects in the treatment of acute upper respiratory tract infections, including sinusitis[85] and a randomised trial of the same preparation in children with acute respiratory viral infections was well tolerated and effective.[86] (See the Andrographis monograph for more details of these trials.)

Toxicology and other safety data

Toxicology

The acute oral toxicity of Eleutherococcus is very low. The LD_{50} of the root in mice was $31\,g/kg$.[87] The LD_{50} of the fluid extract in rats was found to be $10\,mL/kg$.[53] No toxic manifestations or deaths were found when Eleutherococcus was fed to rats over their whole lifetime at many times the normal human dose.[87] Rats receiving $10\,mg/kg$ of eleutherosides each day for 2 months showed no evidence of toxic effects.[88] Eleutherococcus did not cause spontaneous mutations in the fruit fly, and reduced the mutagenic effect of N-nitrosomorpholine.[89]

Contraindications

The evidence for contraindications is somewhat contradictory. Although Eleutherococcus has been applied in respiratory and bowel infections,[85,86] there is a tradition in Russia not to use it in the acute phase of infections. Again reports of efficacy in hypertension[81] contradict regulatory and research caution regarding its safety for this condition (at least for readings in excess of $180/90\,mmHg$).[7,90] In the absence of better information it may be prudent to limit the use of the remedy (especially in higher doses) in acute infections and hypertension, other than in formulations with proven safety and efficacy, such as Kan Jang.

Special warnings and precautions

The use of high doses of Eleutherococcus may account for the occasional reports of insomnia, palpitations, tachycardia and hypertension. Hence caution should be exercised with high doses.

Interactions

Eleutherococcus has been found in different reports both to decrease[91] and to increase serum plasma digoxin concentration.[92] A 74-year-old man was found to have elevated serum digoxin, which remained high after digoxin therapy was discontinued. The patient was taking a 'Siberian ginseng' product. Testing of serum digoxin levels was undertaken with and without consumption of the product and indicated it was responsible for the apparent elevation. The capsules were analysed and did not contain any digoxin or digitoxin.[93] These findings were unable to confirm whether Eleutherococcus caused a real increase in serum digoxin levels, as opposed to

an interference with the test method used. Whatever interactive effects are found for Eleutherococcus, it seems unlikely that these will involve perturbation of the CYP540 enzyme system as the plant's constituents appear not to affect standard measures of this activity.[94,95]

The concomitant application in rats of a standardised fixed combination of extracts from Andrographis and Eleutherococcus with warfarin did not produce significant effects on the pharmacokinetics of warfarin, and practically no effect on its pharmacodynamics.[96]

Use in pregnancy and lactation

Category B1 – no documented increase in frequency of malformation or other harmful effects on the fetus from limited use in women. No evidence of increased fetal damage in animal studies. Feeding experiments with several animal species have found no evidence of teratogenicity or other adverse effects in pregnancy.[97]

Eleutherococcus is likely to be compatible with breastfeeding.

A report of an association between Eleutherococcus ('pure Siberian ginseng') and neonatal androgenisation[98] has been dismissed when the suspected product was instead found to contain *Periploca sepium*.[99,100] A pharmacological study of Eleutherococcus in rats observed no androgenicity.[101]

Effects on ability to drive and use machines

No negative influence is expected.

Side effects

'Ginseng Abuse Syndrome' has been described in the USA, but this study had many flaws.[102] Most notably it did not differentiate between Panax and Eleutherococcus. It is likely that the side effects described, such as insomnia, diarrhoea and hypertension, were due to very high doses of Panax (see also the ginseng monograph).

Russian studies on Eleutherococcus have noted a general absence of side effects. However. care should be exercised in patients with cardiovascular disorders since insomnia, palpitations, tachycardia and hypertension have been reported in a few cases. Side effects are more likely if normal doses are exceeded.[103]

Overdosage

Not known (see above).

Regulatory status in selected countries

Eleutherococcus is official in the *Chinese Pharmacopoeia* (English edition, 1992), the *British Pharmacopoeia* (2012), the *European Pharmacopoeia* (2012) and the *United States Pharmacopeia–National Formulary* (USP34–NF29, 2011).

Eleutherococcus is covered by a positive Commission E monograph and can be used as a tonic to counter exhaustion, to increase stamina, to enhance performance and concentration and to assist convalescence.

Eleutherococcus is not on the UK General Sale list (although 'ginseng' is listed, which probably refers to *Panax ginseng* (Korean ginseng)).

Eleutherococcus does not have GRAS status. However, it is freely available as a 'dietary supplement' in the USA under DSHEA legislation (1994 Dietary Supplement Health and Education Act). Ginseng* has been present as an ingredient in products offered over-the-counter (OTC) for use as an aphrodisiac. The FDA however advises that 'based on evidence currently available, any OTC drug product containing ingredients for use as an aphrodisiac cannot be generally recognised as safe and effective'.

Eleutherococcus is not included in Part 4 of Schedule 4 of the Therapeutic Goods Act Regulations of Australia and is freely available for sale.

---

*The listing in the Code of Federal Regulations (Part 310 – New Drugs) lists 'ginseng' in addition to Korean ginseng, and so is likely to include Eleutherococcus.

References

1. *American Herb Association Newsletter.* 1987.
2. Hu SY.. In: Chang HM, Yeung HW, Tso WW, eds. *Advances in Chinese Medicinal Materials Research.* Singapore: World Scientific; 1985. pp. 28–31.
3. European Scientific Cooperative on Phytotherapy. *The ESCOP Monographs , 2nd ed, Supplement.* 2009. pp. 110–120.
4. Bensky D, Gamble A. *Chinese Herbal Medicine Materia Medica.* Seattle: Eastland Press; 1986. pp. 235–236.
5. Chang HM, But PP. *Pharmacology and Applications of Chinese Materia Medica,* vol. 1. Singapore: World Scientific Publishing; 1987. pp. 725–735.
6. Cicero AF, Derosa G, Brillante R, et al. *Arch Gerontol Geriatr Suppl.* 2004;9: 69–73.
7. Panossian A, Wagner H. *Phytother Res.* 2005;19(10):819–838.
8. German Federal Minister of Justice. *German Commission E for Human Medicine Monograph.* Bundes-Anzeiger (German Federal Gazette) no. 11, dated 17.01.1991.
9. British Herbal Medicine Association. *British Herbal Compendium,* vol. 1. Bournemouth: BHMA; 1992. pp. 89–91.
10. Halstead BW, Hood LL. *Eleutherococcus senticosus. Siberian ginseng: An Introduction to the Concept of Adaptogenic Medicine.* USA: Oriental Healing Arts Institute; 1984. pp. 2, 71–73.
11. Szolomicki S, Smochowiec L, Wojciki J, et al. *Phytother Res.* 2000;14(1):30–35.
12. Segiet–Kujawa E, Kaloga M. *J Nat Prod.* 1991;54(4):1044–1048.
13. Hikino H, Takahashi M, Otake K, et al. *J Nat Prod.* 1986;49(2):293–297.
14. Wagner H, Heur YH, Obermeier A, et al. *Planta Med.* 1982;44(4):193–198.
15. Brekhman II, Dardymov IV. *Ann Rev Pharmacol.* 1969;9:419–430.
16. Davydov M, Krikorian AD. *J Ethnopharmacol.* 2000;72(3):345–393.
17. Steinmann GG, Esperester A, Joller P. *Arzneimittelforschung.* 2001;51(1):76–83.
18. Nishibe S, Kinoshita H, Takeda H, et al. *Chem Pharm Bull.* 1990;38(6):1763–1765.

19. Wagner H, Proksch A, Riess-Maurer I, et al. *Arzneimittelforschung.* 1984;34(6): 659–661.
20. Fulder S. *The Root of Being: Ginseng and the Pharmacology of Harmony.* London: Hutchinson & Co; 1980. p. 137.
21. Golotin VG, Gonenko VA, Zimina VV, et al. *Vopr Med Khim.* 1989;35(1):35–37.
22. Farnsworth NR, Kinghorn AD, In: Wagner H, Farnsworth NR, eds. *Economic and Medicinal Plant Research,* vol. 1. London: Academic Press; 1985. p. 202.
23. Fulder S. *The Root of Being: Ginseng and the Pharmacology of Harmony.* London: Hutchinson & Co; 1980. pp. 161, 255.
24. Chubarev VN, Rubtsova ER, Filatova IV, et al. *Farmakol Toksikol.* 1989;52(2): 55–59.
25. Saito H, Nishiyama N, Kamegaya T, et al.. In: Chang HM, Yeung HW, Tso WW, eds. *Advances in Chinese Medicinal Materials Research.* Singapore: World Scientific; 1985. pp. 687–688.
26. Streuer M, Jansen G, Winterhoff H, et al. *International Congress on Phytotherapy.* Munich; September 10–13, 1992.
27. Winterhoff H, Gumbinger HG, Vahlensieck U, et al. *Pharm Pharmacol Lett.* 1993;3:95–98.
28. Lewis W, Zenger VE, Lynch RG. *J Ethnopharmacol.* 1983;8(2):209–214.
29. Abramova JI, Chorny ZH, Natalenko VP, et al. *Lek Sredstva Dalnego Vostoka.* 1972;11:106–108. [Article in Russian].
30. Medon PJ, Ferguson PW, Watson CF. *J Ethnopharmacol.* 1984;10(2):235–241.
31. Bezdetko GN, Brekhman II, Dardymov IV, et al. *Vopr Med Khim.* 1973;19(3): 245–248.
32. Kimura Y, Sumiyoshi M. *J Ethnopharmacol.* 2004;5(2–3):447–453.
33. Panossian A, Wikman G, Kaur P, et al. *Phytomedicine.* 2009;16(6–7):617–622.
34. Minkova M, Pantev T. *Acta Physiol Pharmacol Bulg.* 1987;13(4):66–70.
35. Miyanomae T, Frindel E. *Exp Hematol.* 1988;16(9):801–806.
36. Ben-Hur E, Fulder S. *Am J Chin Med.* 1981;9(1):48–56.
37. Dzhioev FK. *Voprosy Onkologii.* 1965;11(9):51. (T651–T653).

38. Hacker B, Medon PJ. *J Pharm Sci.* 1984;73(2):270–272.
39. Strel'chuk SI. *Tsitol Genet.* 1987;21(2):136–139. 142.
40. Farnsworth NR, Kinghorn AD, Soefarto DD, et al. In: Wagner H, Farnsworth NR, eds. *Economic and Medicinal Plant Research,* vol. 1. London: Academic Press; 1985. p. 197.
41. Baranov AI. *J Ethnopharmacol.* 1982;6(3):339–353.
42. Farnsworth NR, Kinghorn AD, Soefarto DD, et al. In: Wagner H, Farnsworth NR, eds. *Economic and Medicinal Plant Research,* vol. 1. London: Academic Press; 1985. pp. 197, 203.
43. Raman P, Dewitt DL, Nair MG. *Phytother Res.* 2008;22(2):204–212.
44. Leonova EV, Bregman TV. *Zdravookhr Beloruss.* 1979;3:13–16. [Article in Russian].
45. Bazaz'ian GG, Liapina LA, Pastorova VE, et al. *Fiziol Zh USSR.* 1987;73(10):1390–1395. [Article in Russian].
46. Afanasjeva TN, Lebkova NP. *Biull Eksp Biol Med.* 1987;103(2):212–215.
47. Molokovskii DS, et al. *Probl Endokrinol Mosk.* 1989;35(6):82–87.
48. Niu HS, Liu IM, Cheng JT, et al. *Planta Med.* 2008;74(2):109–113.
49. Sievenpiper JL, Arnason JT, Leiter LA, et al. *J Am Coll Nutr.* 2004;23: 248–258.
50. Farnsworth NR, Kinghorn AD, Soefarto DD, et al.In: Wagner H, Farnsworth NR, eds. *Economic and Medicinal Plant Research,* vol. 1. London: Academic Press; 1985. p. 183.
51. Farnsworth NR, Kinghorn AD, Soefarto DD, et al.Wagner H, Farnsworth NR, eds. *Economic and Medicinal Plant Research,* vol. 1. London: Academic Press; 1985. pp. 195, 201.
52. Kaemmerer K, Fink J. *Prakt Tierarzt.* 1980;61:748.
53. Farnsworth NR, Kinghorn AD, Soefarto DD, et al. In: Wagner H, Farnsworth NR, editors. *Economic and Medicinal Plant Research,* vol. 1. London: Academic Press; 1985. pp. 196–197.
54. Pearce PT, Zois I, Wynne KN, et al. *Endocrinol Japon.* 1982;29(5):567–573.

55. Farnsworth NR, Kinghorn AD, Soefarto DD, et al. In: Wagner H, Farnsworth NR, editors. *Economic and Medicinal Plant Research*, vol. 1. London: Academic Press; 1985. pp. 166–167.

56. Arushanian EB, Baida OA, Mastiagin SS, et al. *Eksp Klin Farmakol.* 2003;66(5):10–13.

57. Arushanian EB, Shikine IB. *Eksp Klin Farmakol.* 2004;67(4):64–66.

58. Fulder S. *The Root of Being: Ginseng and the Pharmacology of Harmony*. London: Hutchinson & Co; 1980. pp. 189, 192, 246–248, 255.

59. Winther K, Ranlov C, Rein E, et al. *J Neurol Sci.* 1997;150(1):90.

60. Farnsworth NR, Kinghorn AD, Soefarto DD, et al. In: Wagner H, Farnsworth NR, eds. *Economic and Medicinal Plant Research*, vol. 1. London: Academic Press; 1985. pp. 167. 171, 172.

61. Farnsworth NR, Kinghorn AD, Soefarto DD, et al. In: Wagner H, Farnsworth NR, editors. *Economic and Medicinal Plant Research*, vol. 1. London: Academic Press; 1985. p. 178.

62. Asano K, Takahashi T, Miyashita M, et al. *Planta Med.* 1986;52(3):175–177.

63. McNaughton L, Egan G, Caelli G. *Int Clin Nut Rev.* 1989;9(1):32–35.

64. Gaffney BT, Hugel HM, Rich PA. *Life Sci.* 2001;70(4):431–442.

65. Gaffney BT, Hugel HM, Rich PA. *Med Hypotheses.* 2001;56(5):567–572.

66. Novozhilov GN, Silchenko KI. *Fiziol Chel.* 1985;11(2):303–306.

67. Dardymov IV, Berdyshev VV, Golikov PP, et al. *Lek Sredvesta Dalnego Vostoka.* 1966;7:133–140.

68. Fulder S. *The Root of Being: Ginseng and the Pharmacology of Harmony*. London: Hutchinson & Co; 1980. p. 249.

69. Farnsworth NR, Kinghorn AD, Soefarto DD, et al. In: Wagner H, Farnsworth NR, eds. *Economic and Medicinal Plant Research*, vol. 1. London: Academic Press; 1985. p. 173.

70. Goulet ED, Dionne IJ. *Int J Sport Nutr Exerc Metab.* 2005;15(1):75–83.

71. Eschbach LF, Webster MJ, Boyd JC, et al. *Int J Sport Nutr Exerc Metab.* 2000;10(4):444–451.

72. Dowling EA, Redondo DR, Branch JD, et al. *Med Sci Sports Exerc.* 1996;28(4):482–489.

73. Bohn B, Nebe CT, Birr C. *Int J Immunopharmacol.* 1988;10(S1):67. Abstract WS18-5 *5.

74. Szolmicki S, Samochowiec L, Wojcicki J, et al. *Phytother Res.* 2000;14(1):30–35.

75. Kuo J, Chen KWC, Cheng IS, et al. *Chin J Physiol.* 2010;53(2):105–111.

76. Meyer-Wegener J, Paulus M. *Med Welt.* 1997;48(11):493–496.

77. Williams M. *Int J Altern Complement Med.* 1995;13:9–12.

78. Kupin VI, Polevaia EB. *Vopr Onkol.* 1986;32(7):21–26.

79. Fulder S. *The Root of Being: Ginseng and the Pharmacology of Harmony*. London: Hutchinson & Co; 1980. pp. 201–202.

80. Komosh N, Laktionov K, Antoshechkina M. *Phytother Res.* 2006;20(5):424–425.

81. Farnsworth NR, Kinghorn AD, Soefarto DD, et al. In: Wagner H, Farnsworth NR, editors. *Economic and Medicinal Plant Research*, vol. 1. London: Academic Press; 1985. pp. 179–191.

82. Kaloeva ZD. *Farmakol Toksikol.* 1986;49(5):73.

83. Vereshchagin IA. *Antibiotiki.* 1978;23(7):633–636.

84. Hartz AJ, Bentler S, Noyes R, et al. *Psychol Med.* 2004;34(1):51–61.

85. Gabrielian ES, Shukarian AK, Goukasova GI, et al. *Phytomed.* 2002;9(7):589–597.

86. Shakhova EG, Spasov AA, Ostrovskii OV, et al. *Vestnik Otorinolaringol.* 2003;3:48–50.

87. Farnsworth NR, Kinghorn AD, Soefarto DD, et al. In: Wagner H, Farnsworth NR, editors. *Economic and Medicinal Plant Research*, vol. 1. London: Academic Press; 1985. pp. 164–166.

88. Dardymov IV, Suprunov NI, Sokolenko LA. *Lek Sredstva Dalnego Vostoka.* 1972;11:66–69.

89. Sakharova TA, Revazova YA, Barenboim GM, et al. *Khim Farm Zh.* 1985;19:311–312.

90. Dalinger OI. Cited in: de Smet PAGM, Keller K, Hansel R, et al., eds. *Adverse Effects of Herbal Drugs*, vol. 2. Berlin: Springer-Verlag; 1993. pp. 163–164.

91. Izzo AA, Di Carlo G, Borrelli F, et al. *Int J Cardiol.* 2005;98(1):1–14.

92. Hu Z, Yang X, Ho PC, et al. *Drugs.* 2005;65(9):1239–1282.

93. MacRae S. *Can Med Assoc J.* 1996;155:293–295.

94. Donovan JL, DeVane CL, Chavin KD, et al. *Drug Metab Dispos.* 2003;31:519–522.

95. Henderson GL, Harkey MR, Gershwin ME, et al. *Life Sci.* 1999;65(15):209–214.

96. Hovhannisyan AS, Abrahamyan H, Gabrielyan ES, et al. *Phytomedicine.* 2006;13(5):318–323.

97. Farnsworth NR, Kinghorn AD, Soefarto DD, et al. In: Wagner H, Farnsworth NR, eds. *Economic and Medicinal Plant Research*, vol. 1. London: Academic Press; 1985. pp. 179–182, 193, 195.

98. Koren G, Randor S, Martin S, et al. *JAMA.* 1990;264(22):2866.

99. Awang DVC. *JAMA.* 1991;266(3):363.

100. Awang DVC. *JAMA.* 1991;265(14):1828.

101. Waller DP, Martin AM, Farnsworth NR, et al. *JAMA.* 1992;267(17):2329.

102. Siegel RK. *JAMA.* 1979;241(15):1614–1615.

103. Farnsworth NR, Kinghorn AD, Soefarto DD, et al. In: Wagner H, Farnsworth NR, eds. *Economic and Medicinal Plant Research*, vol. 1. London: Academic Press; 1985. pp. 179–182, 187, 193, 195.

St John's wort

(*Hypericum perforatum* L.)

Synonyms

Hypericum, hardhay (Engl), Hyperici herba (Lat), Johanniskraut, Sonnenwendkraut, Hartheu (Ger), herb de millepertuis (Fr), iperico (Ital), prikbladet perikon (Dan).

What is it?

The dried aerial parts of *Hypericum perforatum*, gathered during the flowering period or shortly before, are used medicinally. The generic name of the herb derives from the Greek meaning to 'overcome an apparition' and in earlier times homes would have a plant hanging over the door to ward off evil spirits. This species of Hypericum (*H. perforatum*) is referred to as perforate St John's wort due to the perforated appearance of the leaves when they are held up to the light (these are in fact oil glands). *H. perforatum* is not a weed in its native Europe, Asia and North Africa, but has become a weed in most temperate regions of the world. *H. perforatum* and other species of the genus have been used as a remedy since ancient times, particularly to treat ulcers, burns, wounds, abdominal pains and bacterial diseases. Recently it has received considerable attention in clinical trials for the treatment of depression. Shortly after came the finding that certain extracts of the herb have the capacity to reduce the bioavailability of a wide range of conventional medical drugs.

Effects

Moderate antidepressant activity; useful for wound healing; antiviral activity with potential applicability to disorders caused by enveloped viruses.

Traditional view

Hypericum was considered primarily for the nervous system, particularly for nervous afflictions (excitability, menopausal neurosis and hysteria) and disorders of the spine, spinal injuries, neuralgia, sciatica and muscular rheumatism. It was also used for its supposed diuretic and astringent properties, to treat urinary problems, diarrhoea, dysentery, parasitic infestations, jaundice, haemorrhages, menorrhagia and bed wetting. Hypericum ointment and infused oil were used on a wide range of wounds including ulcers, swellings, bruises and even on tumours.[1,2] In Greece the herb was used externally for the treatment of shingles.[3]

Summary actions

Nervine, antidepressant, vulnerary, antiseptic, antiviral.

Can be used for

Indications supported by clinical trials

Treatment of mild-to-moderate depression (high level evidence), particularly when side effects from standard antidepressant drugs become intolerable to the patient; adjunct to standard drug treatment in severe depression (this extrapolation from trial data is now controversial because of claimed interactions); treatment of anxiety; adjunct to light therapy for seasonal affective disorder; orofacial and genital herpes; premature ejaculation; psychological symptoms of menopause; premenstrual syndrome; obsessive-compulsive disorder; social phobia; psychological symptoms associated with irritable bowel syndrome; aerobic endurance in athletes; topically for wound healing and reducing scar formation; topical treatment of subacute mild-to-moderate atopic dermatitis.

Traditional therapeutic uses

Physiological afflictions of the nervous system: spinal injuries, neuralgia, sciatica; muscular rheumatism; mild psychological disorders: excitability, menopausal anxiety and nervousness. Hypericum ointment and infused oil for the treatment of dermatitis, wounds, bruises and shingles.

May also be used for

Extrapolations from pharmacological studies

Treatment and prevention of acute and chronic infections caused by enveloped viruses (e.g. cold sores, genital herpes, chicken pox, shingles, glandular fever, cytomegalovirus infection and viral hepatitis); wound healing; conditions requiring increased nocturnal melatonin plasma levels (e.g. circadian rhythm-associated sleep disorders); alcoholism; may also have potential as an anticancer treatment and as a photosensitising agent in photodynamic therapy; improving resistance to stress; as a neuroprotective agent in cognitive and learning disorders; and as a potential adjunct for treatment of metabolic syndrome.

Other applications

Inclusion in skin care products, particularly for sensitive skin.[4]

Preparations

Dried or fresh herb for infusion, liquid extract, capsule and tablets for internal use.

Infused oil of Hypericum is made by mixing the flowers with a good-quality fixed oil (such as olive oil) in a well-sealed vessel in the presence of sunlight over several weeks. The action of the sunlight produces red oil containing hypericin derivatives, hyperforin, xanthones, flavonoids and the breakdown products of hyperforin.

Dosage

- 2 to 5 g/day of dried herb or the equivalent of 1.0 to 2.7 mg/day of total hypericin (TH)
- Hypericum tablets or capsules (for example 1.5 g, standardised to contain 0.9 mg TH): 3 to 4 per day
- The volume of liquid extract prescribed depends upon the level of TH in the extract; typical doses are 3 to 6 mL per day of 1:2 liquid extract; 7.5 to 15 mL/day of 1:5 tincture.

Doses at the higher end of this range have been utilised in the treatment of depression, HIV infection and other chronic viral infections. For the short-term treatment of acute viral infections, even higher doses may be necessary.

Duration of use

No restriction, but at least 4 weeks of treatment is required to assess the antidepressant effect. (See the Special warnings section.)

Summary assessment of safety

Adverse effects are rare from the use of Hypericum at normal dosages. Avoidance of excessive exposure to sunlight or artificial UVA light is advisable in patients taking high doses. Hypericum should be used cautiously in patients with known photosensitivity. Clinicians should avoid dispensing the sediment from Hypericum extracts. (Refer to the Side effects section.) Hypericum has the potential to reduce the effects of a range of drugs. (See under Interactions and Appendix C.)

Technical data

Botany

Hypericum is a member of the Clusiaceae (alternative name Guttiferae) family[5,6] and grows to approximately 1 m with opposite and paired branches. The leaves are opposite, sessile, up to 2 cm long, oblong and contain numerous translucent glandular dots that are visible against the light. The yellow flowers contain five petals with many stamens protruding. The fruit is a capsule.[7,8]

Key constituents

- Naphthodianthrones (0.05% to 0.6%), including hypericin and pseudohypericin.[9] The upper level of naphthodianthrones is usually much lower than this quoted value, approximately 0.2%
- Flavonoids (such as biapigenin,[10] quercetrin[11] and rutin[12]) and xanthones;[10] phenolics (phloroglucinol derivatives) including hyperforin and adhyperforin;[11] procyanidins;[13] essential oil.[14]

Collectively the naphthodianthrones, hypericin and pseudohypericin are called 'total hypericin' (TH) and are responsible for the red colour of Hypericum extracts. The naphthodianthrones show a restricted solubility in almost all solvents, but more than 40% of the amount present is extractable from the crude herb when preparing a tea with water at 60 to 80°C.[15] This increased solubility suggests the presence of factors in the herb that modify the solubility of the naphthodianthrones. Accordingly, potassium salts of hypericin and pseudohypericin have been identified as 'soluble' pigments in *Hypericum* species.[16] Due to their varying solubility in different solvents, most preparations are standardised for TH content (usually 0.3% hypericin), although there was a move by some manufacturers to standardise for hyperforin (usually 2% to 5%), as attention turned to this compound in terms of antidepressant activity.[17–22] However, hyperforin is typically unstable in extracts of St John's wort, especially in solution (and even in the dry extracts found in tablets and capsules) and rapidly decomposes at an acidic pH.[23] Tinctures and fluid extracts (galenicals) of Hypericum that are older than a few months contain no hyperforin at all.[24]

Pharmacodynamics

Antiviral and antiretroviral activity

Hypericin, and to a lesser extent pseudohypericin, have been the subject of intense research for their antiviral properties. A review article by Kubin and colleagues[25] has been published on this topic. Hypericin and pseudohypericin have demonstrated activity against several enveloped viruses in vitro, including vesicular stomatitis virus, herpes simplex virus types 1 and 2, parainfluenza virus, vaccinia virus,[26] murine cytomegalovirus,[27] duck hepatitis B virus,[28] bovine viral diarrhoea virus, influenza virus type A, parainfluenza virus type 3, radiation leukaemia virus, Moloney murine leukaemia virus, Friend leukaemia virus, vesicular stomatitis virus, Sendai virus, Sindbis virus, equine infectious anaemia virus, bovine immunodeficiency virus and human cytomegalovirus.[25] These compounds were inactive against non-enveloped (naked) viruses such as human rhinovirus, adenovirus and poliovirus.[26,29]

This suggests that the mechanism of viral inactivation is dependent upon the presence of a viral lipid envelope.[29]

The antiviral activity was enhanced by exposure to light[27] and is directed at both the virions and virus-infected cells.[30] Hypericin and pseudohypericin appear to inactivate the viral fusion function via the generation of singlet oxygen upon illumination,[31] which could also occur in vivo in the absence of light if driven by chemically generated excited states.[32] Hypericin and pseudohypericin also interfere with more than one stage in the virus replication cycle (see also below).[33]

Both hypericin and pseudohypericin demonstrated potent activity, in vitro and in vivo (by oral administration or injection),[34,35] against several retroviruses, including HIV.[36] The antiretroviral activity was enhanced by exposure to light.[30,33] The ring structure, the quinone and phenolic groups were deemed necessary for the antiretroviral activity.[36]

The antiretroviral effect was postulated to be achieved in a number of ways:

- By causing photochemical alterations of the capsid, which inhibits the release of reverse transcriptase and prevents reverse transcription of the genome within the target cell[32]
- By inhibiting intracellular transmission of the HIV-induced cytopathic signal[37,38]
- By interfering with processing of gag-encoded precursor polyproteins needed for core maturation[34]
- By impairing the assembly or processing of intact virions[34]
- By inhibiting the signalling pathway that has an immunosuppressive effect on the host immune system.[39]

The antiretroviral activity is probably due to a combination of the photodynamic and lipophilic properties of these compounds: hypericin binds cell membranes and crosslinks virus capsid proteins resulting in a loss of infectivity and an inability to retrieve the reverse transcriptase activity from the virion.[40]

Light-independent inhibition of HIV-1 was demonstrated for highly purified fractions of chloroform extracts of Hypericum.[41] Through bioassay-guided fractionation, 3-hydroxylauric acid found in field-grown *H. perforatum* was identified as inhibiting HIV-1 activity, with little to no cytotoxicity. Similarly, light-independent anti-HIV-1 activity was also observed for Hypericum that lacked detectable levels of naphthodianthrones.

A recent review noted in vitro studies where hypericin inhibited human cytomegalovirus, inhibited the adsorptive ability of foot-and-mouth virus to host cells in a model of BHK-21 cells, with maximal inhibitory rate of 59.7%, and exerted a dose-dependent activity against porcine reproductive and respiratory syndrome virus in a model of Marc-145 cells.[42] No information was provided about light conditions.

Despite promising results from in vitro studies, the review by Kubin and colleagues suggested tests in mice indicate that the efficacy of hypericin on enveloped viruses requires light illumination for effective in vivo virucidal activity.[25] They noted that this was a controversial area, with some results showing positive in vivo antiviral activity in the absence of light. It is possible that marked antiviral activity from the use of Hypericum is only achieved for parts of the body that have access to light, such as the skin. (See the trial in patients with herpes simplex later in this monograph.)

A phase I dose escalation study of patients with chronic hepatitis C virus failed to show any significant antiviral activity. Hypericin was given orally in liquid doses of 0.05 or 0.10 mg/kg for 8 weeks. Seven of 12 patients treated with the 0.05 mg/kg dosage, and all seven treated with the 0.1 mg/kg dosage. experienced photosensitivity reactions judged to be probably related to hypericin, including paraesthesia, dermatitis, darkened colour of exposed skin and pruritic nodules.[43]

Similarly, a phase I dose escalation study of hypericin as a potential antiretroviral drug against HIV was unable to confirm its value in this context. In fact, phototoxic reactions severe enough to cause participants to discontinue treatment were observed. Thirty HIV-infected patients with CD4 counts less than 350 cells/mm[3] were treated with intravenous hypericin (0.25 or 0.5 mg/kg twice weekly or 0.25 mg/kg three times weekly) or oral hypericin (0.5 mg/kg/day). Of the 30 patients who were enrolled, 16 discontinued treatment early because of toxic effects. Severe cutaneous phototoxicity was observed in 11 of 23 evaluable patients, and dose

	R
Hypericin	H
Pseudohypericin	OH

Hyperforin

escalation could not be completed. Virological markers and CD4 cell count did not significantly change.[44]

Antidepressant activity

The exact mechanisms of action and key constituents of Hypericum that play a role in its antidepressant activity have yet to be fully elucidated. Hypericin was previously thought to be the only active constituent in depression,[45–48] but more recent interest has focused on other constituents including hyperforin, an unstable compound shown in in vitro and in vivo studies to have antidepressant activity.[17–22] The flavonoids have also received attention in this context.[49,50] However, the total extract appears to be more effective than isolated constituents[51] in terms of the antidepressant effect of Hypericum, and most of the data to date suggest that multiple mechanisms exhibited by several groups of active compounds may be involved in the antidepressant action of Hypericum.[52,53]

Support for hyperforin as a key antidepressant component is derived from several sources. In vitro research found that the potency of Hypericum products at inhibiting uptake of serotonin depended on their hyperforin content.[54] Furthermore, the effects of two different Hypericum extracts in behavioural despair and learned helplessness in a rodent model closely correlated with their hyperforin content.[18] A randomised, controlled trial comparing the clinical efficacy and safety of 900 mg/day of two different extracts of Hypericum found the low-hyperforin extract (0.5%) was ineffective over placebo compared with the high-hyperforin extract (5%) over a 42-day period.[20] However, there is still considerable debate concerning the relevance of hyperforin to the antidepressant effects. One review of the evidence for different compounds in depression cited six studies using hyperforin-free Hypericum extracts that were able to demonstrate clinical efficacy.[11] Specifically, clinical studies have clearly demonstrated low-hyperforin extracts (1.5% to 3%) to be superior to placebo or equivalent to fluoxetine in the treatment of mild-to-moderate depression.[55] In addition, many positive findings were reported from clinical trials on Hypericum for the treatment of depression prior to 1998, when the extraction process used to make the most clinically tested extract was modified to target higher levels of hyperforin.[11]

Evidence for the relevance of other constituents to the antidepressant activity has been demonstrated using the tail suspension test in mice, where step by step removal of either hyperforin or hypericin did not result in a loss of pharmacological activity.[56] An extract fraction containing a high amount of flavonoids significantly reduced immobility time in the forced swimming test. The effect was comparable to that of imipramine.[49]

The pathophysiological mechanisms underlying the complex disorder of depression are still not well understood. As well as neurotransmitter deficiency, an inflammatory response (elevated pro-inflammatory cytokines), and activation of the hypothalamic-pituitary-adrenal (HPA) axis (elevated levels of corticotropin-releasing hormone, ACTH (adrenocorticotropic hormone) and cortisol) have also been observed in depressed patients. Hence, the following mechanisms that have been observed for Hypericum extracts and/or its constituents are of some relevance, albeit keeping in mind the limitations of in vitro models.

In vitro and ex vivo studies

An extract of Hypericum inhibited synaptic uptake of noradrenaline, serotonin and dopamine, and GABA (gamma-aminobutyric acid) reuptake.[57–59] It is unusual to find this action on all three uptake systems.

It also exhibited a dose-dependent beta-adrenoceptor downregulation equal to that induced by desipramine.[60]

Hypericum extract and hypericin have also demonstrated the following properties using in vitro models:

- Significant receptor affinity for adenosine (non-specific), GABA-A, $GABA_B$, benzodiazepine, inositol triphosphate[61]
- Reduced expression of serotonin receptors[62]
- Inhibition of catechol-O-methyltransferase[63]
- Inhibition of monoamine oxidase (MAO)-A and MAO-B activity although this inhibition was found to be weak[58]
- A suppression of interleukin-6 release for a Hypericum extract in a whole blood culture system.[64]

In terms of the individual constituents of Hypericum, the following has been observed:

- Hypericum extract and hypericin inhibited dopamine-beta-hydroxylase in vitro.[65] Hypericin showed high affinity for the D_3 dopamine receptor.[48] It demonstrated potent binding inhibition to the human corticotropin-releasing factor$_1$ (CRF_1) receptor,[66] but it was subsequently observed that of hypericin, pseudohypericin and hyperforin, only pseudohypericin selectively antagonised CRF in recombinant Chinese hamster ovary cells.[67] Hypericin also potentiated neurotransmitter binding at the GABA-A, benzodiazepine and serotonin receptors[68] and showed an affinity for NMDA (N-methyl-D-aspartate) receptors[61] and sigma receptors.[69]
- Hyperforin is a potent uptake inhibitor of serotonin (5-HT), dopamine, noradrenaline, GABA and L-glutamate,[70–74] possibly by causing an elevation of the intracellular sodium concentration, which is probably in turn due to activation of sodium conductive pathways.[17]
- In isolated hippocampal neurons in the rat, hyperforin modulated voltage- and ligand-gated ion channels known to be involved in neurotransmitter release.[75] At nanomolar concentrations, hyperforin induced significant inhibition of various ion channels. In the case of P-type Ca^{2+} channels, it was established that hyperforin acted via interaction with calmodulin or through calmodulin-activated pathways involving at least one second messenger.[52]
- Hyperforin has been shown to activate non-selective cation channels, suggesting that it may represent a new mechanism for preclinical antidepressant activity.[76]
- Hyperforin modified specific membrane structures in different ways, decreasing the flexibility of fatty acids in the membrane hydrocarbon core, but fluidising the hydrophilic region of membrane phospholipids.[77]
- The non-hypericin fraction of Hypericum inhibited MAO-A in vitro, unlike hypericin and the flavonols.[78,79] The xanthones, flavones and flavonols were found to be potent and selective MAO-A inhibitors and the coumarins affected MAO-B in vitro. Amentoflavone demonstrated

binding activity at the benzodiazepine receptor in vitro and significantly inhibited binding at serotonin receptors 5-HT_{1D} and 5-HT_{2C}, and dopamine D_3 receptors.[80]

An extract of Hypericum exhibited suppression of interleukin-6 in blood samples ex vivo.[81,82] This suppression may assist in deactivating the HPA axis, leading to inhibition of elevated corticotrophin-releasing factor and other adrenal regulatory hormones. These changes could be linked to antidepressant activity.[83]

In vivo studies

Hypericum extract has shown the following in various animal models:

- Downregulation of beta-adrenoceptor density in the frontal cortex after subchronic administration in various rodent models.[58,71,81,83,84] (Note that the downregulation of these receptors in vivo is expected on subchronic administration of antidepressants, and is not in contradiction to the inhibition of uptake observed in vitro.) Subchronic treatment of rats with Hypericum extract led to a significant downregulation of beta-receptors.[58] A hyperforin-enriched (38%) CO_2 extract also led to a significant beta-receptor downregulation after subchronic treatment.[71] Downregulation of central beta-adrenergic receptors was shown in rat frontal cortex after 2 weeks' administration of Hypericum lipophilic CO_2 extract (containing about 26.2% hyperforin and 3% adhyperforin) and also a methanolic extract. Treatment with hypericin led to a significant downregulation (13%) of beta adrenergic receptors in the frontal cortex after 8 weeks only, while hyperforin and hyperoside were ineffective.[84]
- Upregulation of central serotonergic receptors from cerebral tissue, which is consistent with effects caused by synthetic antidepressants.[83,85] Subchronic treatment of rats with Hypericum extract (240 mg/kg orally for 14 days) led to a significant upregulation of 5-HT2 receptors in the frontal cortex, with the effect on serotonergic receptors varying according to the type of extract: a methanolic extract (LI 160) led to a significant increase in receptor density compared with a (non-significant) decrease in receptor density found with a hyperforin-enriched CO_2 extract.[60] In rats treated daily for 26 weeks with a Hypericum extract (2700 mg/kg, LI 160), the number of both 5-HT_{1A} and 5-HT_{2A} receptors were significantly increased by 50% compared with controls.[85]
- An effect on opioid systems in mesolimbic regions in the CNS in the rat brain, either by a direct or indirect mechanism.[86]
- Inhibition of synaptic reuptake of neurotransmitters: treatment with the LI 160 extract (3 g/kg orally via diet) reduced corticosterone and prolactin responses to the 5-HT2A receptor agonist, 2,5-dimethoxy-4-iodophenyl-2-aminopropane, suggesting that LI 160 may modify brain 5-HT function in the rat, possibly by reducing the sensitivity of central 5-HT2A receptors.[87] Acute treatment of rats with LI 160, hyperforin and hypericin all caused significant increases in plasma corticosterone, associated

with significant increases in brain cortical tissue 5-HT content, suggesting that the corticosterone responses may be mediated via a 5-HT2 mechanism. When subchronic and acute treatment using two different doses of LI 160 were compared, plasma corticosterone levels were significantly decreased, suggesting a downregulation or desensitisation of post-synaptic 5-HT2 receptors. LI 160 and hyperforin treatments decreased plasma prolactin responses to the dopamine antagonist, haloperidol, suggesting that this may be associated with a dopamine-mediated mechanism of action.[88]

- Improved resistance to stress and prevention of exhaustion of the HPA system in rats. In rats exposed to stress, Hypericum extract (3 mg or 6 mg/day, oral for 30 days) reduced adrenal weight and ACTH concentration.[89]
- Modulation of HPA axis function in the rat. Imipramine (15 mg/kg), hypericin (0.2 mg/kg), hyperoside (0.6 mg/kg), isoquercitrin (0.6 mg/kg) and miquelianin (0.6 mg/kg) administered orally to male rats daily (for 2 weeks) significantly downregulated circulating plasma levels of ACTH and corticosterone by 40% to 70 %, but not after chronic treatment (8 weeks).[50] Sub-chronic treatment with an extract of Hypericum (LI 160, 75 mg/day) in the rat resulted in significantly reduced corticosterone and cortisol in brain frontal cortex tissue, although the changes were not reflected in serum.[90]
- A photosensitising effect for hypericin, since Hypericum treatment has lowered the amount of light necessary to obtain a clinical antidepressant effect.[91]
- The antidepressant-like effect of Hypericum extract may be mediated by interaction with sigma receptors, and to some extent by increased serotonergic neurotransmission.[92] Intraperitoneal pretreatment of rats with 20 mg/kg of the sigma receptor antagonist rimcazole completely suppressed the anti-immobility effect of a Hypericum extract (250 mg/kg, oral). Intracerebroventricular pretreatment with 5,7-dihydroxytryptamine, which produced a marked depletion of brain serotonin, also reduced the anti-immobility effect.[92]

In summary, while the exact role of neurochemical mechanisms underlying the in vivo actions of Hypericum and its constituents are not well defined, current evidence suggests that they are unlikely to exert their central antidepressant effects via the same neurochemical mechanisms as conventional, pharmacologically related drugs. Current data suggest that hyperforin, quercetin, the biflavones amentoflavone and biapigenin and the naphthodianthrones hypericin and pseudohypericin pass the blood-brain barrier poorly in animals, rendering the value of in vitro studies uncertain. Moreover, a review of the data related to entry and diffusion within the CNS of the main Hypericum compounds concluded that pharmacologically effective doses result in brain concentrations of the main compounds too low to be effective on neurotransmitter receptors, the very mechanisms by which central effects are elicited with antidepressant drugs.[93] Some components of Hypericum might interact with some central targets not yet evaluated in vitro, or even act peripherally, influencing central transmission. Despite the uncertainties over mechanisms and active agents in the CNS, pharmacological studies in humans have certainly demonstrated effects in the brain. Subsequent effects on centrally determined hormone levels have also been observed in some of these studies (see below).

In a double blind, crossover, placebo-controlled study over 4 weeks in 12 older healthy volunteers, Hypericum extract (2.7 mg/day TH equivalent) induced an increase in deep sleep during the total sleeping period, as evidenced by EEG and visual analysis. The interference with REM sleep phases, which is typical for tricyclic antidepressants and MAO inhibitors, did not occur for Hypericum. Continuity of sleep, onset of sleep, intermittent wake-up phases and total sleep duration were not improved by Hypericum, which implies it does not exert a sedative activity.[94]

A shielding effect on the CNS was suggested for Hypericum extracts with a high hyperforin content in a randomised, double blind, placebo-controlled parallel-group trial (phase I). The study evaluated the central pharmacodynamic effects of two Hypericum extracts (900 mg/day for 8 consecutive days) with different contents of hyperforin (0.5% and 5.0%), but an identical hypericin content. The 5% hyperforin extract showed a marked tendency to produce higher increases at the delta, theta, and alpha1 frequency values and significantly outperformed placebo in quantitative EEG (qEEG) power performance in the delta and beta-1 frequency values.[22]

A single blind study compared the CNS effects of two commercially available extracts of Hypericum (including LI 160, 0.9 mg hypericin) with those of placebo in a group of healthy young volunteers (n=35) using quantitative EEG. Alpha2 increases of up to 32% were observed, which may indicate an interaction with serotonergic uptake, and later increases in beta-2, which may be correlated with GABA binding and NMDA agonism. Both preparations tended to decrease the latency of the cognitive potential P300, indicating an improvement in mental performance.[95]

In a double blind, randomised, placebo-controlled, crossover study, 16 healthy volunteers (11 men and 5 women; mean age, 31±5 years) were administered escalating doses of a high-hyperforin Hypericum extract or placebo for 7 days. No effect was observed on plasma concentrations of noradrenaline (norepinephrine) and its main metabolite, dihydroxyphenylglycol, whereas plasma dihydroxyphenylacetic acid (the main metabolite of dopamine) increased in every person (p=0.04). These findings may suggest a novel mode of action, or an inhibitory effect on dopamine beta-hydroxylase.[96]

Several human trials have investigated the effects of Hypericum extracts on cortisol, prolactin and/or growth hormone concentrations. One Hypericum extract high in hyperforin (600 mg/day) was suggested to influence central neurotransmitters, thereby causing cortisol stimulation in a dose-dependent manner in 12 healthy volunteers. Clear cortisol stimulation was observed from 30 up to 90 minutes after the herbal extract application, which was greater than placebo. A small but statistically significant elevation in growth hormone values occurred after a 300 mg dose. No prolactin stimulation was observed.[97]

Similarly, a single-blind study of acute oral administration of several doses (600, 900 and 1200 mg) of a similar Hypericum extract in 12 healthy male volunteers observed a significant stimulatory effect on serum ACTH secretion at the time of administration, and during 5 h thereafter, whereas cortisol and prolactin secretions were not significantly influenced.[98]

A single dose of a methanolic extract of Hypericum (LI 160) was investigated in a double blind, crossover trial, again in 12 healthy male volunteers. A significant increase in plasma growth hormone and a significant decrease in plasma prolactin were observed relative to placebo, while plasma cortisol levels were unchanged, suggesting that this dose of Hypericum may increase some aspects of brain dopamine function in humans.[99]

The effect of two doses of Hypericum extract (LI 160) was measured on evening salivary cortisol and noradrenaline (norepinephrine)-mediated melatonin in 20 healthy male volunteers who were randomly given a lower (600 mg/day) or higher dose (1800 mg/day) for 7 days. Treatment significantly increased salivary cortisol throughout the whole collection period in the lower dose group, but had no discernible effect in the higher dose group. Salivary melatonin was not increased in either group following treatment. It was suggested that Hypericum may enhance salivary cortisol via a U-shaped dose-response relationship and that this may be mediated through a 5-HT2 mechanism.[100]

A pilot study (unblinded) of acute treatment of six healthy male volunteers with 2700 mg Hypericum extract (LI 160, equivalent to 8.1 mg hypericin) for 1 day found mean salivary cortisol to be significantly increased compared with the control group. In the subsequent main study (a double blind, balanced order, crossover design, at the same dosage), growth hormone increased significantly compared with placebo (p<0.01) and plasma prolactin was significantly lowered relative to placebo (p<0.01). Plasma hormone levels were associated with a rise in plasma hyperforin, but not with hypericin, although no significant correlation was found. It was suggested that the extract may effect plasma hormonal changes via both 5-HT- and dopamine-mediated mechanisms, but does not involve noradrenaline (norepinephrine). The data also suggest that hyperforin may be more important than hypericin for effecting these changes following acute treatment.[88]

Anxiolytic activity

In vitro studies suggest that Hypericum components can interact with receptors that mediate anxiolytic effects. For example, hypericin reduced GABA-activated chloride currents in vitro, while pseudohypericin had the opposite effect.[101] Both hypericin and pseudohypericin inhibited the activation of NMDA receptors.[101]

In vivo studies reporting on the anxiolytic effects of whole extracts of *Hypericum* have revealed mechanisms that may be of relevance. Further details of these studies are provided here as follows:

- Benzodiazepine receptor activation[101] and alteration of stress-induced augmented 5-HT levels by decreasing precursor availability to the brain, suggesting that the serotonergic system is involved[102]
- Production of an increase in both thymus and spleen indices, suggesting adaptogenic effects mediated by the

interrelationship between the immune, oxidative defence and neuroendocrine systems[103]

- Inhibition of intraneuronal 5-HT metabolism under adverse conditions[104]
- Prevention of the corticosterone-induced decrease in hippocampal cell proliferation (see below).[105]

Anxiolytic activity was exhibited for a Hypericum extract (0.54% TH) administered orally to rats at the dose of 10 mL/kg, but not by protohypericin or a fraction containing hypericin and pseudohypericin. The activity was blocked by pretreatment with the benzodiazepine antagonist flumazenil, suggesting benzodiazepine receptor activation may be involved.[101]

Anxious/depressive-like behaviour, induced in a mouse model by 7 weeks of corticosterone administration, was reversed by exogenous administration of a methanolic extract of Hypericum (0.34% hypericin, 4.1% hyperforin, 5% flavonoids) at a dose of 30 mg/kg ip for 3 weeks. Treatment with Hypericum also prevented the corticosterone-induced decrease in hippocampal cell proliferation and ameliorated the associated reduced spine density, suggesting that morphological adaptations occurring in mature hippocampal neurons might underlie resilient responses to chronic stress and contribute to the therapeutic effects of Hypericum.[105]

The above mechanistic studies are supported by a number of models consistently demonstrating anxiolytic activity for Hypericum extracts.

A 50% ethanolic extract of Hypericum (100 and 200 mg/kg, oral) administered to rats for 3 consecutive days showed consistent and significant anxiolytic activity for all the experimental paradigms used, and resulted in a significant increase in social interaction.[106]

An infused Hypericum lyophilised aqueous extract devoid of hyperforin showed a clear sedative effect at doses ranging from 10 to 100 mg/kg administered intraperitoneally to mice, and at 5 mg/kg produced an anxiolytic effect.[107] Hypericum (100 and 200 mg/kg, oral) showed significant antistress activity, qualitatively comparable to *Panax ginseng* (100 mg/kg, oral), against a variety of behavioural and physiological perturbations induced by chronic stress over 14 days in albino rats. Adrenal gland and spleen weights were attenuated dose-dependently by Hypericum and Panax.[108]

Oral administration of *Hypericum* (LI 160 at 62.5 to 500 mg/kg) exerted anxiolytic-like effects in rats for a specific subset of defensive behaviours, particularly those related to generalised anxiety. Acute treatment (125 mg/kg) impaired elevated T-maze inhibitory avoidance, indicating an anxiolytic effect. Neither acute nor chronic treatment (250 mg/kg) impaired escape performance.[109]

Putative anxiolytic effects of Hypericum extract were demonstrated in induced hyperthermia in mice, where oral administration of doses of 250 and 500 mg/kg significantly reduced body temperature (deltaT) while higher (750 and 1000 mg/kg) and lower doses (125 mg/kg) had no effect. Among the individual constituents, hypericin (0.1 mg/kg, oral) administered 60 min prior to testing significantly decreased deltaT (p<0.05).[110]

Anxiolytic activity of Hypericum was suggested by findings from acute, subchronic (7 days), and chronic (21 days) administration of LI 160 (150 and 300 mg/kg) to mice

submitted to the mouse defence test battery. The dose of 300 mg/kg for 21 days reduced flight reaction to the presence of a predator, suggesting a possible anti-panic effect. However, perceived risk assessment (the main index of anxiety) was not affected, suggesting that both effects were only mild.[111]

Hypericum extract (LI 160) administered orally to rats (150 to 500 mg/kg) 24, 18 and 1 h before the forced swim test demonstrated anxiolytic and anti-panic effects, with no impact on locomotor activity. Subacute treatment (300 mg/kg) exerted a partial anxiolytic-like effect, while administration of 300 mg/kg for 7 days induced anxiolytic (decreased inhibitory avoidance) and anti-panic effects (increased one-way escape).[112]

Neuroprotective and cognition-enhancing activities

In vitro and in vivo studies suggest that Hypericum extracts and hyperforin have cognition-enhancing and memory-facilitating properties, as well as neuroprotective effects.[113] Mechanisms of potential relevance to the neuroprotective activity of Hypericum and its components are summarised here as follows:

- Antioxidant and anti-inflammatory effects: inhibition by hyperforin of cyclo-oxygenase (COX)-1 and 5-lipoxygenase (5-LOX) in vitro[114] and inhibition of 5-LOX in vivo;[115] cytoprotective effects in glutamate-induced cell death;[116] decreased intracellular reactive oxygen species (ROS) and ROS generation in vitro;[117] decreased reactive astrocyte proliferation in vivo;[118] decreased protein tyrosine nitration in vivo;[119] reduced lipid peroxidation in vitro (free radical scavenging activity);[120] superoxide inhibition in vitro;[121] alteration of brain oxidative parameters including glutathione in vivo[122]
- Release of hippocampal acetylcholine by an indirect, calcium-dependent mechanism in vivo[123]
- N-methyl-D-aspartic acid (NMDA) receptor antagonism in vitro[124]
- Activation of transient receptor protein (TRP)C6 channels in vitro[125] with an induction of neuronal axonal sprouting in a TRPC6-dependent manner in vitro[125]
- Alteration of amyloid precursor protein (APP) processing: increased neuroprotective soluble APP-alpha fragment production in vitro,[113] disassemblage of amyloid-beta fibrils in a concentration-dependent manner in vitro[113] and in vivo;[119] improved microglial viability in vitro, and thereby possible attenuation of amyloid-beta-mediated toxicity in Alzheimer's disease;[126] reduced formation of amyloid-induced reactive oxygen species in microglia in vitro.[126]

The implication of these findings for Alzheimer's disease have been expanded in a comprehensive review by Griffith and colleagues, published in 2010, of the neurobiological effects of hyperforin.[113]

Results from further in vivo studies of Hypericum or its components demonstrate improvements in learning, memory retention and spatial memory, protective effects against memory impairment generated by amyloid-beta and prevention of the deleterious effects of stress on memory and learning.

Oral administration of Hypericum extract (50 mg/kg/day) and hyperforin sodium salt (1.25 mg/kg/day) to rats considerably improved learning ability in conditioned avoidance response models, and memory retention of the acquired responses. A single oral dose (1.25 mg/kg) of hyperforin, but not the total Hypericum extract (25 mg/kg), improved memory acquisition and consolidation and almost completely reversed scopolamine-induced amnesia in mice.[127] It was suggested by the authors that Hypericum extract could be a novel type of antidepressant with memory enhancing properties, while pure hyperforin may be a more potent anti-dementia agent than antidepressant.

Similarly, Hypericum was proposed as a possible treatment for the depression commonly associated with dementia. This was based on findings that acute administration of a Hypericum extract (1% TH, 3% hyperforin) to mice at doses of 4 to 25 mg/kg ip enhanced retrieval memory, but failed to reverse scopolamine-induced amnesia. Pretreatment of the animals with a range of neurotransmitter receptor antagonists revealed the involvement of adrenergic and serotonergic 5-HT$_{1A}$ receptors in the facilitatory effect of Hypericum extract on retrieval memory.[128]

Pretreatment of Wistar rats with a 12:1 Hypericum extract (1% TH, 3% hyperforin) at doses of 4 to 12 mg/kg, ip, subsequent to the administration of 1.4 mg/kg of scopolamine to impair retrieval memory, resulted in an antioxidant effect through altering brain malondialdehyde, glutathione peroxidase and/or glutathione level/activity.[122] The authors suggested that, since oxidative stress is implicated in the pathophysiology of dementia, low doses of Hypericum extract may be of value for patients exhibiting elevated brain oxidative status.

Other studies in rats have suggested that Hypericum has the potential to prevent the deleterious effects of stress on learning and memory disorders. Administration of an extract (350 mg/kg/day, oral for 21 days) standardised to 0.3% TH content prevented non-spatial and/or spatial memory impairments due to chronic restraint stress and exogenous corticosterone at 5 mg/kg/day for 21 days. It also significantly improved recognition memory (p<0.01) compared with controls.[129] These results were subsequently confirmed under the same conditions in male Wistar rats with another Hypericum extract, standardised to 0.2 mg TH, at the same dose. The extract significantly improved hippocampus dependent spatial working memory (p<0.01) and alleviated some other negative effects of stress on cognitive function.[130] In a follow-up study, Hypericum was found to significantly (p<0.05) increase levels of the synaptic plasticity proteins neuromodulin (GAP-43) and synaptophysin in the hippocampus and prefrontal cortex, which may account for its effect of alleviating stress- and corticosterone-related memory impairments.[131]

Acute administration of a standardised 50% ethanolic extract of Hypericum (100 and 200 mg/kg/day, oral for 3 days) to rats demonstrated a possible nootropic action comparable with that induced by piracetam (500 mg/kg).[132,133] Memory retention was facilitated, but a minimal effect was observed on learning acquisition in various learning and memory paradigms.

The effects of acute (500 mg/kg) and chronic (200 mg/kg/day for 3 days) oral administration of Hypericum extract (80% ethanol extract, 1% TH, 3% hyperforin, >20% flavonoids) and hyperforin were tested on prepulse inhibition (PPI) of an acoustic startle response in rats, a paradigm for sensorimotor gating processes. Disruption of PPI resulted with both the chronic dose of the extract and hyperforin, suggesting potential for a possible limitation of cognitive disturbance in psychotic and Huntington's disease patients manifesting PPI deficit.[134]

In an early randomised, double blind trial, the effect of Hypericum extract (2.7 mg/day TH equivalent) was compared with maprotiline on resting EEG and evoked potentials in 24 healthy volunteers. Results indicative of cognitive function were observed, particularly for the Hypericum treatment.[135]

Anticancer activity

The constituents of Hypericum receiving the most research attention for potential anticancer activity are hypericin and, more recently, hyperforin. The results of in vitro, in vivo and clinical studies are outlined separately below. Much of the recent interest in hypericin in the context of cancer has focused on its role as a photosensitiser in photodynamic therapy (PDT), an increasingly accepted and promising therapeutic modality for the treatment of many types of tumours. Studies on PDT are included separately and only briefly, because of their lesser relevance to the potential herbal use of Hypericum.

Hypericin has demonstrated potent antitumour activity in vitro against several tumour cell lines. Early mechanistic experiments demonstrated that H directly inhibits epidermal growth factor receptor and protein tyrosine kinase activity.[136] (Epidermal growth factor is a cellular plasma membrane receptor possibly involved in the loss of inhibitory constraint on cell growth, a factor in tumour formation.) Phosphorylation of proteins on tyrosine residues is a key biochemical reaction mediating a large variety of cellular signals, including control of the cell cycle and cell differentiation. Enhanced protein tyrosine kinase activity is also involved in the transformation of normal cells into tumour cells.

In a study on bovine vascular endothelial cells, non-photoactivated hypericin inhibited several key steps of the angiogenic process, including bovine endothelial cell proliferation, formation of tubular-like structures, migration and invasion, as well as extracellular matrix degrading urokinase.[137]

Other in vitro research has found that the hypericins in the lipophilic extract of Hypericum induced apoptosis in cultured T24 and NBT-II bladder cancer cell lines, suggesting that pure hyperforin does not seem to contribute significantly to the cytotoxicity activity.[138]

In vivo studies have supported antimetastatic activity for hypericin in the absence of light. Intraperitoneal injection of 10 mg/kg hypericin significantly reduced the growth rate of metastases in two murine models: breast adenocarcinoma (DA3) and squamous cell carcinoma (SQ2). Long-term animal survival in DA3 tumour-excised groups increased from 15.6% in controls to 34.5% following supplementary treatment with hypericin. In mice bearing SQ2 tumour metastases, therapy with hypericin increased animal survival from 17.7% in controls to 46.1%.[139]

Significant reduction in the growth of a human prostatic carcinoma cell line and the number of metastases was observed with a Hypericum methanolic extract (containing

0.3% TH and 3.8% hyperforin) in orthotopically implanted nude mice.[140] Treatment administered intraperitoneally at a dose of 15 mg/kg for 25 days inhibited tumour growth by 70%. Regional lymph node metastasis was observed in 100% of controls compared with 30% of the mice treated with Hypericum (p<0.01), with no side effects observed in any of the treated mice.

Photodynamic therapy

Hypericin is probably the most powerful photosensitiser found in nature,[141] and as such has shown promise in PDT, which involves administration of a non-toxic photosensitising drug that accumulates in the tumour. In the presence of oxygen and on illumination with visible light, the photosensitiser generates ROS toxic to the tumour cells, causing tumour cell death by apoptosis and/or necrosis and tissue destruction.[42,142] Other possibly interrelated mechanisms for tumour shrinkage include damage of the tumour-associated vasculature, with resulting tumour infarction, and/or activation of immune responses against tumour cells.[42]

Hypericin (10 nM to 1 μM) showed strong phototoxic effects and induced apoptosis in a dose-dependent fashion in both primary cell cultures and cell lines of human oesophageal cancer. Its phototoxicity was comparable to that of delta-aminolevulinic acid, which is already being used for the photodynamic therapy of gastrointestinal cancer.[143] A number of other studies have demonstrated that hypericin possesses a powerful in vitro photocytotoxic activity. These have been extensively reviewed in several recent articles.[25,42,142]

Positive cytotoxic results have been reported from in vitro studies with hypericin-PDT for cell lines including human bladder cancer cells,[144] human epidermoid carcinoma cells (A431),[145] human umbilical endothelial cells and human glioma cancer cells U-87MG and U-373MG, hepatic hepatoblastoma cells, paediatric hepatocellular carcinoma HepG2 cells, human lung SpcA1 cancer cells, human lung cancer cells A549, MDA231 human mammary carcinoma cells, human renal carcinoma cells and rhabdomyosarcoma cells.[42] Hypericin-PDT was shown to induce apoptosis or necrosis in rat bladder transitional cell carcinoma cells, depending on the concentration of hypericin.[146] Light activation was mandatory for the expression of good cytotoxic activity of hypericin.[42]

Hypericin-PDT has been proposed as a potential adjuvant therapy for melanoma.[147] In vitro assays have shown that an exposure to 1 μM UVA-activated hypericin does not bring about cell death, whereas 3 μM of UVA (400 to 315 nm)-activated hypericin induced a necrotic mode of cell death in pigmented human melanoma cells and melanocytes, and an apoptotic mode of cell death in non-pigmented melanoma cells and keratinocytes.[148]

In vivo investigations have shown that PDT with hypericin successfully inhibits growth of transplanted tumour cells of different histological origin in various mouse tumour models,[142,149–152] and results obtained with hypericin in the RIF tumour mouse model are among the best achieved, compared with other photosensitisers.[142]

Topical treatment with hypericin by intralesional injection was investigated in eight patients with squamous cell carcinoma (SCC) and 11 patients with basal cell carcinoma (BCC). Patients with SCC were given 40 to 100 μg hypericin intralesionally three to five times per week for 2 to 4 weeks; patients with BCC were treated with 40 to 200 μg hypericin three to five times per week for 2 to 6 weeks. Following administration, the hypericin was irradiated with visible light. There was selective tumour targeting: penetration in the surrounding tissues did not induce necrosis or cell loss, and the generation of a new epithelium at the surface of the malignancy was noticed.[153]

The potential of hypericin-PDT treatment was confirmed in a patient with recurrent mesothelioma. Local hypericin was applied 8 weeks after the systemic administration of haematoporphyrin derivatives (HDP). Subsequent light illumination had no efficacy in the HDP-photosensitised area, but there was tumour destruction for both administered photosensitisers.[154]

Hyperforin

Hyperforin has also exhibited antitumour, antiangiogenic and pro-apoptotic activity against various cancer cell lines in both in vitro and in vivo research. Although the mechanisms remain to be fully elucidated, in vitro studies have revealed that several pathways are involved, including promotion of pro-apoptotic effects,[155–158] inhibition of P-gp (P-glycoprotein),[159] inhibition of invasion and metastasis.[158,160–162]

Hyperforin inhibited the growth of leukaemia K562 and U937 cells, brain glioblastoma cells LN229 and normal human astrocytes in vitro. Cytocidal effects of hypericin and its cooperation with hyperforin on leukaemic (K562, U937) cell growth inhibition indicated a synergistic interaction.[155]

Hyperforin was found to stimulate apoptosis in B cell chronic lymphocytic leukaemia cells (CLL) ex vivo and displayed anti-angiogenic properties.[157] Ex vivo treatment of CLL cells with hyperforin markedly impaired the activity of P-gp.[159] The activity of breast cancer resistance protein was inhibited by hyperforin, which also exhibited the potential to revert multi-drug resistance in addition to its pro-apoptotic properties.[159]

Hyperforin inhibited angiogenesis in vitro in bovine aortic endothelial cells and in vivo in the chorioallantoic membrane assay. The phytochemical inhibited the growth of endothelial cells in culture and their invasive capabilities, and produced a complete inhibition of urokinase and a remarkable inhibition of matrix metalloproteinase 2.[163]

With hyperforin treatment in vivo, the growth of Kaposi's sarcoma – a highly angiogenic tumour – was strongly inhibited in mice, with the resultant tumours reduced in size and in vascularisation.[161] Injected hyperforin significantly inhibited MT-450 mammary carcinoma cell tumour growth in Wistar rats, induced apoptosis of tumour cells and reduced tumour vascularisation.[164]

Hyperforin inhibited the growth of autologous MT-450 breast carcinoma in immunocompetent Wistar rats to a similar extent to the cytotoxic drug paclitaxel, without any signs of acute toxicity.[158] Treatment with equimolar concentrations of hyperforin or paclitaxel was initiated 15 days after tumour injection, with daily subcutaneous injections over a period of 2 weeks.

Antibacterial activity

Hyperforin is considered to be the main antibacterial constituent of Hypericum,[165,166] although evidence exists that hypericin, but not the flavonoids, can significantly inhibit the growth of selected micro-organisms.[167] Extracts of other Hypericum species with a low level of hypericin and hyperforin were also found to possess some antimicrobial activity,[168] suggesting that, while these are the main antimicrobial components, they are probably not the only ones responsible for such activity. Hyperforin is the main ingredient of a complex preparation of polyphenolic components, mostly from dianthrone and flavonoid groups, isolated by water-alkali extraction of Hypericum. This preparation has shown antimicrobial properties and has been proposed to be more stable than hyperforin itself.[169]

A variety of preparations of Hypericum have demonstrated antibacterial activity in vitro against more than 40 microorganisms including Staphylococcus Oxford, Staphylococcus aureus, Streptococcus mutans, Streptococcus sanguis, Escherichia coli, Proteus vulgaris, Bacillus cereus, Bacillus subtilis and Nocardia gardene.[169,170] Extracts of the aerial parts have shown activity against Helicobacter pylori (MIC 1.95 to 250 μg/mL).[166] A comprehensive review of the antibacterial activity of Hypericum published in 2010 reported that methanolic/ethanolic extracts have been found to possess more pronounced activity than aqueous extracts.[170] The highest inhibitory properties against Enterococcus faecium, Bifidobacterium animalis, Lactobacillus plantarum and E. coli isolated from the human large intestine were obtained with a 30% ethanol solution, compared with 10% ethanol and pure water extracts.[170] The essential oil has also demonstrated potent antibacterial activity in vitro against a variety of bacterial strains, although it occurs at quite low levels in the herb.[170,171–173] Water-soluble formulations of hypericin have also shown promise as sensitisers in antibacterial photodynamic therapy for inactivating Staphylococcus aureus infections in wounds.[174]

The infused oil of Hypericum has antibacterial activity. Three lipophilic ointments containing this oil (30%, 40% and 50%) demonstrated inhibition of bacterial growth against Streptococcus pyogenes, Streptococcus viridans, Micrococcus luteus ATCC 9341 and Moraxella catarrhalis, but not Lactobacillus acidophilus, with the antibacterial effect correlated with the quantity of oil.[175]

The antibacterial activity of Hypericum against methicillin-resistant Staphylococcus aureus (MRSA) has been demonstrated by several research groups.[165,166,176] Hyperforin at concentrations of 0·1 to 100 mg/mL showed antibacterial activity against resistant Staphylococcus aureus.[165] Aqueous solutions of Hypericum teas were also found to be effective against MRSA (MIC 1.3 to 2.5 mg herb per mL).[166] However, subsequent research supported the superiority of the ethanolic extract against eight clinical and one standard strain of MRSA, with the most pronounced effect observed for 0.5 mg/mL of extract.[177] The extracts were more effective against MRSA than methicillin-sensitive S. aureus.

Some of the literature indicates that Hypericum extracts and its components have a higher antibacterial activity against Gram-positive (MIC 0.1 to 1.0 μg/mL) than Gram-negative bacteria.[166,170,178] However, other research groups have found activity against both Gram-positive and Gram-negative bacteria.

Methanol-acetone extracts from the aerial parts of two subspecies of Hypericum (H. perforatum L. subsp. perforatum, H. perforatum L. subsp. veronense (Schrank) Ces.) were found to be active against two Gram-positive bacteria (Staphylococcus aureus and Enterococcus faecalis) and two Gram-negative bacteria (E. coli and Pseudomonas aeruginosa).[168]

Aqueous extracts were also effective against both Gram-positive (S. aureus ATCC 12600) and Gram-negative bacteria (E. coli ATCC 8677 and P. aeroginosa ATCC 9721). Seasonal variation in antimicrobial activity was noted, with samples collected later in the summer (August) conferring good antimicrobial activity, while those collected in July were inactive.[179] Nikolic and Zlatkovic observed that the antimicrobial activity reached two maximum values during the harvesting season, the first during the budding period, and the second during the period of mass flowering when hyperforin is accumulated in the flowers.[169]

Antifungal activity

Several in vitro studies have investigated the antifungal activity of the flavonoids, essential oil and/or ethanolic extracts of H. perforatum. An investigation of the six known flavonoids in the herb showed 6″-O-acetyl quercetin 3-O-beta-D-alloside, quercitrin and quercetin were inhibitory towards the growth of the phytopathogenic fungus Helminthosporium sativum, with MIC values of 25, 50 and 100 μg/mL, respectively, while, 6″-O-acetyl quercetin, 3-O-beta-D-alloside and quercitrin also inhibited the growth of Fusarium graminearum Schw. (MIC 100 μg/mL).[170]

Ethanolic extracts of Hypericum have shown fungistatic activity against the fungi Fusarium oxysporum and Penicillium canescens, with the concentration high of 45 mg/mL ethanolic extract showing the highest fungistatic activity using a spore counting method.[180] Activity was also demonstrated against Penicillium canescens, Fusarium oxysporum, Alternaria alternata, Aspergillus glaucus and Phialophora fastigiata using the disk diffusion method, at amounts of 20 to 25 mg/disk.[181] The essential oil and water-soluble fraction of an alcohol extract of Hypericum both exhibited in vitro antifungal activity against Microsporum gypseum, Trichophyton rubrum, Aspergillus flavus, Curvularia lunata and Fusarium vasinfectum.[182]

Wound healing/anti-inflammatory activities

The wound healing effect of Hypericum may be attributable to its antibacterial and/or anti-inflammatory activities. When pure constituents were tested in vitro for anti-inflammatory activity in RAW264.7 macrophage cells, flavonoids, amentoflavone, hyperforin and light-activated pseudohypericin all displayed activity, but the anti-inflammatory activity observed for whole plant extracts was light-independent.[183]

Hyperforin has been found to act as a dual inhibitor of 5-lipoxygenase (5-LOX) and cyclo-oxygenase (COX)-1 in intact cells.[114] Extracts of Hypericum have shown inhibitory effects on COX-2 expression in vitro.[184] In two different human epithelial cell lines, alveolar A549/8 and colon DLD-1 cells, H. perforatum extract concentration-dependently inhibited human inducible nitric oxide synthase (iNOS) expression, which resulted from transcriptional inhibition.[185] Hyperforin inhibited the generation of ROS as well as the release of leucocyte elastase (degranulation) in human isolated polymorphonuclear leucocytes challenged by the G protein-coupled receptor ligand N-formyl-methionyl-leucyl-phenylalanine.[117]

In embryonic fibroblasts from fertilised chicken eggs, Hypericum extract was shown to increase the stimulation of fibroblast collagen production and the activation of fibroblast cells that play a role in wound repair by closing the damaged area.[186]

In vivo research using pleural exudate formation in carrageenan-treated rats showed that hyperforin significantly suppressed leukotriene B4 formation, suggesting it may act as a novel type of 5-LOX inhibitor.[115] Hyperforin (4 mg/kg) was administered ip 30 minutes before carrageenan. Topical Hypericum extracts provoked a dose-dependent reduction of croton-oil-induced ear oedema in mice (lipophilic extract > ethyl acetate fraction > hydroalcoholic extract). The pure compounds amentoflavone, hypericin, hyperforin dicyclohexylammonium (DHCA) salt and adhyperforin exhibited anti-inflammatory activity that was more potent than or comparable to indomethacin, whereas isoquercitrin and hyperoside were less active.[187] The lipophilic extract contained no hyperoside, hypericin or pseudohypericin, but contained 27% hyperforin and 5.2% adhyperforin.

In early research, oral administration of Hypericum tincture (0.1 mL of 1:10 tincture) demonstrated improved wound healing in rats. This activity was believed to be due to the facilitation of the collagen maturation phase of wound healing, enhanced new skin growth and an influence on epithelial cell proliferation and migration.[188]

A standardised 50% aqueous ethanolic extract of the Indian variety of *H. perforatum* showed significant anti-inflammatory and analgesic activity in animal models at oral doses of 100 and 200 mg/kg.[189] Additionally, the Hypericum extract potentiated the anti-inflammatory activity of indomethacin (20 mg/kg, ip) and analgesic activities of pentazocine (10 mg/kg, ip) and aspirin (25 mg/kg, ip).

Topical application of Hypericum ointment and its metabolite hyperforin inhibited the allostimulatory capacity of epidermal cells in vivo and the proliferative effect of T lymphocytes on epidermal cells isolated from treated skin, as well as the proliferation of peripheral blood mononuclear cells in vitro, in a dose-dependent manner. This may provide a rationale for the traditional treatment of inflammatory skin disorders with Hypericum extracts.[190]

Hypericum extract (containing 0.27% TH and 2.5% of hyperforin) administered orally to mice at 200 mg/kg significantly inhibited the formation of carrageenan-induced paw oedema (p<0.05). The extract inhibited both iNOS and COX-2 expression, suggesting that the anti-inflammatory effect could be in part related to modulation of COX-2 expression.[184]

In order to determine the active wound healing ingredients, the aerial parts of Hypericum were extracted with ethanol. The ethanolic extract was then submitted to successive solvent extractions with n-hexane, chloroform and ethyl acetate. The ethyl acetate sub-extract was found to be the most active, inhibiting wounds by between 17.9% and 100% in an excision model and between 9.4% and 100% in an incision model. Based on this, the flavonoids and hypericins were suggested as the active components.[191]

Hypericum extract (50 to 300 mg/kg/day, ip) was found to have a protective effect on inflammatory bowel disease induced in rats by 2,4,6-trinitrobenzene sulphonic acid, which the authors postulated was probably due to anti-inflammatory and antioxidant mechanisms.[192] Blood glutathione levels significantly increased for all doses of Hypericum (p<0.001).

Spasmolytic activity

A strong association has been suggested between depression and urinary incontinence. In vitro research found Hypericum extract, hyperforin and, to a lesser extent, the flavonoid kaempferol inhibited excitatory transmission of the rat urinary bladder and also directly inhibited smooth muscle contractility. This could involve opioid receptors, at least in part, as the effect was significantly reduced by the opioid receptor antagonist naloxone.[193]

Spasmolytic activity was also demonstrated in mice for Hypericum crude ethanol extract, ethyl acetate extract, aqueous extract/infusion (50 g dried powdered herb in 500 mL hot water for 15 minutes) administered as a 1% aqueous solution ip (10 mL/kg body weight) for each extract. All extracts significantly reduced intestinal motility.[194] A crude extract of Hypericum at a dose of 500 mg/kg caused a 20% protection against castor oil-induced diarrhoea in mice and a 60% protection at 1000 mg/kg (p<0.05 versus saline).[195]

Sexual function

Findings from in vitro research on Hypericum extract (1 to 300 μM) showed a dose-dependent inhibition of contractions in both the rat and human vas deferens for the whole extract, and for hyperforin but not hypericin or the flavonoids. It was suggested that these results could explain the delayed ejaculation sometimes described in patients receiving Hypericum treatment.[196]

Later in vivo research on the expulsion phase of ejaculation in anesthetised rats suggested that a hyperforin-enriched extract of Hypericum may be a potential treatment for premature ejaculation (see also under Clinical trials).[197]

A study conducted in healthy volunteers (6 men and 6 women) found that 14-day administration of Hypericum extract (LI 160) at 900 mg/day did not significantly alter the concentrations of most circulating androgens (testosterone, dihydrotestosterone, dehydroepiandrosterone sulphate, sex hormone-binding globulin and the combined concentrations of androsterone sulphate and epiandrosterone sulphate) (p>0.05) in men or women.[198] However, the combined concentrations of the 5-alpha-reduced steroids, androsterone sulphate and epiandrosterone sulphate, significantly declined following treatment in all participants (p=0.02) and in the men (p=0.04).

Eye diseases

Intravitreal injection of hypericin demonstrated antitumour activity against proliferative vitreoretinopathy (PVR) in pigmented rabbits.[199] Hypericin in doses of 1 μM, 10 μM and 100 μM significantly inhibited PVR after day 5 (p<0.05).

Histological examination of the hypericin-treated control eyes disclosed no morphological change, and electroretinogram analysis revealed no significant functional change.

The antiangiogenic effects of Hypericum or hypericin were investigated for their potential application in ocular neovascularisation, a leading cause of blindness in ischaemic retinopathies.[200] In a mouse model of oxygen-induced retinopathy, oral administration of Hypericum (15 mg/kg/day) or hypericin (15, 45 or 135 μg/kg/day) for 5 days from post-natal day 12 to day 17 significantly inhibited the degree of retinal neovascularisation, but did not affect the area of retinal vaso-obliteration.

Hypericin was shown to be a highly potent inhibitor of angiogenesis in several ocular models examined in rat eyes.[201] Extensive angiogenesis induced in the cornea and iris by intraocular administration of the fibroblast growth factor (FGF)-2 was effectively inhibited by a minimum of four dose regimens of hypericin (2 mg/kg) administered via the intraperitoneal route at 48h intervals. Maximal inhibition was achieved when treatment with hypericin was initiated 48h prior to inoculation of FGF-2.[201]

Sedative and hypnotic effects

An aqueous ethanolic extract of Hypericum (26.5 mg/kg, oral) induced marked sedation in vivo similar to diazepam controls. None of the isolated fractions from this extract exhibited the same sedative activity as the whole extract.[202]

The effects of Hypericum ethanol extract (A), ethyl acetate extract (B) and aqueous extract/infusion (50g dried powdered herb in 500 mL hot water for 15 minutes) (C) on pentobarbital-induced sleep time, intestinal motility and analgesic activity were investigated in mice, who received a 1% aqueous solution (10 mL/kg body weight, ip) of each extract. Extracts A and B exhibited significant stimulatory and antidepressant effects on the CNS and prolonged pentobarbital-induced sleep, increasing the time up to more than 25min. Extract B exhibited strong analgesic activity. All extracts exhibited spasmolytic activity, significantly reducing intestine motility.[194]

The effect of a single dose of Hypericum was examined at two dosages (0.9 mg TH and 1.8 mg TH equivalent) on the sleep polysomnogram of healthy volunteers using a placebo-controlled, crossover design.[203] At both doses, Hypericum significantly increased the latency to REM sleep (placebo 69 and 64min versus 84min (p=0.030) and 104min (p=0.031) for the low and high doses, respectively), without producing any other effect on sleep architecture. The mean increase in REM latency over placebo was not statistically greater in the participants who received the higher dose of Hypericum (p=0.15).

In an uncontrolled trial with 13 healthy volunteers, a significant increase in nocturnal melatonin plasma concentration was observed after 3 weeks of administration of Hypericum extract (0.5 mg/day TH equivalent).[204]

Models of alcoholism and drug-dependency

In a 2008 review of Hypericum for substance dependence, it was proposed that the inhibitory effects on ethanol withdrawal syndrome may be explained by serotonergic mechanisms or a central inhibition of nitric oxide synthase (NOS).[205] Hypericum extracts (6 to 24 mg/kg) blocked both nicotine (1 mg/kg) and caffeine (16 mg/kg) induced locomotor hyperactivity in mice. These effective doses of Hypericum did not have any significant impact on locomotor activity when administered alone, suggesting that the effect was not related to a non-specific effect such as sedation or muscle relaxation. Additionally, in a second study, pretreatment with L-arginine (1 g/kg) a NO precursor reversed the inhibitory effect of Hypericum (6 mg/kg) on caffeine (16 mg/kg) induced locomotor activity in mice, without producing any significant effect on locomotor activity when administered alone. This implies that the effect may indeed be related to NOS inhibition.

A 2005 review of potential natural treatments for alcoholism reported several preclinical studies indicated Hypericum extracts might reduce the voluntary intake of alcohol in several strains of alcohol-preferring rats. Hyperforin has been suggested to be a compound of relevance in reducing alcohol intake. The ability of extracts of Hypericum to affect serotonergic, dopaminergic and opioidergic systems in mesolimbic regions in the CNS, directly or indirectly, might help to explain this activity.[206]

Oral administration of Hypericum extracts dose-dependently and significantly reduced alcohol intake in two genetic animal models of human alcoholism. Similar results were seen after the rats were deprived of alcohol for 20h and the extract was administered 30 minutes prior to the return of alcohol. Compared with the control group, Hypericum extract (0.6 mg/kg) significantly prevented the alcohol deprivation-induced rebound in alcohol intake.[207]

Doses of a Hypericum CO_2 extract high in hyperforin reduced ethanol intake at 31 or 125 mg/kg, but not at 7 mg/kg. When the opiate receptor antagonist naloxone at 1 mg/kg was combined with the three doses of Hypericum extract, the attenuation of ethanol intake was more pronounced than for the extract alone.[208] Chronic (once a day for 12 days) oral administration to rats of the same Hypericum extract, given alone or combined with naltrexone, markedly reduced ethanol intake (offered 2h/day) at the dose of 125 mg/kg, but not at 7 mg/kg. The effect of 125 mg/kg was observed from the first day of treatment and remained constant across the 12 days.[209] At oral doses of 31 or 125 mg/kg, but not 7 mg/kg, the same Hypericum extract significantly reduced ethanol self-administration in rats.[210]

A randomised, double blind, placebo-controlled, crossover study investigated the interaction of Hypericum extract with alcohol. Thirty-two volunteers received either Hypericum extract (2.7 mg/day TH equivalent) for 7 days or placebo. At the end of the treatment period they underwent several tests following consumption of alcohol. No interaction between Hypericum and alcohol with respect to cognitive capabilities was observed.[211]

A study investigating the effects of Hypericum extract and clonidine on morphine withdrawal syndrome in morphine-dependent rats showed that clonidine was more effective than the lower dose of Hypericum extract (fed to rats orally by a nasogastric tube at 0.4 mL/200g). However, there was no significant statistical difference between the mean frequency of withdrawal signs for Hypericum extract at the dose of 0.8 mL/200g compared with clonidine (0.2 mg/kg, ip), and at

1.2 mL/200 g the Hypericum was significantly stronger than clonidine in attenuating the morphine withdrawal syndrome.[212]

Oral administration of an extract of Hypericum was shown to attenuate nicotine withdrawal signs in mice.[213] Hypericum extract at doses of 125 to 500 mg/kg administered in combination with, or immediately after, nicotine administration (2 mg/kg, four injections daily) abolished the locomotor activity reduction induced by nicotine withdrawal, and also significantly and dose-dependently reduced the total nicotine abstinence score when injected after nicotine withdrawal.

Other activity

In animal models of metabolic syndrome, Hypericum extract was found to significantly lower total cholesterol and low-density lipoprotein cholesterol in normal rats and inhibit weight gain in high-fat- and fructose-fed rats. It also normalised dyslipidaemia and improved insulin sensitivity.[214] Hypericum extract (3% hyperforin and 0.3% TH) was orally administered at the doses of 100 and 200 mg/kg/day for 15 consecutive days. The same extract and doses over 14 days were investigated for antidiabetic activity in alloxan-induced diabetic rats.[215] Treatment with Hypericum led to significant falls (p<0.01) in elevated blood glucose levels and also reversed the weight loss associated with alloxan treatment.

Evidence of persistent thermal and chemical antinociceptive activity of Hypericum mainly mediated by PKC-inhibiting mechanisms was obtained from research in which a dried extract of Hypericum induced an effect that persisted for 120 minutes after oral administration to mice.[216] The presence of hypericin was fundamental to both thermal and chemical antinociception, through inhibition of PKC activity, whereas hyperforin selectively produced a thermal opioid antinociception.

In research by the same group, Hypericum extract (hypericin 0.06 mg/kg, hyperforin 0.978 mg/kg, quercetin 0.249 mg/kg, hyperoside 1.905 mg/kg and amentoflavone 0.016 mg/kg per 30 mg/kg dose of Hypericum) acutely administered at low doses (30 to 60 mg/kg, oral) relieved neuropathic pain and reversed mechanical hyperalgesia in rat models, being effective up to 180 min after injection of oxipl-atin.[217] Hyperforin and hypericin were responsible for this action, whereas flavonoids were ineffective.

Auditory evoked potentials (AEP) provide a correlate of cognitive dysfunction in schizophrenia. In a double blind, randomised, crossover design, treatment with either 1500 mg/day LI 160 or placebo for 1 week in 16 healthy volunteers reversed changes in AEP induced by infusion with ketamine. The influence of ketamine and the effect of Hypericum on the oculodynamic test showed similar (non-significant) trends. Provided that ketamine mimics cognitive deficits in schizophrenia, it was suggested that Hypericum might be effective to treat these symptoms.[218]

Pharmacokinetics

Results for several pharmacokinetic studies of hyperforin in humans were discussed in a 2006 review.[219] It has been shown that the hyperforin plasma concentrations in humans at normal doses of Hypericum extract show inter-individual variability, and may also vary considerably between preparations, mainly due to differences in hyperforin content.[93] For example, after single oral doses of 300, 600, 900 and 1200 mg of WS 5572 (an alcohol/water Hypericum extract containing 5% hyperforin) in healthy volunteers, mean Cmax ranged from 153 to 437 μg/L (0.28 to 0.81 μM). However, the 900 mg dose of the extract yielded a mean Cmax of 246±22 μg/L, much higher than for 900 mg of a different extract (87.1±36.5 μg/L) in healthy volunteers, but lower than 900 mg of LI 160 (1500±200 μg/L) in depressed patients. The results of this study by Biber and colleagues demonstrated that the absorption of hyperforin takes place after a lag time of approximately 1 h, with maximum plasma levels attained within 3 to 3.5 h.[220] No significant difference was found in the mean clearance between the 300 and 600 mg doses, although there was a statistically significant difference between the 300 and 1200 mg doses. Elimination half-lives (9.46, 8.52 and 9.65 h, respectively) were similar for the doses, as was Tmax (3.58, 3.5 and 2.83 h, respectively for the 300, 600 and 1200 mg doses).

In a repeated dose study by the same researchers comparing the same daily dose (900 mg/day) of two Hypericum extracts with different hyperforin contents (WS 5572, 4.5 mg hyperforin and WS 5573, 42.84 mg hyperforin) over a period of 8 days, Tmax values were comparable, but Cmax was 20.7 and 246 ng/mL for the low and high hyperforin tablets, respectively. The area under the concentration-time curve (AUC) values were 254 and 2336 ng×min/mL respectively.[220] The authors speculated that the lower Cmax and AUC values in comparison with the three-dose study outlined above may be due to loss of bioavailability related to the high lipophilicity of hyperforin or its interaction with some extract and/or gastrointestinal tract contents.[220]

A 300 mg dose of Hypericum extract (not defined) was administered in hard and soft capsules and pharmacokinetics were compared.[221] Results for the soft-gel capsules were in good agreement with the findings of Biber and colleagues above.[220] However, with the hard gel capsules, the Cmax of hyperforin was only half the value (84.25 ng/mL, compared with 168.35 ng/mL for the soft-gel formulation).[221] Results of further pharmacokinetic studies are generally in good agreement with earlier findings.[219,222,223]

Two open phase I clinical trials were conducted to obtain pharmacokinetic data for hypericin, pseudohypericin, hyperforin, the flavonoid aglycone quercetin and its methylated form, isorhamnetin, from a Hypericum extract. In each trial, 18 healthy men received 900 mg dry extract of St John's wort (STW 3-VI, Laif 900), either as a single oral dose or as a multiple once daily dose over a period of 14 days. After single dose intake, the key pharmacokinetic parameters were as follows: hypericin AUC 78.33 h×ng/mL, Cmax 3.8 ng/mL, time to reach Cmax (Tmax) 7.9 h, and t1/2 18.71 h; pseudohypericin AUC 97.28 h×ng/mL, Cmax 10.2 ng/mL, Tmax 2.7 h and t1/2 17.19 h; hyperforin AUC 1550.4 h×ng/mL, Cmax 122.0 ng/mL, Tmax 4.5 h and t1/2 17.47 h. Quercetin and isorhamnetin showed two maxima separated by about 3 to 3.5 h. Their parameters were as follows: quercetin AUC 417.38 h×ng/mL, Cmax (1) 89.5 ng/mL, Tmax (1) 1.0 h, Cmax (2) 79.1 ng/mL, Tmax (2) 4.4 h and t1/2 2.6 h; isorhamnetin AUC (0-infinity)

155.72 h×ng/mL, Cmax (1) 12.5 ng/mL, Tmax (1) 1.4 h, Cmax (2) 14.6 ng/mL, Tmax (2) 4.5 h and t1/2 5.61 h. Under steady-state conditions reached during multiple dose administration, similar results were obtained.[223]

Under the same conditions but with a lower dose of 612 mg Hypericum extract (STW-3, Laif 600), hypericin reached a Cmax of 3.14 ng/mL, with a Tmax of 8.1 h, and a t1/2 of 23.76 h; for pseudohypericin Cmax was 8.50 ng/mL, Tmax 3.0 h, t1/2 25.39 h; for hyperforin AUC (0-max) was 1009.0 h × ng/mL, Cmax 83.5 ng/mL, Tmax 4.4 h and t1/2 19.64 h. Similar to the above study, quercetin and isorhamnetin showed two peaks of maximum plasma concentration separated by about 4 h.[222]

Notwithstanding the above, human pharmacokinetic studies of hypericin have predominantly been carried out using the extract LI 160 at doses ranging from 300 to 1800 mg/day.[99,219,224–226] Plasma concentrations of the hypericins were generally found to be lower than hyperforin,[219] with Cmax ranging from 1.3 ng/mL to 91 ng/mL. Hypericin levels peaked at an average of 5.87 h, while the mean Tmax of pseudohypericin was at 3.1 h.[219]

In a phase I trial using synthetic hypericin, oral bioavailability of hypericin after a single dose was measured at 14.6% to 30%.[227]

Current evidence suggests that the acylphloroglucinol hyperforin, the flavonol quercetin and its glycosylated forms and their metabolites, the biflavone amentoflavone and its analogue biapigenin and the naphthodianthrones hypericin and pseudohypericin pass the blood-brain barrier poorly in animals. A recent review by Caccia and colleagues detailed in vitro and in vivo studies of uptake by the brain of the components of Hypericum extracts.[93] Hyperforin was the only component that could be determined in the brain of rodents after oral administration of alcoholic extracts,[219] although even here animal models have revealed its very poor passage across the blood-brain barrier, with a brain-to-plasma ratio <2% to 4%.[93] Findings from these in vivo studies indicate that, after pharmacologically effective doses of Hypericum extracts, brain concentrations of hyperforin are in the low nanomolar range.

Similarly, the penetration of hypericin across the blood-brain barrier seems to be very limited. Pharmacokinetic data on hypericin derived from animal studies using single doses of the pure compound indicate that brain concentrations are well below 50 nM.[228] There was no detectable hypericin in the CSF of non-human primates 48 h after an intravenous dose of 2 to 5 mg/kg. It was estimated that less than 1% of the observed plasma concentration of hypericin (10 μM for up to 12 h) entered the CSF.[93]

There is no information on the concentrations of conjugated and methylated quercetin derivatives reached in the human brain after administration of Hypericum extracts.[93] Amentoflavone protected against hypoxic-ischaemic injury in a rat model, suggesting that it may enter the brain, although after oral treatment of mice with 1000 mg/kg of a Hypericum hydroalcoholic extract and 1 mg/kg authentic amentoflavone, brain concentrations of unchanged compound were below the detection limit. Biapigenin is also suggested to achieve poor blood-brain barrier penetration in rodents, as brain concentrations were less than 2% of the corresponding systemic exposure in mice (0.01 to 0.03 nmol/g).[93]

Clinical trials

Antiretroviral and antiviral activities

In the first reported case studies of HIV-positive patients who had been taking Hypericum preparations (0.35 to 1.2 mg/day TH), nine (of 11) patients demonstrated successful treatment, as evidenced by symptomatic relief of fatigue, nausea, mild peripheral neuropathies and abatement of swollen lymph glands. Changes in CD4 cell counts and p24 antigen levels were slower to occur. One patient became asymptomatic.[229]

In 1990, an uncontrolled study was carried out investigating 26 HIV-positive patients self-administering an over-the-counter Hypericum extract (1 mg/day TH equivalent). At the end of 4 months, p24 antigenaemia disappeared in two of six initially positive patients, both of whom were also using the antiretroviral drug AZT. In 10 patients who had never taken AZT, the mean CD4 cell count increased 13% after 1 month and maintained this increase for 4 months. In those using AZT and Hypericum, CD4 cell counts fell significantly after an initial mild rise. Liver enzyme elevations occurred in five patients, which returned to baseline after 1 month without Hypericum.[230]

In another early uncontrolled trial, 16 HIV patients at various stages of the disease process were treated by intravenous injection and oral doses of Hypericum.[231] Over 40 months of observation, patients showed stable or increasing CD4 cell counts and only two patients encountered an opportunistic infection. None of the known viral complications due to cytomegalovirus, herpes or Epstein-Barr virus were encountered. There were no cases of toxoplasmosis, neurological symptoms or photosensitivity.

A substantial decline in viral load was observed in most of 18 AIDS patients undergoing a similar treatment regime (intravenous injection and oral Hypericum) for 4 to 6 years. In those patients who experienced an increase in viral load, there was no effect on the clinical outcome of viral cytomegalovirus, herpes or Epstein-Barr viral complications.[232] Twenty-four HIV-infected patients in Thailand participated in a study to determine the maximum tolerated effective oral dose (MTD) of hypericin that demonstrated antiviral activity with minimal phototoxic effects. The MTD was found to be 0.05 mg/kg.[233] In a toxicological study involving 10 HIV-positive homosexual men, daily dosages of 0.5, 2.0, 4.0 and 8.0 mg hypericin were each administered for 12 weeks. No early, marked anti-HIV activity was found.[234] There have also been two phase I/II studies of synthetic hypericin in HIV-infected subjects, investigating phototoxicity, pharmacokinetics and antiviral activity by oral or intravenous administration.[232,235] A consistent change in antiviral endpoints was not seen with intermittent intravenous dosing. Pharmacokinetic data indicated that chronic oral dosing would achieve sustained blood levels within an antiretroviral range.[232]

In patients with hepatitis C virus (HCV), purified hypericin had no impact on levels of HCV or liver enzymes.[236] Twelve patients received low-dose hypericin (0.05 mg/kg/day) for 2 months, while the remaining seven received high-dose hypericin (0.1 mg/kg/day) for 2 months. Seven of 12 patients receiving low-dose hypericin and all seven who received the high-dose hypericin developed side effects, predominantly photosensitivity reactions.

A tablet of Hypericum dry extract was compared with placebo in patients suffering from recurrent orofacial herpes (trial 1; 94 patients) or genital herpes (trial 2; 110 patients) in two separate double blind, randomised clinical trials.[237,238] For both trials, the total observation time was 90 days and patients received 3 tablets per day in symptom-free periods and 6 tablets a day during skin outbreaks. Each tablet contained 300 mg of dried extract standardised to contain 0.3% TH. The main measure of efficacy was a symptom score, calculated as a total of the severity ratings of major symptoms (such as presence and number of blisters, intensity of complaints, size of affected area) during the skin outbreak. The total symptom score was significantly lower in the Hypericum group compared with placebo in both trials. Average scores were 20.3 for the herb versus 32.1 for placebo for trial 1 and 15.6 versus 29.4 for trial 2. The herb also led to a superior reduction of the number of patients with herpetic episodes (skin sores) in both trials. Individual symptoms were also noticeably improved by the herbal treatment.

Antidepressant activity

Most studies on Hypericum in the context of depression have been conducted on major depressive disorder (MDD). According to the Diagnostic and Statistical Manual of Mental Disorders IV (DSM-IV),[239] major depression is characterised by at least five of the following symptoms occurring nearly every day over a 2-week period, including either depressed mood or loss of interest or pleasure: depressed mood, markedly diminished interest in most activities, significant weight loss or weight gain, insomnia or hypersomnia, psychomotor agitation or retardation, fatigue or loss of energy, feelings of worthlessness or excessive or inappropriate guilt, diminished ability to think or concentrate or indecisiveness and recurrent thoughts of death or suicide.

The antidepressant activity of many Hypericum extracts in MDD has been established in mild and moderate cases in observational studies, placebo-controlled trials and comparator studies with standard antidepressant medications. Even relatively early meta-analyses of randomised placebo-controlled clinical trials of Hypericum between 1996 and 2000, including up to a total of 2291 patients, reported that extracts of the herb were superior to placebo for the treatment of mild or moderately severe depressive disorders.[240,241,242] In later meta-analyses of placebo-controlled and comparator trials, superiority over placebo and equivalence to conventional antidepressants was also reported (see below).[240,243–246] In a 2000 systematic review of eight randomised controlled trials, Gaster and Holyroyd reported the absolute increase in response rate with Hypericum ranged from 23% to 55% higher than with placebo, but 6% to 18% lower than tricyclic antidepressants.[247] Other systematic reviews reported similar findings to the ones mentioned above.[248–250] Large-scale observational studies of patients with mild-to-moderate depression, including MDD, reported response rates between 65% and 100%.[251]

A Cochrane review published in 2008 of studies comparing Hypericum extracts with placebo or conventional

pharmaceutical antidepressant drugs supported its use in MDD.[243] A total of 29 trials (5489 patients) were included, with 18 of these being placebo-controlled[20,252–268] and 17 active-controlled trials.[256,261–266,269–278] The standard antidepressant drugs were the older tricyclics (maprotiline (one trial), imipramine (three trials) and amitriptyline (one trial)), and selective serotonin reuptake inhibitors (SSRIs, fluoxetine (six trials), sertraline (four trials), paroxetine (one trial) and citalopram (one trial)). The severity of MDD was identified as mild-to-moderate in 19 trials and moderate-to-severe in nine trials. Dosages ranged from 240 to 1800 mg/day Hypericum extract, but were mostly between 500 and 1200 mg/day.

The Hypericum preparations studied in the trials included LI 160 (Jarsin, Lichtwer Pharma, Berlin, Germany), HYP611 (Felis 650, Biocur Arzneimittel GmbH, Holzkirchern, Germany), STW3-1 (Stegerwald Arzneimittelwerk, Darmstadt, Germany), STW3-IV (Stegerwald), STW3-VI (Stegerwald), LoHyp-57 (Dr Werner Loges and Co., GmbH, Winsen, Germany), WS5572 (Schabe Pharmaceuticals, Karlsruhe, Germany), WS5573 (Schwabe), WS5570 (Schwabe), Iperisan (Labaratorio Marjan, Sao Paulo, Brazil), STEI 300 (Steiner Arzneimittel, Berlin, Germany), Ze117 (Max Zeller Sohn, Romanshorn, Switzerland) and Psychotonin Forte (Steigerwald).

The majority of trials were of high quality. Meta-analysis found that for the placebo controlled trials examined, patients receiving Hypericum extracts were significantly more likely to be responders (RR 1.48; 95% CI 1.23 to 1.77), although study results were highly heterogeneous (I^2 75%). For the comparator trials, there were no differences between the groups based on the Hamilton Depression Scale (HAM-D) pooled responder rate (RR) ratio 1.01 (95% CI 0.93 to 1.09; I^2 17% based on an intention-to-treat approach) and on the clinical global impressions (CGI), RR 1.01 (95% CI 0.94 to 1.09). Patients allocated to Hypericum were less likely to drop out of studies due to adverse events than patients allocated to either the older standard antidepressants or SSRIs. Side effects of Hypericum extracts were usually minor and uncommon.

Further details of some of the comparator studies reviewed in mild-to-moderate depression are included here. Hypericum extract LI 160 900 mg/day (2.7 mg/day TH equivalent) had comparable efficacy to amitriptyline 75 mg/day on HAM-D and CGI scores in 149 patients with mild-to-moderate MDD over a 6-week period.[273] In a 6-week comparator trial on mild-to-moderate major depression in 324 outpatients from psychiatric and general medical practices, ZE 117 500 mg/day (equivalent to 1 mg/day hypericin) was therapeutically equivalent to imipramine 150 mg/day, but better tolerated.[274] Similarly, an 8-week trial in 263 patients with moderate MDD found Hypericum extract STEI 300 at a dose of 1050 mg/day (0.2% to 0.3% TH and 2% to 3% hyperforin) to be more effective than placebo and at least as effective as imipramine 100 mg/day in 263 patients.[266] Hypericum extract LoHyp57 at a dose of 800 mg/day was shown to be equivalent to fluoxetine 20 mg/day in mild-to-moderate depression in 149 elderly patients aged 60 to 80 years. Hypericum reduced HAM-D scores from 16.6 to 7.91, while fluoxetine resulted in a reduction from 17.18 to 8.11.[276] In 251 outpatients with moderate-to-severe MDD, Hypericum WS 5572 (hydro-alcoholic extract 3:1 to 7:1 extract ratio; 1 mg to 2.5 mg/day TH) at an initial dose of 900 mg/day, increased to 1800 mg/day after 6 weeks in non-responders, was at least as effective as paroxetine and better tolerated. Hypericum resulted in a 57% reduction in HAM-D scores compared with a 45% reduction for the SSRI.[277]

Placebo-controlled studies covered by the Cochrane review include the following. A 6-week randomised, controlled trial with Hypericum extract WS 5572 at two doses, (600 mg/day and 1200 mg/day, 0.3% TH) in 332 patients with mild-to-moderate major depression found Hypericum to be superior to placebo (p<0.001) at both doses.[254] Hypericum extract STW 3-VI at 900 mg/day for 8 weeks was superior to placebo (p<0.001) in mild-to-moderate depression in 140 outpatients.[258] In a randomised, double blind trial, 102 outpatients with mild-to-moderate depression received either Hypericum extract LI 160 (2.7 mg/day TH equivalent) or placebo. The total Hamilton score in the Hypericum treatment group fell significantly (p<0.001) further after 4 weeks than in the placebo group.[252] The placebo group also responded favourably when switched to active treatment for 2 weeks.

In a study not included in the 2008 Cochrane review, Hypericum extract was found to be superior to placebo in patients with MDD with reversed vegetative signs (RVS) in an exploratory subgroup analysis of a 3-arm study.[279] A total of 135 patients were randomised to 12 weeks' treatment with Hypericum LI 160 (900 mg/day), fluoxetine (20 mg/day) or placebo. Patients with RVS were defined in two steps, according to the DSM-IV. First, patients with melancholy-related vegetative signs were excluded. Secondly, patients had to have at least one score of 2 for items 22 to 26 of the HAMD-28 scale, which are related to hypersomnia and hyperphagia. Twenty-seven patients remained in the group. Post-hoc analysis showed a trend to superiority of Hypericum compared with placebo and fluoxetine. Fluoxetine was not different from placebo.

Severe depression

Whilst most of the research has focused on mild-to-moderate depression, Hypericum extract has also been compared with imipramine for treatment of recurrent MDD in the absence of psychotic symptoms or delusions.[280] At the higher dose of 1800 mg (6:1 extraction ratio 10800 mg/day of herb), the extract LI 160 was found to be as effective as imipramine in improving symptoms of severe depression, and was better tolerated. More recently, Szegedi and colleagues[277] found WS 5572 extract at an initial dose of 900 mg, increased to 1800 mg/day in non-responders, to be at least as effective as paroxetine for moderate-to-severe major depression (HAM-D 17 entry score 22+ and 2+ on the depressive mood item; p=0.08 between groups) and to be better tolerated. The study used a hydro-alcoholic extract containing 3% to 6% hyperforin, equivalent to 2.7 to 5.4 mg, and having a 3:1 to 7:1 extract ratio.

Mild depression

A re-analysis of the original data from two double blind, randomised, placebo-controlled clinical trials and the acute phase of a long-term study found the Hypericum extract WS 5570 to be of benefit during the acute treatment of patients suffering from mild depression (according to DSM criteria), leading to a substantial increase in the probability of remission.[281] The re-analysis included 217 patients who had a pretreatment total score at most 20 points on the 17-item HAM-D. In patients treated with WS 5570, the HAM-D total score decreased by averages of 10.8 (600 mg/day), 9.6 (900 mg/day) and 10.7 (1200 mg/day) points, respectively, between the pretreatment baseline value and the end of acute treatment, compared with 6.8 points for the placebo group (p<0.01 for all pairwise comparisons against placebo). This corresponded to average relative decreases of 49% to 57% for WS 5570 and 36% for placebo. At the end of acute treatment 57% of the patients treated with 600 mg/day, 33% in the 900 mg/day group and 62% in the 1200 mg/day group, as well as 25% in the placebo group were in remission (HAM-D total score no more than 7 points).

Dysthymia versus non-dysthymic patients

A randomised controlled trial compared Hypericum extract PM235 with placebo in patients with minor depressive symptoms or dysthymia. Results suggested a greater sensitivity to Hypericum among non-dysthymic patients.[282] One hundred and fifty patients, aged 25 to 70 years, meeting the (ICD)-10 criteria for mild or moderately severe depressed episodes or with dysthymia, and having a 17-item HAM-D total score between 7 and 17, were randomly assigned to the extract or identical placebo. The active treatment was administered at 270 mg/day in a lower (0.12% hypericin) or a higher (0.18% hypericin) formulation. For the HAM-D, there was a non-significant trend towards a more frequent improvement in the non-dysthymic patients treated with Hypericum (p=0.057). The Beck Depression Inventory (BDI) criteria showed significance (p=0.045) for both doses of Hypericum compared with placebo. Pooling the high- and low-dose groups together, significant reductions for HAM-D and BDI criteria were found among non-dysthymic patients (p=0.03). Significant improvement in response to Hypericum was found in symptoms reflected by a visual analogue scale, again only in non-dysthymic patients (p=0.041). In a secondary analysis, pooling both treated groups concluded that Hypericum had a clinically significant effect in minor depressed patients with HAM-D up to 17. This finding was significant only in non-dysthymic patients.

Relapse prevention

A multicentre, randomised, double blind study showed that Hypericum extract WS 5570 and paroxetine, a potent SSRI, were similarly effective in preventing relapse in a continuation of treatment after recovery from an episode of moderate-to-severe depression, and pointed therefore to an important alternative treatment option for long-term relapse prevention.[283] Patients with a HAM-D (17-item) total score decrease of ≥50% during the 6 weeks of acute treatment were asked to continue the treatment for another 4 months. One hundred and thirty-three adult outpatients who received maintenance doses of 900 (n=33) or 1800 mg/day (n=38) of WS 5570, or 20 (n=28) or 40 mg/day (n=34) of paroxetine were included. Between baseline for the acute phase and the end of continuation treatment, the HAM-D total score decreased similarly in both groups. During maintenance treatment alone (day 154 versus day 42), 61.6% of the patients randomised to Hypericum and 54.6% treated with paroxetine showed an additional reduction (p=0.59) with respect to the HAM-D total score. Remission (HAM-D endpoint total score below 8) occurred in 81.6% (31) of the patients receiving the herbal extract and in 71.4% (30) for paroxetine (p=0.29). In the continuation phase there were 0.006 adverse events per day of exposure for Hypericum and 0.007 events per day for paroxetine.

Hypericum extract STW 3-VI was found to be more efficient at lowering the relapse and recurrence rates of responders when compared with citalopram and placebo.[284] In addition, the duration of response was increased in the group treated with Hypericum. A re-analysis was conducted using data obtained from 154 patients who responded in a randomised, multicentre, double blind, placebo-controlled study to 6 weeks of treatment for an episode of moderate depression with either 20 mg citalopram or 900 mg Hypericum extract.[284] In total, 30 (19.5%) of the 154 responders were diagnosed with a relapse. The number of patients who relapsed was highest in the citalopram group (14 of 54), while patients treated with the Hypericum extract showed the lowest relapse rate (8 of 54). Patients from the placebo group showed a relapse rate of 8 of 46. No difference in the severity of relapse was observed. The duration of response was longest for the Hypericum group (1817 days), intermediate for the citalopram group (1755 days) and shortest for the placebo group (802 days).

Depression with atypical features

A beneficial effect was found for the Hypericum extract LI 160 (600 mg/day) in depression with atypical features in a randomised, double blind, placebo-controlled, multicentre, parallel-group trial involving 200 patients.[285] Patients were recruited if they met the ICD-10 criteria for mild or moderate depression and had been diagnosed with atypical depression (DSM-IV includes the presence of mood reactivity, atypical vegetative features, hypersomnia and hyperphagia, leaden paralysis of the limbs and rejection sensitivity). Using the criterion of an absolute reduction in the HAMD-17, significance was achieved for Hypericum extract (p<0.05). No significant benefit was observed for the sum score of the atypical vegetative items of the HAMD-28. However, the sum score of the hypersomnia items (items 22 to 24) showed a significant superiority for Hypericum. Among moderately depressed patients, there was a highly significant benefit for the primary outcome variable. (A medium effect size of MW 0.64 (0.55, 0.72), p<0.01, was observed in moderately depressed patients compared with a small effect size of Mann-Whitney U test (MW) 0.55 (0.46, 0.65), p=0.25 in only mildly depressed participants.)

Observational studies

A systematic review of 16 large-scale observational studies involving a total of 34 804 patients (minimum of 100 participants per trial, range 101 to 11 296) found response rates (according to physician assessment) to vary between 65% and 100% for Hypericum extracts in the treatment of depressive disorders.[251] The majority of studies focused on mild-to-moderate depression, including MDD, but a limited number of severely depressed patients were included. The total number of different products tested was 12, and the daily extract dose ranged from 360 to 1200 mg. Observation periods ranged from 4 to 6 weeks, with the exception of two studies of 52 weeks. In these two studies, which investigated long-term effects (52 weeks), response rates were 60% and 69%, respectively, and the proportions of patients dropping out due to side effects were 3.4% and 5.7%. The tolerability and acceptability of tested extracts was reported to be very good, with no serious side effects or interactions reported in any study. The proportion of patients dropping out due to side effects varied between zero and 2.8%.

A long-term, open, multicentre study on the Hypericum extract Ze117 concluded it to be safe and effective for the treatment of mild-to-moderate depression over long periods of time, and potentially suitable for relapse prevention.[286] A total of 440 outpatients suffering from mild-to-moderate depression according to ICD-10 were treated for up to 1 year with 500 mg/day. Mean HAM-D scores decreased steadily from 20.58 at baseline to 12.07 at week 26 and to 11.18 at week 52. Mean CGI scores decreased from 3.99 to 2.20 at week 26 and 2.19 at week 52. Thirty of the reported adverse events (6%) were possibly or probably related to the treatment, most notably gastrointestinal and skin complaints. Long-term intake of up to 1 year of the study medication did not result in any changes in clinical chemistry and electrocardiogram recordings.

Juvenile depression

Three open label studies of Hypericum extracts for depressive disorders in children and adolescents have been conducted. One hundred and one children under 12 years with mild-to-moderate depressive symptoms were treated for a minimum of 4 weeks, with an extension to 6 weeks, with parental consent and medical practitioner recommendation.[287] The dosage of Hypericum extract LI 160 ranged from 300 to 1800 mg/day. The number of physicians rating efficacy as 'good' or 'excellent' was 72% after 2 weeks, 97% after 4 weeks and 100% after 6 weeks. (However, the final evaluation included only 76% of the initial sample.) Parental ratings concurred with physician ratings. Tolerability was good and no adverse events were reported.

An 8-week, prospective, open label pilot study examined Hypericum as a treatment for children diagnosed with MDD of at least moderate severity.[288] Of 33 enrolled children (mean age of 10.5±2.9 years) 25 met the response criteria of ≤28 on the Children's Depression Rating Scale-Revised and a CGI severity score ≤2 after 8 weeks of treatment. Patients were initially prescribed 450 mg/day; this dose was increased to 900 mg/day after 4 weeks in 22 children.

Similar findings were reported from an 8-week, open label study evaluating the potential efficacy and safety of Hypericum (900 mg/day, minimum 0.3% hypericin and 3% hyperforin) in adolescents with mild MDD.[289] Of the 11 patients who completed the study, nine (82%) showed significant clinical improvement based on CGI score changes (a treatment response was indicated by a clinical improvement rating of either very much improved or much improved at the final visit). Of the eight non-compliant patients who discontinued the study, four patients (50%) were much improved at week 8, and one patient was very much improved, based on the CGI score change.

Negative trials

Results of clinical trials on Hypericum for depression have not been unanimously favourable. In contrast to the positive results of many placebo-controlled trials,[252–255] Shelton and co-workers[257] found Hypericum (LI 160) to be ineffective for MDD when administered to 200 participants at a dose of 900 mg/day for 4 weeks, increasing to 1200 mg/day for the subsequent 4 weeks. A drug comparison study undertaken by the Hypericum Depression Trial Study Group[262] with an additional placebo arm did not support the superiority of the LI 160 extract of Hypericum over placebo for MDD. However, it is noteworthy that the comparative SSRI was also not superior to placebo in this patient cohort.

Several reasons have been proposed for the discrepancy in the findings between such studies. In their meta-analysis of studies on MDD, Linde and co-workers observed that trials from German-speaking countries reported more favourable findings than trials from other countries, more precise studies showed smaller effects, and higher baseline values were significantly associated with smaller effects sizes.[243]

Other suggested factors for the different findings include a lack of equivalence between preparations trialled.[243] Among the 16 large-scale observational studies in the previously cited review, Linde and Knuppel[251] found the total number of different products was 12, and the daily extract dose ranged from 360 to 1200 mg. However, a meta-analysis of 37 double blind, placebo-controlled trials on Hypericum found little evidence of an association between response and daily dosage and type of extract.[290]

Comparison of different extracts is confounded by several factors. Quantities of key marker constituents such as hypericin, hyperforin and the flavonoids can vary enormously between products. One study of Hypericum products on the German market showed that a number contain only minor amounts of bioactive constituents.[291] Most studies have tested Hypericum products standardised for TH content, as this was previously thought to confer the antidepressant activity. Relatively few specify the hyperforin content, variation in which could potentially account for different findings. An additional limitation is that hyperforin is most unstable in solution and rapidly decomposes at an acidic pH. Galenicals (liquid preparations) of Hypericum that are older than a few months contain no hyperforin at all.[292] Nonetheless, despite these variations, a 2010 review and meta-analysis of Hypericum extracts concluded that LI 160, WS 5572, WS 5570 and Ze 117 have all been shown to be significantly more effective than placebo and have similar efficacy to conventional antidepressants, with LI 160 having been most frequently studied.[293]

Several prognostic factors identified in different studies[251] may also impact on the variability of findings. Although not uniformly observed, these include severity of depression, with those with higher baseline HAM-D scores being less responsive,[290] age (older patients have shown slower improvement in some studies), co-existence of organic disease and concurrent psychotropic co-medication.[294]

On balance, evidence from clinical trials performed on Hypericum extracts support its use as a well-tolerated and effective alternative to standard antidepressants in the treatment of mild-to-moderate MDD, particularly when side effects with the drugs become intolerable to the patient. Patients should be treated long enough and with a sufficiently high daily dose of Hypericum extract, as defined by the various positive studies.

Anxiolytic activity

Anxiolytic clinical activity of Hypericum extracts has been reported in several published case studies as well as in clinical trials investigating a range of conditions, including MDD with co-morbid anxiety, somatoform complaints, obsessive-compulsive disorder, social phobia, irritable bowel syndrome, seasonal affective disorder, sleep disorders, premenstrual syndrome and menopause. (Refer to the relevant sections for further details of these studies.)

In 2001, Davidson and colleagues described three case reports of benefits of Hypericum extract (standardised to 0.3% TH) in generalised anxiety disorder (GAD) diagnosed by DSM-IV criteria.[295] Two of the patients had moderate anxiety and one marked anxiety. Not only did core GAD symptoms improve, but there was an improved ability to cope with daily stress and potential conflicts with others.

In a further three positive case reports by Kobak and colleagues in 2003, all patients were treatment naïve, and responded to initial treatment with Hypericum extracts.[296] In one case, the patient discontinued treatment due to adverse events and subsequently relapsed. In case 1, optimal treatment efficacy (e.g. much improved on both CGI and Patient Global Impressions of Improvement Scale, PGI) was obtained at 1350 mg/day and in cases 2 and 3 at 900 mg/day.

In a multicentre, placebo-controlled double blind trial, the effect of a highly concentrated Hypericum preparation was investigated on 97 depressed outpatients at doses of 200 to 240 mg/day. The preparation showed an anxiolytic effect on the State-Trait Anxiety Inventory of 38% (STAI X1) and 39% (STAI X2), compared with the placebo, which reduced anxiety by only 19% (STAI X1) and 20% (STAI X2).[260]

Superiority was shown for LI 160 on anxiety measured on the Hamilton Anxiety Scale (HAM-A) in an 8-week, randomised, double blind, placebo-controlled, multicentre parallel-group trial evaluating the efficacy of Hypericum extract LI 160 (600 mg/day) in 200 patients who met the ICD-10 criteria for mild or moderate depression and had been diagnosed with atypical depression (p=0.01).[285] LI 160 was also superior to placebo on the Patient Health Questionnaire (PHQ)-9 (p<0.01) and Clinical Global Impressions-Improvement (CGI-I) scale (p=0.01).

A combination of Hypericum and *Piper methysticum* (kava) failed to outperform placebo in a randomised, controlled crossover trial in patients with MDD and co-morbid anxiety.

Standardised Hypericum tablets (3/day, each containing 1.8 g dried herb equivalent containing 990 µg TH, 9 mg hyperforin and 15 mg flavonoid glycosides), and kava (2.66 g three times daily standardised to 50 mg kava lactones) or placebo were administered to 28 participants in a crossover design, with two controlled 4-week phases.[297]

The Hypericum extract LI 160 was found to be superior to placebo in somatisation disorder, independent of depressive symptomatology. In a 6-week multicentre, randomised, controlled trial with 151 patients suffering from somatisation disorder (ICD-10: F45.0), undifferentiated somatoform disorder (F45.1) or somatoform autonomic dysfunctions (F45.3), Hypericum was superior to placebo on the Hamilton Anxiety Scale, sub-factor Somatic Anxiety (HAMA-SOM) (p=0.001).[298]

These findings were subsequently confirmed in a prospective, randomised, placebo-controlled, double blind, parallel group study involving 184 outpatients with somatisation disorder (ICD-10: F45.0), undifferentiated somatoform disorder (F45.1) and somatoform autonomic dysfunction (F45.3), but not major depression.[299] Patients received either 600 mg/day Hypericum extract LI 160 or placebo for 6 weeks. In the intention-to-treat population (n=173) for each of six primary efficacy measures, superiority of Hypericum over placebo was demonstrated (p<0.0001).

In a randomised, controlled trial in patients with social phobia, no significant difference was found between Hypericum and placebo on the Liebowitz Social Anxiety Scale (p=0.27). Forty patients with generalised social anxiety disorder without co-morbid depression were randomised to 12 weeks of treatment with a flexible dose (600 to 1800 mg/day) of Hypericum extract LI 160 (n=20) or placebo (n=20).[300]

Obsessive-compulsive disorder

In an open label exploratory study, 12 patients with a primary DSM-IV diagnosis of obsessive-compulsive disorder (OCD) of at least 12 months' duration were administered a fixed dose of 900 mg/day LI 160 (extended-release formulation) for 12 weeks. A significant change from baseline to week 12 on the Yale-Brown Obsessive Compulsive Scale (Y-BOCS) was observed, with a mean change of 7.4 points (p=0.001). Five (42%) of 12 were rated 'much' or 'very much' improved on the clinician-rated CGI-I scale, six (50%) were 'minimally' improved and one (8%) had 'no change'.[301]

However, such findings were not replicated in a subsequent 12-week randomised controlled trial in 60 patients with OCD using a standardised Hypericum extract (LI 160) at a flexible dose of 600 to 1800 mg/day.[302] There was no significant difference between the mean change on the total Y-BOCS with Hypericum treatment (3.43) and placebo (3.60) (p=0.899), or on any of the subscales.

Seasonal affective disorder

In a postal open label survey of mild-to-moderate seasonal affective disorder (SAD), Hypericum extract LI 160 (900 mg/day) for 8 weeks was compared with the same formulation in addition to light therapy. Significant improvements

were observed in anxiety, loss of libido and insomnia in both groups. No significant between-group differences were observed on any measure except for sleep, which improved more in the Hypericum plus light group (p<0.01). On an 11-item rating scale, the mean score in the 168 patients using Hypericum alone fell from 21.3 at baseline to 13 at endpoint (p<0.001), while the corresponding figures for the 133 patients using Hypericum plus light therapy were 20.6 and 11.8, respectively (p<0.001), suggesting Hypericum may be an effective treatment for SAD.[303]

In an earlier preliminary, single blind trial, 20 patients with SAD were randomised to receive Hypericum extract (2.7 mg/day TH equivalent) combined with either bright or dim light therapy for 4 weeks. A significant reduction of HAM-D scores was observed in both light groups, but with no significant difference between them. The favourable response in the dim light group suggested Hypericum may be an efficient therapy in patients with SAD, as well as in combination with light therapy.[304] In another similar single blind trial, 4 weeks' treatment with Hypericum extract (2.7 mg/day TH equivalent) was associated with a significant reduction in the total Hamilton score. There was no significant additional advantage for bright light treatment over Hypericum.[305]

Menopause-related symptoms

A 12-week monitoring study on a Hypericum liquid (60 drops/day) in 40 patients compared its efficacy to diazepam (6 mg/day) in 20 patients with climacteric anxiety and depression.[306] On the HAM-A, scores reduced by 72% with Hypericum compared with 37% for diazepam. On the Self-rating Depression Scale, scores reduced by 46% and 31% respectively, suggesting a beneficial effect on both anxiety and depression associated with menopause.

In an open, observational study of 111 'pre-' (presumably peri-) and postmenopausal women aged between 43 and 65 years, Hypericum LI 160 was found to significantly improve the psychological (irritability, depressive moods, inner tension, anxiety, sleep and concentration disorders) and somatic symptoms of menopause (hot flushes, sweating, palpitations, dizziness, headaches).[307] The total daily dose was 405 to 675 mg extract, standardised to 0.9 mg hypericin, for 12 weeks. On the self-designed sexuality assessment scale, significant improvements were found in the feeling of attractiveness (p<.0.001) and participants' rating of the importance of sexuality (p<0.001).

A pilot double blind, randomised, controlled trial investigated an ethanolic Hypericum extract (2700 mg/day) against placebo in 47 perimenopausal breast cancer survivors aged 40 to 65 years, experiencing three or more hot flushes per day.[308] After 12 weeks, a non-significant difference favouring the Hypericum group was observed in the daily hot flush frequency (p=0.10). Women on the active treatment reported significantly better menopause-specific quality of life (p=0.01) and significantly fewer sleep problems (p=0.05) compared with the placebo group.

A trial involving 100 women investigated a liquid extract of Hypericum for its impact on hot flushes.[309] The drops, administered three times daily at an unspecified dose, contained hypericin at 0.2 mg/mL. After 8 weeks, the frequency of hot flushes decreased by 54% with Hypericum compared with 32% for placebo (p<0.001), duration decreased 51% and 23%, respectively (p<0.001) and severity decreased 60% and 26%, respectively (p<0.001).

A combination of Hypericum and *Vitex agnus-castus* was studied in a 16-week randomised, controlled trial involving 100 late-perimenopausal and postmenopausal women.[310] No significant effect was found for the herbal combination over placebo on vasomotor symptoms (p=0.42), Greene Climacteric scores (p=0.13) or depressed mood (p<0.42). However, both arms showed significant improvements from baseline on all outcome measures of vasomotor symptoms (p<0.001 and p<0.01 for placebo and study groups, respectively), depressed mood and overall menopausal symptoms measured on the Greene Climacteric Scale, (p<0.001 for both groups). Based on current evidence for their pharmacology, a negative interaction between the two herbs seems unlikely.

Several studies support the benefit of Hypericum in combination with *Actaea racemosa* (black cohosh) for menopausal complaints.[311–315] In a double blind, placebo-controlled trial of 301 women experiencing menopausal complaints with a pronounced psychological component, the combination was significantly superior to placebo (p<0.001).[311] The dosage regime was two tablets twice daily for 8 weeks, reducing to one tablet twice daily for the following 8 weeks. Each tablet contained Hypericum extract equivalent 245 to 350 mg herb, standardised to 0.25 mg TH and Actaea extract equivalent 22.5 to 41.25 mg rootstock, standardised to 1 mg triterpene glycosides. The mean decrease in scores on the Menopause Rating Scale from baseline to week 16 was 50% in the treatment group, compared with 19.6% in the placebo group (p<0.001). The HAM-D score decreased by 41.8% in the treatment group and 12.7% in the placebo group (p<0.001).

A 6-week double blind, randomised controlled trial of the same combination in 179 women found significant improvement of 'psychovegetative' menopausal symptoms such as anxiety, impaired drive, depressive mood, nervousness and irritability, as well as good tolerability and compliance.[312] Symptoms rated on the Kupperman Index (KI) fell from 31.4 to 18.7 (40% reduction) in the treatment group, compared with 30.3 to 22.3 (26% reduction) in the placebo group (p<0.001).

A large-scale prospective, controlled, open label observational study of 6141 women in Germany investigated the effectiveness and safety of Actaea alone for neurovegetative symptoms, and in fixed combination with Hypericum for more pronounced mood complaints.[314] The effectiveness and tolerability profiles of both therapies were supported. For the alleviation of mood symptoms, the fixed combination of Actaea with Hypericum was superior to Actaea alone (p<0.001). The Psych and Hot Flushes subscales showed the greatest improvements for both therapies. Improvement was maintained at 6 and 12 months for both treatments.

A multicentre trial involving 89 symptomatic peri- or postmenopausal women investigated the effect of a combination of Hypericum and Actaea extracts (a 264 mg tablet containing 0.0364 mL extract of Actaea rhizome, equivalent to 1 mg triterpene glycosides, and 84 mg dried extract of Hypericum equivalent to 0.25 mg TH) over 12 weeks.[315] The herbal combination was shown to be superior to placebo for hot flushes (p=0.021) and overall menopausal symptoms rated on the KI (p<0.001).

Premenstrual syndrome

A pilot study involving 19 women suffering at least 6 consecutive months of premenstrual syndrome (PMS) found that Hypericum significantly reduced the severity of symptoms.[316] This open, observational study of Hypericum extract (LI 160) found significant reductions in all outcome measures after treatment for two cycles with Hypericum tablets standardised to 900 µg TH per day. The Mood subscale (as opposed to Pain, Physical and Behaviour), however, showed the most improvement. Hypericum was found to be effective and well-tolerated in alleviating symptoms of moderate-to-severe PMS of 6 months or more duration in 170 women in a randomised, double blind, placebo-controlled study.[317] Hypericum tablets (2.68 mg/day TH, extract not specified) or placebo were administered for 8 weeks (two menstrual cycles). Anxiety (mood swings, anxiety or nervous tension/irritability), hydration (breast tenderness, swelling of extremities or weight gain), depression (depression, crying, forgetfulness or insomnia) and craving (increased appetite, headache or fatigue) were evaluated daily on scale of 1 (not at all) to 6 (extreme). Treatment with Hypericum resulted in significantly lower PMS scores compared with baseline (p<0.001) and compared to placebo (p<0.001). The greatest improvements occurred for symptoms of crying (71%) and depression (52%).

Hypericum (LI 160, 900 mg/day) was found to be superior to placebo for some symptoms of mild PMS in a randomised, double blind, placebo-controlled, crossover study with 36 regularly cycling women aged 18 to 45 years.[318] Hypericum was statistically superior to placebo in improving physical and behavioural symptoms (p<0.05), but not mood- or pain-related symptoms. There was no difference between groups in terms of plasma hormone (FSH, LH, oestradiol, progesterone, prolactin and testosterone) or cytokine (IL-1beta, IL-6, IL-8, interferon-gamma and TNF-alpha) levels, nor weekly reports of anxiety, depression, aggression and impulsivity measured on the State Anxiety Inventory, Beck Depression Inventory, Aggression Questionnaire and Barratt Impulsiveness Scale.

A double blind, placebo-controlled, randomised trial was conducted with 70 university students with premenstrual syndrome.[319] Hypericum (extract not specified) (60 drops for 7 days prior to onset of menstruation) was administered for two complete menstrual cycles. Active treatment resulted in a mean reduction in daily symptom ratings of 46.45% compared with 18.1% for placebo. There were significant reductions in all symptoms between the two groups.

However, superiority over placebo was not found for Hypericum in a placebo-controlled trial conducted in 125 normally menstruating women who experienced recurrent PMS.[320] The primary endpoint was anxiety-related symptoms recorded in a menstrual diary based on Abraham's classification. Although both groups improved significantly in all symptom subgroups (p<0.007 for both groups), there was no difference between treatments (p≥0.57 for all symptom subgroups).

A small study of PMS-like symptoms in late-perimenopausal women investigated the combination of Hypericum (extract equivalent to 5400 mg/day dried herb standardised to contain 2.97 mg TH, 27 mg hyperforin and 54 mg flavonoid glycosides) with Vitex (extract equivalent to dried fruit 1000 mg/day).[321] At the end of the 16-week treatment phase, the herbal combination was significantly superior to placebo on Abraham's Menstrual Symptoms Questionnaire total PMS scores (p=0.02), PMS-D (p=0.006) and PMS-C clusters (p=0.027). The active treatment group also showed significant reductions from baseline in the anxiety (p=0.003) and hydration (p=0.002) clusters.

A case report of premenstrual dysphoric disorder treated with Hypericum extract (900 mg/day) indicated much improvement in symptoms at the 5-month follow-up.[322]

Cognitive activity

In a randomised, double blind trial, the effect of Hypericum extract (2.7 mg/day TH equivalent) was compared with maprotiline on resting EEG and evoked potentials in 24 healthy volunteers. Improved cognitive functions were observed, particularly for Hypericum treatment.[135]

However, no effect on cognitive function was observed in a randomised, double blind, crossover study in 12 healthy male volunteers, administered oral doses of 255 to 285 mg Hypericum extract (900 μg TH content) three times daily for a period of 14 days. No increase was observed in theta power density on qEEG, and Hypericum did not affect heart rate variability.[323]

Hypericum (900 mg or 1800 mg) had no effect on cognitive and psychomotor performance 1, 2 and 4 hours after administration in 13 healthy volunteers in a double blind, placebo-controlled trial in which it was compared with amitriptyline 25 mg. Amitriptyline impaired performance in a battery of psychological tests, while a dose-related impairment was only observed on the digit symbol substitution test with Hypericum.[324]

In a double blind, crossover, repeated-measures design, acute administration of standardised Hypericum extract (900 mg and 1800 mg) to 12 healthy young volunteers showed no nootropic effects. At the higher dose, there was even some evidence it caused impairment of numeric working memory and picture recognition.[325]

Irritable bowel syndrome

Hypericum extract (900 mg/day) was administered to 30 women with irritable bowel syndrome (IBS) and 20 healthy women. After 8 weeks of treatment, HAM-A and HAM-D scores had significantly reduced in the IBS group compared with pretreatment (p<0.05). Low frequency band/high frequency band ratio (a measure of sympathovagal balance) also showed a significant decrease (p<0.05), and gastrointestinal symptoms of pain and bloating were also significantly relieved (p<0.05). These open label results suggested that Hypericum treatment may be of value in the psychological and autonomic reactivity to stress in patients with IBS.[326]

However, these findings were not replicated in a randomised, placebo-controlled trial of Hypericum extract at a dose of 450 mg/day for 12 weeks in 70 participants with an established diagnosis of IBS according to the Rome Criteria II. Both groups reported decreases in overall bowel symptom scores from baseline, with the placebo arm having significantly lower scores at 12 weeks (p=0.03) than Hypericum.[327]

Sexual function

A double blind, randomised, placebo-controlled study of Hypericum extract 160 mg tablets in 50 married men (aged 18 to 50 years) with premature ejaculation found the herb to be statistically superior to placebo in intravaginal ejaculatory latency time (IELT) (p<0.001) after 4 weeks.[328] There was a significant increase in intercourse satisfaction and overall satisfaction in the Hypericum group (p<0.001).

A pilot study found that a hyperforin-containing extract of Hypericum increased the duration of sexual intercourse and improved sexual satisfaction in 16 men (average age 35.0±4.6 years) with and without complaints of premature ejaculation.[329] A rapidly dissolving oral tablet formulated with a 20 mg dose of hyperforin was administered at least 15 to 30 minutes before intercourse over a 4-week period. There was a significant increase in mean IELT time from 246±29 to 331±34 seconds (p<0.002) in participants taking the extract. Fourteen of 16 men (87.5%) reported an improvement in IELT, which was seen in men both with and without premature ejaculation. There was also a significant increase in the average male satisfaction score from 3.8±0.27 to 4.25±0.21 (p<0.03). The female satisfaction score also showed a significant increase from 4.9±0.27 to 5.2±0.23 (p<0.04). No systemic or adverse effects on erectile function or orgasm were reported.

Mean time to ejaculation increased with the administration of hyperforin-containing extract to men with premature ejaculation. Ten male volunteers took the above rapid release formulation for 8 weeks.[330] In five men with mean ejaculatory duration at baseline of less than 90 seconds, four reported a benefit (mean time to ejaculation before and after treatment, 58±12 seconds and 131±23 seconds, respectively). In men with ejaculation times greater than 3 minutes at baseline, the mean sexual intercourse duration increased from 266±30 to 391±34 seconds (p=0.02). No adverse effects on sexual function and systemic side effects were reported. Seven of 10 couples reported subjective global sexual satisfaction improvement for both partners after the herbal extract. Five couples reported more frequent female orgasm.

Attention-deficit hyperactivity disorder

In a small, open trial, Hypericum was investigated for attention-deficit hyperactivity disorder (ADHD) in three 14- to 16-year-old male psychiatric outpatients. Hypericum extract 30 mg/day (extract not specified) was administered for 4 weeks, and a placebo for a further 4 weeks.[331] Patients' mean scores improved on the Conner Scale for hyperactivity (which decreased from 13 to 7), inattention (from 14 to 9) and immaturity factors, and the total score (from 27 to 16). Placebo scores were similar to those at baseline. However,

Hypericum was not associated with an improvement on the Continuous Performance Test. This study is limited by the sample size, but suggests that Hypericum warrants further investigation for the treatment for ADHD.

In an earlier trial, administration of Hypericum for the treatment of ADHD over the course of 8 weeks did not improve symptoms in a randomised, double blind, placebo-controlled trial involving 54 children aged 6 to 17 years who met the DSM-IV criteria for ADHD.[332] Participants were randomised to receive 300 mg/day of Hypericum extract (standardised to 0.3% TH) or placebo. No significant differences were observed in the change of ADHD Rating Scale-IV score, hyperactivity or the CGI. However, it was reported that post-trial testing of the product used found it contained only 0.13% hypericin and 0.14% hyperforin, raising the question of appropriate quality of manufacture as well as adequate dosing.[333]

Wound healing and skin disorders (topical application)

A randomised, controlled trial with 144 women following caesarean section found that topical application of Hypericum cream (20% oily extract in 80% petroleum jelly, oily extract prepared from one part powder of flowering tops in three parts grape seed oil) facilitated wound healing and minimised scar formation, pain and pruritus.[334] Application of the Hypericum cream was commenced 24 h post-surgery and continued for 16 days, three times daily. Significant differences in wound healing on the 10th day, and scar formation on the 40th day postpartum, were demonstrated for the treatment group compared with placebo (p<0.002) and natural history control groups (p<0.008) using the REEDA scale (redness, oedema, ecchymosis, discharge and approximation), the Vancouver Scar Scale (pigmentation, height, pliability and vascularity) and a visual analogue scale. There was no significant difference between placebo and the natural history control groups (p=0.93).

Oily extracts of Hypericum and *Calendula officinalis* were evaluated for their tissue regenerating effect on surgical wounds in 24 women who had undergone caesarean section during childbirth.[335] The extracts were made from plants collected during the months of May to July in rural areas in the countryside of Cagliari (Sardinia) by crushing and maceration in wheat germ oil in the proportion of 320:1000 (flowering tops/oil, g/g). Topical application of a mixture of 70% oily extract of Hypericum and 30% oily extract of Calendula reduced the surface perimeter area of the surgical wound by 37.6±9.9% compared with a reduction of 15.83±4.64% in the control group after twice daily administration for 16 consecutive days.

In a randomised, placebo-controlled, double blind, half-side comparison trial in 21 patients, a cream containing 5% of a lipophilic Hypericum extract (standardised to 1.5% hyperforin) showed a significant superiority over placebo (p<0.05) for the topical treatment of subacute mild-to-moderate atopic dermatitis (mean score on the Score of Atopic Dermatitis Index 44.5).[336] Skin colonisation with *Staphylococcus aureus* was reduced by both verum and placebo, showing a trend to better antibacterial activity for the Hypericum cream (p=0.064).

A phase II, placebo-controlled clinical study found topical hypericin with visible light photodynamic therapy to be an effective and well-tolerated alternative to standard psoralen plus UVA treatment of patch/plaque phase mycosis fungoides and plaque-type psoriasis vulgaris.[337] After 6 weeks of twice-weekly topical applications followed 24 hours later by exposure to visible light at 8 to 20 J/cm^2, several concentrations of hypericin resulted in a significant improvement of treated skin lesions amongst the majority of patients with cutaneous T cell lymphoma and psoriasis, whereas the placebo vehicle was ineffective.

A prospective study investigated the efficacy of PDT after topical application of an extract of Hypericum in actinic keratosis, basal cell carcinoma (BCC) and morbus Bowen (carcinoma in situ) in 34 patients. Eight patients had actinic keratoses (AKs), 21 had BCC and five had Bowen's disease.[338] For an average of 6 weeks, the extract of Hypericum (0.07% TH) was applied on the skin lesions and 10 mm surrounding the lesion in a 1 mm thick layer under an occlusive dressing for 2 hours, followed by irradiation with 75 J/cm^{-2} of red light. Complete clinical response was observed in 50% of patients with the AKs, 28% with superficial BCC and 40% with Bowen's disease. There was only a partial remission seen in patients with nodular BCCs. A complete disappearance of tumour cells was found in the histological preparations of 11% of patients with superficial BCCs and 80% with Bowen's disease. All patients complained of burning and pain sensations during irradiation.

Pain relief

A double blind, randomised, placebo-controlled, single-centre study evaluated the effect of systemic Hypericum extract, 900 mg/day (containing 0.31% TH and 3.0% hyperforin) for 12 weeks in 39 patients with burning mouth syndrome.[339] No significant improvement was noted in pain using a visual analogue scale for either group. However, after 4 weeks of therapy, patients taking the Hypericum extracts reported the burning sensation at significantly fewer oral sites compared with patients on placebo (p=0.036).

A randomised, double blind, placebo-controlled, crossover trial involving 54 patients over 5 weeks reported no significant effect on pain in polyneuropathy, but there was a trend towards a lower total pain score with Hypericum extract (total daily dose of 2.7 mg TH) (p=0.05) compared with placebo. Complete, good or moderate pain relief was experienced by nine patients with Hypericum and two with placebo (p=0.07).[340]

Sleep disorders

The *British Herbal Pharmacopoeia* (1983) lists *Hypericum perforatum* as a herbal sedative.[1]

Sleep disorders, as well as anxiety and depressive agitation, were reduced by Hypericum (Ze 117 extract, 500 mg/day) in patients suffering from mild-to-moderate depression with anxiety symptoms in a multicentre prospective, randomised, double blind trial (n=240) conducted over 6 weeks.[341] There was a marked decrease of depressive agitation (pre/post comparison: 46%), anxiety symptoms (44%) and sleep disorders

(43%) during the therapy with Hypericum, suggesting it is particularly effective in depressive patients suffering from anxiety symptoms.

The effects of treatment with Hypericum extract LI 160 at higher doses (900 mg/day, 2.7 mg/day TH equivalent) on sleep quality and well-being were investigated in a randomised, controlled, crossover trial over a 4-week period with 12 older (59.8±4.8 years), healthy volunteers. Analysis of slow-wave EEG activities showed the herb induced an increase of deep sleep during the total sleeping period, although no benefit was found for onset of sleep, sleep duration or intermittent awakenings, which implies it did not exert sedative activity.[342] The interference with REM sleep phases typical for tricyclic antidepressants and MAO inhibitors did not occur with Hypericum.[94]

As noted earlier, some evidence of an improvement in sleep was observed in an open, observational study of patients with menopausal symptoms involving 111 women aged between 43 and 65 years.[307]

Drug-dependency syndromes

One open label clinical trial suggested a benefit for a Hypericum herbal infusion used in combination with rational psychotherapy of depressive manifestations in 57 outpatients with alcoholism and concomitant digestive problems.[343] After one glass four to five times daily over a period of 2 months, it was concluded that the combination was effective for alcoholism in patients with peptic ulcer disease and chronic gastritis.

Results of a one-arm, phase II feasibility study suggested a role for Hypericum in maintaining smoking cessation. The 12-week quit rate was 37.5% (9/24) in 24 evaluable participants with administration of standardised Hypericum extract, (80% methanol extract standardised to 0.3% TH and a minimum of 4% hyperforin) at an oral dose of 900 mg/day in conjunction with cessation counselling messages.[344]

The effect of Hypericum extract Ze117 (500 mg/day) was compared to a transdermal nicotine patch in an open clinical trial on smoking cessation.[345] Participants in both groups decreased the number of cigarettes smoked per day over the study treatment period, and four (of 17) in the herbal group, compared with six (of 14) on the nicotine patches, succeeded in quitting.

Hypericum extract was investigated for its impact on nicotine withdrawal in a clinical study in which 45 adult smokers were randomised to receive an oral spray containing either Hypericum extract or placebo in addition to nicotine replacement therapy.[346] After 1 month the abstinence rate was identical in both groups. Craving scores, anxiety, restlessness and sleeplessness were lower in the Hypericum treated group.

However, other more rigorous studies have failed to support the benefits of Hypericum extracts in smoking cessation or withdrawal symptoms. In a factorial design, the effects of Hypericum extract (900 mg/day, LI 160) and chromium, alone or in combination, were compared with placebo for smoking cessation over 14 weeks. No significant effect was observed on absolute quit rates or tobacco withdrawal symptoms.[347]

Similarly, a three-arm, dose-ranging randomised, controlled trial found no significant differences in abstinence rates at 12

and 24 weeks between verum and placebo, or attenuation of withdrawal symptoms among abstinent participants. A total of 118 previous smokers were randomly allocated to receive 300 or 600 mg of a Hypericum extract (standardised to 0.3% hypericin) or a matching placebo tablet three times a day, combined with a behavioural intervention for 12 weeks.[348]

In an open, uncontrolled, pilot study, Hypericum extract LI 160 (300 or 600 mg/day for 1 week before and 3 months after a target quit date) plus individual motivational/behavioural support failed to show benefit as an aid to smoking cessation in 28 smokers of 10 or more cigarettes per day.[349] At 3 months, the point prevalence and continuous abstinence rates were both 18%, and at 12 months they were zero.

Other conditions

In a preliminary open trial, low dose Hypericum extract was modestly effective in the short-term treatment of irritability in some patients with autistic disorder.[350] Three male patients with autistic disorder, diagnosed by ICD-10 criteria, were administered Hypericum (extract not specified) 20 mg/day for 4 weeks. Participants were included in the study if their eye contact and expressive language were inadequate for their developmental level, and if they had not tolerated or responded to other psychopharmacological treatments (methylphenidate, clonidine or desipramine). Parent and mentor ratings on the Aberrant Behaviour Checklist, irritability, stereotypy and inappropriate speech factors improved slightly during treatment with Hypericum. Clinician ratings (Psychiatric Rating Scale Autism, Anger and Speech Deviance factors; Global Assessment Scale; Clinical Global Impressions efficacy) did not improve significantly. Limitations of this study included the small sample size, the low dose of Hypericum used and the short trial duration.

One hundred and sixty patients suffering from depression completed a randomised, double blind, multicentre study investigating the electrocardiographic (ECG) effects of high-dose Hypericum treatment (1800 mg extract, 5.4 mg TH) compared with imipramine. Analysis of conduction intervals and pathological findings indicated that, for the treatment of patients with a pre-existing conductive dysfunction or elderly patients, high-dose Hypericum extract was safer with regard to cardiac function than tricyclic antidepressants.[351]

Toxicology and other safety data

Toxicology

Hypericum has very low toxicity. Animals given 2 g/kg per day of dried Hypericum for up to 1 year showed no signs of any toxic changes.[352,353]

Hypericism is a state of sensitivity to sunlight caused by the ingestion of certain *Hypericum* species rich in hypericin-type pigments that are transferred by the bloodstream to the skin. As a disease of livestock, it affects unpigmented portions of the skin of sheep, cattle, horses, goats and swine, depressing the CNS and rendering them hypersensitive to temperature change and handling. Goats are the most resistant.[5,354] *Hypericum perforatum* is more phototoxic to grazing animals if ingested at flowering than when young or dry. The minimum phototoxic dose of foliage for cattle and sheep is approximately 1% and 4% of live weight respectively (about 10 and 40 g/kg). There was a variation observed in susceptibility within a herd.[354] Intragastric doses of 3 g/kg or more of dried *Hypericum perforatum* aerial parts produced photosensitisation in 4- to 6-month-old calves. The first symptoms appeared 3 to 4 h after exposure to the sun. Two calves that had been given the same dose, but not exposed to sunlight, passed soft faeces but showed no other clinical signs. A single dose of 1 g/kg produced no detectable effect when the calves were exposed to sunlight.[355]

There have been no reliable reported cases of hypericism in humans taking oral doses of Hypericum. The usual therapeutic doses of Hypericum extract are about 30 to 50 times below that needed to induce phototoxicity in calves.[356]

Genotoxicity tests showed no mutagenic effects following Hypericum administration.[357,358]

Contraindications

Hypericum is a safe and effective alternative to conventional antidepressants in the treatment of mild-to-moderate depression. However, it is not suited for the treatment of serious depression with psychotic symptoms, suicidal risk or signs and symptoms that are so severe that they do not allow the patient's family or work involvements to continue. However, in these cases, Hypericum may be a valuable adjunct to other therapy such as drug therapy and psychotherapy, despite some concerns expressed regarding its potential negative interactions with antidepressant drugs.

Hypericum should be avoided in patients with known sensitivity to St John's wort or any of its constituents.

(See the Interactions section below and Appendix C for a discussion and list of drugs that are contraindicated with Hypericum, and vice versa.)

Special warnings and precautions

Hypericum is not advisable in cases of known photosensitivity, or in patients taking photosensitising agents. (Refer to the Side effects section below.) It is recommended that patients on higher doses of Hypericum (2.7 mg/day or more of TH equivalent) do not spend excessive amounts of time in the full sun, especially in tropical or subtropical climates, and avoid artificial UVA irradiation. However, total avoidance of sunlight is not advisable, because some activities of Hypericum may be associated with its photosensitising activity.

Avoidance of foods that interact with MAO-inhibiting drugs, such as tyramine-containing foods (cheeses, beer and wine) and drugs such as L-dopa is not necessary. If a significant response in depressive disorders is not apparent after 4 to 6 weeks, the treatment should be discontinued and other forms of treatment implemented.

Clinicians should avoid dispensing the sediment from Hypericum liquid extracts, as it may be linked to adverse events.

Use cautiously in patients with a history of mania or hypomania (as in bipolar disorder) due to the possibility of Hypericum-induced manic episodes.[278,359–366]

Hypericum supplements should be discontinued at least 1 week prior to surgery requiring anaesthetic due to the risk of delayed anaesthesia,[367] or delayed emergence from anaesthesia.[368]

Interactions

See Appendix C for an extensive list of potential herb-drug interactions for Hypericum that are deemed clinically relevant, together with appropriate recommendations. What follows here is a discussion of the likely mechanisms and issues involved in these interactions.

The drug interactions described or speculated in the literature for Hypericum broadly fall into two main categories. The first category is the well-described metabolic or pharmacokinetic interactions, where Hypericum decreases the plasma levels (and hence efficacy) of a variety of drugs. The second category is the pharmacodynamic interactions, where Hypericum is thought to augment or destabilise the effects of prescribed antidepressant drugs, especially the SSRIs (selective serotonin reuptake inhibitors).

Metabolic drug interactions

The metabolic interaction of the herb Hypericum with a range of pharmaceutical drugs is both widely known and well documented. The list of interacting drugs is now quite extensive and includes the anticancer drug irinotecan, the antidepressant amitriptyline, the anticoagulants phenprocoumon and warfarin, the antihistamine fexofenadine, the sedatives alprazolam and midazolam, protease inhibitors, cyclosporin, digoxin, statin drugs, methadone and several oral contraceptives (see also Appendix C).[369] These clinically documented metabolic or pharmacokinetic interactions appear to rely on the capacity of Hypericum to induce faster metabolism of the drug, resulting in lower blood concentrations and compromised drug efficacy.[369] Mechanistic studies suggest that Hypericum is a potent inducer of the cytochrome P450 (CYP) enzyme CYP3A4 (and perhaps other CYPs) and the drug transporter P-glycoprotein (P-gp). This results in increased breakdown and/or reduced intestinal uptake of the drug in question.[369]

It was not long after the first documented cases of the metabolic drug interactions for Hypericum that the evidence emerged that one phytochemical constituent could be largely responsible for this effect. This constituent is hyperforin, a notoriously unstable compound that is only found in some *Hypericum* subspecies, such as *Hypericum perforatum* subsp. *perforatum*.[370] For example, in 2001 a letter by Kroll and co-workers to the journal *Alternative Therapies* already highlighted the importance of hyperforin in causing the drug interactions.[371]

The most compelling case for the culpability of hyperforin came from receptor studies, where it was shown that hyperforin is a potent activator of the pregnane or steroid X receptor. This significant discovery was made in 2000 by two independent research teams.[372,373] The human steroid X receptor (SXR) is activated by a wide range of endogenous and synthetic steroids, and its counterpart in mice is the pregnane X receptor (PXR).[373] However, it is now recognised that the SXR is also activated by other drugs and results in potent induction of CYP3A enzymes, including CYP3A4.[373] In fact PXR and SXR function to protect the body against foreign chemicals or xenobiotics. In an article in the prestigious journal *Science*, the CYP3A system was described as the 'garbage disposal' system of the liver and small intestine.[374] This is cutting edge research and hyperforin has actually helped scientists further understand this newly discovered mechanism. Unlike other nuclear receptors, which are characterised by their high degree of specificity, PXR has apparently evolved to be a broad-specificity xenobiotic sensor.[375]

Hypericum, and specifically hyperforin, also stimulate a second 'garbage disposal' mechanism, namely P-gp, probably again by activating PXR and SXR. P-gp is one of several multidrug resistance (MDR) pumps that are found in many living organisms and act to pump out chemicals from cells. For example, MDRs are one mechanism that bacteria use to become resistant to antibiotics. In fact, another name for P-gp is MDR1. P-gp is said to be 'promiscuous' in that it can recognise and export a diverse range of structurally unrelated compounds from cells. Since the activation of PXR is also known to increase the transcription of the gene *MDR1* that encodes P-gp, it is likely that hyperforin is also the key constituent in Hypericum that induces P-gp.[376] Experimentally, it has been verified that it is indeed hyperforin, and not hypericin, that increases the expression of P-gp in vitro.[376]

The natural conclusion to draw from these findings is that the metabolic drug interactions can be avoided by using a Hypericum preparation that is devoid of hyperforin. However, the prudent clinician would also require verification from clinical studies that this is indeed the case. Fortunately such studies are available.

A clinical study was designed to evaluate the effect on CYP3A function of Hypericum preparations with hyperforin contents ranging from very low to high.[377] The test probe drug midazolam was used to indirectly assess induction of these phase I enzymes after all the herbal products were first administered for 14 days. All Hypericum extracts tested decreased the bioavailability of midazolam. The product containing the highest dose of hyperforin (41 mg/day) did this by 79%, whereas that with the lowest dose (0.13 mg/day) reduced bioavailability by only 21%, which is probably not clinically significant. Overall, a dose-response effect for hyperforin was clearly demonstrated.

Perhaps more significantly, several clinical trials have demonstrated that low-hyperforin Hypericum extracts do not interact with key drugs such as cyclosporin, digoxin and the oral contraceptive pill. In the case of cyclosporin, the effect of two Hypericum preparations on the pharmacokinetics of cyclosporin was investigated in 10 renal transplant patients using a crossover design.[378] The decrease in cyclosporin bioavailability was 52% for the high-hyperforin preparation, but was only a clinically insignificant 7% for the low-hyperforin product. For each preparation, the doses of Hypericum herb were identical, only the hyperforin contents differed.

The pharmacokinetic interactions between a low hyperforin Hypericum extract and alprazolam, caffeine, tolbutamide and digoxin were evaluated in two randomised, placebo-controlled studies with 28 healthy volunteers. The participants received Hypericum extract (240 mg/day containing 3.5 mg hyperforin) or placebo on days 2 to 11. The test drugs were administered on days 1 and 11. No significant differences in bioavailability were found for all the test drugs between the placebo group and the Hypericum group at the end of the study.[379]

In an unpublished study, the effect of a hyperforin-free extract of Hypericum was investigated in 16 women aged between 18 and 43 years taking a low dose oral contraceptive pill.[380] No significant effect on the serum levels of the pill components, namely ethinyloestradiol and 3-keto-desogestrel (the active metabolite of desogestrel) were observed. In addition, intracyclic bleedings were not reported.

If avoiding the use of Hypericum preparations high in hyperforin will alleviate the pharmacokinetic drug interactions, a key question is whether this will compromise the antidepressant activity. An important issue in this regard was highlighted in a review of hyperforin in Hypericum–drug interactions.[55] The issue raised was that the extraction process used to make the most clinically tested extract of Hypericum, namely LI 160, was modified in 1998 to target better levels of hyperforin. This was instituted when research became available suggesting that hyperforin was important for the herb's antidepressant activity. As the review points out, there were no reports of drug interactions with Hypericum prior to 1998, but there were many positive clinical trials for the treatment of depression.[55]

There is still considerable debate concerning the relevance of hyperforin to the antidepressant effects. There are clinical studies that show that low-hyperforin extracts are superior to placebo or equivalent to fluoxetine in the treatment of mild-to-moderate depression. Equally there are clinical studies that demonstrate a low-hyperforin extract was ineffective, compared to a high-hyperforin extract (see earlier). Is it an excess of modern technology, and hence not natural, to be targeting hyperforin during the extraction process? Probably not, since the dry powdered Hypericum herb and the tea, which are both traditional preparations, can deliver clinically significant doses of this phytochemical.[377] (The tea must of course be freshly brewed as hyperforin is quite unstable in solution.)

As just mentioned, hyperforin is unstable in extracts of Hypericum, even in the dry extracts found in tablets and capsules. It is most unstable in solution and rapidly decomposes at an acidic pH.[23] Tinctures and fluid extracts (galenicals) of Hypericum older than a few months contain no hyperforin at all.[381] The most sure and obvious way to avoid the metabolic drug interactions with Hypericum is to use the traditional liquid dosage forms.

As well as the hyperforin content, the actual dose of Hypericum also comes into consideration. A randomised, placebo-controlled, parallel-group study investigated the pharmacokinetic interaction of various Hypericum formulations and doses with digoxin in 96 healthy volunteers.[382] Like the other studies already quoted, this study also found that the interaction with digoxin varied with the hyperforin content in the administered dose. But what the study also highlighted was that the hyperforin dose is a function of two variables, namely the hyperforin percentage in the preparation and the action actual dose of that preparation. When using the same preparation (powdered dried herb in capsules) a clear dose-response relationship was demonstrated for the drug interaction. No effect on digoxin bioavailability compared with placebo was observed for herb doses of 0.5 and 1 g/day, containing daily doses of hyperforin of 2.6 and 5.3 mg, respectively. Significant effects were seen at doses of 2 and 4 g/day of herb (containing 10.6 and 21.1 mg/day hyperforin, respectively), although the authors noted that the effect from 2 g/day was borderline and potentially not clinically relevant.

Pharmacodynamic drug in teractions

The published works on this topic are fewer than the pharmacokinetic interactions. Hence it is rather extraordinary that many writers regard the potential for Hypericum to interact with antidepressant drugs as an accepted truth. The very fact that antidepressant drugs as a broad class are often referred to, rather than the individual classes of drugs, implies that a less than rigorous perspective has been taken.

Monoamine oxidase (MAO) is involved in the metabolism and inactivation of synaptically released neurotransmitters. It inactivates neurotransmitters inside the neuron that have either been synthesised or have resulted from reuptake and it exists in two isoforms, A and B: MAO-A preferentially breaks down adrenaline (epinephrine), noradrenaline (norepinephrine) and serotonin; MAO-B prefers phenylethylamine and benzylamine as substrates. Dopamine, tyramine and tryptamine are metabolised equally well by both forms. Most MAO inhibitors (e.g. phenelzine) inhibit both forms, but some newer drugs, such as moclobemide, inhibit only MAO-A and are considered safer. They cause increased intraneuronal levels of neurotransmitters, which does not necessarily lead to increased levels at receptors. Non-selective MAO inhibitors are not as popular now because of their side effects and well-known interaction with tyramine in foods (e.g. cheeses, red wine, etc).[383] Like tricyclics, the clinical effects of SSRIs in depression probably result more from the delayed postsynaptic adaptive responses than from the acute inhibition of the reuptake of serotonin. These drugs include fluoxetine and sertraline.

Serotonin syndrome is defined as an adverse drug interaction characterised by altered mental status, autonomic dysfunction and neuromuscular abnormalities. It is most frequently caused by the use of SSRIs and MAO inhibitors, leading to excess serotonin availability in the CNS at the serotonin 1A receptor. At least one of these drug classes is always involved. It can also occur with single drug therapy and overdose. Elderly patients are more vulnerable and it is often seen now with SSRI over-medication. The clinical picture is nonspecific and there is no confirmatory test. It can be mistaken for viral illness, anxiety or a neurological disorder.[384]

Is there an inherent issue in prescribing Hypericum with antidepressants? Antidepressant drugs of different classes are often combined, especially by psychiatrists, in patients who are resistant to treatment. This is sometimes called 'augmentation therapy'. The risk of serotonin syndrome from doing this with drugs is infrequent, and so is likely to be even lower (if at all) when Hypericum is combined with antidepressants

(given that the mode of action of Hypericum is unlike conventional drugs; see elsewhere in this monograph and below).

Animal or human studies are most relevant for understanding the mode of action of Hypericum. One study in rats has suggested that the mode of action of Hypericum is more like that of tricyclics than SSRIs.[73] But a human study has shown that amitriptyline (a tricyclic) is quite different in its pharmacological effects compared to Hypericum.[385] Another human study found that effects of Hypericum were quite different to imipramine (another tricyclic). The authors of this study concluded that its effects could be quite novel and possibly linked to dopamine metabolism.[96]

One article in a prestigious pharmaceutical journal described Hypericum as 'nature's Prozac'.[386] However, this was countered by other scientists in a subsequent letter, who stated that there is a paucity of in vivo evidence supporting the proposition that Hypericum impairs any form of monoamine reuptake.[387] In their response the original authors agreed and stated that:[388]

> St John's wort and fluoxetine (Prozac) differ not only in their mode of action … but also in their toxicology ….

An experimental in vivo model found that two different Hypericum extracts (with different hyperforin levels) had no effect on the neuronal activity of the dorsal raphe nucleus of the brain.[389] This contrasted sharply with fluoxetine and sertraline (SSRIs), which markedly depressed such neuronal activity by increasing the synaptic availability of serotonin.

There is currently a paucity of evidence from either in vivo models or from controlled clinical trials that Hypericum interacts pharmacodynamically with any class of antidepressant drugs. However, there are a number of case reports in the literature. These are reviewed below for the major classes of antidepressant drugs.

There are no published adverse reports of pharmacodynamic interactions for Hypericum and tricyclics: neither case reports nor trials. There is a credible clinical study for amitriptyline that showed reduced plasma levels (and hence a pharmacokinetic interaction).[390] Since nortriptyline is basically a metabolite of amitriptyline, this would probably apply for this drug as well. However, all the issues governing the pharmacokinetic interactions with Hypericum will apply (as discussed previously).

The first case report of an alleged interaction between a Hypericum product (unspecified) and an SSRI (paroxetine) was published in 1998.[391] The patient exhibited symptoms of grogginess, incoherence and slow movements, which could hardly be described as serotonin syndrome. The authors incorrectly described Hypericum as a MAO inhibitor. Four case reports of serotonin syndrome in elderly people were described in one published report, as due to an alleged interaction between Hypericum and sertraline.[392] An alleged interaction between Hypericum and paroxetine resembling serotonin syndrome was published in 2000.[393] A manic episode (possibly serotonin syndrome) attributed to an interaction between Hypericum and sertraline was also published in 2000.[394] The quality of all such reports is low.

There are a few case reports in the published literature of adverse pharmacodynamic interactions between Hypericum and novel antidepressant drugs. For example, reports exist of serotonin syndrome attributed to the interaction of Hypericum and the modified cyclics trazodone[395] and nefazodone respectively.[392] An adverse reaction between the selective noradrenaline reuptake inhibitor venlafaxine and Hypericum has also been published.[396] Again the quality of these reports is low.

In conclusion, the research has shown that pharmacokinetic drug interactions should not be an issue for doses of Hypericum less than 2 g/day herb (or its equivalent) or any doses of a Hypericum preparation low in hyperforin (such as a tincture or fluid extract). These preparation and dosage guidelines should be followed whenever there is a requirement to recommend Hypericum to patients taking any of the drug medications known to interact with this herb. In particular, the guidelines should be strictly observed in all patients taking any form of the oral contraceptive pill. However, for depressed patients not taking any of the problem drugs it is best to recommend preparations that deliver a reasonable dose of hyperforin (in the range 15 to 30 mg/day). These will, by necessity, be tablets or capsules containing a dried extract.

In terms of potential pharmacodynamic interactions, the exact mode of action of Hypericum on monoamine neurotransmitters is not fully understood. Results from comparative in vivo studies suggest that its pharmacological profile is quite different to SSRIs and tricyclics. There is currently little convincing evidence from either in vivo studies or controlled clinical trials to support the contention that Hypericum interacts with any class of antidepressant drugs.

On current evidence, the risk of an adverse pharmacodynamic interaction between Hypericum and conventional antidepressant drugs must be rated as quite low. Suggestions of a strong likelihood of such interactions in the literature are tainted by medical politics, since antidepressant drugs are often combined in modern therapy, yet the risk of serotonin syndrome from such practice is regarded as low. If clinically appropriate, it is suggested that Hypericum can be combined with antidepressant drugs under professional supervision. A low dose should be recommended at first both as a caution and to reassure the patient. Due to media attention, and in some cases warnings on labels, many patients are concerned about the drug interaction issues with Hypericum. Sometimes they have also received advice from their medical doctor or psychiatrist on this matter. Hence, all the above recommendations need to take into consideration the fully informed consent of the patient.

Use in pregnancy and lactation

Category B1 – no increase in frequency of malformation or other harmful effects on the fetus from limited use in women. No evidence of increased fetal damage in animal studies (other than minor adverse effects observed at high doses in one study in mice; the relevance of this study to humans is unknown).

A group of 54 pregnant women taking Hypericum extracts was compared with 108 pregnant women either taking other drug therapy for depression or not exposed to any known teratogens. The rates of major malformations were no different from the 3% to 5% risk expected in the general population and were similar across the three groups, with incidences of 5%, 4% and 0% in the Hypericum, disease comparator and healthy groups, respectively. The live birth and prematurity rates were also not different among the three groups. This study provides some evidence of fetal safety with Hypericum in human pregnancy, but is limited by the small numbers.[397]

At 24 weeks of her pregnancy, a woman commenced Hypericum (900 mg/day of a concentrated (6:1) extract) for treatment of depression and took the preparation until 24 hours prior to delivery. She gave birth to a healthy baby, whose physical examination and laboratory results were normal. The woman discontinued taking St John's wort postpartum and initiated breastfeeding. The neonate developed jaundice on day 5. On day 20 the mother resumed Hypericum (300 mg/day of the concentrated extract) and continued breastfeeding. Behavioural assessment of the baby at 4 and 33 days was normal.[398]

Dried herb orally administered to rats (1 g/kg/day) and rabbits (1.5 g/kg/day) did not adversely affect the health of the fetus or of the mother. The fertility of adult animals was not affected.[399] Maternal administration of Hypericum (180 mg/kg/day) for 2 weeks before conception and throughout gestation did not affect the long-term growth and physical maturation of exposed mouse offspring.[400] A significant reduction in litter size and smaller offspring were observed in mice fed Hypericum (136 mg/kg/day) prior to mating and throughout gestation.[401] Prenatal exposure to Hypericum (180 mg/kg/day) in mice reduced male birth weight but did not affect long-term growth and physical development of exposed offspring.[402] Fertility, development of the embryo, prenatal and postnatal development were not influenced by oral administration of a standardised, aqueous methanol extract of Hypericum (4:1 to 7:1) in rats and dogs (0.9 and 2.7 g/kg, for 26 weeks in both species).[403] A lack of toxicity was observed in mothers and offspring in a study in which rats were orally exposed to Hypericum (up to 4.5 g/kg) from gestational day 3 until offspring weaning.[404]

Hypericum is compatible with breastfeeding but caution should be exercised.

Findings of clinical studies support the relative safety of administration of Hypericum extracts during breastfeeding. The constituents of the herb appear to penetrate the breast milk compartment poorly, if at all. A case study confirmed that only hyperforin was excreted into breast milk at a low level, while in the infant's plasma hyperforin and hypericin were below the lower limit of quantification (hypericin 0.20 ng/mL, hyperforin 0.50 ng/mL).[405] Four breast-milk samples from a mother with post-natal depression taking a Hypericum preparation three times a day (LI 160) were analysed over an 18-hour period. No side effects were seen in the mother or infant.[405] However, another study found that infant exposure to hyperforin through milk following maternal administration of 900 mg/day of Hypericum (LI 160) to five mothers was comparable to levels reported in most studies assessing antidepressant or neuroleptic effects.[406] Hyperforin was at the lower limit of quantification in plasma samples analysed from two infants (0.1 ng/mL). Milk/plasma ratios ranged from 0.04 to 0.13. The relative infant doses were 0.9% to 2.5%. No side effects were seen in the mothers or infants.

One clinical study investigating Hypericum intake during lactation found a statistically significant higher frequency of infant side effects (16.6%: colic, drowsiness, lethargy) for the mothers taking Hypericum, compared to the frequency in those not exposed to the herb (two control groups, 0% and 3.3% colic).[407] However, the study was not placebo-controlled. No significant difference was observed in the frequency of maternal reports of decreased milk production among the groups, nor was a difference found in infant weight over the first year of life. It is unclear whether these adverse events were actually attributable to Hypericum due to the small sample size and possible bias resulting from the nature of the (self-selection) reporting method.

The Scientific Committee of ESCOP (European Scientific Cooperative on Phytotherapy) suggests that, in accordance with general medical practice, Hypericum should not be used during pregnancy and lactation without professional advice.[357]

Effects on ability to drive and use machines

No negative influence is expected.

Several reviews[408-410] and clinical trials[411-413] have reported the lack of adverse effects on the ability to drive or operate machinery. In a review of three clinical trials of Hypericum extracts for depression, it was reported that Hypericum was devoid of sedative or anticholinergic effects, and that the ability to drive a car was not affected.[410] This was tested by means of the established psychometric procedure used to assess medical fitness to drive. Hubner investigated the effects of LI 160 at 900 mg/day for 4 weeks in 39 depressed patients and reported no impairment of vigilance or the ability to drive.[411] Similarly, Schmidt and Sommer reported that in a trial with mild-to-moderately depressed patients, the same extract preserved attention and reaction ability and did not interfere with the ability to drive.[412]

A randomised, double blind, placebo-controlled, crossover study investigated the interaction of Hypericum extract with alcohol. Thirty-two volunteers received either Hypericum extract (2.7 mg/day TH equivalent) for 7 days or placebo. At the end of the treatment period they underwent several tests following consumption of alcohol. No interaction between Hypericum and alcohol with respect to cognitive capabilities was observed.[211]

Side effects

General

Adverse events associated with Hypericum tend to be mild and occur rarely. In clinical trials, side effects are often reported no more frequently with Hypericum extracts than in the placebo arm. Data from a meta-analysis of 35 double blind randomised trials showed that dropout and adverse effects rates in patients receiving Hypericum extracts were similar to placebo, lower than for older antidepressants, and slightly lower than for selective serotonin reuptake inhibitors.[414] No serious adverse effects were reported in any study. Hypericum extracts appear to be free of the cardiac

or anticholinergic side effects normally associated with antidepressant medications.[257] In a review of large-scale observational studies with at least 100 patients suffering from depressive disorders, comprising a total of 34804 patients, the percentage of patients reporting side effects ranged between 0% and 5.9%.[251] Hypericum extracts were associated with only mild side effects, the most frequent being gastrointestinal symptoms, followed by increased photosensitivity and skin symptoms. Headaches, palpitations,[266] fatigue and restlessness[247] have also been reported. Anxiety was reported by a small number of participants in trials (5 patients of 2404 patients[294] and 8 of 3250 patients[415]). One clinical trial reported the side effects of muscle and joint stiffness, tremor, sweating, muscle spasms and pain.[278] Frequent urination was reported in 27% of participants taking 900 to 1500 mg Hypericum extract daily for 8 weeks, compared with 11% placebo participants.[262] The most common adverse event (one per 300000 treated cases) among the spontaneous reports in the official German register to year 2000 relate to reactions of the skin exposed to light.[416]

Adverse events from individual case reports often involve concomitant medication or other pathologies, making it difficult to establish a causal connection with the administration of Hypericum extracts. Cases where the link is considered possible are included below.

Photosensitivity

Pharmacokinetic studies suggest that the phototoxic threshold level of hypericin is not reached with the normal doses of Hypericum used for the oral treatment of depression.[414] However, cases of reversible photosensitivity to Hypericum have been reported, including one case of a burning, erythematous eruption that occurred after 4 days of treatment with 33 mg Hypericum extract.[417] Photosensitivity developed in a 61-year-old woman after taking a Hypericum extract for 3 years, which resulted in elevated, itching red lesions in light-exposed areas.[418] The reaction was reversible and confirmed by provocation test. A patient consuming Hypericum at the time of laser treatment developed a severe phototoxic reaction to laser light.[419] In a clinical study, volunteers consuming a threshold dose of Hypericum extract containing 5 to 10 mg hypericin experienced a mild increase in photosensitisation.[416] Mild-to-moderate, reversible photosensitivity developed in participants in two clinical studies of HIV and hepatitis C with oral hypericin in doses from 0.05 to 0.5 mg/kg/day.[43,44,233,236] For example, one of these was a phase I study of intravenous and oral hypericin in HIV-infected adults, in which five of 12 participants receiving the 0.05 mg/kg/day dosing schedule and six of seven receiving the 0.10 mg/kg/day dosing schedule developed phototoxic reactions.[43] However, intravenous hypericin, 0.25 or 0.5 mg/kg twice weekly or 0.25 mg/kg three times weekly, or oral hypericin 0.5 mg/kg daily, caused severe cutaneous phototoxicity in 11 of 23 evaluable HIV-infected patients with CD4 counts less than 350 cells/mm³.[44]

In contrast to these findings, no evidence was found for a phototoxic potential of the Hypericum extract LI 160 in humans when it was administered orally at typical clinical doses up to 1800 mg daily.[420] A prospective randomised study in 72 volunteers of skin types II and III investigated the effect of the Hypericum extract LI 160 on skin sensitivity to ultraviolet B (UVB), ultraviolet A (UVA), visible light and solar-simulated radiation. No significant influence on the erythema index or melanin index was detected in the single-dose (5.4 or 10.8 mg hypericin) or the steady-state studies (5.4 mg hypericin, and subsequently 2.7 mg hypericin, per day for 7 days), with the exception of a marginal influence on UVB-induced pigmentation (p=0.0471) in the single-dose study. These findings were in accordance with previous pharmacokinetic studies that found hypericin serum and skin levels after oral ingestion of Hypericum extract were always lower than the assumed phototoxic hypericin threshold level of 1000 ng/mL.[420]

Other studies supporting this finding found no significant changes of erythema threshold levels following exposure to UV radiation, visible light and solar-simulated radiation with oral LI 160;[421] and no significant change in UVB photosensitivity and a UV light sensitivity that was not, or only marginally increased, with oral intake of Hypericum extract (4.5 to 5.4 mg/day TH equivalent for 7 to 15 days).[422] There was an increased UVA photosensitivity in the subgroup of light sensitive skin types.

Three cases of topical use of Hypericum creams or oil with or without oral administration (dosage unspecified) resulted in phototoxic reaction upon exposure to sunlight or, in one case, after phototherapy commenced.[423] These include erythematobullous dermatosis and facial bullae related to sun exposure, UVB phototherapy-related follicular erythema and urticarial oedema. However, one patient had lupus and another had psoriasis.

In cell cultures, it was found that phototoxic effects with Hypericum extracts in conjunction with visible light and UVA only occurred at high concentrations.[424] Peak hypericin levels in skin blister fluid following administration of an oral dose of 1800 mg or steady-state administration (900 mg daily for 7 days) was at least 20 times below the estimated phototoxic concentration of 100 μg/mL.[165] It has been suggested that the risk of significant photogenotoxic damage incurred by the combination of Hypericum extracts and UVA phototherapy may be low in the majority of individuals.[425]

Other reactions

Four cases of sensory nerve hypersensitivity reactions, with increased sensitivity to heat and cold, and pain in the hands and/or feet were reported.[426] These resolved within 1 to 2 weeks of ceasing the herb. It was suggested that the preparations involved were from the late-harvested herb that contained high levels of resinous constituents that would not normally be ingested.

A possibly related case of subacute toxic neuropathy (nerve damage) was reported. The woman began to experience sharp pains in areas exposed to the sun (face and hands) after 4 weeks' treatment with an over-the-counter preparation of Hypericum (500 mg, concentration undefined). Painful sensitivity on her arms and legs occurred after sunbathing. Her symptoms began to improve and eventually disappeared after she stopped using the product.[427] One case of hyperaesthesia

has been reported following use of Hypericum extract at an unspecified dose.[428]

Delayed emergence from anaesthesia occurred in one patient possibly related to 3 months' ingestion of up to 3 g/day Hypericum. At the time of her procedure she was self-administering Hypericum in tablet form, 1000 mg three times daily.[368]

Elevated thyroid-stimulating hormone was observed in a retrospective case-control study (4 of 37 patients had taken Hypericum).[429] Although there is a probable association with Hypericum intake, further investigation is required. Furthermore, this study has been criticised for design limitations, not adding meaningful scientific information to assess a potential association, and that no association was demonstrated.[430]

As can be expected from such a widely used herb, some unlikely adverse events have been attributed to Hypericum. Multiple side effects in a 47-year-old woman were reported to the Adverse Drug Reaction Advisory Committee in Australia, allegedly related to Hypericum. These included dyspnoea, hyperventilation, palpitations, tremor, flushing, mydriasis and rhinitis, suggestive of an allergic reaction.[428]

Once case of hypertension[431] and another of hypertension with delirium have been reported after ingestion of Hypericum extract (dosage unspecified) for 1 week. In the latter case, the patient had consumed aged cheeses and red wine prior to reaction.[432] However, this erroneously implies that Hypericum is a MAO inhibitor, which suggests a preconceived bias.

Cardiovascular collapse during anaesthesia in one patient was possibly associated with 6 months' administration of Hypericum (dosage unspecified).[433]

A suspected case of withdrawal syndrome occurred in one woman upon cessation of Hypericum tablets (5.4 g/day of herb, corresponding to extract containing 0.3% TH) for 32 days.[434] On discontinuing the Hypericum product she experienced nausea, anorexia, dry retching, dizziness, dry mouth, thirst, cold chills and fatigue within 24 hours. Her symptoms peaked on day 3 and she gradually recovered by day 8. However, this clinical picture is suggestive of a coincidental viral or bacterial infection.

As mentioned above, mania has been reported in 14 cases in patients with and without a history of psychiatric illness, including previous mania. Hypericum products were taken in unspecified, normal and high doses,[360,363–365] in two cases with other products (Ginkgo, valerian, melatonin),[359] and in four cases with or just after pharmaceutical drugs.[361,366] One incidence of psychosis was reported in a patient with Alzheimer's disease and in another two patients with schizophrenia.[435,436] A first episode of psychosis was reported in one patient after taking an extract of Hypericum.[437]

In 26 HIV-positive patients receiving oral Hypericum extracts containing the equivalent of 1 mg/day hypericin for 4 months, mild reversible liver enzyme elevations were observed that returned to baseline levels after 1 month without Hypericum.[230] However, in another clinical study hypericin had no effect on liver enzymes.[43,236] One case report described a patient who experienced hepatotoxicity following ingestion of a Hypericum extract.[438] However, as the authors acknowledge, it is difficult to attribute a causal association between the two events, although the elevation of the liver enzymes were temporally associated with the ingestion of the herb (extract and dose not provided.)

A case of a dynamic ileus associated with the use of Hypericum in a 67-year-old woman has been reported. Her symptoms started 2 weeks after taking the extract, with no other identifiable cause, and resolved gradually and completely after its discontinuation.[358]

One case of sexual dysfunction was reported in a 49-year-old man taking Hypericum tablets (4×0.9 mg/day TH for 1 week).[439] His sexual dysfunction appeared to be drug-induced by both sertraline and Hypericum, as he had previously reported experiencing orgasmic delay, erectile dysfunction and inhibited sexual desire on sertraline. Diminution of libido was reported with Hypericum taken for 9 months in a 42-year-old man with a history of anxiety, depression and OCD.[440] However, his anxiety, depression and tics abated considerably while on the Hypericum extract.

Suicidal and homicidal thoughts in a 51-year-old woman were linked to vitamin C and a Hypericum extract. Within 3 weeks of discontinuing the supplements, the suicidal and homicidal thoughts disappeared. The woman recalled having had similar experience with the same combination previously.[441]

Overdosage

Phototoxicity might be expected to occur with overdose. Typical phototoxic symptoms include rash, pruritus and erythema 24 h after exposure to ultraviolet light.

Convulsions were associated with an overdose of a Hypericum product in a 16-year-old girl who had taken up to 15 tablets/day (300 mg each) in the 2 weeks leading up to admission and an additional 50 tablets just before presentation, for a recent 'depressive episode'.[442] Results of a computed tomography brain scan and cerebrospinal fluid examination were unremarkable, but an EEG confirmed diffuse spike wave activity consistent with generalised epileptic activity. High-performance liquid chromatography was not performed to quantify hypericin in her serum and urine, as these tests were not available in the hospital. A repeat EEG at discharge on day 6 was normal and there were no further seizures in the following 6 months.

Regulatory status in selected countries

Hypericum is official in the *United States Pharmacopeia–National Formulary* (USP34-NF29, 2011).

It does not have GRAS status, but is freely available as a 'dietary supplement' in the USA under DSHEA legislation (Dietary Supplement Health and Education Act of 1994). Hypericum has been present in OTC digestive aid drug products. The FDA, however, advises that: 'based on evidence currently available, there is inadequate data to establish general recognition of the safety and effectiveness of these ingredients for the specified uses'. Hypericum is also being combined with other constituents such as ma huang (Ephedra) and promoted for weight loss. The FDA has issued a warning that this treatment is not safe and/or effective.

Hypericum is covered by a positive Commission E monograph and can be used for psychogenic disturbances, depressive states and excitability. Infused oil of Hypericum can be used internally for dyspeptic complaints and externally for the treatment of wounds, bruises, myalgia and first-degree burns.

In the UK, Hypericum is included on the General Sale List. Hypericum is official in the *British Pharmacopoeia* 2011 and the *European Pharmacopoeia* 2011. Hypericum products have achieved Traditional Herbal Registration in the UK with the traditional indication of relief of symptoms of slightly low mood and mild anxiety.

Hypericum is not included in Part 4 of Schedule 4 of the Therapeutic Goods Regulations in Australia and is freely available for sale. The requirement for listing (automatic registration) is that, if the preparation is not a homeopathic product and the proposed route of administration is oral, the label must include the following warning: St John's Wort affects the way some prescription medicines work. Consult your doctor.

References

1. British Herbal Medicine Association Scientific Committee. *British Herbal Pharmacopoeia.* Cowling: BHMA; 1983. p. 115.
2. Felter H, Lloyd J: *King's American Dispensatory*, rev 3, vol. 2, 1905. Portland: Reprinted by Eclectic Medical Publications; 1983. pp. 1038–1039.
3. Axarlis S, Mentis A, Demetzos C, et al. *Phytother Res.* 1998;12:507–511.
4. Smeh N. *Creating Your Own Cosmetics – Naturally.* Garrisonville: Alliance Publishing Company; 1995. p. 83.
5. Campbell M, Delfosse E. *J Aust Inst Agric Sci.* 1984;50(2):63–73.
6. Mabberley D. *The Plant Book.* Cambridge: Cambridge University Press; 1997. pp. 319–320, 356.
7. Chiej R. *The Macdonald Encyclopedia of Medicinal Plants.* London: Macdonald; 1984. Entry no. 157.
8. Launert E. *The Hamlyn Guide to Edible And Medicinal Plants of Britain and Northern Europe.* London: Hamlyn; 1981. p. 40.
9. Wagner H, Bladt S. In: Wagner H, Bladt S, eds. *The Macdonald Encyclopedia of Medicinal Plants.* London: Macdonald; 1984. Entry no. 157.
10. Nahrstedt A, Butterweck V. *Pharmacopsychiatry.* 1997;30(suppl 2):129–134.
11. Butterweck V, Schmidt M. *Wien Med Wochenschr.* 2007;157(13–14):356–361.
12. Cirak C, Radusiene J, Janulis V, et al. *Nat Prod Commun.* 2010;5(6):897–898.
13. Melzer R, Fricke U, Holzl J. *Arzneimittelforschung.* 1991;41(5):481–483.
14. Franchomme P, Penoel D. *L'aromathérapie Exactement: Encyclopédie De l'utilisation Thérapeutique des Huiles Essentielles.* Limoges: Roger Jollois Editeur; 1990. p. 358.

15. Niesel S, Schilcher H. *Arch Pharm Res*. 1990;323:755.

16. Falk H, Schmitzberger W. *Monatshefte Chem*. 1992;123:731–739.

17. Muller WE, Singer A, Wonnemann M. *Pharmacopsychiatry*. 2001;34 (suppl 1):S98–102.

18. Chatterjee SS, Bhattacharya SK, Wonnemann M, et al. *Life Sci*. 1998;63(6):499–510.

19. Singer A, Wonnemann M, Muller WE. *J Pharmacol Exp Ther*. 1999;290(3):1363–1368.

20. Laakmann G, Schule C, Baghai T, et al. *Pharmacopsychiatry*. 1998;31(suppl 1):54–59.

21. Chatterjee SS, Noldner M, Koch E, et al. *Pharmacopsychiatry*. 1998;31(suppl 1):7–15.

22. Schellenberg R, Sauer S, Dimpfel W. *Pharmacopsychiatry*. 1998;31(suppl 1):44–53.

23. Ang CY, Hu L, Heinze TM, et al. *J Agric Food Chem*. 2004;52(20):6156–6164.

24. Lehmann R. *Personal Communication*. MediHerb; 2004.

25. Kubin A, Wierrani F, Burner U, et al. *Curr Pharm Des*. 2005;11(2):233–253.

26. Andersen D, Weber N, Wood S, et al. *Antiviral Res*. 1991;16(2):185–196.

27. Lopez-Bazzocchi I, Hudson J, Towers G. *Photochem Photobiol*. 1991;54(1):95–98.

28. Moraleda G, Wu T, Jilbert A, et al. *Antiviral Res*. 1993;20:235–247.

29. Tang J, Colacino J, Larsen S, et al. *Antiviral Res*. 1990;13(6):313–325.

30. Hudson J, Harris L, Towers G. *Antiviral Res*. 1993;20:173–178.

31. Lenard J, Rabson A, Vanderoef R. *Proc Natl Acad Sci USA*. 1993;90(1):158–162.

32. Degar S, Prince A, Pascual D, et al. *AIDS Res Hum Retroviruses*. 1992;8(11):1929–1936.

33. Carpenter S, Kraus G. *Photochem Photobiol*. 1991;53(2):169–174.

34. Lavie G, Valentine F, Levin B, et al. *Proc Natl Acad Sci USA*. 1989;86(15):5963–5967.

35. Meruelo D, Lavie G, Lavie D, et al. *Proc Natl Acad Sci USA*. 1988;85(14):5230–5234.

36. Kraus G, Pratt D, Tossberg J, et al. *Biochem Biophys Res Commun*. 1990;172(1):149–153.

37. Takahashi I, Nakanishi S, Kobayashi E, et al. *Biochem Biophys Res Commun*. 1989;165(3):1207–1212.

38. De Witte P, Agostinis P, Van Lint J, et al. *Biochem Pharmacol*. 1993;46(11):1929–1936.

39. Panossian A, Gabrielian E, Manvelian V, et al. *Phytomedicine*. 1996;3(1):19–28.

40. Lavie G, Mazur Y, Lavie D, et al. *Transfusion*. 1995;35(5):392–400.

41. Maury W, Price JP, Brindley MA, et al. *Virol J*. 2009;6:101.

42. Karioti A, Bilia AR. *Int J Mol Sci*. 2010;11(2):562–594.

43. Jacobson JM, Feinman L, Liebes L, et al. *Antimicrob Agents Chemother*. 2001;45(2):517–524.

44. Gulick RM, Mcauliffe V, Holden-Wiltse J, et al. *Ann Intern Med*. 1999;130(6):510–514.

45. Butterweck V, Wall A, Lieflander-Wulf U, et al. *Pharmacopsychiatry*. 1997;30 (suppl 2):117–124.

46. Butterweck V, Petereit F, Winterhoff H, et al. *Planta Med*. 1998;64(4):291–294.

47. Butterweck V, Winterhoff H, Herkenham M. *Mol Psychiatry*. 2001;6(5):547–564.

48. Butterweck V, Nahrstedt A, Evans J, et al. *Psychopharmacology (Berl)*. 2002;162(2):193–202.

49. Butterweck V, Jurgenliemk G, Nahrstedt A, et al. *Planta Med*. 2000;66(1):3–6.

50. Butterweck V, Hegger M, Winterhoff H. *Planta Med*. 2004;70(10):1008–1011.

51. Reichling J, Hostanska K, Saller R. *Forsch Komplementarmed Klass Naturheilkd*. 2003;10(suppl 1):28–32.

52. Krishtal O, Lozovaya N, Fisunov A, et al. *Pharmacopsychiatry*. 2001;34(suppl 1):S74–82.

53. Nahrstedt A, Butterweck V. *J Nat Prod*. 2010;73(5):1015–1021.

54. Schulte-Lobbert S, Holoubek G, Muller WE, et al. *J Pharm Pharmacol*. 2004;56(6):813–818.

55. Madabushi R, Frank B, Drewelow B, et al. *Eur J Clin Pharmacol*. 2006;62(3):225–233.

56. Butterweck V, Christoffel V, Nahrstedt A, et al. *Life Sci*. 2003;73(5):627–639.

57. Muller W. *2nd International Congress on Phytomedicine*. Munich, September 11–14, 1996.

58. Muller WE, Rolli M, Schafer C, et al. *Pharmacopsychiatry*. 1997;30(suppl 2):102–107.

59. Perovic S, Muller WE. *Arzneimittelforschung*. 1995;45(11):1145–1148.

60. Kientsch U, Burgi S, Ruedeberg C, et al. *Pharmacopsychiatry*. 2001;34(suppl 1):S56–60.

61. Cott JM. *Pharmacopsychiatry*. 1997;30(suppl 2):108–112.

62. Muller W, Rossol R. *Nervenheilkunde*. 1993;12:357–358.

63. Thiede H, Walper A. *Nervenheilkunde*. 1993;12:346–348.

64. Thiele B, Brink I, Ploch M. *J Geriatr Psychiatry Neurol*. 1994;7(suppl 1):S60–62.

65. Obry T. Diploma work. Cited in Scientific Committee of ESCOP. *ESCOP Monographs: Hyperici Herba*. Exeter: European Scientific Cooperative on Phytotherapy; 1996.

66. Simmen U, Burkard W, Berger K, et al. *J Recept Signal Transduct Res*. 1999;19 (1–4):59–74.

67. Simmen U, Bobirnac I, Ullmer C, et al. *Eur J Pharmacol*. 2003;458(3):251–256.

68. Curle P, Kato G, Hiller K. Unpublished data. Cited in Scientific Committee of ESCOP. *ESCOP Monographs: Hyperici Herba*. Exeter: European Scientific Cooperative on Phytotherapy; 1996.

69. Raffa RB. *Life Sci*. 1998;62(16):265–270.

70. Jensen AG, Hansen SH, Nielsen EO. *Life Sci*. 2001;68(14):1593–1605.

71. Muller WE, Singer A, Wonnemann M, et al. *Pharmacopsychiatry*. 1998;31(suppl 1):16–21.

72. Wonnemann M, Singer A, Muller WE. *Neuropsychopharmacology*. 2000;23(2):188–197.

73. Misane I, Ogren SO. *Pharmacopsychiatry*. 2001;34(suppl 1):S89–97.

74. Nathan PJ. *J Psychopharmacology*. 2001;15(1):47–54.

75. Chatterjee S, Filippov V, Lishko P, et al. *Life Sci*. 1999;65(22):2395–2405.

76. Treiber K, Singer A, Henke B, et al. *Br J Pharmacol*. 2005;145(1):75–83.

77. Eckert GP, Muller WE. *Pharmacopsychiatry*. 2001;34(suppl 1):S22–25.

78. Demisch L, Holzl J, Gollinik B, et al. *Pharmacopsychiatry*. 1989;22(5):194.

79. Holzl J, Demisch L, Gollinik B. *Planta Med*. 1989;55:643.

80. Nielsen M, Frokjaer S, Braestrup C. *Biochem Pharmacol*. 1988;37(17):3285–3287.

81. Thiele B, Brink I, Ploch M. *Nervenheilkunde*. 1993;12:353–356.

82. Fiebich BL, Hollig A, Lieb K. *Pharmacopsychiatry*. 2001;34(suppl 1):S26–28.

83. Nemeroff CB. *Sci Am*. 1998;278(6):42–49.

84. Simbrey K, Winterhoff H, Butterweck V. *Life Sci*. 2004;74(8):1027–1038.

85. Teufel-Mayer R, Gleitz J. *Pharmacopsychiatry*. 1997;30(suppl 2):113–116.

86. Chen F, Rezvani AH, Lawrence AJ. *Naunyn Schmiedebergs Arch Pharmacol*. 2003;367(2):126–133.

87. Franklin M. *Pharmacopsychiatry*. 2003;36(4):161–164.

88. Franklin M, Cowen PJ. *Pharmacopsychiatry*. 2001;34(suppl 1):S29–37.

89. Makina DM, Taranukhin AG, Chernigovskaya EV, et al. *Bull Exp Biol Med*. 2001;132(6):1180–1181.

90. Franklin M, Reed A, Murck H. *Eur Neuropsychopharmacol*. 2004;14(1):7–10.

91. Buchholzer ML, Dvorak C, Chatterjee SS, et al. *J Pharmacol Exp Ther*. 2002;301(2):714–719.

92. Panocka I, Perfumi M, Angeletti S, et al. *Pharmacol Biochem Behav*. 2000;66(1):105–111.

93. Caccia S, Gobbi M. *Curr Drug Metab*. 2009;10(9):1055–1065.

94. Schulz H, Jobert M. *Nervenheilkunde*. 1993;12:323–327.

95. Dimpfel W, Todorova A, Vonderheid-Guth B. *Eur J Med Res*. 1999;4(8):303–312.

96. Schroeder C, Tank J, Goldstein DS, et al. *Clin Pharmacol Ther*. 2004;76(5):480–489.

97. Schüle C, Baghai T, Ferrera A, et al. *Pharmacopsychiatry*. 2001;34(suppl 1):S127–133.

98. Schule C, Baghai T, Sauer N, et al. *Neuropsychobiology*. 2004;49(2):58–63.

99. Franklin M, Chi J, Mcgavin C, et al. *Biol Psychiatry*. 1999;46(4):581–584.

100. Franklin M, Hafizi S, Reed A, et al. *Pharmacopsychiatry.* 2006;39(1):13–15.

101. Vandenbogaerde A, Zanoli P, Puia G, et al. *Pharmacol Biochem Behav.* 2000;65(4):627–633.

102. Bano S, Dawood S. *Pak J Pharm Sci.* 2008;21(1):63–69.

103. Grundmann O, Lv Y, Kelber O, et al. *Neuropharmacology.* 2010;58(4–5): 767–773.

104. Ara I, Bano S. *Pak J Pharm Sci.* 2009;22(1):94–101.

105. Crupi R, Mazzon E, Marino A, et al. *BMC Complement Altern Med.* 2011;11:7.

106. Kumar V, Jaiswal AK, Singh PN, et al. *Indian J Exp Biol.* 2000;38(1):36–41.

107. Coleta M, Campos MG, Cotrim MD, et al. *Pharmacopsychiatry.* 2001;34 (suppl 1):S20–21.

108. Kumar V, Singh PN, Bhattacharya SK. *Indian J Exp Biol.* 2001;39(4):344–349.

109. Flausino Jr. OA, Zangrossi Jr. H, Salgado JV, et al. *Pharmacol Biochem Behav.* 2002;71(1–2):251–257.

110. Grundmann O, Kelber O, Butterweck V. *Planta Med.* 2006;72(15):1366–1371.

111. Beijamini V, Andreatini R. *Pharmacol Biochem Behav.* 2003;74(4):1015–1024.

112. Beijamini V, Andreatini R. *Pharmacol Res.* 2003;48(2):199–207.

113. Griffith TN, Varela-Nallar L, Dinamarca MC, et al. *Curr Med Chem.* 2010;17(5):391–406.

114. Albert D, Zundorf I, Dingermann T, et al. *Biochem Pharmacol.* 2002;64(12): 1767–1775.

115. Feisst C, Pergola C, Rakonjac M, et al. *Cell Mol Life Sci.* 2009;66(16):2759–2771.

116. Breyer A, Elstner M, Gillessen T, et al. *Phytomedicine.* 2007;14(4):250–255.

117. Feisst C, Werz O. *Biochem Pharmacol.* 2004;67(8):1531–1539.

118. Cerpa W, Hancke JL, Morazzoni P, et al. *Curr Alzheimer Res.* 2010;7(2):126–133.

119. Dinamarca MC, Cerpa W, Garrido J, et al. *Mol Psychiatry.* 2006;11(11):1032–1048.

120. Silva BA, Ferreres F, Malva JO, et al. *Food Chem.* 2005;90(1–2):157–167.

121. Hunt EJ, Lester CE, Lester EA, et al. *Life Sci.* 2001;69(2):181–190.

122. El-Sherbiny DA, Khalifa AE, Attia AS, et al. *Pharmacol Biochem Behav.* 2003;76(3–4):525–533.

123. Kiewert C, Buchholzer ML, Hartmann J, et al. *Neurosci Lett.* 2004;364(3):195–198.

124. Kumar V, Mdzinarishvili A, Kiewert C, et al. *J Pharmacol Sci.* 2006;102(1):47–54.

125. Leuner K, Kazanski V, Muller M, et al. *FASEB J.* 2007;21(14):4101–4111.

126. Kraus B, Wolff H, Heilmann J, et al. *Life Sci.* 2007;81(11):884–894.

127. Klusa V, Germane S, Nöldner M, et al. *Pharmacopsychiatry.* 2001;34 (suppl 1):61–69.

128. Khalifa AE. *J Ethnopharmacol.* 2001;76(1):49–57.

129. Trofimiuk E, Walesiuk A, Braszko JJ. *Pharmacol Res.* 2005;51(3):239–246.

130. Trofimiuk E, Braszko JJ. *Naunyn Schmiedebergs Arch Pharmacol.* 2008;376(6):463–471.

131. Trofimiuk E, Holownia A, Braszko J. *Naunyn Schmiedebergs Arch Pharmacol.* 2011;383(4):415–422.

132. Kumar V, Singh PN, Muruganandam AV, et al. *J Ethnopharmacol.* 2000;72 (1–2):119–128.

133. Rayburn WF, Christensen HD, Gonzalez CL. *Am J Obstet Gynecol.* 2000;183(5):1225–1231.

134. Tadros MG, Mohamed MR, Youssef AM, et al. *J Ethnopharmacol.* 2009;122(3): 561–566.

135. Johnson D, Ksciuk H, Woelk H, et al. *Nervenheilkunde.* 1993;12:328–330.

136. Kil KS, Yum YN, Seo SH, et al. *Arch Pharm Res.* 1996;19(6):490–496.

137. Martinez–Poveda B, Quesada AR, Medina MA. *Eur J Pharmacol.* 2005;516(2):97–103.

138. Skalkos D, Stavropoulos NE, Tsimaris I, et al. *Planta Med.* 2005;71(11):1030–1035.

139. Blank M, Lavie G, Mandel M, et al. *Int J Cancer.* 2004;111(4):596–603.

140. Martarelli D, Martarelli B, Pediconi D, et al. *Cancer Lett.* 2004;210(1):27–33.

141. Vandenbogaerde AL, Kamuhabwa A, Delaey E, et al. *J Photochem Photobiol B.* 1998;45(2–3):87–94.

142. Agostinis P, Vantieghem A, Merlevede W, et al. *Int J Biochem Cell Biol.* 2002;34(3):221–241.

143. Hopfner M, Maaser K, Theiss A, et al. *Int J Colorectal Dis.* 2003;18(3):239–247.

144. Stavropoulos NE, Kim A, Nseyo UU, et al. *J Photochem Photobiol B.* 2006;84(1):64–69.

145. Berlanda J, Kiesslich T, Oberdanner CB, et al. *J Environ Pathol Toxicol Oncol.* 2006;25(1–2):173–188.

146. Kamuhabwa A, Agostinis P, Ahmed B, et al. *Photochem Photobiol Sci.* 2004;3(8):772–780.

147. Davids LM, Kleemann B, Cooper S, et al. *Cell Biol Int.* 2009;33(10):1065–1072.

148. Davids LM, Kleemann B, Kacerovska D, et al. *J Photochem Photobiol B.* 2008;91 (2–3):67–76.

149. Chen B, Xu Y, Roskams T, et al. *Int J Cancer.* 2001;93(2):275–282.

150. Chen B, Zupko I, De Witte PA. *Int J Oncol.* 2001;18(4):737–742.

151. Chen B, Roskams T, Xu Y, et al. *Int J Cancer.* 2002;98(2):284–290.

152. Vandenbogaerde A, De Witte P. *Anticancer Res.* 1995;15(5(A)):1757–1758.

153. Alecu M, Ursaciuc C, Hǎlǎlǎu F, et al. *Anticancer Res.* 1998;18(6B):4651–4654.

154. Koren H, Schenk GM, Jindra RH, et al. *J Photochem Photobiol B.* 1996;36(2): 113–119.

155. Hostanska K, Reichling J, Bommer S, et al. *Eur J Pharm Biopharm.* 2003;56(1): 121–132.

156. Liu JY, Liu Z, Wang DM, et al. *Chem Biol Interact.* 2011

157. Quiney C, Billard C, Faussat AM, et al. *Leukemia.* 2006;20(3):491–497.

158. Schempp CM, Kirkin V, Simon-Haarhaus B, et al. *Oncogene.* 2002;21(8):1242–1250.

159. Quiney C, Billard C, Faussat AM, et al. *Leuk Lymphoma.* 2007;48(8):1587–1599.

160. Dona M, Dell'Aica I, Pezzato E, et al. *Cancer Res.* 2004;64(17):6225–6232.

161. Lorusso G, Vannini N, Sogno I, et al. *Eur J Cancer.* 2009;45(8):1474–1484.

162. Rothley M, Schmid A, Thiele W, et al. *Int J Cancer.* 2009;125(1):34–42.

163. Martinez-Poveda B, Quesada AR, Medina MA. *Int J Cancer.* 2005;117(5):775–780.

164. Schempp CM, Kiss J, Kirkin V, et al. *Planta Med.* 2005;71(11):999–1004.

165. Schempp CM, Pelz K, Wittmer A, et al. *Lancet.* 1999;353(9170):2129.

166. Reichling J, Weseler A, Saller R. *Pharmacopsychiatry.* 2001;34 (suppl 1):116–118.

167. Avato P, Raffo F, Guglielmi G, et al. *Phytother Res.* 2004;18(3):230–232.

168. Cecchini C, Cresci A, Coman MM, et al. *Planta Med.* 2007;73(6):564–566.

169. Nikolic GS, Zlatkovic SZ. *J Med Plants Res.* 2010;43(3):211–224.

170. Saddiqe Z, Naeem I, Maimoona A. *J Ethnopharmacol.* 2010;131(3):511–521.

171. Radulovic N, Stankov-Jovanovic V, Stojanovic G, et al. *Food Chem.* 2007;103(1):15–21.

172. Rancic A, Sokovic M, Vukojevic J, et al. *J Essent Oil Res.* 2005;17:341–345.

173. Saroglou V, Marin PD, Rancic A, et al. *Biochem Syst Ecol.* 2007;35(3):146–152.

174. Engelhardt V, Krammer B, Plaetzer K. *Photochem Photobiol Sci.* 2010;9(3):365–369.

175. Peeva-Naumovska V, Panovsk N, Grdanovska T, et al. <wwwamapseecorg/cmapseec1/Papers/papp067htm>. Accessed 2010.

176. Voss A, Verweij P. *Lancet.* 1999;354(9180):777.

177. Dadgar T, Asmar M, Saifi A, et al. *Asian J Plant Sci.* 2006;5(5):861–866.

178. Conforti F, Statti GA, Tundis R, et al. *Nat Prod Res.* 2005;19(3):295–303.

179. Borchardt JR, Wyse DL, Sheaffer CC, et al. *J Med Plants Res.* 2008;2(5):98–110.

180. Milosevic T, Solujic S, Sukldolak S. *Turk J Biol.* 2007;31:237–241.

181. Maškovi PZ, Mladenovi JD, Cvijovi MS, et al. *Hemijska Industrija.* 2011;65(2):159–164.

182. Khosa RL, Bhatia N. *J Sci Res Plant Med.* 1982;3:49–50.

183. Hammer KD, Hillwig ML, Solco AK, et al. *J Agric Food Chem.* 2007;55(18): 7323–7331.

184. Raso GM, Pacilio M, Di Carlo G, et al. *J Pharm Pharmacol.* 2002;544(10): 1379–1383.

185. Tedeschi E, Menegazzi M, Margotto D, et al. *J Pharmacol Exp Ther.* 2003;307(1):254–261.

186. Ozturk N, Korkmaz S, Ozturk Y. *J Ethnopharmacol.* 2007;111(1):33–39.

187. Sosa S, Pace R, Bornancin A, et al. *J Pharm Pharmacol.* 2007;59(5):703–709.

188. Gurumadhva Rao S, Laxminarayana Udupa A, Saraswathi Udupa L, et al. *Fitoterapia*. 1991;62(6):508–510.

189. Kumar V, Singh PN, Bhattacharya SK. *Indian J Exp Biol*. 2001;39(4):339–343.

190. Schempp CM, Winghofer B, Ludtke R, et al. *Br J Dermatol*. 2000;142(5):979–984.

191. Süntar IP, Akkol EK, Yilmazer D, et al. *J Ethnopharmacol*. 2010;127(2):468–477.

192. Dost T, Ozkayran H, Gokalp F, et al. *Dig Dis Sci*. 2009;54(6):1214–1221.

193. Capasso R, Borrelli F, Capasso F, et al. *Urology*. 2004;64(1):168–172.

194. Jakovljevic V, Popovic M, Mimica-Dukic N, et al. *Phytomedicine*. 2000;7(6):449–453.

195. Khan A-U, Gilani AH. *Pharm Biol*. 2009;47(10):962–967.

196. Capasso R, Borrelli F, Montanaro V, et al. *J Urol*. 2005;173(6):2194–2197.

197. Thomas CA, Tyagi S, Yoshimura N, et al. *Urology*. 2007;70(4):813–816.

198. Donovan JL, Devane CL, Lewis JG, et al. *Phytother Res*. 2005;19(10):901–906.

199. Tahara YR, Sakamoto TR, Oshima YR, et al. *Curr Eye Res*. 1999;19(4):323–329.

200. Higuchi A, Yamada H, Yamada E, et al. *Mol Vis*. 2008;14:249–254.

201. Lavie G, Mandel M, Hazan S, et al. *Angiogenesis*. 2005;8(1):35–42.

202. Birzu M, Carnat A, Privat A, et al. *Phytother Res*. 1997;11:395–397.

203. Sharpley AL, Mcgavin CL, Whale R, et al. *Psychopharmacology*. 1998;139(3):286–287.

204. Demisch L, Sielaff T, Nispel J, et al. *AGNP Symposium, 1991*. Cited in Scientific Committee of ESCOP. *ESCOP Monographs: Hyperici Herba*. Exeter: European Scientific Cooperative on Phytotherapy; 1996.

205. Uzbay TI. *Phytother Res*. 2008;22(5):578–582.

206. Xu BJ, Zheng YN, Sung CK. *Drug Alcohol Rev*. 2005;24(6):525–536.

207. Rezvani A, Yang Y, Overstreet D, et al. *Alcohol Clin Exp Res*. 1988;22(3, suppl):121A.

208. Perfumi M, Santoni M, Cippitelli A, et al. *Alcohol Clin Exp Res*. 2003;27(10):1554–1562.

209. Perfumi M, Mattioli L, Cucculelli M, et al. *J Psychopharmacol*. 2005;19(5):448–454.

210. Perfumi M, Mattioli L, Forti L, et al. *Alcohol Alcohol*. 2005;40(4):291–296.

211. Schmidt U, Harrer G, Kuhn U, et al. *Nervenheilkunde*. 1993;12:314–319.

212. Feily A, Abbasi N. *Phytother Res*. 2009;23(11):1549–1552.

213. Catania MA, Firenzuoli F, Crupi A, et al. *Psychopharmacology*. 2003;169(2):186–189.

214. Husain GM, Chatterjee SS, Singh PN, et al. *Pharmacology*. 2011. Article ID 505247. doi:505210.505402/502011/505247, 2011.

215. Husain GM, Singh PN, Kumar V. *Pharmacologyonline*. 2008;3:889–894.

216. Galeotti N, Vivoli E, Bilia AR, et al. *J Pain*. 2010;11(2):149–159.

217. Galeotti N, Vivoli E, Bilia AR, et al. *Biochem Pharmacol*. 2010;79(9):1327–1336.

218. Murck H, Spitznagel H, Ploch M, et al. *Biol Psychiatry*. 2006;59(5):440–445.

219. Wurglics M, Schubert-Zsilavecz M. *Clin Pharmacokinet*. 2006;45(5):449–468.

220. Biber A, Fischer H, Romer A, et al. *Pharmacopsychiatry*. 1998;31 (suppl 1):36–43.

221. Agrosi M, Mischiatti S, Harrasser PC, et al. *Phytomedicine*. 2000;7(6):455–462.

222. Schulz HU, Schurer M, Bassler D, et al. *Arzneimittelforschung*. 2005;55(1):15–22.

223. Schulz HU, Schurer M, Bassler D, et al. *Arzneimittelforschung*. 2005;55(10):561–568.

224. Bauer S, Stormer E, Graubaum HJ, et al. *J Chromatogr B Biomed Sci Appl*. 2001;765(1):29–35.

225. Kerb R, Brockmoller J, Staffeldt B, et al. *Antimicrob Agents Chemother*. 1996;40(9):2087–2093.

226. Staffeldt B, Kerb R, Brockmoller J, et al. *J Geriatr Psychiatry Neurol*. 1994;7 (suppl 1):S47–53.

227. Mcauliffe V, Gulick RM, Hochster H, et al. *1st National Conference on Human Retroviruses and Related Infections*, December 12–16, 1993, p. 159.

228. Caccia S. *Curr Drug Metab*. 2005;6(6):531–543.

229. James J. *AIDS Treatment News*. 1989;74:1–6.

230. Cooper WC, James J. *International Conference on AIDS*, June 20–23, 1990;6(2):369. Abstract 2063.

231. Steinbeck-Klose A, Wernet P. *International Conference on AIDS* June 6–11, 1993;9(1):470. Abstract PO-B26-2012.

232. Vonsover A, Steinbeck K, Rudich C, et al. *International Conference on AIDS*, July 7–12, 1996;11(1):120. Abstract Mo-B-1377.

233. Pitisuttithum P, Migasena S, Suntharasamai P, et al. *International Conference on AIDS*, July 7–12, 1996;11(1):285. Abstract Tu-B-2121.

234. Furner V, Bek M, Gold J. *International Conference on AIDS*, June 16–21, 1991;7(2):199. Abstract W-B-2071.

235. National Institute of Allergy and Infectious Diseases, AIDS Clinical Trial Group. Protocol ID number: NIAID ACTG 258. Available from AIDSLINE database.

236. [No authors listed]: *TreatmentUpdate*. 2001;12(11):4–5.

237. Mannel M, Koytchev R, Dundarov S. Paper presented at the *3rd International Congress on Phytomedicine*, Munich, October 11–13 2000 (SL–25).

238. Koytchev R, Alken RG, Dundarov S. *Z Phytother*. 1999;20:92.

239. American Psychiatric Association *Diagnostic and Statistical Manual of Mental Disorders*. Washington, DC: American Psychiatric Association; 2000. pp. 356, 411.

240. Linde K, Mulrow CD. *Cochrane Database Sys Rev Abstracts*. 2000;2:CD000448.

241. Linde K, Ramirez G, Mulrow CD, et al. *Br Med J*. 1996;313:253–258.

242. Kim HL, Streltzer J, Goebert D. *J Nerv Ment Dis*. 1999;187(9):532–538.

243. Linde K, Berner MM, Kriston L. *Cochrane Database Syst Rev*. 2008;4:CD000448.

244. Roder C, Schaefer M, Leucht S. *Fortschr Neurol Psychiatr*. 2004;72(6):330–343.

245. Whiskey E, Werneke U, Taylor D. *Int Clin Psychopharmacol*. 2001;16(5):239–252.

246. Rahimi R, Nikfar S, Abdollahi M. *Prog Neuropsychopharmacol Biol Psychiatry*. 2009;33(1):118–127.

247. Gaster B, Holyroyd J. *Arch Intern Med*. 2000;160:152–156.

248. Josey ES, Tackett RL. *Intl J Clin Pharmacol Ther*. 1999;37(3):111–119.

249. Nangia M, Syed W, Doraiswamy PM. *Public Health Nutr*. 2000;3(4A):487–494.

250. Stevinson C, Ernst E. *Eur Neuropsychopharmacol*. 1999;9(6):501–505.

251. Linde K, Knuppel L. *Phytomedicine*. 2005;12(1–2):148–157.

252. Hängsen K-D, Vesper J. *München Med Wochenschr*. 1996;138(3):29–33.

253. Kalb R, Trautmann-Sponsel RD, Kieser M. *Pharmacopsychiatry*. 2001;34(3):96–103.

254. Kasper S, Anghelescu IG, Szegedi A, et al. *BMC Med*. 2006;4:14.

255. Lecrubier Y, Clerc G, Didi R, et al. *Am J Psychiatry*. 2002;159(8):1361–1366.

256. Schrader E. *Int Clin Psychopharmacol*. 2000;15(2):61–68.

257. Shelton RC, Keller MB, Gelenberg A, et al. *JAMA*. 2001;285(15):1978–1986.

258. Uebelhack R, Gruenwald J, Graubaum HJ, et al. *Adv Ther*. 2004;21(4):265–275.

259. Volz H, Eberhardt R, Grill G. *Nervenheilkunde*. 2000;19:401–405.

260. Witte B, Harrer G, Kaptan T, et al. *Fortschr Med*. 1995;113(28):404–408.

261. Bjerkenstedt L, Edman GV, Alken RG, et al. *Eur Arch Psychiatry Clin Neurosci*. 2005;255(1):40–47.

262. Davidson JRT, Hypericum Depression Trial Study Group *JAMA*. 2002;287(14):1807–1814.

263. Fava M, Alpert J, Nierenberg AA, et al. *J Clin Psychopharmacol*. 2005;25(5):441–447.

264. Gastpar M, Singer A, Zeller K. *Pharmacopsychiatry*. 2006;39(2):66–75.

265. Morena RA, Teng CT, De Almeida KM, et al. *Rev Bras Psiquiatr*. 2005;28:29–32.

266. Philipp M, Kohnen R, Hiller KO. *BMJ*. 1999;319:1534–1538.

267. Montgomery SA, Hubner WD, Grigoleit HG. *Phytomedicine*. 2000;7(suppl II):107.

268. Bracher A. *Ärztliche Praxis*. 2001;51(suppl):3–4.

269. Behnke K, Jensen GS, Graubaum HJ, et al. *Advances in Therapy*. 2002;19(1):43–52.

270. Brenner R, Azbel V, Madhusoodanan S, et al. *Clin Ther*. 2000;4:411–419.

271. Harrer G, Hübner WD, Podzuweit H. *Nervenheilkunde*. 1993;12:297–301.

272. Vorbach EU, Arnoldt KH, Hubner WD. *Pharmacopsychiatry*. 1997;30 (suppl 2):81–85.

273. Wheatley D. *Pharmacopsychiatry*. 1997;30(suppl 2):77–80.

274. Woelk H. *BMJ*. 2000;321:535–539.

275. Gastpar M, Singer A, Zeller K. *Pharmacopsychiatry*. 2005;38(2):78–86.

276. Harrer G, Schmidt U, Kuhn U, et al. *Arzneimittelforschung/Drug Res*. 1999;49(4):289–296.

277. Szegedi A, Kohnen R, Dienel A, et al. *BMJ*. 2005;330(7490):503.

278. Van Gurp G, Meterissian GB, Haiek LN, et al. *Can Fam Physician*. 2002;48:905–912.

279. Murck H, Fava M, Alpert J, et al. *Int J Neuropsychopharmacol*. 2005;8(2):215–221.

280. Vorbach EU, Hübner WD, Arnoldt KH. *Nervenheilkunde*. 1993;12:290–296.

281. Kasper S, Gastpar M, Muller WE, et al. *Eur Arch Psychiatry Clin Neurosci*. 2008;258(1):59–63.

282. Randlov C, Mehlsen J, Thomsen CF, et al. *Phytomedicine*. 2006;13(4):215–221.

283. Anghelescu IG, Kohnen R, Szegedi A, et al. *Pharmacopsychiatry*. 2006;39(6):213–219.

284. Singer A, Schmidt M, Hauke W, et al. *Phytomedicine*. 2011;18(8–9):739–742.

285. Mannel M, Kuhn U, Schmidt U, et al. *J Psychiatr Res*. 2010;44(12):760–767.

286. Brattstrom A. *Phytomedicine*. 2009;16(4):277–283.

287. Hubner WD, Kirste T. *Phytother Res*. 2001;15(4):367–370.

288. Findling RL, McNamara NK, O'Riordan MA, et al. *J Am Acad Child Adolesc Psychiatry*. 2003;42(8):908–914.

289. Simeon J, Nixon MK, Milin R, et al. *J Child Adolesc Psychopharmacol*. 2005;15(2):293–301.

290. Linde K, Berner M, Egger M, et al. *Br J Psychiatry*. 2005;186:99–107.

291. Wurglics M, Schubert-Zsilavecz M. *Pharm Unserer Zeit*. 2003;32(3):236–241.

292. Bone K. *e-Monitor*, No. 13. Warwick Queensland: MediHerb. September 2006.

293. Kasper S, Caraci F, Forti B, et al. *Eur Neuropsychopharmacol*. 2010;20(11):747–765.

294. Schakau D, Hiller K, Schultz-Zehden W, et al. *Psychopharmakotherapie*. 1996;3:116–122.

295. Davidson JR, Connor KM. *J Clin Psychopharmacol*. 2001;21(6):635–636.

296. Kobak KA, Taylor L, Futterer R, et al. *J Clin Psychopharmacol*. 2003;23(5):531–532.

297. Sarris J, Kavanagh DJ, Deed G, et al. *Hum Psychopharmacol*. 2009;24(1):41–48.

298. Volz HP, Murck H, Kasper S, et al. *Psychopharmacology (Berl)*. 2002;164(3):294–300.

299. Muller T, Mannel M, Murck H, et al. *Psychosom Med*. 2004;66(4):538–547.

300. Kobak KA, Taylor LV, Warner G, et al. *J Clin Psychopharmacol*. 2005;25(1):51–58.

301. Taylor LH, Kobak KA. *J Clin Psychiatry*. 2000;61(8):575–578.

302. Kobak KA, Taylor LV, Bystritsky A, et al. *Int Clin Psychopharmacol*. 2005;20(6):299–304.

303. Wheatley D. *Curr Med Res Opin*. 1999;15(1):33–37.

304. Martinez B, Kasper S, Ruhrmann B, et al. *Nervenheilkunde*. 1993;12:302–307.

305. Kasper S. *Pharmacopsychiatry*. 1997;30(suppl 2):89–93.

306. Warnecke G. *Z Allg Med*. 1986;62:1111–1113.

307. Grube B, Walper A, Wheatley MD. *Adv Ther*. 1999;16(4):177–186.

308. Al-Akoum M, Maunsell E, Verreault R, et al. *Menopause*. 2009;16(2):307–314.

309. Abdali K, Khajehei M, Tabatabaee HR. *Menopause*. 2010;17(2):326–331.

310. Van Die MD, Burger HG, Bone KM, et al. *Menopause*. 2009;16(1):156–163.

311. Uebelhack R, Blohmer JU, Graubaum HJ, et al. *Obstet Gynecol*. 2006;107 (2 Pt 1):247–255.

312. Boblitz N, Schrader E, Henneicke-Von-Zepelin H-H, et al. *FACT*. 2000;5(1):83–107.

313. Gerhard I, Liske E, Wüstenberg P. *6th Phytotherapy Conference, Berlin*, 1995.

314. Briese V, Stammwitz U, Friede M, et al. *Maturitas*. 2007;57(4):405–414.

315. Chung DJ, Kim HY, Park KH, et al. *Yonsei Med J*. 2007;48(2):289–294.

316. Stevinson C, Ernst E. *Br J Obstet Gynaecol*. 2000;107(7):870–876.

317. Ghazanfarpour M, Kaviani M, Asadi N, et al. *Int J Gynaecol Obstet*. 2011;113(1):84–85.

318. Canning S, Waterman M, Orsi N, et al. *CNS Drugs*. 2010;24(3):207–225.

319. Pak Gouhar M, Mehran A, Ahmadi M, et al. *J Med Plants Res*. 2005;4(15)

320. Hicks SM, Walker AF, Gallagher J, et al. *J Altern Complement Med*. 2004;10(6):925–932.

321. Van Die MD, Bone KM, Burger HG, et al. *J Altern Complement Med*. 2009;15(9):1045–1048.

322. Huang KL, Tsai SJ. *Int J Psychiatry Med*. 2003;33(3):295–297.

323. Siepmann M, Krause S, Joraschky P, et al. *Br J Clin Pharmacol*. 2002;54(3):277–282.

324. Timoshanko A, Stough C, Vitetta L, et al. *Behav Pharmacol*. 2001;12(8):635–640.

325. Ellis KA, Stough CB, Vitetta L, et al. *Behav Pharmacol*. 2001;12(3):173–182.

326. Wan H, Chen Y. *Int J Psychiatry Med*. 2010;40(1):45–56.

327. Saito YA, Rey E, Almazar-Elder AE, et al. *Am J Gastroenterol*. 2010;105(1):170–177.

328. Falahatkar S, Asgari SA, Hosseini Sharifi SH, et al. *J Guilan Uni Med Sci*. 2009;18(69):53–58.

329. Kaufman TWC-SJH. *Internet J Nutr Wellness*. 2007;3(2).

330. Kim DK, Chancellor MB. *Int Braz J Urol*. 2008;34(3):370–371.

331. Niederhofer H. *Nat Prod Res*. 2010;24(3):203–205.

332. Weber W, Vander Stoep A, Mccarty RL, et al. *JAMA*. 2008;299(22):2633–2641.

333. Czap AF. *Altern Med Rev*. 2008;13(2):84.

334. Samadi S, Khadivzadeh T, Emami A, et al. *J Altern Complement Med*. 2010;16(1):113–117.

335. Lavagna SM, Secci D, Chimenti P, et al. *Farmaco*. 2001;56(5–7):451–453.

336. Schempp CM, Windeck T, Hezel S, et al. *Phytomedicine*. 2003;10(suppl 4):31–37.

337. Rook AH, Wood GS, Duvic M, et al. *J Am Acad Dermatol*. 2010;63(6):984–990.

338. Kacerovska D, Pizinger K, Majer F, et al. *Photochem Photobiol*. 2008;84(3):779–785.

339. Sardella A, Lodi G, Demarosi F, et al. *J Oral Pathol Med*. 2008;37(7):395–401.

340. Sindrup SH, Madsen C, Bach FW, et al. *Pain*. 2001;91(3):361–365.

341. Friede M, Henneicke Von Zepelin HH, Freudenstein J. *Pharmacopsychiatry*. 2001;34(suppl 1):S38–41.

342. Schulz H, Jobert M. *J Geriatr Psychiatry Neurol*. 1994;7(suppl 1):S39–43.

343. Krylov AA, Ibatov AN. *Lik Sprava*. 1993;2–3:146–148.

344. Lawvere S, Mahoney MC, Cummings KM, et al. *Complement Ther Med*. 2006;14(3):175–184.

345. Kure C, Tarasuik J, Lloyd J, et al. *3rd International Congress on Complementary Medicine Research*, Sydney, 2008. Abstract P56.

346. Becker B, Bock B, Carmona-Barros R: *Society for Research on Nicotine and Tobacco 9th Annual Meeting*, New Orleans, Louisana USA, 2003.

347. Parsons A, Ingram J, Inglis J, et al. *Drug Alcohol Depend*. 2009;102(1–3):116–122.

348. Sood A, Ebbert JO, Prasad K, et al. *J Altern Complement Med*. 2010;16(7):761–767.

349. Barnes J, Barber N, Wheatley D, et al. *Planta Med*. 2006;72(4):378–382.

350. Niederhofer H. *Phytother Res*. 2009;23(11):1521–1523.

351. Czekalla J, Gastpar M, Hubner WD, et al. *Pharmacopsychiatry*. 1997;30 (suppl 2):86–88.

352. Horsley C. *J Pharmacol*. 1934;50:310–322.

353. Okpanyi SN, Lidzba H, Scholl BC, et al. *Arzneimittelforschung*. 1990;40(8):851–855.

354. Southwell I, Campbell M. *Phytochemistry*. 1991;30:475–478.

355. Araya OS, Ford EJ. *J Comp Pathol*. 1981;91(1):135–141.

356. Seigers C, Biel S, Wilhelm K. *Nervenheilkunde*. 1993;12:320–322.

357. Scientific Committee of ESCOP. *ESCOP Monographs: Hyperici Herba*. Exeter: European Scientific Cooperative on Phytotherapy; 1996.

358. Tran TL. *Curr Clin Strateg*. 1997;125(16):1022–1087.

359. Guzelcan Y, Scholte WF, Assies J, et al. *Ned Tijdschr Geneeskd*. 2001;145(40):1943–1945.

360. Moses EL, Mallinger AG. *J Clin Psychopharmacol*. 2000;20(1):115–117.

361. Nierenberg AA, Burt T, Matthews J, et al. *Biol Psychiatry*. 1999;46(12):1707–1708.

362. Stevinson C, Ernst E. *Int J Clin Pharmacol Ther*. 2004;42(9):473–480.

363. O'Breasail AM, Argouarch S. *Can J Psychiatryol*. 1998;43(7):746–747.

364. Schneck C. *J Clin Psychiatry*. 1998;59(12):689.

365. Fahmi M, Huang C, Schweitzer I. *World J Biol Psychiatry*. 2002;3(1):58–59.

366. Spinella M, Eaton LA. *Brain Inj*. 2002;16(4):359–367.

367. Ciocon JO, Ciocon DG, Galindo DJ. *Geriatrics*. 2004;59(9):20–24.

368. Crowe S, Mckeating K. *Anesthesiology*. 2002;96(4):1025–1027.

369. Zhou S, Chan E, Pan S-Q, et al. *J Psychopharmacol*. 2004;18(2):262–276.

370. Crockett SL, Schaneberg B, Khan IA. *Phytochem Anal*. 2005;16(6):479–485.

371. Kroll DJ, Shaw HS, Wall ME, et al. *Altern Ther Health Med*. 2001;7(6):21–22.

372. Moore LB, Goodwin B, Jones SA, et al. *Proc Natl Acad Sci USA*. 2000;97(13):7500–7502.

373. Wentworth JM, Agostini M, Love J, et al. *J Endocrinol*. 2000;166:R11–R16.

374. Vogel G. *Science*. 2001;291(5501):35–357.

375. Kliewer SA. *J. Nutr*. 2003;133(7 suppl):2444S–2447S.

376. Tian R, Koyabu N, Morimoto S, et al. *Drug Metab Dispos*. 2005;33(4):547–554.

377. Mueller SC, Majcher-Peszynska J, Uehleke B, et al. *Eur J Clin Pharmacol*. 2006;62(1):29–36.

378. Mai I, Bauer S, Perloff ES, et al. *Clin Pharmacol Ther*. 2004;76(4):330–340.

379. Arold G, Donath F, Maurer A, et al. *Planta Med*. 2005;71(4):331–337.

380. Will-Shahab L, Brattström A, Roots I, et al. 2001 Symposium "Phytopharmaka VII": Abstracts of Presentations and Posters, Berlin. p. 15.

381. Lehmann R. *Personal communication*. MediHerb; 2004.

382. Mueller SC, Uehleke B, Woehling H, et al. *Clinical Pharmacol Ther*. 2004;75(6):546–557.

383. Munson PL, Mueller RA, Breese GR. *Principles of Pharmacology: Basic Concepts and Clinical Applications*. New York: Chapman & Hall; 1995.

384. Fennell J, Hussain M. *Ir Med J*. 2005;98(5):143–144.

385. Siepmann M, Kirch W, Krause S, et al. *J Clin Psychopharmacol*. 2004;24(1):79–82.

386. DiCarlo G, Borrelli F, Ernst E, et al. *Trends Pharmacol Sci*. 2001;22(6):292–297.

387. Gobbi M, Mennini T. *Trends Pharmacol Sci*. 2001;22(11):557–559.

388. DiCarlo G, Borrelli F, Ernst E, et al. *Trends Pharmacol Sci*. 2001;22(11):559.

389. Fornal CA, Metzler CW, Mirescu C, et al. *Neuropsychopharmacology*. 2005;25(6):858–870.

390. Johne A, Schmider J, Brockmoller J, et al. *J Clin Psychopharmacol*. 2002;22(1):46–54.

391. Gordon JB. *Am Fam Phys*. 1998;57(5):950. 953.

392. Lantz MS, Buchalter E, Giambanco V. *Geriatr Psychiatry Neurol*. 1999;12(1):7–10.

393. Waksman JC, Heard K, Joliff H, et al. *Clin Toxicol*. 2000;38:521.

394. Barbenel DM, Yusufi B, O'Shea D, et al. *J Psychopharmacol*. 2000;14:84–86.

395. Dermott K. *Clin Psychiatry News*. 1998;26:28.

396. Prost N, Tichadou L, Rodor F, et al. *Presse Med*. 2000;29(23):1285–1286.

397. Moretti ME, Maxson A, Hanna F, et al. *Reprod Toxicol*. 2009;28(1):96–99.

398. Grush LR, Nierenberg A, Keefe B, et al. *JAMA*. 1998;280(18):1566.

399. *Psychotonin M Product Information*, Steigerwald Arzneimittelwerk GmbH, Darmstadt, 1992.

400. Rayburn WF, Gonzalez CL, Christensen HD, et al. *Am J Obstet Gynecol*. 2001;184(2):191–195.

401. Gonzalez C, Stewart J, Rayburn W, et al. *Neurotoxicol Teratol*. 1998;20(3):369.

402. Christensen H, Rayburn W, Coleman F, et al. *Teratology*. 1999;59(6):411.

403. Leuschner J. *2nd International Congress on Phytomedicine*, Munich, September 11–14, 1996. Abstract SL 80.

404. Cada AM, Hansen DK, Laborde JB, et al. *Nutr Neurosci*. 2001;4(2):135–141.

405. Klier CM, Schafer MR, Schmid-Siegel B, et al. *Pharmacopsychiatry*. 2002;35(1):29–30.

406. Klier CM, Schmid–Siegel B, Schafer MR, et al. *J Clin Psychiatry*. 2006;67(2):305–309.

407. Lee A, Minhas R, Matsuda N, et al. *J Clin Psychiatry*. 2003;64(8):966–968.

408. Kasper S. *Pharmacopsychiatry*. 2001;34(suppl 1):S51–55.

409. Lieberman S. *J Womens Health*. 1998;7(2):177–182.

410. Trautmann-Sponsel RD, Dienel A. *J Affect Disord*. 2004;82(2):303–307.

411. Hubner WD, Lande S, Podzuweit H. *J Geriatr Psychiatry Neurol*. 1994;7 (suppl 1):S12–14.

412. Schmidt U, Sommer H. *Fortschr Med*. 1993;111(19):339–342.

413. Sommer H, Harrer G. *J Geriatr Psychiatry Neurol*. 1994;7(suppl 1):S9–11.

414. Knuppel L, Linde K. *J Clin Psychiatry*. 2004;65(11):1470–1479.

415. Woelk H, Burkard G, Grunwald J. *J Geriatr Psychiatry Neurol*. 1993;7 (suppl 1):S34–S38.

416. Schulz V. *Schweiz Rundsch Med Prax*. 2000;89(50):2131–2140.

417. Holme SA, Roberts DL. *Br J Dermatol*. 2000;143(5):1127–1128.

418. Golsch S, Vocks E, Rakoski J, et al. *Hautarzt*. 1997;48(4):249–252.

419. Cotterill JA. *J Cosmet Laser Ther*. 2001;3(3):159–160.

420. Schempp CM, Winghofer B, Muller K, et al. *Phytother Res*. 2003;17(2):141–146.

421. Schempp CM, Muller K, Winghofer B, et al. *Arch Dermatol*. 2001;137(4):512–513.

422. Roots I, Reum T, Brockmoller J, et al. *2nd International Congress on Phytomedicine*, Munich, September 11–14, 1996.

423. Lane-Brown MM. *Med J Aust*. 2000;172(6):302.

424. Bernd A, Simon S, Ramirez Bosca A, et al. *Photochem Photobiol*. 1999;69(2):218–221.

425. Traynor NJ, Beattie PE, Ibbotson SH, et al. *Toxicol Lett*. 2005;158(3):220–224.

426. Baille N. *Modern Phytotherapist*. 1997;3(2):24–26.

427. Bove GM. *Lancet*. 1998;352(9134):1121–1122.

428. Rey JM, Walter G. *Med J Aust*. 1998;169(11–12):583–586.

429. Ferko N, Levine MA. *Pharmacotherapy*. 2001;21(12):1574–1578.

430. Hauben M. *Pharmacotherapy*. 2002;22(5):673–675.

431. Zullino D, Borgeat F. *Pharmacopsychiatry*. 2003;36(1):32.

432. Patel S, Robinson R, Burk M. *Am J Med*. 2002;112(6):507–508.

433. Irefin S, Sprung J. *J Clin Anesth*. 2000;12(6):498–499.

434. Dean AJ, Moses GM, Vernon JM. *Ann Pharmacother*. 2003;37(1):150.

435. Laird RD, Webb MJ. *Herb Pharmacother*. 2001;1(2):81–87.

436. Lal S, Iskandar H. *CMAJ*. 2000;163(3):262–263.

437. Shimizu K, Nakamura M, Isse K, et al. *Hum Psychopharmacol*. 2004;19(4):275–276.

438. Dominguez Jimenez JL, Pleguezuelo Navarro M, Guiote Malpartida S, et al. *Gastroenterol Hepatol*. 2007;30(1):54–55.

439. Assalian P. *J Sex Marital Ther*. 2000;26(4):357–358.

440. Bhopal JS. *Can J Psychiatry*. 2001;46(5):456–457.

441. Nanayakkara PW, Meijboom M, Schouten JA. *Ned Tijdschr Geneeskd*. 2005;149(24):1347–1349.

442. Karalapillai DC, Bellomo R. *Med J Aust*. 2007;186(4):213–214.

(*Silybum marianum* (L.) Gaertn.)

Synonyms

Carduus marianus L. (botanical synonym), milk thistle (Engl), Silybi mariae fructus, Cardui mariae fructus (Lat), Mariendistelfrüchte, Mariendistel, Marienkörner (Ger), chardon-Marie (Fr), carduo mariano (Ital), marietidsel (Dan).

What is it?

St Mary's thistle (milk thistle) is indigenous to the Mediterranean region but has been introduced to most areas of Europe, North and South America and is considered a noxious weed in Australia. The stalk and young leaves have been eaten as a salad vegetable (Culpeper recommended the boiled leaf as a blood cleanser). Although historical references indicate extensive use of St Mary's thistle, even going back 2000 years, its use was revitalised in Germany in the mid-19th century and again in modern practice in the 1930s. Its main active fraction, a flavonolignan complex known as silymarin, has been extensively investigated, particularly as a hepatoprotective agent. Several other novel uses for the silymarin complex have also been identified in recent clinical trials. The leaf of St Mary's thistle is also used medicinally, but this monograph discusses the fruit (seed).

Effects

Scavenges free radicals, increases intracellular concentration of glutathione; stabilises hepatocyte membrane against injury and regulates its permeability, assists in cellular regeneration, increases the proliferation of Kupffer cells.

Traditional view

The seeds of St Mary's thistle were used in Germany for curing jaundice, hepatic and biliary derangements, hepatitis and haemorrhoids, and as a demulcent in catarrh and pleurisy.[1,2] External application of the decoction was recommended for some types of cancer. Dioscorides proposed the seeds as a remedy for snakebite. Culpeper suggested infusion of the fresh root and seeds for breaking and expelling gallstones and to treat dropsy (taken internally and applied externally to the liver).[2] The seeds, or more often the silymarin complex, have recently been adopted in clinical practice for hepatoprotection during chemotherapy, as an adjunct to cancer treatment, and to ameliorate the long-term side effects of cancer treatment.[3]

Summary actions

Hepatoprotective, hepatic trophorestorative, antioxidant, choleretic, galactagogue.

Can be used for

Indications supported by clinical trials

Clinical indications supported by trials using standardised St Mary's thistle extract (70% to 80% silymarin by colorimetric analysis, 50% to 60% by HPLC), otherwise described in this monograph as the silymarin complex or just 'silymarin': non-alcoholic and alcoholic liver damage/disease, including abnormal liver function, alcoholic and Child-Pugh grade A cirrhosis; diabetes secondary to cirrhosis, and other complications of cirrhosis such as bleeding oesophageal varices; fatty liver; exposure to chemical pollutants or xenobiotics (drugs, halogenated hydrocarbons, solvents, paints, glues, anaesthesia); treatment of death cap mushroom poisoning.

The evidence for some of the above applications is controversial. Mixed results have been obtained for treatment of hepatitis, where it should mainly be prescribed for its hepatoprotective properties.

Some support has been obtained for the role of silymarin in improving glycaemic profile and insulin resistance in type 2 diabetes, as an iron chelator in haemochromatosis and beta-thalassemia/thalassemia major, and in promoting lactation in nursing mothers. It has also shown promise as a hepatoprotective agent during chemotherapy, based on results of one clinical trial.

Traditional therapeutic uses

Liver and gallbladder problems.

Despite the common name, milk thistle (which relates to the milky venations on the leaf), only the leaf was attributed with galactagogue properties in some traditional sources.[2]

May also be used for

Extrapolations from pharmacological studies

As a prophylactic for conditions caused by oxidative stress; for complications of hepatitis C; liver problems associated with pregnancy, oral contraceptive use or environmental pollution; for a fetoprotective effect against ethanol ingestion; to prevent gallstone formation; inhibition of cholesterol absorption; may exert a cytoprotective effect on pancreatic tissue, assist in cholestasis and have a role in preventing the complications of diabetes (such as diabetic neuropathy); may be beneficial as an antiallergic and anti–inflammatory agent; may have a chemopreventative activity for some cancers; preventing or reducing hepatotoxicity associated with chemo– or radiotherapy, and as an adjunctive treatment for potentiating chemotherapy and radiation therapy; reducing the side effects of conventional treatment for Alzheimer's disease and hepatotoxicity associated with antituberculosis drugs; possible anti-osteoporotic and selective oestrogen receptor modulator activity. Topically, silymarin may be protective against chemical carcinogen– and UVB radiation–induced skin tumours.

Preparations

Dried seed as a decoction, liquid extract, tablet or capsule for internal use.

Dosage

* 4 to 9 g/day of seed
* 4 to 9 mL/day of 1:1 liquid extract
* Three to four tablets per day containing 200 mg of extract (standardised to at least 140 mg silymarin by colorimetric assay or 100 mg by HPLC).

Higher doses, especially of the tablets, can be used in more severe cases of liver damage. The absorption of silymarin is enhanced by lecithin, and simultaneous dosing with a lecithin supplement is recommended. Extracts with enhanced bioavailability are also available.

Duration of use

There is no restriction on long–term use.

Summary assessment of safety

St Mary's thistle is an extremely safe herb.

Technical data

Botany

Silybum marianum is a member of the Compositae (Asteraceae, daisy) family and in the same tribe as globe artichoke.[4] It is an annual to biennial herb with a 35 to 125 cm stem. The leaves are dark green, oblong, pinnatifid with spiny margins. White veins give the leaves a diffusely mottled appearance. The slightly fragrant, hermaphrodite flower heads are also spiny, deep violet in colour, 1 to 2.5 cm in diameter and sit above an involucre containing rows of spiny bracts. The fruit is an achene, 6 to 7 mm in length and transversely wrinkled, dark in colour, grey–flecked

with a yellow ring near the apex. Attached to the achene is a long white pappus.[5,6]

Key constituents

* Flavonolignans (1.5% to 3%): silybin A and B, isosilybin A and B, silychristin, silydianin and 2,3–dehydro derivatives. These flavonolignans are collectively known as silymarin[7]
* Fixed oil (20% to 30%), flavonoids, taxifolin, sterols.[8]

Silybin (silibin) is also called silibinin (particularly in European literature). The flavonolignans are often incorrectly classified as flavonoids. Based on their structures they would be more correctly named 'flavanolignans'.

The fixed oil can give liquid extracts a milky colour or may sometimes separate in such preparations.

Pharmacodynamics

Antioxidant activity

In vitro research has demonstrated free radical scavenging activity and antioxidant properties exerted by silymarin in a concentration–dependent manner.[9] One possible mechanism for such activity is the in vitro increase by silymarin of activities of the key antioxidant enzymes superoxide dismutase (SOD), catalase, glutathione peroxidase, glutathione reductase, glutathione–S–transferase (GST) and glutathione peroxidase. As a consequence, malondialdehyde (MDA), a marker for lipid peroxidation, was reduced in erythrocytes exposed to exogenous hydrogen peroxide.[10] These findings suggest a role of silymarin in activating the molecular switch for the cell's endogenous protection against oxidative damage, namely the Nrf2/ARE pathway. Some early findings are suggestive of this activity.[11] Silybin also demonstrated free radical scavenger and antioxidant activities in vitro when complexed with molecules that increase its solubility.[12]

Both silybin and silydianin exerted an inhibitory effect on superoxide radical production, peak chemiluminescence and hydrogen peroxide production in stimulated human polymorphonuclear neutrophils in vitro.[13] Oxidative stress induced by a high glucose concentration in human mesangial cell cultures was counteracted by silybin.[14] Silybin (in addition to the finding for silymarin mentioned above) increased the activity of both SOD and glutathione peroxidase in human erythrocytes in vitro. As previously noted, this may explain the protective effect against free radicals and the stabilising effect on the red blood cell membrane, as demonstrated by an increase in the time to full haemolysis.[15] Silybin dihemisuccinate sodium salt demonstrated an inhibitory effect in vitro on radiation–induced deactivation of enzymes and peroxidation of membrane lipids in rat liver microsomes.[16] Silybin inhibited linoleate peroxidation in vitro.[17]

In contrast to other findings, silybin was a potent inhibitor of GST isoenzymes in one in vitro model and displayed a high degree of isoenzyme selectivity.[18]

Intraperitoneal administration of silymarin to rats increased the redox state and total glutathione content of the liver, intestine and stomach, without affecting levels in the kidney, lung and spleen.[19] Although a noticeable effect is observed, the effect of silymarin on lipid peroxidation processes was less

Silybin

Silychristin

Silydianin

marked in patients with chronic diffuse liver diseases than for in vitro experiments.[20]

In vitro research on cultured neural cells demonstrated that a St Mary's thistle extract could promote neuronal differentiation and survival, suggesting potential benefits on the nervous system. The extract also protected cultured rat hippocampal neurons against oxidative stress–induced cell death.[21]

Silymarin and two derivatives, silybin–beta–cyclodextrin and silybin, showed a clear ability to reduce lipid peroxidation in vitro and after oral administration to rats with extrahepatic biliary obstruction.[22] These agents were all administered at doses of 10 to 100 mg/kg/day for 15 days. All three agents inhibited the in vitro and in vivo production of TBARS (thiobarbituric acid reactive substances). Silymarin increased glutathione peroxidase and GST activities in both models.

Silymarin administered in conjunction with praziquantel (PZQ) to mice infected with the larval stage of *Mesocestoides vogae* (Cestoda) showed a strong antioxidant capacity and stimulated the larvicidal effect of PZQ, probably due to the down–regulation of fibrogenesis.[23] Silymarin (30 mg/kg, oral) and PZQ were administered once a day from day 15 post infection for 10 consecutive days. Treatment with silymarin in combination with PZQ downregulated the generation of superoxide anions, prevented lipid peroxidation and stimulated glutathione synthesis and proliferation of hepatocytes in infected livers.

Effects on detoxification mechanisms

St Mary's thistle extracts and components appear to reduce the activity of cytochrome P450 (CYP) enzymes in vitro.

Some evidence for metabolic interactions between silybin and xenobiotics metabolised by CYP3A4 or CYP2C9 was obtained from in vitro studies in human liver microsomes.[24] In human hepatocyte cultures, treatment with silymarin (0.1 and 0.25 mM) significantly reduced the activity of the CYP3A4 isoenzyme (by 50% and 100%, respectively).[25]

In one study, oral administration of silymarin (100 mg/kg/day) to rats resulted in a significant increase of the activity of the mixed function oxidation system (CYP, aminopyrine demethylation and p–nitroanisole demethylation). However, an experimentally induced reduction in the activity of the mixed function oxidation system and glucose–6–phosphatase could not be prevented by pretreatment with silymarin. Also in human volunteers, treatment with silymarin (210 mg/day for 28 days) had no influence on the metabolism of aminopyrine and phenylbutazone.[26]

The protein transporter P–glycoprotein (P–gp) is involved in the clearance of toxic metabolites and xenobiotics from cells into urine, bile and the intestinal lumen. This is in addition to its role as a drug efflux pump at epithelial cells. The influence of silymarin on P–gp has been extensively reviewed in the section on Interactions (see later), and only a summary of findings is included here. In 16 healthy volunteers, silymarin (900 mg/day for 14 days) did not appear to affect digoxin pharmacokinetics, suggesting that it is not a potent modulator of P–gp in vivo.[27] However, while one human study found reduced drug (metronidazole) levels following silymarin, suggesting it may cause an induction of intestinal and perhaps hepatic expression of P–gp and CYP3A4,[28] most findings from in vitro, in vivo and human research point to an inhibition of P–gp by silymarin and its constituents.[29–36] A major implication of silymarin's ability to inhibit P–gp is its potential role in negating multi–drug resistance, which is discussed in the section on cancer below.

Silymarin may prevent the absorption of toxins into hepatocytes, both by occupying binding sites and inhibiting transport proteins at the cell membrane. It has exhibited a regulatory action on cellular and mitochondrial membrane permeability in association with increased membrane stability against xenobiotic injury (see also under Hepatoprotective activity below). The phalloidin–transporting system, which belongs to the organic anion uptake transporters OATP2, is inhibited in a competitive way by silymarin, with no influence on membrane fluidity. OATP2 may represent part of the hepatic equipment that clears the portal blood of bile acids, lipophilic hormones and xenobiotics.[37]

Hence, although it is popularly regarded as a herb that can increase the hepatic clearance of xenobiotics, the balance of evidence suggests that this is not the case for St Mary's thistle. Its role is more to protect the liver from any potential damage that xenobiotic clearance might entail (see also the Interactions section later in this monograph).

Hepatoprotective activity

The pharmacological literature on the hepatoprotective activity of silymarin and silybin is extensive. The following is a selection from publications on this topic. The mechanisms behind the hepatoprotective action of silymarin possibly involve the following:[38]

- Antioxidant activity by scavenging free radicals (reducing reactive oxygen species, ROS), and by increasing the intracellular concentration of glutathione; reduced lipid peroxidation and increased catalase activity.[39]
- Activity at the nuclear level: enhancing the synthesis of ribosomal RNA and proteins and thereby cellular regeneration; a possible steroid–like behaviour on the control of DNA expression.[40] (This is thought to be an important mechanism.)
- Antifibrotic activity by inhibiting NF–kappaB and retarding hepatic stellate cell activation; inducing hepatic stellate cell apoptosis and inhibiting protein kinases and other kinases involved in signal transduction, and possibly interacting with intracellular signalling pathways, or inducing degradation of collagen deposits.[38]
- Toxin blockade via a regulatory action on cellular and mitochondrial membrane permeability in association with an increase in membrane stability against xenobiotic injury, preventing the absorption of toxins into the hepatocytes by occupying binding sites as well as inhibiting many transport proteins at the membrane.[38,41]
- Anti–inflammatory and immune–modulating activity, via decreased expression of hepatic tumour necrosis factor (TNF)–alpha;[42] inhibition of nitric oxide (NO) production and inducible nitric oxide synthase (iNOS) gene expression;[43,44] inhibition of the 5–lipoxygenase pathway in cytoplasm;[45] and possible inhibition of adhesion molecules such as E–selectin.[46]
- Competitive inhibition of the phalloidin–transporting system, belonging to the hepatocyte–specific OATP2.[38,47]

- Improvement of glucose and lipid metabolism, particularly in liver steatosis.[38]
- Reduced tumour promoter activity.

Although relatively high concentrations of silybin are necessary to diminish free radical formation by activated Kupffer cells, significant inhibition of the 5–lipoxygenase pathway occurs at silybin concentrations that can be achieved in vivo. Selective inhibition of leukotriene formation by Kupffer cells could at least partly account for the hepatoprotective properties of silybin.[45]

Some recent in vitro data for the hepatoprotective activity of St Mary's thistle components includes the following. Silybin inhibited interleukin (IL)–1beta–induced production of pro–inflammatory mediators in canine hepatocyte cultures, reinforcing the notion of its hepatoprotective effect.[48] Silybin prevented cholestasis–associated retrieval of the bile salt export pump Bsep in isolated rat hepatocyte couplets by a mechanism probably involving cAMP–induced cytosolic calcium elevations.[49]

The in vivo data demonstrating the hepatoprotective activity of St Mary's thistle and its components is extensive. In earlier research, prior intraperitoneal administration of silymarin protected against the effects of carbon tetrachloride in mice, by decreasing its metabolic activation and acting as an antioxidant.[50] Silymarin and isolated silybin protected against acute administration of liver toxins such as carbon tetrachloride,[51] galactosamine,[52] ethanol,[53] paracetamol,[54] lanthanides and FV3 virus in animal models.[55] Similar protective activity was demonstrated in early research against chronic administration of carbon tetrachloride,[56,57] heavy metals,[58] thioacetamide[59] and several drugs.[60]

One of the key issues with chronic liver damage is the disruption of liver architecture induced by the generation of excessive fibrous tissue. High dose silymarin (200 mg/kg, oral) resolved carbon tetrachloride–induced hepatic fibrosis in rats.[56] In addition, silymarin significantly decreased the elevation of aspartate aminotransferase (AST), alanine aminotransferase (ALT) and alkaline phosphatase in serum, and also reversed the altered expression of alpha–smooth muscle actin in liver tissue. One antifibrotic mechanism for oral silymarin at 50 mg/kg/day was demonstrated in 30 female rats with bile duct occlusion.[61] After 6 weeks, silymarin suppressed expression of profibrogenic procollagen alpha1(I) and TIMP–1, most likely via downregulation of TGF–beta1 mRNA. The lowered hepatic profibrogenic transcript levels correlated with decreased serum levels of the aminoterminal propeptide of procollagen type III. Silymarin treatment reduced granuloma and hepatic fibrosis in the acute phase of experimental schistosomiasis in mice treated intraperitoneally with 10, 20 or 25 doses of silymarin at 10 mg/kg.[62]

Post–treatment of rats with silymarin (25 mg/kg) and *Terminalia chebula* (125 mg/kg) following oral administration of paracetamol (acetaminophen) 500 mg/kg for 1 to 3 days ameliorated the significant elevation of serum triglycerides, total cholesterol, blood urea nitrogen, serum creatinine and AST activity, suggesting that silymarin exhibited good hepato and nephro–protection against paracetamol toxicity.[63] Reduced mortality was demonstrated in mice administered silymarin at doses of 100 or 200 mg/kg for 2 to 4 days following a lethal dose of paracetamol (550 mg/kg, ip), supporting its suggested use as an antidote for paracetamol-induced acute hepatic injury.[64]

Silymarin has shown both prophylactic and curative activities against the toxin of the death cap mushroom (*Amanita phalloides*).[65] It interrupts the enterohepatic recirculation of amanitins, inhibits the binding of alpha–amanitin to hepatocyte membranes, competes with amatoxin for transmembrane transport and inhibits the penetration of amanitin into liver cells.[66,67] Intravenous pretreatment with silybin in animal experiments abolished the morphological changes induced by the toxin and decreased the activities of serum enzymes.[68] (See also under Clinical trials.)

Oral administration of silybin (100 mg/kg) protected against iron–induced hepatic toxicity in rats via an antioxidant mechanism.[69] In addition, silymarin (200 mg/kg, oral) over 2 weeks had a protective effect similar to desferrioxamine on iron overload–induced hepatotoxicity in rats, as manifested by the decreased number of necrotic hepatocytes.[70]

A silybin–phospholipid complex prevented severe oxidative stress and preserved hepatic mitochondrial bioenergetics in a rodent model of nonalcoholic steatohepatitis.[71] Treatment for 7 to 14 weeks with silybin complexed with phospholipids (0.4 g/kg diet) limited glutathione depletion and mitochondrial hydrogen peroxide production, preserved mitochondrial bioenergetics and prevented mitochondrial proton leak and ATP reduction.

Silybin treatment stabilised mitochondrial membrane, inhibited oxidative stress and improved insulin resistance in nonalcoholic fatty liver disease in rats.[72] Intragastric silybin at a dose of 26.25 mg/kg/day significantly protected against high–fat–induced fatty liver in male Sprague–Dawley rats, by stabilising mitochondrial membrane fluidity, reducing the serum content of AST, decreasing hepatic MDA and increasing SOD and glutathione levels.

In a 57–year–old man, silybin therapy by daily intravenous infusion at a dose of 1400 mg for 14 days commenced 8 h after orthotopic liver transplantation (OLT) successfully prevented hepatitis C virus (HCV) liver graft reinfection.[73] At the time of OLT, the patient exhibited a model for end–stage liver disease (MELD) score of 23, Child–Pugh stage C liver cirrhosis and a 25 mm hepatocellular carcinoma in the left lobe. The HCV RNA level measured 182 IU/mL, and it dropped to 127 IU/mL after 48 h. By day 3 onwards, HCV RNA levels were <15 IU/mL and became undetectable by day 9. After 6 months of follow–up, RNA for HCV was still undetectable, and liver histology did not show any cellular inflammation.

A similar result using intravenous silybin therapy was obtained in terms of preventing graft infection in a patient with cirrhosis and end-stage liver failure (Child–Pugh stage C, MELD 20) due to chronic HCV.[74] The 46–year–old male patient with beta–thalassemia was diagnosed with HCV with mixed genotype 1a/4. He was pretreated with silybin (20 mg/kg/day) for 15 days, with an interruption of 2 days in the postoperative period. Baseline viral load was low and decreased to 43 IU/mL on the day of OLT. HCV RNA levels decreased after resuming infusions to 30 IU/mL on day 6 and became unquantifiable (<15 IU/mL) on day 10, and undetectable on day 22 after OLT. Silybin was stopped 25 days after OLT. During 5 months of follow–up, HCV RNA levels remained undetectable.

In early research, silymarin protected against histological changes in the livers of pregnant women and those taking oral contraceptives.[75]

Other anti–toxic effects

Several in vivo studies have found that silymarin ameliorates some of the negative consequences of in utero exposure to ethanol.[76-78] An orally administered complex (one part silybin to two parts phosphatidylcholine) at a dietary dose of 400 mg/kg for 21 days protected the rat fetus from the toxic effects of maternally ingested ethanol.[76] Maternal and fetal gamma-glutamyltranspeptidase (GGT) activity was not elevated in the silybin–treated group, whereas in the ethanol–treated rats it was significantly higher than controls. Fetal mortality was also significantly higher in the ethanol group. Co–administration of a silymarin/phospholipid compound containing 29.8% silybin to the ethanol liquid diet of pregnant Fisher/344 rats at a dose of 400 mg/kg throughout the gestational period protected against the incomplete development of corpus callosum (splenium) in offspring.[77] Silymarin appeared to ameliorate the ethanol–induced learning deficits in pregnant Fischer/344 rats treated with a silymarin/phospholipid compound (containing 29.8% silybin, co–administered at a dose of 400 mg/kg with a liquid diet containing 35% ethanol–derived calories) during days 15 to 21 of the gestational period.[78]

Other gastrointestinal activity

Compared with controls, silybin increased the proliferative activity of Kupffer cells in rats subjected to partial hepatectomy. Phagocytic and bactericidal activities were not modified.[79] Silybin demonstrated anticholestatic activity against paracetamol– and ethinyl oestradiol–induced cholestasis by countering the reduction in bile salt output and bile flow (see also below).[80]

Oral silymarin demonstrated an anticholesterolaemic effect in rats fed a high–cholesterol diet. The effect was similar to the hypocholesterolaemic drug probucol. In addition, silymarin caused an increase in LDL–cholesterol, a decrease in liver cholesterol content and partially prevented the decrease in liver of reduced glutathione. Silybin was not as effective as silymarin.[81]

Silymarin and a polyphenolic fraction (PF) of silymarin administered via the diet (1.0% w/w) for 18 days to male rats fed a high cholesterol diet resulted in an inhibition of cholesterol absorption.[82] This PF of silymarin was obtained by dissolution in acetone followed by precipitation with hexane. Both silymarin and PF significantly reduced cholesterol absorption and caused significant decreases in plasma and VLDL–cholesterol, as well as the content of cholesterol and triacylglycerols in the liver. The level of HDL–cholesterol was significantly increased by silymarin, but not by PF.

Subsequent research by the same group found that polymerised polyphenolics (PP) and silymarin administered via the diet (0.1% to 1.0%) for 3 weeks to female rats fed either a high–cholesterol (1%) or a high–fat (10%) diet caused a dose–dependent decrease in liver cholesterol and VLDL–cholesterol, and an increase in the HDL–cholesterol/VLDL–cholesterol ratio.[83] However, neither silymarin nor PP had any effect on plasma cholesterol content or LDL–cholesterol levels. Only negligible increases of HDL–cholesterol were observed. Both treatments caused moderate dose–dependent increases in blood but not liver glutathione (GSH) content.

Silymarin (50 to 150 mg/kg, ip) prevented 17alpha–ethinyl oestradiol (EO)–induced cholestasis in rats, decreasing both bile–salt–independent and the bile–salt–dependent fractions of the bile flow, and the associated reduction in the bile salt pool size.[84] The extract also counteracted the inhibitory effect of EO on bicarbonate but not GSH output, two major determinants of the bile–salt–independent bile flow.

Silymarin (25 to 150 mg/kg/day for 5 days, ip) induced a dose–dependent increase in bile flow and bile salt secretion.[85] These findings suggest that silymarin increases biliary excretion and the endogenous pool of bile salts by stimulating the synthesis, among others, of hepatoprotective bile salts such as beta–muricholate and ursodeoxycholate.

Silybin (100 mg/kg/day for 7 days, ip, to rats) significantly reduced biliary cholesterol and phospholipid concentrations compared with controls. Bile flow, biliary total bile salt concentration and total liver cholesterol content were unchanged. In gallstone patients and in cholecystectomised patients, oral administration of silymarin (420 mg/day for 30 days) reduced the biliary cholesterol concentration and bile saturation index compared with placebo treatment.[86]

Pre-treatment with silymarin prevented post–ischaemic gastric mucosal injury in rats. The inhibitory activity of silymarin on neutrophil function may contribute significantly to its gastroprotective action.[87]

Cancer overview

Carcinogenesis is a multistep process activated by altered expression of transcription factors and proteins involved in proliferation, cell cycle regulation, differentiation, apoptosis, angiogenesis, invasion and metastasis.[88] The cancer chemopreventative role of silymarin has been established in both in vivo and in vitro cancer models, including skin, breast, lung, colon, bladder, kidney, prostate, ovarian, cervical and hepatocellular carcinomas. This is likely to result from several distinct mechanisms (discussed below under Cancer prevention and Antitumour activity).

A 2010 review stated that most studies performed to date have found beneficial effects of using silymarin and its main active constituent, silybin, as potential cancer therapeutic agents. These effects appear to result from the phytochemical's ability to inhibit cell proliferation, increase apoptosis, decrease angiogenesis, block cell cycle regulators, enhance the expression of cell cycle inhibitors and inhibit transcriptional factors.[89] A limitation of in vitro research in this context is the poor tissue availability of silymarin and its constituents demonstrated in some studies, making extrapolation of these studies to effects in humans of uncertain relevance. Another limitation pointed out by the authors of the 2010 review is that almost all of these studies were performed on cancer cell lines derived from the specific cancer types, rather than primary cell cultures derived from patients' samples.[89]

Some major protein targets of silybin include the anti–apoptotic molecule survivin (a member of the inhibitor of apoptosis family); apoptotic proteins such as caspases; mediators of cell proliferation such as STAT, MAPK, NF–kappaB, ERK and Akt; cell cycle regulators such as Cip1/p21, Kip1/p27 and cyclin D1; the tumour suppressor p53; the oxygen–sensing transcription factor hypoxia inducible factor alpha1; cell death receptors; growth factor and receptors and receptor kinases (for example the epidermal growth factor receptors/receptor protein kinases and vascular endothelial growth factor).[89] In vitro and in vivo studies supporting these propositions have been comprehensively detailed in several recent reviews.[47,88,89,90]

Cancer prevention

In vitro findings show that silybin presents anti–genotoxic activity in human hepatoma cells (HepG2), which suggests potential use as a chemopreventative agent.[91] At a concentration of 200 µM, silybin induced DNA migration, generated oxidised DNA bases, reduced cell viability, decreased the replicative index of the cells and induced oxidative stress. It was able to reduce the genotoxic effect of three different mutagens, bleomycin, benzo(a)pyrene and aflatoxin B1 for both pretreatment and simultaneous treatments, but had no significant effect on DNA damage induction post–treatment.

Silymarin and silybin have demonstrated chemopreventative effects against skin cancer.[88,90] The effects of silymarin against skin carcinogenesis have been attributed to its strong antioxidant and anti–inflammatory action, as well as its inhibitory effect on mitogenic signalling. Silymarin affords strong protection against UV–induced damage in epidermis by decreasing thymine dimer positive cells and upregulating p53 (a key molecule in regulating the DNA repair machinery along with cell cycle regulation and apoptosis).[47] For example, topical application of silymarin prior to carcinogen application resulted in protection against tumour formation in mouse skin.

Topical application or dietary feeding of silybin before or immediately after UVB exposure resulted in a strong protection against photocarcinogenesis in hairless mice, in terms of tumour multiplicity, tumour volume per mouse and size of tumours.[92,93] Silybin also moderately inhibited tumour incidence (5% to 15%) and prolonged the tumour latency period for up to 4 weeks. These effects were attributable to inhibition of DNA synthesis, cell proliferation, cell cycle progression and induction of apoptosis. Silymarin inhibited the carcinogen–caused induction of TNF–alpha mRNA expression.[94,95] A sunscreen containing silymarin applied to the skin of mice prior to UVB exposure prevented the formation of pyrimidine dimers.[96] In another study, in which the free radical–generating tumour promoter benzoyl peroxide was used on DMBA–initiated mouse skin, silymarin showed strong antitumour–promoting effects.[90]

Topical treatment with silymarin (1 mg/cm^2 skin area) in mice exposed to UVB (90 mJ/cm^2) was reported to cause an inhibition of several cellular inflammatory processes.[47] Other relevant anti–inflammatory activity impacting on carcinogenesis includes a possible COX–2 (cyclo-oxygenase-2) selective inhibitory activity. Topical application of silymarin before UVB irradiation resulted in a highly significant inhibition of UVB–caused induction of epidermal COX activity.[90] The silymarin treatment significantly inhibited the expression of iNOS as well as production of NO in UV–treated skin, suggesting its main activity might be inhibition of NF–kappaB.

The antioxidant activity of silymarin has been proposed as one of the mechanisms in preventing a wide range of carcinogen and tumour promoter–induced skin cancers in mice. Silymarin strongly reverses the TPA–caused depletion of epidermal enzyme activities of SOD, catalase and glutathione peroxidase.[90]

Silymarin may have a role in colon cancer prevention. It inhibited microsomal beta–glucuronidase activity in vitro, and both silymarin and silybin inhibited beta–glucuronidase of intestinal bacteria and faeces of healthy humans and patients with colon cancer. Oral administration of silymarin and silybin protected against the increase in beta–glucuronidase activity in rats treated with carbon tetrachloride.[97]

Silymarin significantly decreased the number of aberrant crypt foci (ACF) in an azoxymethane (AOM) induced rat colon cancer model.[98] Dietary administration of silymarin (100, 500 and 1000 ppm in diet), either during or after carcinogen exposure (AOM) for 4 weeks, caused a significant reduction in the frequency of colonic ACF in a dose–dependent manner.[99] In a long–term experiment, dietary feeding of silymarin (100 and 500 ppm) during the initiation or post–initiation phase of AOM–induced colon carcinogenesis reduced the incidence and multiplicity of colonic adenocarcinoma.[88]

Silybin was suggested as a potential human colorectal cancer chemopreventative agent following research demonstrating it achieved high levels in the human colorectal mucosa after administration of doses of 360, 720 or 1440 mg/day for 7 days in colorectal cancer patients.[100] (Refer to the Pharmacokinetics section for further details.)

Effects in preventing other tumours have been observed. Intravesical silybin effectively inhibited the carcinogenesis and progression of bladder cancer in rats initiated by the chemical N–nitroso–N–methylurea NMU by reducing the incidence of superficial and invasive bladder lesions. This effect was without any side effects.[101] Tongue tumorigenesis induced in male rats with the mutagen 4–nitroquinoline 1–oxide was inhibited by silybin, and dietary feeding with 500 ppm silymarin inhibited the incidence of prostatic 3,2'–dimethyl–4–aminobiphenyl (DMAB)–induced adenocarcinoma.[47]

Silymarin and silybin downregulated epidermal growth factor receptor (EGFR) signalling in prostate cancer via inhibition of the expression and secretion of growth factors, inhibition of growth factor binding to and activating of EGFR, and the subsequent impairment of downstream mitogenic events. This resulted in an anticancer efficacy against prostate cancer cells.[90] Dietary administration of silymarin (100 or 500 ppm silymarin for 40 weeks) significantly decreased the incidence of DMAB–induced prostatic adenocarcinoma in male rats, indicating chemopreventative ability possibly through apoptosis induction and modification of cell proliferation.[102]

Other properties of silymarin pertinent to its chemopreventative activity, namely apoptosis induction and inhibition of cell cycle progression, angiogenesis, metastasis and invasion are reviewed in the section on antitumour activity below.

Antitumour activity

The antitumour properties of silybin and its known mechanisms of action have been comprehensively reviewed elsewhere, and are summarised above in the overview.[47,88–90] Only some main findings are highlighted here.

In vivo models of skin cancer have shown that silymarin significantly inhibited tumour growth and caused regression of established tumours.[103] In mice with skin papillomas it resulted in significant reduction of tumour growth and cell proliferation index and enhanced the apoptotic index.[104]

Mechanistic in vitro studies in skin cancer cells have demonstrated that silybin promotes the arrest of the G2–M phase of the cell cycle, inhibits proliferation and growth arrest in the G0–G1 and G2–M phases of the cell cycle, dose–dependently inhibits DNA synthesis and cell growth, inhibits ligand–induced activation of EGFR and inhibits EGFR intrinsic kinase activity.[89] Inhibition of proliferation and promotion of apoptosis by silybin was mediated by a reduction of ERK1/2 activation and an increased activation of JNK1/2 and p38.[104] Other silybin–related anti–skin cancer properties include activation of the apoptotic markers caspases–9, –3 and –7, suppression of the induction of transcriptional factor UVB–induced activator protein 1 (AP1),[105] induction or suppression of NF–kappaB and upregulation of p53.[89]

Further in vitro research using human prostate cancer PC3 cells found that high concentrations (24 to 48 μM) of silymarin and silybin modulated G1 phase cyclins, CDKs and CDKIs for G1 arrest, and the Chk2–Cdc25C–Cdc2/cyclin B1 pathway for G2–M arrest, together with an altered subcellular localisation of critical cell cycle regulators.[106] In prostate cancer cells, silymarin treatment also downregulated androgen receptor–EGFR and NF–kappaB–mediated signalling and induced cell cycle arrest.[90] In vitro studies have further demonstrated that silybin downregulates prostate–specific antigen (PSA) mRNA expression and reduces PSA secretion as well as inhibiting the telomerase activity that mediates cell immortality and carcinogenesis.[107,108] It has also been shown to upregulate insulin–like growth factor–binding protein 3 (IGFBP-3) expression and inhibit proliferation of androgen–independent prostate cancer cells.[109]

Silymarin inhibited androgen receptor mediated signalling and induced differentiation in androgen–dependent LNCaP cells. It also caused growth inhibition in human prostate cancer LNCaP, PC3 and DU145 cells, associated with an induction of G1 arrest and/or G2–M arrest. Silybin inhibited NF–kappaB transcriptional activity in human prostate cancer DU145 cells, and increased their sensitivity for TNF–alpha–induced apoptosis.[90] In vitro, isosilybin A and isosilybin B were reported to be the most effective suppressors of PSA secretion by androgen–dependent LNCaP cells (a cell line established from a metastatic lesion of human prostatic adenocarcinoma),[110] while other researchers found isosilybin B was the most consistent and potent suppressor of human prostate carcinoma cell line growth, compared with other isolated constituents or silymarin extracts.[110]

Dietary feeding of silybin at 0.05% and 0.1% for 60 days strongly inhibited the growth of advanced human prostate tumour xenografts in athymic nude mice, without any apparent signs of toxicity. Silybin exhibited antiproliferative, pro–apoptotic and antiangiogenic efficacy against the prostate tumours.[111,112] In both studies, animals showed no weight loss or reduced food consumption. Administration of silybin to mice engrafted with another androgen–independent cell line (PC3 cells) resulted in similar findings of reduced tumour weight and volume, and associated anti–cancer effects with an increase in plasma IGFBP-3.[113] Dietary silybin inhibited prostate tumour growth and progression in transgenic adeno-carcinoma of the mouse prostate (TRAMP) by modulating the expression of CDKs, CDKIs and insulin–like growth factor 1 (IGF)–1 and IGFBP–3.[114]

A possible mechanism for the antiangiogenic efficacy of silymarin in prostate cancer was suggested by the finding from in vivo research that silybin inhibited microvessel density and vascular endothelial growth factor (VEGF) secretion in pros-tate tumours.[90] Also, in terms of antiangiogenesis, silymarin treatment inhibited the growth and survival of human umbili-cal vein endothelial cells in vitro.[90]

In vitro research demonstrated that silymarin elicited partial oestrogen receptor activation in rat hepatoma cells, with silybin B most likely being responsible for the majority of this action (see also below for MCF-7 cells).[115]

In bladder cancers, in vitro research findings indicate silybin may be effective in decreasing protein and mRNA levels of survivin,[116] and promoting cell cycle arrest and apoptosis.[117] Activation of p53 and caspase–2, leading to mitochondrial permeabilisation, cytochrome c release and cleavage of the cyclin–dependent kinase inhibitor Cip1/p21 are other possible mechanisms.[89,118] These findings have been supported by findings from in vivo studies. Administration of silybin significantly inhibited N-butyl-N-(4-hydroxybutyl) nitrosamine induced urinary bladder carcinogenesis in male mice by causing cell cycle arrest and induction of apopto-sis.[119] It also inhibited the growth of a human bladder tumour xenograft in athymic nude mice by downregulating sur-vivin and increasing p53 expression, together with enhanced apoptosis.[120]

In an orthotopic xenograft model, silybin treatment of immunodeficient mice (0.1% to 4% for 39 days in food pel-lets) resulted in reduced tumour weight, decreased tumour volume and an overall improvement of the gross anatomy of tumour–implanted kidneys compared with vehicle–treated controls.[121]

High concentrations of silymarin ($\geq 80\,\mu$mol/L) induced cervical cancer HeLa cell death in vitro through both apop-totic and necrotic pathways.[122] Silybin inhibited the growth of human ovarian and breast cancer cell lines and DNA synthesis in vitro.[123] It decreased the percentage of cells in the S and G2–M phases of the cell cycle with a concomitant increase in cells in the G0–G1 phases.

One in vivo study demonstrated that silybin strongly inhibited development of mammary tumours as well as lung metastasis in HER–2/neu transgenic mice.[124] However, in another study no effect was found on tumour development in a transgenic adeno-carcinoma mouse model.[125] A silybin–phosphatidylcholine com-plex administered at a dose of 450mg/kg/day by oral gavage to nude mice bearing a tumour xenograft of the human ovarian can-cer cell line A2780 produced a significant tumour weight inhibi-tion of 78%.[126] It was suggested that downregulation of VEGF receptor 3 and upregulation of angiopoietin 2 were the possible mechanisms for the observed antiangiogenic activity. However, dietary supplementation with low–dose silymarin (0.03% to 1%) was observed to enhance mammary carcinogenesis and stimulate the growth of MCF–7 breast cancer cells in female rats.[127]

In both small cell lung carcinoma cells and non–small cell lung carcinoma cells, silybin dose– and time–dependently inhib-ited tumour cell growth and stimulated apoptotic cell death.[89] In a mouse model of urethane–induced lung tumour, adminis-tration of silybin inhibited tumour progression by reducing the cell proliferation, modulating cyclin expression and suppressing expression of angiogenic growth factors (VEGF) and tumour promoting enzymes (such as iNOS and COX–2).[89]

In vitro research on colon cancer cells, ranging from well–differentiated to highly aggressive, has pointed to a number of mechanisms for silybin as an anti–tumour agent, including upregulation of cyclin–dependent kinase inhibitors, promotion of cell cycle arrest and apoptosis, inhibition of cyclin–Cdk pro-moter activity and antiangiogenic activity.[128] These antineoplastic effects were partially mediated by paracrine cytokine interactions between different cell types, involving VEGF.[89]

Coadministration of silymarin extracts has been shown to reduce the toxic effects of cytostatic treatments. For example, the effect of cisplatin (5mg/kg) on glomerular and proximal tubular function as well as proximal tubular morphology was largely ameliorated by silybin (200mg/kg, iv).[129] Pretreatment of male rats with silymarin (50mg/kg) or Silybum seed (0.6g/kg) before a single intraperitoneal injection of 3mg/kg cisplatin prevented tubular damage, suggesting they may pro-tect against cisplatin–induced renal toxicity.[129,130] In the same model, silybin given alone had no effect on renal function. Treated rats had blood urea nitrogen and serum creatinine levels significantly lower than those receiving cisplatin alone, although a mild–to–moderate necrosis was observed.

A high concentration of silymarin or its constituents (100μmol/L), as well as the flavonol quercetin, were reported to protect cardiomyocytes against doxorubicin–induced oxi-dative stress.[131] In oral doses of 70mg/kg or higher, silymarin was reported to reduce radiation–induced liver damage and consequent increases in serum enzyme activities.[132] These effects were attributed to its antioxidant and free radical scav-enging properties.[47] A silybin–phosphatidylcholine complex potentiated the cytotoxicity of the anticancer drug cisplatin in vitro.[133] In vivo, coadministration of the complex at a dose 1350mg/kg resulted in a potentiation of the antitumour activ-ity of cisplatin against A2780 cells in mice. Mice receiving the combination recovered earlier in terms of body weight loss, as compared with the cisplatin–treated mice. An antiangiogenic effect of was also demonstrated. Silybin has also demonstrated synergistic antitumour activity with cisplatin and doxorubicin against both oestrogen–dependent MCF-7 and oestrogen–independent MDF–MB468 breast cancer cells (see also under Interactions).[134-136]

Anti–inflammatory activity and immune–modulating effects

Silybin inhibited arachidonic acid metabolites and arachi-donic acid–induced chemiluminescence of human platelets in vitro.[137] Silybin, silydianin and silychristin inhibited the forma-tion of prostaglandins in vitro and non–competitively inhibited lipoxygenase from soybeans in vitro.[138]

More significantly, studies have demonstrated that silyma-rin is a potent inhibitor of NF–kappaB activation in response to

TNF–alpha.[90] Silymarin blocked TNF–alpha–induced activation of NF–kappaB in vitro in a dose– and time–dependent manner.[139] It inhibited activation of NF–kappaB and the TNF–alpha–induced activation of reactive oxygen intermediates and lipid peroxidation, mitogen–activated protein kinase and c–Jun N–terminal kinase, and abrogated TNF–alpha–induced cytotoxicity and caspase activation.

Silymarin inhibited in vitro T cell proliferation and cytokine production in hepatitis C virus infection.[140] At concentrations between 5 and 40 μg/mL, silymarin dose-dependently inhibited the proliferation and secretion of TNF–alpha, interferon (IFN)–gamma and IL–2 by peripheral blood mononuclear cells stimulated with anti–CD3.

Silymarin demonstrated a neuroprotective effect against lipopolysaccharide (LPS)–induced neurotoxicity in mesencephalic mixed neuron–glia cultures in vitro by inhibiting microglia activation.[141] Silymarin also significantly inhibited the production of inflammatory mediators, such as TNF–alpha and NO, and reduced the damage to dopaminergic neurons. It effectively reduced LPS–induced superoxide generation and NF–kappaB activation, suggesting that the inhibitory effect of silymarin on microglia activation is mediated through an inhibition of NF–kappaB activation.

In early research, oral administration of silymarin resulted in anti–inflammatory activity in carrageenan–induced rat paw oedema. Topical application of silymarin was more effective than intraperitoneal injection in mouse ear inflammation. Silymarin produced a dose–dependent inhibition of leucocyte accumulation in inflammatory exudates after carrageenan injection and reduced the number of neutrophils. However, it was unable to inhibit phospholipase A_2 in vitro.[142]

Parenteral exposure of mice to silymarin resulted in suppression of T lymphocyte function at low doses and stimulation of inflammatory processes at higher doses.[143] Silymarin administration to male BABL/c mice (10 to 250 mg/kg, ip) resulted in significant reductions in the number of CD3+ T lymphocytes at low doses (10 mg/kg) with concomitant decreases in CD4+ cells and expression of IL–2 and IL–4. Expressions of TNF–alpha, iNOS, IL–1beta and IL–6 mRNA were increased dose–dependently.

In vivo exposure to silymarin influenced phenotypic selection processes in the thymus.[144] Using the same model and doses as above, silymarin resulted in an increase in absolute numbers of CD4+ and CD8+ T lymphocytes and increased c–myc expression (an important proto–oncogene in the control of differentiation and function of thymocytes in the thymus), but decreased expressions of IL–2 and IL–4.

Diabetes

The anti–hyperglycaemic properties of silybin suggest a potential role in the treatment of type 2 diabetes. Silybin and its derivative dehydrosilybin were demonstrated to inhibit cellular glucose uptake by directly interacting with glucose transporters (GLUT) in several model systems.[145] Both flavonolignans dose–dependently reduced basal and insulin–dependent glucose uptake by 3T3–L1 adipocytes, with dehydrosilybin showing significantly stronger inhibition. In rat liver microsomes, silybin dose–dependently inhibited glucagon–induced stimulation of gluconeogenesis and glycogenolysis, an effect associated with a reduction of glucose–6–phosphate hydrolysis.[146]

A direct cytoprotective effect of silymarin in pancreatic beta cells was shown in vitro, suggesting that silymarin may be therapeutically beneficial for type 1 diabetes.[147] Silymarin dose–dependently inhibited both cytokine–induced NO production and IL–1beta– and/or IFN–gamma–induced cell death and prevented beta–cell dysfunction in human islets.

Silybin was shown to lower mitochondrial ROS production in perfused rat hepatocytes, suggesting a potential role in diabetic damage.[148] It dose–dependently reduced glycolysis from carbohydrates via an inhibitory effect targeted on pyruvate kinase activity, and demonstrated a dramatic effect upon oxidative phosphorylation, fully mitigating the rise in metabolic flow–driven ROS formation.

Silymarin (70 mg/kg, oral) reduced blood glucose and cholesterol, corrected hypoproteinaemia, inhibited lipoxygenase products in liver tissue, and corrected oxidative phosphorylation disturbances in liver mitochondria in streptozotocin–induced diabetes mellitus in rats.[149]

Silymarin showed a protective effect against pancreatic damage in rats with alloxan–induced diabetes mellitus.[150] It prevented the decrease in the pancreatic activities of antioxidant enzymes (SOD, glutathione peroxidase and catalase) caused by alloxan (150 mg/kg, sc) when both compounds were administered simultaneously (eight oral doses of silymarin, 200 mg/kg each over 48 h). Treatment also restored these enzymatic activities when a single oral daily dose of 200 mg/kg was administered for 9 weeks, 20 days after alloxan intoxication. The same preparation and dosage administered simultaneously or subsequent to alloxan administration resulted in recovery of pancreatic function following alloxan–induced pancreatic damage in rats.[151] Longer–term administration of silymarin protected against the alloxan–induced increase in serum glucose, the decrease in serum insulin and morphological abnormalities in pancreatic tissue (such as islet shrinkage, necrotic areas, loss of cell organisation and so on). The pancreatic tissue, insulin and serum glucose levels of silymarin–treated rats were similar to those of control animals.

A potential role of silymarin has been demonstrated in vivo for the prevention and treatment of diabetic nephropathy. In a rat model, silymarin demonstrated a recuperative effect on renal tissue damage, with results suggesting its effects on oxidative stress may afford protection in this context.[152] Administration of silymarin (200 mg/kg/day for 9 weeks, oral) 20 days after alloxan prevented renal tissue damage and restored the activity and gene expression of the three antioxidant enzymes: SOD, glutathione peroxidase and catalase.

In early research, treatment of diabetic rats with silybin did not affect hyperglycaemia, but prevented the inhibition of protein mono–ADP–ribosylation. Silybin treatment was associated with the prevention of substance P–like immunoreactivity loss in the sciatic nerve, which is typical of diabetic neuropathy. Silybin also prevented the increase in ADP–ribosylation of proteins in sciatic nerve Schwann cells. This latter effect is likely to be indirect and secondary to the improvement of diabetic neuropathy.[153–155]

Findings from in vitro and in vivo studies suggested that silymarin may reduce the burden of advanced glycation end-product (AGE) formation in diabetes and may prevent any resulting complications.[156] In vitro glycation assays demonstrated that silymarin exerted marked inhibition during the late stages of glycation and subsequent crosslinking. Silymarin (50 or 150 mg/kg/day for 12 weeks, oral) in streptozotocin-induced diabetic rats reduced tissue AGE accumulation, tail collagen crosslinking and concentrations of plasma glycated albumin. Levels of oxidative and inflammatory biomarkers were also significantly decreased in silymarin-treated groups, compared with the untreated diabetic group.

Hepatotoxicity caused by antitubercular drugs (ATDs) is more severe in diabetic patients. Coadministration of silymarin (100 mg/kg/day, oral) for 45 days with isoniazid, rifampicin and pyrazinamide was shown to protect against ATD hepatotoxicity in rats with or without streptozotocin-induced diabetes, irrespective of insulin treatment. The silymarin-induced hepatoprotection against ATD-induced liver injury was characterised by near normal levels of marker enzymes, an increase in total proteins and normal hepatic structure.[157]

Other activity

Silymarin demonstrated potent inhibition of cAMP phosphodiesterase in vitro.[158]

The effect of silymarin on corticosteroid secretion was investigated in isolated adrenal cells from an aldosterone-producing adenoma, atrophied adrenal tissue surrounding the adenoma and hyperplastic adrenal tissue from Cushing syndrome patients. The observed dose-dependent effect of silybin on increasing corticosteroid secretion may be attributed to corresponding changes in the activities of cytochrome P450 enzymes and the stimulation of ACTH-induced corticosteroid production, which could result from the antioxidant activity of silybin.[159]

Silybin enhanced the motility of neutrophils inactivated by formyl tripeptide, calcium ionophore, lymphokine or human serum and was effective in enhancing spontaneous motility of leucocytes obtained from healthy volunteers 2 h after administration.[160]

Silybin dose-dependently inhibited f-met peptide and anti-IgE-induced histamine release from human basophils. Further in vitro results suggest a possible antiallergic activity of silybin may be ascribed to a membrane-stabilising effect, possibly related to an interference with calcium influx.[161]

Silybin inhibited RNA and protein synthesis of Gram-positive bacteria in vitro, suggesting a modest antibacterial activity.[162]

In bovine and murine mammary cells, silymarin enhanced cell proliferation and differentiation and was able to increase beta-casein gene expression alone or in association with prolactin, suggesting it may support lactation.[163] (See also the Clinical trials section.)

Evidence exists for an anti-osteoporotic and selective oestrogen receptor modulator activity of silymarin in ovariectomised rats. Administration of silymarin by oral gavage at a dose of 50 mg/kg/day for 12 weeks significantly prevented bone loss in rats induced by ovariectomy, with mild proliferative effects observed in the uterus.[164]

Silymarin attenuated the amyloid-beta plaque burden and improved behavioural abnormalities in an Alzheimer's disease mouse model.[165] Marked suppression of amyloid–beta protein (Abeta) fibril formation and neurotoxicity in PC12 cells was observed after silymarin treatment in vitro. In vivo studies indicated a significant reduction in brain Abeta oligomer deposition and a reduction in anxiety in amyloid precursor protein (APP) transgenic mice that had been prophylactically treated with a diet containing 0.1% silymarin for 6 months.

Silymarin protected spinal cord and cortical cells against oxidative stress and LPS stimulation, suggesting a potential CNS neuroprotective role against toxin– or injury–induced damage.[166] In vitro, silymarin or silybin effectively attenuated peroxide–induced ROS formation, with silymarin being more effective than silybin in mixed neuronal/glial cell cultures from cerebral cortex or spinal cord. In vivo, intrathecal injection of silymarin at 120 μg/rat immediately after spinal cord injury effectively improved hind limb locomotor behaviour.

Silymarin exacerbated renal impairment and p53–mediated tubular apoptosis, but had no effect on tubular necrosis or renal leucocyte infiltration, in glycerol–induced acute kidney injury in rats.[167] Silymarin was injected intraperitoneally (100 mg/kg) concomitant with glycerol injection and 3 h after. Oxidative stress, inflammatory reaction, tubular necrosis as well as p53–mediated tubular apoptosis were all prolonged or exacerbated by treatment with silymarin.

Pharmacokinetics

Most pharmacokinetic studies have shown relatively low bioavailability as such for the flavonolignans. This has led to the development of proprietary products to improve their overall bioavailability.

Phase I crossover studies using three silymarin products indicated that silybin bioavailability varied with product preparation;[168,169] bioavailability seems to depend on several factors including the content of accompanying substances, the dissolution time and the concentration of the preparation itself.[37,170] Approximately 20% to 50% of silymarin is absorbed after oral administration, with about 80% excreted via the bile,[171] while around 10% enters enterohepatic circulation.[37]

The pharmacokinetics of silybin shows fast absorption and elimination. After oral administration of standardised St Mary's thistle extracts, the silymarin flavonolignans are rapidly metabolised and measurable in plasma, mainly in the form of glucuronides.[172] Extensive first–pass phase II metabolism presumably accounts for the low systemic exposures that have been observed with customary doses of silymarin.[173] Silymarin phytochemicals undergo phase I and phase II metabolism, especially multiple phase II conjugation reactions, and are primarily excreted into bile and urine.[174]

The flavonolignans preferentially accumulate in the liver and bile. Six volunteers given 560 mg silymarin (240 mg silybin) registered low maximum serum concentrations (0.2 to 0.6 μg/mL) and low renal excretion (1% to 2% of the silybin dose over 24 h). However, bile collected from cholecystectomised patients given 140 mg silymarin (60 mg silybin) was found to contain 11 to 47 μg/mL, a value approximately 100 times higher than in the serum, despite the lower administered dose,[175] with peak concentrations reached within 2 to 9h. Another study of similar patients showed that, after repeated intake of silymarin, a steady state of silybin elimination was reached by the second day at the latest.[176] Area under the plasma concentration–time curves (AUCs) for total flavonolignans (which reflects parent plus conjugated flavonolignans) have been reported to be 3– to 4–fold and 12– to 36–fold higher for silybin A and silybin B, respectively, compared with AUCs for the parent flavonolignans only, following oral administration of a single oral dose of 600 mg of a standardised extract.[172]

A study conducted in 14 cholecystectomised patients indicated that, in general, there was no relationship between silymarin elimination and bile output, except in two patients: one with pancreatitis and one with liver metastasis, where reduced silybin elimination was linked to a decrease in bile output.[177] However, it has been shown that the pharmacokinetics of silymarin is altered in patients with liver disease (hepatitis C virus (HCV) and non–alcoholic fatty liver disease). This is based on findings from a study in which 20 healthy volunteers and three patient cohorts were administered a single 480 mg oral dose of silymarin, with 14 blood samples obtained over 24h.[173] The AUC values for the sum of total silymarin flavonolignans were 2.4–, 3.3– and 4.7–fold higher for HCV, non–alcoholic fatty liver disease (p≤0.03) and HCV cirrhosis cohorts (p≤0.03), respectively, compared with healthy volunteers.

In a rat model, intravenous silybin was shown to exhibit dose–related pharmacokinetics in the dose range of 10 to 50 mg/kg.[178] All of the unconjugated or total (unconjugated plus conjugated) silybin concentrations in bile were significantly higher than those in plasma, suggesting active hepatobiliary excretion. Co–administration with cyclosporin significantly decreased the AUC in bile, suggesting that active silybin efflux might be partially mediated by P–gp.

Earlier oral pharmacokinetic studies in rats using silymarin and a silybin–phosphatidylcholine complex indicated lower plasma silybin levels and lower biliary excretion for silymarin alone. The relative bioavailability of the complex was 10 times higher than for silymarin.[179] This trend in bioavailability was also observed in healthy human volunteers.[180]

The elimination half–life is generally less than 4h with silymarin and silybin. In four cohorts of eight non-cirrhotic HCV patients, silybin A and silybin B showed low bioavailability at oral doses of 140, 280, 560 or 700 mg silymarin 8 hourly for 7 days.[181] However, with the 5–fold increase in dose, steady-state exposures for silybin A and silybin B increased 11–fold and 38–fold respectively, suggesting the poor bioavailability may be overcome with doses above 700 mg.

In earlier research, the plasma concentrations of unconjugated and conjugated silybin after intake of a single oral dose of a silybin–phosphatidylcholine complex were evaluated in 12 healthy volunteers. It was concluded that silybin undergoes extensive conversion to conjugated derivatives that are retained in the circulation at relatively high concentrations.[182] A contemporary study using the same complex in 14 patients indicated that extrahepatic biliary obstruction is associated with a reduced clearance of conjugated silybin, probably due to impaired excretion of the conjugate in bile.[183] These earlier findings are consistent with the more recent research on straight silymarin quoted above.

Following the administration of single oral doses of a silybin–phosphatidylcholine complex (equivalent to 280 mg silybin) to 20 human volunteers, silybin was absorbed rapidly, with the time to reach peak plasma concentration (Tmax) ranging from 0.67 to 2.67h (mean 1.4h). Other pharmacokinetic parameters included a Cmax of 4.2 μg/mL.[184]

A lack of prostate tissue penetration for silybin was found following oral administration of high–dose (13 g in three divided doses) silybin–phytosome complex.[185] High blood concentrations were achieved transiently in patients with localised prostate cancer, but low levels of silybin were found in prostate tissue. Blood levels 1h after the first silybin–phytosome dose reached a mean value of 19.7 μM, whereas the highest silybin level observed in the harvested prostate tissue was just 496.6 pmol/g. These findings suggest that St Mary's thistle is highly unlikely to exert significant anti–tumour activity in patients with prostate cancer.

High silybin levels were achieved in human colorectal mucosa following repeated administration of a silybin–phosphatidylcholine extract to patients with confirmed colorectal adenocarcinoma.[100] Doses of 360, 720 or 1440 mg silybin daily for 7 days were determined to be safe and achieved levels of silybin of 20 to 141 nmol/g tissue in colorectal tissue, 0.3 to 4 μM in the plasma, and 0.3 to 2.5 nmol/g tissue in the liver. Silybin metabolites were also identified in the plasma.

Clinical trials

The outcomes of many trials have not been consistent, especially those concerned with cirrhosis, hepatitis and alcoholic liver disease (which may have been exacerbated by continued consumption of alcohol). Conflicting findings could also be due to: the range of preparations used, including St Mary's thistle extract, silymarin, silybin, silybin–phosphatidylcholine complex with or without vitamin E; the range of doses (from 240 to 800 mg/day) and the treatment periods, which ranged from 7 days to 6 years.[38]

Several systematic reviews and meta–analyses have been conducted on the potential benefits of silymarin in liver disease. A 2008 systematic review concluded that it is reasonable to employ silymarin as a supportive strategy in the therapy of *Amanita phalloides* poisoning and (alcoholic and Child–Pugh grade A) liver cirrhosis.[186] From an analysis of 19 'double' or 'single blind' trials, the authors reported that, in alcoholic liver disease, aspartate aminotransferase (AST) was significantly reduced in the silymarin–treated groups compared with placebo (p=0.01), and in liver cirrhosis, total mortality was significantly lower with silymarin (p=0.01). A Cochrane meta–analysis of 18 randomised clinical trials assessing silymarin extract in 1088 patients with alcoholic and/or hepatitis B or C virus liver diseases found that silymarin (milk thistle) versus placebo or no intervention had no significant effect on overall mortality (RR 0.78; 95% CI 0.53 to 1.15), complications of liver disease (RR 0.95; 95% CI 0.83 to 1.09) or liver histology.[187] However, liver–related mortality was significantly reduced by milk thistle in all trials (RR 0.50; 95% CI 0.29 to 0.88), but not in high–quality trials (RR 0.57, 95% CI 0.28 to 1.19). Similar results were obtained in the earlier Cochrane meta–analysis that included 13 randomised clinical trials with a total of 915 patients with alcoholic hepatitis and hepatitis B or C.[188] An earlier systematic review of 14 trials found the only statistically significant difference compared with placebo was a greater reduction in ALT levels among patients with chronic liver disease assigned to silymarin extract (–9 IU/L, 95% CI –18 to –1 IU/L; p=0.05).[189]

(See also the Interactions section for a discussion of the possible beneficial effects of St Mary's thistle extracts in combination with pharmaceutical drugs, including relevant clinical trials.)

Non–alcoholic liver damage

In a quite early, uncontrolled study involving 2000 patients suffering from toxic liver damage of differing aetiologies, serum levels of hepatic enzymes were considerably reduced.[190] Symptoms such as nausea, discomfort and skin itching were also improved in 83% of patients. Sixty–seven outpatients with toxic–metabolic liver damage, chronic persistent hepatitis and cholangitis with pericholangitis who were treated with silymarin experienced significant reductions in serum transaminases and bromthalein retention in another early study. On the basis of liver biopsies, patients with chronic persistent hepatitis were deemed to be 'cured' after 3 months of treatment.[191]

Thirty of 49 workers with abnormal liver function and/or haematological values as a result of long–term exposure to organic solvent vapours (toluene and/or xylene) were treated orally with silymarin in an uncontrolled study. Liver function tests and platelet counts significantly improved, with leucocytosis and relative lymphocytosis showing a tendency toward improvement.[192]

In a randomised, double blind, placebo–controlled clinical study, the efficacy of oral silymarin (800 mg/day) in preventing psychotropic drug–induced hepatic damage was evaluated in 90 patients over a 90–day treatment period. Results indicated that silymarin reduced the lipoperoxidative hepatic damage that occurs during treatment with butyrophenones or phenothiazines.[193]

Alcoholic liver disease and cirrhosis

Trials specifically investigating alcohol–related cirrhosis are included in the section below. Results of randomised controlled trials of silymarin in chronic alcoholic liver disease are conflicting and, as noted above, may be confounded by heterogeneity of the degree of disease severity and alcohol intake/abstinence.[37]

In an early, double blind, placebo–controlled clinical trial, silymarin (420 mg/day) improved the biochemical, functional and morphological alterations of the liver in 47 patients with slight acute and subacute liver disease, mostly induced by alcohol abuse, who were treated over 4 weeks.[194] Statistically significant decreases in serum ALT and AST occurred in the treated group (n=47) compared with controls (n=50).

Seventy–two patients with alcoholic liver disease (cirrhosis and hepatitis) began participation in a randomised, double blind, placebo–controlled trial and received silymarin (280 mg/day) or placebo tablets. Twelve patients subsequently dropped out of the trial and 10 patients died during the follow–up period

(15 months). In those who survived, laboratory values and their changes did not differ between silymarin and placebo treatment. However, 22 patients were positive for alcohol ingestion during follow–up. Those who abstained from alcohol exhibited a significant fall in GGT, but without a significant difference between the two groups.[195]

In a double blind, placebo–controlled clinical trial, patients with chronic alcoholic liver disease received 6 months' treatment with silymarin (420 mg/day) or placebo. The measured antioxidant and lipid peroxidation parameters were markedly improved in the silymarin group compared with placebo.[196] One hundred and sixteen patients with histologically proven alcoholic hepatitis (58 with cirrhosis) received either silymarin (420 mg/day) or placebo for 3 months. For those who remained in treatment, significant improvement was observed in both groups, and silymarin was not clinically superior to placebo. The rate of abstinence from alcohol was about 50% in both groups.[197]

In a surveillance study, a St Mary's thistle extract (200 to 400 mg/day corresponding to 80 to 160 mg of silymarin) was administered to 108 patients with alcohol hepatic damage over a 5–week period. Eighty–five per cent of patients responded to treatment with reductions in transaminases and procollagen–III peptide (a fibrosis activity marker).[198] Significant antioxidant activity was verified in a double blind clinical trial involving 36 patients with alcoholic liver disease.[199]

The results of several randomised controlled trials evaluating the effects of Silybum or silymarin on alcoholic and non–alcoholic cirrhosis suggest it may lower transaminases and improve survival benefits, particularly in alcoholic and Child–Pugh grade A liver cirrhosis.[186,200] In non–alcoholic liver cirrhosis, beneficial effects were seen on the frequency of complications,[201] and also in decreased rates of bleeding oesophageal varices.[200] (See also later.) A randomised, double blind clinical trial carried out over 4 years showed a significantly higher survival rate from alcoholic cirrhosis for patients treated with silymarin (420 mg/day, p<0.05). Treatment of non–alcoholic cirrhosis was not as successful.[202] In another double blind, placebo–controlled study, patients with cirrhosis were treated with 420 mg/day of silymarin for 6 months. Serum levels of hepatic enzymes and bilirubin were significantly reduced compared with placebo. These improvements were accompanied by positive histological changes in the livers of patients receiving silymarin.[203]

In a 4–year, double blind, randomised study involving 170 patients with cirrhosis of different aetiologies, it was demonstrated that long–term treatment up to 2 years with 420 mg/day silymarin significantly reduced mortality (p=0.036).[200] This effect was more pronounced in patients with alcoholic cirrhosis. In a prospective crossover study, the cytoprotective effects of either UDCA (ursodeoxycholic acid, 600 mg/day) or silymarin (420 mg/day) were investigated in 27 patients with active cirrhosis. This was followed by an open trial investigating the effects of a combination therapy (UDCA plus silymarin) versus no therapy or UDCA alone. The entire treatment period spanned 25 months, including a 1–month washout period between single treatments. Both UDCA and silymarin decreased serum transaminase levels, whereas only

UDCA significantly diminished serum GGT. Neither agent influenced the functional liver mass when given alone or in combination. Combination therapy did not appear to be more effective than either substance given alone.[204]

In an open, uncontrolled trial, 30 patients affected by chronic ethanol–induced hepatic damage were treated with 450 mg/day of UDCA. After 6 months, a significant decrease of serum hepatic enzymes was noted. The addition of silymarin (400 mg/daily) to UDCA in another 30 patients induced a further improvement in hepatic function.[205]

In an open, controlled study, 60 type 1 diabetic patients with alcoholic cirrhosis received silymarin (600 mg/day) plus standard therapy or standard therapy alone over a 12–month period. In comparison with baseline values, treatment with silymarin reduced lipoperoxidation of cell membranes and insulin resistance and significantly decreased insulin overproduction and the need for exogenous insulin administration. This response was not observed for the untreated group.[206]

Treatment with both silymarin and amino–imidazole–carboxamide phosphate in 60 patients with compensated alcoholic cirrhosis of the liver in a 1 month, double blind, placebo–controlled clinical trial demonstrated hepatoprotective activity, which was accompanied by favourable changes in the parameters of cellular immunoreactivity.[207]

A post–marketing surveillance study documented the effects of treatment with 280 to 420 mg/day silymarin over 12 weeks in 998 patients with chronic liver diseases (fatty infiltration of the liver, hepatitis and cirrhosis of different aetiologies). In addition to clinically relevant decreases in subjective symptoms during treatment (lack of appetite, nausea, upper abdominal pressure), there was a marked decrease of the serum amino-terminal propeptide of procollagen III (a marker of fibrogenesis) values in patient subgroups who had initially elevated levels. This parameter dropped to the normal range in 19% of patients.[208]

Silymarin had no effect on survival or disease progression in alcoholic patients with liver cirrhosis in a randomised, double blind trial comparing 450 mg/day of silymarin with placebo over a 2–year period.[201] However, the frequency of complications was lower in the patients treated with silymarin, p=0.06. A total of 125 patients completed the trial (57 receiving silymarin and 68 receiving placebo). Twenty–nine patients (15 receiving silymarin and 14 receiving placebo) died during the trial. No relevant side effects were observed in any group.

A silymarin preparation at 450 mg/day was evaluated in a randomised, controlled trial in 60 patients with alcoholic liver cirrhosis.[209] After 6 months, the silymarin group showed a small but significant increase in red blood cell glutathione compared with placebo (p<0.001). There were also decreases in lipid peroxidation in peripheral blood cells in the silymarin group (MDA decreased by 33%, p<0.015), and platelet and serum amino–terminal propeptide of procollagen type III values were reduced (p<0.033), but not in the placebo group. There were no significant changes in transaminase levels.

Bleeding oesophageal varices constitute one of the most serious complications of cirrhosis. The total incidence of upper gastrointestinal bleedings reported in two trials showed differences in favour of silymarin (p=0.042): 4.6% versus 9.6% for silymarin and placebo, respectively, and 6.3% versus 13.5%, respectively.[37,200] It was suggested that the decreased rate may reflect an overall improvement in the patients, also evidence by the lower liver–related mortality rate, rather than being a direct effect of silymarin.[37]

Hepatitis

In an early uncontrolled trial, 29 patients with acute progressive hepatitis, active chronic hepatitis or cirrhosis without liver failure were treated with 210 mg/day of silymarin for a period of 3 months. All patients showed an improvement in their general health, and laboratory tests exhibited a trend towards normal values. Serum bilirubin returned to normal in jaundiced patients.[210] Seventy–two patients with similar conditions including fatty liver demonstrated improvement in enzyme levels after silymarin treatment. Treatment duration varied from 6 months for fatty liver and hepatitis (420 mg/day) to up to 4 years for cirrhosis (630 mg/day). Clear–cut results in liver enzyme levels were not achieved for the cirrhosis patients, but the progress of the disease was slowed.[211]

In two small double blind, placebo–controlled clinical trials incorporating 12 and 24 patients with chronic hepatitis treated for 3 months to 1 year, laboratory findings did not reveal any significant differences between silymarin (420 mg/day) and placebo. However, histological changes were improved in some patients treated with silymarin, including a significant improvement in the mesenchymal intralobular reaction (p<0.05). The authors postulated that silymarin may hinder the development of immunological reactions by occupying receptors on the liver cell membrane.[212] In a further randomised, double blind clinical trial, silymarin demonstrated favourable results in the treatment of 180 patients with chronic persistent hepatitis, chronic active hepatitis and hepatic cirrhosis. The trial lasted for 40 days and no side effects were observed.[213]

In a double blind, placebo–controlled clinical trial conducted at two medical centres, 57 patients with acute viral hepatitis received either silymarin (210 mg/day) or placebo for 3 weeks. Significant differences between bilirubin and AST values in the placebo and silymarin groups were observed (higher regression after silymarin treatment). A definite trend in the regression of ALT values in favour of silymarin was also observed. However, the development of immunity was not influenced by silymarin.[214] Similar but significant (p<0.05) results for ALT were observed in a double blind, placebo–controlled trial comprising 77 acute viral hepatitis patients.[215] In a prospective, open, controlled study of 151 acute viral hepatitis patients, silymarin treatment did not demonstrate efficacy (as determined by laboratory findings) compared with no treatment.[216]

In a double blind trial in patients with chronic persistent hepatitis, silybin treatment (silybin complexed with phosphatidylcholine) for 3 months decreased liver enzymes.[217] The same complex reduced parameters related to hepatocellular necrosis in a short–term, double blind study in chronic active hepatitis.[218]

In a randomised, controlled trial that included 105 participants with acute clinical hepatitis regardless of aetiology, silymarin administration resulted in earlier improvement in subjective and clinical markers of biliary excretion.[219] The intervention consisted of 420 mg/day of silymarin or a vitamin placebo for 4 weeks. No adverse events were noted and both silymarin and placebo were well tolerated. Patients randomised to the silymarin group had a quicker resolution of symptoms related to biliary retention: dark urine (p=0.013), jaundice (p=0.02) and scleral icterus (p=0.043). There was a reduction in indirect bilirubin among those assigned to silymarin (p=0.012), but other variables including direct bilirubin, ALT and AST were not significantly reduced.

Hepatitis C

Positive findings have been reported in some, but not all, studies of silymarin on viral load and ALT levels in chronic hepatitis C virus (HCV) infected patients. Other inconsistent benefits in this context include reduced progression from fibrosis to cirrhosis, improved oxidative stress, earlier disappearance of clinical manifestations with a silybin–phosphatidylcholine complex in conjunction with antiviral therapy, and improved symptoms and general well–being. Serum ferritin has also been significantly reduced, and hyperinsulinaemia was significantly reduced by silybin conjugated with vitamin E and phospholipids.

Silymarin supplemental to antiviral therapy improved oxidative stress, but was unable to favourably affect ALT or the sustained virological response in chronic HCV genotype 1 positive patients.[220] Sixteen patients were treated with pegylated interferon (pegIFN) plus ribavirin (RBV) for 6 to 12 months plus placebo for the first 3 months, while the other 16 were treated with the antiviral combination plus silymarin (332 mg/day) for 3 months. In the silymarin group, a more rapid decrease in the MDA level, as well as a marked decrease in SOD and an increase in myeloperoxidase activity after month 12 were found. Randomisation bias was suggested as an explanation for these contradictory findings, as patients in the silymarin group were older with higher fibrosis scores and more severe pre–treatment baseline oxidative stress.

Clinical manifestations of HCV disappeared 7 to 10 days earlier with antiviral therapy in conjunction with a silybin–phosphatidylcholine complex than with pegIFN- alpha–2b and RBV alone.[221] The formulation, containing 40 mg silybin and 80 mg phosphatidylcholine per tablet, was administered at a dose of two capsules twice daily to 20 patients for 3 months in conjunction with the combined antiviral therapy. Cytolytic syndrome resolved in the herbal group and the positive virological response rate was 20% higher, with study withdrawal due to the severe side effects of IFN therapy 10% lower.

Silymarin administration for 1 year improved symptoms and general well–being, but had no effect on HCV viraemia, serum ALT or serum and ultrasound markers for hepatic fibrosis.[222] One hundred and seventy–seven participants with HCV were randomly assigned to receive either silymarin at an average dose of 124.5 mg three times daily, or a low–dose multivitamin and mineral supplement. After 12 months, serum hepatic fibrosis markers, hyaluronic acid, the inflammatory marker YKL-40 and abdominal ultrasound results were similar in both groups and may even have progressed from baseline. After 24 months, both the silymarin and vitamin placebo groups had fewer symptoms and reported they felt

better than prior to participating in the study. They also had no detectable progression of their liver disease over the 24–month period and none developed clinical complications of chronic HCV infection. However, silymarin was not superior to the vitamin supplements in clearing HCV RNA.[223]

Intravenous silybin was found to be a well–tolerated and potent antiviral synergist in patients with HCV, not responding to standard antiviral combination therapy.[224] Sixteen non–responders to full–dose pegIFN/RBV were studied. Intravenous dosing over 4 h of 10 mg/kg/day silybin for 7 days was followed by oral 420 mg/day silymarin in combination with 180 μg/week pegIFN-alpha–2a and 1 to 1.2 g/day RBV. A dose–dependent decrease in viral load was observed: HCV RNA declined on intravenous silybin by 1.32±0.55 log (p<0.001), but increased again in spite of the pegIFN/RBV. ALT also decreased from 162±133 to 118±107 U/L. In a subsequent dose–finding study over 14 days, viral load declined continuously. After the first 7 days the 5 mg/kg dose was marginally effective, whereas the 10 mg/kg, 15 mg/kg and 20 mg/kg daily doses resulted in highly significant decreases in viral load (p<0.001). After a week of combined silybin and pegIFN/RBV therapy, viral load decreased further (p<0.001).[224]

However, 480 mg/day silymarin had no apparent effect on viral load when administered to patients with chronic HCV for 4 weeks in a randomised controlled trial (n=34).[225] There was a statistically significant difference for percentage changes in ALT (p=0.014) and AST (p=0.002) compared with placebo, but not for viral load (p=0.326). No side effects were reported using the herb extract.

Similarly, no clinically meaningful reductions from baseline serum transaminases or HCV RNA titre were observed in patients with well–compensated, chronic non-cirrhotic HCV who had failed IFN–based therapy. They were randomised to receive oral doses of 140, 280, 560 or 700 mg silymarin every 8 h for 7 days. Silymarin up to 2.1 g/day was safe and well tolerated and no drug–related adverse events were reported.[181]

No virological response was observed following administration of silymarin 450 mg/day for 24 weeks, although normalisation of ALT was achieved in 15.3% of HCV patients assigned to silymarin.[226] Patients were randomly assigned to receive a daily combination of ribavirin (600 to 800 mg) plus amantadine (200 mg) and UDCA (500 mg) (n=87) or silymarin 450 mg/day (n=83) for 24 weeks. Normalisation of ALT at the end of treatment was achieved in 58.5% and 15.3% of patients (p<0.001), respectively, and an end of treatment virological response was achieved in 2.4% and 0%, respectively.

The Hepatitis C Antiviral Long–Term Treatment against Cirrhosis (HALT–C) trial investigated the association between silymarin use and subsequent liver disease progression in 1049 non–responders to prior antiviral therapy who had advanced fibrosis or cirrhosis.[227] Silymarin use among patients with advanced hepatitis C–related liver disease was found to be associated with reduced progression from fibrosis to cirrhosis, but had no impact on clinical outcomes. Patients were followed up for liver disease progression. At baseline, 34% of patients had used silymarin, half of whom were current users. Baseline users had less hepatic collagen content on study biopsies at year 1.5 and year 3.5, and had less histo-logical progression over 8.65 years (HR 0.57 95% CI: 0.33 to 1.00; p–trend for longer duration of use was 0.026).

Further, baseline data for the 1145 study participants in HALT–C trial revealed silymarin users had significantly fewer liver–related symptoms (such as fatigue, nausea, liver pain, anorexia, muscle and joint pain) and better general health and quality–of–life parameters than non-users.[228] No difference was observed between users and non-users in terms of ALT or HCV RNA levels.

Treatment with a highly bioavailable silybin product (a standardised silybin and soy phosphatidylcholine complex) was associated with a significant reduction in serum ferritin in patients with chronic hepatitis C, especially among patients with advanced fibrosis.[229] Thirty–seven participants were ran-domised to one of three doses of the complex for 12 weeks. There was a significant decrease in serum ferritin from baseline to the end of treatment (p=0.0005), but no signifi-cant change in serum iron or transferrin–iron saturation. The authors concluded that the formulation could act as a mild iron chelator, addressing the pathogenic aspects of hepatic iron overload in patients with liver disease.

In a study investigating the antioxidant and antifibrotic activity of a silybin–vitamin-E–phospholipid complex to improve insulin resistance and liver damage, 85 outpatients with non–alcoholic fatty liver disease (NAFLD) with or with-out chronic HCV (all genotype 1b and all non–responders to previous antiviral therapy) were treated for 6 months, fol-lowed by another 6 months of follow-up. In all, 53 patients (39 NAFLD and 14 HCV) received active treatment, while the other 32 (20 NAFLD and 12 HCV) served as a control group (no treatment).[230] Each tablet contained 94 mg sily-bin, 194 mg phosphatidylcholine and 90 mg vitamin E (dose 4 tablets per day). Results showed an improvement of liver enzyme levels in the active treatment groups after 6 months, but this persisted for the NAFLD patients only. All indices of liver fibrosis were significantly reduced in both treated groups, with a persistent effect only in the chronic HCV group asso-ciated with NAFLD. Hyperinsulinaemia, present in both groups, was significantly reduced only in the treated patients. Only in the HCV treated patients at 6 and 12 months did the percentage of overweight patients decrease significantly (44%; p<0.01 versus baseline and other group data).[231] Liver stea-tosis was significantly improved in the NAFLD treated group (p<0.01). The authors concluded that silybin conjugated with vitamin E and phospholipids could be used as a complemen-tary approach to the treatment of patients with chronic liver damage.

Poisoning

An early review of 205 cases of clinical poisoning with the death cap mushroom (*Amanita phalloides*) from the period 1971 to 1980 found the combination of penicillin with sily-bin to be associated with increased survival.[232] There are many reports of successful treatment of mushroom poisoning.[233–236] Treatment usually involved intravenous administration of silybin, alone or in combination with penicillin and/or other drugs. There are no side effects from parenteral silybin admin-istration, where as parenteral penicillin can have significant

adverse effects. The clinical picture appears to be markedly mitigated by the early initiation of silybin therapy. A review of 18 cases (1980 to 1981) found a close relationship between the severity of the intoxication and the time elapsed before commencement of silybin therapy.[237] In a review of 87 patients with signs of poisoning with mushrooms and a long period of incubation, a significant reduction of serum transaminases and prothrombin time was found in those on competitive inhibi-tion with silybin or penicillin, as compared with patients only on plasmapheresis.[238] Intravenous infusion of silybin, in combi-nation with normal management techniques, induced a marked reduction in mortality in a multicentre study of 252 cases of intoxication by *Amanita phalloides*.[239]

Silymarin administered during the pre– and postopera-tive period prevented the increase of serum hepatic enzymes induced by the toxic effect of general anaesthesia.[190] Silymarin also improved liver function in patients who had been exposed for many years to halogenated hydrocarbons.[59] Treatment with silymarin (420 mg/day) in patients with occu-pational toxic hepatic damage caused by various toxic sub-stances (mostly solvents, paints and glues) resulted in slight variations in some parameters compared with those treated with placebo. The therapeutic effect of silymarin was more evident when the exposure period to toxins was shorter.[240] Improvement in biochemical parameters was observed in 19 patients on psychotropic drugs after 6 months of silymarin treatment.[241]

Type 2 diabetes

Treatment with silybin (231 mg/day for 4 weeks) in 14 type 2 diabetic patients resulted in significant reduction of red blood cell sorbitol compared with baseline levels. However, silybin treatment had no effect on fasting blood glucose. This suggests that silybin may be an aldose reductase inhibitor and could be valuable in the prophylaxis and treatment of diabetic complications by downregulating the polyol pathway.[242]

Silymarin treatment in type 2 diabetic patients for 4 months had a beneficial effect on improving the glycaemic profile.[243] In a 4–month randomised, double blind clinical trial, 51 type 2 diabetic patients were randomised to receive sily-marin (600 mg/day) plus conventional therapy, or placebo plus conventional therapy. A significant decrease in glycosylated haemoglobin (HbA1c), fasting blood glucose, total choles-terol, LDL–cholesterol, triglyceride, AST and ALT levels were observed in silymarin–treated patients compared with placebo and with baseline values in each group.

A randomised, controlled trial evaluated the adjuvant effect of silymarin in improving long–term and postpran-dial glycaemia and weight control in type 2 diabetic patients treated with glibenclamide.[244] A total of 59 patients, pre-viously maintained on 10 mg/day glibenclamide and diet but with poor glycaemic control, were randomised into three groups. The first two groups were treated with either 200 mg/day silymarin or placebo as adjuncts to glibencla-mide, and the third group was maintained on glibenclamide alone for 120 days. Adjunct use of silymarin with glibencla-mide was found to improve glycaemic control, both fasting and postprandially. Compared with placebo, silymarin treat-ment significantly reduced both fasting and postprandial plasma glucose excursions, in addition to significantly reducing HbA1c levels and BMI after 120 days. No significantly differences were observed for the placebo and glibenclamide alone groups.

A randomised controlled trial investigated the effects of silybin–beta–cyclodextrin (135 mg/day silybin) in 42 outpatients with chronic alcoholic liver disease and concomitant type 2 diabetes.[245] Fasting blood glucose levels decreased significantly (p=0.03) in the active treatment group, while they were virtually unchanged in the placebo group. Plasma triglycerides also dropped significantly in the silybin–beta–cyclodextrin group compared with the placebo group (p<0.01). There was also a trend towards lower mean daily blood glucose levels, HbA1c levels and insulin resistance (HOMA–IR) in the silybin group, although the differences were not significant. MDA decreased significantly only in the patients receiving the active treatment. No clinically relevant side effects were observed in either group.

A randomised controlled trial in 60 patients with diabetes caused by alcoholic liver cirrhosis found that silymarin 600 mg/day significantly reduced mean levels of fasting blood glucose, daily blood glucose, daily glycosuria, HbA1c, daily insulin need, fasting insulinaemia, blood MDA, and basal and glucagon–stimulated C peptide over 6 months, compared with untreated patients and their own baseline values.[246] Results indicated that silymarin can reduce lipoperoxidation of liver cell membranes in cirrhotic diabetic patients, decrease endogenous production of insulin (probably by reducing insulin resistance) and the need for exogenous insulin.

Iron–related disorders

Silybin was investigated for its capacity to reduce iron absorption as a potential adjunct in the treatment of haemochromatosis.[247] In a crossover study, on three separate occasions 10 patients who were homozygous for the C282Y mutation in the HFE gene (and fully treated) consumed a vegetarian meal containing 13.9 mg iron with 200 mL water, 200 mL water and 140 mg silybin or 200 mL tea. Consumption of silybin with a meal resulted in a reduction in the postprandial increase in serum iron (AUC) compared with water and tea, suggesting a beneficial role as an iron chelator.

Silymarin was found to be safe and effective in the treatment of iron–loaded patients with beta–thalassaemia when administered in combination with desferrioxamine in a 3–month randomised, double blind, clinical trial.[248] A total of 59 patients were randomised to receive conventional desferrioxamine therapy in addition to placebo or a silymarin tablet (420 mg/day). The combined therapy was well tolerated and more effective than desferrioxamine alone in reducing serum ferritin levels. Significant improvements in liver alkaline phosphatase and glutathione levels of red blood cells were also observed in the silymarin–treated beta–thalassaemia patients.

Osteoarthritis

The anti–inflammatory effect of silymarin was compared with piroxicam and meloxicam in patients with osteoarthritis of the knee in an 8–week, double blind clinical trial.[249] A total of 220 patients were randomised into five groups, treated with either silymarin (300 mg/day), piroxicam (20 mg/day), meloxicam (15 mg/day) or a combination of silymarin with piroxicam or meloxicam. Silymarin, as well as adjunct use of silymarin with piroxicam, significantly reduced serum levels of IL–alpha1, IL–8, and the complement proteins C3 and C4 after 8 weeks compared with the pretreatment levels. Piroxicam significantly reduced IL–8 compared with pretreatment, while no reductions were seen with meloxicam or for its adjunct use with silymarin.

Hyperlipidaemia

In an open trial, 14 outpatients with type II hyperlipidaemia were treated with silymarin (420 mg/day) for 3 months, followed by a 2–month placebo period and then silymarin treatment for another month. Total cholesterol and HDL–cholesterol levels were slightly decreased, and apolipoprotein levels were somewhat decreased, compared with baseline values. A relative increase in the proportion of cholesterol in the HDL fraction was suggested by the significant decrease of apolipoprotein A–I and A–II values.[250]

Haemodialysis

Oral supplementation with silymarin and vitamin E resulted in a reduction in MDA, an increase in red blood cell glutathione peroxidase and an increase in haemoglobin levels in patients with endstage renal disease on haemodialysis.[251] Eighty patients on haemodialysis were randomised into four groups and received either silymarin 420 mg/day, vitamin E 400 IU/day or both treatments; the fourth group acted as a control. There was a significant increase in glutathione peroxidase levels in all treatment groups compared with controls after 3 weeks, as well as a significant increase in the mean haemoglobin. The combination of silymarin and vitamin E led to a significant reduction in MDA levels (p=0.008).

A study investigating the effects of silymarin administration on TNF–alpha production and haemoglobin concentration in 15 peritoneal dialysis patients found that serum concentrations of TNF–alpha were not significantly reduced (p=0.352) following 2 months of treatment with 210 mg/day silymarin (as three divided doses, extract not specified).[252] However, 40% of patients presented a significant response, and among these responders haemoglobin concentrations were increased significantly after silymarin administration (p=0.048).

In vitro fertilisation

Administration of silymarin to in vitro fertilisation (IVF) patients concomitantly with gonadotropin resulted in reduction of granulosa cell apoptosis, but did not have any effect on the promotion of follicular development, oocyte retrieval or endometrial thickness.[253] In a randomised, controlled trial, 40 healthy women undergoing IVF due to male factor infertility underwent ovulation induction and were assigned to receive silymarin (210 mg/day) or placebo from the beginning of the induction cycle. There was no significant difference between the groups for mean number of follicles (p=0.131), mean number of oocytes retrieved (p=0.209) or endometrial thickness (p=0.673). However, the proportion of total apoptosis in the study group was significantly lower than in the placebo group (p=0.032).

Liver and prostate cancer

A case of spontaneous regression of hepatocellular carcinoma was reported in 1995. In June 1991, 11 months after being diagnosed with inoperable carcinoma of both lobes, the man presented to the hospital. All laboratory parameters were normal except for one liver enzyme, and the liver was clear of the earlier signs of carcinoma. The man claimed to have stopped alcohol and smoking and had been taking silymarin (450 mg/day) for 10 months and glibenclamide (a hypoglycaemic drug).[254]

The traditional Chinese herbal combination, Bushen Jianpi Recipe (BSJPR), was compared with a combination of silymarin and vitamin C on cellular immunity in 117 primary liver cancer patients in a randomised controlled trial over 12 weeks.[255] The clinical benefit rate in the silymarin/vitamin C group (92.7%, 51/55 cases) was higher than that in the BSJPR–treated group (78.0%, 46/59 cases, p=0. 035), although the half–year survival rate was higher in the BSJPR group compared with the silymarin/vitamin C group.

In a 6-month, placebo–controlled, double blind clinical trial in 37 men after radical prostatectomy, a combination of silymarin and selenomethionine at daily doses of 570 mg of silymarin and 240 µg of selenium was shown to significantly reduce two markers of lipid metabolism known to be associated with prostate cancer progression.[256] Blood levels of LDL-cholesterol and total cholesterol decreased, the quality of life score improved, and serum selenium levels increased. The combination had no effect on blood antioxidant status or testosterone levels.

Other conditions

A topical treatment based on a combination of silymarin and methylsulfonylmethane was trialled for 1 month in 46 patients affected by stage I to III erythematous–telangiectactic rosacea. A statistically significant improvement of skin redness, papules, itching, hydration and skin colour occurred (p<0.001), especially in the subtype 1 erythematous-telangiectatic phase.[257]

Silymarin alleviated pruritus associated with intrahepatic cholestasis of pregnancy. However, it did not assist with the biochemical alterations associated with this condition.[258,259]

Silymarin at a dose of 420 mg/day administered to 50 healthy lactating women for 63 days showed a clear galactagogue action, increasing daily milk production by 85.9% compared with 32.1% in the placebo group.[260] No unwanted side effects were reported in either group.

Toxicology and other safety data

Toxicology

The acute toxicology of silymarin is very low. A 2010 review of clinical studies of the various St Mary's thistle extracts in liver diseases reported them to be non–toxic in humans.[37] Hyperbilirubinaemia occurred in prostate cancer patients receiving 91 courses each of a silybin–phytosome complex (daily dose of 2.5 to 20 g) with grade 1 to 2 bilirubin elevations in nine of the 13 patients.[261] The only grade 3 toxicity observed was an elevation of ALT in one patient; no grade 4 toxicity was noted.

Oral doses of 20 g/kg in mice and 1 g/kg in dogs resulted in no mortality or any signs of adverse effects.[262] Long–term studies (100 mg/kg/day for 16 to 22 weeks) also failed to demonstrate toxicity or teratogenic effects.

In 2–year feed studies, exposure of Silybum extract (presumably silymarin) to rats and mice at 0, 12 500, 25 000 or 50 000 ppm (equivalent to average daily doses of approximately 570, 1180 or 2520 mg/kg to males and 630, 1300 or 2750 mg/kg to females) showed no evidence of carcinogenic activity and had no effect on survival. Exposure to Silybum extract resulted in increased incidences of clear cell and mixed cell foci in the liver of female rats and decreases in body weights of exposed groups of male and female mice. Decreased incidences of mammary gland neoplasms occurred in female rats and decreased incidences of hepatocellular neoplasms occurred in the male mice.[263]

Silymarin is capable of inducing DNA damage (measured as strand breaks) and inhibiting human cell growth in vitro. Toxicity was only seen at high micromolar concentrations (levels that are unlikely to be achieved in humans). Neither cytotoxicity nor genotoxicity was associated with the antioxidant enzyme capacity of the test cells.[264]

Contraindications

Known allergy to St Mary's thistle or any of its constituents.

Special warnings and precautions

Caution in patients with known hypersensitivity to plants in the Asteraceae/Compositae family.

It is possible that silymarin and its constituents may reduce or enhance (studies are conflicting) the oral bioavailability of drugs subject to the P–glycoprotein (P–gp) efflux pump. Patients coadministered pharmaceutical drugs with silymarin should be monitored for potential signs of altered drug levels, although the risks are probably quite low. St Mary's thistle and silymarin also have the potential to reduce iron absorption, especially if taken with iron supplements. (See also Appendix C and the Interactions section below.)

Interactions

(See also Appendix C for a summary of recommendations regarding the potential herb–drug interactions for St Mary's thistle that are deemed to be clinically relevant.)

Several clinical studies published in the last decade have investigated potential interaction of Silybum extracts with prescribed drugs. The majority of human clinical herb–drug interaction studies indicate that St Mary's thistle and silymarin are unlikely to interfere with drug metabolism. If they do interact at all, this typically results in increased, not reduced, drug levels. A 2009 review of the herb–drug interactions with silymarin concluded that it has limited effect on the pharmacokinetics of several drugs in vivo, despite decreasing the activity of cytochrome P450 (CYP) enzymes, UDP–glucuronosyltransferase (UGT) and reducing P–gp transport.[174] It should also be noted that the occasional effects observed on P–gp induction are not likely to impact on levels of intravenously administered drugs.

In conjunction with chemotherapy agents, St Mary's thistle or the silymarin complex may in fact favourably impact on treatment outcomes. Early indications from in vitro, in vivo and human studies are encouraging. These are also reviewed below.

Cytochrome P450 enzymes

Some in vitro studies in human hepatocyte cultures have suggested metabolic interactions between silymarin or silybin and xenobiotics metabolised by CYP3A4 and/or CYP2C9.[24,25,265,266] Treatment with silymarin (0.1 and 0.25 mM) significantly reduced the activity of CYP3A4 (by 50% and 100%, respectively) in one study,[25] while in another in vitro model CYP3A4 showed a strong dose–dependent modulation (downregulation) by silybin.[265] However, other in vitro research has found that silymarin did not modify reporter gene activity mediated by CYP3A4 promoters and the pregnane X receptor.[267] A further in vitro study investigating a standardised dry extract from Silybum marianum on the enzyme kinetics of cytochrome P450 isoenzymes (CYP) with primary human hepatocytes and human liver microsomes concluded that herb–drug interactions are possible, but not likely, for CYPs 2C8 and 2C9, and are remote for CYPs 2C19, 2D6 and 3A4.[266] Similarly, using human hepatocytes, silybin and its beta–glycosides did not affect inducible expression of CYP1A2 and CYP3A4 by dioxin and rifampicin, respectively, suggesting they do not interfere with the expression of CYP1A2 and CYP3A4.[268]

As noted earlier, while oral administration of silymarin (100 mg/kg/day) to rats resulted in a significant increase of the activity of the mixed function oxidation system (CYP; aminopyrine demethylation, p–nitroanisole demethylation), in human volunteers treatment with silymarin (210 mg/day for 28 days) had no influence on the metabolism of aminopyrine and phenylbutazone.[26]

A clinical study evaluating the impact of Silybum on human CYP activity using various probe drug cocktails found that Silybum extract (350 mg/day standardised to 80% silymarin) for 28 days had no impact on CYP1A2, CYP2D6, CYP2E1 and CYP3A4.[269] A meta–analysis of three trials involving concurrent use of silymarin (340 to 420 mg/day 12 to 28 days) and the anti–HIV drug indinavir found no impact on drug levels.[270] Silymarin (480 mg/day for 4 or 12 days) had no impact on the metabolism of the anticancer drug

irinotecan in six cancer patients.[271] The authors noted that irinotecan is highly susceptible to CYP3A4 inhibition (which silymarin demonstrates in vitro), and concluded that silybin concentrations after intake of St Mary's thistle are too low to significantly affect the function of CYP3A4 and UGT1A1 in vivo, indicating that the herb is unlikely to alter the disposition of anticancer drugs metabolised by these enzymes.

A similar conclusion (that St Mary's thistle is not a potent CYP3A4 inducer) was reached after a short–term study of the impact of the herbal extract (280 mg administered 10 h and 1.5 h prior to the administration of nifedipine) on the calcium channel blocking drug nifedipine (10 mg) as a CYP3A4 test drug in 16 healthy male volunteers.[272] No significant inhibition of CYP2D6 activity was found with silymarin supplementation in 16 healthy volunteers for 14 days, using the CYP2D6 substrate, debrisoquine (5 mg) as a test drug before and at the end of supplementation. This suggests no interaction with drugs that are CYP2D6 substrates.[273] An earlier in vitro study concluded that, although four flavonolignans (silybin, dehydrosilybin, silydianin and silychristin) displayed dose–dependent inhibition of three specific CYP activities involving CYP2D6, CYP2E1 and CYP3A4, the inhibition was not clinically relevant because of the low concentrations of the individual flavonolignans recorded in human bioavailability studies.[274]

P–glycoprotein

Interference with transporter proteins such as P–gp is another means by which significant herb–drug interactions can occur. P–gp is a molecule that acts as a drug efflux pump at epithelial cells, especially the intestinal wall. Induction of P–gp results in less absorption of any drug that is subject to its effects. In this context, it was found that 900 mg/day of silymarin for 14 days had a small but non–significant impact on reducing digoxin levels in 16 healthy volunteers.[275] An Indian study found that levels of the antibiotic drug metronidazole were significantly reduced by just 140 mg/day of silymarin for 9 days, due to suspected induction of intestinal and perhaps hepatic expression of P–gp and CYP3A4.[29] This is the only human herb–drug interaction study for St Mary's thistle that has found reduced drug levels. (See also Appendix C.)

In contrast, increased drug levels have been demonstrated in some studies. The isoflavone biochanin A and silymarin were found to inhibit P–gp–mediated efflux in human Caco–2 cells, suggesting they could potentially increase the intestinal absorption/bioavailability of co–administered drugs that are P–gp substrates.[35] Silybum extract (80% silymarin) at a dose of 420 mg/day for 14 days increased levels of the beta–blocker talinolol by around 36%.[276] Inhibition of P–gp was suggested as a possible mechanism. The same authors also found that silymarin at the same dose appeared to inhibit the metabolism of the hypotensive drug losartan in individuals with a particular CYP2C9 genotype.[30] This finding is consistent with an animal study that reported silybin (0.3, 1.5 and 6 mg/kg) significantly enhanced the oral bioavailability of loratadine in rats.[33] (The relative bioavailability of loratadine was 1.50– to 1.77–fold greater than that in the control group.)

Drug–induced hepatotoxicity

Preliminary evidence for the involvement of silymarin in attenuation of drug–induced hepatotoxicity was provided in a study in which male Swiss albino mice were treated with silymarin (40 mg/kg, ip) 2 h prior to intraperitoneal administration of rifampicin (20 mg/kg) and/or pyrogallol (40 mg/kg) for 1, 2, 3 and 4 weeks.[277] Silymarin restored the rifampicin and/or pyrogallol–induced alterations in the expression and activities of CYP1A2 and CYP2E1, glutathione, glutathione reductase and glutathione peroxidase, and the degree of lipid peroxidation.

Adjunct to chemotherapy

St Mary's thistle has potential application in oncology settings in preventing or reducing hepatotoxicity associated with chemotherapy or radiotherapy, and possibly potentiating chemotherapy and radiation therapy as an adjunctive treatment.

Drug resistance is one of the main causes of treatment failure and mortality in cancer patients. In vitro research on P–gp function in human breast cancer cell lines suggested that some phytochemicals such as biochanin A and silymarin may reverse multidrug resistance by inhibiting the P–gp function.[29] This was confirmed in subsequent studies in sensitive and multidrug resistant human breast cancer cell lines for silymarin on daunomycin accumulation and doxorubicin cytotoxicity. Silymarin inhibited P–gp–mediated cellular efflux and the mechanism of the interaction involved, at least in part, a direct interaction.[36]

Silybin has shown promise in vitro as a potent sensitiser for apoptosis induced by anticancer drugs. The invasive potential of A2780 and A2780/taxol cells was reduced dramatically by silybin treatment, which also enhanced the sensitivity of A2780/taxol cells to paclitaxel and increased paclitaxel–induced apoptosis and G2/M arrest. This suggests that silybin in combination with paclitaxel may be a beneficial chemotherapeutic strategy, especially in patients with tumours refractory to paclitaxel alone.[278] Other in vitro research findings support the synergistic effects of silymarin on the anti–proliferative activities of two chemotherapy agents, doxorubicin and paclitaxel, in both sensitive and, at higher concentrations, multidrug-resistant colon cancer cells. The authors concluded that silymarin extract alone or in combined chemotherapy may offer a valuable option for treatment of colon tumours, including chemoresistant ones.[279]

In vivo, silymarin reduced, delayed onset or prevented toxic effects of doxorubicin, modulating doxorubicin–induced oxidative stress and p53 expression, while preventing apoptotic and necrotic cell death in the liver.[280] Silymarin was orally administered to mice at 16 mg/kg/day for 14 days, with an approximate LD_{50} dose of doxorubicin (60 mg/kg) administered intraperitoneally on day 12.

In a case study of a 34–year–old female patient with acute promyelocytic leukaemia, treatment with silymarin countered the hepatotoxic effects of chemotherapy.[281] The patient's maintenance methotrexate and 6–mercaptopurine chemotherapy had been intermittent due to her elevated liver enzymes. During 4 months of treatment with silymarin extract (800 mg/day) administered in combination with maintenance chemotherapy, liver enzymes were maintained at normal levels for the first time.

The results of a randomised controlled trial of 50 children (aged 1 to 21 years) with acute lymphoblastic leukaemia (ALL) provide support for the role of silymarin in the prevention or treatment of chemotherapy–associated hepatotoxicity.[282] The children were randomly assigned to herbal treatment or placebo for 28 days during maintenance chemotherapy. The extract contained only two compounds from the flavonolignan complex, namely silybin A and B (target dose for trial participants 5.1 mg/kg/day), together with soy phosphatidylcholine for improved bioavailability. The intravenous chemotherapy drugs administered to the children included vincristine, prednisone, methotrexate and 6–mercaptopurine. No significant differences in frequency of side effects, incidence and severity of toxic reactions, infections or liver parameters were observed at the end of the trial (day 28). However, by day 56 the herbal group had a significantly lower AST (p=0.05) and a trend toward a significantly lower ALT (p=0.07), compared with baseline. AST in the treatment arm was also significantly different to placebo at day 56 (p=0.04). Although not significant, chemotherapy doses had to be reduced in 61% of the herbal group, compared with 72% for placebo. The concurrent use of St Mary's thistle extract did not antagonise the effects of chemotherapy agents used for the treatment of ALL.

Other

In 12 healthy male volunteers, pretreatment with silymarin for 7 days (420 mg/day) had no influence on the pharmacokinetics of 150 mg ranitidine.[283]

Silymarin has been effectively used to reduce the side effects of conventional treatment for Alzheimer's disease. In a 12–week trial, co–administration of silymarin (420 mg/day, extract not specified) to 217 patients reduced the rate of gastrointestinal and cholinergic side effects induced by the anticholinesterase drug tacrine, formerly used for Alzheimer's disease (now withdrawn), without any impact on cognitive status, although it did not prevent tacrine–induced alanine transaminase elevation.[284]

Silybin has demonstrated iron–chelating activity in vitro[285] and in vivo (see previous). As a mild iron chelator, silybin may potentially address the pathogenic effect of hepatic iron overload in patients with liver disease. However, it also has the potential to reduce iron absorption, especially if taken with iron supplements.

Use in pregnancy and lactation

Category B1 – no increase in frequency of malformation or other harmful effects on the fetus from limited use in women. No evidence of increased fetal damage in animal studies.

Oral administration of silymarin extract (100 mg/kg/day from days 8 to 17 in rabbits, 1 g/kg/day from days 8 to 12 in rats) failed to demonstrate teratogenic effects compared with controls.[263] As noted earlier, a silymarin–phospholipid compound demonstrated a foetoprotective effect against ethanol–induced behavioural deficits in rats.[76]

A pregnant woman in her 28th week of gestation was treated with penicillin and silybin for accidental poisoning with an Amanita mushroom. After 5 days at the intensive care unit, mother and unborn child were discharged in a normal physical condition.[286]

Administration of silymarin (300 mg/day) from 13 gestational weeks in conjunction with lamivudine in a woman with an aggravation of her chronic hepatitis B during pregnancy had no adverse effect on the subsequent spontaneous delivery her male baby.[287]

No adverse effects were observed on blood or milk parameters of cows or their offspring following administration of 10 g/day silymarin by an oral drench from 10 days before expected calving to 15 days after calving.[288]

St Mary's thistle is compatible with breastfeeding and has been shown to improve milk production in a clinical trial.

Effects on ability to drive and use machines

No negative influence is expected.

Side effects

Silymarin is reported to have a very good safety profile. Drug monitoring studies evaluating more than 3500 patients using silymarin up to 1995 indicate that adverse effects were seen in 1% of patients and consisted mainly of mild gastrointestinal complaints.[289,290] Similarly, gastrointestinal symptoms were the most common adverse effect reported in a systematic review that included seven randomised clinical trials, six cohort studies and five case reports, involving more than 7000 participants up to 1999. Overall their frequency was low, ranging from 2% to 10% in controlled trials, which was similar to that of placebo. Other adverse effects included dermatological symptoms and headaches, which were also similar in frequency between placebo and treatment groups.[291]

A 2010 review of clinical studies of St Mary's thistle extracts (mainly as silymarin) in liver diseases reported them to be generally non–toxic and without side effects when administered to adults in the oral dose range of 240 to 900 mg/day as two or three divided doses.[37] At higher doses of more than 1500 mg/day, silymarin may produce a laxative effect with an increased bile flow and secretion. A systematic review of clinical studies conducted between 2003 and 2008 reported, no serious side effects attributed to the therapy, and even a slightly lower incidence in the silymarin than in the placebo–treated population.[186] The incidence of side effects in general, and interruption of treatment due to these, was also very low and similar to placebo values. In comparative studies, side effects with an incidence of ≥1% were headaches (silymarin 1.01%; placebo 1.35%) and pruritus (silymarin 1.35%; placebo 3.70%). The side effects reported in open silymarin trials showed a predominance of digestive symptoms (diarrhoea 0.20%, irregular stools 0.10%, nausea 0.13% and dyspepsia 0.08%).

Three adverse event reports exist in the literature to date. Gastroenteritis (intermittent episodes of sweating, nausea, colicky pain, diarrhoea, vomiting and weakness) associated with 'collapse' was reported for a combination product containing St Mary's thistle, with recurrent symptoms after rechallenge.[292] Later reports suggested that the capsules may have been contaminated. Anaphylactic reactions have also been reported (cases after ingestion of tea or standardised extract, respectively).[293,294] One of these was described in a patient with immediate–type allergy to kiwi fruit. St Mary's thistle tea caused facial oedema, swelling of the oral mucosa, marked respiratory distress, bronchospasm and decreased blood pressure in a 54–year–old man. He exhibited a pronounced immediate–type reaction to an extract of St Mary's thistle seed using the skin prick test.

Overdosage

As noted above under Toxicology, for prostate cancer patients who received a total of 91 courses of oral high–dose silybin–phytosome (2.5 to 20 g daily), the most prominent adverse event was hyperbilirubinaemia, with grade 1 to 2 bilirubin elevations in 9 of the 13 patients.[261]

Safety in children

Adverse effects are not expected. Children administered silymarin (200 mg/day for 30 days) showed no adverse clinical or biochemical effects.[295]

Regulatory status in selected countries

Silybum marianum is official in the *United States Pharmacopeia–National Formulary* (USP34-NF29, 2011). It does not have Generally Recognised as Safe (GRAS) status. However, it is freely available as a 'dietary supplement' in the USA under DSHEA legislation (1994 Dietary Supplement Health and Education Act).

Silybum is now on the General Sale List in the UK. St Mary's thistle (milk thistle) products have achieved Traditional Herbal Registration in the UK with the traditional indication of relief of symptoms associated with occasional over indulgence of food and drink, such as indigestion and upset stomach.

St Mary's thistle is covered by a positive Commission E monograph and has the following applications:

- Crude drug: dyspeptic disorders
- Preparations: for toxic liver damage; as supportive treatment in chronic inflammatory liver conditions and liver cirrhosis.

St Mary's thistle is not included in Part 4 of Schedule 4 of the Therapeutic Goods Act Regulations of Australia, and is freely available for sale.

References

1. Madaus G. *Lehrbuch der biologischen Heilmettel*. Band 1. Reprinted Hildesheim, Germany: 1979. pp. 830–836.
2. Grieve M. *A Modern Herbal*, vol. 2. New York: Dover Publications; 1971. p. 797.
3. Greenlee H, Abascal K, Yarnell E, et al. *Integr Cancer Ther*. 2007;6(2):158–165.
4. Mabberley DJ. *The Plant Book*. Cambridge: Cambridge University Press; 1997. pp. 175, 663.
5. Evans WC. *Trease and Evans' Pharmacognosy*. London: WB Saunders; 1996. p. 435.
6. Launert EL. *The Hamlyn Guide to Edible and Medicinal Plants of Britain and Northern Europe*. London: Hamlyn; 1981. p. 200.
7. Wagner H, Bladt S. *Plant Drug Analysis: A Thin Layer Chromatography Atlas*. Berlin: Springer-Verlag; 1996. p. 204.
8. Bisset NG, ed. *Herbal Drugs and Phytopharmaceuticals*. Stuttgart: Medpharm Scientific Publishers; 1994.
9. Asghar Z, Masood Z. *Pak J Pharm Sci*. 2008;21(3):249–254.
10. Kiruthiga PV, Shafreen RB, Pandian SK, et al. *Basic Clin Pharmacol Toxicol*. 2007;100(6):414–419.
11. Velmurugan K, Alam J, Mccord JM, et al. *Free Radic Biol Med*. 2009;46(3):430–440.
12. Basaga H, Poli G, Tekkaya C, et al. *Cell Biochem Funct*. 1997;15(1):27–33.
13. Ignatowicz E, Szaefer H, Zielinska M, et al. *Acta Biochim Pol*. 1997;44(1):127–129.
14. Wenzel S, Stolte H, Soose M. *J Pharmacol Exp Ther*. 1996;279(3):1520–1526.
15. Altorjay I, Dalmi L, Sari B, et al. *Acta Physiol Hung*. 1992;80(1–4):375–380.
16. Gyorgy I, Antus S, Blazovics A, et al. *Int J Radiat Biol*. 1992;61(5):603–609.
17. Valenzuela A, Guerra R, Videla LA. *Planta Med*. 1986(6):438–440.
18. Bartholomaeus AR, Bolton R, Ahokas JT. *Xenobiotica*. 1994;24(1):17–24.
19. Valenzuela A, Aspillaga M, Vial S, et al. *Planta Med*. 1989;55:420–422.
20. Loginov AS, Matiushin BN, Sukhareva GV, et al. *Ter Arkh*. 1988;60(8):74–77.
21. Kittur S, Wilasrusmee S, Pedersen WA, et al. *J Mol Neurosci*. 2002;18(3):265–269.
22. Gonzalez-Correa JA, De La Cruz JP, Gordillo J, et al. *Pharmacology*. 2002;64(1):18–27.
23. Velebny S, Hrckova G, Konigova A. *Parasitol Int*. 2010;59(4):524–531.
24. Beckmann-Knopp S, Rietbrock S, Weyhenmeyer R, et al. *Pharmacol Toxicol*. 2000;86(6):250–256.
25. Venkataramanan R, Ramachandran V, Komoroski BJ, et al. *Drug Metab Dispos*. 2000;28(11):1270–1273.
26. Leber HW, Knauff S. *Arzneimittelforschung*. 1976;26(8):1603–1605.
27. Gurley BJ, Barone GW, Williams DK, et al. *Drug Metab Dispos*. 2006;34(1):69–74.
28. Rajnarayana K, Reddy MS, Vidyasagar J, et al. *Arzneimittelforschung*. 2004;54(2):109–113.
29. Chung SY, Sung MK, Kim NH, et al. *Arch Pharm Res*. 2005;28(7):823–828.
30. Han Y, Guo D, Chen Y, et al. *Eur J Clin Pharmacol*. 2009;65(6):585–591.
31. Jiao Z, Shi XJ, Li ZD, et al. *Br J Clin Pharmacol*. 2009;68(1):47–60.
32. Lee CK, Choi JS. *Pharmacology*. 2010;85(6):350–356.
33. Li C, Lee MY, Choi JS. *Pharmazie*. 2010;65(7):510–514.
34. Repalle SS, Yamsani SK, Gannu R, et al. *Acta Pharm*. 2009;51(1):15–20.
35. Zhang S, Morris ME. *Pharm Res*. 2003;20(8):1184–1191.
36. Zhang S, Morris ME. *J Pharmacol Exp Ther*. 2003;304(3):1258–1267.
37. Abenavoli L, Capasso R, Milic N, et al. *Phytother Res*. 2010;24(10):1423–1432.
38. Valenzuela A, Garrido A. *Biol Res*. 1994;27(2):105–112.
39. Batakov EA. *Eksp Klin Farmakol*. 2001;64(4):53–55.
40. Sonnenbichler J, Scalera F, Sonnenbichler I, et al. *J Pharmacol Exp Ther*. 1999;290(3):1375–1383.
41. Wellington K, Jarvis B. *BioDrugs*. 2001;15(7):465–489.
42. He Q, Kim J, Sharma RP. *Toxicol Sci*. 2004;80(2):335–342.
43. Kang JS, Jeon YJ, Kim HM, et al. *J Pharmacol Exp Ther*. 2002;302(1):138–144.
44. Schumann J, Prockl J, Kiemer AK, et al. *J Hepatol*. 2003;39(3):333–340.
45. Dehmlow C, Erhard J, De Groot H. *Hepatology*. 1996;23(4):749–754.
46. Kang JS, Park SK, Yang KH, et al. *FEBS Lett*. 2003;550(1–3):89–93.
47. Saller R, Melzer J, Reichling J, et al. *Forsch Komplementmed*. 2007;14(2):70–80.
48. Au AY, Hasenwinkel JM, Frondoza CG. *J Vet Pharmacol Ther*. 2011;34(2):120–129.
49. Crocenzi FA, Basiglio CL, Perez LM, et al. *Biochem Pharmacol*. 2005;69(7):1113–1120.
50. Letteron R, Labbe G, Degott C, et al. *Biochem Pharmacol*. 1990;39(12):2027–2034.
51. Vogel G, Trost W, Braatz R, et al. *Arzneimittelforschung*. 1975;25(1):82–89.
52. Schriewer H, Lohmann J, Rauen HM, et al. *Arzneimittelforschung*. 1975;25(10):1582–1585.
53. Valenzuela A, Lagos C, Schmidt K, et al. *Biochem Pharmacol*. 1985;34(12):2209–2212.
54. Campos R, Garrido A, Guerra R, et al. *Planta Med*. 1989;55:417–419.
55. German Federal Minister of Justice. *German Commission E for Human Medicine Monograph*. Bundes-Anzeiger (German Federal Gazette); no. 50, dated 13.03.1986.
56. Tsai JH, Liu JY, Wu TT, et al. *J Viral Hepatol*. 2008;15(7):508–514.
57. Mourelle M, Muriel P, Favari L, et al. *Fundam Clin Pharmacol*. 1989;3:183–191.
58. Barbarino F, Neumann E, Deaciuc I, et al. *Med Interne*. 1981;19(1):347–357.
59. Leng-Peschlow E, Strenge–Hesse AZ. *Z Phytother*. 1991;12:162–174.
60. Martines G, Copponi V, Cagnetta G, et al. *Arch Sci Med (Torino)*. 1980;137(3):367–386.
61. Jia JD, Bauer M, Cho JJ, et al. *J Hepatol*. 2001;35(3):392–398.
62. Mata-Santos HA, Lino FG, Rocha CC, et al. *Parasitol Res*. 2010;107(6):1429–1434.
63. Gopi KS, Reddy AG, Jyothi K, et al. *Toxicol Int*. 2010;17(2):64–66.
64. Hau DK, Wong RS, Cheng GY, et al. *Forsch Komplementmed*. 2010;17(4):209–213.
65. Choppin J, Desplaces A. *Arzneimittelforschung*. 1978;28(1):636–641.
66. Floersheim G, Eberhard M, Tschumi P, et al. *Toxicol Appl Pharmacol*. 1978;46:455–462.
67. Kroncke K, Fricker G, Meier P, et al. *J Biol Chem*. 1986;261(27):12562–12567.
68. Tuchweber B, Sieck R, Trost W. *Toxicol Appl Pharmacol*. 1979;51(2):265–275.
69. Pietrangelo A, Borella F, Casalgrandi G, et al. *Gastroenterol Clin Biol*. 1995;109(6):1941–1949.
70. Najafzadeh H, Jalali MR, Morovvati H, et al. *J Med Toxicol*. 2010;6(1):22–26.
71. Serviddio G, Bellanti F, Giudetti AM, et al. *J Pharmacol Exp Ther*. 2010;332(3):922–932.
72. Yao J, Zhi M, Minhu C. *Braz J Med Biol Res*. 2011
73. Neumann UP, Biermer M, Eurich D, et al. *J Hepatol*. 2010;52(6):951–952.
74. Beinhardt S, Rasoul-Rockenschaub S, Scherzer TM, et al. *J Hepatol*. 2011;54(3):591–592.
75. Martines G, Piva M, Copponi V, et al. *Arch Sci Med (Torino)*. 1979;136(3):443–454.
76. Edwards J, Grange LL, Wang M, et al. *Phytother Res*. 2000;14(7):517–521.
77. Moreland N, La Grange L, Montoya R. *BMC Complement Altern Med*. 2002;2:10.
78. Neese S, La Grange L, Trujillo E, et al. *BMC Complement Altern Med*. 2004;4:4.
79. Magliulo E, Scevola D, Carosi G. *Arzneimittelforschung*. 1979;29(7):1024–1028.
80. Shukla B, Visen P, Patnaik G, et al. *Planta Med*. 1991;57(1):29–33.
81. Krecman V, Skottova N, Walterova D, et al. *Planta Med*. 1998;64:138–142.
82. Sobolová L, Skottová N, Vecera R, et al. *Pharmacol Res*. 2006;53(2):104–112.

83. Skottová N, Vecera R, Urbánek K, et al. *Pharmacol Res.* 2003;47(1):17–26.

84. Crocenzi FA, Sanchez Pozzi EJ, Pellegrino JM, et al. *Hepatology.* 2001;34(2):329–339.

85. Crocenzi FA, Pellegrino JM, Sánchez Pozzi EJ, et al. *Biochem Pharmacol.* 2000;59(8):1015–1022.

86. Nassuato G, Iemmolo R, Strazzabosco M, et al. *J Hepatol.* 1991;12(3):290–295.

87. Alarcon De La Lastra A, Martin M, Motilva V, et al. *Planta Med.* 1995;61(2):116–119.

88. Ramasamy K, Agarwal R. *Cancer Lett.* 2008;269(2):352–362.

89. Cheung CW, Gibbons N, Johnson DW, et al. *Anticancer Agents Med Chem.* 2010;10(3):186–195.

90. Deep G, Agarwal R. *Integr Cancer Ther.* 2007;6(2):130–145.

91. Angeli JP, Barcelos GR, Serpeloni JM, et al. *Mutagenesis.* 2010;25(3):223–229.

92. Mallikarjuna G, Dhanalakshmi S, Singh RP, et al. *Cancer Res.* 2004;64(17):6349–6356.

93. Katiyar S, Korman N, Mukhtar H, et al. *J Natl Cancer Inst.* 1997;89(8):556–566.

94. Zi X, Mukhtar H, Agarwal R. *Biochem Biophys Res Commun.* 1997;239(1):334–339.

95. Agarwal C, Singh RP, Dhanalakshmi S, et al. *Oncogene.* 2003;22(51):8271–8282.

96. Chatterjee M, Agarwal R, Mukhtar H. *Biochem Biophys Res Commun.* 1996;229(2):590–595.

97. Kim D, Jin Y, Park J, et al. *Biol Pharm Bull.* 1994;17(3):443–445.

98. Volate SR, Davenport DM, Muga SJ, et al. *Carcinogenesis.* 2005;26(8):1450–1456.

99. Kohno H, Tanaka T, Kawabata K, et al. *Int J Cancer.* 2002;101(5):461–468.

100. Hoh C, Boocock D, Marczylo T, et al. *Clin Cancer Res.* 2006;12(9):2944–2950.

101. Zeng J, Sun Y, Wu K, et al. *Mol Cancer Ther.* 2011;10(1):104–116.

102. Kohno H, Suzuki R, Sugie S, et al. *Clin Cancer Res.* 2005;11(13):4962–4967.

103. Singh RP, Agarwal R. *Eur J Cancer.* 2005;41(13):1969–1979.

104. Singh RP, Tyagi AK, Zhao J, et al. *Carcinogenesis.* 2002;23(3):499–510.

105. Singh RP, Dhanalakshmi S, Mohan S, et al. *Mol Cancer Ther.* 2006;5(5):1145–1153.

106. Deep G, Singh RP, Agarwal C, et al. *Oncogene.* 2006;25(7):1053–1069.

107. Thelen P, Jarry H, Ringert RH, et al. *Planta Med.* 2004;70(5):397–400.

108. Thelen P, Wuttke W, Jarry H, et al. *J Urol.* 2004;171(5):1934–1938.

109. Zi X, Zhang J, Agarwal R, et al. *Cancer Res.* 2000;60(20):5617–5620.

110. Davis-Searles PR, Nakanishi Y, Kim NC, et al. *Cancer Res.* 2005;65(10):4448–4457.

111. Singh RP, Dhanalakshmi S, Tyagi AK, et al. *Cancer Res.* 2002;62(11):3063–3069.

112. Singh RP, Sharma G, Dhanalakshmi S, et al. *Cancer Epidemiol Biomarkers Prev.* 2003;12(9):933–939.

113. Singh RP, Deep G, Blouin MJ, et al. *Carcinogenesis.* 2007;28(12):2567–2574.

114. Raina K, Blouin MJ, Singh RP, et al. *Cancer Res.* 2007;67(22):11083–11091.

115. Pliskova M, Vondracek J, Kren V, et al. *Toxicology.* 2005;215(1–2):80–89.

116. Tyagi AK, Agarwal C, Singh RP, et al. *Biochem Biophys Res Commun.* 2003;312(4):1178–1184.

117. Tyagi A, Singh RP, Agarwal C, et al. *Carcinogenesis.* 2006;27(11):2269–2280.

118. Tyagi A, Agarwal C, Harrison G, et al. *Carcinogenesis.* 2004;25(9):1711–1720.

119. Tyagi A, Raina K, Singh RP, et al. *Mol Cancer Ther.* 2007;6(12 Pt 1):3248–3255.

120. Singh RP, Tyagi A, Sharma G, et al. *Clin Cancer Res.* 2008;14(1):300–308.

121. Cheung CW, Taylor PJ, Kirkpatrick CM, et al. *BJU Int.* 2007;100(2):438–444.

122. Huang Q, Wu LJ, Tashiro S, et al. *J Asian Nat Prod Res.* 2005;7(5):701–709.

123. Bhatia N, Zhao J, Wolf DM, et al. *Cancer Lett.* 1999;147(1–2):77–84.

124. Provinciali M, Papalini F, Orlando F, et al. *Cancer Res.* 2007;67(5):2022–2029.

125. Verschoyle RD, Brown K, Steward WP, et al. *Cancer Chemother Pharmacol.* 2008;62(2):369–372.

126. Gallo D, Giacomelli S, Ferlini C, et al. *Eur J Cancer.* 2003;39(16):2403–2410.

127. Malewicz B, Wang Z, Jiang C, et al. *Carcinogenesis.* 2006;27(9):1739–1747.

128. Hogan FS, Krishnegowda NK, Mikhailova M, et al. *J Surg Res.* 2007;143(1):58–65.

129. Gaedeke J, Fels LM, Bokemeyer C, et al. *Nephrol Dial Transplant.* 1996;11(1):55–62.

130. Karimi G, Ramezani M, Tahoonian Z. *Evid Based Complement Altern Med.* 2005;2(3):383–386.

131. Chlopcikova S, Psotova J, Miketova P, et al. *Phytother Res.* 2004;18(2):107–110.

132. Kropacova K, Misurova E, Hakova H. *Radiats Biol Radioecol.* 1998;38(3):411–415.

133. Giacomelli S, Gallo D, Apollonio P, et al. *Life Sci.* 2002;70(12):1447–1459.

134. Scambia G, De Vincenzo R, Ranelletti F, et al. *Eur J Cancer.* 1996;32A(5):877–882.

135. Lee SO, Jeong YJ, Im HG, et al. *Biochem Biophys Res Commun.* 2007;354(1):165–171.

136. Tyagi AK, Agarwal C, Chan DC, et al. *Oncol Rep.* 2004;11(2):493–499.

137. Worner P. *Thromb Haemost.* 1981;46(3):584–589.

138. Fiebrich F, Koch H. *Experientia.* 1979;35(12):1548–1560.

139. Manna SK, Mukhopadhyay A, Van NT, et al. *J Immunol.* 1999;163(12):6800–6809.

140. Morishima C, Shuhart MC, Wang CC, et al. *Gastroenterology.* 2010;138(2):671–681.

141. Wang MJ, Lin WW, Chen HL, et al. *Eur J Neurosci.* 2002;16(11):2103–2112.

142. Del La Puerta R, Martinez E, Bravo L, et al. *J Pharm Pharmacol.* 1996;48(9):968–970.

143. Johnson VJ, He Q, Osuchowski MF, et al. *Planta Med.* 2003;69(1):44–49.

144. Johnson VJ, Osuchowski MF, He Q, et al. *Planta Med.* 2002;68(11):961–965.

145. Zhan T, Digel M, Kuch EM, et al. *J Cell Biochem.* 2011;112(3):849–859.

146. Guigas B, Naboulsi R, Villanueva GR, et al. *Cell Physiol Biochem.* 2007;20(6):925–934.

147. Matsuda T, Ferreri K, Todorov I, et al. *Endocrinology.* 2005;146(1):175–185.

148. Detaille D, Sanchez C, Sanz N, et al. *Life Sci.* 2008;82(21–22):1070–1076.

149. Vengerovskii AI, Khazanov VA, Eskina KA, et al. *Bull Exp Biol Med.* 2007;144(1):53–56.

150. Soto C, Recoba R, Barron H, et al. *Comp Biochem Physiol C Toxicol Pharmacol.* 2003;136(3):205–212.

151. Soto C, Mena R, Luna J, et al. *Life Sci.* 2004;75(18):2167–2180.

152. Soto C, Perez J, Garcia V, et al. *Phytomedicine.* 2010;17(14):1090–1094.

153. Gorio A, Donadoni M, Finco C, et al. *Eur J Pharmacol.* 1996;311(1):21–28.

154. Gorio A, Donadoni M, Finco C, et al. *Adv Exp Med Biol.* 1997;419:289–295.

155. Donadoni M, Gavezzotti R, Borella F, et al. *J Pharmacol Exp Ther.* 1995;274(1):570–576.

156. Wu CH, Huang SM, Yen GC. *Antioxid Redox Signal.* 2011;14(3):353–366.

157. Srivastava RK, Sharma S, Verma S, et al. *Meth Find Exp Clin Pharmacol.* 2008;30(10):731–737.

158. Koch H, Bachner J, Loffler E. *Meth Find Exp Clin Pharmacol.* 1985;7(8):409–413.

159. Racz K, Feher J, Csomos G, et al. *J Endocrinol.* 1990;124(2):341–345.

160. Kalmar L, Kadar J, Somogyi A, et al. *Agents Actions.* 1990;29(3–4):239–246.

161. Miadonna A, Tedeschi A, Leggieri E, et al. *Br J Clin Pharmacol.* 1987;24(6):747–752.

162. Lee DG, Kim HK, Park Y, et al. *Arch Pharm Res.* 2003;26(8):597–600.

163. Starvaggi Cucuzza L, Motta M, Miretti S, et al. *J Anim Physiol Anim Nutr (Berl).* 2010;94(1):111–117.

164. El-Shitany NA, Hegazy S, El-Desoky K. *Phytomedicine.* 2010;17(2):116–125.

165. Murata N, Murakami K, Ozawa Y, et al. *Biosci Biotechnol Biochem.* 2010;74(11):2299–2306.

166. Tsai MJ, Liao JF, Lin DY, et al. *Neurochem Int.* 2010;57(8):867–875.

167. Homsi E, De Brito SM, Janino P. *Ren Fail.* 2010;32(5):623–632.

168. Schulz H, Schurer M, Krumbiegel G, et al. *Arzneimittelforschung.* 1995;45(1):61–64.

169. Kim YC, Kim EJ, Lee ED, et al. *Int J Clin Pharmacol Ther.* 2003;41(12):593–596.

170. Voinovich D, Perissutti B, Grassi M, et al. *J Pharm Sci.* 2009;98(11):4119–4129.

171. Mennicke W. *Dtsch Apoth Ztg.* 1975;115(33):1205–1206.

172. Wen Z, Dumas TE, Schrieber SJ, et al. *Drug Metab Dispos.* 2008;36(1):65–72.

173. Schrieber SJ, Wen Z, Vourvahis M, et al. *Drug Metab Dispos.* 2008;36(9):1909–1916.

174. Wu JW, Lin LC, Tsai TH. *J Ethnopharmacol.* 2009;121(2):185–193.

175. Lorenz D, Lucker P, Mennicke W, et al. *Meth Find Exp Clin Pharmacol.* 1984;6(10):655–661.

176. Lorenz D, Mennicke W, Behrendt W. *Planta Med.* 1982;45(4):216–223.

177. Lorenz D, Mennicke W. *Meth Find Exp Clin Pharmacol.* 1981;3(suppl 1):S103–S106.

178. Wu JW, Lin LC, Hung SC, et al. *Drug Metab Dispos.* 2008;36(3):589–596.

179. Morazzoni P, Montalbetti A, Malandrino S, et al. *Eur J Drug Metab Pharmacokinet.* 1993;18(3):289–297.

180. Barzaghi N, Crema F, Gatti G, et al. *Eur J Drug Metab Pharmacokinet.* 1990;15(4):333–338.

181. Hawke RL, Schrieber SJ, Soule TA, et al. *J Clin Pharmacol.* 2010;50(4):434–449.

182. Gatti G, Perucca E. *Int J Clin Pharmacol Ther.* 1994;32(11):614–617.

183. Schandalik R, Perucca E. *Drugs Exp Clin Res.* 1994;20(1):37–42.

184. Li W, Gao J, Zhao HZ, et al. *Eur J Drug Metab Pharmacokinet.* 2006;31(4):265–270.

185. Flaig TW, Glode M, Gustafson D, et al. *Prostate.* 2010;70(8):848–855.

186. Saller R, Brignoli R, Melzer J, et al. *Forsch Komplementmed.* 2008;15(1):9–20.

187. Rambaldi A, Jacobs BP, Gluud C. *Cochrane Database Syst Rev.* 2007(4):CD003620.

188. Rambaldi A, Jacobs BP, Iaquinto G, et al. *Cochrane Database Syst Rev.* 2005(2):CD003620.

189. Jacobs BP, Dennehy C, Ramirez G, et al. *Am J Med.* 2002;113(6):506–515.

190. Fintelmann V. *Med Klin.* 1973;68(24):809–815.

191. Poser G. *Arzneimittelforschung.* 1971;21(8):1209–1212.

192. Szilard S, Szentgyorgyi D, Demeter I. *Acta Med Hung.* 1988;45(2):249–256.

193. Palasciano G, Portincasa P, Palmier V, et al. *Curr Ther Res Clin Exp.* 1994;55(5):537–545.

194. Salmi H, Sarna S. *Scand J Gastroenterol.* 1982;17(4):517–521.

195. Bunout D, Hirsch S, Petermann M, et al. *Rev Med Chil.* 1992;120(12):1370–1375.

196. Muzes G, Deak G, Lang I, et al. *Orv Hetil.* 1990;131(16):863–866.

197. Trinchet J, Coste T, Levy V, et al. *Gastroenterol Clin Biol.* 1989;13(2):120–124.

198. Held C. *Therapiewoche.* 1993;43(39):2002–2006.

199. Feher J, Vereckei A. *Z Gastroenterol.* 1991;29:67.

200. Ferenci P, Dragosics B, Dittrich H, et al. *J Hepatol.* 1989;9(1):105–113.

201. Pares A, Planas R, Torres M, et al. *J Hepatol.* 1998;28(4):615–621.

202. Benda L, Dittrich H, Ferenzi P, et al. *Wien Klin Wochenschr.* 1980;92(19):678–683.

203. Feher J, Deak G, Muzes G, et al. *Orv Hetil.* 1989;130(51):2723–2727.

204. Lirussi F, Nassuato G, Orlando R, et al. *Med Sci Res.* 1995;23(1):31–33.

205. Bettini R, Gorini M. *Clin Ter.* 2002;153(5):305–307.

206. Velussi M, Cernigoi A, De Monte A, et al. *J Hepatol.* 1997;26(4):871–879.

207. Lang I, Nekam K, Deak G, et al. *Ital J Gastroenterol.* 1990;22(5):283–287.

208. Schuppan D, Strösser W, Burkard G, et al. *Z Allgemeinmed.* 1998;74:577–584.

209. Lucena MI, Andrade RJ, De La Cruz JP, et al. *Int J Clin Pharmacol Ther.* 2002;40(1):2–8.

210. Brodanova M, Filip J. *Prak Arzt.* 1976;30(346):354–367.

211. Ravanelli D, Haase W. *Prak Arzt.* 1976;30(355):1592–1612.

212. Kiesewetter E, Leodolter I, Thaler H. *Leber Magen Darm.* 1977;7(5):318–323.

213. Tanasescu C, Petrea S, Baldescu R, et al. *Med Interne.* 1988;26(4):311–322.

214. Magliulo E, Gagliardi B, Fiori G. *Med Klin.* 1978;73(28–29):1060–1065.

215. Plomteux G, Albert A, Heusghem C. *IRCS Med Sci.* 1977;5:259.

216. Bode J, Schmidt U, Durr H. *Med Klin.* 1977;72(12):513–518.

217. Marcelli R, Bizzoni P, Conte D, et al. *Eur Bull Drug Res.* 1992;1(3):131–135.

218. Buzzelli G, Moscarella S, Giusti A, et al. *Int J Clin Pharmacol Ther Toxicol.* 1993;31(9):456–460.

219. El-Kamary SS, Shardell MD, Abdel-Hamid M, et al. *Phytomedicine.* 2009;16(5):391–400.

220. Par A, Roth E, Miseta A, et al. *Orv Hetil.* 2009;150(2):73–79.

221. Tel'nykh Iu V, Maevskaia MV, Glushenkov DV. *Klin Med (Mosk).* 2008;86(11):60–62.

222. Tanamly MD, Tadros F, Labeeb S, et al. *Dig Liver Dis.* 2004;36(11):752–759.

223. Strickland GT, Tanamly MD, Tadros F, et al. *Dig Liver Dis.* 2005;37(7):542–543.

224. Ferenci P, Scherzer TM, Kerschner H, et al. *Gastroenterology.* 2008;135(5):1561–1567.

225. Torres M, Rodriguez-Serrano F, Rosario DJ, et al. *P R Health Sci J.* 2004;23 (suppl 2):69–74.

226. El-Zayadi AR, Attia M, Badran HM, et al. *Liver Int.* 2005;25(4):746–751.

227. Freedman ND, Curto TM, Morishima C, et al. *Aliment Pharmacol Ther.* 2011;33(1):127–137.

228. Seeff LB, Curto TM, Szabo G, et al. *Hepatology.* 2008;47(2):605–612.

229. Bares JM, Berger J, Nelson JE, et al. *J Clin Gastroenterol.* 2008;42(8):937–944.

230. Federico A, Trappoliere M, Tuccillo C, et al. *Gut.* 2006;55(6):901–902.

231. Loguercio C, Federico A, Trappoliere M, et al. *Dig Dis Sci.* 2007;52(9):2387–2395.

232. Floersheim G, Weber O, Tschumi P, et al. *Schweiz Med Wochenschr.* 1982;112(34):1164–1177.

233. Serne EH, Toorians A, Gietema JA, et al. *Neth J Med.* 1996;49:19–23.

234. Mikos B, Biro E. *Orv Hetil.* 1993;134(17):907–910.

235. Hofer JF, Egermann G, Mach K, et al. *Wien Klin Wochenschr.* 1983;95(7):240–243.

236. Carducci R, Armellino MF, Volpe C, et al. *Minerva Anestesiol.* 1996;62(5):187–193.

237. Hruby K, Fuhrmann N, Csomos G, et al. *Wien Klin Wochenschr.* 1983;95(7):225–231.

238. Gasparovic V, Puljevic D, Radonic R, et al. *Lijec Vjesn.* 1991;113(1–2):16–20.

239. Hruby K, Csomós G. *1st IGSC.* Amsterdam: 1989.

240. Boari C, Montanari FM, Galletti GP, et al. *Minerva Med.* 1981;72(40):2679–2688.

241. Saba P, Galeone F, Salvadorini F, et al. *Gazz Med Ital.* 1976;135:236–251.

242. Zhang J, Mao X, Zhou Y. *Chung Kuo Chung Hsi I Chieh Ho Tsa Chih.* 1993;13(12):725–726.

243. Huseini HF, Larijani B, Heshmat R, et al. *Phytother Res.* 2006;20(12):1036–1039.

244. Hussain SA. *J Med Food.* 2007;10(3):543–547.

245. Lirussi F, Beccarello A, Zanette G, et al. *Diabetes Nutr Metab.* 2002;15(4):222–231.

246. Velussi M, Cernigoi AM, Viezzoli L, et al. *Curr Ther Res Clin Exp.* 1993;53(5):533–545.

247. Hutchinson C, Bomford A, Geissler CA. *Eur J Clin Nutr.* 2010;64(10):1239–1241.

248. Gharagozloo M, Moayedi B, Zakerinia M, et al. *Fundam Clin Pharmacol.* 2009;23(3):359–365.

249. Hussain SA, Jassim NA, Numan IT, et al. *Saudi Med J.* 2009;30(1):98–103.

250. Somogyi A, Ecsedi G, Blazovics A, et al. *Acta Med Hung.* 1989;46(4):289–295.

251. Roozbeh J, Shahriyari B, Akmali M, et al. *Ren Fail.* 2011;33(2):118–123.

252. Nazemian F, Karimi G, Moatamedi M, et al. *Phytother Res.* 2010;24(11):1654–1657.

253. Moosavifar N, Mohammadpour AH, Jallali M, et al. *East Mediterr Health J.* 2010;16(6):642–645.

254. Grossmann M, Hoermann R, Weiss M, et al. *Am J Gastroenterol.* 1995;90(9):1500–1503.

255. Wang WH, Zhou RY, Yan ZP. *Zhongguo Zhong Xi Yi Jie He Za Zhi.* 2008;28(7):583–587.

256. Vidlar A, Vostalova J, Ulrichova J, et al. *Biomed Pap Med Fac Univ Palacky Olomouc Czech Repub.* 2010;154(3):239–244.

257. Berardesca E, Cameli N, Cavallotti C, et al. *J Cosmet Dermatol.* 2008;7(1):8–14.

258. Reyes H. *Gastroenterol Clin North Am.* 1992;21(4):905–921.

259. Reyes H, Simon F. *Semin Liver Dis.* 1993;13(3):289–301.

260. Di Pierro F, Callegari A, Carotenuto D, et al. *Acta Biomed.* 2008;79(3):205–210.

261. Flaig TW, Gustafson DL, Su LJ, et al. *Invest New Drugs.* 2007;25(2):139–146.

262. Hahn G, Lehmann HD, Kurten M, et al. *Arzneimittelforschung.* 1968;18:698–704.

263. Toxicology and carcinogenesis studies of milk thistle extract (CAS No. 84604-20-6) in F344/N rats and B6C3F1 mice (Feed Studies). *Natl Toxicol Program Tech Rep Ser.* 2011;(565):1–177.

264. Duthie S, Johnson W, Dobson V. *Mutat Res.* 1997;390(1–2):141–151.

265. Budzinski JW, Trudeau VL, Drouin CE, et al. *Can J Physiol Pharmacol.* 2007;85(9):966–978.

266. Doehmer J, Weiss G, McGregor GP, et al. *Toxicol In Vitro.* 2011;25(1):21–27.

267. Raucy JL. *Drug Metab Dispos.* 2003;31(5):533–539.

268. Kosina P, Maurel P, Ulrichova J, et al. *J Biochem Mol Toxicol.* 2005;19(3):149–153.

269. Gurley BJ, Gardner SF, Hubbard MA, et al. *Clin Pharmacol Ther.* 2004;76(5):428–440.

270. Mills E, Wilson K, Clarke M, et al. *Eur J Clin Pharmacol.* 2005;61(1):1–7.

271. Van Erp NP, Baker SD, Zhao M, et al. *Clin Cancer Res.* 2005;11(21):7800–7806.

272. Fuhr U, Beckmann-Knopp S, Jetter A, et al. *Planta Med.* 2007;73(14):1429–1435.

273. Gurley BJ, Swain A, Hubbard MA, et al. *Mol Nutr Food Res.* 2008;52(7):755–763.

274. Zuber R, Modriansky M, Dvorak Z, et al. *Phytother Res.* 2002;16(7):632–638.

275. Gurley B, Hubbard MA, Williams DK, et al. *J Clin Pharmacol.* 2006;46(2):201–213.

276. Han Y, Guo D, Chen Y, et al. *Xenobiotica.* 2009;39(9):694–699.

277. Upadhyay G, Kumar A, Singh MP. *Eur J Pharmacol.* 2007;565(1–3):190–201.

278. Zhou L, Liu P, Chen B, Wang Y, et al. *Anticancer Res.* 2008;28(2A):1119–1127.

279. Colombo V, Lupi M, Falcetta F, et al. *Cancer Chemother Pharmacol.* 2011;67(2):369–379.

280. Patel N, Joseph C, Corcoran GB, et al. *Toxicol Appl Pharmacol.* 2010;245(2):143–152.

281. Invernizzi R, Bernuzzi S, Ciani D, et al. *Haematologica.* 1993;78(5):340–341.

282. Ladas EJ, Kroll DJ, Oberlies NH, et al. *Cancer.* 2010;116(2):506–513.

283. Rao BN, Srinivas M, Kumar YS, et al. *Drug Metabol Drug Interact.* 2007;22(2–3):175–185.

284. Allain H, Schuck S, Lebreton S, et al. *Dement Geriatr Cogn Disord.* 1999;10(3):181–185.

285. Borsari M, Gabbi C, Ghelfi F, et al. *J Inorg Biochem.* 2001;85:123–129.

286. Schleufe P, Seidel C. *Anasthesiol Intensivmed Notfallmed Schmerzther.* 2003;38(11):716–718.

287. Hung J-H, Chu C-J, Sung P-L, et al. *J Chinese Med Assoc.* 2008;71(3):155–158.

288. Tedesco D, Tava A, Galletti S, et al. *J Dairy Sci.* 2004;87(7):2239–2247.

289. Albrecht M, Frerick H, Kuhn H, et al. *Z Klin Med.* 1992;47:87–92.

290. Grungreiff K, Albrecht M, Strenge-Hesse A. *Med Welt.* 1995;46:222–227.

291. Busby A, Ll Grange, Edwards J, et al. *J Herbal Pharmacother.* 2002;2(1):39–47.

292. ADRAC *Med J Aust.* 1999;170:218–219.

293. Geier J, Fuchs T, Wahl R. *Allergolog.* 1990;13(10):387–388.

294. Mironets VI, Krasovskaia EA, Polishchuk II. *Vrach Delo.* 1990;7:86–87.

295. Mingrino F, Tosti U, Anania S, et al. *Minerva Pediatr.* 1979;31(6):451–456.

Thyme

(*Thymus vulgaris* L.)

Synonyms

Common or garden thyme (Engl), Thymi herba, Folia thymi (Lat), Gartenthymian, Thymianblätter (Ger), thym (Fr), timo (Ital), almindelig timian (Dan).

What is it?

The leaf and flowers of thyme have been used extensively in cooking, particularly in meat dishes and as a flavouring ingredient in teas and liqueurs. The dried flowers have been employed in the same way as lavender, to preserve linen from insects. Thyme oil is used in perfumery, cosmetics, aromatherapy and, more recently, in pest control as a preservative for agricultural commodities such as grains. Thyme extract in combination with other herbs is available in a number of commercial products to treat cough and/or acute bronchitis. Thymol, one of the major constituents of thyme, is commonly used in commercial antiseptic mouth washes.

The thyme monographs in the *British Pharmacopoeia* and the *European Pharmacopoeia* allow the use of whole leaf and flowers of *Thymus zygis* (Spanish thyme) as well as *Thymus vulgaris*.[1]

Effects

Spasmolytic, antiseptic and expectorant for respiratory conditions; antimicrobial and antiviral in topical application for conditions of the skin and mucous membranes.

Traditional view

Traditionally thyme has been considered a major antispasmodic cough remedy, particularly when administered as a cough syrup. Infusion of thyme, sweetened with honey or sugar, would be prescribed for whooping cough, sore throats and catarrh. Thyme tea was used as a carminative for colic, to treat dyspepsia and to control fever in common colds. Thyme oil was used as a rubefacient and counter-irritant in rheumatism and neuralgic pain.[2,3] Eclectic physicians also considered thyme to be an emmenagogue and tonic, and prescribed the tea for hysteria, dysmenorrhoea and convalescence after exhausting illness.[3] Thyme was also used for diarrhoea and enuresis in children and as a gargle for tonsillitis.[4]

Summary actions

Expectorant, spasmolytic, antibacterial, antifungal, antioxidant, anti-inflammatory; rubefacient, antimicrobial, antiviral and antiparasitic in external preparations.

Can be used for

Indications supported by clinical trials

Indications supported by trials using thyme: productive cough, and in combination for acute bronchitis (better evidence for combinations).

Traditional therapeutic uses

Bronchitis, whooping cough, asthma and catarrh or inflammation of the upper respiratory tract; gastrointestinal disorders including dyspepsia, colic, flatulence and diarrhoea, especially in children; as an adjunct in convalescence; topically for tonsillitis and inflammation of the mouth.

May also be used for

Extrapolations from pharmacological studies

Spasmodic conditions of the gastrointestinal tract; adjunct in the treatment of peptic ulcer; topically for fungal and bacterial skin disorders and as a mouthwash to reduce oral bacteria. Thyme may also be useful in the topical treatment of herpes simplex virus type 2.[5]

Other applications

As a flavouring in teas and cough preparations, especially for children;[6,7] steeped in boiling water for inhalation.[8] Thyme oil can be used in toothpastes, soaps, detergents, creams, lotions and perfumes[6] and as an antiseptic agent in lotions, ointments, mouthwashes and ear drops.[9] It can also be used as a component in chest rubs[8] and for healing preparations for oily or damaged skin; for hair and scalp treatments including for preventative hair loss; in bath preparations[9] and in massage oils to ease muscle pain and arthritis.[10,11] The essential oil was effective against head lice in clinical trials.[12] Thyme is one of five plant extracts in a proprietary haemostatic and antibacterial formula.[13]

Preparations

As with all essential oil-containing herbs, use of the fresh plant or carefully dried herb is advised. Keep covered if infusing the herb to retain the essential oil.

Liquid extract, tincture or essential oil for internal use. Infusion, essential oil or extract for topical use.

Typical dosage forms and dosage

Typical adult dosage ranges are:

- 3 to12 g/day of dried aerial parts or by infusion
- 2 to 6 mL/day of a 1:2 liquid extract or equivalent in tablet or capsule form
- 6 to 18 mL/day of a 1:5 tincture.

Topical use: 5% infusion as a gargle or mouthwash.

Duration of use

No problems known with long-term use.

Summary assessment of safety

Allergic reactions are possible, especially from topical use. No major adverse effects are expected from ingestion of thyme.

Technical data

Botany

Thymus vulgaris is a member of the Lamiaceae (Labiatae or mint) family, native to the western Mediterranean and southern Italy, but widely cultivated.[14] It is an evergreen sub-shrub growing up to 25 cm, with a branched stem. The sessile leaves vary from elliptic to linear or diamond-shaped. The small pink to lilac flowers appear in whorls in the upper leaf axils and have a tube-like calyx and tubular corolla with a three lobed lower lip. The fruit consists of a smooth, dark-coloured nutlet and the roots are robust. The whole plant has an aromatic fragrance.[15]

Key constituents

- Essential oil (1% to 2.5%) containing antimicrobial and antioxidant[16,17] phenols, predominantly thymol and/or carvacrol[18] (up to 51% and 4%, respectively, of the essential oil,[19] but varying considerably with the many chemotypes of thyme), and their corresponding monoterpene hydrocarbon precursors (p-cymene and gamma-terpinene), together with thymol methyl ether (1.5% to 2.5%)
- Strongly antioxidant carnosol, rosmanols, galdosol and carnosic acid[20]
- Flavonoids; acetophenone glycosides;[21] salicylates;[22] and a polysaccharide[23] with anti-complementary properties.[24]

Spanish thyme has similar essential oil content and composition to common thyme but contains a higher amount of carvacrol and less thymol methyl ether (0.3%).[25]

Thymol   **Carvacrol**

Adulteration

Adulteration occurs rarely with Moroccan thyme such as *Thymus satureioides* and wild thyme (*T. serpyllium*).[26,27] There are several chemotypes of *T. vulgaris* which do not have high levels of phenols and should be regarded as inferior substitutes. The thyme monograph in the British and European pharmacopoeias requires the essential oil to contain at least 40% thymol and carvacrol combined.[1]

There is innate protection in the herb against aflatoxin contamination,[28] and potentially preservative properties against other fungi[29] and some bacterial strains,[30] especially anaerobes such as *Escherichia coli*,[31] *Campylobacter jejuni*, *Salmonella enteritidis*, *Staphylococcus aureus* and *Listeria*.[32]

Pharmacodynamics

Spasmolytic activity

Extracts of dried thyme inhibited agents that stimulate smooth muscle and also demonstrated a spasmolytic effect on various isolated smooth muscle tissues. The relaxing effect of bradykinin was also potentiated.[33] The phenol (thymol and carvacrol) concentration of these and other thyme extracts used in such studies was found to be very low and could not have been responsible for the observed spasmolytic activity. However, thymol and carvacrol in sufficient doses have demonstrated tracheal relaxant activity.[34] Essential oil of thyme also relaxed tracheal smooth muscle and inhibited the phasic contractions of ileal longitudinal muscle in vitro. The relaxant effect was higher on tracheal muscle than on ileal.[35]

Thyme extracts and its flavonoids demonstrated spasmolytic activity on smooth muscle from ileum, trachea and vas deferens in vitro. Spasm caused by specific receptor agonists (acetylcholine, histamine, L-noradrenaline) as well as by non-specific agents was inhibited. The spasmolytic activity may be due to the inhibition of calcium ion flux by the flavonoids.[36] In a slightly earlier study, the spasmolytic activity of thymol and carvacrol on isolated ileum and trachea was found to be significantly less potent than the thyme flavonoids.[37] More recently, an in vitro study found that thyme extract, but not thymol, inhibited endothelin-induced contractions of isolated rat trachea.[38]

The antispasmodic activity of thyme extract was further investigated in vitro in isolated (organ bath) rat trachea and ileum using acetylcholine, barium chloride, potassium chloride and endothelin as triggers of muscle spasm. A comparison of the effect of a thyme extract with normal thymol content (>0.038%) with that of a thyme extract with a low content (<0.005%) revealed that it was not important for the overall antispasmodic effect. In confirmation of the above findings, thymol alone had no effect on endothelin-induced tracheal spasm, whereas thyme extract did.[39]

Other observations from in vitro experiments revealed that unidentified compounds in thyme slightly interact with beta-2 receptors in rat lung, trachea and uterus, but this mechanism cannot fully explain the spasmolytic activity of the extract.[40]

Expectorant activity

In an early in vitro study, thyme leaf tea exerted an inhibitory effect on the normal transport velocity of isolated ciliated oesophageal epithelium.[41] This suggested a decrease in expectorant activity, which contrasted with very early in vivo work by Gordonoff using thymol and thyme.[42] This in vitro study only assessed one mechanism of expectoration, and an aqueous extract (tea) was used rather than a liquid extract.[43]

Recent in vivo studies do support an expectorant activity for thyme. One such study demonstrated an improvement in expectoration and mucociliary clearance in the mouse trachea, although the mechanism of action was unclear.[40]

Another study examined mucociliary transport in mice, by comparing high-thymol and low-thymol thyme extracts or a saline control administered intragastrically. While both thyme extracts improved mucociliary transport compared with the control, only the extract with high thymol content produced an effect that was statistically significant. This suggests that thymol makes an important contribution to the mucociliary transport enhancing activity of thyme.[39]

Antibacterial activity

The in vitro antibacterial and antifungal activity of thymol is well recognised and no attempt has been made to review this subject comprehensively. Brief exposure to a low concentration of thymol rapidly killed cariogenic and periodontopathogenic bacteria.[44] Thymol has also demonstrated antibacterial activity against other oral bacteria (*Porphyromonas gingivalis*, *Selenomonas artemidis*, *Streptococcus sobrinus*). The principal mode of action appears to be membrane perforation, resulting in rapid efflux of intracellular constituents.[45] Thymol, carvacrol, cinnamaldehyde and eugenol showed inhibitory activity on seven oral bacteria. A synergistic effect was observed with certain combinations (such as eugenol and thymol, eugenol and carvacrol, and thymol and carvacrol).[46] As noted earlier, thymol and carvacrol are found together in oil of thyme. Components of thyme oil were effective against seven standard strains of Gram-positive and Gram-negative bacteria.[47] A broad spectrum of activity was observed for thymol and carvacrol against bacteria involved in upper respiratory tract infections. A synergistic effect for the combination of thymol and carvacrol was also observed.[48]

Essential oil of thyme has demonstrated antibacterial activity in vitro,[49] including against *Clostridium botulinum*, *Escherichia coli*, *Haemophilus influenzae*, *Klebsiella pneumoniae*, *Salmonella typhi*, *Sarcina spp.* and *Staphylococcus aureus et spp.*[50,51] Thyme oil and thymol decreased the growth of *Salmonella typhimurium*, especially under anaerobic conditions. The authors suggested that the phenolic compounds of thyme exert their antibacterial activity by complexing with the bacterial membrane proteins (leading possibly to membrane perforation).[52] Thyme essential oil (1%) in an alcohol-free pharmaceutical mouth-wash formulation was shown to be effective against *Streptococcus mutans*, which is implicated in plaque development.[53]

Aqueous and ethanolic extracts of thyme demonstrated significant inhibition of *Helicobacter pylori* in vitro.[54] One study reported that an extract of thyme substantially reduced the minimum inhibitory concentration (MIC) of tetracycline against methicillin-resistant *Staphylococcus aureus* (MRSA).[55] The investigators reported that the compound in the thyme extract with this activity was the flavonoid baicalein. This appears to be the only report of baicalein in thyme, and it does raise questions about the botanical identity of the extract.

Further to the above comments on the antibacterial mode of action of essential oil components, two studies from one research group demonstrated that thymol and carvacrol decreased unsaturated fatty acids in bacterial membranes during co-culture and caused structural alterations in the cell envelope.[56,57] A later study observed that thymol and carvacrol exerted an antimicrobial activity on *Escherichia coli* via their ability to permeabilise and depolarise the cytoplasmic membrane.[58]

Fungicidal activity

Thymol and carvacrol have demonstrated fungitoxic activity towards *Cryptococcus neoformans* in vitro.[59] They also exhibited strong antifungal activity towards fungal strains known to contaminate food, including *Penicillium spp.* From the range of substances tested, a free hydroxyl group in connection with an alkyl substituent (as in thymol) appeared to render the antifungal activity.[60]

Thyme oil (200 ppm) was a highly effective inhibitory agent against eight different species of dermatophytic fungi in vitro[61] and stopped mycelial growth of *Aspergillus parasiticus* at a concentration of 0.1%. Aflatoxin synthesis was also inhibited.[62] Thymol (250 ppm) was highly effective at inhibiting *Aspergillus flavus* growth and aflatoxin production in vitro.[63]

One study observed that thyme oil inhibited the growth of several pathogenic fungi, including *Rhizoctonia solani*, *Pythium ultimum* var. *ultimum*, *Fusarium solani* and *Colletotrichum lindemuthianum*. The fungicidal activity was attributable to thymol and might be due to degeneration of the fungal hyphae.[64] Thyme oil was fungitoxic to the spores of *Aspergillus flavus*, *A. niger* and *A. ochraceus* in stored grain.[65] Thyme completely inhibited aflatoxin production on lentil seeds during 8 weeks of incubation.[66]

The essential oils of three species of thyme (*Thymus vulgaris*, *T. zygis* subsp. *zygis* and *T. mastichina* subsp. *mastichina*) were evaluated for their antifungal activity.[67] The effect of the essential oils upon germ (filamentation) tube formation, an important virulence factor, was also studied. The mechanism of action was investigated by flow cytometry, after staining with propidium iodide. The essential oils of *T. vulgaris* and *T. zygis* showed similar antifungal activity, which was greater than *T. mastichina*. At the MIC concentrations of the essential oils, propidium iodide rapidly penetrated the majority of the yeast cells, indicating that the fungicidal effect resulted primarily from extensive lesions in the cell membrane. Concentrations below the MIC values significantly inhibited germ tube formation.

The envelope (plasma membrane plus certain cell wall components) of *Candida albicans* is critical to the virulence of the species in terms of adhesiveness and transition to the hyphal form. Thymol altered the morphogenesis of the envelope in vitro and thereby demonstrated an ability to inhibit *C. albicans* from colonisation and infectivity.[68] Thymol also interfered with the initial phases of *C. albicans* biofilm formation as well as inhibiting mature biofilms, both of which are important mechanisms of antifungal activity.[69] Treatment of the yeast *Saccharomyces cerevisiae* with thymol led to cell lysis as a result of the alteration of both the cell membrane and cell wall.[70]

Antiviral activity

An aqueous extract of thyme demonstrated in vitro inhibitory activity against herpes simplex virus (HSV) type 1, HSV type 2 and an acyclovir-resistant strain of the virus, but had no effect on intracellular virus replication.[71] These findings suggest that topical application of thyme extract might have a therapeutic effect on herpes infections. Thyme essential oil also demonstrated high level in vitro virucidal activity against acyclovir-resistant clinical isolates of HSV type 1.[72] This activity was confirmed in a later study for both thyme oil and thymol.[73]

Antioxidant activity

Rosmarinic acid has demonstrated antioxidant activity in vitro, including inhibition of lipid peroxidation, decreased production of the superoxide anion radical[74] and inhibition of the external oxidative effects of polymorphonuclear granulocytes.[75] A biphenyl compound and a flavonoid (eriodictyol) isolated from thyme demonstrated antioxidant activity in vitro by inhibiting superoxide anion production and lipid peroxidation. The biphenyl compound was extremely potent and also protected red blood cells against oxidative haemolysis.[76]

Thymol produced a dose-dependent inhibition of endothelial cell-mediated oxidation of low-density lipoprotein.[77] Thymol, carvacrol and p-cymene-2,3-diol isolated from thyme oil demonstrated antioxidant activity in vitro. p-Cymene-2,3-diol exhibited the strongest activity which was greater than alpha-tocopherol.[78] Another study found thymol and carvacrol exerted the following antioxidant effects in vitro: decreased peroxidation of phospholipid liposomes and scavenging of peroxyl radicals.[79] A methanol extract of thyme demonstrated strong hydroxyl radical-scavenging activity in vitro.[80]

The antioxidant effects of thymol were investigated in a chemiluminescence assay. Thymol was found to interfere with the production of reactive oxygen species, nitric oxide and nitric oxide-derived peroxynitrite released from human neutrophils after activation, suggesting that it is both a possible antioxidant and an anti-inflammatory agent.[81]

Thyme oil possesses an anti-radical activity that is greater than thymol or carvacrol in the 2,2-diphenyl-l-picrylhydrazyl assay. The oil also scavenged hydroxyl and superoxide radicals at low concentrations. Thyme essential oil (0.05%) also exerted antioxidant effects in a linoleic acid emulsion, where it caused a 59.5% inhibition of conjugated diene formation and 72.4% inhibition of the generation of secondary oxidised products from the linoleic acid.[82]

Antimutagenic activity

Luteolin, a flavonoid isolated from thyme, demonstrated antimutagenic activity in vitro against a dietary carcinogen formed during cooking.[83] An extract of thyme demonstrated antimutagenesis with modulating effects on DNA repair in *Escherichia coli*. The antimutagenic activity was a consequence of the stimulation of error-free repair (and not due to the suppression of error-prone repair).[84]

Antiallergic and anti-inflammatory activity

Rosmarinic acid inhibited immunohaemolysis of erythrocytes in vitro, which was due to inhibition of the classic complement pathway (C3-convertase). Oral administration of rosmarinic acid (1 to 100 mg/kg) inhibited passive cutaneous anaphylaxis in the rat.[85] In a study of phenolic compounds, thymol inhibited neutrophil chemotaxis in vitro. A positive correlation was observed between superoxide anion generation in neutrophils and inhibition of neutrophil chemotaxis by phenolic compounds. A free phenolic group is essential for both these anti-inflammatory activities.[86] Thyme oil also inhibited prostaglandin biosynthesis in vitro.[87]

Thyme inhibited an immediate allergic reaction via the inhibition of beta-hexosaminidase release from rat basophilic leukaemia cells in vitro.[88]

Elastase is a serine proteinase released by activated human neutrophils and is considered a marker of inflammatory disease. Thymol was found to inhibit elastase release from stimulated human neutrophils in vitro in a concentration-dependent manner.[89]

Neurological activity

After thymol, carvacrol is the major phenolic constituent of the essential oil of thyme. Carvacrol was screened for pharmacological effects on the central nervous system and found to have anxiolytic activity when administered orally to mice.[90] This study lead researchers to further investigate a possible antidepressant effect for carvacrol in mice. Antidepressant effects were observed in mice after carvacrol administration (12.5 to 50 mg/kg, oral), most likely due to an increase in dopamine levels.[91]

Thymol has an in vitro agonistic influence on the α-1, α-2 and beta-adrenergic receptors of smooth muscle strips from guinea pig stomach and portal vein and displayed spasmolytic activity at concentrations greater than 10^{-6} molar. It was assumed to be capable of an analgesic effect as a result of its activity on α-2 adrenergic receptors in nerve cells.[92]

The antinociceptive activity of an 80% methanolic extract (100 to 1000 mg/kg, ip) of thyme was studied in mice, for both acute pain in the hot plate and tail flick tests and chronic pain in the formalin test. Results showed that both thyme extract and the reference drug dexamethasone exerted analgesic activity at all tested concentrations in all three tests, compared with the control group (p<0.01). Further experiments, in which animals were pre-treated with the opioid antagonist naloxone, suggested that the antinociceptive effect of the thyme partially involved the opioid system.[93]

Other activity

Screening herbs for antithrombotic activity revealed thyme exerted an inhibitory effect on platelets both in vitro and in vivo.[94] A follow-up in vivo study has demonstrated thyme included at 5% in a high fat diet fed to mice for 12 weeks had a significant antithrombotic effect, most likely due to the inhibition of platelets and stimulation of endothelial cells. However, this was not accompanied by a prolongation of bleeding time.[95]

Dietary administration (720 mg, every second day) of essential oils (thyme, clove, nutmeg or pepper) to ageing mice had a marked effect on fatty acid distribution. The proportions of polyunsaturated fatty acids within phospholipids were almost restored to the levels observed in young mice. The saturated fatty acid to polyunsaturated fatty acid (PUFA) ratio decreased from 2.28 to 1.20 for the animals treated with thyme oil. Although antioxidant activity was demonstrated in vitro by the oils, it was not considered responsible for the favourable effect on the PUFA content of tissue.[96]

Thyme essential oil and its constituents carvacrol and thymol displayed inhibitory activity on acetylcholinesterase activity in vitro, with carvacrol being 10-fold more potent than thymol, but two orders of magnitude less potent than the plant alkaloid galantamine used in the treatment of Alzheimer's disease.[97]

The hepatoprotective activity of thymol was investigated against paracetamol- and carbon tetrachloride-induced hepatic damage in mice. Pre-treatment with oral thymol (150 mg/kg) reduced the mortality rate from 100% to 30% in mice receiving oral paracetamol at a dose of 1 g/kg. Thymol also protected against the rise in hepatic enzymes indicative of liver damage (alkaline phosphatase and transaminases) induced by a lower paracetamol dose (640 mg/kg) and oral carbon tetrachloride (1.5 mL/kg).[98]

Thyme oil (diluted 1:1 with olive oil) applied topically appeared to increase the formation of new tissue when studied in rats with burn wounds.[99]

Five monoterpenes from thyme oil (carvacrol, p-cymene, linalool, alpha-terpinene and thymol) used topically at concentrations of 0.05% were shown to have mosquito repellent properties in a human forearm bioassay, with alpha-terpinene and carvacrol being the most potent.[100]

The effects of thyme, and its phenolic compounds thymol and carvacrol, on the activities of xenobiotic-metabolising enzymes (phase I enzymes such as 7-ethoxycoumarin O-deethylase (ECOD) and phase II enzymes such as glutathione S-transferase (GST) and quinone reductase (QR)) were investigated.[101] Mice were fed a diet containing thyme (0.5% or 2%) or treated orally with thymol (50 to 200 mg/kg) or carvacrol (50 to 200 mg/kg) once a day for 7 successive days. Dietary administration of 2% thyme caused slightly but significantly higher ECOD, GST and QR activities by 1.1- to 1.4-fold. Thymol (200 mg/kg) resulted in significantly higher ECOD, GST and QR activities by 1.3- to 1.9-fold, and carvacrol (200 mg/kg) treatment caused significantly higher ECOD, GST and QR activities by 1.3- to 1.7-fold. These results imply that thyme contains bifunctional inducers (substances capable of inducing both phase I and phase II enzymes) and that thymol and carvacrol may account for such effects of thyme. However, the doses used were relatively high and this study might not therefore be clinically relevant.

Pharmacokinetics

A study of the metabolism of thymol and carvacrol in rats indicated that the urinary excretion of metabolites was rapid, with only small amounts excreted beyond 24 h. Although large amounts of both compounds were excreted unchanged (or as conjugates of glucuronide and sulphate), extensive oxidation of the methyl and isopropyl groups also occurred.[102] A study designed to assess the systemic availability and pharmacokinetics of thymol after oral administration was conducted in 12 healthy volunteers. Each person received a single tablet containing 1.08 mg thymol. Thymol was not detected in plasma or urine, but two metabolites were thymol sulphate in both plasma and urine and thymol glucuronide only in urine. The peak plasma concentration of thymol sulphate was 93.1±24.5 ng/mL and was reached after 2.0±0.8 h, with an elimination half-life of 10.2 h. Thymol sulphate was detected up to 41 h after administration. The amounts of thymol sulphate and thymol glucuronide excreted over 24 h corresponded to 16.2±4.5% of the initial dose of thymol.[103]

Clinical trials

Respiratory conditions

In a double blind, randomised study, 60 patients with acute respiratory infection and productive cough received either syrup of thyme or bromhexine for a period of 5 days. There was no significant difference between the two groups based on self-reported symptom relief and both groups made similar gains. A non-statistically significant improvement was observed in the recovery rate of non-smokers compared to smokers in both groups.[104] This study would have benefited from the inclusion of a placebo group.

An open trial investigated the efficacy and safety of a herbal cough syrup combining ivy leaf extract (main ingredient) with a decoction of thyme and aniseed and mucilage from marshmallow root. General practitioners in Switzerland recruited 62 patients between 16 and 89 years of age (mean 50 years) with an irritating cough caused by the common cold (n=29), bronchitis (n= 20) or respiratory tract disease with mucus production (n=15). The treatment was taken for an average of 12 days and the mean daily dose was 10 mL. Outcome measures were changes in symptom scores for both cough and expectoration of mucus, assessed by both the participants and their doctors. All patient scores showed an improvement compared with baseline. Both patients and doctors rated efficacy as good or very good in close to 90% of cases. Only one adverse event was reported, but this was not considered likely to have been caused by the herbal syrup.[105]

Thyme appears in combination with other herbs in several commercial preparations for the treatment of bronchitis. Two commercial combinations that have been clinically studied are discussed below.

One is a syrup containing fluid extracts of thyme (15% of a 1:2 to 2:5 extract) and ivy leaves (1.5% of a 1:1 extract). This preparation was studied in a double blind, placebo-controlled, multicentre trial involving patients suffering from acute bronchitis with a productive cough, at least 10 coughing fits per day and a Bronchitis Severity Score (BSS) of at least 5. Three hundred and sixty-one outpatients were randomly assigned to an 11-day treatment with either the thyme–ivy combination syrup (5.4 mL, three times daily) or a placebo syrup. Results demonstrated a mean reduction of coughing fits on days 7 to 9 relative to baseline of 68.7% for the thyme–ivy combination, compared with 47.6% for placebo (p<0.0001). A 50% reduction in coughing fits was achieved 2 days earlier in the thyme–ivy group than the placebo group. Symptoms of acute bronchitis (BSS) improved rapidly in both groups, but they declined more rapidly in the herbal group. Responder rates for the thyme–ivy group were higher than for placebo at day 4 and at the end of treatment (p<0.0001). The herbal treatment was well tolerated and no serious adverse events were reported.[106]

This formulation was also studied in 1234 children and adolescents in a post-marketing surveillance study. The preparation demonstrated good efficacy and tolerability in this uncontrolled design, with the average BSS value decreasing from 8.8 points to 4.8 after 4 days, and to 1.3 points after 10 days of treatment. [107]

A fixed combination of dry extracts of thyme and cowslip (*Primula veris*) root in tablet form (200 mg thyme extract and 60 mg cowslip extract per tablet) was evaluated in a placebo-controlled study involving 361 outpatients with acute bronchitis and productive cough. The BSS and frequency of coughing fits were used to assess efficacy. This preparation was also found to be beneficial and well-tolerated against placebo over an 11-day treatment period.[108]

Another commercial preparation that has been clinically evaluated is a combination of a fluid extract of thyme and a cowslip root tincture. The clinical efficacy and tolerability of this preparation was investigated in a double blind, randomised, placebo-controlled, multicentre study. One hundred and fifty patients (97 women and 53 men) diagnosed with untreated bronchitis for less than 48 h were randomised and treated with either the combination (5 mL/day) or placebo over 7 to 9 days. In the treatment group the BSS decreased from 12.0±4.4 points at baseline to 1.0±2.1 at study end compared with 11.7±4.3 points at baseline to 6.5±4.8 at study end in the placebo group. Significantly more patients were symptom-free at the end of the study in the treatment group (58.7%) compared with the placebo group (5.3%). Results also demonstrated the therapeutic effect was more significant in the patients with a higher BSS at baseline. Tolerability was rated as good or very good by more than 90% of participants in both groups and no serious adverse events were observed.[109]

Alopecia areata

Thyme essential oil in combination with rosemary, cedar wood and lavender essential oils was studied in a randomised, double blind trial involving 86 patients with alopecia areata. After 7 months of massaging the essential oil blend or placebo into their scalp, 44% of the treatment group reported new hair growth compared with 15% of the control group.[110] This study was poorly designed and results may have been affected by the lack of follow-up of dropouts in the control group.

Case reports

Oral treatment with thymol, in daily doses of 1 to 4 g in two cycles of 64 and 169 days with a 35-day interval, resolved Kaposi's sarcoma in a 20-year-old woman. Heartburn was observed as a side effect.[111] Oral administration of thymol resolved a case of dermatomyositis[112] and a case of progressive scleroderma.[113] Note: Large doses of thymol were used in these case studies and these results could not be expected from normal usage of thyme.

In conjunction with maintaining a continuous state of dryness, thymol was successfully used in the treatment of paronychia and onycholysis.[114] (See also the section on Side effects.)

Vulval lichen sclerosis in two sisters was successfully treated with a cream containing thyme extract. There were no side effects.[115]

A mixture of five herbs (Ankaferd Blood Stopper) with a long tradition of use in Anatolia, Turkey, to topically stop bleeding is undergoing extensive investigation. The formulation comprises *Thymus vulgaris*, *Glycyrrhiza glabra* leaf, *Vitis vinifera*, *Alpinia officinarum* and *Urtica diocia* root.[116] It is currently being used successfully as a haemostatic agent for intractable bleeding not responsive to conventional treatments. There are preliminary clinical trials, several case reports, in vitro and in vivo studies supporting its use. Other possible benefits include antimicrobial, antineoplastic and wound healing activities in certain diseases. The exact mechanism of action remains unknown, but in vitro studies have demonstrated its activity on endothelium, blood cells, angiogenesis, cellular proliferation, vascular dynamics and cell mediators. There are case reports of its successful use as a haemostatic agent in cases of severe gastrointestinal bleeding, after major heart, lung kidney and liver surgery, for postoperative dental bleeding and periodontal surgery, tonsillectomy and in trauma patients with haemophilia A, von Willebrand disease, thrombocytopenia and thrombasthenia.[116]

Toxicology and other safety data

Toxicology

The LD_{50} of thyme essential oil by oral route in rats was reported variously as 2.84 g/kg and 4.7 g/kg.[117,118]

Oral doses (0.5 to 3.0 g/kg) of concentrated thyme extract (equivalent to 4.3 to 26.0 g/kg of thyme) decreased locomotor activity and caused a slight slowing of respiration in mice. An increase in liver and testes weight was observed after chronic administration for 3 months (100 mg/kg equivalent to 0.9 g/kg dried plant per day). Spermatotoxic activity was not demonstrated.[119] Thyme oil had no mutagenic or DNA-damaging activity in the Ames or *Bacillus subtilis* rec-assay.[120] Thymol was not mutagenic in the Ames assay.[121]

Contraindications

None known.

Special warnings and precautions

None required.

Interactions

None known.

In mice fed thyme leaves (0.5% or 2% of diet) or treated with thymol or carvacrol (50 to 200 mg/kg), certain hepatic phase I and phase II detoxification enzymes were moderately induced.[101] The relevance or significance of this finding to human use is uncertain. The minimum inhibitory concentration (MIC) of the antifungal drug amphotericin B against *Candida albicans* in vitro was reduced by 80% when combined with 0.2 µL/mL thyme oil, suggesting a potential advantageous interaction.[122]

Use in pregnancy and lactation

Category B2 – no increase in frequency of malformation or other harmful effects on the fetus from limited use in women. Animal studies are largely lacking.

A study in mice receiving 0.25% thyme essential oil in their feed over 2 weeks and during 4 days of pregnancy observed no influence on the growth and development of 126 embryos.[123]

A 1913 German reference indicated that thyme leaf had been used as an abortifacient.[124] A paste consisting of soap, potassium iodide, thymol and astringents was used topically by doctors into the 1970s to procure abortion via an irritant action. However, it was regarded as carrying a high risk, with a number of maternal deaths attributed to its use.[125] Ingestion of large doses of thymol (>1 g) may produce abortion.[126]

Thyme is considered to be compatible with breastfeeding.

Effects on ability to drive or operate machinery

No adverse effects expected.

Side effects

Occasional cases of airborne contact dermatitis have been reported in farmers and other workers exposed to thyme dust.[127,128,129] One case of systemic allergy to thyme and other Labiates has been reported.[130] Five per cent of patients with crural ulceration were found to be positive on patch testing to thyme oil, perhaps present in dressings and topical treatments.[131] Case reports exist of acute contact dermatitis occurring following the application of a poultice containing a mix of herbs including thyme.[132]

Overdosage

No incidents found in published literature.

Safety in children

Thyme oil should not be applied near the mouth and nose of infants and young children as it can provoke a dangerous reflex breathing spasm.[133] Otherwise no adverse effects from thyme are expected.

Regulatory status in selected countries

Thyme is official in the *British Pharmacopoeia* 2012 and the *European Pharmacopoeia* 2012.

Thyme is included on the UK General Sale List.

It is covered by a positive Commission E monograph and has the following applications:

- Symptoms of bronchitis and whooping cough
- Catarrh of the upper respiratory tract.

Thyme and thyme oil have GRAS status. It is also freely available as a 'dietary supplement' in the USA under DSHEA legislation (Dietary Supplement Health and Education Act of 1994).

Thyme is not included in Part 4 of Schedule 4 of the Therapeutic Goods Regulations of Australia and is freely available for sale.

References

1. *British Pharmacopoeia, vol. IV: Herbal Drugs, Herbal Drug Preparations and Herbal Medicinal Products*, 2012.

2. Grieve M. *A Modern Herbal*, vol. 2. New York: Dover Publications; 1971. pp. 808–813.

3. Felter HW, Lloyd JU. *King's American Dispensatory*, 18th ed., rev 3, vol. 2, 1905. Portland: Reprinted by Eclectic Medical Publications; 1983. pp. 1939–1940.

4. British Herbal Medicine Association Scientific Committee. *British Herbal Pharmacopoeia*. Cowling: BHMA; 1983. pp. 212–213.

5. Koch C, Reichling J, Schneele J, et al. *Phytomedicine*. 2008;15(1–2):71–78.

6. Leung AY, Foster S. *Encyclopedia of Common Natural Ingredients used in Food, Drugs and Cosmetics*, 2nd ed New York: John Wiley; 1996. pp. 492–495.

7. Schilcher H. *Phytotherapy in Paediatrics*. Stuttgart: Medpharm Scientific Publishers; 1997. p. 39.

8. Weiss RF. *Herbal Medicine*. Beaconsfield: Beaconsfield Publishers; 1988. pp. 216–217.

9. Tyler VE, Brady LR, Robbers JE. *Pharmacognosy*, 9th ed. Philadelphia: Lea and Febiger; 1988. pp. 127–129.

10. Smeh NJ. *Creating Your Own Cosmetics – Naturally*. Garrisonville: Alliance; 1995. p. 95.

11. Pharmaceutical Society of Great Britain. *British Pharmaceutical Codex 1934*. London: Pharmaceutical Press; 1934. pp. 748–749.

12. Veal L. *Complement Ther Nurs Midwifery*. 1996;2(4):97–101.

13. Goker H, Haznedaroglu IC, Ercetin S, et al. *J Int Med Res*. 2008;36(1):163–170.

14. Mabberley DJ. *The Plant Book*, 2nd ed Cambridge: Cambridge University Press; 1997. pp. 713–714.

15. Chiej R. *The Macdonald Encyclopedia of Medicinal Plants*. London: Macdonald; 1984. Entry no. 309.

16. Lee KG, Shibamoto T. *J Agric Food Chem*. 2002;50(17):4947–4952.

17. Takacsova M, Pribela A, Faktorova M. *Nahrung*. 1995;39(3):241–243.

18. Cosentino S, Tuberoso CI, Pisano B, et al. *Lett Appl Microbiol*. 1999;29(2):130–135.

19. Hudaib M, Speroni E, Di Pietra AM, et al. *J Pharm Biomed Anal*. 2002;29(4):691–700.

20. Miura K, Kikuzaki H, Nakatani N. *J Agric Food Chem*. 2002;50(7):1845–1851.

21. Wang M, Kikuzaki H, Lin CC, et al. *J Agric Food Chem*. 1999;47(5):1911–1914.

22. Swain AR, Dutton SP, Trusswell AS. *J Am Diet Assoc*. 1985;85(8):950–960.

23. Chun H, Shin DH, Hong BS, et al. *Biol Pharm Bull*. 2001;24(8):941–946.

24. Chun H, Jun WJ, Shin DH, et al. *Chem Pharm Bull (Tokyo)*. 2001;49(6):762–764.

25. Wagner H, Bladt S. *Plant Drug Analysis: A Thin Layer Chromatography Atlas*, 2nd ed Berlin: Springer-Verlag; 1996. p. 155.

26. Blaschek W, Ebel S, Hackenthal E, et al. *HagerROM 2002: Hagers Handbuch der Drogen und Arzneistoffe*. Heidelberg: Springer; 2002.

27. Bisset NG, ed. *Herbal Drugs and Phytopharmaceuticals: A Handbook for Practice on a Scientific Basis*. Stuttgart: Medpharm Scientific; 1994. pp. 470–472, 493–495.

28. Llewellyn GC, Burkett ML, Eadie T. *J Assoc Off Anal Chem*. 1981;64(4):955–960.

29. Soliman KM, Badeaa RI. *Food Chem Toxicol*. 2002;40(11):1669–1675.

30. Manou I, Bouillard L, Devleeschouwer MJ, et al. *J Appl Microbiol*. 1998;84(3):368–376.

31. Marino M, Bersani C, Comi G. *J Food Prot*. 1999;62(9):1017–1023.

32. Smith–Palmer A, Stewart J, Fyfe L. *Lett Appl Microbiol*. 1998;26(2):118–122.

33. Jensen KB, Dyrud OK. *Acta Pharmacol Toxicol*. 1962;19:345–355.

34. Van Den Broucke CO, Lemli JA. *Planta Med*. 1981;41:129–135.

35. Reiter M, Brandt W. *Arzneimittelforschung*. 1985;35(1A):408–414.

36. Van Den Broucke CO, Lemli JA. *Pharm Weekbl Sci*. 1983;5(1):9–14.

37. Van Den Broucke CO. In: Margaris N, Koedam A, Vokou D, eds. *Aromatic Plants: Basic and Applied Aspects*. The Hague: Martinus Nijhoff; 1982. pp. 271–276.

38. Engelbertz J, Schwenk T, Kinzinger U, et al. *Planta Med*. 2008;74(12):1436–1440.

39. Begrow F, Engelbertz J, Feistel B, et al. *Planta Med*. 2010;76:311–318.

40. Wienkötter N, Begrow F, Kinzinger U, et al. *Planta Med*. 2007;73(7):629–635.

41. Muller-Limmroth W, Frohlich HH. *Fortschr Med*. 1980;98(3):95–101.

42. Gordonoff T, Janett F. *Z Ges Exp Med*. 1931;79:486–494.

43. Schilcher H. In: Baerheim Svendsen A, Scheffer JJC, eds. *Essential Oils and Aromatic Plants*. Dordrecht: Martinus Nijhoff; 1985. pp. 217–230.

44. Shapiro S, Meier A, Guggenheim B. *Oral Microbiol Immunol*. 1994;9(4):202–208.

45. Shapiro S, Guggenheim B. *Oral Microbiol Immunol*. 1995;10(4):241–246.

46. Didry N, Dubreuil L, Pinkas M. *Pharm Acta Helv*. 1994;69(1):25–28.

47. Agnihotri S, Vaidya AD. *Indian J Exp Biol*. 1996;3(7):712–715.

48. Didry N, Dubreuil L, Pinkas M. *Pharmazie*. 1993;48(4):301–304.

49. Panizzi L, Flamini G, Cioni PL, et al. *J Ethnopharmacol*. 1993;39(3):167–170.

50. Kalemba D, Kunicka A. *Curr Med Chem*. 2003;10(10):813–829.

51. Vampa G, Albasini A, Provvisionato A, et al. *Plantes Med Phytother*. 1998;22(3):195–202.

52. Juven BJ, Kanner J, Schved F, et al. *J Appl Bacteriol*. 1994;76(6):626–631.

53. Santos RI, Pereira DFA, Teodoro GR, et al. *Latin Am J Pharm*. 2010;29(6):941–947.

54. Tabak M, Armon R, Potasman I, et al. *J Appl Bacteriol*. 1996;80(6):667–672.

55. Fujita M, Shiota S, Kuroda T, et al. *Microbiol Immunol*. 2005;49(4):391–396.

56. Di Pasqua R, Hoskins N, Betts G, et al. *J Agric Food Chem*. 2006;54(7):2745–2749.

57. Di Pasqua R, Betts G, Hoskins N, et al. *J Agric Food Chem*. 2007;55(12):4863–4870.

58. Xu J, Zhou F, Ji BP, et al. *Lett Appl Microbiol*. 2008;47(3):174–179.

59. Viollon C, Chaumont JP. *Mycopathologia*. 1994;128(3):151–153.

60. Pauli A, Knobloch K. *Z Lebensm Unters Forsch*. 1987;185(1):10–13.

61. El-Kady IA, El-Maraghy SSM, Mostafa ME. *Qatar Uni Sci J*. 1993;13(1):63–69.

62. Tantaoui-Elaraki A, Beraoud LJ. *Environ Pathol Toxicol Oncol*. 1994;13(1):67–72.

63. Mahmoud AL. *Lett Appl Microbiol*. 1994;1(2):110–113.

64. Zambonelli A, D'Aulerio AZ, Bianchi A, et al. *J Phytopathol*. 1996;144(9–10):491–494.

65. Paster N, Menasherov M, Ravid U, et al. *J Food Protect*. 1995;58(1):81–85.

66. El-Maraghy SSM. *Folia Microbiol*. 1995;40(5):490–492.

67. Pina-Vaz C, Goncalves Rodrigues A, Pinto E, et al. *J Eur Acad Dermatol Venereol*. 2004;18(1):73–78.

68. Braga PC, Sasso MD, Culici M, et al. *Fitoterapia*. 2007;78(6):396–400.

69. Braga PC, Culici M, Alfieri M, et al. *Int J Antimicrob Agents*. 2008;31(5):472–477.

70. Bennis S, Chami F, Chami N, et al. *Lett Appl Microbiol*. 2004;38(6):454–458.

71. Nolkemper S, Reichling J, Stintzing FC, et al. *Planta Med*. 2006;72(15):1378–1382.

72. Schnitzler P, Koch C, Reichling J. *Antimicrob Agents Chemother*. 2007;51(5):1859–1862.

73. Astani A, Reichling J, Schnitzler P. *Phytother Res*. 2010;24(5):673–679.

74. Huang YS, Zhang JT. *Yao Hsueh Hsueh Pao*. 1992;2(2):96–100.

75. Van Kessel KP, Kalter ES, Verhoef J. *Agents Actions*. 1986;17(3–4):375–376.

76. Haraguchi H, Saito T, Ishikawa H, et al. *Planta Med*. 1996;62(3):217–221.

77. Pearson DA, Frankel EN, Aeschbach R, et al. *J Agric Food Chem*. 1997;45(3):578–582.

78. Schwarz K, Ernst H, Ternes W. *J Sci Food Agric*. 1996;70(2):217–223.

79. Aeschbach R, Loliger J, Scott BC, et al. *Food Chem Toxicol.* 1994;32(1):31–36.

80. Chung SK, Osawa T, Kawakishi S. *Biosci Biotech Biochem.* 1997;61(1):118–123.

81. Braga PC, Sasso MD, Culici M, et al. *Pharmacology.* 2006;76(2):61–68.

82. Stoilova I, Bail S, Buchbauer G, et al. *Nat Prod Commun.* 2008;3(7):1047–1050.

83. Samejima K, Kanazawa K, Ashida H, et al. *J Agric Food Chem.* 1995;43(2):410–414.

84. Vukovic-Gacic B, Simic D. *Basic Life Sci.* 1993;61:269–277.

85. Englberger W, Hadding U, Etschenberg E, et al. *Int J Immunopharmacol.* 1988;10(6):729–737.

86. Azuma Y, Ozasa N, Ueda Y, et al. *J Dent Res.* 1986;65(1):53–56.

87. Wagner H, Wierer M, Bauer R. *Planta Med.* 1986;52:184–187.

88. Tanaka Y, Konishi Y, Takagaki Y, et al. *J Food Hyg Soc Jap.* 1997;38(1):7–11.

89. Braga PC, Sasso MD, Culici M, et al. *Pharmacology.* 2006;77(3):130–136.

90. Melo FHC, Venâncio ET, de Sousa DP, et al. *Fundam Clin Pharmacol.* 2009;24(4):437–443.

91. Melo FHC, Moura BA, de Sousa DP, et al. *Fundam Clin Pharmacol.* 2011;25:362–367.

92. Beer A-M, Lukanov J, Sagorchev P. *Phytomedicine.* 2007;14:65–69.

93. Taherian AA, Babaei M, Vafaei AA, et al. *Pakistan J Pharm Sci.* 2009;22(1):83–89.

94. Yamamoto J, Yamada K, Naemura A, et al. *Nutrition.* 2005;21(5):580–587.

95. Naemura A, Ura M, Yamashita T, et al. *Thromb Res.* 2008;122(4):517–522.

96. Deans SG, Noble RC, Penzes L, et al. *Age.* 1993;16:71–74.

97. Jukic M, Politeo O, Maksimovic M, et al. *Phytother Res.* 2007;21(3):259–261.

98. Janbaz KH, Saeed SA, Gilani AH. *Pakistan J Biol Sci.* 2003;6(5):448–451.

99. Dursun N, Liman N, Ozyazgan I, et al. *J Burn Care Res.* 2003;24(6):395–399.

100. Park BS, Choi WS, Kim JH, et al. *J Am Mosq Control Assoc.* 2005;21(1):80–83.

101. Sasaki K, Wada K, Tanaka Y, et al. *J Med Food.* 2005;8(2):184–189.

102. Austgulen LT, Solheim E, Scheline RR. *Pharmacol Toxicol.* 1987;61(2):98–102.

103. Kohlert C, Schindler G, Marz RW, et al. *J Clin Pharmacol.* 2002;42(7):731–737.

104. Knols G, Stal PC, Van Ree JW. *Huisart Wetens.* 1994;37(9):392–394.

105. Büechi S, Vögelin R, von Eiff MM, et al. *Forsch Komplementarmed Klass Naturheilkd.* 2005;12(6):328–332.

106. Kemmerich B, Eberhardt R, Stammer H. *Arzneimittelforschung.* 2006;56(9):652–660.

107. Marzian O. *MMW Fortschr Med.* 2007;149(27–28 suppl):69–74.

108. Kemmerich B, Eberhardt R, Stammer H. *Arzneimittelforschung.* 2007;57(9):607–615.

109. Gruenwald J, Graubaum HJ, Busch R. *Arzneimittelforschung.* 2005;55(11):669–676.

110. Hay IC, Jamieson M, Ormerod AD. *Arch Dermatol.* 1998;134(11):1349–1352.

111. Buccellato G. *Giorn Ital Derm.* 1964;105:419–430.

112. Buccellato G. *Giorn Ital Derm.* 1965;106:89–94.

113. Buccellato G. *Giorn Ital Derm.* 1965;106:373–376.

114. Wilson JW. *Arch Dermat.* 1965;92:726–730.

115. Hagedorn M. *Z Hautkr.* 1989;64(9):810.813–814.

116. Beyazit Y, Kurt M, Kekilli M, et al. *Altern Med Rev.* 2010;15(4):329–336.

117. Skramlik E. *Pharmazie.* 1959;14:435–445.

118. Opdyke DLJ. *Food Cosmet Toxicol.* 1974;12:1003–1004.

119. Qureshi S, Shah AH, Al-Yahya MA, et al. *Fitotherapia.* 1991;62(4):319–323.

120. Zani F, Massimo G, Benvenuti S, et al. *Planta Med.* 1991;57(3):237–241.

121. Azizan A, Blevins RD. *Arch Environ Contam Toxicol.* 1995;28(2):248–258.

122. Giordani R, Regli P, Kaloustian J, et al. *Phytother Res.* 2004;18(12):990–995.

123. Domaracky M, Rehák P, Juhás S, et al. *Physiol Res.* 2007;56(1):97–104.

124. Watt JM, Breyer-Brandwijk MG. *The Medicinal and Poisonous Plants of Southern and Eastern Africa: Being an Account of Their Medicinal and Other Uses, Chemical Composition, Pharmacological Effects and Toxicology in Man and Animal*, 2nd ed Edinburgh: Livingstone; 1962. pp. 528–529.

125. [No authors listed]. *Br Med J* 2(6027): 70, 1976.

126. Sollmann T. *A Manual of Pharmacology and Its Applications to Therapeutics and Toxicology*, 7th ed. Philadelphia: WB Saunders; 1948. p. 190.

127. Spiewak R, Skorska C, Dutkiewicz J. *Contact Dermatitis.* 2001;44(4):235–239.

128. Golec M, Skórska C, Mackiewicz B, et al. *Ann Univ Mariae Curie Sklodowska Med.* 2003;58(1):195–203.

129. Golec M, Skórska C, Mackiewicz B, et al. *Ann Agric Environ Med.* 2005;12(1):5–10.

130. Benito M, Jorro G, Morales C, et al. *Ann Allergy Asthma Immunol.* 1996;76(5):416–418.

131. Le Roy R, Grosshans E, Foussereau J. *Derm Beruf Umwelt.* 1981;29(6):168–170.

132. Martinez-Gonzalez MC. *Contact Dermatitis.* 2007;56:49–50.

133. Naumann HH. In: Dost FH, Leiber B, eds. *Menthol and Menthol-Containing External Remedies.* Stuttgart: Thieme; 1967. pp. 99–107.

Tribulus leaf

(*Tribulus terrestris* L.)

Synonyms

Caltrops, Puncture vine (Engl), Fructus Tribuli (Lat), (Dan), Gokshura (Sanskrit), Bai ji li (Chin).

What is it?

Tribulus is a prostrate, spreading herb with a fruit bearing sharp, rigid spines – and for this reason is also known as 'puncture vine'. It is regarded as a weed and hepatotoxic to ruminant livestock in many parts of the world, including Australia.

The entire plant, but particularly the fruit, is used in traditional medicine. In recent years, Tribulus leaf or herb (aerial parts) has gained a reputation amongst bodybuilders and athletes as an alternative to anabolic steroids. Attention has also focused on the Bulgarian research using a standardised Tribulus leaf product for the treatment of male and female infertility and for menopausal symptoms and low male libido. The information in this monograph is mainly centred on this research.

Effects

Enhancing effect on male sexual function; improves production and motility of spermatozoa; increases sex hormone production in both men and women; alleviates menopausal symptoms; improves fertility in women.

Traditional view

There is no well-documented information on the traditional use of Tribulus leaf. In Ayurveda, Tribulus fruit is used mainly for diseases of the urinary system (cystitis, painful urination, kidney stones and oedema) and of the reproductive system (spermatorrhoea, gonorrhoea, impotence and uterine disorders after parturition). It is also used to treat gout, cough and heart disease. Tribulus fruit is regarded as a diuretic, with antiseptic and soothing activities on the mucous membranes of the urinary tract, but also as an adaptogen, nervine tonic, aphrodisiac and a rejuvenative tonic for the kidneys, being often combined with Withania. The entire plant, including the root, is also used.[1-3]

In traditional Chinese medicine the fruit is used for skin lesions with itching, for pain and distension in the chest, insufficient lactation due to constrained liver Qi and for swollen, painful eyes.[4]

Summary actions

Tonic, male aphrodisiac, oestrogenic in females (indirectly), androgenic in males (indirectly), fertility agent.

Can be used for

Indications supported by clinical trials

Male infertility, impotence and decreased libido; female infertility, menopausal symptoms (generally low-level evidence from uncontrolled trials).

May also be used for

Extrapolations from pharmacological studies

To restore and build vitality (especially during convalescence or after surgery), assist in responding to stress and improve physical performance.

Preparations

Dried aerial parts for decoction, fluid extract and tablets or capsules.

Dosage

The recommended adult dosage for the hormonal effects is one tablet (containing a standardised concentrate equivalent to 3 to 10 g of dried leaf or aerial parts, providing 100 to 112.5 mg of furostanol saponins (calculated as protodioscin)) three times per day.

There are many products with inferior potency in the marketplace and the researched effects of Tribulus leaf cannot be attributed to these products because of their poor level of active components (see below). Equivalent doses of a fluid extract can also be employed, for example 10 mL/day of a 2:1 extract containing 30 mg/mL of furostanol saponins as protodioscin.

Duration of use

No restriction on long-term use if taken within the recommended dosage.

Summary assessment of safety

No adverse effects are expected.

Technical data

Botany

Tribulus terrestris, a member of the Zygophyllaceae family, is a prostrate, spreading herb. The leaves are opposite, 5 to 8 cm long, containing four to seven pairs of leaflets. The flowers are pale yellow, 1 to 1.5 cm in diameter. The fruit is distinctive: usually hairy and consisting of five cocci (mericarps), each with two long and two short, very sharp, spines.[1,3]

Adulteration

The root or fruit are often substituted for the leaf in modern products, but are unlikely to have the same therapeutic profile. A Tribulus leaf product designated for performance enhancement was found to contain anabolic steroids.[5]

Key constituents

The active components of Tribulus leaf are steroidal saponins, mainly furostanol glycosides (including protodioscin and prototribestin) and small quantities of spirostanol glycosides.[6–8] Several novel furostanol glycosides have recently been isolated from the aerial parts.[9,10] Other constituents include phytosterols, such as, beta-sitosterol.[11] While very small quantities of harmala alkaloids (tryptophan-derived beta-carbolines) are said to occur in some varieties,[12] this is unlikely, and such findings have not been confirmed by recent studies.

The furostanol glycosides are a subdivision of steroidal saponins. They have a sugar group at the carbon-3 (C-3) position and a second sugar group at position C-26. Furostanol glycosides readily convert into spirostanol saponins (with one sugar group at C-3) in the presence of plant enzymes.[13] Such degradation resulting in loss of sugars may occur postharvest, in manufacturing or during experimental analysis. Tribulus leaf contains a higher concentration of steroidal saponins than the fruit, and there is a substantially higher protodioscin content in the leaf of eastern European origin than in the leaf from other geographical locations. (See Analytical studies below.)

Analytical studies

An analytical investigation in 1998 of 20 Tribulus preparations, most available for sale in the USA, found insufficient levels of furostanol saponins in the majority of products except a Bulgarian Tribulus leaf product.[14] Many Tribulus products on the market are quite different in phytochemical profile from the Bulgarian extract. A study conducted in the USA in late 2001 found that the level of protodioscin varied substantially with the plant part (leaf, stem or fruit) and the origin of the Tribulus (Bulgaria, India or China). Only leaf from Bulgaria was high in protodioscin. An analysis of three products selected from the US market found substantial levels of protodioscin only in the product manufactured in Bulgaria. The other two samples (one of which contained Tribulus fruit) were deficient in protodioscin.[15] An eastern European variety of Tribulus (from Slovakia) was found to contain high levels of protodioscin in the leaf but none in the fruit. Leaf samples from Australia and India did not contain protodioscin.[16] Bulgarian research has confirmed that the chemotype occurring in south-eastern Europe and west Asia is rich in protodioscin, unlike samples from India and Vietnam.[17] Prototribestin was also a main saponin component in samples from the former group of countries.

If a Tribulus product is made from the root or fruit of the plant, or is sourced from anywhere else other than eastern Europe, it will probably contain low levels of protodioscin and prototribestin, and will therefore be quite different clinically to the Bulgarian standardised extract. This is despite what might be claimed on the label of such products, because often inferior or inappropriate methods of analysis have been used to measure the furostanol saponins, such as gravimetric or colorimetric techniques. The quality of Tribulus products is best assessed by high performance liquid chromatography, as used in the studies cited above.

Pharmacodynamics

Tribulus leaf standardised extract (TLSE) is a product obtained from the aerial parts of eastern European *Tribulus terrestris* that contains mainly saponins of the furostanol type (not less than 45%, calculated as protodioscin). Hence a typical dose of 750 mg/day contains around 300 mg of protodioscin and prototribestin. Another trade preparation, VT, has also been studied and contains TLSE, vitamins, folic acid and potassium orotate.

Hormonal and sexual activity

Oral doses of TLSE have demonstrated the following effects in vivo:

- Improved libido, weight gain, sexual activity and intracavernous pressure in male rats (2.5 to 10 mg/kg/day),[18] and a pro-erectile effect on the corpus cavernosum smooth muscle of rabbits (tissue isolated after treatment, 2.5 to 10 mg/kg/day)[19]
- Aphrodisiac activity in castrated male rats (5 mg/kg/day) that may be due to androgenic activity.[20] The results of an in vivo study investigating the effect of TLSE on the brain tissue of normal male rats (5 mg/kg/day) added further evidence for this, suggesting that TLSE may have a central effect. The authors proposed that any aphrodisiac activity of TLSE might be mediated by increases in both androgen receptor and nitric oxide synthase (NOS)-containing neurons. (NOS is present in regions of the brain that regulate sexual functions)[21]

- Marked stimulation of spermatogenesis, increased density of Sertoli cells, increased tenacity and viability of spermatozoa and accelerated and emphasised sexual activity in male rats (70 mg/kg/day).[22] Female rats treated with the saponin fraction produced more offspring[23]

- Increased plasma testosterone concentrations compared with controls in male lambs and rams (250 mg/day); acceleration of sexual development, activation of spermatogenesis and stimulation of seminiferous tubule growth in immature male sheep[24]

- Increased testosterone levels, improved semen production and normalised sexual activity in rams with sexual impotence; no morphologic changes in the structure of either testes or epididymides were observed during the treatment period[25]

- Restored libido and sexual reflexes in 71% of male boars displaying absence of libido. Five animals with prolonged poor libido also improved (70 mg/kg/day).[26]

In terms of human pharmacodynamic studies, TLSE (750 mg/day for 5 days) increased serum follicle-stimulating hormone (FSH) and oestradiol compared with baseline values in human female volunteers and increased the level of luteinising hormone (LH) and testosterone in male volunteers,[27] thereby demonstrating increased sex hormone production in both men and women. In contrast, another study found no significant difference in serum testosterone, androstenedione or LH in healthy men (20 to 36 years) administered TLSE, compared with controls. Volunteers were randomly assigned to receive one of two doses of Tribulus extract of Bulgarian origin (corresponding to 6 mg/kg/day or 12 mg/kg/day of saponins) or placebo.[28] This Bulgarian extract was different to the one used in the previous positive studies.

Mechanism of action

It can be hypothesised that saponins from Tribulus appear to increase FSH in menstruating women, which in turn increases levels of oestradiol. They may do this by binding with, but only weakly stimulating, hypothalamic oestrogen beta-receptors, which are part of the negative feedback mechanism of oestrogen control. The weak stimulus (compared with oestrogen) leads the body to interpret that oestrogen levels are lower than they really are, thereby provoking increased production via the normal feedback loop. In the postmenopausal woman, Tribulus might alleviate the symptoms of oestrogen withdrawal via the binding of its steroids to vacant receptors in the hypothalamus (in this low oestrogen situation). This interaction could be sufficient to convince the body that more oestrogen is present in the bloodstream than actually is, calming the hypothalamic response. A similar mechanism via the hypothalamus could apply for men.

The suggestion by Adimoelja[29] that TLSE acts via the in vivo conversion of protodioscin to DHEA (dehydroepiandrosterone) has no basis in fact and should not confuse the discussion regarding the mode of action of this herb.

Tonic activity

TLSE increased non-specific resistance in mice with experimental lung infection, possibly due to the activation of alveolar macrophages.[30] TLSE has been shown to intensify protein synthesis and enhance the activity of some enzymes connected with energy metabolism. VT increased the absorption of iron from the small intestine and inhibited lipid peroxidation during stress.[31]

TLSE (oral, 100 mg/kg/day for 5 days) increased static physical endurance in rats. Treatment with VT (oral, 300 mg/kg/day for 1 month) markedly increased endurance. VT (by injection) accelerated the restoration process after heavy exercise, had a slight protective action on capillary and peritoneal lesions and decreased capillary permeability.[32] The mechanism behind improved endurance was probably not directly connected with the adrenergic system and VT does not stimulate the CNS, with a mode of action different from that of psychostimulants.[30,32] VT improved resistance to stress and endurance in vivo compared with controls. It increased the concentration of dopamine and serotonin metabolites and the levels of noradrenaline (norepinephrine) in the hypothalamus.[33]

VT given for 5 days (equivalent to 270 mg/day TLSE) increased serum concentrations of growth hormone, insulin and aldosterone in human volunteers, without exceeding normal values and with no clinical suggestion of hyperfunction of the respective endocrine glands. Greater increases were seen in the group actively engaged in sports, compared with the untrained group. There were no effects on cortisol, testosterone and prolactin levels.[34]

Pharmacokinetics

Pharmacokinetic studies of TLSE in rats indicated that 12% to 14% of protodioscin is excreted in bile and 6% to 7% in urine (at 24 h) when administered intravenously (50 and 200 mg/kg). After oral administration of the same individual doses, 2% to 4% of protodioscin was excreted in the bile, but protodioscin was not detected in urine.[35]

Clinical trials

Male infertility and impotence

The results of open clinical trials conducted by four Bulgarian research teams, including a total of 363 men, indicated that TLSE had a stimulating effect on sexual function:[36–40]

- Treatment with 750 mg/day for 60 days significantly increased motility and rate of movement of spermatozoa from 38 men with idiopathic oligospermia. In some cases, after repeated treatment at a dose of 1500 mg/day, a normalisation of the sperm profile was observed, accompanied by increased LH and testosterone and decreased oestradiol.

- Two groups of men with oligospermia after varicocele operations were treated with either 750 mg/day for 60 days or 1500 mg/day for 90 days. Significant improvement in sperm motility was observed in both groups. Treatment with 1500 mg also resulted in an increase in ejaculate quantity in all patients.

- Patients with unilateral or bilateral hypotrophy of the testes and oligospermia demonstrated improvements in ejaculate volume, sperm concentration and motility after treatment (1500 mg/day, 60 days). Testosterone levels were also increased. A light palpable pain in the testicular region with slight oedema was reported by patients during the treatment, which abated 2 to 3 months later.

- Treatment of 51 infertile men with 750 mg/day TLSE for 3 months significantly increased ejaculate volume, sperm concentration, motility and velocity. Spermatozoa morphology normalised and ejaculate liquefaction time decreased. Semen immune parameters decreased leucocyte counts, alpha-amylase values (an enzyme involved in ejaculate liquefaction) and secretion of local immunoglobulins. Cholesterol, LDL-cholesterol, triglycerides and VLDL-cholesterol all decreased, and HDL-cholesterol increased. Libido was normalised or enhanced in those reporting poor libido.

- Thirty-one pregnancies were recorded for 100 couples with infertility involving an immunological cause within 12 months of initiating TLSE treatment. The average time taken to conceive was 5.2 months. Prior to treatment sperm number and quality varied, but all men and 74% of women had abnormal results for sperm-agglutinating antibody tests. The dosage used was 750 mg/day for men and 750 mg/day from days 21 to 27 of the menstrual cycle for women until conception occurred.

- Improvement in sperm profile was not observed in patients with chronic prostatitis (750 to 1500 mg/day).

- Of 14 patients suffering reduced libido, 12 showed considerable improvement after 30 days (1500 mg/day) and one patient was slightly improved after 60 days. Libido was improved in 27 of 36 patients with chronic prostatitis. The other nine patients, who all had chronic prostatitis for over 5 years, demonstrated no improvement. Libido was incidentally improved in patients with hypotrophy of the testes and idiopathic oligospermia.

- Libido and sexual activity were improved in some patients with Klinefelter's syndrome (genetic hypogonadism), Noonan syndrome (a multifaceted disorder that includes cryptorchidism) and simple cryptorchidism.

- TLSE was well tolerated in all of the above studies.

Tribulus has been part of a number of herbal formulations successfully used in uncontrolled clinical trials in India and Russia to treat sexual dysfunction or sexual inadequacy in men. The main formulations contained 7% to 12.5% of Tribulus by weight. Improvement in sexual function was observed in convalescing postmyocardial infarction male patients,[41] and in leprosy patients experiencing testicular and epididymal changes. Patients with oligospermia showed objective improvement.[42] Impotence and loss of libido improved in male diabetics.[43] Improvement was also observed in men with impotence.[44,45] Sperm count and motility increased in approximately 60% to 70% of subfertile and oligospermic men.[46,47]

Female infertility

In an open study involving infertile women, TLSE (750 to 1500 mg) was administered every day for 2 to 3 months (Group 1), only on days 5 to 14 of the menstrual cycle for 2 to 3 months (Group 2), or used in the preovulatory phase in combination with a conventional ovulation stimulant for 3 months (Group 3).[26] Group 1 did not show improvement in the ovulation parameters measured and side effects were observed, especially when the treatment was abruptly terminated. Of the 36 women in Group 2, 6% experienced normalised ovulation with resultant pregnancy, 61% demonstrated normalised ovulation without pregnancy and 33% demonstrated no effect from the treatment. Parallel control studies on a comparable cohort were carried out utilising three ovulation stimulants. The best results were obtained with 62 women treated using epimestrol: 39% had normalised ovulation with pregnancy, 35% had normalised ovulation without pregnancy and 26% demonstrated no effect from treatment. No side effects were recorded for the TLSE group, compared with incident rates of 6.5%, 10.6% and 38% in women treated with various ovulation stimulants. For the 20 women treated with TLSE and an ovulation stimulant (Group 3), the effect from their combined use was better than treatment with either agent alone.

Menopause

In an open label study, 98% of 50 menopausal women experienced symptom improvement after TLSE treatment, but not after placebo. Fifty-two per cent of patients were experiencing natural menopause and 48% had postoperative symptoms after removal of their ovaries. Predominant symptoms included hot flushes, sweating, insomnia and depression. The dosage prescribed varied, but generally a maintenance dose of 500 to 750 mg/day of TLSE was reached after higher initial doses. Treatment did not result in significant changes in FSH, LH, prolactin, oestradiol, progesterone and testosterone, although FSH tended to be lower.[26]

Body composition and exercise performance

A purported standardised extract of Tribulus leaf given for 8 weeks at a daily dose of 3.2 mg/kg did not enhance body composition or exercise performance in eight resistance-trained men when coupled with a resistance-training programme in a randomised, double blind, placebo-controlled trial. The authors conceded that the lack of improvement in body composition in both groups may be attributed to the fact that these men were already lean and may not have consumed enough protein or calories to gain lean body mass. In addition, the method chosen to assess exercise performance was not the most objective measure available.[48] The dose of extract used was low (240 to 260 mg/day) compared with previous studies and the origin and quality of the extract is uncertain.

A randomised, placebo-controlled clinical trial involving 22 elite Australian rugby league players found that an undefined Tribulus extract (450 mg/day for 5 weeks) had no significant impact on muscular strength, body composition and the testosterone/epitestosterone ratio (used in performance-enhancing drug tests).[49] Again the dose used was relatively low and the protodioscin content of the extract was uncertain.

Toxicology and other safety data

Toxicology

LD_{50} values for oral administration of Tribulus leaf extract in both mice and rats were greater than 10g/kg, indicating very low toxicity. No lethality, change in behaviour or changes in biochemical indices were observed in rats given oral doses ranging from 75 to 300mg/kg for 30 and 90 days or in dogs receiving 75mg/kg for 180 days.[50] There was no evidence of induced carcinogenicity after oral administration of Tribulus leaf extract at 50 or 150mg/kg/day for 93 weeks in rats.[51]

'Tribulus staggers' is a unique neuromuscular disorder in sheep. Although its cause was suggested to be due to the accumulation of harmala alkaloids over a period of time, their presence in the plant was not confirmed using more sophisticated analytical techniques.[12,52] A photosensitisation reaction known as 'geeldikkop' has been reported in livestock after consumption of Tribulus.[53–55] Cholestasis is believed to play a role in the development of this disorder, probably due to a novel pathway of steroidal saponin metabolism specific to ruminants. These reactions have not been observed in humans and are furthermore highly unlikely at the recommended therapeutic dosage.

Contraindications

None required on current evidence. Tribulus should not be used during pregnancy or lactation without professional advice.

Special warnings and precautions

While it is unlikely that normal doses of Tribulus in humans would cause the cholestasis observed in ruminants after grazing on this plant, saponin-containing herbs such as Tribulus are best kept to a minimum in patients with pre-existing cholestasis.

Use of Tribulus leaf is unlikely to impact tests for performance-enhancing drugs, although the intake of supplements containing this herb has been used as a defence in doping cases. To test this hypothesis, two female volunteers ingested 1500mg/day TLSE for 2 consecutive days.[56] None of the tested steroid hormone parameters revealed a significant variation or exceeded the World Anti-Doping Agency limits. However, testing in both men and women over a longer period of time, say up to several months, would provide more certainty on this issue.

Interactions

None known.

Use in pregnancy and lactation

Category B3 – no increase in frequency of malformation or other harmful effects on the fetus from limited use in women. Evidence of increased fetal damage in animal studies exists, although the relevance to humans is unknown.

According to traditional Chinese medicine Tribulus fruit should be used with caution in pregnancy.[4]

Preliminary experiments with penned ewes fed *Tribulus terrestris* leaf from days 85 to 130 of gestation indicated that lamb survival was decreased. Intravenous infusion of the ewe with an ethanolic extract of Tribulus was noted to sometimes cause a decrease of fetal heart rate. In another experiment, five ewes began consuming 300 to 400g of dried powdered *Tribulus terrestris* leaf (which was equivalent to at least 900 to 1200g of the fresh plant) at days 103 to 112 of gestation and were then exposed to it for the next 18 to 44 days. No consistent change in fetal blood pressure or heart rate was observed following the ingestion of Tribulus. The incidence of fetal breathing movements was significantly lower compared with the lucerne-fed group. This may indicate there was an effect on the functional maturation of some pathways in the central nervous system. Despite this, fetal growth and postnatal survival were not impaired.[57]

Tribulus is compatible with breastfeeding but caution should be observed.

Effects on ability to drive and use machines

No adverse effects expected.

Side effects

As with all herbs rich in saponins, oral use may cause irritation of the gastric mucous membranes and reflux. A case of gynaecomastia in a 21-year-old male attributed to *Tribulus terrestris* (product unspecified) has been described.[58] Given the possibility that such a product could have been adulterated with hormones or other agents, the connection with Tribulus must be regarded as tenuous.

Overdosage

A case has been reported of purported hepatotoxicity, nephrotoxicity and neurotoxicity in an Iranian man who consumed an unspecified large amount of a Tribulus product ('Tribulus water') over a period of 2 days.[59] In their justification of attributing the patient's condition to Tribulus consumption, the authors inappropriately quoted the published effects of Tribulus on ruminant livestock (geeldikkop and Tribulus staggers; see under Toxicology). However, these conditions are unique to ruminants and develop over a much longer period of time, as was pointed out in a subsequent letter to the editor.[60] There is also conjecture that Tribulus staggers is due to fungal contamination of the plant. More plausible explanations for the patient's condition can be ascribed to either microbial contamination of the 'Tribulus water' or the patient's past history of kidney stones (the reason why he began taking the Tribulus). Moreover, there was no information provided in the case report regarding the plant part, quality and composition (and even identity) of the Tribulus product involved.[60]

Safety in children

No information available.

Regulatory status in selected countries

Tribulus leaf is not on the UK General Sale List.

Tribulus leaf does not have GRAS status. However, it is freely available as a 'dietary supplement' in the USA under DSHEA legislation (1994 Dietary Supplement Health and Education Act).

Tribulus leaf is not included in Part 4 of Schedule 4 of the Therapeutic Goods Act of Australia and is freely available for sale.

References

1. Kapoor LD. CRC *Handbook of Ayurvedic Medicinal Plants*. Boca Raton: CRC Press; 1990. p. 325.
2. Frawley D, Lad V. *The Yoga of Herbs: An Ayurvedic Guide to Herbal Medicine*, 2nd ed Santa Fe: Lotus Press; 1988. pp. 169–170.
3. Thakur RS, Puri HS, Husain A. *Major Medicinal Plants of India*. Lucknow: Central Institute of Medicinal and Aromatic Plants; 1989. pp. 506–509.
4. Bensky D, Gamble A. *Chinese Herbal Medicine Materia Medica*. Seattle: Eastland Press; 1986. pp. 607–608.
5. Geyer H, Mareck–Engelke U, Reinhart U, et al. *Dtsch Z Sportmed*. 2000;51(11):378–382.
6. Gjulemetowa R, Tomowa M, Simowa M, et al. *Pharmazie*. 1982;37(4):296.
7. Tomova M, Gyulemetova R, Zarkova S, et al. *Int Conf Chem Biotechnol Biol Act Nat Prod (Proc)* 1st. 1981;3:298–302.
8. Yan W, Ohtani K, Kasai R, et al. *Phytochemistry*. 1996;42(5):1417–1422.
9. Conrad J, Dinchev D, Klaiber I, et al. *Fitoterapia*. 2004;75(2):117–122.
10. De Combarieu E, Fuzzati N, Lovati M, Mercalli E. *Fitoterapia*. 2003;74(6):583–591.
11. Mahato SB, Sahu NP, Ganguly AN, et al. *J Chem Soc Perk Trans*. 1981;1(9):2405–2410.
12. Bourke CA, Stevens GR, Carrigan MJ. *Aust Vet J*. 1992;69(7):163–165.
13. Hostettmann K, Marston A. *Chemistry & Pharmacology of Natural Products: Saponins*. Cambridge: Cambridge University Press; 1995. pp. 76–96.
14. Obreshkova D, Pangarova T, Milkov S, et al. *Pharmacia*. 1998;45(2):11.
15. Ganzera M, Bedir E, Khan IA, et al. *J Pharm Sci*. 2001;90(11):1752–1758.
16. Lehmann RP, Penman KG, Halloran KG, et al. *Rev Fitoterapia*. 2002;2(S1):217. Abstract B006.
17. Dinchev D, Janda B, Evstatieva L, et al. *Phytochemistry*. 2008;69(1):176–186.
18. Gauthaman K, Ganesan AP, Prasad RN. *J Altern Complement Med*. 2003;9(2):257–265.
19. Adaikan PG, Gauthaman K, Prasad RNV. *Aging Male*. 2001;4(3):163–169.
20. Gauthaman K, Adaikan PG, Prasad RN. *Life Sci*. 2002;71(12):1385–1396.

21. Gauthaman K, Adaikan PG. *J Ethnopharmacol*. 2005;96(1–2):127–132.
22. Zarkova S. *Rev Port Ciencias Vet*. 1984;79(470):117–126.
23. Tomova M, Gyulemetova R, Zarkova S, et al. *Int Conf Chem Biotechnol Biol Act Nat Prod (Proc)*. 1981;3:298–302.
24. Georgiev P, Dimitrov M, Vitanov S, et al. *Vet Sb*. 1988;3:20–22.
25. Dimitrov M, Georgiev P, Vitanov S, et al. *Vet Med Nauki*. 1987;24(5):102–110.
26. Zarkova S. *Tribestan: Experimental and Clinical Investigations*. Sofia, Bulgaria: Chemical Pharmaceutical Research Institute. www.bpg.bg/tribestan/table.phtml Accessed July 2009.
27. Milanov S, Maleeva E, Taskov M. *MBI: Medicobiol Inform*. 1985;4:27–29.
28. Neychev VK, Mitev VI. *J Ethnopharmacol*. 2005;101(1–3):319–323.
29. Adimoelja A. *Int J Androl*. 2000;23 (suppl 2):82–84.
30. Toshkov A, Dimov V, Zarkova S. *MBI: Medicobiol Inform*. 1985:28–31.
31. Taskov M. *MBI: Medicobiol Inform*. 1988;1:3.
32. Taskov M. *MBI: Medicobiol Inform*. 1988;1:4–9.
33. Tyutyulkova N, Taskov M, Manolova B. *MBI: Medicobiol Inform*. 1988;6:27–30.
34. Taskov M, Milanov S, Maleeva A. *MBI: Medicobiol Inform*. 1988;1:24–26.
35. Dikova N, Ognyanova V. *Anniversary Scientific Session: 35 Years Chemical Pharmaceutical Research Institute*. Sofia, Bulgaria, 1983. pp. 1–7.
36. Protich M, Tsvetkov D, Nalbanski B, et al. *Akush Ginekol (Sofia)*. 1983;22(4):326–329.
37. Kumanov F, Bozadjieva E, Andreeva M, et al. *Savrem Med*. 1982;33(4):211–215.
38. Viktorov IV. In: Zarkova S, ed. *Tribestan: Experimental and Clinical Investigations*. Sofia, Bulgaria: Chemical Pharmaceutical Research Institute; 1982. www.bpg.bg/tribestan/table.phtml. Accessed July 2009.
39. Nikolova V, Stanislavov R. *Dokl Bolg Akad Nauk*. 2000;53(12):113–116.
40. Stanislavov R, Nikolova V. *Dokl Bolg Akad Nauk*. 2000;53(10):107–110.

41. Nikolaeva LF, Dedov II Kurbanov VA. *Kardiologiia*. 1986;26(7):82–85.
42. Nigam P, Mukhija RD, Gupta AK, et al. *Hansenol Int*. 1984;9(1–2):10–20.
43. Sathyanathan TJ. *Indian Med Gaz*. 1985;119(6):196–197.
44. Sankaran JR. *J Natl Integ Med Assoc*. 1984;26(11):315–317.
45. Misra DN, Shukla GD. *Indian Med Gaz*. 1984;118(10):322–324.
46. Pardanani DS, Delima RJ, Rao RV, et al. *Indian J Surg*. 1976;38:34–39.
47. Dandapat MC, Mohapatro SK, Patro SK. *Indian Med Gaz*. 1985;119(1):14–17.
48. Antonio J, Uelmen J, Rodriguez R. *Int J Sport Nutr Excer Metab*. 2000;10(2):208–215.
49. Rogerson S, Riches CJ, Jennings C, et al. *J Strength Cond Res*. 2007;21(2):348–353.
50. Tanev G, Zarkova S. Cited in Zarkova S. *Tribestan: Experimental and Clinical Investigations*. Sofia, Bulgaria: Chemical Pharmaceutical Research Institute. www.bpg.bg/tribestan/table.phtml. Accessed July 2009.
51. Gendzhev Z. *Tr Nauchnoizsled Khim Farm Inst*. 1985;15:241–250.
52. Lehmann R, Penman K. *Private communication*. 2002
53. Tapia MO, Giordano MA, Gueper HG. *Vet Hum Toxicol*. 1994;36(4):311–313.
54. Glastonbury JR, Doughty FR, Whitaker SJ, et al. *Aust Vet J*. 1984;61(10):314–316.
55. Waller G.R.Yamasaki K, eds. *Saponins Used in Food and Agriculture. Advances in Experimental Medicine and Biology*, vol. 405. New York: Plenum Press; 1996. pp. 381–382.
56. Saudan C, Baume N, Emery C, et al. *Forensic Sci Int*. 2008;178(1):e7–e10.
57. Walker D, Bird A, Flora T, et al. *Reprod Fertil Dev*. 1992;4(2):135–144.
58. Jameel JK, Kneeshaw PJ, Rao VS, Drew PJ. *Breast*. 2004;13(5):428–430.
59. Talasaz AH, Abbasi MR, Abkhiz S, et al. *Nephrol Dial Transplant*. 2010;25(11):3792–3793.
60. Schmidt M, Thomsen M, Bone K. *Nephrol Dial Transplant*. 2011;26(9):3065–3066. Author reply pp. 3066–7.

Turmeric

(*Curcuma longa* L.)

Synonyms

Curcuma domestica Val. (botanical synonym), Indian saffron (Engl), Kurkumawurzelstock, Gelbwurzel (Ger), rhizome de curcuma, safran des Indes (Fr), gurkemeje (Dan), jianghuang (Chin), shati (Sanskrit).

What is it?

The rhizome of *Curcuma longa* L. (turmeric) has been used as a medicine, spice and colouring agent for thousands of years. A native of India and South-East Asia, it is now cultivated in many countries, but India still accounts for a large percentage of current world production. Turmeric was listed in an Assyrian herbal dating from about 600 BC and was also mentioned by Dioscorides.

The yellow pigment curcumin is a key active component in turmeric. It has been extensively investigated and possesses a promiscuous pharmacology, demonstrating interaction with a wide range of biochemical pathways. Curcumin has been shown to influence a variety of molecular targets, including transcription factors, cytokines, growth factors, kinases and other enzymes. It has also demonstrated a considerable repertoire of anticancer and chemopreventative effects, although the former are mainly in vitro.

Effects

Anti-inflammatory (curcumin is a dual inhibitor of arachidonic acid metabolism, among other such effects); antioxidant (particularly by reducing lipid peroxidation and priming Nrf2/ARE); favourably influences cardiovascular function; antimicrobial (particularly by topical application); inhibits carcinogenesis and tumour promotion; exerts an array of tissue protective effects, including neuroprotective and hepatoprotective activity.

Traditional view

Turmeric has a long list of traditional health uses across many cultures. In India, it is regarded as a stomachic, tonic and blood purifier[1] and used for poor digestion, fevers, skin conditions, vomiting in pregnancy and liver disorders. Externally, it is applied for conjunctivitis, skin infections, cancer, sprains, arthritis, haemorrhoids and eczema.[1,2] Indian women also apply it to their skin to reduce hair growth.[3] Another common use is to promote wound healing.

In traditional Chinese medicine (TCM) different applications are attributed to the 'rhizome' and 'tuber'. Turmeric 'rhizome' is said to be a *Blood* and *Qi* (vital energy) stimulant with analgesic properties. It is used to treat chest and abdominal pain and distension, jaundice, frozen shoulder, amenorrhoea due to blood stasis and postpartum abdominal pain due to stasis. It is also applied to wounds and injuries.[4] The 'tuber' has similar properties, but is used in hot conditions, as it is considered to be more cooling. One particular application is viral hepatitis.[5]

Traditional Thai medicinal uses include gastrointestinal ulcer, anal haemorrhage, vaginal haemorrhage, skin disease, ringworm, insect bites and to prevent gonorrhoea and the common cold.[6]

In earlier Western herbal medicine, turmeric was regarded as an aromatic digestive stimulant and as a cure for jaundice.[7]

Summary actions

Anti-inflammatory, antioxidant, hypolipidaemic, choleretic, cholagogue, antimicrobial, carminative, depurative, anticarcinogenic, antitumour, radioprotective, neuroprotective, hepatoprotective, nephroprotective, cardioprotective, vasoprotective.

Can be used for

Indications supported by clinical trials

From clinical trials on curcumin: rheumatoid arthritis (small, uncontrolled), postoperative inflammation, osteoarthritis, precancerous conditions (internal use, uncontrolled), tropical pancreatitis (with piperine), induction of gallbladder contraction, stabilisation of inflammatory bowel disease, HIV-associated chronic diarrhoea (uncontrolled), idiopathic orbital inflammatory syndrome (uncontrolled), chronic anterior uveitis (uncontrolled), psoriasis (topical, uncontrolled), monoclonal gammopathy.

From clinical trials on turmeric: osteoarthritis (and in combination), elevated blood lipids (uncontrolled), precancerous lesions (topical or internal, uncontrolled), irritable bowel syndrome (uncontrolled).

Traditional therapeutic uses

Topically for skin disorders and to promote healing; internal use for poor digestion and liver function.

May also be used for

Extrapolations from pharmacological studies

Inflammatory conditions such as asthma, infection, eczema, psoriasis; long-term prevention and treatment of cardiovascular disease, adjunct in the treatment of hyperlipidaemia; prevention of cancer and as an adjunct to cancer treatment; to improve gastric and hepatic function; as a clinically targeted antioxidant. Topically for inflammation, skin diseases and skin infections.

Preparations

Dried root as a decoction; liquid extract, tablets, capsules, oleoresin or essential oil for internal or external use. The powdered root is also used externally.

There are many phytopharmaceutical preparations available containing either pure curcumin or, more typically, a mixture of the three key curcuminoids extracted and isolated from turmeric. Some of these preparations claim enhanced bioavailability for curcuminoids.

Dosage

Turmeric can be taken as the powdered rhizome or the 1:1 liquid extract prepared using 45% ethanol or higher. The dose for the liquid extract is 5 to 14 mL/day, best taken in four to five equal doses throughout the day. A heaped teaspoon of powdered turmeric (about 4 g) can be mixed with water or milk to form a slurry and consumed one to two times daily. A teaspoon of lecithin can be added to improve absorption. Taking turmeric as a powder may be more desirable for anti-inflammatory effects, since aqueous extracts devoid of essential oil or curcumin also have shown some activity. Turmeric extracts should be stored in dark glass away from direct sunlight due to the decomposition of curcumin on exposure to light.

Duration of use

May be taken in the long term within the recommended dosage.

Summary assessment of safety

No adverse effects from ingestion of turmeric are expected when consumed within the recommended dosage.

Technical data

Botany

Turmeric, a member of the Zingiberaceae (ginger) family, is a perennial herb growing up to 1 m high with large tufted leaves. The leaf blade is long and tapers to the base. Pale yellow flowers containing three petals appear close to ground level. The rhizome is oblong or cylindrical and often short-branched. Its external colour is brown and internally ranges from yellow to yellow-orange.[8,9] The rhizome consists of two parts: an egg-shaped primary rhizome and several cylindrical and branched secondary rhizomes growing from the primary rhizome. These two parts were once differentiated in the Western trade as C. rotunda and C. longa.[10] In TCM this differentiation is retained, the primary rhizome being called the 'tuber' and the secondary rhizome the 'rhizome'.[5]

Adulteration

Confusion with Curcuma xanthorrhiza (Javanese turmeric) or C. zedoaria (zedoary) occurs rarely.[9,11] C. aromatica is often used as a medicinally interchangeable species in TCM.[4,12]

Powdered turmeric is sometimes adulterated with synthetic dyes.[13]

Key constituents

* Essential oil (0.3% to 5%), containing sesquiterpene ketones (65% including ar-turmerone), zingiberene (25%), phellandrene, sabinene, cineole, borneol[14]
* Yellow pigments (3% to 6%) known as diarylheptanoids or curcuminoids, including curcumin (diferuloylmethane) and demethoxylated curcumins.[14,15]

ar-Turmerone

	R^1	R^2
Curcumin	OCH$_3$	OCH$_3$
Desmethoxycurcumin	OCH$_3$	H
Bisdesmethoxycurcumin	H	H

Diarylheptanoids

Pharmacodynamics

The clinical relevance of the numerous in vitro pharmacological studies on curcumin (or its intravenous use) is uncertain, especially in the context of oral (but not topical) use of turmeric. This is because curcumin appears to undergo rapid biotransformation during and after gastrointestinal absorption. (See also the Pharmacokinetics section.) The biotransformation products of curcumin need to be further studied, since oral doses of curcumin have exerted significant activity in several experimental models and clinical trials.

Owing to the extensive pharmacological work on curcumin, this monograph has drawn substantially from published reviews. It is likely that in many cases what is referred to as 'curcumin' in a published work is in fact the natural mixture of curcuminoids extracted from turmeric. Sometimes this is explicitly stated, and if so it has been noted in this monograph.

Anti-inflammatory activity of curcumin

The anti-inflammatory activity of curcumin was first reported in 1971.[16] In an extension of this work,[17] it was reported that oral doses of curcumin possess significant anti-inflammatory action in both acute and chronic animal models. Curcumin was as potent as phenylbutazone and almost as potent as cortisone in the acute test (carrageenan oedema), but only about half as potent as phenylbutazone in chronic tests.[17]

NF-kappaB is one of the key transcription factors responsive to curcumin. It suppresses NF-kappaB activation by a variety of factors in vitro, including (TNF)-alpha and phorbol esters. A range of cells have been used in these studies, including mouse macrophages, embryonic kidney cells and tumour cell lines. The mechanism appears to be via reduced IkappaB-alpha phosphorylation and degradation, suggesting that curcumin acts a step above IkappaB kinase (IKK) in the NF-kappaB activation pathway. In fact many of the observed pharmacological influences of curcumin are NF-kappaB-dependent, not just the anti-inflammatory effects. Curcumin also suppresses activation of the serine/threonine protein kinase Akt and its association with IKK, suggesting its effects on NF-kappaB may be a downstream consequence of influence on upstream targets.[18]

Curcumin modulates the inflammatory response in vitro by downregulating the impact of cyclo-oxygenase-2 (COX-2), lipoxygenase (LOX) and inducible nitric oxide synthase (iNOS). The inhibition of COX-2 and iNOS expression is likely accomplished by curcumin's suppression of NF-kappaB activation.[19] In other words, curcumin probably inhibits the transcription of these proteins, rather than their enzymatic activities. Curcumin also inhibited inflammation and arachidonic acid (AA) metabolism in vivo in mouse skin epidermis via downregulation of COX and LOX.[20]

However, curcumin has been also shown to directly influence the activity of LOX in vitro, thereby inhibiting inflammatory leukotriene formation. Such activity has been demonstrated in vivo in skin after topical application to mouse epidermis and in the rat colonic mucosa after ingestion of 0.2% dietary curcumin. Curcumin may also regulate LOX through the inhibition of transforming growth factor (TGF)-alpha signalling.[21]

Several studies have demonstrated the in vitro suppression of cytokine production by curcumin, including interleukin (IL)-6 and IL-8. These observations may be secondary to the suppression of intermediary signalling pathways such as NF-kappaB by curcumin.[18] Downregulation of protein kinase C may be another mechanism.[19]

Peroxisome proliferator-activated receptor (PPAR)-gamma is a nuclear receptor and transcription factor involved in cell cycle control, proliferation and differentiation, exerting anti-inflammatory, anticancer and insulin-sensitising actions. It is highly expressed in adipose tissue and colonic mucosa, where tight control of proliferation, differentiation and apoptosis is vital for homeostasis and prevention of oncogenesis; here PPAR-gamma may have a tumour suppressor function. It is activated by prostaglandins and possibly by dietary components such as linolenic and linoleic acids. Curcumin induces and activates PPAR-gamma in rat hepatic stellate cells, a liver cell type responsible for fibrosis in liver injury that contributes to chronic liver damage and cirrhosis. PPAR-gamma activity is also enhanced in other cell lines by curcumin.[18]

In health, fibroblasts produce low levels of matrix metalloproteinases (MMPs) that remain largely in latent form and mediate physiological extracellular matrix turnover. In inflammatory disease, MMPs are overexpressed and become activated, causing unchecked tissue destruction, fibrosis and further increases in immune cell activation. MMPs also play a key role in tumour progression. Curcumin downregulates MMP production in various cell types in vitro. For example, in human fibrosarcoma cells, it decreases invasion, migration and production of MMP-2 and MMP-9, and in human and rabbit peripheral blood mononuclear cells it reduces MMP-9. Recently, it has been shown to reduce MMP-9 in human intestinal epithelial cells.[18]

Slaked lime is traditionally mixed with powdered turmeric for topical application as an anti-inflammatory agent.[22] This process probably increases the water solubility of curcumin through salt formation. The anti-inflammatory action of sodium curcuminate (0.1 to 0.5 mg/kg, ip) was investigated in rats in early research as an experimental model of this traditional use.[23] Sodium curcuminate exhibited considerably higher anti-inflammatory activity than either curcumin (1 to 10 mg/kg, ip) or hydrocortisone (10 mg/kg, ip) in acute and chronic tests. This was confirmed in a later study, which also found that curcumin and sodium curcuminate were more potent than phenylbutazone in acute and chronic models.[24] However, curcumin was only one-tenth as active as ibuprofen at reducing subacute inflammation.[25]

NSAIDs (non-steroidal anti-inflammatory drugs) such as phenylbutazone can cause gastric ulceration. In earlier research curcumin was found to have a lower ulcerogenic index (0.60) than a nearly equivalent active dose of phenylbutazone (1.70).[17] However, curcumin given orally for 6 consecutive days to rats caused gastric ulceration at a dose of 100 mg/kg, but not at 50 mg/kg.[26] In contrast, lower doses of curcumin in guinea pigs protected against gastric ulceration from phenylbutazone[27] but not histamine.[28] Ulceration caused by high doses of curcumin is associated with a marked reduction in mucin secretion.[26]

Several recent studies in various rodent disease models provide strong preclinical evidence for the anti-inflammatory activity of curcumin. For example, in multidrug-resistant gene-deficient (MDR) mice, which spontaneously develop colitis, addition of curcumin to their diet significantly reduced intestinal inflammation. Other investigators used 2,4-dinitro-chlorobenzene-induced colitis in rats to show a dose-dependent improvement in disease activity parameters following dietary curcumin that was of equal potency to sulfasalazine treatment. Curcumin was associated with a reduction in colonic NF-kappaB, iNOS and various measures of oxidative stress, for example myeloperoxidase and lipid peroxidation.[18] In two rat models of experimentally induced pancreatitis, curcumin (200 mg/kg, as a single iv dose) decreased inflammation by markedly decreasing activation of NF-kappaB, iNOS and other inflammatory factors.[29]

Curcumin may also possess an indirect anti-inflammatory activity via the adrenal cortex, although results are conflicting. Curcumin was less effective in adrenalectomised rats,[17] whereas sodium curcuminate maintained its activity.[24] A single dose of sodium curcuminate did not alter plasma cortisol levels,[16] but prolonged doses of curcumin doubled plasma cortisol.[25] It is possible that curcumin and sodium curcuminate may be acting via different mechanisms.

Anti-inflammatory activity of turmeric extracts and essential oil

Injected doses of the petroleum ether extract of turmeric, and two fractions isolated from it, demonstrated significant anti-inflammatory activity when compared against hydrocortisone and phenylbutazone in acute and chronic tests.[30] Successive extraction of turmeric with petroleum ether followed by 50% alcohol and then water gave yields of 2%, 9% and 10% respectively.[31] These fractions, representing 21% by weight of the components of turmeric, were then compared for anti-inflammatory activity. In both acute and chronic tests, the aqueous extract was significantly more active and was often more active than reference drugs such as hydrocortisone and oxyphenbutazone. Unfortunately no fraction was chemically characterised and the doses were administered by intraperitoneal injection, both factors which make the relevance of these findings to the action of oral doses of turmeric difficult to interpret.

Topical application of aqueous extract of turmeric delayed corneal wound healing in rabbits indicative of 'cortisone-like' anti-inflammatory activity.[32] An aqueous-alcoholic extract was inactive, but this also corresponded to a much lower dose of turmeric. Since curcumin is relatively insoluble in water this local 'cortisone-like' effect must be due to other components of turmeric.

A diethyl ether extract of turmeric inhibited platelet aggregation and altered eicosanoid biosynthesis in human platelets (see below).[33] This research suggests that turmeric may have anti-inflammatory activity partly due to its inhibition of AA uptake and release from membrane phospholipids.

Oral doses of the essential oil of turmeric were studied in adjuvant arthritis in rats.[34] Significant anti-inflammatory activity was found in this long-term test at a dose of 0.1 mL/kg. The essential oil also has antihistaminic properties,[35] which may explain the anti-inflammatory effect observed in a short-term test.[34] An oil-depleted extract of turmeric demonstrated anti-inflammatory properties in a well-validated rat model of rheumatoid arthritis.[36] The extract contained 40.6% total curcuminoids. It was effective when given 4 days prior to arthritis induction (4 mg/kg/day curcuminoids, ip), but not if administered after. An extract containing 93.6% total curcuminoids was more effective. Joint inflammation was reduced by 48% on day 3 and by 45% on day 23 when oral doses were administered 4 days prior (120 mg/kg/day curcuminoids).

Antiplatelet activity

Agents that cause a relative inhibition of platelet aggregation may be useful in the prevention and treatment of cardiovascular degeneration. In early research, sodium curcuminate had no effect on in vitro platelet aggregation stimulated by ADP, adrenaline (epinephrine) or collagen.[24] However, curcumin inhibited ADP-, collagen- and adrenaline- (epinephrine-) induced platelet aggregation in vitro and ex vivo with about the same activity as aspirin.[37] Unlike aspirin, curcumin did not decrease prostacyclin synthesis in rat thoracic aorta in vitro. The suggestion that curcumin selectively inhibits thromboxane production was supported by a contemporary publication.[38] In this study, curcumin was found to inhibit thromboxane production from platelets in vitro and ex vivo. Also, it was found that increasing doses of curcumin (25 to 200 mg/kg, ip) progressively protected against collagen- or adrenaline- (epinephrine-) induced thrombosis in mice, whereas increasing doses of aspirin beyond a certain level (15 mg/kg, ip) afforded decreased protection. This again suggests a thromboxane-inhibiting, but prostacyclin-sparing, activity for curcumin.

In further work, curcumin inhibited platelet aggregation induced by arachidonate, adrenaline (epinephrine) and collagen in vitro. It inhibited thromboxane B_2 production from exogenous radiolabelled arachidonate in washed platelets (with a concomitant increase in the formation of 12-LOX products), reduced the incorporation of arachidonate into platelet phospholipids, and inhibited the liberation of free arachidonic acid.[39] A similar in vitro study found that curcumin suppressed platelet aggregation induced by adrenaline (epinephrine), platelet activating factor, collagen and arachidonic acid.[40] In this study, curcumin inhibited thromboxane A_2 and intracellular calcium influx, but had no effect on protein kinase C. The sesquiterpene ketone ar-turmerone has also demonstrated an ability to inhibit platelet aggregation induced by collagen and AA in vitro.[41] The compound had no effect on thrombin-induced platelet aggregation or platelet activating factor, but was significantly more effective than aspirin in inhibiting collagen-induced platelet aggregation.

A diethyl ether extract of turmeric inhibited AA- but not ADP- and collagen-induced platelet aggregation in vitro and also inhibited thromboxane production from exogenous AA in washed platelets.[33] The turmeric extract also reduced the incorporation of AA into platelet phospholipids and AA release under appropriate stimulation. The chemical content of the diethyl ether extract was not investigated. The author noted that a low incidence of cardiovascular disease is observed in the regions where spices such as turmeric are regularly consumed. Chinese research found that turmeric extract and curcumin enhanced fibrinolytic activity and inhibited platelet aggregation, but the essential oil was devoid of these activities.[4]

Most of these investigations were in vitro, and it remains to be established if either curcumin or turmeric possesses significant clinical antiplatelet activity.

Antioxidant activity

The antioxidant activity of curcumin has been extensively studied over more than 30 years. Earlier research focused on its direct antioxidant activity in vitro. Curcumin inhibited in vitro lipid peroxide formation in liver homogenates from oedemic mice[16] and was also an inhibitor of lipid peroxidation in brain tissue.[42] Lipid peroxidation induced by air on linoleic acid was inhibited by curcumin and related diarylheptanoids extracted from turmeric.[43] These natural curcuminoids also inhibited haemolysis and lipid peroxidation of mouse erythrocytes induced by hydrogen peroxide, but were not as active as vitamin E.[44] Curcumin had a weaker scavenging effect than vitamin C on active oxygen radicals generated by polymorphonuclear leucocytes, but was stronger than vitamin E.[45] However, curcumin had the strongest scavenging effect on hydroxyl radicals.

Curcumin was as effective as the antioxidant BHA in inhibiting lipid peroxidation.[46] Curcumin protected DNA against single-strand breaks induced by singlet oxygen. The observed antioxidant activity was both time- and dose-dependent. The protective ability of curcumin was higher than that of lipoate, alpha-tocopherol and beta-carotene.[47] Curcumin reduced experimentally generated nitrite in vitro. This NO-scavenging activity was also exhibited by other curcuminoids.[48]

More significantly, curcumin also appears to activate other cellular antioxidants such as heme oxygenase-1, NADPHquinone oxidoreductase-1 and glutathione by stimulating PKC activation of the antioxidant response element (ARE)-Nrf2 signalling pathway.[49] Nuclear factor-erythroid-2-related factor (Nrf2) plays a crucial role in the coordinated induction of those genes encoding many stress-responsive and cytoprotective enzymes (including the antioxidant enzymes mentioned above), and related proteins. The simplistic view of antioxidants as mere chemical reactants with free radicals has been challenged by the discovery of Nrf2, which instead delineates critical gene regulatory roles for important 'antioxidant' phytochemicals.

A 2008 review noted that curcumin in vitro upregulated Nrf2-ARE-regulated pathways in a variety of cell lines.[50] At 0.05% in the diet it increased expression, nuclear translocation and ARE binding of Nrf2 in the liver and lungs of mice, and increased hepatic phase II detoxification pathways. In rats curcumin (200 mg/kg, oral) increased the DNA binding of the Nrf2-ARE complex in the liver and reduced dimethylnitrosamine-induced hepatotoxicity.[50]

Capsaicin and curcumin were fed to rats on a diet containing 8% by weight of coconut oil, olive oil, peanut oil or cod liver oil for 8 weeks. Macrophages isolated from treated animals produced lower levels of reactive oxygen species (ROS) compared with macrophages from the control groups fed the oil alone. A hydroalcoholic extract of turmeric administered orally to mice (4 mg/kg/day, delivering 0.4 mg/kg/day curcumin) for 4 weeks resulted in a decrease in both plasma and liver lipid peroxide levels, compared to controls.[51] Turmeric extract (equivalent to 20 mg/day curcumin, oral) for 45 days dramatically decreased blood lipid peroxide levels in an uncontrolled study involving 18 healthy men.[52]

The efficacy of curcumin in preventing cataract formation was tested ex vivo in a rat model. Lenses from curcumin-treated rats were much more resistant to oxidant-induced opacification than were lenses from control animals.[53] In another study, one group of rats treated with naphthalene, a known opacification agent, were also supplemented with 0.005% of dietary curcumin.[54] Curcumin produced significantly less opacity of the lens compared to the rats given only naphthalene. In a more recent study, rats treated with curcumin (75 mg/kg, oral) and then administered selenium showed no lens opacities and exhibited significantly less oxidative damage than control animals.[55]

An aqueous extract of turmeric was also found to be an effective inhibitor of oxidation in vitro. An unidentified water-soluble antioxidant from turmeric extended 80% protection to DNA against oxidative injury and had potential as an antipromoter. The active component may have been an antioxidant protein, which has recently been isolated.[56] However, this constituent probably does not account for the in vivo antioxidant activity of turmeric, since it would not be present in ethanolic extracts and is probably not absorbed after oral doses.

Hepatoprotective and nephroprotective activities

Curcumin has demonstrated hepatoprotective effects, which appear to be linked to antioxidant activity. Curcumin inhibited the formation of ROS and apoptosis in human hepatocytes treated with methylglyoxal and induced heme oxygenase-1 in vitro.[57] Curcumin inhibited collagen synthesis and hepatic stellate cell activation in vitro and in vivo, and may therefore help prevent hepatic fibrosis.[58,59] The hepatoprotective activity of curcumin has been demonstrated in vivo using various hepatotoxic agents, including carbon tetrachloride,[60] alcohol,[61] cadmium,[62] N-nitrosodiethylamine[63] and chloroquine.[64] Curcumin normalised hepatic glutathione,[65] glutathione-S-transferase and gamma-glutamyltransferase in response to damage in rats.[66] Additionally, it appears to block the endotoxin-mediated activation of NF-kappaB and suppress the expression of cytokines, chemokines, COX-2 and iNOS in Kupffer cells ex vivo.[67] A recent study concluded that curcumin improved survival and minimised oxidative stress, cellular injury and inflammation in induced hepatic failure in rats due to reduced NF-kappaB binding and iNOS expression.[68] Intraperitoneal doses of 200 or 400 mg/kg/day were given 48 h prior to the first of two doses of thioacetamide. Survival was much better in the curcumin treated animals, as compared with controls. However the higher dose of curcumin produced more significant results.

Oral administration of curcumin (30 mg/kg, oral) reduced iron-induced hepatic damage in rats by lowering lipid peroxidation.[69] Dietary turmeric (1%) lowered lipid peroxidation in normal rats (compared with controls) by enhancing the activities of antioxidant enzymes (superoxide dismutase (SOD), catalase, glutathione peroxidase).[70] A similar study demonstrated that dietary turmeric reduced iron-induced lipid peroxidation and triacylglycerol deposition in the liver ex vivo.[71] After finding a protective effect for turmeric extract against carbon tetrachloride-induced hepatotoxicity in mice, the various constituents of turmeric were examined for in vitro hepatoprotective activity.[72] Curcumin and related diarylheptanoids (curcuminoids) exhibited considerable intrinsic activity; that is, activity that was not due to their metabolites.

Curcumin may also have nephroprotective properties due to its antioxidant and anti-inflammatory activities. Curcumin reduced nephrotoxicity in gentamicin-treated rats.[73] Animals treated with gentamicin only exhibited significantly higher levels of the drug (39%) in renal cortex, 31% less glutathione and a 27% reduction in the activity of SOD. Curcumin at a dose of 200 mg/kg/day for 10 days significantly curtailed these effects. Another study published in the same year investigated the effects of curcumin on cyclosporine-induced nephrotoxicity in vivo.[74] Curcumin (15 mg/kg/day, oral, administered concurrently) significantly attenuated renal dysfunction and reduced oxidative stress by restoring glutathione, SOD and catalase levels to normal. Curcumin and its metabolite tetrahydrocurcumin have also demonstrated nephroprotective active in additional in vivo models.[75]

Neuroprotective activity

Curcumin (200 to 300 mg/kg, ip) demonstrated neuroprotective potential in cerebral ischaemia reperfusion injury in rats, an effect thought to be largely mediated by antioxidant mechanisms.[76,77] Additionally, an in vivo study evaluated the neuroprotective effects of curcumin (200 mg/kg/day, ip) on neural death in the hippocampus following transient forebrain ischaemia in rats.[78] Immediate treatment, treatment after 3 h and treatment after 24 h all significantly reduced neural damage, as assessed 7 days after injury. Treatment with curcumin increased glutathione, SOD and catalase activities. Rats pretreated with curcumin were protected against cerebral oedema caused by infection.[79] The authors theorised that the effects may be associated with antioxidant activity together with an inhibition of cytokine production. Intraperitoneal curcumin (30 mg/kg) demonstrated the possible ability to chelate lead (lead acetate 20 mg/kg) in vivo, as evidenced by its reduction of the neurotoxic activity of this metal in rats.[80]

The possible preventative role of curcumin in Alzheimer's disease (AD) is receiving considerable research attention. A review found that curcumin was able to target at least eight anti-amyloid toxicity mechanisms in vitro. Findings from experiments using animal models suggest that curcumin suppressed beta-amyloid plaque accumulation.[81] For example, dietary curcumin lowered oxidative brain damage and plaque build-up in two models of AD. A report using direct multiphoton microscopy to observe amyloid plaque in an AD mouse model showed the ability of curcumin to enter the brain, bind plaque and reduce plaque size by 30%.[81]

Cardioprotective and vasoprotective activities

The effects of both turmeric and curcumin have been evaluated on myocardial ischaemia reperfusion injury in vivo. The cardioprotective effects of turmeric were evaluated using the whole extract (100 mg/kg, oral) in rats with ischaemia-induced myocardial infarction.[82] Turmeric reduced oxidative stress by restoring antioxidant status and improved ventricular function. In another study, curcumin was found to reduce myocardial infarct size, serum creatine phosphokinase and lactate dehydrogenase activity.[83] Additionally, glutathione peroxidase and SOD activity were significantly increased. Hence curcumin appeared to exert protective effects on myocardial ischaemic injury due to its exogenous and endogenous antioxidant capabilities. A single oral dose (15 mg/kg) of curcumin pre- and post-ischaemic injury led to decreased levels of xanthine oxidase, superoxide anion, lipid peroxides and myeloperoxidase, and increased SOD, catalase, glutathione peroxidase and glutathione-S-transferase.[84]

Two recent reviews have focused on the cardioprotective role of curcumin.[85,86] Curcumin reduced doxorubicin-induced cardiotoxicity in rats and exerted protective activity in two different in vivo models of congestive heart failure.[85] A favourable modulating effect in cardiac remodelling following pressure overload or myocardial ischaemia was noted from other studies.[86]

Hypolipidaemic activity

Curcumin upregulated low-density lipoprotein (LDL) receptors in vitro in murine macrophages.[87] Two-thirds of LDL clearance is mediated through these receptors, and in many cases high LDL-cholesterol is a result of either their mutation (familial hypercholesterolaemia) or suppression. Curcumin increased LDL uptake by up to 13 times more than controls.[87] A subsequent study using the human hepatoma cell line HepG2 found that curcumin effected a 7-fold increase in LDL receptor mRNA and regulated gene expression controlling lipid/cholesterol homeostasis.[88]

Early toxicity studies on rats to establish the safety of turmeric extracts as a colouring agent also found that liver levels of total cholesterol were somewhat lower than normal.[89] A subsequent study revealed that turmeric extract and curcumin counteracted the increase in liver cholesterol in rats induced by cholesterol feeding.[90] Dietary levels of curcumin as low as 0.1% significantly reduced the rises in serum and liver cholesterol in rats fed cholesterol, but did not lower serum cholesterol in rats fed a normal diet.[91] It was also observed that curcumin increased the faecal excretion of bile acids and cholesterol in both the normal and hypercholesterolaemic rats and counteracted the rise in body and liver weights caused by cholesterol intake. These findings would suggest that turmeric might raise the ratio of HDL-cholesterol to total cholesterol, and this was verified in a subsequent study on hyperlipidaemic rats.[92] Triglyceride levels were also significantly lower with turmeric treatment. Turmeric and curcumin had no effect on cholesterol levels of plasma, liver and egg yolk in hens fed a diet containing cholesterol.[93]

Oral administration of the ethanolic extract of turmeric (1.66 mg/kg) significantly reduced oxidation in erythrocyte and liver microsome membranes in rabbits fed a high fat diet.[94] These particular cell membranes are commonly affected in the atherosclerotic process, and a reduction in oxidative stress might help protect against some of the consequences of atherosclerotic changes. In another study, dietary curcumin (0.2%) produced a 10% to 14% decrease in the cholesterol content of erythrocyte membranes.[95] This study observed an increased osmotic fragility of erythrocytes in hypercholesterolaemic rats, which curcumin appeared to reduce by improving the lipid profile. A whole extract of turmeric (1.66 mg/kg containing 10% curcuminoids, oral) significantly reduced both oxidative stress and the formation of fatty streaks in rabbits fed a high cholesterol diet.[96]

Dietary curcumin (0.5%) decreased serum total cholesterol by 21% and LDL-cholesterol by 42.5% in rats fed a high cholesterol diet.[97] Additionally, HDL-cholesterol was increased by 50% and the activities of aspartate aminotransferase (AST) and alanine aminotransferase (ALT) were significantly reduced compared to control animals. The effects of a combination of dietary curcuminoids (curcumin 73.4%) were investigated on lipid metabolism in rats.[98] Concentrations of hepatic cholesterol and plasma VLDL were significantly lower in the group fed 1% curcuminoids, and hepatic acyl-CoA oxidase activity was significantly higher.

The activity of hepatic cholesterol 7-alpha-hydroxylase (the rate-limiting enzyme of bile acid biosynthesis) was significantly elevated in rats fed curcumin. Serum and liver microsomal cholesterol contents were also significantly higher. However, the simultaneous stimulation of cholesterol synthesis by curcumin suggests that this may not be the key mechanism behind its hypocholesterolaemic action, which may be largely due to interference with exogenous cholesterol absorption.[99]

In experimentally induced diabetic rats maintained on a 0.5% curcumin-containing diet for 8 weeks, blood cholesterol was lowered significantly, exclusively as the LDL-VLDL fraction. Significant decreases in blood triglyceride and phospholipids were also observed. Hepatic cholesterol 7-alpha-hydroxylase activity was markedly higher, suggesting a higher rate of cholesterol catabolism.[100]

Effects on the digestive tract

Early in vivo research demonstrated that the essential oil of turmeric[101] and curcumin[102] increased bile secretion, but the aqueous extract of turmeric was inactive. Curcumin and the essential oil were each about half as active as sodium deoxycholate administered the same way.[103] Sodium curcuminate induced a stimulation of bile flow, although the concentration of solids in the bile was somewhat decreased.[104] At higher doses, total excretion of bile salts, bilirubin and cholesterol were enhanced. Such a finding is consistent with animal feeding experiments with curcumin, which also found increased bile acid and cholesterol excretion.[91]

Mice with pre-established cholesterol gallstones were fed a diet containing curcumin (0.5%) for 5 or 10 weeks. A regression of gallstones occurred in 45% after 5 weeks and in 80% after 10 weeks, compared to controls. Biliary cholesterol decreased and phospholipids and bile acids increased over the duration of feeding.[56] Feeding a lithogenic diet supplemented with 0.5% curcumin for 10 weeks reduced the incidence of gallstone formation by 74% compared to mice fed the lithogenic diet alone. Biliary cholesterol concentration, lithogenic index and the cholesterol/phospholipid ratio of bile were also reduced.[105]

A test meal of 0.5 g/kg of turmeric in rabbits did not show any change in the volume, acid or pepsin content of gastric secretions, but the mucin content was considerably increased.[106] This contrasts with studies using high doses of curcumin that found ulceration in association with a marked decrease in mucin secretion.[26] Oral doses of 0.5 g/kg of an ethanolic extract of turmeric produced significant protection against ulceration caused by stress, pyloric ligation, indomethacin and reserpine in rats.[107] Turmeric extract increased gastric wall mucus production and also enhanced its cytoprotective quality. More recent studies have attempted to shed further light on how curcumin protects and heals the gastric mucosa. Curcumin prevented glutathione depletion, lipid peroxidation and protein oxidation in indomethacin-induced acute gastric ulceration in rats.[108] Interestingly, both oral and intraperitoneal administration of curcumin prevented gastric ulceration. The authors propose that this may involve the action of curcumin on MMP-2 and -9, which are involved in normal tissue remodelling and wound healing. In another study, curcumin was found to offer 82% protection against the development of indomethacin-induced gastric ulcers at an ip dose of 25 mg/kg.[109] Turmeric may also protect against gastric ulceration by blocking the H2 histamine receptor.[110] However, this study was conducted in vitro. Curcumin has also been shown to inhibit the induction of pro-inflammatory cytokines induced by *Helicobacter pylori* in vitro.[111]

Curcumin is a chelator of hepatic iron in vivo. In a recent study, mice fed dietary curcumin exhibited a reduction in ferritin protein in the liver.[112]

Curcuminoids may also display spasmolytic activity. Studies on the smooth muscle of isolated guinea-pig ileum and rat uterus demonstrated that the force of contraction was significantly reduced.[113]

Antimicrobial activity

An alcoholic extract of turmeric, its essential oil and curcumin inhibited the growth of Gram-positive bacteria in vitro.[114] However, the antibacterial activity of turmeric is much weaker than conventional antibiotics.[115] The essential oil of turmeric has significant antifungal activity at dilutions of 1 in 500.[116]

An interesting discovery is that low concentrations of curcumin are highly toxic to Salmonella in the presence of visible light.[117] This phototoxic effect was thought to be due to unstable intermediates, probably free radicals formed during irradiation. Since an *Escherichia coli* strain with DNA repair capacity was largely resistant to curcumin phototoxicity, this implies that light in combination with curcumin is genotoxic and may be mutagenic. The authors concluded that the observed phototoxicity makes curcumin a potential photosensitising drug that may be useful in the phototherapy of psoriasis, cancer and bacterial and viral infections. This finding was confirmed by other workers who observed that curcumin is more phototoxic to Gram-positive bacteria than to Gram-negative bacteria.[118] Oxygen is required for the phototoxic effect and results suggested that hydrogen peroxide might be the toxic intermediate.

An extract of turmeric rhizome has demonstrated antimicrobial activity against strains of methicillin-resistant *Staphylococcus aureus* (MRSA) in vitro.[119] Turmeric also significantly decreased the minimum inhibitory concentrations (MICs) of ampicillin and oxacillin, thereby restoring their activity against MRSA. The ethyl acetate extract (MIC 1 to 4 mg/mL) demonstrated the most potent antibacterial activity, compared with the methanol and water extracts. Turmeric oil (the hexane extract of the rhizome) at in vitro dilutions of 1:40 to 1:320 inhibited 15 isolates of dermatophytes. At dilutions of 1:40 to 1:80 it also inhibited four isolates of pathogenic fungi (curcumin was inactive). Six isolates of yeasts were insensitive to turmeric oil and curcumin. Turmeric oil (diluted to 1:80) applied topically on the 7th day following dermatophytosis induction using *Trichophyton rubrum* in guinea pigs resulted in an improvement within 2 to 5 days after application. The lesion disappeared at days 6 to 7.[120] Curcumin inhibited human immunodeficiency virus (HIV) type-1 integrase in vitro[121] and is a modest inhibitor of the HIV-1 and HIV-2 proteases.[122]

In vitro and in vivo tests have demonstrated an antiviral activity for curcumin against herpes simplex virus (HSV) type 2.[123] In the in vivo component of this test, 15 μL of curcumin (100 mg/mL) was instilled vaginally in anaesthetised rats, followed by inoculation with the virus. Of the animals treated with curcumin only 33.3% developed the infection compared to 75% of control animals.

Antiparasitic activity

A 2010 review summarised the published research on *Curcuma* species as parasiticidal agents.[124] Much of this research has been conducted using turmeric or its curcuminoids. Curcuminoids were active against *Plasmodium falciparum* (the malaria parasite) in vitro at 3 to 4.2 μg/mL, concentrations almost 300 times higher than the control drug chloroquine. However, curcumin administered orally at 100 mg/kg/day for 5 days decreased parasitaemia of *P. berghei*-infected mice by 80% to 90%. Synergistic in vivo studies of curcumin with artemisinin have yielded mixed results. Moderate activities against leishmania and schistosoma parasites have also been demonstrated in vitro and in vivo for curcumin. Research is continuing for a variety of other parasites.

Cancer prevention

Chemoprevention is the use of non-toxic agents to intervene in the multistage process of carcinogenesis. There is a substantial body of research demonstrating the chemopreventative properties of curcumin and curcuminoids. This is likely to result from several distinct mechanisms, as was summarised in a comprehensive review[125]:

> Curcumin inhibits tumour initiation by blocking the metabolic activation of carcinogens or by stimulating their detoxification. It also exerts antitumour-promoting effects by suppressing

inflammatory signalling mainly mediated by COX-2 and iNOS that are under the control of NF-kappaB and other transcription factors. Curcumin also acts in the progression stage of carcinogenesis by inhibiting metastasis and angiogenesis, which are crucial for the survival and spread of tumour cells. Furthermore, curcumin has antiproliferative effects that are attributed to its capability to induce apoptosis of precancerous and malignant cells or inhibit the cell cycle progression.

The same review summarised the in vitro and in vivo data supporting these propositions.[125] Inhibition of carcinogen activation by downregulation of cytochrome P450 activity or expression by curcumin has been demonstrated in liver cell lines and in rats and mice. Stimulation of carcinogen detoxification by induction or upregulation of phase II enzymes has also been observed, especially in vivo (rats and mice). Relevant anti-inflammatory activity impacting on carcinogenesis includes suppression of COX-2 and iNOS expression or activity in a variety of cell lines, including macrophages and human epithelial cells. Oncogene expression or activation has been inhibited, mainly in mouse skin cells, and potentiation of tumour suppressor function via increased p53 accumulation or phosphorylation has also been observed in vitro for a range of cell lines.[125] Another review noted that these activities of curcumin have also been demonstrated in several in vivo models, together with additional relevant mechanisms, including inhibition of NF-kappaB and MAPK (mitogen-activated protein kinase).[126]

(Other activities of curcumin relevant to its chemopreventative activity, namely apoptosis induction and inhibition of cell cycle progression, angiogenesis, metastasis and invasion, are reviewed in the section on Antitumour activity.)

A 2008 review noted that curcumin activates Nrf2 (nuclear-factor-erythroid-2-related factor 2) which plays a crucial role in the coordinated induction of those genes encoding many stress-responsive and cytoprotective enzymes and related proteins.[50] These include phase II detoxification enzymes and antioxidant enzymes such as SOD. Nrf2 has been shown to be an important modulator of tumour susceptibility in animal models of carcinogenesis.[127]

The review noted above also summarised the anticarcinogenic effects of curcumin demonstrated in animal studies.[125] The mouse skin carcinogenesis model allows study of molecular alterations associated with the multistep process of malignant transformation (namely initiation, promotion and progression). Topical application of curcumin has exhibited antipromotion activity against 12-O-tetradecanylphorbol-13-acetate-induced tumour promotion in such models. Curcumin also prevented the development of carcinogen-induced liver, colorectal, oral, oesophageal, gastric, duodenal, lung, mammary and immune cell tumours. Curcumin doses were typically administered via the diet at 0.2% to 2%.[125] A 2008 review additionally noted chemopreventative activity for curcumin in chemically induced prostate and oral cancer.[128]

Cancer preventative activity has also been shown for turmeric in various experimental models. Both curcumin and aqueous extract of turmeric protected against DNA damage induced by fuel smoke condensate in human lymphocytes.[129] Turmeric at 1% in the diet of mice reduced benzo(a) pyrene (BAP)-induced stomach tumours and also reduced the incidence of spontaneous mammary tumours.[130] A dose-dependent decrease in binding of BAP metabolites to calf thymus DNA was observed in the presence of turmeric, curcumin and aqueous turmeric extract, but not in the presence of curcumin-free aqueous turmeric extract. Further studies using mouse liver microsomes indicate that curcuminoids inhibit BAP-DNA adduct formation.[131]

It has been demonstrated that turmeric, like curcumin, increases the activity of the phase II carcinogen-detoxifying enzyme glutathione-S-transferase in the stomach, liver and oesophagus of mice.[132] Glutathione levels were also significantly elevated and the in vivo mutagenic effect of BAP in mouse bone marrow cells was suppressed. Curcuminoids are probably responsible for this activity.[133]

Curcuminoids and turmeric caused dose-dependent inhibition of nitrosomethylurea formation in vitro.[134] Nitrosamines are formed in cured meats via the reaction of secondary amines with nitrites added during manufacturing and are potent carcinogens.

Oral administration of turmeric to mice from 2 months of age caused a suppression of both mammary tumour virus-related reverse transcriptase activity and preneoplastic changes in mammary glands. Feeding turmeric from 6 months of age resulted in a 100% inhibition of mammary tumours.[135] In another study, turmeric (0.15%) was added to the diet of mice with a mutation of the APC gene.[136] Mice with this gene defect usually develop numerous intestinal adenomas by 15 weeks of age. However, tumour formation in the treatment group was reduced by approximately 63%.

Catechin in drinking water and dietary turmeric significantly inhibited the tumour burden and tumour incidence in two tumour models: experimentally induced forestomach tumour in mice and oral mucosal tumour in golden hamsters. Chemoprevention with both catechin and turmeric inhibited the gross tumour yield and burden more effectively in the two tumour models than either treatment alone.[137] Turmeric (2% or 5%) in the diet again significantly inhibited BAP-induced forestomach tumours in mice, and this was dose- and time-dependent. The 2% diet also significantly suppressed skin tumours in mice. The 5% turmeric diet for 7 consecutive days resulted in a 38% decrease in hepatic cytochrome b5 and cytochrome P450 levels. Glutathione content was increased by 12% and glutathione-S-transferase activity was enhanced by 32% in the liver.[138]

Antitumour activity

Curcumin is a potent cytotoxic agent in vitro against a wide variety of tumour cell lines of different tissue origin. Its activity is dependent on the cell type, the concentration of curcumin (IC_{50} range of 2 to 40μg/mL) and the time of exposure.[139] Studies in colon adenocarcinoma cell lines demonstrated that curcumin inhibited cell proliferation, causing cell cycle arrest, and induced apoptosis. Similar effects have been observed in breast, kidney, lung, pancreatic, gastric, ovarian, cervical, hepatocellular, lymphoid, myeloid, melanoma, oral epithelial and prostate cell lines derived from a variety of malignant tumours.[140] Curcumin has also shown growth inhibitory effects in vitro in human prostate, leukaemia, breast, large intestine, bone and bladder cancer cell lines. In this diverse range of studies, curcumin has been observed to exert variable effects on the cell cycle, probably dependent on the cell origin and tissue type.[140] A 2009 reviewed noted more than 100 in vitro studies where curcumin has demonstrated antiproliferative effects against cancer cell lines.[141]

Further mechanistic studies of curcumin have revealed a range of in vitro cytotoxic effects on cancer cell lines. The 2009 review mentioned above summarised the current knowledge.[141] Curcumin modulates the growth of tumour cells through regulation of multiple cell signalling pathways including aspects of the cell proliferation pathway (cyclin D1, c-myc), cell survival pathway (Bcl-2, Bcl-xL, cFLIP), caspase activation pathway (caspase-8, -3, -9), tumour suppressor pathway (p53, p21), death receptor pathway (DR4, DR5), mitochondrial pathways and the protein kinase pathway (JNK, Akt, AMPK). Several other pathways where curcumin is also active are reviewed. The authors noted that the reason why curcumin kills tumour cells and is generally not toxic to normal cells is not fully understood. Several reasons have been suggested, including enhanced curcumin uptake by tumour cells, the low glutathione in tumour cells (making them more sensitive to curcumin's effects) and the fact most tumour cells express constitutively active NF-kappaB that is important for their survival, whereas normal cells do not. Concerning the last point, curcumin can therefore inhibit tumour cell biochemistry by suppressing NF-kappaB-regulated gene products.[141]

The in vivo antitumour activity of curcumin has been investigated using tumour cells transplanted into normal animals (the xenograft model). Reduced tumour incidence or size and enhanced survival have been shown in several studies, generally for curcumin administered via injection or orally. Examples of models include Dalton's lymphoma cells in mice (50mg/kg, ip) HL60 leukaemia and SGC7901 lymphoma in nude mice (50 to 200mg/kg, oral), glioblastoma in mice (100mg/kg, intratumoral), human breast cancer cells in nude mice (2%, dietary), colorectal cancer cells in mice (40mg/kg, iv), squamous cell carcinoma cell lines in mice (topical application), pancreatic cells in nude mice (40mg/kg, iv), LNCaP prostate cancer cells in mice (2%, dietary) and ovarian cancer cells in athymic mice (500mg/kg, oral).[128] Another review also noted activity in xenograft models of hepatic and pulmonary cancers.[142]

Some antitumour activity has also been demonstrated for turmeric. A turmeric extract prepared with 50% ethanol inhibited the cell growth of normal mammalian cells and was cytotoxic to lymphoma cells at a concentration of 0.4mg/mL.[143] The active constituent was proposed as curcumin, which was cytotoxic to the lymphoma cells at a concentration of 4μg/mL. Injections of both turmeric extract and curcumin reduced the development of tumours and enhanced survival in mice injected with lymphoma cells.[143] Earlier work reported that a turmeric extract exhibited cytotoxicity to mammalian cells in vitro by arresting mitosis and altering chromosome morphology.[144]

Several studies have examined the antimetastatic potential of curcumin. One review suggested that curcumin possesses pronounced activity.[139] In one model it was found to inhibit pulmonary metastasis of melanoma cells in mice, with inhibition of MMPs. Curcumin was also highly antimetastatic against prostate cells in vitro and in vivo. In a human breast cancer xenograft model, the administration of curcumin markedly decreased metastasis to the lung and suppressed the expression of a number of factors including NF-kappaB, MMP-9 and COX-2. Curcumin also reduced the metastasis of tumours in LEC rats, which develop tumours of the kidney and liver due to aberrant copper metabolism.[139] Antimetastatic properties have also been demonstrated for curcumin in vitro.[125]

Angiogenesis, the formation of new blood vessels from the host vasculature, is critical for tumour growth and metastasis. A review noted that in vitro experiments have shown curcumin to be a direct inhibitor of angiogenesis. It also down-regulates various proangiogenic proteins such as vascular endothelial growth factor and basic fibroblast growth factor.[145] Curcumin's in vitro antiangiogenic effect is also in part due to its inhibitory effect on signal transduction pathways (including those involving protein kinase C and the transcription factors NF-kappaB and AP-1) and on two groups of proteinases involved in angiogenesis (MMPs and the urokinase plasminogen activator family). Curcumin also blocks cell adhesion molecules in vitro.[145] However, all these effects need to be established in vivo.

A review observed that curcumin is a potentially significant chemosensitiser in cancer chemotherapy.[146] Relevant key properties include reversal of MDR and blocking of NF-kappaB. Sensitisation of a variety of chemoresistant cell lines after treatment with curcumin has been demonstrated. Tetrahydrocurcumin, a major metabolite of curcuminoids in humans, is also active as an MDR inhibitor.[146] These findings need to be replicated in vivo.

Curcumin inhibits P-glycoprotein (P-gp) in vitro.[147] P-gp is an ATP-dependent drug efflux pump that is linked to the development of MDR in cancer cells. The inhibition of P-gp by curcumin may provide a novel approach for reversing multidrug resistance in tumour cells,[148] as MDR is a major cause of chemotherapy failure in cancer patients. Curcumin has been shown to reverse the MDR in many cancer cell lines, including gastric and cervical in vitro.[149–152]

Activity in cystic fibrosis models

Cystic fibrosis (CF) is caused by mutations in the cystic fibrosis transmembrane conductance regulator (CFTR) gene. Therefore compounds that can improve the function of the CFTR chloride channel may be of value in the treatment of this disorder. Deletion of phenylalanine 508 (deltaF508) accounts for nearly 70% of all mutations, and is responsible for the misfolding and retention of the CFTR protein in the endoplasmic reticulum.[153] A promising report demonstrated that curcumin corrected the defects in deltaF508 CF mice and was able to rectify the characteristic nasal potential difference defect and improve survival.[154] A subsequent investigation attempted to reproduce and extend this preclinical data.[155] Various curcumin preparations and treatment regimens were used, including that used above.[154] However, these different researchers failed to reproduce the initial results. A more recent study also found that curcumin failed to induce the maturation of deltaF508 CFTR, or induce chloride secretion in vitro and in vivo.[156] However, other subsequent

studies have been positive,[157–160] although more research is needed to understand if this intriguing effect of curcumin has clinical relevance.

Antidepressant activity

Turmeric is a major ingredient in Xiaoyao-san, a traditional Chinese medicinal formula used for the treatment of depression and related illness. Consequently recent investigations have attempted to validate the antidepressant effects of turmeric and curcumin in vivo. Oral administration of an aqueous extract of turmeric (140 to 560 mg/kg) for 14 days demonstrated dose-dependent improvements in tail suspension and swimming tests in mice.[161] Additionally, the 560 mg/kg dose was found to be more effective than the reference antidepressant fluoxetine. Doses of 140 mg/kg or above significantly inhibited monoamine oxidase MAO-A activity in a dose-dependent manner, and 560 mg/kg produced an observable MAO-B inhibitory activity.

Curcumin at oral doses of 5 and 10 mg/kg for 14 days also reduced the duration of immobility in both the tail suspension and swimming tests.[162] At doses of 10 mg/kg it was also able to produce a marked increase of serotonin and noradrenaline levels in both the frontal cortex and the hippocampus. Dopamine levels were also increased in the frontal cortex and the striatum. Like turmeric, curcumin was found to inhibit MAO activity. A subsequent study investigated the effects of curcumin at oral doses of 1.25 to 10 mg/kg for 14 days and found that it significantly reduced immobility time in the swim test and reversed behavioural abnormalities associated with the bilateral olfactory bulbectomy model.[163] This model induces low levels of serotonin and noradrenaline (norepinephrine) in the hippocampus, which were completely reversed by curcumin administration. The potential of curcumin as an antidepressant was the subject of a 2009 review.[164]

Skeletal muscle activity

Sepsis, injury and cancer can result in muscle wasting, mainly due to proteolysis. This phenomenon is partially regulated by the activation of NF-kappaB. A 2009 review examined in vivo evidence suggesting that curcumin may prevent loss of muscle mass during sepsis and endotoxaemia and may stimulate muscle regeneration after traumatic injury.[165] There are only a few studies. The most recent found that treatment of rats with curcumin (600 mg/kg, ip) blocked the sepsis-induced increase in muscle protein breakdown associated with NF-kappaB activation.[166] Another study in rats found that curcumin (10 to 60 μg/kg, ip) dose-dependently inhibited lipopolysaccharide-induced loss of muscle wasting and protein in mice.[167] A much earlier study observed that curcumin (10 to 40 μg/kg, ip) stimulated muscle regeneration after traumatic injury in mice.[168] The review did note that in other publications curcumin failed to prevent muscle atrophy caused by unloading, experimental cancer and muscular dystrophy.[165]

Pulmonary activity

Several studies have investigated the impact of curcumin on lung injury and fibrosis and these were the subject of a recent review.[169] Oral treatment with curcumin demonstrated beneficial activity in radiation, paraquat-, cyclophosphamide-, bleomycin- and amioderone-induced lung fibrosis in rats. Negative effects of nicotine-induced (rats) and endotoxic (mice) lung injury were also partially countered by oral curcumin. Doses were typically 200 to 300 mg/kg.[169]

Radioprotective activity

A review noted that oral pre- or post-treatment of mice with 5 to 20 mg/kg curcumin reduced the frequency of micronucleated polychromatic erythrocytes following exposure to gamma irradiation. In another study, oral administration of 400 μmol to mice reduced radiation-induced chromosomal damage. Feeding of 1% curcumin in the diet protected against radiation-induced mammary tumours in rats, and a dose of 200 mg/kg ameliorated radiation-induced mucositis. Radiation-induced delayed wound healing was reduced by curcumin (100 mg/kg, oral in mice) in several studies, together with enhanced overall survival.[170]

Curcumin has also demonstrated radiosensitising activity in vitro against various cancer cell lines.[170]

Antiallergic activity

A 2008 review explored the role of curcumin in the treatment of allergies. While it was claimed that curcumin has antiallergic activity in hypersensitivity reactions types I to IV in animal models, relatively few studies were reviewed.[171] Antiasthmatic activity was demonstrated in ovalbumin-induced airway hypersensitivity in guinea pigs and in a murine model of latex allergy. Curcumin was also active in a murine model of allergic aspergillosis.

Other activity

Turmeric (4 g/kg) and curcumin (0.4 g/kg) induced significant increases in hepatic levels of glutathione-S-transferase and acid-soluble sulphydryl after 14 or 21 days in lactating mice and translactationally exposed mouse pups. Cytochrome b5 and cytochrome P450 levels were also significantly elevated in the mice and their pups.[172] (See also the Cancer prevention section for an additional discussion of the effect of curcumin on phase II detoxifying enzymes.)

Curcumin can influence various cytochrome P450 (CYP) enzyme activities in vivo after toxic insult. In one study, rats were fed a curcumin rich diet (0.05, 0.5 and 5 g/kg diet) with or without the injection of carbon tetrachloride ($CCl_{(4)}$).[173] With curcumin only, all CYP enzymes remained unchanged, other than in the group fed 5 g/kg. Injection of $CCl_{(4)}$ drastically decreased CYP activity, but treatment with curcumin ameliorated this effect for all the CYP enzymes tested (1A, 2B, 2C and 3A), except CYP2E1. In a similar study, CYP enzymes were experimentally suppressed with a bacterial endotoxin.[174] Injection of curcumin significantly blocked the suppression of CYP3A2 and, in contrast to the study above, also inhibited the suppression of CYP2E1.

Turmeric has been utilised as a wound-healing agent since antiquity. Recent in vivo studies demonstrated that pretreatment with curcumin significantly enhanced wound contraction, decreased healing time, increased the synthesis of collagen, hexosamine, DNA and NO and improved fibroblast

and vascular densities in irradiated full excise wounds in mice.[175–177] A study investigating the healing potential of a paste containing fresh turmeric demonstrated that it was as effective as honey for the healing of full thickness wounds in rabbits.[178] Both treatment groups were significantly superior to the control group. (See also the Clinical trials section on this topic.)

Curcumin extended the lifespan of two different strains of fruit fly (*Drosophila melanogaster*), an effect that was accompanied by protection against oxidative stress, improvement in locomotion and chemopreventative activity.[179]

In human peripheral blood mononuclear cells, curcumin dose-dependently inhibited the responses to phytohaemagglutinin and mixed lymphocyte reaction. It dose-dependently inhibited the proliferation of rabbit vascular smooth muscle cells stimulated by fetal calf serum. Curcumin had a greater inhibitory effect on platelet-derived growth factor-stimulated proliferation than on serum-stimulated proliferation. It may therefore be beneficial in the prevention of the pathological changes associated with atherosclerosis and re-stenosis.[180]

Pharmacokinetics

Most investigations have examined the pharmacokinetics of curcumin or curcuminoids, rather than turmeric. There have been several reviews of this topic.[181–183] One such review concluded that the bioavailability of curcumin is poor due to low absorption, rapid metabolism (including reduction and conjugation immediately upon absorption by enterocytes) and rapid systemic elimination.[181]

The pharmacokinetic properties of curcumin have in fact been investigated since the 1970s. In the first ever published study, the uptake, distribution and excretion of curcumin was studied in rats.[184] When administered orally as a single dose of 1 g/kg, 65% to 85% of curcumin passed through the gastrointestinal tract unchanged and was found in the faeces. Only traces appeared in the urine and a small amount of curcumin was found in the bile, liver, kidneys and body fat. After intravenous injection, curcumin was actively transported into bile, but the majority was rapidly metabolised by the liver.

This poor bioavailability of curcumin was confirmed in a subsequent study on rats, which found that 38% of the administered 400 mg dose remained unchanged in the digestive tract.[185] Only traces were found in body tissues and no curcumin was detected in urine. A subsequent in vitro study suggested that curcumin undergoes transformation to a less polar, colourless compound(s) during absorption from the intestine,[186] a finding confirmed using radiolabelled curcumin.[187] While significant levels of radioactivity were absorbed, only traces of curcumin could be measured in body tissues. Subsequently, curcumin glucuronide, dihydrocurcumin glucuronide, tetrahydrocurcumin glucuronide and tetrahydrocurcumin were confirmed as the major metabolites of curcumin in mice, as noted in a 2000 review.[188]

Several subsequent rodent studies have yielded similar findings.[180,182] A relatively recent study in rats quantified the oral bioavailability of curcumin at 1%.[189] After oral administration of curcumin (500 mg/kg), Cmax was measured at 0.06 μg/mL, with a Tmax of 41.7 min.

A dose-escalation pilot study was designed to evaluate the pharmacokinetic properties of turmeric in humans.[190] Fifteen patients with advanced, treatment-resistant colorectal cancer received turmeric extract (440 to 2200 mg/day, containing 36 to 180 mg of curcumin) for up to 4 months. Curcumin demonstrated low bioavailability. Neither curcumin nor its metabolites were detected in blood or urine. In a phase I clinical trial, high dose curcumin (3.6 g/day for up to 4 months) produced low concentrations of detectable metabolites in blood and urine. However, it engendered 62% and 57% decreases in inducible PGE_2 production in blood samples taken on days 1 and 29 of treatment, respectively (compared with levels observed pre-dose, $p<0.05$).[191]

Another trial investigating the pharmacological effects of curcumin in women with colorectal cancer concluded that a daily dose of 3.6 g curcumin for 7 days achieved pharmacologically effective levels in the colon and rectum, but with negligible systemic distribution.[192] Twelve patients with hepatic metastases from colorectal cancer received 450 to 3600 mg of curcumin daily for 1 week prior to surgery. Levels of curcumin and its metabolites were measured in portal and peripheral blood, bile and liver tissue. Curcumin was poorly available, with very low levels of both the parent compound and its metabolites detected in serum.[193] In a dose escalation study, 24 volunteers received 500 to 8000 mg of curcumin, with no detectable levels found in blood. However, low levels of curcumin were detected in two participants who had been administered doses of 10 or 12 g.[194] The authors suggested that curcumin may be effective for the chemoprevention of colorectal cancer, given that systemic bioavailability is not essential for this, and a substantial amount of curcumin reaches the colon.

In an investigation in 12 healthy volunteers given 10 or 12 g of curcumin, only one person had detectable free curcumin at any of the 14 time points tested over 72 h.[195] However, curcumin glucuronides and sulphates were detected in all participants. The average Cmax value for these derivatives was 2.3 μg/mL for the 10 g dose and Tmax was 3.29 h.

Given the low concentrations of curcumin and its metabolites observed after oral doses, investigations have been initiated to improve its bioavailability. When curcumin was given alone at a dose of 2 g/kg to rats, only moderate serum concentrations were achieved over a 4 h period.[196] Concomitant administration of piperine at 20 mg/kg increased the bioavailability by 154%. Administration of 20 mg of piperine to 10 healthy volunteers increased the relative bioavailability of curcumin by 20 times. However, the absolute bioavailability of curcumin under these conditions was still less than 10% and the elimination half-life was still relatively rapid at 0.41±0.17 h.

Ways to enhance bioavailability were also included in one pharmacokinetic review.[181] Three key strategies are possible: adjuvants (such as piperine), nanoparticles and enhanced lipid solubility (liposomes, micelles and phospholipid complexes).

In another study on piperine included in the review, six healthy male volunteers took 2 g of curcumin with or without 5 mg of piperine. In this study, piperine only doubled the absorption of curcumin but it did improve its brain uptake by 48%. It appeared to act mainly by inhibiting glucuronidation. Studies on curcumin, nanoparticles are relatively few and this area is still in its infancy.

In terms of enhanced lipid solubility, a proprietary formulation of curcumin combined with a fraction of turmeric essential oil (probably as a micellar emulsification) demonstrated enhanced bioavailability in a human trial.[197] Results indicated that the relative bioavailability of this formulation was 6.93-fold compared to normal curcumin and about 6.3-fold compared with a curcumin-lecithin-piperine formulation.

Curcumin as a proprietary phospholipid complex (chemically bound to phosphatidylcholine (lecithin)) exhibited enhanced bioavailability (5-fold) compared to normal curcumin in rats.[198] The same formulation yielded a total curcuminoid absorption that was 29 times higher than normal curcumin in a randomised, double blind, crossover human study.[199] However, only phase II metabolites could be detected in plasma. The major plasma curcuminoid after administration of the phospholipid complex was demethoxycurcumin, which is more potent than curcumin in some in vitro anti-inflammatory assays.

While the phase II metabolites of curcumin are likely to have less activity than curcumin, it is conceivable that they could release curcumin at tissue sites. Moreover, one review also noted that tetrahydrocurcumin, a major metabolite of curcumin (in this case the reduced form) detected in the rat studies, also possesses significant chemopreventative activity.[75] Its serum concentration was 20 times that of curcumin following the administration of curcumin. It is also worth noting that, despite its poor bioavailability, curcumin has still demonstrated significant pharmacological activity in experimental models after oral dosing. However, attempts to use natural means to enhance the bioavailability of curcumin are still a positive development. Missing from the experimental work to date is any understanding of the bioavailability of curcumin from different turmeric extracts. Thus far, only the isolated curcuminoid fraction of turmeric has been extensively studied, as outlined above.

Clinical trials

Anti-inflammatory activity

In a 2-week, double blind trial involving 18 rheumatoid arthritis patients, curcumin (1200 mg/day) was compared with 300 mg/day phenylbutazone. A significant symptom improvement occurred with the curcumin, but phenylbutazone gave greater improvement, possibly because it also has analgesic activity.[200] When postoperative inflammation was used as a model for evaluating anti-inflammatory activity, curcumin (1200 mg/day for 5 days) was found to have similar activity to 300 mg/day phenylbutazone (in terms of improvement of typical postoperative symptoms) and greater activity than a placebo in a double blind clinical trial involving 45 patients.[201] In both trials above, use of curcumin was devoid of significant side effects.

In a double blind, placebo-controlled, crossover trial, 42 osteoarthritis (OA) patients received either a herb/mineral preparation or placebo for 3 months. After a 15-day wash-out period the patients were transferred to the other treatment for a further 3-month period. The preparation consisted of turmeric, *Withania somnifera*, *Boswellia serrata* and a zinc complex. Treatment with the herb/mineral preparation produced a significant drop in pain severity (p<0.001) and disability score (p<0.05). Radiological assessment did not show any significant changes in either group. The treatment was well tolerated.[202]

In a single blind, controlled clinical trial, 107 patients with knee OA were randomised to receive ibuprofen 800mg/day or turmeric extract 2g/day (containing 1g of curcuminoids) for 6 weeks.[203] The primary clinical outcomes were pain on level walking and on climbing stairs, as assessed by a numerical rating scale, and the time taken to walk 100m and go up and down a flight of stairs. Both turmeric and the drug resulted in significant improvements from baseline for all of these measures, with no significant difference between treatment effects in the two groups. However, the number of patients was inadequate to establish the equivalence of the treatments.

The activity of a proprietary curcumin phospholipid complex (delivering 200mg/day curcumin) was assessed in a controlled trial involving 50 patients with knee OA.[204] Results demonstrated a significant decrease in the mean WOMAC scores (assessing pain, stiffness and physical function) in the group receiving the curcumin preparation. In addition, walking ability was also significantly increased and oedema significantly reduced compared to the untreated control group (p<0.05). Assessment of those patients with elevated C-reactive protein (CRP) found this parameter was also significantly reduced by the curcumin complex. This trial was hampered by the lack of a placebo control group, although the change observed in the objective CRP measurement is encouraging.

The same proprietary phospholipid complex (delivering 200mg/day curcumin) was further evaluated in an open label clinical trial involving 100 patients with radiologically confirmed knee OA over 8 months (in what appears to be a continuation of the above trial with additional patient recruitment).[205] As the authors noted, the study represents the most extensive (to date) clinical evaluation of curcumin as an anti-inflammatory agent. Unfortunately, a full clinical interpretation of their striking findings is again hampered by the lack of a placebo control group (50 patients acted as untreated controls and 50 received the curcumin preparation). However, in the context of this trial, the 'untreated' group received the best available conventional treatment, including physiotherapy and conventional drugs. Another drawback of the trial design was statistical significance was assessed against baseline values, rather than as a difference from the control group. Significant decreases (p<0.05) from baseline after 8 months of treatment with the curcumin phospholipid complex were noted for the WOMAC score (and all its subscores), inflammatory markers (interleukins (IL)-1beta and IL-6, erythrocyte sedimentation rate, soluble CD40 ligand and soluble vascular cell adhesion molecule (sVCAM)-1)), use of NSAIDs, painkillers, gastrointestinal complications (probably because of the reduced use of NSAIDs), use of other drugs, use of non-drug treatments, distal oedema, hospital admissions, consultations and tests, and management costs. Significant increases (p<0.05) were observed for treadmill walking distance and the Karnofsky Performance Scale Index. The only significant improvement

in the control group was for treadmill walking distance (p<0.05). The changes in objective inflammatory parameters known to be significant in OA, particularly IL-1beta, IL-6 and sVCAM-1, represent a promising outcome.

Hypolipidaemic activity

An early uncontrolled clinical trial involving 16 patients in China found that 12 weeks of turmeric extract (equivalent to about 50g/day of turmeric) lowered plasma cholesterol levels by 49mg/dL (1.3mmol/L) and triglycerides by 62mg/dL.[4] The therapeutic effect was at least equal to clofibrate. Another early, uncontrolled study with 90 patients found cholesterol and triglyceride levels were reduced by turmeric in almost all cases.[4] It was observed in both studies that use of turmeric also partially ameliorated symptoms of angina pectoris.

In a series of case studies, 200mg of turmeric extract (containing 20mg curcumin) was given to healthy men aged between 27 and 67 years for 45 days.[52] A significant decrease of up to 60% in serum lipid peroxides was noted. A follow-up study, using the same dose and study design for 60 days in 30 healthy volunteers, demonstrated a 25% to 50% decrease in HDL and LDL peroxides, again with no side effects.[206] Results were significantly better in patients exhibiting higher peroxide levels at baseline.

Apolipoprotein A (apo A) appears to play a protective role in the pathogenesis of atherosclerosis, whereas high levels of apolipoprotein B (apo B) are generally considered to be associated with increased uptake of cholesterol-laden LDL particles. An uncontrolled study by the same research group above investigated the effect of turmeric on apo A and apo B levels in 30 healthy men and women aged between 24 and 70 years.[207] Participants received a hydro-alcoholic extract of turmeric containing 20mg of curcumin for 30 days. Results demonstrated that turmeric significantly reduced apo B from an average 109.25mg/dL to 90.75mg/dL (p<0.05) and LDL-cholesterol by 38.4% (p<0.01). It increased apo A by 24% (p<0.01) and HDL-cholesterol by 72% (p<0.01). In addition there was also a marked decrease in the apo B/apo A ratio after 30 days (p< 0.01). This research team also reported on fibrinogen levels both before and after 15 days of treatment with the same extract and dosage in eight patients with abnormally high levels. Plasma fibrinogen fell significantly from an average 535.6mg/dL to 271.1mg/dL (p<0.05).[208] These studies suggest that turmeric may potentially decrease the risk of cardiovascular disease. However, the designs of these studies have several flaws, most notably the lack of a placebo control group. An early proof of principle study in 10 healthy volunteers found that curcumin (500mg/day) for 7 days significantly lowered serum lipid peroxides and total cholesterol from baseline.[209] HDL-cholesterol was increased by 29%. Interestingly, two later placebo-controlled trials found no impact of curcumin on serum lipids for either quite high (4g/day) or low (45 to 180mg/day) doses.[210,211] Whether the turmeric extract used above is more active than isolated curcumin remains to be tested.

Anticancer or preventative activity

In an open study, 58 patients with submucous fibrosis (a condition linked to oral cancer and associated with betel nut chewing) received one of the following treatments each day for 3 months: turmeric essential oil (600 mg) mixed with turmeric extract (3 g), turmeric oleoresin (600 mg) mixed with turmeric extract (3 g) or turmeric extract (3 g). Thirty-nine patients completed the treatment and results were compared with those for 32 healthy volunteers. All three treatments normalised the number of micronucleated cells in both exfoliated oral mucosal cells and in circulating lymphocytes. Turmeric oleoresin was more effective at reducing the number of micronuclei in oral mucosal cells (p<0.001) than the other two treatments. The decrease in micronuclei in circulating lymphocytes was comparable in all three treatment groups.[212]

A phase I study evaluated the cancer preventative effect of high doses of curcumin in five high-risk precancerous conditions.[213] Biopsies were performed at the very beginning and conclusion of the study. The curcumin dose was started at 500 mg/day and gradually increased to a maximum dose of 12 g/day over a 3-month period if no toxicity was evident. Histological improvement of precancerous lesions was seen in one of two patients with bladder cancer, two of six patients with Bowen's disease of the skin, one of four patients with cervical intraepithelial neoplasia (CIN), two of seven patients with oral leukoplakia and one of six patients with gastric epithelial metaplasia. However, one patient with CIN and another with oral leukoplakia progressed to malignancies. Oral doses of curcumin were shown to be safe and non-toxic up to 8 g/day for 3 months.

Japanese men (n=85) with elevated prostate-specific antigen (PSA) who were found to not have prostate cancer and prostatic intraepithelial neoplasia on systematic biopsy were randomised to receive either a placebo or a combination of isoflavones (40 mg/day) and curcumin (100 mg/day) for 6 months in a double blind trial.[214] In the subgroup of patients with PSA >10 ng/mL, the phytochemical treatment resulted in a significant reduction in PSA (p=0.02) compared with the placebo treatment. This finding probably reflects an anti-inflammatory activity that might ultimately reduce the risk of subsequent development of prostate cancer.

Turmeric given at a dose of 1.5 g/day for 30 days to 16 chronic smokers significantly reduced the urinary excretion of mutagens in an uncontrolled trial. There was no change in the urinary mutagen excretion after 30 days in six non-smokers who served as controls. Turmeric exerted no significant adverse effect on serum aspartate aminotransferase and alanine aminotransferase, blood glucose, creatinine and lipid profile.[215] An uncontrolled study involving people at high risk of palatal cancer due to reverse smoking demonstrated that turmeric (1 g/day) for 9 months had a significant impact on the regression of precancerous lesions. The treatment also decreased micronuclei and DNA adducts in oral epithelial cells.[216] (Reverse smoking is a practice where the burning end of the cigarette is kept in the mouth and causes a high incidence of oropharyngeal carcinoma.)

In an uncontrolled trial, a 50% ethanolic extract of turmeric and an ointment containing curcumin produced symptomatic relief in 62 patients with oral cancer and leukoplakia who had failed to respond to conventional treatments.[217] There was a reduction in the odour of the lesions

in 90% of cases and also reduction in itching and exudation. Pain intensity and the thickness of the lesion were reduced in a small number of patients (10%).

Two trials in colorectal cancer patients reviewed in the Pharmacokinetics section also included some preliminary clinical outcomes. In the trial in 15 patients given turmeric extract, stable disease was observed in five, with a substantial reduction in carcinoembryonic antigen levels in one.[189] In the second trial where curcumin was given at up to 3.6 g/day, two of 15 patients exhibited stable disease.[190]

Twenty-five patients with advanced pancreatic cancer received 8 g/day curcumin until disease progression, with restaging assessed every 2 months.[218] Evaluation of 21 patients revealed that curcumin was detectable in plasma as glucuronide and sulphate conjugates, albeit at low steady-state levels. Significant clinical activity was observed in two patients: one experienced ongoing stable disease for >18 months and another had a brief but marked tumour regression (73%) accompanied by significant increases in serum cytokine levels. Curcumin downregulated expression of NF-kappaB, COX-2 and phosphorylated STAT3 (signal transducer and activator of transcription 3) in peripheral blood mononuclear cells from the patients (most of whom exhibited baseline levels considerably higher than those found in healthy volunteers).

Fourteen patients with advanced and metastatic breast cancer participated in an open label phase I trial of docetaxel combined with curcumin.[219] A standard intravenous dose of docetaxel was administered (100 mg/m^2) every 3 weeks for six cycles. Curcumin was given orally in escalating doses from 500 mg/day for 7 days around each docetaxel infusion. The maximum tolerated dose of curcumin under these conditions was 8 g/day, with 6 g/day recommended for future phase II studies. No progressive disease was observed in the 14 patients, and nine were evaluable for tumour response. One patient had only evaluable bone lesions that were stable, and according to the RECIST criteria, another five patients had a partial response. The other three exhibited stable disease for at least 6 weeks after the last cycle of treatment. The authors concluded that their study demonstrated the feasibility, safety and tolerability of the combination.

Digestive tract

The safety and efficacy of turmeric for the treatment of dyspepsia (abdominal pain, epigastric discomfort, flatulence or belching) were tested in a three-way, randomised, double blind, placebo-controlled trial over 7 days.[220] Forty-one patients were in the placebo group, 36 received a herbal formula for flatulence and 39 received 2 g/day of turmeric powder. An 87% favourable outcome was recorded for the turmeric group, which was significantly different to the 53% improvement for the placebo group (p=0.003). Mild side effects were observed with similar frequencies in all three groups.

A partially blinded, randomised, pilot study was initiated to investigate the efficacy of a standardised extract of turmeric (method of standardisation not specified) in 207 volunteers with self-reported irritable bowel syndrome (IBS).[221] Patients were divided into two groups and received either one or two tablets a day containing 72 mg of turmeric extract (corresponding to about 1.8 g of turmeric root) for 8 weeks. IBS prevalence decreased by 53% and 60% in the lower and higher dose groups, respectively, compared with baseline. Post-study analysis also revealed that abdominal discomfort was reduced by 22% and 25%, respectively. This trial was hampered by the lack of a placebo group, as a substantial placebo effect can be expected in IBS.

Twenty patients with tropical pancreatitis (a form of chronic pancreatitis) were randomised to receive either oral curcumin (1500 mg/day) and piperine (15 mg/day) or placebo for 6 weeks in a pilot trial, with 15 returning for evaluation. The curcumin preparation significantly reduced lipid peroxidation from baseline levels (p<0.01). However, no effect on pain was noted.[222]

Curcumin appears to induce gallbladder contraction. A double blind, randomised, crossover trial was undertaken in 12 healthy volunteers to compare the effects of curcumin (20 mg) and placebo on gallbladder volume.[223] An ultrasound was performed periodically for up to 2 h after ingestion of the curcumin or placebo. The peak reduction in gallbladder volume by curcumin in the 2 h observation period was 29%, statistically significant compared with placebo. A follow-up randomised, single blind, 3-phase, crossover trial was conducted with 12 healthy volunteers to determine the dose needed to increase gallbladder contraction by 50%.[224] It was concluded that 40 mg of curcumin can increase contraction by 50% in 2 h. The study failed to show a linear dose-response effect, although the effect on gallbladder contraction did increase with increasing doses.

An open label pilot study produced preliminary data to suggest that curcumin might be effective in inflammatory bowel disease.[225] Five patients with ulcerative proctitis received curcumin at 1100 mg/day for 1 month, then at 1650 mg/day for another month. Stool quality was greatly improved and frequency was significantly reduced. Two patients were able to eliminate their concomitant medications altogether, while another two patients were able to reduce them (including one patient who was able to eliminate prednisone). CRP and ESR were normalised by the completion of the study. Five patients with Crohn's disease were also included in the trial. They received 1080 mg/day of curcumin for 1 month, followed by 1440 mg/day for another 2 months. The Crohn's disease activity index, CRP and ESR fell significantly in four patients. Following these trials, a Japanese double blind, placebo-controlled trial involving 89 patients investigated the efficacy of curcumin for maintaining remission in ulcerative colitis.[226] Patients were randomised to receive 2 g/day curcumin, together with sulfasalazine or mesalazine, or placebo plus the sulfasalazine or mesalazine. At the end of the 6-month study period, 4.65% of patients in the curcumin group had relapsed during treatment compared with 20.51% in the placebo group (p=0.040). There was also a significant difference in recurrence rates based on intention-to-treat analysis (p=0.049). Curcumin significantly improved the clinical activity index (p=0.038) and endoscopic index (p=0.0001) compared to baseline, suggesting that the treatment influenced disease pathology. Only mild side effects such as nausea and bloating were observed in some patients.

The effect of turmeric (1000 mg/day) was compared with that of an antacid formulation in 50 patients over 6 weeks in an open label study of the treatment of gastric ulcer.[227] The liquid antacid formula was significantly superior to turmeric at inducing ulcer healing (p<0.05). In a joint Vietnam-Sweden prospective, double blind, two-centre study, turmeric at a dose of 6 g/day (as suggested in the *Vietnamese Pharmacopoeia*) was compared with placebo in 118 patients suffering from duodenal ulcer.[228] Follow-up endoscopy and/or radiography were performed after 28±4 days and 56±4 days. Turmeric was not superior to placebo in healing duodenal ulcer after either 4 or 8 weeks of treatment. After 8 weeks, the ulcer-healing rate of turmeric was 27% compared to 29% for placebo. Both treatments were well tolerated. A later open label study examined the efficacy of turmeric in 25 patients with peptic ulcer disease diagnosed via endoscopy.[229] Oral doses of turmeric powder (600 mg, 5 times a day) cleared ulcers in 48% of patients after 4 weeks, 72% of patients after 8 weeks, and 76% of patients after 12 weeks of treatment. No significant changes were noted in liver or kidney function.

An open label crossover study investigated whether turmeric added to the diet has beneficial effects on intestinal motility and colonic fermentation, as assessed by breath hydrogen.[230] Eight healthy subjects fasted for 12 h and ingested curry and rice with or without turmeric. The test meal provided 500 mg of turmeric, containing 8.25 mg of curcuminoids. Curry with turmeric significantly increased the area under the curve of breath hydrogen and shortened small-bowel transit time, compared with curry not containing turmeric. This suggests that dietary turmeric increases bowel motility and colonic carbohydrate fermentation.

HIV/AIDS

Following pharmacological research that suggested curcumin might weakly inhibit the LTR (long terminal repeat) of HIV-1, a clinical study was undertaken. Eighteen HIV-positive patients took an average of 2 g/day curcumin for an average of 127 days.[231] There was a significant increase in CD4 (p=0.029) and CD8 (p=0.009) lymphocyte counts. However, a follow-up phase I/II open study in HIV-positive patients using doses of 2.7 g and 4.8 g/day of curcumin failed to show any benefit on viral loads or CD4 count.[232] It was suggested that the poor bioavailability of curcumin may have been a factor behind this negative result.[233]

Eight patients with HIV-associated chronic diarrhoea with no identifiable pathogenic cause received an average dose of 1862 mg/day of curcumin and were followed for a mean of 41 weeks in an uncontrolled pilot study.[234] All patients exhibited resolution of their diarrhoea and normalisation of stool quality in 13±9.3 days. At the end of the follow-up period, the mean number of bowel movements per day had dropped from 7.0±3.6 to 1.7±0.5 (p=0.006). Seven of eight patients exhibited considerable weight gain while on curcumin and five of six experienced resolution of bloating and abdominal pain. Mean symptom severity fell from 7.8±1.6 to 1.6±0.5 (p=0.0001). There was no interference observed with antiretroviral therapy.

Eye disorders

Eight patients suffering from idiopathic inflammatory orbital pseudo-tumours were treated with oral curcumin (1125 mg/day) for 6 to 22 months in an uncontrolled study.[235] Idiopathic orbital inflammatory syndrome is a rare eye condition characterised by swelling of ocular tissue and is often associated with pain, restricted movement, vision disturbances, nausea, vomiting and headaches. Of the five patients who completed the study, four achieved a complete recovery. The other patient exhibited a complete regression of swelling, but some restriction of movement remained.

An open label clinical trial was conducted in India to investigate the efficacy of curcumin in chronic anterior uveitis.[236] The 32 patients who completed the study (of 53 initially enrolled) had been divided into two groups: group A (18 patients) received curcumin alone (1125 mg/day), while group B (14 patients) received curcumin (1125 mg/day) together with antitubercular treatment due to their strong positive PPD (purified protein derivative) reaction. Both groups used topical mydriatics (atropine/cyclopentolate 1%) as needed. Curcumin treatment was continued for 12 weeks, but the antitubercular treatment was sustained for 1 year. Improvements in both groups were noted after just 2 weeks of treatment, with a 100% response rate in group A at 12 weeks. Group B patients had a lower (but still high) response rate of 86%. Follow-up of all patients over the next 3 years indicated a recurrence rate of 55% in group A and 36% in group B. These results were comparable to corticosteroid treatment, but with significantly fewer side effects.

A later uncontrolled trial examined the efficacy of oral doses of a curcumin-phospholipid complex (delivering 240 mg/day curcumin) as an adjunctive treatment over 12 months in 106 patients (from 122 enrolled) with chronic anterior uveitis.[237] Compared with before curcumin, the number of relapses was substantially fewer (p<0.001). The patients with autoimmune anterior uveitis seemed to be the most responsive. Overall the treatment was well tolerated and reduced eye discomfort after just a few weeks in more than 80% of the trial participants. Only one patient could not tolerate the treatment due to gastrointestinal side effects.

Genetic diseases

Familial adenomatous polyposis (FAP) is an autosomal-dominant disorder characterised by the development of numerous colorectal adenomas and eventually colorectal cancer. NSAIDs and COX-2 inhibitors can regress the adenomas. Five patients with FAP who had undergone prior colectomy (four with retained rectum and one with an ileoanal pouch) were given 1440 mg/day curcumin and 60 mg/day quercetin orally in an uncontrolled pilot study.[238] After a mean of 6 months of treatment, all five patients exhibited a decrease in the number (by 60.4%) and size (by 50.9%) of rectal polyps compared with baseline (p<0.05). Minimal adverse side effects and no laboratory abnormalities were noted.

Déjérine-Sottas disease (hereditary motor and sensory polyneuropathy type III) is an autosomal-dominant or -recessive disease of the peripheral nervous system caused by myelin sheath defects. A dose-escalation safety trial of oral curcumin in a 15-year-old girl with Déjérine-Sottas disease (point mutation Ser72Leu) complicated by severe weakness, scoliosis and respiratory impairment was undertaken.[239] The patient received 50 mg/kg/day oral curcumin for the first 4 months and 75 mg/kg/day thereafter, to complete a 12-month trial. Outcome measures included muscle strength, pulmonary function, upper/lower extremity disability, neurophysiological studies and health-related quality of life. After 12 months, the patient experienced no adverse events and reported good compliance. There was little improvement in objective outcome measures. Knee flexion and foot strength increased slightly, but hand and elbow strength decreased. Pulmonary function, hand function and measures of upper/lower extremity disability were stable or reduced. Her neurophysiological findings were unchanged. Parent-reported quality of life improved for most domains, especially self-esteem, during the 12 months of treatment. Patient-reported quality of life, assessed at the final visit, mirrored these results, with overall feelings of happiness and contentment.

A Thai study investigated the impact of curcuminoids (500 mg/day) in 21 patients with beta-thalassaemia/HbE in an uncontrolled trial.[240] At baseline, levels of malonyldialdehyde (MDA), SOD and glutathione peroxidase in red blood cells and non-transferrin bound iron in serum were all elevated compared with normal values, indicative of increased oxidative stress. The level of reduced glutathione in red blood cells was lower than normal. All of these parameters were significantly improved (various p values) after 12 months of curcuminoid treatment and retreated towards baseline levels 3 months after treatment withdrawal. However, curcuminoids did not impact the lower Hb levels and red blood cell counts in this patient cohort.

The promising results for curcumin in cystic fibrosis models await verification in controlled clinical trials.

Clinical antioxidant activity

Additional studies have demonstrated clinical antioxidant activity. Hyperglycaemia leads to increased oxidative stress that can result in vascular endothelial dysfunction. In a partially blinded, placebo-controlled, three-arm clinical trial, 72 type 2 diabetic patients with endothelial dysfunction were randomised to receive a proprietary curcuminoid extract (delivering 300 mg/day curcumin), atorvastatin (10 mg/day) or placebo for 8 weeks.[241] Sixty-seven patients completed the trial. Compared with baseline, there was a significant improvement in endothelial function (as assessed by a measure of arterial vascular tone) and reductions in MDA, endothelin-1, IL-6 and TNF-alpha for both the curcumin and atorvastatin groups, with no change for placebo.

Groundwater arsenic (As) contamination is a health hazard in some areas of the world. A survey of 286 people from five villages in West Bengal, India found high blood levels of As and extensive DNA damage (as a result of As-induced oxidative stress).[242] These villagers were randomly selected to take curcumin with piperine (952 mg/day and 48 mg/day, respectively) or a placebo for 3 months. After 3 months there was a significant reduction in DNA damage for the villagers taking the curcumin formulation, as compared with placebo (p<0.001). There were also significant reductions in lymphocyte intracellular reactive oxygen species production and lipid peroxidation (MDA), together with increases in catalase, SOD, glutathione, glutathione-S-transferase, glutathione peroxidase and glutathione reductase, with respect to placebo (all p<0.001).

Alzheimer's disease

A review of the potential of curcumin in AD noted that epidemiological studies in India, where turmeric consumption is widespread, suggest it has one of the lowest prevalence rates of AD in the world.[243] In addition, an epidemiological study in Singapore found an association between curry consumption and preserved cognitive function. The association was assessed in a population-based cohort involving 1010 Singapore citizens aged 60 to 93 years in 2003.[244] Those who consumed curry occasionally and often/very often had significantly better Mini-Mental State Examination scores than people who never or rarely consumed curry. The most common curry dish in Singapore is the yellow curry rich in turmeric, with green and red curries seldom consumed.

In a three-arm, double blind, placebo-controlled, trial, 34 patients with AD were randomly assigned to receive curcumin (1 or 4g/day) or placebo for 6 months.[245] Results for 27 patients were analysed and indicated that there was no difference between the groups, although the lack of cognitive decline in the placebo group may have precluded any ability to detect the activity of curcumin. Also, the trial was underpowered. Moreover, the true value of curcumin/turmeric in AD might be as a preventative (see the Pharmacodynamics section).

Skin conditions

A randomised, placebo-controlled, double blind clinical trial involving 33 patients with oral lichen planus found that curcuminoids at 2000mg/day for 7 weeks had no observable effect above the placebo treatment.[246] However, all patients also received 60mg/day prednisone for the first week, which may have masked any impact of curcumin.

Phosphorylase kinase (PhK) integrates signalling pathways involved in cell migration and proliferation. An open label study found that PhK was highly elevated in 10 untreated psoriasis patients and was substantially and significantly reduced to near normal in 10 patients using a topical curcumin (as a 1% gel preparation).[247] A small uncontrolled trial in 12 patients with psoriasis given oral curcuminoids (4.5g/day) for 12 weeks found that two of the eight patients who completed the trial had responded to treatment.[248] A larger placebo-controlled trial is necessary, as suggested by the authors.

A US dermatologist described the outcomes of a number of cases treated with topical curcumin as the same gel preparation referred to above.[249] A resolution rate of 70% was observed in 647 consecutive psoriasis patients treated with topical curcumin, in a protocol that also included topical steroids, avoidance of precipitating factors (not specified) and treatment of infections. A higher concentration of curcumin used as the sole therapeutic agent prevented or decreased scar tissue formation following surgery in another 220 patients.

Other case observations with the curcumin gel included reduced inflammation and scarring from burns and scalds, together with accelerated healing and an improvement in the texture of photodamaged skin (after a minimum of 3 to 6 months of application). Topical curcumin was also observed to be clinically effective in decreasing solar-induced erythema in photosensitivity and rosacea, and in improving solar-induced telangiectasia. In photodamaged skin with actinic keratoses and solar lentigenes, curcumin gel was observed to induce repair of these lesions.

A paste consisting of turmeric and neem (Azadirachta indica) was used for the treatment of scabies in 814 patients. It resulted in cure in 97% within 3 to 15 days of treatment. No toxic or adverse reactions were observed.[250]

Other conditions

The efficacy of a product containing 480mg curcumin and 20mg quercetin per capsule was investigated in 43 dialysis-dependent kidney transplant recipients.[251] Patients were randomised into three groups: low dose (one capsule/day), high dose (two capsules/day) and placebo, and treated for 1 month immediately after transplant surgery. Early graft function appeared to be higher in the high dose group (as evidenced by lower serum creatinine levels). Acute rejection after 6 months was zero in the high dose group, compared with 14.3% in both the low dose and placebo groups. Neurotoxicity (as assessed by tremor) was also lowest in the high-dose group.

Ingestion of 6g of turmeric powder had no significant impact on glucose levels during a standard 75g oral glucose tolerance test, as assessed in 14 healthy volunteers in a placebo-controlled, crossover trial.[252] However, insulin levels were significantly higher (p<0.02 at 120min).

A combination of turmeric and Tinospora cordifolia (each at a dose equivalent to 6g/day from a combination of powder and extract) for 6 months significantly reduced hepatotoxicity (p<0.0001) in an open label, controlled study of 508 patients receiving extended anti-tubercular drug cocktail medication.[253]

Twenty-six men and women (average age of 68 years) with monoclonal gammopathy of undefined significance (MGUS) received curcuminoids (4g/day) for 6 months in a single blind, placebo-controlled, crossover clinical trial.[254] Patients with a baseline serum paraprotein level of <20g/L did not show a response to curcumin. Before crossover, five of 10 patients with serum paraprotein >20g/L experienced a 12% to 30% decrease in response to curcuminoids. This decrease remained stable in most patients until they were crossed over to placebo, of which point two showed a rebound. There also may have been a decrease in bone resorption in some participants receiving curcuminoids (MGUS is associated with increased risk of fracture). The authors suggested that, due to the risk of MGUS progressing to multiple myeloma, these promising results warrant further investigation. However, a subsequent letter suggested that immunosuppression is a risk factor for MGUS progression; hence caution should be exercised with the use of turmeric or curcumin in this condition.[255]

Toxicology and other safety data

Toxicology

The following LD$_{50}$ data have been recorded for various fractions of turmeric, indicating low toxicity:

Substance	Route, model	LD$_{50}$	Reference
Turmeric petroleum ether extract	Oral, rats	12.2 g/kg	30
Turmeric oleoresin	Oral, mice and rats	>10 g/kg	256
Turmeric oil	Oral, rats	>5 g/kg	257
Turmeric essential oil	Dermal, rabbits	>5 g/kg	257

In acute toxicity studies, no toxic effects were observed when either turmeric powder (2.5 g/kg and 30% of diet), an ethanol extract (0.3 to 3 g/kg) or curcumin (1 to 5 g/kg) was orally administered to mice, rats, guinea pigs and monkeys.[10,17,184,258,259]

No toxic effects were observed in chronic oral toxicity studies of turmeric powder (0.1 to 10% of diet and 500 mg/kg/day) for up to 52 weeks; a hydroalcoholic extract (4 mg/kg/day) for 4 weeks; a petroleum ether extract (1 and 2 g/kg) for 4 weeks; and curcumin (0.1 to 2% of diet; 400 to 800 mg/kg) for 8 to 13 weeks, in mice, rats and monkeys.[10,30,51,256,260,261]

Reduced weight gain due to decreased food intake was observed in rats fed turmeric powder (10% of diet) for 8 weeks. This effect was not found in the groups fed lower concentrations and was attributed to a change in the taste of the food.[260] However, reduced weight gain without an apparent reduction in food intake, together with hair loss, were observed in another study involving rats fed the same dietary concentration of turmeric for 4 to 7 weeks.[262]

Turmeric extract (0.05% to 0.25% of diet) and turmeric powder (0.2% to 5% of diet) caused some cases of hepatotoxicity when fed to mice for 14 days or longer.[263,264] The mouse is probably a susceptible species for turmeric-induced toxicity. Guinea pigs fed turmeric (500 mg/kg/day) or its alcohol extract (70 mg/kg/day) for 90 days showed no significant changes from controls, apart from reduced liver weight.[10]

Oral administration of a concentrated ethanolic extract of turmeric (100 mg/kg/day) for 90 days to mice significantly increased sperm motility, heart, lung and caudae epidiymis weights, and significantly decreased red and white blood cell levels. No spermatotoxic effects were observed.[259] Subcutaneous injection of an alcohol extract (0.1 mL/day) to immature male rats for 10 days resulted in a significant decrease in testis weight and testosterone concentration.[265]

Administration of turmeric (4 g/kg) and curcumin (0.4 g/kg) for 14 to 21 days to lactating mice significantly elevated cytochrome b5 and P450 levels in mothers and pups.[172]

Curcumin increased the formation of stomach ulcers in rats at a dose of 100 mg/kg, but not at 50 mg/kg, after oral administration for 6 days.[26] Lower doses of curcumin and turmeric have been shown to protect against ulceration.[27,107] The ulcerogenic effect was attributed to the reduced mucin secretion that also occurred at the higher dosage.[26]

Thyroid enlargement, pericholangitis and epithelial changes in the kidney and bladder were observed in pigs fed turmeric oleoresin (296 and 1551 mg/kg/day) for 102 to 109 days. Reduced weight gain due to decreased food intake was observed only in the higher dose group.[266] Turmeric oleoresin consists mainly of curcuminoids and essential oil.

Turmeric oil (1.8 and 3 mL/day for 1 and 2 months, respectively) was without toxic effects in nine healthy volunteers, apart from one allergic reaction.[267] Phase I dose-escalation studies of curcuminoids indicated that single high oral doses (up to 12 g/day) were well tolerated.[213] (See also the Clinical trials section for further information on the safety of high oral doses of curcuminoids.)

Undiluted turmeric oil was slightly irritating to rabbit skin after topical application, but was not irritating or photosensitising in hairless mice. Turmeric essential oil (4% in petroleum) was not irritating to the skin or sensitising in human volunteers.[257]

A turmeric ethanolic extract and curcumin demonstrated cytotoxic effects after direct contact with mammalian cells in vitro, including chromosomal separation and breakage, mitotic arrest and growth inhibition.[143,144,268,269] A turmeric methanolic extract demonstrated chromosomal damage in vivo in mice after intraperitoneal administration at a dose of approximately 6 g/kg of turmeric.[270] However, turmeric powder, the ethanolic extract, oleoresin and curcumin were not mutagenic in vitro in the Ames test.[271,272] Turmeric powder (0.5% of the diet and 1.25 to 5 g/kg) and curcumin (0.015% of the diet) were not mutagenic in vivo after oral administration.[10,260,273] Absence of mutagenicity in vitro was also reported for a turmeric ethanolic extract, following activation with caecal microorganisms.[274] A turmeric ethanolic extract exhibited mutagenic activity in the Ames test in one study,[275] but not in another.[271]

Contraindications

According to the Commission E, turmeric is contraindicated in biliary tract obstruction and should be used only after seeking professional advice if gallstones are present.[276] Allergic reactions are possible, but are considered to be rare.

Special warnings and precautions

High doses greater than 15 g/day should not be prescribed long-term or concomitantly with antiplatelet or anticoagulant medication.[277] Care should be exercised with women wishing to conceive and patients complaining of hair loss. Turmeric has traditional use as a topical depilatory[3,265] and hair loss has been reported in feeding experiments with rats.[262] However, the relevance of this research to human use is uncertain.

Patients applying topical doses of turmeric or curcumin should not be exposed to excessive sunlight, as curcumin has demonstrated phototoxic effects in vitro.

Interactions

High doses (greater than 15 g/day) of turmeric should not be prescribed concomitantly with antiplatelet or anticoagulant medication. Antiplatelet activity has been demonstrated for in vitro and in vivo studies (mainly with curcumin) suggesting turmeric may potentiate the effects of these medications.

A 2010 review of potential herb-drug interactions for turmeric or curcumin noted that the data were mainly from experimental models.[278] Using the in vitro Caco-2 cell model of the intestinal lining in conjunction with probe drugs, it has been observed that curcumin can inhibit P-gp activity and reduce CYP3A4 activity. Inhibition of P-gp and CYP3A4 by curcumin has also been observed in rats, along with inhibition of the enterocytic phase II enzyme UDP-glucuronosyltransferases in mice.

An investigation in rabbits using the quinolone antibiotic norfloxacin found that curcumin (60 mg/kg/day, oral for 3 days) increased the bioavailability of the drug.[279]

A randomised, open label trial in 12 healthy volunteers found that a 6-day treatment with curcumin (300 mg/day) significantly reduced the bioavailability of a single 50 mg dose of the P-gp substrate talinol.[280] The authors suggested that other mechanisms might have been at play, since any P-gp inhibition by curcumin should have increased the bioavailability of talinol.

A randomised, crossover study involving healthy Thai women found that cayenne (Capsicum annuum) inhibited iron absorption from a rice-based meal containing vegetables and iron-fortified fish sauce.[281] Despite its higher polyphenol content, addition of turmeric (0.5 g dry powder containing 50 mg of polyphenols) to the test meal did not inhibit iron absorption.

A study using the probe drug caffeine in 16 healthy men found that curcumin (1000 mg/day for 14 days) significantly reduced CYP1A2 by 28.6% ($p < 0.0001$), while CYP2A6 was increased by 48.9% ($p < 0.0001$).[282]

(See also Appendix C for a summary of recommendations regarding the potential herb-drug interactions for turmeric that are deemed to be clinically relevant.)

Use in pregnancy and lactation

Category A - no proven increase in the frequency of malformation or other harmful effects on the fetus despite consumption by a large number of women as an item of diet. Turmeric decoction is traditionally used in Ayurvedic medicine to treat vomiting of pregnancy.[1] In the traditional medicine of Indonesia[283] and Fiji,[284] turmeric is given at parturition.

Oral administration of high doses of turmeric extract (100 mg/kg/day and 200 mg/kg/day) did not exhibit significant anovulatory activity in rabbits, but oral administration of the same doses to mice during the first week of pregnancy reduced the number of implantations and number of pups delivered at term. No teratogenic effects were observed.[285] However, when turmeric (0.5% of diet) or curcumin (0.015% of diet) were fed to mice for 12 weeks, there were no significant effects on the pregnancy rate, number of live and dead embryos and number of implantations.[10,259] Similarly, no reproductive toxicity or teratogenic effects were observed in rats fed turmeric (50 mg/kg/day) for 52 weeks[255] or rats and rabbits fed curcumin (600 mg/kg/day and 1600 mg/kg/day) from days 6 to 15 post-coitus.[10]

Oral administration of very high doses (15 g/kg) of Curcuma spp. used in TCM (C. aromatica, C. zedoaria or C. wenyujin) prevented implantation or led to abortion in mice.[286] Similar antifertility effects were demonstrated with the essential oil administered by intraperitoneal, subcutaneous or intravaginal routes in mice and rabbits.[287] It is uncertain whether this research has any relevance to women wishing to conceive.

Turmeric rhizome decoction and extract had a stimulant effect on isolated uteri of mice and guinea pigs and on uterine fistulae of rabbits.[288]

Turmeric is compatible with breastfeeding, and in Fijian traditional medicine turmeric is taken by new mothers to promote lactation.[284]

Effects on ability to drive and use machines

No adverse effect expected.

Side effects

Turmeric at 10% of diet caused some hair loss in rats and may have this effect in humans.[261] Two cases of allergic contact dermatitis (due to curcumin in one case[289] and occupational use of turmeric in the other[264]) have been reported. A 2001 review of the literature concluded that allergic reactions to turmeric are rare.[290]

Generally turmeric and curcumin have been well tolerated in clinical trials after oral and topical administration. One incident of localised itchiness was reported in a trial following topical application.[217] Frequent bowel movements and mild gastric discomfort may occur in individual patients,[4] especially at the high curcumin doses used in recent clinical trials. Eleven healthy volunteers ingested cinnamon bark followed by turmeric rhizome, each for 4 weeks and providing 55 mg/day oxalate.[291] Compared with cinnamon and the control group, the consumption of turmeric significantly increased urinary oxalate levels and may adversely impact on kidney stone risk.

Overdosage

No incidents found in the published literature.

Safety in children

No information available but adverse effects are not expected.

Regulatory status in selected countries

Turmeric is official in the Pharmacopoeia of the People's Republic of China (English Edition, 1997). It was official in the second edition of the *Indian Pharmacopoeia* (1966) but was not included in the third edition (1985).

Turmeric is covered by a positive Commission E monograph and can be used for the treatment of dyspeptic conditions.

Turmeric is not on the UK General Sale List.

Turmeric and turmeric oleoresin have GRAS status. It is also freely available as a 'dietary supplement' in the USA under DSHEA legislation (1994 Dietary Supplement Health and Education Act).

Turmeric is not included in Part 4 of Schedule 4 of the Therapeutic Goods Act Regulations of Australia and is freely available for sale.

References

1. Chopra RN, Chopra IC, Handa KL, et al. *Chopra's Indigenous Drugs of India*, 2nd ed. Caluctta: Academic Publishers; 1958. Reprinted 1982. pp. 325–327.

2. Nadkarni KM, Nadkarni AK. *Indian Materia Medica*, vol 1. Bombay: Popular Prakashan Private; 1976. pp. 414–418.

3. Goh CL, Ng SK. *Contact Derm.* 1987;17(3):186.

4. Chang HM, But PP. *Pharmacology and Applications of Chinese Materia Medica*, vol 2. Singapore: World Scientific; 1987. pp. 936–939.

5. Bensky D, Gamble A. *Chinese Herbal Medicine Materia Medica*. Seattle: Eastland Press; 1986. pp. 390–391.

6. Farnsworth NR, Bunyapraphatsara N, eds. *Thai Medicinal Plants*. Bangkok: Medicinal Plant Information Centre; 1992.

7. Grieve M. *A Modern Herbal*, vol 2. New York: Dover Publications; 1971. pp. 822–823.

8. Kapoor LD. *Handbook of Ayurvedic Medicinal Plants*. Boca Raton: CRC Press; 1990. pp. 149–150.

9. Bisset NG, ed. *Herbal Drugs and Phytopharmaceuticals*. Stuttgart: Medpharm Scientific Publishers; 1994. pp. 173–175.

10. Govindarajan VS. *Crit Rev Food Sci Nutr.* 1980;12(3):199–301.

11. Sen AR, Gupta PS, Dastidar NG. *Analyst.* 1974;99:153–155.

12. Raghuveer KG, Govindarajan VS. *J Assoc Off Anal Chem.* 1979;62:1333–1337.

13. Salmen R, Pedersen BF, Malterud KE. *Z Lebensm Unters Forsch.* 1987;184:33–34.

14. Wagner H, Bladt S. *Plant Drug Analysis: A Thin Layer Chromatography Atlas*, 2nd ed. Berlin: Springer-Verlag; 1996. p. 159.

15. Food and Agriculture Organisation of the United Nations. *FAO Food and Nutrition Papers* 1990;49:75–78.

16. Srimal RC, Khanna NM, Dhawan BN. *Indian J Pharmacol.* 1971;3:10.

17. Srimal RC, Dhawan BN. *J Pharm Pharmacol.* 1973;25(6):447–452.

18. Epstein J, Sanderson IR, Macdonalt TT. *Br J Nutr.* 2010;103(11):1545–1557.

19. Jurenka JS. *Altern Med Rev.* 2009;14(2):141–153.

20. Huang MT, Lysz T, Ferraro T, et al. *Cancer Res.* 1991;51(3):813–819.

21. Rao CV. *Adv Exp Med Biol.* 2007;595:213–226.

22. Nadkarni KM, Nadkarni AK. *Indian Materia Medica*, vol. 1. Bombay: Popular Prakashan Private; 1976. p. 417.

23. Ghatak N, Basu N. *Indian J Exp Biol.* 1972;10(3):235–236.

24. Mukhopadhyay A, Basu N, Ghatak N, et al. *Agents Actions.* 1982;12(4):508–515.

25. Srivastava R, Srimal RC. *Indian J Med Res.* 1985;81:215–223.

26. Gupta B, Kulshrestha VK, Srivastava RK, et al. *Indian J Med Res.* 1980;71:806–814.

27. Sinha M, Mukherjee BP, Mukherjee B, et al. *Indian J Pharmacol.* 1974;6:87–90.

28. Bhatia A, Singh GB, Khanna NM. *Indian J Exp Biol.* 1964;2:158–160.

29. Gukovsky I, Reyes CN, Vaquero EC, et al. *Am J Physiol Gastrointest Liver Physiol.* 2003;284:G85–G95.

30. Arora RB, Basu N, Kapoor V, et al. *Indian J Med Res.* 1971;59(8):1289–1295.

31. Yegnanarayan R, Saraf AP, Balwani JH. *Indian J Med Res.* 1976;64(4):601–608.

32. Mehra KS, Mikuni I, Gupta V, et al. *Tokai J Exp Clin Med.* 1984;9(1):27–31.

33. Srivastava KC. *Prostagland Leukot Essent Fatty Acids.* 1989;37(1):57–64.

34. Chandra D, Gupta SS. *Indian J Med Res.* 1972;60:138–142.

35. Gupta SS, Modh PR. *Indian J Pharmacol.* 1969;1:22–25.

36. Funk JL, Oyarzo JN, Frye JB, et al. *J Nat Prod.* 2006;69(3):351–355.

37. Srivastava R, Puru V, Srima RC, et al. *Arzneimittelforschung.* 1986;36:715–717.

38. Srivastava R, Dikshit M, Srimal RC, et al. *Thromb Res.* 1985;40:413–417.

39. Srivastava KC, Bordia A, Verma SK. *Prostagland Leukot Essent Fatty Acids.* 1995;52(4):223–227.

40. Shah BH, Nawaz Z, Pertani SA, et al. *Biochem Pharmacol.* 1999;58(7):1167–1172.

41. Lee HS. *Bioresour Technol.* 2006;97(12):1372–1376.

42. Sharma OP. *Biochem Pharmacol.* 1976;25:1811–1812.

43. Toda S, Miyase T, Arichi H, et al. *Chem Pharm Bull.* 1985;33:1725–1728.

44. Toda S, Ohnishi M, Kimura M, et al. *J Ethnopharmacol.* 1988;23:105–108.

45. Zhao BL, Li XJ, He RG, et al. *Cell Biophys.* 1989;14:175–185.

46. Shalini VK, Srinivas L. *Mol Cell Biochem.* 1987;77:3–10.

47. Subramanian M, Sreejayan Rao MN, et al. *Mutat Res.* 1994;311(2):249–255.

48. Sreejayan Rao MN. *J Pharm Pharmacol.* 1997;49(1):105–107.

49. Rushworth SA, Ogborne RM, Charalambos CA, et al. *Biochem Biophys Res Commun.* 2006;341(4):1007–1016.

50. Surh YJ, Kundu JK, Na HK. *Planta Med.* 2008;74(13):1526–1539.

51. Miquel J, Martinez M, Diez A, et al. *Age.* 1995;18(4):171–174.

52. Ramirez–Bosca A, Soler A, Gutierrez J, et al. *Age.* 1995;18:167–169.

53. Awasthi S, Srivatava SK, Piper JT, et al. *Am J Clin Nutr.* 1996;64(5):761–766.

54. Pandya U, Saini MK, Jin GF. *Toxicol Lett.* 2000;115(3):195–204.

55. Padmaja S, Raju TN. *Indian J Exp Biol.* 2004;42(5):601–603.

56. Selvam R, Subramanian L, Gayathri R, et al. *J Ethnopharmacol.* 1995;47(2):59–67.

57. McNally SJ, Harrison EM, Ross JA. *Transplantation.* 2006;81(4):623–626.

58. Kang HC, Nan JX, Park PH. *J Pharm Pharmacol.* 2002;54(1):119–126.

59. He YJ, Shu JC, Lv X, et al. *Zhonghua Gan Zang Bing Za Zhi.* 2006;14(5):337–340.

60. Kamalakkannan N, Rukkumani R, Varma PS, et al. *Basic Clin Pharmacol Toxicol.* 2005;95(1):15–21.

61. Rukkumani R, Aruna K, Varma PS, et al. *J Pharm Pharm Sci.* 2004;7(2):274–283.

62. Eybl V, Kotyzova D, Bludovska M. *Toxicol Lett.* 2004;151(1):79–85.

63. Sreepriya M, Bali G. *Fitoterapia.* 2005;76(9):549–555.

64. Pari L, Amali DR. *J Pharm Pharm Sci.* 2005;8(1):115–123.

65. Sreepriya M, Bali G. *Mol Cell Biochem.* 2006;284(1–2):49–55.

66. Shukla Y, Arora A. *Nutr Cancer.* 2003;45(1):53–59.

67. Nanji AA, Jokelainen K, Tipoe GL, et al. *Am J Physiol Gastrointest Liver Physiol.* 2003;284(2):G321–G327.

68. Shapiro H, Ashkenazi M, Weizman N, et al. *J Gastroenterol Hepatol.* 2006;21(2):358–366.

69. Reddy AC, Lokesh BR. *Toxicology.* 1996;107(1):39–45.

70. Reddy AC, Lokesh BR. *Food Chem Toxicol.* 1994;32(3):279–283.

71. Asai A, Nakagawa K, Miyazawa T. *Biosci Biotechnol Biochem.* 1999;63(12):2118–2122.

72. Kiso Y, Suzuki Y, Watanabe N, et al. *Planta Med.* 1983;49:185–187.

73. Ali BH, Al-Wabel N, Mahmoud O, et al. *Fundam Clin Pharmacol.* 2005;19(4):473–477.

74. Tirkey N, Kaur G, Vij G, et al. *BMC Pharmacol.* 2005;5:15.

75. Osawa T. *Adv Exp Med Biol.* 2007;595:407–423.

76. Thiyagarajan M, Sharma SS. *Life Sci.* 2004;76(8):969–985.

77. Ghoneim AI, Abdel-Naim AB, Khalifa AE, et al. *Pharmacol Res.* 2002;46(3):273–279.

78. Al-Omar FA, Nagi MN, Abdulgadir MM, et al. *Neurochem Res.* 2006;31(5):611–618.

79. Luo F, Huang R, Yang YJ, et al. *Zhonghua Er Ke Za Zhi.* 2003;41(12):940–944.

80. Daniel S, Limson JL, Dairam A, et al. *J Inorg Biochem.* 2004;98(2):266–275.

81. Cole GM, Teter B, Frautschy SA. *Adv Exp Med Biol.* 2007;595:197–212.

82. Mohanty I, Singh Arya D, Dinda A. *Life Sci.* 2004;75(14):1701–1711.

83. Cheng H, Liu W, Ai X. *Zhong Yao Cai.* 2005;28(10):920–922.

84. Manikandan P, Sumitra M, Aishwarya S. *Int J Biochem Cell Biol.* 2004;36(10):1967–1980.

85. Wongcharoen W, Phrommintikul A. *Int J Cardiol.* 2009;133(2):145–151.

86. Srivastava G, Mehta JL. *J Cardiovasc Pharmacol Ther.* 2009;14(1):22–27.

87. Fan C, Wo X, Qian Y, et al. *J Ethnopharmacol.* 2006;105(1–2):251–254.

88. Peschel D, Koerting R, Nass N. *J Nutr Biochem.* 2006;18(2):113–119.

89. Bhuvaneswaran C, Kapur OP, Sriramachari S, et al. *Food Sci.* 1963;12:182–185.

90. Srinivasan M, Aiyar AS, Kapur OP, et al. *Indian J Exp Biol.* 1964;2:104–106.

91. Rao SD, Sekhara CN, Satyanarayana MN, et al. *J Nutr.* 1970;100:1307–1316.

92. Dixit VP, Jain P, Joshi SC. *Indian J Physiol Pharmacol.* 1988;32:299–304.

93. Keshavarz K. *Poult Sci.* 1976;55:1077–1083.

94. Mesa MD, Aguilera CM, Ramirez-Tortosa CL, et al. *Nutrition.* 2003;19(9):800–804.

95. Kempaiah RK, Srinivasan K. *Mol Cell Biochem.* 2002;236(1–2):155–161.

96. Quiles JL, Mesa MD, Ramirez-Tortosa CL, et al. *Arterioscler Thromb Vasc Biol.* 2002;22(7):1225–1231.

97. Arafa HM. *Med Sci Monit.* 2005;11(7):BR228–BR234.

98. Asai A, Miyazawa. T. *J Nutr.* 2001;131(11):2932–2935.

99. Srinivasan K, Sambaiah K. *Int J Vitam Nutr Res.* 1991;61(4):364–369.

100. Babu PS, Srinivasan K. *Mol Cell Biochem.* 1997;166(1–2):169–175.

101. Grabe F. *Arch Exp Pathol Pharmacol.* 1935;176:673–676.

102. Jentzsch K, Gonda T, Holler H. *Pharm Acta Helv.* 1959;34:181–188.

103. Ramprasad C, Sirsi M. *J Sci Industr Res.* 1956;15C:262–265.

104. Ramprasad C, Sirsi M. *J Sci Industr Res.* 1957;16C:108–110.

105. Hussain MS, Chandrasekhara. N. *Indian J Med Res.* 1992;96:288–291.

106. Mukerji B, Zaidi SH, Singh GB. *J Sci Industr Res.* 1961;20C:25–28.

107. Rafatullah S, Tariq M, Al-Yahya MA, et al. *J Ethnopharmacol.* 1990;29:25–34.

108. Swarnakar S, Ganguly K, Kundu P, et al. *J Biol Chem.* 2005;280(10):9409–9415.

109. Chattopadhyay I, Bandyopadhyay U, Biswas K, et al. *Free Radic Biol Med.* 2006;40(8):1397–1408.

110. Kim DC, Kim SH, Choi BH, et al. *Biol Pharm Bull.* 2005;28(12):2220–2224.

111. Foryst-Ludwig A, Neumann M, Schneider-Brachert W, et al. *Biochem Biophys Res Commun.* 2004;316(4):1065–1072.

112. Jiao Y, Wilkinson J, Pietsch CE, et al. *Free Radic Biol Med.* 2006;40(7):1152–1160.

113. Itthipanichpong C, Ruangrungsi N, Kemsri W, et al. *J Med Assoc Thai.* 2003;86 (suppl 2):S299–S309.

114. Lutomski J, Kedzia B, Debska W. *Planta Med.* 1974;26:9–19.

115. Basu AP. *Indian J Pharm.* 1971;33:131.

116. Banerjee A, Nigam SS. *J Res Indian Med Yoga Homoeopathy.* 1978;13:63–70.

117. Tonnessen HH, De Vries H, Karlsen J, et al. *J Pharm Sci.* 1987;76:371–373.

118. Dahl TA, McGowan WM, Shard MA, et al. *Arch Microbiol.* 1989;151:183–185.

119. Kim KJ, Yu HH, Cha JD, et al. *Phytother Res.* 2005;19(7):599–604.

120. Apisariyakul A, Vanittanakom N, Buddhasukh D. *J Ethnopharmacol.* 1995;49(3):163–169.

121. Mazumder A, Raghavan K, Weinstein J, et al. *Biochem Pharmacol.* 1995;49(8):1165–1170.

122. Sui Z, Salto R, Li J, et al. *Biochem Pharmacol.* 1993;1(6):415–422.

123. Bourne KZ, Bourne N, Reising SF, et al. *Antiviral Res.* 1999;42(3):219–226.

124. Haddad M, Sauvain M, Deharo E. *Planta Med.* 2011;77(6):672–678.

125. Surh YJ, Chun KS. *Adv Exp Med Biol.* 2007;595:149–173.

126. López-Lázaro M. *Mol Nutr Food Res.* 2008;52(suppl 1):S103–S127.

127. Khor TO, Yu S, Kong AN. *Planta Med.* 2008;74(13):1540–1547.

128. Kunnumakkara AB, Anand P, Aggarwal BB. *Cancer Lett.* 2008;269(2):199–225.

129. Shalini VK, Srinivas L. *Mol Cell Biochem.* 1990;95:21–30.

130. Nagabhushan M, Bhide SV. *J Nutr Growth Cancer.* 1987;4(2):83–90.

131. Deshpande SS, Maru GB. *Cancer Lett.* 1995;96(1):71–80.

132. Aruna K, Sivaramakrishnan VM. *Indian J Exp Biol.* 1990;28:1008–1011.

133. Susan M, Rao MN. *Arzneimittelforschung.* 1992;42(7):962–964.

134. Nagabhushan M, Nair UJ, Amonkar AJ, et al. *Mutat Res.* 1988;202(1):163–169.

135. Bhide SV, Azuine MA, Lahiri M, et al. *Breast Cancer Res Treat.* 1994;30(3):233–242.

136. Mahmoud NN, Carothers AM, Grunberger D, et al. *Carcinogenesis.* 2000;21(5):921–927.

137. Azuine MA, Bhide SV. *J Ethnopharmacol.* 1994;44(3):211–217.

138. Azuine MA, Bhide SV. *Nutr Cancer.* 1992;17(1):77–83.

139. Kuttan G, Kumar KB, Guruvayoorappan C, et al. *Adv Exp Med Biol.* 2007;595:173–184.

140. Strimpakos AS, Sharma RA. *Antioxid Redox Signal.* 2008;10(3):511–545.

141. Ravindran J, Prasad S, Aggarwal BB. *AAPS J.* 2009;11(3):495–510.

142. Anand P, Sundaram C, Jhurani S, et al. *Cancer Lett.* 2008;267(1):133–164.

143. Kuttan R, Bhanumathy P, Nirmala K, et al. *Cancer Lett.* 1985;29:197–202.

144. Goodpasture CE, Arrighi FE. *Food Cosmet Toxicol.* 1976;14:9–14.

145. Bhandarkar SS, Arbiser JL. *Adv Exp Med Biol.* 2007;595:185–195.

146. Limtrakul P. *Adv Exp Med Biol.* 2007;595:269–300.

147. Nabekura T, Kamiyama S, Kitagawa S. *Biochem Biophys Res Commun.* 2005;327(3):866–870.

148. Zhou S, Lim LY, Chowbay B. *Drug Metab Rev.* 2004;36(1):57–104.

149. Tang XQ, Bi H, Feng JQ, et al. *Acta Pharmacol Sin.* 2005;26(8):1009–1016.

150. Anuchapreeda S, Leechanachai P, Smith MM, et al. *Biochem Pharmacol.* 2002;64(4):573–582.

151. Chearwae W, Anuchapreeda S, Nandigama K, et al. *Biochem Pharmacol.* 2004;69(10):2043–2052.

152. Chearwae W, Wu CP, Chu HY, et al. *Cancer Chemother Pharmacol.* 2006;57(3):376–388.

153. Mall M, Kunzelmann K. *Bioessays.* 2005;27(1):9–13.

154. Egan ME, Pearson M, Weiner SA, et al. *Science.* 2004;304(5670):600–602.

155. Song Y, Sonawane ND, Salinas D, et al. *J Biol Chem.* 2004;279(39):40629–40633.

156. Grubb BR, Gabriel SE, Mengos A, et al. *Am J Respir Cell Mol Biol.* 2006;34(3):355–363.

157. Yu YC, Miki H, Nakamura Y, et al. *J Cyst Fibros.* 2011;10(4):243–252.

158. Wang G. *J Biol Chem.* 2011;286(3):2171–2182.

159. Cartiera MS, Ferreira EC, Caputo C, et al. *Mol Pharm.* 2010;7(1):86–93.

160. Bernard K, Wang W, Narlawar R, et al. *J Biol Chem.* 2009;284(45):30754–30765.
161. Yu ZF, Kong LD, Chen Y. *J Ethnopharmacol.* 2002;83(1–2):161–165.
162. Xu Y, Ku BS, Yao HY, et al. *Eur J Pharmacol.* 2005;518(1):40–46.
163. Xu Y, Ku BS, Ya HY, et al. *Pharmacol Biochem Behav.* 2005;82(1):200–206.
164. Kulkarni S, Dhira Akula KK. *Sci World J.* 2009;9:1233–1241.
165. Alamdari N, O'Neal P, Hasselgren PO. *Nutrition.* 2009;25(2):125–129.
166. Poylin V, Fareed MU, O'Neal P, et al. *Mediators Inflamm.* 2008:13. ID: 317851.
167. Jin B, Li YP. *J Cell Biochem.* 2007;100(4):960–969.
168. Thaloor D, Miller KJ, Gephart J, et al. *Am J Physiol.* 1999;277(2 Pt 1):C320–C329.
169. Venkatesan N, Punithavathi D, Babu M. *Adv Exp Med Biol.* 2007;595:379–405.
170. Jagetia GC. *Adv Exp Med Biol.* 2007;595:301–320.
171. Kurup VP, Barrios CS. *Mol Nutr Food Res.* 2008;52(9):1031–1039.
172. Singh A, Singh SP, Bamezai R. *Cancer Lett.* 1995;96(1):87–93.
173. Sugimoto K, Nagata J, Yamagishi A, et al. *Gastroenterology.* 2006;78(19):2188–2193.
174. Cheng PY, Wang M, Morgan ET. *J Pharmacol Exp Ther.* 2003;307(3):1205–1212.
175. Jagetia GC, Rajanikant GK. *J Surg Res.* 2004;120(1):127–138.
176. Jagetia GC, Rajanikant GK. *J Wound Care.* 2004;13(3):107–109.
177. Jagetia GC, Rajanikant GK. *Plast Reconstr Surg.* 2005;115(2):515–528.
178. Kundu S, Biswas TK, Das P, et al. *Int J Low Extrem Wounds.* 2005;4(4):205–213.
179. Lee KS, Lee BS, Semnani S, et al. *Rejuvenation Res.* 2010;13(5):561–570.
180. Huang HC, Jan TR, Yeh SF. *Eur J Pharmacol.* 1992;221(2–3):381–384.
181. Anand P, Kunnumakkara AB, Newman RA, et al. *Mol Pharm.* 2007;4(6):807–818.
182. Sharma RA, Steward WP, Gescher AJ. *Adv Exp Med Biol.* 2007;595:453–470.
183. Villegas I, Sánchez-Fidalgo S, Alarcón de la Lastra C. *Mol Nutr Food Res.* 2008;52(9):1040–1061.
184. Wahlström B, Blennow G. *Acta Pharmacol Toxicol (Copenh).* 1978;43:86–92.
185. Ravindranath V, Chandrasekhara N. *Toxicology.* 1980;16:259–265.
186. Ravindranath V, Chandrasekhara N. *Toxicology.* 1981;20:251–257.
187. Ravindranath V, Chandrasekhara N. *Toxicology.* 1982;22:337–344.
188. Lin JK, Pan MH, Lin-Shiau SY. *Biofactors.* 2000;13(1–4):153–158.
189. Yang KY, Lin LC, Tseng TY, et al. *J Chromatogr B Analyt Technol Biomed Life Sci.* 2007;853(1–2):183–189.
190. Sharma RA, McLelland HR, Hill KA, et al. *Clin Cancer Res.* 2001;7(7):1894–1900.
191. Sharma RA, Euden SA, Platton SL, et al. *Clin Cancer Res.* 2004;10(20):6847–6854.
192. Garcea G, Berry DP, Jones DJ, et al. *Cancer Epidemiol Biomarkers Prev.* 2005;14(1):120–125.
193. Garcea G, Jones DJ, Singh R, et al. *Br J Cancer.* 2004;90(5):1011–1015.
194. Lao CD, Ruffin MT, Normolle D, et al. *BMC Complement Altern Med.* 2006;6:10.
195. Vareed SK, Kakarala M, Ruffin MT, et al. *Cancer Epidemiol Biomarkers Prev.* 2008;17(6):1411–1417.
196. Shoba G, Joy D, Joseph T, et al. *Planta Med.* 1998;64:353–356.
197. Antony B, Merina B, Iyer VS, et al. *Indian J Pharm Sci.* 2008;70(4):445–449.
198. Marczylo TH, Verschoyle RD, Cooke DN, et al. *Cancer Chemother Pharmacol.* 2007;60(2):171–177.
199. Cuomo J, Appendino G, Dern AS, et al. *J Nat Prod.* 2011;74(4):664–669.
200. Deodhar SD, Sethi R, Srimal RC. *Indian J Med Res.* 1980;71:632–634.
201. Satoskar RR, Shah SJ, Shenoy SG. *Int J Clin Pharmacol.* 1986;24:651–654.
202. Kulkarni RR, Patki PS, Jog VP, et al. *J Ethnopharmacol.* 1991;22(1–2):91–95.
203. Kuptniratsaikul V, Thanakhumtorn S, Chinswangwatanakul P, et al. *J Altern Complement Med.* 2009;15(8):891–897.
204. Belcaro G, Cesarone M, Dugall M, et al. *Panminerva Med.* 2010;52(2):1–8.
205. Belcaro G, Cesarone MR, Dugall M, et al. *Altern Med Rev.* 2010;15(4):337–344.
206. Ramirez-Bosca A, Carrion Gutierrez MA, Soler A, et al. *Age.* 1997;20(3):165–168.
207. Ramirez-Bosca A, Soler A, Carrion MA, et al. *Mech Ageing Dev.* 2000;119(1–2):41–47.
208. Ramirez-Bosca A, Soler A, Carrion MA, et al. *Mech Ageing Dev.* 2000;114(3):207–210.
209. Soni KB, Kuttan R. *Indian J Physiol Pharmacol.* 1992;36(4):273–275.
210. Alwi I, Santoso T, Suyono S, et al. *Acta Med Indones.* 2008;40(4):201–210.
211. Baum L, Cheung SK, Mok VC, et al. *Pharmacol Res.* 2007;56(6):509–514.
212. Hastak K, Lubri N, Jakhi SD, et al. *Cancer Lett.* 1997;116(2):265–269.
213. Cheng AL, Hsu CH, Lin JK, et al. *Anticancer Res.* 2001;21(4B):2895–2900.
214. Ide H, Tokiwa S, Sakamaki K, et al. *Prostate.* 2010;70(10):1127–1133.
215. Polasa K, Raghuram TC, Krishna TP, et al. *Mutagenesis.* 1992;7(2):107–109.
216. Krishnaswamy K, Raghuramulu N. *Indian J Med Res.* 1998;108:167–181.
217. Kuttan R, Sudheeran PC, Joseph CD. *Tumori.* 1987;73:29–31.
218. Dhillon N, Aggarwal BB, Newman RA, et al. *Clin Cancer Res.* 2008;14(14):4491–4499.
219. Bayet-Robert M, Kwiatkowski F, Leheurteur M, et al. *Cancer Biol Ther.* 2010;9(1):8–14.
220. Thamlikitkul MD, Bunyapraphatsara N, Dechatiwongse T, et al. *J Med Assoc Thai.* 1989;72(11):613–620.
221. Bundy R, Walker AF, Middleton RW, et al. *J Altern Complement Med.* 2004;1(6):1015–1018.
222. Durgaprasad S, Pai CG, Vasanthkumar *Indian J Med Res.* 2005;122(4):315–318.
223. Rasyid A, Lelo A. *Aliment Pharmacol Ther.* 1999;13(2):245–249.
224. Rasyid A, Rahman AR, Jaalam K, et al. *Asia Pac J Clin Nutr.* 2002;11(4):314–318.
225. Holt PR, Katz S, Kirshoff R. *Dig Dis Sci.* 2005;50(11):2191–2193.
226. Hanai H, Iida T, Takeuchi K, et al. *Clin Gastroenterol Hepatol.* 2006;4(12):1502–1506.
227. Kositchaiwat C, Kositchaiwat S, Havanondha J. *J Med Assoc Thai.* 1993;76(11):601–605.
228. Van Dau N, Ngoc Ham N, Huy Khac D, et al. *Phytomedicine.* 1998;5(1):29–34.
229. Prucksunand C, Indrasukhsri B, Leethochawalit M, et al. *Southeast Asian J Trop Med Public Health.* 2001;32(1):208–215.
230. Shimouchi A, Nose K, Takaoka M, et al. *Dig Dis Sci.* 2009;54(8):1725–1729.
231. Copeland R, Baker D, Wilson H. *Proc Int Conf AIDS.* 1994;10(2):216.
232. Hellinger JA, Cohen CJ, Dugan ME, et al. *3rd Conf Retro Opportun Infect.* 1996; Jan 28–Feb 1:78.
233. Gilden D, Smart T. *GMHC Treat Issues.* 1996;10(2):9.
234. Conteas CN, Panossian AM, Tran TT, et al. *Dig Dis Sci.* 2009;54(10):2188–2191.
235. Lal B, Kapoor AK, Agrawal PK, et al. *Phytother Res.* 2000;14(6):443–447.
236. Lal B, Kapoor AK, Asthana OP, et al. *Phytother Res.* 1999;13(4):318–322.
237. Allegri P, Mastromarino A, Neri P. *Clin Ophthalmol.* 2010;4:1201–1206.
238. Cruz-Correa M, Shoskes DA, Sanchez P, et al. *Clin Gastroenterol Hepatol.* 2006;4(8):1035–1038.
239. Burns J, Joseph PD, Rose KJ, et al. *Pediatr Neurol.* 2009;41(4):305–308.
240. Kalpravidh RW, Siritanaratkul N, Insain P, et al. *Clin Biochem.* 2010;43(4–5):424–429.
241. Usharani P, Mateen AA, Naidu MU, et al. *Drugs R D.* 2008;9(4):243–250.
242. Biswas J, Sinha D, Mukherjee S, et al. *Hum Exp Toxicol.* 2010;29(6):513–524.
243. Ringman JM, Frautschy SA, Cole GM, et al. *Curr Alzheimer Res.* 2005;2(2):131–136.
244. Ng TP, Chiam PC, Lee T, et al. *Am J Epidemiol.* 2006;164(9):898–906.
245. Baum L, Lam CW, Cheung SK, et al. *J Clin Psychopharmacol.* 2008;28(1):110–113.

246. Chainani-Wu N, Silverman Jr S, Reingold A, et al. *Phytomedicine*. 2007;14(7–8):437–446.

247. Heng MC, Song MK, Harker J, et al. *Br J Dermatol*. 2000;143(5):937–949.

248. Kurd SK, Smith N, VanVoorhees A, et al. *J Am Acad Dermatol*. 2008;58(4):625–631.

249. Heng MC. *Int J Dermatol*. 2010;49(6):608–622.

250. Charles V, Charles SX. *Trop Geogr Med*. 1992;44(1–2):178–181.

251. Shoskes D, Lapierre C, Cruz-Corerra M, et al. *Transplantation*. 2005;80(11):1556–1559.

252. Wickenberg J, Ingemansson SL, Hlebowicz J. *Nutr J*. 2010;9:43.

253. Adhvaryu MR, Reddy N, Vakharia BC. *World J Gastroenterol*. 2008;14(30):4753–4762.

254. Golombick T, Diamond TH, Badmaev V, et al. *Clin Cancer Res*. 2009;15(18):5917–5922.

255. Vermorken AJ, Zhu J, Van de Ven WJ. *Clin Cancer Res*. 2010;16(7):2225.

256. Francis FJ. *Food Chem Safety*. 2002:173–206.

257. Opdyke DLJ, Letizia C. *Food Chem Toxicol*. 1983;21(6):839–840.

258. Shankar TNB, Shantha NV, Ramesh HP, et al. *Indian J Exp Biol*. 1980;18(1):73–75.

259. Qureshi S, Shah AH, Ageel AM. *Planta Med*. 1992;58(2):124–127.

260. Vijayalaxmi *Mutat Res*. 1980;79(2):125–132.

261. Sambaiah K, Ratankumar S, Kamanna VS, et al. *J Food Sci Technol*. 1982;19:187–190.

262. Patil TN, Srinivasan M. *Indian J Exp Biol*. 1971;9(2):167–169.

263. Deshpande SS, Lalitha VS, Ingle AD, et al. *Toxicology Lett*. 1998;95(3):183–193.

264. Kandarkar SV, Sawant SS, Ingle AD, et al. *Indian J Exp Biol*. 1998;36(7):675–679.

265. Rao AJ, Kotagi SG. *IRCS Med Sci*. 1984;12:500–501.

266. Billie N, Larsen JC, Hansen EV, et al. *Food Chem Toxicol*. 1985;23:967–973.

267. Joshi J, Ghaisas S, Vaidya A, et al. *J Assoc Physicians India*. 2003;51:1055–1060.

268. Blasiak J, Trzeciak A, Malecka-Panas E, et al. *Teratog Carcinog Mutagen*. 1999;19(1):19–31.

269. Donatus IA, Vermeulen S, Vermeulen NPE. *Biochem Pharmacol*. 1990;39(12):1869–1875.

270. Jain AK, Tezuka H, Kada T, et al. *Curr Sci*. 1987;56:1005–1006.

271. Nagabhushan M, Bhide SV. *Nutr Cancer*. 1986;8(3):201–210.

272. Jensen NJ. *Mutat Res*. 1982;105(6):393–396.

273. Abraham SK, Kesavan PC. *Mutat Res*. 1984;136(1):85–88.

274. Shah RG, Netrawali MS. *Bull Environ Contam Toxicol*. 1998;40(3):350–357.

275. Mahmoud I, Alkofahi A, Abdelaziz A. *Int J Pharmacognosy*. 1992;30(2):81–85.

276. German Federal Minister of Justice. *German Commission E for Human Medicine Monograph*. Bundes-Anzeiger (German Federal Gazette), no. 223, dated 30.11.1985: no 164, dated 01.09.1990.

277. Blaschek W, Ebel S, Hackenthal E, et al. *HagerROM 2002: Hagers Handbuch der Drogen und Arzneistoffe*. Heidelberg: Springer; 2002.

278. Colalto C. *Pharmacol Res*. 2010;62(3):207–227.

279. Pavithra BH, Prakash N, Jayakumar K. *J Vet Sci*. 2009;10(4):293–297.

280. Juan H, Terhaag B, Cong Z, et al. *Eur J Clin Pharmacol*. 2007;63(7):663–668.

281. Tuntipopipat S, Judprasong K, Zeder C, et al. *J Nutr*. 2006;136(12):2970–2974.

282. Chen Y, Liu WH, Chen BL, et al. *Ann Pharmacother*. 2010;44(6):1038–1045.

283. Dharma AP. *Indonesian Medicinal Plants*. Jakarta: Balai Pustaka; 1987. pp. 148–149.

284. Cambie RC, Ash J. *Fijian Medicinal Plants*. Australia: CSIRO; 1994. 64–65.

285. Garg SK. *Planta Med*. 1974;26(3):225–227.

286. Chen ZZ, Yang DH, Zhou SQ, et al. *Zhong Cao Yao*. 1980;11(9):409–411.

287. An YS, Sung E, Yue YG, et al. *Shengzhi Yu Biyun*. 1983;3(1):57–58, 47.

288. Zhang YZ. *Chin Med J*. 1955;5:400.

289. Hata M, Sasaki E, Ota M, et al. *Contact Dermatitis*. 1997;36(2):107–108.

290. Lucas CD, Hallagan JB, Taylor SL. *Adv Food Nutr Res*. 2001;43:195–216.

291. Tang M, Larson-Meyer DE, Liebman M. *Am J Clin Nutr*. 2008;87(5):1262–1267.

Valerian

(*Valeriana officinalis* L.)

Synonyms

European valerian, all heal (Engl), Valerianae radix (Lat), Baldrianwurzel, Katzenwurzel, Balderbrackenwurzel (Ger), racine de valériane (Fr), valeriana, amantilla (Ital), baldrion (Dan).

What is it?

Species of Valeriana have enjoyed a long history of use in many herbal traditions as mild sedatives. Scientific studies have verified anxiolytic and hypnotic effects, but the exact biochemical mechanisms and active components are not completely understood. Although the root and rhizome of *Valeriana officinalis* L. is favoured by the European tradition, research has demonstrated that other species of Valeriana are also active; in particular, Mexican valerian (*Valeriana edulis* Nutt. ex Torr & Gray, or *V. mexicana* DC) is rich in active constituents. Indian valerian (*V. wallichii* DC or *V. jatamansi* Jones) is also used in herbal medicine. Japanese valerian (*V. fauriei* Briq.) is substantially different from all of these species and will not be considered here. Surprisingly, valerian and its oil have also been utilised in perfumery (valerian root has a strong and characteristic odour).

Effects

Improves subjective sleep quality, lowers periods of wakefulness, increases slow-wave sleep (consolidates non-REM sleep); reduces anxiety; relaxes smooth muscle.

Traditional view

Valerian has been an important in traditional medicine since the time of Dioscorides and Galen, where it was seen to have 'warming' or metabolic stimulating features. Its main applications in Graeco-Roman times were as a diuretic, carminative, menstrual stimulant and expectorant, and it was only briefly referred to as having any hypnotic action. It was also applied topically for cleansing and healing wounds and infections. After this time, valerian was seen as valuable for certain kinds of epilepsy with a reputation for an influence on the cerebrospinal system, in particular as a sedative in conditions of nervous unrest, stress and neuralgia. It has been employed as a sedative and spasmolytic in Europe since the sixteenth century and was officially recognised as such in the nineteenth and early twentieth centuries in North America and across much of the world. Valerian was used to promote sleep, particularly by the civilian population in Britain during World War II. In Europe,

oil of valerian was a popular remedy for cholera.[1,2] Paradoxical characteristics of valerian include its reputation as a stimulant and tonic in early European tradition, with use in depression and low-grade, unresolved, feverish conditions, and the North American Eclectic use as a cerebral stimulant in chorea, hysteria (with mental depression, despondency) and low forms of fever where a nervous stimulant was required. (The activity here was suggested as aiding cerebral circulation.) In contrast, it was also employed to relieve irritability, nervous headache and pain, and favour rest and sleep.[3]

Both *V. officinalis* and *V. wallichii* have been utilised in Ayurvedic traditional medicine for hysteria, neurosis and epilepsy. Indian valerian was also regarded as a carminative and spasmolytic.[4]

Reference has also been made to extensive use of valerian to treat shell shock after World War I.

Summary actions

Anxiolytic, mild sedative, hypnotic, spasmolytic.

Can be used for

Indications supported by clinical trials

Subjective difficulties with sleep, restlessness, nervous tension; may be useful for the treatment of depression or anxiety, especially in combination with other herbs, in particular *Hypericum perforatum*.

Traditional therapeutic uses

To promote sleep and as an anxiolytic for nervous unrest, stress, neuralgia, shell shock; epilepsy; as a tonic remedy in convalescing from illness; to relieve digestive and other spasms of smooth muscle.

May also be used for

Extrapolations from pharmacological studies

Alleviation of the symptoms of benzodiazepine withdrawal.

Preparations

Root/rhizome as a decoction; liquid extract, tincture, capsules and tablets for internal use.

Dosage

- 3 to 9 g/day dried root/rhizome
- 2 to 6 mL/day of 1:2 liquid extract, 5 to 15 mL/day of 1:5 tincture or equivalent solid doses.

The Commission E recommends that valerian root can be used for external application (for example as a bath additive), probably as a sedative and to promote sleep.

Duration of use

May be used long term.

Summary assessment of safety

No adverse effects from ingestion of valerian are expected when consumed within the recommended dosage range.

Technical data

Botany

Valeriana officinalis, a member of the Valerianaceae family, is a herbaceous plant growing to about 1 m. *Valeriana officinalis* is a collective term and includes subspecies and varieties. Polypoidy occurs in the species, ranging from diploid to octoploid types. The leaves are opposite, pinnate and mostly sessile, although the basal ones are petiolate and the leaflets are sometimes irregularly toothed. The flowers are hermaphrodite, arranged in a terminal cymose inflorescence with a many-toothed calyx and a pink, five-lobed corolla. The fruit is one-seeded with a leathery persistent calyx. It has a short, unbranched rhizome, rarely with stolons and rootlets with hollow centres.[5-7]

Key constituents

The *European Pharmacopoeia* defines valerian root as from *Valeriana officinalis* (European valerian) and containing not less than 5 mL/kg of essential oil.[8] The root and rhizome typically contain:

- Iridoids (0.5% to 2%), known as valepotriates (valeriana epoxy-triesters) including valtrate, isovaltrate, didrovaltrate and acevaltrate[9,10]
- Essential oil (0.35% to 1%), containing monoterpenes (mainly borneol, bornyl acetate), sesquiterpenes (beta-bisabolene, valerenal (fresh root)) and carboxylic compounds (esters of valerianic/isovaleric acid)[9]
- Non-volatile cyclopentane sesquiterpenes known as valerenic acid and its derivatives;[9] flavonoids, amino acids,[11] lignans,[12] low levels of GABA.[13] (See also under Sedative and anxiolytic activity.)

Valeriana edulis (Mexican valerian) contains 3% to 8% iridoids (and a larger valtrate/isovaltrate content); *Valeriana wallichii* (Indian valerian) contains 3% to 6% iridoids.[9] Valerenic acid and acetoxyvalerenic acid are unique to *V. officinalis*.[14] Studies in The Netherlands indicate there is seasonal variation in the content of these compounds in valerian roots.[15]

Valepotriates are unstable compounds: they are thermolabile and decompose rapidly under acid or alkaline conditions or in alcoholic solutions to form baldrinals.[16] These baldrinals, which can also form in dried valerian root or its extracts, can further decompose into inactive products. The characteristic odour of dried valerian is due to the isovaleric acid released by decomposing valepotriates.[17]

	R¹	R²	R³
Valtrate	acetyl	isovaleryl	isovaleryl
Isovaltrate	isovaleryl	acetyl	isovaleryl

isovaleryl = $(CH_3)_2CH-CH_2-CO-$
acetyl = $CHOCH_3$

	R
Valerenal	CHO
Valerenic acid	COOH

Pharmacodynamics

Some valepotriates have shown pronounced cytotoxicity in vitro[18] and this has caused concern in the past over the safety of valerian. However, subsequent research has indicated that the valepotriates are not cytotoxic when given orally; the unstable valepotriates do not survive the acidity of the stomach and form safe decomposition products.[19]

Sedative and anxiolytic activity

Valeriana officinalis contains several groups of compounds that demonstrate sedative activity. While much of the early research concentrated on the effects of the essential oil,[20,21] it was later proposed that this makes only a minor contribution to overall activity.[22] In fact, research as early as the 1950s demonstrated the essential oil was not primarily responsible for valerian's sedative activity.[23] More recently, however, valerian 'odorant' was shown to significantly prolong phenobarbital-induced sleeping time in rats that could smell (though not in anosmic ones). On EEG, significant shortening in sleep latency and prolongation of total sleep time were observed with valerian inhalation.[24] (The potential soporific effects of valerian odour increase the problems of double blinding in clinical trials, as is noted below. In some recent cases placebo capsules have been given a valerian odour to improve blinding: the above finding casts doubt on this strategy.)

Initial disappointment with the effects of the essential oil led to the search for other compounds, with the valepotriates being discovered about 10 years later.[25] Attention next focused on these[17] and then their decomposition products.[26] Subsequent investigations gave priority to valerenic acid and its derivatives as important sedative components that were unique to European valerian.[14] Being quite water soluble, these compounds could explain the activity of the aqueous extract of valerian noted in clinical trials.

More recently, several flavonoids that demonstrate CNS sedative activity have been identified in *V. officinalis* and *V. walichii*.[27] Specifically, the flavonoids 6-methylapigenin (an anxiolytic that binds to benzodiazepine binding sites),[28] hesperidin and linarin (which synergistically have significant sedative and sleep-enhancing effects)[29] have been isolated from *V. officinalis*.[30] However, these pharmacological findings were demonstrated in rats and mice after ip injection, casting some doubt on their relevance to the oral use of valerian, since flavonoid glycosides are typically not greatly absorbed as such (see Chapter 2). Furthermore, the 6-methylapigenin was found only at very low levels in the herb (60 μg/g).

When the valepotriates were compared with chlorpromazine (an antipsychotic drug), it was shown that their sedative effect was weaker but, unlike chlorpromazine, they actually improved coordination: while tests of the valepotriates on cats showed no decrease in reactivity, there were decreases in anxiety and aggression.[31] Diazepam increased the toxicity of alcohol, but no such effect occurred with valepotriates.[32]

Intraperitoneal administration of valerenic acid (50 to 100 mg/kg) demonstrated non-specific central depressant properties in tests conducted on mice and compared with diazepam, chlorpromazine and pentobarbital. A decrease in motility and prolongation of pentobarbital-induced sleeping time were observed. Other isolated sesquiterpenoid compounds such as valerenolic acid and valeranone did not cause impairment of performance. The activity resembled central nervous depression, rather than muscle relaxation or a neuroleptic effect.[21]

A study found that valepotriates (12 mg/kg, ip) reversed the anxiogenic effect of acute diazepam withdrawal in dependent rats, whereas 6 mg/kg failed to reverse these symptoms.[33] Later studies of an aqueous valerian extract revealed pronounced sedative effects in mice (10, 20 and 200 mg/kg, oral, of a 5:1 to 6:1 extract), as demonstrated by reduced motility and increased sleeping time. However, a direct comparison with diazepam and chlorpromazine revealed only a relatively moderate sedative activity for valerian.[34]

A study comparing four different valerian extracts in mice and rats found that none displayed sedative or myorelaxant effects up to oral doses of 1000 mg/kg.[35] In contrast, results obtained in the elevated plus maze test revealed a pronounced anxiolytic effect for the 45% methanolic and 35% ethanolic extracts, but not the 70% ethanolic extract (100 to 500 mg/kg for all extracts, oral). A refined 35% ethanolic extract also demonstrated antidepressant activity.

Valerian (as a 50% ethanolic extract equivalent to 100 mg/kg herb, ip) and valerenic acid (3 mg/kg, ip) demonstrated potent anxiolytic activity in rats in the elevated plus maze test.[13] The activity was comparable to diazepam (1 mg/kg, ip). The authors suggested that valerenic acid was the primary anxiolytic component in valerian.

The sedative effects of the valepotriates in humans were demonstrated in German clinical research conducted in the late 1960s.[36,37] A more recent example follows.

A randomised, double blind, placebo-controlled study examined the effects of valepotriates (300 mg/day; 80% didrovaltrate, 15% valtrate, 5% acevaltrate) or placebo on poor sleepers with a benzodiazepine dependency. Compared with normal sleepers and those taking placebo, participants in the valerian group showed significantly *higher* sleep latency (p<0.05). However, valerian users were also found to have improved slow-wave sleep and deep sleep, and decreased stage 2 non-REM sleep. Stages 3 and 4 non-REM sleep were similar in all groups. During the second week of the trial, sleep was rated better by those taking valerian than by those taking placebo.[38]

Interaction with neurological receptors

Research on agents with sedative or anxiolytic activity often explores potential interactions with receptors that can mediate such effects. Much of this information regarding valerian or its components is presented below. Conflicting results are apparent and any interpretation or extrapolation of this largely in vitro work needs to be conducted with caution because of the many uncertainties involved.

Both valerian and valerenic acid bind to GABA-A receptors in vitro,[39] specifically the beta-3 GABA-A receptor.[40] Valerenic acid is an allosteric modulator of this receptor,[41] potentiating the effects of GABA at lower concentrations in vitro and inhibiting them at higher concentrations.[42] Valerian extract also stimulated glutamic acid decarboxylase activity in vitro.[43] An aqueous extract of valerian induced the release of radiolabelled GABA in rat brain synaptosomes. The release was Na^+ dependent, Ca^{2+} independent and sensitive to certain transport inhibitors, suggesting reversal of the GABA carrier. The increase in GABA release appears to be independent of Na^+,K^+-ATPase activity and membrane potential. Further in vitro work showed that the amount of GABA present in aqueous extracts of valerian is sufficient to account for this release from synaptosomes, since valerian extract increased the release of radiolabelled GABA by the same mechanism as exogenous GABA.[44] A comparison of three different valerian extracts on the release of GABA in rat brain synaptosomes in vitro found the aqueous and aqueous-alcoholic extracts stimulated release, but the pure ethanolic extract did not. GABA was absent from the ethanol extract and present in the others.[45]

In an early study, a hydroalcoholic extract of valerian (but not the aqueous extract) demonstrated a dose-dependent inhibition of binding to adenosine receptors, indicating a sedative effect.[46] In a more recent study, polar extracts of valerian appear to bind to adenosine A1 receptors, while non-polar extracts rich in isovaltrate have been shown to act as antagonists or inverse agonists at the same site[47] (this might be compatible with the preference for water-based extracts in traditional use). In vitro studies suggest that activation of A1 and GABA-A receptors is mediated by different components of valerian; the two mechanisms may contribute independently to valerian's sleep-inducing effect.[48] A lignan isolated from valerian bound the human A1 adenosine receptor in micromolar and submicromolar concentrations,[49] activity that is supported by the finding that a proprietary valerian extract acts as an A1 receptor agonist in a concentration-dependent manner in vitro,[50] and a valerian-hops extract acted as an A1 receptor agonist in rats.[51] Both valerian and valerenic acid appear to be partial agonists of $5\text{-}HT_{5A}$ receptor in vitro.[52]

Using an in vitro cell culture model of the blood-brain barrier, valerenic acid and its derivatives did not exhibit significant transport by passive diffusion, instead probably relying on an unknown and relatively slow transport system.[53] Hence, as noted above, in vitro receptor studies need to be interpreted with caution.

Other activity

Valerian extract was found to have neuroprotective activity in vitro against the toxicity of amyloid beta peptide; this activity may be mediated by signalling pathways involving Ca^{2+}.[54] Neuroprotective activity of valerian has also been demonstrated against common neurotoxic agents in vitro[55] and for an in vitro model of Parkinson's disease.[56]

Orally administered ethanolic and aqueous extracts of valerian (50, 100 and 200 mg/kg) to guinea pigs demonstrated antihypertensive, coronary spasmolytic and bronchospasmolytic activities, similar to those exhibited by the calcium-channel blocker nifedipine.[57] Direct spasmolytic activity has been demonstrated in vitro on isolated human non-pregnant uterine muscle.[58]

Intraperitoneal administration of valerian root extract or valerenic acid demonstrated anticonvulsant activity in mice against picrotoxin (but not pentetrazol and harman) with an ED_{50} of between 4.5 and 6 mg/kg.[59] The aqueous extract of valerian (500 mg/kg, ip) demonstrated anticonvulsant activity in a rat model of temporal lobe epilepsy.[60] This effect was thought to be partially mediated through the activation of the adenosine system.

Pharmacokinetics

Following incubation of valerian with freshly prepared rat hepatocytes, analysis revealed considerable metabolism of sesquiterpenes and iridoids through O-deacetylation. Acetoxyvalerenic acid decreased 9-fold, while hydroxyvalerenic acid increased 9-fold. Valerenic acid did not appear to change appreciably. The valepotriates didrovaltrate, isovaltrate and valtrate decreased 2-, 18- and 16-fold, respectively.[61] The main decomposition products of valtrate and isovaltrate included the metabolites baldrinal and homobaldrinal, whereas the decomposition products of dihydrovaltrate did not.[62] Human digestion has the same decomposing effect on these key constituents. This is not an inherent problem, since the initial decomposition products of valepotriates are active as sedatives.[26] Oral, intravenous and intraduodenal administration of radiolabelled didrovaltrate in mice demonstrated that it is only absorbed in the unchanged form to a small extent.[63]

After administration of valerenic acid to rats, the hepatic formation of seven valerenic acid glucuronides was observed, which were excreted into bile.[64]

Six healthy adults (aged 22 to 61 years, five men and one woman) received a single 600 mg dose of valerian extract (about 2.7 g of dried root) at 8 a.m. Blood samples were collected for 8 h after administration.[65] The maximum serum concentration (Cmax) of valerenic acid for five of the six volunteers occurred after 1 to 2 h and ranged from 0.9 to 2.3 ng/mL. Valerenic acid serum concentrations were measurable for at least 5 h after the valerian dose. One participant showed a peak plasma value at 1 h and a second peak at 5 h. The elimination half-life for valerenic acid was about 1.1 h. The area under the concentration time curve (AUC), as a measure of valerenic acid exposure, was variable and not correlated with age or weight. Assuming that valerenic acid serum concentrations correlate with the pharmacological activity of valerian, the timing of the valerenic acid peak concentration is consistent with the standard recommendation to take valerian 30 min to 2 h before bed.

Further work has been published by the same research group. The pharmacokinetics of valerenic acid was determined in a group of 16 elderly women after receiving a single nightly valerian dose (300 mg of extract) and after 2 weeks of valerian dosing.[66] There was not a statistically significant difference in Cmax, time to maximum concentration (Tmax), AUC, elimination half-life (t1/2) and oral clearance after a single dose compared with multiple dosing. There was considerable inter- and intra-subject variability in the pharmacokinetic parameters. Cmax and AUC decreased and t1/2 increased with increased body weight. The authors suggested that the large variability in the pharmacokinetics of valerenic acid may contribute to inconsistencies in the effect of valerian as a sleep aid.

Clinical trials

Sleep quality

The consensus view that valerian is an effective treatment for sleep problems has been questioned by recent reviews of the clinical trial data. In a 2006 systematic review, the authors found 370 articles and listed 16 that met their inclusion criteria.[67] They concluded that valerian may improve sleep quality, but the methodological problems even in the included studies limited the ability to draw firm conclusions. In a 2007 review supported by the US National Institutes of Health (selecting 36 studies, including 17 in German) the conclusions were less positive, and the authors found no convincing evidence of efficacy in sleep. They added concerns about the poor quality of published studies, including the failure to account for the distinctive aroma of valerian root in designing double blind studies and the use of non-robust outcomes. They noted also that none of the most recent studies, which were also the most methodologically rigorous, found significant effects of valerian on sleep.[68]

A 2010 systematic review and meta-analysis again found methodological shortcomings in some of the 18 included studies and concluded that, although studies choosing qualitative dichotomic outcomes (for example, was sleep quality improved or not?) tended to be positive, suggesting that valerian could be effective for subjective improvement of insomnia, its efficacy has not been established by quantitative or objective measurements.[69] In contrast, the assessment report on *Valeriana officinalis* from the Committee on Herbal Medicinal Products (HMPC) of the European Medicines Agency concluded that: '…the evidence available from literature and from clinical trials with valerian root extracts in adults confirms that aqueous-ethanolic extracts of valerian root have a clinical effect in sleep disturbances as assessed by subjective ratings as well as by means of validated psychometric scales and EEG recordings… There is quite strong evidence from both clinical experience and sleep EEG studies that the treatment effect increases during treatment over several weeks'.[70]

Whilst objective measurements provide valuable information, it has been argued that from the user's point of view subjective experience may be a more realistic assessment of sleep quality.[71] If so, this needs to be more clearly articulated in claims for the remedy. The following examples of clinical trials are among the highly rated studies featuring in the reviews cited above.

In Leathwood and Chauffard's classic valerian research from Switzerland in the 1980s, 128 volunteers tested three sets of tablets over three non-consecutive nights: freeze-dried aqueous valerian extract (400 mg, approximately 3:1), a proprietary preparation containing an equivalent amount of valerian extract and a hops extract (200 mg, extract ratio unknown), and placebo. The valerian extract did not contain valepotriates or essential oil, but presumably contained valepotriate decomposition products and valerenic acid derivatives. Based on a subjective assessment by patients, the researchers found that valerian shortened sleep latency (p<0.05) and improved sleep quality, without increasing sleepiness the next morning, compared with placebo. Further analysis of results indicated that the group of volunteers who rated themselves as good sleepers were largely unaffected by valerian, but the poor or irregular sleepers reported a significant improvement (p<0.05). Interestingly, valerian did not increase the frequency of 'more sleepy than usual (the next morning)' responses.[71–73]

Leathwood and Chauffard also conducted a double blind, placebo-controlled study on eight poor sleepers, in this case combining an objective measurement of sleep latency with subjective assessment. Dried aqueous valerian extract corresponding to 1.3 g of root taken 1 h before retiring reduced sleep latency (as the average time taken to fall asleep) from 15.8 to 9 min. Participants also reported significant improvements in sleep quality and depth, without increased sleepiness the next morning. The authors commented that results for valerian compared favourably with those from studies of conventional sleeping agents. Higher doses of valerian 1 h before retiring were not as beneficial as the 1.3 g dose.[74]

In a later trial by other researchers, the efficacy and tolerability of a valerian tablet were evaluated against placebo in the treatment of insomnia. This randomised, double blind study was conducted on 121 patients diagnosed with insomnia not due to organic causes. Patients were studied over 4 weeks and the daily dosage of aqueous-ethanolic valerian extract was 600 mg (equivalent to about 2400 mg of dried root and rhizome), taken in the evening. Clinicians rated sleep improvement as higher following valerian therapy than after placebo. Patients also preferred valerian, and at the 28-day mark there was a significant improvement in the feeling of being rested after sleep for valerian treatment. Subjective sleep quality also improved significantly in the valerian group. In both the valerian and the placebo groups, the rate of side effects was 3.3% and the drop-out rate was also 3.3%.[75,76] Note that the dosage used was reasonably high and the paradoxical stimulation that valerian can induce in some patients was not observed at this high dose. Improvements in sleep latency time and sleep quality were also observed in 80 elderly patients treated with 270 mg/day of an aqueous dried valerian extract (5:1 to 6:1) for 14 days.[77]

In a double blind, placebo-controlled, crossover study of the effect of *V. edulis* on children with IQ of less than 70 and significant sleep problems, valerian (20 mg/kg) was found to reduce sleep latency and time spent awake and increase total sleep time and sleep quality, compared with baseline. No significant changes from baseline occurred with placebo. Valerian capsules (500 mg dried, whole, crushed root, containing 5.52 mg valtrate/isovaltrate) or placebo (25 mg whole root valerian extract, preparation not specified) capsules were administered nightly before bed for 2 weeks. This study was small (n=5), short (2 weeks), male-only, involving a heterogeneous group of subjects (different disabilities and medications), and subjectively evaluated by parents.[78]

Several trials have measured objective parameters (especially EEG traces) EEG in volunteers or poor sleepers provided with single doses of valerian, often compared with placebo or conventional drugs. One such trial yielding positive results is reviewed below.

A small randomised, double blind, placebo-controlled, cross-over study was conducted in 16 patients with previously established psychophysiological insomnia (ICSD code 1A1), confirmed by polysomnographic recording. A mix of measures of sleep quality was used, including regular polysomnographic recordings. Subjective parameters such as sleep quality, morning feeling, daytime performance, perceived duration of sleep latency and sleep period time were assessed by means of questionnaires. After a single dose of valerian, no effects on sleep structure and subjective sleep assessment were observed. After multiple-dose treatment, sleep efficiency showed a significant increase for both placebo and valerian in comparison with baseline polysomnography. There were, however, significant differences between valerian and placebo for parameters describing slow-wave sleep. In comparison with the placebo, slow-wave sleep latency was reduced after administration of valerian (21.3 versus 13.5 min, respectively, $p<0.05$). The reported time in bed was increased after long-term valerian treatment, compared with baseline (9.8 versus 8.1%, respectively, $p<0.05$). At the same time point, a tendency for shorter subjective sleep latency, as well as a higher correlation coefficient between subjective and objective sleep latencies, was observed under valerian treatment.[79]

Some of the strongest papers with negative outcomes identified in the above reviews relate to the use of objective measures. Two of these trials are described below.

In a randomised, double blind, placebo-controlled, three-way crossover study, participants took 300 or 600 mg of a valerian dry root extract (3:1 to 6:1, 70% ethanol) or placebo. Prior to the study, sleep EEG was recorded during an adaptation night. Sixteen sleep-disturbed participants aged 50 to 64 years slept overnight in a sleep laboratory. EEG sleep was recorded for each person throughout the night, and a psychometric evaluation was performed in the morning. Test periods were separated by a 6-day washout period. Results showed no significant effect between valerian 300 mg, valerian 600 mg or placebo on any EEG parameter or psychometric measure.[80]

The effect of an aqueous valerian extract on sleep quality was investigated in two groups of healthy, young volunteers, some of whom slept at home (subjective assessment) and the others in a sleep laboratory (objective assessment). In the home study, both doses of valerian extract (450 mg, 900 mg) reduced perceived sleep latency and wake time after sleep onset. A dose-dependent effect was suggested by the results. In the sleep laboratory where the higher dose was used, no significant differences from placebo were obtained. However, the direction of the changes corresponded to those observed under home conditions.[81] It has been suggested that the lack of significant changes in the objective sleep parameters may have been due to the selection of participants: young people with normal sleep quality, rather than those with disturbed sleep.[82]

Other clinical studies have yielded some novel findings. A small, pilot trial investigated the effect of treatment with valerian on the symptom severity of restless legs syndrome (RLS). Over 8 weeks, 37 patients received valerian or placebo.[83] The dried root of valerian (0.8 g/day) was provided in capsules, and contained 0.58 mg of total valerenic acids per capsule (1.16 mg/day). The single dose of herb or placebo was taken 60 min before bed. Patients made subjective assessments at baseline and at the completion of treatment.

Patients in both the valerian and placebo groups experienced an improvement in sleep quality and RLS severity over the duration of the study. Although the valerian group showed a greater improvement for the majority of sleep quality and RLS scores, there was no statistically significant difference between the groups. Further analysis evaluated the efficacy of valerian in the subgroup of sleepy versus non-sleepy participants. 'Sleepy' was defined as a score of 10 or greater on the Epworth Sleepiness Scale. Significant differences were found between sleepy and non-sleepy groups in sleepiness scores before and after valerian treatment. A strong positive association between changes in sleepiness and RLS symptom severity was found in the valerian group. These results suggest that valerian may be beneficial for people who have severe RLS that affects unrecovered sleep and causes excessive sleepiness during the day.

Residual sedative effects were examined in a controlled study involving 20 healthy volunteers who were assigned to four treatment groups and received the following medication as a single dose: tablets of valerian and hops, valerian syrup, flunitrazepam or placebo. Objectively measurable impairment of performance on the morning after medication occurred only in the flunitrazepam group. Fifty per cent of volunteers in the flunitrazepam group reported mild side effects, compared with 10% from the other groups. Subjective perception of sleep quality was improved in all three medication groups compared with placebo. A very slight impairment of vigilance after taking valerian syrup was statistically significant, as was retardation in the processing of complex information for the tablets. It was suggested that these herbal treatments offer a viable alternative to benzodiazepines with regard to reducing any impairment of vigilance on the morning after ingestion.[84]

Combination products and sleep quality

Valerian has also been combined with other herbal extracts including *Melissa officinalis* (lemon balm), passionflower and hops for the treatment of sleep disorders. The combination of valerian and hops has been studied for more than 30 years in clinical trials. For example, in an early double blind, placebo-controlled study, a combination of valerian extract (240 mg/day) and hops extract (400 mg/day) reduced noise-induced disturbance of sleep stage patterns (slow-wave sleep and REM) in sleep-disturbed people, compared with baseline values. The authors suggested that the initial treatment of severe insomnia with strong sleeping pills could be followed by a period of herbal use before discontinuation of therapy.[85]

A more recent study of good methodological quality (although small) compared a combination of valerian and hops extracts against the same valerian extract on its own. Using a double blind, placebo-controlled design, 30 patients were randomised to receive either 500 mg valerian extract (5.3:1, 45% methanol) and 120 mg hops extract (6.6:1, 45% methanol), 500 mg valerian extract alone or placebo as a single daily dose for 4 weeks.[86] Only the combination was significantly superior to placebo in terms of reducing objectively measured sleep latency (the primary trial outcome) from 56.5 min at baseline to 12.0 min. (The authors assigned a p value of 0.10

or less as significant, taking into account the small number of patients and the individual instability of the sleep parameters.) Analysis of the secondary outcomes revealed statistically significant superiority for the combination over placebo for percentage of slow-wave sleep (stages 3 and 4) and clinical global impression.

A single-dose study of a valerian and hops liquid combination (fresh plant tinctures) also yielded positive results in a recent randomised, double blind, placebo-controlled trial using an EEG-derived parameter for sleep quality.[87,88]

The draft assessment report of the HMPC on valerian and hops in combination reviewed six clinical trials and concluded that: '... preclinical and clinical evidence are sufficient to support a well-established use of several fixed combinations of valerian root dry extract and hops dry extract to treat patients suffering from non-organic sleep disorders'.[89]

The effect of a herbal preparation (dried aqueous-ethanolic extracts of valerian (160 mg, no valepotriates detected; 4.5:1) and lemon balm (80 mg, 5.5:1)) on objective sleep parameters was compared with a sedative drug (triazolam) and placebo in 20 volunteers, including both good and poor sleepers. The herbal preparation induced a significant increase ($p < 0.05$) in sleep efficiency in stages 3 and 4 (slow-wave sleep). It was apparent that poor sleepers benefited more from the treatment, as indicated by the significant increase in delta sleep. There was no shortening of sleep latency or wake time. Rebound effects were not observed for either the herbal preparation or triazolam.[90]

A randomised, double blind, placebo-controlled, multicentre trial investigated the use of the same herbal preparation in 68 ambulatory patients with light insomnia. Those in the test group received two tablets, each containing dried aqueous-ethanol extracts of valerian (160 mg, 4.5:1) and lemon balm (80 mg, 5.5:1) twice a day for a period of 3 weeks. In the treatment group, improvement in the primary test criteria (sleep quality, daily condition, initiative, and change in condition) occurred after 2 weeks. The valerian and lemon balm combination also improved accompanying indicators such as time to fall asleep, total duration of sleep, concentration and performance ability. There were no hangover, withdrawal or rebound phenomena in the treated group.[91]

The same combination of valerian and lemon balm extracts was found to be beneficial in the treatment of restlessness and dyssomnia in children less than 12 years old.[92] (Dyssomnia is a broad category of sleep disorders characterised by either insomnia or hypersomnia (excessive sleepiness).) In an uncontrolled, multicentre, postmarketing surveillance study, patients were treated for at least 4 weeks with a maximum daily dose of four tablets. A total of 918 patients were evaluated. Restlessness and dyssomnia were reduced from moderate or severe to either mild or absent in most of the patients. The benefit was assessed as very good or good by parents (60.5%) and investigators (67.7%). There were no herb-related adverse effects observed. However, since this trial lacked a control group its value is more in demonstrating the safety of the combination in children.

Twenty healthy volunteers took two tablets of a herbal combination three times on the day before their sleep was evaluated, or a matching placebo, in a double blind, randomised trial.[93] The total daily dose of each herbal extract was 360 mg St John's wort (*Hypericum perforatum*), 168 mg valerian and 192 mg passionflower, corresponding to around 2 g, 0.9 g and 1 g of equivalent dried herb, respectively. The herbal formulation significantly improved sleep quality. This was manifested as improved sleep continuity and reductions in sleep latency, wakefulness, the period of the first sleep cycle (especially non-REM sleep) and the REM latency. For example, REM latency (the time until REM sleep begins) was reduced from 98 to 72 min ($p = 0.005$). These effects were compensated by an increase in non-REM sleep (deep sleep) in the second sleep cycle. The following day a positive trend was observed in terms of mood and some aspects of anxiety, but there was no deterioration (or improvement) of cognitive performance from the herbal treatment.

Other conditions

The effect of valerian on activation, performance and mood of healthy volunteers under social stress conditions was investigated in a single-dose, double blind, placebo-controlled design. An undefined valerian extract (200 mg) favourably influenced subjective feelings of somatic arousal, despite high physiological activation during a call-up procedure in which participants were asked to solve mental arithmetic problems. No sedative effects were demonstrated, which suggested that valerian has thymoleptic activity.[94]

A number of clinical trials have investigated the use of a combination of valerian and St John's wort for the treatment of depression or anxiety. Some of these trials are outlined below.

The combination was shown to have equivalent benefits to the drug amitriptyline in a randomised, controlled, double blind study. One hundred and forty-seven outpatients aged between 20 and 65 were given a daily dose of 450 to 900 mg of valerian and St John's wort extracts (containing 0.45 to 0.9 mg total hypericin) or 75 to 150 mg of amitriptyline over 6 weeks. Benefit was observed in 82% of patients in the herbal group compared with 77% in the amitriptyline group. The total Hamilton Depression Score was reduced from 24.2 to 8.4 after 6 weeks with herbal treatment and from 24.3 to 8.9 after the drug. Statistical analysis showed that the herbal treatment was equivalent in benefit to amitriptyline, but without the high frequency of side effects such as dry mouth and lethargy.[95] In an earlier double blind trial involving 93 patients, this herbal combination demonstrated significant improvement compared to the antidepressant desipramine, as assessed by physicians after 6 weeks of treatment ($p = 0.0004$).[96] There was also a significant improvement in the Physical Complaint Inventory compared with the drug treatment ($p = 0.0021$).

The same combination (at a dose containing 0.3 to 0.6 mg/day total hypericin) was also shown in another double blind study to be significantly more effective than diazepam after 2 weeks of treatment in 100 patients suffering from moderate anxiety. Fewer side effects were observed in the herbal treatment group (4%), compared with diazepam treatment (14%).[97] A comparable reduction in symptoms of fear and depressive mood was observed for a valerian-St

John's wort combination in comparison to amitriptyline. This double blind, multicentre trial treated 162 patients diagnosed with fear and depression.[98] In a drug monitoring study that included 5682 patients, only 1.1% of patients reported side effects with the valerian-St John's wort combination.[99]

A double blind, placebo-controlled, three-way crossover trial investigated a valerian and St John's wort extract combination and St John's wort extract alone for their effects on safety-related performance in 12 volunteers tested over 10 days. The two herbal products were shown to be comparable to placebo in terms of performance and well-being. The effect after simultaneous intake of alcohol was not greater than that for alcohol alone.[100]

Toxicology and other safety data

Toxicology

Valerian extract (extracted with ether and then 90% ethanol to produce a 9.5:1 concentrate) exhibited an LD_{50} of 3.3 g/kg after ip injection to mice.[101] The oral LD_{50} of the essential oil was 15 g/kg in mice.[102] Studies involving large doses of valerian extract (600 mg/kg/day; undefined extract strength, 1.5% valtrates) over 30 days in rats showed unremarkable adverse effects.[103] A month of exposure to *Valeriana officinalis* did not produce any oxidative damage to the CNS in a murine model.[104]

No acute toxicity was found for valtrate, didrovaltrate and acevaltrate in mice after oral administration up to 4.6 g/kg.[31] Oral treatment of mice with doses of 500, 1000 and 2000 mg/kg/day of valerian extract/root combination for 7 days resulted in increased aberrations in chromosomes in the testis, induced spermatozoa abnormalities and affected erythrocyte ratios adversely in the femur (this last finding only at the highest dose).[105] These findings need to be repeated before any definitive conclusions can be drawn about the impact of valerian on male fertility.

Valepotriates developed mutagenic activity only in the presence of S9 mix in the Salmonella/microsome test and the SOS chromotest. Baldrinal and homobaldrinal showed mutagenic effects in both tests with and without metabolic activation.[62] The cytotoxic potential of valerian constituents and valerian tinctures was investigated in two human in vitro cancer cell lines. Valepotriates of the diene type (valtrate, isovaltrate, acevaltrate) demonstrated the highest toxicity. In comparison, valepotriates of the monoene type were 2- to 3-fold less toxic. The decomposition products baldrinal and homobaldrinal were 10 to 30 times less toxic. Valerenic acids also showed low toxicity. A clear relationship between valepotriate content and in vitro toxicity was established for fresh tinctures (*V. officinalis*, *V. edulis* subsp. *procera*, *V. wallichii*; all 1:5). A significant reduction in cytotoxicity was observed for the same tinctures stored at room temperature for 2 months. These stored tinctures had lower concentrations of valepotriates, which had decomposed.[106]

Contraindications

None known.

Special warnings and precautions

None required.

Interactions

Speculative suggestions of interactions have been made in the cases of antiepileptic prescriptions,[107] anaesthetics[108,109] and various other sedative drugs.[110] However, these are generally not well supported by other evidence. A single animal study suggests a potential interaction between the antipsychotic haloperidol and valerian: a potential marker for oxidative stress (hepatic delta-aminolevulinic acid dehydratase activity) was inhibited after supplementation with both medications, while levels remained unchanged when administered singly.[111]

In vitro studies found that valerian modulates CYP 3A4[112,113] and other metabolic enzymes.[114] However, a human study found that 1000 mg of valerian administered nightly to healthy adults for 2 weeks did not alter drug metabolism via the CYP3A4 or 2D6 pathways.[115] A second study in 12 healthy human volunteers found that 28 days of valerian supplementation had no effect on phenotypic ratios for CYP3A4/5, CYP1A2, CYP2E1 or CYP2D6.[116]

A brief episode of acute delirium occurred in a woman taking loperamide (an opioid-based antidiarrhoeal agent), St John's wort and valerian.[117] Hand tremor, dizziness and muscular fatigue were reported in a 40-year-old male patient treated with lorazepam who additionally self-prescribed valerian and passionflower.[118]

Compounding effects on mental symptoms in alcohol abusers have been adduced from a 51-year-old woman consuming alcohol (about 0.3 gallon/day of wine for more than 2 years), valerian tablets (about 2 to 4 g/day, 2 years) and Ginkgo (unknown amount, unknown duration) who presented with fainting and psychosis. Alcohol intake was increased prior to the incident.[119]

Use in pregnancy and lactation

Category B1 - no increase in frequency of malformation or other harmful effects on the fetus from limited use in women. No evidence of increased fetal damage in animal studies.

No problems were noted in three cases of intentional overdose with 2 to 5 g of valerian during weeks 3 to 10 of pregnancy.[120] Very high oral doses of valerian (2.79 g/kg/day) reduced placental weights at days 1 to 8 and days 8 to 15 of gestation in rats. Fetal weights showed no significant changes compared with controls. Implantation loss and litter size were not significantly different from controls and major malformations were relatively rare. The herb was administered as an ethanol extract and the dose administered was the highest possible at which ethanol remained below the teratogenic threshold.[121]

There was no alteration in the fertility of female rats after oral administration of a mixture of valepotriates (6 to 24 mg/day, for 30 days). In another study, the valepotriate mixture was given from the first to the 19th day of pregnancy (6 to 24 mg/day) and did not exert fetotoxicity or affect external formation. However, internal examination revealed an increase in the number of retarded ossifications at the higher doses (12 and 24 mg/kg).[122]

In a review of the Swedish Medical Birth Register from 1995 to 2004, valerian was one of the most commonly reported herbs used during pregnancy. An analysis of the database found no evidence of unfavourable outcomes associated with valerian use, although the number of exposures was too low to detect rare outcomes.[123]

Valerian is compatible with breastfeeding but caution should be observed.

Effects on ability to drive and use machines

No adverse effect is expected. Evidence from clinical trials indicates that valerian does not cause excessive sedation. A randomised, controlled, double blind trial involving 102 male and female volunteers showed no effect on reaction time, alertness and concentration on the morning after intake of 600 mg root extract. The primary criterion was median reaction time measured with the Vienna Determination Test. Secondary criteria were an alertness test, a two-handed coordination test, sleep quality and safety. The single administration of valerian did not impair reaction time, concentration and coordination. After 14 days of treatment the effect of valerian on reaction time was no different from placebo.[124]

In an Australian study, nine healthy volunteers received single doses of valerian root (1000 mg or 500 mg), the drug triazolam (0.25 mg) or placebo in a double blind, placebo-controlled, crossover trial.[125] Results confirmed that while triazolam had a detrimental effect on cognitive processes, the valerian was without effect. Another study compared even higher doses of valerian (600, 1200 and 1800 mg of a 5:1 extract) with 10 mg diazepam and placebo in a clinical trial of similar design.[126] Again an impairment of performance occurred for the benzodiazepine drug, whereas the valerian had no impact on any parameters tested. A third study found that valerian (400 mg and 800 mg) was not different from placebo on any measure used of psychomotor performance or sedation.[127]

As noted earlier, residual sedative effects were examined in a controlled study involving 20 healthy volunteers assigned to receiving either tablets of valerian and hops, valerian syrup, flunitrazepam or placebo. Objectively measurable impairment of performance on the morning after medication occurred only in the flunitrazepam group.[84]

Side effects

In some individuals, valerian can aggravate a sensation of tiredness or drowsiness, particularly in higher doses, but this is usually more a case of an increased awareness of the body's needs rather than a negative depressant effect. A few people find valerian stimulating and should avoid its use.

There are few confirmed human cases where valerian is strongly associated with adverse effects and, given the variability of some commercial examples, identification of suspect products is rare. A literature search of clinical trial data confirmed that there were few adverse effects reported in the short term.[128] A remarkable finding of one study (that demonstrated efficacy of long-term use of valerian in reducing insomnia in a randomised, placebo-controlled, crossover trial) was the extremely low number of adverse events during the valerian treatment periods, substantially less than placebo.[79]

Only one minor stomach reaction was observed in randomised, double blind, controlled clinical trial with a valerian-hop product.[129] In another sleep study, 600 mg/day valerian extract was at least as efficacious as 10 mg/day oxazepam in a double blind, randomised study in 202 subjects. Over 6 weeks adverse events occurred in 28.4% of patients receiving valerian extract and 36% of patients under oxazepam, and were all rated mild to moderate.[130] Three cases of 'vivid dreams' were the only side effect reported in 19 people observed taking valerian over 6 weeks in a controlled study.[131]

One publication contained unusual reports of toxic reactions to valerian root in Israel.[132] These included nephrotoxicity, headaches, chest tightness, mydriasis, abdominal pain and tremor. In the absence of additional information, the linking of these adverse reactions to valerian intake is highly suspect.

Reports of an association of valerian intake with liver damage in four cases[133] were not sustained, but the impression has been left in the literature.[134] (The products, which included other herbs, may have contained germander masquerading as skullcap.[133]) Since then, acute hepatitis was reported in 1999 in a woman taking homeopathic medications and valerian tea. Viral markers were negative and there was no evidence of autoimmune liver disease. A link to valerian intake was not established.[135] In one case report of hepatotoxicity associated with valerian, a 27-year-old woman reported ingesting a 600 mg valerian root daily for 3 months. She presented with epigastric pain, fatigue and hepatomegaly. Laboratory tests revealed elevated liver enzymes and bilirubin with no other signs of pathology. She was instructed to stop the valerian, whereafter symptoms improved within 3 days. Four weeks later liver function tests were within normal range.[136] Another case of a mild, reversible idiosyncratic hepatotoxic reaction has been attributed to consumption of valerian tea and extracts.[137]

Minor short-term hepatotoxic reactions to valerian have also been impugned from observations of reactions to a proprietary mixture combining valerian with hyoscine and cyproheptadine. However, direct evidence was not found, and the other components of the formula make any such assessment unsafe.[138]

A patient taking multiple medications experienced serious cardiac complications and delirium following a surgical procedure.[139] He had self-medicated for 'many years' with valerian root extract (0.53 to 2 g per dose, five times daily). However, due to his multiple medications, valerian cannot be credibly causally linked to his symptoms.

Overdosage

The following effects have been reported when excessive valerian is taken: blurred vision, change in heartbeat, excitability, headache, nausea, restlessness, uneasiness.[140] Traditional texts also refer to large doses causing headache, stupor, mental excitement, visual illusions, giddiness, restlessness, agitation and even spasmodic movements.[1,3] However, in the first well-documented case of valerian overdose, the patient, who had consumed 20 times the recommended therapeutic dose, presented with mild symptoms all of which resolved within 24h. The authors described the overdose as benign.[141]

In contrast to this, a 1998 letter described 24 patients who were treated in a medical unit after taking an overdose of over-the-counter 'valerian products'. The amounts of valerian ingested were estimated in 23 patients and ranged from 0.15 to 4.5g. Six patients developed vomiting. The clinical problems were mainly CNS depression and anticholinergic poisoning. One patient required ventilatory support and developed aspiration pneumonia; in 17 patients liver function tests were performed and were all normal. All patients made a complete recovery.[142] However, a closer reading of the letter shows that the culprit was not valerian at all. As well as containing valerian, the product also contained the drugs hyoscine hydrobromide and cyproheptadine hydrochloride, which readily explain the symptoms observed on overdose.

Injection of an alcoholic valerian extract in one case of abuse led to transient fevers, pains and stiffness, headache and mild liver function abnormalities. These were probably due to the presence of endotoxin in the injected material. The person involved recovered over the following 3 days.[143]

Safety in children

It is recommended that use of valerian is avoided in children less than 3 years of age.[144] Valerian was safely administered (with lemon balm) in a clinical trial involving children less than 12 years (average age 8.3 years), with 21.6% younger than 6 years.[92]

The efficacy and tolerability of a valerian extract were also investigated in an open, observational study involving children aged to 6 to 12 years.[145] An average daily dosage of two tablets (range 1 to 4), each containing 300mg of 5:1 extract, was administered to 130 children suffering from nervous sleep disturbances and/or nervous tension over a period of 4 weeks. Therapeutic efficacy was estimated by parents and clinicians as good to very good in 95% of cases. One side effect (tiredness in the morning) was reported in only one case, which disappeared after dose adjustment.

Regulatory status in selected countries

European valerian is official in the *European Pharmacopoeia* (2011), the *British Pharmacopoeia* (2011) and the *United States Pharmacopeia-National Formulary* (USP34-NF29, 2011).

Valerian is covered by a positive Commission E monograph and has the following applications: restlessness and sleeping disorders based on nervous conditions.

Valerian is on the UK General Sale List. Valerian and valerian combination products have achieved Traditional Herbal Registration in the UK with the traditional indication of aiding sleep and for the temporary relief of symptoms of mild anxiety.

Valerian does not have GRAS status. However, it is freely available as a 'dietary supplement' in the USA under DSHEA legislation (1994) Dietary Supplement Health and Education Act).

Valerian is not included in Part 4 of Schedule 4 of the Therapeutic Goods Act Regulations of Australia and is freely available for sale.

References

1. Grieve M. *A Modern Herbal*, vol. 2. New York: Dover Publications; 1971. pp. 824–829.
2. *Culpeper's Complete Herbal and English Physician*. 1826. Reprinted by Harvey Sales; 1981. pp. 188–189.
3. Felter HW, Lloyd JU. *King's American Dispensatory*. 18th ed. rev 3, vol. 2. 1905. Portland: Reprinted by Eclectic Medical Publications; 1983. pp. 2041–2043.
4. Chopra RN, Chopra IC, Handa KL, et al. *Chopra's Indigenous Drugs of India*. 2nd ed. 1958. Calcutta: Reprinted by Academic Publishers; 1982. pp. 253–255.
5. Chiej R. *The Macdonald Encyclopedia of Medicinal Plants*. London: Macdonald; 1984. Entry no. 323.
6. Launert EL. *The Hamlyn Guide to Edible and Medicinal Plants of Britain and Northern Europe*. London: Hamlyn; 1981. pp. 180–181.
7. Evans WC. *Trease and Evans' Pharmacognosy*, 16th ed. Edinburgh: Saunders/Elsevier; 2009. pp. 335–337.
8. *European Pharmacopoeia*. 3rd ed. Strasbourg: European Department for the Quality of Medicines within the Council of Europe; 1996. pp. 1702–1703.
9. Wagner H, Bladt S. *Plant Drug Analysis: A Thin Layer Chromatography Atlas*, 2nd ed. Berlin: Springer-Verlag; 1996. pp. 342–344.
10. Wang PC, Hu JM, Ran XH, et al. *J Nat Prod*. 2009;72(9):1682–1685.
11. Santos MS, Ferreira F, Faro C, et al. *Planta Med*. 1994;60(5):475–476.
12. Bodesheim U, Holzl J. *Pharmazie*. 1997;52(5):386–391.
13. Murphy K, Kubin ZJ, Shepherd JN, et al. *Phytomedicine*. 2010;17(8–9):674–678.
14. Hansel R, Schultz J. *Dtsch Apoth Ztg*. 1982;122:215–219.
15. Bos R, Woerdenbag JH, Scheffer JJC. *Planta Med*. 1993;59(7 suppl):A698.
16. De Smet P.A.G.M.Keller K, Hansel R, editors. *Adverse Effects of Herbal Drugs*, vol. 3. Berlin: Springer-Verlag; 1997. p. 166.
17. Houghton PJ. *J Ethnopharmacol*. 1988;22(2):121–143.
18. Bounthanh C, Bergmann C, Beck JP, et al. *Planta Med*. 1981;41(1):21–28.
19. Braun R, Dittmar W, Hubner E, et al. *Planta Med*. 1984;50(1):1–4.
20. Hendriks H, Geertsma HJ, Malingre TM. *Pharm Weekbl*. 1981;116(43):1316.
21. Hendriks H, Bos R, Woerdenbag HJ, et al. *Planta Med*. 1985;51(1):28–31.
22. Wagner H, Bladt S. *Plant Drug Analysis*. New York: Springer-Verlag; 1984. p. 264.
23. Gstir--ner F, Kleinbauer E. *Pharmazie*. 1958;13(7):415–420.
24. Komori T, Matsumoto T, Motomura E, et al. *Chem Senses*. 2006;31(8):731–737.
25. Thies PW, Funke S. *Tetrahedron Lett*. 1966;11:1155–1162.
26. Wagner H, Jurcic K, Schaette R. *Planta Med*. 1980;39(4):358–365.
27. Fernández SP, Wasowski C, Loscalzo LM, et al. *Eur J Pharmacol*. 2006;539(3):168–176.

28. Fernández SP, Wasowski C, Paladini AC, et al. *Eur J Pharmacol.* 2005;512(2–3):189–198.

29. Fernández S, Wasowski C, Paladini AC, et al. *Pharmacol Biochem Behav.* 2004;77(2):399–404.

30. Marder M, Viola H, Wasowski C, et al. *Pharmacol Biochem Behav.* 2003;75(3):537–545.

31. Von Eickstedt KW, Rahman S. *Arzneimittelforschung.* 1969;19(3):316–319.

32. Von Eickstedt KW. *Arzneim Forsch.* 1969;19(6):995–997.

33. Andreatini R, Leite JR. *Eur J Pharmacol.* 1994;260(2–3):233–235.

34. Leuschner J, Muller J, Rudmann M. *Arzneimittelforschung.* 1993;43(6):638–641.

35. Hattesohl M, Feistel B, Sievers H, et al. *Phytomedicine.* 2008;15(1–2):2–15.

36. Dziuba K. *Med Welt.* 1968;35:1866–1868.

37. Jauch H. *Med Klin.* 1969;64(10):437–439.

38. Poyares DR, Guilleminault C, Ohayon MM, et al. *Prog Neuropsychopharmacol Biol Psychiatry.* 2002;26(3):539–545.

39. Yuan CS, Mehendale S, Xiao Y, et al. *Anesth Analg.* 2004;98(2):353–358.

40. Benke D, Barberis A, Kopp S, et al. *Neuropharmacology.* 2009;56(1):174–181.

41. Trauner G, Khom S, Baburin I, et al. *Planta Med.* 2008;74(1):19–24.

42. Khom S, Baburin I, Timin E, et al. *Neuropharmacology.* 2007;53(1):178–187.

43. Awad R, Levac D, Cybulska P. *Can J Physiol Pharmacol.* 2007;85(9):933–942.

44. Santos MS, Ferreira F, Cunha AP, et al. *Planta Med.* 1994;60(3):278–279.

45. Ferreira F, Santos MS, Faro C, et al. *Rev Port Farm.* 1996;46(2):74–77.

46. Balduini W, Cattabeni F. *Med Sci Res.* 1989;17(15):639–640.

47. Lacher SK, Mayer R, Sichardt K, et al. *Biochem Pharmacol.* 2007;73(2):248–258.

48. Sichardt K, Vissiennon Z, Koetter U, et al. *Phytother Res.* 2007;21(10):932–937.

49. Schumacher B, Scholle S, Hölzl J, et al. *J Nat Prod.* 2002;65(10):1479–1485.

50. Vissiennon Z, Sichardt K, Koetter U, et al. *Planta Med.* 2006;72(7):579–583.

51. Dimpfel W, Brattström A, Koetter U. *Eur J Med Res.* 2006;11(11):496–500.

52. Dietz BM, Mahady GB, Pauli GF, et al. *Brain Res Mol Brain Res.* 2005;138(2):191–197.

53. Neuhaus W, Trauner G, Gruber D, et al. *Planta Med.* 2008;74(11):1338–1344.

54. Malva JO, Santos S, Macedo T. *Neurotox Res.* 2004;6(2):131–140.

55. Sudati JH, Fachinetto R, Pereira RP, et al. *Neurochem Res.* 2009;34(8):1372–1379.

56. De Oliveria DM, Barreto G, De Andrade DV, et al. *Neurochem Res.* 2009;34(2):215–220.

57. Circosta C, De Pasquale R, Samperi S, et al. *J Ethnopharmacol.* 2007;112(2):361–367.

58. Occhiuto F, Pino A, Palumbo DR, et al. *J Pharm Pharmacol.* 2009;61(2):251–256.

59. Hiller KO, Zetler G. *Phytother Res.* 1996;10(2):145–151.

60. Rezvani ME, Roohbakhsh A, Allahtavakoli M, et al. *J Ethnopharmacol.* 2010;127(2):313–318.

61. Simmen U, Saladin C, Kaufmann P, et al. *Planta Med.* 2005;71(9):890.

62. Von Der Hude W, Scheutwinkel-Reich M, Braun R. *Mutat Res.* 1986;169(1–2):23–27.

63. Wagner H, Jurcic K. *Planta Med.* 1980;38(4):366–376.

64. Maier-Salamon A, Trauner G, Hiltscher R, et al. *J Pharm Sci.* 2009;98(10):3839–3849.

65. Anderson GD, Elmer GW, Kantor ED, et al. *Phytother Res.* 2005;19(9):801–803.

66. Anderson GD, Elmer GW, Taibi DM, et al. *Phytother Res.* 2010;24(10):1442–1446.

67. Bent S, Padula A, Moore D, et al. *Am J Med.* 2006;119(12):1005–1012.

68. Taibi DM, Landis CA, Petry H, et al. *Sleep Med Rev.* 2007;11(3):209–230.

69. Fernández-San-Martín MI, Masa-Font R, Palacios-Soler L, et al. *Sleep Med.* 2010;11(6):505–511.

70. European Medicines Agency. Assessment Report on *Valeriana officinalis* L., Radix; London: 29 November, 2007.

71. Leathwood PD, Chauffard F. *J Psychiatr Res.* 1982/1983;17(2):115–122.

72. Leathwood PD, Chauffard F, Heck E, et al. *Pharmacol Biochem Behav.* 1982;17(1):65–71.

73. Leathwood PD, Chauffard F, Munoz-Bos R. *6th European Congress on Sleep Research.* Zurich: 23–26 March, 1982.

74. Leathwood PD, Chauffard F. *Planta Med.* 1985;51(2):144–148.

75. Vorbach EU, Arnold KH. *6th Phytotherapy Conference.* Berlin: October 5–7, 1995.

76. Vorbach EU, Gortelmeyer R, Bruning J. *Psychopharmakotherapie.* 1996;3:109–115.

77. Kamm-Kohl AV, Jansen W, Brockman P. *Med Welt.* 1984;35:1450–1454.

78. Francis AJ, Dempster RJ. *Phytomedicine.* 2002;9(4):273–279.

79. Donath F, Quispe S, Diefenbach K, et al. *Pharmacopsychiatry.* 2000;33(2):47–53.

80. Diaper A, Hindmarch I. *Phytotherapy Res.* 2004;18(10):831–836.

81. Balderer G, Borbely AA. *Psychopharmacology.* 1985;87(4):406–409.

82. Schulz H, Stolz C, Muller J. *Pharmacopsychiatry.* 1994;27(4):147–151.

83. Cuellar NG, Ratcliffe SJ. *Altern Ther Health Med.* 2009;15(2):22–28.

84. Gerhard U, Linnenbrink N, Georghiadou C, et al. *Schweiz Rundsch Med Prax.* 1996;85(15):473–481.

85. Muller-Limmroth W, Ehrenstein W. *Med Klin.* 1977;72:1119–1125.

86. Koetter U, Schrader E, Käufeler R, et al. *Phytotherapy Res.* 2007;21(9):847–851.

87. Ross SM. *Holist Nurs Pract.* 2009;23(4):253–256.

88. Dimpfel W, Suter A. *Eur J Med Res.* 2008;13(5):200–204.

89. European Medicines Agency. Assessment Report on *Valeriana officinalis* L., Radix and *Humulus lupulus* L., Flos: London; 14 May, 2009.

90. Dressing H, Riemann D, Low H, et al. *Therapiewoche.* 1992;42(12):726–736.

91. Dressing H, Kohler S, Muller WE. *Psychopharmakotherapie.* 1996;3(3):123–130.

92. Muller SF, Klement S. *Phytomedicine.* 2006;13(6):383–387.

93. Giesler M, Thum A, Haag A, et al. *Planta Med.* 2007;73(9):979. Abstract P500.

94. Kohnen R, Oswald WD. *Pharmacopsychiatry.* 1988;21:447–448.

95. Hiller KO, Rahlfs V. *Forsch Komplementarmed.* 1995;2:123–132.

96. Steger W. *Z Allg Med.* 1985;61:914–918.

97. Panijel M. *Therapiewoche.* 1985;35(41):4659–4668.

98. Kniebel R, Burchard JM. *Z Allg Med.* 1988;64:689–696.

99. Quandt J. *Therapiewoche.* 1994;44:292–299.

100. Herberg KW. *Therapiewoche.* 1994;44(12):704–713.

101. Rosecrans JA, Defeo JJ, Youngken Jr HW. *J Pharm Sci.* 1961;50:240–244.

102. Skramlik E. *Pharmazie.* 1959;14:435–445.

103. Fehri B, Aiache JM, Boukef K, et al. *J Pharm Belg.* 1991;46(3):165–176.

104. Fachinetto R, Villarinho JG, Wagner C, et al. *Prog Neuropsychopharmacol Biol Psychiatry.* 2007;31(7):1478–1486.

105. Al-Majed AA, Al-Yahya AA, Al-Bekairi AM, et al. *Food Chem Toxicol.* 2006;44(11):1830–1837.

106. Bos R, Hendriks H, Scheffer JJC, et al. *Phytomedicine.* 1998;5(3):219–225.

107. Spinella M. *Epilepsy Behav.* 2001;2(6):524–532.

108. Ang-Lee MK, Moss J, Yuan CS. *JAMA.* 2001;286(2):208–216.

109. Chaplin Jr RL, Jedynak J, Johnson D, et al. *AANA J.* 2007;75(6):431–435.

110. Ugaide M, Reza V, Gonzalez-Trujano ME, et al. *J Pharm Pharmacol.* 2005;57(5):631–639.

111. Dalla Corte CL, Fachinetto R, Colle D, et al. *Food Chem Toxicol.* 2008;46(7):2369–2375.

112. Hellum BH, Nilsen OG. *Basic Clin Pharmacol Toxicol.* 2008;102(5):466–475.

113. Lefebvre T, Foster BC, Drouin CE. *J Pharm Pharm Sci.* 2004;7(2):265–273.

114. Hellum BH, Hu Z, Nilsen OG. *Basic Clin Pharmacol Toxicol.* 2007;100(1):23–30.

115. Donovan JL, DeVane CL, Chavin KD, et al. *Drug Metab Dispos.* 2004;32(12):1333–1336.

116. Gurley BJ, Gardner SF, Hubbard MA, et al. *Clin Pharmacol Ther.* 2005;77(5):415–426.

117. Khawaja IS, Marotta RF, Lippmann S. *Psychiatr Serv.* 1999;50(7):969–970.

118. Carrasco MC, Vallejo JR, Pardo-de-Santayana M, et al. *Phytother Res.* 2009;23(12):1795–1796.

119. Chen D, Klesmer J, Giovanniello A, et al. *Am J Addict.* 2002;11(1):75–77.

120. Czeizel AE, Tomcsik M, Timar L. *Obstet Gynecol.* 1997;90(2):195–201.

121. Yao M, Brown-Woodman PDC, Ritchie H. *Birth Defects Res (Part A).* 2003;67: 141–147. Abstract 9.

122. Tufik S, Fujita K, Seabra Mde L, et al. *J Ethnopharmacol.* 1994;41(1–2):39–44.

123. Holst L, Nordeng H, Haavik S. *Pharmacoepidemiol Drug Saf.* 2008;17(2):151–159.

124. Kuhlmann J, Berger W, Podzuweit H, Schmidt U. *Pharmacopsychiatry.* 1999;32(6):235–241.

125. Hallam KT, Olver JS, McGrath C, et al. *Hum Psychopharmacol.* 2003;18(8): 619–625.

126. Gutierrez S, Ang-Lee MK, Walker DJ, et al. *Pharmacol Biochem Behav.* 2004;78(1):57–64.

127. Glass JR, Sproule BA, Herrmann N, et al. *J Clin Psychopharmacol.* 2003;23(3): 260–268.

128. Pallesen S, Bjorvatn B, Nordhus IH, et al. *Tidsskr Nor Laegeforen.* 2002;122(30):2857–2859.

129. Schmitz M, Jackel M. *Wien Med Wochenschr.* 1998;148(13):291–298.

130. Ziegler G, Ploch M, Miettinen-Baumann A, et al. *Eur J Med Res.* 2002;7(11):480–486.

131. Wheatley D. *Hum Psychopharmacol.* 2001;16(4):353–356.

132. Boniel T, Dannon P. *Harefuah.* 2001;140(8):780–783. [805].

133. MacGregor FB, Abernethy VE, Dahabra S, et al. *BMJ.* 1989;299(6708):1156–1157.

134. Shepherd C. *BMJ.* 1993;306(6890):1477.

135. Mennecier D, Saloum T, Dourthe PM, et al. *Presse Med.* 1999;28(18):966.

136. Cohen DL, Del Toro YJ. *Clin Gastroenterol.* 2008;42(8):961–962.

137. Vassiliadis T, Anagnostis P, Patsiaoura K, et al. *Sleep Med.* 2009;10(8):935.

138. Chan TY, Tang CH, Critchley JA. *Postgrad Med J.* 1995;71(834):227–228.

139. Garges HP, Varia I, Doraiswamy PM. *JAMA.* 1998;280(18):1566–1567.

140. USP Drug Information. *US Pharmacopeia Patient Leaflet, Valerian (Oral).* The United States Pharmacopeial Convention; Rockville: 1998.

141. Willey LB, Mady SP, Cobaugh DJ, et al. *Vet Hum Toxicol.* 1995;37(4):364–365.

142. Chan TY. *Int J Clin Pharmcol Ther.* 1998;36:569.

143. Mullins ME, Horowitz BZ. *Vet Hum Toxicol.* 1998;40(5):290–291.

144. Schilcher H. *Phytotherapie in der Kinderheilkunde,* 2. Aufl. Stuttgart: Wissenschaftlische Verlagsgesellschaft; 1992. pp. 60–61.

145. Hintelmann C. *Z Phytother.* 2002;23:60–61.

(Salix spp. including *S. alba* L., *S. daphnoides* Vill., *S. purpurea* L. and *S. fragilis* L.)

Synonyms

White willow, European willow.

What is it?

The name willow bark is synonymous with the development of one of the most successful and widely used synthetic drugs, namely aspirin. The German scientist Felix Hoffman was investigating a way to reduce the gastric irritant effects of salicylic acid (originally isolated from willow bark) and produced the synthetic derivative acetylsalicylic acid in 1897. This was a serendipitous discovery because the key pharmacological properties of aspirin are largely mediated by the acetyl group he added to make the molecule. Ironically, aspirin was still active as a gastric irritant, but by a different mechanism to salicylic acid.

The stem barks from many species of willow are used medicinally, especially *Salix alba, S. daphnoides, S. purpurea* and *S. fragilis*. Recent clinical trials indicate that a high-potency standardised willow bark extract has analgesic activity, but with fewer side effects than standard drug treatments. Pharmacokinetic studies have demonstrated that this activity cannot be due to salicin alone and other yet unidentified constituents and mechanisms also probably contribute to the observed clinical effects.

Effects

Exerts analgesic and anti-inflammatory effects by an uncertain mechanism, but unlike aspirin, is not a potent inhibitor of platelet aggregation or the enzyme cyclo-oxygenase (COX).

Traditional view

Dioscorides in the first century AD prescribed willow bark to patients suffering from rheumatism.[1] Willow bark was traditionally used for inflammatory disorders such as rheumatism, gouty arthritis and ankylosing spondylitis.[2] It was also considered to be a tonic, astringent bitter and an antiperiodic (antimalarial) useful for dyspepsia, chronic mucus discharges, influenza, fevers, convalescence from acute diseases, worm infestation, chronic diarrhoea and dysentery, neuralgia, mild headache and passive haemorrhages.[2,3-5] During the 18th and 19th centuries in America, willow bark was commonly recommended as a febrifuge. Native Americans also used willow bark for lumbago and as a poultice for headache.[6] It was noted in 1876 that native South Africans had long used willow bark for treating rheumatic diseases.[7]

On 25 April 1763, the Oxfordshire clergyman Reverend Edward Stone submitted a comprehensive report to the Royal Society in London indicating he had found, by clinical experience, that the bark of the willow tree was efficacious in the treatment of a variety of fevers. He described 50 cases treated for ague (fever) and intermittent disorders and noted that the results were uniformly satisfactory. Stone administered 20 to 60 grains (1.3 to 3.9 g) of dried, powdered bark every 4 h to the patients.[8] Further medical reports of the antipyretic and analgesic effects of willow bark emerged in Europe from 1772 to 1803.[7]

Summary actions

Anti-inflammatory, analgesic, antirheumatic, antipyretic.

Can be used for

Indications supported by clinical trials

Temporary relief of acute or chronic musculoskeletal pain, including low back pain and osteoarthritis (good evidence).

Traditional therapeutic uses

As an antipyretic for fever management; as a treatment and preventative for headache.

Preparations

Willow bark standardised extract (WBSE) prepared from the dried root and typically containing 15% total salicin, in tablet or capsule form; dried bark as a decoction or liquid extract for internal use.

Dosage

- 800 to 1600 mg/day of WBSE containing 120 to 240 mg of salicin for anti-inflammatory and analgesic uses, as supported by clinical trial data
- 3.5 to 7 mL/day of a 1:2 liquid extract or equivalent doses (e.g. 9 to 17.5 mL/day) of a 1:5 tincture for traditional uses.

Duration of use

May be taken long term.

Summary assessment of safety

Few adverse effects from ingestion of willow bark are expected, provided the warnings and contraindications are observed. Stomach pains, nausea, headache, tiredness and allergic reaction are rarely reported as adverse reactions. Any potentiation of antiplatelet drugs is likely to be mild.

Technical data

Botany

Willow bark is a member of the Salicaceae family. *Salix alba* is a deciduous tree, up to 26 m tall, with ascending branches and a deeply fissured grey bark. The leaves are alternate, shortly petiolate, up to 11 cm long, lanceolate from a wedge-shaped base, with silky whitish appressed hairs on both sides. The flowers appear with the leaves, arranged in dense cylindrical catkins; the male ones are up to 5 cm long with two stamens, anthers yellow; the female ones are up to 4 cm; 6.5 cm in fruit. The fruit is a capsule.[9]

Adulteration

No adulterants have been documented. Other species of Salix low in salicin are possible substitutes.

Key constituents

Willow bark contains salicin and salicin esters (including salicortin, 2'-O-acetylsalicortin, fragilin (2'-O-acetylsalicin) and tremulacin), other phenolic glucosides, flavonoids, polyphenols, oligomeric procyanidins and condensed tannins.[5,10]

The total salicin content (after hydrolysis) varies according to the species: *S. daphnoides* and *S. fragilis* (2% to 10%), *S. purpurea* (3% to 8.5%) and *S. alba* (0.5% to 1%).[10] Salicin is a phenolic glucoside consisting of the aglycone saligenin (also known as salicyl alcohol) and glucose.

Pharmacodynamics

The clinical use of willow bark as an antipyretic and analgesic was first documented from 1763 to 1803. By the mid-19th century, active principles were being isolated from this herb and others with similar activity: salicin from willow bark (1826 to 1829), salicylaldehyde from *Spiraea ulmaria* (meadowsweet, 1831) and methyl salicylate from wintergreen (*Gaultheria spp.*, 1843). Salicylic acid was prepared from these isolated constituents (1835 to 1843) and in 1874 a factory was set up for its large-scale production. The activity of salicylic acid was confirmed clinically for the treatment of rheumatic disorders in 1876. In the same year, successful treatment with salicin was described for eight patients with acute and subacute rheumatism. Unfortunately salicin was largely overlooked and the cheaper salicylic acid remained the focus of pharmaceutical attention. As the use of salicylic acid and its salts increased, the problem of the severe gastric side effects became more evident. The German pharmaceutical company Bayer began looking for a version of salicylic acid with a better side effect profile, and between 1893 and 1897 Felix Hoffman developed an improved way of producing acetylsalicylic acid. He tested it on his father, whose chronic arthritis improved markedly.[11] In 1899 acetylsalicylic acid was commercially released with the name aspirin, apparently from the former botanical name for meadowsweet. Despite early reports, adverse reactions to aspirin were largely ignored until the 1950s.[7] The irony is that salicin, which is inactive until it travels past the stomach, is a much gentler substance on the digestive tract than either salicylic acid or aspirin.

The differing pharmacologies of the various salicylate derivatives and willow bark

Many articles seem to regard willow bark as a kind of herbal aspirin. But there are important differences between aspirin and the salicylate compounds in willow bark, as can be seen from the chemical diagrams below.

In terms of pharmacology, aspirin is regarded as a potent inhibitor of COX-1 and COX-2 because it contains an acetyl group that causes irreversible acetylation of COX, completely inactivating this enzyme system. Aspirin therefore has analgesic and anti-inflammatory activities via this mechanism (COX-2 inhibition), but is also noted to cause gastric damage and inhibit platelet function (COX-1 inhibition).[11,12]

Specifically, platelet function is inhibited by reducing the production of thromboxane A_2 (a prostaglandin) by COX-1.

Salicylic acid

Aspirin

Salicin

Because aspirin irreversibly inactivates COX by acetylation, and because platelets cannot make new proteins such as COX (they have no nucleus), the effect of aspirin persists for the lifetime of the platelet (7 to 10 days). Even low doses of aspirin can therefore have profound blood-thinning effects.[12]

Unlike aspirin, salicylic acid has only a weak inhibitory effect on isolated COX-1 or COX-2[13-15] that, despite some arguments to the contrary,[16] is unlikely to be the mechanism behind any clinically significant anti-inflammatory activity. This means that salicylic acid or sodium salicylate will have little antiplatelet (blood thinning) effects, especially since they lack the acetyl group. However, a high dose of salicylic acid can still irritate the stomach, but this is because it is a phenol, not because of any significant effects on COX-1 inhibition.

Salicin, the major salicylate compound in willow bark, appears naturally designed to minimise this gastric irritation. It effectively delivers salicylic acid into the bloodstream, but it does this in a novel way. Salicin is carried unchanged (and hence is stomach friendly) to the distal ileum or colon where gut flora remove the sugar and convert it into salicyl alcohol. The salicyl alcohol is absorbed and oxidised in the blood, tissue and liver to give salicylic acid/salicylate. Salicin provides a more sustained release of salicylate than sodium salicylate itself.[17] (For more details on the pharmacokinetics of salicin, see below and Chapter 2.)

COX-1 is constitutively expressed, whereas COX-2 is inducible by pro-inflammatory agents such as endotoxin and cytokines. Hence, although it has little direct effect on inhibiting COX-2 activity once it is formed, salicylic acid could exert anti-inflammatory and analgesic activity by inhibiting COX-2 production. It has been reported that aspirin and sodium salicylate equipotently suppress COX-2 induction at therapeutic concentrations.[11]

As an elaboration of this possible inhibition of COX-2 induction, an interesting insight has been added to the aspirin and salicylate discussion by Wu.[18] It is proposed that aspirin is a less potent inhibitor of COX-2 than COX-1, and the theory that aspirin exerts its anti-inflammatory action via inhibition of COX-2 is inconsistent with experimental and clinical findings. Specifically, aspirin has a relatively short half-life in circulating blood (around 20 min) and is rapidly deacetylated to yield salicylate. Hence any long-term anti-inflammatory effect of aspirin must be derived from salicylate. Despite its low anti-COX activity, salicylate exerts a substantial anti-inflammatory effect and markedly inhibits inflammatory prostaglandin biosynthesis in intact cells and animals.[15] Based on their in vitro experiments, Wu and team have proposed that salicylate does indeed act by inhibiting the COX-2 production that would normally follow from pro-inflammatory signals to the cell. The specific mechanism suggested is the inhibition of RSK1/2 (ribosomal S6 kinase 1/2), which is a key factor mediating COX-2 transcription.[19] Also, salicylate appears to have direct analgesic effects in the CNS by unknown mechanisms.[11]

To investigate the differing actions of willow bark and aspirin on platelet function, 35 patients were given either willow bark extract (WBSE delivering 240 mg/day of salicin) or placebo under double blind conditions. Another 16 patients were given 100 mg/day of aspirin.[20] The maximum arachidonic-acid-induced platelet aggregation readings were as follows: willow bark $61.0 \pm 21.6\%$, placebo $78.0 \pm 15.4\%$ and aspirin $12.7 \pm 9.1\%$. Hence, the inhibitory effect of willow bark extract on platelet aggregation was far less than aspirin and only marginally stronger than placebo (but was still significantly different, $p = 0.04$). This confirms that willow bark is not a substitute for aspirin for clinically relevant antiplatelet activity. However, since the mild effect was statistically significant, WBSE should be used cautiously (under supervision) with warfarin and antiplatelet drugs.

It is likely that not just the salicylate compounds in WBSE contribute to its analgesic activity. A study involving 10 healthy volunteers found that a single dose of WBSE (providing 240 mg of salicin) resulted in blood salicylate levels of around $1.4 \, \mu g/mL$. In contrast, blood salicylate levels of 35 to $50 \, \mu g/mL$ have been reported after taking just 500 mg of aspirin.[21] Clearly, the clinically observed analgesic effects from willow bark (see later) must come from more than just the effects of salicylate.[21]

Based on research on willow bark and related herbs, it has been suggested that lipoxygenase and hyaluronidase inhibition and free radical scavenging effects, all from other components in willow bark, contribute to its overall anti-inflammatory and analgesic effects. (See below for a further discussion on this topic.) This implies that many of the side effects, interactions and contraindications for aspirin, such as interactions with methotrexate, spironolactone and furosemide, are unlikely to apply for willow bark.[22,23]

Anti-inflammatory activity

Salicin, other constituents of willow bark and willow bark extract did not inhibit prostaglandin synthesis from sheep seminal vesicles in vitro. Salicin and salicortin produced a marginal inhibition of lipoxygenase.[24] A hexane extract of willow bark inhibited COX-1 and COX-2 by greater than 60% in an in vitro assay,[25] but the hexane extract of willow bark would represent a small fraction of its total content. Indeed, clinical studies suggest that willow bark extract does not cause the same gastrointestinal side effects as aspirin, and clinically relevant inhibition of COX-1 or COX-2 activity is considered to be unlikely, as discussed above.[26]

Tremulacin demonstrated anti-inflammatory activity, inhibited peritoneal leucocyte migration and writhing response in several experimental models (via injection), and inhibited leukotriene B_4 biosynthesis in vitro.[27] Salicin inhibited the spasmodic action of prostaglandin $F_{2\alpha}$ on isolated rabbit non-pregnant myometrium.[28] Tremulacin also inhibited contraction of isolated ileum induced by histamine or SRS-A (slow-reacting substance of anaphylaxis – now defined as a group of leukotrienes) and inhibited the release of these substances from isolated tissue and cells.[29] Metabolites of salicin and tremulacin have also demonstrated anti-inflammatory activity in vitro.[30]

The effects of an ethanolic extract of willow bark were evaluated in an established in vitro assay test model using primary human monocytes.[31] IC_{50} values obtained for inhibition of lipopolysaccharide (LPS)-induced release of prostaglandin E_2 (PGE_2), reflecting COX-2-mediated release, were $47\,\mu g/mL$ and $0.6\,\mu g/mL$ for the willow bark extract and a rofecoxib-like research compound, respectively. However, there was no direct inhibitory effect from willow bark on COX-1 and COX-2 activity. The willow bark extract also inhibited the LPS-induced release of tumour necrosis factor-alpha, interleukin-1beta and interleukin-6, with IC_{50} values of 180, 33 and $86\,\mu g/mL$, respectively. Interestingly, both salicin and salicylate had no effect on any of the parameters tested.

Recently a standardised willow bark extract was examined to clarify its possible mechanism of action as an anti-inflammatory agent.[32] Various aspects were investigated in two inflammation models: the 6-day air pouch model in rats, representing the acute state, and adjuvant-induced arthritis, representing the chronic state. Parameters assessed included leucocytic infiltration, levels of cytokines and prostaglandins in blood, effects on COX-1 and/or COX-2 enzyme output and effects on free radical production. The extract was compared at two dosage levels, together with comparable anti-inflammatory doses of aspirin as a non-selective COX inhibitor and celecoxib as a selective COX-2 inhibitor. All doses were administered orally. On a mg/kg basis, the willow bark extract was at least as effective as aspirin in reducing inflammatory exudates, inhibiting leucocytic infiltration and preventing a rise in cytokines. It was more effective than aspirin in suppressing leukotrienes and equally effective in suppressing prostaglandins. For COX-2 output (in terms of PGE_2 production), willow bark was a slightly more effective inhibitor than aspirin, but much less than celecoxib. Willow bark also significantly raised reduced glutathione levels, an effect that would help limit lipid peroxidation. Based on these findings, the authors supported previous assertions that other constituents of willow bark extract, such as the polyphenols, contribute to its anti-inflammatory activity.[32]

This hypothesis was supported by an investigation of five chemical fractions of a willow bark extract using in vitro and in vivo models.[33] All the studied models pointed to the contribution of complex polyphenols and flavonoids to the observed anti-inflammatory activity of the whole extract. In particular, Fraction E (containing mainly procyanidins) was considerably more active than Fraction D (which largely contained salicin) after oral dosing in the carrageenan-induced rat paw oedema model.

Other activity

Willow bark extract has demonstrated antioxidant activity in several in vitro systems, including the scavenging of free radicals.[34,35] Unlike aspirin and sodium salicylate, salicin did not suppress lymphocyte transformation in vitro.[36]

Pharmacokinetics

Salicin derivatives (e.g. salicortin, tremulacin) are first probably converted into salicin in the stomach or small intestine. Salicin is then mainly carried to the distal ileum or colon, where gut flora conversion into its aglycone (salicyl alcohol) occurs. Salicyl alcohol is absorbed and oxidised in blood, tissue and liver to form salicylic acid. Salicylic acid is then converted to salicylic acid conjugates or to gentisic acid by hepatic transformation for excretion via the urine. From the excretion data, it was concluded that 86% of an administered dose of salicin was absorbed.[37,38] A 4 g oral dose of salicin was rapidly metabolised, reaching a peak plasma level of salicylate in just under 2 h. This peak plasma level was maintained for several hours. Comparison of the salicylate plasma levels obtained from both sodium salicylate and salicin demonstrated that the curve for salicin is slightly lower and flatter, indicating a longer half-life for salicin. The maximum plasma concentration of free salicylate from 4 g of salicin was $100\,\mu g/mL$, whereas 2 g of sodium salicylate yielded $150\,\mu g/mL$.[37] (For a more detailed discussion see Chapter 2.)

Clinical trials

A combination of feverfew (600 mg/day) and willow bark (600 mg/day) reduced the frequency and duration of migraine headaches in a prospective, open label clinical trial.[39] For more details see the feverfew monograph.

The following clinical trials were conducted using a potent extract of WBSE. In most cases S. daphnoides and S. purpurea were prescribed, although other species of willow can probably be used, provided the full spectrum of phytochemicals is present and sufficient salicin content is provided.

A Cochrane Collaboration systematic review examining herbal medicine for low back pain concluded that willow bark seemed to reduce pain more than placebo, but the quality of clinical trial reporting was poor and additional trials against standard treatments are needed.[40,41] A systematic review of the efficacy of willow bark for musculoskeletal pain found that there was moderate evidence to support willow bark in low back pain and that further trials were required in arthritis.[42] Only minor adverse events were noted for willow bark in the review.

Trials included in these reviews are summarised below.

A small, randomised, double blind, pilot study involving 21 patients indicated a clinically relevant analgesic effect from 2160 mg/day of WBSE, containing 240 mg/day of salicin, taken over a 2-week period. The mean reduction in the WOMAC pain score was significantly greater in the willow bark group compared with placebo (40% versus 18%, respectively).[43] The WOMAC (Western Ontario and McMaster Universities) Osteoarthritis Index is a test questionnaire that assesses symptoms and functional disability in patients with knee and hip osteoarthritis.

A trial of double blind, placebo-controlled design involving 78 patients tested the efficacy of willow bark for osteoarthritis of the knee and/or hip joint.[21] After a washout period of 4 days, patients received 1360 mg/day of WBSE or placebo for 2 weeks. The active treatment corresponded to an intake of 240 mg/day of salicin, the identical-looking placebo consisted of cellulose and lactose. An analgesic effect was observed by monitoring the change in the WOMAC pain score. This was reduced by 14% from baseline values after 2 weeks' treatment with willow bark, compared with an increase of 2% in the placebo group ($p < 0.05$). Adverse effects were reported less frequently in the willow bark group than from those taking placebo. Patient diary VAS (visual analogue scales) for pain and physical function confirmed the positive result for willow bark extract and the final overall assessments (by patients and investigators) demonstrated the superiority of willow bark extract over placebo. The analgesic effect of willow bark was mild, estimated to be 40% lower than standard NSAID (non-steroidal anti-inflammatory drug) treatment over the same time period (based on the documented WOMAC pain score reduction after diclofenac treatment at 150 mg/day). However, the analgesic effect of WBSE could increase with longer treatment times (see below).

A randomised, double blind, three-group trial compared oral treatment with one of two doses of WBSE or placebo (lactose) over 4 weeks.[44] A total of 191 patients with acute exacerbation of chronic low back pain completed the study. The primary outcome measure was the proportion of patients who were pain-free, without having taken the rescue analgesic medication tramadol for at least 5 days during the final week of the study. The numbers of pain-free patients in the last week of treatment were 39% in the high-dose group (1600 mg/day of extract containing 240 mg of salicin), 21% in the low-dose group (800 mg/day of extract containing 120 mg of salicin) and 6% in the placebo group. In addition, significantly more patients in the placebo group required tramadol during each week of the study than those taking WBSE ($p < 0.001$). A dose-dependent analgesic effect was therefore observed for the WBSE, even though patients in the high-dose group had more severe and prolonged pain at baseline. Furthermore, a statistically significant response in the high-dose group was evident after only 1 week of treatment, and the smaller effect seen in the low-dose group was significantly different from placebo by the end of the second week. One patient in the low-dose group exhibited a severe allergic reaction that was attributed to willow bark extract.

A postmarketing surveillance study confirmed the efficacy of WBSE (containing 240 mg/day of salicin for 4 weeks) in the treatment of low back pain. Forty per cent of patients were pain-free at the end of the treatment period irrespective of whether or not they received additional conventional treatments.[45] Another open, randomised, postmarketing study compared WBSE with rofecoxib (a selective COX-2 inhibitor) in patients with acute exacerbations of low back pain.[46] After 4 weeks' treatment there was no difference between the two products in terms of pain, the need for additional analgesics and side effects. Each group consisted of 114 patients who received either 1600 mg/day of WBSE containing 240 mg of salicin or 12.5 mg/day of rofecoxib.

In a randomised, double blind, parallel group trial, the therapeutic efficacy and tolerance of WBSE was compared against diclofenac sodium (a conventional NSAID) in patients with knee or hip arthritis.[47] From the 79 patients enrolled, 59 completed the study. The patients were randomly allocated to one of three groups, receiving either 150 mg/day of diclofenac sodium or willow bark extract in two different doses (corresponding to 90 or 180 mg/day salicin, respectively). No additional analgesic NSAID medication was allowed during the study period, lasting over 3 weeks. Outcome measures used were evaluation of pain intensity by a VAS, evaluation of functional capacity and pain intensity during different activities, impairment of daily activity, estimation of whether pain was localised or diffuse, amount of oedema and the intensity and duration of stiffness of the observed joint. Results indicated a good tolerance for the willow bark extract and statistically supported its therapeutically relevant analgesic activity. In terms of pain intensity, an effect comparable to diclofenac sodium was demonstrated.

Specific results for the trial included the following:

- Pain intensity (VAS) was reduced by 48% for the NSAID and by 39.5% and 31.3% for the two willow bark groups, respectively
- Functional capacity was significantly ($p < 0.05$) improved in all groups (after NSAID treatment 100% of patients were grouped in the lowest ratings of 1 or 2 compared with 90% for the higher dose of willow bark)
- The percentage of symptom-free patients (with various daily activities) increased by similar amounts for all groups.

Not all clinical trials on WBSE have been positive. A 2004 publication contained data for two small randomised, placebo-controlled, double blind trials in patients with osteoarthritis and rheumatoid arthritis, respectively.[48] The osteoarthritis study suggested that the willow bark extract showed no relevant efficacy above placebo. Similarly, the small rheumatoid arthritis trial did not demonstrate a significant therapeutic effect above placebo.

Two large-scale observational studies supporting the safety and efficacy of WBSE in the management of osteoarthritis and chronic low back pain in a clinical setting were presented at conferences. The first study, presented at a Berlin conference in early 2004, involved 922 physicians and 4731 patients in Germany.[49] Over 6 to 8 weeks, patients with arthritis or back pain took various doses of WBSE (an average of around three tablets/day) and rated their pain intensity from 1 to 10 (with 10 representing pain of the highest intensity). Most of the patients had previously been taking antirheumatic drugs, but had typically discontinued these because of either a lack of efficacy or side effects. During the observation period, only 15.5% needed supplementary antirheumatic drugs in addition to the willow bark. Average pain intensity reduced from 6.4 to 3.7 points in the first 4 weeks of treatment and fell further to 2.7 after 8 weeks, with 97% of patients reporting a reduction in pain and 18% reporting no pain at all. Side effects were judged as minor and occurred in only 1.3% of patients. These were mainly abdominal pain or an allergic skin rash.

The second study was undertaken in Switzerland and involved 204 physicians and 807 patients.[50] Most patients suffered osteoarthritis (44%) or chronic back pain (36%); in 69% of patients the problem had existed for more than 6 months. In 55% of patients the willow bark was prescribed on its own, whereas in 39% it was combined with the conventional medications that the patients were already taking. The average daily dosage of WBSE was 3.4 tablets at the beginning of the study and 2.8 at the end. Throughout the 6 to 8 week observation period, mean pain intensity decreased from 6.4 points to 3.3 and at the final visit 15% of patients were pain free. A substantial reduction of physical impairment was also observed. Suspected adverse reactions occurred in 4.5%

of patients and none of them were rated as serious. More than two-thirds of patients rated the tolerability of the willow bark extract as better than conventional antirheumatic drugs. The WBSE used in these two observational studies was standardised to contain 60 mg of salicin per tablet.

Professor Reinhard Saller, a rheumatologist based in Zurich, was interviewed concerning these two studies and his clinical perspective on willow bark extract.[51] He highlighted the high tolerability demonstrated for WBSE in the trials and emphasised that the studies provided useful information concerning its effective dose in a clinical setting. When questioned on the relative value of willow bark extract versus NSAIDs, he suggested that the herbal product had a large advantage because its complex of active principles had an overall modulating effect. The mixture of actives neither provoked a complete blockage nor a maximal stimulation of biochemical phenomena. This resulted in a broader spectrum of action and a greater tolerability than NSAIDs, which he then advised the patients to use on a limited 'as required' basis once they had started willow bark. Given the current disillusionment with COX-2 inhibitors, Professor Saller stressed the advantages of using willow bark extract, which had complex and multiple activities.[52]

Toxicology and other safety data

Toxicology

In acute toxicity studies, the LD_{50} of a liquid willow bark ethanolic extract was 28 mL/kg in mice.[53] No toxic effects were observed in rats orally administered a combination of willow bark and Primula extracts for 13 weeks.[54]

Contraindications

Willow bark is contraindicated in those with known allergy, in sensitivity or hypersensitivity to salicylates, and in glucose-6-phosphate dehydrogenase (G6PD) deficient patients (in this condition salicylic acid causes haemolytic anaemia).

Special warnings and precautions

Use with caution in lactating women and in patients combining willow bark with anticoagulants or synthetic salicylates. Willow bark cannot be substituted for aspirin for the prevention of stroke or myocardial infarction. Clinicians should be aware of the unlikely possibility of Reye's syndrome. (Refer to Safety in children section below.)

Because of the tannin content of this herb, use cautiously in highly inflamed or ulcerated conditions of the gastrointestinal tract. In principle, the use of tannins is inappropriate in extreme constipation, iron deficiency anaemia and malnutrition.

The following conditions should be approached with caution when using herbal analgesics: concurrent prescription of powerful analgesics; pain in children; neurological disease;

depression and psychosis; history of allergic or anaphylactic reactions.

Interactions

Willow bark may mildly add to the effects of antiplatelet drugs and may interact with anticoagulants, including warfarin. The clinical study previously noted observed very mild, but significant, antiplatelet activity in patients after the consumption of willow bark extract (standardised to 240 mg/day of salicin) for 4 weeks.[20]

Use in pregnancy and lactation

Category B1 – no documented increase in frequency of malformation or other harmful effects on the fetus from limited use in women. No evidence of increased fetal damage in limited animal studies.

A combination of willow bark and Primula root extracts did not exert teratogenic effects in rabbits and no negative effects were observed on reproductive function in female rats.[54] Salicylates can cross the placenta and acetylsalicylic acid (aspirin) has been shown to be teratogenic in animals, although there is no conclusive evidence that aspirin causes malformations in humans.[55] Moreover, the salicylates in willow bark do not have the same pharmacology as aspirin.

Willow bark is not advisable during lactation because salicylates are excreted in the breast milk[55] and hypersensitivity reactions might occur.

Effects on ability to drive and use machines

No adverse effects expected.

Side effects

A 2002 review of clinical trials found that 3.8% to 35.8% of 420 patients treated with willow bark extracts (containing 120 mg/day or 240 mg/day of salicin) reported mild adverse events compared to 2.8% to 35.2% of patients who received placebo.[52] In an earlier review, mild adverse events were reported in 3.7% of 733 patients and volunteers treated with three different preparations containing willow bark.[56] The adverse events reported included stomach ache, nausea, headache, dizziness, tiredness, sweating, skin rash and allergic reactions.[52,56]

High doses of tannins lead to excessive astringency on mucous membranes, which has an irritating effect. Gastrointestinal side effects due to willow bark have been attributed to the high tannin content, rather than the salicylate glycosides.[57] Oral administration of salicin (1.4 g/kg) to rats did not cause gastric injury.[58]

Acute salicylate poisoning is not expected from the use of willow bark, as the salicylate dose administered in the form of salicylate glycosides is relatively low. Hypersensitivity reactions, which include symptoms such as rhinitis, urticaria, bronchoconstriction, asthma and collapse, can occur from a few milligrams of aspirin and therefore are possible from the administration of willow bark, but the danger is not classed as high.[57] One case of anaphylaxis attributed to a dietary supplement containing willow bark and other ingredients has been reported[59] and another case was noted for WBSE in a clinical trial (see above).[43]

A patient with G6PD deficiency presented with acute massive intravascular haemolysis. The patient had been taking a diuretic medication and a herbal combination that contained *Salix caprea*. As salicin is metabolised to salicylic acid, and salicylic acid is a known inducer of haemolysis in G6PD-deficient patients, it was speculated that the herbal preparation might be responsible for the reaction. However, the herbal preparation was not analysed for its salicin content.[60]

Overdosage

No incidents have been found in the published literature for willow bark. Overdose resulting from acute ingestion of aspirin (6.5 to 9.8 g) usually produces a serum salicylate level of 300 mg/L or greater.[61] More than 50 g/day of pure salicin would need to be ingested in order to achieve this blood level of salicylate.[21]

Safety in children

Clinicians should be aware of the possibility of Reye's syndrome, an acute sepsis-like illness encountered exclusively in children below 15 years of age. The cause is unknown, although viral agents and drugs, especially salicylate derivatives, have been implicated.[62] However, it is unknown if the salicylates in willow bark are capable of causing this reaction and no cases have been documented.

Regulatory status in selected countries

Willow bark does not have GRAS status in the USA. However, it is freely available as a 'dietary supplement' in the USA under DSHEA legislation (Dietary Supplement Health and Education Act of 1994).

In the UK willow bark is included on the General Sale List and in Germany is covered by a positive Commission E monograph. Willow bark is official in the *European Pharmacopoeia* (2011) and is the topic of an ESCOP monograph.

In Australia willow bark is not included in Part 4 of Schedule 4 of the Therapeutic Goods Regulations and is freely available for sale.

References

1. Calixto JB, Beirith A, Ferreira J, et al. *Phytother Res*. 2000;14:401–418.
2. British Herbal Medicine Association Scientific Committee. *British Herbal Pharmacopoeia*. Bournemouth: BHMA; 1983.
3. Felter HW, Lloyd JU. *King's American Dispensatory*. 18th ed., 3rd rev, 1905. Portland: Reprinted Eclectic Medical Publications; 1983.
4. Culbreth DMR. *A Manual of Materia Medica and Pharmacology*. First published 1922. Portland: Reprinted Eclectic Medical Publications; 1983.
5. British Herbal Medicine Association. *British Herbal Compendium*. Bournemouth: BHMA; 1992.
6. Vogel VJ. *American Indian Medicine*. Norman: University of Oklahoma Press; 1970.
7. Hedner T, Everts B. *Clin Rheumatol*. 1998;17:17.
8. Stone E. *Philos Trans R Soc Lond* 1763;53:195. Cited in Hedner T, Everts B. *Clin Rheumatol* 17:17, 1998.
9. Launert E. *The Hamlyn Guide to Edible and Medicinal Plants of Britain and Northern Europe*. London: Hamlyn; 1981. p.126.
10. American Herbal Pharmacopeia. *Willow Bark – Salix spp.: Analytical, Quality Control, and Therapeutic Monograph*. Santa Cruz: American Herbal Pharmacopeia; December 1999.
11. Vane JR, Botting RM. *Thromb Res*. 2003;110:255–258.
12. Patrono C, Baigent C. *Mol Interv*. 2009;9(1):31–39.
13. Binder M, Zeiller P. *Fortschr Med*. 1993;111(33):530–532.
14. Gray PA, Warner TD, Vojnovic I, et al. *Br J Pharmacol*. 2002;137(7):1031–1038.
15. Wu KK. *Biochem Pharmacol*. 1998;55(5):543–547.
16. Giuliano F, Mitchell JA, Warner TD. *J Pharmacol Exp Ther*. 2001;299(3):894–900.
17. Reimeier C, Schneider I, Schneider W, et al. *Arzneimittelforschung*. 1995;45(2):132–136.
18. Wu KK. *Circulation*. 2000;102(17):2022–2023.
19. Wu KK. *Thromb Haemost*. 2006;96(4):417–422.
20. Krivoy N, Pavlotzky E, Chrubasik S, et al. *Planta Med*. 2001;67:209–212.
21. Schmid B, Ludtke R, Selbmann HK, et al. *Phytother Res*. 2001;15(4):344–350.
22. Bliddal H, Rosetzky A, Schlichting P, et al. *Osteoarthritis Cartilage*. 2000;8:9–12.
23. Altman RD, Marcussen KC. *Arthritis Rheum*. 2001;44(11):2531–2538.
24. Meier B. *Z Phytother*. 1990;11:50.
25. Lohmann K, et al. *Phytomedicine*. 2000;7(suppl 2):99.
26. Wagner I, Greim C, Laufer S, et al. *Clin Pharmacol Ther*. 2003;73(3):272–274.
27. Cheng GF, et al. *Phytomedicine*. 1994;1:209–211.
28. Smith ID, et al. *Prostaglandins*. 1975;10:41.
29. Yang DX, et al. *Yao Xue Xue Bao*. 1995;30:254.
30. Albrecht M. *Planta Med*. 1990;56:660.
31. Fiebich BL, Chrubasik S. *Phytomedicine*. 2004;11(2–3):135–138.
32. Khayyal MT, El-Ghazaly MA, Abdallah DM, et al. *Arzneimittelforschung*. 2005;55(11):677–687.
33. Nahrstedt A, Schmidt M, Jaggi R, et al. *Wien Med Wochenschr*. 2007;157(13–14):348–351.
34. Kahkonen MP, et al. *J Agric Food Chem*. 1999;47:3954.
35. Rohnert U, Schneider W, Elstner EF. *Z Naturforsch C*. 1998;53(3–4):241–249.
36. Opelz G, Terasaki PI. *Lancet*. 1973;2:478.
37. Steinegger E, Hovel H. *Pharm Acta Helv*. 1972;47:222.
38. Fotsch G, Pfeifer S, Bartoszek M, et al. *Pharmazie*. 1989;44(8):555–558. [Article in German].
39. Shrivastava R, Pechadres JC, John GW. *Clin Drug Investig*. 2006;26(5):287–296.
40. Gagnier JJ, van Tulder MW, Berman B, et al. *Spine*. 2007;32(1):82–92.
41. Gagnier JJ, van Tulder M, Berman B, Bombardier C. *Cochrane Database Syst Rev*. 2006;2:CD004504.
42. Vlachojannis JE, Cameron M, Chrubasik S. *Phytother Res*. 2009;23(7):897–900.

43. Schaffner W.. In: Chrubasik S, Wink M, eds. *Rheumatherapie mit Phytopharmaka*. Stuttgart: Hippokrates Verlag; 1997. pp. 125–127.

44. Chrubasik S, Eisenberg E, Balan E, et al. *Am J Med*. 2000;109(1):9–14.

45. Chrubasik S, Künzel O, Black A, et al. *Phytomedicine*. 2001;8(4):241–251.

46. Chrubasik S, Kunzel O, Model A, et al. *Rheumatology (Oxford)*. 2001;40(12): 1388–1393.

47. Lardos A, Schmidlin CB, Fischer M, et al. *Zeit Phytother*. 2004;25:275–281.

48. Biegert C, Wagner I, Ludtke R, et al. *J Rheumatol*. 2004;31(11):2121–2130.

49. Werner G, Scheithe K. *Congress Phytopharmaka and Phytotherapy*. Berlin: February 26–28, 2004.

50. Zenner-Weber MA. *Gemeinsamer Kongress der Schweizerischen Gesellschaft für Rheumatologie und für Physikalische Medizin und Rehabilitation*. Locarno: September 16–17, 2004.

51. Saller R. *Rev Med Suisse*. 2005;1(14):971.

52. Marz RW, Kemper F. *Wien Med Wochenschr*. 2002;152(15–16):354–359.

53. Leslie G. *Medita*. 1978;10:31–37.

54. Leslie G, Salmon G. *Swiss Med*. 1979; 1:43–45.

55. E-MIMS. Version 4.00.0457. *Havas MediMedia International*, 2000.

56. Scientific Committee of ESCOP (European Scientific Cooperative on Phytotherapy). *ESCOP Monographs: Salicis cortex*. European Scientific Cooperative on Phytotherapy, UK, July 1997, ESCOP Secretariat.

57. Hansel R, Haas H. *Therapie mit Phytopharmaka*. Berlin: Springer-Verlag; 1984. pp. 234–235.

58. Akao T, Yoshino T, Kobashi K, et al. *Planta Med*. 2002;68(8):714–718.

59. Boullata JI, McDonnell PJ, Oliva CD. *Ann Pharmacother*. 2003;37(6):832–835.

60. Baker S, Thomas PS. *Lancet*. 1987;1(8540):1039–1040.

61. Munson PL, Mueller RA, Breese GR, eds. *Principles of Pharmacology: Basic Concepts and Clinical Applications*. New York: Chapman & Hall; 1995. p. 1167.

62. Isselbacher KJ, Podolsky DK. [CD–ROM]. In: Harrison TR, Fauci AS, eds. *Harrison's Principles of Internal Medicine*, 14th ed. New York: McGraw–Hill; 1998.

Synonyms

Hamamelis (Engl), Hamamelidis folium, Hamamelidis cortex (Lat), virginische Zaubernub, Hamamelis, Hexenhasel (Ger), noisietier de la sorcière, hamamélis (Fr), amamelide (Ital), troldnød (Dan).

What is it?

Witchhazel is an American shrub that was used by the Native Americans as a poultice for the treatment of painful swellings and tumours. Pond's Extract of Witchhazel was once a very popular general household remedy for burns, scalds, insect bites and inflammatory conditions of the skin. The name Hamamelis was adopted from a Greek word to indicate its resemblance to an apple tree. The parts normally used therapeutically are the leaves and bark, which have similar properties. The distilled twig of witchhazel (hamamelis water) is still a popular topical remedy.

Effects

Improves vascular tone; astringent and anti-inflammatory to mucosa; protects against oxidative stress and ultraviolet radiation when used topically; haemostyptic.

Traditional view

Witchhazel was used to treat vascular disorders including haemorrhoids, varicose veins, phlebitis, haemorrhages and other conditions associated with poor venous tone or congestion. Other uses included reproductive disorders, such as dysmenorrhoea, menorrhagia and metrorrhagia; acute and chronic diarrhoea in children and adults; renal complaints associated with poor venous tone including haematuria; irritation of the bladder; muscular soreness; aching and bruised sensation (whether from cold, exposure, bruises, strains or physical exertion); and as a gargle for chronic pharyngitis and inflammation of the gums.[1]

Summary actions

Astringent, anti-inflammatory, haemostyptic.

Can be used for

Indications supported by clinical trials

Topical use for haemorrhoids; topical use for mild abrasions and skin inflammation. In oral combination with Hydrastis for the treatment of varicose veins (short-term open trial).

Traditional therapeutic uses

Haemorrhoids, varicose veins (topical use as well); diarrhoea, mucous colitis; topical use for bruises and localised, inflamed swellings.

May also be used for

Extrapolations from pharmacological studies

The dual inhibition of leukotriene and platelet-activating factor (PAF) production in vitro suggests potential therapeutic benefits in the treatment of disorders such as asthma, ulcerative colitis and Crohn's disease. However, these findings first need to be confirmed in vivo.

Other applications

Use in antiageing or antiwrinkle skin preparations[2] and also as a skin toner.[3]

Preparations

Dried bark and leaves as a decoction, liquid extract, tablets, capsules and suppositories for internal use. Decoction, extract and distilled extract for topical use.

Dosage

- 2 g of the dried leaf or bark three times per day or as an infusion
- 7 to 14 mL/day of 1:2 liquid extract of leaf or equivalent doses in other forms
- Hamamelis water BPC for local application, or as a cream or ointment
- 0.1 to 1 g in suppositories applied one to three times daily.

Duration of use

May be taken long term for external applications. Caution should be exercised with long term oral intake due to the presence of tannins.

Summary assessment of safety

No significant adverse effects from the ingestion of witchhazel are expected. It may cause irritation of the stomach in a small number of susceptible individuals and topical application can cause contact allergy in rare cases.

Technical data

Botany

Hamamelis virginiana L., a member of the Hamamelidaceae family, is a deciduous shrub that grows to approximately 2 m in height and is native to North America. The shrub consists of several crooked branching trunks 10 to 15 cm in diameter and up to 2 m in height, with a smooth grey bark. The alternate, ovoid, glabrous leaves have crenate margins, are 7 to 12 cm long and about 7 cm in width on short petioles. The yellow flowers consist of four sepals, four petals, four stamens and two styles and are grouped in two or three axillary glomerules with short peduncles. The fruit is a dehiscent, woody, bilocular capsule containing two dark-coloured glossy edible seeds that are ejected up to 4 m away when ripe. The medicinally useful parts of the plant are gathered in spring.[4,5]

Adulteration

Adulteration occurs rarely, but occasionally witchhazel leaf and bark are substituted with that of the hazel *Corylus avellana*.[6]

Key constituents

- A mixture of tannins (3% to 10%), including hamamelitannin, condensed catechins, gallotannins and procyanidins[7]
- Essential oil, flavonoids.[7]

The bark contains significantly higher levels of phenylpropanoids and sesquiterpenoids in the volatile fractions compared with the leaves, which contain higher amounts of monoterpenoids.[8] The bark is richer in hydrolysable tannins (mainly hamamelitannin) and the leaves mainly contain condensed tannins (procyanidins).

An analysis conducted in 2003 found 4.77% (w/w) of hamamelitannin in samples of bark, compared to less than 0.04% in the leaves.[9] The procyanidins (present in the bark at about 5%) are composed predominantly of epicatechin and epigallocatechin as chain extension units. Terminal chain units were catechin and gallocatechin.[10]

Pharmacodynamics

Anti-inflammatory effects

Hamamelitannin and galloylated proanthocyanidins isolated from witchhazel bark were found to be potent inhibitors of 5-lipoxygenase in vitro. The procyanidins also inhibited lyso-PAF:acetyl-CoA acetyltransferase and thus inhibited the production of PAF. These results demonstrate a dual inhibitory activity in vitro against inflammatory mediators by the procyanidins present in witchhazel.[11]

Oral administration of an aqueous ethanolic extract of witchhazel leaf (200 mg/kg) significantly inhibited the chronic phase of adjuvant arthritis-induced rat paw swelling. It was inactive against the acute phase and against carrageenan-induced rat paw oedema.[12] A witchhazel bark concentrate displayed radical scavenging properties, inhibited alpha-glucosidase and human leucocyte elastase in vitro and exhibited strong anti-inflammatory effects in the croton oil ear oedema test in the mouse. The extract contained mainly oligomeric to polymeric procyanidins.[13]

The anti-inflammatory effect of an aftersun lotion containing 10% witchhazel distillate, the vehicle, and the prior aftersun lotion were tested in 20 healthy volunteers using a modified UVB erythema test as a model of inflammation. Test areas on the back were treated with the lotions for 48 h following irradiation and compared with an untreated, irradiated control area. Erythema suppression ranged from 20% to 27% at 7 and 48 h respectively for the witchhazel treated areas. A suppression of 11% to 15% was recorded in the fields treated with the vehicle and prior aftersun lotion. Witchhazel led to a highly significant reduction in erythema when compared with the prior aftersun lotion (p=0.00039), the vehicle (p=0.00001) or untreated, irradiated skin (p=0.00001).[14] In a later study, an anti-inflammatory effect was also demonstrated for several aftersun lotions containing 10% witchhazel distillate.[15]

Anti-irritant activity

Topical application of procyanidins from witchhazel bark reduced transepidermal water loss and erythema formation in healthy volunteers. In this preliminary evaluation, an irritant

Hamamelitannin

contact dermatitis was induced in the volunteers using a repeated short-time occlusive irritation test. The experimental irritation and the treatment continued over a period of 3 days. Results also indicated that the procyanidins significantly reduced skin inflammation.[16]

Antioxidant activity

Hamamelitannin demonstrated in vitro antioxidant activity and protected murine skin fibroblasts from damage induced by UVB irradiation. It protected murine fibroblasts against external active oxygen radicals generated by UVB irradiation by associating with the cell surface through its sugar moiety.[17] Further tests indicated that hamamelitannin has higher protective activity against cell damage induced by superoxide anions than gallic acid (its functional moiety).[18]

In earlier work, hamamelitannin increased the survival rate of fibroblasts compared with controls. Hamamelitannin inhibited superoxide anion radicals at a much lower concentration than ascorbic acid. Further test results supported the superoxide scavenging activity of hamamelitannin.[19] Witchhazel extract demonstrated strong active oxygen-scavenging activity and protected against cell damage induced by active oxygen. The authors recommended witchhazel as a potential topical antiageing or antiwrinkle material for the skin.[2] Witchhazel bark extract and hamamelitannin demonstrated a strong ability to scavenge the peroxynitrite ion in vitro.[20]

Vasoconstrictive activity

Vasoconstrictive activity has been demonstrated for administration of witchhazel leaf preparations in isolated rabbit arteries.[21,22] The activity was not blocked by alpha- or beta-sympatholytic agents.[22] Topical application of a witchhazel leaf extract produced a significant reduction in skin temperature in 30 volunteers. The lowered skin temperature was interpreted as a vasoconstrictive activity.[23]

Antimicrobial activity

A witchhazel concentrate exhibited significant antiviral activity against herpes simplex virus type 1 in vitro.[10] Methanol extract of witchhazel leaves demonstrated an inhibitory effect against anaerobic and facultative aerobic bacteria associated with periodontitis. As an example, the best activity was demonstrated against *Eikenella corrodens* and two strains of *Actinomyces odontolyticus*, with a minimum inhibitory concentration (MIC) of 32 mg/L, which compared well to the drug spiramycin (MIC 2 mg/L). The methanol extract showed better antibacterial activity than the decoction (MIC 128 mg/L) for the above bacteria.[24] (Note that 1 mg/L is the same as 1 µg/mL.)

Witchhazel distillate (obtained from witchhazel leaf and bark by steam distillation, followed by the addition of ethanol) exhibited topical antimicrobial activity in healthy volunteers. This was demonstrated by the use of two standard tests. Antimicrobial activity against anaerobes was much less than that against aerobes. Quantitative comparison with other antiseptic agents such as chlorhexidine digluconate 1% and fuchsine 0.5% indicated a relatively weak activity for witchhazel distillate. The antimicrobial activity could be considered an additional benefit to the main effects of relief of inflammation, barrier-stabilisation and hydration.[25]

Pharmacokinetics

No data available.

Clinical trials

Haemorrhoids and venous tone

In an uncontrolled study, 50 patients with painful skin lesions in the anogenital area were treated with a salve containing witchhazel bark distillate (5%), zinc oxide and vitamins A and D. After a week the healing process was completed in 40 patients.[27] In an uncontrolled trial on 75 patients with itching, painful and bleeding haemorrhoids, application of a salve containing witchhazel bark resulted in a majority of patients becoming free from symptoms after 3 weeks of treatment.[28] A comparison of this witchhazel bark salve with two other salves (one containing corticosteroids) was undertaken in a double blind trial in 90 patients with grade 1 haemorrhoids. Several patients receiving the witchhazel salve had also received sclerotherapy. All three preparations demonstrated similar efficacy, except that the witchhazel was superior in terms of relief of symptoms, with greater reduction in itching and soreness and less frequent bleeding.[29]

In a similar double blind clinical trial, 90 patients with first-degree haemorrhoids were treated with witchhazel bark ointment and two ointments containing synthetic agents, one of which additionally contained a corticosteroid. Treatment was of 21 days' duration, with follow-up examinations on the third, 14th and 21st days of treatment. Four typical symptoms (pruritus, bleeding, burning sensation and sore sensation) were evaluated by both physician and patient. All three ointments proved highly effective. No major differences were found between the three treatment groups, but, in the case of some of the test parameters (itch) a positive tendency in favour of the witchhazel ointment was observed.[30]

The therapeutic effect of witchhazel on venous tone was studied in patients with varicose veins in an open trial. Four groups were each given different medications and studied by plethysmography for the next 5 h. In the untreated controls, venous tone decreased during rest. A reference drug had no effect and the increase in venous tone induced by the ingestion of a high dose of a Hamamelis-Hydrastis mixture was equivalent to that induced by 150 mg of oligomeric procyanidins.[31]

Dermatological conditions

Application of witchhazel leaf cream twice daily for 2 weeks in an uncontrolled study resulted in complete healing or considerable improvement in 37 patients with various forms of eczema or atopic neurodermatitis.[32]

Thirty-six patients with endogenous eczema and 80 patients with toxic degenerative eczema were treated in a double blind, placebo-controlled trial with either witchhazel salve (25% water distillate from leaf and twigs) or a control preparation. The witchhazel salve was superior to placebo in the treatment of atopic dermatitis, but of no benefit in the treatment of primary irritant contact dermatitis.[33] Twenty-two patients with atopic dermatitis were treated with a standardised witchhazel salve on one arm and a non-steroidal anti-inflammatory cream (containing bufexamac) on the other over a 3-week period.

Both treatments showed a clear improvement in the symptoms investigated: redness, scaling, lichenification, pruritus and infiltration. The salve contained 25 g of water distillate (from 4 g of fresh leaf and twigs) per 100 g of salve, which was also standardised for hamamelis ketone (0.75 mg).[34]

Hamamelis distillate cream (5.35 g Hamamelis distillate containing 0.64 mg ketone/100 g) was compared with 0.5% hydrocortisone cream and an unmedicated cream base in a double blind, randomised trial in 72 patients with moderately severe atopic eczema over a period of 14 days. All treatment regimens significantly reduced itching, erythema and scaling after 1 week. The hydrocortisone cream proved superior to the hamamelis distillate, which was no more effective than the unmedicated base.[35] In a previous study by the same authors, creams containing various concentrations of Hamamelis distillate (containing 0.64 to 2.56 mg Hamamelis ketone per 100 g) were compared with a chamomile cream and a 1% hydrocortisone cream on human volunteers who had erythema induced by UV irradiation and cellophane tape stripping of the horny layer. A mild anti-inflammatory effect was demonstrated for the hamamelis cream, especially if incorporated into a phospholipid base. Although less active than hydrocortisone cream, hamamelis cream was superior to the unmedicated cream base.[36] The anti-inflammatory activity described here could, at least in part, be due to a vasoconstrictor activity.[37]

A lotion containing witchhazel distillate and essential oil of *Melissa officinalis* improved itching and redness in patients with intertrigo (dermatitis caused by friction on skin surfaces in contact with each other) in an open label trial.[38] A case was reported where treatment with witchhazel extract healed a sodium hypochlorite-induced skin burn. Sodium hypochlorite is used as an irrigating solution for endodontic treatment (e.g. during root canal preparation), but can cause serious complications after inadvertent use (in this case, leakage onto the patient's chin, which went unnoticed underneath the rubber dam). Witchhazel extract was applied topically twice a day for 2 weeks. The burning sensation stopped in 3 days, the scab fell off in 7 days, but the tenderness continued for 10 more days. The skin discoloration caused by the burn had disappeared after 3 months.[39]

A mild anti-inflammatory effect for standardised witchhazel salve (25 g distillate from 4 g fresh leaf and twigs, 0.75 mg of ketone, all per 100 g), compared with its neutral ointment base, was demonstrated by instrumental testing and transcutaneous oxygen measurement in 22 healthy people and five patients with dermatosis.[40]

An observational study collected data on the safety, tolerability and clinical effects of a witchhazel ointment containing the distillate in 309 children up to the age of 11 years with minor skin complaints including nappy (diaper) rash. Compared with baseline there was a significant improvement in signs and symptoms after a median treatment period of 8 days. Use of the ointment was well tolerated and yielded similar outcomes to topical use of dexpanthenol (derived from pantothenic acid, vitamin B5).[41]

Analgesic activity

A randomised open study in 300 mothers examined the effectiveness of hamamelis water, ice or Epifoam in achieving analgesia for episiotomy associated with forceps delivery. All three agents were equally effective at achieving analgesia on the first day. Approximately one-third of the mothers derived no benefit from any of the treatments.[42]

Toxicology and other safety data

Toxicology

A methanol extract and a tincture of witchhazel bark showed dose-dependent inhibition of mutagenicity in the Ames assay. Tannin-free samples did not display any activity. Fractionation yielded two active fractions, both of which contained oligomeric procyanidins. The antimutagenic effect increased with an increasing degree of polymerisation in the procyanidins.[43] In a study of 18 substances for mutagenic potential in vitro, witchhazel was not identified as a mutagen.[44]

Catechin and a low-molecular weight procyanidin fraction (at concentrations up to 166 μg/mL) caused only slight increases of OTM (olive tail moment, an indicator of DNA damage) in Hep G2 hepatoma cells. (Hep G2 cells have retained the activities of various phase I and phase II enzymes and reflect the metabolism of genotoxins better than bacteria or metabolic incompetent mammalian cells.) Hamamelitannin and the procyanidin fraction with higher molecular weight had a much greater increase in this parameter. However, treatment of the cells with these compounds (at concentrations up to 166 μg/mL) prior to exposure to the mutagen benzo(a)pyrene led to a reduction of induced DNA damage. In investigating this protective activity, it was found that detoxification by glutathione-S-transferase was induced by catechin and the low-molecular weight procyanidin fraction. These compounds may have inactivated the ultimate metabolite of benzo(a)pyrene by the formation of an adduct.[45]

Contraindications

None known.

Special warnings and precautions

Care should be exercised with long term oral use due to the presence of tannins.

Interactions

Tannins can inhibit the absorption of minerals and B vitamins.

Use in pregnancy and lactation

Category B2 – no increase in frequency of malformation or other harmful effects on the fetus from limited use in women. Animal studies are lacking.

Witchhazel is compatible with breastfeeding.

Effects on ability to drive and use machines

No adverse effects expected.

Side effects

Irritation of the stomach may occur in susceptible patients after oral doses.[6] Contact dermatitis caused by the topical use of witchhazel has been reported in rare cases.[46] In a study of 1032 consecutively tested patients, four were found to react to an ointment containing a 25% extract of witchhazel. Two of these patients had reacted positively to the wool fat in the ointment base.[47]

Overdosage

No effects known.

Safety in children

No information available for oral use, but adverse effects are not expected. The safety of topical application of distilled witchhazel was demonstrated in an observational study in children (see above).

Regulatory status in selected countries

Witchhazel leaf is official in the *European Pharmacopoeia* (2011) and distillate made from witchhazel twig is official in the *United States Pharmacopeia–National Formulary* (USP34-NF 29, 2011).

Witchhazel leaf and bark are covered by positive Commission E monographs and both have the following applications: mild damage to the skin, local inflammation of the skin and mucous membranes, haemorrhoids and varicose veins.

Witchhazel is not on the UK General Sale List.

Witchhazel does not have GRAS status. However, it is freely available as a 'dietary supplement' in the USA under DSHEA legislation (1994 Dietary Supplement Health and Education Act). Witchhazel has been defined as an astringent active ingredient in over-the-counter (OTC) skin protectant drug products for relief of minor skin irritations due to insect bites, minor cuts and minor scrapes and in OTC anorectal drug products. These OTC products, in a form suitable for topical administration, are generally recognised as safe and effective if they meet the requirements outlined in the Code of Federal Regulations. The FDA, however, advises that 'based on evidence currently available, there is inadequate data to establish general recognition of the safety and effectiveness of these ingredients for the specified uses'.

Witchhazel is not included in Part 4 of Schedule 4 of the Therapeutic Goods Act Regulations of Australia and is freely available for sale.

References

1. Felter HW, Lloyd JU. *King's American Dispensatory*, ed 18, rev 3, vol. 2, 1905. Portland: Reprinted by Eclectic Medical Publications; 1983, pp. 974–976.
2. Masaki H, Sakaki S, Atsumi T, et al. *Biol Pharm Bull*. 1995;18(1):162–166.
3. Smeh NJ. *Creating Your Own Cosmetics – Naturally*. Garrisonville: Alliance Publishing Company; 1995. p. 142.
4. Grieve M. *A Modern Herbal*, vol. 2. New York: Dover Publications; 1971. p. 851.
5. Chiej R. *The Macdonald Encyclopedia of Medicinal Plants*. London: Macdonald; 1984. Entry no. 148.
6. Bisset NG, ed. *Herbal Drugs and Phytopharmaceuticals: A Handbook for Practice on a Scientific Basis*. Stuttgart: Medpharm Scientific Publishers; 1994. pp. 243–247.
7. Bisset NG, ed. *Herbal Drugs and Phytopharmaceuticals*. Stuttgart: Medpharm Scientific Publishers; 1994. pp. 245–247.
8. Engel R, Gutmann M, Hartisch C, et al. *Planta Med*. 1998;64:251–258.
9. Wang H, Provan GJ, Helliwell K. *J Pharm Biomed Anal*. 2003;33(4):539–544.
10. Dauer A, Rimpler H, Hensel A. *Planta Med*. 2003;69(1):89–91.
11. Hartisch C, Kolodziej H, Von Bruchhausen F. *Planta Med*. 1997;63:106–110.
12. Duwiejua M, Zeitlin IJ, Waterman PG, et al. *J Pharm Pharmacol*. 1994;46(4):286–290.
13. Erdelmeier CA, Cinatl Jr J, Rabenau H, et al. *Planta Med*. 1996;62(3):241–245.
14. Hughes-Formella BJ, Bohnsack K, Rippke F, et al. *Dermatology*. 1998;196:316–322.
15. Hughes-Formella BJ, Filbry A, Gassmueller J, et al. *Skin Pharmacol Appl Skin Physiol*. 2002;15(2):125–132.
16. Deters A, Dauer A, Schnetz E, et al. *Phytochemistry*. 2001;58(6):949–958.
17. Masaki H, Atsumi T, Sakurai H. *J Dermatol Sci*. 1995;10(1):25–34.
18. Masaki H, Atsumi T, Sakurai H. *Biol Pharm Bull*. 1995;18(1):59–63.
19. Masaki H, Atsumi T, Sakurai H. *Free Radic Res Commun*. 1993;19(5):333–340.
20. Choi HR, Choi JS, Han YN, et al. *Phytother Res*. 2002;16(4):364–367.
21. Bernard P, Balansard P, Balansard G, et al. *J Pharm Belg*. 1972;27(4):505–512.
22. Balansard P, Faure F, Balansard G, et al. *Therapie*. 1972;27(5):793–799.
23. Diemunsch AM, Mathis C. *STP Pharma*. 1987;3:111–114.
24. Iauk L, Lo Bue AM, Milazzo I, et al. *Phytother Res*. 2003;17(6):599–604.
25. Gloor M, Reichling J, Wasik B, et al. *Forsch Komplementarmed Klass Naturheilkd*. 2002;9(3):153–159.
26. Habtemariam S. *Toxicon*. 2002;40(1):83–88.
27. Seeberger J. *Z Allg Med*. 1979;55(29):1667–1668.
28. Moosmann EB. *Fortschr Med*. 1991;109(116):5–6.
29. Moosmann EB. *Fortschr Med*. 1991;109(116):7–8.
30. Knoch HG, Klug W, Hübner WD. *Fortschr Med*. 1992;110(8):69–74.
31. Royer RJ, Schmidt CL. *Sem Hop*. 1981;57(47–48):2009–2013.
32. Wokalek H. *Deut Dermatol*. 1995;5:498–506.
33. Pfister R. *Fortschr Med*. 1981;99(31–32):1264–1268.
34. Swoboda M, Meurer J. *Z Phytother*. 1991;12:114–117.
35. Korting HC, Schafer-Korting M, Klovekorn W, et al. *Eur J Clin Pharmacol*. 1995;48(6):461–465.
36. Korting HC, Schafer-Korting M, Hart H, et al. *Eur J Clin Pharmacol*. 1993;44(4):315–318.
37. Hormann HP, Korting HC. *Phytomedicine*. 1994;1(2):161–171.
38. Schindera I, Falch B. *Forsch Komplementarmed*. 1999;6(suppl 2):31–32.
39. Serper A, Ozbek M, Calt S. *J Endod*. 2004;30(3):180–181.
40. Sorkin B. *Phys Med Rehabil*. 1980;21(1):53–57.
41. Wolff HH, Kieser M. *Eur J Pediatr*. 2007;166(9):943–948.
42. Moore W, James DK. *J Obstet Gynecol*. 1989;10(1):35–39.

43. Dauer A, Metzner P, Schimmer O. *Planta Med*. 1998;64:324–327.

44. McGregor DB, Brown A, Cattanach P, et al. *Environ Mol Mutagen*. 1988;11(1):91–118.

45. Dauer A, Hensel A, Lhoste E, et al. *Phytochemistry*. 2003;63(2):199–207.

46. Granlund H. *Contact Dermatitis*. 1994;31:195.

47. Bruynzeel DP, Van Ketel WG, Young E, et al. *Contact Dermatitis*. 1992;27(4): 278–279.

(*Withania somnifera* (L.) Dunal)

Synonyms

Winter cherry, Indian ginseng (Engl), ashwagandha (Sanskrit), blærebæger (Dan).

What is it?

Withania somnifera is an important herb from the Ayurvedic medical system used for the treatment of debility, emaciation, impotence and premature ageing. Not surprisingly, it has been dubbed the 'Indian ginseng'. Its Indian name, ashwagandha, is said to refer to the 'smell and strength of a horse' and possibly alludes to its reputed aphrodisiac properties, although it could also relate to the smell of the root. Pharmacological research on Withania has stressed its antitumour and adaptogenic actions, reinforcing its comparison with *Panax ginseng*. However, Withania occupies an important place in the herbal materia medica because, while it is not as potent as Panax, it lacks the potential stimulating effects of the latter. In fact, it has a mild sedative action as indicated by its specific name '*somnifera*'. It is therefore ideally suited to the treatment of overactive but debilitated patients, in whom Panax might tend to aggravate the overstimulation. Many parts of the plant have been used in traditional medicine, including the leaves, bark and root. Except where specified in this monograph, 'Withania' refers to use of the root.

Effects

Adaptogen (helping to conserve adaptation energy as defined in Selye's general adaptation syndrome); tonic (helping to boost levels of adaptation energy); modulates the immune system; glucocorticoid-like anti-inflammatory and antiproliferative activity; potentially has cytotoxic, cancer chemopreventative and radiosensitising activities.

Traditional view

In Ayurveda, the roots are said to have aphrodisiac, tonic, depurative and anthelmintic properties, besides being useful in *vata* and *kapha* conditions and for inflammation, psoriasis, bronchitis, asthma, ulcers, scabies, wasting in children, insomnia, senile debility and as a tonic for the elderly.[1,2] Withania is described as a 'medharasayan' or promoter of learning and memory retrieval.[3] In Unani, the roots are noted to have tonic, aphrodisiac and emmenagogue properties and are used in asthma, inflammation, leucoderma, bronchitis, lumbago, arthritis and to promote conception.[1] In the Middle East,

Withania root is used as a sedative and hypnotic and is also taken for rheumatic pains.[4]

Summary actions

Tonic, adaptogen, mild sedative, anti-inflammatory, immune modulator, anti-anaemic, antitumour (possibly, in high doses).

Can be used for

Indications supported by clinical trials

Anxiety; reduction of the negative physiological effects of stress; improvement in well-being; growth promotion in children and anti-anaemic activity; improvement in conditions associated with ageing, including muscle strength and function; adjunct in type 2 diabetes and for modification of cardiovascular risk factors; rheumatoid arthritis (uncontrolled trial); improvement of stamina in athletes (uncontrolled trial); low testosterone and fertility in men (uncontrolled trials).

Traditional therapeutic uses

Asthma, bronchitis; psoriasis; arthritis, rheumatic pains; insomnia; senile debility; promotion of conception.

In India, Withania is given with pungent or heating herbs such as ginger and long pepper to increase its tonic effects.

May also be used for

Extrapolations from pharmacological studies

Debility and nervous exhaustion, especially due to stress; convalescence after acute illness or extreme stress, impotence due to devitalisation; chronic diseases, especially those marked by inflammation (e.g. connective tissue diseases); as a general tonic for disease prevention; may be useful for depressed white blood cell count, especially if caused by cytotoxic drugs; possibly as prophylactic against cancer; to assist in withdrawal from addictive drugs.

Preparations

Dried root as a decoction, liquid extract, capsules or tablets for internal use.

Dosage

- 3 to 8g/day of dried root by decoction
- 3 to 8mL/day of 1:1 liquid extract or equivalent in other dosage forms.

Withania combines well with a low dose of *Panax ginseng* and adrenal restorative herbs such as licorice and Rehmannia.

Duration of use

No problems known with long-term use.

Summary assessment of safety

No adverse effects from ingestion of Withania are expected.

Technical data

Botany

Withania somnifera, a member of the Solanaceae (nightshade) family, is a small-to-medium perennial shrub that grows 1 to 1.5m in height. It has ovate hair-like branches with simple, alternate leaves, up to 10cm long. The small, greenish-yellow flowers (approximately 1cm) are borne together in short axillary clusters. The red fruit (6mm in diameter) is smooth, spherical and enclosed in the inflated and membranous calyx. The root is long and tuberous.[5]

Adulteration

Withania coagulans has been reported to be both a substitute and an adulterant of *W. somnifera*.[6]

Key constituents

- Steroidal compounds, including lactones (withaferin A, sitoindoside IX, X (carbon-27 glycowithanolides)) and acylsteryl glucosides (sitoindosides VII, VIII)[7]
- Alkaloids: tropane-type (tropine, pseudotropine), other alkaloids (including isopelletierine, anaferine).[8]

Withania is also said to be rich in iron, but there is no recent verification of this.[9]

Pharmacodynamics

Adaptogenic and tonic activity

Adaptogens increase the ability of the body to cope with stress. They therefore help to conserve energy, whereas a tonic boosts energy reserves and promotes health in a non-specific manner. In experimental models, adaptogenic effects can be assessed by subjecting an animal to stress, while tonic effects might be assessed by the long-term influence of a substance on the development, health and offspring of a test animal. For Withania it is possible that significant glucocorticoid-like tonic and adaptogenic effects may result from the complex of the many steroidal withanolides found in the root. Traditional use emphasises the tonic properties of Withania.

Several experiments using in vivo models demonstrated that Withania could counter the deleterious effects of chronic stress.[10–14] Oral pretreatment with Withania (5, 10 and 20mg/kg) for 3, 7 and 14 days resulted in protection against stress-induced stomach ulcers in rats.[15] A methanol extract of Withania given orally reduced the ulcer index, volume of gastric secretion and acidity in experimentally induced ulceration. The antiulcer effect of Withania treatment was comparable to ranitidine.[16]

Several herbs including Withania were evaluated for their protective effects against cyclophosphamide neutropenia in

Withanolides

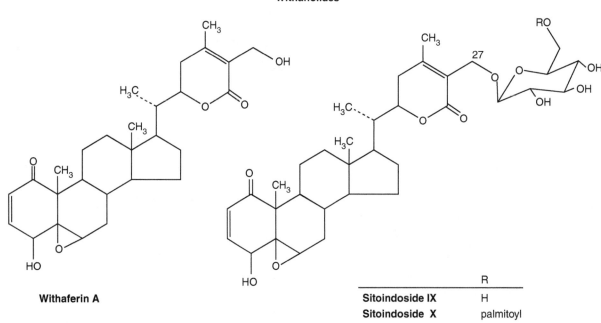

Withaferin A

	R
Sitoindoside IX	H
Sitoindoside X	palmitoyl

mice. The dosage used was 100 mg/kg as a decoction, given for 15 days prior to a single dose of cyclophosphamide. Results are tabulated below:

		Day 0	Day 3
Control	Total count	7800	4390
	Neutrophils	3960	1440
Withania	Total count	11 180	8030
	Neutrophils	7020	5060

Withania significantly increased white blood cell and neutrophil counts both before and after treatment with cyclophosphamide (day 3 after gave the lowest counts). There were no deaths in the Withania group compared with 10% mortality in other groups.[17]

The reduction in interferon-gamma and granulocyte macrophage colony stimulating factor induced by treatment with cyclophosphamide in mice was reversed by oral treatment with Withania extract.[18] Administration of bone marrow cells from donor mice treated with Withania extract increased spleen nodular colonies in irradiated mice, compared with those receiving unmedicated bone marrow cells.[18] Oral treatment with Withania also reversed the neutropaenia induced by paclitaxel in mice.[19]

Oral administration of an aqueous fraction of Withania root reduced the depletion of T cells in chronically stressed mice. The expression of Th1 cytokines was also increased by Withania.[20] Withania aqueous extract (7:1) at a once daily oral dose of 100 mg/kg resulted in a significant selective up-regulation of the Th1 response in mice. There was an increase in CD4+ and CD8+ counts compared with controls and cyclosporin treatment, with a faster recovery of CD4+ T cells in the immune suppressed animals.[21]

Young rats were fed whole plant of Withania or root of *Asparagus racemosus* at oral doses of 100 mg/kg for 8 months. The weight gain for Withania-treated rats was 257%, compared with 195% for *Asparagus racemosus* and 161% for controls. Animals were alert and in good health. While there was no difference in number and size of pregnancies, average body weight of offspring was 70 g for Withania compared with 45 g for controls. This study was followed up with a second short-term study over 4 weeks at 250 mg/kg in adult rats. No weight gain was seen, which indicates that Withania's anabolic effect was only exerted in the growth phase. However, other interesting effects in this short-term study were noted. Body temperature was reduced by 1.7°C and liver weight increased for the Withania group. Plasma cortisol was also significantly lower and adrenal weight reduced following Withania treatment.[22] This may reflect the 'steroid-like' activity of Withania constituents. An anabolic effect at oral doses of 100 mg/kg has been demonstrated.[23]

A pharmacological comparison of Withania and *Panax ginseng* demonstrated that Withania had similar potency to Panax in terms of adaptogenic, tonic and anabolic effects. Significant increases in swimming time were shown by both Withania and Panax (100 mg/kg per day, oral administration for 7 days)

compared with the control group. Following oral administration of aqueous suspensions of the powdered herb at 1 g/kg for 7 days, the increase in body weight seen in the Withania-treated group was greater than that for animals treated with Panax. Gain in wet weight of the levator ani muscle was significant for both the Withania ($p<0.01$) and Panax groups ($p<0.001$), possibly indicating anabolic effects.[24]

Chronic stress induces hyperglycaemia, glucose intolerance, increased plasma corticosterone levels, gastric ulceration, sexual dysfunction, cognitive deficit, depression and immune suppression in male rats. Pretreatment with Withania reduced these changes. A concentrated fraction of Withania root containing 30% sitoindosides VII to IX and withaferin A was administered orally.[25] In an earlier study using the same chronic stress model, pretreatment with glycowithanolides (sitoindosides VII to X and withaferin A, 10 to 50 mg/kg, oral doses) also had an antistress effect on the frontal cortex and striatum. Glycowithanolides tended to normalise the stress-induced increase in superoxide dismutase activity and lipid peroxidation, and enhanced the activities of catalase and glutathione peroxidase, thereby exerting an antioxidant effect.[26]

A fraction of Withania root devoid of withanolides has also demonstrated adaptogenic activity. Pretreatment had a positive effect on liver function parameters in rats exposed to swimming-induced stress. An oral dose of 25 mg/kg of this withanolide-free fraction produced similar results to 100 mg/kg of a complete extract of Withania root.[27] In an earlier study, oral administration of this fraction demonstrated adaptogenic activity in a range of tests including swimming performance time, swimming-induced gastric ulceration and hypothermia, immobilisation-induced gastric ulceration, auto-analgesia and hypoxia time. Stress-induced hypertrophy of the adrenal glands was also reduced by the treatment.[28]

Sitoindosides protected rats against stress-induced stomach ulcers. Sitoindosides IX and X (50 to 200 mg/kg) by oral administration produced significant antistress activity in mice and rats and augmented learning acquisition and memory retention in both young and old rats.[29] An aqueous-methanolic extract of Withania and a combination of sitoindosides VII, VIII and withaferin A also exhibited significant antistress activity. An antidepressant effect was observed after intraperitoneal administration of sitoindosides VII and VIII to mice subjected to the swimming test.[30]

Withania extract significantly increased the total white blood cell count in normal mice and reduced leucopenia induced by a sublethal dose of gamma radiation. Treatment increased the bone marrow cellularity significantly and normalised the ratio of normochromatic and polychromatic erythrocytes in mice after radiation exposure.[31]

Immune function

Several positive effects of Withania on immune function have been observed in various models of chronic stress (see above for details). In addition, Withania extract protected mice from a lethal dose of *Listeria monocytogenes* when administered prophylactically. Withania also prevented the myelo-suppression and splenomegaly caused by sublethal infection with *L. monocytogenes*. This was attributed to increased numbers of granulocyte-macrophage progenitors. It also reduced the effect of Listeria infection via enhanced proliferation of lymphocytes, increased interferon-gamma levels and higher myeloid progenitors in bone marrow.[32] Oral treatment of immunised mice with Withania extract increased antibody titres to *Bordetella pertussis* (the cause of whooping cough). Mortality was reduced and overall health improved in Withania-treated animals exposed to intracerebral challenge with *Bordetella pertussis*.[33] Aqueous extracts of Withania root and Withania leaf by oral administration both successfully reduced Salmonella infection in mice, as indicated by increased survival rates and lower bacterial load in vital organs compared with control animals.[34]

Withania alcoholic extract significantly inhibited the experimentally induced suppression of chemotactic activity and production of interleukin-1 and tumour necrosis factor-alpha (TNF-alpha) by macrophages obtained from carcinogen-treated mice ($p<0.005$). Withania extract was co-administered (100 mg/kg per day) by oral administration with the carcinogen (ochratoxin A) for 17 weeks.[35]

A significant modulation of immune reactivity after orally administered Withania extract was observed in mice with myelosuppression induced by three different immunosuppressive drugs (cyclophosphamide, azathioprine and prednisolone). In addition, significant increases in haemoglobin concentration ($p<0.01$), red blood cell count ($p<0.01$), white blood cell count ($p<0.05$), platelet count ($p<0.01$) and body weight ($p<0.05$) were observed in Withania-treated mice compared with untreated controls. In a model of immunostimulation, treatment with Withania was accompanied by significant increases in haemolytic antibody responses.[36]

Sitoindosides IX and X (100 to 400 mg/mouse) produced significant mobilisation and activation of peritoneal macrophages, phagocytosis and increased activity of the lysosomal enzymes secreted by activated macrophages. Withaferin A demonstrated immunosuppressive effects, in contrast to the immunostimulating activity found for Withania extracts.[29] A steroidal withanolide isolated from roots of *Withania somnifera*[37] demonstrated immunomodulating activity by inhibiting proliferation of murine spleen cells in vitro.[38]

A standardised extract of Withania (30 mg/kg for 15 days, oral) increased Th1-mediated immune responses in mice.[39] The extract also strongly activated macrophage function ex vivo and in vitro. Withanolide A, a major constituent of the extract, was suggested to be responsible for the Th1 effect, based on its activity on mouse splenocyte cultures.

Antitumour activity

In a recent review it was suggested that the antitumour activity of Withania could possibly result from several mechanisms demonstrated in experimental models, including regulation of cell cycle proliferation, increased tumour apoptosis, inhibition of angiogenesis, NF-kappaB suppression and enhanced immune activity.[40]

In terms of cytotoxic activity in vitro, much of the research focus has been on withaferin A, the most active compound in this regard.[40,41–44] Apoptosis is a major mechanism behind its activity and has been demonstrated on a variety of cell lines.

The compound has also demonstrated in vivo antitumour activity[40,45] as well as antigenotoxicity.[46]

Withaferin A induced a mitotic arrest in the metaphase of dividing Ehrlich ascites carcinoma cells.[47] It also caused disappearance of Ehrlich ascites tumours in mice, and treated mice were resistant to rechallenge with the tumour cells. Such a response was explained as both a direct effect of withaferin A and an induced immune response.[48]

A study of the in vitro mode of action of withaferin A and withanolide D postulated that the cell death of sarcoma-180 tumour cultures was due to inhibition of RNA synthesis.[49] (Several chemotypes of Withania exist; withaferin A is the major withanolide found in leaves of one chemotype and withanolide D is the major one found in another.[50])

Withaferin A produced mitotic arrest in the metaphase of dividing normal human lymphocytes stimulated by phytohaemagglutinin. The membrane system of cells at interphase was also damaged.[51] However, the mechanism of action of the antitumour and radiosensitising properties of withaferin A cannot be explained wholly by effects on the cell cycle or macromolecular synthesis.[52,53] Mouse sarcoma-180 solid and ascites tumour cells treated in vitro and in vivo with withaferin A were also affected in a similar way to the above study.[54] Withaferin A has also demonstrated potent inhibition of angiogenesis in vitro and in vivo.[55] The latter was at ip doses between 7 and 200 μg/kg/day in mice, representing a potency around 500-fold higher than its antitumour activity.

Both withaferin A and withanolide E exhibited specific immunosuppressive effects on human B and T lymphocytes in vitro. Intraperitoneal administration of withanolide E was also active against several animal tumour systems. Withaferin A and withanolide D predominate in the leaves of *Withania somnifera* and it is mainly the leaves of Withania which were traditionally used to treat cancerous growths.[56] However, the root does contain significant quantities of withaferin A.

Withania extracts have also shown antitumour activity in vitro and in vivo.[57,58] For example, a Withania extract at 150 mg/kg, ip, inhibited more than 50% of tumour growth in various murine models.[57] The same extract was also active orally at doses of 100 to 400 mg/kg in mice with Ehrlich ascites tumours. A study investigating the effects of Withania, gamma radiation and hyperthermia on sarcoma in mice found that Withania root (500 mg/kg/day for 10 days, ip) produced an 18% rate of response. Although radiation and heat treatment had greater individual effects on the tumours, Withania increased their impact on tumour regression and growth delay when administered concomitantly. The study concluded that Withania had a tumour inhibitory effect and acted as a radiosensitiser.[59] Withania given at 200 mg/kg (whole plant) orally to mice significantly decreased mortality from urethane-induced lung cancers. It countered the decrease in body weight due to the tumours and also decreased their incidence, number and size.[60] A withanolide sulphoxide was isolated from Withania root that had marked activity across a range of cancer cell lines.[61]

Withania extracts and root powder have also demonstrated chemopreventative activity. Oral administration of Withania in combination with paclitaxel stabilised membrane bound enzyme (ATPases) profiles, decreased lipid peroxidation and reduced cell proliferation in benzo(a)pyrene-induced experimental lung cancer in mice. (Alterations of these enzyme activities in membrane and tissues is a consequence of tumour formation caused by benzo(a)pyrene.[62,63]) Powdered Withania root (2.5 to 5% w/w of diet) demonstrated a chemopreventive effect against forestomach and skin carcinogenesis in mice. Treatment with Withania inhibited phase I and activated phase II and antioxidant enzymes in the liver. Aqueous alcoholic extract of Withania (as a pretreatment and continuing treatment) decreased the incidence and number of skin lesions in experimentally induced squamous cell carcinoma in mice. The level of antioxidant enzymes, such as superoxide dismutase and glutathione-S-transferase, in the skin lesions was sustained in the Withania-treated group. An antitumour effect was also demonstrated by Withania extract as a pre-treatment and continuing treatment in experimentally induced fibrosarcoma in mice. Antioxidant enzymes in the liver were supported by Withania treatment. This dose of standardised Withania extract provided approximately 8 mg/kg of total withanolides per day.[64]

Anti-inflammatory activity

Anti-inflammatory activities have been observed using in vitro models. An ethanolic extract of Withania demonstrated anti-inflammatory activity, such as suppression of lipopolysaccharide-induced cytokine and nitric oxide production in peripheral blood mononuclear cells from normal volunteers and patients with rheumatoid arthritis.[65] Withaferin A inhibited NF-kappaB in cellular models of cystic fibrosis inflammation.[66] Both glucosamine and a Withania extract demonstrated variable anti-inflammatory responses in a validated explant model of in vitro human cartilage damage.[67,68] Explants from around 50% of patients tested showed favourable effects, suggesting there is a subset of responders.

Anti-inflammatory activity has also been demonstrated in vivo, albeit using rather high doses. The body weight loss induced by adjuvant arthritis in rats was corrected by 1 g/kg Withania given orally over 15 days. Some of the inflammation and bony degenerative changes were also decreased.[69] The effect of Withania on experimentally induced granuloma in rats was compared with cortisone and phenylbutazone. Withania (in relatively high doses) was the most effective treatment at decreasing the glycosaminoglycan content of the granuloma.[70] Withania root powder (1 g/kg, oral) reduced adjuvant-induced inflammation in rats. It also attenuated the inflammation occurring during a delayed-type hypersensitivity response. No effect on the humoral immune response was observed.[71] A follow-up study using the same model and doses found Withania caused significant reductions in inflammation-induced elevations of lipid peroxides, glycoproteins and urinary bone collagen metabolites.[72]

Withania root powder (500 to 1000 mg/kg, oral doses) demonstrated marked prevention of inflammatory responses in an experimental rat model of gouty arthritis.[73] Analgesic and antipyretic activities were also found for these doses in vivo, but without the induction of gastric damage (unlike the control drug indomethacin).

CNS activity

One interesting property of Withania root is its activity on the central nervous system (CNS). Despite the fact that it is a tonic herb, it has demonstrated neuroprotective, sedative and antiepileptic effects, and is also a cognition enhancer (confirming traditional use). These effects may be partly modulated by the alkaloids (note that these are not to be confused with particular tropane alkaloids found in stramonium and belladonna, which can cause marked side effects). Withania may also have some value in addiction, but clinical trials confirming this interesting aspect of its pharmacology are lacking to date.

In high doses, alkaloids from Withania exhibited prolonged hypotensive, bradycardic and respiratory stimulant actions and had a depressant effect on higher cerebral centres.[74] Sedative effects have also been demonstrated.[75] The complex of alkaloids from Withania was only twice as active as the total extract from the root,[74,76] indicating the presence of other components with synergistic or contributive activity.

An in vitro study found a methanolic extract of Withania contains a component that interacts with the GABA-A receptor and enhances the binding of flunitrazepam (a benzodiazepine drug) to this receptor.[77] This indicates a possible sedative activity similar to that postulated for some steroid hormones and could also be related to the antiepileptic activities summarised in Table 1. Anxiolytic and antidepressant activity was demonstrated in rats after oral administration of glycowithanolides (sitoindosides VII to X and withaferin A, 20 to 50 mg/kg).[78] Oral doses of Withania extract (100 to 500 mg/kg) have also demonstrated anxiolytic effects in a rat model.[79] At the ineffective dose of 50 mg/kg, Withania still potentiated the anxiolytic action of diazepam.

Research on the neuroprotective, antidegenerative, antiepileptic and antiaddictive activities of Withania is summarised in Table 1.[80–98]

Cardiovascular activity

Withania root powder (0.75 to 1.5 g/day) added to the diet of hypercholesterolaemic rats significantly decreased total lipids, total cholesterol and triglycerides. Increases were noted for plasma high-density lipoprotein cholesterol levels, HMG-CoA reductase activity and bile acid content of bile. In these animals, administration of Withania resulted in increased bile acid, cholesterol and neutral sterol excretion. Lipid peroxidation was also decreased. An increase in HMG-CoA reductase activity, along with increased cholesterol elimination, might be due to increased hepatic bile acid production. This would lead to a decline in body cholesterol levels.[99]

A cardioprotective effect was demonstrated for various oral doses of Withania extract (ranging from 25 to 300 mg/kg) in the following rat models: ischaemia-reperfusion injury, isoprenaline-induced myonecrosis and doxorubicin-induced toxicity.[100–102] Antioxidant effects may have contributed to the activity. Cardioprotective effects were also later observed for ischaemia-reperfusion injury after oral doses (50 mg/kg of extract in rats).[103]

Other activity

Oral administration of ethanol extract of Withania (65 mg/kg) improved bone calcification and strength in calcium-deficient ovariectomised rats.[104]

Table 1 Key neurological activities of Withania and its components

Neurological activity	Model	Preparation and dosage (if relevant)	Finding	Reference
Neuroprotective	Focal cerebral ischaemia-reperfusion injury in rats	Oral doses of an aqueous ethanolic Withania extract (1 g/kg) for 15 or 30 days as a pretreatment	No effect for 15 days, but a significant reduction in the cerebral lesion for 30 days' pretreatment, with reduced oxidative stress (malondialdehyde generation)	Chaudhary et al (2003)[80]
	Streptozotocin-induced diabetes in mice	Oral doses of Withania extract (20 mg/kg) for 30 days	Reduced oxidative brain damage and corresponding improvements in memory impairment, motor dysfunction and blood glucose	Parihar et al (2004)[81]
	Huntington's disease rat model (3-nitropropionic acid-induced cerebral dysfunction)	Oral doses of Withania extract, (100 and 200 mg/kg) for 14 days	Significant improvement in behavioural, biochemical and enzymatic changes	Kumar et al (2009)[82]
Antidegenerative/ neuroprotective	Rat model of Alzheimer's disease	Oral doses of an aqueous Withania extract (20 and 50 mg/kg) containing equimolar amounts of sitoindosides VII-X and withaferin A for 14 days	Reversal of cognitive deficit and cholinergic markers induced by ibotenic acid	Bhattacharya et al (1995)[3]
	Rat model of reserpine-induced tardive dyskinesia	Oral doses of Withania extract at 50 and 100 mg/kg for 28 days	Progressive reduction in orofacial dyskinesia and cognitive dysfunction. Reversal of changes in brain superoxide dismutase and catalase suggesting an antioxidant effect	Naidu et al (2006)[83]
	Rat model of 6-hydroxy-dopamine-induced Parkinsonism	Oral doses of Withania extract (100 to 300 mg/kg)	Dose-dependent reversal of neurological and oxidative stress parameters	Ahmad et al (2005)[84]
	Rat model of haloperidol-induced tardive dyskinesia	Oral doses of withanolides (100 to 200 mg/kg)	Inhibition of dyskinetic signs and cerebral antioxidant effects	Bhattacharya et al (2002)[85]
	MPTP-induced Parkinsonism in mice	Oral doses of Withania extract (100 mg/kg)	Protective action on behavioural and antioxidant parameters	Sankar et al (2007)[86]
	Haloperidol-induced catalepsy in mice	Oral doses of Withania extract (1.7 to 8.5 mg/kg) for 1 and 7 days	Dose-dependent reduction in cataleptic scores in both acute and chronic studies that was more effective than scopolamine (1 mg/kg)	Nair et al (2008)[87]
	MPTP-induced Parkinsonism in mice	Oral doses of Withania extract (100 mg/kg) for 7 or 28 days	Improved motor function and levels of dopamine, glutathione and glutathione peroxidase	RajaSankar et al (2009)[88]
	Beta-amyloid-induced memory deficits in mice	Oral doses of withanoside IV (10 μmol/kg)	Improvements in memory deficits and neuronal loss	Kuboyama et al (2006)[89]
Antiepileptic	Pentylenetetrazole (PTZ)-induced kindling in mice	Oral doses of Withania extract (100 mg/kg)	Protection against convulsions, but with less potency than diazepam (1 mg/kg, ip)	Kulkarni et al (1996)[90]
	Epilepsy rat model (electrical stimulation)	Pretreatment with oral doses of Withania extract (100 mg/kg)	Reduction in seizure severity	Kulkarni et al (1995)[91]
	PTZ-induced seizure in mice	Pretreatment with oral doses of Withania extract (30 to 200 mg/kg) with or without pentobarbitone	Withania alone dose-dependently protected against convulsions. Withania enhanced the protective effect of pentobarbitone suggesting it may act at the barbiturate-modulating centre on the GABA-A receptor	Kulkarni et al (1993)[92]

(Continued)

Table 1 (Continued)

Neurological activity	Model	Preparation and dosage (if relevant)	Finding	Reference
	Lithium-pilocarpine-induced seizure in rats	Pretreatment with oral doses of Withania extract (50 to 200 mg/day) for 7 days	Reduced mortality and additive protective effect to benzodiazepine drugs	Kulkarni et al (1998)[93]
	PTZ-induced seizure in mice	Oral doses of Withania extract (50 to 200 mg/kg) with or without diazepam	Withania at 100 or 200 mg/kg increased seizure threshold, but not at 50 mg/kg. Co-administration of 50 mg/kg Withania with a subprotective dose of either GABA or diazepam increased seizure threshold, suggesting GABA-A receptor modulation	Kulkarni et al (2008)[94]
Antiaddictive	Morphine tolerance and dependence in mice	Oral doses of Withania extract (100 mg/kg) for 9 days	Chronic treatment with Withania inhibited the development of tolerance to the analgesic effect of morphine (p<0.01). Withania also suppressed signs of naloxone-induced withdrawal	Kulkarni et al (1997)[95]
	Morphine tolerance and dependence in mice	Pretreatment with sitoindosides VII-X and withaferin A (10 to 150 mg/kg, ip)	Reversal of morphine-induced inhibition of gastrointestinal transit time (p<0.05) and inhibition of morphine-induced analgesia (p<0.05)	Ramarao et al (1995)[96]
	Morphine tolerance and dependence in rats	Withania extract (50 or 100 mg/kg, ip) 30 min before each morphine dose for 14 days	Withania reduced the severity of withdrawal syndrome when given in conjunction with morphine, but not when given only during withdrawal. Co-treatment also prevented the reduction of spine density in the nucleus accumbens shell	Kasture et al (2009)[97]
	Ethanol dependence in rats	Oral doses of Withania extract (200 or 500 mg/kg)	Increased ethanol-induced anxiolysis and a marked reduction in ethanol withdrawal anxiety	Gupta et al (2008)[98]

Oral doses of Withania extract enhanced serum T4 (thyroxine) levels in female mice,[105] and both T3 and T4 in male mice (1.4 g/kg of aqueous extract).[106] At the same dose it also ameliorated metformin-induced hypothyroidism in a mouse model (dexamethasone-induced) of type 2 diabetes.[107] Withania extract (200 and 400 mg/kg, oral) for 5 weeks improved hyperglycaemic parameters and countered the rise in insulin resistance in a rat model of diabetes (streptozotocin-induced).[108]

Withania alkaloids are spasmolytic in vitro for intestinal, uterine, bronchial and arterial smooth muscle, with a similar mode of action to papaverine.[75]

Intraperitoneal administration of a mixture of sitoindosides VII to X and withaferin A at doses of 10 and 20 mg/kg/day for 3 weeks to rats induced a dose-related increase in superoxide dismutase, catalase and glutathione peroxidase activities in the frontal cortex and striatum. These effects were generally significant on days 14 and 21 and activity were comparable to the test antioxidant deprenyl (2 mg/kg/day).[109]

Oral administration of glycowithanolides (sitoindosides VII to X and withaferin A) in graded doses (10 to 50 mg/kg)

reduced the increase in hepatic lipid peroxidation and liver enzymes caused by iron-induced hepatotoxicity in rats.[110] Co-administration of high doses of Withania extract with lead acetate decreased the oxidative damage caused by lead in liver and kidney of mice.[111] Treatment with Withania for 48 days healed lesions in the liver and kidney induced by the fungicide carbendazim.[112] A withanolide-free fraction of Withania protected against carbon-tetrachloride-induced hepatotoxicity in rats.[27] Withania extract also protected bladder cells from cyclophosphamide-induced toxicity in mice.[113]

Withania is used externally in rural parts of India as an antidote to snakebite. A glycoprotein isolated from Withania root inhibited the hyaluronidase activity of cobra and viper venoms in vitro.[114] While the methanolic and aqueous extracts of Withania demonstrated only modest antimalarial activity in vitro,[115] oral doses of the root at 600 mg/kg significantly inhibited parasitaemia in mice inoculated with the rodent malaria parasite.[116]

Pharmacokinetics

No data available.

Clinical trials

Tonic activity

A double blind clinical trial compared the effect of milk fortified with Withania against placebo (lactose powder in milk) in 58 children aged 8 to 12 years. The dose of Withania was 2g/day over a period of 60 days. For the Withania-treated children there was a significant increase in mean corpuscular haemoglobin and serum albumin. Blood haemoglobin, serum iron, body weight and strength of hand grip also showed increases that were not statistically significant. There were no significant changes for any of these parameters in the control group. The authors concluded that Withania is a growth promoter with anti-anaemic activity in children.[9]

The effect of Withania on parameters of ageing was studied in 101 healthy male patients aged 50 to 59 years under double blind conditions. The men were given 3g of Withania root or 3g of starch per day for 1 year. Compared with the placebo control group, Withania was responsible for a significant increase in haemoglobin (p<0.001) and red blood cell count (p<0.02), and also significantly increased seated stature (p<0.05) and hair melanin content (less greying, p<0.1). It countered the decrease in nail calcium (p<0.05) and also decreased serum cholesterol (p<0.1) and erythrocyte sedimentation rate (p<0.02). About 71% of the men receiving Withania reported an improvement in sexual performance.[117]

Withania (1g/day) was administered to trainee mountaineers over 29 days in an uncontrolled trial that included a 5200m altitude gain through trekking and 6 days' training at that height, including a climb to 6400m and subsequent descent. Psychological and physiological parameters were tested at various altitudes. Withania improved sleep patterns, responsiveness, alertness and state of awareness, together with physical capabilities.[118]

Administration of Withania to 28 healthy elderly men and women (60 to 75 years of age) modestly improved muscle strength and muscle functional performance in an uncontrolled trial. The dosage was described as two 500mg capsules daily for 3 months, possibly as the dried root. (Sarcopenia is defined as muscle mass more than two standard deviations below the sex-specific young-normal mean.) Muscle strength in biceps, measured using the MRC scale, increased from 4.5 to 4.7 (statistical significance not stated). (The MRC scale, developed by the Medical Research Council in Britain, runs from 0 (no movement) to 5 (normal power).) The results for the Timed Up and Go test improved from 13.5 to 11.8 seconds. (This test measures the time taken to stand up from a standard armchair, complete a walk, turn around and sit down again.)[119] Higher doses might lead to more marked results in sarcopenia.

Using a double blind, placebo-controlled design, 130 chronically stressed patients were randomised to receive either 125mg of a proprietary Withania root and leaf extract (corresponding to about 1g of starting material) four times daily (n=30), 125mg twice daily (n=35), 250mg twice daily (n=35) or a placebo (n=30) for 60 days.[120] The dried extract was specified to contain at least 8% withanolides and up to 2% withaferin A and possessed a similar profile to root alone. A high dropout rate of 32 participants occurred and hence a per-protocol analysis was used, rather than intention-to-treat. There were significant improvements from baseline for well-being in all the Withania-treated groups (p<0.001), as assessed by a modified Hamilton Anxiety Scale (mHAM-A). By day 60, the reductions in mHAM-A were quite marked, of the order of around 70%, and the decrease was greatest in the group receiving 250mg Withania extract twice daily. For the various biochemical parameters tested, similar changes from baseline were observed for all the Withania-treated groups, again with results most marked for those receiving 250mg twice daily. For this patient group there was a significant reduction in serum cortisol (measured in the morning) of 30.5% and an increase in serum dehydroepiandrosterone sulphate of 32.5%. Significant reductions from baseline were also measured for C-reactive protein (35.2%), fasting blood glucose (6.1%), total cholesterol (13.1%), triglycerides (11.7%) and LDL-cholesterol (17.4%). HDL-cholesterol increased by 17.3% and haemoglobin by 9.1%. (See below for another clinical study on cardiovascular risk parameters.) There were small but significant reductions in pulse rate and blood pressure. Many of these parameters were also significantly different to placebo (p<0.05 to p<0.001). There were no adverse effects reported.

Male fertility

Results from two uncontrolled clinical trials from the one research group in India suggest that Withania might exert beneficial effects in male fertility. However, these results need to be confirmed in suitably designed and controlled studies. One trial investigated the impact of Withania (5g/day of root powder in milk) for 3 months in 75 infertile men.[121] While there was a 'control' group of 75 normal untreated men, their inclusion was to establish normal levels of the various parameters tested, rather than act as a control for any treatment effect from Withania. The Withania-treated group consisted of three subgroups: 25 men with relatively normal semen profile (although much poorer than the control group), 25 with low sperm concentration and 25 men with low sperm motility. The herbal treatment resulted in significant increases from baseline for sperm motility and concentration in all three subgroups (p<0.01), although values were still substantially lower than the normal controls. Compared with the start of treatment there was a significant reduction (p<0.01) in semen lipid peroxides and protein carbonyl groups for all three subgroups and an improvement (p<0.01) in semen antioxidant parameters (superoxide dismutase, catalase and glutathione). Seminal plasma levels of vitamins A, E and C and of fructose were also improved from baseline (p<0.01). Interestingly, serum luteinising hormone (LH) and testosterone increased in all subgroups (p<0.01), while a fall in follicle-stimulating hormone (FSH) and prolactin (p<0.01) was most marked in the subgroup with low sperm count.

In the other trial, 60 apparently infertile men with normal sperm parameters received the above dose of Withania for 3 months.[122] The men were again classified into three subgroups: 20 heavy smokers, 20 under psychological stress and 20 with infertility of unknown aetiology. Again the various parameters measured were assessed against an untreated healthy control group. Compared with baseline, significant improvements were noted for sperm liquefaction and concentration in all three subgroups (p<0.01 to p<0.05). Semen volume was not changed in any subgroup and sperm motility improved only in the smokers and stressed men. Morning (8 a.m.) and afternoon (4 p.m.) serum cortisol levels were significantly lower in all subgroups following Withania treatment (results were quite marked for the afternoon readings, with 36% to 48% reductions). Antioxidant parameters in semen were generally improved. LH and testosterone were significantly higher in all subgroups and FSH and prolactin were lower (except for prolactin in the subgroup with unknown aetiology).

Anxiety

In a double blind, placebo-controlled trial, 39 patients diagnosed with generalised anxiety disorder according to the ICD-10 were randomised to receive either Withania extract (1000 mg/day, probably from about 6 to 8 g of root) or placebo for 6 weeks.[123] The first follow-up was at 2 weeks, at which time the dose was lowered or increased according to the clinical response and adverse effects reported. Subsequent dose changes to individual requirements occurred at weekly intervals if needed, within the range of 500 to 2500 mg/day of extract. The average dose by the end of the trial was 1,250 mg. The primary treatment outcome was change in the HAM-A score. Patients were evaluated at week 2 (six dropouts) and week 6 (19 dropouts). The mean HAM-A score dropped in both groups, but more in the herbal group, which trended towards a significant benefit compared with placebo (at week 2 p=0.098, at week 6 p=0.062) despite the low patient numbers. There was no difference in the adverse effects reported by both groups, except for perhaps greater drowsiness for Withania.

Canada Post employees with moderate or severe anxiety of longer than 6 weeks were randomised to receive either naturopathic care (n=41) or psychotherapy (n=40) for 12 weeks.[124] Naturopathic care consisted of dietary counselling, relaxation techniques, a standard multivitamin and Withania extract (600 mg/day standardised to 1.5% withanolides). The psychotherapy group received psychotherapy, a matched relaxation technique and a placebo. Seventy-five participants were followed for 8 or more weeks. By the end of the trial, final Beck Anxiety Inventory scores had decreased by 56.5% in the Withania/naturopathy group, compared with 30.5% in the placebo/psychotherapy group. This difference in treatment effects was significant (p=0.003). Significant differences favouring Withania/naturopathy treatment were also observed for mental health, concentration, fatigue, social functioning and overall quality of life. No serious adverse reactions were observed in either group.

Arthritis

Withania (4 to 9 g/day) was beneficial for patients with acute rheumatoid arthritis (and some cases of non-articular rheumatism and chronic rheumatoid arthritis with acute exacerbations) in an uncontrolled trial conducted in the late 1960s.[125]

A 32-week randomised, double blind, placebo-controlled clinical study in 90 patients found a reduction in pain and improvement in WOMAC scores for patients with osteoarthritis of the knee treated with an Ayurvedic formulation. The formulation contained Withania, Boswellia, ginger and turmeric. (WOMAC is a measure of osteoarthritis; a reduction in this score indicates an analgesic effect.)[126]

Other activity

Withania (3 g/day for 30 days) decreased blood sugar levels from baseline in six patients with type 2 diabetes in an open label trial. The hypoglycaemic effect at around 12% reduction (p<0.01) was similar to that obtained in the control group (n=6) treated with glibenclamide. In addition, Withania appeared to increase diuresis, as evidenced by decreased serum potassium and increased urinary excretion of sodium (but not potassium). In another group of six hypercholesterolaemic patients, Withania significantly decreased (p<0.01) serum total cholesterol (by 10%), triglycerides (by 15%) and LDL- and VLDL-cholesterol compared with baseline values. Lipid profiles remained largely unchanged in the untreated control group (n=6). The mean calorie and fat intakes of the treatment groups were higher than those of the control groups.[127]

A preparation containing extracts of Withania, *Tinospora cordifolia*, *Emblica officinalis* and *Ocimum sanctum* produced good symptomatic improvement within 6 months in patients with HIV infection in an open trial. Mean viral load decreased and there was an increase in mean CD4 cell count. The strength of the extracts (and hence the dried herb equivalent) was not disclosed.[128]

In an uncontrolled pilot study, five volunteers took 6 mL of an aqueous-ethanolic Withania extract in milk twice daily for 4 days.[129] Compared with baseline, peripheral blood samples showed a marked increase in the number and activation of CD4 T cells and activity of CD56+ natural killer (NK) cells.

Withania root powder or extract has been used in preliminary and uncontrolled settings with cancer patients in India, although details are limited. An encouraging response was observed in advanced oral carcinoma (Withania extract and radiotherapy): tumours disappeared in three patients and the response in the other three patients was good. Blood glutathione levels decreased.[52,130] Treatment with Withania powder improved the life status of neuroblastoma patients (after surgery) and some laryngeal carcinoma patients (who received radiotherapy). It was also beneficial for recovery of neural deficit after encephalitis.[131]

Toxicology and other safety data

Toxicology

A single intraperitoneal injection of 1100 mg/kg of alcohol extract of Withania root in mice did not produce any deaths within 24h, but dosages beyond this level resulted in mortality (100% mortality with a 1500 mg/kg dose). The acute LD_{50} within 24h was 1260 mg/kg. Subacute toxicity studies with repeated intraperitoneal injections of this extract at a dose of 100 mg/kg for 30 days in rats did not result in any mortality. An increase in haemoglobin and a non-significant increase in red blood cell count were observed. Significant reductions in the weights of spleen, thymus and adrenals were also observed in male rats at the end of the experiment. Levels of DNA, RNA, protein and alkaline and acid phosphates within the liver were normal, but the acid phosphatase content of peripheral blood showed a significant increase from controls.[132] An LD_{50} of more than 1g/kg was measured for an aqueous extract of Withania root by oral administration in mice and rats.[133]

No toxic effects were observed in rats and mice orally administered Withania root aqueous extract (50 to 1000mg/kg/day) for up to 4 weeks[133] or in rats orally administered an undefined Withania root extract at 100mg/kg/day for 180 days.[134] Catecholamine levels increased in cardiac and aortic tissues and decreased in the adrenal glands when this extract (100 and 200mg/kg/day) was administered orally for 30 days.[134]

Oral administration of Withania whole plant extract (200mg/kg/day) for 7 months had no significant effect on mortality in mice.[60] Histopathological lesions were observed in the liver, lungs and kidneys of mice fed very high doses of Withania whole plant (20% w/w of diet, about 5g/rat/day) for 10 to 14 days.[135] However, organ histopathology was not observed when rats were orally administered a Withania whole plant decoction at 250mg/kg/day for 4 weeks. Adrenal weight decreased and liver and lung weights increased. Also no toxic effects were observed when the decoction was orally administered at a dose of 100mg/kg/day for 8 months.[22]

Male rats orally administered a methanol extract of Withania root at dose of 3g/kg dry extract 33:1 (much greater than the human therapeutic dose) for 7 days failed to ejaculate during the treatment period and for at least 7 days after and demonstrated reduced sexual performance, with sexual vigour and behaviour indicative of penile erectile dysfunction and reduced libido. There was no significant effect on serum liver enzymes, urea nitrogen, seminal fluid pH or the gross appearance and weight of the reproductive organs, liver, kidneys or adrenal glands. It was concluded that the effects were not due to changes in testosterone levels or toxicity.[136] In contrast, healthy men (aged 50 to 59 years) prescribed therapeutic doses of Withania (3g/day) for 1 year in a randomised, double blind, placebo-controlled clinical trial reported an increase in their sexual performance.[117]

Contraindications

None known.

Special warnings and precautions

None required.

Interactions

Withania extract may enhance the effect of benzodiazepines. Oral administration of Withania extract (100mg/kg) to rats reduced the effective dose of benzodiazepines, while providing a protective effect in experimentally induced epilepsy.[137] Withania enhanced the binding of a benzodiazepine to the GABA-A receptor in vitro.[77] However, this interaction is speculative and the doses used in the experimental model were relatively high.

Use in pregnancy and lactation

Category B1 – no increase in frequency of malformation or other harmful effects on the fetus from limited use in women. No evidence of increased fetal damage in animal studies.

A review of traditional Ayurvedic literature noted that Withania (part and dose undefined) was listed as an abortifacient in three of the five sources checked. However, the definition of abortifacient was very broad and included emmenagogue, ecbolic (uterine contractor) and 'antimetabolite'.[138] A 1952 publication noted that Withania root powder was used in Casablanca for abortion.[139] In West Pakistan, Withania root is used to cause abortion. It has also been employed to tone the uterus in women who habitually miscarry and to remove retained placenta.[140] In contrast, another traditional source notes its use as a nutrient and tonic for pregnant women[5] and the animal study below would suggest that it is safe during pregnancy. The confusion over safety in pregnancy from traditional use may arise from the use of different plant parts. Withania leaf has a very different phytochemical content compared with the root.[141,142]

Rats orally administered Withania whole plant decoction (100mg/kg/day) for 8 months had comparable litter sizes and frequency of pregnancy to controls, but produced progeny with higher average body weight (indicating perhaps tonic activity).[22] Withania root powder (25mg/day for 10 days) administered orally to male and female mice that were later paired for mating resulted in decreased litter size and produced some infertility.[140] (This indicates a potential antifertility effect but does not imply harm during pregnancy.)

Withania use is compatible with breastfeeding. Withania is used to promote lactation in Ayurvedic medicine and the traditional medicine of South-East Asia.[5,143] One teaspoon (0.5g) of Withania powder may be given twice daily with milk for insufficient lactation.[144]

Withania improved milk yield and quality in lactating cows.[145,146] Rats orally administered Withania whole plant decoction (100mg/kg/day) throughout their lactation period produced offspring with higher average body weight.[22]

Effects on ability to drive and use machines

No negative influence is expected at the recommended dosage.

Side effects

High doses have been reported to cause gastrointestinal upset, diarrhoea and vomiting,[147] which may be due to the steroidal saponin content. Few side effects have been noted in clinical trials.

A 32-year-old woman developed symptoms of thyrotoxicosis (weight loss, palpitations, confusion) while taking capsules containing Withania for symptoms of chronic fatigue.[148] She was reportedly not taking any other treatments and her thyroid-stimulating hormone (TSH) was tested at <0.01mU/L and serum thyroxine at 33.9pmol/L. All symptoms and abnormal laboratory values resolved spontaneously after discontinuing the herb. The reported dose was 500 mg/day of Withania, possibly of a dry extract. This case report might testify to the thyroid-stimulating properties of Withania observed in animal studies.

Overdosage

No incidents found in published literature.

Safety in children

Adverse events were not reported in a randomised, double blind, placebo-controlled trial in which healthy children were orally administered 2 g/day of Withania for 60 days.[9] Withania is traditionally used in Ayurvedic medicine to treat failure to thrive in children.[5]

Regulatory status in selected countries

Withania was official in the second edition of the *Indian Pharmacopoeia* (1966) but was not included in the third edition (1985).

Withania is not covered by a Commission E monograph and is not on the UK General Sale List.

Withania does not have GRAS status. However, it is freely available as a 'dietary supplement' in the USA under DSHEA legislation (1994 Dietary Supplement Health and Education Act).

Withania is not included in Part 4 of Schedule 4 of the Therapeutic Goods Act Regulations of Australia and is freely available for sale.

References

1. Thakur RS, Puri HS, Husain A. *Major Medicinal Plants of India*. Lucknow: Central Institute of Medicinal and Aromatic Plants; 1989. pp. 531–535.
2. Atal CK, Schwarting AE. *Econ Bot*. 1961;15(3):256–263.
3. Bhattacharya SK, Kumar A, Ghosal S. *Phytother Res*. 1995;9(2):110–113.
4. Miller AG, Morris M. *Plants of Dhofar*. The Office of the Adviser for Conservation of the Environment, Diwan of Royal Court Sultanate of Oman; 1988. p. 274.
5. Kapoor LD. CRC *Handbook of Ayurvedic Medicinal Plants*. Boca Raton: CRC Press; 1990. pp. 337–338.
6. American Herbal Pharmacopeia *Ashwagandha Root – Withania somnifera: Analytical, Quality Control, and Therapeutic Monograph*. Santa Cruz: American Herbal Pharmacopoeia; 2000.
7. Wagner H, Norr H, Winterhoff H. *Phytomedicine*. 1994;1:63–76.
8. Atal CK, Gupta OP, Raghunathan K, et al. *Pharmacognosy and Phytochemistry of Withania Somnifera (Linn) Dunal (Ashwagandha)*. New Delhi: Central Council for Research in Indian Medicine and Homoeopathy; 1975. pp. 47–53.
9. Venkataraghavan S, Seshadri C, Sundaresan TP, et al. *J Res Ayu Sid*. 1980;1:370–385.
10. Archana R, Namasivayam A. *J Ethnopharmacol*. 1999;64(1):91–93.
11. Dadkar VN, Ranadive NU, Dhar HL. *Ind J Clin Biochem*. 1987;2:101–108.
12. Jain S, Shukla SD, Sharma K, et al. *Phytother Res*. 2001;15(6):544–548.
13. Saksena AK, Singh SP, Dixit KS, et al. *Planta Med*. 1989;55:95.
14. Singh A, Saxena E, Bhutani KK. *Phytother Res*. 2000;14(2):122–125.
15. Roy U, Mukhopadhyay S, Poddar MK, et al. *International Seminar – Traditional Medicine*. Calcutta: November 7–9, 1992. p. 141.
16. Bhatnagar M, Sisodia SS, Bhatnagar R. *Ann N Y Acad Sci*. 2005;1056:261–278.
17. Thatte UM, Chhabria SN, Karandikar SM, et al. *J Postgrad Med*. 1987;33(4):185–188.
18. Davis L, Kuttan G. *Immunopharmacol Immunotoxicol*. 1999;21(4):695–703.
19. Gupta YK, Sharma SS, Rai K, et al. *Indian J Physiol Pharmacol*. 2001;45(2):253–257.
20. Khan B, Ahmad SF, Bani S, et al. *Int Immunopharmacol*. 2006;6(9):1394–1403.
21. Bani S, Gautam M, Sheikh FA, et al. *J Ethnopharmacol*. 2006;107(1):107–115.
22. Sharma S, Dahanukar S, Karandikar SM. *Indian Drugs*. 1986;23(3):133–139.
23. Singh N, Nath R, Lata A, et al. *Int J Crude Drug Res*. 1982;20(1):29–35.
24. Grandhi A, Mujumdar AM, Patwardhan B. *J Ethnopharmacol*. 1994;44(3):131–135.
25. Bhattacharya SK, Muruganandam AV. *Pharmacol Biochem Behav*. 2003;75(3):547–555.
26. Bhattacharya A, Ghosal S, Bhattacharya SK. *J Ethnopharmacol*. 2001;74(1):1–6.
27. Singh B, Chandan BK, Gupta DK. *Phytother Res*. 2003;17(5):531–536.
28. Singh B, Saxena AK, Chandan BK, et al. *Phytother Res*. 2001;15(4):311–318.
29. Ghosal S, Lal J, Srivastava R, et al. *Phytother Res*. 1989;3(5):201–206.
30. Bhattacharya SK, Goel RK, Kaur R, et al. *Phytother Res*. 1987;1(1):32–37.
31. Kuttan G. *Indian J Exp Biol*. 1996;34(9):854–856.
32. Teixeira ST, Valadares MC, Goncalves SA, et al. *Int Immunopharmacol*. 2006;6(10):1535–1542.
33. Gautam M, Diwanay SS, Gairola S, et al. *Int Immunopharmacol*. 2004;4(6):841–849.
34. Owais M, Sharad KS, Shehbaz A, et al. *Phytomedicine*. 2005;12(3):229–235.
35. Dhuley JN. *J Ethnopharmacol*. 1997;58(1):15–20.
36. Ziauddin M, Phansalkar N, Patki P, et al. *J Ethnopharmacol*. 1996;50(2):69–76.
37. Menssen HG, Stapel G. *Planta Med*. 1973;24(1):8–12.
38. Bähr V, Hänsel R. *Planta Med*. 1982;44(1):32–33.
39. Malik F, Singh J, Khajuria A, et al. *Life Sci*. 2007;80(16):1525–1538.
40. Winters M. *Altern Med Rev*. 2006;11(4):269–277.
41. Oh JH, Lee TJ, Kim SH, et al. *Apoptosis*. 2008;13(12):1494–1504.
42. Mandal C, Dutta A, Mallick A, et al. *Apoptosis*. 2008;13(12):1450–1464.
43. Malik F, Kumar A, Bhushan S, et al. *Apoptosis*. 2007;12(11):2115–2133.
44. Srinivasan S, Ranga RS, Burikhanov R, et al. *Cancer Res*. 2007;67(1):246–253.
45. Stan SD, Hahm ER, Warin R, et al. *Cancer Res*. 2008;68(18):7661–7669.
46. Panjamurthy K, Manoharan S, Menon VP, et al. *J Biochem Mol Toxicol*. 2008;22(4):251–258.
47. Shohat B, Gitter S, Lavie D. *Int J Cancer*. 1970;5(2):244–252.
48. Shohat B, Joshua H. *Int J Cancer*. 1971;8(3):487–496.
49. Chowdhury K, Neogy RK. *Biochem Pharmacol*. 1975;24:919–920.
50. Chakraborti SK, De BK, Bandyopadhyay T. *Experientia*. 1974;30(8):852–853.
51. Shohat B, Ben-Bassat M, Shaltiel A, et al. *Cancer Lett*. 1976;2(2):63–70.
52. Devi PU. *Indian J Exp Biol*. 1996;34(10):927–932.
53. Devi PU, Akagi K, Ostapenko V, et al. *Int J Radiat Biol*. 1996;69(2):193–197.
54. Shohat B, Shaltiel A, Ben-Bassat M, et al. *Cancer Lett*. 1976;2(2):71–77.

55. Mohan R, Hammers HJ, Bargagna-Mohan P, et al. *Angiogenesis*. 2004;7(2):115–122.

56. Shohat B, Kirson I, Lavie D. *Biomedicine*. 1978;28(1):18–24.

57. Malik F, Kumar A, Bhushan S, et al. *Eur J Cancer*. 2009;45(8):1494–1509.

58. Sumantran VN, Boddul S, Koppikar SJ, et al. *Phytother Res*. 2007;21(5):496–499.

59. Devi PU, Sharada AC, Solomon FE. *Indian J Exp Biol*. 1993;31(7):607–611.

60. Singh N, Singh SP, Nath R, et al. *Int J Crude Drug Res*. 1986;24(2):90–100.

61. Mulabagal V, Subbaraju GV, Rao CV, et al. *Phytother Res*. 2009;23(7):987–992.

62. Senthilnathan P, Padmavathi R, Magesh V, et al. *Mol Cell Biochem*. 2006;292 (1–2):13–17.

63. Senthilnathan P, Padmavathi R, Magesh V, et al. *Cancer Sci*. 2006;97(7):658–664.

64. Prakash J, Gupta SK, Kochupillai V, et al. *Phytother Res*. 2001;15(3):240–244.

65. Singh D, Aggarwal A, Maurya R, et al. *Phytother Res*. 2007;21(10):905–913.

66. Maitra R, Porter MA, Huang S, et al. *J Inflamm (Lond)*. 2009;6(1):15.

67. Sumantran VN, Chandwaskar R, Joshi AK, et al. *Phytother Res*. 2008;22(10):1342–1348.

68. Sumantran VN, Kulkarni A, Boddul S, et al. *J Biosci*. 2007;32(2):299–307.

69. Begum VH, Sadique J. *Indian J Exp Biol*. 1988;26(11):877–882.

70. Begum VH, Sadique J. *Biochem Med Metab Biol*. 1987;38(3):272–277.

71. Rasool M, Varalakshmi P. *Vascul Pharmacol*. 2006;44(6):406–410.

72. Rasool M, Varalakshmi P. *Fundam Clin Pharmacol*. 2007;21(2):157–164.

73. Rasool M, Varalakshmi P. *Chem Biol Interact*. 2006;164(3):174–180.

74. Malhotra CL, Das PK, Dhalla NS, et al. *Indian J Med Res*. 1961;49:448–460.

75. Malhotra CL, Mehta VL, Prasad K, et al. *Indian J Physiol Pharmacol*. 1965;9:9–15.

76. Fugner A. *Arzneimittelforschung*. 1973;23(7):932–935.

77. Mehta AK, Binkley P, Gandhi SS, et al. *Indian J Med Res*. 1991;94:312–315.

78. Bhattacharya SK, Bhattacharya A, Sairam K, et al. *Phytomedicine*. 2000;7(6):463–469.

79. Gupta GL, Rana AC. *Indian J Physiol Pharmacol*. 2007;51(4):345–353.

80. Chaudhary G, Jagannathan NR, Gupta YK. *Clin Exp Pharmacol Physiol*. 2003;30(5–6):399–404.

81. Parihar MS, Chaudhary M, Shetty R, et al. *J Clin Neurosci*. 2004;11(4):397–402.

82. Kumar P, Kumar A. *J Med Food*. 2009;12(3):591–600.

83. Naidu PS, Singh A, Kulkarni SK. *Phytother Res*. 2006;20(2):140–146.

84. Ahmad M, Saleem S, Ahmad AS, et al. *Hum Exp Toxicol*. 2005;24(3):137–147.

85. Bhattacharya SK, Bhattacharya D, Sairam K, et al. *Phytomedicine*. 2002;9(2):167–170.

86. Sankar SR, Manivasagam T, Krishnamurti A, et al. *Cell Mol Biol Lett*. 2007;12(4):473–481.

87. Nair V, Arjuman A, Gopalakrishna HN, et al. *Phytother Res*. 2008;22(2):243–246.

88. RajaSankar S, Manivasagam T, Sankar V, et al. *J Ethnopharmacol*. 2009;125(3):369–373.

89. Kuboyama T, Tohda C, Komatsu K. *Eur J Neurosci*. 2006;23(6):1417–1426.

90. Kulkarni SK, George B. *Phytother Res*. 1996;10(5):447–449.

91. Kulkarni SK, George B. *Indian Drugs*. 1995;32(1):37–49.

92. Kulkarni SK, Sharma A, Verma A, et al. *Indian Drugs*. 1993;30(7):305–312.

93. Kulkarni SK, George B, Mathur R. *Indian Drugs*. 1998;35(4):208–215.

94. Kulkarni SK, Akula KK, Dhir A. *Indian J Exp Biol*. 2008;46(6):465–469.

95. Kulkarni SK, Ninan J. *J Ethnopharmacol*. 1997;57(3):213–217.

96. Ramarao P, Rao KT, Srivastava RS, et al. *Phytother Res*. 1995;9(1):66–68.

97. Kasture S, Vinci S, Ibba F, et al. *Neurotox Res*. 2009;16(4):343–355.

98. Gupta GL, Rana AC. *Indian J Exp Biol*. 2008;46(6):470–475.

99. Visavadiya NP, Narasimhacharya AV. *Phytomedicine*. 2007;14(2–3):136–142.

100. Mohanty I, Gupta SK, Talwar KK, et al. *Mol Cell Biochem*. 2004;260(1–2):39–47.

101. Mohanty I, Arya DS, Dinda A, et al. *Basic Clin Pharmacol Toxicol*. 2004;94(4):184–190.

102. Hamza A, Amin A, Daoud S. *Cell Biol Toxicol*. 2008;24(1):63–73.

103. Mohanty IR, Arya DS, Gupta SK. *Clin Nutr*. 2008;27(4):635–642.

104. Nagareddy PR, Lakshmana M. *J Pharm Pharmacol*. 2006;58(4):513–519.

105. Panda S, Kar A. *J Ethnopharmacol*. 1999;67(2):233–239.

106. Panda S, Kar A. *J Pharm Pharmacol*. 1998;50(9):1065–1068.

107. Jatwa R, Kar A. *Phytother Res*. 2009;23(8):1140–1145.

108. Anwer T, Sharma M, Pillai KK, et al. *Basic Clin Pharmacol Toxicol*. 2008;102(4):498–503.

109. Bhattacharya SK, Satyan KS, Ghosal S. *Indian J Exp Biol*. 1997;35(3):236–239.

110. Bhattacharya A, Ramanathan M, Ghosal S, et al. *Phytother Res*. 2000;14(7):568–570.

111. Chaurasia SS, Panda S, Kar A. *Pharmacol Res*. 2000;41(6):663–666.

112. Akbarsha MA, Vijendrakumar S, Kadalmani B, et al. *Phytomedicine*. 2000;7(6):499–507.

113. Davis L, Kuttan G. *Cancer Lett*. 2000;148(1):9–17.

114. Machiah DK, Girish KS, Gowda TV. *Comp Biochem Physiol C Toxicol Pharmacol*. 2006;143(2):158–161.

115. Kirira PG, Rukunga GM, Wanyonyi AW, et al. *J Ethnopharmacol*. 2006;106(3):403–407.

116. Dikasso D, Makonnen E, Debella A, et al. *Ethiop Med J*. 2006;44(3):279–285.

117. Kuppurajan K, Rajagopalan SS, Sitaraman R, et al. *J Res Ayu Sid*. 1980;1:247–258.

118. Roy AS, Acharya SB, De AK, et al. *International Seminar – Traditional Medicine*. Calcutta: November 7–9, 1992. p. 161.

119. Mishra S, Ravi B. *Neuromuscul Disord*. 2006;16(suppl 1):S176–S177. Abstract M-P-16.12.

120. Auddy B, Hazra J, Mitra A, et al. *J Am Nutraceutical Assoc*. 2008;11(1):50–56.

121. Ahmad MK, Mahdi AA, Shukla KK, et al. *Fertil Steril*. 2009 [Epub ahead of print].

122. Mahdi AA, Shukla KK, Ahmad MK, et al. *Evid Based Complement Alternat Med*. 2011. Article ID 576962, 9 pages.

123. Andrade C, Aswath A, Chaturvedi SK, et al. *Indian J Psychiatry*. 2000;42(3):295–301.

124. Cooley K, Szczurko O, Perri D, et al. *PLoS One*. 2009;4(8):e6628.

125. Bector NP, Puri AS, Sharma D. *Indian J Med Res*. 1969;56:1581–1583.

126. Chopra A, Lavin P, Patwardhan B, et al. *J Clin Rheumatol*. 2004;10(5):236–245.

127. Andallu B, Radhika B. *Indian J Exp Biol*. 2000;38:607–609.

128. Usha PR, Naidu MU, Raju YS. *Drugs R D*. 2003;4(2):103–109.

129. Mikolai J, Erlandsen A, Murison A, et al. *J Altern Complement Med*. 2009;15(4):423–430.

130. The Hindu Business Line 8/11/1994. In: Premila MS: *Ayurvedic Herbs: A Clinical Guide to the Healing Plants of Traditional Indian Medicine*. New York: Haworth Press; 2006. pp. 326–327.

131. Singh N. *Curr Med Pract*. 1981;25:50.

132. Sharada AC, Soloman FE, Devi PU. *Int J Pharmacog*. 1993;31(3):205–212.

133. Rege NN, Thatte UM, Dahanukar SA. *Phytother Res*. 1999;13(4):275–291.

134. Dhuley JN. *J Ethnopharmacol*. 2000;70(1):57–63.

135. Arseculeratne SN, Gunatilaka AA, Panabokke RG. *J Ethnopharmacol*. 1985;13(3):323–335.

136. Ilayperuma I, Ratnasooriya WD, Weerasooriya TR. *Asian J Androl*. 2002;4(4):295–298.

137. Kulkarni SK, George B, Mathur R. *Phytother Res*. 1998;12(6):451–453.

138. Casey RCD. *Indian J Med Sci*. 1960;14:590–600.

139. Merzouki A, Ed-derfoufi F, Molero Mesa J. *J Ethnopharmacol*. 2000;73(3):501–503.

140. Garg LC, Parasar GC. *Planta Med*. 1965;13:46–47.

141. Singh S, Kumar S. *Withania somnifera: The Indian Ginseng Ashwagandha*. Lucknow: Central Institute of Medicinal and Aromatic Plants (CIMAP); 1998. pp. 131–177.

142. Lehmann R, Penman K. *Information on File*. Australia: MediHerb Research Laboratory; 2003.

143. World Health Organization. *The Use of Traditional Medicine in Primary Health Care: A Manual for Health Workers in South-East Asia.* New Delhi: WHO Regional Office for South-East Asia, New Delhi, WHO Regional Office for South-East Asia; 1990. pp. 96–97.

144. World Health Organization. *The Use of Traditional Medicine in Primary Health Care: A Manual for Health Workers in South-East Asia.* : WHO Regional Office for South-East Asia, New Delhi, WHO Regional Office for South-East Asia; 1990. p. 132.

145. Shelukar PS, Dakshinkar NP, Sarode DB, et al. *Indian Vet J.* 2000;77(7):605–607.

146. Shelukar PS, Dakshinkar NP, Sarode DB. *Indian Vet J.* 2001;78(3):249–250.

147. Chandha E, ed. *The Wealth of India: A Dictionary of Indian Raw Materials and Industrial Products,* vol. 10. Council of Scientific and Industrial Research, New Delhi, 1976. Cited in American Herbal Pharmacopoeia. *Ashwagandha Root – Withania somnifera: Analytical, Quality Control, and Therapeutic Monograph.* Santa Cruz: American Herbal Pharmacopeia; April 2000.

148. Van der Hooft CS, Hoekstra A, Wintr A, et al. *Ned Tijdschr Geneeskd.* 2005;149(47):2637–2638.

Appendix A: Glossary of herbal actions

Adaptogenic	A substance that increases the body's resistance or adaptation to physical, environmental, emotional or biological stressors and promotes normal physiological function.
Adrenal tonic or restorative	A substance that improves the tone, histology and function of the adrenal glands (especially the cortex).
Alterative	*See Depurative*
Analgesic	A substance that relieves pain.
Anaphrodisiac	A substance that reduces libido (usually in males).
Anodyne	*See Analgesic*
Antacid	A substance that counteracts or neutralises acidity in the gastrointestinal tract.
Anthelmintic	A substance that kills or assists in the expulsion of intestinal worms.
Antiallergic	A substance that tones down the allergic response, often by stabilising mast cells.
Antiandrogenic	A substance that inhibits or modifies the action of androgens (male sex hormones).
Antianaemic	A substance that prevents or corrects anaemia (that is a reduction in the number of circulating red blood cells or in the quantity of haemoglobin).
Antiarrhythmic	A substance that prevents or is effective against arrhythmias (that is any variation from the normal rhythm or rate of the heart beat).
Antiasthmatic	A substance that prevents or relieves asthma attacks.
Antibacterial	A substance that inhibits the growth of bacteria (bacteriostatic) or destroys bacteria (bactericidal).
Anticariogenic	A substance that reduces the incidence of dental caries (tooth decay).
Anticatarrhal	A substance that reduces the formation of catarrh or phlegm (pathological mucus secretion).
Anticoagulant	A substance that reduces the rate of blood coagulation.
Anticonvulsant	A substance that tends to prevent or arrest seizures (convulsions).
Antidepressant	A substance that alleviates depression.
Antidiabetic (see also *Hypoglycaemic*)	A substance that alleviates diabetes or the effects of diabetes.

Antidiarrhoeal	A substance that alleviates diarrhoea.
Antiecchymotic	A substance that prevents or alleviates bruising.
Anti-oedematous	A substance that prevents or alleviates oedema (fluid retention).
Antiemetic	A substance that reduces nausea and vomiting.
Antifibrotic	A substance that reduces the excessive formulation of fibrous connective tissue (e.g. in scleroderma).
Antifungal	A substance that inhibits the growth of or destroys fungi.
Antihaemorrhagic	A substance that reduces or stops bleeding when taken internally.
Antihyperhidrotic	A substance that reduces excessive sweating.
Anti-inflammatory (see also *Antiallergic, Antirheumatic, Anti-oedematous, Immune depressant*)	A substance that reduces inflammation.
Antilithic	A substance that reduces the formation of calculi (stones) in the urinary tract.
Antimicrobial (see also *Antibacterial, Antifungal, Antiparasitic, Antiviral, Antiprotozoal*)	A substance that inhibits the growth of or destroys micro-organisms.
Antiobesity	A substance that assists in the reduction of body weight.
Antioxidant	A substance that protects against oxidation and free radical damage.
Anti-PAF	A substance that inhibits the activity of platelet-activating factor (PAF). (PAF is a potent platelet aggregating agent and inducer of systemic anaphylactic symptoms.)
Antiparasitic	A substance that inhibits the activity of or kills parasites, especially protozoa.
Antiplatelet	A substance that reduces platelet aggregation (and hence prolongs bleeding time and may prevent thrombus formation).
Antiprostatic	A substance that reduces symptoms from the prostate gland.
Antiprotozoal	A substance that kills protozoa or inhibits their growth and activity.
Antipruritic	A substance that relieves or prevents itching.
Antipsoriatic	A substance that tends to relieve the symptoms of psoriasis.
Antipyretic	A substance that reduces or prevents fever.
Antirheumatic	A substance that prevents or relieves rheumatic symptoms.
Antiseptic	See *Antimicrobial*
Antispasmodic	See *Spasmolytic*
Antithyroid	A substance that reduces the activity of the thyroid gland.
Antitumour	A substance that has activity against a malignant tumour.
Antitussive	A substance that reduces the amount or severity of coughing.
Antiulcer	A substance that prevents or relieves ulceration (usually in the gastrointestinal tract).
Antiuraemic	A substance that reduces the levels of urea in the blood (especially in kidney failure).
Antiviral	A substance that inhibits the growth of or destroys viruses.
Anxiolytic	A substance that alleviates anxiety.

Aperient	A mild laxative
Aphrodisiac	A substance that stimulates sexual desire or libido.
Aromatic digestive	A substance that is generally pleasant tasting and/or smelling that assists digestion. They are warming to the body and are also known as warming digestive tonics.
Astringent	A substance that causes constriction of mucous membranes and exposed tissues, usually by precipitating proteins. This has the effect of producing a barrier on the mucus or exposed surfaces.
Bitter tonic (also known as a *Bitter*, see also *Digestive stimulant*, *Gastric stimulant*)	A substance that is bitter tasting and stimulates the upper gastrointestinal tract via the bitter-sensitive taste buds of the mouth and/or by direct interaction with gastrointestinal tissue. Bitters have a promoting effect on all components of upper digestive function, namely the stomach, liver and pancreas. In addition to appetite and digestion they improve general health and immune function.
Bladder tonic	A substance that improves the tone and function of the bladder and reduces post-void residual urine.
Bronchospasmolytic	A substance that reduces spasm in the lower respiratory tract.
Cancer preventative (see also *Antitumour*)	A substance that prevents the incidence of cancer.
Cardioprotective	A substance that protects cardiac tissue against hypoxia (oxygen deficiency) and decreases the risk of heart damage.
Cardiotonic	A substance that improves the force of contraction of the heart.
Carminative	A substance that relieves flatulence and soothes intestinal spasm and pain, usually by relaxing intestinal muscle and sphincters. They are also added to herbal formulations to ease the intestinal spasm or pain that may be caused by laxative herbs.
Cathartic	A substance that assists or induces evacuation of the bowel and has a strong laxative action.
Cholagogue	A substance that increases the release of stored bile from the gallbladder.
Choleretic	A substance that increases the production of bile by the liver.
Circulatory stimulant	A substance that improves blood flow through peripheral body tissues. Circulatory stimulants are warming and they support vitality in the body tissues.
CNS stimulant	A substance that stimulates the central nervous system, increasing alertness.
Cognition enhancing	A substance that facilitates learning, memory or concentration.
Collagen stabilising	A substance that stabilises collagen and protects collagen from degradation. Connective tissue tone is thereby improved.
Counter-irritant	A substance that produces a superficial inflammation of the skin in order to relieve a deeper inflammation (e.g. in muscles, joints and ligaments).
Demulcent	A substance that has a soothing effect on mucous membranes (e.g. within the respiratory, digestive and urinary tracts).
Depurative	A substance that improves detoxification and aids elimination to reduce the accumulation of metabolic waste products within the body. They were formerly known as alteratives or blood purifiers and are largely used to treat chronic skin and musculoskeletal disorders.
Diaphoretic	A substance that controls a fever often by promoting sweating. They are also known as sudorifics.
Diuretic	A substance that increases urinary output.
Diuretic depurative	A substance that assists detoxification of the body by the kidneys.
Dopaminergic agonist	A substance that binds to and activates dopamine receptors.
Emetic	A substance that causes vomiting.
Emmenagogue	A substance that initiates and promotes the menstrual flow. Several of these herbs are also regarded as abortifacients.

Emollient	A substance used to soothe, soften or protect skin.
Expectorant	A substance that improves the clearing of excess mucus from the lungs by either altering the production and viscosity of mucus or improving the cough reflex.
Febrifuge	See *Antipyretic*
Female tonic	A substance that improves the tone, vigour and function of the female reproductive system.
Galactagogue	A substance that increases breast milk production.
Gastric stimulant (see also *Bitter tonic* and *Digestive stimulant*)	A substance that stimulates the function of the stomach.
General body tonic	See *Tonic*
Haemostatic	See *Styptic*
Healing promoter	A substance that promotes the healing of tissue.
Hepatic (*Hepatic tonic*)	A substance that improves the tone, vigour and function of the liver. This term is vague and other more specific terms are preferable.
Hepatoprotective	A substance that protects the hepatocytes (liver cells) against toxic damage.
Hepatotrophorestorative	A substance that restores the integrity of liver tissue.
Hypnotic	A substance that induces drowsiness and sleep. They are also known as soporifics.
Hypocholesterolaemic (see also *Hypolipidaemic*)	A substance that reduces the level of cholesterol in the blood.
Hypoglycaemic	A substance that reduces the level of glucose in the blood.
Hypolipidaemic	A substance that reduces the lipid level (cholesterol and triglycerides) of blood.
Hypotensive (see also *Peripheral vasodilator*)	A substance that reduces blood pressure.
Immune depressant	A substance that reduces immune function and is used particularly where part of the immune system is overactive.
Immune enhancing	A substance that enhances immune function.
Immune modulating	A substance that modulates and balances the activity of the immune system.
Laxative	A substance that facilitates evacuation of the bowel.
Local anaesthetic	A substance that removes sensation or pain when applied locally.
Lymphatic	A substance that assists detoxification by its effect on lymphatic tissue and often also improves immune function. They are often used when the lymph glands (nodes) are enlarged or tender.
Male tonic	A substance that improves the tone, vigour and function of the male reproductive system.
Metabolic stimulant	A substance that boosts basal metabolic rate.
Mucolytic	A substance that helps break up and disperse sticky mucus in the respiratory tract.
Mucoprotective	A substance that protects the mucous membranes, especially in the context of the gastric lining.
Mucous membrane tonic	A substance that improves the tone, vigour and function of the mucous membranes (particularly of the respiratory tract).
Mucous membrane trophorestorative	A substance that restores the integrity of mucous membranes (e.g. in the respiratory and digestive tracts).
Nervine tonic (*Nervine*)	A substance that improves the tone, vigour and function of the nervous system. Nervine tonics relax and energise the nervous system.

Neuroprotective	A substance that helps prevent damage to the brain or spinal cord from ischaemia, stroke, convulsions or trauma.
Nootropic	See *Cognition enhancing*
Nutrient	A substance that has a nutritive effect in the body.
Orexigenic	A substance that stimulates appetite.
Oestrogen modulating	In the context of use of herbs, a substance that acts by subtle, poorly understood mechanisms to promote oestrogen production and/or effects in the body. The activity may involve interaction with secondary oestrogen receptors such as those in the hypothalamus. They are used to balance hormonal effects, promote fertility and alleviate menopausal symptoms.
Ovarian tonic	A substance that improves the tone, vigour and function of the ovaries.
Oxytocic	A substance that causes contraction of the uterine muscle in association with giving birth.
Parturifacient	A substance that induces labour and assists in the efficient delivery of the fetus and placenta.
Partus preparatory	A substance taken in preparation for labour and childbirth. Treatment usually begins in the second trimester.
Peripheral vasodilator	A substance that dilates or widens the peripheral blood vessels and thereby improves circulation to peripheral tissues and may assist in reducing blood pressure.
Progesterogenic	A substance that promotes the effect or production of progesterone.
Prolactin inhibitor	A substance that inhibits the secretion of prolactin.
Pungent	A hot-tasting substance that acts upon a common group of nerve cell receptors having the effect of warming the body and improving digestion and circulation.
Refrigerant	A substance that has cooling properties, particularly when applied to the skin.
Rubefacient	See *Counter-irritant*. Rubefacients are mild counter-irritants.
Sedative (mild)	A substance that reduces activity, particularly in the nervous system, and decreases nervous tension. It may alleviate pain, anxiety or spasm and induce sleep.
Sexual tonic	A substance that improves the tone, vigour and function of the sexual organs.
Sialagogue	A substance that increases the secretion of the salivary glands.
Skeletal muscle relaxant	A substance that relaxes skeletal muscle tone.
Spasmolytic	A substance that reduces or relieves smooth muscle spasm (involuntary contractions).
Stimulant	A substance that heightens the function of an organ or system: for example, a central nervous stimulant increases the activity of the central nervous system, particularly behavioural alertness, agitation, or excitation. The term has a second, more subtle, meaning derived from the Thomsonian system (an early branch of herbal therapy in the USA): a substance capable of increasing the action or energy of the living body.
Styptic	A substance that stops bleeding when applied locally.
Thymoleptic (see also *Antidepressant*)	A substance that elevates mood.
Thyroid stimulant	A substance that enhances the activity of the thyroid gland.
Tissue perfusion enhancing	A substance that enhances the flow of nutrients into a tissue.
Tonic (also known as *General body tonic*; see also other specific body tonics)	A substance that improves the tone, vigour and function of the whole body. Tonics can give a boost in energy.
Trophorestorative	A substance that has a healing and restorative action on a specific organ or tissue.
TSH antagonist	A substance that blocks the activity of TSH (thyroid-stimulating hormone).

Urinary antiseptic	A substance that inhibits the growth of or destroys micro-organisms within the urinary tract.
Urinary demulcent	A substance that has a soothing effect on mucous membranes of the urinary tract.
Uterine antihaemorrhagic	A substance that reduces the menstrual flow when taken internally.
Uterine sedative	A substance that reduces the activity of the uterine muscle.
Uterine tonic	A substance that increases the tone of the uterine muscle.
Vasoconstrictor	A substance that constricts or narrows the blood vessels.
Vasodilator	A substance that dilates or widens the blood vessels.
Vasoprotective	A substance that protects the integrity of the blood vessels, especially the fine and more delicate ones.
Venotonic	A substance that improves the tone and function of the veins.
Vermifuge	See *Anthelmintic*
Vulnerary (see also *Antiulcer*, *Astringent*, *Demulcent*)	A substance that promotes the healing of wounds when applied locally.

967

Appendix B: Toxic or potentially toxic herbs

These herbs should not be taken during pregnancy and lactation and are generally not recommended for internal use under any circumstances, the last point with a few exceptions, specifically Convallaria, Lobelia, boldo, poke root, Rauwolfia and Gelsemium.

Abrus precatorius seed and root	jequirity
Aconitum species	aconite
Acorus calamus	sweet flag
Adonis vernalis	
Ammi visnaga	
Apocynum	
Aristolochia (all or any species)	snakeroot, birthwort
Arnica (all or any species), other than for external use	Arnica
Arum maculatum	cuckoopint, lords and ladies
Belladonna	deadly nightshade
Brugmansia	
Brunfelsia uniflora	manaca, mercury
Calotropis	
Catha edulis	khat
Chenopodium ambrosioides	wormseed oil
Cicuta virosa	cowbane
Cinchona	quinine bark
Colchicum	
Convallaria	lily of the valley
Coronilla	
Crotalaria (all or any species)	
Croton (all or any species)	cascarilla, Croton
Cynoglossum officinale	hound's tongue
Daphne mezereum	mezereum
Datura	jimson weed
Digitalis	foxgloves
Dryopteris filix-mas	male fern
Duboisia	
Echium vulgare	viper's bugloss
Erysimum	
Euonymus europaeus	European spindle tree
Galanthus	snowdrop
Gelsemium	
Heliotropium (all or any species)	heliotrope
Helleborus (all or any species)	hellebore
Hyoscyamus	henbane
Lantana camara	Lantana
Lathyrus sativus, other than the cooked seed	grass pea

Lithospermum (all or any species)	
Lobelia	
Mandragora	mandrake
Menispermum canadense	yellow parilla
Mentha pulegium	pennyroyal
Oleander	
Opuntia cylindrica	San Pedro cactus
Papaver somniferum	opium poppy
Peganum harmala	wild rue
Petasites (all or any species)	butterbur
Peumus boldus	boldo
Phytolacca decandra (P. americana)	poke root, pokeweed
Podophyllum resin	
Pteridium aquilinum	bracken fern
Rauwolfia	
Ricinus communis, other than the fixed oil of the seed	castor tree
Robinia pseudoacacia, other than the leaf and flower	false acacia
Schoenocaulon officinale (Sabadilla officinarum, Veratrum officinale)	Sabadilla
Scopolia carniolica	
Semecarpus anacardium (Anacardium orientale), other than the seed	marking nut tree

Senecio (all or any species)	
Solanum (all or any species) except stems of Solanum dulcamara (bittersweet) and potatoes	
Sophora secundiflora	mescal bean
Spigelia marilandica	pink root, worm grass
Staphisagria	
Strophanthus	
Strychnos	nux vomica
Strychnos gaulthieriana	
Strychnos ignatii (Ignatia amara)	Ignatious bean
Symphytum (all or any species)	comfrey
Tamus communis fruit and root	black bryony
Tanacetum vulgare (except in preparations containing 0.8% or less of oil of tansy)	tansy
Teucrium (all or any species)	germander
Thevetia	
Toxicodendron radicans (Rhus toxicodendron)	poison ivy
Tussilago farfara	coltsfoot
Virola sebifera	cuajo negro, camaticaro
Yohimbe (yohimbine)	

Appendix C: Potential herb–drug interactions for commonly used herbs

Herb	Drug	Potential interaction	Basis of concern	Recommended action
Baical Skullcap *Scutellaria baicalensis*	Losartan	May increase drug levels.	Clinical trial with healthy volunteers (water-based extract,[A] dried herb equivalent: 12 g/day).[1]	Monitor (low level of risk at typical doses).
	Rosuvastatin	May decrease drug levels.	Clinical study with healthy volunteers using 150 mg/day of isolated constituent (baicalin).[2]	Monitor (low level of risk).[B]
Barberry *Berberis vulgaris*	Drugs that displace the protein binding of bilirubin, e.g. phenylbutazone	May potentiate effect of drug on displacing bilirubin.	Theoretical concern based on in vitro data and in vivo animal study (high dose of berberine by injection reduced bilirubin serum protein binding).[3]	Monitor (low level of risk).
Bilberry *Vaccinium myrtillus*	Warfarin	Potentiation of bleeding.	**Herb alone** Antiplatelet activity observed in healthy volunteers (173 mg/day of bilberry anthocyanins).[4] Case report of postoperative bleeding (bilberry extract undefined).[5] **Herb and drug** Case report (patient reported to consume 'large amounts of bilberry fruits every day for five years').[6]	Monitor at high doses (>100 mg/day anthocyanins, low level of risk).
Black Cohosh *Cimicifuga racemosa*	Statin drugs, e.g. atorvastatin	May potentiate increase in liver enzymes, specifically ALT.	Case report.[7] Also based on a projection of the idiosyncratic hepatotoxic potential of the herb.	Monitor (low level of risk).
Bladderwrack *Fucus vesiculosus*	Hyperthyroid medication, e.g. carbimazole	May decrease effectiveness of drug due to natural iodine content.[8]	Theoretical concern, no cases reported.	Contraindicated unless under close supervision.
	Thyroid replacement therapies, e.g. thyroxine	May add to effect of drug.	Theoretical concern linked to a case report where 'kelp' caused hyperthyroidism in a person not taking thyroxine.[9]	Monitor (low level of risk).
Bugleweed *Lycopus virginicus* *Lycopus europaeus*	Radioactive iodine	May interfere with administration of diagnostic procedures using radioactive isotopes.[10]	Case report.	Contraindicated.

Herb	Drug	Potential interaction	Basis of concern	Recommended action
	Thyroid hormones	Should not be administered concurrently with preparations containing thyroid hormone.[11]	Theoretical concern based on deliberations of German Commission E.	Contraindicated.
Cat's Claw *Uncaria tomentosa*	HIV protease inhibitors	May increase drug level.	Case report, in a patient with cirrhosis being evaluated for a liver transplant.[12]	Monitor (low level of risk).
Cayenne (Chilli Pepper) *Capsicum spp.* (See also Polyphenol-containing herbs)	ACE inhibitor	May cause drug-induced cough.	Case report (topical capsaicin). Theoretical concern since capsaicin depletes substance P.[13]	Monitor (very low level of risk).
	Theophylline	May increase absorption and drug level.	Clinical study (healthy volunteers, chilli-spiced meal). Absorption and drug level lower than during fasting.[14]	Monitor (low level of risk).
Celery Seed *Apium graveolens*	Thyroxine	May reduce serum levels of thyroxine.	Case reports.[15]	Monitor (very low level of risk). Take as many hours apart as possible.
Coleus *Coleus forskohlii*	Antiplatelet medication	May potentiate effects of drug.	Theoretical concern based on in vivo animal studies of standardised Coleus extract and the active constituent forskolin.[16]	Monitor (low level of risk).
	Hypotensive medication	May potentiate effects of drug.	Theoretical concern based on ability of high doses of forskolin and standardised Coleus extract to lower blood pressure in normotensive and hypertensive animals.[17,18] Clinical data from weight management trials: no effect on blood pressure in three trials, trend toward lower blood pressure in one small study.[19,20] No experimental or clinical studies conducted with hypotensive medication.	Monitor (low level of risk).
	Prescribed medication	May potentiate effects of drug.	Theoretical concern based on ability of forskolin to activate increased intracellular cyclic AMP in vitro.[21]	Monitor (low level of risk).
Cranberry *Vaccinium macrocarpon*	Midazolam	May increase drug levels.	Clinical trials with healthy volunteers: effect on drug levels conflicting – increased (double strength juice,[C] 240 mL tds; defined as a weak interaction[D])[22] and no effect (cranberry juice,[E] 200 mL tds).[23]	Monitor (low level of risk).
	Warfarin	May alter INR (most frequently increase).	Case reports (where reported the dosage was frequently high: up to 2000 mL/day, juice strength undefined; 1.5-2 quarts (1420-1893 mL)/day of cranberry juice cocktail; 113 g/day, cranberry sauce).[24–31] Clinical trials: no significant effect found in atrial fibrillation patients (250 mL/day cranberry juice cocktail),[32] in patients on warfarin for a variety of indications (8 oz (236 mL)/day cranberry juice cocktail),[33] but increase observed in healthy volunteers (juice concentrate equivalent to 57 g of dry fruit/day).[34] No alteration of prothrombin time in patients on stable warfarin therapy (480 mL/day cranberry juice)[35] or of thromboplastin time in healthy volunteers (600 mL/day cranberry juice[E]).[23] *See also Footnote C.*	Monitor (low level of risk at typical doses).

Herb	Drug	Potential interaction	Basis of concern	Recommended action
Dan Shen *Salvia miltiorrhiza*	Midazolam	May decrease drug levels.	Clinical trial with healthy volunteers.[36]	Monitor (medium level of risk).
	Warfarin	May potentiate effect of drug.	Case reports: increased INR.[37–39]	Contraindicated.
Devil's Claw *Harpagophytum procumbens*	Warfarin	May increase bleeding tendency.	Case report (purpura) containing very few details.[40] Unlikely to occur.	Monitor (very low level of risk).
Dong Quai *Angelica sinensis* *Angelica polymorpha*	Warfarin	May potentiate effect of drug.	Case reports: increased INR and PT;[41] increased INR and widespread bruising.[42]	Monitor (low level of risk).
Echinacea *Echinacea angustifolia* *Echinacea purpurea*	HIV protease inhibitors, e.g. darunavir	May decrease drug levels.	Clinical trial (*E. purpurea* root; HIV-infected patients): no effect overall, but some patients showed a decrease by as much as 40%. All maintained an undetectable viral load.[43]	Monitor (low level of risk).
	Immunosuppressant medication	May decrease effectiveness of drug.[44,45]	Theoretical concern based on immune-enhancing activity of Echinacea. No adverse events reported.	Contraindicated.
	Midazolam	Decreases drug levels when drug administered intravenously.[F]	Clinical study (*E. purpurea* root, 1.6 g/day).[46]	Monitor (medium level of risk) when drug administered intravenously.
Evening Primrose Oil *Oenothera biennis*	Phenothiazines	May decrease effectiveness of drug.	Reports of worsening epilepsy in schizophrenics. No causal association demonstrated and no effect observed in later trials.[47]	Monitor (very low level of risk).
Garlic *Allium sativum* (See also Hypoglycaemic herbs)	Antiplatelet and anticoagulant drugs, e.g. aspirin, warfarin	Aspirin: May increase bleeding time. Warfarin: May potentiate effect of drug. Large doses could increase bleeding tendency.	Concern may be overstated, as antiplatelet drugs are often coadministered with warfarin. **Herb alone** Case reports of increased bleeding tendency with high garlic intake. In three of the four cases the bleeding occurred after surgery.[48–51] Anecdotal: garlic taken shortly before testing interferes with platelet aggregation in control subjects.[52] *Single-dose studies excluded.* Clinical studies (3 g/day or less of fresh garlic): inhibited platelet aggregation in three trials (about 2.4-2.7 g/day, patients and healthy volunteers),[53–55] but no effect on platelet aggregation in one trial (about 1.8 g/day, patients);[56] decreased serum thromboxane in one trial (3 g/day, healthy volunteers).[57] *See Footnote G.* Clinical studies (4.2-5 g/day of fresh garlic, patients and healthy volunteers): no effect on platelet aggregation, fibrinogen level, prothrombin time, whole blood coagulation time.[58–60] Clinical studies (8-10 g/day of fresh garlic): inhibited platelet aggregation and increased clotting time (healthy volunteers).[61,62]	Monitor at doses equivalent to ≥3 g/day fresh garlic (low level of risk). Stop taking at least 1 week before surgery.

Herb	Drug	Potential interaction	Basis of concern	Recommended action
			Herb and drug Aspirin: No published studies. Clopidogrel: Garlic tablet ('odourless', dose undefined) added to improve drug therapy, reduced platelet hyperactivity in two patients.[52] Warfarin: Two cases of increased INR and clotting times, very few details (garlic pearls, garlic tablets: dosage undefined).[63] Clinical trial: no effect in healthy volunteers (enteric-coated tablets equivalent to 4 g/day of fresh garlic).[34]	
	HIV protease inhibitors, e.g. saquinavir	Decreases drug level.	Two clinical studies (garlic extract, standardised for allicin content) with healthy volunteers;[64,65] large variability (in one study,[65] decrease (15%) was not significant).	Monitor (medium level of risk).
Ginger *Zingiber officinale*	Antacids	May decrease effectiveness of drug.	Theoretical concern since ginger increases gastric secretory activity in vivo (animals).[44]	Monitor (low level of risk).
	Antiplatelet and anticoagulant drugs, e.g. phenprocoumon, warfarin	Phenprocoumon: May increase action of drug. Warfarin: Increased risk of spontaneous bleeding.	Case report (dosage undefined): increased INR.[66] Concern based on antiplatelet activity and potential to inhibit thromboxane synthetase. **Herb alone** Clinical studies: inhibition of platelet aggregation (5 g, divided single dose, dried ginger) in healthy volunteers,[67] and coronary artery disease patients (10 g, single dose, dried ginger),[68] but no effect in healthy volunteers (2 g, single dose, dried ginger),[69] or coronary artery disease patients (4 g/ day, dried ginger);[68] inhibition of platelet thromboxane production in healthy volunteers (5 g/day, fresh ginger).[70] **Herb and drug** Case report: bleeding (ginger dosage undefined).[71] No pharmacokinetic or pharmacodynamic effect demonstrated in a clinical trial with healthy volunteers (3.6 g/day, dried ginger).[72]	Monitor at doses equivalent to <4 g/day dried ginger (low level of risk). Monitor at doses equivalent to <4 g/day dried ginger (very low risk). Contraindicated unless under close supervision at doses equivalent to >4 g/day dried ginger.
	Nifedipine	May produce a synergistic antiplatelet effect.	Clinical study (1 g/day, dried ginger) in healthy volunteers and hypertensive patients.[73]	Contraindicated.
Ginkgo *Ginkgo biloba*	Anticonvulsant medication, e.g. carbamazepine, sodium valproate	May decrease the effectiveness of drug.	Case reports, two with well-controlled epilepsy,[74] others anecdotal and uncertain.[75–77]	Monitor (medium level of risk). Increasing the intake of vitamin B6 may be advisable for patients taking anticonvulsants.[H]
	Antiplatelet and anticoagulant drugs, e.g. aspirin, cilostazol, clopidogrel, ticlopidine, warfarin	Prolongation of bleeding and/or increased bleeding tendency.	Concern based on antiplatelet activity. **Herb alone** Rare case reports of bleeding.[78–80] Clinical studies: results not indicative of clinically-relevant antiplatelet or anticoagulant effects (see also monograph).[81]	Monitor (low level of risk).

Herb	Drug	Potential interaction	Basis of concern	Recommended action
			Herb and drug Retrospective population-based study in Taiwan: the relative risk of haemorrhage associated with the combined use of Ginkgo extract with drugs (clopidogrel, cilostazol, ticlopidine, warfarin) was not significant.[82] Aspirin: Two case reports (bleeding).[78] Clinical studies: no additional effect on platelet function, platelet aggregation or bleeding time.[83–85] Cilostazol: Clinical studies with healthy volunteers (Ginkgo 50:1 extract: single dose 120 mg, equivalent to 6 g of dried leaf), bleeding time prolonged; no change in platelet aggregation or clotting time, and no significant correlation between prolongation of bleeding time and inhibition of platelet aggregation;[86] no effect on pharmacokinetics, platelet aggregation or bleeding time (Ginkgo extract (undefined): 160 mg/day).[87] Clopidogrel: Clinical study with healthy volunteers (Ginkgo 50:1 extract: single dose 120 mg, equivalent to 6 g of dried leaf), no effect on platelet aggregation, bleeding times.[86] Ticlopidine: Case report.[79] Clinical study with healthy volunteers (Ginkgo 50:1 extract: single dose 80 mg, equivalent to 4 g of dried leaf), no significant additional effect on bleeding time or platelet aggregation[88] and at the higher dose (120 mg/day) did not affect drug levels.[89] Warfarin: Case report (bleeding).[78] Clinical studies (healthy volunteers and patients): no additional effect on INR, platelet aggregation, coagulation parameters or plasma drug level.[72,90,91] *See also Footnote J.*	
	Antipsychotic medication, e.g. haloperidol, olanzapine, clozapine	May potentiate the efficiency of drug in patients with schizophrenia.	Randomised, controlled trials (Ginkgo 50:1 extract: 120-360 mg/day, equivalent to 6-18 g/day of dried leaf).[92–95]	Prescribe cautiously. Reduce drug if necessary in conjunction with prescribing physician.
	Benzodiazepines, e.g. diazepam, midazolam	May alter drug level.	Diazepam: Clinical trial in healthy volunteers found no effect (Ginkgo 50:1 extract: 240 mg/day, equivalent to 12 g/day of dried leaf).[96] Midazolam: Clinical trials: effect on drug levels conflicting – increased (defined as a weak interaction[D])[97] and decreased (most rigorous results; Ginkgo 50:1 extract: 240 mg/day, equivalent to 12 g/day of dried leaf).[98]	Monitor (low level of risk).

Herb	Drug	Potential interaction	Basis of concern	Recommended action
	HIV non-nucleoside transcriptase inhibitors, e.g. efavirenz	May decrease drug levels.	Case report.[99]	Monitor (medium level of risk).
	Hypoglycaemic drugs, e.g. glipizide, metformin, pioglitazone, tolbutamide	Glipizide: May cause hypoglycaemia.	Observation from aborted trial: hypoglycaemia occurred in volunteers with normal glucose tolerance within 60 minutes.[100] Ginkgo 50:1 extract was administered as a single dose of 120 mg, equivalent to 6 g of dried leaf.[101]	Monitor (low level of risk).
		Metformin: May enhance action of drug.	Clinical trial: elimination half-life was increased at doses of metformin 850 mg, three times a day. Effect not significant at doses to 500 mg, twice a day. Ginkgo 50:1 extract was administered as a single dose of 120 mg, equivalent to 6 g of dried leaf.[100]	Monitor at doses of metformin >1 g/day (medium level of risk). Reduce drug if necessary in conjunction with prescribing physician.
		Pioglitazone: May increase drug level.	Clinical trial with healthy volunteers (Ginkgo 50:1 extract: 120 mg/day, equivalent to 6 g/day of dried leaf).[102]	Monitor (low level of risk).
		Tolbutamide: May decrease effectiveness of drug.	Clinical trial with healthy volunteers (high dose of Ginkgo 50:1 extract: 360 mg/day, equivalent to 18 g/day of dried leaf).[97]	Monitor (low level of risk).
	Nifedipine	May increase drug levels or side effects.	Clinical studies: mixed results found for mean plasma drug level – increase (120 mg/day, equivalent to 6 g/day of dried leaf)[103] and no effect (240 mg/day, equivalent to 12 g/day of dried leaf).[104] However, at the higher dose, maximal plasma drug level and heart rate was increased with adverse drug reactions for participants with highest plasma drug levels (headache, dizziness, hot flushes).	Monitor at doses <240 mg/day, equivalent to <12 g/day of dried leaf (medium level of risk). Contraindicated for higher doses.
	Omeprazole	May decrease drug levels.	Clinical trial with healthy volunteers (Ginkgo 50:1 extract: 280 mg/day, equivalent to 14 g/day of dried leaf).[105]	Monitor (low level of risk).
	Talinolol	May increase drug levels.	Clinical trial with healthy volunteers.[106]	Monitor (low level of risk).
Golden Seal *Hydrastis canadensis*	Drugs which displace the protein binding of bilirubin, e.g. phenylbutazone	May potentiate effect of drug on displacing bilirubin.	Theoretical concern based on in vitro data and in vivo animal study (high dose of berberine by injection reduced bilirubin serum protein binding).[3]	Monitor (low level of risk).
	Midazolam	May increase drug level.	Clinical trial (defined as a weak interaction[D]).[107]	Monitor (low level of risk).
Green Tea *Camellia sinensis* (See also Polyphenol-containing herbs and Tannin-containing herbs)	Boronic acid-based protease inhibitors, e.g. bortezomib	May decrease efficacy of drug.	Theoretical concern based on in vitro data and in vivo animal study (green tea constituent: EGCG).[108]	Contraindicated at high doses (around 600 mg/day EGCG or 1 g/day green tea catechins).[K] More information required for doses below this level.

Herb	Drug	Potential interaction	Basis of concern	Recommended action
	Folate	May decrease absorption.	Clinical study with healthy volunteers.[109] Clinical significance unclear, as was a one-day study (not ongoing administration), with 50 mg of green tea catechins administered before, during and up to 2 hours after folate (for a total of 250 mg of catechins).	If taken simultaneously, may need to increase dose of folate. The effect may be relatively small, more information is required.
	Statin drugs, e.g. simvastatin	May increase plasma level and side effect of drug.	One case reported of muscle pain (side effect). Pharmacokinetic evaluation indicated green tea (1 cup) increased the bioavailability of simvastatin in this patient.[110]	Monitor (low level of risk).
	Warfarin	May inhibit effect of drug: decreased INR.	Case report (brewed green tea: 0.5-1 gallon/day).[111]	Monitor (very low level of risk).
Hawthorn *Crataegus monogyna Crataegus laevigata* (*C. oxyacantha*) (See also Tannin-containing herbs)	Digoxin	May increase effectiveness of drug.	Very early clinical studies indicate a (beneficial) synergistic effect.[112,113] Pharmacokinetics not affected in a clinical study.[114]	Monitor (low level of risk).
	Hypotensive drugs including beta-blockers	May increase effectiveness of drug.	Three controlled clinical trials: two demonstrated hawthorn causes a slight reduction in blood pressure in patients with heart conditions.[115–117]	Monitor (low level of risk).
Hypoglycaemic herbs, e.g. fenugreek (*Trigonella foenum-graecum*), garlic, *Gymnema sylvestre*, goat's rue (*Galega officinalis*), psyllium (*Plantago ovata, P. psyllium, P. indica*) (See also Ginkgo, Korean ginseng, St John's wort, St Mary's thistle)	Hypoglycaemic drugs, including insulin	May potentiate hypoglycaemic activity of drug.	In uncontrolled trials, high dose, long-term administration of Gymnema extract (equivalent to 10-13 g/day dried leaf) reduced insulin and hypoglycaemic drug requirements in diabetics.[118,119] Hypoglycaemic effects of fenugreek (15-100 g/day dried and/or defatted seed) observed in type 1 and type 2 diabetics including those on therapeutic and subtherapeutic doses of hypoglycaemic drugs.[120–125]	Prescribe cautiously and monitor blood sugar regularly. Warn patient about possible hypoglycaemic effects. Reduce drug if necessary in conjunction with prescribing physician.
			Hypoglycaemic effects observed in many well-controlled clinical trials for psyllium (10.2-15 g/day, more than 6 weeks) in type 2 diabetics. Drug dosage adjustments were not required.[126–129] *See also footnote L.* In one small, uncontrolled trial, nearly 70% of type 1 diabetics experienced hypoglycaemic episodes. Reductions in insulin dosage may have been required had the trial been of longer duration (10.8 g/day of husk, about 1 week).[130] (There is also clinical evidence that high fibre diets (10-60 g/day) worsen control of type 2 diabetes in patients who are poorly controlled with oral hypoglycaemic drugs.[131])	

Herb	Drug	Potential interaction	Basis of concern	Recommended action
			Several trials have found no effect for garlic on blood glucose in type 2 diabetes, although in a double blind, placebo-controlled trial (using enteric-coated tablets), a reduction in the dosage of oral hypoglycaemic drugs was required (these patients had fasting blood glucose above 8.0 mmol/L).[132]	
Kava *Piper methysticum*	CNS depressants, e.g. alcohol, barbiturates, benzodiazepines	Potentiation of drug effects.	Theoretical concern based on deliberations of German Commission E[11] and the anxiolytic activity of kava.[44] Two apparent case reports (kava+benzodiazepines).[133,134] Clinical trials with healthy volunteers: no additional side effects observed for kava (extract containing 240 mg/day of kava lactones)+benzodiazepine,[135] and kava (extract containing 210 mg/day of kava lactones)+alcohol.[136]	Monitor (low level of risk).
	L-Dopa and other Parkinson's disease treatments	Possible dopamine antagonist effects.	Case reports.[137] (See also a discussion of this issue in the kava monograph.)	Contraindicated unless under close supervision.
Korean Ginseng *Panax ginseng*	Antihypertensive medications including nifedipine	General: May decrease effectiveness of drug.	Theoretical concern. Clinical significance unclear.[44] Assessment of 316 hospital patients found ginseng to have a contrary effect only in a very small percentage: blood pressure increase in 5% of hypertensives; increase in 3% and decrease in 2% of normotensives; decrease in 6% of hypotensives.[138] No information on concurrent medications. (See also discussion in monograph.) **Herb and drug** Clinical trials: *decreased* blood pressure in essential hypertension,[139] and coronary artery disease[140] but no effect in white coat hypertension[139] and essential hypertension.[141]	Monitor (very low level of risk).
		Nifedipine: May increase drug levels.	Clinical trial.[103]	Monitor (low level of risk).
	Antiplatelet and anticoagulant drugs	General: May potentiate effects of drug.	**Herb alone** Two epidemiological studies in Korea: long-term intake (3-5 years) prolonged plasma clotting times (APTT),[142,143] and decreased platelet aggregation.[142] (Dosage in Korea is generally high.) Clinical trial (healthy volunteers): inhibited platelet aggregation, but no effect on coagulation (PT, APTT).[144]	Monitor (low level of risk).
		Warfarin: May decrease effectiveness of drug.	**Herb and drug** One case reported (decreased INR)[145] but clinical significance unclear. No effect demonstrated in three clinical trials (healthy volunteers and patients) for INR, prothrombin time and platelet aggregation.[146–148]	Monitor (low level of risk).

Herb	Drug	Potential interaction	Basis of concern	Recommended action
	CNS stimulants	May potentiate effects of drug.[44]	Theoretical concern. Clinical significance unclear.	Monitor (low level of risk).
	Hypoglycaemic drugs, including insulin	May potentiate hypoglycaemic activity of drug.[45]	Theoretical concern based on clinically observed hypoglycaemic activity of ginseng in newly diagnosed type 2 diabetics.[149] Clinical significance unclear. No effect on insulin sensitivity or beta-cell function after very high doses in newly diagnosed type 2 diabetics or those with impaired glucose tolerance.[150] Korean red ginseng (2.7 g/day) reduced the requirement for insulin in about 40% of diabetics in a small uncontrolled trial.[151] No adverse effects in three trials of type 2 diabetics well controlled with diet and/or oral hypoglycaemic drugs.[152–154]	Monitor (low level of risk).
	MAO inhibitors, e.g. phenelzine	Headache and tremor, mania.	Case reports.[155,156] However, identity of the ginseng was not confirmed and is disputed by some authors.	Monitor (uncertain level of risk)
	Sildenafil	Potentiation of drug possible.	Theoretical concern based on in vitro studies which show ginseng increases nitric oxide release from corpus cavernosum tissue.[157,158]	Monitor (very low level of risk).
	Warfarin – *See Antiplatelet and anticoagulant drugs above*			
Laxative (anthraquinone-containing) herbs eg. aloe resin (*Aloe barbadensis*, *Aloe ferox*), senna (*Cassia spp.*), cascara (*Rhamnus purshiana*, *Rhamnus purshianus*), yellow dock (*Rumex crispus*)	Antiarrhythmic agents	May affect activity if potassium deficiency resulting from long-term laxative abuse is present.	German Commission E and ESCOP recommendation.[11,159]	Avoid excessive doses of laxatives. Maintain patients on a high potassium diet.
	Cardiac glycosides	May potentiate activity, if potassium deficiency resulting from long-term laxative abuse is present.	German Commission E and ESCOP recommendation.[11,159]	Monitor (low level of risk at normal doses).
	Potassium depleting agents, e.g. thiazide diuretics, corticosteroids, licorice root (*Glycyrrhiza glabra*)	May increase potassium depletion.	German Commission E and ESCOP recommendation.[11,159]	Avoid excessive doses of laxatives. Maintain patients on a high potassium diet.
Licorice *Glycyrrhiza glabra*	Antihypertensive medications other than diuretics	General: May decrease effectiveness of drug.	When consumed in high doses, licorice can cause pseudoaldosteronism and high blood pressure. **Herb alone** Hypertension demonstrated in case reports, usually from long-term intake and/or very high dose.[160] Clinical studies (up to 200 g/day of licorice): dose-dependent relationship found between licorice and increase in blood pressure, more pronounced effect in hypertensive patients than in normotensive volunteers, adverse effect greater in women, and effect shown for dose as low as 50 g/day of licorice (75 mg/day of glycyrrhetinic acid =130 mg/day of glycyrrhizin[M]) taken for 2 weeks.[161–163] Other studies show variation of effects on blood pressure (*see Footnote N*) – renal function may be a factor.[164]	Avoid long-term use at doses >100 mg/day glycyrrhizin unless under close supervision.[P] Place patients on a high potassium diet.

Herb	Drug	Potential interaction	Basis of concern	Recommended action
			Herb and drug Case report (high dose of licorice). Patient still hypertensive despite treatment with drugs.[165]	
		ACE-inhibitor: May mask the development of pseudoaldosteronism.	Case report (patient consumed licorice (200-240 mg/day glycyrrhizin)). Drug dosage was reduced, leading to pseudoaldosteronism.[166] *See Footnote Q.*	Avoid long-term use at doses >100 mg/day glycyrrhizin unless under close supervision.[P] Place patients on a high potassium diet.
	Cilostazol	May cause hypokalaemia, which can potentiate the toxicity of the drug.	Case report (patient taking 150 mg/day of glycyrrhizin). Serum potassium levels were stable prior to administration of drug.[167]	Monitor (medium level of risk). Place patients on a high potassium diet.
	Digoxin	May cause hypokalaemia, which can potentiate the toxicity of the drug.	**Herb alone** Hypokalaemia demonstrated in case reports and clinical studies, usually from long-term intake and/or very high dose, however effect has been demonstrated in sensitive individuals at low doses (licorice containing 100 mg/day of glycyrrhizin). Side effects would be common at 400 mg/day of glycyrrhizin.[160,168,169] **Herb and drug** Case report (patient taking herbal laxative containing licorice (1.2 g/day) and rhubarb (*Rheum spp.*, 4.8 g/day)). In addition to digoxin, patient was also taking a potassium-depleting diuretic.[170]	Avoid long-term use at doses >100 mg/day glycyrrhizin unless under close supervision.[P] Place patients on a high potassium diet.
	Diuretics	Spironolactone (potassium-sparing diuretic): reduced side effects of drug.	Clinical study: in women with PCOS addition of licorice (containing about 463 mg/day glycyrrhizin) reduced side effects related to the diuretic activity of drug.[171]	Monitor (low level of risk at normal doses).
		Thiazide and loop (potassium-depleting) diuretics: The combined effect of licorice and the drug could result in excessive potassium loss.[11]	**Herb alone** Hypokalaemia demonstrated in case reports and clinical studies, usually from long-term intake and/or very high dose,[160,168,169] however effect has been demonstrated in patients for ongoing treatment with glycyrrhizin (80-240 mg/day).[172] **Herb and drug** Case reports, usually from long-term intake and/or very high dose,[165,168,173–179] however effect has been demonstrated for ongoing treatment at glycyrrhizin doses of 80 mg/day.[172] Clinical trial (confectionery containing 40 mg/day of glycyrrhizin): decreased plasma potassium, with 20% of healthy volunteers hypokalaemic in the first week.[180]	Contraindicated unless under close supervision at doses >40 mg/day glycyrrhizin.
	Immuno-suppressives, e.g. sirolimus	May decrease drug clearance.	Population pharmacokinetic study with 112 Chinese adult renal transplant recipients: clearance of sirolimus decreased in those patients with abnormal ALT values who were taking glycyrrhizin formulations (route and dosage unknown).[181]	Monitor (medium level of risk) in hepatically impaired patients.

Herb	Drug	Potential interaction	Basis of concern	Recommended action
	Midazolam	May decrease drug level.	Clinical study with healthy volunteers (potassium salt of glycyrrhizin, equivalent to 287 mg/day of glycyrrhzin).[182]	Monitor (low level of risk at normal doses).
	Omeprazole	May decrease drug level.	Clinical study with healthy volunteers (potassium salt of glycyrrhizin, equivalent to 287 mg/day of glycyrrhizin).[183]	Monitor (low level of risk at normal doses).
	Potassium-depleting drugs other than thiazide and loop diuretics, e.g. corticosteroids, stimulant laxatives	The combined effect of licorice and the drug could result in excessive potassium loss.	**Herb alone** Hypokalaemia demonstrated in case reports and clinical studies, usually from confectionery intake (high dose), however effect has been demonstrated in sensitive individuals at low doses (licorice containing 100 mg/day of glycyrrhizin). Side effects would be common at 400 mg/day of glycyrrhizin.[160,168] *See also Prednisolone below.*	Avoid long-term use at doses >100 mg/day glycyrrhizin unless under close supervision.[P] Place patients on a high potassium diet.
	Prednisolone	May potentiate the action or increase levels of drug.	Two clinical studies (oral administration of glycyrrhizin or glycyrrhetinic acid;[M] prednisolone administered intravenously): increased drug level[184] and increased prednisolone/prednisone ratio[R] in urine and plasma.[185] Dosage was high: 200 mg/day glycyrrhizin,[184] and 400 mg/day glycyrrhetinic acid (=700 mg/day glycyrrhizin).[185]	Monitor (low level of risk) when drug administered intravenously.
Marshmallow Root *Althaea officinalis*	Prescribed medication	May slow or reduce absorption of drugs.	Theoretical concern based on absorbent properties of marshmallow root.	Take at least 2 hours away from medication.
Meadowsweet *Filipendula ulmaria* (See also Tannin-containing herbs)	Warfarin	May potentiate effects of drug.	Theoretical concern based on in vivo animal study demonstrating anticoagulant activity (dosage unavailable).[186]	Monitor (very low level of risk).
Phellodendron *Phellodendron amurense*	Drugs that displace the protein binding of bilirubin, e.g. phenylbutazone	May potentiate effect of drug on displacing bilirubin.	Theoretical concern based on in vitro data and in vivo animal study (high dose of berberine by injection reduced bilirubin serum protein binding).[3]	Monitor (low level of risk).
Polyphenol-containing[S] or Flavonoid-containing herbs especially cayenne (*Capsicum annuum*), chamomile (*Matricaria recutita*), cocoa, green tea (*Camellia sinensis*), lime flowers (*Tilia cordata*), rosemary (*Rosmarinus officinalis*), St Mary's thistle (*Silybum marianum*), vervain (*Verbena officinalis*). (See also Tannin-containing herbs)	Immuno-suppressives, e.g. cyclosporin	Decreases drug levels, due to impaired absorption or increased metabolism.	Three case reports, in transplant patients (2 L/day of herbal tea; 1-1.5 L/day of chamomile tea; 'large quantities' of fruit tea containing hibiscus extract and a drink containing black tea). Confirmed by rechallenge in one case, but no signs of rejection.[187]	Monitor (medium level of risk). Also advisable not to take simultaneously.
	Iron	Inhibition of non-haem iron[T] absorption.	Clinical study (included herb teas (German chamomile, vervain, lime flower, peppermint; all 3 g/300 mL), beverages (e.g. black tea, coffee, cocoa)): effect dependent on polyphenol content (per serving: 20-400 mg).[188] *See also Footnote U.* Timing of intake may be important. *See also Footnote V.*	In anaemia and where iron supplementation is required, do not take simultaneously with meals or iron supplements.

Herb	Drug	Potential interaction	Basis of concern	Recommended action
			Mixed results in other studies (healthy volunteers): rosemary (32.7 mg of polyphenols)[189] and cayenne (high dose: 14.2 g, fresh weight,[W] containing 25 mg polyphenols)[190] caused inhibition; chamomile[191] and turmeric (2.8 g, fresh weight, containing 50 mg polyphenols)[190] did not. See also Footnote X.	
			Results for green tea have been conflicting: two studies found no effect (healthy volunteers and those with anaemia),[192,193] two studies (healthy volunteers) found an effect.[189,194] Two epidemiological studies (French and Japanese populations) found mixed results for serum ferritin and haemoglobin, although risk of iron depletion or anaemia was not increased.[195,196] Clinical study (150-300 mg/day EGCG): decreased absorption in healthy women with low iron stores administered together with iron. Results significant only at higher dosage.[197]	
			Concentrated extract of St Mary's thistle reduced iron absorption in haemochromatosis patients.[198]	
Psyllium *Plantago ovata* *Plantago psyllium* *Plantago indica* (See also Hypoglycaemic herbs)	Carbamazepine	Decreases plasma drug level.	Clinical study (psyllium husk),[199] although no adverse effect observed in one case report.[200]	Take at least 2 hours away from medication.
	Digoxin	May decrease absorption of drug.	Decreased bioavailability found for digoxin and 'crude' (undefined) dietary fibre,[201] but no effect was found on digoxin levels in two clinical studies (psyllium husk).[202,203] Slight decrease in absorption (15%) found in healthy volunteers when psyllium husk[Y] (15 g) and digoxin taken concomitantly but when given 30 minutes apart the decrease was much smaller (3%).[204]	Take at least 2 hours away from medication.
	Iron	Inhibition of non-haem iron absorption.	**Iron from test meal** Clinical studies: absorption decreased by 8% (5 g/day for 2 meals, psyllium undefined) in healthy volunteers;[205] no effect overall in type 2 diabetics, although significant differences among participants (14 g/day, for 6 weeks, psyllium undefined).[206]	In anaemia and where iron supplementation is required, do not take simultaneously with meals or iron supplements.

Herb	Drug	Potential interaction	Basis of concern	Recommended action
			Iron from diet Clinical studies: no change in serum iron in two trials with patients (6 g/day, for 4-5 weeks, psyllium undefined;[207] maximum tolerated dose, generally less than 25 g/day, for 4 months, psyllium husk);[208] iron absorption decreased in non-anaemic adolescent girls, but iron balance was positive (25 g/day, for 3 weeks, psyllium husk);[209] slight decrease in plasma iron in obese patients without effects on other iron parameters during first period of treatment (30 days), without further modification on long-term treatment of 6 months (6 g/day, psyllium undefined).[210]	
	Lithium	May decrease absorption of drug.	Case report (psyllium husk),[211] and clinical study with healthy volunteers (psyllium husk).[212] Hydrophilic psyllium may prevent lithium from ionising.	Take at least 2 hours away from medication.
	Prescribed medication	May slow or reduce absorption of drugs.	Theoretical concern based on absorbent properties of psyllium. No effect found on absorption or prothrombin time in healthy volunteers when psyllium husk (14 g) and warfarin were taken concomitantly.[213] In a crossover trial, psyllium husk (6 g) was administered with orlistat[Z] three times a day and found to reduce the subsequent side effects. Single dose of psyllium (12 g) at bedtime was also effective in reducing the side effects.[214]	Take at least 2 hours away from medication,[AA] except for orlistat which may be taken at the same time.
	Thyroxine	May decrease efficacy of drug.	Clinical study: decreased efficacy found in 12 hypothyroid patients consuming dietary fibre (one patient: whole grain cereal+psyllium laxative); some patients stabilised by decreasing or removing the fibre from their diet.[215] Clinical study (healthy volunteers, 3.4 g/day, for 4 days, psyllium husk): decrease in absorption not significant.[216]	Take as many hours apart as possible. May require dose reduction or cessation of herb.
Schisandra *Schisandra chinensis*	Immuno-suppressives, e.g. tacrolimus	May increase drug levels.	Observations in some renal and liver transplanted recipients. Clinical studies: markedly increased drug levels in healthy volunteers[217] and transplant recipients,[218,219] given *S. sphenanthera* extract, providing 67.5 mg/day of deoxyschisandrin.[BB]	Monitor (low level of risk at normal doses).
	Midazolam	May increase drug levels.	Increased drug level (defined as a moderate interaction[D]), increase in sleeping time and increase in mild to moderate adverse effects found in healthy volunteers, given *S. chinensis* extract, providing 22.5 mg/day of deoxyschisandrin.[BB,220]	Monitor (medium level of risk at normal doses).
	Prescribed medication	May accelerate clearance from the body.	Theoretical concern based on in vivo animal studies demonstrating enhanced phase I/II hepatic metabolism.[221,222]	Monitor (medium level of risk).

Herb	Drug	Potential interaction	Basis of concern	Recommended action
	Talinolol	May increase drug levels – possible effect on inhibiting P-gp.	Increased drug level and decreased clearance found in healthy volunteers given *S. chinensis* extract, providing 33.75 mg/day of deoxyschisandrin.[BB,106]	Monitor (low level of risk at normal doses).
Siberian Ginseng *Eleutherococcus senticosus*	Digoxin	May increase plasma drug levels.	Case report: apparent increase in plasma level, but herb probably interfered with digoxin assay[CC] (patient had unchanged ECG despite apparent digoxin concentration of 5.2 nmol/L).[223] In a later clinical trial no effect observed on plasma concentration.[224]	Monitor (very low level of risk).
Slippery Elm Bark *Ulmus rubra*	Prescribed medication	May slow or reduce absorption of drugs.	Theoretical concern based on absorbent properties of slippery elm.	Take at least 2 hours away from medication.
St John's Wort[DD] *Hypericum perforatum* (See also Tannin-containing herbs)	Amitriptyline	Decreases drug levels.[225]	Clinical study.	Monitor (medium level of risk).
	Anticonvulsants, e.g. carbamazepine, mephenytoin, phenobarbitone, phenytoin	May decrease drug levels via CYP induction.[226–228]	Theoretical concern. An open clinical trial demonstrated no effect on carbamazepine pharmacokinetics in healthy volunteers.[229] Case report: increase in seizures in patient taking several antiepileptic drugs, two of which are not metabolised by cytochrome P450.[230] Clinical study (healthy volunteers; clinical significance unclear): increased excretion of a mephenytoin metabolite in extensive metabolisers, but not in poor metabolisers.[231] *See Footnote EE.*	Monitor (low level of risk).
	Antihistamine, e.g. fexofenadine	Decreases drug levels.	Clinical studies.[232,233]	Monitor (medium level of risk).
	Antiplatelet and anticoagulant drugs, e.g. clopidogrel, phenprocoumon, warfarin	Clopidogrel: May potentiate effects of drug.	Clinical study: increased responsiveness (decreased platelet aggregation) in hyporesponsive volunteers and patients,[234–236] possibly via the formation of the active metabolite (CYP3A4 activity was increased) thus providing a beneficial effect in these patients. This is a complex situation, with the meaning of clopidogrel resistance/hyporesponsiveness debated.[234,237])	In patients with known clopidogrel resistance: Monitor (medium level of risk). In other patients: Monitor (risk is unknown).
		Phenprocoumon: Decreases plasma drug levels.	Clinical study.[238]	Contraindicated.
		Warfarin: Decreases drug levels and INR.	Case reports (12: decreased INR (9), increased INR (3)).[239–241] Clinical study with healthy volunteers (decreased drug level and INR).[146]	Contraindicated.
	Benzodiazepines, e.g. alprazolam, midazolam, quazepam	Decreases drug levels, and is probably dependent upon the hyperforin content.[242]	Alprazolam: Mixed results for drug levels in two clinical studies (similar amounts of hyperforin) – no effect[243] and decrease.[244]	Monitor (medium level of risk).
			Midazolam: Four clinical studies, effect not regarded as clinically relevant for low (< 1 mg/day) hyperforin extracts.[233,242,245,246]	Hyperforin-rich extracts: Monitor (medium level of risk).

Herb	Drug	Potential interaction	Basis of concern	Recommended action
				Low-hyperforin extracts: Monitor (low level of risk).
			Quazepam: Decreased drug levels, but no effect on pharmacodynamic (sedative) effects.[247]	Monitor (low level of risk).
	Calcium channel antagonists, e.g. nifedipine, verapamil	Decreases drug levels.	Nifedipine: Clinical studies.[103,248] Verapamil: Clinical study.[249]	Contraindicated.
	Cancer chemotherapeutic drugs, e.g. irinotecan, imatinib	Decreases drug levels.	Clinical studies.[250–253]	Contraindicated.
	Digoxin	Decreases drug levels.	Clinical studies (several studies showed decrease, one study showed no effect)[243,254–256] but effect is dependent upon dose of herb and the hyperforin content.[256]	Contraindicated at doses equivalent to >1 g/day dried herb, especially for high-hyperforin extracts.
	Finasteride	May decrease drug levels.	Clinical study with healthy volunteers.[257]	Contraindicated.
	HIV non-nucleoside transcriptase inhibitors, e.g. nevirapine	Decreases drug levels.	Case report.[258]	Contraindicated.
	HIV protease inhibitors, e.g. indinavir	Decreases drug levels.	Clinical study.[259]	Contraindicated.
	Hypoglycaemic drugs, e.g. gliclazide, tolbutamide	Gliclazide: May reduce efficacy of drug by increased clearance.	Clinical study with healthy volunteers, but glucose and insulin response to glucose loading were unchanged.[260]	Monitor (low level of risk).
		Tolbutamide: May affect blood glucose.	Two clinical studies (healthy volunteers):[243,245] no effect on pharmacokinetics, but there was an increased incidence of hypoglycaemia in the trial using hyperforin-rich extract.[245]	Monitor (low level of risk).
	Immuno-suppressives, e.g. cyclosporin, tacrolimus	Decreases drug levels.	Cyclosporin: Case reports,[261–269] case series,[270,271] clinical studies.[233,272] Interaction is dependent upon the hyperforin content.[264,272] Tacrolimus: Case report and clinical studies.[273–275]	Contraindicated especially for high-hyperforin extracts.
	Ivabradine	May decrease drug levels.	Clinical trial with healthy volunteers. No pharmacodynamic effect was observed.[276]	Monitor (medium level of risk).
	Methadone	Decreases drug levels, possibly inducing withdrawal symptoms.	Case reports.[277]	Contraindicated.
	Methylphenidate	May decrease efficacy.	Case report,[278] but clinical significance unclear.	Monitor (low level of risk).

Herb	Drug	Potential interaction	Basis of concern	Recommended action
	Omeprazole	May decrease drug levels.	Clinical trial.[279]	Monitor (low level of risk).
	Oral contraceptives	May increase metabolism of drug.	Breakthrough bleeding reported which was attributed to increased metabolism of drug.[239,261] Clinical significance unclear. Cases of unwanted pregnancies have been reported.[280,281] Contradictory results for effect on bioavailability, hormone levels and ovulation demonstrated in three clinical studies, although some breakthrough bleeding occurred.[282–284] In one clinical trial an extract low in hyperforin did not affect plasma contraceptive drug levels or cause breakthrough bleeding.[285] Clinical trial: clearance of levonorgestrel at emergency contraceptive doses increased (not statistically significant).[286] Clinical study: antiandrogenic effect of contraceptive not affected.[287]	Hyperforin-rich extracts: Monitor (medium level of risk). Low-hyperforin extracts: Monitor (very low level of risk).
	Oxycodone	Decreases drug levels.	Clinical trial with healthy volunteers.[288]	Monitor (medium level of risk).
	SSRIs, e.g. paroxetine, trazodone, sertraline and other serotonergic agents, e.g. nefazodone, venlafaxine	Potentiation effects possible with regard to serotonin levels.	Case reports: clinical significance unclear.[289–294]	Monitor (very low level of risk).
	Statin drugs	May decrease effect and/or drug levels.	Atorvastatin: Clinical study, serum LDL-cholesterol increased by 0.32 mmol/L which corresponds to a decrease in effect of drug in patients by about 30%. Serum total cholesterol was also increased.[295] Pravastatin: Clinical study, no effect on plasma level in healthy volunteers.[296] Rosuvastatin: Case report.[297] Simvastatin: Two clinical studies, decrease in drug levels in healthy volunteers,[296] and small increases in serum total cholesterol and LDL-cholesterol in patients.[298]	Monitor blood cholesterol regularly (medium level of risk).
	Talinolol	May decrease drug levels.	Clinical study with healthy volunteers.[299]	Monitor (medium level of risk).
	Theophylline	May decrease drug levels.	Case report.[300] No effect observed in clinical study.[301]	Monitor (low level of risk).
	Voriconazole	Decreases drug levels.	Clinical study.[302]	Monitor (medium level of risk).
	Zolpidem	May decrease drug levels (but with wide inter-subject variability).[FF]	Clinical study (healthy volunteers).[303]	Monitor (low level of risk).

Herb	Drug	Potential interaction	Basis of concern	Recommended action
St Mary's Thistle *Silybum marianum* (See also Polyphenol-containing herbs)	Hypoglycaemic drugs, including insulin	May improve insulin sensitivity.	Controlled trials: improved glycaemic control and reduced insulin requirements in patients with type 2 diabetes and cirrhosis (silymarin: 600 mg/day),[304] improved glycaemic control in diabetics treated with hypoglycaemic drugs (silymarin: 200 and 600 mg/day);[305,306] but no effect on glucose metabolism in NAFLD patients including those with insulin resistance (silymarin: 280 and 600 mg/day).[307,308]	Prescribe cautiously and monitor blood sugar regularly. Warn patient about possible hypoglycaemic effects. Reduce drug if necessary in conjunction with prescribing physician.
	Immuno-suppressives, e.g. sirolimus	May decrease drug clearance.	Population pharmacokinetic study with 112 Chinese adult renal transplant recipients: clearance of sirolimus decreased in those patients with abnormal ALT values who were taking silymarin formulations (route and dosage unknown).[181]	Monitor (medium level of risk) in hepatically impaired patients.
	Metronidazole	May decrease absorption of drug by increasing clearance.	Clinical study with healthy volunteers (silymarin: 140 mg/day).[309]	Monitor (medium level of risk).
	Nifedipine	May delay the absorption rate of drug.	Clinical study with healthy volunteers (silymarin: 280 mg/day), but bioavailability unchanged.[310]	Monitor (low level of risk).
	Ornidazole	May increase drug levels.	Clinical study with healthy volunteers (silymarin: 140 mg/day).[311]	Monitor (medium level of risk).
	Talinolol	May increase drug levels.	Clinical study with healthy volunteers (silymarin: 420 mg/day).[312]	Monitor (low level of risk).
Tannin-containing or OPC-containing herbs eg agrimony (*Agrimonia eupatoria*), bearberry (*Arctostaphylos uva-ursi*), cranesbill root (*Geranium maculatum*), grape seed extract (*Vitis vinifera*), green tea (*Camellia sinensis*), hawthorn (*Crataegus spp.*), lemon balm (*Melissa officinalis*), meadowsweet (*Filipendula ulmaria*), peppermint (*Mentha x piperita*), Pelargonium (*Pelargonium sidoides*), pine bark (*Pinus massoniana*), raspberry leaf (*Rubus idaeus*), sage (*Salvia fruticosa*), St John's wort (*Hypericum perforatum*), willow bark (*Salix spp.*) (See also Polyphenol-containing herbs)	Minerals, especially iron	Iron: May reduce absorption of non-haem iron[T] from food. Zinc: May reduce absorption from food. Clinical studies with healthy volunteers: results conflicting for effect on zinc (undefined tea,[326] black tea[194] consumed at or immediately after food).	Clinical studies in healthy volunteers, administration during or immediately following the meal [188,313–320] (black tea, typical strength: 0.8-3.3 g/100 mL;[188,313–317,319] sorghum[GG] (0.15% tannins)[318]), and in women with iron deficiency anaemia (IDA)[321] (black tea: 1-2×150 mL of 1:100 infusion containing 78 mg of tannins per 150 mL).[321] Iron absorption reduced to a greater extent in those with IDA.[321] However, the results from single test meals may exaggerate the effect of iron inhibitors and enhancers.[322] Effects were not significant in a 14-day study.[194] Cases of IDA resistant to treatment: heavy black tea drinkers (2 cases, 1.5-2 L/day).[323,324] Epidemiological studies (12, to 2002) found mixed results, but some evidence of an association between drinking black tea and poor iron status.[322] Clinical study in patients with haemochromatosis (black tea: 250 mL with meal).[325]	Take at least 2 hours away from food or medication. Take at least 2 hours away from food or medication.
Turmeric (*Curcuma longa*)	Talinolol	May decrease drug levels.	Clinical study with healthy volunteers (300 mg/day of curcumin).[327]	Monitor at high doses (≥300 mg/day curcumin, low level of risk).

Herb	Drug	Potential interaction	Basis of concern	Recommended action
Valerians Mexican Valerian (*Valeriana edulis*), Valerian (*Valeriana officinalis*)	CNS depressants or alcohol	May potentiate effects of drug.	Theoretical concern expressed by US Pharmacopeial Convention.[328] However a clinical study found no potentiation with alcohol.[329] Case report of adverse effect with benzodiazepine drug[330] – herb dosage undefined but likely high (tablet contained valerian and passionflower (*Passiflora incarnata*)).	Monitor (very low level of risk).
Willow Bark *Salix alba, Salix daphnoides, Salix purpurea*, Salix fragilis. (See also Tannin-containing herbs)	Warfarin	May potentiate effects of drug.	Herb alone Clinical study observed very mild but statistically significant antiplatelet activity (extract containing 240 mg/day of salicin).[331]	Monitor (low level of risk).

CODE FOR RECOMMENDED ACTION

Contraindicated: Do not prescribe the indicated herb.

Monitor: Can prescribe the indicated herb but maintain close contact and review the patient's status on a regular basis. Note that where the risk is assessed as medium, self-prescription of the herb in conjunction with the drug is not advisable.

Abbreviations:
ACE: angiotensin-converting enzyme; **ALT:** alanine transaminase, also known as glutamic pyruvic transaminase (GPT); **AMP:** adenosine monophosphate; **APTT:** activated partial thromboplastin time; **CNS:** central nervous system; **CYP:** cytochrome P450; **ECG:** electrocardiogram/graph; **EGCG:** epigallocatechin gallate; **GAS:** ginseng abuse syndrome; **HIV:** human immunodeficiency virus; **IDA:** iron deficiency anaemia; **INR:** international normalized ratio; **NAFLD:** nonalcoholic fatty liver disease; **OPC:** oligomeric procyanidin; **PCOS:** polycystic ovary syndrome; **PT:** prothrombin time; **SSRI:** selective serotonin reuptake inhibitor; **tds:** three times per day; **>:** greater than; **≥:** greater than or equal to; **<:** less than.

Footnotes:
*This chart contains information the authors believe to be reliable or that has received considerable attention as posing potential issues. However, speculative and theoretical concerns expressed by many other authors have not been included. Due to the focus on safety, positive interactions between herbs and drugs, and the effect of drugs on the bioavailability of herbs are generally not included.

A. Research paper describes administration of Scutellaria radix. Trial authors confirm this was root of Baical skullcap (*Scutellaria baicalensis*).[332]

B. Analysis of Baical skullcap root samples from Japan found the baicalin content varied from 3.5 to 12%. For a dose of 150 mg/day of baicalin, 1.2-4.3 g/day of dried root would be required.[333]

C. Single-strength (freshly squeezed, 100%) cranberry juice is highly acidic and astringent, making it unpalatable. For this reason, cranberry juice is usually diluted and sweetened (often known as cranberry juice drink). Cranberry juice cocktail usually contains 25% cranberry juice, although can be up to 35%. Cranberry juice drinks contain about 10% cranberry juice. Cranberry sauce is about half the strength of cranberry juice cocktail, about the same strength as juice drinks. Cranberry juice can be concentrated to a dry powder (unsweetened and usually up to 25:1) and used in tablets and capsules. Juices can be prepared by diluting juice concentrates yielding a concentrated juice (e.g. double strength juice, at twice the strength of single-strength, squeezed juice). It is likely that unless defined, cranberry juice referred to in case reports and clinical studies is juice drink containing around 10% cranberry juice.

D. Refer to Assessment of Risk and Recommended Action above for definition of the extent of this interaction.

E. The cranberry 'juice' administered was similar in concentration to a reference cranberry 'juice' containing about 25% cranberry juice,[334] but with a higher concentration of anthocyanins, and lower in catechins and organic acids. *See also note C.*

F. No effect overall when midazolam was administered orally: oral clearance and area under the drug concentration-time curve were unchanged.

G. These four trials used tablets containing a concentrated, standardised extract. A dosage of 900 mg/day of dry extract was equivalent to about 2.7 g/day of fresh garlic,[335] and was said to contain 12 mg/day of alliin,[53,61] although there is some doubt as to the amount of allicin released from this brand of tablet from around 1995 to 2000.[336]

H. Ginkgotoxin (4'-O-methylpyridoxine) is present in substantial amounts in Ginkgo seed, and convulsions arising from ingestion of Ginkgo seed have been documented in Japan (infants are particularly vulnerable). Ginkgotoxin is known to inhibit vitamin B6 phosphorylation, which may lead to increased neuronal excitability.[337] Poisoning by ginkgotoxin can be counteracted by vitamin B6,[337] in cases of poisoning it is administered by intravenous injection.[338,339] Ginkgotoxin is present in very small amounts in standardised Ginkgo leaf extracts,[340] but is below the detection limits in human plasma after oral doses (240 mg of 50:1 extract, equivalent to 12 g of dried leaf).[341] According to the manufacturer, despite the extensive use of this special extract (more than 150 million daily doses per year for more than two decades) no cases of epileptic seizure have been attributed to this extract.[341] (Ginkgo preparations associated with the above case reports were undefined.) Strictly speaking this is a potential adverse effect (rather than a herb–drug interaction) as there is no pharmacokinetic data indicating an interaction for coadministration of Ginkgo and anticonvulsants in humans. An interaction is suggested though, because Ginkgo has been found to induce CYP2C19 activity (see entry for omeprazole), an enzyme involved in the metabolism of some anticonvulsants.

J. Analysis of over 320 000 patients in a German adverse drug reaction reporting system (1999-2002) found no increase in prevalence of bleeding during Ginkgo intake compared to periods without Ginkgo in those taking anticoagulant or antiplatelet medication.[342] In a trial involving 3069 healthy volunteers treated for an average of 6.1 years, there were no statistically significant differences between placebo and Ginkgo in the rate of major bleeding or the incidence of bleeding in individuals taking aspirin. (Compliance during the trial was however low (at the end of the trial, about 60% were taking Ginkgo/placebo).)[343] In Korea, Ginkgo extract is administered with ticlopidine for the prevention of ischaemic stroke or acute coronary syndrome.[344]

K. The in vitro study found a pronounced anticytotoxic effect for a concentration of 2.5-5 µM of EGCG, and when applied as green tea polyphenols a very substantial effect occurred at a EGCG concentration of 1 µM (the other polyphenols may contribute to the activity).[108] A pharmacokinetic study with healthy volunteers found a EGCG plasma concentration of 0.7 µM after a dose of 580 mg of EGCG, and a EGCG plasma concentration of 0.5 µM after a dose of 1 g of green tea polyphenols.[345]

L. Better gastric tolerance to metformin was noted in the psyllium group of one trial.[126]

M. Glycyrrhetinic acid is the aglycone of glycyrrhizin. Glycyrrhizin is the glycoside and contains the aglycone (glycyrrhetinic acid) and a sugar unit.

N. No effect on blood pressure in healthy volunteers in two studies (130 mg/day of glycyrrhetinic acid = 227 mg/day of glycyrrhizin, for 14 days;[164] licorice (266 mg/day of glycyrrhizin) for 56 days;[346] including where plasma renin levels were high (3.1 ng/mL/h),[346] but in another study, blood pressure increased in healthy volunteers taking 546 mg/day of glycyrrhizin for 4 weeks, only for those with plasma renin activity greater than 1.5 ng/mL/h.[347]

P. This is a guide, based on a recommendation from the German Commission E for long-term consumption of licorice as a flavouring. Glycyrrhizin is also known as glycyrrhizinic acid and glycyrrhizic acid.

Q. ACE-inhibitors cause mild natriuresis (an increase in sodium excretion in the urine) and occasionally hyperkalaemia. The mechanism of the interaction is not known, although it may involve opposing effects on 11beta-hydroxysteroid dehydrogenase type 2 (glycyrrhizin inhibiting, ACE-inhibitor promoting), thus affecting mineralocorticoid receptor activity. Reduction of drug dosage revealed the existing hypokalaemia caused by this dosage of glycyrrhizin.

R. A higher prednisolone/prednisone ratio indicates decreased conversion of prednisolone (active) to prednisone (inactive). Glycyrrhetinic acid (GA) is the aglycone of glycyrrhizin (GL). GL is the glycoside and contains the aglycone (GA) and a sugar unit.

S. The word tannin has a long established and extensive usage although it is considered in more recent years to lack precision. Polyphenol is the preferred term when considering the properties at a molecular level. Plant polyphenols are broadly divisible into proanthocyanidins (condensed tannins) and polymers of esters based on gallic and/or hexahydroxydiphenic acid and their derivatives (hydrolysable tannins).[348] The terms 'tannin' and 'polyphenol' are sometimes used interchangeably. For example, the results of a clinical study are described: 'polyphenols present in tea and coffee inhibited iron absorption in a dose-dependent manner'. The 'polyphenol' content was measured using a spectrophotometric method for the determination of 'tannins and other polyphenolics'.[320] Depending on the analytical method used, it is possible that the polyphenol content may actually be the content of tannins or tannins + polyphenols.[349] It is recommended that both sections of this chart be considered: Polyphenol-containing or Flavonoid-containing herbs, and Tannin-containing or OPC-containing herbs.

T. Haem iron is derived from haemoglobin and myoglobin mainly in meat products. Non-haem iron is derived mainly from cereals, vegetables and fruits.

U. At an identical concentration of total polyphenols, black tea was more inhibitory than all the herb teas excluding peppermint: black tea was of equal inhibition to peppermint tea.[188] The type of polyphenols present, as well as the concentration, may affect iron absorption.

V. Another clinical study also found a dose-dependent effect, and the reduced absorption was most marked when coffee was taken with the meal or 1 hour later. No decrease in iron absorption occurred when coffee was consumed 1 hour before the meal.[319]

W. Administered in freeze-dried form (4.2 g), which would be expected to have a lower inhibitory effect than with the use of fresh chilli, as freeze drying probably decreased the ascorbic acid content (ascorbic acid enhances iron absorption).[190]

X. The different results for cayenne and turmeric under the same experimental conditions, suggest it is not only the quantity of polyphenol present that determines the inhibition, but also for example, the structure of the polyphenol (and hence mechanism of iron binding).[190]

Y. Plant part defined in other publication.[350]

Z. Orlistat inhibits gastric and pancreatic lipases in the lumen of the stomach and small intestine which leads to decreased absorption of dietary fat, and the subsequent excretion of the unabsorbed fats in faeces. No systemic absorption is required to exert its therapeutic effect.

AA. This procedure has been adopted in clinical trials where hypocholesterolaemic drugs (statins) were coadministered.[351,352]

BB. Fructus Schisandra is defined as the fruit of *Schisandra chinensis* or *Schisandra sphenanthera* in traditional Chinese medicine. The major constituents are dibenzocyclooctene lignans. Several factors including harvest season, origin of herb and extraction solvent affect the levels of the individual lignans. Aqueous or ethanolic extracts of *S. chinensis* are not likely to contain more than 2.5 mg/g of deoxyschisandrin.[353,354] A maximum dose of *S. chinensis* extract equivalent to 4 g/day, would provide 10 mg/day of deoxyschisandrin.

CC. Eleutherosides (from Siberian ginseng) and ginsenosides (from Korean ginseng) have some structural similarity with digoxin. Because of this similarity interference with serum digoxin measurements is possible, as confirmed when mice fed these herbs demonstrated digoxin activity in their serum. More specific assays are able to negate the interference.[355]

DD. As noted for several drugs, the hyperforin content of the St John's wort preparation, as well as the dosage of herb, affects the extent of the interaction. All types of preparations can contain hyperforin, including dry extracts used in tablets and capsules. Hyperforin is however, unstable – particularly when in solution.[356] Tinctures and liquid extracts made using a standard ethanol content (45%) contain negligible amounts of hyperforin. Liquid extracts using a higher ethanol content (such as 60%) will contain a higher initial amount of hyperforin than standard liquid extracts. Over time the hyperforin content is substantially reduced and after a few months tinctures and liquid extracts contain no hyperforin.[357]

EE. Genetic polymorphisms are important in determining differences in the response to drugs, and may influence interactions. There are many genetic variants of the CYP genes, including the CYP2C19 gene. Phenotypes of CYP2C19 have been classified functionally as extensive metabolisers and poor metabolisers, the latter having a deficiency of CYP2C19 activity.[183,358]

FF. In 3 of the 14 volunteers a small increase in AUC was observed after administration of St John's wort.

GG. Sorghum also contains phytate. Both phytate and polyphenol inhibit nutrients such as iron.[359,360]

General reference

Braun L. *Herb Drug Interaction Guide for Pharmacists*. FH Faulding, August 2000; Fugh-Berman A. *Lancet*. 2000 355(9198):134–138.

References

1. Yi SJ, Cho JY, Lim KS, et al. *Basic Clin Pharmacol Toxicol*. 2009;105(4):249–256.
2. Fan L, Zhang W, Guo D, et al. *Clin Pharmacol Ther*. 2008;83(3):471–476.
3. Chan E. *Biol Neonate*. 1993;63(4):201–208.
4. Pulliero G, Montin S, Bettini V, et al. *Fitoterapia*. 1989;60(1):69–75.
5. Duterte M, Waugh S, Thanawala R. *Am J Gastroenterol*. 2007;102(Suppl 2):S350.
6. Aktas C, Senkal V, Sarikaya S, et al. *Turk J Geriatr*. 2011;14(1):79–81.
7. Patel NM, Derkits RM. *J Pharm Pract*. 2007;20(4):341–346.
8. de Smet P.A.G.M.Keller K, Hansel R, editors. *Adverse Effects of Herbal Drugs*, vol. 3. Berlin: Springer-Verlag; 1997.
9. Miller LG. *Arch Intern Med*. 1998;158(20):2200–2211.
10. de Smet P.A.G.M.Keller K, Hansel R, editors. *Adverse Effects of Herbal Drugs*, vol. 2. Berlin: Springer-Verlag; 1993.
11. Blumenthal M, ed. *The Complete German Commission E Monographs: Therapeutic Guide to Herbal Medicines*. Austin: American Botanical Council; 1998.
12. Lopez Galera RM, Ribera Pascuet E, Esteban Mur JI, et al. *Eur J Clin Pharmacol*. 2008;64(12):1235–1236.
13. Hakas JF. *Ann Allergy*. 1990;65(4): 322–323.
14. Bouraoui A, Toum A, Bouchoucha S, et al. *Therapie*. 1986;41(6):467–471.
15. Moses G. *Australian Prescriber*. 2001;24(1):6.
16. de Souza NJ. *J Ethnopharmacol*. 1993;38(2–3):177–180.
17. de Souza NJ, Dohadwalla AN, Reden J. *Med Res Rev*. 1983;3(2):201–219.
18. Dubey MP, Srimal RC, Nityanand S, et al. *J Ethnopharmacol*. 1981;3(1):1–13.
19. Sabinsa Corporation. *ForsLean® Product Information*. Available from <www.forslean.com>; Accessed November 2004.
20. Henderson S, Magu B, Rasmussen C, et al. *J Int Soc Sports Nutr*. 2005;2(2):54–62.
21. Seamon KB, Daly JW. *J Cyclic Nucleotide Res*. 1981;7(4):201–224.
22. Ngo N, Yan Z, Graf TN, et al. *Drug Metab Dispos*. 2009;37(3):514–522.
23. Lilja JJ, Backman JT, Neuvonen PJ. *Clin Pharmacol Ther*. 2007;81(6):833–839.
24. Medicines and Healthcare Products Regulatory Agency, Committee on Safety of Medicines. *Current Problems in Pharmacovigilance*. vol. 30. October 2004, p. 10.
25. Rindone JP, Murphy TW. *Am J Ther*. 2006;13(3):283–284.
26. Sylvan L, Justice NP. *Am Fam Physician*. 2005;72(6):1000.
27. Paeng CH, Sprague M, Jackevicius CA. *Clin Ther*. 2007;29(8):1730–1735.
28. Welch JM, Forster K. *J Pharm Technol*. 2007;23(2):104–107.
29. Mergenhagen KA, Sherman O. *Am J Health Syst Pharm*. 2008;65(22): 2113–2116.
30. Griffiths AP, Beddall A, Pegler S. *J R Soc Promot Health*. 2008;128(6):324–326.
31. Hamann GL, Campbell JD, George CM. *Ann Pharmacother*. 2011;45(3):e17.
32. Li Z, Seeram NP, Carpenter CL, et al. *J Am Diet Assoc*. 2006;106(12):2057–2061.
33. Ansell J, McDonough M, Zhao Y, et al. *J Clin Pharmacol*. 2009;49(7):824–830.
34. Mohammed Abdul MI, Jiang X, Williams KM, et al. *Br J Pharmacol*. 2008;154(8):1691–1700.
35. Mellen CK, Ford M, Rindone JP. *Br J Clin Pharmacol*. 2010;70(1):139–142.
36. Qiu F, Wang J, Zhang R, et al. *Brit J Clin Pharmacol*. 2010;69(6):656–662.
37. Tam LS, Chan TYK, Leung WK, et al. *Aust NZ J Med*. 1995;25(3):258.
38. Yu CM, Chan JCN, Sanderson JE. *J Intern Med*. 1997;241(4):337–339.
39. Izzat MB, Yim APC, El-Zufari MH. *Ann Thorac Surg*. 1998;66(3):941–942.
40. Shaw D, Leon C, Kolev S, et al. *Drug Saf*. 1997;17(5):342–356.
41. Page RL, Lawrence JD. *Pharmacotherapy*. 1999;19(7):870–876.
42. Ellis GR, Stephens MR. *BMJ*. 1999;319(7210):650.
43. Moltó J, Valle M, Miranda C, et al. *Antimicrob Agents Chemother*. 2011;55(1):326–330.
44. Mills S, Bone K. *Principles and Practice of Phytotherapy: Modern Herbal Medicine*. Edinburgh: Churchill Livingstone; 2000.
45. Newall CA, Anderson LA, Phillipson JD. *Herbal Medicines – A Guide for Health–Care Professionals*. London: Pharmaceutical Press; 1996.
46. Gorski JC, Huang SM, Pinto A, et al. *Clin Pharmacol Ther*. 2004;75(1):89–100.
47. Mills S, Bone K. *The Essential Guide to Herbal Safety*. USA: Churchill Livingstone; 2005.
48. Rose KD, Croissant PD, Parliament CF, et al. *Neurosurgery*. 1990;26(5): 880–882.
49. Burnham BE. *Plast Reconstr Surg*. 1995;95(1):213.
50. German K, Kumar U, Blackford HN. *Br J Urol*. 1995;76(4):518.
51. Carden SM, Good WV, Carden PA, et al. *Clin Experiment Ophthalmol*. 2002;30(4):303–304.
52. Manoharan A, Gemmell R, Hartwell T. *Am J Hematol*. 2006;81(9):676–683.
53. Legnani C, Frascaro M, Guazzaloca G, et al. *Arzneim Forsch*. 1993;43(2): 119–122.
54. Kiesewetter H, Jung F, Jung EM, et al. *Eur J Clin Pharmacol*. 1993;45(4):333–336.
55. Kiesewetter H, Jung F, Jung EM, et al. *Clin Investig*. 1993;71(5):383–386.
56. Harenberg J, Giese C, Zimmermann R. *Atherosclerosis*. 1988;74(3):247–249.
57. Ali M, Thomson M. *Prostaglandins Leukot Essent Fatty Acids*. 1995;53(3):211–212.
58. Luley C, Lehmann-Leo W, Moller B, et al. *Arzneim Forsch*. 1986;36(4):766–768.
59. Scharbert G, Kalb ML, Duris M, et al. *Anesth Analg*. 2007;105(5):1214–1218.
60. Jain RC. *Am J Clin Nutr*. 1977;30(9):1380–1381.
61. Lawson LD. *FASEB J*. 2007;21(6):A1126.
62. Gadkari JV, Joshi VD. *J Postgrad Med*. 1991;37(3):128–131.
63. Sunter W. *Pharm J*. 1991;246:722.
64. Piscitelli SC, Burstein AH, Welden N, et al. *Clin Infect Dis*. 2002;34(2): 234–238.
65. Hajda J, Rentsch KM, Gubler C, et al. *Eur J Pharm Sci*. 2010;41(5):729–735.
66. Kruth P, Brosi E, Fux R, et al. *Ann Pharmacother*. 2004;38(2):257–260.
67. Verma SK, Singh J, Khamesra R, et al. *Indian J Med Res*. 1993;98:240–242.
68. Bordia A, Verma SK, Srivastava KC. *Prostaglandins Leukot Essent Fatty Acids*. 1997;56(5):379–384.
69. Lumb AB. *Thromb Haemost*. 1994;71(1):110–111.
70. Srivastava KC. *Prostaglandins Leukot Essent Fatty Acids*. 1989;35(3): 183–185.
71. Lesho EP, Saullo L, Udvari-Nagy S. *Cleve Clin J Med*. 2004;71(8):651–656.
72. Jiang X, Williams KM, Liauw WS, et al. *Br J Clin Pharmacol*. 2005;59(4):425–432.
73. Young HY, Liao JC, Chang YS, et al. *Am J Chin Med*. 2006;34(4):545–551.
74. Granger AS. *Age Ageing*. 2001;30(6): 523–525.
75. Gregory PJ. *Ann Intern Med*. 2001;134(4):344.
76. Kupiec T, Raj V. *J Anal Toxicol*. 2005;29(7):755–758.
77. Bruhn JG. *Phytomedicine*. 2003;10(4):358.
78. Bent S, Goldberg H, Padula A, et al. *J Gen Intern Med*. 2005;20(7):657–661.

79. Griffiths J, Jordon S, Pilon K. *Canadian Adverse Reaction Newsletter.* 2004;14(1):2–3.

80. Pedroso JL, Henriques Aquino CC, Escórcio Bezerra ML, et al. *Neurologist.* 2011;17(2):89–90.

81. Bone KM. *Mol Nutr Food Res.* 2008;52(7):764–771.

82. Chan AL, Leung HW, Wu JW, et al. *J Altern Complement Med.* 2011;17(6): 513–517.

83. DeLoughery TG, Kaye JA, Morris CD, et al. *Blood.* 2002;100(11) [Abstract #3809].

84. Gardner CD, Zehnder JL, Rigby AJ, et al. *Blood Coagul Fibrinolysis.* 2007;18(8):787–793.

85. Wolf HR. *Drugs R D.* 2006;7(3):163–172.

86. Aruna D, Naidu MU. *Br J Clin Pharmacol.* 2007;63(3):333–338.

87. Yeo C, Cho H, Park S, et al. *Clin Pharm Ther.* 2010;87:S43.

88. Kim BH, Kim KP, Lim KS, et al. *Clin Ther.* 2010;32(2):380–390.

89. Lu WJ, Huang JD, Lai ML. *J Clin Pharmacol.* 2006;46(6):628–634.

90. Engelsen J, Nielsen JD, Winther K. *Thromb Haemost.* 2002;87(6):1075–1076.

91. Lai CF, Chang CC, Fu CH, et al. *Pharmacotherapy.* 2002;22(10):1326.

92. Zhang XY, Zhou DF, Su JM, et al. *J Clin Psychopharmacol.* 2001;21(1):85–88.

93. Zhang XY, Zhou DF, Zhang PY, et al. *J Clin Psychiatry.* 2001;62(11):878–883.

94. Atmaca M, Tezcan E, Kuloglu M, et al. *Psychiatry Clin Neurosci.* 2005;59(6): 652–656.

95. Doruk A, Uzun O, Ozsahin A. *Int Clin Psychopharmacol.* 2008;23(4):223–237.

96. Zuo XC, Zhang BK, Jia SJ, et al. *Eur J Clin Pharmacol.* 2010;66(5):503–509.

97. Uchida S, Yamada H, Li XD, et al. *J Clin Pharmacol.* 2006;46(11):1290–1298.

98. Robertson SM, Davey RT, Voell J, et al. *Curr Med Res Opin.* 2008;24(2):591–599.

99. Wiegman DJ, Brinkman K, Franssen EJ. *AIDS.* 2009;23(9):1184–1185.

100. Kudolo GB, Wang W, Javors M, et al. *Clin Nutr.* 2006;25(4):606–616.

101. Personal communication from trial author. Kudolo GB. 29 February 2008.

102. Wang W, Javors M, Blodgett J, et al. *Diabetes.* 2007;56(Suppl 1):A560.

103. Smith M, Lin KM, Zheng MD. *Clin Pharmacol Ther.* 2001;69(2):P86. [Abstract #PIII–89].

104. Yoshioka M, Ohnishi N, Koishi T, et al. *Biol Pharm Bull.* 2004;27(12):2006–2009.

105. Yin OQ, Tomlinson B, Waye MM, et al. *Pharmacogenetics.* 2004;14(12):841–850.

106. Fan L, Mao XQ, Tao GY, et al. *Xenobiotica.* 2009;39(3):249–254.

107. Gurley BJ, Swain A, Hubbard MA, et al. *Clin Pharmacol Ther.* 2008;83(1):61–69.

108. Golden EB, Lam PY, Kardosh A, et al. *Blood.* 2009;113(23):5927–5937.

109. Alemdaroglu NC, Dietz U, Wolffram S, et al. *Biopharm Drug Dispos.* 2008;29(6):335–348.

110. Werba JP, Giroli M, Cavalca V, et al. *Ann Intern Med.* 2008;149(4):286–287.

111. Taylor JR, Wilt VM. *Ann Pharmacother.* 1999;33(4):426–428.

112. Wolkerstorfer H. *MMW.* 1966;108(8):438–441.

113. Jaursch U, Landers E, Schmidt R, et al. *Med Welt.* 1969;27:1547–1552.

114. Tankanow R, Tamer HR, Streetman DS, et al. *J Clin Pharmacol.* 2003;43(6): 637–642.

115. Iwamoto M, Ishizaki T, Sato T. *Planta Med.* 1981;42(1):1–16.

116. Leuchtgens H. *Fortschr Med.* 1993;111(20–21):352–354.

117. Walker AF, Marakis G, Simpson E. *Br J Gen Pract.* 2006;56(527):437–443.

118. Shanmugasundaram ER, Rajeswari G, Baskaran K, et al. *J Ethnopharmacol.* 1990;30(3):281–294.

119. Baskaran K, Kizar Ahamath B, Radha Shanmugasundaram K, et al. *J Ethnopharmacol.* 1990;30(3):295–300.

120. Sharma RD, Raghuram TC, Rao NS. *Eur J Clin Nutr.* 1990;44(4):301–306.

121. Sharma RD, Raghuram TC. *Nutr Res.* 1990;10(7):731–739.

122. Sharma RD, Sarkar A, Hazra DK, et al. *Nutr Res.* 1996;16(8):1331–1339.

123. Madar Z, Abel R, Samish S, et al. *Eur J Clin Nutr.* 1988;42(1):51–54.

124. Raghuram TC, Sharma RD, Sivakumar B, et al. *Phytother Res.* 1994;8:83–86.

125. Kassaian N, Azadbakht L, Forghani B, et al. *Int J Vitam Nutr Res.* 2009;79(1):34–39.

126. Ziai SA, Larijani B, Akhoondzadeh S, et al. *J Ethnopharmacol.* 2005;102(2):202–207.

127. Sartore G, Reitano R, Barison A, et al. *Eur J Clin Nutr.* 2009;63(10):1269–1271.

128. Anderson JW, Allgood LD, Turner J, et al. *Am J Clin Nutr.* 1999;70(4):466–473.

129. Rodriguez-Moran M, Guerrero-Romero F, Lazcano-Burciaga G. *J Diabetes Complications.* 1998;12(5):273–278.

130. Florholmen J, Arvidsson-Lenner R, Jorde R, et al. *Acta Med Scand.* 1982;212(4):237–239.

131. Scott AR, Attenborough Y, Peacock I, et al. *BMJ.* 1988;297(6650):707–710.

132. Sobenin IA, Nedosugova LV, Filatova LV, et al. *Acta Diabetol.* 2008;45(1):1–6.

133. Almeida JC, Grimsley EW. *Ann Intern Med.* 1996;125(11):940–941.

134. Cartledge A, Rutherford J. Rapid response (electronic letter), *BMJ* 12 Feb 2001. Available from bmj.com/cgi/eletters/322/7279/139#12643, downloaded 21/2/02.

135. Herberg KW, Winter U. *2nd International Congress on Phytomedicine.* Munich: September 11–14, Abstract P-77, 1996.

136. Herberg KW. *Blutalkohol.* 1993;30(2): 96–105.

137. Schelosky L, Raffauf C, Jendroska K, et al. *J Neurol Neurosurg Psychiatry.* 1995;58(5):639–640.

138. Yamamoto M, Tamura Y, Kuashima K, et al. [Cited in: Han KH, Choe SC, Kim HS, et al.] *Am J Chin Med.* 1998;26(2):199–209.

139. Han KH, Choe SC, Kim HS, et al. *Am J Chin Med.* 1998;26(2):199–209.

140. Chung IM, Lim JW, Pyun WB, et al. *J Ginseng Res.* 2010;34(3):212–218.

141. Rhee MY, Kim YS, Bae JH, et al. *J Altern Complement Med.* 2011;17(1):45–49.

142. Lee JH, Park HJ. *J Ginseng Res.* 1998;22(3):173–180.

143. Lee JH, Kim SH. *Korean J Nutr.* 1995;28(9):862–871.

144. Shin KS, Lee JJ, Kim YI, et al. *J Ginseng Res.* 2007;31(2):109–116.

145. Janetzky K, Morreale AP. *Am J Health Syst Pharm.* 1997;54(6):692–693.

146. Jiang X, Williams KM, Liauw WS, et al. *Br J Clin Pharmacol.* 2004;57(5):592–599.

147. Lee SH, Ahn YM, Ahn SY, et al. *J Altern Complement Med.* 2008;14(6):715–721.

148. Lee YH, Lee BK, Choi YJ, et al. *Int J Cardiol.* 2010;145(2):275–276.

149. Sotaniemi EA, Haapakoski E, Rautio A. *Diabetes Care.* 1995;18(10):1373–1375.

150. Reeds DN, Patterson BW, Okunade A, et al. *Diabetes Care.* 2011;34(5): 1071–1076.

151. Okuda H, Yoshida R. *Proceedings of the Third International Ginseng Symposium.* Seoul, Korea: Korea Ginseng Research Institute; 1980. pp. 53–57.

152. Ma SW, Benzie IF, Chu TT, et al. *Diabetes Obes Metab.* 2008;10(11):1125–1127.

153. Vuksan V, Sung MK, Sievenpiper JL, et al. *Nutr Metab Cardiovasc Dis.* 2008;18(1):46–56.

154. Tetsutani T, Yamamura M, Yamaguchi T, et al. *Ginseng Rev.* 2000;28:44–47.

155. Jones BD, Runikis AM. *J Clin Psychopharmacol.* 1987;7(3):201–202.

156. Shader RI, Greenblatt DJ. *J Clin Psychopharmacol.* 1988;8(4):235.

157. Gillis CN. *Biochem Pharmacol.* 1997;54(1):1–8.

158. Kim HJ, Woo DS, Lee G, et al. *Br J Urol.* 1998;82(5):744–748.

159. *ESCOP Monographs: The Scientific Foundation for Herbal Medicinal Products,* 2nd ed. Exeter, ESCOP, European Scientific Cooperative on Phytotherapy, 2003.

160. Stormer FC, Reistad R, Alexander J. *Food Chem Toxicol.* 1993;31(4):303–312.

161. Sigurjonsdottir HA, Franzson L, Manhem K, et al. *J Hum Hypertens.* 2001;15(8):549–552.

162. Sigurjonsdottir HA, Manhem K, Axelson M, et al. *J Hum Hypertens.* 2003;17(2):125–131.

163. Sigurjonsdottir HA, Ragnarsson J, Franzson L, et al. *J Hum Hypertens.* 1995;9(5): 345–348.

164. Sobieszczyk P, Borlaug BA, Gornik HL, et al. *Clin Sci.* 2010;119(10):437–442.

165. Brouwers AJ, van der Meulen J. *Ned Tijdschr Geneeskd.* 2001;145(15): 744–747.

166. Iida R, Otsuka Y, Matsumoto K, et al. *Clin Exp Nephrol.* 2006;10(2):131–135.

167. Maeda Y, Inaba N, Aoyagi M, et al. *Intern Med.* 2008;47(14):1345–1348.

168. Shintani S, Murase H, Tsukagoshi H, et al. *Eur Neurol.* 1992;32(1):44–51.

169. Bernardi M, d–Intimo PE, Trevisani F, et al. *Life Sci.* 1994;55(11):863–872.

170. Harada T, Ohtaki E, Misu K, et al. *Cardiology.* 2002;98(4):218.

171. Armanini D, Castello R, Scaroni C, et al. *Eur J Obstet Gynecol Reprod Biol.* 2007;131(1):61–67.

172. Kurisu S, Inoue I, Kawagoe T, et al. *J Am Geriatr Soc.* 2008;56(8):1579–1581.

173. Heidemann HT, Kreuzfelder E. *Klin Wochenschr.* 1983;61(6):303–305.

174. Chataway SJ, Mumford CJ, Ironside JW. *Postgrad Med J.* 1997;73(863):593–594.

175. Folkersen L, Knudsen NA, Teglbjaerg PS. *Ugeskr Laeger.* 1996;158(51):7420–7421.

176. Famularo G, Corsi FM, Giacanelli M. *Acad Emerg Med.* 1999;6(9):960–964.

177. Nielsen I, Pedersen RS. *Lancet.* 1984;323(8389):1305.

178. Conn JW, Rovner DR, Cohen EL. *JAMA.* 1968;205(7):492–496.

179. Sontia B, Mooney J, Gaudet L, et al. *J Clin Hypertens.* 2008;10(2):153–157.

180. Hukkanen J, Ukkola O, Savolainen MJ. *Blood Press.* 2009;18(4):192–195.

181. Jiao Z, Shi XJ, Li ZD, et al. *Br J Clin Pharmacol.* 2009;68(1):47–60.

182. Tu JH, He YJ, Chen Y, et al. *Eur J Clin Pharmacol.* 2010;66(8):805–810.

183. Tu JH, Hu DL, Dai LL, et al. *Xenobiotica.* 2010;40(6):393–399.

184. Chen MF, Shimada F, Kato H, et al. *Endocrinol Jpn.* 1991;38(2):167–174.

185. Conti M, Frey FJ, Escher G, et al. *Nephrol Dial Transplant.* 1994;9(11):1622–1628.

186. Liapina LA, Koval'chuk GA. *Izv Akad Nauk Ser Biol.* 1993;4:625–628.

187. Nowack R, Nowak B. *Nephrol Dial Transplant.* 2005;20(11):2554–2556.

188. Hurrell RF, Reddy M, Cook JD. *Br J Nutr.* 1999;81(4):289–295.

189. Samman S, Sandstrom B, Toft MB, et al. *Am J Clin Nutr.* 2001;73(3):607–612.

190. Tuntipopipat S, Judprasong K, Zeder C, et al. *J Nutr.* 2006;136(12):2970–2974.

191. Olivares M, Pizarro F, Hertrampf E, et al. *Nutrition.* 2007;23(4):296–300.

192. Kubota K, Sakurai T, Nakazato K, et al. *Nippon Ronen Igakkai Zasshi.* 1990;27(5):555–558.

193. Mitamura T, Kitazono M, Yoshimura O, et al. *Nippon Sanka Fujinka Gakkaai Zasshi.* 1989;41(6):688–694.

194. Prystai EA, Kies CV, Driskell JA. *Nutr Res.* 1999;19(2):167–177.

195. Mennen L, Hirvonen T, Arnault N, et al. *Eur J Clin Nutr.* 2007;61(10):1174–1179.

196. Imai K, Nakachi K. *BMJ.* 1995;310(6981):693–696.

197. Ullmann U, Haller J, Bakker GC, et al. *Phytomedicine.* 2005;12(6–7):410–415.

198. Hutchinson C, Bomford A, Geissler CA. *Eur J Clin Nutr.* 2010;64(10):1239–1241.

199. Etman MA. *Drug Dev Indust Pharm.* 1995;21(16):1901–1906.

200. Ettinger AB, Shinnar S, Sinnett MJ, et al. *J Epilepsy.* 1992;5(3):191–193.

201. Brown DD, Juhl RP, Warner SL. *Am J Cardiol.* 1977;39(2):297.

202. Nordstrom M, Melander A, Robertsson E, et al. *Drug Nutr Interact.* 1987;5(2): 67–69.

203. Walan A, Bergdahl B, Skoog M–L. *Scand J Gastroenterol.* 1977;12(Supp 45):111.

204. Reissell P, Manninen V. *Acta Med Scand Suppl.* 1982;668:88–90.

205. Rossander L. *Scand J Gastroenterol Suppl.* 1987;129:68–72.

206. Sierra M, García JJ, Fernández N, et al. *Eur J Clin Nutr.* 2002;56(9):830–842.

207. Dennison BA, Levine DM. *J Pediatr.* 1993;123(1):24–29.

208. Burton R, Manninen V. *Acta Med Scand Suppl.* 1982;668:91–94.

209. Kawatra A, Bhat CM, Arora A. *Eur J Clin Nutr.* 1993;47(4):297–300.

210. Enzi G, Inelmen EM, Crepaldi G. *Pharmatherapeutica.* 1980;2(7):421–428.

211. Perlman BB. *Lancet.* 1990;335(8686):416.

212. Toutoungi M, Schulz P, Widmer J, et al. *Therapie.* 1990;45(4):358–360.

213. Robinson DS, Benjamin DM, McCormack JJ. *Clin Pharmacol Ther.* 1971;12(3): 491–495.

214. Cavaliere H, Floriano I, Medeiros-Neto G. *Int J Obes Relat Metab Disord.* 2001;25(7):1095–1099.

215. Liel Y, Harman-Boehm I, Shany S. *J Clin Endocrinol Metab.* 1996;81(2):857–859.

216. Chiu AC, Sherman SI. *Thyroid.* 1998;8(8):667–671.

217. Xin HW, Wu XC, Li Q, et al. *Br J Clin Pharmacol.* 2007;64(4):469–475.

218. Jiang W, Wang X, Xu X, et al. *Int J Clin Pharmacol Ther.* 2010;48(3):224–229.

219. Jiang W, Wang X, Kong L. *Immunopharmacol Immunotoxicol.* 2010;32(1):177–178.

220. Xin HW, Wu XC, Li Q, et al. *Br J Clin Pharmacol.* 2009;67(5):541–546.

221. Ko KM, Ip SP, Poon MK, et al. *Planta Med.* 1995;61(2):134–137.

222. Lu H, Liu GT. *Zhongguo Yao Li Xue Bao.* 1990;11(4):331–335.

223. McRae S. *Can Med Assoc J.* 1996;155(3):293–295.

224. Cicero AF, Derosa G, Brillante R, et al. *Arch Gerontol Geriatr Suppl.* 2004(9): 69–73.

225. Johne A, Schmider J, Brockmoller J, et al. *J Clin Psychopharmacol.* 2002;22(1):46–54.

226. Australian Therapeutic Goods Administration. Media Release, March 2000.

227. Breckenridge A. Message from Committee on Safety of Medicines, 29 February. London, 2000, Medicines Control Agency.

228. Henney JE. *JAMA.* 2000;283(13):1679.

229. Burstein AH, Horton RL, Dunn T, et al. *Clin Pharmacol Ther.* 2000;68(6): 605–612.

230. *Drug Safety Update.* November 2007;1(4):p 7. Available from <www. mhra.gov.uk/Publications/Safetyguidance/ DrugSafetyUpdate/index.htm> Accessed 18.04.08.

231. Wang LS, Zhu B, Abd El-Aty AM, et al. *J Clin Pharmacol.* 2004;44(6):577–581.

232. Wang Z, Hamman MA, Huang SM, et al. *Clin Pharmacol Ther.* 2002;71(6):414–420.

233. Dresser GK, Schwarz UI, Wilkinson GR, et al. *Clin Pharmacol Ther.* 2003;73(1):41–50.

234. Lau WC, Gurbel PA, Carville DG, et al. *J Am Coll Cardiol.* 2007;49(9, Suppl 1):343A–344A.

235. Lau WC, Welch TD, Shields TA, et al. *J Am Coll Cardiol.* 2010;55(10, Suppl 1):A171. [E1600].

236. Lau WC, Welch TD, Shields T, et al. *J Cardiovasc Pharmacol.* 2011;57(1):86–93.

237. Fitzgerald DJ, Maree A. *Hematology Am Soc Hematol Educ Program.* 2007(1): 114–120.

238. Maurer A, Johne A, Bauer S, et al. *Eur J Clin Pharmacol.* 1999;55(3):A22.

239. Yue QY, Bergquist C, Gerden B. *Lancet.* 2000;355(9203):576–577.

240. Barnes J, Anderson LA, Phillipson JD. *J Pharm Pharmacol.* 2001;53(5):583–600.

241. Uygur Bayramıçlı O, Kalkay MN, Oskay Bozkaya E, et al. *Turk J Gastroenterol.* 2011;22(1):115.

242. Mueller SC, Majcher-Peszynska J, Uehleke B, et al. *Eur J Clin Pharmacol.* 2006;62(1):29–36.

243. Arold G, Donath F, Maurer A, et al. *Planta Med.* 2005;71(4):331–337.

244. Markowitz JS, Donovan JL, DeVane CL, et al. *JAMA.* 2003;290(11):1500–1504.

245. Wang Z, Gorski JC, Hamman MA, et al. *Clin Pharmacol Ther.* 2001;70(4): 317–326.

246. Mueller SC, Majcher–Peszynska J, Mundkowski RG, et al. *Eur J Clin Pharmacol.* 2009;65(1):81–87.

247. Kawaguchi A, Ohmori M, Tsuruoka S, et al. *Br J Clin Pharmacol.* 2004;58(4):403–410.

248. Wang XD, Li JL, Lu Y, et al. *J Chromatogr B Analyt Technol Biomed Life Sci.* 2007;852(1–2):534–544.

249. Tannergren C, Engman H, Knutson L, et al. *Clin Pharmacol Ther.* 2004;75(4): 298–309.

250. Mathijssen RH, Verweij J, de Bruijn P, et al. *J Natl Cancer Inst.* 2002;94(16):1247–1249.

251. Mansky PJ, Straus SE. *J Natl Cancer Inst.* 2002;94(16):1187–1188.

252. Smith PF, Bullock JM, Booker BM, et al. *Blood.* 2004;104(4):1229–1230.

253. Frye RF, Fitzgerald SM, Lagattuta TF, et al. *Clin Pharmacol Ther.* 2004;76(4): 323–329.

254. Johne A, Brockmoller J, Bauer S, et al. *Clin Pharmacol Ther.* 1999;66(4): 338–345.

255. Durr D, Stieger B, Kullak-Ublick GA, et al. *Clin Pharmacol Ther.* 2000;68(6):598–604.

256. Mueller SC, Uehleke B, Woehling H, et al. *Clin Pharmacol Ther.* 2004;75(6):546–557.

257. Lundahl A, Hedeland M, Bondesson U, et al. *Eur J Pharm Sci.* 2009;36(4–5): 433–443.

258. de Maat MMR, Hoetelmans RMW, Mathot RAA, et al. *AIDS.* 2001;15(3):420–421.

259. Piscitelli SC, Burstein AH, Chaitt D, et al. *Lancet.* 2000;355(9203):547–548.

260. Xu H, Williams KM, Liauw WS, et al. *Br J Pharmacol.* 2008;153(7):1579–1586.

261. Bon S, Hartmann K, Kuhn M. *Schweiz Apoth.* 1999;16:535–536.

262. Ahmed SM, Banner NR, Dubrey SW. *J Heart Lung Transplant.* 2001;20(7):795.

263. Ruschitzka F, Meier PJ, Turina M, et al. *Lancet.* 2000;355(9203):548–549.

264. Mai I, Kruger H, Budde K, et al. *Int J Clin Pharmacol Ther.* 2000;38(10):500–502.

265. Karliova M, Treichel U, Malago M, et al. *J Hepatol.* 2000;33(5):853–855.

266. Rey JM, Walter G. *Med J Aust.* 1998;169(11–12):583–586.

267. Barone GW, Gurley BJ, Ketel BL, et al. *Transplantation.* 2001;71(2):239–241.

268. Barone GW, Gurley BJ, Ketel BL, et al. *Ann Pharmacother.* 2000;34(9): 1013–1016.

269. Moschella C, Jaber BL. *Am J Kidney Dis.* 2001;38(5):1105–1107.

270. Beer AM, Ostermann T. *Med Klin.* 2001;96(8):480–483.

271. Breidenbach T, Kliem V, Burg M, et al. *Transplantation.* 2000;69(10):2229–2230.

272. Mai I, Bauer S, Perloff ES, et al. *Clin Pharmacol Ther.* 2004;76(4):330–340.

273. Bolley R, Zulke C, Kammerl M, et al. *Transplantation.* 2002;73(6):1009.

274. Mai I, Stormer E, Bauer S, et al. *Nephrol Dial Transplant.* 2003;18(4):819–822.

275. Hebert MF, Park JM, Chen YL, et al. *J Clin Pharmacol.* 2004;44(1):89–94.

276. Portoles A, Terleira A, Calvo A, et al. *J Clin Pharmacol.* 2006;46(10):1188–1194.

277. Eich-Hochli D, Oppliger R, Golay KP, et al. *Pharmacopsychiatry.* 2003;36(1): 35–37.

278. Niederhofer H. *Med Hypotheses.* 2007;68(5):1189.

279. Wang LS, Zhou G, Zhu B, et al. *Clin Pharmacol Ther.* 2004;75(3):191–197.

280. Information from the MPA (Medical Products Agency, Sweden) and the MCA (Medicines Control Agency, UK), 2000–2002.

281. Schwarz UI, Buschel B, Kirch W. *Br J Clin Pharmacol.* 2003;55(1):112–113.

282. Murphy PA, Kern SE, Stanczyk FZ, et al. *Contraception.* 2005;71(6):402–408.

283. Hall SD, Wang Z, Huang SM, et al. *Clin Pharmacol Ther.* 2003;74(6):525–535.

284. Pfrunder A, Schiesser M, Gerber S, et al. *Br J Clin Pharmacol.* 2003;56(6):683–690.

285. Will-Shahab L, Bauer S, Kunter U, et al. *Eur J Clin Pharmacol.* 2009;65(3): 287–294.

286. Murphy P, Bellows B, Kern S. *Contraception.* 2010;82(2):191.

287. Fogle RH, Murphy PA, Westhoff CL, et al. *Contraception.* 2006;74(3):245–248.

288. Nieminen TH, Hagelberg NM, Saari TI, et al. *Eur J Pain.* 2010;14(8):854–859.

289. Gordon JB. *Am Fam Phys.* 1998;57(5):950–953.

290. Dermott K. *Clinical Psychiatry News.* 1998;26(3):28.

291. Barbenel DM, Yusuf B, O'Shea D, et al. *J Psychopharmacol.* 2000;14(1):84–86.

292. Lantz MS, Buchalter E, Giambanco V. *J Geriatr Psychiatry Neurol.* 1999;12(1): 7–10.

293. Prost N, Tichadou L, Rodor F, et al. *Presse Med.* 2000;29(23):1285–1286.

294. Waksman JC, Heard K, Jolliff H, et al. *Clin Toxicol.* 2000;38(5):521.

295. Andren L, Andreasson A, Eggertsen R. *Eur J Clin Pharmacol.* 2007;63(10):913–916.

296. Sugimoto K, Ohmori M, Tsuruoka S, et al. *Clin Pharmacol Ther.* 2001;70(6): 518–524.

297. Gordon RY, Becker DJ, Rader DJ. *Am J Med.* 2009;122(2):e1–e2.

298. Eggertsen R, Andreasson A, Andren L. *Scand J Prim Health Care.* 2007;25(3):154–159.

299. Schwarz UI, Hanso H, Oertel R, et al. *Clin Pharmacol Ther.* 2007;81(5):669–678.

300. Nebel A, Schneider BJ, Baker RK, et al. *Ann Pharmacother.* 1999;33(4):502.

301. Morimoto T, Kotegawa T, Tsutsumi K, et al. *J Clin Pharmacol.* 2004;44(1): 95–101.

302. Rengelshausen J, Banfield M, Riedel KD, et al. *Clin Pharmacol Ther.* 2005;78(1):25–33.

303. Hojo Y, Echizenya M, Ohkubo T, et al. *J Clin Pharm Ther.* 2011;36(6):711–715.

304. Velussi M, Cernigoi AM, de Monte A, et al. *J Hepatol.* 1997;26(4):871–879.

305. Hussain SA. *J Med Food.* 2007;10(3): 543–547.

306. Huseini HF, Larijani B, Heshmat R, et al. *Phytother Res.* 2006;20(12):1036–1039.

307. Hashemi SJ, Hajiani E, Sardabi EH. *Hep Mon.* 2009;9(4):265–270.

308. Deng YQ, Fan XF, Li JP. *Chin J Integr Med.* 2005;11(2):117–122.

309. Rajnarayana K, Reddy MS, Vidyasagar J, et al. *Arzneim Forsch.* 2004;54(2):109–113.

310. Fuhr U, Beckmann-Knopp S, Jetter A, et al. *Planta Med.* 2007;73(14): 1429–1435.

311. Repalle SS, Yamsani SK, Gannu R, et al. *Acta Pharm Sci.* 2009;51(1):15–20.

312. Han Y, Guo D, Chen Y, et al. *Xenobiotica.* 2009;39(9):694–699.

313. Rossander L, Hallberg L, Bjorn-Rasmussen E. *Am J Clin Nutr.* 1979;32(12): 2484–2489.

314. Disler PB, Lynch SR, Charlton RW, et al. *Gut.* 1975;16(3):193–200.

315. Brune M, Rossander L, Hallberg L. *Eur J Clin Nutr.* 1989;43(8):547–557.

316. Derman D, Sayers M, Lynch SR, et al. *Br J Nutr.* 1977;38(2):261–269.

317. Hallberg L, Rossander L. *Hum Nutr Appl Nutr.* 1982;36(2):116–123.

318. Chung KT, Wong TY, Wei CI, et al. *Crit Rev Food Sci Nutr.* 1998;38(6):421–464.

319. Morck TA, Lynch SR, Cook JD. *Am J Clin Nutr.* 1983;37(3):416–420.

320. Layrisse M, García-Casal MN, Solano L, et al. *J Nutr.* 2000;130(9):2159–2195. [Erratum in: J Nutr 130(12): 3106, 2000].

321. Thankachan P, Walczyk T, Muthayya S, et al. *Am J Clin Nutr.* 2008;87(4):881–886.

322. Nelson M, Poulter J. *J Hum Nutr Diet.* 2004;17(1):43–54.

323. Gabrielli GB, De Sandre G. *Haematologica.* 1995;80(6):518–520.

324. Mahlknecht U, Weidmann E, Seipelt G. *Haematologica.* 2001;86(5):559.

325. Kaltwasser JP, Werner E, Schalk K, et al. *Gut.* 1998;43(5):699–704.

326. Ganji V, Kies CV. *Plant Foods Hum Nutr.* 1994;46(3):267–276.

327. Juan H, Terhaag B, Cong Z, et al. *Eur J Clin Pharmacol.* 2007;63(7):663–668.

328. U.S.P. Drug Information, US Pharmacopeia Patient Leaflet, Valerian (Oral). Rockville: The United States Pharmacopeial Convention; 1998.

329. Herberg KW. *Therapiewoche.* 1994;44(12):704–713.

330. Carrasco MC, Vallejo JR, Pardo-de-Santayana M, et al. *Phytother Res.* 2009;23(12):1795–1796.

331. Krivoy N, Pavlotzky E, Chrubasik S, et al. *Planta Med.* 2001;67(3):209–212.

332. Personal communication from trial author Yu KS. 2 February 2010.

333. Makino T, Hishida A, Goda Y, et al. *Nat Med.* 2008;62(3):294–299.

334. Product information for Cranberry Classic juice drink. Available from <www.oceanspray.com.au> Accessed November 2009.

335. Warshafsky S, Kamer RS, Sivak SL. *Ann Intern Med.* 1993;119(7 Pt 1):599–605.

336. Lawson LD, Wang ZJ, Papadimitriou D. *Planta Med.* 2001;67(1):13–18.

337. Leistner E, Drewke C. *J Nat Prod.* 2010;73(1):86–92.

338. Kajiyama Y, Fujii K, Takeuchi H, et al. *Pediatrics.* 2002;109(2):325–327.

339. Hasegawa S, Oda Y, Ichiyama T, et al. *Pediatr Neurol.* 2006;35(4):275–276.

340. Arenz A, Klein M, Fiehe K, et al. *Planta Med.* 1996;62(6):548–551.

341. Kuenick C. *Dtsch Apoth Ztg.* 2010;150(5):60–61.

342. Gaus W, Westendorf J, Diebow R, et al. *Methods Inf Med.* 2005;44(5):697–703.

343. DeKosky ST, Williamson JD, Fitzpatrick AL, et al. *JAMA.* 2008;300(19):2253–2262.

344. Kim TE, Kim BH, Kim J, et al. *Clin Ther.* 2009;31(10):2249–2257.

345. Henning SM, Niu Y, Liu Y, et al. *J Nutr Biochem.* 2005;16(10):610–616.

346. Mattarello MJ, Benedini S, Fiore C, et al. *Steroids.* 2006;71(5):403–408.

347. Kageyama Y, Suzuki H, Saruta T. *Endocrinol Jpn.* 1991;38(1):103–108.

348. Haslam E, Lilley TH. *Crit Rev Food Sci Nutr.* 1988;27(1):1–40.

349. Price ML, Butler LG. *J Agric Food Chem.* 1977;25(6):1268–1273.

350. Ewerth S, Ahlberg J, Holmstrom B, et al. *Acta Chir Scand Suppl.* 1980;500:49–50.

351. Moreyra AE, Wilson AC, Koraym A. *Arch Intern Med.* 2005;165(10):1161–1166.

352. Agrawal AR, Tandon M, Sharma PL. *Int J Clin Pract.* 2007;61(11):1812–1818.

353. Halstead CW, Lee S, Khoo CS, et al. *J Pharm Biomed Anal.* 2007;45(1):30–37.

354. Zhu M, Chen XS, Wang KX. *Chromatographia.* 2007;66(1–2):125–128.

355. Dasgupta A, Wu S, Actor J, et al. *Am J Clin Pathol.* 2003;119(2):298–303.

356. Ang CYW, Hu L, Heinze TM, et al. *J Agric Food Chem.* 2004;52(20):6156–6164.

357. MediHerb Research Laboratories, 2004.

358. Tomlinson B, Hu M, Lee VW. *Mol Nutr Food Res.* 2008;52(7):799–809.

359. Lynch SR. *Nutr Rev.* 1997;55(4):102–110.

360. Gillooly M, Bothwell TH, Charlton RW, et al. *Br J Nutr.* 1984;51(1):37–46.

General prescribing guidelines

- Exercise great caution when prescribing herbs for patients taking drugs with a narrow therapeutic window. These drugs may become dangerously toxic or ineffective with only relatively small changes in their blood concentrations. Examples include digoxin, warfarin, antirejection (immunosuppressive) drugs, many anti–HIV drugs, theophylline, phenytoin and phenobarbital. These patients need to be monitored on a frequent, regular basis.

- Exercise great caution when prescribing herbs for patients taking drugs:
  - if heart, liver, or kidney function is impaired
  - in elderly patients
  - in pregnant women
  - in those who have received an organ transplant
  - in those with a genetic disorder that disturbs normal biochemical functions.

These patients need to be monitored on a frequent, regular basis.

- Care should be exercised with patients who exhibit long-term use of laxative herbs or potassium-losing diuretics.

- Critical drugs should be taken at different times of the day from herbs (and food) to reduce chemical or pharmacokinetic interactions. They should be separated by at least 1 h, preferably more.

- Stop all herbs approximately 1 week before surgery. St Mary's thistle may help reduce the toxic after-effects of anaesthetic drugs, so it can be taken up to the day before, and then again after surgery (it will not interact with the anaesthesia – see monograph).

- Carefully monitor the effects of drugs such as antihypertensives and antidiabetic drugs when combining with herbal remedies. The herbs may make them more or less effective. In the ideal situation the dose of the drug could be adjusted.

- Interactions may be dose related for the herb and the drug, for example, St John's wort and digoxin (see monograph).

Assessment of risk and recommended action

The best information about HDIs comes from case observations (detailed and validated if possible) and clinical studies. Assessment of the risk of an adverse effect from a potential herb–drug interaction (as done for the table in this appendix) considers several factors:[1,2]

- The quality of the evidence, such as probable causality from case reports (probable/possible/unlikely) and confirmation and ideally repeated results from clinical studies with clinically relevant endpoints.[A]
  - A well-documented case report (especially with a positive rechallenge) does not always constitute a lower level of evidence than a negative result from a controlled trial. This is provided that all other possible causes have been considered and adequately dealt with
  - The quality of the publication should also be considered – a poster from a scientific meeting is regarded as a lower level of evidence than well-documented case reports and controlled trials (due to lack of peer review). Is the pharmacokinetic study placebo-controlled?[B]
  - Theoretical concerns based on pharmacological activity are considered the lowest quality of evidence and are often speculative at best.

- The incidence of the interaction (what is the chance that the interaction occurs? How many well–documented cases are reported compared to the extent of use of the herb?)

- The seriousness of the potential adverse reaction, for example in order of increasing importance:
  - An insignificant clinical effect from an increased drug level without clinical symptoms or an increase in INR (international normalised ratio)[C] up to 4 in the case of warfarin
  - Transient inconvenience (<2 days) without residual symptoms such as fatigue, nausea
  - Failure of therapy for nonserious disease such as decreased effects from an antacid drug

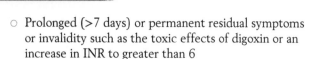

○ Prolonged (>7 days) or permanent residual symptoms or invalidity such as the toxic effects of digoxin or an increase in INR to greater than 6

○ Failure of life–saving therapy such as failure of therapy with antiretroviral drugs or cyclosporin

○ Death or severe side effects

By considering these factors and the totality of evidence, the risk of a herb–drug interaction would range from very low (such as where evidence is poor or lacking and the effect is clinically irrelevant) to contraindicated (such as where the evidence consists of controlled, published interaction studies with a clinically relevant endpoint, the adverse outcome is clinically very relevant, including decreasing plasma levels of drugs being prescribed for serious conditions). An altered plasma drug level in healthy volunteers or even patients without a substantial clinical effect would be considered low or medium risk.

Probe drugs

Studies using probe drugs (which assess individual cytochrome P450 enzyme activity, and hence potential interactions for drugs that utilise that enzyme) are only included in the chart where the drug is currently used clinically. For example, midazolam (a benzodiazepine, used clinically as a sedative and frequently in anaesthesia) is metabolised by CYP3A4 and can be used to assess the interaction of other drugs and herbs with this enzyme (e.g. another drug or herb may inhibit or induce CYP3A4 resulting in increased or decreased plasma drug levels, respectively). A number of drugs are used as probes for CYP3A4 activity such as nifedipine and alprazolam. Other examples of probe drugs included in the chart due to their therapeutic activity include tolbutamide (for CYP2C9 activity), omeprazole (CYP2C19) and talinolol (P-glycoprotein). (P-glycoprotein helps transport molecules across biological membranes and hence can affect the absorption and elimination of a drug.) Although there are a large number of cytochrome P450 enzymes, more than 90% of the metabolism of drugs is due to the activity of CYP1A2, CYP2C9, CYP2C19, CYP2D6, CYP2E1 and CYP3A4. For a comprehensive review of the effect of herbs on probe drugs in clinical trials the reader is referred to the following systematic review: Kennedy DA, Seely D. *Expert Opin Drug Saf* 9(1): 79-124, 2010.

Midazolam is used clinically as a sedative and frequently in anaesthesia. Such studies ideally need to have administered the herb for at least 7 days and investigated drug clearance by using the area under the serum concentration–time curve (AUC).

The US Food and Drug Administration has defined the clinical significance of an interaction that causes an increased plasma level of oral midazolam. The interaction is weak (hence low risk) if the increase in the AUC is between 1.25–and 2-fold; AUC changes ranging from 2- to 5-fold are moderate (hence medium risk) and greater than a 5-fold increase is a strong interaction and may result in contraindication.[3] An increase below 1.25-fold, in other words an increase in the plasma level of midazolam by up to 25%, means no interaction has occurred (i.e. it is clinically insignificant).

HDI chart examples: how the recommended action is determined

CONTRAINDICATED

ST JOHN'S WORT AND DIGOXIN

• Three clinical studies (two controlled with placebo) found St John's wort extract high in hyperforin sharply decreased drug levels. The decrease in drug levels increased with increasing doses of St John's wort.

The evidence is considered to be strong and the adverse outcome is potentially serious, in addition to the drug having a narrow therapeutic window (small changes in blood levels may have considerable pharmacological effect).

DAN SHEN AND WARFARIN

• Three case reports of bleeding complications and elevated INR values (above 5.5) were observed. INR returned to normal target range after cessation of herb. Dan shen was the only substance introduced after the INR was initially stabilised.

Reasonably strong case report evidence and adverse effects considered serious.

BLADDERWRACK AND HYPERTHYROID MEDICATION

BUGLEWEED AND THYROID HORMONES

ECHINACEA AND IMMUNOSUPPRESSANT MEDICATION

Although the evidence is based on theoretical concerns only, the adverse effect from the potential interaction is considered great enough for a suggested contraindication.

MONITOR (MEDIUM LEVEL OF RISK)

ST JOHN'S WORT AND AMITRIPTYLINE

• Clinical study (not controlled with placebo) with patients found a decrease in drug levels.

Evidence considered moderate, given the wide use of the herb. Assigned a medium rather than a low risk due to seriousness of potential adverse outcome.

GARLIC AND HIV PROTEASE INHIBITORS

• Clinical study (2000; not controlled with placebo) with healthy volunteers found an allicin-producing garlic tablet caused significant decrease (from baseline) in plasma drug concentration.

• A probe drug study (2010) also with healthy volunteers taking an allicin-producing garlic tablet, found a non–significant decrease overall in AUC (15%) with large variability (AUC increased in several volunteers).

Evidence considered moderate, as there is an absence of case reports despite the fact that garlic is widely consumed in the diet. Assigned medium rather than low risk due to potential adverse outcome.

GINKGO AND HIV NON–NUCLEOSIDE TRANSCRIPTASE INHIBITORS

• Case report: ingestion of Ginkgo coincided with decreasing drug level.

This is the first case reported for this interaction. The decrease in drug levels coincided approximately when 'the patient appeared to be using Ginkgo'. The long history of stable drug levels prior to the ingestion of Ginkgo, and the patient not taking medications other than antiretroviral therapy are suggestive of a causal effect. Patient 'successfully switched to alternative antiretroviral therapy'. Despite the lack of strong causality, assigned medium due to potential adverse outcome.

MONITOR (LOW LEVEL OF RISK)

ST JOHN'S WORT AND OMEPRAZOLE

- Clinical study with healthy volunteers found that St John's wort extract caused significant decrease in plasma drug concentration.

Evidence considered preliminary or moderate at best. Assigned low due to a lack of seriousness of effects from a potential interaction.

ST JOHN'S WORT AND ANTICONVULSANTS

- Theoretical concern raised in 2000 by regulators on the basis that St John's wort may induce cytochrome P450, the pathway by which some drugs including anticonvulsants are metabolised, thereby potentially increasing their breakdown and reducing their blood concentrations.
- No effect on carbamazepine pharmacokinetics found in a 2000 clinical study with healthy volunteers (not controlled with placebo).
- One case reported with few details in 2007 in which an increase in the frequency and severity of seizures was reported in a patient taking several anticonvulsants, two of which are not metabolised by cytochrome P450.
- A probe drug study (2004) found increased excretion of a mephenytoin metabolite in some volunteers – those with a CYP2C19 wild-type genotype (extensive metabolisers). In poor metabolisers (mutant genotype; having a deficiency of CYP2C19 activity) there was no significant alteration. (Mephenytoin is almost exclusively metabolised by CYP2C19.) The clinical significance is unknown, as plasma drug levels of mephenytoin were not measured.

Evidence considered low, with a clinical study supporting a lack of interaction despite the theoretical concern. Due to the recognised ability of St John's wort to interact with some drugs metabolised via cytochrome P450 (particularly CYP3A4), and the importance of maintaining stable blood levels of anticonvulsants this interaction

was assigned low rather than very low risk. The 2008 case report does not support the theoretical concern (different metabolism). Additional and well-documented case reports would be required to alter the risk assessment.

GINKGO AND TOLBUTAMIDE

- Clinical study with healthy volunteers found a high dose of Ginkgo (50:1 extract: 360 mg/day, equivalent to 18 g/day of dried leaf) decreased the area under concentration versus time curve by 16% (statistically significant, but being less than a 20% decrease this is not regarded as clinically significant). No statistically significant differences found for other pharmacokinetic parameters.
- To assess the effect on the pharmacodynamics of tolbutamide, volunteers were also given a 75 g oral dose of glucose. When combined with Ginkgo the blood glucose lowering effect of tolbutamide was less than with tolbutamide alone, but the difference was not even statistically significant.

The decrease in exposure to tolbutamide caused by a high dose of Ginkgo did not have a significant effect on the ability of tolbutamide to lower glucose in healthy volunteers. Assigned low risk until information in diabetic patients becomes available.

MONITOR (VERY LOW LEVEL OF RISK)

SIBERIAN GINSENG AND DIGOXIN

- One case report: possibly increased plasma concentration of drug but ECG (electrocardiogram) unchanged. The possibility that the herb may have interfered with the digoxin measurement was also raised, and later supported.
- No effect on plasma concentration of drug in later controlled clinical trial.

The case report provides minimal evidence, with a lack of clinical relevance (ECG results) and the possibility of testing interference. The clinical trial results reduce the strength of evidence.

DEVIL'S CLAW AND WARFARIN

- One poorly documented case report.

Minimal evidence with too few details. No other evidence exists to suggest this interaction.

Notes

A. An example of a clinically relevant endpoint is the increase in serum LDL-cholesterol caused by St John's wort in patients taking atorvastatin. In the absence of trials using clinical endpoints how then is the risk assessed? The pharmacokinetics and/or pharmacodynamics are considered, but how much of a pharmacokinetic change should be considered clinically relevant? This issue, in the context of drug–drug interactions, is currently a topic for debate.[4] Tests of statistical significance such as the p value for parameters such as the peak plasma concentration are not necessarily clinically relevant.[3,5]

In interaction trials where clinically relevant endpoints have not been measured, the Food and Drug Administration has provided guidelines to assess the relevance of the pharmacokinetic results. A decrease of 20% up to an increase of 25% in drug exposure (e.g. peak plasma concentration, AUC) does not result in relevant changes of drug effect and no clinically significant interaction is present. (Technically, the 90% confidence interval for the geometric mean ratio of the herb–drug phase to the drug phase needs to be within 0.8 to 1.25.[3]) This limit has been considered too conservative, with a recommendation that the no-effect limit be expanded to ranging from a decrease of 30% up to an increase of 43% in drug exposure (i.e. the ratio falls within 0.7 to 1.43).[6] The FDA no-effect limit does not constitute a hard and fast rule however, as for example, the therapeutic index of the drug should still be considered.[7] Not all clinical studies however provide the information to assess the no-effect limit.

B. A herb–drug interaction can have a pharmacodynamic basis such as similar or opposing pharmacological effects, for example the effect on INR (international normalised ratio), and/or a pharmacokinetic basis (making the drug more or less available to the body).

C. The target therapeutic range for oral anticoagulation is an INR (international normalised ratio) between 2.5 and 3.0 depending on the condition. A rise in INR increases the risk of bleeding (for example, when INR is well above 5.0). A decrease in INR is also considered undesirable as a low INR may increase the risk of clotting.

References

1. Mills S, Bone K, eds. *The Essential Guide to Herbal Safety*. USA: Churchill Livingstone; 2005. pp. 50–88.
2. De Smet PA. *Br J Clin Pharmacol*. 2007;63(3):258–267.
3. *Guidance for industry: drug interaction studies: study design, data analysis and implications for dosing and labeling*. Draft published September 2006. Available from <http://www.fda.gov/ohrms/dockets/dockets/06d0344/06d–0344–c000008–01–vol1.pdf> Accessed November 2011.
4. Fuhr U. *Eur J Clin Pharmacol*. 2007;63(10):897–899.
5. Greenblatt DJ. *Cardiovasc Ther*. 2009;27(4):226–229.
6. Mueller SC, Majcher-Peszynska J, Mundkowski RG, et al. *Eur J Clin Pharmacol*. 2009;65(1):81–87.
7. Butterweck V, Derendorf H. *Clin Pharmacokinet*. 2008;47(6):383–397.

Appendix D: Herbs and children: basic dosage rules

Given the difficulties with metabolism of xenobiotics in young children, it is acknowledged in conventional medicine that dosing in young children is an imprecise affair. The following quotation from *Neonatal and Pediatric Pharmacology: Therapeutic Principles in Practice*, a major textbook in the field, is relevant:[1]

> Optimal tailoring of a drug's *(and we can also read herb's)* dose to the newborn infant and child is a delicate obligation of the treating physician. All suggestions and dosing rules that have been proposed reveal the complexity of the problem. No universal dosage rule can be recommended.

So with that in mind, and the need to be flexible and to use our judgement, the various dosing rules (including briefly how they were developed) are discussed below.[2]

Dosage rules are based on age, weight and, more recently (in the last few decades), the sophisticated concept of body surface area. Most experts agree that body surface area is probably the most valid concept to use in terms of dosage calculations, but the computations can be very complex. There are some simple dosage rules that approximate body surface area (BSA) and can be used as a good substitute in the clinic (see later). The earlier dosage rules used age as the basis for calculation, and Dilling's rule, which is simply the age in years divided by 20 as the fraction of the adult dose, is the oldest. Dilling's rule is said to date from the 8th century, so even as long ago as this it was recognised that a dosage rule for children was needed. This is a very simple rule; in fact, it is overly simplistic and not recommended. Note that in the context of this and other dosage rules, the 'adult dose' is the dose for an adult under similar circumstances.

One of the most commonly used age-based rules, which is more sophisticated and reasonable to use, is Young's rule. The formula is age in years divided by age plus 12 as the fraction of the adult dose. It is debated whether Young's rule becomes valid at the age of 1 or 2, so that is why its applicable range is variously given as children aged 1 to 12 years or children age 2

to 12. A very useful age-based rule for infants is Fried's rule, which is age in months divided by 150 as the fraction of the adult dose. It dictates quite low doses to infants. For example, in the case of a neonate up to 1 month, only 1/150th of the adult dose is given. Fried's rule is a conservative dosage rule, but it should be considered for children up to about 2 years. Where this rule cuts out and another rule cuts in requires some discretion, and the discretionary aspects of Fried's rule will be discussed later. Another age-based rule that is less useful is Gabius' rule which is a simple fixed relationship between age and the fraction of the adult dose: 1 year is 1/12th, 2 years is 1/8th and 3 years 1/6th and so on.

More relevant and useful are the weight-based rules; the first such rule was said to have been proposed by Clark in the 1930s, less than 100 years ago. Only at that time were we becoming sophisticated about understanding dosage rules for children, so this is a very recent phenomenon. Clark's rule was developed in the days before metric weights were widely used in medicine and so was based on pounds. It is weight in pounds divided by 150 as the fraction of the adult dose. This rule is not very sophisticated and not that useful. A much better rule, that represents a refinement of Clark's rule, was developed by Augsberger in the 1960s. He added a factor of 10, in recognition of the faster metabolism of children. The rule is one and a half times the weight in kilograms plus 10 as the percentage of the adult dose. If a child weighs 20 kg, the calculation is 1½ times 20, which equals 30, plus 10, giving 40. Hence, the percentage of the adult dose from Augsberger's rule for this example is 40%. As noted previously, most experts agree that BSA is the best parameter to use in any dosage calculation. Augsberger's rule has been shown to be a good approximation to a body surface area curve in children.[3]

A group of anaesthetists at Salisbury Hospital in the UK have come up with a very simple rule that closely approximates BSA calculations.[3] Anaesthetists, of course, have to know about giving the right doses to children. The rule is

Table 1 Dosage comparisons for the different rules

Child age (weight)	Fried (a)	Young (a)	Gabius (a)	Augsberger (w)	Salisbury (w/bsa)
6 months (8 kg)	4	NA	NA	22	16
1 year (10.5 kg)	8	8	8	26	21
2 years (12.5 kg)	NA	14	12	29	25
4 years (16 kg)	NA	25	25	34	32
7 years (23 kg)	NA	37	33	45	46
10 years (32 kg)	NA	45	40	58	64

Values are expressed as p of adult dose. a=age-based calculation, bsa = body surface area, w=weight-based calculation.

Table 2 Summary of key dosage rules

Young's rule	age/(age+12) is the FRACTION of the adult dose where age=age in years
Fried's rule	(age in months/150) is the FRACTION of the adult dose used for infants up to 24 months
Augsberger's rule	((1.5×weight(kg))+10) is the PERCENTAGE of the adult dose
Salisbury rule	weight(kg)×2 (if weight <30 kg) is the PERCENTAGE of the adult dose weight(kg)+30 (if weight >30 kg) is the PERCENTAGE of the adult dose

weight in kg times 2 as the percentage of the adult dose if the weight of the child is less than 30 kg, and weight plus 30 if the weight is greater than 30 kg. This is called the Salisbury rule. So for a 20 kg child the dose is 40% (20 times 2) of the adult dose. However, for a 35 kg child the dose is 65% (35 plus 30) of the adult dose.

Table 1 provides a comparison of the calculations from the different dosage rules expressed as a percentage of the adult dose. Naturally, the weights of different children vary for any given age, so average weights were used for the purpose of comparison. For the Fried, Young and Gabius rules, and there is an (a) indicating they are based on age. For the Augsberger and Salisbury rules, there is a (w) to indicate they are based on weight, although for the Salisbury rule BSA is added, because that is actually what it aims to approximate. Looking first at the example of a 10-year-old child (average weight 32 kg), the table indicates that there is not a large variation from the various rules that are applicable. The Augsberger and Salisbury rules are in quite good agreement at around 60% of the adult dose. Gabius' and Young's rule tend to be around 40% and probably predict doses that are too low. This is where the age-based rules probably break down: for an older child they tend to lead to underdosing. Looking now at a very young child, say 6 months, there are marked differences. Young's and Gabius' rules do not apply. Fried's rule predicts 4% of the adult dose, Augsberger's predicts 22% and the Salisbury rule indicates 16%. Probably the most accurate rule in this context is the 16% from the Salisbury rule, but we need to take into account that infants have a very high degree of uncertainty because of the factors discussed previously.

Consequently, Fried's rule is recommended as the starting point for dosage in such young patients. The dose can be subsequently adjusted upwards, depending on the response of the patient. But it should be adjusted to no more than that indicated by the Salisbury rule.

The key dosage rules are summarised in Table 2 and the summary recommendations are as follows: for children aged 2 years or older, Augsberger's or the Salisbury rule can be used. For infants less than 2 years, caution dictates that Fried's rule should be used as the dosage starting point, working on the basis of beginning with the minimum effective dosage. This is especially the case when using alcohol-based extracts. The dose can then be increased if necessary towards that predicted by the Salisbury rule, but applying Augsberger's rule to infants is not recommended because it will typically result in overdosing.

While infants do tend to have a reduced capacity to metabolise alcohol, it is usually fully developed by the age of 2 or 3. However, alcohol-based extracts can be given to young children without any associated problems if the above dosage guidelines are observed. As long as these rules are followed, it is safe to give an ethanolic extract to children of any age.

References

1. Sumner JY, Jacob VA, eds. *Neonatal and Pediatric: Pharmacology Therapeutic Principles in Practice* (3rd ed.). USA: Lippincott Williams & Wilkins; 2004. p. 37.
2. Santich R, Bone KM. *Healthy Children: Optimising Children's Health with Herbs.* Warwick: Phytotherapy Press; 2008.
3. Lack JA, Stuart-Taylor ME. *Br J Anaesth.* 1997;78:601–605.

Appendix E: Herbal clinical trial papers: how to read them

Clinicians are faced with an ever-increasing amount of reading material as more research that is clinical is published on herbal medicine. This appendix is designed to assist in the reading of clinical trials and covers the following issues:

- What a randomised controlled trial is
- Why they are important (but are not without limitations)
- A comparison between herbal and conventional medicine in published literature
- The structure of a clinical trial paper
- How to identify a badly written paper
- What to look for when you decide to keep reading
- How to interpret the trial dosages and their relevance to the products you use.

What are randomised controlled trials?

In the hierarchy of generating scientific evidence, randomised controlled trials (RCTs) are considered the gold standard.[1] A randomised clinical trial involves at least one test treatment (such as a herbal medicine) and one control treatment (a placebo or standard treatment, such as a drug). Patients are allocated to the treatment groups by a random process (use of a random-numbers table) to eliminate selection bias and confounding variables. (Note: the toss of a coin, patient social security numbers, days of the week and medical record numbers are considered unacceptable methods for randomisation). For randomisation to be successful, the allocation must remain concealed. In RCTs, some form of blinding or masking is also usually applied. Although the definitions vary, a trial can be considered double blind when the patient, investigators and outcome assessors are unaware of a patient's assigned treatment throughout the duration of the trial. Blinding helps eliminate biases other than selection bias, such as differences in the care provided to the two groups, withdrawals from the trial and how the outcome is assessed and analysed. In some

cases, double blinding cannot be implemented and a single blind design may be used.

There are numerous reasons suggested as to why phytotherapy should be subjected to the same degree of scientific scrutiny as conventional medicine. Such reasons include the need to become accepted by governments and conventional medicine, to help us determine if the therapy is safe and effective and to give patients a reasonable idea of the potential success rate.[1,2,3]

This is not to say RCTs are without criticism. There are circumstances in which such a trial would be unethical. RCTs do not address why a treatment works, how participants are experiencing the treatment and/or how they give meaning to these experiences. They may not illustrate benefits other than the specific effects measured, explain the effects of the patient-practitioner relationship or take into consideration the patients' beliefs and expectations. Statistically significant results may be produced that have no clinical significance or importance to patients or their caregivers. Outcome measures may focus on the physical while ignoring issues related to meaning, purpose and spirituality (for example, quality of life measures in terminally ill patients). This is also not to say that RCTs are the 'only game in town'. Epidemiological and social research methods with appropriate designs also provide valuable information.[1,2,4–7]

Despite its gold standard status, there is also no guarantee that a RCT will be well conducted, or will produce meaningful results (see later) and often once published results are open to distortion and misinterpretation.[8]

CAM versus conventional medicine in the published literature

Before looking at the structure of clinical trials and how they should be read, it is worth examining the published literature in perspective: what can be said about the quality of information that is published and is there a difference between how complementary and alternative medicine (CAM) is handled compared with conventional/orthodox/mainstream medicine?

An analysis of 207 randomised trials found that trials of complementary therapies often have relevant methodological weaknesses. Reporting and handling of drop-outs and withdrawals was a major problem in all therapies reviewed. (The data analysed here was originally collected for previously published systematic reviews on homeopathy (published 1997), herbal medicine (St John's wort for depression (1998), Echinacea for common cold (1999), acupuncture (for asthma (1996) and recurrent headaches (1999).) Larger trials published more recently in journals listed in Medline and in English exhibited better methodological quality, but stringent quality restrictions would result in the exclusion of a majority of trials. However, the average methodological quality of the complementary medicine trials reviewed was not necessarily worse than trials in conventional medicine.[9] (It would be interesting to have this analysis repeated using more recent systematic reviews containing more rigorous trials of herbal medicines such as for Ginkgo and St John's wort.)

A randomised, controlled, double blind study investigated the hypothesis that the process of peer review favours an orthodox form of treatment over an unconventional therapy. A short report describing a randomised, placebo-controlled trial of appetite suppressants ('orthodox'=hydroxycitrate, 'alternative'=homeopathic sulphur) was randomly sent to 398 reviewers. Reviewers showed a wide range of responses to both versions of the paper, with a significant bias in favour of the orthodox version. Authors of technically good unconventional papers may therefore be at a disadvantage when subject to the peer review process. However, the effect is probably too small to preclude publication of their work in peer-reviewed orthodox journals.[10]

Publication bias is a recognised phenomenon in mainstream medicine (MM), so does it exist in complementary and alternative medicine (CAM)? An analysis of controlled trials of CAM found that more positive outcome trials than negative outcome trials are published. (The analysis looked at journals aimed specifically at a CAM readership and journals that specialised primarily in mainstream medical topics.) The only exception to this was in the highest impact factor MM-journals (this means that the publication bias in favour of a positive outcome for CAM clinical trials did not occur in those mainstream medicine journals with the highest citation rate). In non-impact factor CAM-journals, positive studies were of poorer methodological quality than the corresponding negative studies. (CAM therapies in this investigation included herbal medicine, homeopathy, chiropractic, osteopathy, spinal manipulation and acupuncture. The analysis used systematic reviews and meta-analyses from 1990 to October 1997.) Considerable bias may also be caused by using Medline as a single source of information, although this is not unique to CAM (an investigation of mainstream medicine publications found that European journals may be underrepresented in Medline).[11] An investigation of trials published in four prominent Medline-indexed CAM journals from 1995 to 2000 found that the bias towards the publication of a positive outcome persisted in 2000, although it was less strong than in 1995.[12]

What to look for when reading a clinical trial paper

A trial often seeks to question, rather than confirm, its own hypothesis. The authors of a study set out to demonstrate a difference between the two arms of their study (e.g. a herbal medicine compared with placebo, herbal medicine compared with a drug or a comparison of two different dosages of herb) and do it in the following way 'Let's assume there's no difference; now let's try to disprove that theory'.[13] This is why the results are presented as 'there was/was not a statistically significant difference between [the herb] and placebo'.

The standard (and best) presentation for papers published in medical journals includes:[14]

- Introduction (why the authors decided to do this particular piece of research)
- Methods (how they did it and how they chose to analyse their results)
- Results (what they found)
- Discussion (what they think the results mean).

The design of the methods section is important in estimating the quality of the trial. Having worked through the methods section, you should be able to tell yourself:[14,15]

- What sort of study was performed
- On how many participants
- Where the participants came from
- What treatment was offered
- How long the follow up period was
- What outcome measures were used.

When scanning clinical trials (abstracts and full papers!) it is best to start with the conclusion section: was the outcome positive or negative? What herb was trialled? Then go to the method: what objective parameter was measured? What was the form and dosage of the herb? In the methods section it really helps when it is spelled out as 'the aim of this randomised study was to [assess the effectiveness of ...], the secondary objectives were to assess ...'.

Some characteristics of poorly conducted/written clinical trials:

- Abstract/summary not clearly written, conclusion not easy to find
- Method not clearly outlined
- Who received what and when; was there a washout period (crossover trials) and when did it occur? Was there a follow-up and when did it occur?
- Dosage:
  - Not clearly outlined; e.g. dried herb equivalent not outlined – only the extract or concentrate or active constituent dosage given; 'patients received one capsule of the plant extract'
  - Placebo not clearly outlined or inappropriate:
    - misleading information, e.g. 'ginger extract is a preparation (250 mg of Zingiberis Rhizoma per capsule)' when further investigation of the product (e.g. via company/product website) indicates 'capsules contain 250 mg of a concentrated pure ginger material'

○ Duration of treatment not specified
  ▪ Raw data presented but not summarised or the numbers do not add up (e.g. numbers conflicting between results and discussion/conclusion sections)
  • Very small number of trial participants
  • Side effect rate given but not explained (e.g. were the side effects mild or serious and were they related to the treatment?)
  • Drop-out numbers not given (and where given, explanation for drop-outs not given, i.e. was it related to the treatment?)
  • Abbreviations not explained; information, figures or tables missing.

Checklist for reading RCTs

The following points illustrate the type of questions to ask from a clinical trial paper. Examples are outlined below.

(a) What clinical question did the study address?
  • Treatment of depression, prevention of atherosclerosis

(b) Was the study conducted with patients with pre-existing disease or healthy volunteers?
  • A memory test in elderly patients with age-associated memory impairment assessing the efficacy of Ginkgo provides different information from that obtained from young healthy volunteers

(c) Were the participants studied in the trial relevant to your practice?
  • Results involving Inuit (native Canadians) may not be relevant to western societies
  • Results from participants of a social group that abstains from alcohol, or women not taking the contraceptive pill
  • An assessment of St John's wort involving severely depressed patients (which might be more appropriately treated with intensive psychotherapy)

(d) What treatment was considered?
  • Herbal treatment, diet modification, use of compression stockings

(e) What parameters were measured and what is the clinical relevance?

(The best quality papers outline why that parameter is relevant, so you do not have to go searching to understand the connection).

In a clinical trial assessing the efficacy of a standardised willow bark extract, the primary outcome measure was the pain dimension of the WOMAC Osteoarthritis Index, a reduction in this score indicates an analgesic effect. It would be useful to compare the reduction observed from willow bark (14%) with that obtained from a standard drug (diclofenac, 19%).

'Softer' outcome measures include patient and physician assessments, although it is better if this information is also objectively evaluated.
  • In the above willow bark trial, patient and physician overall assessments used the visual analogue scale (which assesses pain and physical function).

Here are some examples where the measured parameter may not be clinically relevant:
• Use of inappropriate endpoints (i.e. not a direct measure of clinical benefit):
  ○ only measuring serum PSA (prostate-specific antigen) in a trial investigating saw palmetto liposterolic extract for benign prostatic hyperplasia would not be as useful as measuring urinary symptoms, pain and quality of life
  ○ in HIV, CD4 count alone has been found not to correlate with survival – a combination of several markers gives a better indication.[16]
• Trials assessing pharmacological/physiological effects may increase the understanding of the mode of action of the treatment but may not provide immediately useful clinical information:
  ○ measurement of biological markers (TNF alpha and IL-1beta) in patients treated with saw palmetto liposterolic extract to test the hypothesis that infiltrating cells are associated with progression of benign prostatic hyperplasia
  ○ after 6 months of saw palmetto treatment a difference occurred in nuclear morphometric descriptors, suggesting the herbal blend alters the DNA chromatin structure and organisation in prostate epithelial cells a possible molecular basis for tissue changes and therapeutic effect of the compound is suggested
  ○ serum of women given phyto-oestrogens to ingest stimulated prostacyclin release in human endothelial cells (ex vivo) phyto-oestrogens might produce a beneficial cardiovascular effect
  ○ in vivo gene expression within peripheral leukocytes evaluated in healthy nonsmoking subjects who consumed Echinacea pattern showing an anti-inflammatory and antiviral response
  ○ Panax ginseng, at doses of 200 mg of the extract daily, increases the QTc interval (an electrocardiographic (ECG) parameter, not immediately clinically significant) and decreases diastolic blood pressure 2 h after ingestion in healthy adults on the first day of therapy→increases in ECG parameters may have clinical implications as they increase the risk of ventricular tachyarrhythmias.
• Mechanism of a potential herb-drug interaction:
  ○ high-dose treatment with St John's wort extract induced CYP3A activity in healthy volunteers as evidenced by increased 6-beta-hydroxycortisol excretion. Induction of this enzyme most likely contributes to the decreased bioavailability observed upon co-administration of various drugs with St John's wort extract. The D-glucuronic acid pathway appeared unaffected by St John's wort. (Note: Although this trial did not tell us anything immediately clinically relevant, some trials investigating cytochrome P450 enzymes are relevant, such as those that demonstrate an interaction between St John's wort and specific drugs such as omeprazole, irinotecan, verapamil).

- For another purpose such as using a herb as a test agent:
  - oral treatment with a *Ginkgo biloba* extract (Gibidyl Forte(R)) dilated forearm blood vessels causing increments in regional blood flow without changing blood pressure levels in healthy participants→the increments in blood flow may be used as a biological signal for pharmacokinetic studies.

(f) Was the route of administration relevant to herbal practice?
- Injection of a polysaccharide is not relevant in terms of results or practice, but injection of an active constituent might be relevant in terms of results (e.g. blood levels of the active may relate back to oral intake of a herb, providing the active from the herb gets into the bloodstream in that form (and is not altered by passage through the liver or gut) although it is not relevant to practice (injection of the active is not an option for herbal practitioners)).

(g) Was the preparation relevant to the products you use?
- The levels of active constituent may be too high to be achieved by a herbal product – a trial investigating soy protein will not be relevant to a soy product standardised for isoflavone content, as the protein level is likely to be very low in the latter
- To use the results of a trial administering triterpene fraction of gotu kola it would be necessary to know the content of these constituents in the herb/extract
- Efficacy of *Pygeum africanum* in benign prostatic hyperplasia is interesting but Pygeum is difficult to obtain as it is an endangered species
- Freshly expressed juice of Echinacea aerial parts will give different results than liquid extracts prepared from dried Echinacea root
- A supercritical carbon dioxide extract of chamomile will have a different phytochemical profile and hence pharmacological activity than an aqueous ethanol extract
- Products containing red clover isoflavones will not be translatable to low ethanolic liquid extracts as these constituents are present in low quantities.

(h) Was the dosage relevant to herbal practice?
- The daily dose of herbs prescribed was well below the normal therapeutic limit (hence more like a homeopathic protocol)
- Exceedingly high dosages require a safety judgment on the part of the practitioner, e.g. a 2002 trial of hawthorn used 1,800 mg/day of 5:1 dry extract=9 g/day dried herb (the usual dosage is around 3 to 6 g/day); a standardised ginger extract used a dose equivalent to 40 mg/day of gingerol, a good quality 1:2 liquid extract contains approx. 5 mg/mL=8 mL/day which is too high to prescribe for safety and compliance reasons!).

Note: A clinical trial does not necessarily determine the optimum dose, but provides information that for a given dose of a given herbal preparation a certain percentage of patients will be likely to respond i.e. [herbal preparation] at xx mg/day given for a period of yy weeks improved [the disease/disorder] in ZZ% of patients.

(i) Was the choice of placebo suitable?

- In assessing the effect of phyto-oestrogens, wheat may not be an inactive control for comparison with soy grits
- Olive oil may not be suitable to compare with evening primrose oil for the treatment of rheumatoid arthritis, as it too may have benefit.

(j) Was the blinding successful?
A well-designed trial will report the methods used to produce the double blinding. An analysis of the methodological quality of controlled trials published in 1995 found that trials for which no double blinding was reported produced larger estimates of effects.[17] It is not enough for the trial to describe itself as double blind, the success of the blinding should be evaluated and reported. (One way would be to ask the patients and clinicians at the end of trial which treatment they thought they had received.) Evaluation of blinding is rarely done in trials of conventional medicine (a recent analysis found only 7% for general medicine trials)[18] let alone in CAM trials. The evaluation of blinding has also been questioned. Trial participants asked to guess their treatment might be influenced by outcome (e.g. marked therapeutic or adverse effects). Assessments of blinding success would be more reliable if carried out before the clinical outcome has been determined. But in the case of a comparative treatment (no placebo) clinicians' predictions may be a measure of pre-trial hunches and inseparable from the blinding effectiveness.[19,20]

An example of evaluation of blinding in a randomised, comparative trial between St John's wort (*Hypericum perforatum*) and sertraline for major depressive disorder is outlined below.[21]

> At the end of 8 weeks, the proportion of patients guessing their treatment correctly was 55% for sertraline, 29% for Hypericum, and 31% for placebo (p=0.02 for differences between treatment groups). Correct guesses for clinicians totalled 66% for sertraline, 29% for Hypericum, and 36% for placebo (p=0.001 for differences between treatment groups). The change (mean) in HAM-D total score from baseline to week 8 did not differ for patients who were in the sertraline group and either had guessed the correct treatment (−11.6; 95% CI, −13.1 to −10.1) or had not (−11.9; 95% CI, −13.9 to −9.9).

This assessment was criticised, with the conclusion that the blinding was compromised. Clinicians who believed in the strength of sertraline treatment may have inadvertently let this bias affect their ratings. HAM-D is regarded as a clinician-rated measure (it would have been better to measure this against the clinician's guesses rather than the patient's guesses) – better yet, assess the other score (CGI-I, Clinical Global Impressions) which is a better measure of treatment effect).[22,23]

(k) Was the treatment beneficial?
This will be a comparison of the results of the two groups, but most well-designed clinical trials now also report the difference between the two treatments using statistics, which is often expressed with a p value. The p value is the probability that any particular outcome would have arisen by chance. Standard practice usually

regards a p value less than one in twenty (expressed as p<0.05) as 'statistically significant' and a p value less than one in 100 (p<0.01) as 'statistically highly significant', and p<0.001 more highly significant again. So if you read 20 clinical papers that reported a significant outcome of p<0.05 then it is likely that the outcome for one trial was not significant but due to chance:[24]

- Nonstatistical results: 'complete healing of duodenal ulcer occurred in 35% of those receiving deglycyrrhizinised licorice compared with 12% of those receiving placebo'
- Statistical: 'the occurrence of radiation-induced acute dermatitis of grade 2 or higher was significantly lower (41% vs 63%; p<0.001) with the use of topical Calendula than trolamine'

(A cautionary note about statistics. A recent analysis found that statistical errors occurred in two leading scientific and medical journals. In 12% of cases, the significance level could have changed by one or more orders of magnitude. The conclusion would change from significant to nonsignificant in about 4% of the errors.[25])

(l) What was the side effect rate, side effect severity and drop-out rate?

Did it differ between the two groups?

- In a trial comparing chaste tree with fluoxetine for premenstrual dysphoric disorder, although the number of patients experiencing side effects was similar, sexual dysfunction was reported by two patients in the fluoxetine group while none of the chaste tree group experienced this side effect).

More information

The above checklist helps the reader to obtain information from the clinical trial paper, but critical appraisal (such as assessing the scientific validity and practical relevance) of the trial involves a whole lot more and is beyond the scope of this discussion. More information on critical appraisal can be found from well written books devoted to the topic,[26,27] and some examples include:

- did the study enrol too few patients?
- were the trial participants representative of all those with the disease or all those for whom the therapy is intended?
- was the treatment duration too short or the follow up period too long?
- have confounding variables been eliminated?
- did the efficacy result from the treatment or from another factor?
- was the drop-out rate too high?
- what do the statistics really tell you? A p value in the nonsignificant range tells you that either there is no difference between the groups or there were too few participants to demonstrate the difference if it existed.

Published research of other designs have not been discussed here (e.g. controlled (nonrandomised) trials, postmarketing surveillance trials, uncontrolled trials, cohort and case-controlled

trials, surveys, case reports, pharmacokinetic studies and herb-drug interactions) but many of the same principles apply. A higher level of rigour (and regarded as a higher level of evidence) can be found in systematic reviews and meta-analyses. (A systematic review summarises the available evidence on a specific clinical question with attention to methodological quality. A meta-analysis is a quantitative systematic review involving the application of statistics to the numerical results of several trials which all addressed the same question.) Systematic reviews and meta-analyses are useful in that they summarise the available clinical trial results. Meta-analyses are particularly valuable because by pooling the trial results they provide greater statistical power to measure a difference between the treatment and the control group.[28] Narrative (nonsystematic) reviews, as employed for the monographs in this book, may provide a useful overview of the literature but do not employ the same rigour as systematic reviews (they are not standardised or as objective). But even these more rigorous studies (systematic reviews and meta-analyses) are not beyond criticism and subjectivity.[29]

Clinical trial papers: how to calculate dosage

Extraction or concentration ratio

The strength of a herbal liquid preparation is usually expressed as a ratio.

Example:

1:2 means 1 g of dried herb was used to produce 2 mL of liquid extract

For solid dose preparations, the concentration ratio is the ratio of the starting herbal raw material to the resultant finished concentrated extract (also known as a concentrate or dry extract or native extract). The finished extract is always expressed as 1 and comes second.

Example:

4:1 means 4 g of dried herb was used to produce 1 g of concentrated extract that went into a tablet or capsule

1:1 liquid extract	1 g dried herb produced 1 mL of 1:1 liquid extract
1:2 liquid extract	1 g dried herb produced 2 mL of 1:2 liquid extract
1:3 tincture	1 g dried herb produced 3 mL of 1:3 tincture
1:5 tincture	1 g dried herb produced 5 mL of 1:5 tincture
2:1 concentrated extract	2 g dried herb produced 1 g of 2:1 concentrated extract *also written as:* 1 g of 2:1 concentrated extract was produced from 2 g dried herb

Note: These ratios apply to extracts made from dried herb (not fresh herb).

Converting back to the dried herb (known as 'dried herb equivalent') is a useful way for comparing doses between different strengths of herbal liquids or between liquids and tablets.

Note: This conversion is commonly done when reviewing clinical papers for example, or comparing herbal products, but does not apply to standard texts such as the *British Herbal Pharmacopoeia* (BHP) 1983. The reason for the latter inconsistency relates to how the information was gathered (a survey of dosage recommendations by those practising at the time, and the reproduction of earlier pharmacopoeial information). For more information, refer to Chapter 6 or *A Clinical Guide to Blending Liquid Herbs* (pages 20 to 22).[30] This discrepancy in the BHP, however, does not negate the validity of using the dried herb equivalent.

Often there is insufficient information provided to accurately determine the dose of herb evaluated in a trial. Many trial authors seem to think that a trade name is sufficient for defining a product (despite the fact that unlike drugs, information about the content of the herbal products is not always readily available). In response to a question, one author said he could not define the product (even by name), as he had merely requested the herb from the hospital pharmacy.

Worse still, authors may not even indicate that a concentrated extract was administered, with readers assuming the dosage to be equivalent to dried herb. A clinical trial published in *JAMA* (*Journal of the American Medical Association*) 2002 indicated in the abstract that 'the daily dose of *H. perforatum* could range from 900 to 1500 mg', implying a dried herb dosage. The Methods section indicated 'Hypericum and matching placebo were provided by Lichtwer Pharma (Berlin) ... The Lichtwer extract (LI-160) was selected ... '. The extract was standardised to between 0.12% and 0.28% hypericin, but unfortunately for readers the concentration ratio was not defined. Given it was the Lichtwer extract, this is likely to have a concentration ratio of 6:1. So the 900 to 1500 mg daily dose range referred to above probably translates to the equivalent of 5.4 to 9 g of dried herb. Products often change over time also, so the concentration ratio of a particular product needs to be determined at the time it was evaluated.

It is best to assume that clinical trials are evaluating concentrated extracts and look for the product definition (most often in the Methods section if not in the abstract) before considering how to use the information in the clinic.

Rules to consider before calculating dosage

When working out extraction and concentration factors, first consider the dosage form (starting with dried herb, liquid extract or concentrated extract).

If the amount of concentrated extract is known, first work out the dried herb equivalent and then calculate a relevant liquid extract or tablet dosage. Multiply the weight of concentrate by the first number in the ratio:

$$\text{weight of 5:1 concentrate} \times 5 = \text{dried herb equivalent}$$

Once the dried herb equivalent is known this can be converted to a liquid extract by multiplying by the second number of the ratio:

$$\text{dried herb equivalent} \times 2 = \text{dosage in mL of 1:2 liquid extract}$$

Examples:

Product	Extraction/Dilution Ratio	Concentration Ratio
1:1 liquid extract	1	–
1:2 liquid extract	2	–
1:3 liquid extract	3	–
1:5 liquid extract	5	–
2:1 concentrated extract	–	2
4.5:1 concentrated extract	–	4.5
5:1 concentrated extract	–	5

The table below illustrates how to calculate doses cited in clinical trials and convert them to products, such as standardised liquid extracts and tablets. The first column contains a statement from the methods section of the cited clinical trial and the subsequent columns show how to convert the dosage first to the dried herb equivalent (or active constituent level) and then to liquid extract or tablet dosages where relevant. Notes explaining the calculations are provided in italics.

Clinical Trial Details	Clinical Trial Dosage Converted to Dried Herb Equivalent/Active Constituent Dosage	Equivalent Liquid Extract and/or Tablet Dosage
Trial Type: meta-analysis; psyllium for hypercholesterolaemia[31] Treatment with 5.1 g psyllium twice daily produces significant net reductions in serum total and LDL-cholesterol concentrations.	*weight x no. times per day →* 5.1 g of psyllium twice daily = 10.2 g/day of psyllium	–

Trial Type: postmarketing surveillance study; globe artichoke for irritable bowel syndrome[32] Patients were treated with Hepar-SL forte, a high-dose standardised aqueous-alcohol extract of artichoke leaf (*Cynara scolymus*). One 400 mg capsule contained 320 mg ALE (artichoke leaf extract). The average ratio of raw material (native extract) was 4.5:1. The recommended dosage was 2 capsules three times daily.	Two capsules three times per day *no. capsules x no. times per day x weight of concentrated extract →* = 2 × 3 x 320 mg/day of 4.5:1 extract = 1,920 mg/day of 4.5:1 extract *weight x concentration factor →* = 1,920 × 4.5 mg/day of dried herb = 8,640 mg/day of dried herb = 8.64 g/day of dried herb	8.64 g/day of dried herb *dried herb equivalent x extraction factor →* = 8.64 × 2 mL/day of 1:2 liquid extract = 17.2 mL/day of 1:2 liquid extract
Trial Type: randomised, double blind, placebo-controlled; willow bark for osteoarthritis[33] Coated tablets containing 340 mg of extract (*Salix purpurea × daphnoides* corresponding to 60 mg salicin) were provided. Patients were treated with either willow bark extract or placebo (two tablets twice daily).	Two tablets twice daily *no. tablets × no. times per day x weight of active constituent →* = 2 × 2 × 60 mg/day of salicin = 240 mg/day of salicin	Prescribe willow bark tablets standardised for salicin content to provide 240 mg/day of salicin = 4 tablets/day of tablets containing 60 mg/tablet of salicin (4 × 60=240)
Trial Type: randomised, double blind, placebo-controlled; hawthorn for congestive heart failure NYHA class II[34] Patients were treated with either 240 mg/day Crataegus extract WS 1442 (80 mg t.i.d.) or matching placebo for 12 weeks. One capsule of WS 1442 contains 80 mg WS 1442 dry extract from hawthorn leaves with flowers (5:1), adjusted to 15 mg oligomeric procyanidins (OPCs).	3 × 80 mg/day WS 1442 *no. capsules × weight of concentrated extract →* = 240 mg/day of 5:1 dry extract *weight × concentration factor →* = 240 × 5 mg/day of dried herb = 1200 mg/day of dried herb = 1.2 g/day of dried herb Also, One capsule contained 15 mg OPC *no. capsules × weight of active constituent →* = 3 × 15 mg/day of OPCs = 45 mg/day of OPCs	1.2 g/day dried herb *dried herb equivalent × extraction factor →* = 1.2 × 2 mL/day of 1:2 leaf liquid extract = 2.4 mL/day of 1:2 leaf liquid extract Or, 45 mg/day OPCs = 4.5 mL/day of leaf liquid extract containing 10 mg/mL of OPCs (4.5 × 10=45) Prescribe hawthorn tablets standardised for OPC content to provide 45 mg/day of OPC = 3 tablets/day of tablets containing 15 mg/tablet of OPC (3 × 15=45)
Trial Type: randomised, double blind, placebo-controlled; fennel cream for idiopathic hirsutism[35] The groups were treated with a cream containing 1% or 2% fennel extract or placebo. The patients used the cream twice a day on their face. Crushed fennel seeds were extracted with ethanol, the solvent was removed under reduced pressure yielding 8%.	8% yield → 8 g concentrate obtained from 100 g dried herb = 12.5:1 concentrate *concentration factor →* = 12.5 of dried herb equivalent 1% cream = 1 g of concentrate in 100 g cream = 12.5 g of dried herb in 100 g cream 2% cream = 2 g of concentrate in 100 g cream = 25 g of dried herb in 100 g cream	1% cream = 12.5 g dried herb in 100 g cream *dried herb equivalent × extraction factor →* = 12.5 × 2 mL of 1:2 liquid extract in 100 g cream = 25 mL of 1:2 liquid extract* in 100 g cream 2% cream = 25 g of dried herb in 100 g cream *dried herb equivalent × extraction factor →* = 50 mL of 1:2 liquid extract* in 100 g cream

*When making creams, particularly with this volume of extract, it is best to reduce the alcohol content with gentle and slow heat, to preserve the quality of the extract, produce a cream of appropriate consistency and reduce the chance of the alcohol stinging the skin. The concentrated extract used in this trial had the alcohol removed by reduced pressure which may have also removed the essential oil (although the authors stated that they analysed for anethole content (a major constituent of fennel essential oil) – they did not define how much was present). Different results may be obtained using extracts which better preserve the essential oil content.

References

1. Levin JS, Glass TA, Kushi LH, et al. *Med Care.* 1997;35(11):1079–1094.
2. Verhoef MJ, Casebeer AL, Hilsden RJ. *J Altern Complement Med.* 2002;8(3):275–281.
3. Harlan Jr. WR. *J Altern Complement Med.* 2001;7(suppl 1):S45–S52.
4. Cohen SR, Mount BM. *J Palliat Care.* 1992;8(3):40–45.
5. Jonas WB, Goertz C, Ives J, et al. *JAMA.* 2004;291(18):2192.
6. Herman J. *J Clin Epidemiol.* 1995;48(7):985–988.
7. Riegelman RK, Hirsch RP. *Studying a Study and Testing a Test: How to Read the Health Science Literature*, 3rd ed Boston: Little Brown; 1996. p. 73.
8. Greenhalgh T. *How to Read a Paper.* London: BMJ Books; 2001. p. 48.

9. Linde K, Jonas WB, Melchart D, et al. *Int J Epidemiol.* 2001;30(3):526–531.

10. Resch KI, Ernst E, Garrow J. *J R Soc Med.* 2000;93(4):164–167.

11. Pittler MH, Abbot NC, Harkness EF, et al. *J Clin Epidemiol.* 2000;53:485–489.

12. Schmidt K, Pittler MH, Ernst E. *Swiss Med Wkly.* 2001;131(39–40):588–591.

13. Greenhalgh T. *How to Read a Paper.* London: BMJ Books; 2001. pp. 42, 47.

14. Greenhalgh T. *How to Read a Paper.* London: BMJ Books; 2001. p. 39.

15. Greenhalgh T. *How to Read a Paper.* London: BMJ Books; 2001. p. 73.

16. Greenhalgh T. *How to Read a Paper.* London: BMJ Books; 2001. p. 100.

17. Schulz KF, Chalmers I, Hayes RJ, et al. *JAMA.* 1995;273(5):408–412.

18. Fergusson D, Glass KC, Waring D, et al. *BMJ.* 2004;328(7437):432.

19. Altman DG, Schulz KF, Moher D. *BMJ.* 2004;328(7448):1135.

20. Sackett DL. *BMJ.* 2004;328(7448):1136.

21. Hypericum Depression Trial Study Group. *JAMA.* 2002;287(14):1807–1814.

22. Jonas W. *JAMA.* 2002;288(4):446.

23. Spielmans GI. *JAMA.* 2002;288(4):446–447.

24. Greenhalgh T. *How to Read a Paper.* London: BMJ Books; 2001. p. 87.

25. Garcia–Berthou E, Alcaraz C. *BMC Med Res Methodol.* 2004;4(1):13.

26. Greenhalgh T. *How to Read a Paper.* London: BMJ Books; 2001.

27. Riegelman RK, Hirsch RP. *Studying a Study and Testing a Test: How to Read the Health Science Literature*, 3rd ed. Boston: Little Brown; 1996.

28. Greenhalgh T. *How to Read a Paper.* London: BMJ Books; 2001. pp. 120–122, 128–133.

29. Teagarden JR. *Pharmacotherapy.* 1989;9(5):274–281.

30. Bone K. *A Clinical Guide to Blending Liquid Herbs: Herbal Formulations for the Individual Patient.* St. Louis: Churchill Livingstone; 2003. pp. 20–22.

31. Anderson JW, Davidson MH, Blonde L, et al. *Am J Clin Nutr.* 2000;71(6): 1433–1438.

32. Walker AF, Middleton RW, Petrowicz O. *Phytother Res.* 2001;15(1):58–61.

33. Schmid B, Ludtke R, Selbmann HK, et al. *Phytother Res.* 2001;15(4):344–350.

34. Zapfe Jr. G. *Phytomedicine.* 2001;8(4): 266–272.

35. Javidnia K, Dastgheib L, Mohammadi Samani S, et al. *Phytomedicine.* 2003; 10(6–7):455–458.

Actions index

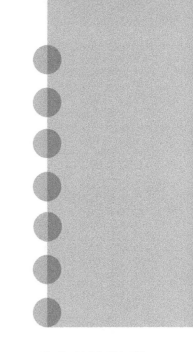

A

Adaptogens, 151, 168–169, 179–180, 278–279, 292, 294, 312, 329–330, 332, 381, 384–385, 602, 628, 630–631, 665–666, 818
Anabolic effects, 821
Analgesics, 30, 142, 271–272, 274, 364, 373, 423, 481, 509, 511, 560, 590–591, 660, 699, 702, 755, 772, 783, 786–787, 847, 935–936, 946
Anthelmintic activity, 29, 566
Anthraquinone laxatives, 48–50, 193, 199
Antiallergic agents, 198, 242–243, 320–321, 364, 395, 444, 525, 553, 566, 727, 760, 888, 910
Antianaemic activity, 517, 949
Antiandrogenic activity, 804
Antiarrhythmic activity, 509, 517, 671
Antiarthritic agents, 393, 427, 433–434, 441, 443–447, 509, 546, 566, 766–767, 957
Anticatarrhals, 242, 245–246, 248–249, 332, 399–400, 475, 553, 753
Anticathartic activity, 581
Anticholestatic activity, 649
Anticoagulant activity, 777–778
Anticonvulsants, 512, 702
Antidepressant activity, 273–274, 278–279, 338, 596, 726–727, 826, 829–831, 840–843, 848, 909, 929
Antidiabetic activity, 345, 360, 386, 388, 399, 406–407, 410–411, 540–542, 546, 596, 615, 628, 643, 720, 755, 801, 821, 869–870, 875–876
Antidiarrhoeal activity, 399, 403–404, 475
Anti-ecchymotic agents, 373
Antiemetics, 196, 578–580, 584t–588t, 649, 783, 790
Antifibrotic effects, 660

Antifungal activity, 401, 501, 651, 764, 773, 776–777, 785, 835, 885, 887–888
Antigonadotropic activity, 455–456
Antihaemorrhagic activity, 799
Antihypertensives, 222–223
Anti-inflammatories, 25, 141–142, 159–160, 169, 185, 197, 242–243, 282, 309, 317, 320, 332, 364, 373–375, 386, 393, 395, 405–406, 419, 423, 431, 441–444, 467–468, 475–477, 481, 501, 504, 509–511, 517, 525, 531, 540, 542, 553–555, 566, 568–570, 578, 581–582, 590, 602, 651, 657, 660, 676, 685, 719–720, 722–723, 747–749, 755, 760, 762–763, 787, 795, 799, 804, 808–809, 835–836, 868–870, 885, 888, 900–903, 911–912, 935, 937–938, 944, 949, 953
Antiirritant activity, 944–945
Antilithics, 263
Antimalarial agents, 361–362
Antimicrobial agents, 28–30, 361–362, 373, 375, 394–395, 400–403, 402t–403t, 407–408, 451, 478–479, 493, 502–503, 525, 531, 553–554, 559, 570–571, 583, 661, 704, 726, 742, 744, 764, 772–773, 776–777, 783, 785–786, 835, 885, 887, 900, 906–907, 945
Antimutagenic activity, 888
Antioedema activity, 373, 419–420, 441, 467, 469, 477, 600, 617, 685–688, 747–749, 818
Antioxidants, 33, 37, 141, 180, 233, 254, 365, 381, 386, 419, 421, 431, 479, 560, 596, 600, 652, 654, 671, 675–676, 764, 861–863, 885, 888, 900–901, 904, 915–916, 945
Antiparasitic activity, 29, 400–403, 402t–403t, 583, 661, 753–755, 757, 772, 776, 785–786, 885, 907

Antiplatelet agents, 227–228, 231, 375, 408, 421, 504, 517, 550, 560, 578, 582, 654, 755, 777–778, 900, 903–904
Antiproliferative activity, 519
Antiprostatic activity, 760
Antipyretics, 364, 799, 935–936
Antiretroviral activity, 827–829, 839–840
Antirheumatic activity, 427, 509–513, 760, 935
Antiseptic agents, 142, 201–202, 248–249, 263, 317, 320, 373, 558, 783
Antispasmodics, *see Spasmolytics*
Antistress effects, 601–602, 628, 638, 818, 820–822
Antithrombotic activity, 704, 742
Antithyroid activity, 454–456
Antitoxic activity, 865
Antitussives, 243, 248–249, 719, 727, 783
Antiulcer activity, 475, 478, 480, 581, 693, 721–722, 743
Antiurolithic activity, 407
Antiviral activity, 29, 169, 217, 381, 384, 387, 501, 525, 531, 553, 719–720, 725–726, 777, 826–829, 839–840, 885, 888
Antpruritic activity, 783
Anxiolytics, 272–273, 275–276, 279, 281, 330, 475, 481, 519–520, 596, 657, 660, 699, 701–702, 705–707, 826, 831–832, 843–844, 923, 925, 929, 957
Aphrodisiacs, 804, 894
Aquaretics, 261–263
Aromatics, gastrointestinal activity, 192, 196
Astringents, 141, 317, 393, 419, 553, 671, 742

B

Biliary activity, 210, 212, 214, 399, 407, 649

Bitters, 39–42, 84–85, 104, 150–151, 184, 193–194, 196–197, 202, 212, 320, 649
Bronchodilating herbs, 249
Bulk laxatives, 25, 189

C

Cancer preventive activity, 30–31, 34, 52, 175–178, 216, 271, 333, 362–363, 375, 386, 401, 405, 423, 430, 435, 444, 462–463, 480, 493, 503–505, 519, 547–548, 554, 570, 583, 616, 628, 632–634, 640–641, 661, 688, 703–704, 719–720, 724–725, 744, 747, 749–750, 772, 774–776, 778, 787, 809–810, 820–821, 833–835, 866–868, 877, 900, 907–909, 912–913, 949, 952–953
Cardioprotective activity, 34, 188, 190, 220, 224–231, 233–234, 363–364, 385, 387–388, 395, 404–405, 411–412, 421, 423, 454, 509, 511–512, 518–519, 547, 582, 590, 596, 600–601, 634, 639–640, 671, 673–674, 678t–680t, 747, 749, 764, 821, 900, 953
Cardiotonic activity, 628, 671
Carminative herbal remedies, 29, 184, 195, 197, 475, 557, 578, 581, 783, 900
Chemotherapy adjunct, 179–181, 360, 388–389, 430, 724–725, 799, 879
Choleretics/cholagogues, 184, 196, 199, 204, 210–212, 218–219, 283, 363, 501–502, 504–505, 649, 651, 653, 728, 783, 861, 900
Cognitive function, 233, 284–286, 596, 602, 613–615, 628, 631–632, 636–638, 657, 699, 726, 832–833, 846

Conditions index

General index

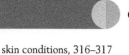

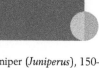